Robotic Urologic Surgery

Peter Wiklund • Alexandre Mottrie
Mohan S Gundeti • Vipul Patel
Editors

Robotic Urologic Surgery

Third Edition

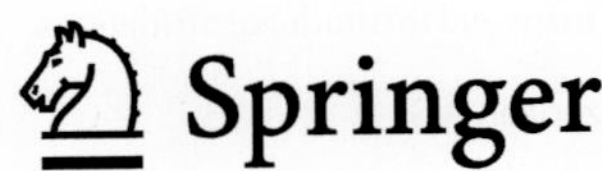

Editors
Peter Wiklund
Department of Urology
Icahn School of Medicine at Mount Sinai
New York, USA

Alexandre Mottrie
Department of Urology
ORSI Academy
Aalst, Belgium

Mohan S Gundeti
Pediatric Urology
University of Chicago Medicine and
Biological Sciences
Chicago, IL, USA

Vipul Patel
Urology
Global Robotics Institute
Celebration, FL, USA

ISBN 978-3-031-00362-2 ISBN 978-3-031-00363-9 (eBook)
https://doi.org/10.1007/978-3-031-00363-9

This Springer imprint is published by the registered company Springer Nature Switzerland AG
The registered company address is: Gewerbestrasse 11, 6330 Cham, Switzerland

This book is dedicated to my wife, Sejal, and my children, Ela (17 years) and Evan (15 years), who have been my inspiration in life.

Recognition and thanks to our sets of parents Ranchhodbhai and Savitaben Patel and Prabodh and Chhaya Dharia whose support has allowed us to grow both personally and professionally.

Also, appreciation to the members of the team and supporting cast without whom the journey would not have been possible. A special thanks to my colleagues Marcio Moschovas and Ashley Fialkowski who have worked tirelessly to ensure the completion and quality of this book.

A special thank you to my associate editors, Drs. Alexander Mottrie, Peter Wiklund, and Mohan Gundeti who worked tirelessly and used their expertise to make this textbook possible.

Vipul Patel MD.

Preface

Robotic surgery is a breakthrough in minimally invasive approach that amplifies a surgeon's vision and dexterity to treatment of diseases across many surgical specialties. Where human dexterity is limited, the robotic arm takes over and seamlessly scales, filters, and translates the precise movements of the hand with greater precision and less collateral damage. We see the future ahead, and the applications of robotics are poised to grow exponentially as advances continue in the fields of machine learning, artificial intelligence, and advanced imaging.

Since the first edition of the book in 2007, the practice of Robotic Urologic Surgery has undergone a significant evolution. Something that was initially based on theory and possibilities now presents concrete solutions. The early adopters have now amassed a significant amount of experience, allowing the new surgeons to benefit from a significantly shorter learning curve. The question is no longer whether robotic surgery is feasible, viable, or the right way forward, but how to further improve the surgical outcomes and quality of life for the patient. The field of urology has led the way in robotics for over two decades now and continues to be the sub-specialty of innovation and exploration.

The first edition of our book focused mainly on robotic prostatectomy as this was believed to be the best indication for robotics technology. The current edition shows a greater breadth of applications in urology as robotics has expanded into other organ systems and procedures. Robotic surgery in urology is now a mature practice, widely implemented for the improvement of patient care.

This third edition of "Robotic Urologic Surgery," consistent with the goals of the initial endeavor 15 years ago, is not only a compilation of the knowledge and experiences of the best robotic surgeons around the world but is also an incorporation of the recent advances in machine learning, artificial intelligence, and advanced imaging. We are very grateful to the contributors who have shared their expertise and to all urologists who have **adopted** this book and given valuable insight.

As Albert Einstein said, "To raise new questions, new possibilities, to regard old questions from a new angle, requires creative imagination and marks real advances in science". We hope this third edition of Robotic Urologic Surgery answers questions that arise on robotic surgery and raises new questions that will spearhead further advances and improved techniques in the field of robotic surgery; For Man and Machine in collaboration are here to stay!

Celebration, FL

Vipul Patel

Contents

Part I

Robotic Surgery Book

History of Robotic Surgery

Jonathan Noël, Sunil Reddy, Camilo Giedelman, Rigby C. D. Swarovski-Adams, Evan Patel, and Richard M. Satava

1 Introduction

Since the mid-twentieth century, during the "Information Age," there has been an exponential growth of information technology. The substitution of information for physical objects, the hallmark of this period, laid the foundation for the development of the field of minimally invasive surgery. Digitization of information allowed the surgeon to move from open surgery to laparoscopic and eventually robotic surgery [1].

The benefits of minimally invasive surgery have been seen with decreased blood loss, shorter hospital stays, smaller incisions, less pain, and improved visualization among others. There have been limitations also, such as increased cost, steep learning curve, and operative time. Robotics has helped address some of these limitations of the laparoscopic approach such as surgical fatigue (ergonomics) and learning curve. Open surgery was the Industrial Age, where the surgeon directly touched and felt the tissues and moved the tip of the instruments. Laparoscopic surgery was the transition: half in the Industrial Age, where the surgeon still moved the tip of the instruments, and half in the Information Age, where the visual feedback was the electronic image (information) of the organs on the monitor. The robot completes the transition to the Information Age. In less than two decades, the robotic approach has even become the gold standard of surgical treatment for localized prostate cancer. How did we get to this point?

The word "robot" is from the Czech word "robota" which means forced labor; it is Slavic root "rab" meaning "slave." The word was further popularized by Isaac Asimov in his short story *Runaround* where he coined the term "robotics" in 1942. In 1951, while working for the Atomic Energy Commission, Raymond Goertz designed the first teleoperated master–slave manipulator to handle hazardous waste material. The first industrial robot was known as Unimate and was a 6-axis articulating robot used for die cast handling and spot welding in General Motors (GM) assembly lines. Since 1988, robots have continued to develop from machines capable of performing simple operations to those of today that can perform highly sophisticated tasks, as seen in Fig. 1.

2 Origins of Modern Robotics

The modern history of robotic surgery began with the Programmable Universal Machine for Assembly (PUMA) 560®, a robot which was developed in 1978 by the same company that manufactured the Unimate. In 1985, Dr. Yik San Kwoh used the PUMA 560 to hold a stereotactic frame for brain biopsies. In 1988, Sir John Wickham and Brian Davies of the Imperial College London used this system to perform a transurethral resection of prostate (TURP). Integrated Surgical Supplies Ltd (Sacramento, USA) constructed two models with similar features: Probot®, a robot designed specifically for transurethral prostatectomy, and Robodoc®, a robotic system for more precision in hip replacement operations. The latter system was converted into the first robot approved by the FDA.

J. Noël (✉)
Department of Urology, Guy's & St Thomas' NHS Foundation Trust, London, UK

S. Reddy
Global Robotics Institute, Celebration, FL, USA

C. Giedelman
Clinica Marly, Bogotá, Colombia

R. C. D. Swarovski-Adams
Winchester College, Hampshire, UK

E. Patel
Lake Highland Preparatory School, Orlando, FL, USA

R. M. Satava
Department of Surgery, University of Washington Medical Center, Seattle, WA, USA

P. Wiklund et al. (eds.), *Robotic Urologic Surgery*, https://doi.org/10.1007/978-3-031-00363-9_1

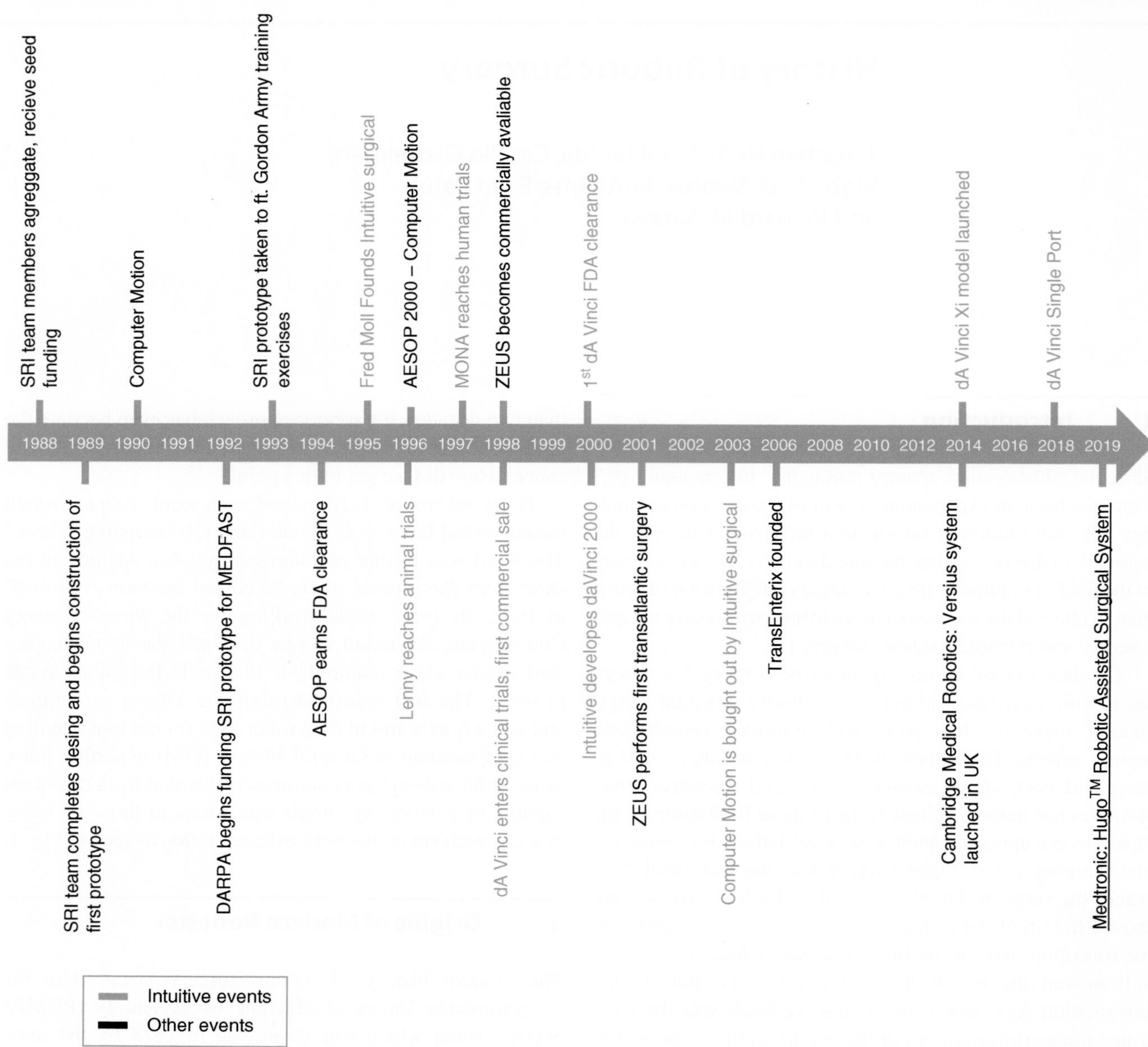

Fig. 1 Timeline of developments in robotic surgery

2.1 Probot® System for TURP

The Probot bore similarity to ROBODOC, in that precision of the coring action was preplanned based on a scan, in this case ultrasound. The system had 7 degrees of freedom (DOF) coupled to a motorized component to automate TURP. Software allowed the surgeon to fully override and adjust it anytime, and the robot helped reduce the strain on the surgeon's neck that came from looking through an eyepiece without video assistance. The goal was to make the procedure safer and shorter to limit fluid irrigant absorption which mostly accounted for morbidity and mortality of TURP during the 1980s–1990s. In their feasibility study, the procedure would take five minutes and coagulation could occur by means of the surgeon manually. This was the first time an active robot had been used to remove tissue from a patient [2]. A safety frame allowed the resecting instrument to stay within predefined limits of the verumontanum and bladder neck. Their results showed the Probot system to be as good as traditional method of TURP, with respect to urinary flow rates [3]. However, the dependence of Probot on preoperative TRUS, inaccuracies of TRUS estimation, and the need for manual electrocautery for hemostasis hindered adoption of this machine [2].

2.2 ROBODOC

The ROBODOC (Integrated Surgical Systems, Sacramento, CA, USA) was developed in the 1980s and was an orthopedic surgical system that assisted in hip and knee replacement surgeries. This robot was the creation of late veterinary surgeon Howard "Hap" A. Paul and orthopedic surgeon William Bargar, both from the University of California. CT scan data overlayed with computer-assisted design/computer-assisted manufacturing (CAD/CAM) technology could produce a customized orthopedic implant. A five-axis robotic arm with a milling device connected to the tip of the arm via a force torque sensor, ROBODOC could then mill the bone cavity to the corresponding dimension, serving as a rasp. Human trials in 1992 showed its feasibility and superiority [4] as a radiographically superior implant fit and through elimination of intra-operative femoral fractures after total hip arthroplasty. In 1994, the ROBODOC was commercialized in Europe and in 2008 received 510(k) FDA approval for use in the USA. In 2014, THINK Surgical Inc. acquired ROBODOC and used it as the core technology for its next generation TSolution One® Surgical System which received FDA approval in 2019. It never gained wide adoption in part due to studies showing no significant difference compared to conventional TKA [5].

2.2.1 Stanford Research Institute and National Aeronautics and Space Administration

In 1986, Colonel Dr. Richard Satava joined the Stanford Research Institute (SRI) where Philip Green was developing a telemanipulator system for hand surgery. The team combined several technologies to create an early "virtual reality," one of which was VPL Inc.'s DataGlove, a hand gesture interface tool that could be used to measure hand position and orientation as well as provide haptic feedback. Another was a head-mounted display (HMD) which was developed by NASA-Ames Research Center's Michael McGreevey and Stephen Ellis, who were utilizing HMDs to allow 3D visualization of data for NASA's planetary exploration missions. 3D audio was added to the HMD by Scott Fisher to further immerse users, coining it "telepresence" as seen in Fig. 2. This concept allowed surgeons' hands to have a computer interface with their patient in another room.

While laparoscopy gained popularity, the loss of three-dimensional visualization and the hindrance of dexterity due to the fulcrum effect made it advantageous for patients but challenging for many surgeons [6]. A workstation was created with instrument handles instead of gloves, an arm rest, and a monitor located 5–15 degrees below the horizontal (see Fig. 3) [7]. The system allowed for haptic feedback through force-sensing elements on end effectors and motion prohibition when resistance was met [8, 9].

2.2.2 Defence Advanced Research Projects Agency

Dr. Satava was recruited by the Surgeon General of the Army, Alcide LaNoue, to join Defense Advanced Research Projects Agency (DARPA) and develop the telepresence system for military use during the 1990s. The imperative was to reduce mortality of soldiers who had sustained battlefield casualties by at least 50%. The premise was to change access to trauma care "from the golden hour to the golden minute" through telepresence surgery. Data analyzed from the Vietnam war had revealed that life-threatening wounds were a major contribution to mortality and had not changed since the Civil war [10].

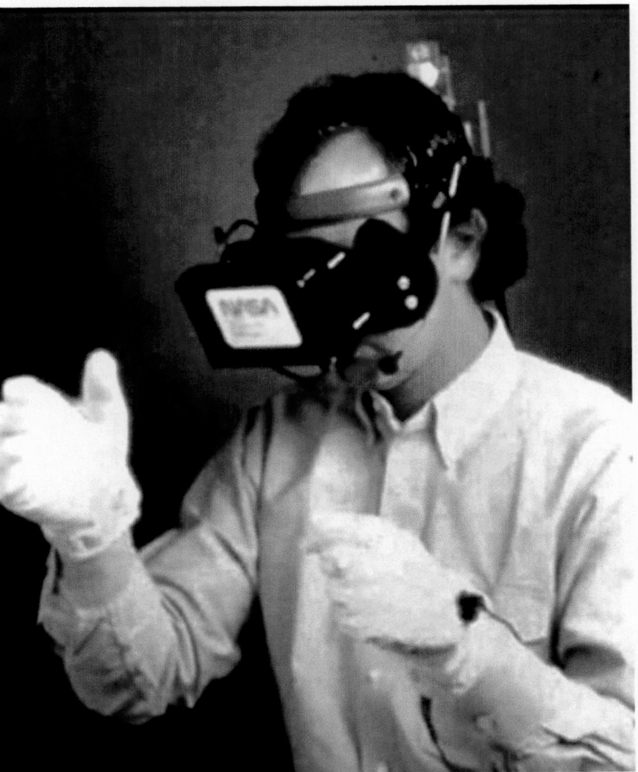

Fig. 2 Head-mounted display (HMD) with DataGlove interface demonstrated by Dr. Scott Fisher (From George & Satava et al., Origins, Journal of the Society of Laparoscopic & Robotic Surgeons)

The DARPA project of a telepresence surgeon for the wounded soldier would be possible by positioning a surgical console workstation in a Mobile Advanced Surgical Hospital (MASH). The remote Robotic Surgical Unit (manipulator arms) would be mounted in an armored vehicle (mobile operating room) in the forward battlefield to perform critical lifesaving surgical tasks (damage control surgery) until the patient arrived at a MASH for definitive care. This vehicle was known as the medical forward advanced surgical treatment (MEDFAST) vehicle. The concept envisioned that, when a soldier was critically wounded, the soldier would be placed in a portable intensive care unit for life support and transport (LSTAT or "trauma pod"), which would be immediately inserted into the MEDFAST, so a surgeon would be able to operate with bedside assistance from a medic. The MEDFAST also integrated telepresence into non-surgical technology

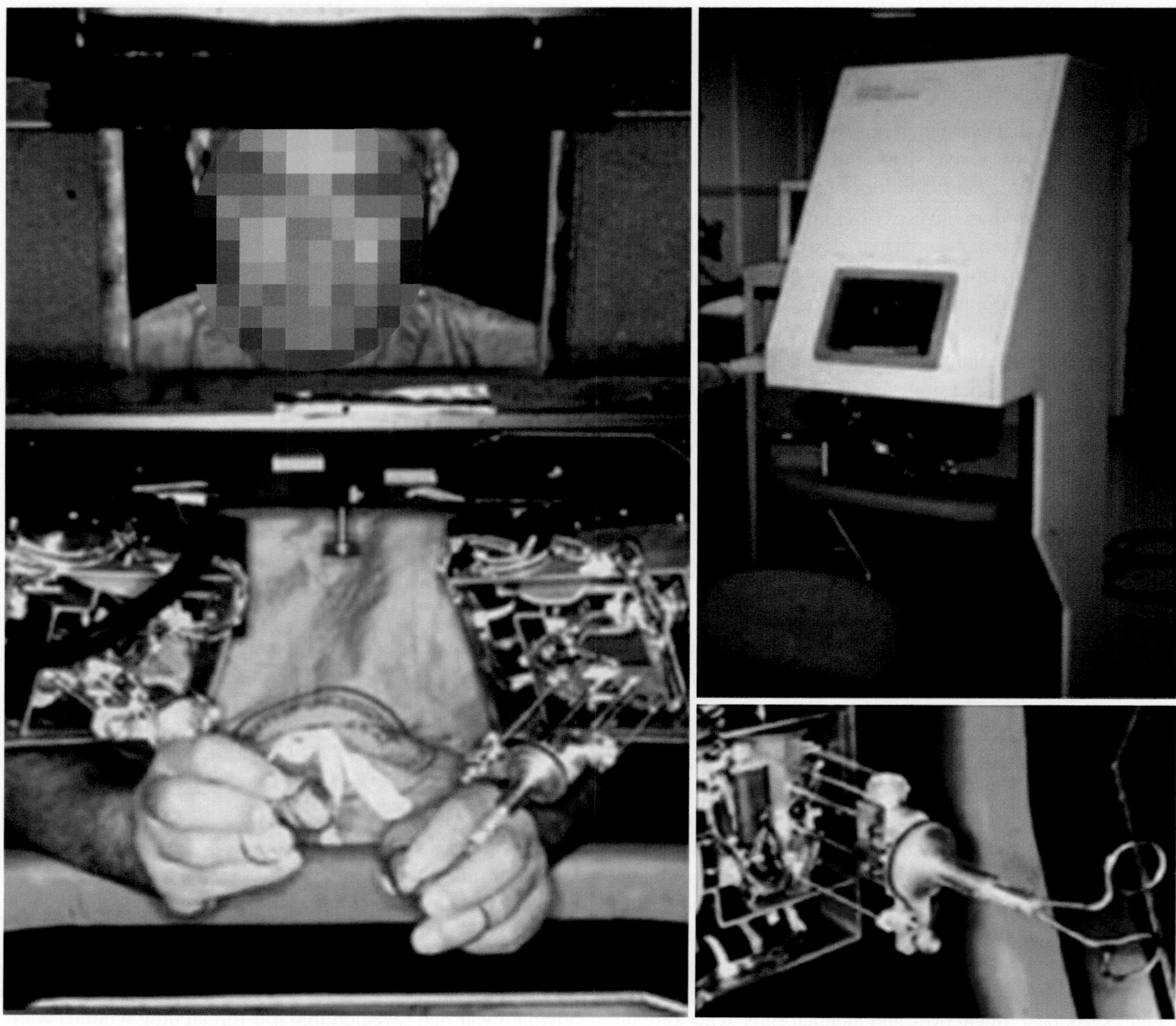

Fig. 3 Early prototype of surgical workstation (ergonomic design, armrest to stabilize arms, instruments handles)

of anesthesia, remote monitoring, radiography, and life support, to ensure that full operating room capabilities could be deployed in the battlefield. The first prototype was completed and demonstrated in October 1994 to the Secretary of Defence William Perry at the Annual Convention of the Association of the US Army in Washington, DC. The subsequent development was the creation and demonstration by Oak Ridge National Laboratory of robotic surgical scrub and circulating nurses—integrated with the surgical robotic system and suitable for automatically performing tool changes and dispensing various surgical supplies, thus completing the total capabilities of a remote, mobile operating room. Due to political reasons the DARPA program came to a halt, and the intellectual property of the SRI telepresence system was eventually pitched to venture capitalists and acquired by Intuitive Surgical, Inc. for commercialization [11].

3 First Telerobotic Commercial Systems

3.1 AESOP (Automated Endoscopic System for Optical Positioning)

Around the same time SRI was working on their "telepresence" system. Computer Motion Inc. (Goleta, CA, USA) was founded by Yulun Wang, Ph.D., in 1989. Wang would eventually go on to develop an automatic endoscopic system for optimal positioning (AESOP®), which was a robotic arm designed to hold a laparoscopic camera. Following this commercial success, Computer Motion then independently developed Hermes and then the Zeus robotic surgery system [12].

The HERMES system was a software interface that was developed to control devices through voice command, offering the concept of a "smart operating room." Computer Motion focused its research on the AESOP arm, which maneuvered an endoscope intracorporeally using verbal commands. The surgeon positioned the camera while controlling the other two arms with conventional laparoscopy or by coupling it to the ZEUS system [13]. The development of the arm was carried out under a NASA SBIR (Small Business Innovation Research) contract. NASA funded these derivatives of technological enterprise with the aim of eventually helping astronauts work remotely on repairs of orbiting space shuttles [14].

AESOP began in 1994, with the Model 1000, which was the world's first FDA-approved general-purpose surgical robot. In 1996, Computer Motion Inc. continued with the improvements until reaching model AESOP 3000 (Fig. 4).

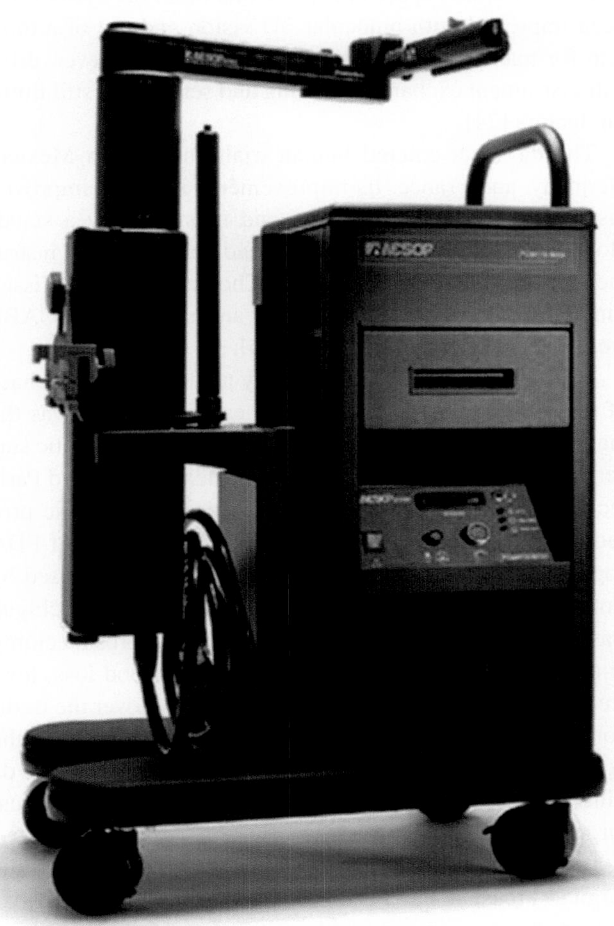

Fig. 4 AESOP (Automated Endoscopic System for Optical Positioning)

Computer Motion used the FDA's 510K process instead of class III approval, allowing it to be released to the market several years faster and set a precedent for future competition to use [15].

In 1998, *the Journal of Thoracic Cardiovascular Surgery* published an article where the feasibility of AESOP was evidenced in minimally invasive mitral valve repair [16].

AESOP's success is illustrated by its adoption into more than 1000 hospitals and represents the beginning of robotic surgery's global impact.

3.2 ZEUS System

In 1993, Computer Motion Inc. began working on the Zeus surgical robot, whose first prototype was available in 1995 and was tested in an animal model in 1996. The system consisted of 3 AESOP "arms" (two instrument holders and the camera holder) plus a surgical console to control the arms. Two years later, in 1998, the ZEUS Robotic Surgical System performed its first minimally invasive microsurgical procedures on humans, including endoscopic coronary artery bypass grafting (E-CABG) [17], tubal reanastomosis, and other complex procedures such as heart valve surgery. In 2000, the ZEUS was equipped to hold 28 different surgical instruments, and in 2001, it received FDA approval [14–18].

Jacques Marescaux used this robot in September 2001 to perform the first transatlantic remote laparoscopic cholecystectomy from New York. The patient was in Strasbourg, France (Fig. 5). This was a major landmark for surgery. The main drawback of the ZEUS system was the large size of robotic arms, which limited operating room space and caused frequent collisions between the trocars [19, 20].

The ZEUS system, seen in Fig. 6, was discontinued in 2003 after Computer Motion was acquired by rival Intuitive Surgical; later it would develop the Da Vinci Surgical System [21].

3.3 Computer Motion vs. Intuitive Surgical

In 2000, Computer Motion filed lawsuits against its rival company in medical robotics, Intuitive Surgical, for allegedly infringing Computer Motion's patents related to robotic surgery.

In June 2000, Intuitive Surgical went public, and on March 7, 2003, Computer Motion and Intuitive Surgical were merged into one company. This was done in part to try to resolve the litigation between the companies, but in so doing, it increased the effectiveness and usability of such technology. Shortly after the merger, ZEUS was phased out in favor of Intuitive Surgical's Da Vinci system [11].

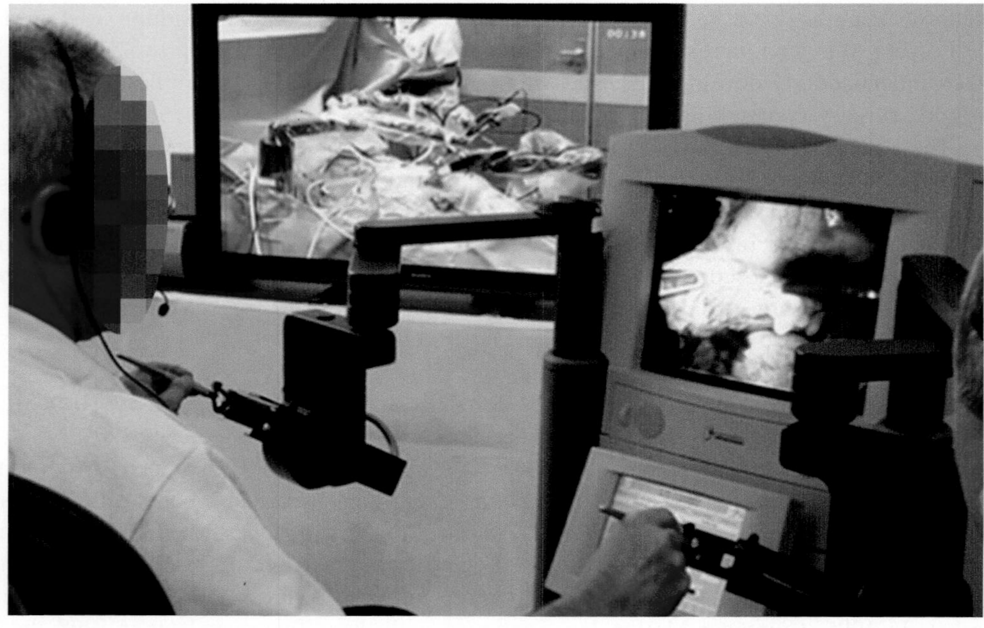

Fig. 5 Dr. Marescaux performing the first transatlantic remote laparoscopic cholecystectomy in New York on a patient in Strasbourg, France

4 Intuitive Surgical: Mona to DaVinci (FDA Approved 2000)

In 1995, the company Intuitive Surgical Inc. (Sunnyvale, CA, USA) was founded by Frederic H. Moll, John Dreund, and Robert Younge after negotiating for SRI's intellectual property with the aim of developing a complete surgical robotics project. In 1996, the company started with a prototype known as "Lenny" (after Leonardo da Vinci) and was used in animal trials; however, its limitations in visualization and mechanical reliability precluded use in humans. As the company's prototypes became more advanced, they were named using da Vinci themes; "Leonardo" and another "Mona." The final version of the prototype was nicknamed the "da Vinci," which was the final marketing label [14]. "Mona" prototype was the precursor robot with a control console and independent exchangeable arms. On March 3, 1997, the first procedures, two cholecystectomies, were performed by bariatric surgeons Dr. Jaques Himpen and Dr. Guido Leman out of St. Blasius General Hospital in Belgium [14]. The following day the creation of two arteriovenous fistulas was performed by Dr. Marc Bosiers using Mona.

Starting in 1997, various procedures of general surgery, gynecology, and urology were carried out, and in 1999, Intuitive Surgical began marketing this system in Europe while awaiting FDA approval in the USA [21]. The da Vinci surgical system obtained FDA approval in 2000 to perform laparoscopic abdominal surgery procedures in the USA [22, 23].

On September 16, 1998, using Mona, Dr. Guy-Bernard Cadière performed a band gastroplasty and published the report in *Obesity Surgery* which highlighted the safety, feasibility, and ergonomic advantages of robotic surgery, especially in confined spaces [21]. By this time, the system had been improved with binocular 3D vision and use of a third arm for manipulation of the optical system; however, difficult instrument exchange coupling and setup were still limiting factors [24].

The da Vinci entered human trials in 1998 in Mexico, Germany, and France. Its improvements included improved visualization, range of motion, and most notably a standalone robot which replaced the need for mounting instrument manipulators to the table. Cholecystectomy, Nissen fundoplication, mitral valve repair, and eventually a CABP were performed using the system [5].

Leipzig Heart Center in Germany made the first purchase of the da Vinci in late 1998 where cardiac surgery was the main focus. By 2001, over 140 different types of robotic surgery had been performed in Brussels, Mexico City, and Paris including cardiac, bariatric, gynecologic, and urologic procedures. On July 17, 2000, the da Vinci received full FDA approval through the same 510K expedited process used by Computer Motion. The Vattikuti Institute in Detroit, Michigan was the first to document the robotic-assisted prostatectomy in the year 2000, which offered decreased blood loss, lowered pain scores, and shortened hospital stays over the traditional open retropubic approach [25–27]. Rather than the expected implementation in cardiovascular surgeries, the da Vinci found robust adoption in urologic and gynecological surgeries.

In spite of the growth in robotic surgery in almost all the surgical areas, it has been the urology field where it has caused the main impact, with vast expansion and excellent results in different types of interventions: simple prostatec-

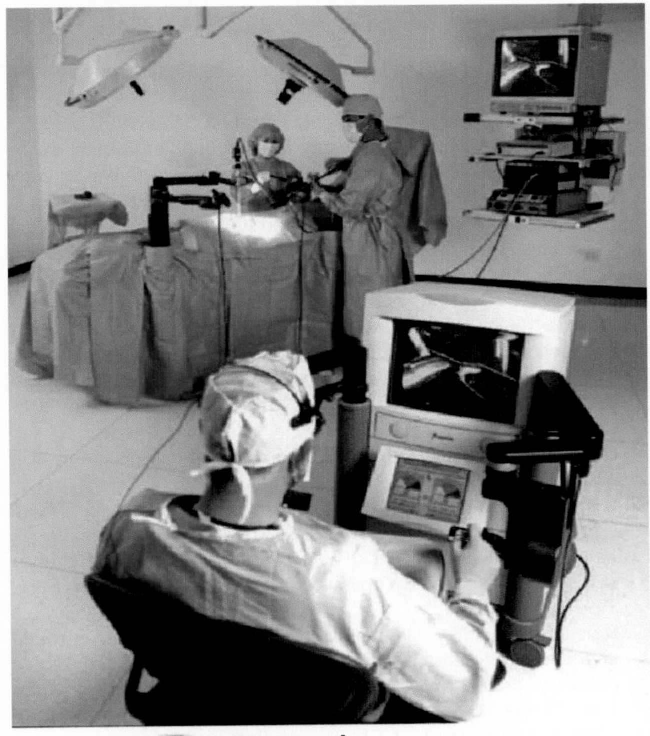

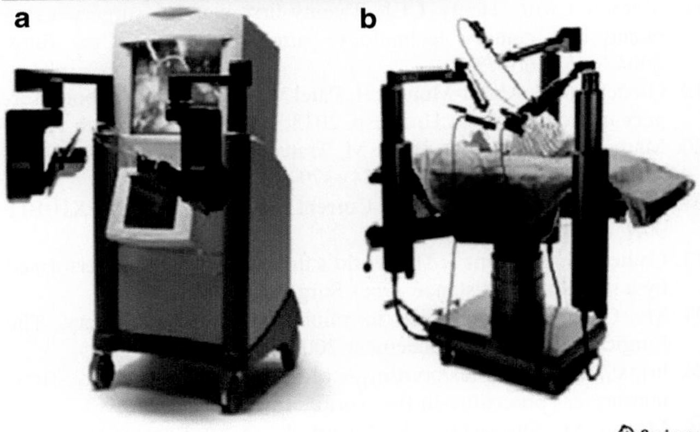

Fig. 6 Zeus system in OR. (**a**) surgeon console and (**b**) robotic arms (from Lealghezzi et al. 2016)

tomy, radical prostatectomy, partial nephrectomy, live donor nephrectomy, and pyeloplasty, among others. The first robotic radical prostatectomy was realized by Binder in Germany, while Abbou and his colleagues, in France, were the first ones in publishing it in the literature [25–27]. The group of Guillonneau and his colleagues reported the first nephrectomy [28] and robotic lymphadenectomy as a treatment for prostate cancer [29].

Technological advances continue to impact the modern practice of urology, none more so in recent years than the development of robotic surgery. Since the first publication of a series of patients undergoing robot-assisted radical prostatectomy in 2001, the field has seen a dramatic increase in the

Table 1 Timeline of the da Vinci® surgical system in general surgery

Year	Author	Surgery
1997	Cadiére	Cholecystectomy
1998	Cadiére	Adjustable gastric band
1999	Cadiére	Nissen fundoplication
2000	Horgan	Roux-en-Y gastric bypass
	Giulianotti	Total gastrectomy in malignant disease
	Hashizume	Colectomy in malignant disease
	Hashizume	Splenectomy
	Hashizume	Unilateral and bilateral inguinal hernia repair
2001	Weber	Colectomy in benign disease
	Horgan	Adrenalectomy
	Giulianotti	Liver resection
	Giulianotti	Distal pancreatectomy and duodenopancreatectomy
	Melvin	Heller's esophagomyotomy
	Melvin	Transthoracic esophagomyotomy in malignant disease
2002	Ballantyne	Ventral and incisional hernioplasty
2003	Horgan	Transhiatal esophagectomy in malignant disease
	Giulianotti	Anterior resection of the rectum
2007	Kang	Thyroidectomy in malignant disease

From Leal Ghezzi, T., & Campos Corleta, O. (2016). *30 Years of Robotic Surgery. World Journal of Surgery, 40(10), 2550–2557.* https://doi.org/10.1007/s00268-016-3543-9

use of robotic surgery for urologic procedures. In the USA, 42% and 63% of all radical prostatectomies in 2006 and 2007, respectively, were performed with robot assistance. This number is likely to increase to 85% for the year 2009.

The minimally invasive nature of these procedures allows for better precision, decreased blood loss, shorter hospital stay, decreased morbidity, and shorter convalescence while preserving functional and oncologic outcomes. Additionally, the application of robotic surgery has spread beyond radical prostatectomy to include radical cystectomy, nephrectomy, partial nephrectomy, adrenalectomy, and other upper urinary tract surgery (pyeloplasty, ureteral reimplant, etc.). Robotic surgery has even seen dramatic growth in pediatric urologic and general surgery applications (Table 1).

5 Current Status of New Platforms and Future

Haptic feedback and sound will add a dimension of reality, but the challenge is providing information to more than 20 nerve endings for sensation in the hand. For instance, computers judging 1 mm two-point discrimination and proprioception with the need to display this to the user present exciting future endeavors.

5G wireless networks will allow for faster information transfer with 100-fold increase in bandwidth, speed, and significant decrease of latency to 1 ms, making remote telesurgery safer and for longer distances. However, the bedside cart will need to be upgraded with additional software to accommodate telesurgery since most of the control of the manipulators reside in the console in the current systems. A necessary consideration is security and reliability of the communication network, though the current 5G systems use blockchain for security and 7-nines reliability.

Single-port technology of robotic systems has become widely available in the USA, and this is discussed in a separate chapter. Patients should respond positively to less scars for the same procedure. The long-term outcomes of such minimal access surgery in cancer are still being evaluated [30].

Lastly, artificial intelligence is on the forefront and will be integrated into robotic surgical systems in unique ways.

6 Conclusion

Robotics is a cutting-edge technology that manipulates information in the service of the surgeon. Its high impact is given by the ease to develop almost any urologic procedure, a shorter learning curve, greater ergonomics, and proven better results than other approaches.

The next step is to continue with the exploration of how to achieve an increasingly better, more accurate dissection that more closely matches our expectations to patients' expectations.

References

1. Patel VR. Robotic urologic surgery, evolution of robotic surgery: past, present, and future. Springer; 2012.
2. Hemal AK, Menon M, editors. Robotics in genitourinary surgery, vol. 655. London: Springer; 2011. https://doi.org/10.1007/978-1-84882-114-9_59.
3. Davies BL, Hibberd RD, Ng WS, Timoney AG, Wickham JE. The development of a surgeon robot for prostatectomies. Proc Inst Mech Eng H. 1991;205(1):35–8. https://doi.org/10.1243/PIME_PROC_1991_205_259_02.
4. Bargar WL, Bauer A, Börner M. Primary and revision total hip replacement using the Robodoc system. Clin Orthop Relat Res. 1998;354:82–91. https://doi.org/10.1097/00003086-199809000-00011.
5. Song EK, Seon JK, Yim JH, Netravali NA, Bargar WL. Robotic-assisted TKA reduces postoperative alignment outliers and improves gap balance compared to conventional TKA knee. Clin Orthop Relat Res. 2013;471:118–26.
6. Satava RM. Surgical robotics: the early chronicles: a personal historical perspective. Surg Laparosc Endosc Percutan Tech. 2002;12(1):6–16. https://doi.org/10.1097/00129689-200202000-00002.
7. George EI, Brand TC, LaPorta A, Marescaux J, Satava RM. Origins of robotic surgery: from skepticism to standard of care. JSLS. 2018;22(4):e2018.00039. https://doi.org/10.4293/JSLS.2018.00039.
8. Jensen JF, Hill JW. Surgical manipulator for a telerobotic system. Google Patents, CA2222150A1, 1998.
9. Green PS. Surgical system. Google Patents, US6788999B2, 2005.
10. Zajtchuck R, Jenkins DP, Bellamy RF. Textbook of military medicine: part 1. Warfare, weaponry and the casualty, vol. 5. Washington, DC: Office of the Surgeon General of the Army; 1998. p. 64–72.
11. Brand T. A chronicle of robotic assisted surgery and the Department of Defense: from DARPA to the MTF. Presentation given at Western Urologic Forum in Vancouver BC, March 2018; 2017.
12. Sánchez-Martín FM, Rodríguez F. Historia de la robótica: de Arquitas de Tarento al Robot da Vinci. (Parte II). Actas Urológicas Españolas. 2007;31(3):185–96.
13. Pugin F, Bucher P, Morel P. History of robotic surgery: from AESOP(R) and ZEUS(R) to da Vinci(R). J Visc Surg. 2011 Oct;148(5 Suppl):e3–8.
14. Shah J, Vyas A. The history of robotics in surgical specialties. Am J Robot Surg. 2014;1(1):12–20.
15. George E, Brand T, Satava R. Origins of robotic surgery: from skepticism to standard of care. JSLS. 2018;22(4):e2018.00039.
16. Falk V, Walther T, Mohr FW. Robot-assisted minimally invasive solo mitral valve operation. J Thorac Cardiovasc Surg. 1998;115(2):470–1.
17. Reichenspurner H, Damiano R. Use of the voice-controlled and computer-assisted surgical system ZEUS for endoscopic coronary artery bypass grafting. J Thorac Cardiovasc Surg. 1999;118(1):11–6.
18. Marohn CMR, Hanly CEJ. Twenty-first century surgery using twenty-first century technology: surgical robotics. Curr Surg. 2004;61(5):466–73.
19. Giedelman C, Abdul-Muhsin H, Patel V. The impact of robotic surgery in urology. Actas Urol Esp. 2013;37(10):652–7.
20. Marescaux J, Leroy J, Smith M. Transatlantic robot-assisted telesurgery. Nature. 2001;413(6854):379–80.
21. Intuitive Surgical Inc - ISRG Current report filing (8-K) EXHIBIT 99.1. Sec.edgar-online.com
22. Cadiere G, Himpens J. The world's first obesity surgery performed by a surgeon at a distance. Obes Surg. 1999;9(2):206–9.
23. Mc Guiness A. Robotics in minimally invasive surgery. The Surgical Technologist December 2000, pp 11–16.
24. https://bariatrictimes.com/my-experience-performing-the-first-telesurgical-procedure-in-the-world/
25. Menon M, Shrivastava A, Tewari A, et al. Laparoscopic and robot assisted radical prostatectomy: establishment of a structured program and preliminary analysis of outcomes. J Urol. 2002;168:945–9.
26. Leal Ghezzi T, Campos Corleta O. 30 Years of robotic surgery. World J Surg. 2016;40(10):2550–7. https://doi.org/10.1007/s00268-016-3543-9.
27. Abbou C, Hoznek A, et al. Laparoscopic radical prostatectomy with a remote controlled robot. J Urol. 2001;165:1964.
28. Guillonneau B, Jayet C, et al. Robot assisted laparoscopic nephrectomy. J Urol. 2001;166:200.
29. Guillonneau B, Cappele O, et al. Robotic assisted, laparoscopic pelvic lymph node dissection in humans. J Urol. 2001;165:1078.
30. Moschovas MC, Bhat S, Sandri M, Rogers T, Onol F, Mazzone E, Roof S, Mottrie A, Patel V. Comparing the approach to radical prostatectomy using the multiport da Vinci Xi and da Vinci SP robots: a propensity score analysis of perioperative outcomes. Eur Urol. 2021;79(3):393–404. https://doi.org/10.1016/j.eururo.2020.11.042.

Current and Upcoming Robotic Surgery Platforms and Adjunctive Technologies

Nikhil Sapre, Taimur T. Shah, and Prokar Dasgupta

1 Introduction

Over the last 30 years, laparoscopic surgery has transformed care of patients in urological surgery. However, laparoscopy is limited by its 2-dimensional (2D) vision, ergonomics, and limited range of motion. This has meant several aspects such as operating in a narrow field in the pelvis, and complex reconstruction remains challenging with a significant learning curve. The advent of robotic assistance has overcome several limitations of laparoscopy with its 3-dimensional (3D) vision, better dexterity and range of movement, HD visualization, motion scaling, and tremor filtration. Robotic assistance has increased the utilization of laparoscopy significantly changing the landscape of urological surgery. In urology, it has been used to perform pelvic surgery such as radical prostatectomy, cystectomy, and urinary diversion as well as upper tract surgery such as radical and partial nephrectomy, adrenalectomy, and pyeloplasty. More recently, we have seen robot-assisted laparoscopic surgery in female and functional urology as well as reconstructive urology. Robot assistance and autonomous systems are also being applied to BPH surgery, ureteroscopic stone surgery, and ultrasound-guided prostate biopsies.

Robot-assisted laparoscopy was first used in urology at Frankfurt, Germany, using the da Vinci surgical system (Intuitive Surgical Inc., Sunnyvale, CA, USA) [1] to perform radical prostatectomy. Since then, innovation in robot-assisted laparoscopy has seen several versions of this system enter the market from the original Si system to the current models such as Xi and SP (single-port) systems. Some patents for the da Vinci system expired in 2019 paving way for new platforms to enter the market.

N. Sapre · T. T. Shah
Department of Urology, Guys Hospital, London, UK

P. Dasgupta (✉)
Department of Urology, Guys Hospital, London, UK

MRC Centre for Transplantation, Guy's Hospital, King's College London, London, UK

In this chapter, we summarize the various robotic platforms available in the market currently as well as systems in development which are likely to enter the market in the near future. We also discuss various adjunct technologies that are in use on these robotic platforms for pre-operative planning as well as intra-operative guidance.

Finally, we discuss how precision robotics, connectivity, and surgical data science are being used to expand the horizons of robotic surgery.

2 Robotic Platforms

Table 1 summarizes the currently approved robotic assistance systems currently available in the market [2].

2.1 da Vinci Surgical System

Approved by the FDA in 2000, this is the main surgical system in the market and is used in adult cardiac, general, gynecology, head and neck, and urological surgery as well as in pediatric surgery [3]. This master–slave robotic system consists of a surgeons console system, which is used to control interactive robotic arms at the patient-side cart (Figs. 1 and 2). The robotic arms have EndoWrist technology and seven degrees of freedom and can act as retraction, cutting, or electrosurgical tools. Four generations of this system have since been released including the da Vinci, S, Si, and Xi. In 2018, the da Vinci SP (single-port) system was approved by the FDA.

The Xi system has an end-mounted camera that can be positioned in any port, thinner robotic arms, better endowrist joints, and longer instrument shafts allowing more efficient multiquadrant procedures.

The SP system patient cart utilizes a single robotic arm with a 2.5 cm cannula, through which an oval 12 × 10-mm 3D-HD fully wristed endoscope and three 6-mm wristed and elbowed instruments can reach up to 24 cm depth. The can-

P. Wiklund et al. (eds.), *Robotic Urologic Surgery*, https://doi.org/10.1007/978-3-031-00363-9_2

Table 1 Currently approved robotic surgical systems

Robotic system	Surgeon console	Controller	Key features
da Vinci Xi	Closed	Finger loops	8 mm camera port and 8 mm instruments 10 uses per instrument Three instrument arms Port hopping camera Dual console
da Vinci SP	Closed	Finger loops	Single-port Single robotic arm through a 2.5 cm cannula with 360° of rotation 12 mm articulating camera Three 6 mm instrument arms
Senhance	Open/3D glasses	Laparoscopic handles	10 mm camera Four independent robotic arms (10 mm, 5 mm, 3 mm) Infrared eye tracking for camera control Haptic feedback Dock free design Reusable instruments
Revo-I	Closed	Finger loops	10 mm camera 7.4 mm instruments with 20 uses each Excessive force use warning
Versius	Open/3D glasses	Joystick handles	10 mm camera and 5 mm instruments Haptic feedback Portable independent arms, individually mounted in separate patient-side carts Surgeon can be in sitting or standing position Dock free design
Avatera	Open	Finger loops	10 mm camera with 5 mm instruments Only consists of 2 components Single use instruments
Hinotori	Semi-open	Finger loops	Dock free design Only approved for use in Japan

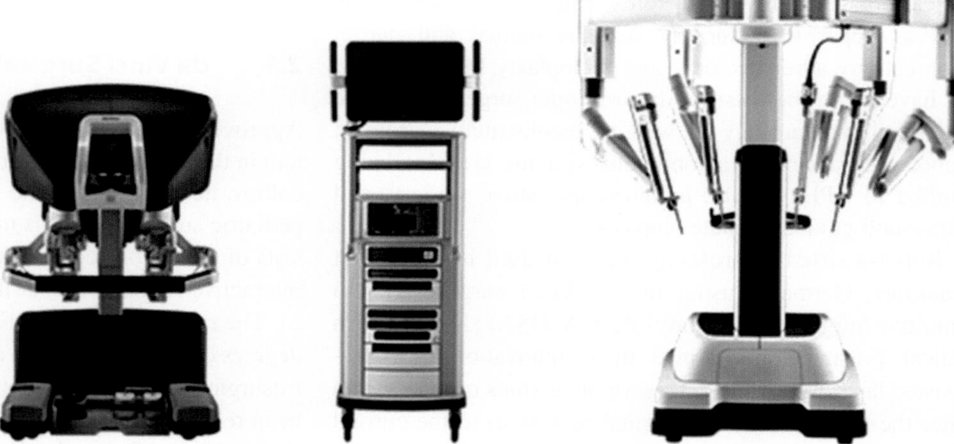

Fig. 1 The three components of the DaVinci Xi system and the surgeons console, visual tower, and patient cart on a single extendable and maneuverable boom

nula and the boom can rotate 360° allowing excellent vision. The surgeon console of the SP system, while similar to multi-port model, has additional features that allow the surgeon to move the entire robotic arm in addition to moving the instruments separately. The navigation interface also allows the surgeon to tract the position of each instrument during surgery. Many surgeons have since published their experience and outcomes of robot-assisted laparoscopic radical prostatectomy (RALP), robot-assisted radical cystectomy (RARC), robot-assisted radical nephrectomy (RARN) and robot-assisted partial nephrectomy (RAPN), robot-assisted pyeloplasty, and other reconstructive procedures using the SP system [4–8].

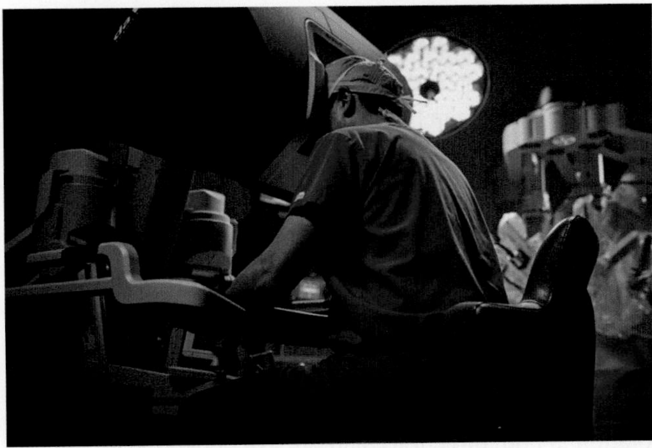

Fig. 2 Surgeon sitting at the DaVinci Xi closed console

2.2 Senhance

Initially developed by the Sofar (Milan, Italy) and originally named the ALF-X, the Senhance surgical system (TransEnterix Surgical Inc., Morrisville, NC, USA) has been approved by FDA for general and gynecology procedures. It has CE Mark certification for all abdominal and non-cardiac thoracic procedures and recently its use for various urological procedures was described in Europe [9, 10]. It has a remote console unit called a cockpit, up to four independent robotic arms in separate patient carts. It provides 3D HD vision, haptic feedback, camera control using surgeon's eye movements via infrared eye tracking system and reusable laparoscopic tools.

2.3 Revo-I

The Revo-I is approved for use in Korea and is based on a similar platform to the da Vinci system. It consists of a four-arm patient cart with 7.4 mm wristed instruments, a closed surgeon console, and a HD vision cart with a 10 mm endoscope. It has been used to perform retzius-sparing RALP in the first human trial in 17 patients with acceptable peri-operative, early oncological, and continence outcomes [11]. Specifically, there were no conversions to open to laparoscopic surgery.

2.4 Versius

The Versius surgical system (Cambridge Medical Robotics Ltd, Cambridge, UK) received the European CE Mark in March 2019. The robotic arms, which have shoulders, elbows, and wrists, are individually mounted in separate patient-side carts allowing for optimization of port placements [12] (Fig. 3). Instruments are sleek at 5 mm diameter

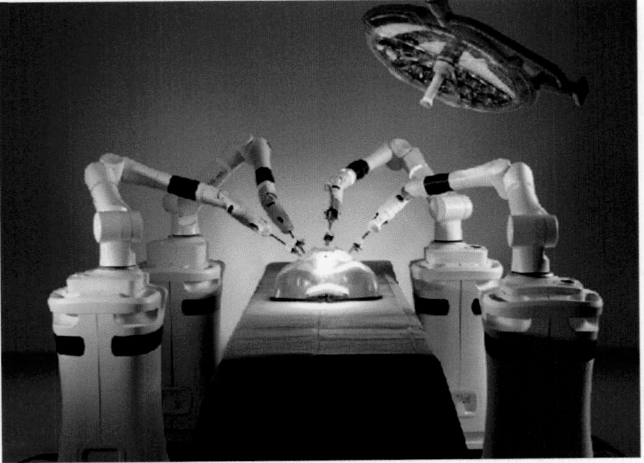

Fig. 3 CMR robot dockless individual patient arms

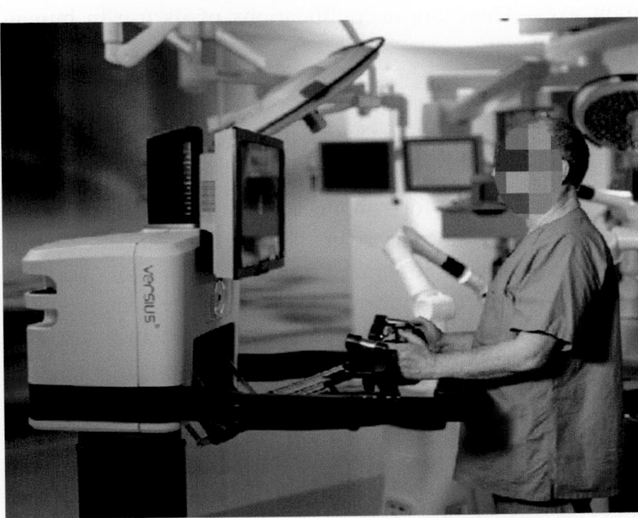

Fig. 4 Surgeon standing at the CMR robot console

and are controlled through a joystick on the console. The open-console design with 3D HD vision allows for excellent communication between the console surgeon and the bedside team. The ability of the surgeon to be upright in the sitting and standing position allows for excellent ergonomics (Fig. 4). The system has been used in a preclinical setting, where multiple surgeons successfully performed prostate surgeries, renal surgeries, and pelvic lymph node dissection (PLND) on cadavers and porcine models [13].

2.5 Avatera

The Avatera system (Avateramedical GmbH, Jena, Germany) consists of only two components. The surgical robot has four robot arms, which controls up to 3, 5 mm avatera instruments, which provide seven degrees of freedom and a 10 mm HD endoscope. The open-console control unit includes a microscope-like eyepiece, an integrated and flexible seat, and easy handling via haptic, manual input devices and foot-switches. All instruments are single use eliminating the need for sterilization.

2.6 Hinotori

The Hinotori system (Medicaroid Corporation, Kobe, Japan) is approved for human use in Japan only with plans for expansion internationally [14]. The surgeon cockpit is a semi-open console with microscope-like eyepiece, which provides a 3D HD view and loop-like handles, which control the wristed robotic arms. The operative unit has four robotic arms, which have multiple joints with movement in eight axes. There are no publications of its use in human studies yet.

2.7 Future Robotic Surgical Systems

The global market for robotic surgery is $13.3 billion by 2026 [15]. It is not surprising that many companies have developed surgical robotic systems to enter this lucrative market. Multiport robotic systems recently launched include the Hugo RAS system (Medtronic, Dublin, Ireland), a modular, open-console surgical robot; and in development the BITRACK system (Rob Surgical, Barcelona, Spain), a three-arm, open-console system, the Tumai surgical robot (MicroPort, Shanghai, China), Verb surgical (Johnson & Johnson, USA), Virtuoso Surgical system (Nashville, TN, USA). The Single-Port Orifice Robotic Technology (SPORT) surgical system now rebranded as ENOS (Titan Medical, Toronto, Canada) is a robotic single access system with a flexible camera and two multi-articulated instruments [16] and is expected to compete with the da Vinci SP if it receives FDA clearance for commercial use.

2.8 Other Robotic Systems in Urology

The use of robotics is not only confined to laparoscopic surgery but has also been utilized within the fields of benign prostatic hypertrophy (BPH), urolithiasis, and diagnostic with a different method of application in each system.

Aquablation is a minimally invasive robotic system for the treatment of BPH using high-pressure saline. The aim being to destroy prostatic tissue through non-thermal hydrodissection, the system is made up of a conformal planning unit (CPU), a robotic hand-piece, and a console. Prior to commencing treatment, the prostate and ablation zone is mapped out in advance with the required depth and angle of the water jet selected. The high-velocity jet is controlled by the surgeons foot pedal and will proceed along the pre-defined ablation map [17].

Since 2010, ELMED (Ankara, Turkey) has been working on a system specifically designed for Robotic flexible ureterorenoscopy (FURS) called the Avicenna Roboflex. The robot consists of the surgeon's console and the robotic arm which controls the flexible ureterorenoscope with different attachments available for the various endoscope manufacturers. The robotic arm is controlled from the console using a joystick and wheel which allow for very accurate and fine movements in all directions such as forward/backward, 220° rotation in both directions, and 262° of deflection bilaterally. The entire procedure can be performed from a sitting position, outside of radiation field. The laser fiber and the irrigation speed of the fluid can both be controlled from the console [18].

Robotic systems have also been developed for automated prostate cancer biopsies such as the transperineal biopsy iSR'obot Mona Lisa from Biobot Surgical Ltd., Singapore. It incorporates fusion of the pre-biopsy MRI with real-time transrectal ultrasound images to construct a 3D model of the prostate. As with other MRI-fusion systems the images are contoured prior to biopsies taking place; however, in the case of the iSR'obot™ Mona Lisa a software-controlled robotic arm mounted to the operation table that takes biopsies according to the pre-defined plan up to a sampling density of every 1 mm [19].

3 Adjunct Technologies for Robotic Surgical Systems

3.1 Instruments

3.1.1 Robotic Staplers and Sealers

The EndoWrist Stapler, a fully wristed endoscopic linear stapler, which can be introduced into the operative field through a 12 mm port, places more control in the hands of the console surgeon. It is equipped with *SmartClamp* technology, which detects whether the jaws can adequately close on the target tissue for the given staple height and informs the surgeon accordingly. It also notifies the surgeon and prevents firing when it detects that no reload or a spent reload is installed accidentally. The use of this system has been published in colorectal, thoracic, and upper gastrointestinal surgery but more evidence to document its equivalence to laparoscopic linear staplers are needed especially in urological surgery such as RARC and urinary diversion [20, 21].

The vessel sealer extend is another instrument compatible with the da Vinci Xi surgical system that has independent grasping, dissecting, cutting, and sealing functions. Its wristed technology with 60° articulation can cut and seal vessel or bundles of tissue up to 7 mm with orthogonal transection at right angles and is manipulated directly by a surgeon utilizing a console. Used with the Erbe VIO dV generator system, a generator inserted in the vision cart of the da Vinci system, the energy and bipolar effect can be regulated, as with other instruments [22].

3.1.2 Magnetic Retraction System

Levita™ Magnetic Surgical System (LMSS) (Levita Magnetics, San Mateo, CA) is designed to magnetically grasp and retract the target tissue. It works by attaching a spring-loaded grasper, characterized by a small magnetic end, to the targeted tissue, subsequently controlling it using an external stronger magnet. This eliminates the need for a dedicated trocar and shafted instrumentation that may clutter the operative field. This may be especially useful in single-port surgery or reducing the number of ports in multiport surgery. Steinberg et al. [23] reported the feasibility of LMSS in 15 patients undergoing single-port RALP without any additional assistant ports or conversion to open surgery. They found that LMSS improved tissue exposure and ergonomics in single-port surgery, thus mimicking multiport surgery. Others have reported the safety and feasibility of LMSS during robotic upper tract surgery [24]

3.2 3-Dimensional Pre-operative Planning

Conventional surgical planning based on cross-sectional imaging requires complex cognitive processing to convert 2D images into a 3D reconstruction to guide intra-operative decision-making. The use of virtual 3D models and 3D printing has evolved to enable the surgeon to create a roadmap for more precise surgery. In urology, this has been applied principally to RALP and RAPN.

The current 3D model reconstructions utilize machine learning algorithms to convert cross-sectional images into a 3D image segmentation of the scan, which is then validated by engineers to create a final 3D rendered model. Startups such as Innersight Labs from academic institutions in the United Kingdom are paving the way for this technology to be used in patient selection, planning, and intra-operative guidance.

For RAPN, better surgical planning using 3D models can be useful in patients with complex anatomy such as ectopic or horseshoe kidneys [25] and may have a role in reducing warm ischemia times and better preservation of renal function by allowing selective and super-selective clamping [26].

Porpiglia et al. [27] in their study of 101 patients showed that nephrometric scores obtained using 3D models were lower for half of the cases than when scored using conventional 2D CT images. Interestingly, their study also showed that the scores obtained using 3D information were better predictors of postoperative complications, which they attributed to better perception of tumor depth and its relationships with intra-renal structures.

Bianchi et al. [28] showed that during RAPN, the 3D-guided plan allows the surgeon to perform selective clamping in higher proportion of patients compared with the standard 2D-guided approach without increasing intra-operative and postoperative complications.

Such 3D reconstructions can actually be 3D printed to give surgeons a sense of touch and potentially reduce positive margins during RALP [29] or RAPN. Furthermore, these technologies can also be used for purposes of urology training, patient counseling, and patient consent.

3.3 Virtual and Augmented Reality and Artificial Intelligence

MIMIC technologies (Seattle, USA), the leading firm for virtual reality robotic simulators, has both standalone simulation systems such as the dV-trainer and FlexVR as well as the da Vinci skills simulator, a simulator co-developed by MIMIC and Intuitive which connects a simulation computer directly to the da Vinci console to allow for simulation directly on the console [30].

Although virtual reality simulators are used for training to improve a surgeon's skill set and shorten the learning curve, there is no high quality evidence of skills transfer from simulation to clinical surgery on real patients [31]. Some studies have used virtual reality models to show that it can aid the identification of the renal artery during RAPN, and plan and guide various surgical steps during RARP for peripherally placed and advanced tumors [12, 32].

3D reconstructed images from cross-sectional imaging may be superimposed onto in-vivo anatomy to allow better surgical navigation using data from fused virtual reality images as well as real-time in-vivo observations. Such augmented reality (AR) models have been developed and used for surgical navigation in RALP and RAPN [33–35].

Porpiglia et al. [35] demonstrated that using hyper accuracy 3D (HA3D) AR models during RAPN of complex renal masses can lead to lower rates of global ischemia with less violation of the collecting system and lower drop of the estimated renal plasma flow at 3 months. Their tumor enucleation rate was also higher using HA3D models than intra-operative ultrasound (US) guidance.

Using HA3D models in 30 patients undergoing RARP, Pulliati et al. showed 100% and 79% accuracy in predicting the location of the index lesion and ECE, respectively, using histopathological specimens as gold standard [33]. Their team also developed elastic HA3D AR models of the prostate that allowed identification of ECE with 100% accuracy compared to 47% with the 2D MRI cognitive models [34].

In the field of robotics, artificial intelligence (AI) has so far been used mainly to assess surgical performance. Baghdadi et al. [36] used machine learning and logistic regression algorithms to train a model for computerized assessment of PLND during RARC. Compared to an expert panel of surgeons, the model was 83.3% accurate in assessing the quality of the lymph node clearance. Another study showed that automated performance metrics using an AI model could distinguish surgeon expertise in various areas such as time, movement efficiency, camera manipulation, and tissue trauma during vesicourethral anastomosis of RALP [37].

3.4 Image-Guided Surgery

3.4.1 USS Guidance

The introduction of the drop-in ultrasound controlled by the ProGrasp forceps allows the surgeon to optmize the intra-operative assessment of the extent of the tumor, allowing for precise tumor excision and enucleation [38]. This is a useful tool especially when resecting endophytic tumors. Contrast-enhanced ultrasonography (CEUS), which uses microbubble-based contrast agents with existing ultrasound techniques, allows for enhanced evaluation of macrovascular and microvascular structures, potentially allowing for selective clamping and reducing warm ischemia times [39]. Rao et al. [40] have described a novel technique of occlusion angiography using intra-operative contrast-enhanced ultrasound scan (CEUS) for zero-ischemia RAPN in five patients. However, more studies are needed to assess whether this technology will consistently translate to better functional and oncological outcomes.

3.4.2 Fluorescent Dyes

Fluorescence imaging in robotic surgery relies on detection of variable uptake of a molecular marker in different tissues, which can be detected by a high-resolution endoscope using near infrared (NIFR) light spectrum. Indocyanine green (ICG) is the most commonly used fluorescent dye in robotic urological surgery, as it can be detected using NIRF [41]. ICG has been used for guidance in selective clamping for nephron sparing during RAPN [42]; assess tissue vascularity during robot-assisted ureteral reconstruction [43, 44], precise dissection of prostatic neurovascular bundle [45], identification of lymph nodes during lymphadenectomy for renal cancer [46], and during RARP and robotic PLND [47].

Renal tumors are hypofluorescent after ICG administration as they are deficient in the transporter bilitranslocase which is present in normal renal parenchyma [46]. However, Manny et al. [48] showed that this property cannot reliably identify malignant renal lesions. In their study of 100 RAPN cases, they were able to identify malignant tumors with a positive predictive value of 87% and negative predictive value of 52%.

The risks of blood loss and suboptimal views leading to potential positive surgical margins on the off-clamp approach and risk of reperfusion injury and nephron loss in the on-clamp approach have driven the interest in selective arterial clamping [49]. ICG-based fluorescence imaging has been used to help identify the arterial supply to the tumor and adequacy of selective clamping to improve the functional outcomes [41]. In this large series of 318 patients undergoing ICG-guided RAPN, the authors showed that ICG-guided surgery is a promising tool for guiding the surgeon strategy of global versus selective during robot-assisted partial nephrectomy especially in cases with challenging vascular supply or impaired renal function. They reported a trifecta rate of 80%; however, their study lacked a control group. Other studies have also shown that ICG-guided selective clamping during RAPN shows promise with lower glomerular filtration rate (GFR) reduction compared to global clamping [49–51]. Other potential uses of ICG-guided RAPN lie in localization of completely endophytic tumors and assessment of potential positive margin due to differing fluorescence of malignant and benign renal tissue [41, 52].

The use of ICG-guidance during ureteral reconstruction has helped in identification of the ureter in cases of inflammation and fibrosis as well as allow precise marking of diseased or strictured segments of the ureter allowing complete resection and guiding subsequent reconstruction. This may help prevent recurrences while allowing maximal preservation of the healthy ureter in cases such as complex pyeloplasty, ureteric reimplantation, ureteroureterostomy, and uretero-ileal stricture repairs post urinary diversion [43, 44].

Patel et al. demonstrated that ICG-guidance revised 30% of neurovascular bundle dissections [45] during RALP. Further studies are needed to assess if this can translate to better functional outcomes of continence and erectile function. Similarly, ICG-guided PLND has been explored for lymphatic mapping with an aim to reduce the morbidity associated with extensive PLND but with suboptimal results to conventional PLND [53]. Others have reported improved results with ICG bound to fluorescent radiotracers with the hybrid ICG-^{99m}Tc-nanocolloid tracer capable of identifying 80.4% of the lymph nodes detected by the combined pre-operative lymphoscintigraphy and SPECT/CT [54].

3.4.3 Gamma Probes and Sentinel Lymph Nodes

Laparoscopic gamma probes have enabled identification and resection of sentinel lymph nodes in robotic surgery. While the original probes have limitations of their length, movement, and being only been able to be controlled by the assistant, more recent trials have reported drop-in gamma probe that can be controlled by the ProGrasp robotic forceps for sentinel lymph node dissection during RALP [55]. When used for intra-operative identification and excision of metastatic lymph nodes in robotic salvage PLND, ^{99m}Technetium-prostate-specific membrane antigen (PSMA) and ^{111}Indium-PSMA revealed a sensitivity of 83.6% and 92.3%, specificity of 100% and 93.5%, respectively [56, 57].

3.5 Intra-operative Pathological Processing

3.5.1 NeuroSAFE

To optimize oncological outcomes while maintaining functional outcomes, NeuroSAFE, a frozen section-navigated nerve sparing during RALP, was first described by the Martini-Klinik in Hamburg, Germany [58] While some have reported positive reports on the benefits of NeuroSAFE [16, 59, 60], others retrospective series do not show a clear benefit and highlight the logistical problems of NeuroSAFE [61, 62]. Randomized controlled trials are currently underway to prospectively evaluate this technique [63].

3.5.2 Confocal Microscopy

Intra-operative pathological processing can be resource and time intensive limiting its use in routine practice. Newer technologies have emerged such as confocal LASER microendoscopy (CLE) [64] which uses intravenous fluorescein in vivo assessment of prostatic and periprostatic tissue using LASER probes and ex vivo fluorescence confocal microscopy (FCM), which uses lasers to provide rapid histopathological confirmation with high accuracy compared to traditional hematoxylin and eosin staining. Lopez et al. published an initial report showing the feasibility of using CLE (Mauna Kea Technologies, Paris, France) to identify prostate pedicles and neurovascular bundles [64]. Two other studies show a 91–100% accuracy of FCM (MAVIG GmbH, Munich, Germany; Caliber I.D.; Rochester, NY, USA) in differentiating benign and malignant prostate on intra-operative biopsies [65, 66]. While these technologies show initial promise, more studies are needed to assess their feasibility and impact on avoidance of positive margins while maintaining functional outcomes.

4 Future Directions

4.1 Connectivity

A unique aspect of robotic surgery that has been lacking is a robust support for telepresence surgery over large distances. There is an unmet need for this in terms of training, mentoring, performing surgery in remote locations and to allow complex sub-specialist procedures to be performed remotely by highly skilled surgeons. A limitation has been our global communication infrastructure with robotic surgery needing very low latency high bandwidth networks to remove and perceptible delay. Over the past decade, there has been significant development of high bandwidth wired and now wireless networks such as 5G. AI may also be able to augment this process using predictive movement models to give the surgeon-console signal enough time to cover very long distances [67].

4.2 Surgical Data Science

The surgical data science initiative workshop in 2016 defined surgical data science as an emerging scientific field with the objective of improving the quality of interventional healthcare and its value through capturing, organization, analysis, and modeling of data [68]. This may be applied not only in the robotic operative theater for decision support but also for performance assessment and surgical training.

While a robotic surgical system may help with many assistance functions, the surgeon will always remain the one making the decisions. A future where the robot gathers and processes data from sensors, videos, images, and haptic feedback and provides assistance and feedback to the surgeon in real time to aid decision-making is very likely.

Similarly, data science registries could provide performance feedback to the surgeon and culture of continuous measurement, assessment, and improvement using evidence from data is likely to become a key component of surgical practice and quality assurance for institutions.

In surgical practice, poor technical skills as well as poor non-technical skills such as judgement and decision-making are both associated with adverse surgical outcomes [69, 70]. Data collected from simulation training and real-time operating theater performance can be used in the future to provide targeted feedback and facilitate assessment, learning, and improvement of technical skills as well context-specific decision-making [71–73].

4.3 Precision and Soft Robotics

Current versions of the da Vinci do not provide haptic feedback, resulting in the surgeon having to rely on visual cues to assess tension on tissues. Some emerging robotic surgical systems on the market have incorporated haptic feedback technology into their systems. Surgeons and engineers continue to enhance haptic feedback in the form of force or tactile feedback and these developments may have a role in further reducing intra-operative injury [74]. Improvements in motion scaling and tremor filters are likely to make surgery more dextrous. While fully autonomous surgery is still some while away, increasing automation in established surgical systems is likely to lead to further incremental improvements in delivering precision robotic surgery. While this will be challenging, especially in tasks that require contextual understanding, simpler tasks such as suturing are more likely to have incremental automation applied to them. At each step, we will need to ensure through research that these systems are ready for clinical use.

Current robotic systems are made from rigid structures limiting their access to certain sites. Soft robotics uses flexible systems where their stiffness can be controlled to overcome these barriers. A team at Kings College, London, through the STIFFness controllable Flexible and Learnable manipulator for surgical OPerations (STIFF FLOP) project, have developed a soft-robotic arm that can be squeezed through a 12 mm Trocar-port, reconfigure and stiffen itself to perform tasks. This also allows greater flexibility and incorporation of haptic feedback in robotic surgery.

Increasing automation, in future, may have the advantages of further reducing the learning curve in robotic surgery, reducing dependence on surgical volume to achieve outcomes and thus making these technologies available to areas where they current may not be [75].

5 Discussion

The past decade of robotics technological advances has been dominated by Intuitive and the Da Vinci system. It has led to the widespread adoption of robotic-assisted laparoscopic surgery across all urological subspecialities. The next decade will bring much change in this field with new devices and companies entering the market. Each system will have its own pros and cons. In addition to these advances in 3D modeling, intra-operative imaging, real-time fusion of cross-sectional imaging, ICG, haptics, Neurosafe, and remote telepresence have the potential to improve many surgical steps and also lead to better outcomes for the patients. Ultimately it will be the clinical results, cost, and how easily these new technologies are integrated into the surgical plan that will lead to their success.

References

1. Binder J, Kramer W. Robotically-assisted laparoscopic radical prostatectomy. BJU Int. 2001;87(4):408–10.
2. Koukourikis P, Rha KH. Robotic surgical systems in urology: What is currently available? Investig Clin Urol. 2021;62(1):14–22.
3. DaVinci Surgical System's world. Available online: www.intuitivesurgical.com.
4. Heo JE, et al. Pure single-site robot-assisted pyeloplasty with the da Vinci SP surgical system: initial experience. Investig Clin Urol. 2019;60(4):326–30.
5. Kang SK, et al. Robot-assisted laparoscopic single-port pyeloplasty using the da Vinci SP(R) system: initial experience with a pediatric patient. J Pediatr Urol. 2019;15(5):576–7.
6. Kaouk J, et al. Step-by-step technique for single-port robot-assisted radical cystectomy and pelvic lymph nodes dissection using the da Vinci((R)) SP surgical system. BJU Int. 2019.
7. Agarwal DK, et al. Initial experience with da Vinci single-port robot-assisted radical prostatectomies. Eur Urol. 2020;77(3):373–9.
8. Billah MS, et al. Single port robotic assisted reconstructive urologic surgery-with the da Vinci SP surgical system. Transl Androl Urol. 2020;9(2):870–8.
9. Samalavicius NE, et al. Robotic surgery using Senhance((R)) robotic platform: single center experience with first 100 cases. J Robot Surg. 2020;14(2):371–6.
10. Kastelan Z, et al. Extraperitoneal radical prostatectomy with the Senhance Surgical System robotic platform. Croat Med J. 2019;60(6):556–9.
11. Chang KD, et al. Retzius-sparing robot-assisted radical prostatectomy using the Revo-i robotic surgical system: surgical technique and results of the first human trial. BJU Int. 2018;122(3):441–8.
12. Kobayashi S, et al. Assessment of surgical skills by using surgical navigation in robot-assisted partial nephrectomy. Int J Comput Assist Radiol Surg. 2019;14(8):1449–59.
13. Thomas BC, et al. Preclinical evaluation of the versius surgical system, a new robot-assisted surgical device for use in minimal access renal and prostate surgery. Eur Urol Focus. 2021;7(2):444–52.
14. Medicaroid. Hinotori robotic assisted surgery system [Internet]. Kobe: Medicaroid; 2020. Accessed 2021 April 9. http://www.medicaroid.com/en/product/hinotori/
15. Insights on the Surgical Robotic Systems Global Market to 2026 - Industry Analysis and Forecasts. Research and Markets. Accessed 2021 April 9. https://www.researchandmarkets.com/r/hsc5zl
16. Schlomm T, et al. Neurovascular structure-adjacent frozen-section examination (NeuroSAFE) increases nerve-sparing frequency and reduces positive surgical margins in open and robot-assisted laparoscopic radical prostatectomy: experience after 11,069 consecutive patients. Eur Urol. 2012;62(2):333–40.
17. Taktak S, et al. Aquablation: a novel and minimally invasive surgery for benign prostate enlargement. Ther Adv Urol. 2018;10(6):183–8.
18. Rassweiler J, et al. Robot-assisted flexible ureteroscopy: an update. Urolithiasis. 2018;46(1):69–77.
19. Miah S, et al. A prospective analysis of robotic targeted MRI-US fusion prostate biopsy using the centroid targeting approach. J Robot Surg. 2020;14(1):69–74.
20. Gutierrez M, Ditto R, Roy S. Systematic review of operative outcomes of robotic surgical procedures performed with endoscopic linear staplers or robotic staplers. J Robot Surg. 2019;13(1):9–21.
21. Johnson CS, et al. Performance of da Vinci Stapler during robotic-assisted right colectomy with intracorporeal anastomosis. J Robot Surg. 2019;13(1):115–9.
22. Galetta D, et al. New stapling devices in robotic surgery. J Vis Surg. 2017;3:45.
23. Steinberg RL, et al. Magnet-assisted robotic prostatectomy using the da Vinci SP robot: an initial case series. J Endourol. 2019;33(10):829–34.
24. Fulla J, et al. Magnetic-assisted robotic and laparoscopic renal surgery: initial clinical experience with the levita magnetic surgical system. J Endourol. 2020;34(12):1242–6.
25. Raman A, et al. Robotic-assisted laparoscopic partial nephrectomy in a horseshoe kidney. a case report and review of the literature. Urology. 2018;114:e3–5.
26. Porpiglia F, et al. Hyperaccuracy three-dimensional reconstruction is able to maximize the efficacy of selective clamping during robot-assisted partial nephrectomy for complex renal masses. Eur Urol. 2018;74(5):651–60.

27. Porpiglia F, et al. Three-dimensional virtual imaging of renal tumours: a new tool to improve the accuracy of nephrometry scores. BJU Int. 2019;124(6):945–54.
28. Bianchi L, et al. The impact of 3D digital reconstruction on the surgical planning of partial nephrectomy: a case-control study. Still time for a novel surgical trend? Clin Genitourin Cancer. 2020;18(6):e669–78.
29. Chandak P, et al. Three-dimensional printing in robot-assisted radical prostatectomy - an Idea, Development, Exploration, Assessment, Long-term follow-up (IDEAL) Phase 2a study. BJU Int. 2018;122(3):360–1.
30. MIMIC Technolgies. Available at mimicsimulation.com. Accessed April 9 2021.
31. Moglia A, et al. A systematic review of virtual reality simulators for robot-assisted surgery. Eur Urol. 2016;69(6):1065–80.
32. Mehralivand S, et al. A multiparametric magnetic resonance imaging-based virtual reality surgical navigation tool for robotic-assisted radical prostatectomy. Turk J Urol. 2019;45(5):357–65.
33. Porpiglia F, et al. Augmented-reality robot-assisted radical prostatectomy using hyper-accuracy three-dimensional reconstruction (HA3D) technology: a radiological and pathological study. BJU Int. 2019;123(5):834–45.
34. Porpiglia F, et al. Three-dimensional elastic augmented-reality robot-assisted radical prostatectomy using hyperaccuracy three-dimensional reconstruction technology: a step further in the identification of capsular involvement. Eur Urol. 2019;76(4):505–14.
35. Porpiglia F, et al. Three-dimensional augmented reality robot-assisted partial nephrectomy in case of complex tumours (PADUA >/=10): a new intraoperative tool overcoming the ultrasound guidance. Eur Urol. 2020;78(2):229–38.
36. Baghdadi A, et al. A computer vision technique for automated assessment of surgical performance using surgeons' console-feed videos. Int J Comput Assist Radiol Surg. 2019;14(4):697–707.
37. Chen J, et al. Use of automated performance metrics to measure surgeon performance during robotic vesicourethral anastomosis and methodical development of a training tutorial. J Urol. 2018;200(4):895–902.
38. Di Cosmo G, et al. Intraoperative ultrasound in robot-assisted partial nephrectomy: state of the art. Arch Ital Urol Androl. 2018;90(3):195–8.
39. Alenezi AN, Karim O. Role of intra-operative contrast-enhanced ultrasound (CEUS) in robotic-assisted nephron-sparing surgery. J Robot Surg. 2015;9(1):1–10.
40. Rao AR, et al. Occlusion angiography using intraoperative contrast-enhanced ultrasound scan (CEUS): a novel technique demonstrating segmental renal blood supply to assist zero-ischaemia robot-assisted partial nephrectomy. Eur Urol. 2013;63(5):913–9.
41. Diana P, et al. the role of intraoperative indocyanine green in robot-assisted partial nephrectomy: results from a large, multi-institutional series. Eur Urol. 2020;78(5):743–9.
42. Bjurlin MA, et al. Near-infrared fluorescence imaging: emerging applications in robotic upper urinary tract surgery. Eur Urol. 2014;65(4):793–801.
43. Lee Z, et al. Use of indocyanine green during robot-assisted ureteral reconstructions. Eur Urol. 2015;67(2):291–8.
44. Tuderti G, et al. Transnephrostomic indocyanine green-guided robotic ureteral reimplantation for benign ureteroileal strictures after robotic cystectomy and intracorporeal neobladder: step-by-step surgical technique, perioperative and functional outcomes. J Endourol. 2019;33(10):823–8.
45. Kumar A, Samavedi S, Bates A. Use of intra-operative indocyanine green and Firefly technology to visualize the "landmark artery" for nerve sparing robot assisted radical prostatectomy. Eur Urol Suppl. 2015;2(14):eV36.
46. Tobis S, et al. Near infrared fluorescence imaging with robotic assisted laparoscopic partial nephrectomy: initial clinical experience for renal cortical tumors. J Urol. 2011;186(1):47–52.
47. van den Berg NS, et al. Multispectral fluorescence imaging during robot-assisted laparoscopic sentinel node biopsy: a first step towards a fluorescence-based anatomic roadmap. Eur Urol. 2017;72(1):110–7.
48. Manny TB, Krane LS, Hemal AK. Indocyanine green cannot predict malignancy in partial nephrectomy: histopathologic correlation with fluorescence pattern in 100 patients. J Endourol. 2013;27(7):918–21.
49. Mattevi D, et al. Fluorescence-guided selective arterial clamping during RAPN provides better early functional outcomes based on renal scan compared to standard clamping. J Robot Surg. 2019;13(3):391–6.
50. Borofsky MS, et al. Near-infrared fluorescence imaging to facilitate super-selective arterial clamping during zero-ischaemia robotic partial nephrectomy. BJU Int. 2013;111(4):604–10.
51. Krane LS, Hemal AK. Surgery: Is indocyanine green dye useful in robotic surgery? Nat Rev Urol. 2014;11(1):12–4.
52. Simone G, et al. "Ride the green light": indocyanine green-marked off-clamp robotic partial nephrectomy for totally endophytic renal masses. Eur Urol. 2019;75(6):1008–14.
53. Chennamsetty A, et al. Lymph node fluorescence during robot-assisted radical prostatectomy with indocyanine green: prospective dosing analysis. Clin Genitourin Cancer. 2017;15(4):e529–34.
54. KleinJan GH, et al. Multimodal hybrid imaging agents for sentinel node mapping as a means to (re)connect nuclear medicine to advances made in robot-assisted surgery. Eur J Nucl Med Mol Imaging. 2016;43(7):1278–87.
55. Meershoek P, et al. Robot-assisted laparoscopic surgery using DROP-IN radioguidance: first-in-human translation. Eur J Nucl Med Mol Imaging. 2019;46(1):49–53.
56. Maurer T, et al. (99m)Technetium-based prostate-specific membrane antigen-radioguided surgery in recurrent prostate cancer. Eur Urol. 2019;75(4):659–66.
57. Rauscher I, Eiber M, Maurer T. PSMA-radioguided surgery for salvage lymphadenectomy in recurrent prostate cancer. Aktuelle Urol. 2017;48(2):148–52.
58. Beyer B, et al. A feasible and time-efficient adaptation of NeuroSAFE for da Vinci robot-assisted radical prostatectomy. Eur Urol. 2014;66(1):138–44.
59. Mirmilstein G, et al. The neurovascular structure-adjacent frozen-section examination (NeuroSAFE) approach to nerve sparing in robot-assisted laparoscopic radical prostatectomy in a British setting - a prospective observational comparative study. BJU Int. 2018;121(6):854–62.
60. Fromont G, et al. Intraoperative frozen section analysis during nerve sparing laparoscopic radical prostatectomy: feasibility study. J Urol. 2003;170(5):1843–6.
61. Heinrich E, et al. Clinical impact of intraoperative frozen sections during nerve-sparing radical prostatectomy. World J Urol. 2010;28(6):709–13.
62. Gillitzer R, et al. Intraoperative peripheral frozen sections do not significantly affect prognosis after nerve-sparing radical prostatectomy for prostate cancer. BJU Int. 2011;107(5):755–9.
63. Dinneen E, et al. NeuroSAFE robot-assisted laparoscopic prostatectomy versus standard robot-assisted laparoscopic prostatectomy for men with localised prostate cancer (NeuroSAFE PROOF): protocol for a randomised controlled feasibility study. BMJ Open. 2019;9(6):e028132.
64. Lopez A, et al. Intraoperative optical biopsy during robotic assisted radical prostatectomy using confocal endomicroscopy. J Urol. 2016;195(4 Pt 1):1110–7.
65. Puliatti S, et al. Ex vivo fluorescence confocal microscopy: the first application for real-time pathological examination of prostatic tissue. BJU Int. 2019;124(3):469–76.
66. Rocco B, et al. Real-time assessment of surgical margins during radical prostatectomy: a novel approach that uses fluorescence

confocal microscopy for the evaluation of peri-prostatic soft tissue. BJU Int. 2020;125(4):487–9.
67. Kim SSY, Dohler M, Dasgupta P. The Internet of Skills: use of fifth-generation telecommunications, haptics and artificial intelligence in robotic surgery. BJU Int. 2018;122(3):356–8.
68. Maier-Hein L, et al. Surgical data science for next-generation interventions. Nat Biomed Eng. 2017;1(9):691–6.
69. Birkmeyer JD, et al. Surgical skill and complication rates after bariatric surgery. N Engl J Med. 2013;369(15):1434–42.
70. Nathwani JN, et al. Relationship between technical errors and decision-making skills in the junior resident. J Surg Educ. 2016;73(6):e84–90.
71. Vedula SS, Ishii M, Hager GD. Objective assessment of surgical technical skill and competency in the operating room. Annu Rev Biomed Eng. 2017;19:301–25.
72. Greenberg CC, et al. Surgical coaching for individual performance improvement. Ann Surg. 2015;261(1):32–4.
73. Singh P, et al. A randomized controlled study to evaluate the role of video-based coaching in training laparoscopic skills. Ann Surg. 2015;261(5):862–9.
74. Okamura AM. Haptic feedback in robot-assisted minimally invasive surgery. Curr Opin Urol. 2009;19(1):102–7.
75. Svoboda E. Your robot surgeon will see you now. Nature. 2019;573(7775):S110–1.

Robot-Assisted Radical Prostatectomy: Development of Nerve-Sparing Techniques at Vattikuti Urology Institute

Anudeep Mukkamala, Wooju Jeong, Michael Gorin, and Mani Menon

1 Introduction

Continued innovation of the robot-assisted radical prostatectomy (RARP) since 2001 has resulted in an effective, high quality surgical treatment for prostate cancer. Complete recovery of sexual function, however, remains challenging to achieve. Multiple approaches have been tested with varying levels of success: preserving the prostatic fascia, dissecting the prostate antegrade versus retrograde, and athermal techniques along the neurovascular bundles/cavernosal nerves. In 2007, a pivotal study at Vattikuti Urology Institute (VUI) on the outcomes of the Vattikuti Institute Prostatectomy (VIP) with Veil of Aphrodite nerve sparing demonstrated a potency rate of 70% at 12 months [1, 2]. Other groups around the world have developed and published their nerve-sparing approaches with varied rates of success (range of potency from the reference) [3–7]. Despite these efforts, a paper published by Capogrosso et al. in 2019 demonstrated that potency rate has not overall significantly changed in 20+ years, as illustrated in Fig. 1 [8]. Therefore, opportunities remain to continue building, innovating, and developing on prior techniques to achieve complete recovery of sexual function.

2 Historical Perspective

Radical prostatectomy for the treatment of prostate cancer has evolved dramatically from its initial introduction by Hugh Hampton Young as an open perineal surgery in 1905 to its current iteration as a robot-assisted retropubic procedure with nerve-sparing techniques designed to achieve maximal oncologic control with complete recovery of sexual function. First popularized by Mani Menon in 2001, RARP revolutionized the field of urology with major improvements in hospital stay (1 day, down from 3 weeks), blood loss (100 mL, down from >1 L), and erectile dysfunction (up to 40% recovery, improved from complete loss of erections) [7]. Efforts since its introduction have centered on improving sexual function without compromising oncologic outcomes.

Surgeons at the VUI have continued to hone and refine the RARP with nerve-sparing approaches such as the Veil of Aphrodite [9, 10] (2006) and the Super Veil [2] (2009) technique to improve post-operative sexual function. While the initial Veil approach develops the plane of dissection between the prostate capsule and the prostate fascia at the 1 o'clock and 5 o'clock positions and the 6 o'clock and 11 o'clock positions, the Super Veil approach extends the dissection anteriorly thereby preserving the prostatic fascia between the 11 o'clock and 1 o'clock positions, the pubovesical ligaments and the dorsal venous complex. At 1 year, 70% of patients undergoing the VIP with Veil technique achieved potency with or without use of phosphodiesterase (PDE5) inhibitors [4]. Performing Super Veil resulted in 94% of patients achieving sexual potency with the use of PDE5 inhibitors at 1 year [2].

Promising advances for RARP with nerve-sparing have also been reported at other institutions, including use of local hypothermia with an endorectal cooling balloon (ECB) system [4]; flexible CO_2 laser fiber-guided dissection 2010 [11]; and use of dehydrated human amnion/chorion membrane (dHACM) wrap around the neurovascular bundles to improve potency [12]. Trials utilizing augmented reality to improve RARP are currently being investigated, with preliminary data [13] showing feasibility and accuracy (2018).

A. Mukkamala · W. Jeong (✉) ·
Vattikuti Urology Institute, Henry Ford Health System, Detroit, MI, USA

M. Gorin
Urology Associates & UPMC Western Maryland, Cumberland, MD, USA

Department of Urology, University of Pittsburgh School of Medicine, Pittsburgh, PA, USA

M. Menon
Urology, Mount Sinai Ichan School of Medicine, New York, USA

P. Wiklund et al. (eds.), *Robotic Urologic Surgery*, https://doi.org/10.1007/978-3-031-00363-9_3

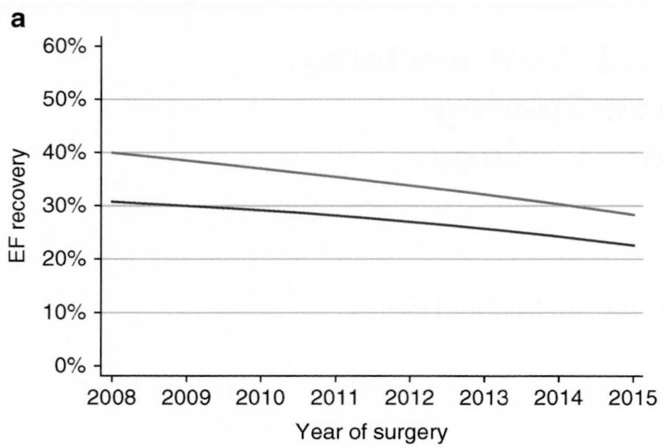

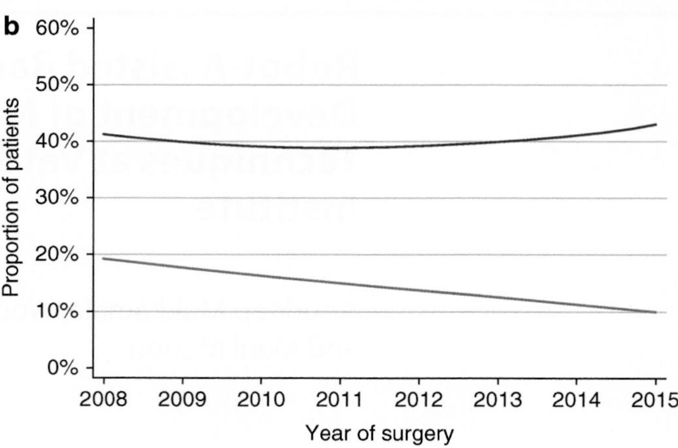

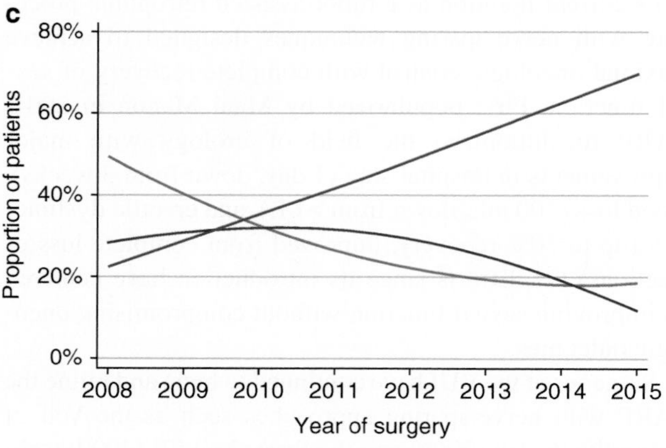

Fig. 1 (**a**) Unadjusted rate of patients reporting erectile function recovery at 12 (blue line) and 24 (orange line) mo after radical prostatectomy (RP). (**b**) Rate of patients reporting regular use of phosphodiesterase type 5 inhibitors at 12 (blue line) and 24 (orange line) mo assessment. (**c**) Rate of patients treated with different surgical approach: open RP (blue line); laparoscopic RP (orange); robot-assisted RP (dark orange)

3 Indications/Contraindications

Indications for RARP with nerve-sparing [14]:

- Fully potent preoperatively (SHIM >17)
- Preservation of urinary continence
- Organ-confined cancer
- Clinical T1/T2a/T2b disease
- Gleason score ≤7
- PSA ≤10 ng/mL

Contraindications for RARP with nerve-sparing [14]:

Absolute
- Locally advanced disease (T3c lesions)
- Palpable disease at the apex
- Gleason Grade 5 disease
- PSA >20 ng/mL
- Preoperative impotence

Relative
- Intraoperative difficulties with mobilization of the neurovascular bundles
- Palpable localized disease (T2c, other than at apex)
- PSA serology between 10 and 20 ng/mL
- Greater than 50% Gleason Grade 4 disease on biopsy
- Perineural invasion on biopsy
- Presence of cancer in three needle cores from the same prostate lobe on sextant biopsy

4 Nerve-Sparing Approaches

4.1 Standard Nerve-Sparing Technique

The prostate pedicle is exposed once the base of the seminal vesicle is retracted superomedially and lies anterior to the neurovascular bundles. The pedicles provide only a prostatic blood supply and are controlled by either clipping or individual cauterization using a bipolar robotic instrument.

Incisions are made on the prostatic fascia anterior and parallel to the neurovascular bundles. Careful sharp and blunt dissection is performed to separate the neurovascular tissue from the prostate posterolaterally, mostly at 5 or 7 o'clock position. The assistant or fourth robotic instrument retracts the prostate to provide counter retraction to expose the dissection plane.

4.2 Nerve-Sparing Technique: The "Veil of Aphrodite"

The first decision for potency preservation to consider is sparing the cavernosal nerves during RARP by incising the prostate fascia anteriorly. Surgeons at the VUI first developed the lateral prostatic fascia sparing technique termed "Veil of Aphrodite" for the RARP in 2005, with results [1, 15] showing significant improvement in sexual potency rates regardless of preoperative SHIM score after Veil technique compared with standard nerve-sparing approach: 13 to 22%, 31 to 61%, and 39 to 73%.

Although the classical concept is that two neurovascular bundles are located near the posterolateral aspect at the 5 and 7 O'Clock positions of the protate, the cavernosal nerves form "veils" that extend from the posterolateral at the base of te prostate to the anterolateral at the apex of the prostate. The veils of cavernosal nerves are spared by incising the prostate fascia anterolaterally and entering the plane deep to the venous sinuses of the Santorini plexus, starting infero-laterally where the prostatic fascia reflects off the prostate at the base of the seminal vesicles and proceeds in an antegrade fashion (Fig. 2).

Careful sharp and blunt dissection of the neurovascular bundle and contiguous prostatic fascia is then performed using the cold scissors, to mobilize the entire prostatic fascia

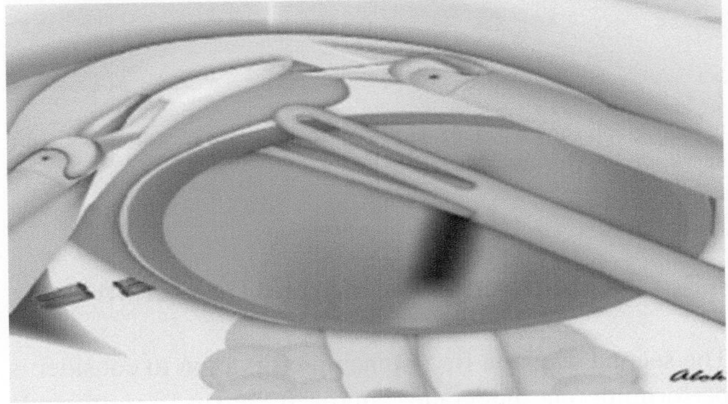

Fig. 2 Plane of dissection for veil of Aphrodite

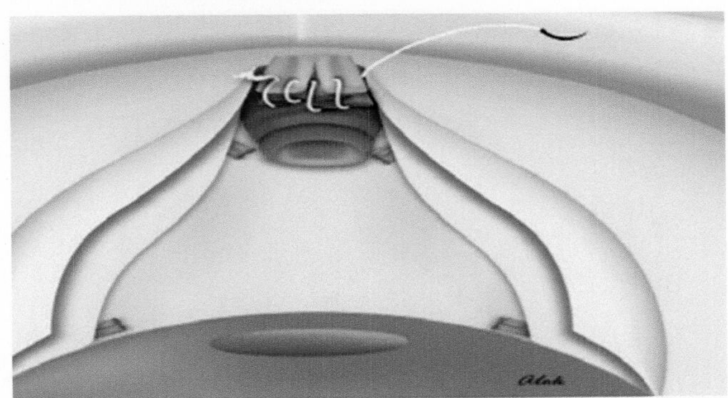

Fig. 3 Control of dorsal venous complex and completed veil of Aphrodite after removal of specimen

and the ipsilateral pubourethral ligaments. This "veil" plane is mostly avascular except the anterior apex of the prostate where the fascia is fused with the puboprostatic ligaments and covers the dorsal venous plexus. The ultimate result is an intact "veil" of periprostatic tissue extending from the pubourethral ligaments to the bladder neck (Fig. 3). In case patients have the difficult plane to enter, possibly from the fibrosis after biopsy, the dissection can be performed retrograde and enter the fascia on the anterolateral surface of the prostate at the 10 o'clock or 2 o'clock positions to develop the veil plane.

Robot-Assisted Radical Prostatectomy with Veil Nerve-sparing technique (Vattikuti Institute Prostatectomy) video performed by Dr. Mani Menon (Jan 2009):

https://www.youtube.com/watch?v=QOqjt3-3sqA

The mean distance between the resection margin and the tumor was 0.3 mm with Veil nerve sparing and 1.4 mm with conventional nerve sparing [16]. The photomicrograph of the Veil of Aphrodite shows the plane of dissection is clearly outside of the prostate capsule without capsular incision or positive margin (Fig. 4a). With staining with S-100 for the neural structures, the prostate fascia is on the prostate gland with the nerves at the conventional nerve-sparing side (Fig. 4b), while no nerve with an intact capsule is observed at the Veil nerve-sparing side, indicating that periprostatic nerve bundles were preserved in situ in Veil nerve sparing.

Figure 5 demonstrates the preoperative and postoperative SHIM scores between the conventional "standard" nerve-sparing group and the "Veil" nerve-sparing group from the initial series of 34 Veil nerve-sparing patients. Benefits of Veil nerve-sparing technique with respect to improved post-operative SHIM score and quality of erections satisfactory for intercourse. 86% of Veil nerve-sparing patients postoperatively achieved potency of SHIM score over 21 with or without PDE5 inhibitor, and 97% of patients were able to have intercourse postoperatively.

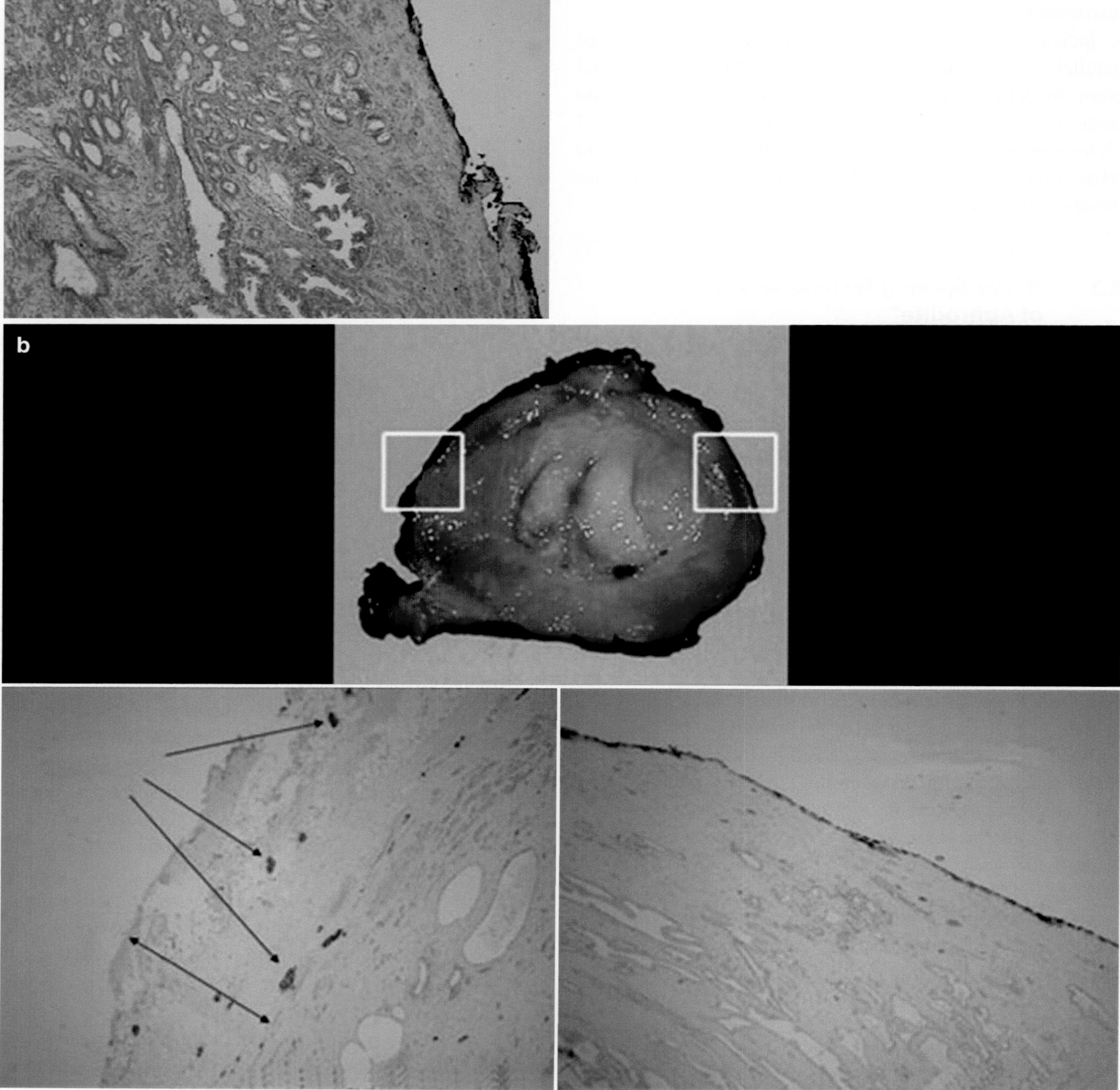

Fig. 4 Photomicrograph of the Veil of Aphrodite (**a**) showing the plane of dissection on the capsule of the prostate. Hematoxylin and eosin, ×100. Compared to the conventional nerve sparing (**b** bottom left), photomicrograph shows lack of nerves on the prostate specimen with Veil nerve sparing (**b** bottom right). S-100, X200

Later, the authors updated the potency outcomes for 154 patients with Veil nerve sparing [9]. This series reported 96% patients had intercourse postoperatively. 69% patients had normal erection of SHIM score over 21 and 45% had used PDE5 inhibitors.

4.3 Antegrade vs Retrograde Dissection

The second decision for potency preservation to consider is performing an antegrade approach versus a retrograde approach to nerve sparing during RARP. The first descrip-

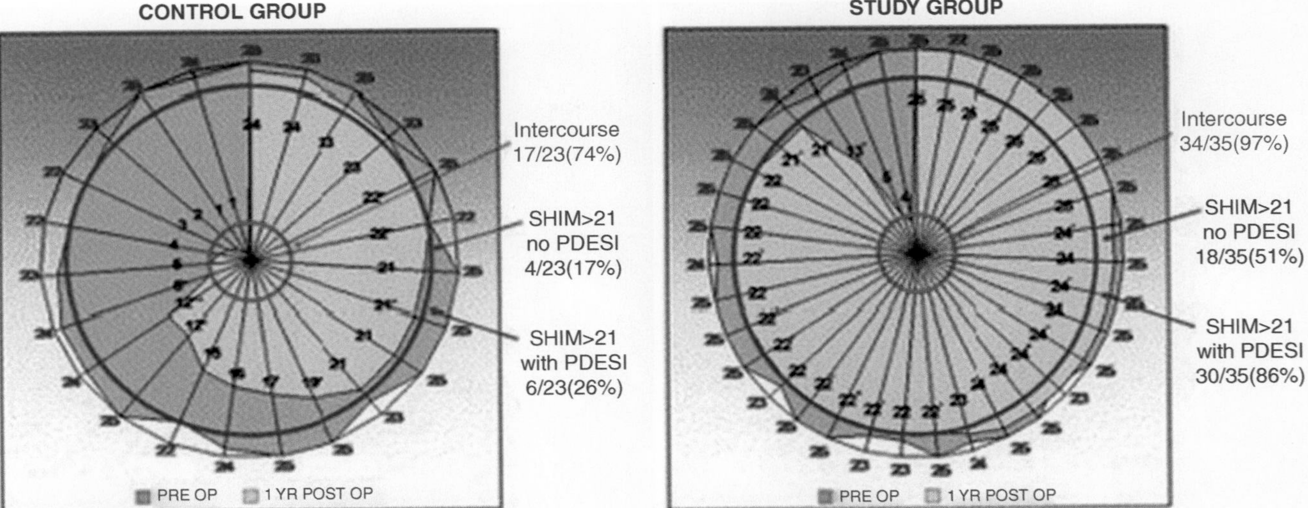

Fig. 5 Every spoke in this graph represents an individual patient. * patients on PDESI, double ** patient on vaccum erection device, *PDESI* phosphodiesterase 5 inhibitors

tion of Vattikuti Institute Prostatectomy (VIP) technique was a retrograde dissection starting from the apex of the prostate after DVC ligation, which was changed to antegrade dissection as a standard technique for VIP [17]. The authors claimed that this early apical dissection provided enormous help to identify the apex at the time of specimen detachment. Later, the difference in approaches was described by Patel et al. in 2012 to evaluate oncologic and functional outcomes after RARP [18]. While the positive margin rate was similar between antegrade and retrograde dissections, the potency rate was significantly higher with the retrograde approach.

4.4 Athermal vs Thermal Dissection

The third decision for potency preservation to consider is performing an athermal versus thermal dissection near the neurovascular bundles and cavernosal nerves during RARP. Menon et al. proposed athermal dissection of NVB using Hem-O-Lok clips and sharp dissection using cold scissors, to avoid electro-cautery during the dissection [1, 17]. Ahlering et al. published their results in 2008, demonstrating the effect of thermal energy on the return of sexual activity [19]. Potency was defined as "erections hard enough for vaginal penetration with or without the use of PDE-5 inhibitors." In the thermal dissection/cautery group, 14.7% of patients were potent after 9 months (UNS-10%; BNS-16.7%) and 63.2% were potent at 24 months (UNS-50%; BNS-67.9%), as compared to 69.8% after 9 months (UNS-56.3%; BNS-72.8%) and 92% after 24 months (UNS-83.3%; BNS-92%) for the athermal dissection/cautery free group.

4.5 Puboprostatic Ligament Preservation/Super Veil Technique

The fourth decision for potency preservation to consider is preserving the puboprostatic ligaments and performing a tension-free dissection of the neurovascular bundle during RARP [2]. With favorable anatomy, the dissection complex formed an avascular "hood," the so-called Super Veil. This technique was proposed to the highly selected patients with low-risk prostate cancer, and at a medial follow-up of 18 months, 94% had an erection strong enough for penetration with a median SHIM score of 18. According to Asimakopoulos et al., performing a pubovesical complex (PVC) sparing technique is feasible and may be effective in improving early functional outcomes [20]. The preliminary data from this trial showed that 73% of patients were potent (defined as IIEF score > 17) with or without PDE5 inhibitors at 3 months.

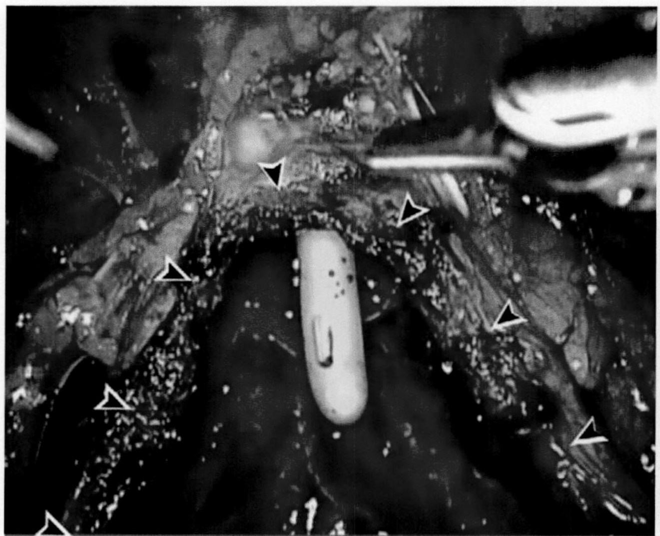

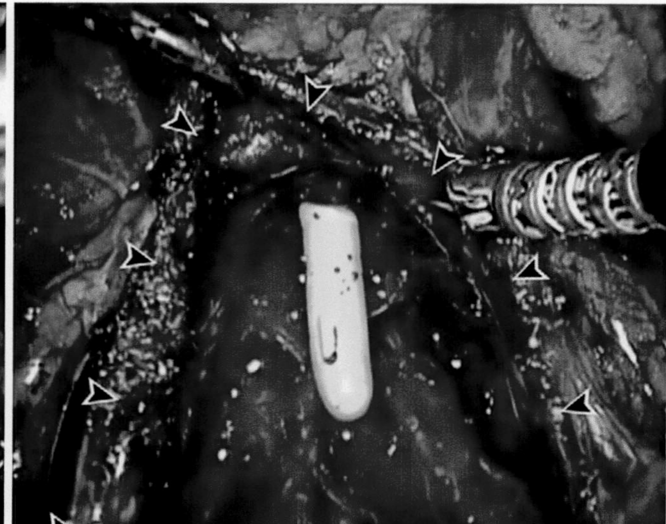

Operative photos

4.6 Menon Precision Prostatectomy

As a nerve-sparing approach in development, the Menon Precision Prostatectomy (MPP) is a novel technique designed to maximize extirpation of prostatic tissue without affecting functional reserve. In brief, this procedure involves removal of all prostatic tissue except for a 5–10 mm rim of prostate capsule ("remnant") on the side contralateral to the dominant lesion. An IDEAL Stage 0 study was performed by Sood et al. in 2019 to provide preliminary data (Fig. 6) for the current Phase III randomized clinical trial underway at the Vattikuti Urology Institute (VUI) evaluating this focal therapy approach for the treatment of prostate cancer [21]. Prior to the MPP, patients who are biopsy-naïve will undergo a transperineal saturation biopsy along with capsular biopsies, while patients who have had a prior prostate biopsy will only undergo capsular biopsies focusing on the remnant side. This method of thorough sampling will minimize the chances of leaving significant cancer behind at the time of robotic MPP.

As a fail-safe measure, the remnant prostatic capsule will be biopsied intraoperatively to ensure absence of cancer. If cancer is present on frozen section, a standard RARP will instead be performed. Based on early clinical trials, there is preliminary data ($n = 8$) showing that the MPP had multiple benefits over focal/hemi-ablation, most importantly 100% potency within 12 months. Upcoming data from patients being enrolled in the Phase III clinical trial ought to shed further light on functional and oncologic outcomes after MPP. In particular, it is important to be aware that preservation of sexual potency may come at the cost of oncologic control in MPP-eligible patients, many of whom will need follow-up biopsies given high likelihood of clinically significant disease in remnant tissue.

5 Future Strategies

Novel approaches to nerve-sparing techniques for the RARP remain on the horizon, with the possible adoption of augmented reality (AR) technology for prostatic surgery [22]. An early study published in 2020 demonstrated the effectiveness of a 3D model with AR to guide nerve sparing during RARP, with AR-3D technology changing the nerve-sparing approach in 38.5% of men on patient-based analysis and 34.6% of sides on side-based analysis. The theorized benefits of AR-3D technology include improved identification of the index prostate cancer, meticulously tailored dissection to the index lesion, and modification of the extent of nerve sparing. Other efforts to help integrate mpMRI and clinical data for surgical planning of RARP are currently being investigated [23].

6 Conclusions

In summary, robotic technology and nerve-sparing approaches have transformed the field of urology—and urologic oncology in particular—in tremendous ways. The ideal outcome of oncologic control with complete recovery of sexual potency after RARP remains elusive. However, as described above, multiple innovative nerve-sparing approaches including ret-

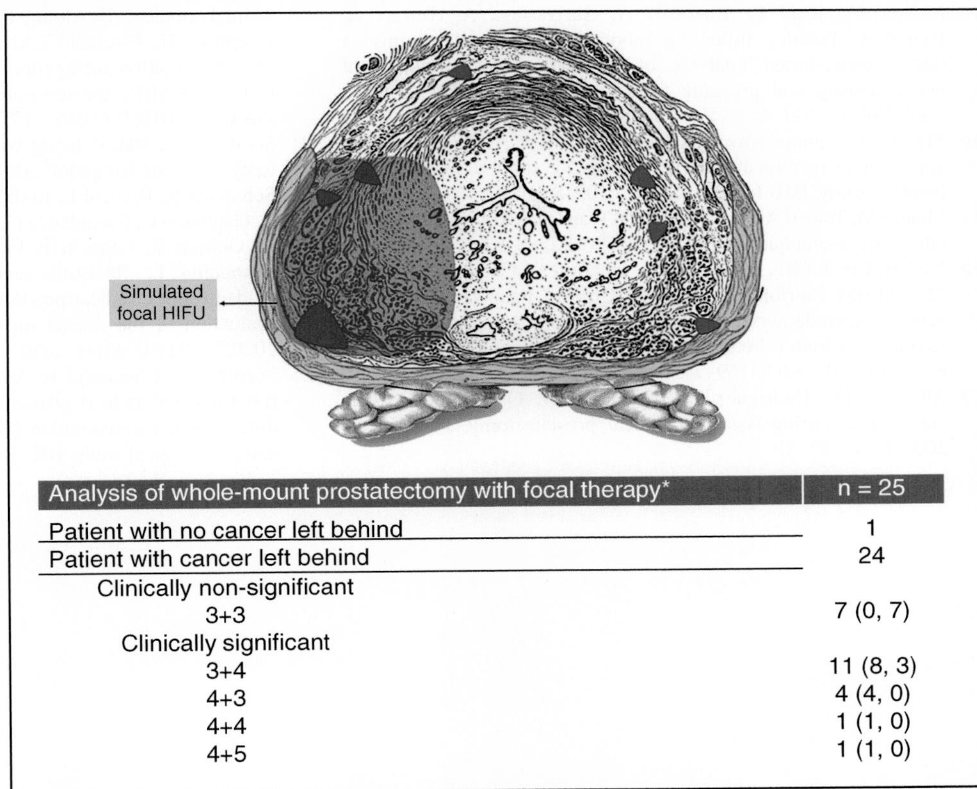

Analysis of whole-mount prostatectomy with focal therapy*	n = 25
Patient with no cancer left behind	1
Patient with cancer left behind	24
Clinically non-significant	
3+3	7 (0, 7)
Clinically significant	
3+4	11 (8, 3)
4+3	4 (4, 0)
4+4	1 (1, 0)
4+5	1 (1, 0)

Fig. 6 Simulation, pictorial representation, and outcomes of focal HIFU in the whole-mount radical prostatectomy specimens of patients eligible for focal therapy; $n = 25$ patients (IDEAL stage 0 study) (reproduced with permission from Sood et al., BMJ surgery, interventions & health technologies, 2019). * patients fulfilling the criteria of 40 g prostate weight for focal HIFU; only the dominant nodule was treated in this simulation—where the dominant nodule was within 5 mm of the edge of prostate capsule, a part of the dominant nodule was considered not treated in this simulation. 14 patients had dominant nodules within 5 mm of edge, hence, a part of dominant nodule was considered untreated; 10 patients had dominant nodule completely treated, but had additional nodules

rograde dissection, going cautery-free near the neurovascular bundles, sparing the endopelvic fascia, and puboprostatic ligament preservation have been performed at multiple institutions with varying degrees of success in improving potency recovery. Thorough analysis of the MPP clinical trial data will be helpful in integrating current knowledge with future nerve-sparing strategies to achieve clinical excellence in the treatment of prostate cancer.

References

1. Menon M, Shrivastava A, Kaul S, Badani KK, Fumo M, Bhandari M, Peabody JO. Vattikuti Institute prostatectomy: contemporary technique and analysis of results. Eur Urol. 2007;51(3):648–58.
2. Menon M, Shrivastava A, Bhandari M, Satyanarayana R, Siva S, Agarwal PK. Vattikuti Institute prostatectomy: technical modifications in 2009. Eur Urol. 2009;56:89–96.
3. Patel VR, Schatloff O, Chauhan S, Sivaraman A, Valero R, Coelho RF. The role of the prostatic vasculature as a landmark for nerve sparing during robot-assisted radical prostatectomy. Eur Urol. 2012;61:571–6.
4. Finley DS, Osann K, Skarecky D, Ahlering TE. Hypothermic nerve-sparing radical prostatectomy: rationale, feasibility, and effect on early continence. Urology. 2009;73:691–6.
5. Chien GW, Mikhail AA, Orvieto MA, Zagaja GP, Sokoloff MH, Brendler CB. Modified clipless antegrade nerve preservation in robotic-assisted laparoscopic radical prostatectomy with validated sexual function evaluation. Urology. 2005;66:419–23.
6. Kumar A, Samavedi S, Bates A, Coelho R, Rocco B, Marquinez J. Using indocyanine green and near-infrared fluorescence technology to identify the "landmark artery" during robot-assisted radical prostatectomy. Videourology. 2015;85(1):29–31.
7. Costello AJ. Considering the role of radical prostatectomy in 21st century prostate cancer care. Nat Rev Urol. 2020;17(3):177–88.
8. Capogrosso P, Vertosick EA, Benfante NE, Eastham JA, Scardino PJ, Vickers AJ, Mulhall JP. Are we improving erectile function recovery after radical prostatectomy? Analysis of patients treated over the last decade. Eur Urol. 2019;75(2):221–8.
9. Kaul S, Savera A, Badani KK, Fumo M, Bhandari A, Menon M. Functional outcomes and oncological efficacy of Vattikuti Institute prostatectomy with Veil of Aphrodite nerve-sparing: an analysis of 154 consecutive patients. BJU Int. 2006;97:467–72.
10. Shigemura K, Yamanaka N, Yamashita M. Veil nerve-sparing technique and postoperative urinary continence in open antegrade radical prostatectomy. Urol Int. 2012;89(3):283–9.
11. Cheetham PJ, Truesdale MD, Lee DJ, Landman JM, Badani KK. Use of a flexible carbon dioxide laser fiber for precise dissection of the neurovascular bundle during robot-assisted laparoscopic prostatectomy. J Endourol. 2010;24:1091–6.
12. Patel VR, Samavedi S, Bates AS, Kumar A, Coelho R, Rocco B. Dehydrated human amnion/chorion membrane allograft nerve wrap around the prostatic neurovascular bundle accelerates early return to continence and potency following robot-assisted radical prostatectomy: propensity score-matched analysis. Eur Urol. 2015;67:977–80.
13. Porpiglia F, Fiori C, Checcucci E, Amparore D, Bertolo R. Augmented reality robot-assisted radical prostatectomy: preliminary experience. Urology. 2018;115:184.
14. Gontero P, Kirby R. Nerve-sparing radical retropubic prostatectomy: techniques and clinical considerations. Prostate Cancer Prostatic Dis. 2005;8(2):133–9.

15. Menon M, Kaul S, Bhandari A, Shrivastava A, Tewari A, Hemal A. Potency following robotic radical prostatectomy: a questionnaire-based analysis of outcomes after conventional nerve sparing and prostatic fascia sparing techniques. J Urol. 2005;174(6):2291–6.
16. Martini A, Cumarasamy S, Haines KG III, Tewari AK. An updated approach to incremental nerve sparing for robot-assisted radical prostatectomy. BJU Int. 2019;124(1):103–8.
17. Menon M, Tewari A, Peabody J, VIP Team. Vattikuti Institute prostatectomy: technique. J Urol. 2003;169(6):2289–92.
18. Ko YH, Coelho RF, Sivaraman A, Schatloff O, Chauhan S, Abdul-Muhsin HM, Carrion RJ, Palmer KJ, Cheon J, Patel VR. Retrograde versus antegrade nerve sparing during robot-assisted radical prostatectomy: which is better for achieving early functional recovery? Eur Urol. 2013;63(1):169–77.
19. Ahlering TE, Rodriguez E, Skarecky DW. Overcoming obstacles: nerve-sparing issues in radical prostatectomy. J Endourol. 2008;22(4):745–50.
20. Asimakopoulos AD, Annino F, D'Orazio A, Pereira CF, Mugnier C, Hoepffner JL, Piechaud T, Gaston R. Complete periprostatic anatomy preservation during robot-assisted laparoscopic radical prostatectomy (RARP): the new pubovesical complex-sparing technique. Eur Urol. 2010;58(3):407–17.
21. Sood A, Abdollah F, Jeong W, Menon M. The precision prostatectomy: "waiting for godot". Eur Urol Focus. 2020;6(2):227–30.
22. Schiavina R, Bianchi L, Lodi S, Cercenelli L, Chessa F, Bortolani B, Gaudiano C, Casablanca C, Droghetti M, Porreca A, Romagnoli D, Golfieri R, Giunchi F, Fiorentino M, Marcelli E, Diciotti S, Brunocilla E. Real-time augmented reality three-dimensional guided robotic radical prostatectomy: preliminary experience and evaluation of the impact on surgical planning. Eur Urol Focus. 2020;31: S2405-4569(20)30217-0.
23. Porpiglia F, Checcucci E, Amparore D, et al. Augmented-reality robot-assisted radical prostatectomy using hyper-accuracy three-dimensional reconstruction (HA3D™) technology: a radiological and pathological study. BJU Int. 2019;123(5):834–45.

Robotic Training, Certification, and Ongoing Evaluation of Robotic Skills

Richard M. Satava

1 Introduction

Technology and surgical practice are in the fourth generation of Surgery: Robotic-assisted Minimally Invasive Surgery (RAMIS). The three previous generations are: Open surgery, endoluminal surgery (flexible endoscopy), and laparoscopic surgery, each one building a new niche and even spawning new "specialties," thus the need for continuous training at all levels of surgeons: novice initiates, current practitioners and even senior surgeons. In the author's career, all three "generations" were "new" technologies with unique challenges and required initial training and retraining, as the technologies allowed opportunity for "less invasive" surgery, there was improvement in reduced pain, shorter hospital stay, lower cost, and improved outcomes. Repeatedly, it became time for retraining in the "new" technology—and currently, it is RAMIS. Some fundamental principles and basic skills remain the same (allowing the surgeon to build upon accumulated knowledge and psychomotor skills), yet there is a need for adaptation and adopting to the new technology. And while the first three generations made major evolutionary changes, RAMIS is a totally disruptive change and uniquely representative of the Information Age (Digital Age).

Not only does the surgeon need new knowledge in medicine and surgery, but also must learn (at least superficially) many of the new digital (non-medical) technologies (computers, information science, mechanical engineering, and soon telecommunications). For the first time ever, the surgeon does not "see" or even "touch" the patient during the surgical procedure. The surgeon looks at a video monitor (not the patient's organs, tissues, etc.) and does not "directly manipulate" instruments; rather the surgeon receives visual information (image on the monitor) and sends information using electronic "handles" (input device) to move the instruments. The RAMIS is essentially an "information system," allowing the manipulation of instruments with more accuracy and precision than the unaided hands. But it is also the only surgical system that can connect with the internet, the Internet of Things (IoT), supercomputers, artificial intelligence, remote surgery sites, and yet to discover next generation of surgery (see FUTURE section). Just as flexible endoscopy (and its inherent technologies) was the transition from "traditional" Industrial Age open surgery to the Information Age minimally invasive surgery, RAMIS is the transition from Information Age minimally invasive surgery to a future of non-invasive surgery. With each transition, the complexity (and hence the need for training) increases.

All surgical education, and especially RAMIS, has undergone an entirely new approach to education and training, such that the following principles apply to not only RAMIS but to surgical education in general.

Changes from earlier education have suddenly changed, rather than evolving slowly over time. Traditional training consisted of knowledge gained from books in the library or didactic lectures in a lecture hall plus technical clinical skills observed and practice on a cadaver or patient. And assessment of knowledge was through standardized testing and oral examinations, while technical clinical skills were mainly assessed through observation and subjective opinion of performance. Engagement for learning/practicing was episodic and opportunistic, principally reliant upon the various diseases which presented to the hospital or surgeon. This recent paradigm shift rapidly occurred during the final decades of the twentieth century.

2 Current Status

Information Age training has expanded the educational experience enormously by adding (not replacing) traditional methods and has introduced advanced technologies and learning principles, with as much patient-centered focus as there is a focus upon the needs of the surgical trainee. And while formal education/training previously ended upon com-

R. M. Satava (✉)
Department of Surgery, University of Washington School of Medicine, Seattle, WA, USA
e-mail: rsatava@uw.edu

P. Wiklund et al. (eds.), *Robotic Urologic Surgery*, https://doi.org/10.1007/978-3-031-00363-9_4

pletion of residency, the current direction is upon planned continuous professional development CPD) and life-long learning - not specific learning at specific times of a career. There is a new emphasis on formal training for remediation and, because such rapid surgical technological changes are occurring, there is the need for learning new surgical technologies and techniques. This is in counter-distinction to former surgical education, where knowledge and skills learned during residency were sufficient for an entire career. Thus, there is a need (requirement?) for continuous evaluation and self-evaluation of RAMIS training.

The onset of online learning, which has been heralded by the inception of the Internet and personal mobile telecommunication, has resulted in learning at any time, from any place, about any subject, with any real-time or archived information, and near-limitless opportunities through the Internet. With the onset of the COVID-19 pandemic, education is presented through telemedicine with remote individual learning or through webinars or conferences. Other adaptations include remote applicant interviews and the concept of hybrid classrooms. Training is not only one-way transfer from teacher to student but has become highly interactive, especially with automatic real-time feedback.

One of the most important new aspects of current medical practice is that of "evidence-base medicine," which has the foundational principles being that medical practice must be conducted through scientifically verified evidence derived by the scientific method—thus changing from subjective opinion-based practice to objectively proven evidence-based practice. For surgical technical skills training, in 1996, Reznick et al. [1, 2] introduced one of the first curriculum using objective scoring of skills performance called objective structured assessment of technical skills (OSATS) for surgical residents. Numerous new curricula followed, based upon the OSATS methodology. With the introduction of laparoscopic surgery, the Society of American Gastrointestinal and Laparoscopic Surgeons (SAGES) created the Fundamentals of laparoscopic Surgery (FLS), which was later required by all surgeons by the American Board of Surgery.

One of the more important new methodologies in RAMIS surgical training was introduced in 2002 by Gallagher and O'Sullivan's book is proficiency-based progression (PBP) skills training [3]. This is predicated upon a rigorously defined curriculum with objective outcomes measures, metrics and milestones, and then setting benchmarks values, which are derived from the mean of the performance of experienced (expert) surgeons performing the surgical skills curriculum, thus setting the values of performance which the learners must achieve before performing surgical procedure(s) upon patients This has been accomplished because of the introduction of surgical simulators, which allow the learner to practice surgical skills/procedures with "permission to fail" without harm to a patient, and continuing to practice their skills until performing without errors for two consecutive trials. Then and only then may the learner progress to the next task or procedure. Using this methodology, Satava et al., developed and then validated a RAMIS curriculum called the Fundamentals of Robotic Surgery (FRS) [4]. Initial attempts were to use the FLS physical models; however, a new 3D model was created to optimize training of the "wrist" of the RAMIS systems. Regardless of future training, robotic or otherwise, the key issues with any surgical educational curriculum can be summated as: "Evidence-based medicine requires evidence-based education."

The latest addition to RAMIS training assessment is video review of performance, especially using crowd-sourced assessment of technical skills (C-SATS) [5] methodology. While there are a number of variations of video review of surgical skills performance, all methods require submission of the whole (or a portion of) a procedure training on a simulator or of an actual clinical surgical procedure. A panel of raters - surgeons, faculty, educators, or a professionally trained group of non-medical professionals (the "crowd")—are selected to review a "critical and/or representative" portion of the procedure to score with a validated checklist, such as the Global Evaluative Assessment of Robotic Skills (GEARS). Such a panel has the experience to objectively and rapidly quantify technical performance and evaluate the level of expertise (Novice, Intermediate, Expert) of the subject. The report that is generated can be used as feedback to the learner, or as evidence of technical performance for hospital privileging committees. The issue of certification is addressed below.

3 Future Trends

One certainty is that the current rapid technological innovation will continue, and likely at an even more accelerated pace. The next generation for RAMIS to transition to will be non-invasive surgery. While most of the infrastructure for this to happen is in place, the missing element is the next generation of "instruments." An indication of one pathway will be non-invasive "directed energy." Today there are a few early examples. In general surgery, there is the use of high-intensity focused ultrasound (HIFU) which is used for transcutaneous, non-invasive ablation of solid tumors (benign and malignant) in many of the subspecialties; in the neurosurgery, transcranial HIFU is used for solid tumors in the brain and for eradication of foci of excitation in various motion abnormalities, like epilepsy, Parkinsonism and other dyskinesias. In addition, there are new applications using photon-ics (of which lasers are one example). Photo-biomodulation (light that can induce apoptosis or angiogenesis) is in research phases. In addition, devices are available to provide instantaneous diagnosis through Raman spectroscopy or mass spectroscopy; combining both diagnosis and treatment in a single device is referred to as Directed Energy for Diagnosis and Therapy (DEDAT) [6]. Although current prototype systems are handheld, future versions would require the use of robotics to provide the precision and systems integration for artificial intelligence enhanced image guidance. In the farther future, research on brain–machine interfaces (BMI), based upon current research success with implantable neural prostheses linked to prosthetic arms [7], suggests a distant future where remote robotic arms will be controlled by a surgeon's thoughts. In the immediate future, the next generations of telecommunications (5-G and 6-G) will have such massive bandwidth, low latency, and high reliability that remote telesurgery can become a reality, depending more upon business models, regulations, opportunities, and acceptance than on technological capabilities. Such innovative systems will clearly require special training for their use.

Although there currently are computer-based simulators, they are limited to basic skills, simple tasks, or elementary procedures and often at low visual fidelity. The next-generation surgical simulators will be significantly more complex, having high visual realism, interactivity, and feedback based upon very realistic tissue properties, and major improvement in haptic sensation. The stand-alone simulators, as well as RAMIS systems (which will have the option for integrated simulation), can be connected to the internet, providing access to real-time augmentation by supercomputers, artificial intelligence (AI), computational analytics, and feedback to improve not only technical skills but perception and decision making. There will be the opportunity to perform pre-operative planning and surgical rehearsal upon the patient-specific 3D reconstructed CT scan, permitting the surgeon to plan and practice various surgical approaches to customize and optimize the surgical outcome.

The above connectivity will bring an AI "virtual mentor" during simulation training, as well be available during surgical procedures, for guidance, alerts, or consultation. There will be automatic collecting of information (in all formats), intra-operatively for archiving the procedure into personalized Big Data, analyzed by computational analytics and retrievable and immediately useable—for situational awareness, predicting possible outcomes, answers to inquiries/request, the electronic medical record (EMR), etc. There is research in automating certain simple tasks (suturing, knot tying, etc), to support the surgeon especially in very difficult or inaccessible locations, which will likely be implemented in the near future, though complex surgery performed autonomously by a robot is in far distant future—if at all.

4 Certification

It is critical at first to distinguish between certification, credentials, and privileging. Certification is "confirmation that a certain level of achievement has been reached"—this is normally awarded (a certificate) by an accredited authority to a surgeon after high stakes examination, such as one of the many surgical "boards," which is forwarded to the Hospital Credentials Committee. Credentials is "any document used as a proof of identity or qualifications to serve as a recommendation or qualification for a person, a person's actions, etc."—these are collected by the Credentials Committee and forwarded to the Hospital Privileging Committee. Privileging is "to be entitled *to* a special right or benefit; to authorize or permit something"—in healthcare, this is awarded by the hospital (or institution) through their Privileging Committee to which the surgeon is applying for permission to practice. It is the Privileging Committee that reviews all the documents and information (letters of recommendation, credentials, license to practice surgery, educational (including fellowship and CME) and employment records, etc.) needed to recommend that the applicant surgeon met the qualifications to be permitted to the requested scope of practice of surgery at the hospital.

Initially, the certification process began with training during the residency until the Program Director and Chair of Surgery determined that the surgeon was ready to graduate. Before the practice of "Surgery" was divided into the current major specialties (Neurosurgery, Urology, Orthopedics, General Surgery, etc.) and then further divided into subspecialties (bariatric, hepatobiliary, colorectal, hernia, trauma, etc.), after completion of residency in "Surgery" the surgeon was "trained" to literally any type of surgery. Training and evaluation in the major specialties evolved to the additional evidence needed for competence, resulting in certification by the major specialty societies/boards. Current status, with multiple subspecialties, requires proof of graduation from one of the major specialties, and further evidence from the major specialty and/or proof of completion of a subspecialty fellowship. At this time, the issue of whether RAMIS is an additional subspecialty, or if it remains a part of the major specialties is under discussion. Although RAMIS is acknowledged as needing additional training, the question remains whether a separate fellowship is required, or robotic training is required as part of every specialty and subspecialty. Wherein lies the conundrum of what constitutes "training" in RAMIS and hence what (if any) formal certification is required for the Privileging Committees.

The current status appears to be determined by the local hospitals—what will they accept as qualifications to perform robotic surgery. What the difficulty is the determination of amount of time and/or cases of non-patient training (frequently in a simulation laboratory or center), in addition to the number of surgical cases during completion of training. The minimal most thorough and advanced training appears to be the following:

1. One week of laboratory training, with both: (1) instructions for use (IFU) of the robotic system, as required by the FDA for any surgical device; and (2) RAMIS technical surgical skills training, conducted by surgical faculty, which can include basic skills (usually on a simulator), followed by procedure training on a high-fidelity simulator, animal model and/or cadaver. [NOTE: This can be a dedicated week, or spread over multiple weeks—the total hours for training have not been clarified] This can be the initial part of a fellowship, or within a surgical residency, depending upon the resources and programming of the residency].
2. Observation followed by acting as bedside first assistant during RAMIS procedures, with gradual increase of performing steps of the procedure.
3. Resident/fellow as a primary surgeon with faculty assisting as a preceptor, with increasing responsibility for the resident/fellow.
4. Resident/fellow as primary surgeon, with faculty (as a preceptor) available as needed.
5. Proctoring first 2–3 cases (proctor observing and conducting formal evaluation on behalf of Privileging Committee).
6. After privileges granted: Minimum of 25 cases/year, with at least 2 cases/month—averaged as 6 cases/3 months (this is based upon data indicating that skills degradation reaches a maximum by 2 weeks).
7. Some suggest addition of submission of 1 procedure videotaped/3 months for an independent video review by an independent panel of peer for the first 3 years, preferably by the C-SATS model of review.

The long-term evaluation is unclear, though there is some early evidence that submission of a minimal number of cases for video review every year for evaluation, especially for feedback from video review panel for quality improvement not only individual surgeons but the hospital robotic program performance should be monitored at least annually.

Suggestions for exploration of future program opportunities based upon emerging technologies include:

Technology to provide real-time outcomes and milestone assessment (intra-operatively or post-operatively?)

Comparison of outcomes to peer-performance—local/national

Development of much larger/comprehensive personal/institutional database of performance (big data)

Scheduled reporting of deidentified video-review performance of robotic surgery evaluations

5 Conclusions

Technology innovation is a major force in robotic surgery of all kinds. The non-medical information technologies can radically increase innovation and turn current potential robotic opportunities (telesurgery, pre-operative planning and surgical rehearsal, addition of AI and haptics, transition to non-invasive surgery, etc.) into realities within the next decade. However, every significant increase in technology will require a complimentary development of surgical education, training, and assessment. The new tools of evidence-based education (Proficiency-based progression methods, objective assessment of skills (including C-SATS type of video review, surgical simulators)) will significantly enhance surgical training. Life-long learning and continued professional development will be necessary to keep up with the rapid pace of change.

Acknowledgments None.

Conflict of Interest None.

References

1. Faulkner H, Regehr G, Martin J, Reznick R. Validation of an objective structured assessment of technical skills for surgical residents. Acad Med. 1996;71:1363–5.
2. Reznick R, Regehr G, MacRae H, Martin J, McCulloch W. Testing technical skill via an innovative bench station examination. Am J Surg. 1997;173:226–30.
3. Gallagher AG, O'Sullivan GC. Fundamentals of surgical simulation: principles and practice (Improving medical outcomes – zero tolerance). London: Springer; 2012.
4. Satava RM, Stefanidis D, Levy JS, et al. Proving the effectiveness of the fundamentals of robotic surgery (FRS) skills curriculum: a single-blinded, multispecialty, multi-institutional randomized control trial. Ann Surg. 2020;272(2):384–92. https://doi.org/10.1097/SLA.0000000000003220.
5. Chen C, White L, Kowalewski T, et al. C-SATS video assessment of technical skills. J Surg Res. 2014;187(1):65–71. https://doi.org/10.1016/j.jss.2013.09.024.
6. Satava RM. Future directions in robotic surgery. In: Rosen J, Hannaford B, Satava R, editors. Surgical robotics. Boston, MA: Springer; 2011. https://doi.org/10.1007/978-1-4419-1126-1_1.
7. Lebedev M, Nicolelis M. Brain-machine interfaces: from basic science to neuroprostheses and neurorehabilitation. Physiol Rev. 2017;97(2):767–837. https://doi.org/10.1152/physrev.00027.2016.

Preparation of the Operating Room, Back Table, and Surgical Team

Travis Rogers and Cathy Corder

1 Introduction

In order for hospitals and physicians to remain competitive, ongoing training and the use of new technology are necessary to keep pace with the ever-evolving healthcare world. Robotic surgery is a perfect example of how technology has revolutionized the surgical field.

Establishing a robotic surgery program requires a structured plan and key elements in place to allow successful development. Once the decision has been made by your hospital to become a robotic facility, there are several "next steps" that need to be taken before starting the program per se. The establishment of an economic model is crucial for a robotic program. Development of the business plan requires an evaluation of the direct costs (such as buying the robotic system) and of the associated material, staff recruitment, and/or staff training. Possible operating room (OR) modifications could be necessary to support the console and the other equipment. Meanwhile, a robotic surgical team needs to be established aiming to create and maintain the standards necessary to make the program successful.

The beginning of a robotic program is challenging as multiple members of the team are learning the technology and their personal roles. Although the learning curve can be considered less challenging than pure laparoscopic for the surgeon himself, there are so many other aspects that need to be developed at the beginning of the experience. Robot preparation, docking and undocking, use of disposable and new instruments, assisting at the bedside far from the console: all the different people involved in the robotic program have their own role and learning curve which can affect the overall outcomes.

In this chapter, we will discuss the essential elements involved in the preparation of the robotic operating room, the back table, and the robotic surgical team.

T. Rogers (✉) · C. Corder
Global Robotics Institute, Advent Health, Celebration, Fl, USA

2 Preparation of the Operating Room

A robotic operating room reserved and dedicated for robotic surgeries is advisable. This will avoid the timely and arduous task of transferring the robot between rooms, which may lead to increased setup times, chances of mechanical or wiring damages, and decreased productivity. A robotic OR needs larger spaces due to the surgical console and surgical cart. Farther, there is a potential need for specific robotic assistants used in addition to the regular OR staff, particularly at the beginning of the learning curve. It is recommended to maintain a specific number of stock due to the short life of many disposable instruments and the need for extra instruments in case of possible malfunctioning.

Therefore, OR planning should include time and room availability, room layout, availability of proper receptacles and circuits, imaging (either monitor or 3D room projection), and access to supplies. Having a dedicated robot room(s) enhances productivity, quickens turnover time, and limits potential damage to the robot in transport. With these aspects in mind, state-of-the-art operating theaters were designed to accommodate the specific needs of the surgical robot, OR team, and the patient. These rooms provided incorporation of additional imaging modalities and the ability to broadcast out educational live surgical cases to training physicians [1, 2].

Here are described particularities of a robotic OR that should be attended:

- *Robotic operating theaters need larger rooms*; around 60 m^2 feet is considered optimal for a robotic system to fit in comfortably. Smaller rooms will make personal flow and placement of equipment complicated.
- *LCD screens and appropriate technological controls are advisable.*
- *Keeping all the electrosurgical units together can avoid scattering of the cables.* A tower to hold all the cables and units can facilitate the circulation and avoid accidents inside the OR.

P. Wiklund et al. (eds.), *Robotic Urologic Surgery*, https://doi.org/10.1007/978-3-031-00363-9_5

- Make sure to have available an OR table that allows steep Trendelenburg and reverse Trendelenburg.
- *Group apparatus according to their use.* It will make location of replacements or extra instruments easier and faster.
- *If possible, make available wall gas for pneumoperitoneum.* Gas tanks occupy space in the OR and often require hanging before finishing the case. During the longer cases, especially in the beginning of the learning curve, it is not uncommon to go through 2–4 tanks of gas. Occasionally tanks that are thought to be full are discovered to be empty after changing.

Because robotic surgery is expensive but continues to grow, there is a need to improve its cost-competitiveness. Diminishing operative costs is of utmost importance and is enhanced with reduced operative time and faster turnover. In this regard, any modifications of procedure or technology that lower operative time are essential. Simple modifications can optimize OR productivity such as:

Time-oriented surgical goals for trainees. Trainees can significantly increase operative times when in learning curve. The establishment of time-oriented surgical goals (e.g., 30 min for vesical-urethral anastomosis, then the proctor assumes the console) can decrease surgical times besides making surgery safer for the patient [3].

Having a dedicated anesthesia and OR team can determine significant reduction in operative times. As those teams surpass their learning curves, operative times reduce as well.

Create a presurgery robot-specific inspection checklist so that everything will be available and ready when the patient arrives in the room. Specifically, this checklist must include basic laparoscopic and robotic instruments that are crucial to initiate the surgical procedure: light cable connected to the light source and to the camera; white balance, focus, and the robotic scope alignment; suction and irrigation; insufflator tubing connected to the insufflators which is turned on to allow the surgeon to see that there is proper flow of CO_2; an extra tank of CO_2 if wall gas is not available; the Veress needle checked to make sure the tip retracts properly; both the handheld and robotic electrocautery tested to make sure they are functional; and, finally, a sterile open tray should be available in the room.

If wall gas is not available, monitor quantity of gas remaining in the CO_2 tank to allow for anticipation of a change. It is also advisable to employ an insufflator system with two tanks of gas so they can be switched when the first one gets low and then replace the first empty tank.

Maintain enough instruments to perform at least two cases, so that back-to-back procedures will not have to wait for equipment to be cleaned.

Custom packs and minimal instrument sets can help to reduce the turnover time. The cost of the pack that contains everything needed for robot draping is close to the cost of opening each item individually. The savings are seen in the time it takes to open one pack versus several individual items.

Have available and sterile all types of individual instruments that can be necessary during the procedure, such as positioning supplies, robotic instruments, drapes, scopes, light cords, and even camera heads.

Reducing turnover times is also essential for improving productivity and having a dedicated team for that is a key point. As with all surgeries, optimization is critical to ensure consistency between cases and to maximize efficiency. Determining personal function in every step of the turnover is essential [1–4].

Surgeon Surgeon is responsible for positioning the patient, performs surgical site assessment, makes incisions, places ports, and docks robotic arms. At the end of the procedure the surgeon closes the port sites and goes to speak with the family and sees the next patient.

First Assistant First assistant helps to set up back table, check presurgery inspection, and assist preparing the patient, gathers and inspects robotic and auxiliary instrumentation as well as prepares them for insertion. At the end of the surgery the first assistant can help in undocking the patient cart, clearing the back table, and assisting in the turnover process.

Surgical Scrub The scrub tech sets up the back table before the patient gets into the room, drapes the patient cart, assists the surgeon with incisions, port placement, and docking the cart. During the procedure the surgical scrub maintains all necessary sterile supplies on the back table and anticipates what to give the assistant for the next step in the surgical procedure.

Circulator Circulator gets the patient from the preoperative suite, positions and prepares the patient, prepares auxiliary equipment (energy source, gas, etc.), and positions the patient cart. At the end of the procedure, they remove the patient cart from the patient as well as undrape it, cleans the system, and takes the patient to recovery.

3 Preparation of the Back Table

In the beginning, preparing the back table for a robotic procedure is trial and error. Until the surgeon becomes skilled with robotic surgery, this will be a learning experience for everyone. Depending on the previous experience of the main surgeon, it will be necessary to keep laparoscopic or open surgery instruments on the table for eventual conversion.

Occasionally, both types of instruments will be necessary even if they obviously will not be used.

Once the surgeon works through the learning curve, it will be easy to make a robotic case preference card. A custom procedure pack should also be prepared. Prepare packs with supplies as base robotic instrument trays can help to decrease the room turnover time. Instruments that must be used by every surgeon using the robot can be put into a basic tray.

The items necessary to support a robotic program include:

- A dedicated robotic/laparoscopic room.
- Reusable robotic accessories (e.g., sterile adapters, scopes, light guide cables, trocars).
- Limited life reusable robot instrumentation that can be used on as few as eight or as many as 20 cases depending on which instrument it is (e.g., needle drivers, forceps, scissors, cautery tools).
- Disposable robotic supplies (e.g., drapes, cannula seals).
- Additional smaller (5 mm) ports and instruments which are necessary for pediatric programs as well as bariatric trocars for extremely obese patients.

As the surgical technique is refined, use of only one or two instruments (e.g., curved cautery scissors and bipolar Maryland grasper) becomes more common, thereby saving cost and time. In addition to the supplies provided by the robot vendor, other equipment and materials are required including insufflators, a suction irrigator, a scope warmer, video equipment, clips, sutures, trocars, and basic laparoscopic instruments (scissors, graspers, clip appliers, needle drivers). Examples of robotic and laparoscopic instruments used during robot-assisted laparoscopic radical prostatectomy (RALP) are listed in Table 1 and displayed in Fig. 1.

Table 1 Surgical instruments for robotic-assisted radical prostatectomy

Laparoscopic instruments and trocars	Robotic instruments	Sutures
• Laparoscopic scissors • Laparoscopic needle driver • Laparoscopic Weck Hem-o-lok clip appliers and disposable clips • Laparoscopic grasper • Long suction tip (5 mm) • Endocatch bag • Laparoscopic trocars (5 and 12MM Surgiquest) • Veress needle • S retractors • Facial closure device	• Monopolar • Long bipolar grasper • Robotic needle drivers • ProGrasp • Monopolar and bipolar cord • Robotic trocars (8 mm)	• 2-0 *Quill Monoderm* VLM 2005 (DVC) • 2-0 *Quill Monoderm* VP 2000 (double arm cut in half, bladder neck reconstruction) • 2-0 *Quill Monoderm* VLM 2005 (Rocco/Posterior Reconstruction) • 2-0 *Quill Monoderm* VP 2000 (Double arm, anastomosis)

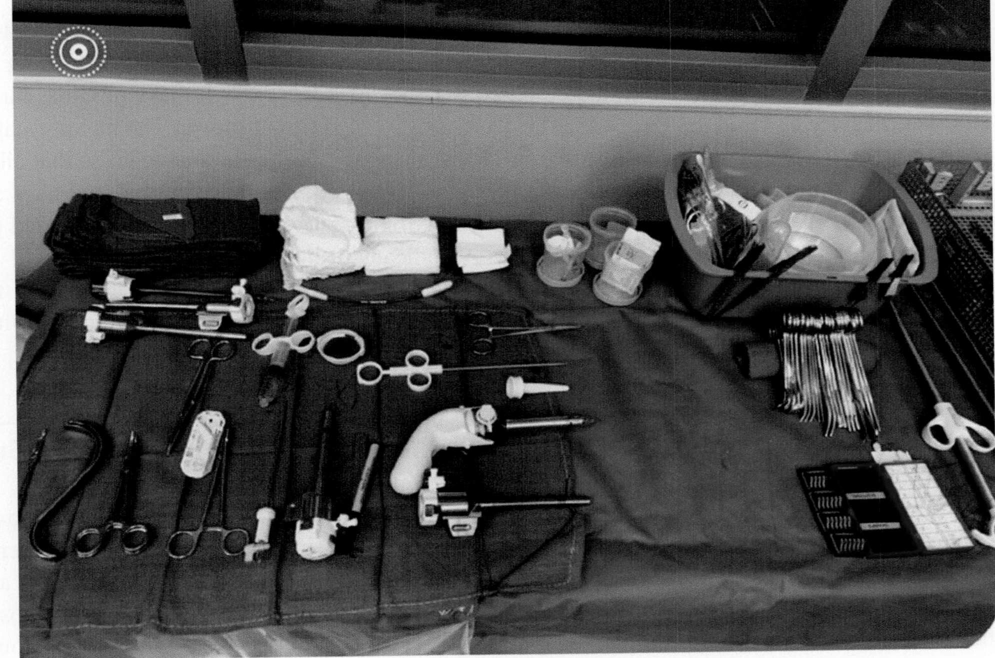

Fig. 1 Basic back table including laparoscopic and robotic Xi instrumentation. Laparoscopic and robotic instrumentation left to right: robotic and disposable trocars, Weck hem-o-lok disposable clips, Weck Hem-o-lok laparoscopic clip applier (10 mm Large). In the basket: Medtronic MicroFrance graspers ×2, suction tip 45 cm, needle driver, EndoWrist monopolar scissor, EndoWrist ProGrasp forceps, EndoWrist long bipolar grasper, EndoWrist large needle driver ×2, Ethicon Endocatch bag

4 Troubleshooting

Malfunction of the robotic system is rare and is mostly secondary to inappropriate setup or skipping fundamental steps in preparing the robot or docking. It can impair surgical times and even put the patient at risk. It is important to always have an experienced and well-trained team to overcome any difficulty. Here are a few basic situations and the troubleshooting tips to deal with them.

- **Dark Image or Pool Color:** Check default settings on camera control unit (CCU) and redo black and white balance. If it does not work, replace endoscope or light cable and redo white and black balance.
- **Flickering Image:** Turn system off and reset vision cable connections and/or camera cable at CCU; then turn on again. Replace camera cable. If noise happens only when cautery is applied, separate energy source units.
- **Blurry Image:** Clean endoscope, review focus from focus controller or camera head, review focus from surgeon console, change endoscope or camera head.
- **EndoWrist Instrument Not Engaging:** Remove and reset instrument arm or EndoWrist instrument, try another instrument in that arm, replace sterile adapter, and drape and reset arm.
- **EndoWrist Cautery Not Responding to Footswitch:** Check cable connections, grounding pad, AC power connection. If that does not work, attach generator to standard exterior foot pedal.

5 The Surgical Team

The creation of a functioning robotics team is imperative to the success of the program. The ability of the operating room staff can make or break a program; therefore, consistency of staff is necessary to avoid delays.

A proper OR setup includes at least two surgeons, a surgical scrub, circulating nurse, and anesthesia personnel. With the widespread use of the devices equipped with a fourth arm, the second assistant became unnecessary. A dedicated team of surgeons and OR staff is crucial to the successful implementation of a robotic program. Constantly changing assistants, nurses, and anesthesiologists delays the turnover and operative time, increasing cost [1–7].

The *first assistant* must be an individual that has forethought into the procedure to ensure timely and efficient cooperation. Contrary to traditional open surgery, robotic surgery implies that the leading surgeon does not have direct contact with the patient, being completely immersed in the console, making the surgeon extremely dependent on the assistant. Usually, robotic surgeons feel more dependent on the assistant then when performing pure laparoscopic procedures. Thereby, there must exist a perfect coordination between the team. A complete knowledge of the anatomy and the surgical steps is also mandatory for the assistant to provide adequate traction and exposure of the surgical field according to the surgeon's preferences and to place vascular clips or vascular clamps. Because of this, it is extremely important that the bedside surgeon or the surgical technician has good laparoscopic skills. The first assistant will be responsible for the establishment of pneumoperitoneum, safe port placement, exposure and manipulation of tissue, suctioning, passage of suture and retrieval of needles, bagging of specimens, and port closure. Knowing profoundly all the surgical steps can greatly reduce operative times and can be achieved with mentoring and careful study of recorded cases. Unlike open or other endoscopic surgeries, many robotic surgeries, especially radical prostatectomy, are nearly impossible to perform without an accomplished first assistant [1, 2, 4].

There are not specific particularities to robotic surgery regarding anesthesia, when comparing to laparoscopic surgery. Especially in the early stages of the program when cases are likely to be of longer duration, an *anesthesiologist* familiar with laparoscopic anesthesia is critical to patient safety. The steep Trendelenburg position used by many teams coupled with the intraperitoneal approach can create difficulties with high ventilatory pressures and carbon dioxide retention and can also lead to facial and corneal edema. Anesthetic techniques to deal with these problems should be familiar to the team [1–7].

Finally, the *scrub* and *circulating nurses* play important roles in the background of the procedures [8]. The surgical scrub should coordinate with the assistant during the entire procedure, providing sutures and instruments and helping taking care of the camera. A team able to efficiently prepare the robotic system, including the draping and calibration of lenses, will make possible earlier start times and more rapid case turnover. The nursing staff should rehearse with the rest of the surgical team so that all parties know what equipment is regularly needed and have available instruments, sutures, and catheters that are needed less frequently. Efficiency and decreased learning time will be facilitated with a devoted, well-trained, and consistent team. Initial consistency will increase efficiency and facilitate education of future team members [1–7].

6 Training of the Surgical Team

Once a robotics program has been established, the focus shifts toward training. Proper training of the next generation of robotics surgeons is a key aspect to maintaining a successful program. Most hospitals generally require completing a Robotic Training course, taught by representatives of the robotic company, for credentialing. All surgeons and supporting OR staff must complete this basic robotics course which emphasizes the various parts of the robot, robot setup, and basic use of the console. For OR staff, the course focuses on robot setup, draping, proper maintenance, and troubleshooting. Staff training may be most beneficial in a community setting where there are no rotating students. Everyone on the team should attend this in-service training [7].

A "dry run" is also advisable before the first case. During this dry run, everyone on the team should have the chance to perform his role: set up the room the way it will be for the case, set up the back table with instruments, position the patient on the OR table safely, and place the equipment and instruments in the adequate location. Use this walk through to fine-tune your procedure and never stop fine-tuning. For the initial cases, it is advisable to have a robotic company representative present in the operating room. In the event a surgeon or any other member of the robotic team has a question or problem, troubleshooting with a representative can occur immediately.

When the robotic program first starts, the team is often asked to stay late to finish cases, which eliminates staff changes mid-case in the beginning of the learning curve. They may find themselves working without breaks or even lunch because the team is small and specialized. The ideal team will have an extra trained person or facilitator. That person can help with turnover, give breaks or lunches, run for supplies, or prepare the instruments for the next case. Everyone on the team needs to recognize how important they are to the success of the program. Surgical fellows, residents, physician assistants, and even the surgeons should be able to take over for any member of the team.

After the first few cases it is important to meet as a team and discuss what went wrong and how to make it better. But more importantly, talk about what went right and congratulate for a job well done. Inviting the staff for educational meetings as well as social events can also help to create the "team spirit," crucial for a successful robotic program [7].

The surgical team should continue to maintain their robotic competencies by completing online modules provided by the robotic company, robotic in services, as well as attending any robotic educational conferences available to them and by using an established list of robotic competencies developed by their institution. Certificates of completion should then be put in all staff education folders.

7 Conclusion

Robotic Surgery is rapidly becoming the benchmark for many different surgical procedures. The number of companies having surgical robots is constantly growing. No matter what system your institution has or may change to in the future, following the outline in this chapter can lead to a successful and safe robotics program.

References

1. Palmer KJ, Lowe GJ, Coughlin GD, Patil N, Patel VR. Launching a successful robotic surgery program. J Endourol. 2008;22(4):819–24.
2. Patel VR. Essential elements to the establishment and design of a successful robotic surgery program. Int J Med Robot. 2006;2(1):28–35.
3. Rebuck DA, Zhao LC, Helfand BT, Casey JT, Navai N, Perry KT, et al. Simple modifications in operating room processes to reduce the times and costs associated with robot-assisted laparoscopic radical prostatectomy. J Endourol. 2011;25(6):955–60.
4. Rocco B, Lorusso A, Coelho RF, Palmer KJ, Patel VR. Building a robotic program. Scand J Surg. 2009;98(2):72–5.
5. Sarle RC, Guru KA, Peabody J. Training: preparing the robotics team for their first case. In: Patel VR, editor. Robotic urologic surgery. London: Springer; 2007. p. 41–6.
6. Menon M, Shrivastava A, Tewari A, et al. Laparoscopic and robot assisted radical prostatectomy: establishment of a structured program and preliminary analysis of outcomes. J Urol. 2002;168:945.
7. Matsunaga GS, Costello AJ, Skarecky DW, Ahlering TE. Essential elements of building a robotics program. In: Patel VR, editor. Robotic urologic surgery. London: Springer; 2001. p. 28–33.
8. Corder CJ, Coelho RF, Guglielmetti GB. Preparation of the operating room, back table, and surgical team. In: Gharagozloo F, et al., editors. Robotic surgery. 2nd ed. Springer; 2021. p. 1183–8.

The Role of Bedside Assistant in Robotic Urological Surgery

Fikret Fatih Onol, Ananthakrishnan Sivaraman, and John Andrich

1 Introduction

Robotic surgery is primarily based on an efficient team which includes the console surgeon (CS), bedside assistant (BA), anesthesiologist/CRNA, surgical technologist, and circulating nurse. Teamwork in robotic surgery should correlate to a pit stop in a Formula 1 race. Each member has a specific role to play strictly adhering to the protocols. A delay in milliseconds by one person can cost the trophy for the racer. The bedside assistant plays a key role which cannot be underestimated as even a small error in assistance can potentially lead to a catastrophe. The assistant should anticipate and enhance the actions of the console surgeon. The prerequisites to be a BA are, first, a great passion toward surgery and robotics, second, basic training in laparoscopy, and third, knowledge about the surgery and mechanism of the robotic surgical system.

The reappraisal of every surgical video by the console surgeon along with the bedside assistant greatly improves their coordination in the surgery and thereby improving speed and efficiency of the surgery as a whole. By actively participating in the bedside assistance in robotic surgery, one can refine his or her laparoscopic skills and the lack of tactile sensation for the CS can be bridged by the BA at times. It is always prudent for the CS to walk through the surgical steps with his or her team prior to the surgery in complicated or uncommonly performed cases.

F. F. Onol (✉)
Orlando Veterans Affairs Medical Center, Orlando, FL, USA

A. Sivaraman
Chennai Urology and Robotics Institute Hospital, Chennai, India

J. Andrich
AdventHealth Global Robotics Institute, Celebration, FL, USA

2 Preoperative Preparation

2.1 Room Setup

The operating room must be spacious enough to accommodate the robotic system (patient cart, vision cart, and console). Optimal temperature and humidity should be maintained in the operating room. Sterile draping of the robotic arms should be done before starting the surgery. The robotic team should be aware of the proper placement of patient table, carts (vision cart, patient cart, and anesthesia cart), instrument trolley, etc., for each surgery specifically. Vision cart or standalone monitors should be placed ergonomically for the bedside assistant. All the cables between the carts and console should be properly tucked and guarded to avoid accidental dislodgement. A dedicated cart for robotic endoscopes (30° and 0° if needed) should be present.

The main instrument table should be arranged by the surgical technologist who lays out the following (using robotic-assisted laparoscopic radical prostatectomy as an example):

1. Veress needle/Hasson's cannula
2. Robotic and assistant trocars
3. Anti-fog solution or hot water in sterile flask
4. Laparoscopic instruments—scissor, needle holder, grasper, and bariatric suction tip with irrigator
5. Hem-o-lok clip applier with clips
6. Necessary suture materials for the surgery
7. Monopolar cable, bipolar cable
8. Tubings for insufflation, suction, irrigation
9. Robotic instruments—monopolar curved scissors, bipolar dissecting forceps (Maryland/Long/Fenestrated), Prograsp, and 2 large needle drivers.

Emergency table should be kept ready with the following instruments:

1. Vascular clamps
2. Rescue stitch with hem-o-lok clip

P. Wiklund et al. (eds.), *Robotic Urologic Surgery*, https://doi.org/10.1007/978-3-031-00363-9_6

3. Tissue sealants
4. Open surgical instruments in case of conversion

Each member of the team should be aware of the surgery and possible intraoperative complications. A short discussion by the bedside assistant to the OR team prior to initiating surgery plays a major role for assuring a safe and effective operation.

2.2 Patient Positioning

The positioning of the patient in robotic surgery should be done right at the start, as after docking, repositioning of the patient cannot be done without undocking. Ideal positioning of the patient ensures proper exposure of the operating area without compromising the safety of the patient. The anesthesiologist or CRNA should be familiar with the possible complications of OR table position (full Trendelenburg for example) and should be ready to address it and discuss with the surgical team. The BA should check adequate cushioning of pressure points, and make sure that the patient's position is supported sufficiently to prevent sliding of the patient during surgery (like shoulder supports in Trendelenburg position and side supports in lateral position) and allows adequate range of movement of the robotic arms without causing any inadvertent injury to the patient.

3 Intraoperative Role with Console Surgeon

This section will be directly referring to the da Vinci Xi surgical system and robotic prostatectomy technique we perform, which was described by Patel et al. [1, 2].

3.1 Starting the Surgery

3.1.1 Trocar Placement

As the patient is now completely secured to the operating table and our anesthesiology team has completed intubation, we can begin trocar placement. An important note for the robotic assistant before an incision is made relates to the patient's past surgical history. Prior open abdominal surgery may preclude easy trocar placement due to the presence of adhesions. Ideally, the patient's surgical history is addressed at their initial visit and a decision can be made for general surgery consultation prior to scheduling surgery. With this done ahead of time, the surgeon and assistant can have more confidence in safe trocar placement. One last note prior to trocar insertion is reviewing patient's BMI and body habitus. Having immediate access to bariatric trocars for morbidly obese patients will prevent wasted operating time.

After Universal Protocol is completed with a "time-out," an approximately 3 cm supraumbilical incision is made in the midline. This incision will serve as eventual robotic camera location as well as direct visualization for trocar placement. Minimal blunt dissection is done along with cautery to allow bolstering bilateral fascial suture placement. Upward traction on these sutures will allow Veress needle placement to achieve pneumoperitoneum. An 8 mm bladeless da Vinci Xi trocar is placed along with subsequent camera insertion.

We now utilize the 30° robotic laparoscope for the remaining trocar placement. The robotic assistant will make an 8 mm incision about 8–10 cm from the camera location in horizontal line or just inferior with the umbilicus. The assistant's last incision will be for a 12 mm insufflation trocar, made another 8 cm laterally in the same line with the previous incision although in obese patients it may be more prudent for this incision to be made slightly inferior, for better reach to the pelvis. A fascial suture will be necessary for this incision and can either be placed with a suture passer now or at the end of the case. The surgeon will make the remaining two 8 mm incisions lateral and left of the supraumbilical incision in line with contralateral incisions just made by the assistant. The surgeon will also, with guidance from the assistant, make the 5 mm incision for the other accessory port located in the right subcostal area inferior to the ribs and medial to the right robotic trocar. Each bladeless trocar is placed perpendicular to the patient's abdomen with a twisting or screwing motion. For radical prostatectomy, the operating table will need to be in at least 25° Trendelenburg. Achieving this position prior to docking is crucial to thus avoid redocking unless a compatible integrated table motion bed is being used. The patient is now ready for robot docking.

3.1.2 Docking the Robot

Continuing with a case of radical prostatectomy, 4 separate trocars will require cannula trocar placement with the robot. The bedside assistant should communicate with the circulating nurse and the anesthesia team to maintain sterility during deployment for docking and positioning of the da Vinci Surgical System, making sure that all external monitors and overhead OR lights are not colliding with the robotic arms [3]. Correct trocar placement starts with supination of the nondominant hand while continuously holding the trocar itself and gently pressing against the skin of the patient. This serves as both a guide for the robot to dock and protection for the patient's skin. The dominant hand will then control the desired robotic arm either by using the port clutch button or the "grab and move" feature. The "grab and move" feature was introduced with the Xi robot and allows robotic arm movement by grabbing anywhere along the gray arm. This allows all robot joints to move freely and once movement has ceased, the arm will lock

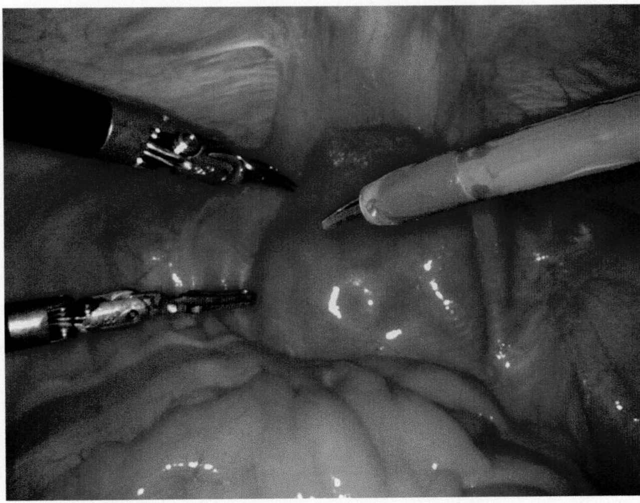

Fig. 1 Three instrument view

into place. The dominant hand will then use the port clutch for fine movement along with the wing clip to fit into place with the trocar.

The camera port should be docked first by the robotic assistant (arm #3 in this case) to allow for targeting. The subsequent trocars are then docked to the robot. The surgeon will utilize robotic arm #1 for the ProGrasp forceps and robotic arm #2 for the monopolar curved scissors. The fourth arm of the robot will utilize one of the bipolar instruments, Maryland bipolar forceps, or long bipolar grasper, for example. The da Vinci Xi cautery settings are important to review prior to beginning surgery.

Once all instruments are introduced into the abdomen, "burping" the trocars allows for less tension on the skin and centering of the instruments for maximum working space. Besides burping of the trocars, the Xi robot features a guide to maximizing working space located at the top of each robotic arm. The 4 letter word, F-L-E-X, is on each robotic arm and if the arm is rotated between the L and E letters, the surgeon will then have maximum mobility. Centering the camera to display the three-instrument view (Fig. 1) signals the surgeon to initiate the robotic portion of the surgery. The other 2 aforementioned trocars (5 mm and 12 mm) will be utilized for suctioning and Hem-o-lok clipping, respectively. The 12 mm portal entry is also used for introducing/removing sutures, laparoscopic scissors for suture cutting, as well as providing traction with laparoscopic graspers.

3.2 Robotic Assisting Techniques

The following section will include important techniques for the robotic assistant to master.

3.2.1 Substitution of Robotic Instruments

After docking has been completed, the tip of the instrument will then need guidance to the cannula opening using one hand while the other hand is fitting the housing of the instrument into the robotic arm adapter. An important note is that the instrument itself should be closed and the wrist straightened before attempting insertion. Instrument exchange starts with pressing both buttons located at the instrument housing and then physically pulling the instrument out of the trocar. LED colors are important to note as flashing green lights indicate "Guided Tool Change" is possible. This process allows quicker reset of the new instrument back to the location the previous instrument occupied without needing visualization.

3.2.2 Exposure and Countertraction

The next set of robotic assistant techniques to cover encompass basic surgery principles. Exposure and countertraction are hallmarks of surgery regardless of approach and are especially important for robotic bedside assisting. The robotic assistant needs familiarity with laparoscopic instruments such as laparoscopic grasper and suction/irrigator for example. The suction/irrigator is typically thought of as the name implies but also is a great tool for providing exposure. Throughout a robotic radical prostatectomy, the suction can help with difficult aspects of the surgery such as neurovascular bundle dissection and the posterior dissection involving Denonvillier's fascia simply by creating better exposure and/or providing traction. Right-sided neurovascular bundle dissection is aided by the assistant once the surgeon has developed the appropriate plane. The suction is then advanced into the plane and lateral traction is applied by the assistant (Fig. 2). Similarly with posterior dissection, once the correct plane is developed by the surgeon, the assistant advances the

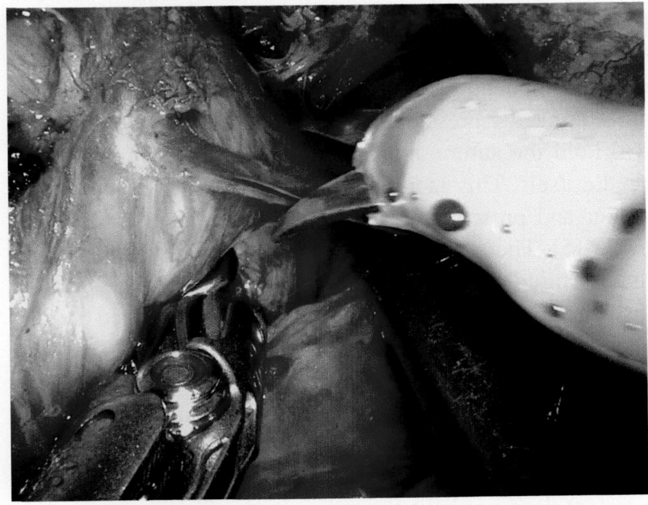

Fig. 2 Nerve spare

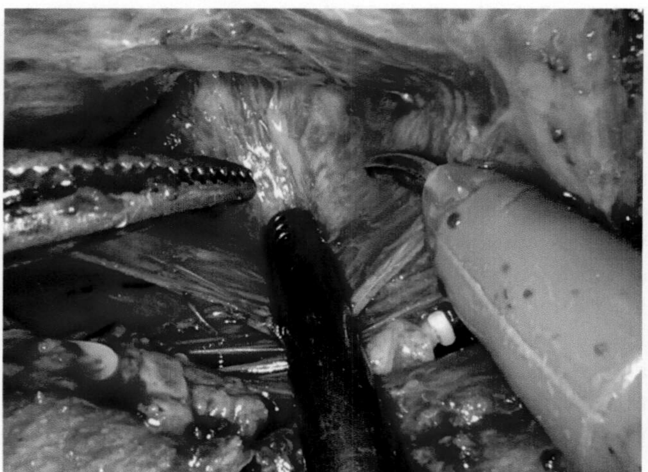

Fig. 3 Posterior dissection

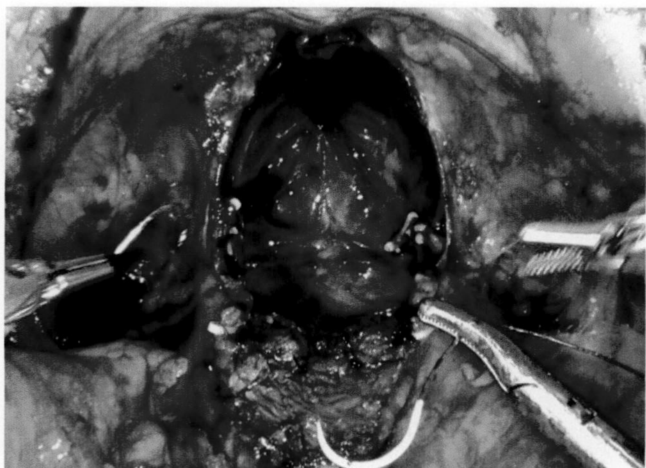

Fig. 4 Needle present

suction into the space and inferior traction is applied (Fig. 3). Forceful traction can cause trauma to the rectum; thus, it is important for the assistant to know how to gauge appropriate traction.

Surgical field cleaning is another task accomplished through the use of the suction/irrigator. A surgical field with excess blood darkens the surgeon's field of view and can cause unnecessary errors. Suctioning throughout surgery is a technique that sounds straightforward enough but can easily be overdone. A fine balance exists between over- and under-suctioning. The goal should be to suction just enough to keep the immediate field clear [4].

3.2.3 Introduction and Extraction of the Needle

Needle presentation and extraction are another set of basic robotic principles crucial for the robotic beside assistant to master. This technique starts with communication between the surgeon and robotic assistant to how exactly the needle should be presented on the laparoscopic needle driver. This will vary depending on the surgeon. For a standard procedure on needle presentation, the laparoscopic needle driver will hold the suture approximately 1–2 cm away from the needle itself. This facilitates the introduction of the needle holder and preserves the integrity of the membrane of the trocar [5]. The robotic assistant will then present the suture into the middle of the surgical field just inferior to the robotic instruments and then cease movement (Fig. 4). Once the surgeon grabs hold of the needle, the robotic assistant will then release the suture and withdraw the laparoscopic needle driver. Importance is placed on the assistant allowing the surgeon to take the needle for himself instead of the assistant presenting the needle to one of the robotic arms directly. The assistant does not have the same depth of vision as the surgeon; thus, this technique will provide quicker exchange and less fumbling of the suture.

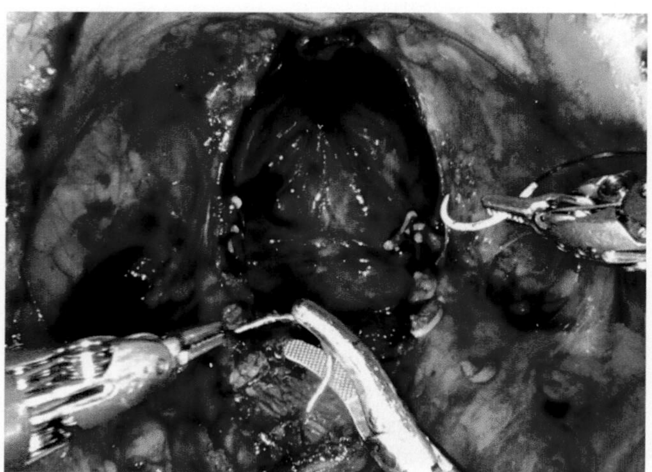

Fig. 5 Needle extract

Once suturing is completed or if another suture is required, needle extraction will occur in a similar fashion although the laparoscopic needle driver will this time grasp the needle itself. The surgeon will hold the finished suture approximately 1–2 cm away from the needle and present the needle with the half circle shape opening toward the camera (Fig. 5). The robotic assistant will then either allow the next suture to be taken by the surgeon as discussed earlier, or if no further suture is needed, the assistant will open the needle driver and allow the surgeon to place the needle within the opening (Fig. 5). After closure of the needle driver, the robotic assistant will withdraw the needle and transfer the instrument itself to the scrub nurse with verbal communication of the needle being received outside of the patient.

3.2.4 Hem-o-lok Positioning

Endoscopic Hem-o-lok ligation is one of the more difficult techniques for the bedside assistant to master. This is particularly true for robotic prostatectomy as the tissue being ligated is denser in comparison to a single vessel in other procedures. Hem-o-lok clip placement is completed through the 12 mm assistant trocar and allows the surgeon to preserve the neurovascular bundles athermally (Fig. 6). Experienced assistants will typically be able to tell the difference in clip failure from bulkier tissue versus equipment malfunction or assistant error. An experienced assistant must also communicate the reasoning for clip failure not only to the surgeon but to the OR staff. Improving clip success can be as simple as using a new set of clips or using a new clip applier. With regard to physical placement of the polymer clips, greater success is achieved when traction is provided either from the surgeon or the assistant themselves (Fig. 7). Orientation/angle of the clip is crucial as well and can be the difference between success and failure.

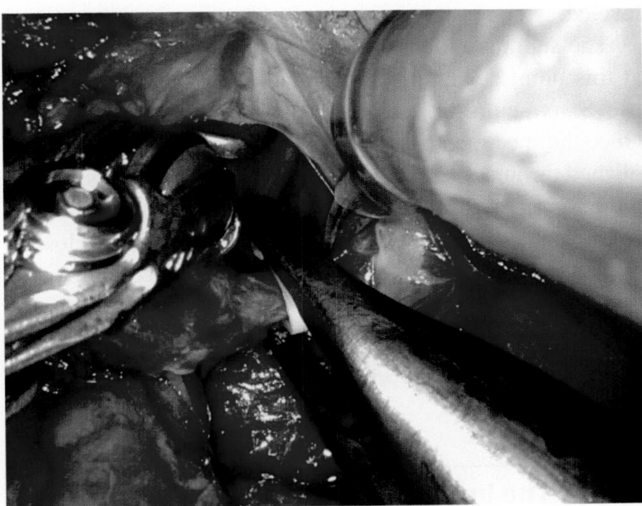

Fig. 6 Hemolock, neurovascular bundle

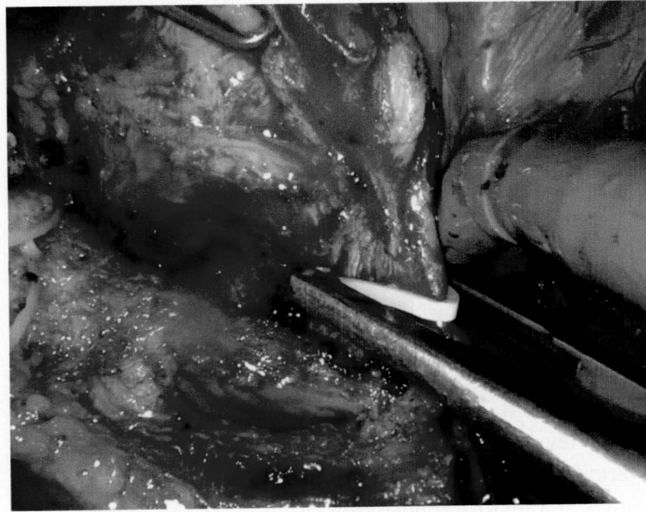

Fig. 7 Hemolock clip

3.2.5 Catheter Management

Foley catheter manipulation is the final technique to review for the bedside assistant. Catheter manipulation begins with deflation of the balloon as the surgeon is performing anterior dissection between the bladder neck and base of the prostate gland. While the surgeon is continuing dissection, it is important for the assistant to have Kelly forceps when ready with lubricant. Once the surgeon has developed the correct plane and can see the catheter, the assistant must retract the catheter until the tip of the catheter is in view. The surgeon will grab hold of the bladder opening of the catheter with the ProGrasp forceps and then retract the prostate gland toward the abdominal wall. The assistant can now use the Kelly forceps to grasp the catheter just distal to the meatus. Lubricant will allow minimal sliding of the Kelly forceps to keep constant traction on the prostate internally but will also avoid trauma to the foreskin or glans penis externally. Catheter management will continue once this area of dissection is complete with a simple retraction of the catheter. As the surgery progresses to dorsal venous complex suturing, the assistant will periodically check the catheter for difficulty with retraction. An important note is that the catheter should be past the area of suturing as each suture pass can potentially limit catheter placement later in the surgery if not in the appropriate plane.

Presentation of the catheter tip is helpful for the surgeon during posterior reconstruction and visualization of the rhabdosphincter. Just having the catheter tip visible helps with the location of the rhabdosphincter and at the same time showcases the anatomy of the proximal urethra for anastomotic closure. Catheter management continues with repetitive presentation and retraction of the catheter tip during anastomotic closure. Importance is placed on timing of the presentation or retraction of the catheter tip to coincide with suturing. Incorrect timing can lead to prolonged operative times or mistakenly suturing through the catheter. The final step is to introduce a new foley catheter after all suturing is completed to confirm the absence of catheter trauma.

3.3 Team Interaction During Surgery: *Verbal and Nonverbal Communication*

Communication is one of the more overlooked topics when it comes to reviewing surgical skills. It is paramount for the bedside assistant to communicate both verbally and nonverbally with the surgeon and the rest of the OR staff when needed. Feeling comfortable with the surgeon is the basis of good communication technique. Comfortability will grow with experience and especially collaboration between the surgeon and the assistant. In the case of robotic surgery, the console where the surgeon sits for the case is located away from the operating table and sometimes can be in another room adjacent to the operating room. This is particularly important regarding nonverbal communication. Although the da Vinci Xi robot has microphones allowing straightforward communication between the surgeon and assistant, there are many instances in which direct verbal communication is unnecessary.

Earlier in this chapter we discussed the three-instrument view which can be used by both the surgeon and the assistant to signify progression to the next step of surgery (Fig. 1). The assistant utilizes this view after docking the robot and introducing the instruments into the abdomen (this implies the surgeon can now start). The surgeon commonly utilizes this view for instrument exchange, camera cleaning, and completion of the surgery. These are simple instances that do not require verbal communication but are yet important, nonetheless. Further instances of nonverbal communication are also accomplished by the assistant always being prepared for the next step in the surgery. For example, sometimes the PA (bedside assistant) can proactively perform the suction task when he or she evaluates this is needed according to what is shown in the shared view, without the surgeon always requesting it [6]. The assistant should be skilled to the degree that functions like this are automatic.

Although nonverbal communication can be effective, it should never replace verbal communication. There are moments throughout surgery in which a quick verbal statement can help avoid an adverse event. This would be no different than in any other surgery but should still rely on the relationship between the surgeon and the assistant. There are certain relationships that will require more verbal communication and some that require more nonverbal communication but understanding the appropriate amount of each is important.

3.4 Closing the Surgery: Undocking and Port Removal

Undocking will first begin with instrument removal which should always be achieved after the three-instrument view occurs. After all instruments are removed, including the camera, the robotic arms are released from the trocars in the opposite fashion as they were installed. The wing flap located on the robotic arm is depressed and then the port clutch is depressed as well to physically move the arm away from the trocar (this can also be accomplished with the previously mentioned grab and move feature as well).

Once all robotic arms are undocked, the circulating nurse may reverse the robot away from the operating table. The assistant in this case must watch carefully and guide the nurse on proper robot height to avoid contacting the patient. While the patient is still in Trendelenburg position, the robotic camera is inserted into the right lateral accessory trocar for visualization of specimen bag transfer from the 5 mm accessory port to the supraumbilical robotic trocar. Once transferred, the specimen bag is clamped with a hemostat or Kelly forceps and the robotic camera is moved back to the same supraumbilical trocar. Next, removing all trocars under vision is important to confirm no internal hemorrhage is present that may require cauterization or fascial suturing with a suture passer. The first trocars removed are both left robotic trocars, followed by the right robotic trocar, and the 5 mm subcostal assistant trocar. Lastly, removal of the 12 mm accessory trocar and tying off the fascial suture must occur right as the insufflation is turned off to avoid abdominal contents getting trapped in the fascial suture. The robotic camera is then removed from the supraumbilical trocar and handed off the surgical field while the operating table is leveled.

The supraumbilical incision may need further dissection at this point depending on prostate size. The assistant will use S retractors to provide visualization for the surgeon. Once the specimen bag is removed, fascial closure is accomplished through five interrupted figure of eight knots. Again, the assistant will utilize the S retractors along with suture following through completion of fascial closure. Subcutaneous skin closure is then accomplished with a running, absorbable monofilament suture. This same suture is used for the lateral incisions as well, although in an interrupted fashion. Surgical skin glue is then administered over each incision.

4 The Impact of Bedside Assistant on Surgical Outcomes

Although the important role of the bedside assistant in robotic-assisted urologic surgery has been described above, the literature has mainly focused on the performance and outcomes of the CS. However, a successful robotic-assisted surgery depends on a successful team, and the BA represents a major part of such success. A remote interaction between the CS and BA makes the role of the BA critical. Cooperation and harmony between the two are fundamental to avoid time loss and prevent mistakes and complications.

There is a scarcity of literature analyzing the impact of bedside assistant on robotic urologic surgery outcomes. A summary of these studies has been presented in Table 1. These studies were conducted in different patient populations operated on by surgeons and assistants at varying experience levels and used different robotic systems (3-arm vs. 4-arm), thus making it difficult to reliably compare the outcomes among different studies

Table 1 Summary of contemporary studies that examine the impact of bedside assistant experience on surgical outcomes

Study [reference]	Study period	Cohort	Robotic system and technique	Study groups	Outcome measures	Methodology	Findings
Yu et al. 2021 [15] Prospective	Mar. 2016–Nov. 2016	92 RALPs 3 centers	Not specified	14 console surgeons	Global Evaluative Assessment of Robotic Skills (GEARS)	Association between BA- OSATS and CS- GEARS scores, Multivariable linear regression model to control for patient factors	Significant correlation between BA- OSATS and CS- GEARS score in the neurovascular bundle step in surgeons with prior >100 RALP experience
				22 bedside assistants	Objective Structured Assessment of Technical Skills (OSATS)		
Mangano et al. 2021 [11] Retrospective	2017–2018	116 RALPs *Single surgeon beyond learning curve*	Four-Arm Da Vinci Xi Transperitoneal, 6-port technique	BA-bedside and console experience ($n = 38$)	OT, EBL, LOS, Catheterization days, PSM rate	Statistical comparison of outcomes measures	OT:193 vs 195 vs 198 min, $p = 0.80$), EBL: 189 vs 190 vs 213 mL, $p = 0.32$), LOS: 5.43 vs 5.87 vs 5.26 days, $p = 0.39$), days of catheterization: 12.28 vs 13.53vs 13.18, $p = 0.34$), PSM rate: 32.3% vs30.3% vs 31.3%, $p = 0.17$).
				BA-only bedside experience ($n = 38$)			
				BA-inexperienced ($n = 40$)			
Garbens et al. 2020 [9] Retrospective	2013–2015	170 RALPs *Single surgeon in initial learning curve*	Transperitoneal posterior approach	Non-expert BA (PGY2–3 or PA w/o experience) $N = 111$	Primary: PSM status Secondary: console time, EBL, LOS	Multivariable regression analysis to determine predictors for primary and secondary outcomes	PSM rate: 37% vs 10% ($p = 0.03$) EBL: 441 vs 296 mL ($p < 0.0001$) LOS: 42 vs 31 h ($p = 0.004$) Expert BA not predictor of console time, LOS Expert BA significant predictor of PSM
				Expert BA (PA w/ experience) $N = 59$			
Albo et al. 2020 [5] Retrospective	2013–2016	129 RALPs *Single surgeon >1000 case experience*	Four-Arm Da Vinci Si Transperitoneal, 6-port technique	Two non-expert BAs in their learning curve Group 1: first 20 cases	OT, EBL, LOS, Catheterization days, PSM rate, Complications	Linear regression analysis to assess the relationship between BA experience and surgical outcomes. Uni- and multivariate logistic regression analysis to explore relationship between categorical variables.	Experience of the BA, patient age, BMI not predictive of OT, EBL, and LOS No relationship between the experience of the BA and PSMs or complications. Risk of complications increased if prostate weight >50 g (OR 15.5) and high ISUP grade (OR 10.7) High clinical stage (OR 9.1), age (OR 9.7), and BMI (OR 7.2) increased the risk of PSMs.
				Group 2: 21–40 cases			
				Group 3: >40 cases			

(continued)

Table 1 (continued)

Study [reference]	Study period	Cohort	Robotic system and technique	Study groups	Outcome measures	Methodology	Findings
Cimen et al. 2019 [8] Retrospective	2009–2015	36 RALPs *Two beginner surgeons*	Same Transperitoneal posterior approach	Surgeon 1 + beginner BA ($n = 20$) Surgeon 2 + expert BA (>150 cases) ($n = 16$)	Trocar insertion time, Robot docking time, Console surgery time, Anesthesia time, Specimen extraction time, EBL, LOS, Complication rates	Comparative analysis of variables	All surgical times significantly shorter in group 2 No significant difference in EBL, LOS, complication and PSM rates
Abu-Ghanem et al. 2017 [10] Retrospective	2011–2015	106 RALPs *Single surgeon beyond learning curve of 108 cases*	Transperitoneal approach	Group 1 BA (PGY1–3 residents) ($n = 44$) Group 2 BA (PGY4–5 residents) ($n = 43$) Group 3 BA (senior surgeon) ($n = 19$)	OT, EBL, LOS, Complication rates	Univariate analysis and Spearman's correlation tests to assess the relationship between the variables of interest	No correlation found between the assistant's seniority and OT, EBL and LOS. No influence of assistant on Immediate post-operative complications.
Nayyar et al. 2016 [7] Retrospective	2006–2013	222 robotic procedures *Single center* 82 RALPs 100 pyeloplasty 12 partial nephrectomy 18 ureterolithotomy 10 cystectomy	Not specified	Two BAs First half of BAs (inexperienced stage) Second half of BAs (experienced stage)	OT, EBL, Complications	Linear regression used to assess the possible cutoff level for the learning curve in terms of reduction in operative time for BAs.	For all procedures, mean OT reduced from 138.06 to 124.32 min ($P = 0.001$) and mean EBL decreased from 191.93 to 187.61 mL ($p = 0.57$) in second half Most significant OT decrease observed in robotic pyeloplasty (102 vs 82 min for first and second half, respectively, $P = 0.001$) OT and EBL did not drop significantly in RALP
Mitsinikos et al. 2017 [12] Retrospective	2011–2013	162 RAPNs *Three hospitals*	Transperitoneal	Teaching vs non-teaching hospital Teaching: PGY2–3 residents ($n = 112$) Non-teaching: attending surgeon ($n = 50$)	OT, WIT, EBL, LOS, Change in eGFR, 90-day readmission, PSM	Comparative analysis of variables, 2 cohorts matched based on R.E.N.A.L. nephrometry score	OT longer in teaching hospitals (229 vs 213 min, $p = 0.011$) WIT comparable (21 vs. 20.5 min, $p = 0.276$) Trend toward lower PSM in teaching hospitals (3.6% vs 10%, $p = 0.079$)

Table 1 (continued)

Study [reference]	Study period	Cohort	Robotic system and technique	Study groups	Outcome measures	Methodology	Findings
Potretzke et al. 2016 [13] Retrospective	2011–2014	414 RAPNs *Four experienced surgeons*	Not specified	Two BA groups: Junior-level (PGY2–3 residents or nurse) (n = 115) Senior-level (PGY4–5 residents or fellow) (n = 299)	OT, WIT, EBL, LOS, Complications, PSM	Multivariate analyses to assess for a relationship between the level of BA experience and outcomes	Operative time 9.3 min longer in the junior-level group (p = 0.051) No differences in outcomes between the junior and senior assistant groups, including for operative time, EBL, WIT, LOS, presence of a postoperative complication, and surgical margin status

RALP robotic-assisted laparoscopic prostatectomy, *RAPN* robotic-assisted partial nephrectomy, *BA* bedside assistant, *OT* operative time, *EBL* estimated blood loss, *LOS* length of stay, *PSM* positive surgical margin, *WIT* warm ischemia time, *PGY* post-graduate year, *BMI* bod mass index, *OR* odds ratio

4.1 Impact on Operative Time (OT)

Nayyar et al. performed a retrospective analysis of 222 urologic robotic procedures performed by two teams of CS and BA [7]. They split the data into two chronological halves, assuming that the assistant was inexperienced in the first half and had become experienced by the second half. They demonstrated that with increasing experience of the BA, mean OT for all procedures showed a significant reduction. Maximum reduction was noted for pyeloplasty which was the most commonly performed surgery. However, the reduction in OT was not statistically significant in the subset of 82 RALP cases.

Cimen et al. compared the outcomes of two CSs who performed RALP with an inexperienced and experienced BA, respectively, and found that trocar placement, robotic docking, console surgery, and specimen extraction times were significantly shorter in the experienced BA group [8]. The surgeons were in their initial learning curve; hence, the authors attributed this difference to the experience of the assistant. In contrast, Garbens et al. did not find a significant difference in the console times when a novice or expert BA assisted the same CS during his initial 170 RALP cases [9].

Abu-Ghanem et al. reported that BA seniority (PGY 1–3 vs. PGY 4–6 residents vs. senior surgeon) had no influence on surgery times in a cohort of consecutive 106 RALPs operated by a single surgeon beyond his learning curve [10]. In another single surgeon series, Mangano et al. analyzed 116 RALPs assisted by three BAs randomly distributed based on availability, one with bedside and console experience, one with relevant bedside experience only, and one basically inexperienced. There were no statistically significant differences between the three BAs in terms of mean operative time (198 vs. 195 vs. 193 mins, respectively, p = 0.8), as well as other perioperative parameters [11].

Mitsinikos et al. investigated the impact of BA on robotic-assisted partial nephrectomy (RAPN) outcomes in 162 cases [12]. They compared outcomes in two teaching hospitals where PGY-2 or PGY-3 residents served as BA vs. a non-teaching hospital where a senior surgeon had assisted all cases. The two cohorts were matched for R.E.N.A.L. nephrometry score. The total OT, but not warm ischemia time, was longer in the teaching hospitals (229 vs. 213 min, respectively, p = 0.011). Likewise, Potretzke et al. found a mean 9.3 min. Longer OT with a junior-level (PGY 2 or 3) vs. a senior-level (PGY 4 or 5, or fellow) BA in a cohort of 414 consecutive RAPNs [13]. However, warm ischemia time was not significantly different between the BA groups (21.3 vs. 20.9 min, p = 0.843).

4.2 Impact on Perioperative Outcomes and Complications

The majority of studies have shown no benefit in terms of the quality or experience of the BA as they pertain to perioperative outcomes [10–13]. Estimated blood loss, length of stay, days of catheterization, and postoperative complication rates in RALP were similar between different BA groups [10, 11]. In a series of 129 RALPs, Albo et al. analyzed the effect of learning curve of two inexperienced BAs on perioperative outcomes and found that blood loss, hospital stay, catheterization time, and complication rates were comparable in their first 20, 21–40, and >40 procedures [5]. However, the aforementioned studies examined single surgeons who were well beyond their learning curve.

In contrast, other series that included surgeons early in their learning curve have shown that an experienced BA can improve operative outcomes [8, 9]. Garbens et al. examined the effect of expert (physician assistants or advanced nurse practitioners who had completed formal bedside training followed by a period of apprenticeship) vs. non-expert BAs (residents in their second and third years of training or physician assistants without formal laparoscopic or bedside training) on operative outcomes [9]. The series began with the first RALP performed by the surgeon after fellowship and involved his initial 170 cases. The expert and non-expert BA groups were similar in terms of patient demographics and cancer characteristics. The authors found almost 150 ml lower blood loss and shorter hospital stay in the expert BA group. Furthermore, the use of an expert assistant was associated with a 60% decrease in positive margin rates than when surgery was performed with a non-expert assistant. Considering that more than 80% of urologists in the USA perform less than 10 prostatectomies per year and these urologists account for approximately 40% of the total number of prostatectomies performed [14], Garbens et al. emphasized the importance of an experienced BA in common urological practice.

However, all studies above suffer from retrospective design, small sample size, and lack of cost analysis and long-term outcomes. The only prospective, multicenter study scored the performance of 14 CSs and 22 BAs by using objective skill assessment tools, and tested the relationship between assistant and surgeon technical performance in 92 RALP cases [15]. The dissection of the prostatic pedicle and neurovascular bundle (NVB) step were used for quantification of CS and BA performance. Interestingly, CS scores were disproportionally affected by the technical ability of the BA in surgeons who had completed >100 RALP cases completed at the outset of the study. After controlling for patient age and BMI, prostate volume, tumor stage, and nerve-sparing presence, assistant's performance remained a significant predictor of console surgeon's performance. The authors argued that the expectations of more experienced surgeons from their assistants to anticipate ahead and move with a similar pace and familiarity may be exaggerated, and this may negatively impact the surgeon's performance when the technical gap between CS and BA is large. Nevertheless, this study did not take into account the RALP steps other than NVB preservation.

4.3 Impact on Oncological Outcomes

Cancer-specific survival data were not available in any of the series. Positive surgical margin (PSM) rate was the only examined oncological parameter in both RALP and RAPN studies [5, 8, 9, 11–13]. In most series, PSM rates were not affected by the presence of an experienced or inexperienced BA [5, 8, 11–13]. In contrast, Garbens et al. found a significantly lower percentage of PSMs (20% vs. 37%, $p = 0.03$) in RALP surgeries that involved an experienced assistant [9]. In their multivariate analysis, the use of an expert BA, PSA at diagnosis, and prostate size were significant predictors of PSM status. They hypothesized that the expert BA can optimize visualization in situations where significant bleeding obscures visualization of important structures and results in suboptimal identification of tissue planes, thereby resulting in lower surgical margin rates. They also argued that the expert assistants may provide more optimal tissue retraction allowing for improved visualization and dissection of correct tissue planes as they are more familiar with the steps of the surgical procedure.

In summary, currently available data on the impact of bedside assistant on robotic surgery outcomes are derived from small, retrospective studies that reported conflicting results. It was generally argued that it is the console surgeon's experience which dictates perioperative outcomes and a less experienced assistant can be safely incorporated into this kind of surgery. However, others showed a benefit from experienced BAs in improving the surgical outcomes of a novice surgeon, including oncological outcomes such as PSM rates. As a BA is essential to complete any robotic urological procedure, it is important that the BA has sufficient experience to anticipate problems, reduce conflicts with the CS and the bedside team, and act in a timely manner in situations where patient safety may be compromised.

5 Conclusions

A skilled bedside assistant is an essential part of an effective urologic robotic surgery team. The bedside assistant represents a vital bridge between the console surgeon and the patient, and executes critical roles in preoperative preparation as well as intraoperative assistance and troubleshooting. Successful bedside assistance requires understanding the key steps of the operation, facilitating the flow of surgery, and timely management of unanticipated circumstances. The ability to work in harmony with the console surgeon depends on effective communication and repetitive execution. There is scarce literature that examined the impact of the experience of bedside assistant on robotic urological surgery outcomes. In general, perioperative outcomes and complication rates did not differ significantly with utilization of a novice vs. experienced assistant when the console surgeon was beyond his learning curve. Some studies demonstrated a benefit from an experienced bedside assistant in improving the surgical outcomes of a beginner surgeon. It is possible that the small number of cases and retrospective nature of these studies might have prevented from quantifying the effect of assistant experience on surgical outcomes. Roles and responsibilities of the robotic bedside assistant will continue to evolve; however, their position as a vital bridge between the console surgeon and the patient will remain.

References

1. Onol FF, Ganapathi HP, Rogers T, Palmer K, Coughlin G, Samavedi S, Coelho R, Jenson C, Sandri M, Rocco B, Patel V. Changing clinical trends in 10 000 robot-assisted laparoscopic prostatectomy patients and impact of the 2012 US Preventive Services Task Force's statement against PSA screening. BJU Int. 2019;124(6):1014–21.
2. Bhat KRS, Moschovas MC, Onol FF, Rogers T, Reddy SS, Corder C, Roof S, Patel VR. Evidence-based evolution of our robot-assisted laparoscopic prostatectomy (RALP) technique through 13,000 cases. J Robot Surg. 2021;15(4):651–60. https://doi.org/10.1007/s11701-020-01157-5.
3. Van der Horst S, Voli C, Polanco IA, et al. Robot-assisted minimally invasive esophagectomy (RAMIE): tips and tricks from the bedside assistant view-expert experiences. Dis Esophagus. 2020;33:1–7.
4. Yuh B. The bedside assistant in robotic surgery – keys to success. Urol Nurs. 2013;33(1):29–32.
5. Albo G, De Lorenzis E, Gallioli A, Boeri L, Zanetti SP, Longo F, Rocco B, Montanari E. Role of bed assistant during robot-assisted radical prostatectomy: the effect of learning curve on perioperative variables. Eur Urol Focus. 2020;6(2):397–403.
6. Tiferes J, Hussein AA, Bisantz A, et al. Are gestures worth a thousand words? Verbal and nonverbal communication during robot-assisted surgery. Appl Ergon. 2019;78:251–62.
7. Nayyar R, Yadav S, Singh P, Dogra PN. Impact of assistant surgeon on outcomes in robotic surgery. Indian J Urol. 2016;32(3):204–9.
8. Cimen HI, Atik YT, Altinova S, Adsan O, Balbay MD. Does the experience of the bedside assistant effect the results of robotic surgeons in the learning curve of robot assisted radical prostatectomy? Int Braz J Urol. 2019;45(1):54–60.
9. Garbens A, Lay AH, Steinberg RL, Gahan JC. Experienced bedside-assistants improve operative outcomes for surgeons early in their learning curve for robot assisted laparoscopic radical prostatectomy. J Robot Surg. 2021;5(4):619–26. https://doi.org/10.1007/s11701-020-01146-8.
10. Abu-Ghanem Y, Erlich T, Ramon J, Dotan Z, Zilberman DE. Robot assisted laparoscopic radical prostatectomy: assistant's seniority has no influence on perioperative course. J Robot Surg. 2017;11(3):305–9.
11. Mangano MS, Lamon C, Beniamin F, De Gobbi A, Ciaccia M, Maccatrozzo L. The role of bedside assistant during robot assisted radical prostatectomy: Is more experience better? Analysis on perioperative and clinical outcomes. Urologia. 2021;88(1):9–13.
12. Mitsinikos E, Abdelsayed GA, Bider Z, Kilday PS, Elliott PA, Banapour P, Chien GW. Does the level of assistant experience impact operative outcomes for robot-assisted partial nephrectomy? J Endourol. 2017;31(1):38–42.
13. Potretzke AM, Knight BA, Brockman JA, Vetter J, Figenshau RS, Bhayani SB, Benway BM. The role of the assistant during robot-assisted partial nephrectomy: does experience matter? J Robot Surg. 2016;10(2):129–34.
14. Savage CJ, Vickers AJ. Low annual caseloads of United States surgeons conducting radical prostatectomy. J Urol. 2009;182(6):2677–9.
15. Yu N, Saadat H, Finelli A, Lee JY, Singal RK, Grantcharov TP, Goldenberg MG. Quantifying the "assistant effect" in robotic-assisted radical prostatectomy (RARP): measures of technical performance. J Surg Res. 2021;260:307–14.

Anesthetics in Robotics

Ruban Thanigasalam, Joshua Makary, Scott Leslie, Ryan Downey, Michael Paleologos, and Joanne Irons

1 Introduction

Over the last two decades, robotic surgery has become increasingly preferred over laparoscopic and open techniques. It provides the perioperative advantages of minimally invasive surgery, while the dexterity afforded by endowrist instruments has expanded the indications of robotic surgery to even the most complex pelvic operations. Urological surgeons in particular have transitioned to robotic surgery for major procedures with a 2018 study revealing the highest proportion of robotic assistance was seen in radical prostatectomy and pyeloplasty [1].

The rise of robotic surgery requires anesthetists to also familiarize themselves with the management of these patients. Currently anesthetists unlike robotic surgeons do not complete a formal training program/fellowship specifically in managing robotic surgery patients. For this reason, anesthetists are encouraged to discuss anesthetic concerns with the robotic surgeon pre-operatively to prevent potentially foreseeable issues and complications from occurring. A recent survey of American anesthetists identified that the three most common reported anesthetic complications in robotic surgery include facial/airway edema, brachial plexus injury, and corneal abrasion [2].

In this chapter, we will evaluate anesthetic issues associated with robotic surgery and provide the reader with strategies to avoid and manage them.

R. Thanigasalam (✉) · J. Makary · S. Leslie
Institute of Academic Surgery, Royal Prince Alfred Hospital, Sydney, NSW, Australia

The University of Sydney, Sydney, NSW, Australia

R. Downey · M. Paleologos · J. Irons
The University of Sydney, Sydney, NSW, Australia

Department of Anaesthesia, Royal Prince Alfred Hospital, Sydney, NSW, Australia

2 Pre-operative Considerations

As with any major surgery requiring a general anesthetic, a thorough pre-operative evaluation of the medical history and physical examination are required. Particularly important considerations prior to robotic surgery include intraoperative airway access, pneumoperitoneum, and patient positioning. Especially the Trendelenburg position that is required for most robotic pelvic procedures.

An appreciation of the physiological response to positioning during robotic surgery is required to assess if the patient can safely tolerate the procedure. Patients being considered for robotic surgery with significant cardiac/respiratory conditions (refer to Table 1), morbid obesity, raised intracranial pressure (ICP), other intracranial pathology, and glaucoma are a particularly high-risk group due to the Trendelenburg position and pneumoperitoneum used intraoperatively [3].

In our institution, patients with glaucoma or neurosurgical pathology are referred pre-operatively to ophthalmology and neurosurgical specialists as required to ensure these conditions are optimized. Similarly, patients with cardiac/respiratory disease may benefit from specialist review and pre-operative assessment. Through this multi-disciplinary approach, both the surgeon and anesthetist can ensure the likelihood of complications related to these comorbidities is reduced.

Initially designed to focus on improving post-operative care, enhanced recovery after surgery (ERAS) is a protocol that now also includes guidelines for pre-operative optimization [4, 5]. We will explore the ERAS protocol and its relevance to both pre- and post-operative care later in this chapter.

Table 1 High-risk cardio-respiratory conditions

High-risk conditions
• Severe valvular pathology (particularly aortic stenosis)
• Severe heart failure (both left and right sided)
• Ischemic heart disease/previous myocardial infarction
• Significant arrhythmia
• Severe respiratory disease (COPD, poorly controlled asthma)

P. Wiklund et al. (eds.), *Robotic Urologic Surgery*, https://doi.org/10.1007/978-3-031-00363-9_7

3 Intraoperative considerations

3.1 Airway and Ventilation

The standard for airway management is endotracheal intubation. This is usually achieved using an oral cuffed endotracheal tube that additionally prevents aspiration of gastric contents that may occur with the steep Trendelenburg position. Because of the significant patient movement that occurs during positioning it is recommended that the position of the endotracheal tube be checked not only before but also after positioning the patient [6].

Facial and airway edema is seen more frequently in robotic surgery patients secondary to the Trendelenburg position. Consequently, prior to extubating the patient, an assessment for airway edema should be undertaken to ensure airway patency. This can be carried out in the form of a "leak test" that involves listening for air escaping around the endotracheal tube as the cuff is deflated. In addition, endotracheal tube ties can increase the risk of airway edema and should be avoided [3].

Robotic surgery can present unique issues with ventilation. Both the steep Trendelenburg and pneumoperitoneum cause decreased functional residual capacity due to splinting of the diaphragm. This in turn can result in higher inspiratory pressures and impaired ventilation [7, 8]. To counteract these pulmonary physiological changes and avoid atelectasis it has been suggested to maintain positive end-expiratory pressure between 4 and 7 cm H_2O and to keep the maximal airway pressure below 35 cm H_20. Furthermore, altering the inspiratory: expiratory ratio from 1–2:1 to 1:2 is a reasonable alternative in achieving improved gas exchange and a lower partial pressure of carbon dioxide PCO_2 [9].

A degree of hypercarbia is common during robotic surgery and requires appropriate management. Caution is required when titrating the tidal volume as barotrauma can arise due to the elevated inspiratory pressures [3, 10]. In our institution, we use a volume guaranteed pressure mode of ventilation to reduce peak airway pressures. Measures that can be taken by the surgeon to assist with difficulty in ventilation include reducing the steepness/angle of Trendelenburg and lowering the pressure of pneumoperitoneum. This may need to be considered in the morbidly obese or those with restrictive lung disease [11].

3.2 Pneumoperitoneum

Pneumoperitoneum is required during robotic surgery to obtain appropriate visualization of abdominal and pelvic organs. The physiological impact this has on airway and ventilation has been discussed but equally important are the changes that can occur in relation to cardiac output. Pneumoperitoneum leads to an increased intra-abdominal pressure (IAP). Small increases in IAP actually lead to increased venous return and cardiac output; however, more significant increases (i.e., >10 mmHg) can increase systemic vascular resistance and decrease cardiac output. An even higher IAP of >20 mmHg is associated with significant decreases in mean arterial pressure and cardiac output [12].

For these reasons, in our institution the IAP is usually maintained at the lowest level to achieve satisfactory surgical conditions (typically 12–15 mmHg). The practice of conducting robotic surgery with low-pressure pneumoperitoneum although ideal, may impact on the surgeon's ability to visualize the surgical field. Improvements in the equipment used to maintain low-pressure pneumoperitoneum address this issue and can provide low pressure but high flow insufflation, an example of such a device is the *AirSeal intelligent flow system* which relies on valveless trocar system technology [13]. In addition to the cardiovascular benefits of low-pressure pneumoperitoneum, the incidence of post-operative ileus may also be decreased [14, 15].

Generally, the gas used for insufflation is CO_2 and the relative hypercarbia seen in robotic surgery can be partially attributed to its solubility and rapid absorptivity. These properties are also advantageous in reducing the likelihood of catastrophic venous gas embolism [16]. Nonetheless, gas embolism should be considered and promptly managed in the case of sudden hemodynamic compromise. Particularly during robot-assisted laparoscopic prostatectomy (RALP), a degree of gas embolus can be expected during ligation of the dorsal venous complex, especially considering a higher IAP (up to 20 mm Hg) is often required to safely complete the ligation. A 2010 study conducted intraoperative transesophageal echocardiograms in both patients undergoing RALP and open retropubic prostatectomy, they observed that 40% and 80% of patients, respectively, developed venous gas embolism. Reassuringly, none of these patients displayed signs of hemodynamic compromise [17].

3.3 Monitoring

Intraoperative access to the patient undergoing robotic surgery is limited due to the robot itself occupying much of the space above the patient. Additionally, the sterile operative field further restricts access to the patient. The difficulty in accessing the patient, specifically the face is a likely factor in the relatively high rate of corneal abrasion. In a review of 1500 RALP procedures, one institution found the rate of corneal abrasion was 3% but were able to reduce this to 1% by switching from using eye tape to eye pads [18]. Eye injuries can also occur from gastric/oral secretions tracking up the face secondary to the gravitational effect of Trendelenburg. To mitigate against this risk, the mouth can be sealed around the endotracheal tube using waterproof dressings/tapes. Additionally, the limited patient access mandates careful placement of monitoring equipment prior to the commencement of surgery. Monitoring or IV access lines typically need to be longer to provide remote access distant from the patient. Arterial lines are not always required but should be considered in patients with comorbidities that place them in a high-risk category for GA.

Once abdominal ports are placed and the robotic arms engaged it is critical the patient remains immobile. This is achieved with neuromuscular blockers to keep the patient paralyzed, any movement by the patient intraoperatively can be disastrous and potentially cause injury to intra-abdominal organs and blood vessels. Equally important is for the patient to remain securely positioned to avoid slipping. In open/laparoscopic surgery the proceduralist is positioned adjacent to the operating table and is likely to observe changes in the patient position such as slipping. In contrast, robotic surgeons are removed from the operating table for the majority for the case and are less likely to notice inadvertent changes in patient positioning. Non-slip mats, bean bags, tape, and straps can all be used to secure the patient [3, 6]. When straps are used caution should be exercised in avoiding overtightening as this may lead to pressure injuries.

3.4 Trendelenburg

The Trendelenburg position involves tilting the operating table "head down." This position is employed during robotic surgery particularly on pelvic organs as it allows for improved exposure by allowing the bowel to slide away from the pelvis. As previously alluded to, the Trendelenburg position leads to increased ICP and intra-ocular pressure [6]. Thus, patients with pre-existing elevated ICP, glaucoma, retinal detachment, and ventriculoperitoneal shunts may require further pre-operative planning and multi-disciplinary input. To mitigate these challenges and also to avoid cerebral/airway edema, it has been suggested to avoid aggressive IVF while the patient remains in this position [19]. Equally important in reducing the complications of Trendelenburg is minimizing the time that the surgery is conducted in this position. For potentially prolonged cases such as cystectomy it is not uncommon for the bed to be leveled at regular intervals. In our institution for extended cases that continue beyond 4 hours, a "second time-out" is conducted which provides an opportunity for the surgeon, anesthetist, and nursing staff to discuss any relevant concerns. The feasibility of implementing a "second time-out" has been previously reported; however, further studies are required to assess the benefits including any potential reduction in complications [20].

A recent case–control study of 67 urological patients compared two groups with different degrees of Trendelenburg tilt. The control group angle was set at 30°, and the mean angle in the reduced tilt group was 20.5°. The authors of this study demonstrated that robotic pelvic surgeries can be safely performed with a reduced Trendelenburg tilt and also noted the advantages of decreased hemodynamic and respiratory stress [21]. The modified Z Trendelenburg position is a variant of the traditional position but with the head maintained at a horizontal position which creates a "Z" shape (Fig. 1).

A prospective randomized controlled study examined the differences in physiological parameters between the standard Trendelenburg position (angle set at 23°) and the modified Z version. A significant reduction in IOP and blood pressure in favor of the modified Z Trendelenburg position was observed for the majority of cases [22]. In summary, minimizing length of surgery, avoiding aggressive IVF replacement, and reducing steepness of the operating table can reduce the complications associated with Trendelenburg.

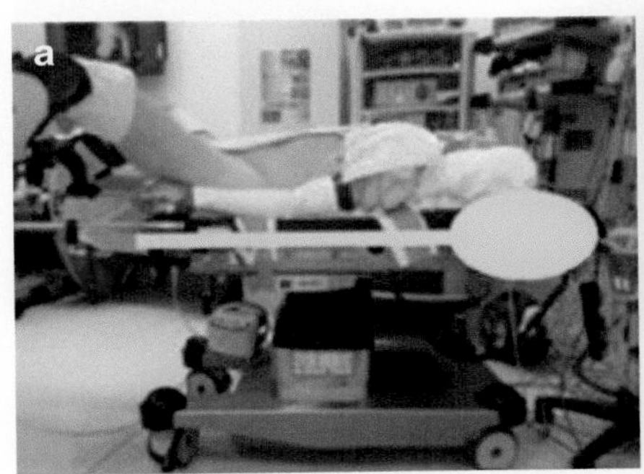

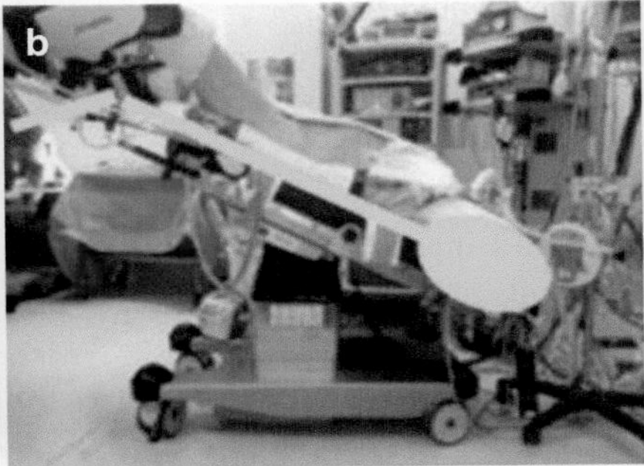

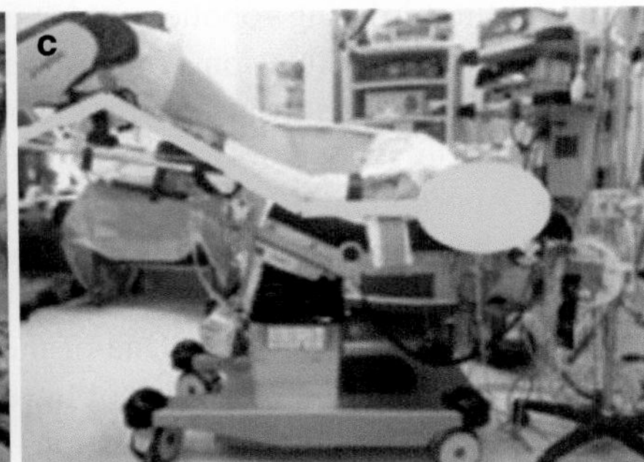

Fig. 1 Courtesy of Raz et al. [22]. (**a**) Horizontal supine position with legs in lithotomy position. (**b**) Head down in 23° Trendelenburg position. (**c**) Modified Z Trendelenburg position with horizontal head and shoulders

3.5 Fluid Balance

Because of the aforementioned unique physiological perturbations that robotic surgery patients experience, the fluid balance management significantly differs from patients undergoing GA in a standard supine position. As previously mentioned to avoid complications such as facial/airway edema it is advised to limit the delivery of IVF while the patient remains in Trendelenburg [9]. The decreased urine output that results from limiting IVF also provides an added benefit of improving vision in the surgical field, particularly in RALP after the bladder neck has been dissected.

While the administration of IVF is initially restricted, toward the end of a RALP procedure when the urethrovesical anastomosis is being performed, IVF replacement can be increased. Similarly in other robotic cases such as cystectomy when the patient's position is reverted back to a supine leveled position, IVF should be administered to encourage urine production and avoid renal impairment. This is important to consider given decreased renal perfusion is expected intraoperatively secondary to the effects of pneumoperitoneum and decreased cardiac output. Evidence of renal impairment can be seen during routine post-operative blood investigations that reveal a transiently elevated serum creatinine [6]. Another benefit of adequate urine output at the completion of surgery is the reduced likelihood of blood clots occluding the urinary catheter. In summary we suggest limiting fluid administration intraoperatively while the patient is subject to the extreme positioning associated with surgery and later increasing the rate of IVF toward the end of the case and maintain a clear urine output.

3.6 Neuropraxia

Nerve injuries to both upper and lower limbs have previously been reported during robotic surgery and a significant portion of closed claims can be attributed to this [23]. The combination of Trendelenburg and lithotomy position is commonly used during robotic surgery and care should be taken to avoid overextension of the lower limbs and ensure appropriately placed stirrups. Stirrups should ideally provide adequate ankle support to reduce the pressure on the calf muscles. Appropriate lithotomy positioning should reflect a natural rather than exaggerated position to avoid injuring susceptible nerves such as the common peroneal, femoral, and obturator nerves [24, 25]. One of the main factors that have been linked to increased risk of lower limb neuropathy is prolonged surgical time >2 h duration [24, 26].

Brachial plexus injuries can also occur and are often secondary to slipping during changes in patient positioning. Depression of the acromioclavicular joint is thought to be at least partially responsible for brachial plexus injuries [27]. In one high volume robotic surgery institution, the arms had been positioned in abduction, with bean bags and shoulder girdle restraints utilized to prevent patient slipping. However, this was associated with several cases of brachial plexus injury. Subsequent modifications in patient positioning included keeping arms adducted and using shoulder padding. Brachial plexus injuries were prevented in the subsequent 2674 cases [28]. In agreeance with the findings of this study, the most recent advice from the American Society of Anaesthetics practice advisory also suggests limiting arm abduction [29]. In summary, by avoiding restraints that place pressure on the shoulder girdle and keeping the arms well secured and adducted there is a reduced likelihood of brachial plexus injury.

3.7 Pressure Injuries and Compartment Syndrome

Adequate padding, especially at bony prominences is necessary to prevent the formation of pressure sores (Refer to Fig. 2). Monitoring equipment and IV lines in contact with the patient are also potential sites of pressure injuries but easily preventable [3]. Compartment syndrome of the lower limbs or *"Well leg"* syndrome is a severe complication that can occur with prolonged steep Trendelenburg and lithotomy. Risk factors for developing this include extended length

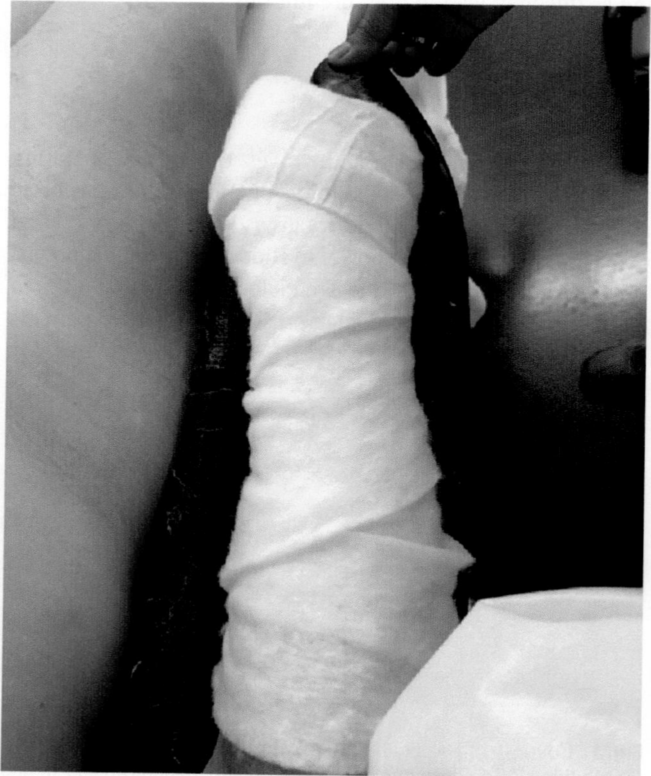

Fig. 2 Padding applied and gel pad beneath forearm

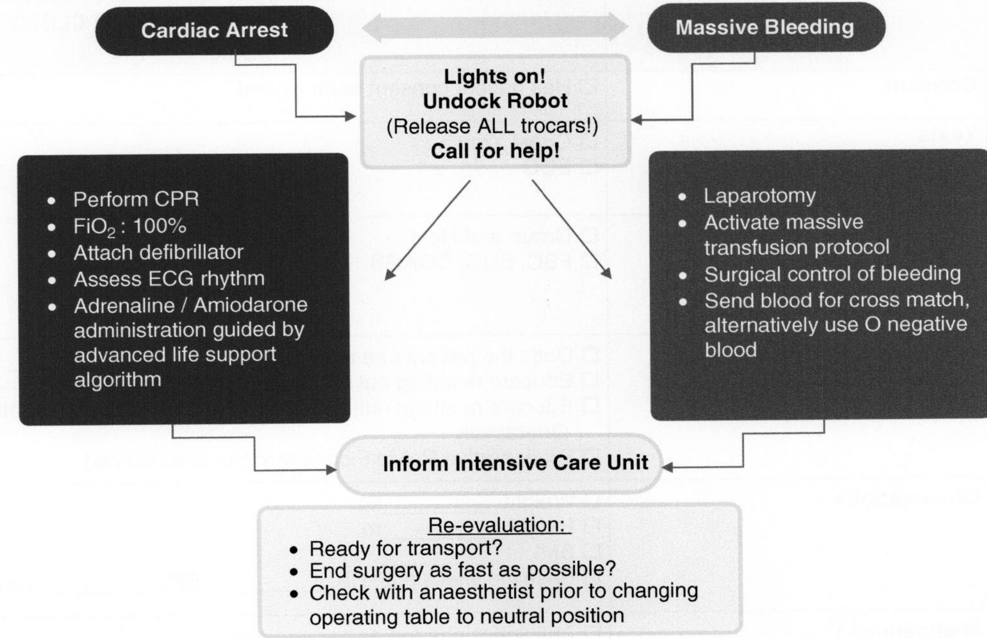

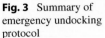

Fig. 3 Summary of emergency undocking protocol

of surgery, obesity, hypotension, and peripheral vascular disease. Steps that can be taken to avoid compartment syndrome of the lower limbs include leveling the bed periodically, intermittent pneumatic compression of the calves, and ensuring the stirrups used provide adequate padding and ankle support to increase the surface area in contact with the lower limb. In patients at risk of lower limb ischemia in Trendelenburg, placing a pulse oximeter on the great toe will detect changes in blood flow to the lower limbs and may trigger earlier reversal of identifiable aggravating factors [16].

3.8 Emergency Undocking

Estimates for the rate of conversion from robotic to an open procedure vary from 1.3 to 4.3% [30, 31]. The proportion of these cases which represent emergency undocking is not clear but despite it being a relatively rare occurrence, the whole surgical team (surgeon, surgical assistant, anesthetist, scrub/anesthetic nurses, and theater orderly/assistants) should familiarize themselves with local protocols in place for emergency undocking. The indications for emergency undocking include but are not limited to anesthetic concerns, cardiac/respiratory arrest, surgical complications (massive hemorrhage), and failure of the robotic equipment. A clear understanding of roles and communication is required by all members of the surgical team to ensure emergency undocking occurs in a safe but prompt manner [32]. Experienced and well-rehearsed teams have reportedly been able to progress through the emergency undocking process in less than 30 s [19].

Cardiopulmonary resuscitation is a challenge in robotic surgery due to the patient's position and bulkiness of the robotic cart. Although not ideal, it is important to be aware that DC defibrillation shocks **CAN** be delivered, while the robotic arms remain docked [19]. A flow diagram summarizing the emergency undocking protocol is shown in Fig. 3.

3.9 Enhanced Recovery After Surgery (ERAS)

The management of a surgical patient of course does not end immediately after the procedure. Arguably as important as the procedure itself is the pre-operative planning and post-operative care provided. An advantage of robotic surgery when compared to an open approach is the decreased length of stay (LOS) [33]. This is a result of the minimally invasive nature of the procedure but also post-operative management protocols play a role in ensuring patients recover more rapidly. ERAS is defined as a multi-modal and multi-disciplinary care pathway that influences the pre-/intra-/post-operative management of surgical patients.

Pre-operatively, patients should be screened in a pre-admission clinic and receive education across several domains including adequate nutrition, smoking cessation, pain management, and early mobilization (Refer to Fig. 4). From a detailed social history, issues that may hamper recovery post-discharge can be anticipated and support services organized depending on the patient's individual circumstances. Intraoperatively improved thermoregulation can be

ASSESSMENT	PRE ADMISSION CLINIC Date: ____/____/____
Consent	☐ Has patient consent been signed
Tests	☐ Chest Xray ☐ ECG
Pathology	☐ Group and Hold ☐ FBC, EUC, COAGS
Mobilisation / Physiotherapy / Oxygen Therapy	☐ Does the patient use any mobility aides_____________ ☐ Educate re sitting out of bed the night of surgery ☐ Educate re sitting out of bed, ambulation and deep breathing exercises post-Operatively ☐ Preoperative Pelvic Floor exercises commenced
Observations	☐ Weight _________kg ☐ Height _________m ☐ BMI __________ ☐ Baseline vital signs: HR: ________ BP: ________ Oxygen Sats: ________
Medications / VTE Prophylaxis	☐ Antibiotics charted as per surgeon ☐ Bowel Prep ☐Yes ☐ No ☐ Instructions given ☐ Educate patient on TED stockings which will be provided in TPU ☐ Educate patient on VTE prophylaxis ☐ Anticoagulants to cease on ___/___/___ (Patient educated re same)
Pain Management	☐ Education: Post-op pain control
Wounds / Drains	☐ Patient educated regarding presence of IDC post-operatively ☐ Patient educated regarding +/- drain post-operatively
Nutrition	Patient educated re: ☐ No solid food from 24:00hrs pre-operatively (Clear Fluids for 24hrs if Bowel Prep) ☐ Clear Fluids up to 2 hours pre-operatively ☐ Strictly NBM once patient has left home
Pressure Area Care (Waterlow Score)	
Falls Risk Assessment	
Current Support Services and Referrals to be made	☐ ERAS booklet given to patient - ☐ Surgeon ☐ Nurse ☐ Patient has read booklet ☐ Do you have any current support services in place? ____________ ☐ Will you need a community nurse to help with IDC care? ____________ ☐ Will you require any services post operatively? ____________ ☐ How will you be getting home? ____________ ☐ Social Worker ☐ Compacks ☐ Community Nurses ☐ Occupational Therapy ☐ Physiotherapy

Fig. 4 Example of RALP ERAS (pre-operative component)

achieved by reducing the patient's time exposed and raising the operating theater temperature. The choice of analgesia administered intraoperatively also plays a role in allowing earlier mobilization and for these reasons, epidural and patient-controlled analgesia are usually avoided.

The key elements of ERAS in the post-operative stage include minimizing opiates, encouraging early mobilization, early feeding, nausea and ileus prophylaxis and venous thromboembolism (VTE) prophylaxis [4] (**Refer to** Fig. 5). A cohort study of 110 patients undergoing radical cystec-

Operation Performed:						☐ No PLND ☐ PLND ☐ Extended PLND				
ASSESSMENT	**DAY OF SURGERY** Date: ___/___/___	AM	PM	ND	Vari-ance	**DAY 1 POST-OPERATIVE** Date: ___/___/___	AM	PM	ND	Vari-ance
Procedures / Investigations						☐ EUC ☐ FBC ☐ Discharge Referral Written				
Hygiene	☐ Post-op sponge					☐ Assisted shower				
Mobilisation / Physiotherapy	☐ Sit out of bed 1-2hrs					☐ Sit out of bed for 2hrs ☐ AM and ☐ PM ☐ Ambulate 100 metres x2 ☐ ☐				
Observations	☐ Standard observations as per protocol ☐ 1/24 Urine Output for 24hrs ☐ SFBC (input / output) ☐ BSL as per protocol ☐ Assess pain and nausea ☐ Enter height and weight					☐ Standard observations as per protocol ☐ 4/24 Urine Output ☐ Continue monitoring all output on FBC ☐ BSL as per protocol ☐ Assess pain and nausea				
Medications / VTE Prophylaxis	☐ IV antibiotics TDS ☐ Coloxyl & Senna BD ☐ Movicol BD ☐ Regular Oxycodone / Naloxone combination ☐ Regular Meloxicam ☐ Regular Paracetamol ☐ PRN oral analgesia ☐ TED stockings ☐ Heparin 5000u BD					☐ Cease IV antibiotics after 24 hours ☐ Coloxyl & Senna BD ☐ Movicol BD ☐ Regular Oxycodone / Naloxone combination ☐ Regular Meloxicam ☐ Regular Paracetamol ☐ PRN oral analgesia ☐ TED stockings ☐ Heparin 5000u BD ☐ Discharge scripts In progress				
Wounds / Drains	☐ Review wound ☐ Drain(s) in situ ☐Y ☐N How many: ________ ☐ Free drainage or 4/24 revac ☐ Change drainage bags at 24:00hrs + record					☐ Review wound ☐ Drain(s) in situ ☐Y ☐N How many: ________ ☐ Free drainage or 4/24 revac ☐ Change drainage bags at 24:00hrs+ record				
IV Therapy / Access	☐ IVC Day___ ☐ Position______ ☐ Cease IV Therapy post 1st litre if patient tolerating diet					☐ Remove IVC once IV antibiotics ceased				
Elimination	☐ IDC secured with STAT-LOCK ☐ Passing flatus ☐Y ☐N ☐ Bowel motion ☐Y ☐N					☐ IDC remains secured ☐ Change IDC to long leg bag ☐ IDC + leg bag education ☐ Passing flatus ☐Y ☐N ☐ Bowel motion ☐Y ☐N				
Nutrition	☐ Clear fluids and progress to light diet **if** tolerated					☐ Full diet				
Pressure Area Care (Waterlow Score)										
Falls Risk Assessment										

Fig. 5 Example of RALP ERAS (post-operative component)

tomy showed a significant reduction in LOS in favor of the ERAS group when compared to conventional care (4 vs 8 days) [5]. A larger study specifically assessing the impact of ERAS on robotic-assisted radical cystectomy patients also demonstrated a decreased LOS without significant differences in readmission rates [34]. RALP patients also benefit from ERAS in reducing LOS by 2.5 days based on a recent systematic review and meta-analysis [35]. Crucial to achieving these improved patient outcomes is the collaboration between surgeons and anesthetists in correctly implementing ERAS protocols.

3.10 VTE Prophylaxis

As previously mentioned, ERAS protocols contain recommendations for the management of VTE prophylaxis. Variations in VTE prophylaxis regimen exist based on the patient's VTE risk. Major risk factors that alter the VTE prophylaxis regimen include previous/family history of deep vein thrombosis (DVT)/pulmonary embolus (PE), prolonged surgery (>2 h), and presence of active cancer. Other minor risk factors include age, obesity, and chronic venous insufficiency [36].

Low molecular weight heparin (LMWH) and low dose unfractionated heparin (LDUH) are the most commonly used forms of pharmacological VTE prophylaxis. Multiple studies have reported on the outcomes of both of these anticoagulants with both demonstrating similar efficacy [37]. Other important considerations in prescribing either LMWH/LDUH include dosage and duration of treatment. Obese patients in particular seem to benefit from a reduction in VTE risk with appropriate weight adjusted dosing [38]. A systematic review of 1728 patients demonstrated continuing LMWH post-discharge in patients undergoing major abdominal/pelvis surgery resulted in a significant reduction in VTE events [39]. The most recent American Society of hematology VTE prophylaxis guidelines for cancer patients support the use of extended pharmacological VTE prophylaxis for major abdominal/pelvic surgery [40]. For radical cystectomy patients, the standard of care is to continue pharmacological VTE prophylaxis for 28 days post-operatively [41]. Post RALP, pharmacological VTE prophylaxis post-discharge is not usually necessary but can be considered if the patient is deemed high risk of VTE.

Early ambulation and mechanical VTE prophylaxis are also paramount in reducing the post-operative VTE risk. Both European and American VTE prophylaxis guidelines suggest the combination of pharmacological and mechanical VTE prophylaxis is superior to a single VTE prophylaxis modality. When mechanical prophylaxis is used the preference is for intermittent pneumatic compression rather than graduated compression stockings [38, 40].

3.11 Analgesia

Post robotic surgery side effects include abdominal pain, shoulder tip pain, and ileus [6]. Compared to an open procedure, robotic surgery patients generally have smaller midline incisions and subsequently a reduced requirement for analgesia. Multi-modal analgesia including paracetamol, NSAIDs (assuming normal renal function), limited use of opiates and local/regional anesthesia (for example, erector spinae/transversus abdominus plane block) is common and usually sufficient in managing pain particularly in the context of ERAS [4].

Epidurals are infrequently used given the preference to encourage early mobilization as part of the post op recovery and the expected short length of admission. There may be cases where it is determined an epidural is required, it should however not be used intraoperatively as the Trendelenburg positioning may lead to cardiac instability from potential high block [19]. Spinal anesthesia may also be used as part of a multi-modal analgesia plan. However, anesthetists should first determine if the patient has been administered prophylactic anticoagulation. European Surgical Association (ESA) guidelines on VTE prophylaxis suggest if neuraxial anesthesia is planned that prophylactic anticoagulation be commenced post-operatively [42]. A significant common issue post RALP is abdominal pain due to bladder spasms. There is limited evidence suggesting intravesical local anesthetic is beneficial in reducing catheter related discomfort [43]. A small-scale 2013 study comparing RALP patients receiving intravesical ropivacaine and placebo suggested patients in the treatment arm had similar pain scores but required smaller doses of NSAIDs [44].

References

1. Juo Y-Y, Mantha A, Abiri A, Lin A, Dutson E. Diffusion of robotic-assisted laparoscopic technology across specialties: a national study from 2008 to 2013. Surg Endosc. 2018;32(3):1405–13.
2. Souki FG, Rodriguez-Blanco YF, Polu SR, Eber S, Candiotti KA. Survey of anesthesiologists' practices related to steep Trendelenburg positioning in the USA. BMC Anesthesiol. 2018;18(1):117.
3. Carey BM, Jones CN, Fawcett WJ. Anaesthesia for minimally invasive abdominal and pelvic surgery. BJA Educ. 2019;19(8):254–60.
4. Azhar RA, Bochner B, Catto J, Goh AC, Kelly J, Patel HD, et al. Enhanced recovery after urological surgery: a contemporary systematic review of outcomes, key elements, and research needs. Eur Urol. 2016;70(1):176–87.
5. Daneshmand S, Ahmadi H, Schuckman AK, Mitra AP, Cai J, Miranda G, et al. Enhanced recovery protocol after radical cystectomy for bladder cancer. J Urol. 2014;192(1):50–5.
6. Awad H, Walker CM, Shaikh M, Dimitrova GT, Abaza R, O'Hara J. Anesthetic considerations for robotic prostatectomy: a review of the literature. J Clin Anesth. 2012;24(6):494–504.
7. Fahy BG, Barnas GM, Nagle SE, Flowers JL, Njoku MJ, Agarwal M. Effects of Trendelenburg and reverse Trendelenburg postures on lung and chest wall mechanics. J Clin Anesth. 1996;8(3):236–44.

8. Suh MK, Seong KW, Jung SH, Kim SS. The effect of pneumoperitoneum and Trendelenburg position on respiratory mechanics during pelviscopic surgery. Korean J Anesthesiol. 2010;59(5):329–34.
9. Lee JR. Anesthetic considerations for robotic surgery. Korean J Anesthesiol. 2014;66(1):3–11.
10. Berger JS, Alshaeri T, Lukula D, Dangerfield P. Anesthetic considerations for robot-assisted gynecologic and urology surgery. J Anesth Clin Res. 2013;4(8):345.
11. Sprung J, Whalley DG, Falcone T, Warner DO, Hubmayr RD, Hammel J. The impact of morbid obesity, pneumoperitoneum, and posture on respiratory system mechanics and oxygenation during laparoscopy. Anesth Analg. 2002;94(5):1345–50.
12. Perrin M, Fletcher A. Laparoscopic abdominal surgery. Contin Educ Anaesth Crit Care Pain. 2004;4(4):107–10.
13. George AK, Wimhofer R, Viola KV, Pernegger M, Costamoling W, Kavoussi LR, et al. Utilization of a novel valveless trocar system during robotic-assisted laparoscopic prostatectomy. World J Urol. 2015;33(11):1695–9.
14. Rohloff M, Cicic A, Christensen C, Maatman TK, Lindberg J, Maatman TJ. Reduction in postoperative ileus rates utilizing lower pressure pneumoperitoneum in robotic-assisted radical prostatectomy. J Robot Surg. 2019;13(5):671–4.
15. Rohloff M, Peifer G, Shakuri-Rad J, Maatman TJ. The impact of low pressure pneumoperitoneum in robotic assisted radical prostatectomy: a prospective, randomized, double blinded trial. World J Urol. 2021;39(7):2469–74.
16. Hayden P, Cowman S. Anaesthesia for laparoscopic surgery. Contin Educ Anaesth Crit Care Pain. 2011;11(5):177–80.
17. Hong JY, Kim JY, Choi YD, Rha KH, Yoon SJ, Kil HK. Incidence of venous gas embolism during robotic-assisted laparoscopic radical prostatectomy is lower than that during radical retropubic prostatectomy. Br J Anaesth. 2010;105(6):777–81.
18. Danic MJ, Chow M, Alexander G, Bhandari A, Menon M, Brown M. Anesthesia considerations for robotic-assisted laparoscopic prostatectomy: a review of 1,500 cases. J Robot Surg. 2007;1(2):119–23.
19. Irvine M, Patil V. Anaesthesia for robot-assisted laparoscopic surgery. Contin Educ Anaesth Crit Care Pain. 2009;9(4):125–9.
20. Song JB, Vemana G, Mobley JM, Bhayani SB. The second "time-out": a surgical safety checklist for lengthy robotic surgeries. Patient Saf Surg. 2013;7(1):19.
21. Aggarwal D, Bora GS, Mavuduru RS, Jangra K, Sharma AP, Gupta S, et al. Robot-assisted pelvic urologic surgeries: is it feasible to perform under reduced tilt? J Robot Surg. 2020.
22. Raz O, Boesel TW, Arianayagam M, Lau H, Vass J, Huynh CC, et al. The effect of the modified Z trendelenburg position on intraocular pressure during robotic assisted laparoscopic radical prostatectomy: a randomized, controlled study. J Urol. 2015;193(4):1213–9.
23. Mills JT, Burris MB, Warburton DJ, Conaway MR, Schenkman NS, Krupski TL. Positioning injuries associated with robotic assisted urological surgery. J Urol. 2013;190(2):580–4.
24. Warner MA, Warner DO, Harper CM, Schroeder DR, Maxson PM. Lower extremity neuropathies associated with lithotomy positions. Anesthesiology. 2000;93(4):938–42.
25. Litwiller JP, Wells RE Jr, Halliwill JR, Carmichael SW, Warner MA. Effect of lithotomy positions on strain of the obturator and lateral femoral cutaneous nerves. Clin Anat. 2004;17(1):45–9.
26. Koç G, Tazeh NN, Joudi FN, Winfield HN, Tracy CR, Brown JA. Lower extremity neuropathies after robot-assisted laparoscopic prostatectomy on a split-leg table. J Endourol. 2012;26(8):1026–9.
27. Maerz DA, Beck LN, Sim AJ, Gainsburg DM. Complications of robotic-assisted laparoscopic surgery distant from the surgical site. Br J Anaesth. 2017;118(4):492–503.
28. Devarajan J, Byrd JB, Gong MC, Wood HM, O'Hara J, Weingarten TN, et al. Upper and middle trunk brachial plexopathy after robotic prostatectomy. Anesth Analg. 2012;115(4):867–70.
29. Practice advisory for the prevention of perioperative peripheral neuropathies 2018: an updated report by the American society of anesthesiologists task force on prevention of perioperative peripheral neuropathies. Anesthesiology. 2018;128(1):11–26.
30. Capmas P, Suarthana E, Larouche M. Conversion rate of laparoscopic or robotic to open sacrocolpopexy: are there associated factors and complications? Int Urogynecol J. 2021;32(8):2249–56.
31. Ko OS, Weiner AB, Smith ND, Meeks JJ. Rates and predictors of conversion to open surgery during minimally invasive radical cystectomy. J Endourol. 2018;32(6):488–94.
32. O'Sullivan OE, O'Sullivan S, Hewitt M, O'Reilly BA. Da Vinci robot emergency undocking protocol. J Robot Surg. 2016;10(3):251–3.
33. Coughlin GD, Yaxley JW, Chambers SK, Occhipinti S, Samaratunga H, Zajdlewicz L, et al. Robot-assisted laparoscopic prostatectomy versus open radical retropubic prostatectomy: 24-month outcomes from a randomised controlled study. Lancet Oncol. 2018;19(8):1051–60.
34. Collins JW, Adding C, Hosseini A, Nyberg T, Pini G, Dey L, et al. Introducing an enhanced recovery programme to an established totally intracorporeal robot-assisted radical cystectomy service. Scand J Urol. 2016;50(1):39–46.
35. Zhao Y, Zhang S, Liu B, Li J, Hong H. Clinical efficacy of enhanced recovery after surgery (ERAS) program in patients undergoing radical prostatectomy: a systematic review and meta-analysis. World J Surg Oncol. 2020;18(1):131.
36. Caprini JA. Thrombosis risk assessment as a guide to quality patient care. Dis Mon. 2005;51(2-3):70–8.
37. Matar CF, Kahale LA, Hakoum MB, Tsolakian IG, Etxeandia-Ikobaltzeta I, Yosuico VE, et al. Anticoagulation for perioperative thromboprophylaxis in people with cancer. Cochrane Database Syst Rev. 2018;7(7):Cd009447.
38. Venclauskas L, Maleckas A, Arcelus JI, Force ftEVGT. European guidelines on perioperative venous thromboembolism prophylaxis: surgery in the obese patient. Eur J Anaesthesiol. 2018;35(2):147–53.
39. Felder S, Rasmussen MS, King R, Sklow B, Kwaan M, Madoff R, et al. Prolonged thromboprophylaxis with low molecular weight heparin for abdominal or pelvic surgery. Cochrane Database Syst Rev. 2019;8(8):Cd004318.
40. Lyman GH, Carrier M, Ay C, Di Nisio M, Hicks LK, Khorana AA, et al. American Society of Hematology 2021 guidelines for management of venous thromboembolism: prevention and treatment in patients with cancer. Blood Adv. 2021;5(4):927–74.
41. Pariser JJ, Pearce SM, Anderson BB, Packiam VT, Prachand VN, Smith ND, et al. Extended duration enoxaparin decreases the rate of venous thromboembolic events after radical cystectomy compared to inpatient only subcutaneous heparin. J Urol. 2017;197(2):302–7.
42. Venclauskas L, Llau JV, Jenny J-Y, Kjaersgaard-Andersen P, Jans Ø. Force ftEVGT. European guidelines on perioperative venous thromboembolism prophylaxis: day surgery and fast-track surgery. Eur J Anaesthesiol. 2018;35(2):134–8.
43. Pournajafian A, Ghodraty MR, Shafighnia S, Rokhtabnak F, Khatibi A, Tavoosian S, et al. The effect of intravesical diluted bupivacaine on catheter-related bladder discomfort in young and middle-aged male patients during postanaesthetic recovery. Turk J Anaesthesiol Reanim. 2020;48(6):454–9.
44. Fuller A, Vanderhaeghe L, Nott L, Martin PR, Pautler SE. Intravesical ropivacaine as a novel means of analgesia post-robot-assisted radical prostatectomy: a randomized, double-blind, placebo-controlled trial. J Endourol. 2013;27(3):313–7.

The Role of Virtual Reality, Telesurgery, and Teleproctoring in Robotic Surgery

Barbara Seeliger, Justin W. Collins, Francesco Porpiglia, and Jacques Marescaux

1 Introduction

Computer interfaces and Internet connections have led to significant technological advances, which impact our everyday life, as well as surgical practice. The SARS-CoV-2 pandemic has catalyzed the set-up of a telemedicine infrastructure in many healthcare systems worldwide, and remote workplaces have become increasingly common. Will tomorrow's surgeons be able to simultaneously provide teaching across multiple continents, based on protected and secured connections? Will they not only virtually scrub in, but operate from home too?

Technological progress is paving the way for this change in surgical paradigm, and upcoming developments in digital surgery are highly anticipated.

2 Virtual and Augmented Reality in Robotic Surgery

Virtual Reality (VR) applications that immerse users into a digital version of reality are based on a synthetic three-dimensional (3D) environment. Augmented Reality (AR) is closely related, and superimposes VR data onto the real-world environment, through a variety of available displays. Three essential characteristics of VR and AR include immersion, presence, and interaction. These digital technologies allow the automation of repetitive tasks and support medical education and training.

The use of VR has the potential to develop and improve surgical skills and reduce procedure errors [1]. **VR simulators** allow to familiarize surgeons with robotic systems and to shift robotic surgery training outside of the operating room (OR). Various sets of VR exercises are available for several robotic surgical platforms. Despite a growing evidence for skill transfer to the OR from laparoscopic VR simulators, equivalent data is scarce for robotic VR simulators. Consequently, a recent systematic review and meta-analysis addressed the transferability of surgical skills acquired on robotic VR simulators to the OR, as well as the predictability of intraoperative performance from robotic VR simulator performance [2]. Out of more than 14,000 articles on **robotic VR simulation training**, only 8 pertained to these inclusion criteria (skill transferability: 5, predictability: 3). The limited available data support the use of robotic VR simulators for surgical skill acquisition and assessment. Significant positive correlations between robotic VR simulator and intraoperative technical surgical performance were observed in two of three studies. Quantitative analysis showed a positive combined correlation ($r = 0.67$, 95% CI [0.22, 0.88]). In addition to technical skills, non-technical aspects such as cognitive training and clinical decision-making should also be investigated to assess robotic VR simulator training benefits and limitations [2]. More studies are necessary to correlate robotic surgery training modalities to intraoperative performance and operative outcomes.

By taking patient-specific data into account, procedures can be tailored to individual characteristics. Dedicated software allows for 3D reconstructions of tomographic imaging studies, yielding **patient-specific virtual models** from computed tomography (CT) or magnetic resonance imaging (MRI) [3–5]. A clear understanding of normal and pathologic patient anatomy is key for any type of surgery. Different methods are available to obtain a **3D reconstruction** of

Supplementary Information The online version contains supplementary material available at [https://doi.org/10.1007/978-3-031-00363-9_8].

B. Seeliger
IHU-Strasbourg, Institute of Image-Guided Surgery/IRCAD, Research Institute Against Digestive Cancer/University of Strasbourg/Strasbourg University Hospitals, Strasbourg, France

J. W. Collins
Division of Surgery and Interventional Science, Research Department of Targeted Intervention, University College London, London, UK

F. Porpiglia
Division of Urology, Department of Oncology, San Luigi Gonzaga Hospital, University of Turin, Orbassano (Torino), Italy

J. Marescaux (✉)
IRCAD, Research Institute Against Digestive Cancer/University of Strasbourg, Strasbourg, France

P. Wiklund et al. (eds.), *Robotic Urologic Surgery*, https://doi.org/10.1007/978-3-031-00363-9_8

tomographic images. Direct volume rendering (DVR), commonly integrated into radiological workstations, creates a 3D reconstructed view, which makes the anatomy easier to understand. However, DVR is unsuitable for computing organ volumes or simulating a surgical resection. To do so, a surface rendering (SR) technique has to be used. SR is based on organ segmentation, which is a delineation of all structures of interest. It allows for an interactive visualization of the reconstructed anatomy, including navigation features such as zooming in and out, rotating the virtual model, and transparent views selectively showing the chosen structures [4, 6]. Even anatomical variants which are potentially missed when screening CT or MRI images in conventional slices become apparent in SR 3D reconstructions. As a result, these reconstructions best meet surgical needs, allowing for patient-specific virtual surgical exploration and surgical strategy planning by means of individual procedure simulation [5].

These 3D anatomical models provide an **individual virtual reality environment**. The VR simulation of a procedure on the patient-specific digital clone allows trainers and trainees to discuss and come to an agreement upon the ideal operative approach. These digital clones are easy to share with experts around the world, if desired. The comprehensive visualization of the target anatomy can be shared to **obtain a second opinion** on the same 3D model, which minimizes the potential difference in interpretation based on 2D slices. In a pioneering study (Argonaute, 2004), the same 3D reconstruction could be viewed virtually by several surgeons in different locations, in order to allow joint decision-making [7] (Fig. 1/Video 1).

As an example, a liver tumor occasionally appears to be located in one specific segment in standard tomographic images, whereas segmental vessel occlusion in the virtual model reveals that the affected segment is indeed a different one. **Surgical planning** based on a virtual model provided valuable assistance and led to a change in operative strategy in approximately 10% of more than 100 liver resections [5]. In the Visible Patient software, which is based on research of the IRCAD research and development team, additional virtual surgical tools such as selective vascular clamping allow to **simulate resections**. This makes it possible to identify liver tumors with regard to the vascular territory and its respective segments (Fig. 2/Video 2). As a result, resections can be optimized for an organ-sparing approach with safe margins [8, 9].

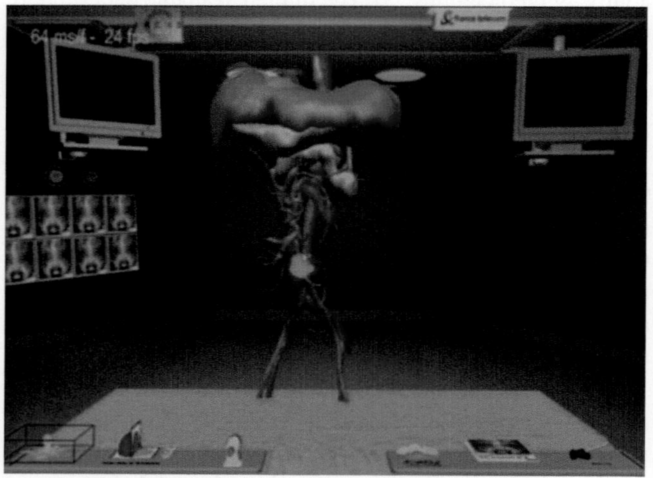

Fig. 1 Teleconference with interactive visualization of the virtual 3D model within the Argonaute project. The model can be rotated, and organ systems can be shown or hidden individually, in order to facilitate the remote assessment of liver tumors by several experts (see Video 1)

When the ideal operative strategy has been defined, a virtual environment allows to **simulate the individual intervention**. The ability to repeatedly rehearse procedures allows to enhance surgical training and prepares for the real surgical procedure [10]. **Repetition with deliberate practice** is key for skill acquisition [11]. In other disciplines, rehearsing is a much more common practice than in surgery. Movie production is based on the separate study of scenes, which are practiced and recorded until perfection, even in an arbitrary order under a director's guidance, and then compiled into the final film. Surgery is somewhat different and more like a musical piece, which has to be performed at once in the predefined order. When playing an instrument, compositions are divided into passages which are practiced and repeated until perfection. The oeuvres are rehearsed individually, within smaller groups, and with the entire orchestra. Only then, the complete piece is performed on stage in the intended order. During practice, musicians get input from their teachers and orchestral conductors. The time has come to integrate such practice routines into the preparation of similarly complex surgical procedures, which not only rely on procedural skills, but also include different tasks for each team member and necessitate team interaction.

The **combination of simulation with surgical planning** will thus lead to optimal care delivery [10], and rehearsal in the form of preliminary virtual operations should become mandatory for complex operations. Expert assistance provides valuable feedback during procedure rehearsals, where the specialist can be local or remotely connected. With virtual procedure simulation environments, discussion of the ideal surgical approach is again accessible for validation by a second expert. The preplanned surgical strategy with anticipated port positioning, procedural steps, resection planes, etc., then provides intraoperative guidance.

3D reconstruction in a pediatric urology case series, including congenital malformations and Wilms' tumors, facilitated the understanding of complex anatomical relationships and diagnosis of anatomical anomalies. Virtual surgical planning included the assessment of the renal vasculature, individual vessel clip applications, and 3D

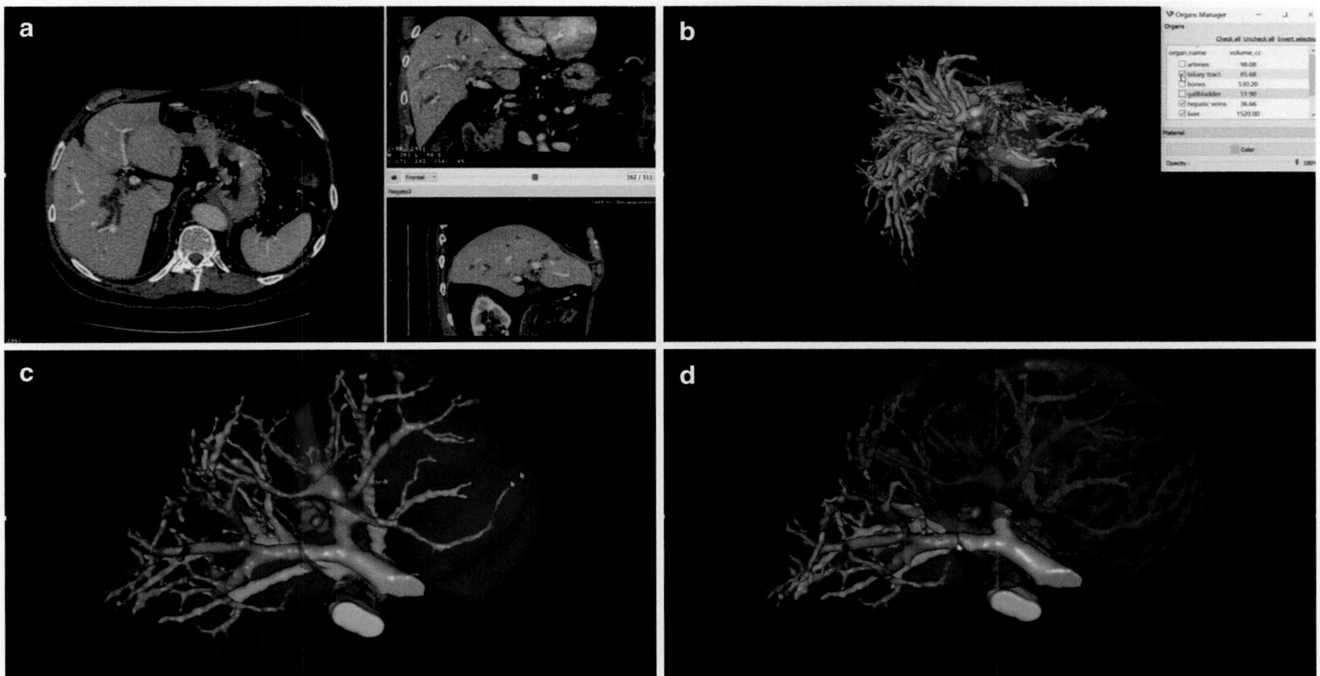

Fig. 2 This central cholangiocarcinoma was interpreted as right-sided from the CT scan alone (**a**). The 3D model allows to focus on the relevant anatomy (**b**). Once the hepatic and portal veins have been selected (**c**), vascular clamping can be simulated, demonstrating the need for a change in operative strategy to perform a left hemi-hepatectomy instead of a right-sided one (**d**) (see Video 2)

model volume measurements for the renal tumor and remnant after organ-sparing surgery. Patient-specific stepwise procedural planning allowed for an accurate partial nephrectomy simulation [4]. Such a simulation of resection according to the vascular territory making it possible to check which segment can be preserved in a parenchyma-sparing approach is shown in Fig. 3. Video 3 shows the preoperative CT scan and 3D reconstruction of a bilateral nephroblastoma in a child, with planning of a function-preserving bilateral partial nephrectomy, as well as the reconstructed postoperative CT scan.

Individual VR models can be displayed **intraoperatively**, with various software solutions available for 3D reconstruction. Intuitive Surgical offers Iris [12], a visualization service segmenting and labeling anatomical structures to generate a 3D model from patient deidentified CT scans. In a recent multi-institutional propensity score-matched analysis assessing 3D-image-guided robot-assisted partial nephrectomy (3D-IGRAPN), the risk for major complications was significantly lowered and perioperative outcomes improved using virtual 3D models of the tumoral kidneys obtained with the Synapse 3D® Kidney analysis® application software (Fujifilm, Japan). The trifecta (namely, the combination of negative surgical margins, 90% preservation of eGFR at the first clinical visit postoperatively (3–6 months), and absence of perioperative complications) achievement rate was significantly higher in the 3D-IGRAPN group [13].

The da Vinci platforms' built-in computer interfaces allow to connect a mobile device to display 3D reconstructions and navigate manually within any of these VR models. With the use of TilePro, the VR models are then shown in a **side-by-side image within the console display** next to the live video feed, and can also be visualized on the auxiliary screen for the rest of the OR team [5].

As a future perspective, artificial intelligence (AI)-based software will allow automatized reconstructions even in real time in the operating room. For automatized 3D reconstructions, the implementation of an AI approach was recently proposed as a means to avoid time-consuming manual segmentation [14] (Fig. 4).

Similarly, **3D-printed models** based on virtual 3D imaging models support the understanding of the relevant anatomy and surgical planning. In a urological study focused on robot-assisted radical prostatectomy and partial nephrectomy (RARP and RAPN), 3D-printed models were perceived as a useful tool, as evaluated by urologists (from trainees to experts) and patients regarding the understanding of the disease and the planned intervention [3]. The 3D-printed models allowed for a quick understanding of the specific case, and they were superior to virtual 3D models and standard CT in terms of vascular anatomy in particular [15]. While 3D-printed models can be used for ex vivo procedure training, the virtual models have the advantage of a fusion with the real-time stereoscopic intraoperative view, resulting in an

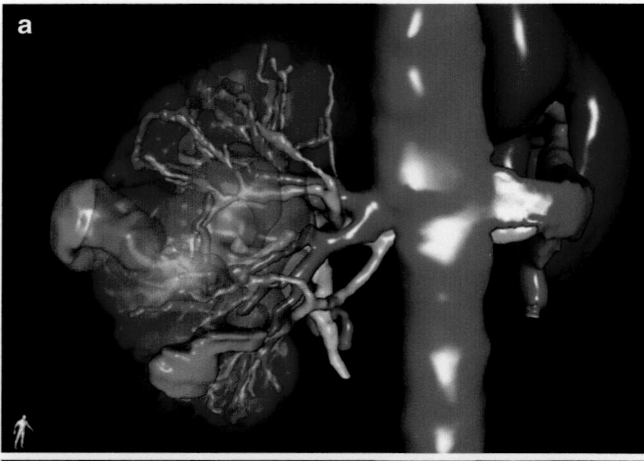

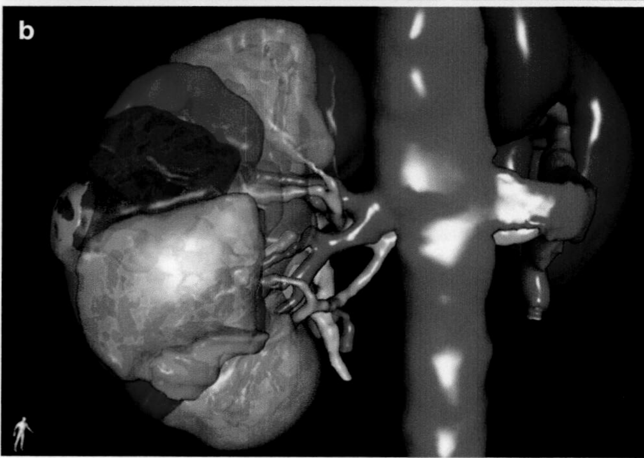

Fig. 3 3D reconstruction for a patient with multiple tumors in the right kidney (**a**). Virtual clip application on the segmental arterial branches makes it possible to visualize each segment in a different color (**b**). Image courtesy Visible Patient online service

augmented reality view [9]. With a transparency adjustment of the virtual image, the overlay improves the orientation and identification of anatomical landmarks. The precise overlay (registration) is still a challenge, as respiratory motions, peritoneal gas insufflation, and organ deformation via surgical manipulation have to be taken into account for an AR view throughout any procedure [5]. The more stable the target organ during a procedure, the easier the AR overlay. In a pioneering study for laparoscopy, AR assistance was first described in adrenalectomy [16]. With the use of a video mixer, the 3D reconstruction was manually merged with the video feed from the integrated camera in the surgical light (external view), as well as with the laparoscopic view. The AR view was then displayed onto an additional video screen and adapted during the procedure, supporting the identification of the dissection planes, the adrenal gland with a Conn's adenoma, and the relevant vasculature [16] (Fig. 5).

In a subsequent adrenalectomy series (12 right-sided and 3 left-sided procedures), AR superimposition was more precise on the right side (maximal error of 2 mm) than on the left side. In the anterior left adrenal approach, splenic mobilization and organ retraction represented a challenge for the live manual interactive AR overlay with a computer scientist [6]. The virtual and augmented reality approach developed at the Institute for Research against Digestive Cancer (IRCAD) was applied to various clinical settings and minimally invasive procedures, including endocrine [17], colorectal [18, 19], hepatobiliary, and pancreatic surgery [8–10, 20–22].

With a focus on urologic cancers, a collaboration with a team of bioengineers was started 4 years ago by Porpiglia et al. to define the "high-definition 3D models" [23]. Hyperaccuracy three-dimensional (HA3D) reconstruction also relies on the clinical expertise (of urologists and radiologists), with a professional software authorized for medical use managed by the engineers. The 3D models were merged with the camera images in a manual overlapping of the images, performed by an assistant of the surgeon with the use of a 3D professional mouse. Their AR display in the da Vinci surgical console via the integrated TilePro software provided intraoperative AR guidance during robotic surgery [24].

This technology was applied both in prostate and kidney cancer surgery (Fig. 6, Videos 4/5). In prostate cancer surgery, the AR images allowed to correctly identify the tumor location in a static phase of the intervention [25]. Subsequently, with the development of elastic virtual models, it was also possible to overlap these models during a dynamic phase of the intervention, such as the nerve-sparing phase, in which the tissue shapes are deformed by the surgical action [26]. The implementation of AR guidance for the modulation of surgical resection on the neurovascular bundle reduced the risk of positive surgical margins. Concerning renal cancer surgery, the 3D AR images allowed to identify the arterial branches of the renal pedicle, thereby helping with the pedicle dissection and allowing to perform a higher rate of selective clamping.

In addition, these AR images demonstrated their usefulness during the extirpative phase during partial nephrectomy for endophytic tumors. The availability of AR technology allowed to project hidden lesions precisely on the organ surface. Lastly, after tumor removal, AR guidance allowed to identify intraparenchymal structures involved in the resective phase, such as violated calyces or arteries and veins bleeding into the resection bed, which gave the surgeon the opportunity to manage them selectively [27].

The next step in the evolution of AR-guided robotic surgery is the automatic overlay of 3D virtual images. The advent of AI in particular will help to recognize some structures as landmarks inside the operative field (artificial landmarks such as the urinary catheter during prostatectomy, or natural landmarks such as the kidney shape during partial nephrectomy). After an algorithm training phase, AI-based

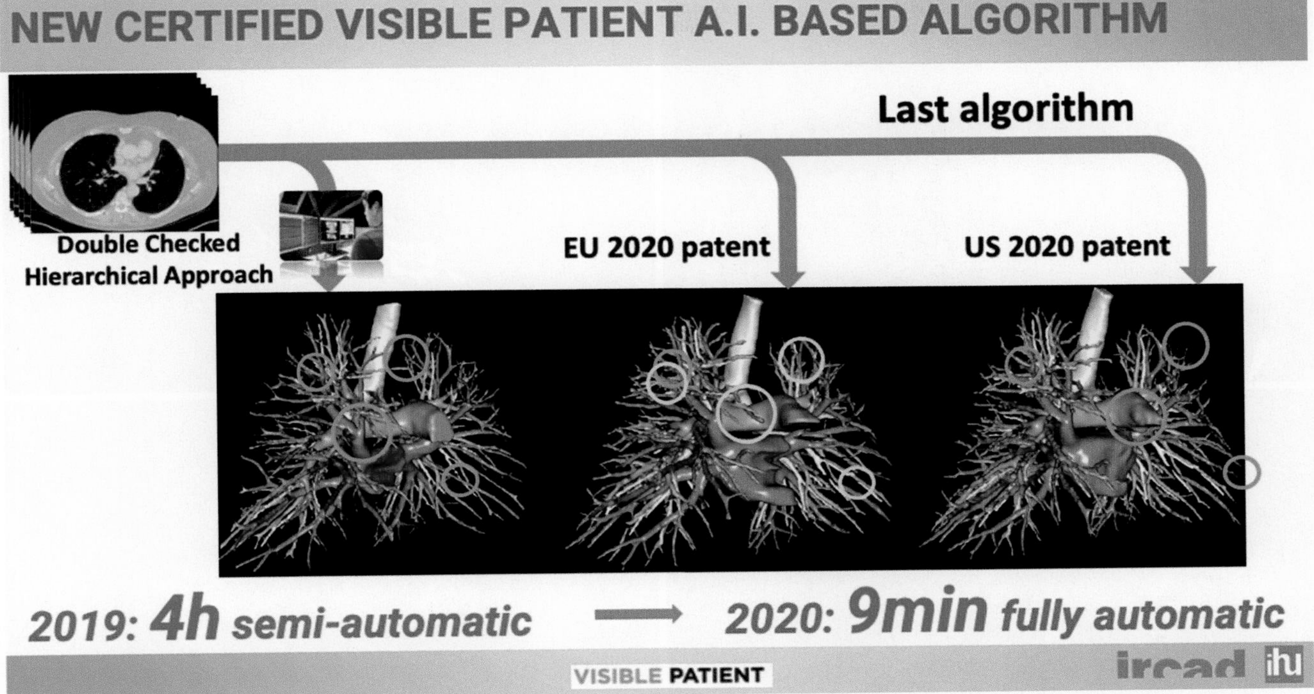

Fig. 4 Significantly reduced duration for 3D reconstructions with the implementation of artificial intelligence-based algorithms

software will allow to anchor the 3D models to the real anatomy automatically, hence avoiding the need for any manual assistance [28]. Recently presented pioneering experiences demonstrated promising findings for both kidney and prostate cancer surgeries. Indeed, the automatically overlapped 3D AR images correctly identified the tumor during the intervention [29].

Port placement for robotic surgery has to be planned by taking individual robotic arm movements into account. More and more robotic surgical systems reach the market, and surgical access must be adapted for each one, according to the specific platform. VR models and AR overlay of the target anatomy support access planning via a "see-through" view, as shown for laparoscopic adrenalectomy [16], liver segmentectomy [9] (Fig. 7), or to obtain an optimal triangulation despite the constraints of intercostal port positioning in a trans-thoracic approach for liver surgery [22]. For the Versius® Surgical Robotic System (CMR Surgical Ltd, United Kingdom), the subcostal port position can be adopted from the posterior retroperitoneoscopic adrenalectomy (PRA) approach as standardized by Professor Martin Walz, Germany [30] (Fig. 8).

Augmented reality is a critical step forward to the **automatization of robotic interventions**, for which the robot needs to learn to see in transparency what the camera does not show. Twenty years of experience on AR taught us about the challenges of registration accuracy, in particular of real-time deformable registration to fuse the digital model with the manipulated organs in a live video feed. Three main approaches were reported to address the limitations of current registration solutions, namely manual alignment (operator-dependent, for small deformations only), automatic rigid registration (for small deformations), and deformable registration (for strong deformations, technically challenging and requiring organ-specific parameter tuning) [31].

To resolve such challenges, a **hybrid operating room** was built at IHU Strasbourg, a facility equipped with medical imaging (CT, MR, cone-beam CT, ultrasound, fluoroscopy) and/or guidance systems in addition to full surgical capabilities. A hybrid OR allows for dynamic planning, guidance, and control via various human-machine interfaces intraoperatively [32]. However, it is neither in the interest of surgeons nor patients to undergo repetitive intraprocedural irradiation for continuous imaging updates. Additionally, there is little compatibility of large-footprint medical imaging such as CT, cone-beam CT, and MRI with current robotic surgical systems. Unlike in interventional cardiology or percutaneous procedures (e.g., ablation therapies), these technical challenges make general and urological surgery too complex for a routine integration of robotic laparoscopy into hybrid ORs. **Ultrasound** is an imaging modality that is much less expensive and more readily available. It carries a great potential for 3D reconstructed views, automated robotic needle placement, and integration with AI for diagnosis and treatment, particularly in percutaneous interventions.

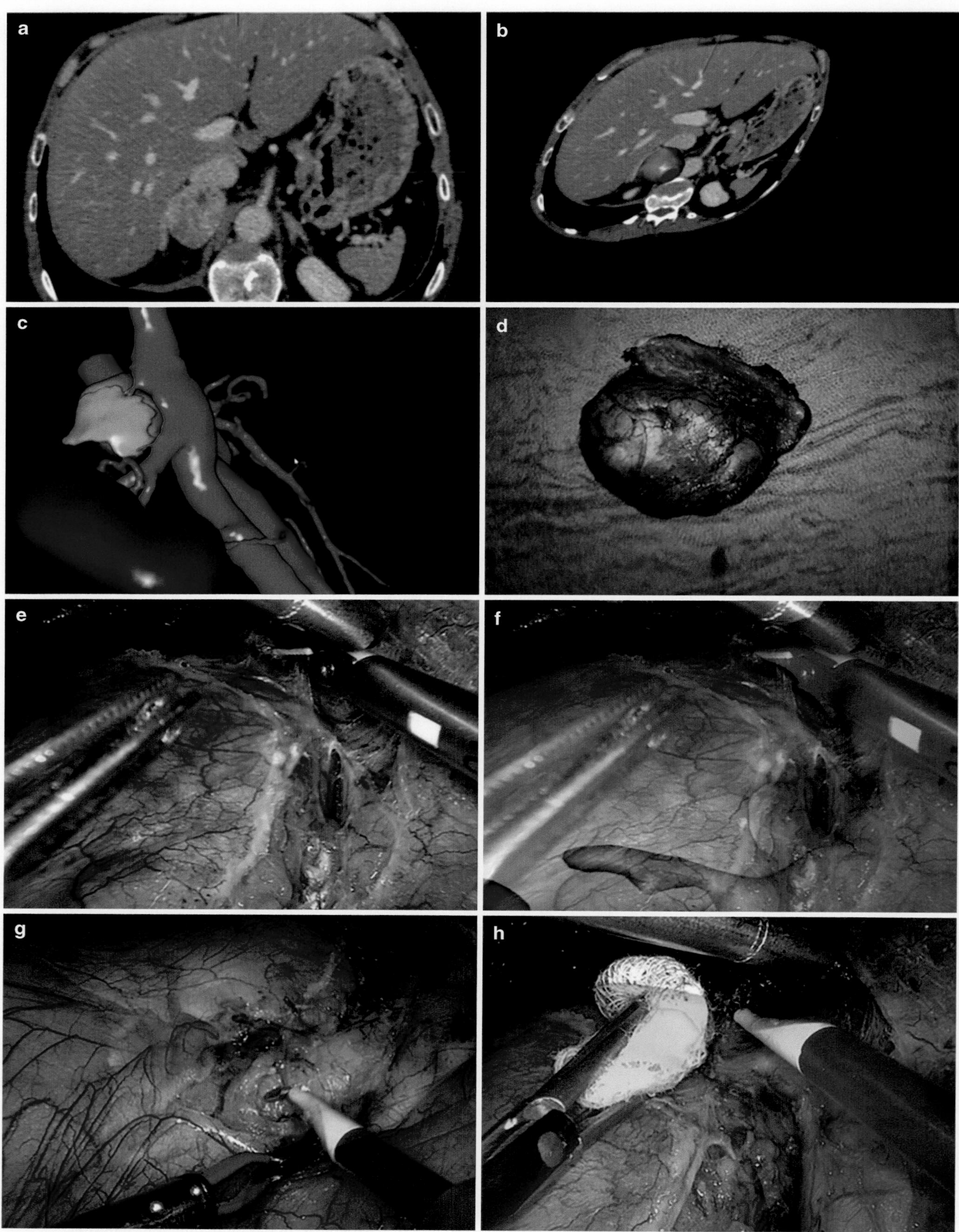

Fig. 5 Augmented reality-assisted laparoscopic right adrenalectomy. The contrast-enhanced CT scan (**a**) is reconstructed in 3D with the display focused on the relevant anatomy (**b**, **c**). The 3D volumes of the adrenal gland and lesion are congruent with the resected specimen (**d**). The intraoperative view (**e**) can be supplemented with augmented reality guidance at any given step of the dissection (**f**, **g**, **h**)

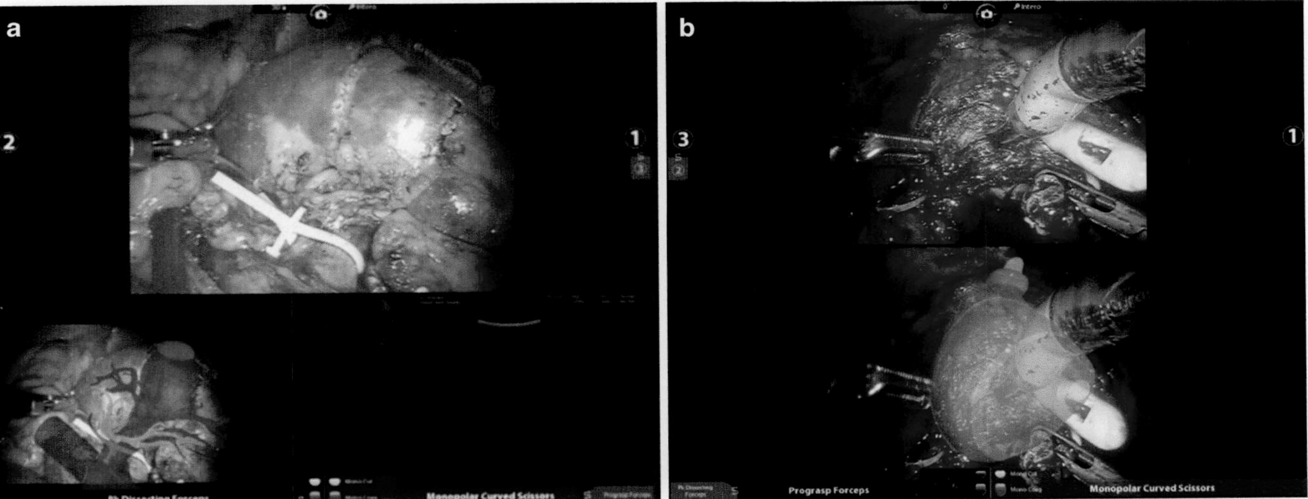

Fig. 6 Intraoperative augmented reality (AR) guidance in robotically assisted partial nephrectomy (**a**) and radical prostatectomy (**b**) (Videos 4 and 5 for the digital version)

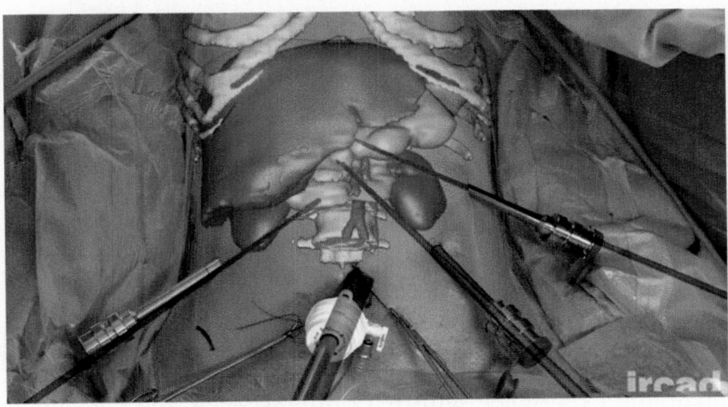

Fig. 7 AR-guided robotic port placement guided by projecting the virtual model onto the patient via an external beamer above the patient [9]

Ablation procedures such as radiofrequency ablation and cryoablation, among others, are much more suitable for robotization than laparoscopic approaches. Ablation therapies are increasingly being reported for prostatic [33], renal parenchyma-sparing, and adrenal procedures [34–36] to a lesser extent. Aquablation of benign prostatic hyperplasia is the first procedure to incorporate features of **autonomous robot-assisted surgery in clinical trials,** and it is categorized at the level of conditional autonomy. Biplanar transrectal ultrasound (TRUS) is used for manual mapping of the target resection areas. The machine subsequently delivers the saline at a high velocity to autonomously perform prostatic resection according to the mapping. A 3D reconstructed model built from TRUS images is also the basis for dosimetric planning and needle trajectories of the EUCLIDIAN system for autonomous robot-assisted prostate brachytherapy [33].

For small benign adrenal tumors, partial adrenalectomy can replace total adrenalectomy if the lesion can be removed completely [37–39]. Partial adrenalectomy is increasingly performed for steroidogenic function preservation with low rates of adrenal insufficiency and recurrence [39–43]. When a partial adrenalectomy is envisaged, periadrenal dissection exposes the gland at the price of division of the abundant arterial network reaching the adrenal capsule. Devascularization of the future remnant has to be avoided, and as a result, the intraoperative view of the gland is limited. Intraoperative measurements with a flexible ruler and CT-calculated volumes showed a considerable discrepancy [44]. Intraoperatively, the adrenal glands can be hidden from view, particularly in an abundance of retroperitoneal adipose tissue commonly encountered in Cushing's syndrome (Fig. 9). Virtual 3D reconstructed models provide valuable guidance to ensure complete tumor removal while preserving a maximum of adjacent healthy adrenal gland. See-through vision with AR approaches based on 3D image reconstructions, as well as a near-infrared light tissue penetration depth of several millimeters (<1 cm) in fluorescence imaging, are promising tools for partial adrenalectomy.

Fluorescence image-guided surgery (FIGS) is a navigation modality based on the use of near-infrared (NIR) light sources that interact with an intravenously or locally administered fluorophores such as indocyanine green (ICG). During NIR light illumination, the fluorophore is excited and emits a fluorescent signal, which is then captured by a designated camera system [45]. The view captured in the NIR range is overlaid onto the standard visible light video feed. As a result, FIGS represents an enhanced reality imaging modality.

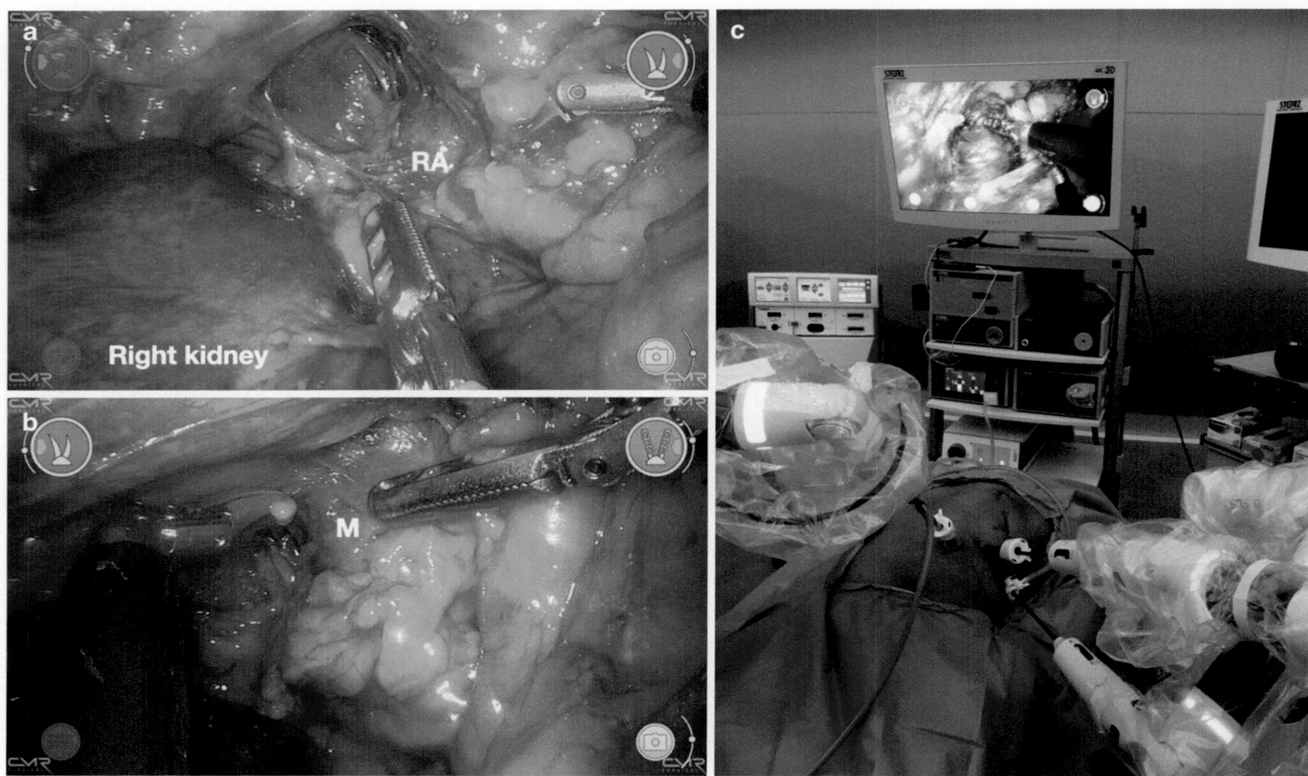

Fig. 8 Translation of the posterior retroperitoneoscopic adrenalectomy (PRA) technique to a new robotic surgical system. (**a**) intraoperative view of the retroperitoneum, dorsal view onto the right kidney and normal adrenal tissue (RA). (**b**) Exposure of the right adrenal metastasis (M). (**c**) Prone positioning and right-sided port placement derived from the PRA technique

FIGS allows for **augmented reality registration**, as reported via the use of fluorescent fiducials in kidneys [46]. A near-infrared fluorescence 3D visual tracking system, including 3D surface reconstruction, is the basis for bowel anastomoses performed by the **Smart Tissue Autonomous Robot** (STAR) [33]. With a near-infrared visualization technology (Firefly mode) and the Iris navigation tool, both AR imaging modalities are integrated into the da Vinci robotic systems (Intuitive Surgical, Inc., Sunnyvale, CA, United States). The Firefly mode can be activated from the surgeon console. Several other manufacturers plan to integrate fluorescence imaging into their robotic platforms over time.

In addition, fluorescence guidance is continuously gaining interest during minimally invasive adrenal surgery. Since its first description [47], a handful of studies reported its use [48, 49]. ICG-enhanced imaging was felt to contribute to procedural safety and efficacy, based on the superior visualization of the adrenal glands during **robotic adrenalectomy** [50]. Separate fluorescence characteristics were recently described for different pathological adrenal conditions [51]. The contrast between different fluorescence patterns allows for an enhanced **tissue distinction** between tumor and normal adrenal gland, as well as retroperitoneal tissue. Due to a favorable experience with ICG fluorescence, the Cleveland Clinic group incorporated it within their routine robotic adrenal surgery practice [51].

Most studies assessed adrenal fluorescence data qualitatively and subjectively [51, 52], which is valid to discriminate the adrenal glands from surrounding tissues. However, the interpretation of fluorescence signals can be biased. When moving the camera closer to the target, fluorescence signal intensity increases due to its relationship inversely to the square of the camera-to-target distance (inverse-square law in optics). Additionally, a residual fluorescence signal from a previous injection can limit qualitative assessment upon reinjection [45].

In contrast, a quantitative assessment of fluorescence signal intensity dynamics over time allows for a more objective documentation [51], and is a prerequisite for **perfusion assessment**. ICG injection in perfusion assessment is based on the fluorescence signal arrival in the target tissue resulting in distinct perfusion curves, which can only be visualized by quantitative fluorescence imaging [42, 45]. However, it is currently not integrated into commercially available systems. At the IRCAD, a quantitative software-based approach

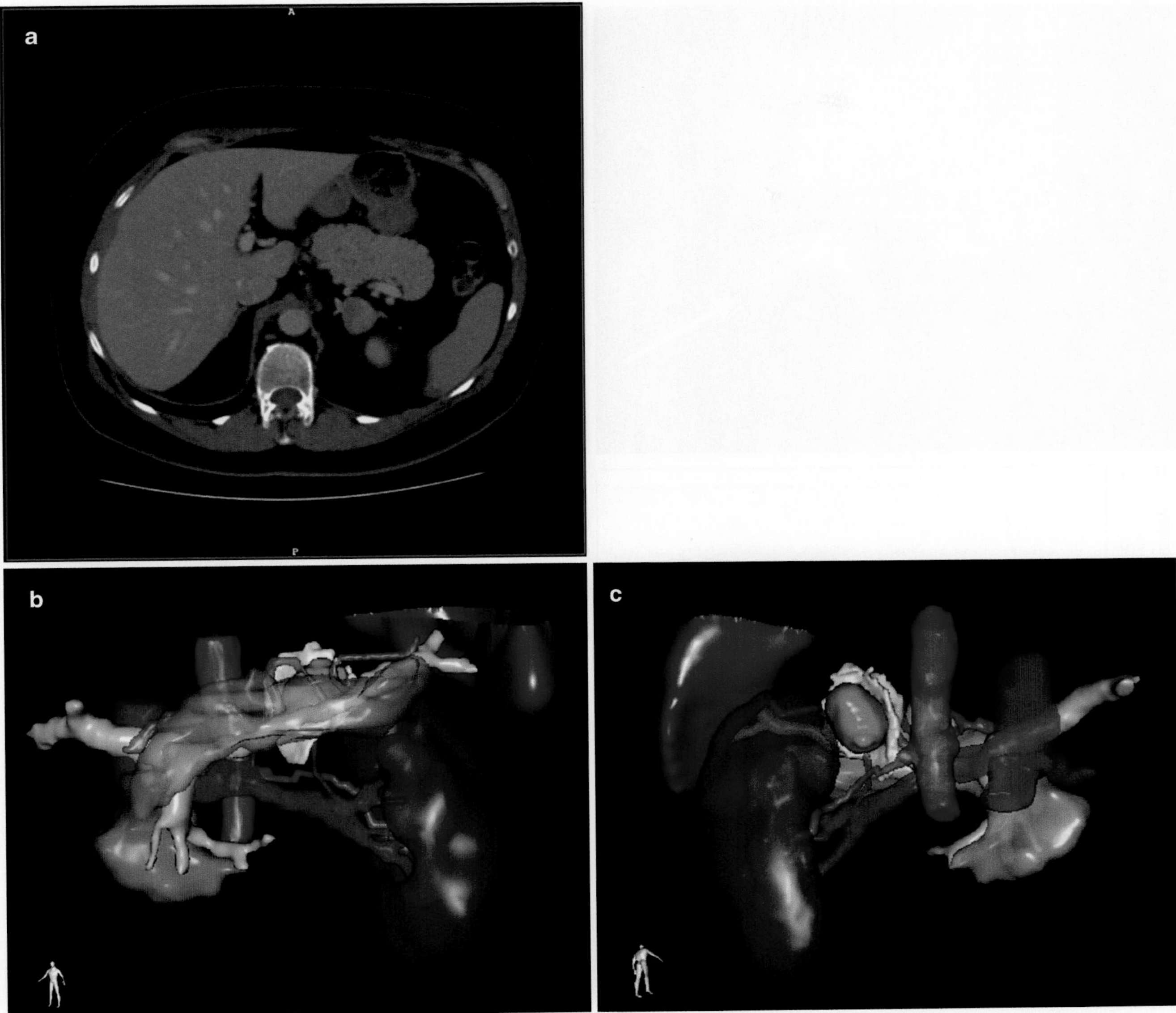

Fig. 9 Cushing's adenoma within the left adrenal gland. (**a**) standard axial CT view, (**b**) anterior 3D model view, (**c**) posterior 3D model view as in posterior retroperitoneoscopic adrenal surgery

was thus developed to allow a measurement of the dynamic evolution of fluorescence signal intensity over time [42, 45]. This dynamic fluorescent signal intensity evolution captured with a static camera is independent of the camera-to-target distance, and the arrival speed of the fluorescence signal after intravenous dye injection represents tissue perfusion. These data can be translated into a color-coded perfusion cartography for an intraoperative overlay.

In a bilateral posterior retroperitoneoscopic approach, the proprietary software was used to assess fluorescence dynamics simultaneously for both adrenal glands. It allowed to calculate bilateral perfusion cartographies and to superimpose them onto the images of the corresponding left and right camera systems [42, 45]. In the enhanced reality view after adrenal gland division without any circumferential dissection, the remnant segments with an impaired perfusion could easily be distinguished from the ones with regular perfusion, with the ipsilateral kidney serving as a reference for normal fluorescent signal arrival speed (Fig. 10). Quantitative evaluation of adrenal remnant perfusion was congruent between FIGS and contrast-enhanced intraoperative CT scan measurements and it has the potential to be a surrogate marker for cellular integrity [42]. Quantitative FIGS provides an evaluation of organ perfusion, and it is independent of residual fluorescence signal intensity when multiple fluorophore injections are administered [42, 45].

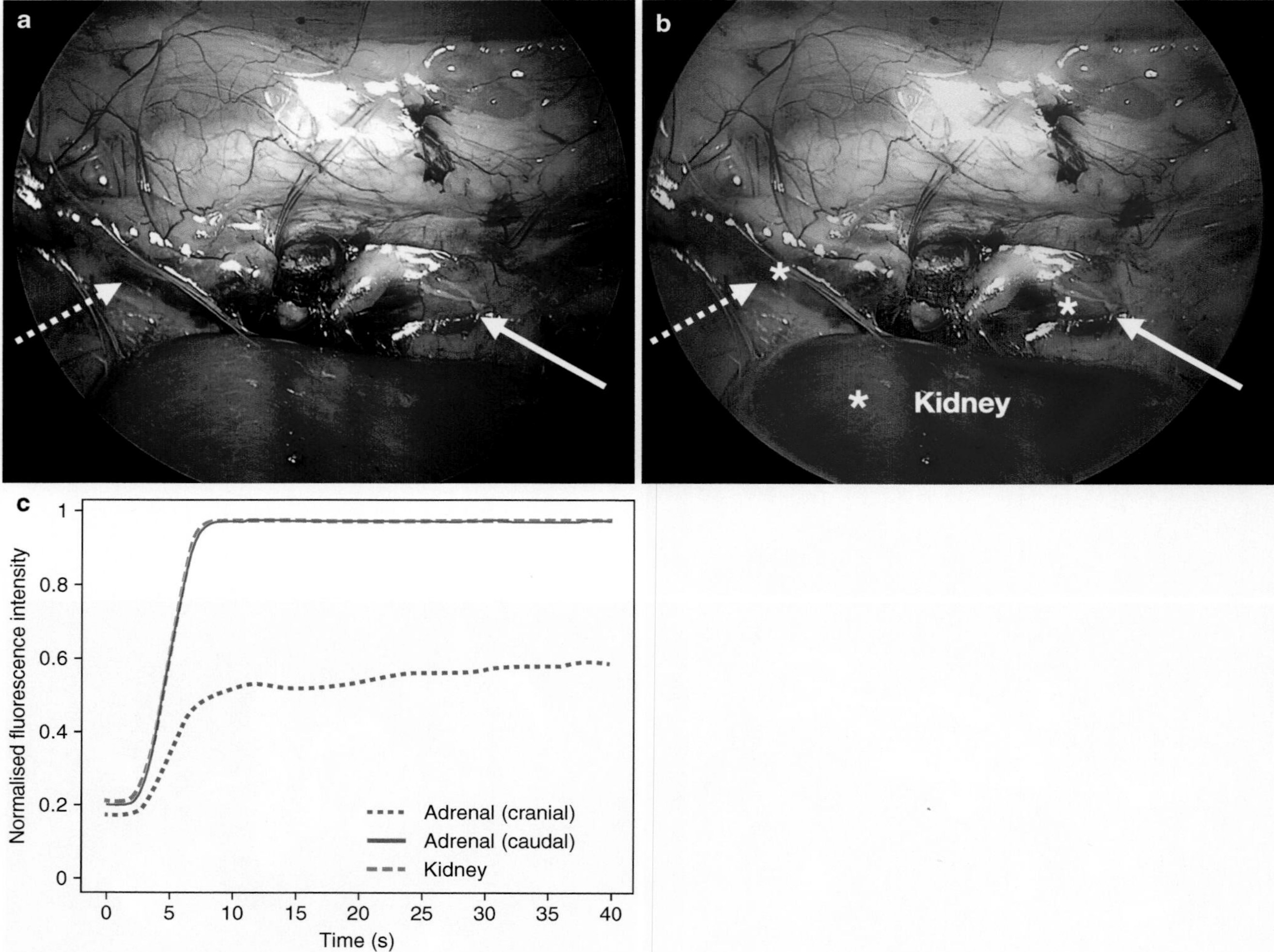

Fig. 10 Intraoperative white light (**a**) and enhanced reality view (**b**) of a left adrenal gland divided in its middle. Asterisks mark measuring points for representative perfusion curves. On the right (**c**), corresponding perfusion curves are shown for the cranial and caudal parts of the adrenal gland and the kidney. The cranial adrenal segment (dotted arrow) shows decreased perfusion (blue), whereas caudal perfusion (solid arrow, red) is equal to that of the kidney (Published in [42])

3 Telesurgery

Telesurgery is defined as a procedure performed by a surgeon operating from a remote location. Telepresence means that someone appears to be present or to have an effect at a location other than the actual place where the person is situated [11]. The initial impulse for the development of multipurpose robotic systems was to perform **long-distance surgery**, in order to minimize harm for the surgical team while decreasing trauma casualties in battlefield settings. The military intended to provide immediate surgical control at the site of injury, as opposed to evacuation of the wounded to the closest mobile army surgical hospital (MASH). A telepresence surgeon's workstation would be operated from the MASH, and the remote surgical unit transported to the patient in an armored vehicle [53].

The **Lindbergh Operation** was a world premiere in the quest for the globalization of surgical procedures via long-distance robotic telesurgery, using the ZEUS system (Computer Motion, United States). The system components were connected across the Atlantic Ocean at a distance of 6200 km via a high-speed fiberoptic connection. The time delay inherent to long-distance transmissions was defined during preliminary studies. A safe maximum threshold for the latency between the command of an action and its return on the screen was determined (330 ms). In order to allow for a safe surgical procedure, this latency was further limited to a level that was virtually imperceptible to the human eye (155 ms). Consequently, the surgical team steering the console in New York was able to perform a robotic cholecystectomy in a patient in Strasbourg, with telemanipulation of the 2 instrument arms, and electrosurgery activation via voice commands to the on-site surgical team in Strasbourg [54, 55]. Soon afterwards, the world's first national telesurgical service was established in Canada, connecting a teaching hospital to a community medical center. A total of 22 remote telesurgical procedures were performed by two surgeons, including 13 laparoscopic fundoplications, 7 colorectal resections, and 2 inguinal hernia repairs, with a similar latency [56]. Despite this novelty and significant technological requirements, no major intraoperative complications were come across, and postoperative recovery was uneventful [54–56]. **Telerobotic assistance** provided "on the job" training to the community hospital surgeon, allowing the expert surgeon to switch from performing the early procedures to assisting the later fundoplication case series [56]. These pioneering cases demonstrated that long-distance surgery was safe and feasible. However, it implied substantial costs, considering the expense of robotic surgical systems and telecommunication infrastructures. As technology advances, its implementation gets more cost-effective. A few decades afterwards, a multitude of teleoperated surgical systems is now commercially available or about to enter the marketplace. When compatible, a single robotic console at an expert center could be connected to a number of bedside units located at various community hospitals [56].

Both high bandwidth and low latency are essential for optimal data transmission and telesurgical performance. The evolution of networks used for surgery included satellite, Integrated Services Digital Network (ISDN), ATM (used in the Lindbergh operation), Internet Protocol/Virtual Private Network (IP/VPN used in the Canadian series), and current wireless networks [57]. The advent of **fifth-generation cellular networks (5G)** brings about a technology standard for broadband connectivity with a low latency. Download speeds can reach the gigabit per second (Gbit/s) range, and broadband capacity will further increase during the rollout of 5G networks. In combination with near-instantaneous latency (1–2 ms), 5G is suitable for remote telesurgery and will even allow the integration of virtual and augmented reality. The use of high frequencies of up to 30GHz provides the high data transmission rate. However, with these shorter wavelengths, the range is influenced by a worse penetration of objects. Consequently, 5G high bands have a 100× faster data rate, a 10× lower latency, but overcome a 60× shorter distance when compared to LTE (Long-term evolution/4G) [57].

Despite an increasing amount of newspaper articles and announcements on company websites, peer-reviewed scientific publications regarding the most recent telesurgical procedures using a 5G network are still awaited. 5G availability provides a more economical solution than the ATM technology, and 5G networks will become the backbone for a **democratized robotic telesurgery**. A 2021 review [57] summarized the scientific publications on 5G use in surgery, with its use for remote robotic camera control [58], telementoring (at a 4 and 6 km distance) [59], a vocal cord procedure on a cadaver (15 km distance) [60], remote laparoscopic surgery in an animal model (3000 km) [61], and one case series of remote spinal surgery (120–3000 km) [62]. In only two of these studies, remote telesurgery was performed in vivo, and their network connection was reported as stable [61, 62]. In porcine laparoscopic long-distance surgery, the mean total latency was 264 ms (258–278 ms), as opposed to a wired Internet connection with 206 ms (204–210 ms). Whereas the delays from surgical robot servoing, mechanical response, imaging and image processing, and video codec were equal, the observed latency difference was due to a shorter mean round-trip delay via the wired Internet connection (5G: 114 ms; wired connection 56 ms) [61]. With 3000 versus 6200 km of distance covered, these round-trip delays are nearing the one achieved via ATM transport during the Lindbergh Operation (78–80 ms) [54]. In spine surgery case series with distances ranging from 120 to 3000 km for the various hospitals involved, the mean network latency was reported as 28 ms, without listing the involved components [62]. Although modern networks reduce signal latency, it remains an issue. Instrument motion scaling has been proposed to improve safety and efficiency in robotic surgery that is subject to a latency. Not surprisingly, delays of 500 ms and 750 ms significantly increased task time, as well as the number of errors. In these high latency settings, improvements in instrument path motion were observed with the implementation of negative robotic instrument motion scaling, and the error profile was equivalent to the no-latency scenario for 2 out of 3 users [63].

5G-based advanced robotic telesurgery is an area of ongoing research, and it is paving the way for further telesurgery progress, along with other opportunities for 5G use in telementoring and telehealth. Transcontinental telesurgery demonstrated that the technological advances of robotic platforms allow for telepresence surgery from remote locations, irrespective of the geographical distance between surgeons and patients on the Earth. The concept of remote surgery reaches another dimension when envisaging **space travel** and outposts on other planets. Due to weight limitations in space travel, a telesurgery robotic patient-side module would have to be considerably more lightweight than current robotic systems. Space surgery was explored in experimental settings of simulated microgravity and aboard spacecraft. In open surgery, microgravity leads to the floating of mobile bowel and body fluids, which can disperse throughout the cabin. As a result, a sealed laparoscopic approach is more suitable in weightlessness [64]. The feasibility of endoscopic surgery in weightlessness was demonstrated in the porcine model on parabolic flights, including laparoscopy, thoracoscopy, creation of bleeding, and observation of blood spread without gravity [65]. The rich history of urological investigations in spaceflight is detailed in a 2017 review, with interesting issues such as urolithiasis, infections and antibiotic treatment, urological interventions, and fertility in weightlessness [66]. As there is no means to timely get an expert surgeon to a patient beyond Earth orbit or vice versa, surgical care on spaceflights relies on remote assistance, including telementoring and—potentially—robotic telesurgery. Advanced surgical care will be required in future long-duration missions to the Moon or Mars, whereas it is not practiced in space missions in low Earth orbit. A similar isolation from medical care as in spaceflights exists in the Antarctic and enclosed undersea environment research stations, from which rescue missions are challenging. During the NEEMO 9 mission, extreme communication latencies of over 2 s were tested, representing the Earth-to-Moon communication time-of-flight. This resulted in the duration of 10 min to accomplish a single knot-tying [67]. Communication lag time increases with the target distance from the Earth, so that teleoperated surgical robots can only be controlled in proximity to the Earth. Support further out in space has to rely on telementoring in a middle range, which transforms to offline consultancy telemedicine with the long-distance delay [68].

4 Telementoring/Teleproctoring

Remote procedural collaboration technology allows both telementoring (remotely delivered supervised surgical skills training via telepresence) and teleproctoring (remotely delivered proctorship for licensing and/or revalidation assessments) [11]. Over the last two decades, videoconference equipment evolved from an expensive technology for the happy few towards an opportunity for virtually everyone, democratized via the Internet and smartphone applications.

Next steps include the establishment of the necessary infrastructure (Internet access and 5G networks) worldwide, which might be delayed in rural and low-income areas which would most benefit from remote teaching and interventions. Worldwide, 313 million surgical procedures take place each year. However, only 6% of these operations are performed in countries where one-third of the world's population lives. Many people die from conditions that necessitate surgical care (32.9% of deaths worldwide in 2010), and 143 million additional lifesaving and disability-preventing operations would be required. In low- and lower-middle-income countries, 9 out of 10 people lack access to basic surgical care, resulting in high case-fatality rates from common treatable surgical conditions [69].

Robotic surgery equipment is mainly available in larger centers, and may represent an additional factor of centralization [70]. The worldwide dissemination of robotic telesurgery might have to wait for new low-cost business models for robot accessibility other than in privileged first-world environments. In contrast to remote telesurgery, which relies on an equally skilled local back-up team to complete the procedure in case of failure of the network and/or robotic system, telementoring and teleproctoring are becoming increasingly available. At the IRCAD, an entirely virtual university program has targeted teleeducation and tele-accreditation (WebSurg), telemanipulation, and telesurgery over the past two decades [71, 72]. In 2007, a mobile videoconferencing robot was used for robotic telementoring to provide live remote laparoscopic training guidance (including an intercontinental connection between France and the United States) [73] (Video 6). Nowadays, integrated operating room solutions offered by various companies provide telementoring tools (Fig. 11). A recent systematic review indicates that the safety and efficacy profile of telementoring is similar to on-site mentoring [74].

Telementoring has the potential to deliver surgical expertise to underserved areas and to allow for a global reach of expertise to facilitate the teaching of advanced surgical skills. However, a successful delivery requires a shared understanding of set-up requirements, including legal and ethical implications, how the service will be delivered, and how to audit outcomes to allow for continuous incremental improvements [11]. Both the preceptor and preceptee should have appropriate training and agreement on how the service will be run prior to implementation, as underlined equally for on-site preceptorship [75]. A checklist of the requirements for the successful implementation of telementoring is shown in Fig. 12.

Future research into the beneficial effects of collaboration will likely result in new thinking strategies. If benefits to patient outcomes and improved safety are confirmed, both legal and reimbursement issues will be more easily resolved [76].

Telementoring and teleproctoring will impact the worldwide democratization of surgery at two levels of expertise: the global dissemination of basic surgical techniques, as well as the targeted expansion of specialized interventions.

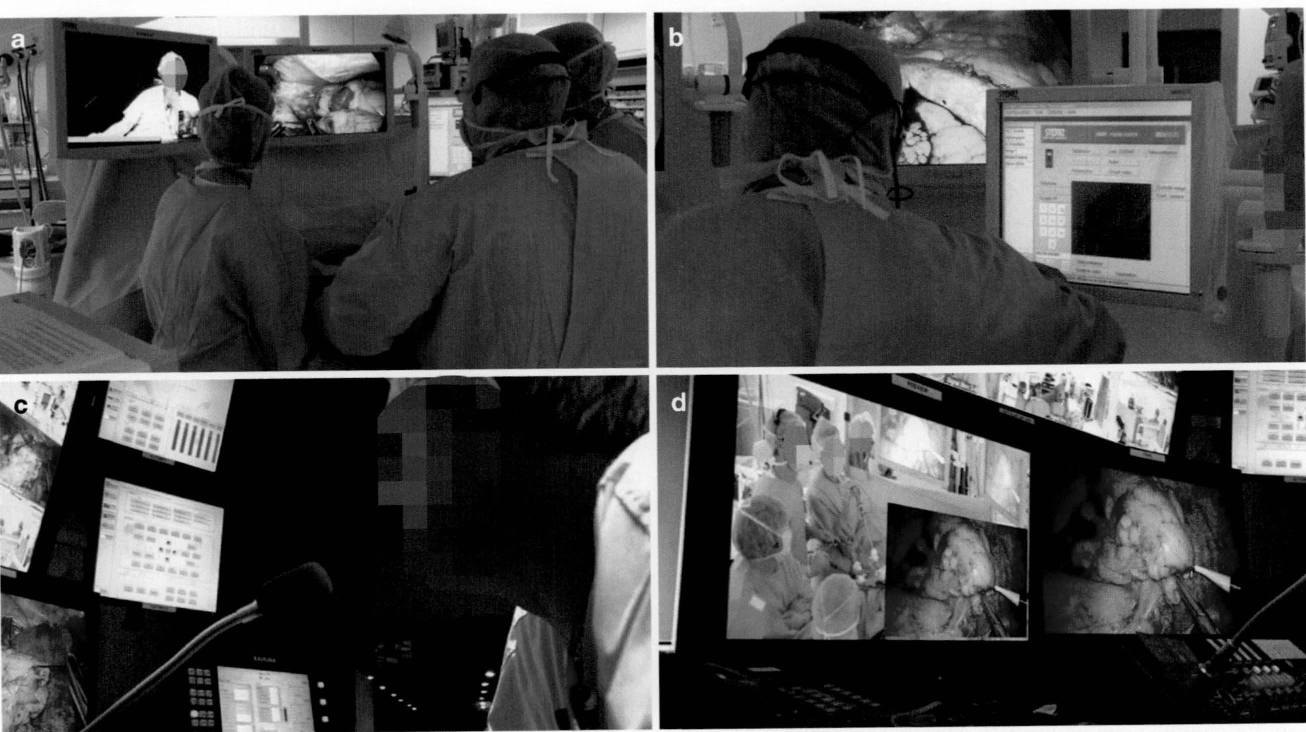

Fig. 11 Telementoring provided from IRCAD to the University Hospitals of Strasbourg for a laparoscopic sleeve gastrectomy (**a**, **b**) and laparoscopic colorectal surgery (**c**, **d**)

TELEMENTORING SET-UP, PLANNING AND SAFETY CHECKLIST

Before installing the service ▸▸▸▸▸▸▸▸ Before patients involved ▸▸▸▸▸▸▸▸▸▸ Before patient leaves operating room

SET-UP

- ☐ **Local IT contact confirmed**
  - Sufficient bandwidth (>5MbS)
  - Good audio-visual links
  - Secure connection
  - Stable connection available
  - Enable firewall traversal, appropriate ports
- ☐ **Equipment required**
  - Laptop
  - Video converter
  - External camera(s)
  - Telestration/image overlay/VR and AR options
- ☐ **Telepresence software licence**
- ☐ **Test connectivity**
  - Ability to view video streams on laptop
  - Video resolution for use case – between 720p at 20fps to 1080p at 30fps
  - Drops ≤ 1 drop per hour
  - RTD <250ms between centres
- ☐ **Hospital organisation confirms**
  - Protocols for telepresence services
  - Legal implications/GDPR/HIPAA compliance

DELIVERY

- ☐ OR team trained in telepresence
- ☐ Communication terminology
- ☐ TTT certified telementor identified
- ☐ Telepresence service agreement signed between trainer and trainee

- ☐ Teleconference with trainer
- ☐ Review: procedural phases, visual cues, tasks and errors
- ☐ Review: patient Hx, imaging, MDT
- ☐ Agree op plan and telepresence schedule for the planned operation

- ☐ Informed consent form for patients
- ☐ Informed consent form for OR team

AUDIT

- ☐ **Surgeon records in the notes**
  - Name of the procedure
  - Length of time of the operation
  - Whether there were any telepresence problems to be addressed
- ☐ **Connectivity**
  - Good image quality
  - Good audio
  - Drops ≤ 1 drop per hour
- ☐ **Telepresence functionality**
  - Telepresence software functioned
- ☐ **Trainer followed agreed protocols**
  - Trainer and trainee discussed case before the operation
  - Available for WHO checklist 'time out'
  - Present for port placement
  - Available for agreed op plan timings
- ☐ **Trainee followed agreed protocols**
  - Trainee followed agreed operative plan
  - Satisfactorily followed telementorship guidance during the operation

THIS CHECKLIST NOT INTENDED TO BE COMPREHENSIVE, ADDITIONS AND MODIFICATIONS TO FIT LOCAL PRACTICE ARE TO BE ENCOURAGED

Fig. 12 Telepresence set-up, planning, and safety checklist (modified version of figure published in [11])

5 Global Dissemination of Basic Techniques

In a new era of global health, the *Lancet* Commission on Global Surgery targeted the global health goal to ensure access to safe and affordable surgical care for all. Scaling up basic surgical care promotes global health, welfare, and economic growth. Access to affordable and timely essential surgery, with a high surgical volume and low perioperative mortality, is one among several core indicators. By the year 2030, in order to reach the target of at least 20 surgical, anesthetic and obstetric physicians per 100,000 people in all countries, an additional 1.27 million providers will need to be trained, costing more than $45 billion, as 44% of the world's population lives in countries below this specialist surgical workforce density threshold. In addition to a major international surgical workforce shortage, a gross inequity results from its maldistribution [69].

Experts are used to traveling in order to provide humanitarian aid, perform procedures, and train local teams in order to overcome knowledge gaps and lack of local infrastructures [11]. On the other hand, visitors are welcomed and taught in training centers such as the IRCAD, in order to disseminate standard-of-care surgical skills. However, such travels, often halfway around the world, entail logistical and financial hurdles, even prior to COVID-19 restrictions. Telepresence is a means for expert surgeons to provide mentoring of novice surgeons who are performing new procedures in remote locations. For many community surgeons, the completion of a training period at a distant site is not a viable option, entailing a slowed adoption of advanced laparoscopic skills in the global surgical community [56]. In 1999, remote knowledge translation via telementoring was already successfully used for laparoscopic surgery aboard a naval vessel [77] or in a mobile surgical truck in the rainforest [78], and is of no less relevance today for rural areas within the United States [79].

6 Targeted Expansion of Specialized Interventions

An organized educational program is of paramount importance to achieve proficiency in complex procedures, in contrast to simple ones. Adrenal surgery carries a significant potential for morbidity and mortality, and it is subject to a clear volume-outcome effect [70]. The European guidelines recommend a minimum volume threshold of 6 adrenalectomies per year per surgeon to ensure sufficient experience, and >20 adrenalectomies per year for adrenocortical cancer surgery [80]. Although the threshold of 6 annual adrenalectomy procedures is low, only 55–65% of patients were operated on by a surgeon performing ≥6 adrenalectomies annually, which corresponded to a third of surgeons, as reported in a recent study on 4189 unilateral adrenalectomies over a 6-year period in the UK. Twenty-one percent of procedures in this study were performed for malignancy, and the majority of unilateral adrenalectomies were minimally invasive approaches (76%). Robotic surgery was increasingly performed over the 6-year study period, although it represented <5% of procedures [70].

Despite the existence of convincing data favorable to posterior retroperitoneoscopic adrenalectomy (PRA), its dissemination was slowed down by the lack of surgical familiarity with the altered view on the anatomy and the posterior operative field, patient positioning and set-up, as well as the different dissection technique via the creation of the working space in the retroperitoneum [45, 81, 82]. Due to the relative rarity of adrenal diseases when compared to colon cancer as an example, on-the-job training opportunities are limited. Sufficiently high case numbers for state-of-the-art training are available in specialized centers only [45, 83]. Ideally, on-site observation of an experienced surgeon-mentor precedes hands-on experience of the surgeon-learner under supervision, with involvement of the entire local OR team [82]. Time constraints and long-distance travels for the mentor make implementation of complex procedures in remote areas challenging. When on-site supervision in the surgeon-learner's institution is unavailable, distant preceptorship via broadband Internet access and videoconferencing equipment is a valid option.

Remote telementoring has proven to be safe and effective when introducing PRA to Melbourne, Australia [82]. The surgeon-learner was trained in advanced laparoscopy and had >10 years of adrenal surgery experience before undergoing a dedicated training period in a high-volume center in the United States, and a surgical workshop with an internationally renowned expert who developed and standardized the PRA technique. The Australian OR team had the necessary equipment available and was prepared including video review of the PRA procedures to be implemented via a distant preceptorship support. Consequently, the first three PRAs were performed via audiovisual telementoring without any technical events and without any intraoperative or postoperative complications. The transcontinental visual or audio lag between the United States and Australia was minimal or absent, and the connection quality (via Skype) was perceived as excellent, despite the use of inexpensive standard laptop/desktop computers without advanced telecommunication systems [82]. PRA telementoring was continued in further collaborations [84]. If no local mentor is available, the telepresence of an experienced surgeon during the implementation of a new technique eases stress on the operating team and provides a valuable safety net [82]. Recently, telementoring was used for the integration of transurethral enucleation of the prostate using bipolar energy into an expert endourologist's portfolio [85].

References

1. Yeung AWK, Tosevska A, Klager E, Eibensteiner F, Laxar D, Stoyanov J, et al. Virtual and augmented reality applications in medicine: analysis of the scientific literature. J Med Internet Res. 2021;23(2):e25499.
2. Schmidt MW, Koppinger KF, Fan C, Kowalewski KF, Schmidt LP, Vey J, et al. Virtual reality simulation in robot-assisted surgery: meta-analysis of skill transfer and predictability of skill. BJS Open. 2021;5(2):zraa066.
3. Porpiglia F, Bertolo R, Checcucci E, Amparore D, Autorino R, Dasgupta P, et al. Development and validation of 3D printed virtual models for robot-assisted radical prostatectomy and partial nephrectomy: urologists' and patients' perception. World J Urol. 2018;36(2):201–7.
4. Lachkar AA, Soler L, Diana M, Becmeur F, Marescaux J. 3D imaging and urology: why 3D reconstruction will be mandatory before performing surgery. Arch Esp Urol. 2019;72(3):347–52.
5. Mascagni P, Longo F, Barberio M, Seeliger B, Agnus V, Saccomandi P, et al. New intraoperative imaging technologies: innovating the surgeon's eye toward surgical precision. J Surg Oncol. 2018;118(2):265–82.
6. Nicolau S, Soler L, Mutter D, Marescaux J. Augmented reality in laparoscopic surgical oncology. Surg Oncol. 2011;20(3):189–201.
7. Le Mer P, Soler L, Pavy D, Bernard A, Moreau J, Mutter D, et al. Argonaute 3D: a real-time cooperative medical planning software on DSL network. Stud Health Technol Inform. 2004;98:203–9.
8. Mutter D, Dallemagne B, Bailey C, Soler L, Marescaux J. 3D virtual reality and selective vascular control for laparoscopic left hepatic lobectomy. Surg Endosc. 2009;23(2):432–5.
9. Pessaux P, Diana M, Soler L, Piardi T, Mutter D, Marescaux J. Towards cybernetic surgery: robotic and augmented reality-assisted liver segmentectomy. Langenbeck's Arch Surg. 2015;400(3):381–5.
10. Marescaux J, Clement JM, Tassetti V, Koehl C, Cotin S, Russier Y, et al. Virtual reality applied to hepatic surgery simulation: the next revolution. Ann Surg. 1998;228(5):627–34.
11. Collins JW, Ghazi A, Stoyanov D, Hung A, Coleman M, Cecil T, et al. Utilising an accelerated delphi process to develop guidance and protocols for telepresence applications in remote robotic surgery training. Eur Urol Open Sci. 2020;22:23–33.
12. Intuitive Surgical. Iris 2021. Available from: https://www.intuitive.com/en-us/products-and-services/da-vinci/vision/iris
13. Michiels C, Khene ZE, Prudhomme T, Boulenger de Hauteclocque A, Cornelis FH, Percot M, et al. 3D-Image guided robotic-assisted partial nephrectomy: a multi-institutional propensity score-matched analysis (UroCCR study 51). World J Urol. 2021. https://doi.org/10.1007/s00345-021-03645-1.
14. Heitz A, Weinzorn J, Noblet V, Naegel B, Charnoz A, Heitz F, et al., editors. Lubrav: a new framework for the segmentation of the lung's tubular structures. 2021 IEEE 18th international symposium on biomedical imaging (ISBI). IEEE; 2021. https://doi.org/10.1007/s00345-021-03645-1.
15. De Hauteclocque A, Michiels C, Sarrazin J, Faessel M, Mosillo L, Percot M, et al. Intérêt de modèles tridimensionnels virtuels et physiques pour évaluation de la complexité tumorale rénale et la planification opératoire des néphrectomies partielles (étude UroCCR-63: 3D-planning). Prog Urol. 2019;29(13):757–8.
16. Marescaux J, Rubino F, Arenas M, Mutter D, Soler L. Augmented-reality-assisted laparoscopic adrenalectomy. JAMA. 2004;292(18):2214–5.
17. D'Agostino J, Diana M, Vix M, Nicolau S, Soler L, Bourhala K, et al. Three-dimensional metabolic and radiologic gathered evaluation using VR-RENDER fusion: a novel tool to enhance accuracy in the localization of parathyroid adenomas. World J Surg. 2013;37(7):1618–25.
18. Franchini Melani AG, Diana M, Marescaux J. The quest for precision in transanal total mesorectal excision. Tech Coloproctol. 2016;20(1):11–8.
19. Guerriero L, Quero G, Diana M, Soler L, Agnus V, Marescaux J, et al. Virtual reality exploration and planning for precision colorectal surgery. Dis Colon Rectum. 2018;61(6):719–23.
20. Pessaux P, Diana M, Soler L, Piardi T, Mutter D, Marescaux J. Robotic duodenopancreatectomy assisted with augmented reality and real-time fluorescence guidance. Surg Endosc. 2014;28(8):2493–8.
21. Soler L, Nicolau S, Pessaux P, Mutter D, Marescaux J. Real-time 3D image reconstruction guidance in liver resection surgery. Hepatobiliary Surg Nutr. 2014;3(2):73–81.
22. Hallet J, Soler L, Diana M, Mutter D, Baumert TF, Habersetzer F, et al. Trans-thoracic minimally invasive liver resection guided by augmented reality. J Am Coll Surg. 2015;220(5):e55–60.
23. Porpiglia F, Fiori C, Checcucci E, Amparore D, Bertolo R. Hyperaccuracy three-dimensional reconstruction is able to maximize the efficacy of selective clamping during robot-assisted partial nephrectomy for complex renal masses. Eur Urol. 2018;74(5):651–60.
24. Porpiglia F, Fiori C, Checcucci E, Amparore D, Bertolo R. Augmented reality robot-assisted radical prostatectomy: preliminary experience. Urology. 2018;115:184.
25. Porpiglia F, Checcucci E, Amparore D, Autorino R, Piana A, Bellin A, et al. Augmented-reality robot-assisted radical prostatectomy using hyper-accuracy three-dimensional reconstruction (HA3D) technology: a radiological and pathological study. BJU Int. 2019;123(5):834–45.
26. Porpiglia F, Checcucci E, Amparore D, Manfredi M, Massa F, Piazzolla P, et al. Three-dimensional elastic augmented-reality robot-assisted radical prostatectomy using hyperaccuracy three-dimensional reconstruction technology: a step further in the identification of capsular involvement. Eur Urol. 2019;76(4):505–14.
27. Porpiglia F, Checcucci E, Amparore D, Piramide F, Volpi G, Granato S, et al. Three-dimensional augmented reality robot-assisted partial nephrectomy in case of complex tumours (PADUA >/=10): a new intraoperative tool overcoming the ultrasound guidance. Eur Urol. 2020;78(2):229–38.
28. Checcucci E, Autorino R, Cacciamani GE, Amparore D, De Cillis S, Piana A, et al. Artificial intelligence and neural networks in urology: current clinical applications. Minerva Urol Nefrol. 2020;72(1):49–57.
29. Amparore D, Checcucci E, Piazzolla P, Piramide F, De Cillis S, Piana A, Verri P, Manfredi M, Fiori C, Vezzetti E, Porpiglia F. Indocyanine Green Drives Computer Vision Based 3D Augmented Reality Robot Assisted Partial Nephrectomy: The Beginning of "Automatic" Overlapping Era. Urology. 2022 Jan 19:S0090-4295(22)00029-2. https://doi.org/10.1016/j.urology.2021.10.053. Epub ahead of print. PMID: 35063460.
30. Walz MK, Alesina PF, Wenger FA, Deligiannis A, Szuczik E, Petersenn S, et al. Posterior retroperitoneoscopic adrenalectomy--results of 560 procedures in 520 patients. Surgery. 2006;140(6):943–8. discussion 8–50
31. Modrzejewski R, Collins T, Seeliger B, Bartoli A, Hostettler A, Marescaux J. An in vivo porcine dataset and evaluation methodology to measure soft-body laparoscopic liver registration accuracy with an extended algorithm that handles collisions. Int J Comput Assist Radiol Surg. 2019;14(7):1237–45.
32. Gimenez M, Gallix B, Costamagna G, Vauthey JN, Moche M, Wakabayashi G, et al. Definitions of computer-assisted surgery and intervention, image-guided surgery and intervention, hybrid operating room, and guidance systems: strasbourg international consensus study. Ann Surg Open. 2020;1(2):e021.

33. Connor MJ, Dasgupta P, Ahmed HU, Raza A. Autonomous surgery in the era of robotic urology: friend or foe of the future surgeon? Nat Rev Urol. 2020;17(11):643–9.
34. Seyam R, Khalil MI, Kamel MH, Altaweel WM, Davis R, Bissada NK. Organ-sparing procedures in GU cancer: part 1-organ-sparing procedures in renal and adrenal tumors: a systematic review. Int Urol Nephrol. 2019;51(3):377–93.
35. Abu-Ghanem Y, Fernandez-Pello S, Bex A, Ljungberg B, Albiges L, Dabestani S, et al. Limitations of available studies prevent reliable comparison between tumour ablation and partial nephrectomy for patients with localised renal masses: a systematic review from the European Association of Urology Renal Cell Cancer Guideline Panel. Eur Urol Oncol. 2020;3(4):433–52.
36. Ierardi AM, Carnevale A, Angileri SA, Pellegrino F, Renzulli M, Golfieri R, et al. Outcomes following minimally invasive imagine-guided percutaneous ablation of adrenal glands. Gland Surg. 2020;9(3):859–66.
37. Colleselli D, Janetschek G. Current trends in partial adrenalectomy. Curr Opin Urol. 2015;25(2):89–94.
38. Lorenz K, Langer P, Niederle B, Alesina P, Holzer K, Nies C, et al. Surgical therapy of adrenal tumors: guidelines from the German Association of Endocrine Surgeons (CAEK). Langenbeck's Arch Surg. 2019;404(4):385–401.
39. Kaye DR, Storey BB, Pacak K, Pinto PA, Linehan WM, Bratslavsky G. Partial adrenalectomy: underused first line therapy for small adrenal tumors. J Urol. 2010;184(1):18–25.
40. Lowery AJ, Seeliger B, Alesina PF, Walz MK. Posterior retroperitoneoscopic adrenal surgery for clinical and subclinical Cushing's syndrome in patients with bilateral adrenal disease. Langenbeck's Arch Surg. 2017;402(5):775–85.
41. Walz MK, Peitgen K, Diesing D, Petersenn S, Janssen OE, Philipp T, et al. Partial versus total adrenalectomy by the posterior retroperitoneoscopic approach: early and long-term results of 325 consecutive procedures in primary adrenal neoplasias. World J Surg. 2004;28(12):1323–9.
42. Seeliger B, Alesina PF, Walz MK, Pop R, Charles AL, Geny B, et al. Intraoperative imaging for remnant viability assessment in bilateral posterior retroperitoneoscopic partial adrenalectomy in an experimental model. Br J Surg. 2020.
43. Walz MK, Iova LD, Deimel J, Neumann HPH, Bausch B, Zschiedrich S, et al. Minimally Invasive Surgery (MIS) in children and adolescents with pheochromocytomas and retroperitoneal paragangliomas: experiences in 42 patients. World J Surg. 2018;42(4):1024–30.
44. Brauckhoff M, Stock K, Stock S, Lorenz K, Sekulla C, Brauckhoff K, et al. Limitations of intraoperative adrenal remnant volume measurement in patients undergoing subtotal adrenalectomy. World J Surg. 2008;32(5):863–72.
45. Seeliger B, Walz MK, Alesina PF, Agnus V, Pop R, Barberio M, et al. Fluorescence-enabled assessment of adrenal gland localization and perfusion in posterior retroperitoneoscopic adrenal surgery in a preclinical model. Surg Endosc. 2020;34(3):1401–11.
46. Kong SH, Haouchine N, Soares R, Klymchenko A, Andreiuk B, Marques B, et al. Robust augmented reality registration method for localization of solid organs' tumors using CT-derived virtual biomechanical model and fluorescent fiducials. Surg Endosc. 2017;31(7):2863–71.
47. Manny TB, Pompeo AS, Hemal AK. Robotic partial adrenalectomy using indocyanine green dye with near-infrared imaging: the initial clinical experience. Urology. 2013;82(3):738–42.
48. Kahramangil B, Berber E. The use of near-infrared fluorescence imaging in endocrine surgical procedures. J Surg Oncol. 2017;115(7):848–55.
49. Pathak RA, Hemal AK. Intraoperative ICG-fluorescence imaging for robotic-assisted urologic surgery: current status and review of literature. Int Urol Nephrol. 2019;51(5):765–71.
50. Colvin J, Zaidi N, Berber E. The utility of indocyanine green fluorescence imaging during robotic adrenalectomy. J Surg Oncol. 2016;114(2):153–6.
51. Kahramangil B, Kose E, Berber E. Characterization of fluorescence patterns exhibited by different adrenal tumors: determining the indications for indocyanine green use in adrenalectomy. Surgery. 2018;164(5):972–7.
52. Moore EC, Berber E. Fluorescence techniques in adrenal surgery. Gland Surg. 2019;8(Suppl 1):S22–S7.
53. George EI, Brand TC, LaPorta A, Marescaux J, Satava RM. Origins of robotic surgery: from skepticism to standard of care. JSLS. 2018;22(4)
54. Marescaux J, Leroy J, Gagner M, Rubino F, Mutter D, Vix M, et al. Transatlantic robot-assisted telesurgery. Nature. 2001;413(6854):379–80.
55. Marescaux J, Leroy J, Rubino F, Smith M, Vix M, Simone M, et al. Transcontinental robot-assisted remote telesurgery: feasibility and potential applications. Ann Surg. 2002;235(4):487–92.
56. Anvari M. Remote telepresence surgery: the Canadian experience. Surg Endosc. 2007;21(4):537–41.
57. Börner Valdez L, Datta RR, Babic B, Müller DT, Bruns CJ, Fuchs HF. 5G mobile communication applications for surgery: an overview of the latest literature. Artif Intell Gastrointest Endosc. 2021;2(1):1–11.
58. Jell A, Vogel T, Ostler D, Marahrens N, Wilhelm D, Samm N, et al. 5th-Generation mobile communication: data highway for surgery 4.0. Surg Technol Int. 2019;35:36–42.
59. Lacy AM, Bravo R, Otero-Pineiro AM, Pena R, De Lacy FB, Menchaca R, et al. 5G-assisted telementored surgery. Br J Surg. 2019;106(12):1576–9.
60. Acemoglu A, Peretti G, Trimarchi M, Hysenbelli J, Krieglstein J, Geraldes A, et al. Operating from a distance: robotic vocal cord 5G telesurgery on a cadaver. Ann Intern Med. 2020;173(11):940–1.
61. Zheng J, Wang Y, Zhang J, Guo W, Yang X, Luo L, et al. 5G ultra-remote robot-assisted laparoscopic surgery in China. Surg Endosc. 2020;34(11):5172–80.
62. Tian W, Fan M, Zeng C, Liu Y, He D, Zhang Q. Telerobotic spinal surgery based on 5G network: the first 12 cases. Neurospine. 2020;17(1):114–20.
63. Orosco RK, Lurie B, Matsuzaki T, Funk EK, Divi V, Holsinger FC, et al. Compensatory motion scaling for time-delayed robotic surgery. Surg Endosc. 2021;35(6):2613–8.
64. Panesar SS, Ashkan K. Surgery in space. Br J Surg. 2018;105(10):1234–43.
65. Campbell MR, Kirkpatrick AW, Billica RD, Johnston SL, Jennings R, Short D, et al. Endoscopic surgery in weightlessness: the investigation of basic principles for surgery in space. Surg Endosc. 2001;15(12):1413–8.
66. Leapman MS, Jones JA, Coutinho K, Sagalovich D, Garcia MM, Olsson CA, et al. Up and away: five decades of urologic investigation in microgravity. Urology. 2017;106:18–25.
67. Doarn CR, Anvari M, Low T, Broderick TJ. Evaluation of teleoperated surgical robots in an enclosed undersea environment. Telemed J E Health. 2009;15(4):325–35.
68. Haidegger T, Sandor J, Benyo Z. Surgery in space: the future of robotic telesurgery. Surg Endosc. 2011;25(3):681–90.
69. Meara J, Leather A, Hagander L. Global Surgery 2030: evidence and solutions for achieving health, welfare, and economic development [published online April 21, 2015]. Lancet. 2015;
70. Gray WK, Day J, Briggs TWR, Wass JAH, Lansdown M. Volume-outcome relationship for adrenalectomy: analysis of an administrative dataset for the Getting It Right First Time Programme. Br J Surg. 2021;108(9):1112–9.
71. Marescaux J, Soler L, Mutter D, Leroy J, Vix M, Koehl C, et al. Virtual university applied to telesurgery: from teleeducation to telemanipulation. Stud Health Technol Inform. 2000;70:195–201.

72. Mutter D, Vix M, Dallemagne B, Perretta S, Leroy J, Marescaux J. WeBSurg: an innovative educational Web site in minimally invasive surgery--principles and results. Surg Innov. 2011;18(1):8–14.
73. Sereno S, Mutter D, Dallemagne B, Smith CD, Marescaux J. Telementoring for minimally invasive surgical training by wireless robot. Surg Innov. 2007;14(3):184–91.
74. Erridge S, Yeung DKT, Patel HRH, Purkayastha S. Telementoring of surgeons: a systematic review. Surg Innov. 2019;26(1):95–111.
75. Feliciano DV, Delaney CP, Schauer P, Takanishi DM Jr, Alford LA, Medlin W, et al. Upgrading your surgical skills through preceptorship. J Am Coll Surg. 2021;233(3):487–93.
76. Collins J, Akre O, Challacombe B, Karim O, Wiklund P. Robotic networks: delivering empowerment through integration. BJU Int. 2015;116(2):167–8.
77. Cubano M, Poulose BK, Talamini MA, Stewart R, Antosek LE, Lentz R, et al. Long distance telementoring. A novel tool for laparoscopy aboard the USS Abraham Lincoln. Surg Endosc. 1999;13(7):673–8.
78. Rosser JC Jr, Bell RL, Harnett B, Rodas E, Murayama M, Merrell R. Use of mobile low-bandwith telemedical techniques for extreme telemedicine applications. J Am Coll Surg. 1999;189(4):397–404.
79. Wachs JP, Kirkpatrick AW, Tisherman SA. Procedural telementoring in rural, underdeveloped, and austere settings: origins, present challenges, and future perspectives. Annu Rev Biomed Eng. 2021;23:115–39.
80. Fassnacht M, Dekkers OM, Else T, Baudin E, Berruti A, de Krijger R, et al. European Society of Endocrinology Clinical Practice Guidelines on the management of adrenocortical carcinoma in adults, in collaboration with the European Network for the Study of Adrenal Tumors. Eur J Endocrinol. 2018;179(4):G1–G46.
81. Vrielink OM, Wevers KP, Kist JW, Borel Rinkes IHM, Hemmer PHJ, Vriens MR, et al. Laparoscopic anterior versus endoscopic posterior approach for adrenalectomy: a shift to a new golden standard? Langenbeck's Arch Surg. 2017;402(5):767–73.
82. Miller JA, Kwon DS, Dkeidek A, Yew M, Hisham Abdullah A, Walz MK, et al. Safe introduction of a new surgical technique: remote telementoring for posterior retroperitoneoscopic adrenalectomy. ANZ J Surg. 2012;82(11):813–6.
83. Brunt LM. SAGES Guidelines for minimally invasive treatment of adrenal pathology. Surg Endosc. 2013;27(11):3957–9.
84. Treter S, Perrier N, Sosa JA, Roman S. Telementoring: a multi-institutional experience with the introduction of a novel surgical approach for adrenalectomy. Ann Surg Oncol. 2013;20(8):2754–8.
85. Amato M, Eissa A, Puliatti S, Secchi C, Ferraguti F, Minelli M, et al. Feasibility of a telementoring approach as a practical training for transurethral enucleation of the benign prostatic hyperplasia using bipolar energy: a pilot study. World J Urol. 2021;39(9):3465–71.

The Role of Artificial Intelligence and Machine Learning in Surgery

Runzhuo Ma, Justin W. Collins, and Andrew J. Hung

1 Introduction

Artificial intelligence (AI) has pervaded nearly every aspect of our life: from Internet search engines, social media channels, facial recognition, to self-driving cars, or even language translation. Of its various definitions, it commonly refers to the general ability of a machine (usually, a computer) to independently replicate intellectual processes typical of human cognition in deciding on an action in response to its perceived environment to achieve a predetermined goal [1].

The intersection of AI and medicine has resulted in remarkable accomplishments in the past few years: image diagnostic algorithms on par with or even better than humans, accurate prediction of 1-year mortality for palliative care based on big data, and an AI clinician optimizes treatment strategies for sepsis in the ICU, just to name a few [2–5].

Surgery is no exception to this trend. AI, and its associated computer science techniques, such as machine learning, deep learning, reinforcement learning, and computer vision, have been extensively used in the surgical field in recent years, across areas such as preoperative surgical candidate selection, surgical assessment and training, surgical outcome prediction, intelligent intraoperative assistance, and eventually, autonomous surgery. Collectively, these applications have been referred to *Surgical AI*. In this chapter, we will go into various aspects of *Surgical AI* and delineate its progress during the past few years.

R. Ma · A. J. Hung (✉)
Catherine and Joseph Aresty Department of Urology, Center for Robotic Simulation and Education, USC Institute of Urology, University of Southern California, Los Angeles, CA, USA

J. W. Collins
Division of Surgery and Interventional Science, Research Department of Targeted Intervention, University College London, London, UK

Wellcome/ESPRC Centre for Interventional and Surgical Sciences (WEISS), University College London, London, UK

Division of Uro-oncology, University College London Hospital, London, UK

2 Artificial Intelligence for Surgeons

AI may seem mysterious at first, but they are actually deeply related to traditional statistical models and should be recognizable to physicians. Generally speaking, by the scope of its ability, AI can be classified as *narrow*, *general*, and *super* AI (Fig. 1).

- Most if not all AI in use now are *narrow AI*, which means they are designed to solve one specific task, like AlphaGo, who specializes in Go and successfully beat the best human player [6].
- *General AI*, in theory, should be able to solve any tasks humans can do, even the ones we have not thought of.
- Then *Super AI* is defined by its ability to solve any intellectual tasks better than humans.

Since the latter two AI concepts are still in the theoretical stage and have not existed in reality, in this chapter, the term *AI* only refers to *narrow AI*.

As a subfield of AI, *machine learning (ML)* involves the development and deployment of algorithms that, instead of being explicitly programed to assign specific outputs (actions) in response to specific inputs (perceived environment), analyze the data and its properties on its own to determine the actions, thus constantly learning from data [7, 8].

ML algorithms can be further classified as either *supervised learning* (labeled) or *unsupervised learning* (unlabeled), depending on whether outputs are labeled by humans [1]. Supervised learning (i.e., Naïve Bayes classification, support vector machines, and random forests) is often used to predict clinical outcomes, whereas unsupervised learning (i.e., *k*-means clustering, principal component analysis, and autoencoders) is often used to search for patterns within complex data, such as genomics [1].

Deep learning (DL), on the other hand, refers to the model structure. It is a form of artificial neural networks inspired by the human biological nervous system. These models consist of multiple layers, as each layer receives, pro-

P. Wiklund et al. (eds.), *Robotic Urologic Surgery*, https://doi.org/10.1007/978-3-031-00363-9_9

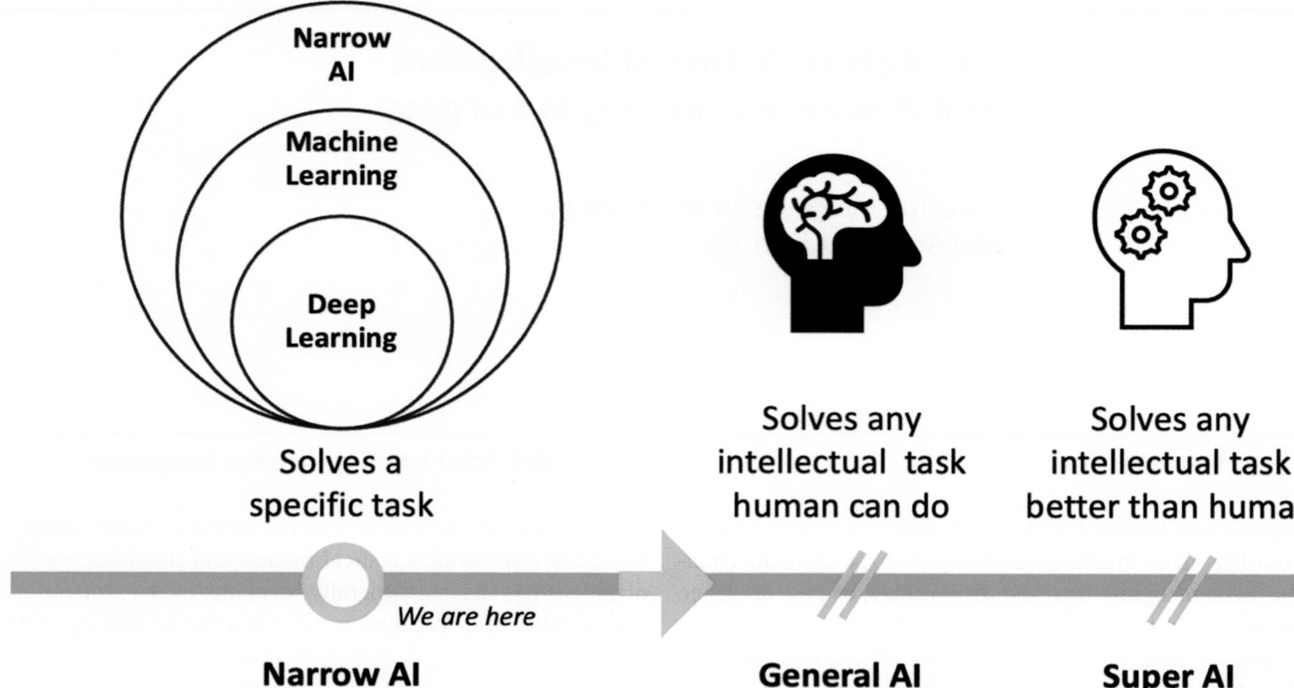

Fig. 1 Artificial intelligence (AI) and machine learning

cesses, and outputs information to the next layer [9]. The input into the first layer is the data set of interest, while the output of the last layer is the outcome of interest. DL is often used in image analysis.

Reinforcement learning (RL) also refers to the model structure; however, it is generally in an interactive feedback loop as the model receives either a reward or penalty for its action. The model eventually learns the best action with each turn. Two forms of RL have been reported in the literature—*implicit imitation learning*, which learns from experts' action directly, and *inverse RL*, which learns through inferring experts' intention [10]. RL has the potential to be used for autonomous surgery [9].

Computer vision is about machine discovers and learns information from videos or images in a way similar to human beings [11]. Some of the greatest successes of AI applications in medicine come from computer vision, including diagnostic pathology, radiology, and autonomous surgery.

Natural language processing is a subfield of AI that emphasizes building a computer's ability to parse and comprehend human written and spoken language [11]. In healthcare, it is mainly used in digging through electronic health records.

One advantage of these ML algorithms is their flexibility to deal with different sources of input (Fig. 2). Recent advances in surgical technology and electronic healthcare databases have been generating big volumes, various kinds of data in the surgical field, including surgical video, audio, instrument kinematics, surgeon biometrics, and detailed patient characteristics [12]. The combination of ML and "big data" have produced and will continuously produce a huge impact in medicine.

3 AI in Surgical Candidate Selection

With a large amount of data available from medical imaging and electronic health records, ML has shown the ability to aid preoperative surgical candidate selection.

The first application of AI in this field is to *facilitate accurate preoperative diagnosis*, which could avoid unnecessary surgery. For example, preoperatively distinguishing benign renal masses (e.g., oncocytoma and angiomyolipoma) from renal cell carcinoma can be challenging, yet remaining fundamental to treatment choices. Some studies suggest ML models have appeared to be on par or even better than imaging experts in this area [13, 14]. Feng et al. used quantitative texture analysis to differentiate small benign lesions (i.e., lipid-poor angiomyolipoma) from renal cell carcinoma based on preoperative CT [15]. The model utilized support vector machine to establish discriminative classifiers and achieved an AUC of 0.955 [15]. Nityanand et al. utilized three different algorithms, namely random forest, logistic regression, and support vector machine, to facilitate Bosniak classification of cystic renal masses based on CT [16]. All models achieved moderate sensitivity (0.56–0.67) and high specific-

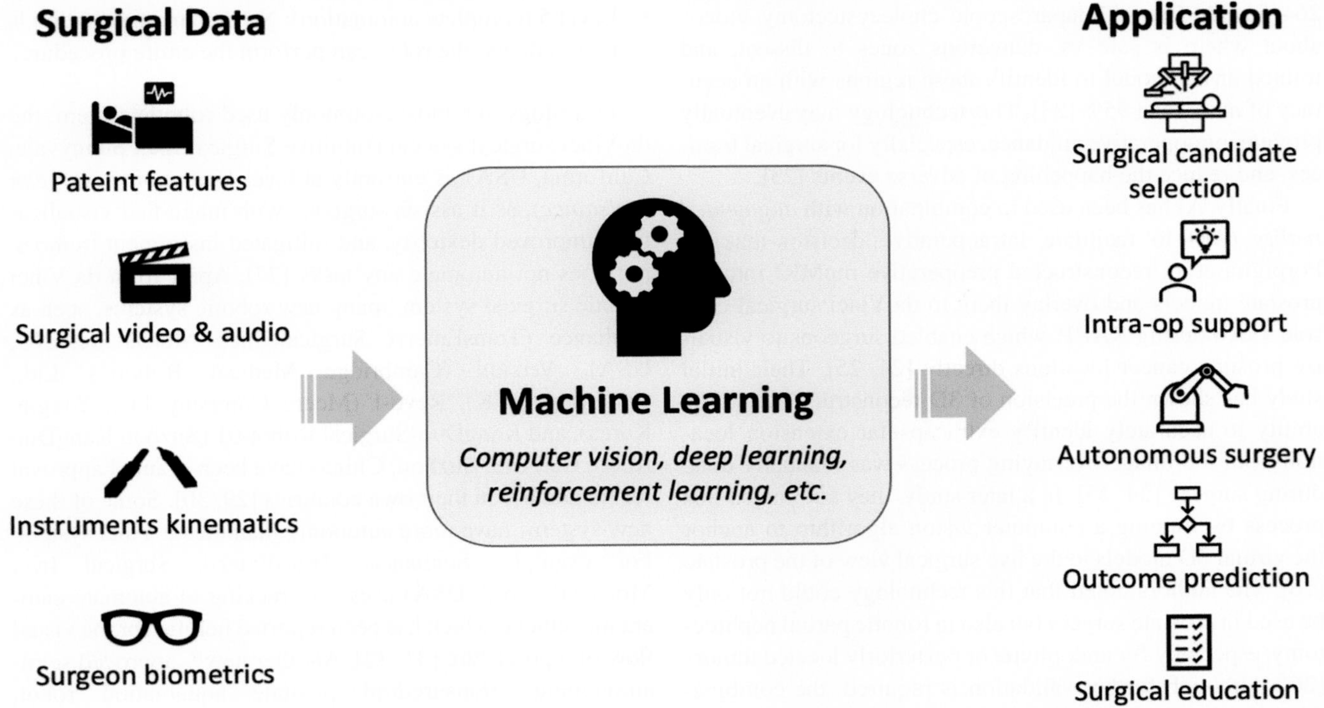

Fig. 2 Machine learning applications in the surgical field

ity (0.91–0.93) in distinguishing benign (Bosniak I or II) vs. potentially malignant lesions (Bosniak IIF, III, or IV) [16]. Furthermore, several studies aimed to identify low Fuhrman nuclear grade (I and II) from high-Fuhrman nuclear grade (III and IV) renal cell carcinoma preoperatively, in order to facilitate decision-making between active surveillance vs. surgery [17, 18]. By unenhanced CT, one study achieved an AUC of 0.71, while by three-phase CT, another study achieved an AUC of 0.87 [17, 18].

The second application of AI is to *predict surgical morbidity and mortality* by preoperative risk factors. For example, radical cystectomy is complicated and associated with as high as 8% postoperative mortality rate [19]. Identifying appropriate surgical candidates is of huge importance to decrease surgical mortality. Using an ML model, Klén et al. identified strong preoperative risk factors for early (<90 days) postoperative mortality following radical cystectomy and constructed a user-friendly risk table [20].

Finally, AI can learn from existing data and *inform a patient of management strategies chosen by patients with similar conditions*. Based on the large-scale clinical registry data, the Michigan Urological Surgery Improvement Collaborative (MUSIC) group trained an ML algorithm that can yield individualized treatment options for new prostate cancer patients [21]. The group created a web-based platform, namely askMUSIC (http://ask.musicurology.com), to inform patients of the percentage of choices among active surveillance, radical prostatectomy, radiation therapy, and androgen deprivation therapy made by other prostate cancer patients with similar demographic and clinicopathologic features. In their validation cohort, the AUC of prediction achieved 0.81. Though the intention of this study is to provide data-driven information for patients facing difficult treatment choices, the methodology also has the potential to be used in the development of AI treatment decision algorithm.

4 AI in Intelligent Intraoperative Assistance

Decision-making is an important aspect of a successful surgery. With the advantage of powerful computing ability and compatibility with a wide range of data sources, AI has the potential to provide a variety of intelligent assistance to facilitate intraoperative decision-making.

Utilizing shortwave Raman spectroscopy data, an AI algorithm has been trained to differentiate malignant kidney tumors from normal kidney tissue with high accuracy (92.5%) under laboratory settings [22]. Since this technology does not require any special lighting condition changes in the operation room, it has the potential to expedite the process of surgical margin check-in partial nephrectomy and even replace traditional frozen section pathology [22].

Another aspect AI has been used in intraoperative assistance is to *identify surgical anatomy*. Altieri et al. annotated

264 frames from 63 laparoscopic cholecystectomy videos about where is safe vs. dangerous zones to dissect, and trained an AI model to identify these regions with an accuracy of more than 95% [23]. This technology may eventually provide intraoperative guidance, especially for surgical trainees, and reduce the happening of adverse events [23].

Finally, AI has been used in combination with *augmented reality (AR)* to facilitate intraoperative decision-making. Porpiglia et al. reconstructed preoperative mpMRI into 3D prostate models and overlay them to da Vinci surgical console video during RARP, which enabled surgeons to visualize prostate cancer locations directly [24, 25]. Their initial study has shown the precision of 3D reconstruction and the ability to accurately identify extracapsular extension locations, but the image-overlaying process was manually done during surgery [24, 25]. In a later study, they automated this process by training a computer vision algorithm to anchor the virtual 3D models to the live surgical view of the prostate [26]. The authors noted that this technology could not only be used in prostate surgery but also in robotic partial nephrectomy, especially for endophytic or posteriorly located tumors [26]. Although further validation is required, the combination of AI and 3D AR promises to advance intraoperative navigation, and help to optimize the balance between oncological control and sexual function preservation [27].

5 AI in Autonomous Surgery

5.1 Autonomy

Similar to autonomous driving, there are *different levels of autonomy* in surgical robots. One commonly accepted framework classifies the autonomy of robotic surgery from level 0 (no automation) to level 5 (full automation) [28].

- Level 0 (no autonomy): The operator is in charge of all duties, including monitoring, producing performance alternatives, choosing which option to perform (decision-making), and carrying out the decision.
- Level 1 (robot assistance): The operator keeps constant control of the system while the robot assists in certain ways.
- Level 2 (task autonomy): The operator maintains discrete control of the system, and the robot can automatically accomplish specified tasks initiated by the operator.
- Level 3 (conditional autonomy): The surgeon chooses and approves the surgical plan, and the robot executes the procedure automatically but under the supervision of a human surgeon.
- Level 4 (high autonomy): The robot can make decisions on its own, but only with the help of a competent operator.
- Level 5 (complete automation): No human intervention is required, and the robot can perform the entire procedure.

In urology, the most commonly used robotic system, the da Vinci surgical system (Intuitive Surgical Inc., Sunnyvale, California, USA), is currently at level 1 autonomy (*surgeon assistance*), as it assists surgeons with magnified visualization, improved dexterity, and mitigated instrument tremors, but does not automate any tasks [27]. Apart from da Vinci robotic surgical system, many new robotic systems, such as Senhance (TransEnterix Surgical Inc., Morrisville, NC, USA), Versius (Cambridge Medical Robotics Ltd., Cambridge, UK), Revo-I (Meere Company Inc., Yongin, Korea), and KangDuo-Surgical Robot-01 (Suzhou KangDuo Robot Co., Ltd, Suzhou, China) have been granted approval for human use in their own countries [29, 30]. Some of these new systems have more autonomy than the da Vinci system. For example, Senhance (TransEnterix Surgical Inc., Morrisville, NC, USA) uses eye-tracking to automate camera movement, which has been reported helpful for the visual flow of a procedure [31, 32]. Another newly approved semi-autonomous transurethral prostate aquablation robot, Aquablation™ (Procept BioRobotics, Redwood Shores, CA, USA), expands the application of surgical robots to endourology [33]. Surgeons only need to create a procedural plan by contouring the tissue to be removed, and then the robot will autonomously resect tissues with high pressure, non-heated saline. Studies have shown comparable operation time and symptom relief to conventional transurethral resection of the prostate (TURP), but with fewer complication rates (25.9% vs. 41.5%, $p < 0.02$) [33]. Besides, this system is especially useful in patients with large prostate volumes (80–150 ml), where TURP operated by the surgeon is usually challenging [34]. This novel system should be deemed as an example of level 2 autonomy (*task autonomy*). Ongoing studies are mostly exploring the feasibility of level 2 automation (*task autonomy*), in which robots perform repetitive tasks (e.g., camera positioning and tissue retraction), enabling surgeons to concentrate more on the critical aspects of a procedure.

The rapid growth of surgical robots provides a new opportunity to incorporate AI into the operating room. The abundant, diverse data derived from surgical robots serve as nutritious soil to develop, train, and validate AI algorithms. AI, in return, has the unique ability to learn from prior experience and process new data, which enables a self-perpetuating cycle, much like how surgeons grow in their daily practice. To be more specific, computer vision and reinforcement learning are the most commonly used models in autonomous surgery—the former one can perceive the surgical environment and identify surgical planes, and the latter one can learn surgical techniques from surgeons' demonstration or in a trial-and-error manner [9]. A traditional theory in robot autonomy is the "sense-think-act paradigm" [28, 35].

5.2 Sense

In current practice, the most important "sense" during robotic surgery is vision. To achieve autonomous vision, two aspects need to be addressed—automatic camera positioning and vision recognition.

Automatic Camera Positioning Wang et al. developed an auto-tracking algorithm to navigate robotic camera based on its kinematic relationships with robotic instrument arms [36]. However, this approach is limited by the requirement of accurate instrument/camera coordinates, which is difficult to acquire in some robotic systems. The other way is by video input. Rivas-Blanco et al. used reinforcement learning to train a magnet-manipulated camera to automatically navigate based on vision information of instruments movement, and the system was validated through an in-vivo experiment in a pig [37]. The drawback of this method is the possible occlusion of instruments or vision markers during the surgery. To solve this problem, Sun et al. developed a predictive model based on computer vision to predict instruments' trajectories in case they are occluded by blood [38]. By the prediction, the robotic camera can automatically adjust to the appropriate position, thus solving the difficulty of automating camera navigation when vision is partially occluded [38]. Another study by Wagner et al. developed a cognitive camera with learning ability, which can optimize camera position tailored to the surgeon's need [39]. The system's performance and efficiency improved along with the increase in experience [39].

Visual Recognition Samiei et al. exploited computer vision strategies to recognize different anatomical structures during surgery [40]. By combining AI with their novel molecular chemical imaging endoscope, which comprises molecular spectroscopy and digital imaging, the algorithm successfully discriminated anatomical structures like ureter, lymph node, blood vessels, and nerve bundles with an AUC $\geq$0.90 in live porcine models [40]. The advantage of their technique is no need for a contrast agent or special lighting conditions. This technology has the potential to enhance surgeons' ability to differentiate structures, avoid iatrogenic injuries, and enable autonomous robot vision. Another aspect of visual recognition is recognizing the position of instruments. Seemingly easy at first, this task is actually challenging. A recent pixel-wise instrument segmentation technique, developed by deep neural network architectures, has shown promise in this aspect [41]. Another study by Sun et al. further reduced the computational burden of the algorithm, making it more feasible to perform in real time [42].

5.3 Think

Trajectory planning is important. After sensing outside signals, the robot needs to make a reasonable plan about how to move instruments to achieve the determined task while not colliding with other instruments or surrounding tissues. Current research suggests planning trajectory during static conditions is relatively easy, but planning trajectory in a dynamic environment can be difficult [43]. To solve this problem, Baek et al. combined reinforcement learning with a probabilistic roadmap [44]. Taking advantage of reinforcement learning's ability to deal with uncertainty, the algorithm achieved collision-free pathway planning in real time to automate dissection tasks [44].

5.4 Act

During the action phase, it is essential for an autonomous system to control and adjust tissue tension spontaneously. Thananjeyan et al. used reinforcement learning to optimize tensioning policies during a pattern cutting task and compared this algorithm with the traditional fixed and analytic algorithm [45]. They concluded the reinforcement learning algorithm outperformed the traditional method in both performance and robustness of tension adjustment [45]. Another group further developed the reinforcement learning algorithm by allowing multipoint grasping, rather than one-point grasping, which improved the performance and robustness of the model further [46].

5.5 Training AI Model

Much like training a surgeon, the process of training an AI requires repetitive practice. As mentioned before, reinforcement learning (RL) is the most commonly used model in autonomous surgery. The learning process happens through trial and error, demonstration, or a hybrid of the two approaches [9]. Shin et al. compared models learning from experts' surgical demonstration vs. from trial and error, and found that experts' demonstration helped the model learn faster than purely data-driven, highlighting the profound role of expert surgeons in the learning process of AI [47]. Another study from Pedram et al. conjoined these two methods and found that with an initial selection of simple and intuitive features instructed by surgeons, the mixed machine learning algorithm can be trained successfully in multiple tissue dynamic circumstances [48]. This synergic learning model may serve as an efficient tool to lessen the time cost of surgeons training AI while still keeping the best performance of the system.

6 AI in Surgical Outcome Prediction

Outcome prediction is no new thing in the surgical field. By traditional statistical models (e.g., logistic regression and Cox regression), multiple prediction nomograms have been established to estimate patient outcomes [49, 50]. The advantage of AI models is their potential to improve prediction accuracy, their freedom from strict statistical assumptions, and their flexibility of data distributions [51]. Due to these advantages, AI can combine novel intraoperative surgical data and traditional patient features to predict postoperative outcomes in a more accurate fashion.

For example, Hung et al. used intraoperative robotic system data (e.g., energy usage and camera pedal counts) and kinematic data (e.g., instruments velocity and wrist articulation), namely automated performance metrics (APMs), to train an ML model which accurately predicted postoperative length of hospital stay after RARP [52, 53]. The same group then utilized APMs combining with patient features to predict urinary continence recovery after RARP [54]. The predictive accuracy was moderate, and intriguingly the top ten predictive features all came from APMs [54]. These results were further validated in a bi-institutional study [55]. Furthermore, APMs have been reported correlating with intraoperative outcomes of RAPN, and the next step would be to predict postoperative outcomes [56]. These studies highlight the significant impact of surgical performance on surgical outcomes and indicate the huge potential of AI models in digging intraoperative data.

Another example is that Soguero-Ruiz et al. used natural language processing (NLP) to automatically comb through EMRs (i.e., operative reports and progress notes) to accurately predict anastomotic leak after colorectal resections [57]. The model achieved a sensitivity of 100% and a specificity of 72% [57]. This technology could detect the catastrophic complication before actually happening, winning time for effective management.

However, AI also has its limitations. First, it sacrifices the transparency of the model. Most AI algorithms operate like a "black box," which makes humans unable to interpret what is going on inside the model [58]. Thus, AI has mostly been used for the prediction of outcomes rather than the inference of the biological process [51]. Second, overfitting is a concern. Big data increases the chance of confounders, and the implicit nature of AI models amplifies the chance of "false positive" findings. Careful preselection of variables should be carried out to avoid false discovery.

7 AI in Surgical Education

Conventional surgical skill assessment and performance evaluation are performed manually, which is time-consuming and prone to observer biases. AI provides an ideal solution to both problems. Utilizing big data (i.e., video footage and instrument kinematics) derived from surgery, ML models are starting to play an important role in novel surgical assessment. However, there are also risks to application in training, which include data and privacy issues, transparency, biases, accountability, and liabilities [59].

7.1 Video Segmentation

Surgical videos have educational value [60]. By reviewing surgical videos, formative assessment can be provided, surgical techniques can be improved, and patient outcomes can be enhanced [61]. However, organizing and finding the relevant clip from surgical videos is usually time consuming, which becomes the main hurdle for routinely utilizing videos to improve surgical techniques [62].

ML has the potential to reduce the time cost of surgical video review by automatically segmenting and identifying critical steps [63]. For example, Zia et al. applied a machine-learning model to automate the segmentation of RARP into 12 surgical steps [64]. Compared with expert annotations, the model correctly annotated most RARP steps with less than 200 s error [64].

Khalid et al. utilized an ML model to classify surgical tasks of JHU-ISI Gesture and Skill Assessment Working Set (JIGSAWS), which comprises da Vinci robotic suturing, knot-tying, and needle-passing tasks on a bench-top model [65]. The model achieved highly accurate results (precision 91% and recall 94%) [65]. Using the same dataset, Wang and Majewicz Fey predicted the surgical task type with similar accuracy [66]. However, their ML approach only requires 1–3 s for data interpretation, making it especially useful for active summative feedback.

AI has even been shown to be able to recognize the most basic movements in surgery at the gesture level. Luongo et al. trained deep-learning-based computer vision algorithms to identify different dissection gestures with an AUC of 0.87 [67].

A more recent study used computer vision to identify important clinical clips of surgery. Mascagni et al. trained an algorithm based on an expert annotated critical safety view of laparoscopic cholecystectomy to automatically locate important video clips with 91% accuracy [68].

Overall, using the ML method to segment surgical videos may drive the workflow toward standardization, efficiency, and objectiveness.

7.2 Automated Surgical Skills Assessment

Surgical data usually has three layers: kinematics, video footage, and surgeons' biometrics. Studies have been using AI models to analyze these data aiming to quantify expertise.

Instrument kinematic metrics generally measure instrument motion such as traveling distance, moving velocity, acceleration/deceleration, Endowrist® articulation, and jerk (a derivative of acceleration with respect to time) [69, 70]. In laboratory settings, Fard et al. used ML analysis of raw kinematic tool movements in JIGSAWS to predict expertise with >90% accuracy [71]. In clinical settings, Hung et al. showed that expert surgeons performed significantly better than novices during RARP in nearly all these metrics (e.g., shorter instrument path length, less time, and faster velocity) [53]. Utilizing ML models, the group re-ranked eight surgeons based on the most important kinematic metrics and found the new ranking correlated with continence-recovery better than the ranking by surgeon experience [54]. Chen et al. utilized kinematic metrics at stitch and sub-stitch levels to predict expertise [72]. They found that sub-stitch metrics could better distinguish experts from novices [72].

With the development of minimal invasive surgery, surgical videos have become easily accessible. Using AI to analyze surgical videos can be an effective way of surgical assessment. Baghdadi et al. automated the assessment of pelvic lymph node dissection by computer vision algorithms [73]. Their model achieved an accuracy of 83.3% compared to the scores experts gave [73]. In an intriguing study, Jin et al. extracted instrument kinematic metrics from surgical video [74]. They first detected the instrument by leveraging region-based convolutional neural networks in real-world laparoscopic surgical videos, and then successfully extracted instrument movement ranges and economy of motion. They finally inspected the relationship of these extracted metrics with surgical quality scores given by experts and found apparent associations between them [74].

Another approach to assessing surgeon proficiency is by *biometrics*, which represents the internal responses of surgeons. AI has shown promise in this field.

Richstone et al. recorded surgeons' eye data during surgery, including eye movement, blinking, fixation and saccade, and pupil size change during simulation tasks and renal surgery, and then utilized linear discriminate analysis and nonlinear network analyses to distinguish experts from novice surgeons [75]. In the simulated surgical setting, the models achieved an accuracy of >90%; while in the live operating room setting, the accuracy was >80% [75]. Another study by Koskinen et al. found that by pupil diameter change alone on a suture level, the ML model support vector machine classifier can distinguish expertise with 75% accuracy, while adding blinking rate and further segmenting the eye data into sub-suture granularity failed to improve prediction accuracy [76].

7.3 Automated Training Feedback

Studies using AI to provide useful real-time feedback are still in the infancy state, represented by the exploratory nature of most research. Opportunities to change the status quo lie in this field and are waiting for researchers to explore. Fawaz et al. developed a new model based on convolutional neural network to classify surgical skills by extracting latent patterns in the trainees' motions performed during robotic surgery [77]. The novelty of this model is that it utilized a technique called class activation map, which can pinpoint which parts of the surgery determined the predictive results most, thus allowing trainees to understand where to focus practicing on [77].

8 Challenges and Future Directions

Despite the promise of machine learning, there are still formidable obstacles and limitations [59].

Data and Privacy ML models usually need a large amount of data for initial training, ongoing validation, and further improvement. This amount of data may need to be shared across multiple institutions and potentially across the nation. Data privacy is a big concern during this process, especially if compromised by a cyber-attack [78]. Issues related to data privacy need to be addressed with hospitals having agreed protocols that follow rules and guidance established by the Data Protection Officer for surgeons and patients. Data can be improved by collecting data in a standardized way (Table 1). In robotic surgical training, this can be achieved with standardized robotic curricula, train-the-trainer courses, and agreed metrics that define surgical training at a granular level that can be aligned with telemetry data and more easily interpreted in computer vision analysis [53, 79–81].

Transparency and Reproducibility The accuracy of supervised ML models highly relies on labels annotated by humans. Thus, transparency of how the model was trained is important for others to critically evaluate the model [82]. Besides, most ML algorithms operate like a "black box," lacking transparency like traditional statistical models, which means if anything goes off, humans may not be able to

Table 1 General guidelines for anonymizing data to protect privacy (adapted from Collins et al. [59])

How to anonymize data to safeguard privacy?
1. Data deidentification is a **shared duty** for everyone who works with it.
2. The **data protection officer (DPO)** is in charge of all data protection compliance issues.
3. All data that is to be **gathered, approved, and maintained** in accordance with the organization's data protection office's requirements.
4. A **DPO's tasks** include: • Informing and counseling organizations on their data protection duties. • Monitoring compliance with the legislation and related policies, as well as personnel knowledge and training. • Providing procedures, guidance, and advice to support this policy, such as for Data Protection Impact Assessments (DPIAs). • Assisting the Information Commissioner's Office as the organization's initial point of contact (ICO). • Handling third-party subject access requests and official requests for personal data. • Losses and unlawful disclosures of personal data are being investigated.
5. **Organizational accountability** is required under GDPR to implement the following measures: • Governance issues on a broad scale. • Impact assessments on privacy. • By design, there are privacy safeguards.
6. **Legality**: Data processing must be done for a specified reason that the user has agreed to, and it must match how it is described.
7. **Reason limitations**: Data will only be used for a specific purpose that the user has given clear agreement to.
8. **Data minimization**: Think about what data you have and why you have it. Capture only the information you require.
9. **Data accuracy**: Ensure that the data is correct, and that it is kept in a fashion that allows the user to change or delete it (securely).
10. **Limitations on storage**: Data that is no longer needed should be deleted. To safeguard users' identities, data should be pseudonymized if maintained for longer than necessary.
11. **Integrity**: Processors must secure user data from unauthorized access or loss. Encryption of user data and privacy by default design is ideal.

explain why. Transparency and reproducibility will be aided by the adoption of standardized performance metrics for key index procedures. To achieve this, metrics will need to be open source and culminated together in data registries in established robotic surgery networks [83]. The development of research networks that share open-source material is already established in areas of healthcare such as diagnostic imaging [84].

Bias and Inequality It has been reported that AI technologies have the potential for algorithmic bias and may bring medical inequality by reinforcing discriminatory practices based on race, sex, or other features. Transparency of training data and of model interpretability would enable evaluation for potential biases. Machine learning could be a solution to resolve recognized biases [85]. A recent Delphi consensus view concluded that AI could avoid certain biases that may occur in human assessments, but maybe worse in other areas. Among the Delphi panelist, there was 100% consensus that both confirmation bias and interpretation bias would be better or at least the same with AI. Whereas there was concern that both prediction bias and information bias could be worse or equivalent with AI [59].

Accountability and Liability If a patient suffers from an adverse event due to AI-based technology, it is not presently clear who would be responsible. With the utilization of AI algorithms to facilitate medical diagnosis, treatment strategy, and even operational procedures, the responsibility will shift from the physician mainly to a shared liability among the physician, the vendor providing the software, the developer who built the algorithm, and even the source for the training data [86].

The implementation of AI into medicine, or specifically the surgical field, is not simply a technical question but a multidimensional question that must involve a multidisciplinary team to solve. For the surgeon, the ideal role is to be a critical link between patients, data scientists, and regulators. After all, no one knows better than a physician what a patient needs and what technology may benefit them eventually.

9 Conclusions

The intersection of AI and surgery is a swiftly evolving field, harboring the potential to optimize surgical safety and quality. Predictive machine learning models have been used for preoperative surgical patient selection, intraoperative intelligent assistance, and postoperative outcome prediction. Reinforcement learning empowers surgical robots to learn procedures autonomously through expert demonstrations, trial-and-error, or a hybrid of these two approaches, which is extremely useful in autonomous surgery design. Various studies have used AI models to provide objective and efficient surgical assessment, with the fundamental goal of providing timely and meaningful surgical feedback. With the rapid development of computer science and surgical techniques, the story of applying AI in the surgical field has just begun.

References

1. Goldenberg SL, Nir G, Salcudean SE. A new era: artificial intelligence and machine learning in prostate cancer. Nat Rev Urol. 2019;16:391–403. https://doi.org/10.1038/s41585-019-0193-3.
2. Nam JG, Park S, Hwang EJ, Lee JH, Jin K-N, Lim KY, et al. Development and validation of deep learning–based automatic detection algorithm for malignant pulmonary nodules on chest

radiographs. Radiology. 2018;290:218–28. https://doi.org/10.1148/radiol.2018180237.
3. Gulshan V, Peng L, Coram M, Stumpe MC, Wu D, Narayanaswamy A, et al. Development and validation of a deep learning algorithm for detection of diabetic retinopathy in retinal fundus photographs. JAMA. 2016;316:2402–10. https://doi.org/10.1001/jama.2016.17216.
4. Komorowski M, Celi LA, Badawi O, Gordon AC, Faisal AA. The Artificial Intelligence Clinician learns optimal treatment strategies for sepsis in intensive care. Nat Med. 2018;24:1716–20. https://doi.org/10.1038/s41591-018-0213-5.
5. Avati A, Jung K, Harman S, Downing L, Ng A, Shah NH. Improving palliative care with deep learning. BMC Med Inform Decis Mak. 2018;18:122. https://doi.org/10.1186/s12911-018-0677-8.
6. Silver D, Huang A, Maddison CJ, Guez A, Sifre L, van den Driessche G, et al. Mastering the game of Go with deep neural networks and tree search. Nature. 2016;529:484–9. https://doi.org/10.1038/nature16961.
7. Duda RO, Hart PE, Stork DG. Pattern classification. 2nd ed. Wiley; 2000.
8. Bishop CM. Pattern recognition and machine learning. 1st ed. Springer; 2006.
9. Esteva A, Robicquet A, Ramsundar B, Kuleshov V, DePristo M, Chou K, et al. A guide to deep learning in healthcare. Nat Med. 2019;25:24–9. https://doi.org/10.1038/s41591-018-0316-z.
10. Kassahun Y, Yu B, Tibebu AT, Stoyanov D, Giannarou S, Metzen JH, et al. Surgical robotics beyond enhanced dexterity instrumentation: a survey of machine learning techniques and their role in intelligent and autonomous surgical actions. Int J CARS. 2016;11:553–68. https://doi.org/10.1007/s11548-015-1305-z.
11. Chen J, Remulla D, Nguyen JH, Aastha D, Liu Y, Dasgupta P, et al. Current status of artificial intelligence applications in urology and their potential to influence clinical practice. BJU Int. 2019;124:567–77. https://doi.org/10.1111/bju.14852.
12. Levin M, McKechnie T, Kruse CC, Aldrich K, Grantcharov TP, Langerman A. Surgical data recording in the operating room: a systematic review of modalities and metrics. Br J Surg. 2021;108:613–21. https://doi.org/10.1093/bjs/znab016.
13. Xi IL, Zhao Y, Wang R, Chang M, Purkayastha S, Chang K, et al. Deep learning to distinguish benign from malignant renal lesions based on routine MR imaging. Clin Cancer Res. 2020;26:1944–52. https://doi.org/10.1158/1078-0432.CCR-19-0374.
14. Kunapuli G, Varghese BA, Ganapathy P, Desai B, Cen S, Aron M, et al. A decision-support tool for renal mass classification. J Digit Imaging. 2018;31:929–39. https://doi.org/10.1007/s10278-018-0100-0.
15. Feng Z, Rong P, Cao P, Zhou Q, Zhu W, Yan Z, et al. Machine learning-based quantitative texture analysis of CT images of small renal masses: differentiation of angiomyolipoma without visible fat from renal cell carcinoma. Eur Radiol. 2018;28:1625–33. https://doi.org/10.1007/s00330-017-5118-z.
16. Miskin N, Qin L, Matalon SA, Tirumani SH, Alessandrino F, Silverman SG, et al. Stratification of cystic renal masses into benign and potentially malignant: applying machine learning to the bosniak classification. Abdom Radiol. 2021;46:311–8. https://doi.org/10.1007/s00261-020-02629-w.
17. Kocak B, Durmaz ES, Ates E, Kaya OK, Kilickesmez O. Unenhanced CT texture analysis of clear cell renal cell carcinomas: a machine learning-based study for predicting histopathologic nuclear grade. AJR Am J Roentgenol. 2019;212:W1–8. https://doi.org/10.2214/AJR.18.20742.
18. Lin F, Cui E-M, Lei Y, Luo L-P. CT-based machine learning model to predict the Fuhrman nuclear grade of clear cell renal cell carcinoma. Abdom Radiol (NY). 2019;44:2528–34. https://doi.org/10.1007/s00261-019-01992-7.
19. Gandaglia G, Popa I, Abdollah F, Schiffmann J, Shariat SF, Briganti A, et al. The effect of neoadjuvant chemotherapy on perioperative outcomes in patients who have bladder cancer treated with radical cystectomy: a population-based study. Eur Urol. 2014;66:561–8. https://doi.org/10.1016/j.eururo.2014.01.014.
20. Klén R, Salminen AP, Mahmoudian M, Syvänen KT, Elo LL, Boström PJ. Prediction of complication related death after radical cystectomy for bladder cancer with machine learning methodology. Scand J Urol. 2019;53:325–31. https://doi.org/10.1080/21681805.2019.1665579.
21. Auffenberg GB, Ghani KR, Ramani S, Usoro E, Denton B, Rogers C, et al. askMUSIC: leveraging a clinical registry to develop a new machine learning model to inform patients of prostate cancer treatments chosen by similar men. Eur Urol. 2019;75:901–7. https://doi.org/10.1016/j.eururo.2018.09.050.
22. Haifler M, Pence I, Sun Y, Kutikov A, Uzzo RG, Mahadevan-Jansen A, et al. Discrimination of malignant and normal kidney tissue with short wave infrared dispersive Raman spectroscopy. J Biophotonics. 2018;11:e201700188. https://doi.org/10.1002/jbio.201700188.
23. Altieri M, Hashimoto D, Rivera AM, Namazi B, Alseidi A, Okrainec A, et al. Using artificial intelligence to identify surgical anatomy, safe zones of DISSection, and dangerous zones of DISSection during laparoscopic cholecystectomy. J Am Coll Surg. 2020;231:e21–2. https://doi.org/10.1016/j.jamcollsurg.2020.08.054.
24. Porpiglia F, Checcucci E, Amparore D, Autorino R, Piana A, Bellin A, et al. Augmented-reality robot-assisted radical prostatectomy using hyper-accuracy three-dimensional reconstruction (HA3D™) technology: a radiological and pathological study. BJU Int. 2019;123:834–45. https://doi.org/10.1111/bju.14549.
25. Porpiglia F, Checcucci E, Amparore D, Manfredi M, Massa F, Piazzolla P, et al. Three-dimensional elastic augmented-reality robot-assisted radical prostatectomy using hyperaccuracy three-dimensional reconstruction technology: a step further in the identification of capsular involvement. Eur Urol. 2019;76:505–14. https://doi.org/10.1016/j.eururo.2019.03.037.
26. Porpiglia F, Checcucci E, Amparore D, Piana A, Piramide F, Volpi G, et al. Extracapsular extension on neurovascular bundles during robot-assisted radical prostatectomy precisely localized by 3d automatic augmented-reality rendering. J Urol. 2020;203:e1297. https://doi.org/10.1097/JU.0000000000000980.012.
27. Ma R, Vanstrum EB, Lee R, Chen J, Hung AJ. Machine learning in the optimization of robotics in the operative field. Curr Opin Urol. 2020;30:808–16. https://doi.org/10.1097/MOU.0000000000000816.
28. Yang G-Z, Cambias J, Cleary K, Daimler E, Drake J, Dupont PE, et al. Medical robotics—regulatory, ethical, and legal considerations for increasing levels of autonomy. Sci Robot. 2017;2:eaam8638. https://doi.org/10.1126/scirobotics.aam8638.
29. Koukourikis P, Rha KH. Robotic surgical systems in urology: What is currently available? Investig Clin Urol. 2021;62:14–22. https://doi.org/10.4111/icu.20200387.
30. Fan S, Dai X, Yang K, Xiong S, Xiong G, Li Z, et al. Robot-assisted pyeloplasty using a new robotic system, the KangDuo-Surgical Robot-01: a prospective, single-centre, single-arm clinical study. BJU Int. 2021;128(2):162–5. https://doi.org/10.1111/bju.15396.
31. deBeche-Adams T, Eubanks WS, de la Fuente SG. Early experience with the Senhance®-laparoscopic/robotic platform in the US. J Robot Surg. 2019;13:357–9. https://doi.org/10.1007/s11701-018-0893-3.
32. Cadeddu JA. Re: early experience with the Senhance®-laparoscopic/robotic platform in the US. J Urol. 2019;202:642–3. https://doi.org/10.1097/01.JU.0000576800.80970.1c.
33. Gilling P, Barber N, Bidair M, Anderson P, Sutton M, Aho T, et al. WATER: a double-blind, randomized, controlled trial of Aquablation® vs transurethral resection of the prostate in benign

prostatic hyperplasia. J Urol. 2018;199:1252–61. https://doi.org/10.1016/j.juro.2017.12.065.
34. Desai M, Bidair M, Bhojani N, Trainer A, Arther A, Kramolowsky E, et al. WATER II (80-150 mL) procedural outcomes. BJU Int. 2019;123:106–12. https://doi.org/10.1111/bju.14360.
35. Panesar S, Cagle Y, Chander D, Morey J, Fernandez-Miranda J, Kliot M. Artificial intelligence and the future of surgical robotics. Ann Surg. 2019;270:223–6. https://doi.org/10.1097/SLA.0000000000003262.
36. Wang Z, Zi B, Ding H, You W, Yu L. Hybrid grey prediction model-based autotracking algorithm for the laparoscopic visual window of surgical robot. Mech Mach Theory. 2018;123:107–23. https://doi.org/10.1016/j.mechmachtheory.2018.01.015.
37. Rivas-Blanco I, López-Casado C, Pérez-del-Pulgar CJ, García-Vacas F, Fraile JC, Muñoz VF. Smart cable-driven camera robotic assistant. IEEE Trans Hum-Mach Syst. 2018;2:183–96. https://doi.org/10.1109/THMS.2017.2767286.
38. Sun Y, Pan B, Fu Y, Cao F. Development of a novel intelligent laparoscope system for semi-automatic minimally invasive surgery. Int J Med Robot Comput Assist Surg. 2020;16:879. https://doi.org/10.1002/rcs.2049.
39. Wagner M, Bihlmaier A, Kenngott HG, Mietkowski P, Scheikl PM, Bodenstedt S, et al. A learning robot for cognitive camera control in minimally invasive surgery. Surg Endosc. 2021;35:5365–74. https://doi.org/10.1007/s00464-021-08509-8.
40. Samiei A, Miller R, Lyne J, Smith A, Stewart S, Gomer H, et al. Molecular chemical imaging endoscope, an innovative imaging modality for enhancing the surgeon's view during laparoscopic procedures. J Urol. 2019;201:e282–3. https://doi.org/10.1097/01.JU.0000555510.24601.ef.
41. Shvets A, Rakhlin A, Kalinin AA, Iglovikov V. Automatic instrument segmentation in robot-assisted surgery using deep learning. 2018 17th IEEE international conference on machine learning and applications (ICMLA), 2018:624–8. https://doi.org/10.1109/ICMLA.2018.00100.
42. Sun Y, Pan B, Fu Y. Lightweight deep neural network for real-time instrument semantic segmentation in robot assisted minimally invasive surgery. IEEE Robot Autom Lett. 2021;6:3870–7. https://doi.org/10.1109/LRA.2021.3066956.
43. Osa T, Sugita N, Mitsuishi M. Online trajectory planning and force control for automation of surgical tasks. IEEE Trans Autom Sci Eng. 2018;15:675–91. https://doi.org/10.1109/TASE.2017.2676018.
44. Baek D, Hwang M, Kim H, Kwon D. Path planning for automation of surgery robot based on probabilistic roadmap and reinforcement learning. 2018 15th international conference on ubiquitous robots (UR), 2018:342–7. https://doi.org/10.1109/URAI.2018.8441801.
45. Thananjeyan B, Garg A, Krishnan S, Chen C, Miller L, Goldberg K. Multilateral surgical pattern cutting in 2D orthotropic gauze with deep reinforcement learning policies for tensioning. 2017 IEEE international conference on robotics and automation (ICRA), 2017:2371–8. https://doi.org/10.1109/ICRA.2017.7989275.
46. Nguyen TT, Nguyen ND, Bello F, Nahavandi S. A new tensioning method using deep reinforcement learning for surgical pattern cutting 2019:1339–1344. https://doi.org/10.1109/ICIT.2019.8755235.
47. Shin C, Ferguson PW, Pedram SA, Ma J, Dutson EP, Rosen J. Autonomous tissue manipulation via surgical robot using learning based model predictive control. 2019 International conference on robotics and automation (ICRA) 2019:3875–81. https://doi.org/10.1109/ICRA.2019.8794159.
48. Pedram SA, Ferguson PW, Shin C, Mehta A, Dutson EP, Alambeigi F, et al. Toward synergic learning for autonomous manipulation of deformable tissues via surgical robots: an approximate Q-learning approach. 2020 8th IEEE RAS/EMBS international conference for biomedical robotics and biomechatronics (BioRob) 2020:878–84. https://doi.org/10.1109/BioRob49111.2020.9224421.
49. Bandini M, Fossati N, Briganti A. Nomograms in urologic oncology, advantages and disadvantages. Curr Opin Urol. 2019;29:42–51. https://doi.org/10.1097/MOU.0000000000000541.
50. Morlacco A, Modonutti D, Motterle G, Martino F, Dal Moro F, Novara G. Nomograms in urologic oncology: lights and shadows. J Clin Med. 2021;10:980. https://doi.org/10.3390/jcm10050980.
51. Bzdok D, Altman N, Krzywinski M. Statistics versus machine learning. Nat Methods. 2018;15:233–4. https://doi.org/10.1038/nmeth.4642.
52. Hung AJ, Chen J, Che Z, Nilanon T, Jarc A, Titus M, et al. Utilizing machine learning and automated performance metrics to evaluate robot-assisted radical prostatectomy performance and predict outcomes. J Endourol. 2018;32:438–44. https://doi.org/10.1089/end.2018.0035.
53. Hung AJ, Chen J, Gill IS. Automated performance metrics and machine learning algorithms to measure surgeon performance and anticipate clinical outcomes in robotic surgery. JAMA Surg. 2018;153:770–1. https://doi.org/10.1001/jamasurg.2018.1512.
54. Hung AJ, Chen J, Ghodoussipour S, Oh PJ, Liu Z, Nguyen J, et al. A deep-learning model using automated performance metrics and clinical features to predict urinary continence recovery after robot-assisted radical prostatectomy. BJU Int. 2019;124:487–95. https://doi.org/10.1111/bju.14735.
55. Hung AJ, Ma R, Cen S, Nguyen JH, Lei X, Wagner C. Surgeon automated performance metrics as predictors of early urinary continence recovery after robotic radical prostatectomy – a prospective Bi-institutional study. Eur Urol Open Sci. 2021;27:65–72. https://doi.org/10.1016/j.euros.2021.03.005.
56. Saum G, Reddy SS, Runzhuo M, Hwang DH, Jessica N, Hung AJ. An objective assessment of performance during robotic partial nephrectomy: validation and correlation of automated performance metrics with intraoperative outcomes. J Urol. 2021;205:1294–302. https://doi.org/10.1097/JU.0000000000001557.
57. Soguero-Ruiz C, Hindberg K, Rojo-Alvarez JL, Skrovseth SO, Godtliebsen F, Mortensen K, et al. Support vector feature selection for early detection of anastomosis leakage from bag-of-words in electronic health records. IEEE J Biomed Health Inform. 2016;20:1404–15. https://doi.org/10.1109/JBHI.2014.2361688.
58. Hung AJ. Can machine-learning algorithms replace conventional statistics? BJU Int. 2019;123:1–1. https://doi.org/10.1111/bju.14542.
59. Collins JW, Marcus HJ, Ghazi A, Sridhar A, Hashimoto D, Hager G, et al. Ethical implications of AI in robotic surgical training: a Delphi consensus statement. Eur Urol Focus. 2021; https://doi.org/10.1016/j.euf.2021.04.006.
60. Ma R, Reddy S, Vanstrum EB, Hung AJ. Innovations in urologic surgical training. Curr Urol Rep. 2021;22:26. https://doi.org/10.1007/s11934-021-01043-z.
61. Prebay ZJ, Peabody JO, Miller DC, Ghani KR. Video review for measuring and improving skill in urological surgery. Nat Rev Urol. 2019;16:261–7. https://doi.org/10.1038/s41585-018-0138-2.
62. Mazer L, Varban O, Montgomery JR, Awad MM, Schulman A. Video is better: why aren't we using it? A mixed-methods study of the barriers to routine procedural video recording and case review. Surg Endosc. 2021;36(2):1090–7. https://doi.org/10.1007/s00464-021-08375-4.
63. Hashimoto DA. Surgeons and machines can learn from operative video: will the system let them? Ann Surg. 2021;274(1):e96. https://doi.org/10.1097/SLA.0000000000004899.
64. Zia A, Guo L, Zhou L, Essa I, Jarc A. Novel evaluation of surgical activity recognition models using task-based efficiency metrics. Int J Comput Assist Radiol Surg. 2019;14:2155–63. https://doi.org/10.1007/s11548-019-02025-w.
65. Khalid S, Goldenberg M, Grantcharov T, Taati B, Rudzicz F. Evaluation of deep learning models for identifying surgical

actions and measuring performance. JAMA Netw Open. 2020;3:–e201664. https://doi.org/10.1001/jamanetworkopen.2020.1664.
66. Wang Z, Majewicz FA. Deep learning with convolutional neural network for objective skill evaluation in robot-assisted surgery. Int J Comput Assist Radiol Surg. 2018;13:1959–70. https://doi.org/10.1007/s11548-018-1860-1.
67. Luongo F, Hakim R, Nguyen JH, Anandkumar A, Hung AJ. Deep learning-based computer vision to recognize and classify suturing gestures in robot-assisted surgery. Surgery. 2020; https://doi.org/10.1016/j.surg.2020.08.016.
68. Mascagni P, Alapatt D, Urade T, Vardazaryan A, Mutter D, Marescaux J, et al. A computer vision platform to automatically locate critical events in surgical videos: documenting safety in laparoscopic cholecystectomy. Ann Surg. 2021;274(1):e93–5. https://doi.org/10.1097/SLA.0000000000004736.
69. Chen J, Cheng N, Cacciamani G, Oh P, Lin-Brande M, Remulla D, et al. Objective assessment of robotic surgical technical skill: a systematic review. J Urol. 2019;201:461–9. https://doi.org/10.1016/j.juro.2018.06.078.
70. Ghasemloonia A, Maddahi Y, Zareinia K, Lama S, Dort JC, Sutherland GR. Surgical skill assessment using motion quality and smoothness. J Surg Educ. 2017;74:295–305. https://doi.org/10.1016/j.jsurg.2016.10.006.
71. Fard MJ, Ameri S, Ellis RD, Chinnam RB, Pandya AK, Klein MD. Automated robot-assisted surgical skill evaluation: predictive analytics approach. Int J Med Robot Comput Assist Surg. 2018;14:e1850. https://doi.org/10.1002/rcs.1850.
72. Chen AB, Liang S, Nguyen JH, Liu Y, Hung AJ. Machine learning analyses of automated performance metrics during granular sub-stitch phases predict surgeon experience. Surgery. 2021;169:1245–9. https://doi.org/10.1016/j.surg.2020.09.020.
73. Baghdadi A, Hussein AA, Ahmed Y, Cavuoto LA, Guru KA. A computer vision technique for automated assessment of surgical performance using surgeons' console-feed videos. Int J Comput Assist Radiol Surg. 2019;14:697–707. https://doi.org/10.1007/s11548-018-1881-9.
74. Jin A, Yeung S, Jopling J, Krause J, Azagury D, Milstein A, et al. Tool detection and operative skill assessment in surgical videos using region-based convolutional neural networks. 2018 IEEE winter conference on applications of computer vision (WACV), 2018:691–699. https://doi.org/10.1109/WACV.2018.00081.
75. Richstone L, Schwartz MJ, Seideman C, Cadeddu J, Marshall S, Kavoussi LR. Eye metrics as an objective assessment of surgical skill. Ann Surg. 2010;252:177–82. https://doi.org/10.1097/SLA.0b013e3181e464fb.
76. Koskinen J, Bednarik R, Vrzakova H, Elomaa A-P. Combined gaze metrics as stress-sensitive indicators of microsurgical proficiency. Surg Innov. 2020;27:614–22. https://doi.org/10.1177/1553350620942980.
77. Ismail Fawaz H, Forestier G, Weber J, Idoumghar L, Muller P-A. Accurate and interpretable evaluation of surgical skills from kinematic data using fully convolutional neural networks. Int J CARS. 2019;14:1611–7. https://doi.org/10.1007/s11548-019-02039-4.
78. Price WN, Cohen IG. Privacy in the age of medical big data. Nat Med. 2019;25:37–43. https://doi.org/10.1038/s41591-018-0272-7.
79. Collins JW, Levy J, Stefanidis D, Gallagher A, Coleman M, Cecil T, et al. Utilising the Delphi process to develop a proficiency-based progression train-the-trainer course for robotic surgery training. Eur Urol. 2019;75:775–85. https://doi.org/10.1016/j.eururo.2018.12.044.
80. Collins JW, Ghazi A, Stoyanov D, Hung A, Coleman M, Cecil T, et al. Utilising an accelerated Delphi process to develop guidance and protocols for telepresence applications in remote robotic surgery training. Eur Urol Open Sci. 2020;22:23–33. https://doi.org/10.1016/j.euros.2020.09.005.
81. Hashimoto DA, Rosman G, Witkowski ER, Stafford C, Navarette-Welton AJ, Rattner DW, et al. Computer vision analysis of intraoperative video: automated recognition of operative steps in laparoscopic sleeve gastrectomy. Ann Surg. 2019;270:414–21. https://doi.org/10.1097/SLA.0000000000003460.
82. He J, Baxter SL, Xu J, Xu J, Zhou X, Zhang K. The practical implementation of artificial intelligence technologies in medicine. Nat Med. 2019;25:30–6. https://doi.org/10.1038/s41591-018-0307-0.
83. Collins J, Akre O, Challacombe B, Karim O, Wiklund P. Robotic networks: delivering empowerment through integration. BJU Int. 2015;116:167–8. https://doi.org/10.1111/bju.13032.
84. Project MONAI n.d.. https://monai.io/ (accessed July 8, 2021).
85. Char DS, Shah NH, Magnus D. Implementing machine learning in health care – addressing ethical challenges. N Engl J Med. 2018;378:981–3. https://doi.org/10.1056/NEJMp1714229.
86. Topol EJ. High-performance medicine: the convergence of human and artificial intelligence. Nat Med. 2019;25:44–56. https://doi.org/10.1038/s41591-018-0300-7.

Part II

Prostate

Robotic Simple Prostatectomy

Ram A. Pathak, Marcio C. Moschovas, David D. Thiel, and Ashok K. Hemal

1 Background

Management of bladder outlet obstruction (BOO) secondary to benign prostatic hyperplasia (BPH) is dependent on the degree of lower urinary tract symptoms (LUTS). Oftentimes, medical management is prescribed initially. As LUTS progress and become more severe, dual therapy with a combination alpha-blocker and a 5-alpha reductase inhibitor is recommended based on the findings of the Medical Therapy of Prostate Symptoms (MTOPS) trial [1]. Surgery, however, can be considered initially and is recommended in patients with renal insufficiency due to BPH, catheter dependence, recurrent urinary tract infections, recurrent gross hematuria, or cystolithiasis [2]. There is a multitude of surgical options ranging from minimally invasive surgical therapies (MIST) to open or robotic prostate removal. Treatment is not innocuous and can have significant perioperative morbidity [3]. To assist clinicians in triaging patients to the appropriate surgical therapy, an amendment to the 2018 AUA Guidelines for BPH published in 2020 strongly encourages urologists to rely on prostate size and morphology when determining treatment [4]. For large prostates (>80 g), laser enucleation of the prostate or simple prostatectomy remains the only recommended options. Herein, we will discuss the role of robotic simple prostatectomy in the management of LUTS attributed to BPH.

Since the initial publication of laparoscopic simple prostatectomy [5], several studies have cemented the superiority of the laparoscopic technique over the open approach with respect to estimated blood loss (EBL), continuous bladder irrigation (CBI) time, duration of catheterization, and length of hospital stay (LOS) [6, 7]. Shortly thereafter, the robotic technique became popularized [8–10]. Data from a multi-institutional series of 487 patients undergoing robotic simple prostatectomy solidified this approach, demonstrating superior functional outcomes defined by International Prostate Symptom Score <8 and maximum flow rate >15 with a minimal intraoperative complication rate (3.2%) [11]. A recent comprehensive review of the literature was performed illustrating several nuances in surgical technique over the past 20 years [12]. In this chapter, we will review some of the more popularized approaches and examine specific surgical innovations that have contributed to the manner in which we perform the procedure today.

2 Preoperative Patient Selection

Patients with symptomatic LUTS in enlarged glands (>80 g) serve as the main indication for performing a simple prostatectomy. An expanded indication can be considered in patients who require concomitant surgery due to symptomatic bladder diverticula, inguinal hernia repair, cystolithotomy, or other pelvic pathology. A thorough patient history and examination is integral due to the inherent risk of prostate cancer, especially in elderly patient. If required, we routinely perform prostate biopsy in a risk-stratified manner employing shared decision-making with both provider and patient input. Usually, these patients are referred to with appropriate imaging studies. CT Urogram is indicated in patients with a history of hematuria, stone disease, or recurrent UTI. Select patients can undergo multi-parametric MRI to further stratify the risk of prostate cancer.

R. A. Pathak · A. K. Hemal (✉)
Atrium Health Wake Forest Baptist, Winston-Salem, NC, USA

M. C. Moschovas
Advent Health, Celebration, FL, USA

D. D. Thiel
Mayo Clinic Florida, Jacksonville, FL, USA

P. Wiklund et al. (eds.), *Robotic Urologic Surgery*, https://doi.org/10.1007/978-3-031-00363-9_10

3 Patient Positioning and Port Placement (Standard Transperitoneal Approach)

Patients are routinely positioned in dorsal lithotomy and arms tucked with care to pad all pressure points. Alternatively, patients can be placed in supine position with the robot (Xi®) docked perpendicularly. The operating table is tilted in Trendelenburg position to about 25–28°. Side-docking can also be utilized with the patient in supine position. For patients undergoing a multi- or single-port extra-peritoneal technique, the Trendelenburg position is not necessary.

Port placement [13] is similar to robotic radical prostatectomy which includes a central camera port (above or below the umbilicus), flanking robotic trocars with an additional left robotic trocar approximately 3–4 cm cranial to the anterior superior iliac spine (ASIS). A 12-mm and 5-mm assistant port are placed 3–4 cm above the right ASIS and lateral and cranial to the camera port, respectively (Fig. 1). For patients undergoing an extra-peritoneal multi-port approach, a 2–3 cm periumbilical incision is made and dissection is carried to the posterior rectus sheath. A balloon dilator is then utilized and under direct visualization, the space of Retzius is developed. Port placement can be done under direct vision in a similar template as above. For single-port, a similar incision is made as the extra-peritoneal approach; however, the bladder is incised and the robot is docked in a trans-vesical manner [14].

Instruments that are required for this case include monopolar scissors, Maryland bipolar forceps, ProGrasp™ forceps, and one of two needle drivers (SutureCut™). If available, the surgeon may also use a robotic Tenaculum forceps but 0 PDS stay sutures can suffice just as well.

4 Surgical Technique

A multitude of techniques and approaches have been described when performing robotic simple prostatectomy [12] with no Level I evidence of one technique or approach showing superiority over another. With respect to approach, the first step in the decision tree (Fig. 2) is to decide if the surgery will be performed in an extraperitoneal or transperitoneal approach. The extraperitoneal approach may be preferred in patients with a hostile abdomen due to significant prior surgical history. Although the dissection ***to*** the adenoma may differ, the technique of dissecting and extracting the adenoma is similar.

4.1 Transperitoneal

Bladder mobilization is initiated by incising medial to the medial umbilical ligaments and the space of Retzius is exposed. The dissection is carried until the peri-prostatic fat is visualized. The fat overlying the prostate is dissected off the prostate exposing the superficial venous complex which is ligated. There is no need to do any further apical dissection, ligate the dorsal venous complex or incise the endopelvic fascia as is commonly done in radical prostatectomy. At this point, an incision can either be made at the prostatic capsule, bladder neck, or 1–2 cm proximal to the bladder neck depending on surgeon preference (Fig. 3). Typically, for significant intravesical protrusion, a greater visualization of the bladder is required and therefore a more generous, proximal bladder neck incision should be made.

Inevitably, at this step, surgeons can encounter a median lobe. Elevation of the median lobe using stay sutures allows

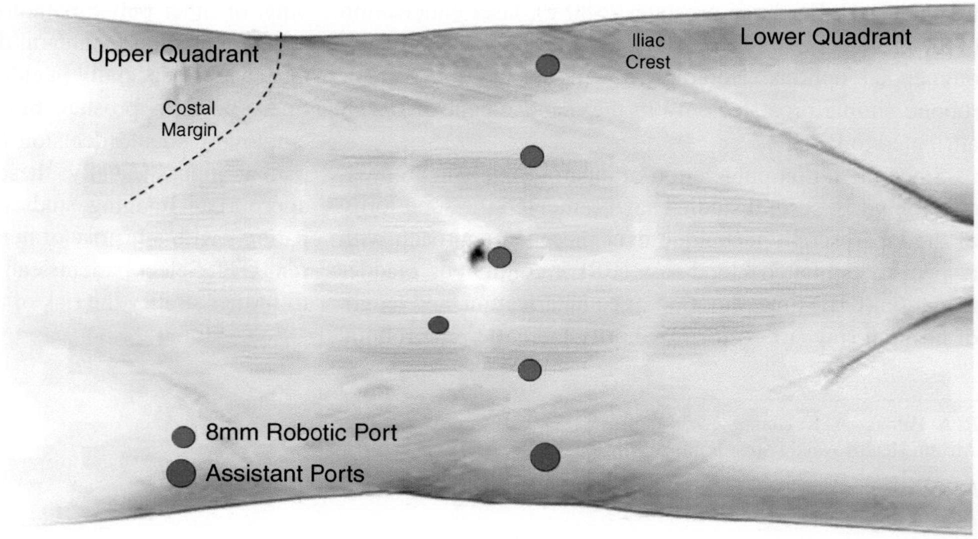

Fig. 1 Port placement for robotic simple prostatectomy. Port placement for robotic simple prostatectomy is shown above. Four 8mm robotic trocars are placed with one 12mm and one 5mm assistant port

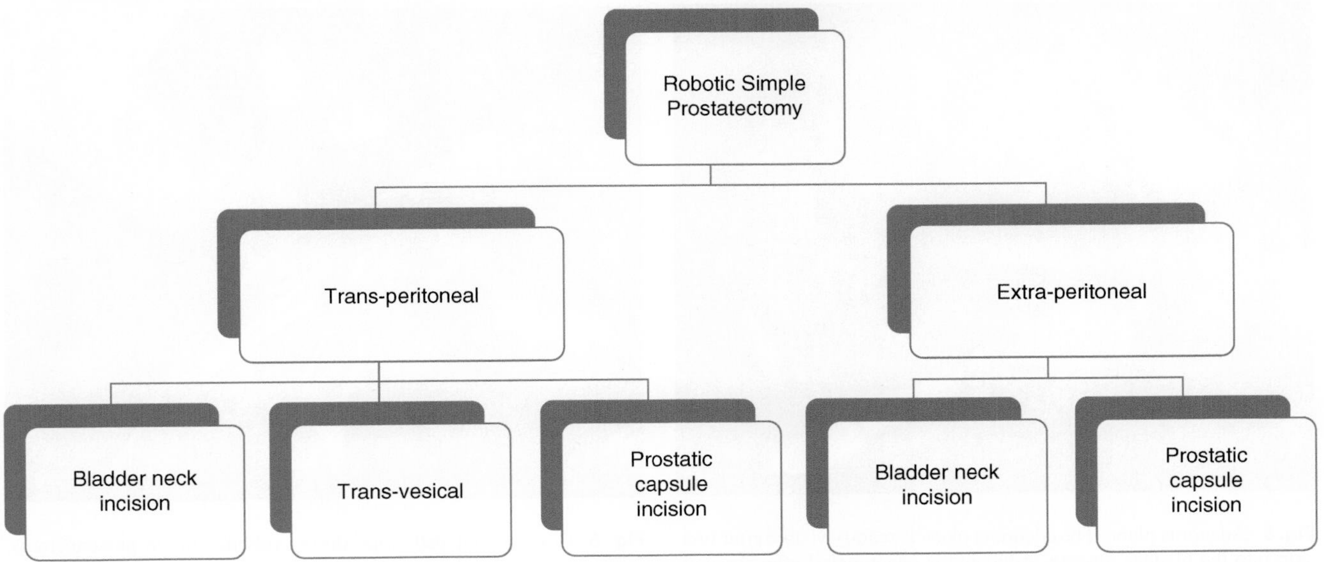

Fig. 2 Decision tree algorithm for approach to robotic simple prostatectomy. A multitude of approaches can be adopted when performing robotic simple prostatectomy dependent on concomitant pathology, prostate morphology, and patient characteristics

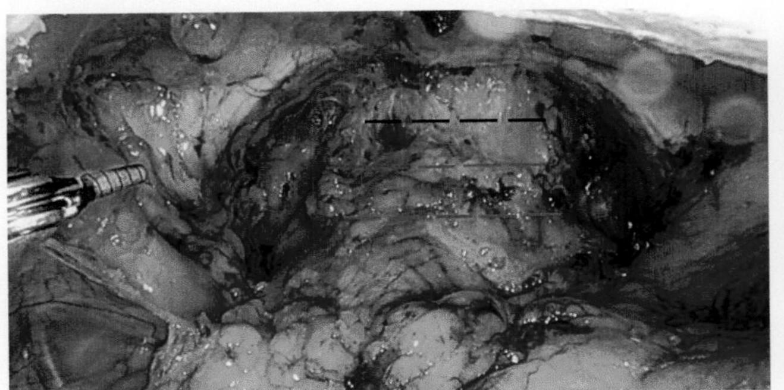

Fig. 3 Prostatic incision vs. bladder neck incision vs. proximal bladder neck incision. Black-dotted line: Prostatic capsule incision. Red-dotted line: Bladder neck incision. Blue-dotted line: Proximal bladder neck incision

identification of the trigone and clear visualization of the bilateral ureteral orifices. It also permits identification of the posterior bladder wall mucosa and overlying median lobe or intravesical protrusion (Fig. 4). After making an incision on the bladder mucosa the shiny, white adenoma is visualized and the posterior plane established (Fig. 5). This plane is developed with a combination of both sharp and blunt dissection utilizing cautery where needed. Posterior dissection is completed at the level of the anatomic capsule and then lateral and anterolateral dissection may ensue. However, more practically, toggling between posterior, lateral, and anterior dissection is routinely done, especially in large glands with limited working space. The EndoWrist® instruments facilitate this dissection by maintaining the various angles of the anatomic capsule. Focal coagulation can assist with hemostasis and following the correct plane. Continuous application of sequential stay sutures or manipulation with a robotic Tenaculum forceps is needed to facilitate dissection.

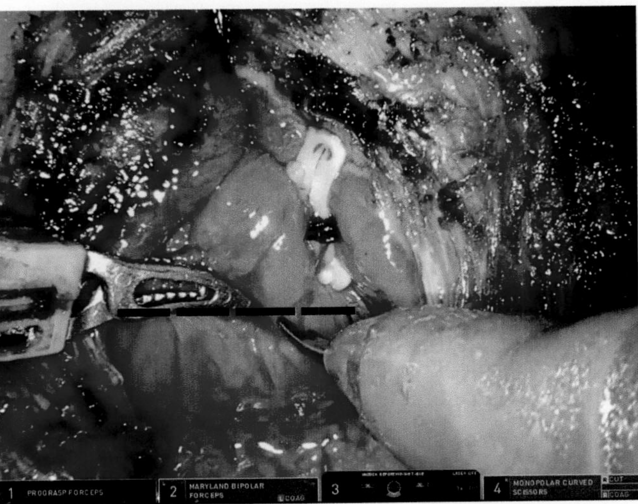

Fig. 4 Incision overlying the posterior bladder wall. An incision is made approximately second/third anterior from the posterior bladder neck on the mucosal overlying the median lobe

When approaching the distal prostatic urethra, first ensure the foley catheter is advanced. The assistant should grab the prostatic capsule anteriorly while the third arm is retracting the prostate cranially. The urethra can be seen by incising the distal most aspect of the anterior commissure. The urethra can then be divided sharply at the apex, freeing the specimen

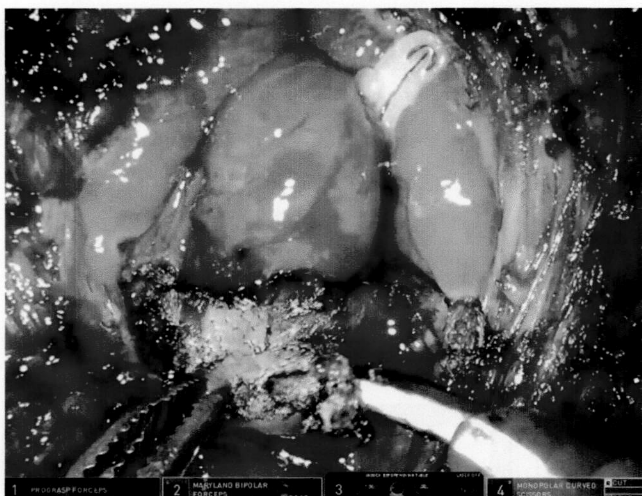

Fig. 5 Adenoma plane. The adenoma plane is readily visible after incision into the bladder mucosa. Adenoma is encountered after the incision is made and is characterized by white shiny tissue

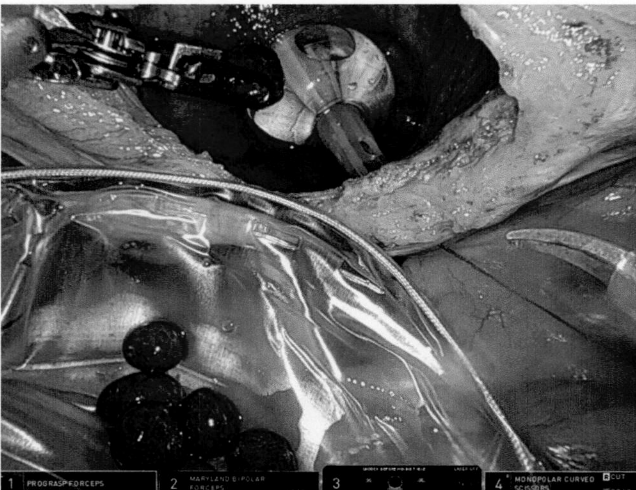

Fig. 6 Concomitant pathology during robotic simple prostatectomy. Stones are removed from the bladder and placed into a specimen retrieval bag

from the capsule of the prostate. The specimen can be placed in a retrieval bag or alternatively taken out piece-meal to avoid a large extraction incision.

After removal of the adenoma, the potential space should be inspected to ensure adequate hemostasis. This may be achieved by using focal bipolar cautery or running sutures. A complete circumferential anastomosis is preferred [9] using 3–0 barbed suture in a running fashion similar to the vesico-urethral anastomosis in radical robotic prostatectomy. The surgeon should take particular attention to identifying the effluxing ureteral orifice so as not to injure these vital structures. Often with this technique, there is no need for a 3-way catheter and continuous bladder irrigation. The urethral catheter should remain for a minimum of 3–5 days.

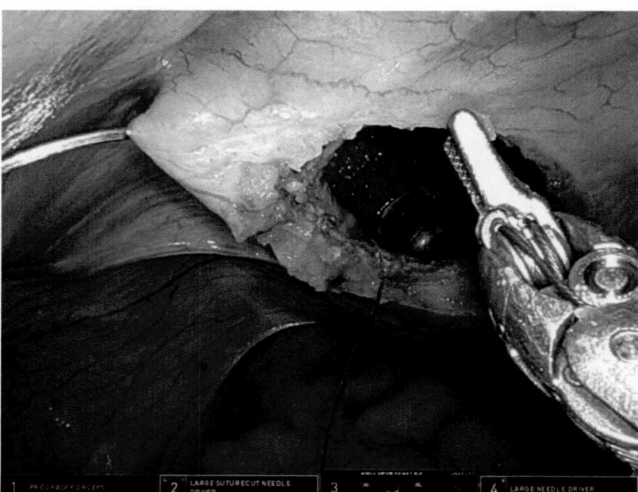

Fig. 7 Longitudinal incision on the wall of the bladder. A longitudinal incision is made on the bladder exposing the foley catheter balloon and prostate

4.2 Transvesical

The transperitoneal, transvesical approach is ideal for patients who need concomitant diverticulum surgery (especially posteriorly located) or in patients with multiple bladder stones (Fig. 6). This approach allows facile identification of the additional pathology.

A generous, longitudinal incision is made in the posterior bladder exposing the Foley catheter and bladder mucosa (Fig. 7). Stay sutures are used to maintain exposure to the prostate (Fig. 8). The prostate is identified and the mucosa overlying the prostate is incised. The remainder of the operation is identical to the technique described above. Closure of the bladder is done in 2 layers. CBI is not necessary and the catheter should remain for about 5–7 days.

4.3 Extraperitoneal

The extraperitoneal approach is ideal in patients who have had prior surgery and the concern for scar tissue is high. Disadvantages of this approach are limited working space and significant difficulty in establishing the proper plane in patients with history of laparoscopic inguinal hernia repair with mesh.

A 2–3 cm infraumbilical incision is made exposing the posterior rectus sheath. Next, a balloon dilator is used to develop the space of Retzius. Ports can be placed in a similar

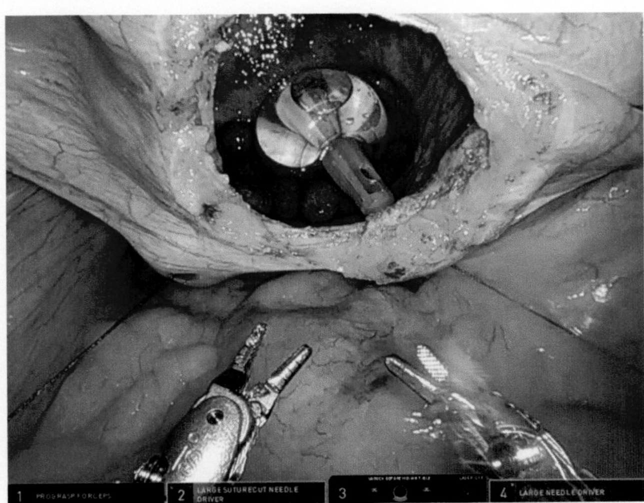

Fig. 8 Use of stay sutures on bladder. Stay sutures are used to maintain exposure to the prostate during robotic simple prostatectomy

template with similar spacing as the intraperitoneal approach. After developing this space, the prostate is readily identified and an incision on the prostate or bladder neck can be made. Technique of removing the adenoma is similar to the above.

5 Commentary

Several alternatives have supplanted transurethral resection of the prostate secondary to the minimal perioperative morbidity profile of these newer treatments. However, as the prostate gland approaches 80 g, the AUA guidelines propose simple prostatectomy or enucleation as the preferred management strategy [4]. A relatively higher perioperative morbidity profile has made open simple prostatectomy less favorable [15], paving way for the minimally invasive robotic approach.

The initial technique of laparoscopic simple prostatectomy was published in 2002 [5]; however, estimated blood loss was 800 ml while operative time was approximately 225 min. When examining this technique over a follow-up of 6 years and 60 patients, estimated blood loss decreased to 331 ml with a mean operative time of 138 min [16]. Despite a superior perioperative complication profile, operative time remained high. The laparoscopic approach remained challenging due to a narrow operative field in the pelvis, difficulty in intracorporeal suturing, and limited ergonomics of laparoscopic instruments [10].

The robotic approach has largely supplanted the laparoscopic approach by overcoming these challenges. Improved dexterity and ergonomics of robotic instruments make the procedure technically easier for the surgeon. After being first described in a series of 7 patients in 2008 [8], the robotic approach was adapted to larger [17] and more complex cases [10]. Adoption of the robotic platform outpaced the laparoscopic approach by almost a 3:1 from 2012 to 2014 [11]. A key technical advance to robotic simple prostatectomy was the introduction of the urethro-vesical anastomosis. Both incomplete [18] and 360° [9] complete urethro-vesical anastomosis have been described. Both approaches minimize the need for continuous bladder irrigation hastening postoperative recovery while decreasing the length of stay [10].

A recent multi-institutional study reported functional outcomes and complication profiles of 1330 minimally invasive robotic simple prostatectomies, finding a median improvement in IPSS of 19 (23 → 4) and a median improvement in Qmax of 17 ml/s (5 ml/s → 22 ml/s) [11]. The 90-day perioperative complication rate was exceedingly low with 1.3% of patients experiencing a Grade 3 or higher complication.

5.1 Concomitant Pelvic Pathologies

Robotic simple prostatectomy can be a highly versatile operation as it can treat a variety of pelvic pathologies concomitantly. In a series of 20 patients undergoing robotic simple prostatectomy [10], the authors performed 6 concomitant procedures: inguinal hernia repair in two patients, cystolithotomy in three patients, and bladder diverticulectomy in one patient. The feasibility of performing adjunctive procedures at the same time of robotic simple prostatectomy is highly conducive. In fact, the robotic approach is preferential in these circumstances compared to a transurethral approach. In a large National Inpatient Sample (2002–2012) database consisting of 35,171 patients, bladder diverticulum was found in 5% of patients and 17% of patients underwent concomitant cystolithotomy [19]. In a series of 65 patients undergoing robotic bladder diverticulectomy, 4 patients successfully underwent concomitant robotic simple prostatectomy [20]. For these cases, a transvesical approach and identification of the diverticular neck or incision into the diverticulum itself [21] may be preferred. For diverticula located adjacent to the ureteral orifice, a double J stent is placed to minimize the risk of ureteral injury.

5.2 Prostate Adenocarcinoma

Active surveillance is the mainstay therapeutic management strategy for low-risk adenocarcinoma of the prostate. Typically, LUTS can be managed by medical therapy. However, in cases where LUTS persists despite maximal medical therapy, a therapeutic dilemma exists with respect to the patient's diagnosis of cancer: radical prostatectomy may incur unwanted side effects of urinary incontinence and/or erectile dysfunction and endoscopic enucleation techniques result in higher postoperative PSA compared to patients without cancer [22] and uncertainty and anxiety of posttreatment PSA follow-up exist [23].

Pathak and Hemal [24] describe a series of 12 patients who underwent a novel surgical procedure—robotic total prostatectomy (RTP) to combat the cancer diagnosis and treat the symptoms from the enlarged gland. The essence of the surgery is to resect the central, transitional, *and* peripheral zones to the level of the pseudocapsule. Technically, the procedure varies from simple prostatectomy as the dissection occurs at the level anterior to the anterior Denonvillier's fascia. This allows preservation of the musculofascial plate, without violation to the seminal vesical and ampulla of the vas deferens. Final pathology revealed adenocarcinoma in 11/12 patients (92%) with negative surgical margins. Mean postoperative PSA at 3 months was 0.03 with no patients requiring adjunctive hormonal or radiotherapy [24].

Moschovas et al. also addressed this conundrum by performing a modified simple prostatectomy in 34 patients with a full-nerve sparing technique, intrafascial dissection, and seminal vesical sparing [25]. Fifty percent of the patients harbored malignancy and AUA symptom score improved in 97% of patients.

5.3 Single-Port Platform Approach to Simple Prostatectomy

Recently, the da Vinci single-port platform has been used to popularize the simple prostatectomy operation. A GelPoint™ port is placed directly into the bladder dome. The robot is docked and the procedure is performed using a transvesical approach as described above. Kaouk et al. first described this technique initially in 10 patients. Minimal blood loss and hospital stay were reported in a series of 10 patients [26]. Advantages of this approach include not requiring steep Trendelenberg, minimal CO_2 absorption by maintaining pneumovesicum, and optimum working space.

5.4 Conclusion

Robotic simple prostatectomy remains a highly efficient and durable procedure for maximum improvement to a patient's voiding symptomatology and should be considered the standard approach for tackling enlarged prostate glands with or without concomitant pathology. The postoperative functional outcomes are excellent with many patients resolving the need for chronic catheterization. Compared to the open approach, utilizing the robotic platform has obviated the need for prolonged length of stay and excessive blood loss. An important technical advancement is performing a complete urethrovesical anastomosis precluding the need for continuous bladder irrigation. Moreover, robotic simple prostatectomy has a minimal learning curve for those surgeons proficient in robotics.

References

1. McConnell JD, Roehrborn CG, Bautista OM, et al. The long-term effect of doxazosin, finasteride, and combination therapy on the clinical progression of benign prostatic hyperplasia. N Engl J Med. 2003;349(25):2387–98.
2. Foster HE, Barry MJ, Dahm P, et al. Surgical management of lower urinary tract symptoms attributed to benign prostatic hyperplasia: AUA Guideline. J Urol. 2018;200:612.
3. Pathak RA, Broderick GA, Igel TC, et al. Impact of minimally invasive benign prostatic hyperplasia therapies on 30- and 90-day postoperative office encounters. Urology. 2017;99:186–91.
4. Parsons JK, Dahm P, Kohler TS, et al. Surgical management of lower urinary tract symptoms attributed to benign prostatic hyperplasia: AUA Guideline amendment 2020. J Urol. 2020;204:799.
5. Mariano MB, Graziottin TM, Tefilli MV. Laparoscopic prostatectomy with vascular control for benign prostatic hyperplasia. J Urol. 2002;167:2528–9.
6. Baumert H, Ballaro A, Dugardin F, et al. Laparoscopic versus open simple prostatectomy: a comparative study. J Urol. 2006;175:1691–4.
7. McCullough TC, Heldwein FL, Soon SJ, et al. Laparoscopic versus open simple prostatectomy: an evaluation of morbidity. J Endourol. 2009;23:129–33.
8. Sotelo R, Clavijo R, Carmona O, et al. Robotic simple prostatectomy. J Urol. 2008;179:513–5.
9. Dubey D, Hemal AK. Robotic-assisted simple prostatectomy with complete urethrovesical reconstruction. Indian J Urol. 2012;28:231–2.
10. Patel MN, Hemal AK. Robot-assisted laparoscopic simple anatomic prostatectomy. Urol Clin North Am. 2013;31:385–92.
11. Autorino R, Zargar H, Mariano M, et al. Perioperative outcomes of robotic and laparoscopic simple prostatectomy: a European-American multi-institutional analysis. Eur Urol. 2014;68:86–94.
12. Moschovas MC, Timoteo F, Lins L, et al. Robotic surgery techniques to approach benign prostatic hyperplasia disease: a comprehensive literature review and the state of art. Asian J Urol. 2021;8:81–8.
13. Pathak RA, Patel M, Hemal AK. Comprehensive approach to port placement templates for robot-assisted laparoscopic urologic surgeries. J Endourol. 2017;31:1269–76.
14. Kaouk J, Sawczyn G, Wilson C, et al. Single-port percutaneous transvesical simple prostatectomy using the SP robotic system: initial clinical experience. Urology. 2020;141:171–3.
15. Gratzke C, Schlenker B, Seitz M, et al. Complications and early postoperative outcome after open prostatectomy in patients with benign prostatic enlargement: results of a prospective multicenter study. J Urol. 2007;177:1419–22.
16. Mariano M, Tefilli M, Graziottin T, et al. Laparoscopic prostatectomy for benign prostatic hyperplasia – a six-year experience. Eur Urol. 2005;49:127–32.
17. Singh I, Hudson J, Hemal AK. Robot-assisted laparoscopic prostatectomy for a giant prostate with retrieval of vesical stones. Int Urol Nephrol. 2010;42:615–9.
18. Coelho RF, Chauhan S, Sivaraman A, et al. Modified technique of robotic-assisted simple prostatectomy: advantages of a vesico-urethral anastomosis. BJU Int. 2012;109:426–33.

19. Pariser J, Pearce S, Patel S, et al. National trends of simple prostatectomy for benign prostatic hyperplasia with an analysis of risk factors for adverse perioperative outcomes. Urology. 2015;86:721–6.
20. Liu S, Pathak RA, Hemal AK. Robot-assisted laparoscopic bladder diverticulectomy: adaptation of techniques for a variety of clinical presentations. Urology. 2021;147:311–6.
21. Davidiuk AJ, Meschia C, Young P, et al. Robotic-assisted bladder diverticulectomy: assessment of outcomes and modifications of technique. Urology. 2015;85:1347–51.
22. Otsubo S, Yokomizo A, Mochida O, et al. Significant of prostate-specific antigen-related factors in incidental prostate cancer treated by holmium laser enucleation of the prostate. World J Urol. 2015;33:329–33.
23. Tan H, Marks L, Hoyt M, et al. The relationship between intolerance of uncertainly and anxiety in men on active surveillance for prostate cancer. J Urol. 2016;195:1724–30.
24. Pathak RA, Hemal AK. Management of low-risk prostate cancer in patients with enlarged glands and lower urinary tract symptoms: Robotic total prostatectomy, a novel technique. World J Urol. 2020;38(4):829–36.
25. Moschovas MC, Bhat S, Fikret O, et al. Modified simple prostatectomy: an approach to address large volume BPH and associated prostate cancers. J Robot Surg. 2020;14:543–8.
26. Kaouk J, Sawczyn G, Wilson C, et al. Single-port percutaneous transvesical simple prostatectomy using the SP robotic system: initial clinical experience. Urology. 2020;141:173–7.

Prostate Cancer Screening and Biopsy

K. R. Seetharam Bhat, Siddharth Yadav, Sarah Kind, Sanoj Punnen, and Anup Kumar

1 Introduction

Prostate cancer is the most common cancer and the second most common cause of cancer-related death in the USA [1]. Screening for prostate cancer typically involves clinical digital rectal examination (DRE) with serum prostate-specific antigen (PSA). Recent advances in imaging technology have improved the identification and localization of a potentially malignant lesion. However, a biopsy is still required to confirm and grade the disease.

2 Screening for Prostate Cancer

There is nothing more controversial in the field of urology than the routine screening for prostate cancer. Due to its relatively high cancer-specific survival rates compared to other cancers, we question whether we should routinely screen our patients for prostate cancer. Currently, the most contentious issue is the overdiagnosis of prostate cancer and the inability to identify low-grade prostate cancer that will become clinically significant in the future.

2.1 Digital Rectal Examination

A thorough DRE is recommended when prostate cancer is suspected. It has been a part of the standard screening and is currently recommended by most guidelines. The rectal exam's sensitivity, specificity, and PPV are 81, 40, and 42%, respectively [2]. An abnormal DRE indicates a more aggressive disease with possible high-volume prostate cancer. On secondary analysis of the US cohort, abnormal DRE and abnormal PSA were independently associated with clinically significant prostate cancer (csPCa) and prostate cancer-specific mortality [3].

2.2 Prostrate-Specific Antigen

The use of PSA for prostate cancer screening was described first by Dr. William Catalona in 1991 [4]. PSA and DRE are the most commonly used tools for screening prostate cancer. Though a serum PSA cutoff of 4 ng/ml is used universally by physicians to recommend a prostate biopsy, about 15% of malignancy occurs below this cutoff [5]. Many derivatives and complex calculations based on PSA have been studied to complement PSA to better risk-stratify patients. These include free: total PSA ratio (F/T ratio), PSA density (PSAD), PSA velocity (PSAV), complex PSA (cPSA), etc. Of note is the PSAD, which has been increasingly adopted in deciding when patients need a biopsy. Traditionally, 0.15 ng/ml^3 has been used as a cutoff to predict clinically significant prostate cancer. However, many reports suggest that this value should be lowered and that one should consider biopsy even when PSAD is lower than 0.15 ng/ml^3, especially in small prostates [6, 7].

2.3 Free to Total Ratio

There are two forms of PSA which include a free and a complex form. The PSA produced by prostate cancer cells is mainly in the complex form wherein it is bound to serum proteins such as alpha1 antichymotrypsin, alpha2 macroglobulin, and alpha1 protease inhibitor. A free to total PSA ratio (F/T ratio) less than 25% may indicate malignancy and

K. R. S. Bhat (✉)
Global Robotics Institute, Adventhealth Celebration, Celebration, FL, USA

S. Yadav · A. Kumar
Department of Urology, Robotics and Transplantation, SJH & VMMC, New Delhi, India

S. Kind
Johns Hopkins University, Baltimore, MD, USA

S. Punnen
Department of Urology, Miller School of Medicine, University of Miami, Coral Gables, FL, USA

P. Wiklund et al. (eds.), *Robotic Urologic Surgery*, https://doi.org/10.1007/978-3-031-00363-9_11

can prevent about 20% of unnecessary prostate biopsies [8]. In a recent series, an F/T ratio of less than 15% may have higher predictive accuracy [9].

2.4 Prostate Cancer Antigen 3

Prostate cancer antigen 3 (PCA3) is a gene that is highly expressed in prostate cancer patients. Measuring PCA3 in urine is being used increasingly to evaluate prostate cancer. The sensitivity and specificity of urinary PCA3 were 62 and 75%, respectively, at a cutoff of 35 [27–29]. Patients with the BRCA mutation may have elevated PCA3 in urine even in the absence of prostate cancer [10].

2.5 4K Test

The 4K test involves a nomogram developed by combining the values of total PSA, free PSA, intact PSA, and human kallikrein 2 (tPSA, fPSA, iPSA, and hk2) in serum, along with DRE, prior biopsies, and age to predict the probability of prostate cancer. The 4K test can predict aggressive features such as an extension of cancer outside the gland, tumor volumes >0.5 cm^3, or any Gleason grade ≥4 prostate cancer. The area under curve (AUC) of the 4K test is >0.80 [11] 4 [12]. The 4K test can reduce the number of biopsies by 30–58% and at a cutoff of 7.5%. It only misses clinically significant prostate cancer in 1.3–4.7% of patients [13].

Table 1 enlists other miscellaneous commercially available biomarkers.

In summary, PSA with DRE is commonly used for prostate cancer screening. However, the largest unanswered question is at what PSA cutoff should one biopsy the prostate. Prostate cancer can be present even in PSAs as low as 0.1 ng/ml [22, 23]. For this, PSA density is the most useful. An F/T PSA may add some value to a PSA, but, in the current setting of biomarkers and MRI, it has little added value. PSA velocity has been shown to increase the number of negative or indolent biopsies performed. Judicious use of these PSA derivatives and newer tests such as the 4K may be used to predict clinically significant prostate cancer. Many risk calculators are available, utilizing these tests that can predict clinically significant prostate cancer. However, these calculators are not widely used yet clinically [24, 25].

3 Biopsy of the Prostate Cancer

Biopsy of the prostate has been a part of clinical practice since the beginning of the twentieth century. At first, prostate biopsies were performed using the open perineal technique in 1926. However, given its invasiveness and the morbidity, the procedure never gained widespread acceptance [26]. In 1930, this technique was modified, and transperineal needle aspiration, or punch biopsy, was introduced. However, given the small amount of tissue recovered, it lacked the diagnostic potential and thus, too, was abandoned [27]. In 1937 when a finger-guided transrectal prostate biopsy was described, this became the standard of care and remained so for the next 5 decades [28]. In 1974, Watanabe et al. were the first to image the prostate via the transrectal ultrasound, and the development of an attachable biopsy needle guide allowed the possibility of transrectal ultrasound-guided prostate biopsy in the 1980s [29].

Table 1 Commercially available miscellaneous biomarkers

Biomarkers	Type of biomarker	Specimen collected	Comments
Prostate core mitomic test	Genome-based markers—3.4-kB mitochondrial genome deletion (3.4 mtD)	Prostate biopsy	Sensitivity—84%, Specificity—54%, NPV—91% [14]
ConfirmMDx	Epigenome-based marker—GSTP1, APC, and RASSF1	Prostate biopsy	On repeat biopsy ConfirmMDx [15] • Sensitivity—74.1% • Specificity—60.0% • NPV—88–90%
SelectMDx	Transcriptome-based markers—mRNA expression of HOXC6 and DLX1	Urine following DRE	The NPV to detect csPCa of SelectMDx is 95% [16] SelectMDx test avoids unnecessary biopsies in 38% (biopsy-naïve) [17] Misses only 10% high-grade PCa [17]
Progensa	Transcriptome-based markers—PCA3: noncoding mRNA on chromosome 9q21–22 Third-generation assays calculate PCA3 score (ratio of PCA3 mRNA to PSA mRNA)	Urine following DRE	Uses of Progensa [18–21] • AUC: 0.66–0.69. • Combined with other predictive factors for PCa at biopsy, AUC: 0.71–0.75 • Cutoff scores of 20–35 have been suggested for optimal accuracy

DRE digital rectal exam, *NPV* negative predictive value

3.1 TRUS-Guided Prostate Biopsy

Over the years, several advances in ultrasound imaging technology and the biopsy technique made transrectal ultrasound-guided prostate biopsy the procedure of choice to diagnose prostate cancer. The appearance of the malignant prostate lesion on a TRUS could be hypoechoic, isoechoic, or hyperechoic, none of which are pathognomonic.

3.1.1 Pre-operative Preparation

Once a decision to biopsy has been made, significant coagulopathy, severe immune suppression, and acute prostatitis, which are the contraindications to prostate biopsy, must be ruled out. Patients should be counseled regarding the risks and benefits of the procedure and briefed about the possible complications.

3.1.2 Prostate Biopsy and Anticoagulation

All prescribed medications must be reviewed with a particular focus on anticoagulant/antiplatelet therapy such as aspirin, warfarin, and clopidogrel and novel oral anticoagulants such as dabigatran, rivaroxaban, and apixaban. It is imperative to assess the underlying cause for which anticoagulants/antiplatelets are prescribed and the risk of thrombotic events. A detailed consultation with the treating interventionist/cardiologist can help assess the risk–benefit ratio in patients on long-term anticoagulants/antiplatelets, and an individualized approach is preferred. In a patient with a low risk of thrombosis, discontinuation of anticoagulants/antiplatelets may be considered, whereas those at high risk of thrombosis must be bridged [30].

For patients at low risk of thrombotic events, the anticoagulants/antiplatelets can be safely discontinued without an increased risk of bleeding complications. It is common practice to discontinue aspirin for 5 days and warfarin and clopidogrel for 7–10 days before biopsy, and use can be restarted as soon as 12–24 h after biopsy, balancing the risk of bleeding and thrombosis. A large body of evidence suggests low-dose aspirin can be safely continued in patients undergoing prostate biopsy without an increase in moderate or severe hematuria, rectal bleed, or hematospermia [31, 32]. However, patients on aspirin are 1.36 times more likely to have mild hematuria, which tends to last longer than in patients who discontinue aspirin [31, 32].

There is limited evidence to suggest that individuals at high risk of thrombosis may undergo prostate biopsy while on warfarin and maintain the INR in the therapeutic range of 2–3 [33, 34]. However, in clinical practice, the majority of the patients at high risk of thrombotic events are bridged with unfractionated or low-molecular-weight heparin [35].

In patients with significant post-biopsy bleeding, it is preferable to shift the patient to heparin, as none of these novel oral anticoagulant agents are reversible in action. Caution is also required in patients with deranged renal function as these agents are predominantly cleared through kidneys, and a longer wait time may be required before these patients can safely undergo prostate biopsy [36].

3.1.3 Antibiotic Prophylaxis

Infectious complications are the most frequent cause of post-biopsy hospitalizations and have risen in the past few years [37]. A recent systematic review and meta-analysis found that antibiotic prophylaxis significantly reduces the risk of infectious complications to 5.6%, compared to 11.6%, in the patients randomized to placebo or no antibiotic prophylaxis (RR 0.56) [38]. Unlike other lower urinary tract procedures, antimicrobial prophylaxis is recommended for all patients undergoing prostate biopsy irrespective of the risk factors. Fluoroquinolones have been traditionally the antibiotic prophylaxis of choice in this setting. However, overuse and misuse have resulted in an increase in fluoroquinolone resistance, and their use as a prophylactic antibiotic has been suspended in some European countries. The US FDA has restricted the use of fluoroquinolones, as they can cause long-term disabling joint problems [39]. Additionally, the increased antibiotic resistance for fluoroquinolone is so widespread that the readmission rates following quinolone use were similar to no antibiotic use, suggesting increasing antibiotic resistance due to the widespread use of fluoroquinolone [40, 41]. For these reasons, there has been an increase in the use of either carbapenems/multiple antibiotic combinations or antibiotics based on rectal swab culture for prostate biopsy [42, 43]. The AUA also recommends shortening the fluoroquinolone prophylaxis to a maximum of 24 h, given the potential of severe adverse events. First-, second-, or third-generation cephalosporins and aminoglycoside are recommended alternatives. The 2014 AUA update added trimethoprim-sulfamethoxazole as a prophylactic agent, and the 2021 EAU guidelines also recommend fosfomycin trometamol as a feasible alternative based on the findings of a recent meta-analysis [38, 44, 45].

Another method to tackle infectious complications resulting from antibiotic resistance is augmented prophylaxis, where a combination of antibiotics is used as prophylaxis rather than a single antibiotic. However, indiscriminate use of multiple broad-spectrum antibiotics is bound to result in antibiotic resistance and goes against antibiotic stewardship protocols. In order to overcome these shortcomings, targeted prophylaxis has been evaluated in patients undergoing a prostate biopsy, where rectal swabs are taken in patients being planned for prostate biopsy and cultured. Prophylactic antibiotics are administered based on the swab culture antibiograms. Targeted prophylaxis has been shown to reduce infectious complications when compared to empirical antibiotics and may prevent the development of antibiotic resistance [38, 46].

Thus, targeted prophylaxis, based on the rectal swab-directed antibiotics, prescribed for a full 24 h should be the preferred approach based on the current evidence. Alternatively, antibiotics such as an aminoglycoside, cephalosporin, or fosfomycin trometamol (in regions where fluoroquinolones are not licensed) can be an alternative approach and allow the biopsy to be more spontaneous rather than planned, as the swab-directed approach requires 48 h for the antibiogram to be available. Although effective and recommended, augmented prophylaxis contradicts antibiotic stewardship and requires up-to-date knowledge of the local antimicrobial resistance patterns.

3.1.4 Non-antibiotic Strategies to Reduce Post-biopsy Infections

Many institutions routinely advise self-administration of a cleansing enema prior to the biopsy at home. Although this practice reduces the number of feces in the rectum and provides a superior acoustic window to image the prostate, it has not been found to reduce the rates of infectious complications. The rates of infectious complications or hospitalization were similar between those who received cleansing enemas and those who did not [47]. On-table rectal preparation can be performed by soaking a piece of gauze in a slurry made by mixing 15 ml of commercially available 10% povidone-iodine solution with 5 ml of 1% lidocaine jelly, which is then inserted into the rectum and left in place for 2 min, prior to its removal and proceeding to biopsy [48]. Some authors also advocate rubbing the anterior rectal wall with gauze soaked in povidone-iodine rather than simply inserting it into the rectum to ensure uniform application [49]. A recent meta-analysis evaluated the use of rectal povidone-iodine. It found a statistically significant reduction in the infectious complications in the povidone-iodine group as compared to the control group (60 infections in 930 men in the povidone-iodine group versus 131 in 1006 men in the control group, RR 0.56) [47]. In the light of these findings, recent guidelines recommend rectal cleansing with povidone-iodine prior to transrectal prostate biopsy [45]. Rectal povidone-iodine suppositories placed for 1–2 h or just before the biopsy have been shown to reduce the infectious complications [50, 51]. The mean number of colony-forming units in the rectum, as assessed by the rectal swab, was reduced by 99.9% after the povidone-iodine suppository [50].

3.2 Biopsy Technique

3.2.1 Equipment

Trans-rectal prostate biopsy is usually performed with a grayscale trans-rectal ultrasound machine with a 6–10 MHz probe. The newer machines currently in use at most of the centers are self-programming to allow for the best possible imaging of the prostate. They have both end- and side-firing modes and allow for the simultaneous visualization of the prostate in the transverse and the sagittal planes. To allow for adequate coupling, it is common practice to place the lubricant or sonographic jelly between the probe and the condom covering it and between the condom and the rectal surface.

Biopsies can be performed in the side-firing or end-firing mode. For the side-firing configuration, advancing the probe cephalad inside the rectum images the base of the prostate, whereas withdrawing it images the apex. Imaging the lateral aspects requires rotating the probe. The clockwise rotation images the left side of the prostate, whereas the counter-clockwise rotation visualizes the right lobe. For the end-firing probe, the anus is utilized as the fulcrum. Angling the probe toward the scrotum images the base of the prostate, whereas moving it toward the sacrum visualizes the apex. To image the lateral aspects, lifting the probe toward the ceiling images the left lobe of the prostate, whereas taking it down toward the floor visualizes the right lobe.

Although the side-firing mode is more commonly employed, a few large retrospective studies found higher cancer detection rates in patients undergoing biopsy with the end-firing method than the side-firing method [52, 53]. However, these were refuted by two randomized studies published on the topic, both of which did not find a difference in cancer detection rates among the two configurations [54, 55]. Van der Slot et al. noted higher cancer detection in the end-firing configuration (52.4% vs. 45.6%, $p = 0.066$), which did not reach statistical significance, and the cancer detection rates at the apex were similar between the two groups [55]. However, they noted longer core lengths could be obtained by the end-firing configuration as compared to the side-firing method (151 mm vs. 138 mm), thus suggesting better sampling of the prostate by the end-firing method. Besides cancer detection, side-firing probes tend to have a smaller profile and require rotatory and in-out motion and thus may cause less pain, as compared to the end-firing probe, which has a larger tip and requires fulcrum motion at the anal sphincter [56]. However, with the majority of the probes now having both the modes built in a single probe, these factors may no longer play a part.

3.2.2 Patient Positioning and Imaging the Prostate

The patient is positioned in the left lateral position somewhat diagonally on the operating table, with the buttocks at the edge of the table. The knees and hips are flexed at 90 degrees, and a pillow is placed between the knees to help maintain this position. Keeping the buttocks at the edge or just beyond the edge of the table allows for free unobstructed movement of the ultrasound probe. Occasionally, a right lateral decubitus or a lithotomy position may be required.

The patient is advised to empty the bladder, and the parts are prepared and draped. Perianal skin is then inspected for fissures or other abnormalities, and a digital rectal examination is performed to evaluate for prostate nodules. With the attached biopsy guide and covered with a well-lubricated condom, the ultrasound probe is gently introduced into the rectum, and the prostate is imaged.

The prostate imaging begins from the base and proceeds to the apex. The peripheral zone is scanned for the presence of any hypo- or hyperechoic lesions, which may be suspicious for malignancy. Any nodules felt on the digital rectal examination are also screened with ultrasonography. The volume of the prostate is then calculated using the ellipse, sphere, or the prolate formula.

3.2.3 Anesthesia

Prostate biopsy is usually performed under local anesthesia, either under pelvic plexus block (PPB) or peri-prostatic nerve block (PNB), which is usually augmented with intrarectal local anesthesia (ILRA) and intra-prostatic local anesthesia (IPLA) with or without oral analgesics. Although a combination of sedoanalgesia with PNB or a low-dose spinal anesthesia is likely the most effective way to alleviate prostate biopsy-related pain, a potential increase in the medical cost and the associated additional risk limit their use [57]. Simple intra-rectal instillation of local anesthetic jelly alone provides inferior analgesia as compared to local prostatic block and is no longer recommended. Local anesthetic injection can be performed with a 22G, 25 cm Chiba needle with 5 ml of 2% lidocaine, 2.5 ml on each side of the prostate, either as a pelvic plexus block (PPB) or a peri-prostatic nerve block (PNB). For the PPB, the injection is given directly into the pelvic neurovascular bundle, situated at the tip of seminal vesicles, on each side. As these bundles are not visualized on the grayscale ultrasonography, once the tips of the seminal vesicles are visualized in the parasagittal longitudinal scan, the color Doppler mode is activated to identify the tiny vessels, and the anesthetic is injected inside the pelvic neurovascular plexus, making sure to aspirate before injection to avoid intravascular injections [58, 59]. For PNB, a similar concentration and volume of local anesthetic is injected in an echogenic triangle containing fat formed by the angle between the seminal vesicle and the base of the prostate in the parasagittal longitudinal scan, called as "the Mount Everest sign" [60, 61]. The PNB can be augmented by adding an apical block, where the local anesthetic is injected into a small echogenic triangle between the apex of the prostate and the puborectalis muscle, on either side of the apex [62]. This injection aims to block the sensitive somatic nerves at the apex of the prostate, which are commonly the most painful sites during prostate biopsy. Besides the apical block, the local anesthetic can be injected along the lateral aspects of the prostate to block the nerves coursing along the prostate or direct injections into the prostate parenchyma (intra-prostatic injections) can be made to augment the effects of PNB [63, 64]. A recent meta-analysis has compared the efficacy of local anesthetic techniques described for trans-rectal prostate biopsy and concluded that PPB + ILRA provided the best analgesia under the outpatient settings followed by PNB + IPLA, PPB, PNB + ILRA, and PNB alone [57].

3.2.4 Biopsy Technique

A 16- or an 18-gauge spring-loaded biopsy gun is used to take cores of the prostate tissue. The needle is introduced through the needle guide, and, depending on the configuration, the operator chooses the points to sample. Side-firing and end-firing modes are different and typically follow the ruled puncture path. Upon activation, the biopsy gun advances 0.5 cm and then samples 1.5 cm of tissue with the tip extending 0.5 cm beyond the sampled area. Thus, the tip of the needle must be 0.5 cm from the prostate capsule before activation to sample the peripheral zone adequately. Otherwise, one may end up sampling more of the transition zone, missing the most common location of the tumor. Also, directing the needle path laterally allows sampling the anterolateral part of the peripheral zone. The ultrasound probe must be pressed against the rectal wall. This minimizes the discomfort as the needle traverses the rectal mucosa and may reduce the chances of bleeding. One must also take care not to move the probe while the biopsy needle is in contact with rectal mucosa to avoid unnecessary injury and bleeding (Fig. 1).

3.2.5 Number of Cores

The introduction of sextant biopsy scheme, introduced by Hodge et al., as compared to finger-guided biopsy of palpable nodules or ultrasound-guided biopsy of suspicious lesions significantly increased the cancer detection rates [65]. The original scheme sampled one core each from the base, mid gland, and apex, bilaterally, and missed out on the apical and the lateral regions of the peripheral zone. Increasing the number of cores from 6 to 12 improved the cancer detection rates by 31% and reduced the likelihood of a repeat biopsy by improving the negative predictive value without increasing the likelihood of detecting insignificant cancers [66, 67]. However, further increasing the number of biopsy cores from 12 to 18 or 21 did not have the same effect. The cancer detection rate did not improve on comparing 18- or 21-core biopsy schemes with the 12 core biopsies, and neither did the need for a repeat biopsy [66, 68], but the rate of detection of insignificant cancers was found to be higher in the 21-core protocol as compared to the 12-core protocol [69]. Thus, for the initial biopsy, extended 12-core biopsy protocol provides acceptable cancer detection rates and negative predictive value while maintaining a low detection rate of insignificant cancers.

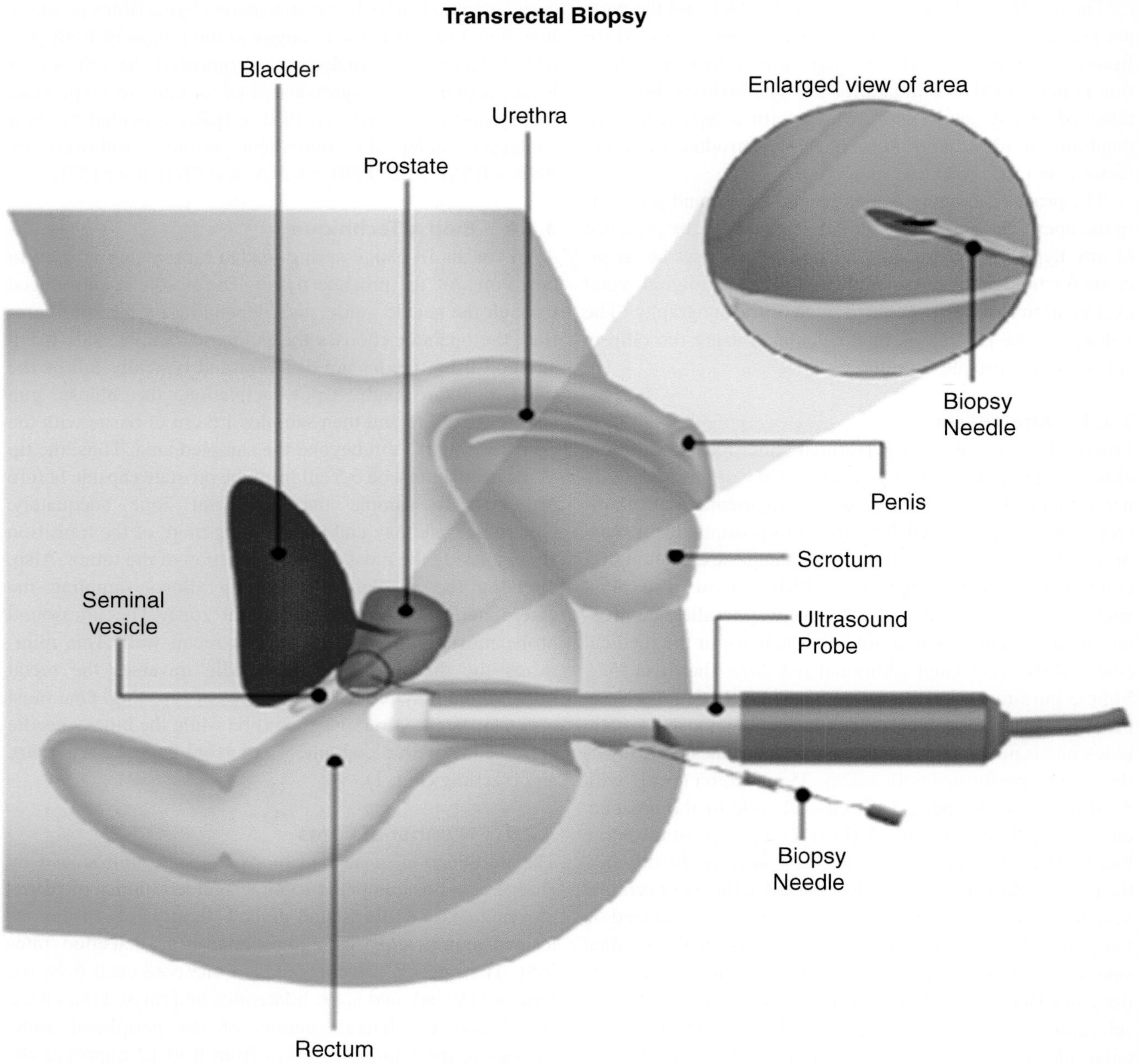

Transrectal Biopsy

Bladder
Urethra
Prostate
Enlarged view of area
Biopsy Needle
Penis
Scrotum
Seminal vesicle
Ultrasound Probe
Biopsy Needle
Rectum

Fig. 1 Illustration demonstrating transrectal biopsy of the prostate

The distribution of the 12 cores must be such to adequately sample the apical and the far lateral regions (anterior horns) of the prostate. Studies evaluating the distribution of cancer in the anterior prostate in the radical prostatectomy specimens found the most common cancer site was the mid gland followed by the apex [70]. The apex is entirely composed of the peripheral zone, and the anterior apex may be missed if not specifically sampled and is the common site of missed cancers detected at repeat biopsy [71]. The laterally directed sampling (far lateral cores) of the peripheral zones allows for adequate sampling of the anterior horns of the peripheral zone and improves the cancer detection rates, as some cancers may only be detected on these cores [72, 73]. These findings suggest the importance of sampling the apical and far lateral regions. Regarding the transition zone sampling, although 15–25% of the cancers are located in the transition zone, only around 2% are exclusively in the transition zone, and the rest can be picked up cores directed at the peripheral zone [74, 75]. Specific sampling of the transition zone at the initial biopsy was not found to improve the cancer detection rates or to reduce the need for repeat biopsy and is not recommended [75, 76].

Thus, an extended 12-core systematic biopsy that incorporates apical and far lateral cores in the template distribution allows for maximum cancer detection while avoiding detection of insignificant cancers or the need for a repeat biopsy is the standard of care.

3.3 Repeat and Saturation Biopsy

A benign biopsy finding in a patient with rising PSA or an abnormal digital examination is a common clinical dilemma. Besides, multifocal high-grade prostatic intra-epithelial neoplasia or atypical small acinar proliferation on the prior biopsy may also mandate a repeat biopsy. The most common site under-sampled in the extended 12-core template is the anterior apex and should be one of the sites of focus on the repeat biopsy [77]. The cancer detection rates are known to fall on each subsequent biopsy. In a cohort of 1051 men with PSA between 4 and 10 ng/ml, the initial cancer detection rate on the sextant biopsy was 22%, which reduced to 10%, 5%, and 4% on the subsequent second, third, and fourth biopsies, respectively [78]. Given the low rate of cancer detection on repeated biopsy, a second biopsy may be contemplated in patients suspected to harbor cancer. However, a third or a fourth biopsy is not warranted. Low cancer detection rates combined with improved cancer detection on the initial extended 12-core biopsy suggest that whenever a repeat biopsy is planned in a patient with a prior negative biopsy, a saturation biopsy (>20 cores) should preferably be undertaken [79]. Repeat saturation biopsies must sample the transition zone and have been shown to detect cancer in 30% of the patients [80].

4 Magnetic Resonance Imaging-Guided Biopsy

Multiparametric magnetic resonance imaging (MP-MRI) helps to identify lesions of the prostate with reasonable accuracy. Various studies on MRI-targeted biopsy conclude that the sensitivity, specificity, a negative predictive value (NPV), and a positive predictive value (PPV) could be between 91% and 93%, 36% and 41%, 89% and 92%, and 51% and 52%, respectively [81–83]. There are three types of MP-MRI-based prostate biopsy, namely, in-bore magnetic resonance imaging-targeted biopsy (MRI-TB), MRI cognitive biopsy (MRI-CB), and MRI fusion biopsy (MRI-FB). While the MRI cognitive biopsy is the easiest and the most cost-effective to perform, it may not be as accurate as the other two modalities. The in-bore MRI-TB, though it theoretically sounds superior as it uses real-time MRI imaging to perform the prostate biopsy, has similar efficacy to the MRI fusion biopsy, which appears to be the middle ground. The ability to accurately target prostatic lesions is the main advantage of the MRI-based technique. However, the data on these techniques in small lesions are limited and, at best, anecdotal. The exact size of the lesion below which the MRI-based techniques have a definite advantage is unknown.

4.1 Multiparametric MRI (MP-MRI)

A combination of high-resolution T2-weighted images (T2WI), dynamic contrast-enhanced MRI (DCE-MRI), and diffusion-weighted imaging (DWI) constitutes the MP-MRI. MP-MRI can be used to evaluate tumors >0.5 cm^3 [84–87]. The prostate imaging reporting and data system (PIRADS) is a scoring system to diagnose prostate cancer was initially proposed in 2012 by the European Society of Urogenital Radiology (ESUR) and has been subsequently revised with the current reiteration being PIRADS v2.1 published in 2019 [88, 89]. The current scoring system utilizes the DWI MRI as the dominant sequence in the peripheral zone and T2-weighted (T2w) MRI as the dominant sequence in the transitional zone. The latest version clarifies the specific use of DCE and b values in DWI, particularly in scores 2 and 3. The changes in T2w are assessed in scores 1 and 2, defining encapsulated nodules and atypical nodules [89].

Final PIRADS v2.1 assessment categories [89]:

1. Very low (clinically significant cancer highly unlikely)
2. Low (clinically significant cancer unlikely)
3. Intermediate (clinically significant cancer equivocal)
4. High (clinically significant cancer likely)
5. Very high (clinically significant cancer highly likely)

The detection rates for prostate cancer using PIRADS v2 for PIRADS 3, 4, and 5 lesions were 35%–39%, 60%–72%, and 91%, respectively. However, the rates of csPCa for PIRADS 3, 4, and 5 were 17%–23%, 34%–49%, and 67%–77%, respectively [90, 91]. Saturation biopsy could potentially be avoided by using PIRADS 3 or above. Using this as the cutoff for MRI-TB, 83.8% of the csPCa were diagnosed, with a false-negative rate of 16.2% [92]. The advantage of using the standardized PIRADS scoring system is that it has moderate interobserver reproducibility with a kappa score of 0.55 [93]. MP-MRI has limited sensitivity to prostate carcinoma (PCa) in the TZ, particularly the presence of concomitant benign prostatic hyperplasia (BPH). This could potentially lead to an error in interpretation. Additionally, in DWI sequence, one can easily interpret BPH nodules as malignant lesions. There are also many benign and premalignant lesions that can mimic prostate cancer, namely, granulomatous prostatitis, adenosis, and prostatic intra-epithelial neoplasia [94].

4.2 MRI-TB

MRI-TB has a sensitivity, specificity, NPV, and PPV between 91% and 93%, 36% and 41% 89% and 92%, and 51% and 52%, respectively [81, 82, 95]. Compared to the standard TRUS biopsy, MRI-TB has more sensitivity in identifying clinically significant prostate cancer (csPca). A combination increases the yield of the biopsy [96].

MRI-TB approaches:

(a) MRI-CB

The surgeon targets the suspicious spots while doing a TRUS biopsy by mentally visualizing the lesions based on prior study of the MRI images. This involves analysis of images and measurement of various distances by recognizing various patterns and 3D spatial reasoning. MRI-CB is superior to the systematic prostate biopsy especially in anterior and apical tumors [97, 98]. It is cheap and can be performed with a simple setup and may be comparable to MRI-FB in expert hands.

(b) MRI-FB

MP-MRI images are superimposed on TRUS images during the prostate biopsy using commercially available systems that overlay MP-MRI scans with real-time ultrasounds. Many systems are available, and they vary based on registration algorithm, navigation strategy, real-time tracking systems, and the method of documentation of the needle track [99]. Each system has its merits and demerits. The most common systems for this purpose include Artemis (Eigen, Grass Valley, California, USA) (Fig. 2), UroNav (Philips Electronics, Amsterdam, the Netherlands), and Urostation (Koelis, LaTronche, France) [100]. Table 2 lists commercially available devices and the basic differences between them.

With more widespread acceptance of transperineal biopsy, these systems have been modified to accommodate transperineal modules to perform MRI-FB transperineally. The BiopSee system was designed to perform transperineal biopsy [101]. Major limitations while using these systems are the added cost and the associ-

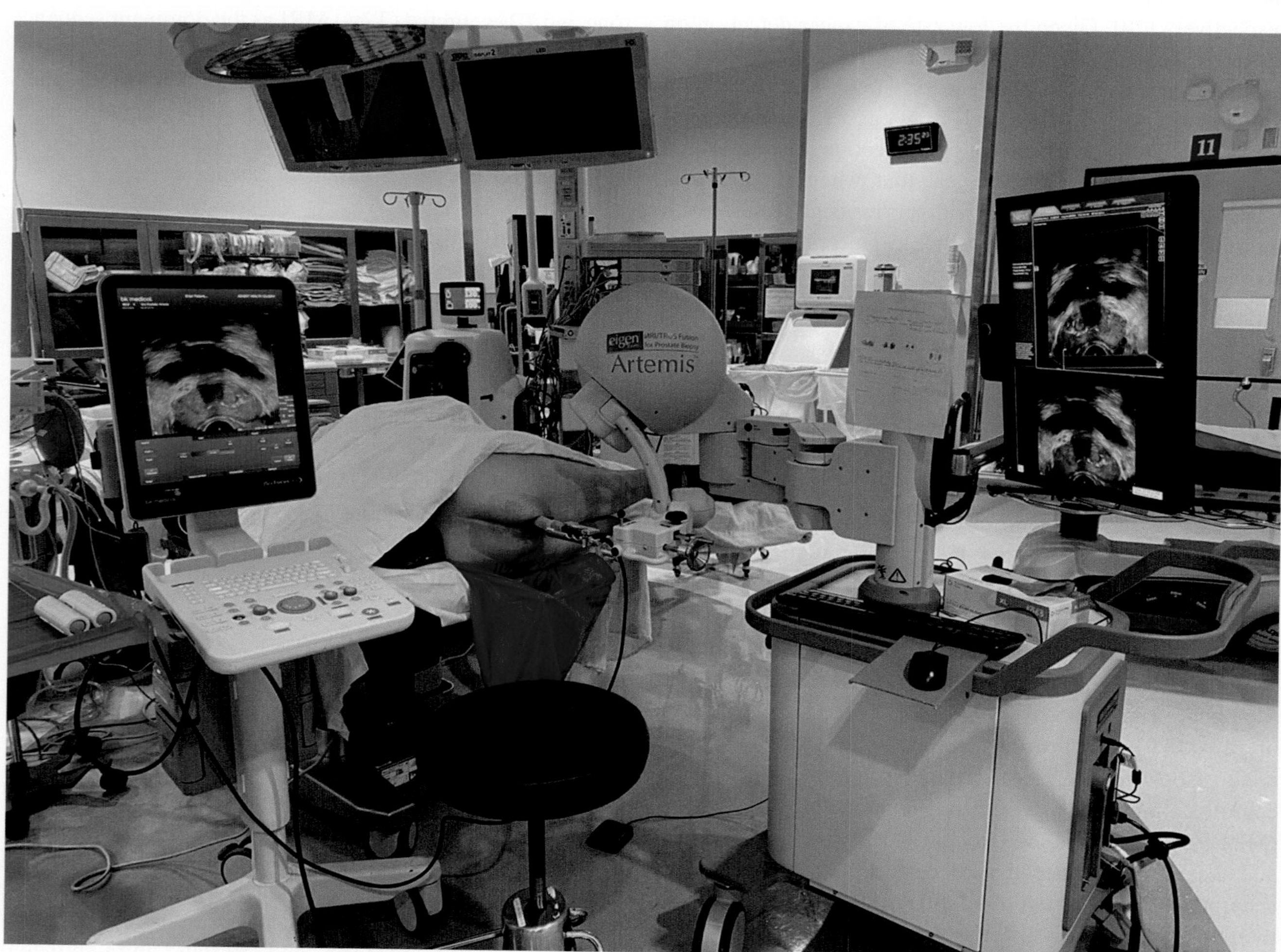

Fig. 2 OR setup of Eigen Artemis system

Table 2 Overview of commercially available MRI-based biopsy systems

Device	Routes	Tracking mechanism	Fusion mechanism	
Artemis	• Transrectal • Transperineal	• Electromagnetic tracking by the mechanical arm with no external trackers • Rigid motion compensation	Rigid and Elastic registration	Biopsy plan can be stored and used to guide the subsequent biopsy or for subsequent focal treatment
Uronav	• Transrectal • Transperineal	• Electromagnetic tracking mechanism	• Elastic registration	Biopsy plan can be stored and used to guide the subsequent biopsy or for subsequent focal treatment
Urostation	• Transrectal • Transperineal	• Organ-based tracking using 3D TRUS	• Rigid and elastic registration	PET/CT can be used for fusion biopsy Biopsy plan can be stored and used to guide the subsequent biopsy or for subsequent focal treatment
Biojet	• Transperineal • Transrectal	• Trackers and angle sensors in the mechanical arm	• Rigid registration	Biopsy plan can be stored and used to guide the subsequent biopsy or for subsequent focal treatment
Real-time virtual sonography	• Transrectal • Transperineal	• Electromagnetic tracking	• Rigid registration	Compatible with many other USC modalities like the B-mode, color Doppler, real-time tissue elastography, and dynamic contrast harmonic imaging
LOGIQ 9	• Transrectal • Transperineal	• Electromagnetic tracking	• Rigid registration	PET/CT can be used for fusion biopsy Automatic motion correction using CIVCO omniTRAX[tm], a plastic support bracket
Fusion Biopsy.2.0	• Transrectal • Transperineal	• Electromagnetic tracking by a robotic arm	• Rigid and elastic registration	Automatic motion compensation
Virtual navigator	• Transrectal • Transperineal	• Electromagnetic two sensors	• Rigid registration	PET/CT/MRI/3D ultrasound fusion
Biopsee	• Transperineal	• Two built-in encoders tracking the TRUS probe • A stepper for the transperineal biopsy	• Rigid registration	Limited by only 2 degrees of freedom motion

PET positron emission tomography, *CT* computer tomography, *MRI* magnetic resonance imaging

ated learning needed. These systems also involve coordination between various specialties, especially the radiologists, to identify and mark the lesion.

Additionally, one needs to be cognizant throughout the procedure, as a faulty segmentation of MP-MRI images and poor registration of the MP-MRI images or transrectal US images can lead to problems and errors during targeting. More than one spatially distributed target may help in overcoming the registration and targeting errors [102].

(c) In-Bore MRI Target Biopsy

MR imaging guidance in MRI gantry is used to target the lesion in real time in this method. This procedure can be performed using the open/closed MRI system or either 1.5T/3T MRI systems. The real advantage of using the in-bore MRI biopsy technique is that it is real time, and any sequence of MRI imaging can perform the biopsy. The most popular device is the DynaTRIM, a portable device used to perform transrectal biopsies [103]. This device uses an adjustable needle guide with three degrees of freedom and is fixed underneath the bed while the patient lies prone. Using the DynaTRIM workstation, the prostate and lesions are identified, and the biopsy is performed transrectally.

The learning curve of this procedure is about 25–30 procedures. The procedure takes about 30 min to perform and may take an additional 15 min for each extra lesion [102].

Recently, the use of the biparametric MRI (BP-MRI) with transverse T2w images and diffusion-weighted images has been suggested to identify suspicious lesions for prostate biopsy, as they are the two main sequences in PIRADS scoring. This cuts down the cost/time to perform the procedure and reduces contrast exposure in these patients. Biparametric MRI has a negative predictive value of 97%, and the only potential drawback is its inability to differentiate between PIRADS scores 3 and 4 in the peripheral zone due to the lack of dynamic contrast-enhanced images. The odds of finding csPCa in PIRADS 3 lesion on BP-MRI are 17% [104].

4.3 Transperineal Biopsy

The drawbacks of the transrectal biopsy have led urologists to explore the transperineal biopsy. The most significant advantage of transperineal biopsy is the reduced use of antibiotics, leading to its increased acceptance by many clinicians [40]. Fluoroquinolones have been the preferred antibiotics used in transrectal prostate biopsy. However, its use has substantial limitations as described above. Transperineal biopsy is relatively a clean procedure as the needle does not pass through the rectum. In a large multicentric study, the readmission rates due to infections following transperineal biopsy were zero [105]. Another advantage of the transperineal biopsy is the increased detection of cancer by about 10% in the anterior zone of the prostate [106–108]. The disadvantages of the transperineal biopsy are the increased rates of urinary retention and the need for general anesthesia [109]. The feasibility of the prostate biopsy transperineally under local anesthesia has been reported [110–112]. In fact, as per the Cambridge Prostate Biopsy (CAMPROBE) trial [113], 87% of the patients preferred the transperineal biopsy under local anesthesia over TRUS biopsy and reported less pain.

Transperineal biopsy may be technically more sound than transrectal biopsy, as the needle passes longitudinally and the biopsy can be confined to the peripheral zone, while in transrectal biopsy, due to the direction of the needle, the biopsy needle can hit the central or transitional zone. Like the TRUS biopsy, transperineal biopsy can also be done using various MRI-based techniques but requires special planning software and equipment. The detection rates of MRI-based transperineal biopsy are similar to template biopsy [114].

4.4 Cost Implications of MRI-TB [115]

The lowest cost of biopsy is that of using standard TRUS biopsy under local anesthesia followed by the cost of TRUS biopsy under sedation, the cost of transperineal template biopsy under general anesthesia, and MRI-FB under sedation and sedation in-bore prostate biopsy (1 vs. 1.9 vs., 2.5 vs. 2.2, $p < 0.001$). However, the cancer detection rates using the above techniques were as follows: TRUS—16% vs. MRI-FB—36% vs. transperineal template biopsy—34%, $p < 0.001$) [116].

In a separate model-based cost analysis MRI, FB had an incremental cost-effectiveness ratio of $1470 per quality-adjusted life-year gained compared to TRUS biopsy [117]. The main drawback is that the cost calculation is based on input parameters and may not be generalized.

Another suggested cost-cutting measure is to use the biparametric MRI (BP-MRI) which is cheaper and is just as cost-effective as the MP-MRI. The main drawback is BP-MRI's inability to correctly classify PIRADS 3 vs. PIRADS 4 in the peripheral zone due to the lack of DCE images, hence mandating the need for biopsy of all PIRADS 3 lesions in the peripheral zone. However, with the BP-MRI, there is a high negative predictive value of 97%, and it takes only 15 min to perform the exam. One added advantage is that ADC maps can be generated using computer software [104]. Another suggested strategy is the use of additional MP-MRI in PIRADS 3 lesion detected by BP-MRI to avoid unnecessary biopsies [118–120].

5 Complications

Like any other procedure, prostate biopsy is associated with a number of complications, although the absolute risk of life-threatening complications is low. A number of adverse events such as hematuria, hematospermia, rectal bleeding, urinary retention, and infectious complications such as urinary tract infection, epididymitis, prostatitis, and sepsis have been reported after transrectal prostate biopsy.

5.1 Bleeding

Bleeding-related complications, such as hematuria, hematospermia, or rectal bleeding, are one of the most frequent and bothersome complications after prostate biopsy. A wide range of patients, 10–84%, report post-biopsy hematuria depending upon the definition used, although only a few (6.2%) report it as a moderate or severe problem [121, 122]. While mild hematuria is common, only a few patients require catheterization (0.4%) or admission (0.14%) [123, 124]. Few authors have reported an increased incidence of hematuria with a higher number of cores sampled, and others have correlated it with larger prostate volumes and transition zone volumes [125, 126]. Hematospermia, similar to hematuria, is also reported by a wide range of patients 1.1–93%, but unlike hematuria, a fourth of the men considered this alarming or concerning [121]. It was found to be associated with anxiety and reduced sexual activity, and lasts for 2–4 weeks or about eight ejaculations [121, 127]. Age, prostate volume, prior transurethral resection of the prostate, and the number of cores were the risk factors associated with hematospermia [121, 126, 128]. The incidence of rectal bleeding varies between 1.3% and 45% and is usually perceived as minor and of little consequence, with major life-threatening rectal bleeding being uncommon [121].

5.2 Post-biopsy Infection

Most infectious complications after prostate biopsy are limited to symptomatic urinary tract infection or low-grade febrile illness, not requiring hospitalization. However, infectious complications are the most common cause of post-biopsy hospital admissions, and an increased incidence has been reported recently [37]. In a multinational, multicenter study, the incidence of febrile UTI was 3.5%, and 3.1% required hospitalization [129]. The recent rise in infectious complications has been attributed mainly to fluoroquinolone resistance [130]. Non-white race, comorbidities, especially diabetes, foreign travel, catheter presence, recent antibiotic use, especially fluoroquinolone, recent hospitalization, and a positive pre-biopsy urine culture have been suggested as the risk factors for infectious complications [121]. Various antibiotic prophylaxis and non-antibiotic prophylaxis strategies to reduce these infectious complications have been detailed above. Targeted prophylaxis is a suitable option in areas with high fluoroquinolone resistance or patients at high risk for post-biopsy infections. It is shown to be effective in preventing life-threatening complications and follows the general principles of antibiotic stewardship, unlike the augmented prophylaxis. Initially, there were particular concerns about the cost-effectiveness of this approach, given the additional cultures and alternative antibiotics required and the low overall incidence of post-biopsy infectious complications. Also, not all patients with fluoroquinolone-resistant *E. coli* on rectal swab cultures developed post-biopsy infections [131]. However, recent studies have shown the efficacy and cost-effectiveness of targeted prophylaxis [132, 133]. In a study by Li et al., by reducing the incidence of infectious complications from 2.42% to 0.23%, targeted prophylaxis reduced the direct cost by 37.5%, and the hospital days avoided per 100 patients was 7.08 days [132]. The number of patients needed to screen to prevent one infection episode was 45.7. Among the non-antibiotic strategies, the number of biopsy cores, peri-prostatic nerve block, the number of injections required for peri-prostatic nerve block, and dipping the biopsy needle into formalin or povidone-iodine between the biopsy cores were not found to reduce post-biopsy infection [47].

5.3 Post-operative Urinary Retention

About 25% of the patients experience worsening of lower tract symptoms after prostate biopsy, but the risk of acute urinary retention is low <2% [121]. Larger prostate size and higher IPSS score are associated with an increased risk of retention and, the majority of the time, the retention is transient and does not require surgical intervention [126]. Although premedication is not necessary for the majority of patients, peri-procedural alpha-blockers can be considered for at-risk patients [121].

6 Take-Home Message

The use of MRI in prior prostate biopsy is the current standard of care and is widely used. The modality used depends on the availability of technology and surgeon preference. With the increasing use of transperineal biopsy, the rates of post-biopsy sepsis have decreased.

References

1. Siegel RL, Miller KD, Fuchs HE, Jemal A. Cancer Statistics, 2021. CA Cancer J Clin. 2021;71(1):7–33. https://doi.org/10.3322/caac.21654.
2. Partin AW, Mangold LA, Lamm DM, Walsh PC, Epstein JI, Pearson JD. Contemporary update of prostate cancer staging nomograms (Partin Tables) for the new millennium. Urology. 2001;58(6):843–8.
3. Halpern JA, Shoag JE, Mittal S, Oromendia C, Ballman KV, Hershman DL, Wright JD, Shih YT, Nguyen PL, Hu JC. Prognostic significance of digital rectal examination and prostate specific antigen in the prostate, lung, colorectal and ovarian (PLCO) cancer screening arm. J Urol. 2017;197(2):363–8.
4. Catalona WJ, Smith DS, Ratliff TL, Dodds KM, Coplen DE, Yuan JJJ, et al. Measurement of prostate-specific antigen in serum as a screening test for prostate cancer. New Eng J Med. 1991;324:1156–61.
5. Thompson IM, Pauler DK, Goodman PJ, Tangen CM, Lucia MS, Parnes HL, et al. Prevalence of prostate cancer among men with a prostate-specific antigen level < or =4.0 ng per milliliter. New Eng J Med. 2004;350(22):2239–46.
6. Nordström T, Akre O, Aly M, Grönberg H, Eklund M. Prostate-specific antigen (PSA) density in the diagnostic algorithm of prostate cancer. Prostate Cancer Prostatic Dis. 2018;21:57–63. https://doi.org/10.1038/s41391-017-0024-7.
7. Yusim I, Krenawi M, Mazor E, Novack V, Mabjeesh NJ. The use of prostate specific antigen density to predict clinically significant prostate cancer. Sci Rep. 2020;10(1):1–6. https://doi.org/10.1038/s41598-020-76786-9.
8. Catalona WJ, Partin AW, Slawin KM, Brawer MK, Flanigan RC, Patel A, et al. Use of the percentage of free prostate-specific antigen to enhance differentiation of prostate cancer from benign prostatic disease: a prospective multicenter clinical trial. JAMA. 1998;279(19):1542–7.
9. Ceylan C, Gazel E, Keleş İ, Doluoğlu Ö, Yığman M. Can the free/total PSA ratio predict the gleason score before prostate biopsy? Curr Urol. 2015;9(1):24–7.
10. Cremers RG, Eeles RA, Bancroft EK, Ringelberg-Borsboom J, Vasen HF, van Asperen CJ, et al. The role of the prostate cancer gene 3 urine test in addition to serum prostate-specific antigen level in prostate cancer screening among breast cancer, early-onset gene mutation carriers. Urol Oncol. 2015;33(5):202.e19–28.
11. Zappala SM, Scardino PT, Okrongly D, Linder V, Dong Y. Clinical performance of the 4Kscore Test to predict high-grade prostate cancer at biopsy: a meta-analysis of us and European clinical validation study results. Rev Urol. 2017;19(3):149–55.
12. Carlsson S, Maschino A, Schröder F, Bangma C, Steyerberg EW, van der Kwast T, et al. Predictive value of four kallikrein markers for pathologically insignificant compared with aggressive prostate cancer in radical prostatectomy specimens: results from the European Randomized Study of Screening for Prostate Cancer section Rotterdam. Eur Urol. 2013;64(5):693–9.
13. Parekh DJ, Punnen S, Sjoberg DD, Asroff SW, Bailen JL, Cochran JS, et al. A multi-institutional prospective trial in the USA confirms that the 4Kscore accurately identifies men with high-grade prostate cancer. Eur Urol. 2015;68(3):464–70.
14. Robinson K, Creed J, Reguly B, Powell C, Wittock R, Klein D, et al. Accurate prediction of repeat prostate biopsy outcomes by a mitochondrial DNA deletion assay. Prostate Cancer Prostatic Dis. 2010;13(2):126–31.
15. Waterhouse RL Jr, Van Neste L, Moses KA, Barnswell C, Silberstein JL, Jalkut M, et al. Evaluation of an epigenetic assay for predicting repeat prostate biopsy outcome in African American men. Urology. 2019;128:62–5.

16. Haese A, Trooskens G, Steyaert S, Hessels D, Brawer M, Vlaeminck-Guillem V, et al. Multicenter optimization and validation of a 2-gene mRNA urine test for detection of clinically significant prostate cancer before initial prostate biopsy. J Urol. 2019;202(2):256–62. https://doi.org/10.1097/JU.0000000000000293.
17. Hendriks RJ, van der Leest MMG, Israël B, Hannink G, YantiSetiasti A, Cornel EB, et al. Clinical use of the SelectMDx urinary-biomarker test with or without mpMRI in prostate cancer diagnosis: a prospective, multicenter study in biopsy-naïve men. Prostate Cancer Prostatic Dis. 2021;24(4):1110–9.
18. Perdon S, Cavadas V, di Lorenzo G, Damiano R, Chiappetta G, del Prete P, et al. Prostate cancer detection in the "grey area" of prostate-specific antigen below 10 ng/ml: head-to-head comparison of the updated PCPT calculator and Chun's nomogram, two risk estimators incorporating prostate cancer antigen 3. Eur Urol. 2011;59(1):81–7.
19. Marks LS, Fradet Y, Lim Deras I, Blase A, Mathis J, Aubin SMJ, et al. PCA3 molecular urine assay for prostate cancer in men undergoing repeat biopsy. Urology. 2007;69(3):532–5.
20. Auprich M, Haese A, Walz J, Pummer K, de La Taille A, Graefen M, et al. External validation of urinary PCA3-based nomograms to individually predict prostate biopsy outcome. Eur Urol. 2010;58(5):727–32.
21. Aubin SMJ, Reid J, Sarno MJ, Blase A, Aussie J, Rittenhouse H, et al. PCA3 molecular urine test for predicting repeat prostate biopsy outcome in populations at risk: validation in the placebo arm of the dutasteride REDUCE trial. J Urol. 2010;184(5):1947–52.
22. Vis AN, Hoedemaeker RF, Roobol M, van der Kwast TH, Schrder FH. Tumor characteristics in screening for prostate cancer with and without rectal examination as an initial screening test at low PSA (0.0-3.9 ng/ml). Prostate. 2001;47(4):252–61.
23. Thompson IM, Pauler DK, Goodman PJ, al. et. Prevalence of prostate cancer among men with a prostate-specific antigen level < or=4.0 ng per milliliter. N Engl J Med. 2004;350:2239–46.
24. Berglund RK, Stephenson AJ, Cronin AM, Vickers AJ, Eastham JA, Klein EA, et al. Comparison of observed biochemical recurrence-free survival in patients with low PSA values undergoing radical prostatectomy and predictions of preoperative nomogram. Urology. 2009;73(5):1098–103.
25. Eastham JA, May R, Robertson JL, Sartor O, Kattan MW. Development of a nomogram that predicts the probability of a positive prostate biopsy in men with an abnormal digital rectal examination and a prostate-specific antigen between 0 and 4 ng/ml. Urology. 1999;54(4):709–13.
26. Young HH, Davis DM. Young's practice of urology. Based on a study of 12,500 cases. South Med J. 1926;19:653.
27. Barringer BS. Prostatic carcinoma. J Urol. 1942;47(3):306–10. https://doi.org/10.1016/S0022-5347(17)70810-5.
28. Astraldi A. Diagnosis of cancer of the prostate: biopsy by rectal route. Urol Cutan Rev. 1937;41:421–2.
29. Watanabe H, Igari D, Tanahasi Y, Harada K, Saito M. Development and application of new equipment for transrectal ultrasonography. J Clin Ultrasound. 1974;2(2):91–8.
30. Daniels P. Therapy Insight: management of urology patients taking long-term warfarin anticoagulation therapy. Nat Clin Pract Urol. 2005;2:343–50.
31. Giannarini G, Mogorovich A, Valent F, Morelli G, de Maria M, Manassero F, et al. Continuing or discontinuing low-dose aspirin before transrectal prostate biopsy: results of a prospective randomized trial. Urology. 2007;70(3):501–5.
32. Carmignani L, Picozzi S, Bozzini G, Negri E, Ricci C, Gaeta M, et al. Transrectal ultrasound-guided prostate biopsies in patients taking aspirin for cardiovascular disease: a meta-analysis. Transfus Apher Sci. 2011;45(3):275–80. https://doi.org/10.1016/j.transci.2011.10.008.
33. Ihezue CU, Smart J, Dewbury KC, Mehta R, Burgess L. Biopsy of the prostate guided by transrectal ultrasound: relation between warfarin use and incidence of bleeding complications. Clin Radiol. 2005;60(4):458–9.
34. Raheem OA, Casey RG, Galvin DJ, Manecksha RP, Varadaraj H, McDermott T, et al. Discontinuation of anticoagulant or antiplatelet therapy for transrectal ultrasound-guided prostate biopsies: a single-center experience. Korean J Urol. 2012;53(4):234–9.
35. Mukerji G, Munasinghe I, Raza A. A survey of the peri-operative management of urological patients on clopidogrel. Ann R Coll Surg Engl. 2009;91(4):313–20.
36. Coscarella M, Motte S, Dalati M-F, Oliveira-E-Silva T, Entezari K, Roumeguere T. New oral anticoagulation drugs and prostate biopsy: a call for guidelines. Ther Adv Urol. 2018;10(12):437–43.
37. Nam RK, Saskin R, Lee Y, Liu Y, Law C, Klotz LH, et al. Increasing hospital admission rates for urological complications after transrectal ultrasound guided prostate biopsy. J Urol. 2013;189(1 Suppl):S12–7. discussion S17–8
38. Pilatz A, Dimitropoulos K, Veeratterapillay R, Yuan Y, Omar MI, MacLennan S, et al. Antibiotic prophylaxis for the prevention of infectious complications following prostate biopsy: a systematic review and meta-analysis. J Urol. 2020;204(2):224–30.
39. FDA Drug Safety Communication: FDA updates warnings for oral and injectable fluoroquinolone antibiotics due to disabling side effects | FDA. [cited 2019 Dec 8]. Available from: https://www.fda.gov/drugs/drug-safety-and-availability/fda-drug-safety-communication-fda-updates-warnings-oral-and-injectable-fluoroquinolone-antibiotics
40. Roth H, Millar JL, Cheng AC, Byrne A, Evans S, Grummet J. The state of TRUS biopsy sepsis: readmissions to Victorian hospitals with TRUS biopsy-related infection over 5 years. BJU Int. 2015;116:49–53. https://doi.org/10.1111/bju.13209.
41. Lange D, Zappavigna C, Hamidizadeh R, Goldenberg SL, Paterson RF, Chew BH. Bacterial sepsis after prostate biopsy - a new perspective. Urology. 2009;74(6):1200–5.
42. Tamma PD, Han JH, Rock C, Harris AD, Lautenbach E, Hsu AJ, et al. Carbapenem therapy is associated with improved survival compared with piperacillin-tazobactam for patients with extended-spectrum β-lactamase bacteremia. Clin Infect Dis. 2015;60(9):1319–25.
43. Duplessis CA, Bavaro M, Simons MP, Marguet C, Santomauro M, Auge B, et al. Rectal cultures before transrectal ultrasound-guided prostate biopsy reduce post-prostatic biopsy infection rates. Urology. 2012;79(3):556–63.
44. Urologic Surgery Antimicrobial Prophylaxis - American Urological Association. [cited 2021 Jun 9]. Available from: https://www.auanet.org/guidelines/archived-documents/antimicrobial-prophylaxis-best-practice-statement
45. EAU. EAU Guidelines on Urological Infections. 2021. p. Table 12/Figure 4.
46. Lydia G, Han TM, Christopher C, Danielle S, Yau LJ, Claudette F, et al. MP66-11 How to prevent prostate biopsy complications: to augment or to swab? J Urol. 2020;203(Suppl 4):e987. https://doi.org/10.1097/JU.0000000000000941.011.
47. Benjamin P, Rajan V, Konstantinos D, Yuhong Y, Imran OM, Steven M, et al. Nonantibiotic strategies for the prevention of infectious complications following prostate biopsy: a systematic review and meta-analysis. J Urol. 2021;205(3):653–63. https://doi.org/10.1097/JU.0000000000001399.
48. Raman JD, Lehman KK, Dewan K, Kirimanjeswara G. Povidone iodine rectal preparation at time of prostate needle biopsy is a simple and reproducible means to reduce risk of procedural infection. J Vis Exp. 2015;103:52670.
49. Costa F, Pontes J Jr, Albertini A, Freire TM, ERC B, Pugliesi F, et al. A randomized controlled trial to investigate the infectious outcomes of intrarectal povidone-iodine cleansing plus formalin

disinfection of needle tip during transrectal ultrasound guided prostate biopsy. J Urol. 2019;201(4S):e271.
50. Park DS, Oh JJ, Lee JH, Jang WK, Hong YK, Hong SK. Simple use of the suppository type povidone-iodine can prevent infectious complications in transrectal ultrasound-guided prostate biopsy. Adv Urol. 2009;2009:750598.
51. Ryu H, Song SH, Lee SE, Song K-H, Lee S. A prospective randomized trial of povidone-iodine suppository before transrectal ultrasonography-guided prostate biopsy. Medicine. 2019;98(12):e14854.
52. Ching C, Moussa A, Li J, Lane B, Zippe C, Jones JS. Does transrectal ultrasound probe configuration really matter? End fire versus side fire probe prostate cancer detection rates. J Urol. 2009;181:2077–82. discussion 2082
53. Paul R, Korzinek C, Necknig U, Niesel T, Alschibaja M, Leyh H, et al. Influence of transrectal ultrasound probe on prostate cancer detection in transrectal ultrasound-guided sextant biopsy of prostate. Urology. 2004;64(3):532–6. https://doi.org/10.1016/j.urology.2004.04.005.
54. Rom M, Pycha A, Wiunig C, Reissigl A, Waldert M, Klatte T, et al. Prospective randomized multicenter study comparing prostate cancer detection rates of end-fire and side-fire transrectal ultrasound probe configuration. Urology. 2012;80(1):15–8. https://doi.org/10.1016/j.urology.2012.01.061.
55. van der Slot MA, Leijte JA, van der Schoot DK, Oomens EHGM, Roemeling S. End-fire versus side-fire: a randomized controlled study of transrectal ultrasound guided biopsies for prostate cancer detection. Scand J Urol. 2020;5(2):101–4.
56. Raber M, Scattoni V, Gallina A, Freschi M, de Almeyda EP, di Girolamo V, et al. Does the transrectal ultrasound probe influence prostate cancer detection in patients undergoing an extended prostate biopsy scheme? Results of a large retrospective study. BJU Int. 2012;109(5):672–7.
57. Kim DK, Lee JY, Jung JH, Hah YS, Koo KC, Lee KS, et al. What is the most effective local anesthesia for transrectal ultrasonography-guided biopsy of the prostate? A systematic review and network meta-analysis of 47 randomized clinical trials. Sci Rep. 2019;9(1):4901.
58. Jindal T, Mukherjee S, Sinha RK, Kamal MR, Ghosh N, Saha B, et al. Transrectal ultrasonography (TRUS)-guided pelvic plexus block to reduce pain during prostate biopsy: a randomised controlled trial. BJU Int. 2015;115(6):892–6.
59. Akpinar H, Tüfek I, Atuğ F, Esen EH, Kural AR. Doppler ultrasonography-guided pelvic plexus block before systematic needle biopsy of the prostate: a prospective randomized study. Urology. 2009;74(2):267–271.e1.
60. Nazir B. Pain during transrectal ultrasound-guided prostate biopsy and the role of periprostatic nerve block: what radiologists should know. Korean J Radiol. 2014;15(5):543–53.
61. Obek C, Onal B, Ozkan B, Onder AU, Yalçin V, Solok V. Is periprostatic local anesthesia for transrectal ultrasound guided prostate biopsy associated with increased infectious or hemorrhagic complications? A prospective randomized trial. J Urol. 2002;168(2):558–61. https://doi.org/10.1016/S0022-5347(05)64679-4.
62. Nguyen CT, Jones JS. Comparison of traditional basal and apical periprostatic block: impact on injection pain and biopsy pain. BJU Int. 2007;99(3):575–8.
63. Mutaguchi K, Shinohara K, Matsubara A, Yasumoto H, Mita K, Usui T. Local anesthesia during 10 core biopsy of the prostate: comparison of 2 methods. J Urol. 2005;173(3):742–5.
64. Bingqian L, Peihuan L, Yudong W, Jinxing W, Zhiyong W. Intraprostatic local anesthesia with periprostatic nerve block for transrectal ultrasound guided prostate biopsy. J Urol. 2009;182(2):474–9.
65. Hodge KK, McNeal JE, Terris MK, Stamey TA. Random systematic versus directed ultrasound guided transrectal core biopsies of the prostate. J Urol. 1989;142(1):71–5.
66. Eichler K, Hempel S, Wilby J, Myers L, Bachmann LM, Kleijnen J. Diagnostic value of systematic biopsy methods in the investigation of prostate cancer: a systematic review. J Urol. 2006;175(5):1605–12.
67. Meng M, v, Elkin EP, DuChane J, Carroll PR. Impact of increased number of biopsies on the nature of prostate cancer identified. J Urol. 2006;176(1):63–8. discussion 69
68. Pepe P, Aragona F. Saturation prostate needle biopsy and prostate cancer detection at initial and repeat evaluation. Urology. 2007;70(6):1131–5.
69. Ploussard G, Nicolaiew N, Marchand C, Terry S, Vacherot F, Vordos D, et al. Prospective evaluation of an extended 21-core biopsy scheme as initial prostate cancer diagnostic strategy. Eur Urol. 2014;65(1):154–61.
70. Babaian RJ, Toi A, Kamoi K, Troncoso P, Sweet J, Evans R, et al. A comparative analysis of sextant and an extended 11-core multisite directed biopsy strategy. J Urol. 2000;163(1):152–7.
71. Moussa AS, Meshref A, Schoenfield L, Masoud A, Abdel-Rahman S, Li J, et al. Importance of additional "extreme" anterior apical needle biopsies in the initial detection of prostate cancer. Urology. 2010;75(5):1034–9.
72. Ravery V, Goldblatt L, Royer B, Blanc E, Toublanc M, Boccon-Gibod L. Extensive biopsy protocol improves the detection rate of prostate cancer. J Urol. 2000;164(2):393–6.
73. Presti JCJ, Chang JJ, Bhargava V, Shinohara K. The optimal systematic prostate biopsy scheme should include 8 rather than 6 biopsies: results of a prospective clinical trial. J Urol. 2000;163(1):163–7.
74. Bazinet M, Karakiewicz PI, Aprikian AG, Trudel C, Aronson S, Nachabé M, et al. Value of systematic transition zone biopsies in the early detection of prostate cancer. J Urol. 1996;155(2):605–6.
75. Pelzer AE, Bektic J, Berger AP, Halpern EJ, Koppelstätter F, Klauser A, et al. Are transition zone biopsies still necessary to improve prostate cancer detection? Results from the tyrol screening project. Eur Urol. 2005;48(6):916–21. discussion 921
76. Terris MK, Pham TQ, Issa MM, Kabalin JN. Routine transition zone and seminal vesicle biopsies in all patients undergoing transrectal ultrasound guided prostate biopsies are not indicated. J Urol. 1997;157(1):204–6.
77. Meng M, v, Franks JH, Presti JCJ, Shinohara K. The utility of apical anterior horn biopsies in prostate cancer detection. Urol Oncol. 2003;21(5):361–5.
78. Djavan B, Zlotta A, Remzi M, Ghawidel K, Basharkhah A, Schulman CC, et al. Optimal predictors of prostate cancer on repeat prostate biopsy: a prospective study of 1,051 men. J Urol. 2000;163(4):1144–9.
79. Scattoni V, Zlotta A, Montironi R, Schulman C, Rigatti P, Montorsi F. Extended and saturation prostatic biopsy in the diagnosis and characterisation of prostate cancer: a critical analysis of the literature. Eur Urol. 2007;52(5):1309–22.
80. Scattoni V, Maccagnano C, Zanni G, Angiolilli D, Raber M, Roscigno M, et al. Is extended and saturation biopsy necessary? Int J Urol. 2010;17(5):432–47.
81. Ahmed HU, El-Shater Bosaily A, Brown LC, Gabe R, Kaplan R, Parmar MK, et al. Diagnostic accuracy of multiparametric MRI and TRUS biopsy in prostate cancer (PROMIS): a paired validating confirmatory study. Lancet. 2017;389(10071):815–22.
82. Thompson JE, van Leeuwen PJ, Moses D, Shnier R, Brenner P, Delprado W, et al. The diagnostic performance of multiparametric magnetic resonance imaging to detect significant prostate cancer. J Urol. 2016;195(5):1428–35.

83. Drost FJH, Osses D, Nieboer D, Bangma CH, Steyerberg EW, Roobol MJ, et al. Prostate magnetic resonance imaging, with or without magnetic resonance imaging-targeted biopsy, and systematic biopsy for detecting prostate cancer: a cochrane systematic review and meta-analysis. Eur Urol. 2020;77:78–94.
84. van As NJ, de Souza NM, Riches SF, Morgan VA, Sohaib SA, Dearnaley DP, et al. A study of diffusion-weighted magnetic resonance imaging in men with untreated localised prostate cancer on active surveillance. Eur Urol. 2009;56(6):981–7.
85. Tamada T, Sone T, Jo Y, Toshimitsu S, Yamashita T, Yamamoto A, et al. Apparent diffusion coefficient values in peripheral and transition zones of the prostate: comparison between normal and malignant prostatic tissues and correlation with histologic grade. J Magn Reson Imaging. 2008;28(3):720–6.
86. Villers A, Puech P, Mouton D, Leroy X, Ballereau C, Lemaitre L. Dynamic contrast enhanced, pelvic phased array magnetic resonance imaging of localized prostate cancer for predicting tumor volume: correlation with radical prostatectomy findings. J Urol. 2006;176(6 Pt 1):2432–7.
87. Girouin N, Mège-Lechevallier F, Tonina Senes A, Bissery A, Rabilloud M, Maréchal J-M, et al. Prostate dynamic contrast-enhanced MRI with simple visual diagnostic criteria: is it reasonable? Eur Radiol. 2007;17(6):1498–509.
88. Barentsz JO, Richenberg J, Clements R, Choyke P, Verma S, Villeirs G, et al. ESUR prostate MR guidelines 2012. Eur Radiol. 2012;22(4):746–57.
89. PI-RADS ® v2.1 PI-RADS ® Prostate Imaging-Reporting and Data System 2019 Version 2.1 PI-RADS ® Prostate Imaging-Reporting and Data System 2019 Version 2.1 Acknowledgements.
90. Kasivisvanathan V, Rannikko AS, Borghi M, Panebianco V, Mynderse LA, Vaarala MH, et al. MRI-targeted or standard biopsy for prostate-cancer diagnosis. N Engl J Med. 2018;378(19):1767–77.
91. Hofbauer SL, Maxeiner A, Kittner B, Heckmann R, Reimann M, Wiemer L, et al. Validation of prostate imaging reporting and data system version 2 for the detection of prostate cancer. J Urol. 2018;200(4):767–73.
92. Pepe P, Garufi A, Priolo GD, Galia A, Fraggetta F, Pennisi M. Is it time to perform only magnetic resonance imaging targeted cores? our experience with 1,032 men who underwent prostate biopsy. J Urol. 2018;200(4):774–8. https://doi.org/10.1016/j.juro.2018.04.061.
93. Rosenkrantz AB, Ginocchio LA, Cornfeld D, Froemming AT, Gupta RT, Turkbey B, et al. Interobserver reproducibility of the PI-RADS version 2 lexicon: a multicenter study of six experienced prostate radiologists. Radiology. 2016;280(3):793–804.
94. de Visschere PJL, Vral A, Perletti G, Pattyn E, Praet M, Magri V, et al. Multiparametric magnetic resonance imaging characteristics of normal, benign and malignant conditions in the prostate. Eur Radiol. 2017;27(5):2095–109.
95. Drost FH, Osses D, Nieboer D, Bangma CH, Steyerberg EW, Roobol MJ, Schoots IG. Prostate magnetic resonance imaging, with or without magnetic resonance imaging-targeted biopsy, and systematic biopsy for detecting prostate cancer: a cochrane systematic review and meta-analysis. Eur Urol. 2020;77(1):78–94.
96. Rouvière O, Puech P, Renard-Penna R, Claudon M, Roy C, Mège-Lechevallier F, et al. Use of prostate systematic and targeted biopsy on the basis of multiparametric MRI in biopsy-naive patients (MRI-FIRST): a prospective, multicentre, paired diagnostic study. Lancet Oncol. 2019;20(1):100–9.
97. Sciarra A, Panebianco V, Ciccariello M, Salciccia S, Cattarino S, Lisi D, et al. Value of magnetic resonance spectroscopy imaging and dynamic contrast-enhanced imaging for detecting prostate cancer foci in men with prior negative biopsy. Clin Cancer Res. 2010;16(6):1875–83.
98. Lee SH, Chung MS, Kim JH, Oh YT, Rha KH, Chung BH. Magnetic resonance imaging targeted biopsy in men with previously negative prostate biopsy results. J Endourol. 2012;26(7):787–91. https://doi.org/10.1089/end.2011.0393.
99. Kongnyuy M, George AK, Rastinehad AR, Pinto PA. Magnetic resonance imaging-ultrasound fusion-guided prostate biopsy: review of technology, techniques, and outcomes. Curr Urol Rep. 2016;17:1–9.
100. Seetharam Bhat KR, Samavedi S, Moschovas MC, Onol FF, Roof S, Rogers T, et al. Magnetic resonance imaging-guided prostate biopsy—A review of literature. Asian J Urol. 2021;8:105–16.
101. Hadaschik BA, Kuru TH, Tulea C, Rieker P, Popeneciu IV, Simpfendörfer T, et al. A novel stereotactic prostate biopsy system integrating pre-interventional magnetic resonance imaging and live ultrasound fusion. J Urol. 2011;186(6):2214–20.
102. Verma S, Choyke PL, Eberhardt SC, Oto A, Tempany CM, Turkbey B, et al. The current state of MR imaging–targeted biopsy techniques for detection of prostate cancer. Radiology. 2017;285(2):343–56. https://doi.org/10.1148/radiol.2017161684.
103. Woodrum D, Gorny K, Greenwood B, Mynderse L. MRI-guided prostate biopsy of native and recurrent prostate cancer. Semin Interv Radiol. 2016;33(03):196–205. https://doi.org/10.1055/s-0036-1586151.
104. Boesen L, Nørgaard N, Løgager V, Balslev I, Bisbjerg R, Thestrup KC, et al. Assessment of the diagnostic accuracy of biparametric magnetic resonance imaging for prostate cancer in biopsy-naive men: the biparametric MRI for detection of prostate cancer (BIDOC) study. JAMA Netw Open. 2018;1(2):e180219.
105. Pepdjonovic L, Tan GH, Huang S, Mann S, Frydenberg M, Moon D, et al. Zero hospital admissions for infection after 577 transperineal prostate biopsies using single-dose cephazolin prophylaxis. World J Urol. 2017;35(8):1199–203.
106. Chang DTS, Challacombe B, Lawrentschuk N. Transperineal biopsy of the prostate-is this the future? Nat Rev Urol. 2013;10:690–702.
107. Roberts MJ, Bennett HY, Harris PN, Holmes M, Grummet J, Naber K, et al. Prostate biopsy-related infection: a systematic review of risk factors, prevention strategies, and management approaches. Urology. 2017;104:11–21.
108. Pepe P, Garufi A, Priolo G, Pennisi M. Transperineal versus transrectal MRI/TRUS fusion targeted biopsy: detection rate of clinically significant prostate cancer. Clin Genitourin Cancer. 2017;15(1):e33–6.
109. Moran BJ, Braccioforte MH, Conterato DJ. Re-biopsy of the prostate using a stereotactic transperineal technique. J Urol. 2006;176(4):1376–81.
110. Stefanova V, Buckley R, Flax S, Spevack L, Hajek D, Tunis A, et al. Transperineal prostate biopsies using local anesthesia: experience with 1,287 patients. Prostate cancer detection rate, complications and patient tolerability. J Urol. 2019;201(6):1121–6. https://doi.org/10.1097/JU.0000000000000156.
111. Gross MD, Shoag JE. Hu JC. Is in-office transperineal biopsy the future of prostate cancer diagnosis? Curr Opin Urol. 2019;29(1):25–6.
112. Kubo Y, Kawakami S, Numao N, Takazawa R, Fujii Y, Masuda H, et al. Simple and effective local anesthesia for transperineal extended prostate biopsy: application to three-dimensional 26-core biopsy. Int J Urol. 2009;16(4):420–3. https://doi.org/10.1111/j.1442-2042.2009.02269.x.
113. Thurtle D, Starling L, Leonard K, Stone T, Gnanapragasam VJ. Improving the safety and tolerability of local anaesthetic outpatient transperineal prostate biopsies: A pilot study of the CAMbridge PROstate Biopsy (CAMPROBE) method. J Clin Urol. 2018;11(3):192–9.
114. Radtke JP, Kuru TH, Boxler S, Alt CD, Popeneciu IV, Huettenbrink C, et al. Comparative analysis of transperineal template satura-

tion prostate biopsy versus magnetic resonance imaging targeted biopsy with magnetic resonance imaging-ultrasound fusion guidance. J Urol. 2015;193(1):87–94.

115. Ho H, Yuen JSP, Mohan P, Lim EW, Cheng CWS. Robotic transperineal prostate biopsy: Pilot clinical study. Urology. 2011 Nov;78(5):1203–8.
116. Altok M, Kim B, Patel BB, Shih YCT, Ward JF, McRae SE, et al. Cost and efficacy comparison of five prostate biopsy modalities: a platform for integrating cost into novel-platform comparative research. Prostate Cancer Prostatic Dis. 2018;21(4):524–32.
117. Venderink W, Govers TM, de Rooij M, Fütterer JJ, Sedelaar JPM. Cost-effectiveness comparison of imaging-guided prostate biopsy techniques: systematic transrectal ultrasound, direct in-bore MRI, and image fusion. Am J Roentgenol. 2017;208(5):1058–63. https://doi.org/10.2214/AJR.16.17322.
118. Washino S, Okochi T, Saito K, Konishi T, Hirai M, Kobayashi Y, et al. Combination of prostate imaging reporting and data system (PI-RADS) score and prostate-specific antigen (PSA) density predicts biopsy outcome in prostate biopsy naïve patients. BJU Int. 2017;119(2):225–33. https://doi.org/10.1111/bju.13465.
119. Ullrich T, Quentin M, Arsov C, Schmaltz AK, Tschischka A, Laqua N, et al. Risk stratification of equivocal lesions on multiparametric magnetic resonance imaging of the prostate. J Urol. 2018;199(3):691–8.
120. Distler FA, Radtke JP, Bonekamp D, Kesch C, Schlemmer HP, Wieczorek K, et al. The value of PSA density in combination with PI-RADS™ for the accuracy of prostate cancer prediction. J Urol. 2017;198(3):575–82.
121. Loeb S, Vellekoop A, Ahmed HU, Catto J, Emberton M, Nam R, et al. Systematic review of complications of prostate biopsy. Eur Urol. 2013;64(6):876–92.
122. Rosario DJ, Lane JA, Metcalfe C, Donovan JL, Doble A, Goodwin L, et al. Short term outcomes of prostate biopsy in men tested for cancer by prostate specific antigen: prospective evaluation within ProtecT study. BMJ (Clinical Research ed). 2012;344:d7894.
123. Pinkhasov GI, Lin Y-K, Palmerola R, Smith P, Mahon F, Kaag MG, et al. Complications following prostate needle biopsy requiring hospital admission or emergency department visits - experience from 1000 consecutive cases. BJU Int. 2012;110(3):369–74.
124. Dodds PR, Boucher JD, Shield DE, Bernie JE, Batter SJ, Serels SR, et al. Are complications of transrectal ultrasound-guided biopsies of the prostate gland increasing? Conn Med. 2011;75(8):453–7.
125. Chowdhury R, Abbas A, Idriz S, Hoy A, Rutherford EE, Smart JM. Should warfarin or aspirin be stopped prior to prostate biopsy? An analysis of bleeding complications related to increasing sample number regimes. Clin Radiol. 2012;67(12):e64–70.
126. Raaijmakers R, Kirkels WJ, Roobol MJ, Wildhagen MF, Schrder FH. Complication rates and risk factors of 5802 transrectal ultrasound-guided sextant biopsies of the prostate within a population-based screening program. Urology. 2002;60(5):826–30.
127. Lee G, Attar K, Laniado M, Karim O. Safety and detailed patterns of morbidity of transrectal ultrasound guided needle biopsy of prostate in a urologist-led unit. Int Urol Nephrol. 2006;38(2):281–5.
128. Berger AP, Gozzi C, Steiner H, Frauscher F, Varkarakis J, Rogatsch H, et al. Complication rate of transrectal ultrasound guided prostate biopsy: a comparison among 3 protocols with 6, 10 and 15 cores. J Urol. 2004;171(4):1471–8.
129. Wagenlehner FME, van Oostrum E, Tenke P, Tandogdu Z, Çek M, Grabe M, et al. Infective complications after prostate biopsy: outcome of the Global Prevalence Study of Infections in Urology (GPIU) 2010 and 2011, a prospective multinational multicentre prostate biopsy study. Eur Urol. 2013;63(3):521–7.
130. Williamson DA, Roberts SA, Paterson DL, Sidjabat H, Silvey A, Masters J, et al. Escherichia coli bloodstream infection after transrectal ultrasound-guided prostate biopsy: implications of fluoroquinolone-resistant sequence type 131 as a major causative pathogen. Clin Infect Dis. 2012;54(10):1406–12.
131. Liss MA, Chang A, Santos R, Nakama-Peeples A, Peterson EM, Osann K, et al. Prevalence and significance of fluoroquinolone resistant Escherichia coli in patients undergoing transrectal ultrasound guided prostate needle biopsy. J Urol. 2011;185(4):1283–8.
132. Li C-K, Tong BCY, You JHS. Cost-effectiveness of culture-guided antimicrobial prophylaxis for the prevention of infections after prostate biopsy. Int J Infect Dis. 2016;43:7–12.
133. Taylor AK, Zembower TR, Nadler RB, Scheetz MH, Cashy JP, Bowen D, et al. Targeted antimicrobial prophylaxis using rectal swab cultures in men undergoing transrectal ultrasound guided prostate biopsy is associated with reduced incidence of postoperative infectious complications and cost of care. J Urol. 2012;187(4):1275–9.

Current Imaging Modalities to Assess Prostate Cancer

Marcelo A. Orvieto, Anup Kumar, Siddharth Yadav, Hugo Otaola Arca, F. Rodrigo Pinochet, and Renato Souper

Abbreviations

ACR	American College of Radiology
ADC	Apparent-diffusion coefficient
AFS	Anterior fibromuscular stroma
AS	Active surveillance
ASCO	American Society of Clinical Oncology
AUA	American Urological Association
BPH	Benign prostatic hyperplasia
bpMRI	Biparametric magnetic resonance imaging
CEUS	Contrast-enhanced ultrasound
csPC	Clinically significant prostate cancer
CT	Computed tomography
CTV	Clinical target volumes
CZ	Central zone
DCE	Dynamic contrast-enhanced
DRE	Digital rectal exam
DWI	Diffusion-weighted imaging
EAU	European Association of Urology
ECE	Extracapsular extension
ERC	Endorectal coil
ESUR	European Society of Urogenital Radiology
FDG	Fluorodeoxyglucose
GG	Grade group
GS	Gleason score
ISUP	International Society of Urological Pathology
LN	Lymph node
LND	Lymph node dissection
MAD	Maximum anteroposterior dimension
MLD	Maximum longitudinal dimension
mpMRI	Multiparametric magnetic resonance imaging
mpUS	Multiparametric US
MRI	Magnetic resonance imaging
MSKCC	Memorial Sloan Kettering Cancer Center
MTD	Maximum transverse dimension
NCCN	National Comprehensive Cancer Network
NPV	Negative predictive value
NVB	Neurovascular bundles
PC	Prostate cancer
PET	Positron emission tomography
PI-RADS	Prostate Imaging-Reporting and Data System
PRECISE	Prostate cancer radiological estimation of change in sequential evaluation
PSA	Prostatic specific antigen
PSAD	Prostatic specific antigen density
PSMA	Prostate-specific membrane antigen
PV	Prostate volume
PZ	Peripheral zone
RECIST	Response Evaluation Criteria in Solid Tumors
RTOG	Radiation Therapy Oncology Group
SD	Standard deviation
SNR	Signal-to-noise ratio
SPECT	Single positron emission computed tomography
SV	Seminal vesicles
SVI	Seminal vesicle invasion
SWE	Shear wave elastography
T1WI	T1-weighted images
T2WI	T2-weighted images
TBx	Targeted biopsy
TP	Transperineal
TR	Transrectal
TRUS	Transrectal ultrasound
TZ	Transitional zone
US	Ultrasound

M. A. Orvieto (✉) · H. O. Arca · F. Rodrigo Pinochet · R. Souper
Clinica Alemana Santiago/Universidad del Desarrollo, Santiago, Chile

A. Kumar
Department of Urology and Renal Transplant, Safdarjung Hospital and VMMC, New Delhi, India

S. Yadav
Safdarjung Hospital and VMMC, New Delhi, India

P. Wiklund et al. (eds.), *Robotic Urologic Surgery*, https://doi.org/10.1007/978-3-031-00363-9_12

1 Ultrasound in Prostate Cancer Diagnosis

1.1 Introduction

Conventional transrectal ultrasound (TRUS) imaging has been studied extensively to assess its performance for PC diagnosis. However, the sensitivity and specificity of conventional TRUS are limited, ranging between 40 and 50% for PC detection, with minimal additional improvement using color/power Doppler [1–3]. Therefore, within the current standard of care, TRUS is used mainly to guide systematic biopsies to general geographic regions of the prostate.

New sonographic modalities such as high-resolution micro-ultrasound, micro-Doppler, sono-elastography, and contrast-enhanced ultrasound (CEUS) have provided promising preliminary findings, either alone or combined with the so-called multi-parametric US. However, these techniques still have limited clinical applicability due to a lack of standardization and large-scale evaluation of inter-observer variability and conflicting results among lesions in the transitional zone [4–6].

1.1.1 High-Resolution Micro-Ultrasound

A novel high-resolution micro-ultrasound system (ExactVu™ system) developed at Sunnybrook Health Sciences Centre operates at 29 MHz compared to 9–12 MHz for a conventional urologic ultrasound. Theoretical spatial resolution at this frequency is between 50 and 70 μm, improving resolution by 300% compared to conventional ultrasound. This system allows identification of anatomic details, ductal anatomy, cellular density, and detection of additional focal lesions usually not seen in conventional US examinations. The focal lesions are stratified based on a standardized PC risk score called "Prostate Risk Identification using Micro-Ultrasound: PRI-MUS," analogous to PI-RADS (Table 1) [5–6]. Thus, micro-ultrasonography allows US real-time guided biopsy of even small suspicious nodules.

Table 1 PRI-MUS™ (prostate risk identification using micro-ultrasound)

Category	Probability of clinically significant prostate cancer (csPC)
PRI-MUS 1	Small regular ducts "Swiss Cheese"
PI-RADS 2	Hyperechoic with/without ductal patches
PI-RADS 3	Mild heterogeneity or Bright Echoes in hyperechoic tissue
PI-RADS 4	Heterogeneous "Cauliflower," "smudgy or mottled," or Bright Echoes ("Starry Sky")
PI-RADS 5	Irregular shadowing or mixed-echo lesions or irregular prostate/PZ border

Micro-ultrasound system is a novel technology, and its data is still preliminary. However, it is inexpensive, accessible, and can improve the sensitivity of TRUS prostate biopsy, thus becoming a convenient alternative to multiparametric magnetic resonance imaging (mpMRI) for imaging and diagnosing PC. Published studies report increased PC detection rate (up to 94%) and an Area Under the Curve (AUC) between 0.60 and 0.80. In addition, initial studies have demonstrated that micro-ultrasound can visualize magnetic resonance imaging (MRI) targets in real time, rather than relying on MRI–TRUS fusion software coupled with conventional TRUS for targeting. Micro-ultrasound, therefore, may have the potential to enhance the accuracy of mpMRI in detecting csPC [7–10].

1.2 Color-Doppler Ultrasound

Conventional color-Doppler ultrasound and power Doppler exhibit a slightly increased PC detection rate when biopsy samples are taken on hypervascular areas, despite normal B-mode appearance [3]. Recently, micro-Doppler imaging techniques have been introduced using adaptative algorithms to eliminate motion artifacts and more pulses dedicated to flow encoding. Preliminary results are encouraging, with a positive correlation between micro-vascularity detected by micro-Doppler imaging and Gleason score (GS) [4]. In addition, micro-Doppler imaging can be performed after ultrasound micro-bubble contrast agent administration allowing temporal summation of the signals.

1.3 Contrast-Enhanced Ultrasound (CEUS)

PC exhibits increased micro-vessel density compared to normal tissue due to the proliferation of pathologic neo-vessels and tumor-associated angiogenesis. This neo-vasculature is typical of small diameter, and it is below the resolution of conventional Doppler imaging; however, micro-bubble contrast agents have demonstrated the ability to enhance sonographic visualization. Therefore, contrast imaging allows accurate guidance of targeted biopsy to areas of increased vascularity [11–13].

The active agents are microbubbles, and their tolerance in clinical practice is excellent, with an incidence of severe anaphylactoid reactions well below that of iodinated contrast media (≈ 0.014%) [12]. Microbubbles are blood pool agents, do not reach the interstitial space or the urine, and do not have renal toxicity. PC exhibits earlier and increased enhancement compared to surrounding benign parenchyma. Furthermore, newer CEUS techniques allow visualization of microvascular anatomy. Vessels that supply tumor areas are more numerous and irregular in configuration than the normal radially oriented vessels extending into the prostate parenchyma from the neurovascular bundles and peri-urethral vascular plexus.

Preliminary studies showed that CEUS improved the detection of the hyper-vascularity of PC nodules, increasing both sensitivities from 54 to 93% and specificity from 79 to 87% for baseline Doppler examination and CEUS examination, respectively [14]. Conventional Doppler imaging is not the most appropriate method to visualize lesions due to some artifacts. Real-time low acoustic power harmonic grayscale imaging is most suitable for prostate CEUS. Using this technique, CEUS demonstrates improved diagnostic accuracy for PC diagnosis compared to pre-contrast imaging, particularly for high-grade (GS ≥ 7), high volume (more than 50% biopsy core involvement), cancer (p = 0.001) (ROC AUC 0.90) [11]. In a large prospective study enrolling 1024 patients, CEUS-targeted biopsies detected 67/326 (20.5%) additional cases of csPC, including 51 patients (15.6%) missed by systematic biopsy [15].

1.4 Prostate TRUS Elastography

Conventional imaging techniques do not provide information about in vivo prostatic elastic properties. PC tissue is stiffer than surrounding healthy prostate tissue due to several changes, including increased cellular density and micro-vascularization, destruction of glandular architecture, and development of stromal reaction combined with collagen deposition in the surrounding prostate parenchyma. This increase in tissue stiffness has been correlated with Gleason score and disease severity [16–19].

Prostate elastography should be performed after a complete B-mode and color-Doppler examination conducted in transverse and sagittal planes to measure prostate volume, identify suspicious areas in the peripheral gland (mostly hypoechoic or hypervascular), and analyze the peri-prostatic space (including the seminal vesicles, SV). Several ultrasound-based methods have been developed to measure in vivo prostate tissue elasticity and provide elasticity maps. In addition, elastography may improve lesion characterization and PC detection, as stiff lesions not visible on conventional TRUS imaging may be detected on elastograms [19].

Two different approaches have been developed. Strain elastography analyzes tissue deformation during mechanical stress and shear wave elastography (SWE) measures the speed at which a shear wave generated via a sonographic pulse travels through tissues with increased propagation seen in stiffer tissues. SWE, unlike strain elastography, does not require manual compression with the TRUS probe. A prospective evaluation of SWE in 50 patients with a 12-core systematic biopsy as the gold standard demonstrated a cancer detection rate of 66% with a sensitivity and specificity of 0.9 and 0.88, respectively. Moreover, stiffness values were significantly higher in confirmed PC with the potential of association with GS [20].

1.5 Multiparametric Ultrasound (mpUS)

The notion of multiparametric US (mpUS) has been introduced as an analogous imaging tool to mpMRI. Grayscale imaging, vascular image techniques, CEUS, and elastography are measurements of anatomic detail, micro-vessel density, and tissue stiffness or cellularity, respectively.

In a prospective study of 78 patients, mpUS had higher sensitivity, negative predictive value, and accuracy than multiparametric MRI (97.4% versus 94.7%, 96.9% versus 92.3%, and 87.2% versus 76.9%, respectively) for detecting localized PC. The mean area under the receiver-operating characteristic curve ± SD for multiparametric TRUS was 0.874 ± 0.043 (95% confidence interval, 0.790–0.959), and 0.774 ± 0.055 (95% confidence interval, 0.666–0.881) for multiparametric MRI [21].

Advanced prostate US imaging techniques have incremental improvements in PC detection, but up to now, none has provided sufficient accuracy when considered on its own. Their combination, especially with elastography and CEUS, is more powerful, but the overall evaluation of patients with a suspicion of PC cannot obviate the utility of mpMRI and the potential of combined information.

2 Role of Computed Tomography (CT) in Prostate Cancer

Abdominal and pelvis CT is recommended to assess lymph node (LN) invasion. Any LN measuring >10 mm in short-axis diameter is considered suspicious for LN metastasis [22]. Recommended size thresholds range from 8 mm to 15 mm. An attempt to standardize these thresholds has been made using Response Evaluation Criteria in Solid Tumors (RECIST) [23].

CT sensitivity for LN detection is low, less than 40% [24, 25]. In a study of 4264 patients, of whom 654 (15.3%) had positive LNs after lymph node dissection (LND), CT was positive in only 105 patients (2.5%) [26]. In a multi-center database of 1091 patients who underwent pelvic LND, CT sensitivity and specificity were 8.8% and 98%, respectively [27].

The size criteria alone does not provide adequate staging. An imaging method utilizing both anatomical and functional information for accurate imaging of the pelvic LN is needed for successful nodal staging.

3 Bone Scan in Prostate Cancer

The current standard imaging test to assess bone metastasis is a whole-body ^{99}mTc-bone scan. It has a role in initial staging, biochemical recurrence, and serial monitoring of treatment response [28]. The bone scan is a low-cost and widely used method, but its diagnostic yield is limited. It can miss bone metastasis in the early stages of the disease. Its specificity is low because it is difficult to distinguish among bone tumors, trauma, degenerative changes, and infection.

The bone scan is significantly influenced by the PSA level, clinical stage, and the International Society of Urological Pathology (ISUP) tumor grade [28, 29]. The mean bone scan positivity rate in 23 different series was 2.3% in patients with PSA levels <10 ng/mL, 5.3% for PSA levels between 10.1 and 19.9 ng/mL, and 16.2% in patients with PSA levels of 20.0–49.9 ng/mL. It was 6.4% in men with organ-confined cancer and 49.5% in men with locally advanced cancers. Detection rates were 5.6% and 29.9% for ISUP grade 2 and >3, respectively. Bone scanning should be performed in symptomatic patients, independent of PSA level, ISUP grade, or clinical stage [26, 32] (Fig. 1).

A systematic review and meta-analysis compared bone scan to prostate-specific membrane antigen–positron emission tomography/computed tomography (PSMA-PET/CT), choline-PET/CT, sodium fluoride (NaF)-PET/CT, and MRI. Results for bone scan showed combined sensitivity and specificity of 86% (95% CI: 76–92%) and 95% (95% CI: 87–98%) at patient level and 59% (95% CI: 55–63%) and 75% (95% CI: 71–79%) at lesion level. Compared with other diagnostic techniques bone scan sensitivity and specificity were inferior in detecting bone metastases [30].

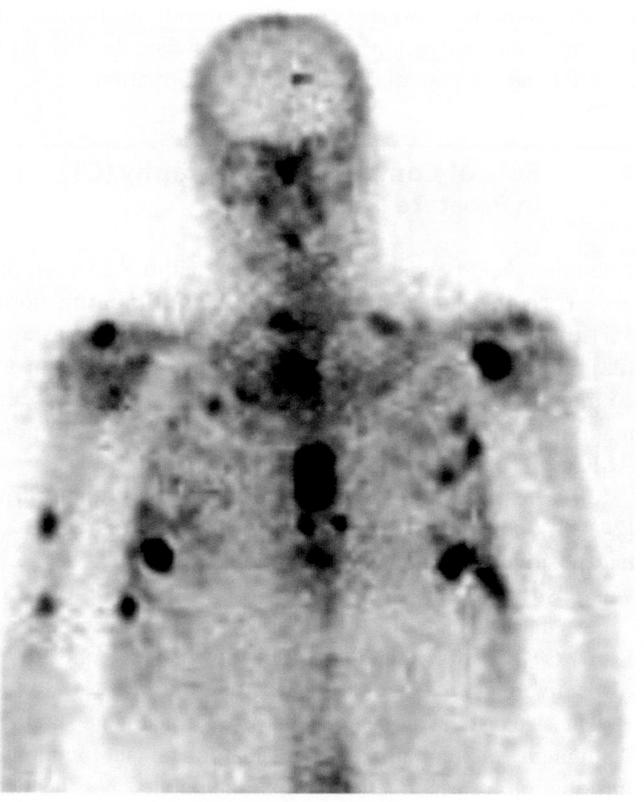

Fig. 1 Bone scan from a patient with Gleason 4 + 5 = 9 PCa and PSA 87 ng/ml showing multiple bone metastases

According to initial risk stratification, National Comprehensive Cancer Network (NCCN) guidelines recommend performing a bone scan in an unfavorable intermediate-, high-, and very high-risk group [31].

4 Magnetic Resonance Imaging (MRI) to Assess Prostate Cancer

4.1 Introduction

Since the 1980s, MRI has been used for the noninvasive evaluation of the prostate. MRI was used at the beginning exclusively to perform loco-regional staging in patients with biopsy-proven PC through anatomic sequences (T1-weighted images (T1WI) and T2-weighted images (T2WI)). However, technological progress, both in software and hardware, led to the development of the mpMRI that combines the above-mentioned anatomic sequences with functional ones, including diffusion-weighted imaging (DWI) (and its derivative, the apparent-diffusion coefficient (ADC) maps) and dynamic contrast-enhanced (DCE) MRI. These technical advances enriched the ability to differentiate clinically significant prostate cancer (csPC) from benign diseases or indolent malignancies. Consequently, clinical applications of prostate MRI went beyond loco-regional staging to image guidance (for biopsy, surgery, focal therapy, and radiation therapy), tumor detection and characterization, risk stratification, surveillance, and assessment of recurrence.

4.2 General Principles of Prostate MRI

4.2.1 Sequences on Prostate MRI

As mentioned above, a variety of anatomic and functional sequences can be performed with MRI to evaluate the prostate. Table 2 summarizes the main utility of each sequence to evaluate the prostate. According to the number and type of sequences performed, it is possible to differentiate two types of MRI protocols:

- **Multiparametric MRI (mpMRI)**: includes anatomical sequences (T1WI/T2WI) and two functional sequences (DWI and DCE).
- **Biparametric MRI (bpMRI)**: includes identical anatomical sequences but only one functional sequence (does

Table 2 Sequences on MRI to evaluate the prostate

Anatomical sequences	
T1-weighted imaging (T1WI)	• Delineate the contour of the gland. • Elucidate the presence of hemorrhage within the prostate and the SV. • Detect lymph node and bone metastasis.
T2-weighted imaging (T2WI)	• It is the fundamental sequence to evaluate the morphology of the CZ, TZ, and PZ. • Identify csPC in the ZT and ZP. • Identify the invasion of SV, extracapsular extension, and lymph node invasion.
Functional sequences	
Diffusion-weighted imaging (DWI)	• Reflect the random movement of water molecules. • Rationale: In healthy tissues, there is a great, random movement of water. On the contrary, water moves with more difficulty in tumor tissues due to the high cellularity (restriction to diffusion). • DWI must include an "ADC map" and "high b-value images." • ADC map – There is an inverse correlation between the Gleason score (GS) and ADC (the lower the ADC, the higher the GS; usually, the csPC has an ADC <1). Hence, ADC improves the identification of csPC. – However, the ADC map should be carefully interpreted due to the considerable overlap between benign prostatic hyperplasia and PC. • High b-value images – b images can be performed with low, intermediate, or high b-values, but the latter is preferred. Although there is no optimal "high b-value," is recommended a value of ≥1400 s/mm^2.
Dynamic contrast-enhanced (DCE)	• Analyze the change in signal intensity in T1WI during the time of the intravenous contrast administration. • Rationale: In healthy tissues, there is an increase in the signal during the passage of the contrast followed by resetting the signal value to normal ranges. Like other malignancies, PC often shows early uptake compared to normal tissue. • Limitation: The kinetics in tumor tissue is quite variable and heterogeneous. – Early uptake alone is not definitive for cancer. – The absence of early uptake does not exclude cancer. • Nowadays, the value of DCE is modest and not firmly established.

ADC apparent-diffusion coefficient, *csPC* clinically significant prostate cancer, *CZ* central zone, *PZ* peripheral zone, *SV* seminal vesicles, *TZ* transitional zone

not include DCE). Given the limited role of DCE, there is a growing interest in performing bpMRI, which would decrease the costs and the time to perform the exam.

4.2.2 Prostate Imaging-Reporting and Data System (PI-RADS)

The Prostate Imaging-Reporting and Data System version 1 (PI-RADS™ v1) are guidelines for prostate mpMRI published in 2012 by the European Society of Urogenital Radiology (ESUR) based on the deliberations of the International Prostate MRI Working Group (organized by the AdMeTech Foundation).

The American College of Radiology (ACR), jointly with ESUR and the AdMeTech Foundation, established the PI-RADS Steering Committee to update and improve the PI-RADS™ v1 that resulted in the development of PI-RADS™ v2 in 2016 [33] and PI-RADS™ v2.1 in 2019 [34]. These updates try to promote global standardization and reduce variation in the acquirement, interpretation, and reporting of prostate mpMRI exams.

The most critical clinical considerations and technical specifications before performing a mpMRI of the prostate are summarized below.

Clinical Considerations [34]

- **Delay After Prostate Biopsy**. A systematic TRUS biopsy may produce hemorrhage (manifested as a hyperintense signal on T1WI) in the PZ and SV, which may confound mpMRI assessment. If the objective of the mpMRI is to detect and characterize csPC, there may be no need to delay mpMRI after prostate biopsy due to the detection of csPC is not likely to be substantially affected by post-biopsy hemorrhage. However, if the purpose of the exam is staging, a delay of at least six weeks between biopsy and MRI should be considered.
- **Improvements at the Bowel Level**. To improve the quality of the images during the mpMRI, it has been proposed to decrease bowel peristalsis with antispasmodic agents (e.g., glucagon, scopolamine bromide, or sublingual hyoscyamine sulfate). Additionally, if the exam is performed without an endorectal coil, bowel preparation with an enema before the exam may be beneficial; however, the enema may also promote peristalsis.
- **Seminal Vesicle Preparation**. Some authors recommend that patients refrain from ejaculation three days before the mpMRI exam to maintain maximum distention of the SV, but an increase in csPC detection has not been firmly established with this routine.

In general, all these measures may be unnecessary, and the incremental cost and potential for adverse drug reactions should be considered. Unfortunately, nowadays, there is no consensus on any of the aspects related to patient preparation.

Technical Specifications [34]

- **Magnetic Field Strength**. Although mpMRI of the prostate can be performed at both 1.5 T and 3 T, most members of the PI-RADS Steering Committee prefer, use, and recommend 3 T for prostate mpMRI, reserving 1.5 T mpMRI for exceptional cases (e.g., patients with an implanted device).
- **Endorectal Coil (ERC)**. An ERC increases the signal-to-noise ratio (SNR) in the prostate at any magnetic field strength but may also increase the time and cost of the exam, deform the gland, introduce artifacts, and be uncomfortable for the patients. However, other technical factors apart from an ERC can influence SNR (e.g., coil design, receiver bandwidth, etc.), and satisfactory results have been obtained with both 1.5 T and 3 T without ERC. Then, the recommendation is to optimize imaging protocols to obtain the best and most consistent image quality possible with the MRI scanner used.

4.3 Structure and Function of the Prostate and Seminal Vesicles on MRI

The prostate is an accessory gland of the male reproductive system with an inverted pyramid shape surrounding the prostatic urethra (a urethral segment extending from the bladder's neck to the external urethral sphincter). It is possible to differentiate the "base of the prostate" as the region directly attached to the urinary bladder neck and the "apex of the prostate" as the distal portion resting against the urogenital diaphragm. A normal gland weighs 15–20 g and has the size of a walnut. Prostate volume (PV) increases with age (mean of 11.5 cc (range 1.6–20.6) in young men; mean of 39.6 cc (range 38–83) at 60 years) [35, 36]. Prostate MRI allows to measure the PV through the ellipsoid formula:

$$PV = MAD \times MLD \times MTD \times 0.52$$

Where …

- PV: prostate volume
- MAD: maximum anteroposterior dimension (on the mid-sagittal T2WI)
- MLD: maximum longitudinal dimension (on the mid-sagittal T2WI)
- MTD: maximum transverse dimension (on the axial T2WI)

Taking PSA and PV is possible to calculate PSA density (PSAD) according to the following formula:

$$PSAD = \frac{PSA}{PV}$$

Where …

- PSAD: prostatic specific antigen density (ng/mL^2)
- PSA: prostatic specific antigen (ng/mL)
- PV: prostate volume (mL)

The prostate produces a liquid medium for the spermatozoa to swim in and provides proteolytic enzymes that increase the likelihood of successful fertilization, constituting 15–20% of the total ejaculation volume [37].

The seminal vesicles (SV) are paired organs of 30 mm length and 15 mm diameter in a young, healthy male, attached to the posterior aspect of the prostate and bladder wall. At the prostate base, the SV join with the ipsilateral vas deferens to form the ejaculatory ducts, which drain in the mid-prostatic urethra, in an elevation called *verumontanum* [38, 39].

Understanding the lymphatic drainage of the prostate is essential to accurately stage PC. The prostate is drained by obturator and intern iliac LN, which disembogue in the external iliac LN. However, it is also described as a direct drain from the prostate to the external iliac LN [40].

4.4 Classification Systems for Prostatic Areas

Defining the different areas of the prostate is of utmost importance to use standard terms when describing findings on MRI reports. Initially, the prostate was structured into two lobes [41]. In 1982, John McNeal described four distinct anatomical regions: peripheral zone (PZ), transition zone (TZ), central zone (CZ), and the anterior fibromuscular stroma (AFS) [38]. PI-RADS™ designs a more complex prostate sector map with 41 regions to enable radiologists, urologists, and pathologists to accurately localize findings described in MRI reports [34].

4.4.1 Zonal Anatomy of the Prostate on MRI (McNeal)

Table 3 contains a detailed anatomical description of each McNeal's area and its characterization on prostate MRI. Comprehending the cellularity, the glandular pattern, and the embryological origin of each prostatic zone is essential to understand the different behavior in prostate MRI [42, 43]. In this regard, the TZ and PZ are derived from the urogenital sinus; however, they have different signal intensities on MRI due to the minor differences in cellularity

Table 3 Summary of the main characteristics of McNeal's zonal anatomy in a non-tumoral prostate [2, 6, 11–13]

	Anatomical description	mpMRI description
Anterior fibromuscular stroma (AFS) (non-glandular tissue)	• AFS is an apron from the bladder neck to the prostatic apex that forms the anterior surface of the prostate.	• T1WI and T2WI: low signal intensity, much like skeletal muscle. • DWI: low signal intensity without restricted diffusion. • DCE: hypovascular relative to the glandular prostate.
Peripheral zone (PZ) (70–80% of the glandular tissue)	• PZ of both sides forms an incomplete ring surrounding the TZ in varying proportion: roughly all the tissue is PZ at the apex, decreasing its presence towards the base.	• T1WI: it is indistinguishable from the rest of the gland. • T2WI: homogeneous high signal intensity that allows differentiation from other zones. • DWI: uniform signal intensity without areas of restricted diffusion. • DCE: uniform enhancement after intravenous contrast administration.
Transition zone (TZ) (5% of the glandular tissue)	• TZ surrounds the prostatic urethra proximal to the verumontanum; it is absent at the prostatic apex. • Benign prostatic hyperplasia can enlarge the TZ until it replaces the entire gland.	• T1WI: it is usually indistinguishable from the rest of the gland but may contain proteinaceous material or blood products that produce foci of hyperintensity. • T2WI: heterogeneous signal intensity that progresses with age and the development of benign prostatic hyperplasia.
Prostatic pseudocapsule or "surgical capsule"	• There is no true capsule between TZ and PZ on histological evaluation. • Corresponds to compressed stromal and fibromuscular tissue from TZ.	• T2WI: thin, dark (low signal intensity) rim at the interface of the TZ with the PZ.
Central zone (CZ) (20% of the glandular tissue)	• CZ is a conical area surrounding the ejaculatory ducts: the base of the cone comprises most of the posteromedial sector of the prostatic base, with the vertex directed toward the verumontanum. • Unlike the TZ, the volume of the CZ decreases with age.	• T2WI: low signal intensity tissue encircling the ejaculatory ducts. • DWI: mildly hyperintense on the high b-value image.
Prostatic capsule	• The prostate lacks a true capsule but has an outer band of concentric fibromuscular tissue inseparable from prostatic stroma, usually called "prostatic capsule." • Then, it is not a true anatomic structure but serves as an essential landmark for assessing the extracapsular extension of cancer.	• T2WI: thin, dark (low signal intensity) rim that is outside the PZ.
Neurovascular bundles (NVB)	• NVBs are two paired longitudinal structures of a triangular section with a posterolateral course to the prostate bilaterally (at 5 and 7 h). • NVBs consist of nerve fibers that supply the corpora cavernosa and arterial branches from the inferior vesical artery and its corresponding veins, which are nestled between three periprostatic fascial planes (prostatic fascia, lateral fascia, and Denonvilliers' fascia).	• T2WI: small and dark (low signal intensity) punctate and tubular structures surrounded by a high signal from adipose tissue. The NVB is less discernible as it moves towards the apex because it becomes intimately adjacent to the prostatic capsule.

ADC apparent-diffusion coefficient, *AFS* anterior fibromuscular stroma, *CZ* central zone, *DWI* diffusion-weighted imaging, *PZ* peripheral zone, *T1WI* T1-weighted images, *T2WI* T2-weighted images, *TZ* transitional zone

and patterns of glandular formation; the CZ is derived from the Wolffian duct [44]. The McNeal's zonal anatomy is visible on MRI due to different embryological origins and its patterns of epithelial cells in each specific zone (Fig. 2). Approximately 70–75% of PC arise in the PZ and only 20–30% in the TZ. Instead, primary CZ cancers are rare. Usually they are a result of direct invasion from the PZ to the CZ [34].

4.5 Assessment and Reporting on Prostate MRI

MRI helps us to identify patients with csPC and, therefore, to decide which patients should undergo a prostate biopsy. csPC is defined in PI-RADS™ v2.1 as Gleason score ≥7, and/or tumor volume ≥0.5 cc, and/or extracapsular extension (ECE) [34]. The probability that the mpMRI

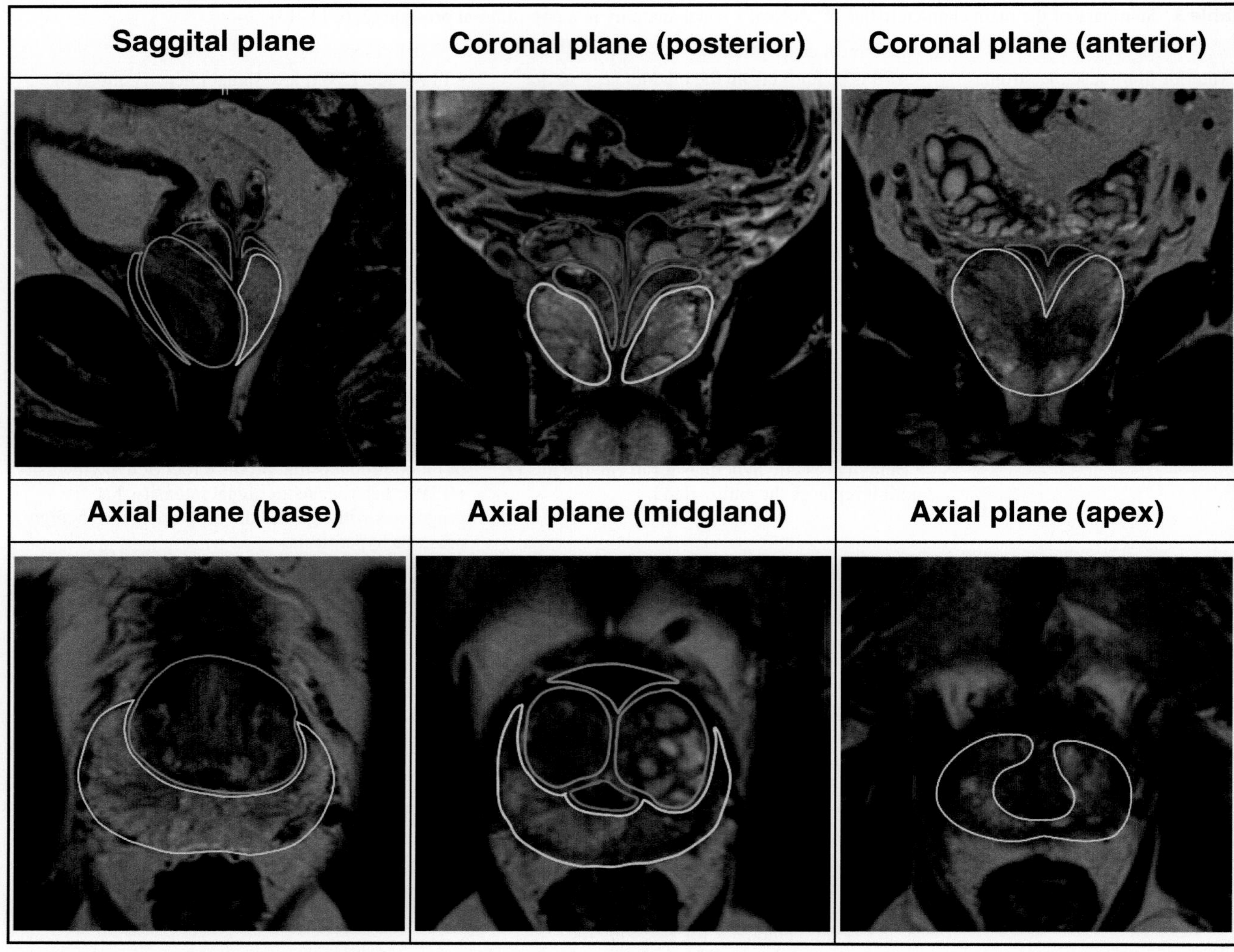

Fig. 2 McNeal's zonal anatomy of the prostate on MRI. Blue = transitional zone; Green: anterior fibromuscular stroma; Purple = seminal vesicles; Red: central zone; Yellow, peripheral zone

(T2WI + DWI + DCE) correlates with the presence of a csPC for each lesion in the prostate gland is assessed with a 5-points scale (Table 4). The assignment of a PI-RADS category should be based only on mpMRI findings (should not consider serum PSA, DRE, or clinical history). In 2019, a systematic review established the probability of csPC according to PI-RADS™ v2.0: 6% of csPC in PI-RADS 1–2, 12% in PI-RADS 3, 48% in PI-RADS 4, and 72% in PI-RADS 5 [46].

According to PI-RADS™ v2.1 assessment categories, patients with PI-RADS 1 or 2 should not be considered for prostate biopsy, whereas patients with PI-RADS 4 or 5 should be strongly considered for a biopsy. In addition, those patients with PI-RADS 3 should be discussed according to factors other than mpMRI alone.

Table 4 PI-RADS™ v2.1 assessment categories

Category	Probability of clinically significant prostate cancer (csPC)
PI-RADS 1	Very low (csPC is highly unlikely to be present)
PI-RADS 2	Low (csPC is unlikely to be present)
PI-RADS 3	Intermediate (the presence of csPC is equivocal)
PI-RADS 4	High (csPC is likely to be present)
PI-RADS 5	Very high (csPC is highly likely to be present)

Generally, there is a primary (dominant) sequence (T2WI or DWI) and a secondary sequence that may upgrade the assessment category (DWI or DCE). In particular, T2WI is the sequence that commands in the TZ, and DWI may upgrade the category in the case of PI-RADS 2 or 3. In the PZ, DWI is the sequence that commands, and, in the case of a PI-RADS 3, DCE may upgrade to PIR-RADS 4 (Fig. 3, Table 5). To assign a PI-RADS category, each prostate lesion must receive a PI-RADS for each sequence. Subsequently, following the established rules for categorization, a single PI-RADS will remain for each prostate lesion.

Considering that PC is often multifocal, according to PI-RADS™ v2.1, up to four lesions with a PI-RADS 3, 4, or 5 may be assigned on the Sector Map. Additionally, the intra-prostatic index lesion (one with the highest PI-RADS category) should be identified. If there are more than four suspicious lesions, only the four with the highest likelihood of csPC should be reported.

To better understand the PI-RADS™ v.2.1 guidelines, please consult the original publication from Turkbey et al. [34].

Many benign signal abnormalities within the prostate can be seen on an MRI exam. For example, **benign prostatic hyperplasia (BPH)** has a heterogeneous signal pattern on MRI. On T1WI, they usually appear isointense to the background prostate. On T2WI, the TZ has been described as "organized chaos" and is composed of well-demarcated or encapsulated nodules (some appearing predominantly hyperintense, while others show heterogeneous or low signal) with intervening areas of low signal intensity [45, 47]. After the administration of contrast, nodules demonstrate variable enhancement, with some demonstrating early hyperenhancement. The PI-RADS™ v2.1 guidelines clarify the distinctions between TZ PC and BPH [34].

Hemorrhage in the PZ and SV is a common finding after a prostate biopsy that appears as a focal or diffuse hyperintense signal on T1WI and iso-hypointense signal on T2WI. **Calcifications** appear as markedly hypointense lesions on all pulse sequences. **Prostatitis** can decrease signal in the PZ on both T2WI and the ADC map and may create a "false positive" on DCE by increasing perfusion. Normal aging or chronic inflammation can evolve to prostatic atrophy, typically associated with hypointense wedge-shaped areas on T2WI and mildly decreased signal (not as low as cancer) on the ADC map. After inflammation, prostatic fibrosis can also be identified by hypointense wedge- or band-shaped areas on T2WI.

Table 5 PI-RADS assessment for prostate lesions on the peripheral and transitional zone

	T2WI	DWI	DCE	Final category
Transitional zone	PI-RADS 1	Any PI-RADS	Any PI-RADS	PI-RADS 1
	PI-RADS 2	PI-RADS $\leq$ 3	Any PI-RADS	PI-RADS 2
		PI-RADS 4–5	Any PI-RADS	PI-RADS 3
	PI-RADS 3	PI-RADS $\leq$ 4	Any PI-RADS	PI-RADS 3
		PI-RADS 5	Any PI-RADS	PI-RADS 4
	PI-RADS 4	Any PI-RADS	Any PI-RADS	PI-RADS 4
	PI-RADS 5	Any PI-RADS	Any PI-RADS	PI-RADS 5
Peripheral zone	Any PI-RADS	PI-RADS 1	Any PI-RADS	PI-RADS 1
	Any PI-RADS	PI-RADS 2	Any PI-RADS	PI-RADS 2
	Any PI-RADS	PI-RADS 3	Negative	PI-RADS 3
			Positive	PI-RADS 4
	Any PI-RADS	PI-RADS 4	Any PI-RADS	PI-RADS 4
	Any PI-RADS	PI-RADS 5	Any PI-RADS	PI-RADS 5

DCE dynamic contrast-enhanced, *DWI* diffusion-weighted imaging, *T2WI* T2-weighted images

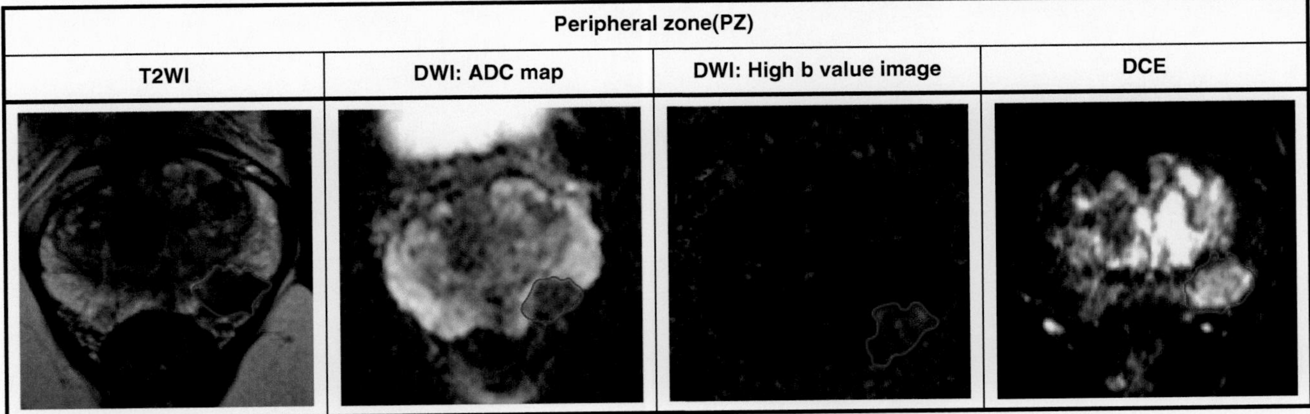

Peripheral zone(PZ)
T2WI
DWI: ADC map
DWI: High b value image
DCE

Fig. 3 The behavior of TZ and PZ lesions in each of the mpMRI sequences. A 65-year-old patient with a focal abnormality of 17 mm in posterolateral midgland peripheral zone of the left prostate lobe that is hypointense in T2WI and presents restricted diffusion and is hypointense on the ADC map (0.540 mm^2/s); bulges adjacent capsule, suspected extracapsular extension (T3a) (PI-RADS 5)

4.6 Role of MRI in Active Surveillance

Active Surveillance (AS) is the standard of care for low-risk PC and highly selected intermediate-risk patients [48–50]. The goal of AS is to avoid overtreatment side effects without compromising survival in those patients who progress.

In the last few years, mpMRI is being introduced in several AS protocols [51] because it has shown a high negative predictive value (NPV) and, thus, a high likelihood of excluding significant PC [52]. In addition, Schoots et al. showed that in patients on AS, a negative MRI will have a reclassification rate of 17% compared with a positive MRI with 39% [53].

One of the major disadvantages of MRI use was the lack of a standardized reporting system, making it difficult to compare different studies and define disease progression. As a result, the European Society of Urogenital Radiology recommended using the PI-RADS [54] and the Prostate Diagnostic Imaging Consensus Meeting panel proposed using 5-point Likert scaling [55]. Fortunately, both systems have similar inter-reader variability and reproducibility [56, 57], so most conclusions of previous literature can still be applied in the same manner.

Regarding the PI-RADS system, nowadays, the most used and well-known grading system, it is known that MRI visibility of disease (PI-RADS 4–5) in AS candidates confers a higher probability of adverse pathology at surgery, which indicates an association between MRI phenotypes and biological features [58]. On the other hand, PI-RADS 3 or less indicates relative safety for AS enrollment and maintenance.

PI-RADS lesion categories at baseline mpMRI during active surveillance enrollment can also be used to predict cancer progression, as shown by Wang et al. [59]. Thus, this information, along with other clinical data, can assist urologists in identifying appropriate candidates for active surveillance.

Prostate Cancer Radiological Estimation of Change in Sequential Evaluation (PRECISE) panel objective was to define patients' conduct and reporting standards on AS having serial MRI scans [60]. Radiologists should assess the likelihood of actual change over time (i.e., change in size or lesion characteristics on one or more sequences) on a 1–5 scale (Table 6). Figure 4 describes the evolution of a PI-RADS 3 lesion during active surveillance.

Patients without radiological progression on MRI (PRECISE 1–3) during AS have a very low likelihood of

Table 6 PRECISE assessment categories

Category	Probability of clinically significant prostate cancer (csPC)
PRECISE 1	Resolution of previous features suspicious on MRI.
PRECISE 2	Reduction in volume and/or conspicuity of previous features suspicious on MRI.
PRECISE 3	Stable MRI appearance: no new focal/diffuse lesions.
PRECISE 4	Significant increase in size and/or conspicuity of features suspicious for prostate cancer.
PRECISE 5	Definitive radiologic stage progression.

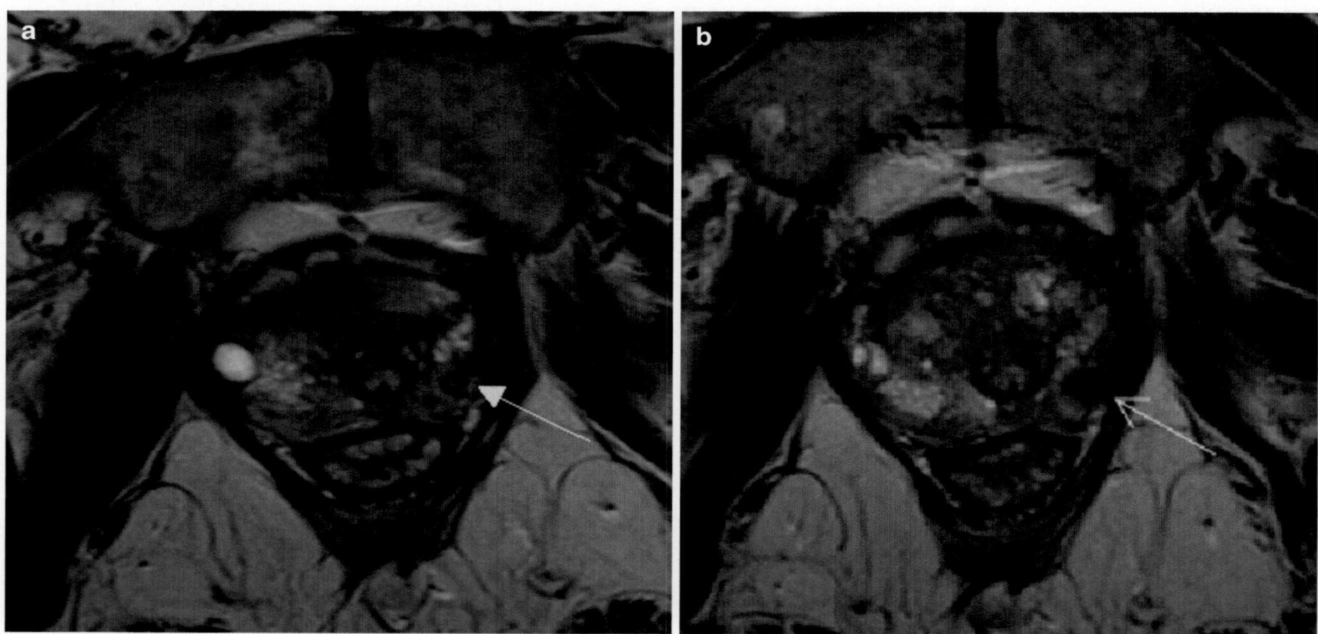

Fig. 4 Evolution of a prostatic lesion during active surveillance. (**a**) Left apex, peripheral zone posterolateral (PZpl) lesion. (**b**) The lesion experienced a 3 mm growth (5 vs. 8 mm) in 18 months. PRECISE 4

clinical progression, and many could, potentially, avoid routine re-biopsy [61].

Against this attractive trend of avoiding routine biopsies, Recabal et al. proved that mpMRI alone missed a clinically relevant proportion of high-grade tumors with lesions resided in areas that were not denoted as regions of interest on mpMRI (17, 12, and 10% of patients with mpMRI PI-RADS score of 3, 4, and 5, respectively) [62]. Also, recent studies suggest that grade progression occurs not infrequently in the absence of image progression on MRI [63].

Stavrinides and colleagues published their outcomes on MRI-based surveillance for their AS cohort. The treatment rate was similar to that reported from standard AS cohorts with comparable follow-up [64]. Nevertheless, concern remains regarding variability in the performance of MRI and MRI-TBx across different practice settings, not allowing to adopt this strategy massively yet.

Regarding baseline and serial biopsies for patients on AS, MRI also plays a significant role. Recently, it has been reported that patients who were on a "Pre-MRI AS Protocol" and then, after the introduction of MRI, underwent TBx if warranted and were significantly more likely to be reclassified and undergo treatment than those who underwent systematic prostate biopsy alone [65]. This statement is confirmed by Schoots et al. in their systematic review and meta-analysis, where they showed that a combined approach of MRI-TBx plus systematic biopsy identified an extra 7% of men who were upgraded compared to TRUS-guided biopsy alone [66].

The ASIST trial objective was to determine if there is a difference in AS failure rate among patients undergoing MRI before initial confirmatory biopsy compared to those who did not [67]. They showed that in patients with Grade Group (GG) 1 PC after confirmatory biopsy, after two years of follow-up, the ones who had a baseline mpMRI before confirmatory biopsy resulted in 50% fewer surveillance failures and less progression to higher-grade cancer. This confirms the value of mpMRI during AS, increasing the chance of detecting patients that are excellent candidates for AS.

MRI-TBx has not only proved its value with the transrectal (TR) approach. For example, the Johns Hopkins group recently published their patients' data on AS undergoing transperineal (TP) biopsy. They showed that patients with PI-RADS 3–4 lesions who underwent MRI-TBx TP biopsies had a significantly higher upgrade rate to GG 2 PC than those who underwent the TR approach [68].

In the last years, AS has gained popularity among treatment options for patients with GG 2 PC. In this setting, MRI plays a vital role, as shown by Stonier [69]. In addition, a positive mpMRI (visible lesion) was associated with higher rates of adverse pathology and upgrading. These reports suggest that mpMRI findings help assess the baseline risk of men with GG2 PC and help select patients who may be good candidates for AS.

In conclusion, mpMRI is useful for detecting clinically significant disease at the initial assessment of men considering AS and facilitates the risk stratification of AS patients by increasing the detection of significant cancer to direct suitable men to active treatment. Potentially, it may reduce the need for additional biopsies in patients with a negative mpMRI.

4.7 Staging Before Local Therapy

MRI can provide details on anatomic staging that help inform decision-making, particularly in patients at higher risk for locally advanced disease based upon clinical factors.

4.7.1 Tumor Staging

Regarding the **T stage**, MRI is helpful to discriminate between a tumor confined to the gland (≤T2 disease) and one that extends beyond the gland (≥T3 disease). In this sense, it is necessary to evaluate the extracapsular extension (ECE) and seminal vesicles invasion (SVI).

ECE should be suspected when (1) there is asymmetry or invasion of the neurovascular bundles; (2) there is bulging of the prostate contour; (3) there are irregular or spiculated prostate margins; (4) there is an obliteration of the rectoprostatic angle; (5) the suspicious lesion has contact with the prostate capsule >1 cm (the more extensive contact size, the greater possibility of ECE); or when (6) there is a rupture of the capsule with evidence of direct tumor extension or invasion of the bladder wall.

The SVI should be suspected when (1) there is focal or diffuse signal hypointensity in T2WI and/or abnormal enhancement of contrast within and/or along with the SV; (2) there is restricted diffusion; (3) there is an obliteration of the angle between the base of the prostate and the SV; or when (4) direct tumor extension from the base of the prostate is seen.

It is also vital to carefully rule out the presence of a **tumor in the apex of the prostate** because its existence can produce a positive margin (in the case of more conservative surgeries) or injure the external sphincter and lead to incontinence (in the case of more radical surgeries). In addition, tumors in this region may also have implications for radiation therapy.

T2WI is the most useful sequence on MRI for the purpose of T staging. Pooled data from a meta-analysis of 9796 patients showed a sensitivity and specificity of 0.57 (95%CI: 0.49–0.64) and 0.91 (95%CI: 0.88–0.93), 0.58 (95%CI: 0.47–0.68) and 0.96 (95%CI: 0.95–0.97), and 0.61 (95%CI: 0.54–0.67) and 0.88 (95%CI: 0.85–0.91), for ECE, SVI, and overall stage T3 assessment, respectively [70].

However, prostate MRI cannot detect microscopic ECE. In this regard, MRI sensitivity and specificity for detecting the pT3 stage were 40% and 95%, respectively, for focal (e.g., microscopic) ECE and 62% and 95% for extensive ECE [71]. Jager et al. reported an ECE detection rate of 14% vs. 100% for an extension radius of <1 mm vs. > 3 mm, respectively [72]. Then, the sensitivity of MRI to detect microscopic ECE increases with the radius of an extension within peri-prostatic fat. It has been demonstrated that the use of high field strength (3T) and functional imaging in addition to T2WI improves sensitivity for ECE or SVI detection [70]. However, the experience of the reader remains of utmost importance [73]. Some studies based on cohorts of men diagnosed with systematic biopsy have suggested that combining MRI findings with clinical and biopsy data could improve the prediction of the pathological stage [74]. However, the generalizability of these findings in the TBx setting is debatable. To improve ECE and SVI prediction, risk calculators have been developed based on MRI findings, clinical data, and prostate biopsy (systematic and targeted) results [75].

Based on the low sensitivity for detecting microscopic ECE, the European Association of Urology (EAU) does not recommend MRI for local staging in low-risk patients (level of evidence (LE): strong), but the examen can be helpful to plan treatment [76].

4.7.2 Lymph Nodes Staging

Pelvic LND is indicated when the probability of LN invasion is >5%. According to the literature, patients with low-risk, intermediate-risk, and high-risk PC have a chance of <5%, 3–20%, and 15–40%, respectively, of LN invasion [76]. LND is the most reliable staging method, but it is an invasive procedure with a high frequency of potential complications, and positive LN can be located outside the template of the performed LND [77].

When the LN is staged, it is recommended to evaluate the following nodal groups bilaterally: common femoral, obturator, external iliac, internal iliac, common iliac, pararectal, presacral, and paracaval and para-aortic up to the level of the aortic bifurcation [34, 78]. The categorization of the LN within the pelvis and retroperitoneum as abnormal on MRI is limited to size, morphology, shape, and enhancement pattern [78]. Usually, LNs with a short axis >8 mm within the pelvis and >10 mm outside the pelvis are considered malignant; however, not all LN harboring metastases are enlarged, and there are enlarged LN without malignant invasion. Therefore, increasing the sensitivity by decreasing these thresholds is possible, but the specificity will also decrease, so the ideal size threshold remains uncertain [79, 80].

The preferred sequences to assess the diameter and morphology of LN are T1WI and T2WI. DWI may detect metastases in normal-sized nodes, but a negative DW cannot rule out the presence of LN metastases [78, 80].

Peabody et al. recently presented a retrospective study with 10,250 patients who underwent radical prostatectomy, with 3924 patients (38.3%) undergoing CT and/or mpMRI before surgery [81]. In this cohort, mpMRI showed a sensitivity, specificity, negative predictive value, and positive predictive value of 19.0%, 97.3%, 95.9%, and 26.7%, respectively.

Because MRI has low sensitivity for detecting positive LN, nomograms combine clinical and biopsy findings to identify patients at higher risk of LN invasion, which should be considered for LND. Some examples of the nomograms using systematic biopsy findings can be the one designed by the Memorial Sloan Kettering Cancer Center (MSKCC) [82], by Briganti et al. [83], or by Gandaglia et al. [84]; however, these instruments may not be sensitive to patients diagnosed with combined MRI-MRI-TBx and systematic biopsy.

Recently nomograms incorporating MRI-TBx biopsy have been developed [75, 85]. Draulans et al. presented a model tested on an external cohort of 187 patients treated with radical prostatectomy, and extended LND showed a C-index of 0.73 (vs. 0.81 in the development cohort); at calibration analysis, the model tended to overpredict the actual risk [85]. Gandaglia et al. presented a model validated in an external multicenter cohort of 487 patients with an area under the curve (AUC) of 0.79 (vs. 0.81 in the development cohort). According to their results, they would have avoided LND in 56% of patients while missing LN invasion in 34% of patients using a threshold of 7% [75].

4.7.3 Metastasis Staging

MRI can detect bone, visceral, and nodal metastases. Bone metastases appear as hypointense lesions on T1WI replacing bone marrow or heterogeneous vs. hyperintense lesions (when fast saturation is used) on T2WI. Generally, bone metastases show restricted diffusion and are hyperintense on high b-value DWI [86].

DWI whole-body and axial MRI are more sensitive than bone scan and targeted conventional radiography in detecting **bone metastases** in high-risk PC [87, 88]. In addition, whole-body MRI is more sensitive and specific than combined bone scan, targeted radiography, and abdominopelvic CT [89]. However, the prognosis and ideal management of patients labeled as metastatic with this more sensitive examination are unknown, chiefly if patients with metastases detectable only by MRI should be managed with systemic therapies as has been done until nowadays or, on the contrary, if they should undergo aggressive local therapies targeting metastasis [90].

4.8 Detection After Local Therapy

PSA persistence (defined as PSA > 0.1 ng/mL at 4–8 weeks after treatment) occurs in 5–20% of patients following radical prostatectomy and evolves to BCR in 74% of cases [91, 92]. Biochemical recurrence (BCR) occurs in 27–53% of patients following local therapy with curative and clinical metastasis in 7–8 years and died in 12–13 years [93, 94].

4.8.1 Imaging in Patients with PSA Persistence After Radical Prostatectomy

Like CT scan and bone scintigraphy, MRI has a low metastasis detection rate in PSA persistence after radical prostatectomy when PSA < 2 ng/mL. On the contrary, prostate-specific membrane antigen (PSMA)-positron emission tomography (PET)/CT scan has shown higher sensitivity and specificity detecting residual cancer with PSA level > 0.2 ng/mL [76].

4.8.2 Imaging in Patients with PSA-Only Recurrence

Assessment of Metastases

The accuracy of whole-body or axial MRI detecting metastases in patients with BCR after RP or RT is not well known [95]. Therefore, the role of MRI in detecting occult bone or LN metastases in patients with BCR requires further evaluation.

Assessment of Local Recurrence after Radical Prostatectomy

The sensitivy of MRI to detect local recurrence in the prostatic fossa directly correlates with the PSA level and its diagnostic ability is limited with a PSA level <0.5 ng/mL [96, 97]. MRI has been demonstrated to be more sensitive than choline-PET/CT detection local recurrences when the PSA level is <1 ng/mL [98]. However, whole-body MRI had a lower performance than PET in detecting regional (16 vs. 9, $p = 0.016$) and distant (12 vs. 6, $p = 0.031$) metastases in a retrospective study with a medium level of 1.5 ng/mL PSA [99].

The sensitivity of anastomotic biopsies is low, especially for PSA levels <1 ng/mL [100]. Additionally, the radiation dose delivered to the prostate surgical bed tends to be uniform since it has not been demonstrated that dose escalation improves the outcome. Hence, salvage radiotherapy is usually based on BCR without local imaging and histological proof of local recurrence [76].

Assessment of Local Recurrence After Radiation Therapy

Given the morbidity of local salvage options, it is necessary to obtain histological proof of the local recurrence before treating the patient [100]. Unlike TRUS that is not reliable in identifying local recurrence after radiotherapy, MRI has shown excellent results and can be used to perform TBx and guide local salvage treatment [100–103]. However, it slightly underestimates the volume of the local recurrence [104]. Choline-PET/CT is an alternative to detect local recurrence in this setting [105] but has not been compared to mpMRI yet.

In summary, MRI has shown excellent results detecting local recurrences and guiding prostate biopsy after radiotherapy. In this regard, and according to the most recent EAU Guidelines for imaging in patients with BCR, MRI should be performed only to localize abnormal areas and guide biopsies in patients fit for local salvage therapy in the scenario of BCR after radiotherapy (LE: weak) [76].

Prostate Magnetic Resonance Imaging for Local Recurrence Reporting (PI-RR)

Experts from the European Society of Urologic Imaging, the European Society of Urogenital Radiology, and individual members of the PI-RADS Steering Committee have recently published Guidelines to standardize the way of reporting PC recurrence after radiation therapy and radical prostatectomy called Prostate Magnetic Resonance Imaging for Local Recurrence Reporting (PI-RR) [106].

PI-RR offers a uniformly structured assessment score based on five assessment categories that summarize the suspicion of local recurrence (Table 7). Thus, PI-RR tries to standardize the acquisition, interpretation, and reporting of mpMRI for PC recurrence. However, PI-RR is based on expert consensus and therefore still requires validation.

4.9 Conclusion

MRI is an invaluable tool in diagnosing, staging, active surveillance, treatment planning, and detection of recurrence in patients with PC. Anatomical and functional sequences on MRI conformed to the so-called mpMRI, constituting a major step forward in increasing this exam's accuracy. However, each sequence included in a protocol must be carefully weighed for incremental clinical utility over additional exam time and costs. A meticulous selection of imaging parameters, appropriate hardware, and adequate patient preparation can optimize image quality.

Table 7 PI-RR assessment categories

Category	Probability of recurrence
PI-RR 1	Very low likelihood of recurrence
PI-RR 2	Low likelihood of recurrence
PI-RR 3	Uncertain likelihood of recurrence
PI-RR 4	High likelihood of recurrence
PI-RR 5	Very high likelihood of recurrence

5 PET Scan in Prostate Cancer

5.1 Introduction

Unlike conventional imaging, such as CT or MRI, which are primarily based on the anatomical size, PET scans bank upon changes at the molecular level, thus having a distinct advantage over conventional imaging.

PET is functional imaging that utilizes positron emitters such as ^{18}F, ^{11}C, ^{68}Ga, etc., to "visualize" a molecular process relatively specific to either the disease or the organ of interest. This tumor or tissue specificity is achieved by attaching these positron emitters to molecules targeting a specific molecular process such as the increase in metabolism in the majority of the tumor tissues (fluorodeoxyglucose, a glucose analog) or the increased utilization of choline (Choline), amino-acids (Fluciclovine) by the prostate tissues. In addition, these positron emitters can also be attached to molecules that target the overexpression of an antigen-specific to either the disease or the organ of interest (prostate-specific membrane antigen). In the past, the role of PET in the evaluation of PC was limited. However, several new PET tracers have emerged in recent years which offer improved diagnostic accuracy and are currently undergoing evaluation to establish their role in the standard diagnostic algorithm in patients with PC.

5.2 ^{18}F-FDG PET/CT

^{18}F-fluorodeoxyglucose (FDG) is the most widely used tracer for PET scans. However, its role in the evaluation of PC is limited. FDG is a glucose analog accumulated in most tumors, demonstrating an increase in the glucose metabolism and up-regulation of glucose transporters [107]. However, on the other hand, PC is characterized by low glucose metabolism and depends on alternate pathways such as the fatty acid pathways or the fructose metabolism for their energy needs [108]. The normal prostate gland usually demonstrates homogenous low-level uptake of FDG [109].

Occasionally, incidental high prostate uptake of FDG may be seen in patients being evaluated for unrelated diseases. The pooled prevalence of incidental high uptake was found to be 1.8% in a systematic review, and 17% of such incidental high uptakes, which were further evaluated and 62% of those who underwent biopsy, were found to be malignant [110]. Thus, it has been suggested that incidental high uptake on FDG PET/CT scans should not be ignored, and at least a serum PSA measurement should be considered [111, 112].

Considerable overlap exists in the levels of FDG accumulation found in normal prostatic tissues, the benign prostatic enlargement, and the malignant diseases, limiting accurate differentiation of the benign from malignant diseases [113, 114]. FDG-PET was found to have low sensitivity and specificity for the detection of the primary disease.

Minamimoto et al. evaluated 50 subjects with elevated PSA with FDG-PET/CT and found the sensitivity, specificity, and positive predictive value of 51.9%, 75.7%, and 42.9%, respectively [115]. However, a larger cohort found the sensitivity to be still lower at 37% when the FDG-PET/CT was used as a screening tool [116]. FDG-PET/CT has also been evaluated in the initial staging of PC, albeit the data is limited. In a cohort of men with high-grade PC, FDG-PET/CT detected only 27% of the patients with histologically proven LN metastasis, and only 6% of the scans showed intra-prostate tracer accumulation [117]. However, the intra-prostatic FDG uptake showed a positive correlation with the Gleason score and the histopathologic T stage, and in addition, the presence of intra-prostatic FDG uptake correlated with poor prognosis [117].

The role of FDG-PET/CT in biochemical recurrence is also limited. For example, in a retrospective study of 91 men with biochemical recurrence following prostatectomy, the overall PET detection rate was only 31%, and the mean PSA levels in FDG-PET/CT positive patients were higher than those with negative results (9.5 ± 2.2 ng/mL vs. 2.1 ± 3.3 ng/mL) [118].

Thus, the ^{18}F-FDG-PET/CT has poor sensitivity as the primary staging investigation in detecting the primary lesion and the LN metastasis and as a restaging investigation while evaluating the patients with biochemical relapse, especially when the PSA level is low. However, FDG PET/CT may help predict the grade and the stage of the disease and the prognosis of the patients.

5.3 ^{11}C- and ^{18}F-Choline-PET/CT

Choline is an essential cell membrane phospholipid and is internalized by choline kinase, an over-expressed enzyme in PC [119]. Three tracers are available for clinical use, ^{11}C-Choline, ^{18}F-Fluoroethylcholine, and ^{18}F-Fluoromethylcholine. The ^{18}F isotopes have a longer half-life, enabling more accessible transport than the ^{11}C isotope, the use of which is limited to centers with an on-site cyclotron. On the other hand, the ^{11}C isotope has lower urinary excretion than the ^{18}F isotopes, enabling theoretically superior prostate imaging. However, both isotopes have demonstrated comparable results [120].

Increased choline uptake within the prostate is observed in benign and malignant pathologies, such as benign prostatic hyperplasia, prostatitis, and PC. Hence, choline-PET cannot reliably differentiate benign from malignant diseases and has a limited role in the localization of PC. For example, in a prospective evaluation of men who underwent ^{11}C-choline-PET/CT before radical prostatectomy, the choline uptake pattern correlated to the histological localization of PC in only 46% of the lesions [121].

For the initial staging of PC, choline-PET/CT is reported to have a higher sensitivity and a similar specificity for the detection of nodal disease as compared to conventional imaging [122]. A positive nodal involvement on choline-PET/CT is of clinical importance, whereas a normal scan cannot exclude micro-metastatic disease. The pooled sensitivity and specificity for detecting pelvic nodal disease are 62% and 92%, respectively [120].

To detect bony metastasis, choline-PET/CT was more sensitive and specific than bone scintigraphy and showed similar sensitivity and higher specificity than sodium fluoride scan [122, 123]. Furthermore, in a meta-analysis comparing choline-PET/CT, bone scintigraphy, MRI, and single positron emission computed tomography (SPECT), choline-PET/CT was found to be most specific of all the investigations for detection of bone metastasis, whereas magnetic resonance imaging had the highest sensitivity [124].

The pooled detection rates of choline-PET/CT for locating the site of relapse in patients with biochemical recurrence were reported as 62%, with a pooled sensitivity and specificity of 89% each [125]. The chances of reporting a positive scan rise with the rising PSA values, with a 19% rate of a positive scan at PSA level 0.2 to 1.0 ng/mL, 46% at PSA level 1 to 3 ng/mL, and 82% at PSA >3 ng/mL [126]. Choline-PET/CT is more accurate in detecting lymph nodal recurrence but somewhat lacks locating prostatic fossa recurrence [127]. Overall, the findings of PET/CT lead to a change in the management in 41–48% of the patients [120].

^{11}C-choline- and ^{18}F-choline-PET/CT have good overall performance in detecting nodal disease in high-risk patients during the initial staging and in patients with biochemical recurrence, especially when the PSA level is high. The current EAU guidelines recommend choline-PET/CT in patients with biochemical recurrence post radical prostatectomy and a PSA level > 1 ng/mL [128].

5.4 ^{18}F-Fluciclovine PET/CT

Trans-1-amino-3^{18}F-fluorocyclobutanecarboxylic acid (^{18}F-fluciclovine), a synthetic non-metabolized leucine amino-acid analog, exploits the increased demand of amino acids in tumor tissues for PC imaging. In contrast to the ^{18}F-FDG, which is excreted via the kidneys and the resultant bladder activity hinders the prostatic imaging, the limited renal excretion and bladder activity of fluciclovine are of particular benefit [129].

^{18}F-fluciclovine PET has a limited role in the initial diagnosis and staging of PC. Non-specific uptake related to benign prostatic hyperplasia limits its use in localizing the primary tumor. Using histopathology as the reference standard, a recent systematic review reported high sensitivity and a variable specificity ranging from 67%–92.5% and 17%–96.6%, respectively, for localizing the primary tumor [130]. The authors explained the high sensitivity because the evaluated patients were already diagnosed cases of PC and proposed that these results may not reproduce in clinical settings.

For the detection of LN metastasis, ^{18}F-fluciclovine showed high specificity (84.8%–100%) but low sensitivity (0%–57.1%) [130]. The authors believed that a certain amount of tumor is required to be detected by ^{18}F-fluciclovine PET. A higher detection rate has been reported for LN $\geq$ 9 mm (83.3%) as compared to those which are $\leq$3 mm (23.7%) [131]. Another meta-analysis, with less stringent inclusion criteria, has shown better results, with a sensitivity and specificity of 83% and 77%, respectively, for the diagnosis of primary carcinoma and 57% and 99% for pre-operative LN staging [132].

^{18}F-fluciclovine has also shown reasonable overall detection rates, ranging from 26–83%, with 78% of the studies reporting >50% detection rates in patients with biochemical recurrence [133]. The pooled sensitivity and specificity for the overall detection of recurrence in a relapsed patient were 68% and 68%, respectively [132]. In general, the detection rates varied with the PSA level, and a detection rate of 55–97% was reported for PSA > 2 ng/mL [133]. A lesion could be detected in 53% of the patients if the PSA was $\leq$0.5 ng/mL, whereas the detection rate was only 29–33% if the PSA was $\leq$0.2 ng/mL. The findings of ^{18}F-fluciclovine impacted the patient management in 59–63% of the patients and impacted the failure-free survival [133]. Nanni et al. compared ^{18}F-fluciclovine-PET/CT with ^{11}C-choline-PET/CT in 89 patients presenting with rising PSA levels post radical prostatectomy and reported superior overall diagnostic performance with ^{18}F-fluciclovine-PET/CT. The overall sensitivity, specificity, and accuracy of fluciclovine-PET/CT were 37%, 67%, and 38%, respectively, whereas for choline-PET/CT were 32%, 40%, and 32%, respectively [134].

The data on ^{18}F-fluciclovine is still emerging, and the dosimetry and the imaging protocol are yet to be standardized. Nevertheless, based on the preliminary data, ^{18}F-fluciclovine appears to be superior to ^{11}C-choline-PET in patients with biochemical recurrence and hence has been approved by the FDA to detect recurrent PC. Although the results are promising, its role in detecting primary tumors and pre-operative LN staging remains to be defined. The current EAU guidelines recommend ^{18}F-fluciclovine-PET/CT as an alternative to choline-PET/CT in patients with biochemical recurrence post radical prostatectomy and a PSA level >1 ng/mL [128].

5.5 ^{68}Gallium Prostate-Specific Membrane Antigen PET/CT

Prostate-specific membrane antigen (PSMA) is a 750-amino acid transmembrane glycoprotein with a small intra-cellular and sizeable extracellular component. It is localized within the apical epithelium of the secretory ducts of benign prostatic tissues. PSMA acts as an enzyme and cleaves α-linked glutamate from N-acetylaspartyl glutamate and γ-linked glutamates from polyglutamate folates, although the physiological significance of this process remains to be defined [135].

PC tissues overexpress PSMA, and instead of being on the apical epithelium, PSMA translocates to the luminal surface of the ducts [136]. Contrary to the name, PSMA is not specific to the prostate and can be found within lacrimal and salivary glands, the kidneys, liver, spleen, and the small intestines [137]. Other tumors such as thyroid, gastric, breast, renal, and colorectal cancers also express PSMA [137]. However, PSMA is over-expressed 100–1000 times in PC tissues compared to other tissues and benign prostatic cells [137]. Also, on binding to its ligand, PSMA is internalized, resulting in enhanced uptake and retention, and both these features result in superior imaging characteristics when used for imaging of PC [138]. Besides, PSMA expression appears to correlate with advanced disease, high Gleason score, high PSA, and castrate-resistant disease; this may result in better imaging quality in patients with aggressive features [139, 140].

5.6 PSMA Targeting Agents

5.6.1 Introduction

PSMA was initially targeted with anti-PSMA monoclonal antibodies, the murine mAb 7E11, which binds to the intracellular domain of PSMA, and the humanized mAb hJ591, which binds to its extracellular domain. 7E11 was radiolabeled with ^{111}In and was developed as a single positron emission tomography (ProstaScint™). However, the overall poor sensitivity gradually phased it out of clinical use [141]. 7E11 was also radiolabeled with ^{90}Y with therapeutic potential. However, high myelotoxicity ultimately stopped further development [142]. The hJ591 was also clinically evaluated for imaging as well as for therapy [143, 144].

These antibody-based imaging agents were marred by long circulation half-life, low signal-to-noise ratio, and poor target tissue uptake. Hence, to overcome imaging shortcomings, small molecule PSMA-peptide inhibitors were developed, which are the current mainstay of PSMA-based imaging and therapeutic modalities. These agents target the extracellular domain of PSMA, have higher PSMA affinity, and are internalized into endosomal recycling system with a rapid blood clearance and low background activity resulting in superior imaging characteristics.

The most widely used PSMA-based tracer is ^{68}Ga-PSMA-N,N′-bis-(2-hydroxy-5-(carboxyethyl)benzyl) ethylenediamine-N,N′-diacetic acid (^{68}Ga-HBED-CC or commonly known as ^{68}Ga-PSMA-11). ^{68}Ga-PSMA-11 belongs to the substance class of peptidomimetic PSMA inhibitors, a class of glutamate-urea-based PSMA inhibitors and has been in clinical use since 2012 [145]. Another promising PSMA specific small molecule imaging agent based on the Glu-urea-Lys structure, similar to Ga-PSMA-11, is 2-(3-{1-carboxy-5-((6-(^{18}F)fluoro-pyridine-3-carbonyl)-amino)-pentyl}-ureido)-pentanedioic acid (^{18}F-DCFPyL).

5.6.2 Physiologic Biodistribution of ^{68}Ga-PSMA

The kidneys excrete unbound 68Ga-PSMA, and this physiologic urinary activity may affect image interpretation and cause a "halo" effect, which is relative photopenia in areas surrounding the areas of high tracer activity such as kidneys and bladder. Because of this halo effect, mild tracer activity in areas surrounding the areas with high tracer activity may not be detected, leading to false-negative results. By this principle, focal physiologic ureteric activity may limit the assessment of small pelvic or retroperitoneal LN, and physiologic urinary bladder activity may activity in mask prostate bed. However, similar limitations caused by urinary physiologic activity are observed with all PET tracers, and ^{68}Ga-PSMA is no exception.

Physiologic uptake of ^{68}Ga-PSMA may also interfere in adequate staging or can be inappropriately reported as metastatic disease. The physiological uptake of PSMA has been demonstrated in lacrimal and salivary glands, the kidneys, liver, spleen, and small intestines, resulting in false-positive or false-negative results [137].

The physiological uptake of ^{68}Ga-PSMA in the liver may obscure liver metastasis, whereas physiologic uptake in the celiac ganglia may be misinterpreted as metastatic retroperitoneal LN and that in the cervicothoracic ganglia may be misinterpreted as bone metastasis [146]. Systemic diseases, such as tuberculosis and sarcoidosis, might also mimic visceral metastasis. Benign bone lesions such as osseous hemangioma, fibrous dysplasia, Paget's disease, and fracture may also show PSMA uptake and may be misreported as metastasis [147]. Several non-prostatic malignancies may demonstrate PSMA uptake, and the most common of them is renal cell carcinoma, particularly clear cell histology followed by chromophobe cell [147]. Of note, 5% of the PC do not demonstrate appreciable PSMA uptake.

5.6.3 ^{68}Ga-PSMA in Localization and Primary Staging of Prostate Cancer

Limited data is available concerning the role of ^{68}Ga-PSMA in the localization of PC. Therefore, ^{68}Ga-PSMA is seldom undertaken and is not recommended for the primary detection of PC in patients with suspicious clinical or biochemical findings. A recent systematic review and meta-analysis evaluated the accuracy of ^{68}Ga-PSMA in patients with suspicion of PC, using histopathology as the reference standard [148]. The authors could identify seven studies with a total of 389 patients, and the mean PSA level of the study group was 12.9 ng/mL. They reported a pooled sensitivity, specificity, positive likelihood ratio, and negative likelihood ratio of 0.97, 0.66, 2.86, and 0.05, respectively, and concluded that ^{68}Ga-PSMA had excellent sensitivity and negative likelihood ratio in the initial detection of PC in patients with clinical or biochemical suspicion [148].

The potential of ^{68}Ga-PSMA for the local staging of PC has been evaluated in biopsy-proven PC patients planned for radical prostatectomy. Fendler et al. evaluated 21 patients with biopsy-proven PC who underwent ^{68}Ga-PSMA before radical prostatectomy [149]. For the detection of primary prostatic cancer, ^{68}Ga-PSMA was found to have a sensitivity, specificity, positive predictive value, negative predictive value, and accuracy of 67%, 92%, 97%, 42%, and 72%, respectively, as compared to the histopathology. PET/CT could correctly detect the SVI with an 86% accuracy, and the tumor spread through the capsule with a 71% accuracy [149]. The intensity of tracer accumulation in primary tumors of patients with PC has been shown to correlate with Gleason score and PSA levels.

Uprimny et al. evaluated 82 patients and noted a significantly lower ^{68}Ga-PSMA uptake in patients with Gleason score 7 or less as compared to those with Gleason score > 7 (median SUV max of 5.9 for Gleason 6, 8.3 for Gleason 7 (3 + 4), 8.2 for Gleason 7 (4 + 3), and 21.2 for Gleason >7; $p < 0.001$) [150]. Also, the patients with PSA ≥ 10.0 ng/mL exhibited significantly higher uptake than those with PSA levels <10.0 ng/mL (median SUV max: 17.6 versus 7.7; $p < 0.001$) [150]. ^{68}Ga-PSMA has been shown to correlate well with the findings of multiparametric MRI for the primary localization of PC [151]. Rhee et al. compared multiparametric MRI and ^{68}Ga-PSMA in 50 histologically confirmed clinically significant lesions and found the sensitivity, specificity, positive predictive value, and negative predictive value for multiparametric MRI as 44%, 94%, 81%, and 76%, respectively, whereas for ^{68}Ga-PSMA were 49%, 95%, 85%, and 88%, respectively [152]. The PSMA-PET/CT yielded a higher specificity and positive predictive value, but a significant proportion of cancers were potentially missed and underestimated by both the imaging modalities [152] (Fig. 5).

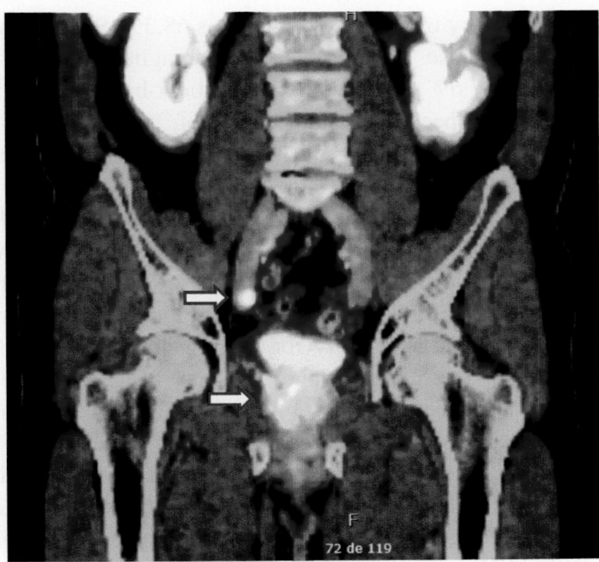

Fig. 5 Staging ^{68}Ga-PSMA PET/CT from a 70-year-old patient demonstrating a large enhancing nodule on the right prostate lobe that extends pass the midline with signs of extraprostatic extension. A single LN involvement is visible on the right external iliac vessels

A combination of ^{68}Ga-PSMA-PET and MRI (^{68}Ga-PSMA-PET/MRI) has also been evaluated for the local staging of PC. PSMA-PET/MRI was able to correctly identify cancer in 97.5% of the patients [153]. Furthermore, the accuracy for overall T staging was 82.5%, for T2 stage was 85%, for T3a stage was 79%, for T3b stage was 94%, and for N1 stage was 93%. In addition, PSMA-PET/MRI changed the therapeutic strategy in 28.7% of the patients with either the onset of systemic therapy/radiotherapy ($n = 16$) or active surveillance ($n = 19$). Therefore, the authors concluded that PSMA-PET/MRI has high accuracy in the initial staging of PC and can change the plan in about a third of the patients [153].

The possible role of ^{68}Ga-PSMA-PET/CT in detecting lymph nodal metastasis during the initial staging is being explored. A prospective multicenter study enrolled 103 patients with newly diagnosed PC with more than 10% Memorial Sloan Kettering Cancer Center (MSKCC) risk for LN metastasis [154]. Ninety-seven extended LND were performed, and 85 LN metastases in 41 patients (42.3%) were found. PET was positive in 17 patients, and per-patient sensitivity, specificity, positive and negative predictive values were 41.5%, 90.9%, 77.3%, and 67.6%, respectively. A PET-based change in the treatment was observed in 12.6% of the patients [154]. Another study retrospectively evaluated 130 patients with high-risk PC staged with ^{68}Ga-PSMA-PET prior to radical prostatectomy and template LND and compared it with morphological imaging [155]. Positive LN at surgery was found in 31.5% of the patients. On the template-based analysis, the authors reported the sensitivity, specificity, and accuracy of ^{68}Ga-PSMA-PET as 68.3%, 99.1%, and 95.2%, and those of morphological imaging as 27.3%, 97.1%, and 87.6%, respectively. On patient-based analysis, the sensitivity, specificity, and accuracy of ^{68}Ga-PSMA-PET were 65.9%, 98.9%, and 88.5%, and those of morphological imaging were 43.9%, 85.4%, and 72.3%, respectively [155]. A recent systematic review, comprising 13 articles and 1597 patients, compared the diagnostic efficiency of ^{68}Ga-PSMA-PET and MRI for staging the LN metastases in patients with PC [156]. ^{68}Ga-PSMA was found to have a higher sensitivity and a comparable specificity for staging pre-operative LN metastases in intermediate- and high-risk PC. The pooled sensitivity and specificity of ^{68}Ga-PSMA-PET were 0.65 and 0.94, respectively, while the corresponding values of MRI were 0.41 and 0.92. Moreover, the area under the symmetric receiver-operating characteristic was higher for ^{68}Ga-PSMA than MRI, indicating a more effective imaging modality in predicting LN metastasis before radical surgery [156].

The efficacy of ^{68}Ga-PSMA-PET/CT has been evaluated to detect bone metastasis as part of initial staging. A recent retrospective review evaluated 1253 men with PC with ^{68}Ga-PSMA-PET/CT with the primary aim to determine the risk of metastasis [157]. The median PSA level was 6.5 ng/mL, and 49.7% had high-risk disease. Metastatic disease was identified in 12.1% of men, including 8.2% with a PSA level of <10 ng/mL and 43% with a PSA level of >20 ng/mL. LN metastases were suspected in 107 men, with 47.7% outside the boundaries of an extended pelvic LND. Skeletal metastases were identified in 4.7%. The chances of detecting metastasis were higher in men with high-risk diseases than those with intermediate-risk PC (19.9% vs. 5.2%) [157].

A prospective randomized multicenter study evaluated men with high-risk PC with either conventional imaging (CT and bone scan) or ^{68}Ga-PSMA-PET/CT with the primary outcome focused on the accuracy of first-line imaging for the identification of pelvic LN or distant metastases, using a predefined reference standard consisting of histopathology, imaging, and biochemistry at 6-month follow-up [158]. PSMA-PET/CT had a 27% greater accuracy than conventional imaging (92% vs. 65%; $p < 0{\cdot}0001$). Also, the sensitivity (85% vs. 38%) and specificity (98% vs. 91%) of PSMA-PET/CT were higher than conventional imaging. Subgroup analysis revealed that PSMA-PET/CT was superior to conventional imaging for the detection of pelvic LN metastasis and distant metastasis. Furthermore, ^{68}Ga-PSMA-PET/CT prompted management change more frequently than conventional imaging (28% vs. 15%) and had fewer equivocal findings (23% vs. 7%). Another prospective multicenter study evaluated 108 patients with an intermediate- and high-risk disease with ^{68}Ga-PSMA-PET/CT as part of initial staging [159].

The findings of Ga-PSMA lead to a change in management in 21% of the patients. Compared to conventional imaging, additional LN and bone/visceral metastasis were found on 25% and 6% of the patients, respectively [159]. Thus, ^{68}Ga-PSMA-PET/CT detects additional lesions over conventional imaging. However, the prognosis and the ideal management of patients diagnosed as metastatic by ^{68}Ga-PSMA-PET/CT are unknown [160]. It is currently unclear whether the patients with metastases, detectable only with PET/CT, should be managed using systemic therapies or whether they should be subjected to aggressive local and metastases-directed therapies [160]. In the absence of prospective studies demonstrating survival benefit, caution must be used when making therapeutic decisions based on ^{68}Ga-PSMA-PET/CT [161].

5.6.4 ^{68}Ga-PSMA in the Restaging of Prostate Cancer

Restaging men with biochemical recurrence after radical treatment is one of the most common clinical indications of ^{68}Ga-PSMA-PET/CT. A single-arm protective study evaluated 635 men with biochemically recurrent PC, either after radical surgery or radiotherapy, who underwent ^{68}Ga-PSMA-PET/CT [162]. ^{68}Ga-PSMA PET localized recurrent PC in 75% of the patients and the detection rates significantly increased with increase in PSA levels: 38% for <0.5 ng/mL, 57% for 0.5 to <1.0 ng/mL, 84% for 1.0 to <2.0 ng/mL, 86% for 2.0 to <5.0 ng/mL, and 97% for ≥5.0 ng/mL. On a per-patient basis, the positive predictive value of ^{68}Ga-PSMA-PET/CT was 84% by histopathologic validation and 92% by the composite reference standard. Two meta-analyses have reported the overall detection rate of ^{68}Ga-PSMA-PET/CT at 74–76% in patients with biochemical relapse and that the pooled estimated rate of positive scans correlates with the PSA levels [163, 164]. ^{68}Ga-PSMA-PET/CT scan also helps identify the affected LN regions before salvage LND in patients with biochemical recurrence [165]. Thirty patients suspected of exclusively nodal PC relapse after primary therapy underwent a template pelvic or retroperitoneal salvage LND after ^{68}Ga-PSMA-PET/CT. The sensitivity, specificity, positive predictive value, negative predictive value, and 68Ga-PSMA-PET/CT accuracy were 93.2%, 100%, 100%, 88.9%, and 95.6%, respectively. The necessary short diameter of tumor deposits in LN metastasis required to reach a detection rate of 50% and 90% was estimated to be ≥2.3 mm and ≥4.5 mm, respectively (Fig. 6).

The findings of ^{68}Ga-PSMA-PET/CT have been shown to impact treatment planning in patients with biochemical recurrence. Two hundred seventy patients with biochemical recurrence post radical prostatectomy and PSA < 1 ng/mL underwent ^{68}Ga-PSMA-PET/CT before radiotherapy as per consensus clinical target volumes (CTVs) based on the Radiation Therapy Oncology Group (RTOG) guidelines [166]. The mean PSA level was 0.48 ng/mL, and 49% of the patients had a positive ^{68}Ga-PSMA-PET/CT result. However, 19% of the patients had at least one PSMA-positive lesion

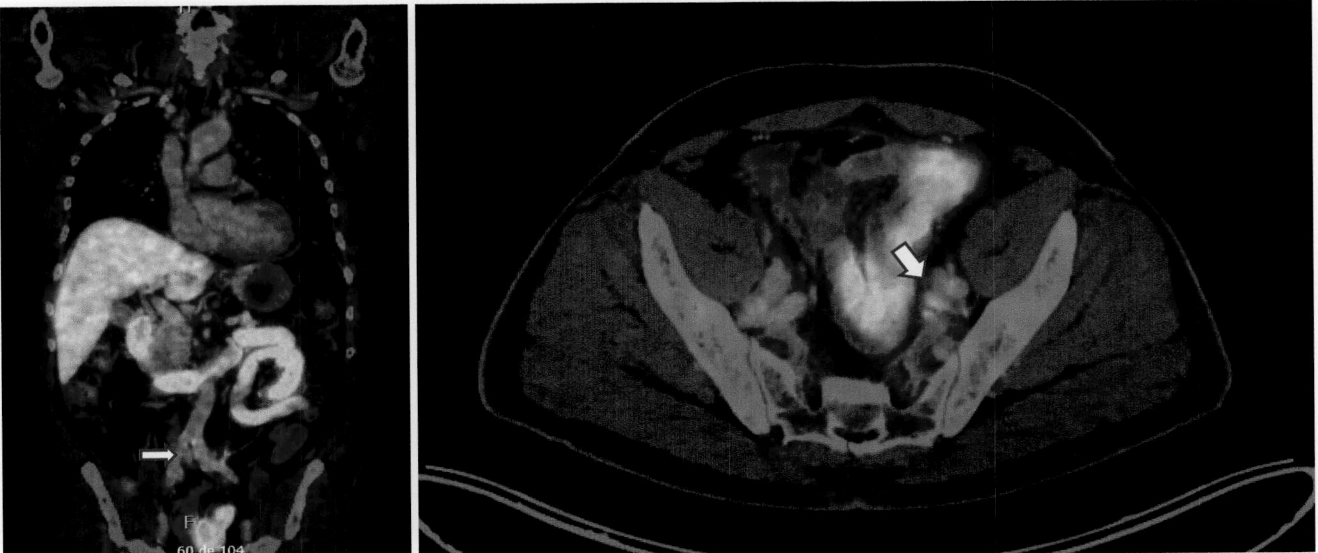

Fig. 6 ^{68}Ga-PSMA PET/CT from a 65-year-old patient who underwent RALP with extended LN dissection 24 months earlier. His PSA has risen to 2.4 ng/ml. PET CT demonstrates saddle uptake of radio-marker on para aortic lymph nodes. Also, some uptake is observed on residual left internal iliac LNs

not covered by the consensus CTVs. In addition, 12% had extra-pelvic PSMA-positive lesions, and 7% had PSMA-positive lesions within the pelvis but not covered by the consensus CTVs. Another study reported a change in the TNM stage in 50.7% of the patients and a change in radiotherapeutic management in 56.3% of the patients with ^{68}Ga-PSMA-PET/CT compared to the conventional imaging in patients with PSA persistence or PSA recurrence post definitive therapy [167]. A meta-analysis that included 15 studies with 1163 patients reported that ^{68}Ga-PSMA-PET/CT findings result in management change in 54% of the patients [168]. In patients with biochemical relapse, ^{68}Ga-PSMA-PET/CT results lead to an increase in the patients being treated with curative intent such as radiotherapy, surgery, focal therapy, or multimodal therapy and a decrease in systemic treatment or no treatment.

5.6.5 ^{68}Ga-PSMA PET/CT Versus Conventional Imaging

Multiple studies have compared ^{68}Ga-PSMA-PET/CT with multiparametric MRI to evaluate men with PC, usually as the initial staging modalities. However, with mixed results, few studies have compared both the imaging modalities for detecting extracapsular extension, SVI, and bladder neck invasion. For example, Celen et al. found that multiparametric MRI had better accuracy than ^{68}Ga-PSMA-PET/CT for detecting extracapsular extension and SVI, whereas both were similar for the detection of bladder neck invasion [169], whereas Muehlematter et al. reported similar detection rates for both the imaging modalities for detecting extracapsular extension and SVI [170].

A recent systematic review compared ^{68}Ga-PSMA-PET/CT and MRI and reported that ^{68}Ga-PSMA-PET/CT had a higher sensitivity and a comparable specificity for staging pre-operative LN metastases in patients with intermediate- and high-risk PC [156] (Fig. 7).

Few studies have compared available imaging for evaluation of bone metastasis—^{68}Ga-PSMA-PET/CT, bone scan (^{99m}Tc-labeled diphosphonate), ^{18}F-sodium fluoride PET scan, and MRI. However, a meta-analysis reported that ^{68}Ga-PSMA-PET/CT had the highest per-patient sensitivity and specificity in detecting bone metastases with PC ([171]). The per-patient pooled sensitivities of 68Ga-PSMA-PET/CT, NaF-PET/CT, MRI, and bone scan were 0.97, 0.96, 0.91, and 0.86, respectively, and the pooled specificities were 1.00, 0.97, 0.96, and 0.95, respectively.

5.6.6 ^{68}Ga-PSMA PET/CT Versus Other PET/CT

^{68}Ga-PSMA-PET/CT and choline-PET/CT are used to detect LN metastasis and distant metastasis in patients with primary and recurrent PC. Although ^{68}Ga-PSMA-PET/CT was found to have higher detection of both LN metastasis and bone metastasis, both imaging modalities tend to miss lesions and complement each other [172]. A meta-analysis did not find a significant difference between ^{68}Ga-PSMA-PET/CT and ^{18}F-choline-PET/CT for staging and restaging performance in patients with PC [173]. The patient-based overall pooled sensitivity, specificity, positive likelihood ratio, negative likelihood ratio, diagnostic odds ratio, and area under the summary receiver-operating characteristic curve of ^{68}Ga-PSMA-PET/CT for staging in PC (13 studies) were 0.92, 0.94, 7.91, 0.14, 79.04, and 0.96, respectively, whereas

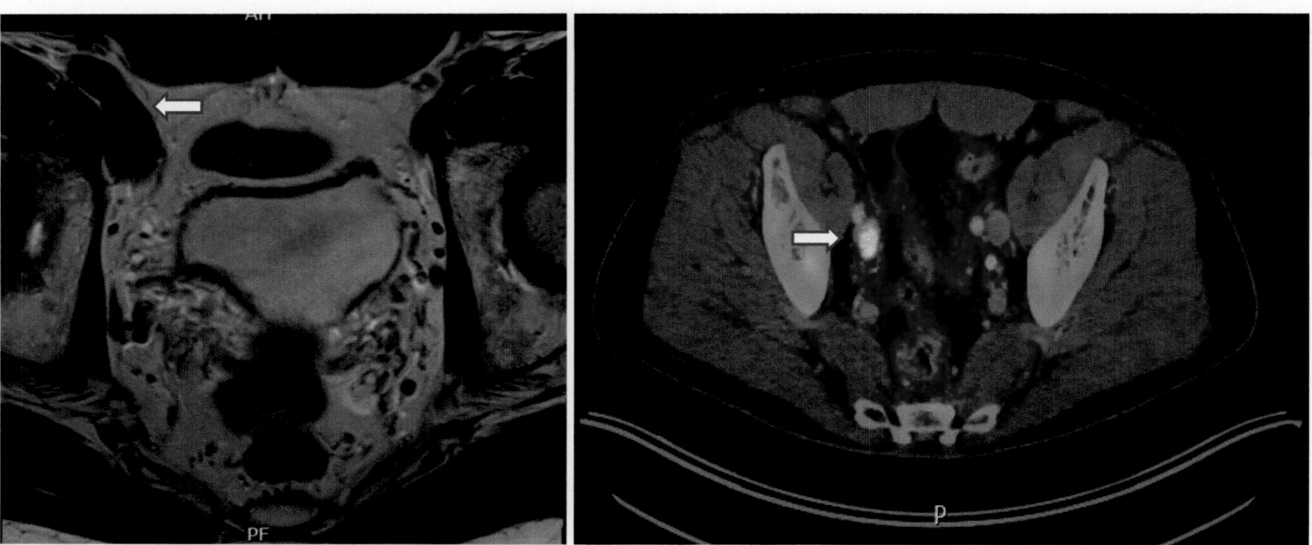

Fig. 7 Staging mp prostate MRI (left) from a 64-year-old patient showing no signs of pelvic LN involvement, whereas ^{68}Ga-PSMA PET/CT (right) from the same patient demonstrates a positive LN on the right external iliac vessels

those of F-choline-PET/CT (16 studies) were 0.93, 0.83, 4.98, 0.10, 68.27, and 0.95, respectively.

Head-to-head comparison studies between ^{68}Ga-PSMA-PET/CT and ^{18}F-fluciclovine-PET/CT are limited but have reported slightly inferior results for ^{18}F-fluciclovine-PET/CT for the detection of pelvic nodal disease, extra-pelvic nodal disease, and bone metastasis [174]. The key advantage of ^{18}F-fluciclovine is its capacity to detect localized foyers in close anatomical relation to the urinary bladder, an area where the physiological accumulation of ^{68}Ga-PSMA-PET/CT hinders the detection [175].

^{68}Ga-PSMA PET/CT is the current imaging modality of choice in patients with biochemical recurrence post definitive therapy. The current EAU guidelines recommend ^{68}Ga-PSMA-PET/CT in patients with biochemical recurrence post radical prostatectomy and a PSA level >0.2 ng/mL [128]. Its role in the primary staging of PC patients is under evaluation. Available data has found ^{68}Ga-PSMA-PET/CT to be superior to conventional imaging in detecting LN metastasis and distant metastasis in intermediate- and high-risk patients. In addition, ^{68}Ga-PSMA-PET/CT findings have been shown to affect management decisions. However, in the absence of prospective studies demonstrating survival benefits, caution must be exercised while making management decisions.

5.7 ^{18}F-DCFPyL PET/CT

2-(3-{1-carboxy-5-((6-(^{18}F)fluoro-pyridine-3-carbonyl)-amino)-pentyl}-ureido)-pentanedioic acid (^{18}F-DCFPyL) is a PSMA specific small molecule imaging agent based on Glu-urea-Lys structure, similar to ^{68}Ga-PSMA-11. Introduced in 2015, ^{18}F-DCFPyL is a second-generation fluorinated PSMA-targeted PET radiotracer and is gradually becoming a front-runner candidate for PSMA PET imaging. ^{18}F labeled small molecules offer a few advantages over those labeled with ^{68}Ga. More favorable dosimetry allows for higher injected radiotracer doses, and lower-energy emitted positrons lead to higher spatial resolution and reduced blurring effects producing superior quality images [176]. Also, the longer half-life (109 min vs. 68 min) allows ^{18}F radiotracers to be produced in cyclotrons in large, centralized batches and then transported to remote locations compared to 68Ga radiotracers that require an on-site generator. These distinct advantages make ^{18}F-DCFPyL a better PSMA-targeted PET radiotracer than ^{68}Ga-PSMA-11, at least in theory.

^{18}F-DCFPyL PET/CT has been evaluated in various clinical scenarios related to PC, and the results have been promising. In patients with intermediate- and high-risk PC, the addition of ^{18}F-DCFPyL PET/CT to the current recommended conventional imaging leads to an upstaging to metastatic disease in 23% of the patients, and 50% of those who were thought to be metastatic were downstaged to non-metastatic disease [177]. Incorporating ^{18}F-DCFPyL PET/CT into the initial conventional imaging workup for PC leads to a change in the pre-specified treatment recommendations in 39% of the patients. In patients with biochemical recurrence, ^{18}F-DCFPyL PET/CT showed a 77.8% overall detection rate, with the PSA stratified detection rates of 47.6%, 50%, 88.9%, and 94% for PSA levels of >0.2 to <0.5, 0.5 to <1.0, 1 to <2.0, and ≥2.0 ng/mL, respectively [178]. A meta-analysis reported a pooled detection rate for ^{18}F-DCFPyL PET/CT as 92%, the detection rate for PSA ≥0.5 ng/mL was

89% whereas that for PSA <0.5 ng/mL was 49% [179]. Dietlein et al. compared ^{18}F-DCFPyL PET/CT with Ga-PSMA PET/CT in 14 patients with biochemical relapse [180]. All suspicious lesions identified by Ga-PSMA PET/CT were also detected with ^{18}F-DCFPyL PET/CT. In three patients, additional lesions were observed using ^{18}F-DCFPyL PET/CT.

^{18}F-DCFPyL PET/CT is a fluorinated PSMA-targeted radiotracer and should have all the essential qualities of PSMA-based imaging with additional benefits of ^{18}F radiotracer such as longer half-life and superior image quality. It has shown promising results in evaluating men with PC in primary as well as recurrent settings. Based on the promising reports, FDA recently approved ^{18}F-DCFPyL PET/CT for use in PC. Ongoing evaluation and research will further help in establishing its role in the diagnostic armamentarium for PC.

Bibliography

Ultrasound

1. Norberg M, Egevad L, Holmberg L, et al. The sextant protocol for ultrasound-guided core biopsies of the prostate underestimates the presence of cancer. Urology. 1997;50:562–6. https://doi.org/10.1016/S0090-4295(97)00306-3.
2. Beerlage HP, Aarnink RG, Ruijter ET, et al. Correlation of transrectal ultrasound, computer analysis of transrectal ultra- sound and histopathology of radical prostatectomy specimen. Prostate Cancer Prostatic Dis. 2001;4:56–62. https://doi.org/10.1038/sj.pcan.4500495.
3. Cheng S, Rifkin MD. Color Doppler imaging of the prostate: important adjunct to endorectal ultrasound of the prostate in the diagnosis of prostate cancer. Ultrasound Q. 2001;17:185–9. https://doi.org/10.1097/00013644-200109000-00008.
4. Correas JM, et al. Advanced ultrasound in the diagnosis of prostate cancer. World J Urol. 2021;39:661.
5. Klotz L. Can high resolution micro-ultrasound replace MRI in the diagnosis of prostate cancer? Eur Urol Focus. 2020;6(2):419–23. https://doi.org/10.1016/j.euf.2019.11.006.
6. Ghai S, Eure G, Fradet V, Hyndman ME, McGrath T, Wodlinger B, Pavlovich CP. Assessing cancer risk on novel 29 MHz micro-ultra- sound images of the prostate: creation of the micro-ultrasound protocol for prostate risk identification (PRIMUS). J Urol. 2016;196(2):562–9.
7. Lughezzani G, et al. Comparison of the diagnostic accuracy of micro-ultrasound and magnetic resonance imaging/ultrasound fusion targeted biopsies for the diagnosis of clinically significant prostate cancer. Eur Urol Oncol. 2019;2:329.
8. Cornud F, et al. MRI-directed high-frequency (29MhZ) TRUS-guided biopsies: initial results of a single-center study. Eur Radiol. 2020;30:4838.
9. Pavlovich C, Hyndman ME, Eure G, et al. A multi-institutional randomized controlled trial comparing novel first generation high resolution micro-ultrasound with conventional frequency ultrasound for transrectal prostate biopsy. J Urol. 2019;201:e394.
10. Klotz L, Lughezzani G, Maffei D, et al. Comparison of micro-ultrasound and multiparametric magnetic resonance imaging for prostate cancer: a multicenter, prospective analysis. Can Urol Assoc J. 2021 Jan;15(1):E11–6. https://doi.org/10.5489/cuaj.6712.
11. Halpern EJ, Gomella LG, Forsberg F, et al. Contrast enhanced transrectal ultrasound for the detection of prostate cancer: a randomized, double-blind trial of dutasteride pretreatment. J Urol. 2012;188:1739–45. https://doi.org/10.1016/j.juro.2012.07.021.
12. Sidhu PS, Cantisani V, Dietrich CF, et al. The EFSUMB guidelines and recommendations for the clinical practice of contrast-enhanced ultrasound (CEUS) in non-hepatic applications: update 2017 (long version). Ultraschall Med. 2018;39:e2–e44. https://doi.org/10.1055/a-0586-1107.
13. Trabulsi EJ, Calio BP, Kamel SI, et al. Prostate contrast enhanced transrectal ultrasound evaluation of the prostate with whole-mount prostatectomy correlation. Urology. 2019;133:187–91. https://doi.org/10.1016/j.urology.2019.07.026.
14. Roy C, Buy X, Lang H, et al. Contrast enhanced color Doppler endorectal sonography of prostate: efficiency for detecting peripheral zone tumors and role for biopsy procedure. J Urol. 2003;170:69–72. https://doi.org/10.1097/01.ju.0000072342.01573.8d.
15. Yunkai Z, Yaqing C, Jun J, et al. Comparison of contrast-enhanced ultrasound targeted biopsy versus standard systematic biopsy for clinically significant prostate cancer detection: results of a prospective cohort study with 1024 patients. World J Urol. 2019;37:805–11. https://doi.org/10.1007/s00345-018-2441-1.
16. Phipps S, Yang THJ, Habib FK, et al. Measurement of tis- sue mechanical characteristics to distinguish between benign and malignant prostatic disease. Urology. 2005;66:447–50. https://doi.org/10.1016/j.urology.2005.03.017.
17. Hoyt K, Castaneda B, Zhang M, et al. Tissue elasticity properties as biomarkers for prostate cancer. Cancer Biomark Sect Dis Markers. 2008;4:213–25. https://doi.org/10.3233/cbm-2008-44-505.
18. Zhang M, Nigwekar P, Castaneda B, et al. Quantitative characterization of viscoelastic properties of human prostate correlated with histology. Ultrasound Med Biol. 2008;34:1033–42. https://doi.org/10.1016/j.ultrasmedbio.2007.11.024.
19. Barr RG, Cosgrove D, Brock M, et al. WFUMB guidelines and recommendations on the clinical use of ultrasound elastography: part 5. Prostate Ultrasound Med Biol. 2017;43:27–48. https://doi.org/10.1016/j.ultrasmedbio.2016.06.020.
20. Ahmad S, et al. Transrectal quantitative shear wave elastography in the detection and characterization of prostate cancer. Surg Endosc. 2013;27(9):3280–7.
21. Zhang M, Tang J, Luo Y, et al. Diagnostic performance of multiparametric transrectal ultrasound in localized prostate cancer: a comparative study with magnetic resonance imaging. J Ultrasound Med Off J Am Inst Ultrasound Med. 2019;38:1823–30.

Computed Tomography Scan

22. Saokar A, et al. Detection of lymph nodes in pelvic malignancies with computed tomography and magnetic resonance imaging. Clin Imaging. 2010;34(5):361–6.
23. Lecouvet FE, et al. Can whole-body magnetic resonance imaging with diffusion-weighted imaging replace Tc 99 m bone scanning and computed tomography for single-step detection of metastases in patients with high-risk prostate cancer? Eur Urol. 2012;62(1):68–75.
24. Harisinghani MG, et al. Noninvasive detection of clinically occult lymph-node metastases in prostate cancer. N Engl J Med. 2003;348:2491.
25. Hovels AM, et al. The diagnostic accuracy of CT and MRI in the staging of pelvic lymph nodes in patients with prostate cancer: a meta-analysis. Clin Radiol. 2008;63:387.

26. Abuzallouf S, et al. Baseline staging of newly diagnosed prostate cancer: a summary of the literature. J Urol. 2004;171:2122.
27. Gabriele D, et al. Is there still a role for computed tomography and bone scintigraphy in prostate cancer staging? An analysis from the EUREKA-1 database. World J Urol. 2016;34:517.

Bone Scan

28. Bjurlin MA, et al. Imaging and evaluation of patients with high-risk prostate cancer. Nat Rev Urol. 2015;12(11):617–28.
29. Briganti A, et al. When to perform bone scan in patients with newly diagnosed prostate cancer: external validation of the currently available guidelines and proposal of a novel risk stratification tool. Eur Urol. 2010;57:551.
30. Zhou J, Gou Z, Wu R, Yuan Y, Yu G, Zhao Y. Comparison of PSMA-PET/CT, choline-PET/CT, NaF-PET/CT, MRI, and bone scintigraphy in the diagnosis of bone metastases in patients with prostate cancer: a systematic review and meta-analysis. Skeletal Radiol. 2019;48(12):1915–24. https://doi.org/10.1007/s00256-019-03230-z.
31. Network (2021) N.C.C. NCCN guidelines version 2.2021 prostate cancer. www.NCCN.org
32. EUA guidelines 2021. www.uroweb.org.

Magnetic Resonance Imaging

33. Weinreb JC, Barentsz JO, Choyke PL, Cornud F, Haider MA, Macura KJ, et al. PI-RADS prostate imaging - reporting and data system: 2015, version 2. Eur Urol. 2016;69:16–40. https://doi.org/10.1016/j.eururo.2015.08.052.
34. Turkbey B, Rosenkrantz AB, Haider MA, Padhani AR, Villeirs G, Macura KJ, et al. Prostate imaging reporting and data system version 2.1: 2019 update of prostate imaging reporting and data system version 2. Eur Urol. 2019;76:340–51. https://doi.org/10.1016/j.eururo.2019.02.033.
35. Turkbey B, Huang R, Vourganti S, Trivedi H, Bernardo M, Yan P, et al. Age-related changes in prostate zonal volumes as measured by high-resolution magnetic resonance imaging (MRI): a cross-sectional study in over 500 patients. BJU Int. 2012;110:1642–7. https://doi.org/10.1111/j.1464-410X.2012.11469.x.
36. Ren J, Liu H, Wang H, Wen D, Huang X, Ren F, et al. MRI to predict prostate growth and development in children, adolescents and young adults. Eur Radiol. 2015;25:516–22. https://doi.org/10.1007/s00330-014-3372-x.
37. Coakley FV, Hricak H. Radiologic anatomy of the prostate gland: a clinical approach. Radiol Clin N Am. 2000;38:15–30. https://doi.org/10.1016/s0033-8389(05)70147-0.
38. McNeal JE. The zonal anatomy of the prostate. Prostate. 1981;2:35–49. https://doi.org/10.1002/pros.2990020105.
39. Selman SH. The McNeal prostate: a review. Urology. 2011;78:1224–8. https://doi.org/10.1016/j.urology.2011.07.1395.
40. Paño B, Sebastià C, Buñesch L, Mestres J, Salvador R, Macías NG, et al. Pathways of lymphatic spread in male urogenital pelvic malignancies. Radiogr Rev Publ Radiol Soc N Am Inc. 2011;31:135–60. https://doi.org/10.1148/rg.311105072.
41. Aaron L, Franco OE, Hayward SW. Review of prostate anatomy and embryology and the etiology of benign prostatic hyperplasia. Urol Clin North Am. 2016;43:279–88. https://doi.org/10.1016/j.ucl.2016.04.012.
42. Fine SW, Reuter VE. Anatomy of the prostate revisited: implications for prostate biopsy and zonal origins of prostate cancer. Histopathology. 2012;60:142–52. https://doi.org/10.1111/j.1365-2559.2011.04004.x.
43. Semple JE. Surgical capsule of the benign enlargement of the prostate. Its development and action. Br Med J. 1963;1:1640–3. https://doi.org/10.1136/bmj.1.5346.1640.
44. Vargas HA, Akin O, Franiel T, Goldman DA, Udo K, Touijer KA, et al. Normal central zone of the prostate and central zone involvement by prostate cancer: clinical and MR imaging implications. Radiology. 2012;262:894–902. https://doi.org/10.1148/radiol.11110663.
45. Kitzing YX, Prando A, Varol C, Karczmar GS, Maclean F, Oto A. Benign conditions that mimic prostate carcinoma: MR imaging features with histopathologic correlation. Radiogr Rev Publ Radiol Soc N Am Inc. 2016;36:162–75. https://doi.org/10.1148/rg.2016150030.
46. Barkovich EJ, Shankar PR, Westphalen AC. A systematic review of the existing prostate imaging reporting and data system version 2 (PI-RADSv2) literature and subset meta-analysis of PI-RADSv2 categories stratified by gleason scores. AJR Am J Roentgenol. 2019;212:847–54. https://doi.org/10.2214/AJR.18.20571.
47. McNeal J. Pathology of benign prostatic hyperplasia. Insight into etiology. Urol Clin North Am. 1990;17:477–86.
48. Sanda MG, Cadeddu JA, Kirkby E, Chen RC, Crispino T, Fontanarosa J, et al. Clinically localized prostate cancer: AUA/ASTRO/SUO guideline. Part II: recommended approaches and details of specific care options. J Urol. 2018;199:990–7. https://doi.org/10.1016/j.juro.2018.01.002.
49. Mottet N, Bellmunt J, Bolla M, Briers E, Cumberbatch MG, De Santis M, et al. EAU-ESTRO-SIOG guidelines on prostate cancer. Part 1: screening, diagnosis, and local treatment with curative intent. Eur Urol. 2017;71:618–29. https://doi.org/10.1016/j.eururo.2016.08.003.
50. Mohler JL, Antonarakis ES, Armstrong AJ, D'Amico AV, Davis BJ, Dorff T, et al. Prostate cancer, version 2.2019, NCCN clinical practice guidelines in oncology. J Natl Compr Cancer Netw. 2019;17:479–505. https://doi.org/10.6004/jnccn.2019.0023.
51. Fam MM, Yabes JG, Macleod LC, Bandari J, Turner RM, Lopa SH, et al. Increasing utilization of multiparametric magnetic resonance imaging in prostate cancer active surveillance. Urology. 2019;130:99–105. https://doi.org/10.1016/j.urology.2019.02.037.
52. Fütterer JJ, Briganti A, De Visschere P, Emberton M, Giannarini G, Kirkham A, et al. Can clinically significant prostate cancer be detected with multiparametric magnetic resonance imaging? A systematic review of the literature. Eur Urol. 2015;68:1045–53. https://doi.org/10.1016/j.eururo.2015.01.013.
53. Schoots IG, Petrides N, Giganti F, Bokhorst LP, Rannikko A, Klotz L, et al. Magnetic resonance imaging in active surveillance of prostate cancer: a systematic review. Eur Urol. 2015;67:627–36. https://doi.org/10.1016/j.eururo.2014.10.050.
54. Barentsz JO, Richenberg J, Clements R, Choyke P, Verma S, Villeirs G, et al. ESUR prostate MR guidelines 2012. Eur Radiol. 2012;22:746–57. https://doi.org/10.1007/s00330-011-2377-y.
55. Dickinson L, Ahmed HU, Allen C, Barentsz JO, Carey B, Futterer JJ, et al. Scoring systems used for the interpretation and reporting of multiparametric MRI for prostate cancer detection, localization, and characterization: could standardization lead to improved utilization of imaging within the diagnostic pathway? J Magn Reson Imaging. 2013;37:48–58. https://doi.org/10.1002/jmri.23689.
56. Vaché T, Bratan F, Mège-Lechevallier F, Roche S, Rabilloud M, Rouvière O. Characterization of prostate lesions as benign or malignant at multiparametric MR imaging: comparison of three scoring systems in patients treated with radical prostatectomy. Radiology. 2014;272:446–55. https://doi.org/10.1148/radiol.14131584.

57. Renard-Penna R, Mozer P, Cornud F, Barry-Delongchamps N, Bruguière E, Portalez D, et al. Prostate imaging reporting and data system and likert scoring system: multiparametric MR imaging validation study to screen patients for initial biopsy. Radiology. 2015;275:458–68. https://doi.org/10.1148/radiol.14140184.
58. Zhai L, Fan Y, Meng Y, Feng X, Yu W, Jin J. The role of Prostate Imaging Reporting and Data System score in Gleason 3 + 3 active surveillance candidates enrollment: a diagnostic meta-analysis. Prostate Cancer Prostatic Dis. 2019;22:235–43. https://doi.org/10.1038/s41391-018-0111-4.
59. Wang AZ, O'Conno LP, Yerram NK, Long L, Zeng J, Mehralivand S, et al. PI-RADS® category as a predictor of progression to unfavorable risk prostate cancer in men on active surveillance. J Urol. 2020;204:1229–35. https://doi.org/10.1097/JU.0000000000001307.
60. Moore CM, Giganti F, Albertsen P, Allen C, Bangma C, Briganti A, et al. Reporting magnetic resonance imaging in men on active surveillance for prostate cancer: the PRECISE recommendations-a report of a european school of oncology task force. Eur Urol. 2017;71:648–55. https://doi.org/10.1016/j.eururo.2016.06.011.
61. Giganti F, Stabile A, Stavrinides V, Osinibi E, Retter A, Orczyk C, et al. Natural history of prostate cancer on active surveillance: stratification by MRI using the PRECISE recommendations in a UK cohort. Eur Radiol. 2021;31:1644–55. https://doi.org/10.1007/s00330-020-07256-z.
62. Recabal P, Assel M, Sjoberg DD, Lee D, Laudone VP, Touijer K, et al. The efficacy of multiparametric magnetic resonance imaging and magnetic resonance imaging targeted biopsy in risk classification for patients with prostate cancer on active surveillance. J Urol. 2016;196:374–81. https://doi.org/10.1016/j.juro.2016.02.084.
63. Chesnut GT, Vertosick EA, Benfante N, Sjoberg DD, Fainberg J, Lee T, et al. Role of changes in magnetic resonance imaging or clinical stage in evaluation of disease progression for men with prostate cancer on active surveillance. Eur Urol. 2020;77:501–7. https://doi.org/10.1016/j.eururo.2019.12.009.
64. Stavrinides V, Giganti F, Trock B, Punwani S, Allen C, Kirkham A, et al. Five-year outcomes of magnetic resonance imaging-based active surveillance for prostate cancer: a large cohort study. Eur Urol. 2020;78:443–51. https://doi.org/10.1016/j.eururo.2020.03.035.
65. Bryant RJ, Yang B, Philippou Y, Lam K, Obiakor M, Ayers J, et al. Does the introduction of prostate multiparametric magnetic resonance imaging into the active surveillance protocol for localized prostate cancer improve patient reclassification? BJU Int. 2018;122:794–800. https://doi.org/10.1111/bju.14248.
66. Schoots IG, Nieboer D, Giganti F, Moore CM, Bangma CH, Roobol MJ. Is magnetic resonance imaging-targeted biopsy a useful addition to systematic confirmatory biopsy in men on active surveillance for low-risk prostate cancer? A systematic review and meta-analysis. BJU Int. 2018;122:946–58. https://doi.org/10.1111/bju.14358.
67. Klotz L, Pond G, Loblaw A, Sugar L, Moussa M, Berman D, et al. Randomized study of systematic biopsy versus magnetic resonance imaging and targeted and systematic biopsy in men on active surveillance (ASIST): 2-year postbiopsy follow-up. Eur Urol. 2020;77:311–7. https://doi.org/10.1016/j.eururo.2019.10.007.
68. Meyer AR, Mamawala M, Winoker JS, Landis P, Epstein JI, Macura KJ, et al. Transperineal prostate biopsy improves the detection of clinically significant prostate cancer among men on active surveillance. J Urol. 2021;205:1069–74. https://doi.org/10.1097/JU.0000000000001523.
69. Stonier T, Tin AL, Sjoberg DD, Jibara G, Vickers AJ, Fine S, et al. Selecting patients with favorable risk, grade group 2 prostate cancer for active surveillance-does magnetic resonance imaging have a role? J Urol. 2021;205:1063–8. https://doi.org/10.1097/JU.0000000000001519.
70. de Rooij M, Hamoen EHJ, Witjes JA, Barentsz JO, Rovers MM. Accuracy of magnetic resonance imaging for local staging of prostate cancer: a diagnostic meta-analysis. Eur Urol. 2016;70:233–45. https://doi.org/10.1016/j.eururo.2015.07.029.
71. Cornud F, Flam T, Chauveinc L, Hamida K, Chrétien Y, Vieillefond A, et al. Extraprostatic spread of clinically localized prostate cancer: factors predictive of pT3 tumor and of positive endorectal MR imaging examination results. Radiology. 2002;224:203–10. https://doi.org/10.1148/radiol.2241011001.
72. Jager GJ, Ruijter ET, van de Kaa CA, de la Rosette JJ, Oosterhof GO, Thornbury JR, et al. Local staging of prostate cancer with endorectal MR imaging: correlation with histopathology. AJR Am J Roentgenol. 1996;166:845–52. https://doi.org/10.2214/ajr.166.4.8610561.
73. Heijmink SWTPJ, Fütterer JJ, Hambrock T, Takahashi S, Scheenen TWJ, Huisman HJ, et al. Prostate cancer: body-array versus endorectal coil MR imaging at 3 T--comparison of image quality, localization, and staging performance. Radiology. 2007;244:184–95. https://doi.org/10.1148/radiol.2441060425.
74. Dell'Oglio P, Stabile A, Dias BH, Gandaglia G, Mazzone E, Fossati N, et al. Impact of multiparametric MRI and MRI-targeted biopsy on pre-therapeutic risk assessment in prostate cancer patients candidate for radical prostatectomy. World J Urol. 2019;37:221–34. https://doi.org/10.1007/s00345-018-2360-1.
75. Gandaglia G, Ploussard G, Valerio M, Mattei A, Fiori C, Roumiguié M, et al. The key combined value of multiparametric magnetic resonance imaging, and magnetic resonance imaging-targeted and concomitant systematic biopsies for the prediction of adverse pathological features in prostate cancer patients undergoing radical prostatectomy. Eur Urol. 2020;77:733–41. https://doi.org/10.1016/j.eururo.2019.09.005.
76. Mottet N, Cornford P, van den Bergh RCN, Briers, E, Expert Patient Advocate, De Santis M, et al. EAU - EANM - ESTRO - ESUR - ISUP - SIOG Guidelines on Prostate Cancer. EAU Guidel Off Arnh Neth 2021. http://uroweb.org/guidelines/compilations-of-all-guidelines/.
77. Hövels AM, Heesakkers RAM, Adang EM, Jager GJ, Strum S, Hoogeveen YL, et al. The diagnostic accuracy of CT and MRI in the staging of pelvic lymph nodes in patients with prostate cancer: a meta-analysis. Clin Radiol. 2008;63:387–95. https://doi.org/10.1016/j.crad.2007.05.022.
78. Thoeny HC, Froehlich JM, Triantafyllou M, Huesler J, Bains LJ, Vermathen P, et al. Metastases in normal-sized pelvic lymph nodes: detection with diffusion-weighted MR imaging. Radiology. 2014;273:125–35. https://doi.org/10.1148/radiol.14132921.
79. Abuzallouf S, Dayes I, Lukka H. Baseline staging of newly diagnosed prostate cancer: a summary of the literature. J Urol. 2004;171:2122–7. https://doi.org/10.1097/01.ju.0000123981.03084.06.
80. Kiss B, Thoeny HC, Studer UE. Current status of lymph node imaging in bladder and prostate cancer. Urology. 2016;96:1–7. https://doi.org/10.1016/j.urology.2016.02.014.
81. Peabody H, Lane BR, Qi J, Kim T, Montie JE, Moriarity A, et al. Limitations of abdominopelvic CT and multiparametric MR imaging for detection of lymph node metastases prior to radical prostatectomy. World J Urol. 2021;39:779–85. https://doi.org/10.1007/s00345-020-03227-7.
82. Prostate cancer nomograms: dynamic prostate cancer nomogram: coefficients | Memorial Sloan Kettering Cancer Center n.d. https://www.mskcc.org/nomograms/prostate/pre_op/coefficients (accessed June 26, 2021).
83. Briganti A, Larcher A, Abdollah F, Capitanio U, Gallina A, Suardi N, et al. Updated nomogram predicting lymph node invasion in patients with prostate cancer undergoing extended pelvic lymph node dissection: the essential importance of percentage of posi-

tive cores. Eur Urol. 2012;61:480–7. https://doi.org/10.1016/j.eururo.2011.10.044.

84. Gandaglia G, Fossati N, Zaffuto E, Bandini M, Dell'Oglio P, Bravi CA, et al. Development and internal validation of a novel model to identify the candidates for extended pelvic lymph node dissection in prostate cancer. Eur Urol. 2017;72:632–40. https://doi.org/10.1016/j.eururo.2017.03.049.
85. Draulans C, Everaerts W, Isebaert S, Van Bruwaene S, Gevaert T, Oyen R, et al. Development and external validation of a multiparametric magnetic resonance imaging and international society of urological pathology based add-on prediction tool to identify prostate cancer candidates for pelvic lymph node dissection. J Urol. 2020;203:713–8. https://doi.org/10.1097/JU.0000000000000652.
86. Messiou C, Collins DJ, Giles S, de Bono JS, Bianchini D, de Souza NM. Assessing response in bone metastases in prostate cancer with diffusion weighted MRI. Eur Radiol. 2011;21:2169–77. https://doi.org/10.1007/s00330-011-2173-8.
87. Gutzeit A, Doert A, Froehlich JM, Eckhardt BP, Meili A, Scherr P, et al. Comparison of diffusion-weighted whole body MRI and skeletal scintigraphy for the detection of bone metastases in patients with prostate or breast carcinoma. Skelet Radiol. 2010;39:333–43. https://doi.org/10.1007/s00256-009-0789-4.
88. Lecouvet FE, El Mouedden J, Collette L, Coche E, Danse E, Jamar F, et al. Can whole-body magnetic resonance imaging with diffusion-weighted imaging replace Tc 99m bone scanning and computed tomography for single-step detection of metastases in patients with high-risk prostate cancer? Eur Urol. 2012;62:68–75. https://doi.org/10.1016/j.eururo.2012.02.020.
89. Pasoglou V, Larbi A, Collette L, Annet L, Jamar F, Machiels J-P, et al. One-step TNM staging of high-risk prostate cancer using magnetic resonance imaging (MRI): toward an upfront simplified "all-in-one" imaging approach? Prostate. 2014;74:469–77. https://doi.org/10.1002/pros.22764.
90. Hicks RJ, Murphy DG, Williams SG. Seduction by sensitivity: reality, illusion, or delusion? The challenge of assessing outcomes after PSMA imaging selection of patients for treatment. J Nucl Med Off Publ Soc Nucl Med. 2017;58:1969–71. https://doi.org/10.2967/jnumed.117.198812.
91. Ploussard G, Staerman F, Pierrevelcin J, Saad R, Beauval J-B, Roupret M, et al. Predictive factors of oncologic outcomes in patients who do not achieve undetectable prostate specific antigen after radical prostatectomy. J Urol. 2013;190:1750–6. https://doi.org/10.1016/j.juro.2013.04.073.
92. Wiegel T, Bartkowiak D, Bottke D, Thamm R, Hinke A, Stöckle M, et al. Prostate-specific antigen persistence after radical prostatectomy as a predictive factor of clinical relapse-free survival and overall survival: 10-year data of the ARO 96-02 trial. Int J Radiat Oncol Biol Phys. 2015;91:288–94. https://doi.org/10.1016/j.ijrobp.2014.09.039.
93. Zagars GK, Pollack A. Kinetics of serum prostate-specific antigen after external beam radiation for clinically localized prostate cancer. Radiother Oncol J Eur Soc Ther Radiol Oncol. 1997;44:213–21. https://doi.org/10.1016/s0167-8140(97)00123-0.
94. Pound CR, Partin AW, Eisenberger MA, Chan DW, Pearson JD, Walsh PC. Natural history of progression after PSA elevation following radical prostatectomy. JAMA. 1999;281:1591–7. https://doi.org/10.1001/jama.281.17.1591.
95. Eiber M, Holzapfel K, Ganter C, Epple K, Metz S, Geinitz H, et al. Whole-body MRI including diffusion-weighted imaging (DWI) for patients with recurring prostate cancer: technical feasibility and assessment of lesion conspicuity in DWI. J Magn Reson Imaging JMRI. 2011;33:1160–70. https://doi.org/10.1002/jmri.22542.
96. Liauw SL, Pitroda SP, Eggener SE, Stadler WM, Pelizzari CA, Vannier MW, et al. Evaluation of the prostate bed for local recurrence after radical prostatectomy using endorectal magnetic resonance imaging. Int J Radiat Oncol Biol Phys. 2013;85:378–84. https://doi.org/10.1016/j.ijrobp.2012.05.015.
97. Linder BJ, Kawashima A, Woodrum DA, Tollefson MK, Karnes J, Davis BJ, et al. Early localization of recurrent prostate cancer after prostatectomy by endorectal coil magnetic resonance imaging. Can J Urol. 2014;21:7283–9.
98. Kitajima K, Murphy RC, Nathan MA, Froemming AT, Hagen CE, Takahashi N, et al. Detection of recurrent prostate cancer after radical prostatectomy: comparison of 11C-choline PET/CT with pelvic multiparametric MR imaging with endorectal coil. J Nucl Med Off Publ Soc Nucl Med. 2014;55:223–32. https://doi.org/10.2967/jnumed.113.123018.
99. Achard V, Lamanna G, Denis A, De Perrot T, Mainta IC, Ratib O, et al. Recurrent prostate cancer after radical prostatectomy: restaging performance of 18F-choline hybrid PET/MRI. Med Oncol Northwood Lond Engl. 2019;36:67. https://doi.org/10.1007/s12032-019-1291-z.
100. Rouvière O, Vitry T, Lyonnet D. Imaging of prostate cancer local recurrences: why and how? Eur Radiol. 2010;20:1254–66. https://doi.org/10.1007/s00330-009-1647-4.
101. Donati OF, Jung SI, Vargas HA, Gultekin DH, Zheng J, Moskowitz CS, et al. Multiparametric prostate MR imaging with T2-weighted, diffusion-weighted, and dynamic contrast-enhanced sequences: are all pulse sequences necessary to detect locally recurrent prostate cancer after radiation therapy? Radiology. 2013;268:440–50. https://doi.org/10.1148/radiol.13122149.
102. Abd-Alazeez M, Ramachandran N, Dikaios N, Ahmed HU, Emberton M, Kirkham A, et al. Multiparametric MRI for detection of radiorecurrent prostate cancer: added value of apparent diffusion coefficient maps and dynamic contrast-enhanced images. Prostate Cancer Prostatic Dis. 2015;18:128–36. https://doi.org/10.1038/pcan.2014.55.
103. Alonzo F, Melodelima C, Bratan F, Vitry T, Crouzet S, Gelet A, et al. Detection of locally radio-recurrent prostate cancer at multiparametric MRI: Can dynamic contrast-enhanced imaging be omitted? Diagn Interv Imaging. 2016;97:433–41. https://doi.org/10.1016/j.diii.2016.01.008.
104. Dinis Fernandes C, Ghobadi G, van der Poel HG, de Jong J, Heijmink SWTPJ, Schoots I, et al. Quantitative 3-T multiparametric MRI and step-section pathology of recurrent prostate cancer patients after radiation therapy. Eur Radiol. 2019;29:4160–8. https://doi.org/10.1007/s00330-018-5819-y.
105. Ceci F, Castellucci P, Graziani T, Schiavina R, Brunocilla E, Mazzarotto R, et al. 11C-choline PET/CT detects the site of relapse in the majority of prostate cancer patients showing biochemical recurrence after EBRT. Eur J Nucl Med Mol Imaging. 2014;41:878–86. https://doi.org/10.1007/s00259-013-2655-9.
106. Panebianco V, Villeirs G, Weinreb JC, Turkbey BI, Margolis DJ, Richenberg J, et al. Prostate magnetic resonance imaging for local recurrence reporting (PI-RR): international consensus-based guidelines on multiparametric magnetic resonance imaging for prostate cancer recurrence after radiation therapy and radical prostatectomy. Eur Urol Oncol. 2021;S2588-9311(21):00027–4. https://doi.org/10.1016/j.euo.2021.01.003.

Positron Emission Tomography CT

107. Macheda ML, Rogers S, Best JD. Molecular and cellular regulation of glucose transporter (GLUT) proteins in cancer. J Cell Physiol. 2005;20:654–62.
108. Liu Y, Zuckier LS, Ghesani NV. Dominant uptake of fatty acid over glucose by prostate cells: a potential new diagnostic and therapeutic approach. Anticancer Res. 2010;30:369–74.

109. Jadvar H, Ye W, Groshen S, Conti PS. (F-18)-Fluorodeoxyglucose PET-CT of the normal prostate gland. Ann Nucl Med. 2008;22:787–93.
110. Bertagna F, Sadeghi R, Giovanella L, Treglia G. Incidental uptake of 18F-fluorodeoxyglucose in the prostate gland: systematic review and meta-analysis on prevalence and risk of malignancy. Nuklearmedizin. 2014;53:249–58.
111. Kang PM, Seo WI, Lee SS, Bae SK, Kwak HS, Min K, et al. Incidental abnormal FDG uptake in the prostate on 18-fluoro-2-deoxyglucose positron emission tomography-computed tomography. Asian Pac J Cancer Prev. 2014;15:8699–703.
112. Seino H, Ono S, Miura H, Morohashi S, Wu Y, Tsushuma F, et al. Incidental prostate 18F-FDG uptake without calcification indicates possibility of prostate cancer. Oncol Rep. 2014;31:1517–22.
113. Jadvar H. Molecular imaging of prostate cancer with (F-18)-fluorodeoxyglucose PET. Nat Rev Urol. 2009;6:317–23.
114. Jadvar H. Imaging evaluation of prostate cancer with 18Ffluorodeoxyglucose PET/CT: utility and limitations. Eur J Nucl Med Mol Imaging. 2013;40:S5–S10.
115. Minamimoto R, Uemura H, Sano F, Tera H, Nagashima Y, Yamanaka S, et al. The potential of FDG PET/CT for detecting prostate cancer in patients with an elevated serum PSA level. Ann Nucl Med. 2011;25:21–7.
116. Minamimoto R, Senda M, Jinnouchi S, Terauchi T, Yoshida T, Murano T, et al. The current status of an FDG-PET cancer screening program in Japan based on a 4-year (2006–2009) nationwide survey. Ann Nucl Med. 2013;27:46–57.
117. Beauregard JM, Blouin AC, Fradet V, Caron A, Fradet Y, Lemay C, et al. FDG-PET/CT for pre-operative staging and prognostic stratification of patients with high-grade prostate cancer at biopsy. Cancer Imaging. 2015;15:2.
118. Jadvar H, Desai B, Ji L, Conti PS, Dorff TB, Groshen SG, et al. Prospective evaluation of 18F-NaF and 18F-FDG PET/CT in detection of occult metastatic disease in biochemical recurrence of prostate cancer. Clin Nucl Med. 2012;37:637–43.
119. Ramírez de Molina A, Gutiérrez R, Ramos MA, Silva JM, Silva J, Bonilla F, et al. Increased choline kinase activity in human breast carcinomas: clinical evidence for a potential novel antitumor strategy. Oncogene. 2002;21:4317–22.
120. von Eyben FE, Kairemo K. Meta-analysis of ^{11}C-choline and ^{18}F-choline PET/CT for management of patients with prostate cancer. Nucl Med Commun. 2014;35:221–30.
121. Bundschuh RA, Wendl CM, Weirich G, Eiber M, Souvatzoglou M, Trieber U, et al. Tumour volume delineation in prostate cancer assessed by (^{11}C)choline PET/ CT: validation with surgical specimens. Eur J Nucl Med Mol Imaging. 2013;40:824–31.
122. Evangelista L, Cimitan M, Zattoni F, Guttilla A, Zattoni F, Saladini G. Comparison between conventional imaging (abdominal-pelvic computed tomography and bone scan) and (18F)choline positron emission tomography/computed tomography imaging for the initial staging of patients with intermediate- to high-risk prostate cancer: a retrospective analysis. Scand J Urol. 2015;49:345–53.
123. Poulsen MH, Petersen H, Høilund-Carlsen PF, Jakobsen JS, Gerke O, Karstoft J, et al. Spine metastases in prostate cancer: comparison of technetium-99m- MDP whole-body bone scintigraphy, (^{18}F) choline positron emission tomography(PET)/computed tomography (CT) and (^{18}F)NaF PET/CT. BJU Int. 2014;114:818–23.
124. Shen G, Deng H, Hu S, Jia Z. Comparison of choline-PET/ CT, MRI, SPECT, and bone scintigraphy in the diagnosis of bone metastases in patients with prostate cancer: a meta-analysis. Skelet Radiol. 2014;43:1503–13.
125. Fanti S, Minozzi S, Castellucci P, Balduzzi S, Herrmann K, Krause BJ, et al. PET/CT with ^{11}C-choline for evaluation of prostate cancer patients with biochemical recurrence: meta-analysis and critical review of available data. Eur J Nucl Med Mol Imaging. 2016;43:55–69.
126. Giovacchini G, Picchio M, Coradeschi E, Bettinardi V, Gianolli L, Scattoni V, et al. Predictive factors of (^{11}C)choline PET/CT in patients with biochemical failure after radical prostatectomy. Eur J Nucl Med Mol Imaging. 2010;37:301–9.
127. Evangelista L, Zattoni F, Guttilla A, Saladini G, Zattoni F, Colletti PM, et al. Choline PET or PET/ CT and biochemical relapse of prostate cancer: a systematic review and meta-analysis. Clin Nucl Med. 2013;38:305–14.
128. Mottet N, Cornford P, van den Bergh RCN, Briers E, De Santis M, Gillessen S, et al. EAU prostate cancer guidelines 2021. European association of urology website. https://uroweb.org/guideline/prostate-cancer/. Updated 2021. Accessed July 21, 2021.
129. McParland BJ, Wall A, Johansson S, Sørensen J. The clinical safety, biodistribution and internal radiation dosimetry of (^{18}F) fluciclovine in healthy adult volunteers. Eur J Nucl Med Mol Imaging. 2013;40:1256–64.
130. Seierstad T, Hole KH, Tulipan AJ, Stromme H, Lilleby W, Revheim ME, et al. ^{18}F-Fluciclovine PET for assessment of prostate cancer with histopathology as reference standard: a systematic review. PET Clin. 2021;16:167–76.
131. Alemozaffar M, Akintayo AA, Abiodun-Ojo OA, Patil D, Saeed F, Huang Y, et al. ^{18}F fluciclovine PET/CT for preoperative staging in patients with intermediate to high risk primary prostate cancer. J Urol. 2020;204:1–7.
132. Biscontini G, Romagnolo C, Cottignoli C, Palucci A, Fringuelli FM, Caldarella C, et al. ^{18}F-Fluciclovine positron emission tomography in prostate cancer: a systematic review and diagnostic meta-analysis. Diagnostics (Basel). 2021;11:304.
133. Rais-Bahrami S, Efstathiou A, Turnbull CM, Camper SB, Kenwright A, Schuster AM, et al. ^{18}F-Fluciclovine PET/CT performance in biochemical recurrence of prostate cancer: a systematic review. Prostate Cancer Prostatic Dis. 2021;24(4):997–1006. https://doi.org/10.1038/s41391-021-00382-9.
134. Nanni C, Zanoni L, Pultrone C, Schiavina R, Brunocilla E, Lodi F, et al. 18F-FACBC (anti1- amino-3-^{18}F-fluorocyclobutane-1-carboxylic acid) versus ^{11}C-choline PET/CT in prostate cancer relapse: results of a prospective trial. Eur J Nucl Med Mol Imaging. 2016;43:1601–10.
135. Yao V, Berkman CE, Choi JK, O'Keefe DS, Bacich DJ. Expression of prostate-specific membrane antigen (PSMA), increases cell folate uptake and proliferation and suggests a novel role for PSMA in the uptake of the non-polyglutamated folate, folic acid. Prostate. 2010;70:305–16.
136. Bouchelouche K, Turkbey B, Choyke PL. PSMA PET and radionuclide therapy in prostate cancer. Semin Nucl Med. 2016;46:522–35.
137. Silver DA, Pellicer I, Fair WR, Heston WD, Cordon-Cardo C. Prostate-specific membrane antigen expression in normal and malignant human tissues. Clin Cancer Res. 1997;3:81–5.
138. Rajasekaran SA, Anilkumar G, Oshima E, Bowie JU, Liu H, Heston W, et al. A novel cytoplasmic tail MXXXL motif mediates the internalization of prostate-specific membrane antigen. Mol Biol Cell. 2003;14:4835–45.
139. Chang SS. Overview of prostate-specific membrane antigen. Rev Urol. 2004;6:S13–8.
140. Mannweiler S, Amersdorfer P, Trajanoski S, Terrett JA, King D, Mehes G. Heterogeneity of prostate-specific membrane antigen (PSMA) expression in prostate carcinoma with distant metastasis. Pathol Oncol Res. 2009;15:167–72.
141. Petronis JD, Regan F, Lin K. Indium-111 capromab pendetide (ProstaScint) imaging to detect recurrent and metastatic prostate cancer. Clin Nucl Med. 1998;23:672–7.

142. Deb N, Goris M, Trisler K, Fowler S, Saal J, Ning S, et al. Treatment of hormone-refractory prostate cancer with 90Y-CYT-356 monoclonal antibody. Clin Cancer Res. 1996;2:1289–97.
143. Pandit-Taskar N, O'Donoghue JA, Beylergil V, Lyashchenko S, Ruan S, Solomon SB, et al. ^{89}Zr-huJ591 immuno-PET imaging in patients with advanced metastatic prostate cancer. Eur J Nucl Med Mol Imaging. 2014;41:2093–105.
144. Tagawa ST, Milowsky MI, Morris M, Vallabhajosula S, Christos P, Akhtar NH, et al. Phase II study of Lutetium-177-labeled anti-prostate-specific membrane antigen monoclonal antibody J591 for metastatic castration-resistant prostate cancer. Clin Cancer Res. 2013;19:5182–91.
145. Afshar-Oromieh A, Haberkorn U, Eder M, Eisenhut M, Zechmann CM. (68Ga)Gallium-labelled PSMA ligand as superior PET tracer for the diagnosis of prostate cancer: comparison with 18F-FECH. Eur J Nucl Med Mol Imaging. 2012;39:1085–6.
146. Wallitt KL, Dubash S, Tam HH, Khan S, Barwick TD. Clinical PET imaging in prostate cancer. Radiographics. 2017;37:1512–36.
147. Bois F, Noirot C, Dietemann S, Mainta IC, Zilli T, Garibotto V, et al. 68Ga Ga-PSMA-11 in prostate cancer: a comprehensive review. Am J Nucl Med Mol Imaging. 2020;10:349–74.
148. Satapathy S, Sinh H, Kumar R, Mittal BR. Diagnostic accuracy of 68Ga-PSMA PET/CT for initial detection in patients with suspected prostate cancer: a systematic review and meta-analysis. AJR. 2021;216:599–607.
149. Fendler WP, Schmidt DF, Wenter V, Thierfelder KM, Zach C, Stief C, et al. ^{68}Ga-PSMA PET/ CT detects the location and extent of primary prostate cancer. J Nucl Med. 2016;57:1720–5.
150. Uprimny C, Kroiss AS, Decristoforo C, Fritz J, von Guggenberg E, Kendler D, et al. ^{68}Ga-PSMA-11 PET/CT in primary staging of prostate cancer: PSA and Gleason score predict the intensity of tracer accumulation in the primary tumour. Eur J Nucl Med Mol Imaging. 2017;44:941–9.
151. Giesel FL, Sterzing F, Schlemmer HP, Holland-Letz T, Mier W, Rius M, et al. Intra-individual comparison of ^{68}Ga-PSMA-11-PET/CT and multi-parametric MR for imaging of primary prostate cancer. Eur J Nucl Med Mol Imaging. 2016;43:1400–6.
152. Rhee H, Thomas P, Shepherd B, Gustafson S, Vela I, Russell PJ, et al. Prostate specific membrane antigen positron emission tomography may improve the diagnostic accuracy of multiparametric magnetic resonance imaging in localized prostate cancer. J Urol. 2016;196:1261–7.
153. Grubmüller B, Baltzer P, Hartenbach S, D'Andrea D, Helbich TH, Haug AR, et al. PSMA ligand PET/MRI for primary prostate cancer: staging performance and clinical impact. Clin Cancer Res. 2018;24:6300–7.
154. van Kalmthout LWM, van Melick HH, Lavalaye J, Meijer RP, Kooistra A, de Klerk JMH, et al. Prospective validation of Gallium-68 prostate specific membrane antigen-positron emission tomography/computerized tomography for primary staging of prostate cancer. J Urol. 2020;203:537.
155. Maurer T, Gschwend JE, Rauscher I, Souvatzoglou M, Haller B, Weirich G, et al. Diagnostic efficacy of ^{68}Gallium-PSMA positron emission tomography compared to conventional imaging for lymph node staging of 130 consecutive patients with intermediate to high risk prostate cancer. J Urol. 2016;195:1436–43.
156. Wu H, Xu T, Wang X, Yu YB, Fan ZY, Li DX, et al. Diagnostic performance of (68)Gallium labelled prostate-specific membrane antigen positron emission tomography/computed tomography and magnetic resonance imaging for staging the prostate cancer with intermediate or high risk prior to radical prostatectomy: a systematic review and meta-analysis. World J Mens Health. 2020;38:208–19.
157. Yaxley JW, Raveenthiran S, Nouhaud FX, Samaratunga H, Yaxley WJ, Coughlin G, et al. Risk of metastatic disease on (68) gallium-prostate-specific membrane antigen positron emission tomography/computed tomography scan for primary staging of 1253 men at the diagnosis of prostate cancer. BJU Int. 2019;124:401–7.
158. Hofman MS, Lawrentschuk N, Francis RJ, Tang C, Vela I, Thomas P, et al. Prostate-specific membrane antigen PET-CT in patients with high-risk prostate cancer before curative-intent surgery or radiotherapy (proPSMA): a prospective, randomised, multicentre study. Lancet. 2020;395:1208–16.
159. Roach PJ, Francis R, Emmett L, Hsiao E, Kneebone A, Hruby G, et al. The impact of (68)Ga-PSMA PET/CT on management intent in prostate cancer: results of an Australian prospective multicenter study. J Nucl Med. 2018;59:82–8.
160. Hicks RJ, Murphy DG, Williams SG, et al. Seduction by sensitivity: reality, illusion, or delusion? The challenge of assessing outcomes after PSMA imaging selection of patients for treatment. J Nucl Med. 2017;58:1969–71.
161. Cornford P, Grummet J, Fanti S. Prostate-specific membrane antigen positron emission tomography scans before curative treatment: ready for prime time? Eur Urol. 2020; 78:e125–8.
162. Fendler WP, Calais J, Eiber M, Flavell RR, Mishoe A, Feng FY, Nguyen HG, et al. Assessment of 68Ga-PSMA-11 PET accuracy in localizing recurrent prostate cancer: a prospective single-arm clinical trial. JAMA Oncol. 2019;5:856–63.
163. Perera M, Papa N, Christidis D, Wetherell D, Hofman MS, Murphy DG, et al. Sensitivity, specificity, and predictors of positive (68)Ga-prostate-specific membrane antigen positron emission tomography in advanced prostate cancer: a systematic review and meta-analysis. Eur Urol. 2016;70:926–37.
164. von Eyben FE, Picchio M, von Eyben R, Rhee H, Bauman G. (68)Ga-labeled prostate-specific membrane antigen ligand positron emission tomography/computed tomography for prostate cancer: a systematic review and meta-analysis. Eur Urol Focus. 2018;4:686–93.
165. Jilg CA, Drendel V, Rischke HC, Beck T, Vach W, Schaal K, et al. Diagnostic accuracy of Ga-68-HBED-CC-PSMA-ligand-PET/CT before salvage lymph node dissection for recurrent prostate cancer. Theranostics. 2017;7:1770–80.
166. Calais J, Czernin J, Cao M, Kishan AU, Hegde JV, Shaverdian N, et al. (68)Ga-PSMA-11 PET/CT mapping of prostate cancer biochemical recurrence after radical prostatectomy in 270 patients with a PSA level of less than 1.0 ng/mL: impact on salvage radiotherapy planning. J Nucl Med. 2018;59:230–7.
167. Koerber SA, Will L, Kratochwil C, Haefner MF, Rathke H, Kremer C, et al. (68)Ga-PSMA-11 PET/CT in primary and recurrent prostate carcinoma: implications for radiotherapeutic management in 121 patients. J Nucl Med. 2018;60:234–40.
168. Han S, Woo S, Kim YJ, Suh CH. Impact of (68)Ga-PSMA PET on the management of patients with prostate cancer: a systematic review and meta-analysis. Eur Urol. 2018;74:179–90.
169. Çelen S, Gültekin A, Özlülerden Y, Mete A, Sağtaş E, Ufuk F, et al. Comparison of 68Ga-PSMA-I/T PET-CT and multiparametric MRI for locoregional staging of prostate cancer patients: a pilot study. Urol Int. 2020;104:684–91.
170. Muehlematter UJ, Burger IA, Becker AS, Schawkat K, Hötker AM, Reiner CSS, et al. Reiner diagnostic accuracy of multiparametric MRI versus 68 Ga-PSMA-11 PET/MRI for extracapsular extension and seminal vesicle invasion in patients with prostate cancer. Radiology. 2019;293:350–8.
171. Zhou J, Gou Z, Wu R, Yuan Y, Yu G, Zhao Y. Comparison of PSMA-PET/CT, choline-PET/CT, NaF-PET/CT, MRI, and bone scintigraphy in the diagnosis of bone metastases in patients with prostate cancer: a systematic review and meta-analysis. Skelet Radiol. 2019;48:1915–24.
172. Schwenck J, Rempp H, Reischl G, Kruck S, Stenzl A, Nikolaou K, et al. Comparison of 68 Ga-labelled PSMA-11 and 11 C-choline

in the detection of prostate cancer metastases by PET/CT. Eur J Nucl Med Mol Imaging. 2017;44:92–101.

173. Lin CY, Lee MT, Lin CL, Kao CH. Comparing the staging/restaging performance of 68Ga-labeled prostate-specific membrane antigen and 18F-choline PET/CT in prostate cancer: a systematic review and meta-analysis. Clin Nucl Med. 2019;44:365–76.
174. Calais J, Ceci F, Eiber M, Hope TA, Hofman MS, Rischpler C, et al. (18)F-fluciclovine PET-CT and (68)Ga-PSMA-11 PET-CT in patients with early biochemical recurrence after prostatectomy: a prospective, single-centre, single-arm, comparative imaging trial. Lancet Oncol. 2019;20:1286–94.
175. Pernthaler B, Kulnik R, Gstettner C, Salamon S, Aigner RM, Kvaternik H. A prospective head-to-head comparison of 18f-fluciclovine with 68Ga-PSMA-11 in biochemical recurrence of prostate cancer in PET/CT. Clin Nucl Med. 2019;44:e566–73.
176. Sanchez-Crespo A. Comparison of Gallium-68 and Fluorine-18 imaging characteristics in positron emission tomography. Appl Radiat Isot. 2013;76:55–62.
177. Parikh NR, Tsai S, Bennett C, Lewis M, Sadeghi A, Lorentz W, et al. The impact of 18F-DCFPyL PET-CT imaging on initial staging, radiation, and systemic therapy treatment recommendations for veterans with aggressive prostate cancer. Adv Radiat Oncol. 2020;5:1364–9.
178. Mena E, Lindenberg ML, Turkbey IB, Shih JH, Harmon SA, Lim I, et al. 18 F-DCFPyL PET/CT imaging in patients with biochemically recurrent prostate cancer after primary local therapy. J Nucl Med. 2020;61:881–9.
179. Pan KH, Wang JH, Wang CY, Nikzad AA, Kong FQ, Jian L, et al. Evaluation of 18F-DCFPyL PSMA PET/CT for prostate cancer: a meta-analysis. Front Oncol. 2020;10:597422.
180. Dietlein M, Kobe C, Kuhnert G, Stockter S, Fischer T, Schomacker K, et al. Comparison of ((18)F)DCFPyL and ((68)Ga)Ga-PSMA-HBED-CC for PSMA-PET imaging in patients with relapsed prostate cancer. Mol Imaging Biol. 2015;17:575–84.

Pelvic Anatomy and Its Relationship to Radical Prostatectomy Urinary Continence Outcomes

Robert P. Myers, Walter Artibani, Markus Graefen, Arnauld Villers, and Jochen Walz

> The surgical anatomy of the prostate and adjacent tissues involved in radical prostatectomy is complex. Precise knowledge of all relevant anatomic structures facilitates surgical orientation and dissection during radical prostatectomy and ideally translates into both superior rates of cancer control and improved functional outcomes postoperatively. [1]

Loss of urinary control post-radical prostatectomy is devastating. No health-related quality of life (HRQOL) functional outcome is more life-troubling. Patients make lifestyle changes proportional to level of incontinence [2]. Erectile function is key for some and an added benefit, but of less importance than not being wet [3]. Regret at having chosen radical prostatectomy as a treatment alternative has been shown to be significant by EPIC-low urinary domain score [4]. In 17 studies comprising those with urinary incontinence at 1 year. after robot-assisted radical prostatectomy (RARP), only 84% were pad-free in those studies for which pad-free was the measure of full urinary control, and 91% when continence was measured by either no pads or a security pad [5]. HRQOL is significantly greater for no pad requirement vs. 1 pad ($p < 0.0001$) [5]. This data behooves rendering urinary control as soon as possible after surgery. Speeding the process is aided by intraoperative techniques to ensure the desired outcome; that is making no mistakes.

Membranous Urethra Membranous urethra as a term has been common parlance for the urethral segment in the male from apex of prostate to superior surface of the corpus spongiosum. In fresh gross cadaveric dissection, the membranous urethra appears laterally as an endopelvic fascia-enshrouded segment emanating from the apex of the prostate and headed distally between lateral leaves of the levator ani constituting the pelvic diaphragm (Fig. 1). The fascial covering is a distal continuation of endopelvic fascia that also covers not only urethra but also the neurovascular bundles containing the cavernous nerves. Thinking of the membranous urethra as the sphincteric urethra provides much-needed ancillary functional connotation [6]. The Terminologia Anatomica lists "Intermediate part of urethra" as preferred terminology and "Membranous urethra" as secondary [7]. However, in light of radical prostatectomy in this day and age, "membranous urethra" has lost practical utility in favor of "urethral sphinc-

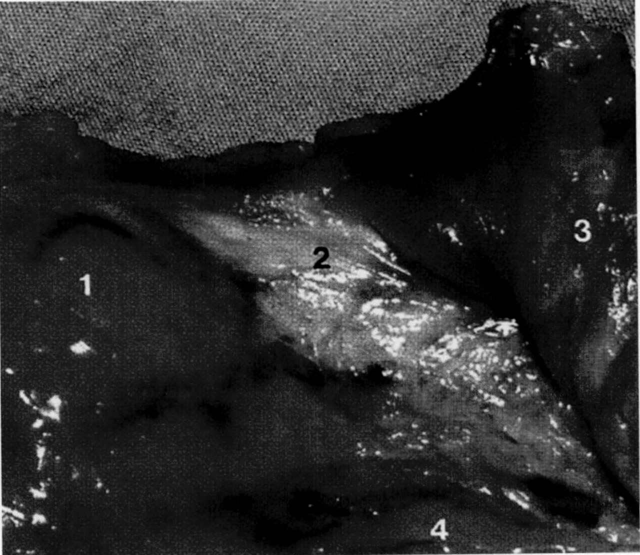

Fig. 1 Lateral view of 1—Prostate, 2—Endopelvic fascia obscures underlying striated urethral sphincter and membranous urethra, 3—Levator ani, bare of fascia, 4—Rectum (From Myers RP. Radical prostatectomy: pertinent surgical anatomy. Atlas of Urol. Clin North Am 1994; 22: 1–18)

R. P. Myers
Department of Urology, Mayo Clinic, Rochester, MN, USA

W. Artibani
Department of Urology, University of Verona, Verona, Italy

M. Graefen
Martini Clinic – Prostate Cancer Centre, Hamburg, Germany

A. Villers
Department of Urology, Centre Hospitalier Régional Universitaire de Lille, Lille, France

J. Walz (✉)
Department of Urology, Institut Paoli-Calmettes Cancer Centre, Marseille, France

P. Wiklund et al. (eds.), *Robotic Urologic Surgery*, https://doi.org/10.1007/978-3-031-00363-9_13

ter" for the urethral stump to which vesico-urethral anastomosis will be performed.

From the standpoint of its smooth muscle and elastic tissue thereby creating a lissosphincter, the sphincteric or membranous urethra extends from seminal colliculus or verumontanum (veru) in the prostatic urethra to the superior surface of the bulb of the penis, not just from apex of the prostate to the bulb. Components consist of external striated urethral sphincter, lissosphincter, urethral mucosal coaptations from multiple invaginations in the resting state, puboperineal levator ani subdivision, officially termed the puboperineales, and intact vascularity and nerve supply, all of which needs to be protected (Figs. 2 and 3 right). The puboperineales (TA) represent the most anteromedial por-

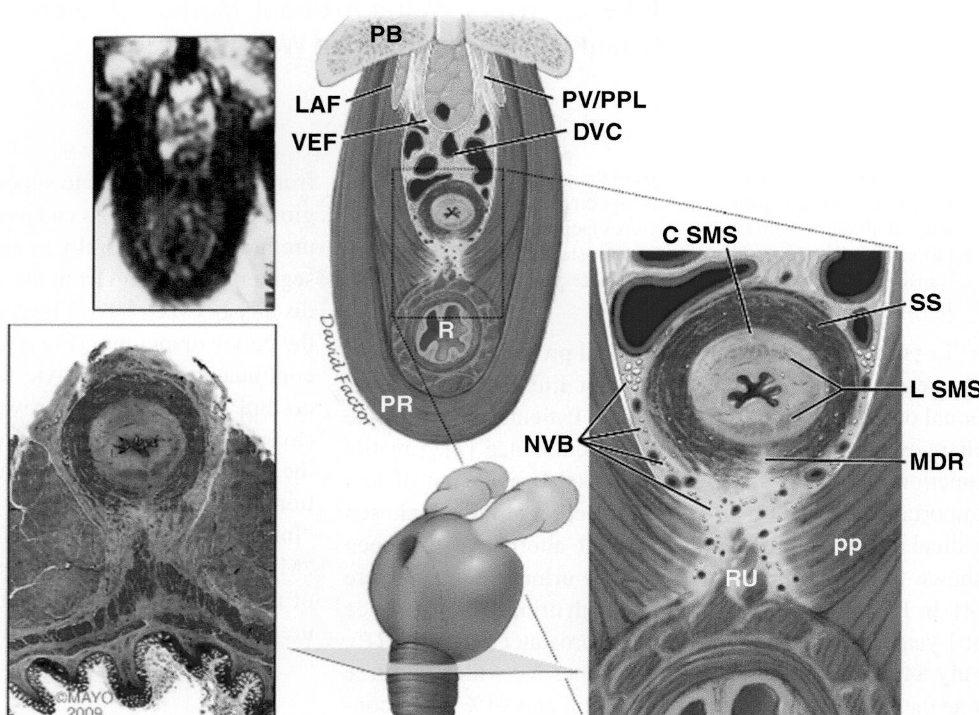

Fig. 2 Axial section of sphincteric or membranous urethra: *DVC* dorsal vascular complex, *LAF* levator ani fascia, *MDR* median dorsal raphe, *NVB* neurovascular bundle, *PB* pubic bone, *PV/PPL* pubovesical/puboprostatic ligament, *pp* puboperinealis muscle, *PR* puborectalis muscle, *R* rectum, *RU* rectourethralis muscle, *SS* striated sphincter (rhabdosphincter), *C SMS* circular smooth muscle sphincter (lissosphincter), *L SMS* longitudinal smooth muscle sphincter (lissosphincter), *U* urethra, *VEF* visceral endopelvic fascia (From Walz J et al. Eur Urol 2010; 57: 179–92)

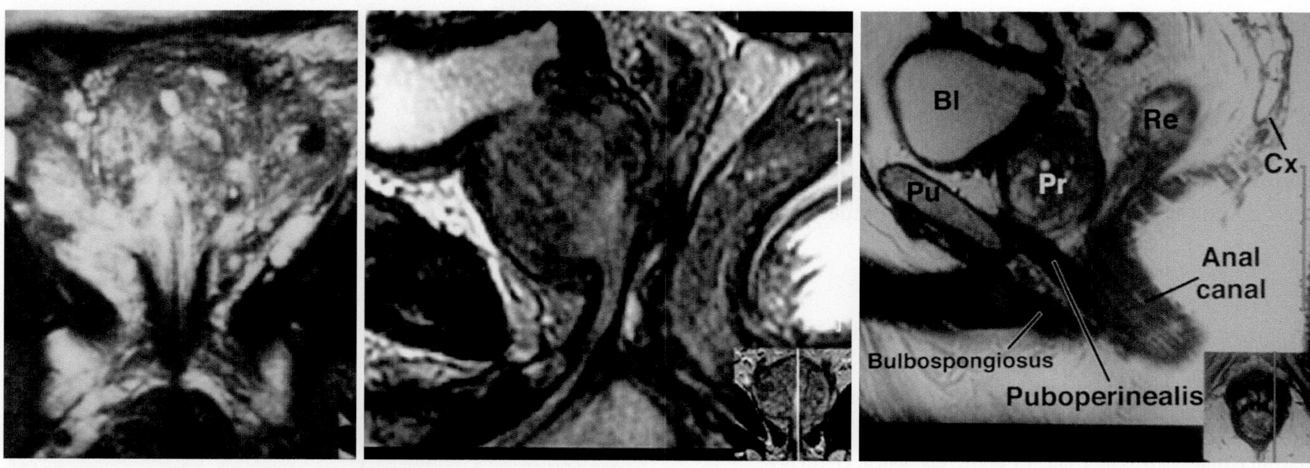

Fig. 3 Left—Coronal MRI-Striated sphincter in urogenital hiatus between levator ani. Middle-Sagittal MRI for MUL. Right—Parasagittal MRI-Puboperinealis (Left—From Myers, R.P.: Anatomy and physiology of the external urethral sphincter: implications for preservation of continence after radical prostatectomy. In: Schröder, F.H. (ed): Recent advances in prostate cancer and BPH. New York: Parthenon, 1997, pp. 81–86. Right—from Myers RP, Cahill D, Devine RM, King BF. Anatomy of radical prostatectomy as defined by magnetic resonance imaging. J Urol 1998; 159: 2148–58)

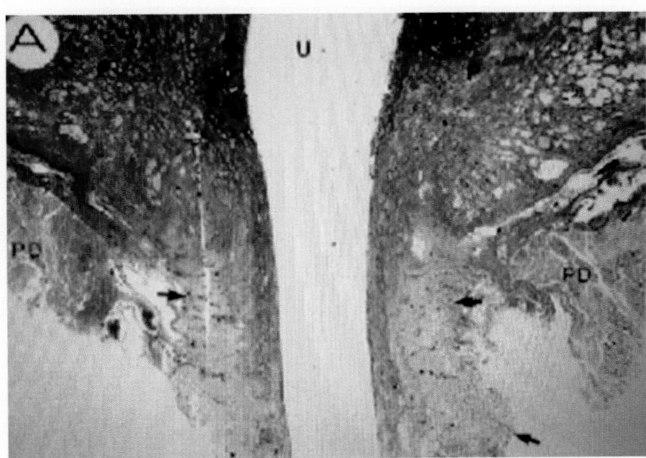

Fig. 4 Coronal Masson trichrome (MT)-Striated sphincter (black arrows) in urogenital hiatus with flanking levator ani as pelvic diaphragm (PD) (From Myers RP, Goellner JR, Cahill DR. Prostate shape, external striated urethral sphincter and radical prostatectomy: the apical dissection. J Urol 1987; 138: 543–50)

tions of the levator ani flanking the membranous urethra. This portion of the levator ani extends from pubis to the perineal body anterior to the rectum and anal canal. They function precisely for quick stop of urination and Kegel exercise [8].

Importantly, distal to the prostate apex, the sphincteric or membranous urethra lies in a urogenital hiatus [9] flanked by pelvic diaphragm (Figs. 3 left and 4). Notably, the membranous urethra is not situated in a urogenital diaphragm as illustrated by a muscle sandwich spanning the pubic rami with superior and inferior fascia enclosing bulbourethral (Cowper's) glands, a configuration that for years has been depicted erroneously in atlases of anatomy, urology textbooks, commercial advertising at urology meetings, and urology news bulletins. Urogenital diaphragm as a term should be confined to the perineal membrane and not infer membranous urethra or a muscle sandwich.

Bladder Neck Urinary control in the male is both proximal in a pre-prostatic sphincter at the bladder neck and distal in what Turner Warwick labeled the "distal continence mechanism," which he described extending from veru to bulb [10]. With bladder neck resected as opposed to preservation, as part of prostate removal, bladder neck function as a continence contributor is lost. No amount of intraoperative dissection, tubularization, or mucosal eversion ever makes it function again as a sphincter. The bladder neck post-surgery is endoscopically observable as a fixed open entity of variable caliber. However, plicating the new bladder opening to the right caliber to meet the urethral stump at the time of anastomosis prevents splaying of the stump lumen distally and may aid in earlier continence recovery. Bladder neck preservation has proved to hasten urinary control at 4 months but not at 1 and 2 years [11]. Importantly, bladder neck size was not associated with EPIC incontinence scores at 6 and 12 weeks [12]. Bladder neck preservation poses the risk of a positive surgical margin demonstrated to be a significantly poor prognostic factor in terms of PSA and clinical failure [13].

Furthermore, preservation of the bladder neck to the greatest possible extent seems to have a positive effect on postoperative orgasm-associated incontinence (climacturia). This side effect has been reported to occur in between 20% and 93% of patients after radical prostatectomy; yet, it is under-reported or non-reported in the vast majority of surgical series [14].

Preservation of Sphincteric or Membranous Urethra The surgical goal is to remove the prostate leaving membranous urethra as a functioning sphincteric urethral stump, protruding proximally to variable degrees from the urogenital hiatus and awaiting vesico-urethral anastomosis. Variable degree means variation in membranous urethral length (MUL). Short vs. long, MUL can be ascertained by preoperative retrograde urethrography (Fig. 5), MRI in midline sagittal or coronal images (Figs. 3 middle and 6) when possible, transperineal ultrasound [15], and endoscopy to observe relationship of veru to sphincter [16] (Fig. 7). In cadaveric study of 33 specimens, MUL was 1.3–2.8 cm (mean 1.72 cm) and mode 1.5 cm in 10 cases [17]. Multiple studies confirm a critical MUL necessary for the patient to be dry [18–21]. Pre-and post-op endorectal coil MUL by MRI were both associated with superior time to post-op urinary continence, the postop measurement ≥13 mm vs <13 mm ($p < .0005$) [19]. A careful review of multiple studies measuring MUL by MRI revealed a mean range of 1.04–1.45 cm and an individual range 0.5–3.43 cm with the conclusion "Every extra millimeter of MUL increased the odds of pad-free continence by 9%" [21].

In a huge meta-analysis study, MUL as a variable was identified together with age, and Charlson Comorbidity Index (≤3 months) as main patient-related factors influencing postprostatectomy urinary incontinence [22]. Clearly, a full-length preservation of the urethral sphincter up to the veru preserves a longer urethral sphincter and may therefore result in better continence.

Useful for preoperative staging, standard multiparametric MRI prostate imaging also includes the routine capturing of T2-weighted coronal and sagittal images allowing the added knowledge of preoperative MUL with ramifications in preoperative patient counseling.

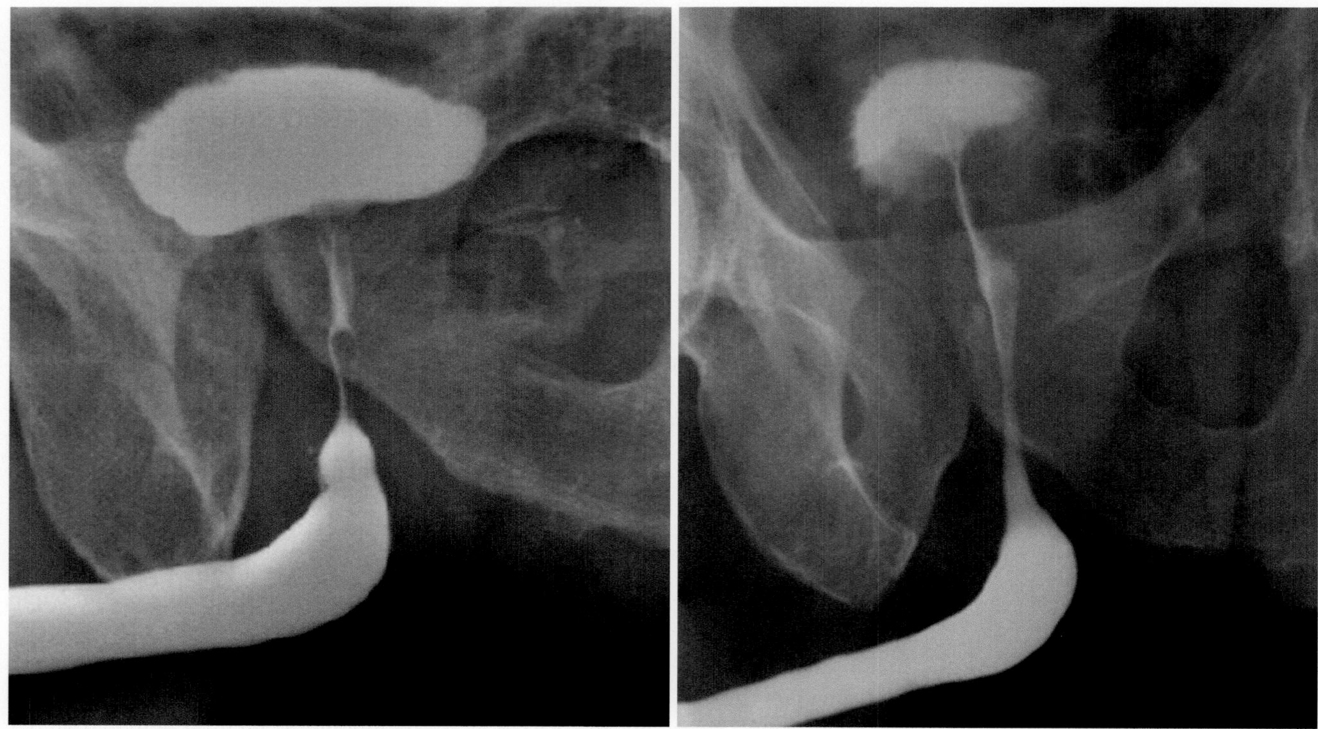

Fig. 5 Retrograde urethrograms. Left—short membranous urethra. Right—long membranous urethra

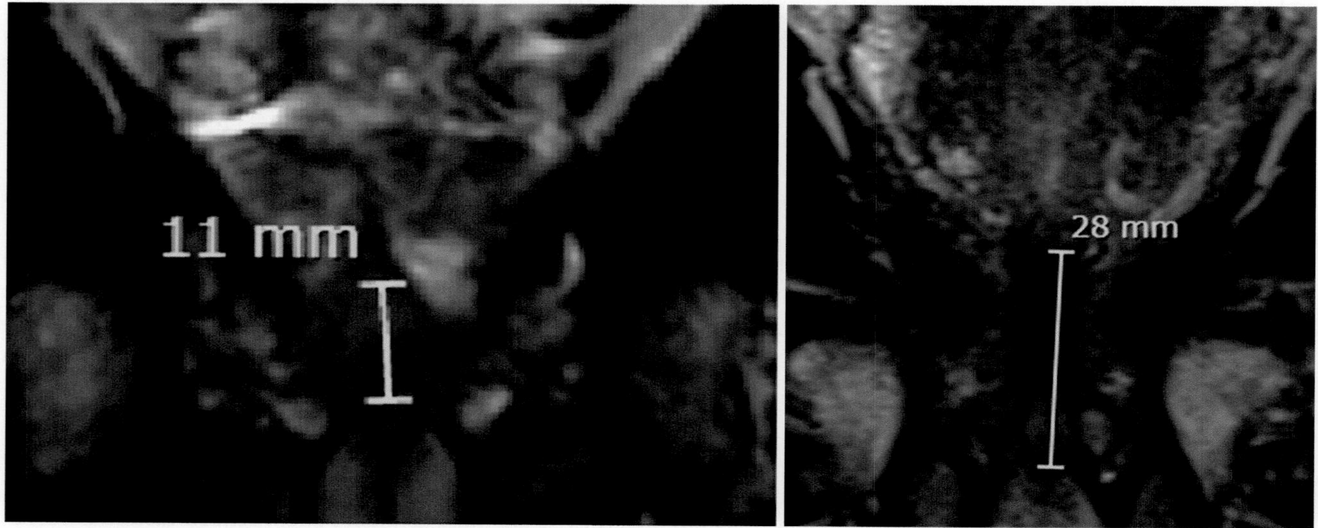

Fig. 6 T2-weighted coronal MRI- MUL 11 mm left, 28 mm right (Courtesy of T. E. Ahlering)

External Striated Urethral Sphincter or Rhabdosphincter Associated with maintaining MUL is preserving external striated sphincter integrity. The striated sphincter inserts on the apex and the anterior surface of the prostate. Histologically, the striated sphincter on axial section is dominant in thickness anterolaterally with tapering toward the midline posteriorly where a fine raphe exists in contact with the posterior termination of Denonvilliers' fascia as it approaches the perineal body. Mirrored in the urethral pressure profile, the cross-sectional diameter of the striated sphincter increases from prostate apex to penile bulb which makes closure capability strongest distally [17].

The external striated urethral sphincter with a demonstrable midline posterior raphe invests the urethra in a near-circular collar of variable cross-sectional dimension from prostate apex to bulb, and in one study was found to have

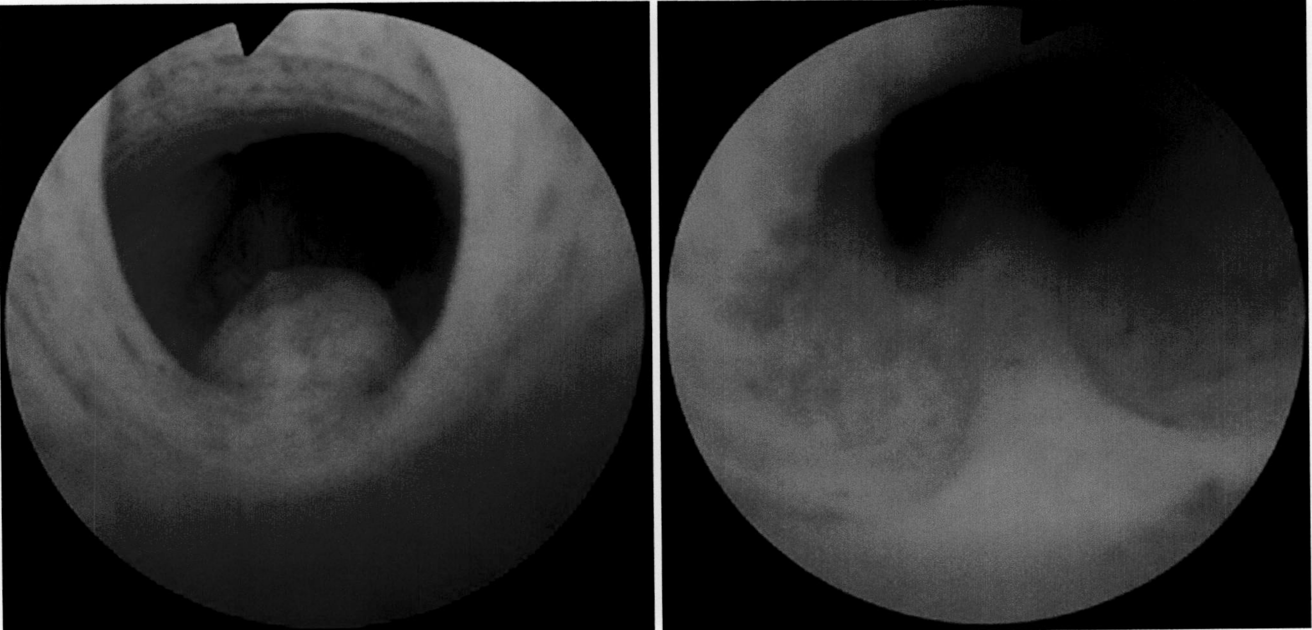

Fig. 7 Endoscopic views—Bulbous urethra to veru. Left—sphincter presumed short. Right—sphincter presumed long

fibers 1/3 the diameter of adjacent levator ani fibers, contains no muscle spindles, by electron micrography and histochemically in cryostat-preserved sections of fresh muscle in 9 subjects composed exclusively of type 1 "slow twitch" fibers designed to maintain tone over long periods without fatigue and no type 2 "fast twitch" fibers, functionally suggesting striated sphincter assistance in post-void urethral closure but not the ability to participate in quick stop like that provided on demand by the puboperineales with their type 2 fibers [23]. At odds is a second study, whereby a disparate subsequent histochemical study showed both type 1 and type 2 fibers, nearly 50–50 by volume, thereby suggesting dual sphincter function. The study was conducted with cadaveric (16–72 h) tissues applying histochemistry without corroboratory electron microscopy, and rendering a challenging result [24]. The only agreement was the finding of no muscle spindles. A third study followed using fresh frozen tissue in 2 subjects with the finding of 100% slow twitch in one subject, and mixed slow twitch/fast twitch in a second subject [25]. These studies suggest a possible dual role in some subjects. Urinary continence has been well demonstrated by pudendal blockade in post-prostatectomy patients thereby making intact smooth muscle and elastic tissue of the membranous urethra the predominant primary continence component at rest with the lissosphincter making the striated sphincter of ancillary support [26].

The adjacent pelvic diaphragm levator ani (the puboperineales) was found to contain both types 1 & 2 fibers, inferring a role of the levator ani in sustaining pelvic support [23]. Mirrored in the urethral pressure profile, the cross-sectional diameter of the striated sphincter increases from prostate apex to bulb showing less continence function from the striated sphincter proximally than distally [17] (Fig. 8). Relevant to proper patient counseling and selection, with advanced age comes atrophy, meaning decreased thickness and volume of the sphincter to some degree, making age an independent predictor of postoperative urinary continence in multivariate analysis [27].

Prostate Apical Shape The membranous urethra as sphincteric urethra meets the apex of the prostate in different ways making optimal urethral transection tricky in light of variably shaped or configured prostate apices. Shape variations include anterior notch, anterior, posterior, unilateral and bilateral projections, and irregular nodular BPH surrounding or extending distally beside the sphincter, and circumferential extension around the sphincter [6] (Fig. 9). Failure to recognize these shapes intraoperatively with corresponding accurate apical dissection risks potentially deleterious MUL shortening in light of imprecise urethral transection. For best results, surgery should be directed to full functional sphincteric urethral length preservation in concert with a particular prostate apical shape [28]. In multivariate analysis, overlap anteriorly or posteriorly of the membranous urethra by the prostate apex as demonstrated on preoperative MRI was the only variable significantly associated with an early return of continence. Circumferential overlap was observed in 38% of all cases, anterior overlap in 25%, posterior overlap in 22% and no overlap in 15% [29]. Significant overlap makes the preservation of both long and short urethral sphincters

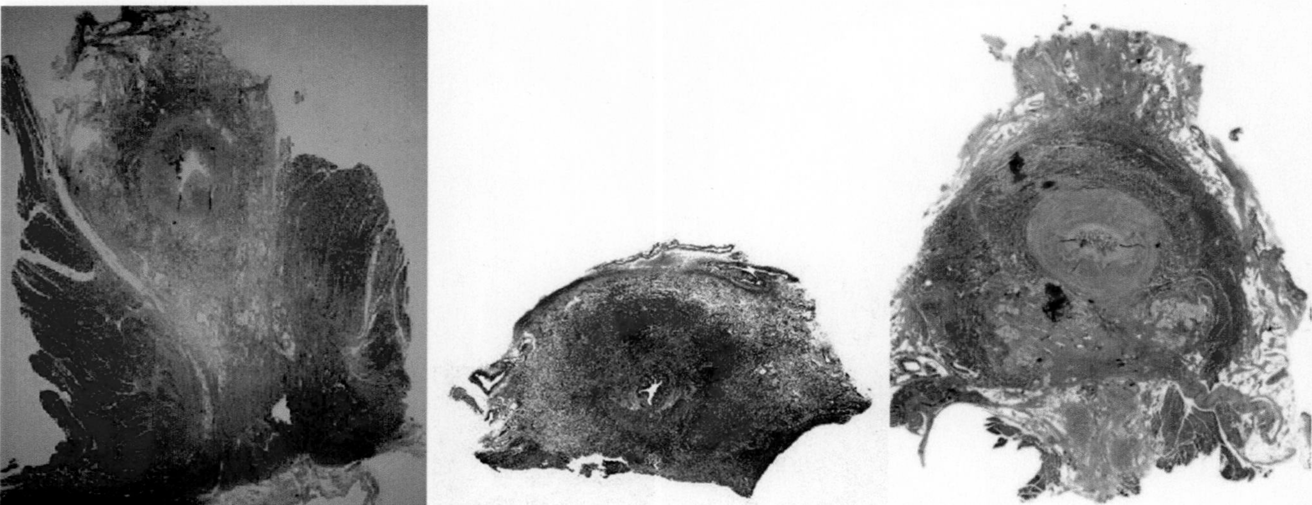

Fig. 8 Axial MT from 3 subjects: Left—high sphincteric urethra with DVC, striated sphincter, lissosphincter, puboperineal levator ani. Middle—Mid-sphincteric urethra with DVC, striated sphincter, lissosphincter, mucosal invaginations. Right—Distal sphincteric urethra with DVC, striated sphincter with bulbourethral glands, lissosphincter, mucosal "seal" (Middle—from Myers RP. Anatomy: Anatomic Considerations for Efficiency and Precision in Robotic-Assisted Radical Prostatectomy. Chap. 1 In: John H, Wiklund P, Witt JH (eds) Atlas of Robotic Prostatectomy, Springer-Verlag Berlin Heidelberg 2013)

difficult and should be considered during dissection and appropriate transection of the urethra at the apex.

Ischioprostatic Ligaments Supporting and flanking the sphincter are two bands of fibrous tissue, the ischioprostatic ligaments [30], in the past dubbed "pillars," [31] at the 10 and 2 o'clock positions, that anchor and provide a measure of rigidity to the sphincter and membranous urethra. Specifically, they potentially factor into countering membranous urethral hypermobility during postoperative healing. The anterior layer of the sphincter's striated muscle inserts into the fibrous bands that constitute the pillars (Fig. 10). The pillar insertion of sphincter should prevent it from posterior displacement on sphincter contraction, an anatomic observation in conflict with transurethral sonomorphologic evaluation [32] and transperineal ultrasound study, both revealing posterior displacement of sphincter toward the perineal body on contraction [33]. These bands have to be transected close to the apex to free the urethral stump. They represent a path for direct extension of prostate cancer from the apical prostate into pillar and striated sphincter (Fig. 11).

Neural Control Nerve supply to the urethral sphincter is complex including somatic innervation from the distal pudendal nerve, intrapelvic from the proximal pudendal nerve, recurrent from the dorsal nerve of the penis, extrapudendal somatic fibers among autonomic fibers that enter the sphincter complex from the inferior hypogastric plexus and neurovascular bundle [34]. Both striated sphincter and lissosphincter innervations have to be supplied in coordinated function with respect to micturition. Significant autonomic afferent denervation of the membranous urethral mucosa was studied and found to be significant in patients postoperatively with impaired membranous urethral sensitivity seemingly associated with urinary incontinence. The conclusion was that afferent autonomic nerve interruption "may have a role in the continence mechanism after nerve-sparing radical retropubic prostatectomy" [35]. Autonomic innervation of the male pelvic floor smooth muscle was found to be notably "dense" posterior to the urethral sphincter [36]. The conclusion from multiple studies is that, when feasible, as much nerve tissue as possible should be saved with respect to achieving urinary continence.

Urinary Continence Preservation Many technical modifications have been proposed and used to preserve sphincteric urethral function with patients able to live without loss of urinary control. These techniques include a urethral suspension stitch [37], preservation of bladder neck [11, 38], and the pubovesical complex including pubovesical/pubprostatic ligaments with detrusor apron [39] left in situ as a reverse perineal prostatectomy [38, 40, 41], nerve-sparing [27, 42–45], MUL optimized, anterior and posterior reconstruction [46, 47], and puboprostatic collar with puboperineoplasty [48, 49].

Although robotic-assisted radical prostatectomy (RARP) was introduced and popularized as a retropubic anterior approach to the prostate to be removed and the urethra to be preserved, the anterior approach now competes with a posterior Retzius-space preserving dissection. Reports employing

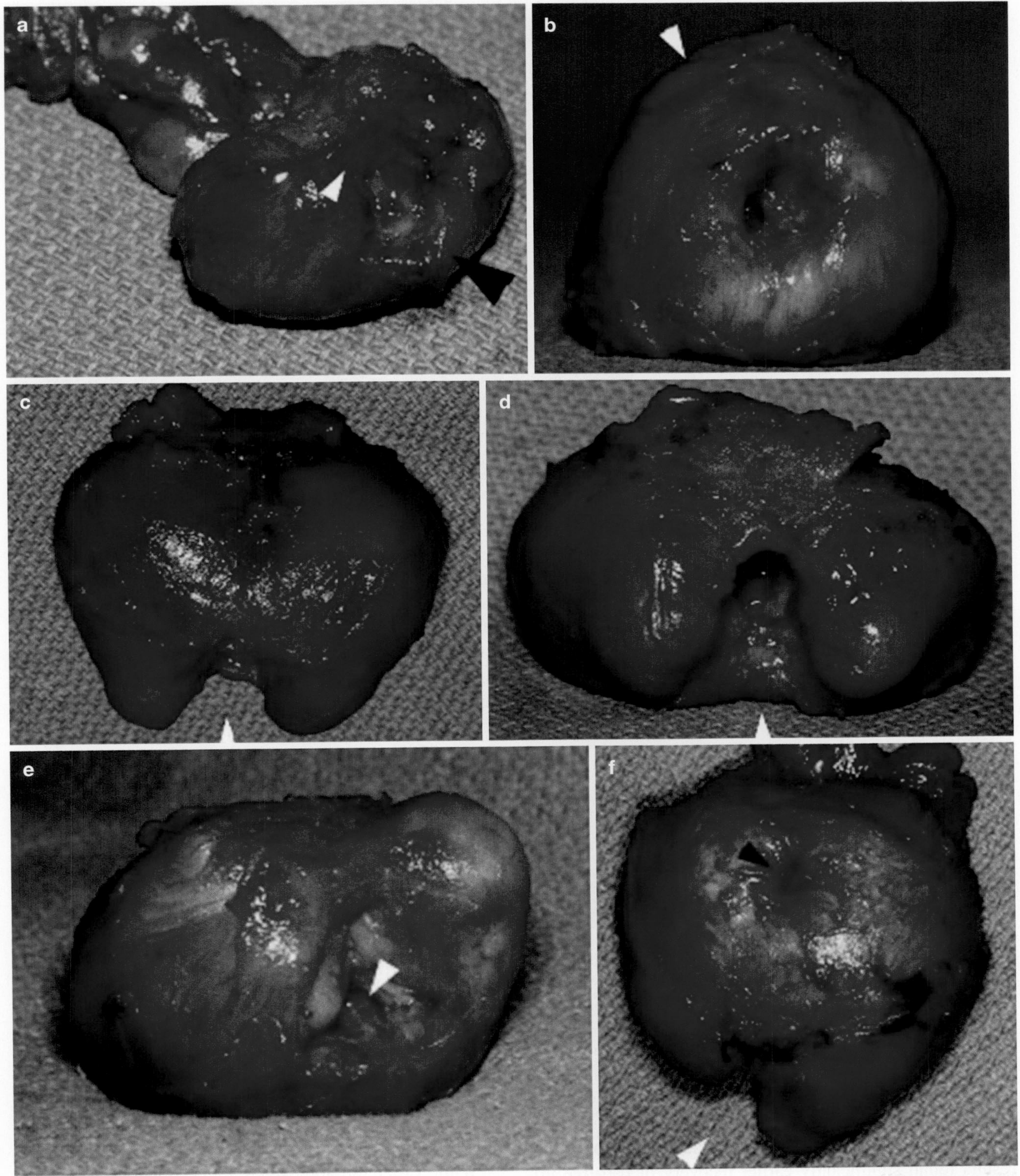

Fig. 9 Radical prostatectomy specimens with difficult dissection apices: (**a**) anterior apical notch with posterior lip. (**b**) "Donut" or circumferential apex. (**c**) Bilateral apical protrusion (top view). (**d**) Same prostate as (**c**). Frontal view. (**e**) Irregular BPH distorts apex. (**f**) Unilateral apical protrusion (From Myers RP. Gross and applied anatomy of the prostate. In: Kantoff PW, Carroll P, D'Amico A. Prostate Cancer, Chap. 1. Philadelphia: Lippincott Williams & Wilkins, 2002, pp. 3–15)

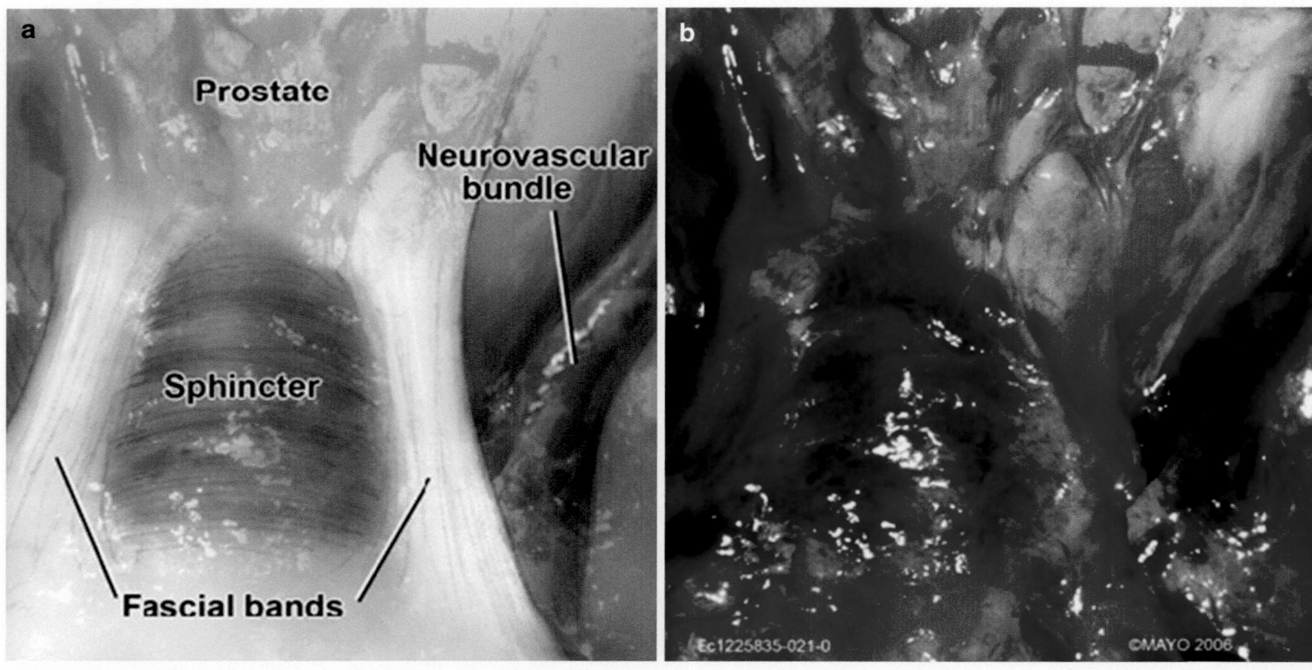

Fig. 10 (a) Fascial bands, ischioprostatic ligaments or "pillars," supporting striated sphincter as illustrated from fresh cadaveric specimen (b)

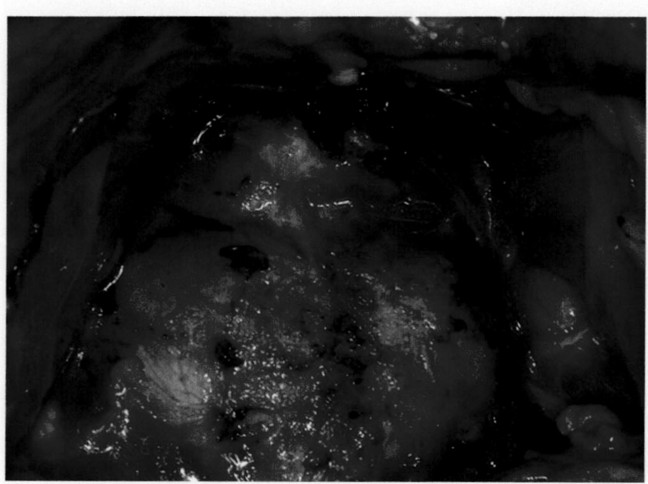

Fig. 11 Looking distally, intraoperative prostate foreground. Prostate cancer (yellow) invading left "pillar" and striated sphincter. Operation aborted

Retzius-sparing RARP (RS-RARP) include 74% pad-free at 7 days in the first 100 patients [50], and 70% pad-free with 92% pad-free exclusive of a "safety liner" at 1 month [41]. As Level 1 evidence in a randomized control trial (RCT) comparing posterior (RS-RARP) vs anterior approaches, results found significantly earlier recovery of pad-free urinary control with a posterior approach: 71% vs 48% at 1 week, 95% vs 86% pad-free at 3 months [51]. Also documented in this study was the finding of significantly reduced measured pad weights and urinary bother scores in those patients undergoing the posterior approach. However, on long-term follow-up, the posterior approach showed no benefit beyond 6 months by urinary function scores [52]. Another RCT utilizing advanced vesico-urethral support including suture anchor of the bladder neck to the arcus tendineus as anterior fixation produced significantly increased continence across all time periods: 24 h, 2, 4, and 8 weeks, and 6 and 12 months [53].

A careful anterior approach, either with a peri-urethral suspension stitch mimicking an open technique [36, 54] or in a propensity score study of modified anterolateral intrafascial dissection with complete nerve bundle preservation vs conventional dissection [27], resulted in equivalent pad-free continence of 92.8% vs. 92%, respectively, at 3 months. An alternate study with preservation of the pubovesical complex utilizing a "tunnel" or "hood" anterior approach resulted in 91% pad-free urinary continence at 3 months while allowing benefit of incremental nerve sparing, dealing with BPH, protection of the ureteral orifices, and a very low 6% PSM rate [55]. An anterior approach in 30 patients utilizing intrafascial dissection of the neurovascular bundles also with preservation of the pubovesical complex resulted in 80% pad-free on catheter removal and 100% pad-free at 1 month [38].

While varied, all approaches are designed and promoted for patients to be pad-free and dry as soon as possible after surgery. A careful review concluded that while "the Retzius-sparing approach seems to provide an earlier return to continence than the traditional anterior transperitoneal approach, no technique has been proved to be superior to other(s) in terms of long-term outcomes" [56]. The focus on nerve sparing has led to more precise or modified apical dissection that could reflect improved continence outcomes rather than the nerve sparing per se [27, 45]. More precise dissection allows greater MUL, but also may prevent injury to an intrapelvic pudendal nerve branch coursing with the long pelvic nerve to enter the striated sphincter [57]. To our knowledge, blood supply to the sphincter may accompany the pudendal innervation of the sphincter but has not been studied. The finding of and avoiding small arteries during dorsal vascular complex (DVC) dissection may be significant with respect to sphincter vascularity and urinary continence postoperatively [50].

Summarizing with additional references, with multiple variables plus and minus comparing postoperative urinary continence, outcome analysis is decidedly problematic in trying to measure what is important anatomically and in technique with respect to prostate removal [56]. Variables include patient age and preoperative AUA symptom score [27], surgeon experience [56], an easier, more anatomically straightforward anterior [36, 58], vs "more demanding" posterior pouch of Douglas (RS-RARP) dissection [41], preserving the detrusor apron-pubovesical complex with features of a reverse perineal prostatectomy [38, 40, 41], fascial collar to invest the remaining urethra after transection [48], the degree of nerve sparing [43], preventing bladder and pelvic "descent" [59]. Once the prostate is removed, skilled tension-free anastomosis of the reconstructed bladder neck to the urethral stump is paramount. Aggressive bladder-to-urethra anastomosis may create a ring of fibrosis, possible stricture, and shortened MUL leading to incontinence. Of note, anastomotic technique in RARP is very safe with Clavien–Dindo Class IIIB stricture formation exceedingly rare involving only one patient in 453 in a series review [27, 38, 41, 50, 52].

In one study MUL preservation technique trumped posterior urethral reconstruction and anterior bladder suspension technique with respect to urinary continence rates [60]. Continued study emphasizes the importance of maximizing MUL [61]. Urethral hypermobility can be countered by DVC control proximal to the prostate apex prior to both apical dissection and urethral transection thereby avoiding direct suture trauma to the underlying urethra, which will then be left undisturbed including its vessels and nerves.

Transvesical single-port RARP as a new platform has proven promising with immediate continence of 64%, 73% at 1 week, 80.9% at 6 weeks, and 100% pad-free with no leakage at 3 months in a limited series of 39 patients (J. Kaouk—personal correspondence).

All studies to date designed to accelerate postoperative urinary control suggest that best results occur when the prostate is removed with the least disturbance to the surrounding anatomy, that is nerves, vessels, and fascia supporting the urethral stump. It should be kept in mind that techniques by a single surgeon in a single institution, however encouraging, do not guarantee reproducibility of results. Anterior dissections followed by assiduous anterior and posterior reconstruction provide urethral stump stability during healing. Interestingly, urethral suspension [37] to restore a proper vesico-urethral junction angle anteriorly is a reminder of the goal in Marshall–Marchetti–Krantz urethropexy in women [62].

Oncologic Safety The importance of avoiding positive margins of resection (PSMs) has become nebulous in light of the fact that PSMs impact biochemical recurrence, local recurrence, and the need for salvage therapy, but are not associated with cancer-specific or overall survival [63]. Despite this, biochemical recurrence, local recurrence, and the need for salvage therapy are disheartening and do not match continued good health for patients found to have negative margins and no future recurrence.

PSMs for radical prostatectomy vary widely based on patient selection, stage, grade, volume of cancer, surgeon experience, and technique in selecting correct planes of dissection. Extrafascial and interfascial dissections are always safer than intrafascial with respect to PSMs. While it has been shown to improve early return of urinary control, intrafascial dissection increases the risk of PSMs. Preoperative staging by multiparametric MRI could help reduce PSMs by allowing, when presumed necessary, to plan wider resection if there is evidence of advanced local disease.

Multiple meta-analysis studies to date reveal increased PSMs for RS-RARP as compared with conventional RARP [64–66]. PSMs are most common at the prostate apex, which should be kept in mind with respect to optimizing MUL.

Conclusion The key to success in producing a happy, pad-free patient boils down to technical steps to provide adequate urethral sphincter length and to prevent urethral hypermobility with maneuvers such as a urethral suspension stitch. Necessary technical precision aside, thorough preoperative imaging to identify and counsel patients with respect to short or marginal length urethras is paramount as this relatively small cohort of patients are at the highest risk for an unsuccessful outcome, and some may want to select treatment other than surgery.

References

1. Walz J, Burnett AL, Costello AJ, Eastham JA, Graefen M, Guillonneau B, et al. A critical analysis of the current knowledge of surgical anatomy related to optimization of cancer control and preservation of continence and erection in candidates for radical prostatectomy. Eur Urol. 2010;57:179–92.

2. Donnellan SM, Duncan HJ, MacGregor RJ, Russell JM. Prospective assessment of incontinence after radical retropubic prostatectomy: objective and subjective analysis. Urology. 1997;49:225–30.
3. Carvalhal GF, Smith DS, Ramos C, Krygiel J, Mager DE, Yan Y, et al. Correlates of dissatisfaction with treatment in patients with prostate cancer diagnosed through screening. J Urol. 1999;162:113–8.
4. Schroeck FR, Krupski TL, Sun L, Albala DM, Price MM, Polascik TJ, et al. Satisfaction and regret after open retropubic or robot-assisted laparoscopic radical prostatectomy. Eur Urol. 2008;54:785–93.
5. Ficarra V, Novara G, Rosen RC, Artibani W, Carroll PR, Costello A, et al. Systematic review and meta-analysis of studies reporting urinary continence recovery after robot-assisted radical prostatectomy [Review]. Eur Urol. 2012;62:405–17.
6. Myers RP. Practical surgical anatomy for radical prostatectomy. Urol Clin North Am. 2001;28:473–90.
7. Federative Committee on Anatomical Terminology. Terminologia anatomica: international anatomical terminology. Stuttgart: Thieme; 1998.
8. Myers RP, Cahill DR, Kay PA, Camp JJ, Devine RM, King BF, et al. Puboperineales: muscular boundaries of the male urogenital hiatus in 3D from magnetic resonance imaging. J Urol. 2000;164:1412–5.
9. Oelrich TM. The urethral sphincter muscle in the male. Am J Anat. 1980;58:229–46.
10. Turner Warwick R. The sphincter mechanisms: their relation to prostatic enlargement and its treatment. In: Hinman Jr F, editor. Benign prostatic hypertrophy, sect IX. New York: Springer; 1983. p. 809–28.
11. Freire MP, Weinberg AC, Lei Y, Soukup JR, Lipsitz SR, Prasad SM, et al. Anatomic bladder neck preservation during robotic-assisted laparoscopic radical prostatectomy: description of technique and outcomes. Eur Urol. 2009;56:972–80.
12. Tyson MD, Ark J, Gregg JR, Johnsen NV, Kappa SF, Lee DJ, Smith JA. The null effect of bladder neck size on incontinence outcomes after radical prostatectomy. J Urol. 2017;198:1404–8.
13. Blute ML, Bostwick DG, Bergstralh EJ, Slezak JM, Martin SK, Amling CL, Zincke H. Anatomic site-specific positive margins in organ-confined prostate cancer and its impact on outcome after radical prostatectomy. Urology. 1997;50:733–9.
14. Capogrosso P, Ventimiglia E, Cazzaniga W, Montorsi F, Salonia A. Orgasmic dysfunction after radical prostatectomy. World J Mens Health. 2017;35:1–13.
15. Mungovan SF, Luiting HB, Graham PL, Sandhu JS, Akin O, Chan L, et al. The measurement of membranous urethral length using transperineal ultrasound prior to radical prostatectomy. Scand J Urol. 2018;52:263–8.
16. Myers RP. Radical prostatectomy: pertinent surgical anatomy. Atlas of Urol Clin North Am. 1994;22:1–18.
17. Myers RP. Male urethral sphincteric anatomy and radical prostatectomy. Urol Clin North Am. 1991;18:211–27.
18. Koraitim MM. The male urethral sphincter complex revisited: an anatomical concept and its physiological correlate. J Urol. 2008;179:1683–9.
19. Coakley FV, Eberhardt S, Kattan MW, Wei DC, Scardino PT, Hricak H. Urinary continence after radical retropubic prostatectomy: Relationship with membranous urethral length on preoperative endorectal magnetic resonance imaging. J Urol. 2002;168:1032–5.
20. Paparel P, Akin O, Sandhu JS, Otero JR, Serio AM, Scardino PT, et al. Recovery of urinary continence after radical prostatectomy: association with urethral length and urethral fibrosis measured by preoperative and postoperative endorectal magnetic resonance imaging. Eur Urol. 2009;55:629–39.
21. Mungovan SF, Sandhu JS, Akin O, Smart NA, Graham PL, Patel MI. Preoperative membranous urethral length measurement and continence recovery following radical prostatectomy: a systematic review and meta-analysis preoperative membranous urethral length measurement and continence recovery following radical prostatectomy: a systematic review and meta-analysis. Eur Urol. 2017;71:368–78.
22. Lardas M, Grivas N, Debray TPA, Zattoni F, Berridge C, Cumberbatch M, et al. Patient- and tumour-related prognostic factors for urinary incontinence after radical prostatectomy for non-metastatic prostate cancer: a systematic review and meta-analysis. Euro Urol Focus. 2021; https://doi.org/10.1016/j.euf.2021.04.020.
23. Gosling JA, Dixon JS, Critchley H, Thompson S-A. A comparative study of the human external sphincter and periurethral levator ani muscles. Br J Urol. 1981;53:35–41.
24. Schrøder HD, Reske-Nielsen E. Fiber types in the striated urethral and anal sphincters. Acta Neuropathol. 1983;60:278–82.
25. Tokunaka S, Murakami U, Fuji H, Okamura K, Miyata M, Hashimoto H, et al. Coexistence of fast and slow myosin isozymes in human external urethral sphincter. A preliminary report. J Urol. 1987;138:659–62.
26. Krahn HP, Morales PA. The effect of pudendal nerve anesthesia on urinary continence after prostatectomy. J Urol. 1965;94:282–5.
27. Moschovas MC, Bhat S, Onol FF, Rogers T, Roof S, Mazzone E, et al. A modified apical dissection and lateral prostatic fascia preservation improves early postoperative functional recovery in robotic-assisted laparoscopic radical prostatectomy: results from a propensity score–matched analysis. Eur Urol. 2020;78:875–84.
28. Schlomm T, Heinzer H, Steuber T, Salomon G, Engel O, Michl U, et al. Full functional-length urethral sphincter preservation during radical prostatectomy. Eur Urol. 2011;60:320–9.
29. Lee SE, Byun S-S, Lee HJ, Song SH, Chang IH, Kim YJ, et al. Impact of variations in prostatic apex shape on early recovery of urinary continence after radical retropubic prostatectomy. Urology. 2006;68:137–41.
30. Müller J. Über die organischen Nerven der erectilen männlichen Geschlectsorgane des Menschen und der Säugethiere (Concerning the autonomic nerves of the male erectile genital organs of man and mammals). Berlin: F. Dummler; 1836.
31. Walsh PC. Urologic surgery: radical retropubic prostatectomy-an anatomic approach with preservation of sexual function. Syracuse, Bristol Laboratories; 1986.
32. Helweg G, Strasser H, Knapp R, Wicke K, Frauscher F, zur Nedden D, et al. Transurethral sonomorphologic evaluation of the male external sphincter of the urethra. Eur Radio1. 1994;4:525–8.
33. Stafford RE, Ashton-Miller JA, Constantinou CE, Hodges PW. A new method to quantify male pelvic floor displacement from 2D transperineal ultrasound images. Urology. 2013;81:685–9.
34. Bessede T, Sooriakumaran P, Takenaka A, Tewari A. Neural supply of the male urethral sphincter: comprehensive anatomical review and implications for continence recovery after radical prostatectomy. World J Urol. 2017;35:549–65.
35. Catarin MV, Manzano GM, Nobrega JA, Almeida FG, Srougi M, Bruschini H. The role of membranous urethral afferent autonomic innervation in the continence mechanism after nerve sparing radical prostatectomy: a clinical and prospective study. J Urol. 2008;180:2527–31.
36. Nyangoh Timoh K, Deffon J, Moszkowicz D, Lebacle C, Creze M, Martinovic J, et al. Smooth muscle of the male pelvic floor: an anatomic study. Clin Anat. 2020;33:810–22.
37. Patel VR, Coelho RF, Palmer KJ, Rocco B. Periurethral suspension stitch during robot-assisted laparoscopic radical prostatectomy: description of the technique and continence outcomes. Euro Urol. 2009;56:472–8.
38. Asimakopoulos AD, Corona Montes VE, Gaston R. Robot-assisted laparoscopic radical prostatectomy with intrafascial dissection of the neurovascular bundles and preservation of the pubovesical complex: a step-by-step description of the technique. J Endourol. 2012;26:1578–85.

39. Myers RP. Detrusor apron, associated vascular plexus, and avascular plane: relevance to radical retropubic prostatectomy—anatomic and surgical commentary. Urology. 2002;59:472–9.
40. Galfano A, Ascione A, Grimaldi S, Petralia G, Strada E, Bocciardi AM. A new anatomic approach for robot-assisted laparoscopic prostatectomy: a feasibility study for completely intrafascial surgery. Euro Urol. 2010;58:457–61.
41. Lim SK, Kim KH, Shin T-Y, Han WK, Chung BH, Hong SJ, et al. Retzius-sparing robot-assisted laparoscopic radical prostatectomy: combining the best of retropubic and perineal approaches. BJU Int. 2014;114:236–44.
42. Reeves F, Preece P, Kapoor J, Everaerts W, Murphy DG, Corcoran NM, et al. Preservation of the neurovascular bundles is associated with improved time to continence after radical prostatectomy but not long-term continence rates: results of a systematic review and meta-analysis [Review]. Eur Urol. 2015;68:692–704.
43. Tewari AK, Srivastava A, Huang MW, Robinson BD, Shevchuk MM, Durand M, et al. Anatomical grades of nerve sparing: a risk-stratified approach to neural-hammock sparing during robot-assisted radical prostatectomy (RARP). BJU Int. 2011;108:984–92.
44. Steineck G, Bjartell A, Hugosson J, Axen E, Carlsson S, Stranne J, et al. Degree of preservation of the neurovascular bundles during radical prostatectomy and urinary continence 1 year after surgery. Euro Urol. 2015;67:559–68.
45. Michl U, Tennstedt P, Feldmeier L, Mandel P, Oh SJ, Ahyai S, et al. Nerve-sparing surgery technique, not the preservation of the neurovascular bundles, leads to improved long-term continence rates after radical prostatectomy. Eur Urol. 2016;69:584–9.
46. Tan GY, Jhaveri JK, Tewari AK. Anatomic restoration technique: a biomechanics-based approach for early continence recovery after minimally invasive radical prostatectomy. Urology. 2009;74:492–6.
47. Vis AN, van der Poel HG, Ruiter AEC, Hu JC, Tewari AK, Rocco B, et al. Posterior, anterior, and periurethral surgical reconstruction of urinary continence mechanisms in robot-assisted radical prostatectomy: a description and video compilation of commonly performed surgical techniques. Eur Urol. 2019;76:814–22.
48. Tewari AK, Bigelow K, Rao S, Takenaka A, El-Tabi N, Te A, et al. Anatomic restoration technique of continence mechanism and preservation of puboprostatic collar: a novel modification to achieve early urinary continence in men undergoing robotic prostatectomy. Urology. 2007;69:726–31.
49. Bianchi L, Maria Turri F, Larcher A, De Groote R, De Bruyne P, De Coninck V, et al. A novel approach for apical dissection during robot-assisted radical prostatectomy: the "collar" technique. Euro Urol Focus. 2018;4:677–85.
50. Galfano A, Trapani DD, Sozzi F, Strada E, Petralia G, Bramerio M, et al. Beyond the learning curve of the Retzius-sparing approach for robot-assisted laparoscopic radical prostatectomy: oncologic and functional results of the first 200 patients with ≥1 year of follow-up. Eur Urol. 2013;64:974–80.
51. Dalela D, Jeong W, Prasad MA, Sood A, Abdollah F, Diaz M, et al. A pragmatic randomized controlled trial examining the impact of the Retzius-sparing approach on early urinary continence recovery after robot-assisted radical prostatectomy. Euro Urol. 2017;72:677–85.
52. Menon M, Dalela D, Jamil M, Diaz M, Tallman C, Abdollah F, et al. Functional recovery, oncologic outcomes and postoperative complications after robot-assisted radical prostatectomy: an evidence-based analysis comparing the Retzius sparing and standard approaches. J Urol. 2018;199:1210–7.
53. Student V Jr, Vidlar A, Grepl M, Hartmann I, Buresova E, Student V. Advanced reconstruction of vesicourethral support (ARVUS) during robot-assisted radical prostatectomy: one-year functional outcomes in a two-group randomised controlled trial. Euro Urol. 2017;71:822–30.
54. Walsh PC. Anatomical radical prostatectomy: evolution of the surgical technique. J Urol. 1998;160:2418–24.
55. Wagaskar VG, Mittal A, Sobotka S, Ratnani P, Lantz A, Falagario UG. Hood technique for robotic radical prostatectomy-preserving periurethral anatomical structures in the space of Retzius and sparing the pouch of Douglas, enabling early return of continence without compromising surgical margin rates. Eur Urol. 2021;80:213–21.
56. Martini A, Falagario UG, Villers A, Dell'Oglio P, Mazzone E, Autorino R, et al. Contemporary techniques of prostate dissection for robot-assisted prostatectomy. Eur Urol. 2020;78:583–91.
57. Hollabaugh RS, Dmochowski RR, Steiner MS. Neuroanatomy of the male rhabdosphincter. Urology. 1997;49:426–34.
58. Ghani KR, Trinh QD, Menon M. Vattikuti Institute prostatectomy-technique in 2012. J Endourol. 2012;26:1558–65.
59. Chang L-W, Hung S-C, Hu J-C, Chiu K-Y. Retzius-sparing robotic-assisted radical prostatectomy associated with less bladder neck descent and better early continence outcome. Anticancer Res. 2018;38:345–51.
60. Hamada A, Razdan S, Etafy MH, Fagin R, Razdan S. Early return of continence in patients undergoing robot-assisted laparoscopic prostatectomy using modified maximal urethral length preservation technique. J Endourol. 2014;28:930–8.
61. Ko YH, Huynh LM, See K, Lall C, Skarecky D, Ahlering TE. Impact of surgically maximized versus native membranous urethral length on 30-day and long-term pad-free continence after robot-assisted radical prostatectomy. Prostate Int. 2020;8:55–61.
62. Quadri G, Magatti F, Belloni C, Barisani D, Natale N. Marshall-Marchetti-Krantz urethropexy and Burch colposuspension for stress urinary incontinence in women with low pressure and hypermobility of the urethra: Early results of a prospective randomized clinical trial. Am J Obstet Gynecol. 1999;181:12–8.
63. Boorjian SA, Karnes RJ, Crispen PL, Carlson RE, Rangel LJ, Bergstralh EJ, et al. The impact of positive surgical margins on mortality following radical prostatectomy during the prostate specific antigen era. J Urol. 2010;183:1003–9.
64. Rosenberg JE, Jung JH, Edgerton Z, Lee H, Lee S, Bakker CJ. Retzius-sparing versus standard robot-assisted laparoscopic prostatectomy for the treatment of clinically localized prostate cancer. BJU Int. 2021;128:12–20.
65. Tai TE, Wu CC, Kang YN, Wu JC. Effects of Retzius sparing on robot-assisted laparoscopic prostatectomy: a systematic review with meta-analysis. Surg Endosc. 2020;34:4020–9.
66. Barakat B, Othman H, Gauger U, Wolff I, Hadaschik B, Rehme CR. Retzius sparing radical prostatectomy versus robot-assisted radical prostatectomy: which technique is more beneficial for prostate cancer patients (MASTER Study)? A systematic review and meta-analysis. Eur Urol Focus. 2021; https://doi.org/10.1016/j.euf.2021.08.003.

Prostate Neurovascular Anatomy and Its Impact on Nerve-Sparing RALP

Anthony J. Costello and Fairleigh Reeves

1 Introduction

A detailed anatomic knowledge of the prostate and pelvic structures informs precise surgical technique for radical prostatectomy. All surgeons performing radical prostatectomy need to have a foundation based on the prostatic neurovascular and sphincteric anatomy. It was the discovery by Walsh and Donker in their seminal paper in 1982 [1], which heralded the ability of surgeons to preserve the neurovascular bundles at radical prostatectomy. Their anatomical insights led to the birth of the nerve sparing procedure as we note today. Prior to their discovery urologists believed that the nerves for erection traveled through the prostate and by removing the prostate impotence was guaranteed after prostatectomy.

Walsh's work represented a rediscovery of the intricate anatomy of the cavernous nerves, that had been thoroughly described over a century earlier by Johannes Müller [2]. This German-language paper by Muller was essentially lost on a practical level and it was not until Walsh described the cavernous nerves nearly 40 years ago now, that this important anatomy became internationally recognized and integrated into surgical practice.

The autonomic cavernous nerves, which are destined for the erectile tissue, do not accompany the blood vessels to the penis but take a much shorter path [2]. It is via the periprostatic neurovascular bundle (NVB) that they course instead (Fig. 1). The NVB transmits other important neurovascular structures including nerve branches to the prostate, rectum, and pelvic floor musculature, and it is not appropriate to use the terms cavernosal or cavernous nerves and "NVB" interchangeably [4].

Walsh's description of the position of the NVB posteromedial to the prostate transformed a procedure that virtually guaranteed impotence, into a procedure where potency could be preserved through the preservation of these NVB structures. NVB (and therefore cavernosal nerve) sparing correlates strongly with improved post-operative potency rates. A systematic review has reported 12-month post-RALP potency rates of 74% (62–90%) for bilateral nerve sparing [5].

This chapter outlines the neurovascular anatomy of the prostate requisite for nerve-sparing RALP.

2 Fascia

An appreciation of the fascia of the pelvis is imperative to the performance of nerve sparing surgery, as the NVB runs through leaves of periprostatic fascia (Fig. 2).

The precise detail of the complex multilayered fascia around the prostate remains controversial [6]. One of the contributing factors to confusion in this area is the variability of the terminology used [7]. For the operating surgeon, the following is a summary of our knowledge to date.

"Endopelvic fascia" is commonly used in prostate surgery to collectively describe the parietal and visceral fascia that lines the pelvis *(pelvic fascia, lateral pelvic fascia, superior pelvic fascia, parietal pelvic fascia, levator fascia, outer layer of periprostatic fascia, parapelvic fascia* [7, 8]). The prostatic fascia *(inner layer of periprostatic fascia, inner layer of lateral pelvic fascia* [7]) forms the medial boundary of the NVB and is applied directly to the prostatic capsule anterolaterally [9].

Posterior to the prostate, between it and the rectum, is Denonvilliers' fasica. Superiorly, Denonvilliers' covers the posterior aspect of the seminal vesicles. Laterally, it merges with the endopelvic fascia at the NVB [7].

A. J. Costello (✉)
The Royal Melbourne Hospital, Parkville, Australia

Department of Surgery, University of Melbourne, Melbourne, Australia

Australian Medical Robotics Academy, North Melbourne, VIC, Australia

F. Reeves
The Urology Centre, Guy's and St Thomas' NHS Foundation Trust, London, United Kingdom

P. Wiklund et al. (eds.), *Robotic Urologic Surgery*, https://doi.org/10.1007/978-3-031-00363-9_14

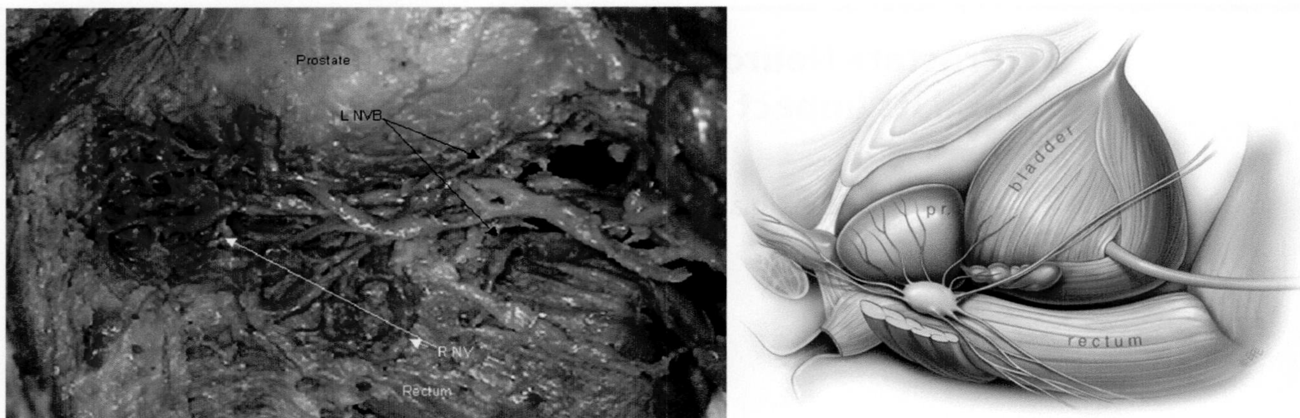

Fig. 1 Neurovascular bundle dissection (left [3]) and schematic (right)

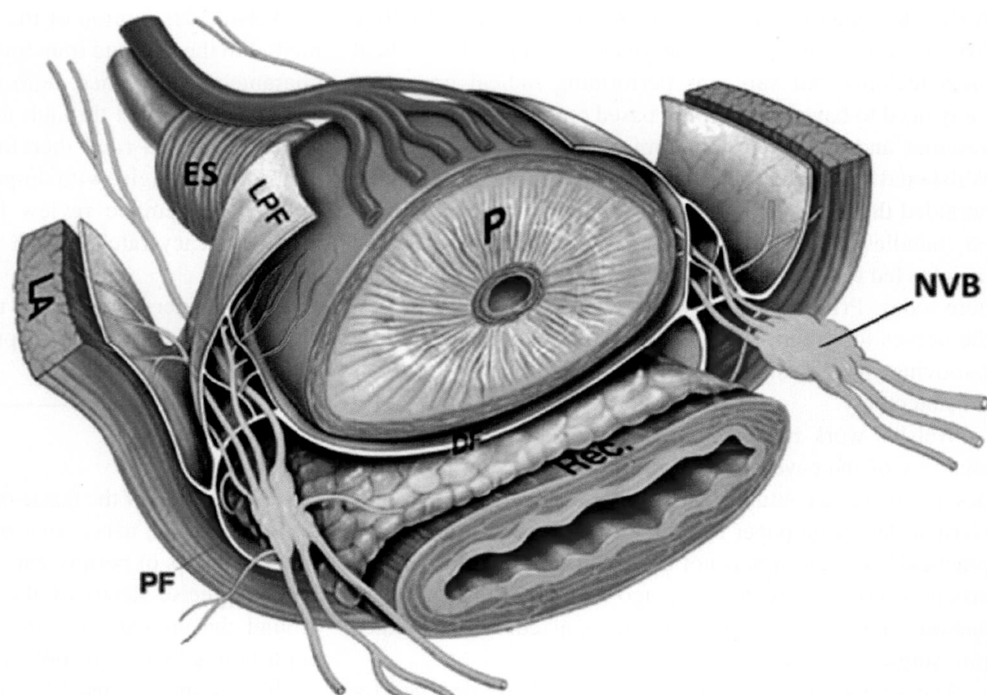

Fig. 2 Illustrative representation of periprostatic autonomic innervations. *DF* Denonviller's Fascia, *LA* Levator ani, *LPF* lateral prostatic fascia, *PF* pararectal fat, *P* rectum and prostate, *Rec* rectum (reprinted from [4])

In McNeal's formative paper on the zonal anatomy of the prostate, the anterior fibromuscular stroma was described as a thick, non-glandular region, continuous with the external urethral sphincter distally and detrusor muscle proximally [10]. Myers later went on to study the detrusor apron in detail, concluding that it should be considered a major component of McNeal's anterior fibromuscular stroma. The detrusor apron ends anteriorly where it forms puboprostatic ligaments that attach to the pubis, anchoring the prostate, urethra and bladder neck, affording stabilization to the urinary continence mechanism [11]. In Li and colleagues' recent celloidin anatomical sections, the detrusor apron is demonstrated overlying the DVC (Fig. 3) [12].

3 Neuroanatomy

The NVB provides an excellent intraoperative landmark for surgeons aiming to preserve the cavernous nerves during RALP, as the individual nerve fibers carried in this structure are extremely fine (measuring 0.04–0.37 mm in diameter). The human hair is a diameter of 0.20 mm [13]. Our work has identified between 6 and 16 nerves in these bundles [3]. Although nerves in the NVB can sometimes be visualized with the assistance of magnification, they are mostly obscured by fibrofatty tissue and blood vessels [13].

The individual nerves within the NVB are vulnerable at multiple points during RALP. They may be subject to direct

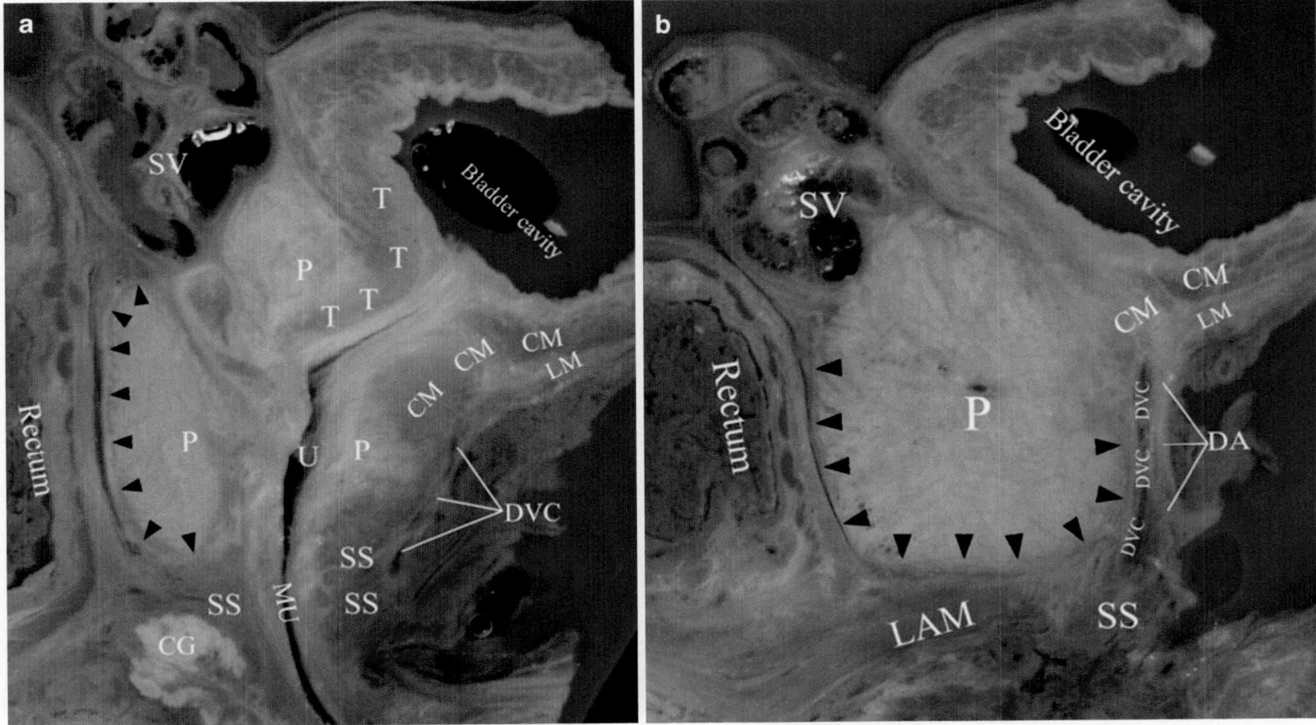

Fig. 3 Sagittal celloidin sections. (**a**) Midsagittal section; (**b**) section through lateral border of striated sphincter. Black triangles indicated the capsule. *CM* circular muscle of detrusor; *SS* striated sphincter; *T* trigone muscle; *LM* longitudinal muscle of detrusor; *LAM* levator ani muscle; *DA* detrusor apron; *DVC* dorsal vascular complex; *P* prostate; *SV* seminal vesicles; *CG* Cowper's glands; *MU* membranous urethra. From [12]

injury by cutting, diathermy or suture ligation or indirect trauma from undue tension leading to a neuropraxia. Areas where maximum care should be exercised during surgical dissection to remove the prostate, include apical dissection, mobilization of the bundles laterally along the mid-prostate, pedicle ligation, and dissection of the seminal vesicles [13]. Our strong belief is that the maximum potential for injury to the cavernous nerves is at the apex where they swing anteromedially on the urethra to run subpubic into the cavernous tissue. It is here where overzealous dissection can injure these delicate nerves.

The NVB originates from the pelvic plexus (also known as *inferior hypogastric plexus*) [14]. The pelvic plexus lies in a sagittal plane lateral to the rectum at the approximate level of S4 and S5 [15]. It varies from 3 to 5.5 cm by 2.5–5 cm high and is a culmination of fibers from the hypogastric plexus which transmits the sympathetic outflow from T10-L2 via the hypogastric nerves, and parasympathetic supply that is delivered via the pelvic splanchnic nerves (S2–4) (Fig. 4). The NVB is commonly understood to carry autonomic fibers, but histological examination has demonstrated that a small percentage of periprostatic nerves are somatic [16]. Note that the ganglion or pelvic plexus where parasympathetic and sympathetic nerves join is situated at the base of the prostate and in some cases slightly more distal than that.

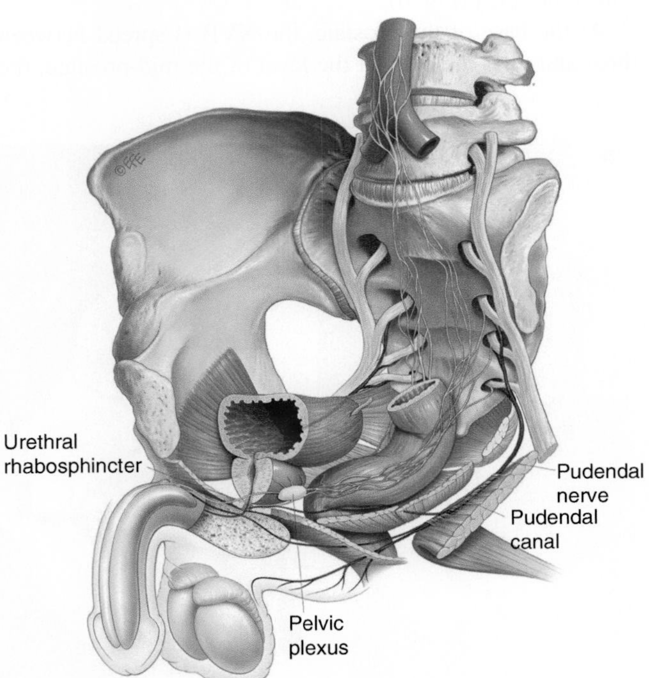

Fig. 4 The pelvic plexus, showing contributions of hypogastric nerve and S2–S4 segments

Three major projections are given off from the pelvic plexus. (1) Anterior: extends across the lateral surface of the seminal vesicle and the inferolateral surface of the bladder; (2) antero-inferior: passes to the vesicoprostatic junction and then obliquely along the lateral surface of the prostate; (3) inferior: the most caudal fibers of the plexus travel between the rectum and the posterolateral surface of the prostate to form the NVB [3].

Fascia creates functional compartmentalization of the NVB, which is not absolute and is less distinct proximally [3] (Fig. 5). There are three or sometimes four major compartments that comprise the neurovascular bundle. The cavernous nerves travel most anteriorly in the NVB. Posteriorly and posterolaterally nerves to the rectum run within the leaves of Denonvilliers' and pararectal fascia. Laterally, levator ani supply travels within the lateral pelvic fascia [3, 12].

Traveling distally, from its origin at the vesicoprostatic junction, at the base of the prostate, the NVB is closely applied to the posterolateral aspect of the prostate [2, 13]. Tiny branches come off the NVB at right angles to enter the prostatic capsular surface alongside tiny arteries and veins. These need to be divided in order properly release the NVB during nerve sparing [13].

Proximally the neurovascular bundle lies close to the inferolateral aspect of the tip of the seminal vesical and the arterial supply to the bladder base [3, 17]. This can be easily appreciated on the celloidoidin section published by Li and colleagues [12] (Fig. 6).

At the base of the prostate, the NVB is spread between three and nine o'clock. At the level of the mid-prostate, the NVB converges to form a more condensed NVB, only to diverge again near the prostatic apex [3]. The position of the NVB is influenced by the presence of BPH. In smaller prostates, the bundles tend to obscure the lateral surface of the prostate. Whereas, as the transition zone of the prostate enlarges with BPH, the peripheral zone is compressed posterolaterally, and the NVB is found tucked more underneath the prostate [13]. Some authors have described a wider spray-like distribution of nerves, rather than a discrete bundle [18]. Certainly, variations can be seen. Histological evaluation however has demonstrated that only a minority of anterolateral nerves are functionally significant parasympathetic fibers [4, 19].

Beyond the apex of the prostate, the cavernous nerves come forward and traverse the urogenital hiatus posterolateral to the prostatic apex. Then, as described by Muller nearly 200 years ago, the minor cavernous nerves penetrate the root of the corpus cavernosum [2]. The main cavernous nerves then continue with the deep artery and vein of the penis [20].

Nerve sparing surgery tends to focus on the extirpation component of radical prostatectomy. However, care must also be paid during reconstruction to ensure the nerves that were once carefully preserved are not later damaged. Posteriorly, in close proximity to the prostatourethral junction is a point of decussation of nerves. Passing a needle here, such as in the reconstruction of the posterior musculofascial plate with a "Rocco stitch" [21], comes close to the junction of the neurovascular bundles, and must be done with care in order to avoid the risk of entrapment of nerves from the neurovascular bundle [13].

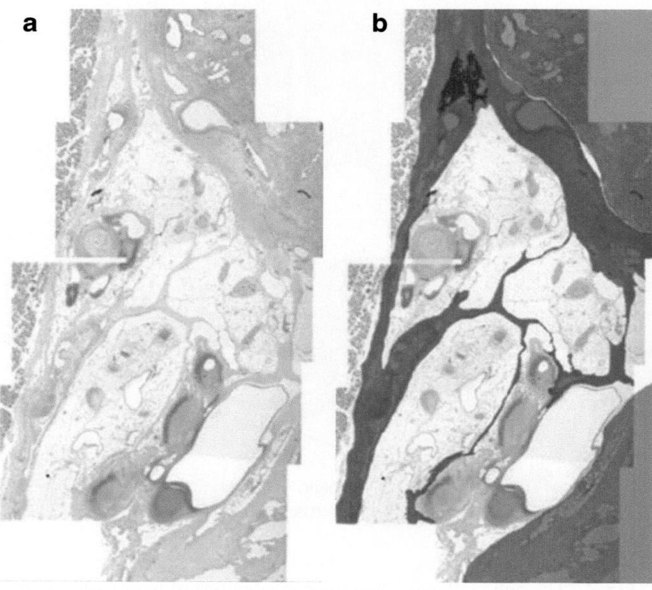

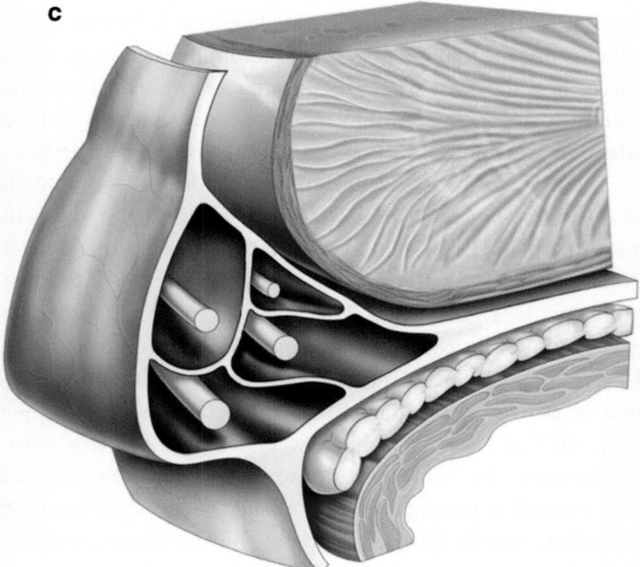

Fig. 5 Compartmental architecture of the neurovascular bundle. (**a**) Left: hematoxylin and eosin slide showing compartmental NVB architecture. (**b**) Right (overlay): prostate (green), fascial bands (blue), nerves (yellow), para-rectal tissue (gray), levator ani musculature (spotted pink) [3]. (**c**) Schematic representation

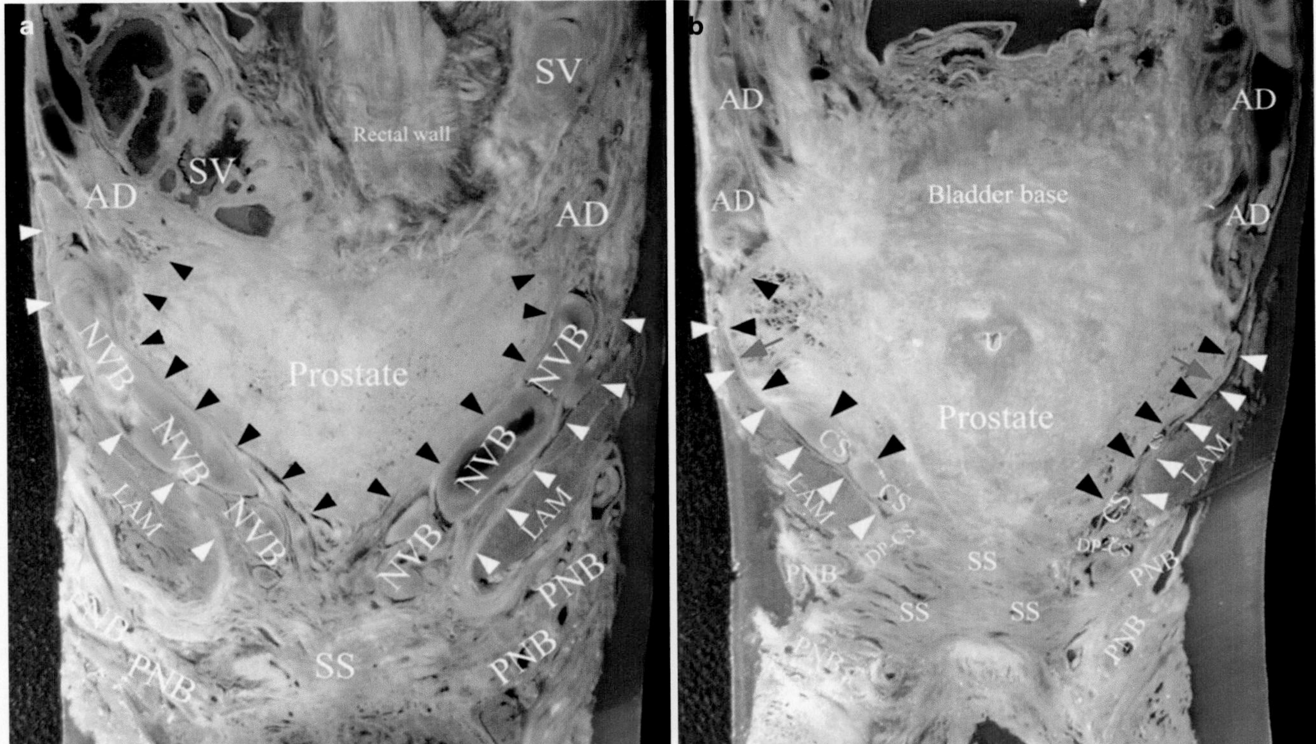

Fig. 6 Coronal celloidin sections. (**a**) Section through seminal vesicles; (**b**) section through the posterior portion of striated sphincter. Note that the capsule and the levator fascia adhered together at the upper lateral aspect (green arrow). Black and white triangles indicated the capsule and the levator fascia respectively. *SS* striated sphincter; *AD* anterior division; *CS* cavernous supply; *DP-CS* the distal part of the cavernous supply; *PNB* pudendal neurovascular bundle; *SV* seminal vesicles; *LAM* levator ani muscle; *U* urthra

In addition to cavernous nerves, nerves essential to continence preservation are potentially at risk during performance of the vesicourethral anastomosis. Pudendal nerve branches to the urinary sphincter have been described as close as 3 mm from the prostate apex [22], and in another study, sphincteric branches of the pudendal nerve were a mean distance of 5.5 mm from the lowest point of the endopelvic fascia [23], thus highly vulnerable to over-enthusiastic posterior anastomotic sutures or a deep Rocco reconstruction.

4 Vascular Anatomy

Arterial supply to the prostate arises from the prostato-vesical artery off the internal iliac. This well-defined trunk has a variable origin and often has anastomotic connections to the internal pudendal and inferior rectal arteries [13]. The prostato-vesical artery passes forward and medially over the antero-inferior surface of the bladder and has its main pedicle located at the junction of the bladder and prostate in close proximity to the seminal vesicle. Although its branching pattern can vary, typically its terminal branches are the inferior vesical and prostatic branches. In some cases, supply to the prostate is received from branches of the superior rectal artery [24].

In addition to nerve sparing, preservation of vascular supply to the erectile tissue must be considered when optimizing functional outcomes. Accessory pudendal arteries pass superior to the pelvic diaphragm before coursing under the pubic bone to enter the penile hilum [6], and as such are at risk during radical prostatectomy. Accessory pudendal arteries have variable origin from the obturator, inferior vesical or external pudendal artery [25]. They are generally seen in the setting of congenital anatomical variation but sometimes correlate with the presence of pudendal atherosclerosis [26]. In some cases, they may provide the sole arterial supply to the corpora [27], thus their injury provides an explanation for vasculogenic impotence after a nerve sparing procedure [28]. For maximal preservation of erectile function post prostatectomy, both nerve sparing and preservation of accessory pudendal arteries should be done where feasible.

Maintaining clear vision within the operative field, through meticulous hemostasis, facilitates precise nerve sparing. A pre-prostatic superficial vein often exists the fascia between puboprostatic ligaments, nestled in preprostatic adipose tissue, which then re-enters vesicovenous plexus. Although it may be absent in 10%, if it is large it may bleed [29].

The key venous structure in radical prostatectomy is the dorsal vascular complex (DVC). Venous bleeding was historically associated with life-threatening bleeding that deterred many surgeons from performing prostatectomy. Recognition and ligation of the DVC is associated with reduced blood loss. It was Walsh who first described the technique of ligation of the dorsal venous complex in 1979 [30]. It was this insight that made surgery much safer for the open radical prostatectomist. Before Walsh described ligation of the dorsal vein, tamponade with a balloon catheter was used along with often unsuccessful attempts to oversew the vein after significant bleeding had occurred. Blood loss of up to 1500 cc was not uncommon.

The DVC is often considered a venous structure but does also include small arteries [31]. It lies anterior to the prostate, cloaked by the DVC, and passes under the pubic arch. An avascular plane lies between the DVC and the prostate at the prostate-urethral junction, providing a landmark for control. To avoid injuring the external urethral sphincter, or neurovascular bundles, one must use caution not to pass ligation sutures distal to the prostate-urethral junction [11]. With the advent of RALP, the DVC ligation technique has been modified to minimize the risk of collateral tissue damage. Exploiting increased intra-abdominal pressure from CO_2 insufflation, and improved vision and dexterity afforded with RALP has enabled surgeons to divide the DVC without initial ligation. This allows the surgeon to precisely select the site of division, maximizing urethral length while ensuring negative apical margin [31]. Hemostasis can then be achieved later with controlled oversewing of any open vessels rather than mass ligation.

5 Application of Anatomical Principles for Optimization of Functional Outcomes

The earliest description of the technique of neurovascular bundle sparing was described by Walsh for open retropubic radical prostatectomy in the 1980s. This technique was adapted by Menon who was trained by Walsh and first popularized the early technique of nerve-sparing robotic prostatectomy. Since the first descriptions of the technique of robotic prostatectomy, there have been many papers published regarding a variety of methods used to avoid injury to the neurovascular bundle in an attempt to preserve potency. In a discussion of the nerve sparing technique at radical prostatectomy, it is of paramount importance that the cart stays behind the horse. The primary aim of radical prostatectomy is to remove all prostate cancer with the specimen. Secondarily, but very importantly, the surgeon's aim is to maintain both potency and continence of the quality of life issues associated with this surgery. The oncological efficacy of robotic prostatectomy must be the principal goal of the surgeon. Walsh and Epstein have published that the maximum average capsular penetration of prostate cancer in pT3 disease is 3 mm [32]. The distance between the prostatic capsule and the fascia surrounding the neurovascular bundle is between 3 and 5 mm. Thus, the surgeon can incrementally go a little wider on the specimen and still preserve the neurovascular bundle.

In 2005 Menon described his technique of the Veil of Aphrodite NVB preservation [33]. Menon suggested that high release of the fascia above the NVB would maximize neural preservation. We do know that the majority of cavernous nerves in the neurovascular bundle lie below the 3 to 9 O'clock level of the prostate. However, the high fascial release described by Menon could potentially produce less traction on the NVB and thus avoid neurapraxia.

Tewari later described risk stratified approach to neural hammock sparing during robot-assisted radical prostatectomy [34]. This thesis was assisted by the insights derived from MRI of the prostate and surrounding fascial tissue. However, there is great variation in the fascial architecture surrounding the prostate and this grading system remains difficult.

Patel and his co-workers in 2012 described an anatomic grading of the extent of nerve sparing during robot-assisted radical prostatectomy [35]. In the paper, they described a nerve sparing score from 5: at least 95% nerve sparing to 1: non-nerve sparing surgery. In the description of optimal nerve sparing (grade 5/5), they highlight the presence of a visual clue. A landmark artery that runs medially at mid prostate to distal apex of the prostate. The artery is used to delineate the course of the neurovascular bundle in a retrograde manner up to the prostatic pedicle. The nerve sparing is performed medial to this artery just outside the prostatic fascia and in the areolar tissue between the prostate and neurovascular bundle. This is a bloodless plane and can be detached without the need for sharp dissection. In the authors' opinion, the technique can be mastered by expert robotic radical prostatectomists. However, it may be difficult to perform for surgeons not as skillful as the lead author of this manuscript. This manuscript is very well illustrated with graphics and histological confirmation of the various layers involved in this anatomically graded nerve sparing.

Another well-described technique of nerve sparing relates to the NeuroSAFE prostatectomy open and robotic methods, popularized by the group at the Martini Clinic in Hamburg, Germany [36]. In this technique, the surgeon requests intraoperative fresh frozen section analysis of the posterolateral aspect of the prostate margin to assess whether cancer extends beyond the capsule. Several authors report evidence from large observation studies of functional outcomes which can be improved and positive surgical margin rate reduced when the neuro-safe technique is used during robotic prostatectomy. However, this technique has not been widely adopted as it is time and resource intense with low sensitivity and specificity and some have said has potentially conflicting oncological results [37, 38].

As the technique has not been widely introduced in the United Kingdom [39], This is due to the lack of level 1 evidence to support the NeuroSAFE robotic prostatectomy method, Dinneen and colleagues propose a randomized trial to test the hypothesis.

In conclusion, most robotic radical prostatectomists do not perform a large number of surgeries and do not have the technical competence of some of the super expert surgeons publishing their techniques. When commencing to perform robotic radical prostatectomy the less experienced surgeon may find it easier to perform a technique of simple retrograde neurovascular bundle preservation and later move to the more complex techniques once proficiency in the simpler technique has been gained.

Although the primary aim of nerve sparing surgery is the preservation of erectile function, there may also be benefits to continence outcomes. Systematic review demonstrated nerve sparing was associated with early return of continence (up to 6 months), but no difference in long-term continence rates [40]. The relationship, however, between nerve sparing and continence outcomes remains controversial. Somatic supply to the external urethral sphincter (rhabdosphincter) is variable. Direct intrapelvic supply to the sphincter may exist in some men [41–44], and in these cases, could account for improved rates of continence return with nerve sparing. However, confounding factors also exist. These include meticulous apical dissection, which may result in preservation of nearby pudendal nerve branches to the sphincter, as well as improved membranous urethral length [45], thereby preserving the external striated rhabdospincter. Decreased collateral tissue damage with vigilant dissection may also result in the preservation of supportive continence structures and urethral vascular integrity [40].

6 Conclusion

Neuroanatomy of the pelvis is complex and varied. We are now fortunate to have a solid foundation of anatomical knowledge that has shaped the current technique of RALP. Ongoing work is warranted to better understand anatomical variations and to develop improved intraoperative monitoring systems to provide more patients access to the best possible functional outcomes after surgery.

References

1. Walsh PC, Donker PJ. Impotence following radical prostatectomy: insight into etiology and prevention. J Urol. 1982;128:492–7.
2. Muller J. Über die organischen Nerven der erectilen männlichen Geschlectsorgane desMenschen und der Säugethiere. (Concerning the autonomic nerves of the male erectile genital organs of man and mammals.). Berlin: F. Dummler; 1836.
3. Costello AJ, Brooks M, Cole OJ. Anatomical studies of the neurovascular bundle and cavernosal nerves. BJU Int. 2004;94:1071–6.
4. Costello AJ, Dowdle BW, Namdarian B, Pedersen J, Murphy DG. Immunohistochemical study of the cavernous nerves in the periprostatic region. BJU Int. 2011;107:1210–5.
5. Ficarra V, Novara G, Ahlering TE, et al. Systematic review and meta-analysis of studies reporting potency rates after robot-assisted radical prostatectomy. Eur Urol. 2012;62:418–30.
6. Walz J, Burnett AL, Costello AJ, et al. A critical analysis of the current knowledge of surgical anatomy related to optimization of cancer control and preservation of continence and erection in candidates for radical prostatectomy. Eur Urol. 2010;57:179–92.
7. Raychaudhuri B, Cahill D. Pelvic fasciae in urology. Ann R Coll Surg Engl. 2008;90:633–7.
8. Rassweiler J, Laguna P, Chlosta P, et al. ESUT expert group on laparoscopy proposes uniform terminology during radical prostatectomy: we need to speak the same language. Eur Urol. 2013;64:97–100.
9. Tewari A, Peabody JO, Fischer M, et al. An operative and anatomic study to help in nerve sparing during laparoscopic and robotic radical prostatectomy. Eur Urol. 2003;43:444–54.
10. McNeal JE. The zonal anatomy of the prostate. Prostate. 1981;2:35–49.
11. Myers RP. Detrusor apron, associated vascular plexus, and avascular plane: relevance to radical retropubic prostatectomy--anatomic and surgical commentary. Urology. 2002;59:472–9.
12. Li X, Wu J, Cai Q, et al. The distribution pattern of periprostatic neurovascular bundles examined with successive celloidin slices. BMC Urol. 2021;21:6.
13. Myers RP. Gross and applied anatomy of the prostate. In: Kantoff PW, Rarroll PR, D'Amico AV, editors. Prostate cancer principles and practice. Philadelphia: Lippincott Williams & Wilkins; 2002.
14. Mauroy B, Demondion X, Drizenko A, et al. The inferior hypogastric plexus (pelvic plexus): its importance in neural preservation techniques. Surg Radiol Anat. 2003;25:6–15.
15. Baader B, Herrmann M. Topography of the pelvic autonomic nervous system and its potential impact on surgical intervention in the pelvis. Clin Anat. 2003;16:119–30.
16. Reeves F, Battye S, Borin JF, Corcoran NM, Costello AJ. High-resolution map of somatic periprostatic nerves. Urology. 2016;97:160–5.
17. Zlotta AR, Roumeguère T, Ravery V, et al. Is seminal vesicle ablation mandatory for all patients undergoing radical prostatectomy? Eur Urol. 2004;46:42–9.
18. Kiyoshima K. Anatomical features of periprostatic tissue and its surroundings: a histological analysis of 79 radical retropubic prostatectomy specimens. Jpn J Clin Oncol. 2004;34:463–8.
19. Ganzer R, Stolzenburg J-U, Wieland WF, Bründl J. Anatomic study of periprostatic nerve distribution: immunohistochemical differentiation of parasympathetic and sympathetic nerve fibres. Eur Urol. 2012;62:1150–6.
20. Paick JS, Donatucci CF, Lue T. Anatomy of cavernous nerves distal to prostate: microdissection study in adult male cadavers. Urology. 1993;42:145–9.

21. Rocco B, Cozzi G, Spinelli MG, Coelho RF, Patel VR. Posterior musculofascial reconstruction after radical prostatectomy: a systematic review of the literature. Eur Urol. 2012.
22. Narayan P, Konety B, Aslam K, Aboseif S, Blumenfeld W, Tanagho E. Neuroanatomy of the external urethral sphincter: implications for urinary continence preservation during radical prostate surgery. J Urol. 1995;153:337–41.
23. Takenaka A, Hara R, Soga H, Murakami G, Fujisawa M. A novel technique for approaching the endopelvic fascia in retropubic radical prostatectomy, based on an anatomical study of fixed and fresh cadavers. BJU Int. 2005;95:766–71.
24. Clegg EJ. The arterial supply of the human prostate and seminal vesicles. J Anat. 1955;89:209–16.
25. Secin FP, Touijer K, Mulhall J, Guillonneau B. Anatomy and preservation of accessory pudendal arteries in laparoscopic radical prostatectomy. Eur Urol. 2007;51:1229–35.
26. Droupy S, Benoit G, Giuliano F, Jardin A. Penile arteries in humans origin-distribution-variations. Surg Radiol Anat. 1997;19:161–7.
27. Breza J, Aboseif S, Lue T, Tanagho EA. Detailed anatomy of penile neurovascular structures: surgical significance. J Urol. 1989;141:437–43.
28. Droupy S, Hessel A, Benoit G, Blanchet P, Jardin A, Giuliano F. Assessment of the functional role of accessory pudendal arteries in erection by transrectal color Doppler ultrasound. JURO. 1999;162:1987–91.
29. Myers RP. Anatomical variation of the superficial preprostatic veins with respect to radical retropubic prostatectomy. J Urol. 1991;145:992–3.
30. Reiner WG, Walsh PC. An anatomical approach to the surgical management of the dorsal vein and Santorini's plexus during radical retropubic surgery. J Urol. 1979;121:198–200.
31. Power NE, Silberstein JL, Kulkarni GS, Laudone VP. The dorsal venous complex (DVC): dorsal venous or dorsal vasculature complex? Santorini's plexus revisited. BJU Int. 2011;108:930–2.
32. Epstein JI, Walsh PC, Carmichael M, Brendler CB. Pathologic and clinical findings to predict tumor extent of nonpalpable (stage T1c) prostate cancer. JAMA. 1994;271:368–74.
33. Kaul S, Bhandari A, Hemal A, Savera A, Shrivastava A, Menon M. Robotic radical prostatectomy with preservation of the prostatic fascia: a feasibility study. Urology. 2005;66:1261–5.
34. Tewari A, Srivastava A, Sooriakumaran P, Grover S, Dorsey P, Leung R. Technique of traction-free nerve-sparing robotic prostatectomy: delicate tissue handling by real-time penile oxygen monitoring. Int J Impot Res. 2012;24:11–9.
35. Schatloff O, Chauhan S, Sivaraman A, Kameh D, Palmer K, Patel VR. Anatomic grading of nerve sparing surgery during robot-assisted radical prostatectomy. Eur Urol. 2012;61:796–802.
36. Eichelberg C, Erbersdobler A, Haese A, et al. Frozen section for the management of intraoperatively detected palpable tumor lesions during nerve-sparing scheduled radical prostatectomy. Eur Urol. 2006;49:1011–6. discussion 1016–1018
37. Kakiuchi Y, Choy B, Gordetsky J, et al. Role of frozen section analysis of surgical margins during robot-assisted laparoscopic radical prostatectomy: a 2608-case experience. Hum Pathol. 2013;44:1556–62.
38. Lepor H, Kaci L. Role of intraoperative biopsies during radical retropubic prostatectomy. Urology. 2004;63:499–502.
39. Dinneen E, Haider A, Allen C, et al. NeuroSAFE robot-assisted laparoscopic prostatectomy versus standard robot-assisted laparoscopic prostatectomy for men with localised prostate cancer (NeuroSAFE PROOF): protocol for a randomised controlled feasibility study. BMJ Open. 2019;9:e028132.
40. Reeves F, Preece P, Kapoor J, et al. Preservation of the neurovascular bundles is associated with improved time to continence after radical prostatectomy but not long-term continence rates: results of a systematic review and meta-analysis. Eur Urol. 2015;68:692–704.
41. Hollabaugh J, Robert S, Dmochowski RR, Steiner MS. Neuroanatomy of the male rhabdosphincter. Urology. 1997;491997:426–34.
42. Akita K, Sakamoto H, Sato T. Origins and courses of the nervous branches to the male urethral sphincter. Surg Radiol Anat. 2003;25:387–92.
43. Karam I, Droupy S, Abd-Alsamad I, et al. The precise location and nature of the nerves to the male human urethra: histological and immunohistochemical studies with three-dimensional reconstruction. Eur Urol. 2005;48:858–64.
44. Reeves F, Everaerts W, Murphy DG, et al. Stimulation of the neurovascular bundle results in rhabdosphincter contraction in a proportion of men undergoing radical prostatectomy. Urology. 2016;87:133–9.
45. O'Donnell PD, Finan BF. Continence following nerve-sparing radical prostatectomy. J Urol. 1989;142:1227–8.

Techniques and Potency Outcomes for Nerve-Sparing RARP

Marcio Covas Moschovas, Mani Menon, Jonathan Noël, and Vipul Patel

1 Introduction

The first report of radical prostatectomy (RP) to treat prostate cancer (PCa) was initially described by Young et al. at the beginning of the 1900s [1]. Since then, multiple authors had described similar techniques with poor functional outcomes due to the limited knowledge of the prostate anatomy until the beginning of the 1980s, when Walsh and Donker described the first report of RP with the nerve-sparing technique. The authors illustrated the technical and anatomic aspects of this surgery and established the anatomic basis of erectile function preservation. The surgical technique innovation was a landmark study for patients and surgeons due to the significant improvement in the potency outcomes following RP [2].

In this scenario, open retropubic RP with nerve-sparing (NS) technique became the gold-standard surgical treatment for localized prostate cancer for years. However, with recent technological advancements and the advent of laparoscopy and robotic surgery, in the United States, robotic-assisted radical prostatectomy (RARP) is the current standard approach [3, 4]. The long-term outcomes of open and robotic RP are similar with experienced surgeons; however, the robotic approach is associated with less blood loss and shorter hospital stay than the open procedure [5].

In 2000, Binder and Kramer described the first robotic-assisted radical prostatectomy (RARP) performed in 10 patients with prostate cancer. The authors used an NS technique combining the Walsh retrograde approach with Campbell's anterograde procedure [6]. Since then, several groups have reported different techniques and outcomes of this surgery. This chapter will describe these NS techniques and anatomical considerations to optimize potency in patients undergoing RARP.

2 Anatomical Considerations of NS-RARP

Some preoperative factors, such as potency (evaluated with SHIM score), comorbidities, and habits, play an essential role in the potency recovery following RP [7, 8]. In addition, different studies of prostate neuroanatomy and physiology performed since the 1980s improved the understanding of the poor outcomes described in the previous RP series. Currently, it is established that potency following RARP is also related to multiple intraoperative factors, and NS technique refinements, with NVB preservation, are crucial to optimize postoperative outcomes [9].

Different neuroanatomical studies of the male pelvis have described that preserving the corpora cavernosa neurovascular supply is an essential factor for erection recovery following RP. These authors have described that maintaining the arterial supply of the pudendal artery and its variants, such as an accessory pudendal artery, optimizes postoperative potency [10]. In addition, sparing the cavernous nerves while dissecting the tip of the seminal vesicles with the athermal technique is also related to better outcomes [11].

Another important factor for potency recovery regards the application of mechanical or thermal energy on the neural bundles during the surgery. Three classifications for peripheral nerve injury have been described according to the damage severity. Neuropraxia is a mild compression usually performed during tissue manipulation and low energy application, which recovers from hours to weeks. Axonotmesis is a moderate to severe injury with up to 24 months of recovery. Neurotmesis is described as a complete nerve transection with no capacity for regeneration [12]. Understanding the neural lesion mechanisms and the outcomes of neural

M. C. Moschovas (✉) · V. Patel
AdventHealth Global Robotics Institute, Celebration, FL, USA

University of Central Florida, (UCF), Orlando, USA

M. Menon
Henry Ford West Bloomfield Hospital, West Bloomfield Township, MI, USA

J. Noël
AdventHealth Global Robotics Institute, Celebration, FL, USA

P. Wiklund et al. (eds.), *Robotic Urologic Surgery*, https://doi.org/10.1007/978-3-031-00363-9_15

damage is essential for the prognosis of potency recovery and patient counseling. Some authors have described the Neuropraxia impacts in the erection outcomes by evaluating patients who had intraoperative NVB counter traction performed by the tableside assistant. According to the study, these patients had worse early potency rates than patients without NVB traction [13]. Other articles also have described the negative impacts and outcomes of electrocautery and thermal injury on cavernous nerves [14].

3 Degrees of Nerve Sparing

Following the pioneer studies of prostate neuroanatomy, some groups have described different types of NVB dissection and preservation, associating anatomic landmarks with tumor characteristics, allowing optimal functional outcomes with a safe oncological dissection. These techniques described degrees of nerve-sparing based on prostatic vasculature landmarks associated with the tumor extension to the NVB.

In this scenario, Tewari et al., in a series of 2317 patients who underwent RARP, divided the grades of NS into four categories, Grade 1 being the best intrafascial preservation and Grade 4 an extrafascial dissection with no preservation [15]. Schatloff et al. upgraded this classification in a series of patients who underwent NS-RARP, reporting five grades of NS based on visual cues using the prostatic artery as a landmark (LA) to delineate the course of NVB. The grades of NS are performed according to the medial or lateral dissection of this LA. Grade 1 indicates no nerve preservation, while Grade 5 indicates ≥95% of preservation [9, 16]. In this study, the author reported 100% of potency rates in patients who were potent before surgery and underwent Grade 5 nerve preservation.

3.1 Intrafascial Dissection

The intrafascial plane is located between the capsule and prostatic fascia at the anterolateral and posterolateral aspects of the prostate. In this plane, the NVB has the optimal preservation with the best outcomes for potency. Potdevin et al. compared interfascial and intrafascial athermal dissection (AIR) in two groups of patients who underwent NS-RARP. According to this study, patients who underwent intrafascial athermal dissection had faster continence recovery. The potency rates at 3, 6, and 9 months in the interfascial group were 16.7%, 43.8%, and 66.7%, respectively, while in the AIR group were 24.2%, 81.8%, and 90.9%. However, these patients have the highest chances of positive surgical margins (when performed in the pT3 disease) compared to the interfascial dissection [17].

3.2 Interfascial Dissection

The interfascial plane is located between the prostatic fascia and the lateral pelvic fascia, allowing partial NS with safe surgical margin rates. In this plane, the lateral prostatic fascia (LPF) is not preserved, and the degree of NVB preservation is inferior compared to the intrafascial approach [18]. Weng and colleagues reported a systematic review and meta-analysis involving 1663 patients (916 intrafascial and 747 interfascial). The author reported advantages for the intrafascial approach in terms of continence (at 6 and 36 months), potency (at 6 and 12 months), positive surgical margins, and biochemical recurrence [19].

3.3 Extrafascial Dissection

The extrafascial plane is located at the external aspect of the lateral prostatic fascia, and its dissection involves complete NVB resection. This is the safest dissection in terms of oncologic outcomes; however, it leads to worse potency recovery [18]. Sergey et al. compared extrafascial with interfascial nerve-sparing in 813 patients who underwent radical prostatectomy (110 extrafascial vs. 703 interfascial). The author described better potency rates for the interfascial group, and the overall positive surgical margins were not statistically significant [20].

4 Techniques for Neurovascular Bundle Preservation

The technique used for neurovascular bundle preservation is one of the crucial aspects of RARP. The different NS approaches described in the literature are derived from the anterograde or retrograde NVB release. Despite the different methods, all techniques have the same basic concept of minimizing neuropraxia and neural damage by avoiding cautery use and traction during the NVB dissection. Some studies described that NVB preservation also improves outcomes for continence [21].

4.1 Anterograde NVB Dissection

After lifting the prostate by the seminal vesicles, the anterograde dissection is performed from the base to apex by accessing the NVB in the space between Denonvilliers fascia, lateral pelvic fascia, and prostate. Then, the prostatic pedicles are controlled with athermal technique and Hem-o-lock clips. Afterward, intra-, inter-, or extrafascial dissection is performed according to the surgeon's preference [4].

4.2 Retrograde NVB Dissection

After dissecting the seminal vesicles and accessing the posterior plane, the levator ani fascia is transected over the prostate to identify the NVB. Then, the plane created (from the apex to the base) is connected with the posterior dissection at the prostate base, performed between the Denonvilliers layers.

Ko YH and colleagues described this technique and compared it to the anterograde approach. In this study, the author described two groups of 172 patients who underwent RARP and concluded that, in patients with optimal preoperative potency, retrograde NS dissection leads to early potency recovery at 3,6, and 9 months compared to the anterograde (80.8%, 90.1%, and 92.9% vs. 65%, 72.1%, and 85.3%, respectively) [22].

Covas Moschovas et al. described a modified retrograde technique with lateral prostatic fascia preservation and minimal apical dissection. In this study, the author reported earlier recovery of continence (46 vs. 70 days) and potency (74 vs. 118 days) for patients who underwent the modified technique compared to the previous retrograde approach [23]. Recently, the same group described their retrograde technique using de da Vinci SP robot. The authors described the step-by-step technique and the modifications necessary to approach NS-RARP with this single-port robot [24–26]. Other authors also reported modified approaches to retrograde dissection, with endopelvic fascia preservation and optimal outcomes [27].

4.3 Veil of Aphrodite

Also known as high anterior release of the prostate, this technique was defined by Menon et al. in 2006 and consisted in developing a plane between the prostatic capsule and prostatic fascia at the seminal vesicle base followed by a bilateral posterior dissection from 1 to 5 o'clock and 6 to 11 o'clock positions [28, 29]. At the end of this dissection, the periprostatic tissue (Veil of Aphrodite) is suspended bilaterally, resembling a curtain from the pubourethral ligament.

Three years later, Menon and colleagues described the Super Veil technique based on technical modifications of the previous approach by expanding the dissection more anteriorly [30]. Ghani and colleagues described the technique outcomes in 85 patients who underwent RARP. The author reported 95% of potency rates in 18 months of follow-up [31].

4.4 Other Techniques

Different authors have described less commonly used techniques to approach NS-RARP, such as hypothermic NS robot-assisted laparoscopic prostatectomy (hRLP) [32], modified clipless antegrade [33], flexible carbon dioxide (CO_2) laser fiber guided [34], potassium titanyl phosphate laser, laparoscopic Doppler ultrasound (LDU) probe in, and transrectal ultrasound (TRUS) guided NSRP [3]. Most of these studies are based on retrospective series with short-term follow-up.

5 Technology Applications to Optimize NS Surgery

5.1 Indocyanine Green (ICG)

The role of indocyanine green application aims the prostatic artery identification during the NS by infusing intracavernous ICG to visualize the contrasted artery with the firefly robotic view. After identifying the landmark artery, the dissection proceeds according to the surgeon's preference, as described earlier in this chapter [35].

5.2 Biological Membranes (BM) for NVB Recovery

The rationale for using BM to accelerate neurovascular recovery is based on previous studies evaluating the healing benefits of these allograft tissues for wound management due to their anti-inflammatory properties [36]. In this scenario, Patel et al. reported the application of dehydrated human amnion/chorion membrane (dHACM) in patients who underwent RARP. The author compared two groups of 58 patients; one group had the NVB covered by the tissue after the prostate removal while the other group had no membrane. In this study, patients with dHACM had better rates of early potency recovery (1.34 months vs. 3.39 months). Afterward, the same group performed another study using dHACM in 235 patients. The author also reported better potency rates at 1, 3, 6, and 9 months for the allograft group [37].

Porpiglia et al. described a similar study using Chitosan (polysaccharide from shellfish exoskeleton) in patients who underwent RARP. Patients with allograft tissue had early potency at 1 and 2 months compared to the control group [38].

5.3 Magnetic Resonance Imaging (MRI) for NS Preservation

The MRI role in the preoperative staging of prostate cancer is already established in the literature. In this scenario, Schiavina et al. described the use of multiparametric MRI to guide NS during RARP comparing two groups of patients who underwent RARP and reported statistically significant lower rates of PSM for patients who underwent preoperative MRI (12.4% vs. 24.1%) [39].

5.4 NeuroSAFE Approach

Initially described by Scholmm et al., this technique is used to evaluate the prostate specimen, soon after the removal for identifying positive margins on the NVB [40]. During this evaluation, the surgery proceeds with lymphadenectomy, hemostasis, and anastomosis. If the microscopic evaluation detects a positive margin, the surgeon expands the NVB dissection on that side. This study was conducted by Scholmm and colleagues evaluating 5392 RARP. The author described lower PSM rates in patients who underwent the NeuroSAFE technique.

5.5 Augmented Reality (AR)

Porpiglia et al. proposed the use of augmented reality in a study with 30 patients who underwent RARP. Although the author described safe and feasible preliminary results, some technological limitations still restrict the application of AR in radical prostatectomies [41].

6 Comparing Different Techniques

In the current literature, no RCTs compared the outcomes of NS techniques in patients who underwent robotic-assisted radical prostatectomy, and there is no consensus on the optimal technique for NVB preservation. Most studies are based on single-surgeon retrospective data with all its inherent risk of bias [42]. The lack of standardized methods for reporting potency outcomes [43] and penile rehabilitation protocols, associated with different preoperative characteristics between the cohorts of the studies, are the main challenges to establishing accurate data on potency recovery between the series of RARP.

In summary, potency outcomes following RP depend on different factors [44]. The literature reporting outcomes for NS-RARP is based mainly on retrospective studies of surgeons with distinct techniques, reporting patients with divergent preoperative demography, describing multiple classifications for potency and penile rehabilitation protocols.

7 Conclusion

Potency outcomes following radical prostatectomy still remain a challenge for patients and surgeons due to its multifactorial etiology. Different techniques to optimize potency recovery have been described in the literature, and pelvic neuroanatomy understanding played a fundamental role in enhancing cavernosal nerve preservation. The literature still lacks well-designed studies comparing the benefits of one technique over the others. However, basic concepts for nerve-sparing are common to all RP techniques, such as minimizing the amount of traction used on dissection, avoiding excessive cautery (energy) during hemostasis, and neural preservation based on anatomical landmarks (arteries and planes of dissection).

References

1. Young HH. Conservative perineal prostatectomy: the results of two years' experience and report of seventy-five cases. Ann Surg. 1905;41(4):549–54957.
2. Walsh PC, Donker PJ. Impotence following radical prostatectomy: insight into etiology and prevention. J Urol. 1982;128:492–7.
3. Kumar A, Patel VR, Panaiyadiyan S, Seetharam Bhat KR, Moschovas MC, Nayak B. Nerve-sparing robot-assisted radical prostatectomy: current perspectives. Asian J Urol. 2021;8(1):2–13. https://doi.org/10.1016/j.ajur.2020.05.012.
4. Martini A, Falagario UG, Villers A, Dell'Oglio P, Mazzone E, Autorino R, Moschovas MC, Buscarini M, Bravi CA, Briganti A, Sawczyn G, Kaouk J, Menon M, Secco S, Bocciardi AM, Wang G, Zhou X, Porpiglia F, Mottrie A, Patel V, Tewari AK, Montorsi F, Gaston R, Wiklund NP, Hemal AK. Contemporary techniques of prostate dissection for robot-assisted prostatectomy. Eur Urol. 2020;78(4):583–91. https://doi.org/10.1016/j.eururo.2020.07.017.
5. Yaxley JW, Coughlin GD, Chambers SK, et al. Robot-assisted laparoscopic prostatectomy versus open radical retropubic prostatectomy: early outcomes from a randomised controlled phase 3 study. Lancet. 2016;388(10049):1057–66.
6. Binder J, Kramer W. Robotically-assisted laparoscopic radical prostatectomy. BJU Int. 2001;87(4):408–10. https://doi.org/10.1046/j.1464-410x.2001.00115.x.
7. Teloken PE, Nelson CJ, Karellas M, Stasi J, Eastham J, Scardino PT, et al. Defining the impact of vascular risk factors on erectile function recovery after radical prostatectomy. BJU Int. 2013;111:653–7.
8. Seetharam Bhat KR, Moschovas MC, Onol FF, Sandri M, Rogers T, Roof S, Rocco B, Patel VR. Trends in clinical and oncological outcomes of robot-assisted radical prostatectomy before and after the 2012 US Preventive Services Task Force recommendation against PSA screening: a decade of experience. BJU Int. 2020 Jun;125(6):884–92. https://doi.org/10.1111/bju.15051.
9. Schatloff O, Chauhan S, Sivaraman A, Kameh D, Palmer KJ, Patel VR. Anatomic grading of nerve sparing during robot-assisted radical prostatectomy. Eur Urol. 2012;61(4):796–802. https://doi.org/10.1016/j.eururo.2011.12.048.

10. Castiglione F, Ralph DJ, Muneer A. Surgical techniques for managing post-prostatectomy erectile dysfunction. Curr Urol Rep. 2017;18(11):90. https://doi.org/10.1007/s11934-017-0735-2.
11. Walz J, Epstein JI, Ganzer R, et al. A critical analysis of the current knowledge of surgical anatomy of the prostate related to optimisation of cancer control and preservation of continence and erection in candidates for radical prostatectomy: an update. Eur Urol. 2016;70:301–11.
12. Chhabra A, Ahlawat S, Belzberg A, Andreseik G. Peripheral nerve injury grading simplified on MR neurography: as referenced to Seddon and Sunderland classifications. Indian J Radiol Imaging. 2014;24(3):217–24. https://doi.org/10.4103/0971-3026.137025.
13. Kowalczyk KJ, Huang AC, Hevelone ND, et al. Step- wise approach for nerve sparing without counter- traction during robot-assisted radical prostatectomy: technique and outcomes. Eur Urol. 2011;60(3):536–47.
14. Ong AM, Su LM, Varkarakis I, Inagaki T, Link RE, Bhayani SB, Patriciu A, Crain B, Walsh PC. Nerve sparing radical prostatectomy: effects of hemostatic energy sources on the recovery of cavernous nerve function in a canine model. J Urol. 2004;172(4 Pt 1):1318–22. https://doi.org/10.1097/01.ju.0000139883.08934.86.
15. Tewari AK, Srivastava A, Huang MW, Robinson BD, Shevchuk MM, Durand M, Sooriakumaran P, Grover S, Yadav R, Mishra N, Mohan S, Brooks DC, Shaikh N, Khanna A, Leung R. Anatomical grades of nerve sparing: a risk-stratified approach to neural-hammock sparing during robot-assisted radical prostatectomy (RARP). BJU Int. 2011;108(6 Pt 2):984–92. https://doi.org/10.1111/j.1464-410X.2011.10565.x.
16. Patel VR, Schatloff O, Chauhan S, et al. The role of the prostatic vasculature as a landmark for nerve sparing during robot-assisted radical prostatec- tomy. Eur Urol. 2012;61(3):571–6.
17. Potdevin L, Ercolani M, Jeong J, et al. Functional and oncologic outcomes comparing interfascial and intrafascial nerve sparing in robot-assisted laparoscopic radical prostatectomies. J Endourol. 2009;23(9):1479–84.
18. Walz J, Burnett AL, Costello AJ, Eastham JA, Graefen M, Guillonneau B, et al. A critical analysis of the current knowledge of surgical anatomy related to optimization of cancer control and preservation of continence and erection in candidates for radical prostatectomy. Eur Urol. 2010;57:179e92.
19. Weng H, Zeng XT, Li S, et al. Intrafascial versus in- terfascial nerve sparing in radical prostatectomy for localized prostate cancer: a systematic review and meta-analysis. Sci Rep. 2017;7(1):1–11.
20. Shikanov S, Woo J, Al-Ahmadie H, Katz MH, Zagaja GP, Shalhav AL, Zorn KC. Extrafascial versus interfascial nerve-sparing technique for robotic-assisted laparoscopic prostatectomy: comparison of functional outcomes and positive surgical margins characteristics. Urology. 2009;74(3):611–6. https://doi.org/10.1016/j.urology.2009.01.092.
21. Murphy DG, Costello AJ. How can the autonomic nervous system contribute to urinary continence following radical prostatectomy? A "boson-like" conundrum. Eur Urol. 2013;63(3):445–7.
22. Ko YH, Coelho RF, Sivaraman A, Schatloff O, Chauhan S, Abdul-Muhsin HM, Carrion RJ, Palmer KJ, Cheon J, Patel VR. Retrograde versus antegrade nerve sparing during robot-assisted radical prostatectomy: which is better for achieving early functional recovery? Eur Urol. 2013 Jan;63(1):169–77. https://doi.org/10.1016/j.eururo.2012.09.051.
23. Covas Moschovas M, Bhat S, Onol FF, Rogers T, Roof S, Mazzone E, Mottrie A, Patel V. Modified apical dissection and lateral prostatic fascia preservation improves early postoperative functional recovery in robotic-assisted laparoscopic radical prostatectomy: results from a propensity score-matched analysis. Eur Urol. 2020 Dec;78(6):875–84. https://doi.org/10.1016/j.eururo.2020.05.041.
24. Moschovas MC, Bhat S, Sandri M, Rogers T, Onol F, Mazzone E, Roof S, Mottrie A, Patel V. Comparing the approach to radical prostatectomy using the multiport da Vinci Xi and da Vinci SP robots: a propensity score analysis of perioperative out-comes. Eur Urol. 2021 Mar;79(3):393–404. https://doi.org/10.1016/j.eururo.2020.11.042.
25. Covas Moschovas M, Bhat S, Onol F, Rogers T, Patel V. Early outcomes of single port robotic radical prostatectomy. Lessons learned from the learning curve experience. BJU Int. 2021;127(1):114–21. https://doi.org/10.1111/bju.15158.
26. Covas Moschovas M, Bhat S, Rogers T, Onol F, Roof S, Mazzone E, Mottrie A, Patel V. Technical modifications necessary to implement the da Vinci single-port robotic system. Eur Urol. 2020 Sep;78(3):415–23. https://doi.org/10.1016/j.eururo.2020.01.005.
27. de Carvalho PA, Barbosa JABA, Guglielmetti GB, Cordeiro MD, Rocco B, Nahas WC, Patel V, Coelho RF. Retrograde release of the neurovascular bundle with preservation of dorsal venous complex during robot-assisted radical prostatectomy: optimizing functional outcomes. Eur Urol. 2020 May;77(5):628–35. https://doi.org/10.1016/j.eururo.2018.07.003.
28. Menon M, Shrivastava A, Kaul S, et al. Vattikuti Institute prostatectomy: contemporary technique and analysis of results. Eur Urol. 2007;51(3):648–58.
29. Kaul S, Savera A, Badani K, Fumo M, Bhandari A, Menon M. Functional outcomes and oncological efficacy of Vattikuti Institute prostatectomy with Veil of Aphrodite nerve- sparing: an analysis of 154 consecutive patients. BJU Int. 2006;97:467e72.
30. Menon M, Shrivastava A, Bhandari M, Satyanarayana R, Siva S, Agarwal PK. Vattikuti Institute prostatectomy: technical modifications in 2009. Eur Urol. 2009;56:89e96.
31. Ghani KR, Trinh QD, Menon M. Vattikuti Institute prostatectomy-technique in 2012. J Endourol. 2012;26(12):1558–65. https://doi.org/10.1089/end.2012.0455.
32. Finley DS, Osann K, Skarecky D, Ahlering TE. Hypothermic nerve-sparing radical prostatectomy: rationale, feasibility, and effect on early continence. Urology. 2009;73:691e6.
33. Chien GW, Mikhail AA, Orvieto MA, Zagaja GP, Sokoloff MH, Brendler CB, et al. Modified clipless antegrade nerve preser- vation in robotic-assisted laparoscopic radical prostatectomy with validated sexual function evaluation. Urology. 2005;66:419e23.
34. Cheetham PJ, Truesdale MD, Lee DJ, Landman JM, Badani KK. Use of a flexible carbon dioxide laser fiber for precise dissection of the neurovascular bundle during robot-assisted laparoscopic prostatectomy. J Endourol. 2010;24:1091e6.
35. Kumar A, Samavedi S, Bates A, Coelho R, Rocco B, Marquinez J, et al. Using indocyanine green and near-infrared fluorescence technology to identify the "landmark artery" during robot-assisted radical prostatectomy. Videourology. 2015;29 https://doi.org/10.1089/vid.2014.0071.vid.2014.0071.
36. Fetterolf DE, Snyder RJ. Scientific and clinical support for the use of dehydrated amniotic membrane in wound management. Wounds. 2012;24(10):299–307.
37. Ogaya-Pinies G, Palayapalam-Ganapathi H, Rogers T, Her-nandez-Cardona E, Rocco B, Coelho RF, et al. Can dehydrated human amnion/chorion membrane accelerate the return to potency after a nerve-sparing robotic-assisted radical pros- tatectomy? Propensity score-matched analysis. J Robot Surg. 2018;12:235e43.
38. Porpiglia F, Manfredi M, Checcucci E, Garrou D, De Cillis S, Amparore D, et al. Use of chitosan membranes after nerve- sparing radical prostatectomy improves early recovery of sexual potency: results of a comparative study. BJU Int. 2019;123:465e73.
39. Schiavina R, Bianchi L, Borghesi M, Dababneh H, Chessa F, Pultrone CV, et al. MRI displays the prostatic cancer anatomy and improves the bundles management before robot-assisted radical prostatectomy. J Endourol. 2018;32:315e21.
40. Schlomm T, Tennstedt P, Huxhold C, Steuber T, Salomon G, Michl U, et al. Neurovascular structure-adjacent frozen-sec- tion

examination (NeuroSAFE) increases nerve-sparing fre- quency and reduces positive surgical margins in open and robot-assisted laparoscopic radical prostatectomy: experi- ence after 11,069 consecutive patients. Eur Urol. 2012;62:333e40.

41. Porpiglia F, Fiori C, Checcucci E, Amparore D, Bertolo R. Augmented reality robot-assisted radical prostatectomy: preliminary experience. Urology. 2018;115:184. https://doi.org/10.1016/j.urology.2018.01.028.
42. Walz J, Epstein JI, Ganzer R, et al. A critical analysis of the current knowledge of surgical anatomy of the prostate related to optimisation of cancer control and preservation of continence and erection in candi- dates for radical prostatectomy: an update. Eur Urol. 2016;70:301–11.
43. Lourenço DB, Amaral BS, Alfer-Junior W, Vasconcellos A, Russo F, Sanchez-Salas R, Bianco B, Wagner AA, Chang P, Moschovas MC, Lemos GC, Carneiro A. Portuguese version of the Expanded Prostate Cancer Index Composite for Clinical Practice (EPIC-CP): psychometric validation and prospective application for early functional outcomes at a single institution. BMC Urol. 2020;20(1):163. https://doi.org/10.1186/s12894-020-00734-y.
44. Bhat KRS, Moschovas MC, Sandri M, Dell'Oglio P, Onol FF, Rogers T, Reddy S, Noel J, Roof S, Sighinolfi MC, Rocco B, Patel VR. A predictive pre- and post-operative nomogram for post-operative potency recovery after robot-assisted radical prostatectomy. J Urol. 2021;206(4):942–51. https://doi.org/10.1097/JU.0000000000001895.

Pneumoperitoneum Physiology

Hal D. Kominsky, Jeffrey A. Cadeddu,
Marcio Covas Moschovas, and Raymond J. Leveillee

1 Introduction

Laparoscopy was initially utilized as a diagnostic procedure and had very limited applications [1]. This technology was revolutionized with the introduction of laparoscopic cholecystectomy in 1990 followed by laparoscopic nephrectomy shortly thereafter [2, 3]. Modern urologic practice routinely incorporates laparoscopy, and more recently robotic surgery, in the treatment of both benign and oncologic disease. Thus, the importance of a surgeon's familiarity with the physiologic principles of pneumoperitoneum and its effects on the patient cannot be understated. This chapter describes the basic physiology of pneumoperitoneum and potential complications arising from its use.

2 Insufflation Agents

Early laparoscopic surgery employed room air or oxygen to establish pneumoperitoneum [4]. These gases proved to be clinically impractical due to the strong potential for venous embolism and intracorporeal combustion. The ideal insufflation gas should:

- Be relatively *inexpensive.*
- Is *noncombustible.*
- Perhaps most importantly, *rapidly dissolve in plasma* [5].

H. D. Kominsky · J. A. Cadeddu
Department of Urology, The University of Texas Southwestern Medical Center, Dallas, TX, USA

M. C. Moschovas
AdventHealth Global Robotics Institute, Celebration, FL, USA

R. J. Leveillee (✉)
Bethesda Center for Advanced Robotics and Urologic Care, Florida Atlantic University Schmidt College of Medicine, Boynton Beach, FL, USA

Options for various gases are discussed below with the following section of the chapter focusing primarily on carbon dioxide effects of pneumoperitoneum.

2.1 Carbon Dioxide

Carbon dioxide (CO_2) is the most commonly used gas at the disposal of the modern laparoscopic and robotic surgeon. It is rapidly absorbed in both blood and tissue. Due to a sharp diffusion gradient, CO_2 quickly evacuates the peritoneal cavity into the surrounding body compartments (fat, bone, visceral organs). While this feature makes CO_2 an excellent option for obtaining pneumoperitoneum, patients are at risk for developing hypercapnia, hypercarbia, and cardiac arrhythmias. The patient population in which these concerns are most relevant are those with chronic obstructive pulmonary disease (COPD). These individuals are particularly sensitive to the acute changes in blood concentrations of CO_2 and may have difficulty with compensatory ventilation required to expel excess gas. Additionally, CO_2 is a well-known stimulant of the sympathetic nervous system, which leads to increased cardiac contractility, heart rate, and systemic vascular resistance. A more robust discussion of these principles comes later in this chapter. Although CO_2 is rapidly absorbed in blood, it can remain in surrounding tissues for several hours or even days [6]. It is prudent that following long operations with CO_2, the surgeon has a low index of suspicion for patients showing signs and symptoms of hypercarbia.

2.2 Helium

Helium (He), an inert and noncombustible gas, emerged as an attractive alternative insufflant to CO_2, particularly in patients who would poorly tolerate hypercarbia. However, due to its lower blood solubility, the risk for air embolus is higher in He compared to that of CO_2. It has been suggested

P. Wiklund et al. (eds.), *Robotic Urologic Surgery*, https://doi.org/10.1007/978-3-031-00363-9_16

that if He is to be used for the procedure, the initial pneumoperitoneum should still be achieved with CO_2 to minimize the risk of air embolus. Similarly, if a patient develops refractory hypercarbia during a surgery utilizing CO_2, the surgical team can switch to He to continue the case [7].

2.3 Nitrous Oxide

Nitrous oxide (NO_2) was popularized as an insufflation agent during the 1970s and 1980s due to its low cost as well as minimal irritation to the peritoneum and lower rate of cardiac-related changes [8, 9]. Importantly, NO_2 is combustible, and reports exist of ***intraoperative explosions*** during laparoscopy, which has greatly limited modern use of this gas for pneumoperitoneum [10, 11]. It is imperative that the use of NO_2 insufflation be restricted to those procedures not utilizing electrocautery.

3 Insufflation Pressure Effects on Organ Systems

3.1 Cardiovascular Effects

The intra-abdominal pressure generated from pneumoperitoneum impacts cardiac function directly in the chest and indirectly with changes to venous return and systemic vascular resistance. Increased intra-abdominal pressure decreases venous return through the inferior vena cava (IVC) as a result of increased venous resistance [12]. This relationship assumes low or normal atrial pressure. In a patient with high atrial pressure, such as in the case of a hypervolemia, the IVC pressure resists the pneumoperitoneum force, and venous return is unaffected or increased [13]. At the same time, increasing peritoneal compartment forces in excess of 20 mmHg transmits pressure to the small capacitance vessels which in turn increase mean systemic pressure. In common practice, most cases are performed at a pressure of 10–12 mmHg, and rarely exceed 15 mmHg.

It has been suggested that pneumoperitoneum actually creates phasic hemodynamic changes observed as a 50% decrease in cardiac index within five minutes of initial insufflation. Then the cardiac index increases as the systemic vascular resistance drops after about 10 minutes [14]. Performing laparoscopy at 15 mmHg can lead to 30% reduction in cardiac output and stroke volume with corresponding 60% decrease in mean atrial pressure [15]. These cardiac changes can be mitigated with pneumoperitoneum at lower pressures [16]. This is relevant for patients with significant cardiac pathology who are particularly sensitive to the hemodynamic dysregulation caused by pneumoperitoneum. When patients have poor cardiac reserve, special attention must be paid to keep insufflation pressure low and balanced with volume status and blood pressure changes during the case [6, 17].

3.2 Renal Effects

Increased intra-abdominal pressure affects renal blood flow. This was empirically demonstrated in 1923 in a bovine model by Thorington and Schmidt, reporting that intra-abdominal pressures exceeding 15 mmHg and 30 mmHg produced oliguria and anuria, respectively [18]. Similarly, in a study of 17 healthy human subjects, Bradley and Bradley showed that an intra-abdominal pressure of 20 mmHg reduced renal blood flow and glomerular filtration rate [19]. Changes in renal function and urine output caused by pneumoperitoneum are most likely the result of multiple factors as demonstrated by several animal studies [20–23]. Diminished renal perfusion, parenchymal compression, and to a lesser extent, hormonal influences from antidiuretic hormone and vasopressin have all been implicated [20, 21, 23, 24]. Of note, decreased cardiac output and ureteral compression do not seem to contribute significantly [21].

Longer duration of laparoscopic cases has been associated with intraoperative oliguria [24, 25]. This phenomenon is reversed upon discontinuation of the pneumoperitoneum at the end of the surgery. Options for the intraoperative management of oliguria include furosemide, mannitol, and dopamine. Vigilant use of these pharmacological agents rather than volume expansion may prevent the patient from experiencing volume overload and edema when treating pneumoperitoneum-related oliguria [26].

3.3 Gastrointestinal Effects

Pneumoperitoneum may lead to diminished blood flow and perfusion of the gastrointestinal system. By measuring intramucosal pH as a surrogate for gastric and splanchnic perfusion, multiple studies have demonstrated the relationship between decreased blood flow to the stomach during prolonged periods of pneumoperitoneum [14, 27]. Caldwell and Ricotta reported on a canine model, wherein they observed decreased visceral blood flow (stomach, small and large intestine, spleen, liver, and kidney) out of proportion to diminished cardiac output as intra-abdominal pressures increased [28]. Although it was theorized that diminished splanchnic blood flow may be a risk factor for bacterial translocation from the peritoneum to the blood [29], this has not borne out in clinical practice.

3.4 Intracranial Pressure Effects

Both experimental and clinical studies have implicated pneumoperitoneum, particularly with CO_2, in the changes of intracranial pressure (ICP) associated with laparoscopic procedures [30–32]. There are multiple reports suggesting that increasing PCO_2 increases ICP [33, 34]. In addition, Schob and colleagues demonstrated a consistent phenomenon of increased ICP with pneumoperitoneum using alternative agents (He, NO_2), but to a lesser severity compared to CO_2 [35].

Multiple theories have been put forth to explain the positive correlation between increasing intra-abdominal pressure and increased ICP. One explanation utilizes the Monroe-Kellie doctrine, or the principle that changing the parameters of one intracranial compartment (parenchymal, cerebrospinal fluid (CSF), and osseous) forces compensatory changes in at least one of the other non-osseous compartments. When there is a rapid change in the pressure within one compartment, as in the case with quick onset of pneumoperitoneum at the beginning of a procedure, there is not enough time for compensatory measures, and the result is increased ICP. An alternative explanation of increased ICP from pneumoperitoneum was suggested by Este-McDonald et al., in which intra-abdominal pressure increase leads to higher intrathoracic pressure, which in turn leads to obstruction of venous outflow from the spinal cord [36]. Higher intravascular volume in the spinal cord transmits to the intracranial compartment and generates higher ICP. Another popular theory speculates that patients experience impaired CSF absorption during laparoscopic surgery, and this has some effect on increasing ICP. This concept was demonstrated in a pig model that showed a 55% reduction in CSF reabsorption after 4 hours of pneumoperitoneum at 15 mmHg [37].

There is a two-phase model proposed by Rosenthal and colleagues [32, 38] that divides the mechanism of ICP increase into an (1) early, passive, venous phase and (2) late, active, arterial phase. The early, passive, venous stage comes about from compression of the IVC, which lowers the CVP. Lower CVP impairs venous drainage from lumbar plexus, which causes a corresponding increase in ICP. In the late arterial stage, hypercarbia brings about vasodilation of the intracranial vessels, and subsequently a rise in ICP. Additionally, the acute elevation in ICP produces a Cushing reflex that releases catecholamines and vasopressin. This leads to increased MAP and SVR while simultaneously decreasing blood flow to the splanchnic circulation. The milieu of hemodynamic alterations leads to a rise in ICP.

The true clinical implications of increased ICP during laparoscopic procedures are not fully understood. To date, there are no reports of patients experiencing any adverse neurological sequelae specifically attributed to intra-abdominal pressure increases from laparoscopic or robotic surgery. In the specific situation of performing laparoscopy on a patient with prior head trauma or with an intracranial lesion, minimizing changes to ICP is prudent. Considerations for these patients include minimal time in the head-down position, low insufflation pressure, and possibly the use of gasless laparoscopy. The use of continuous ICP monitoring during procedures is an option, although not commonly employed in everyday practice.

3.5 Respiratory Effects

The increased intra-abdominal pressure of pneumoperitoneum weakens diaphragmatic excursion, which decreases functional residual capacity and can increase pulmonary dead space. Correspondingly, the peak airway pressure must be increased to maintain constant tidal volume [6]. Motew demonstrated that the average peak airway pressure needed to maintain the same tidal volume increased by 45% when intra-abdominal pressure was increased from 0 mmHg to 20 mmHg [39]. For patients with pulmonary disease, controlling ventilation and use of positive expiratory pressure (PEEP) can counteract the increased dead space and protentional alveolar-perfusion mismatch, which would otherwise result in hypoxemia [40]. However, these tools have not been shown to have clinical significance in patients without lung disease [41].

Additional respiratory parameters altered by pneumoperitoneum include increased chest wall mechanical resistance and decreased pulmonary compliance.

When comparing patients who underwent laparoscopic and open surgery, multiple reports found that after surgery, the laparoscopy patients had better forced expiratory volume in one second (FEV_1), forced vital capacity, peak expiratory flow, and higher blood oxygen saturation compared to match open subjects [42, 43]. The exact reasoning for these observations is not clear.

4 Physiology of Carbon Dioxide Absorption

4.1 Acid–Base Effects of CO_2 Absorption

The absorption of CO_2 from pneumoperitoneum has independent effects on the cardiac and pulmonary systems.

The body has the natural ability to eliminate CO_2 efficiently and effectively using a buffering system. This is done when CO_2 combines with water in red blood cells to form carbonic acid. The carbonic acid quickly dissociates into hydrogen and bicarbonate. The bicarbonate rapidly diffuses into plasma. The hydrogen ion complexes with hemoglobin. This system prevents significant alternations in plasma pH. CO_2 that does not undergo this conversion (about 10% of total blood concentration) is transported to the lungs where it is eliminated through respiration. When CO_2 concentration is increased, as is the case with pneumoperitoneum, pulmonary circulation increases, as the body attempts to evacuate the excess CO_2.

Diffusion of a gas within the body occurs from areas of higher concentration to lower concentration. Multiple factors can influence rates of diffusion, including pressures across different body compartments, gas solubility, distance the gas must travel, gas molecular weight, and body temperature. The diffusion coefficient is an index value for a specific gas that compares the solubility of the gas to the standard diffusion of oxygen. Diffusion coefficients for common gases include O_2 1.00, CO_2 20.30, CO 0.81, N 0.53, and He 0.95. A high diffusion coefficient means that the gas is more rapidly absorbed. This is why CO_2, with a markedly higher diffusion coefficient compared to other gases, makes an excellent choice for pneumoperitoneum during laparoscopy.

In a study comparing blood gas concentrations before and after laparoscopy at 20 mmHg of CO_2 pneumoperitoneum, it was reported that the average P CO_2 increased by 8.6 mmHg and the arterial pH decreased by 0.082 units [44]. When patients underwent laparoscopy at 15–20 mmHg, Montalva and Das noted the development of hypercarbia when minute ventilation was unchanged [45]. Interestingly, when patients were allowed to ventilate spontaneously, they saw a decrease in the CO_2 concentration in the blood. These results demonstrate the body's natural drive to eliminate CO_2 which can be suppressed during controlled ventilation.

Tan and colleagues attempted to quantify the absorption of CO_2 during laparoscopy. By measuring CO_2 elimination, they were able to calculate the average CO_2 absorption of twelve subjects at 15 minutes and 30 minutes after insufflation. They reported that the CO_2 absorption from the peritoneal cavity was 42 mL/min and 39 mL/min, respectively. These results suggest that the absorption of CO_2 actually reaches a steady state. Another study by Mullet et al. demonstrated a plateau in CO_2 absorption at 15–20 minutes in patients undergoing laparoscopy for cholecystectomy and gynecological procedures [46].

4.2 Hemodynamic and Pulmonary Influences of CO_2 Absorption

The hypercarbia from CO_2 absorption produced several hemodynamic changes. The lower blood pH of hypercarbia can cause local myocardial depression and in turn decrease cardiac contractility and heart rate [47]. Low pH in the blood can also have a vasodilatory effect. Conversely, CO_2 is a known stimulant to the sympathetic nervous system; an increased CO_2 concentration can directly increase cardiac contractility and peripheral vascular resistance. Overall, hypercarbia actually creates a state of increased cardiac output, increased heart rate, and mean arterial pressure. Peripherally, the local vasodilation overcomes the sympathomimetic vasoconstriction which results in decreased peripheral vascular resistance [48].

Carbon dioxide diffuses into body tissue until it is eventually eliminated from the lungs [49]. Bone is typically thought to be the largest storage reservoir for CO_2 retention, but muscle can also host a high concentration of the gas because of its high rate of perfusion [50]. Naturally occurring, short-term CO_2 increases are buffered in alveolar and visceral tissue. In the case of a rapid increase of high CO_2 concentration from pneumoperitoneum, the body has an increase in PCO_2 that drives ventilatory changes. Carbon dioxide continues to undergo elimination following laparoscopy as well.

Wallace et al. compared the hemodynamic and pulmonary effects of high- and low-pressure CO_2 pneumoperitoneum. Forty patients undergoing laparoscopic cholecystectomy were randomized to low-pressure insufflation (7.5 mmHg) or high-pressure insufflation (15 mmHg). No differences were observed in terms of PCO_2, end tidal CO_2, peak airway pressure, heart rate, cardiac index, stroke index, or MAP [51]. Slightly different results were reported by Dexter and colleagues, who showed laparoscopy at higher pressure produced a decrease in stroke volume. Cardiac output was favored in the lower pressure laparoscopy group [16].

5 Pneumoperitoneum Effects with Patient Positioning

There are multiple animal and human studies describing the relationship of positioning with pneumoperitoneum [52–54]. Williams and Murr evaluated hemodynamic changes of dogs undergoing pneumoperitoneum, placed at different positions. Cardiac output with the dogs in the horizontal position went from 79% at 15 mmHg to 77% at 30 mmHg. When the dogs were put in the head-down position, cardiac output went to 86% and 82% at 15 mmHg and 30 mm, respectively. In the head-up position, the reductions in cardiac output were 70% and 67% of baseline at the corresponding insufflation pressures, respectively.

Joris et al. observed hemodynamic changes in 15 patients undergoing laparoscopic cholecystectomy at different positions [53]. After induction of anesthesia, while in supine position, patient MAP dropped by 9% and cardiac index fell by 25%. With the patient in head-up position, the investigators found further decreases in MAP and cardiac index by 17% and 14%, respectively. Upon insufflation, the patients experienced a MAP increase of 37% and cardiac index decrease of 18%. Those authors speculated that the reduced cardiac index was a function of increased afterload and decreased venous return. The afterload increase was thought to be a result of both increased abdominal pressure from the pneumoperitoneum and sympathomimetic response from elevated CO_2 concentration in the blood. Similarly, Kelman and colleagues studied how patient positioning affects hemodynamics during pelvic laparoscopy. The baseline cardiac output was higher with the patient's head down compared to the supine position (4.8 L/min vs 3.9 L/min). Once the abdomen was insufflated with 10–20 cmH_2O, cardiac output increased to 5.3 L/min with the head up. Once insufflation pressures reached 30–40 cmH_2O, cardiac output decreased. The authors felt that the central venous pressure increase from the head-down position translated to increased cardiac output but could not be overcome at higher intra-abdominal pressures.

To summarize, patients in the supine position have relatively little change to their cardiac output. When the abdomen is insufflated at a relatively low pressure of pneumoperitoneum (below 15 mmHg), there is minimal change to the cardiac output. Once higher pneumoperitoneum pressures are generated (>20 mmHg), one can expect to observe decreased cardiac output as the patient's venous return is reduced. When the patient is placed in head-down position, cardiac output can be improved, but is still influenced to some degree by intra-abdominal pressure, especially when that pressure is high.

6 Hormone and Immunologic Considerations of Pneumoperitoneum

Abdominal insufflation may contribute to the hormonal and immunologic environment of patients undergoing laparoscopic surgery.

Interleukin-6 (IL-6) is an acute phase reactant, considered to be an early maker of tissue damage and trauma. In the context of comparing laparoscopic and open surgery, blood concentrations of IL-6 appear to be decreased in patients undergoing laparoscopic procedures [55–58]. A similar relationship has been demonstrated for C-reactive protein (CRP) [59, 60], while other studies have found CRP to actually be increased following laparoscopy [61–63].

Chekan et al. measured bacterial clearance rate in mice undergoing laparotomy as well as laparoscopy with pneumoperitoneum using either CO_2 or He. Interestingly, CO_2 pneumoperitoneum displayed the lowest bacterial clearance rate compared to open surgery or pneumoperitoneum using He [64].

Likewise, West and colleagues showed that cells incubated in CO_2 display lower IL-1 and tumor necrosis factor (TNF) levels as well as lower rates of bacterial clearance compared to cells incubated in air or He [65]. They proposed that CO_2 absorption leads to higher levels of intracellular acidification, which in turn impairs macrophage cytokine production.

Sietses randomized patients undergoing laparoscopic cholecystectomy to abdominal insufflation with CO_2, He, or abdominal wall lifting without gas insufflation. The systemic immune response was evaluated, and the investigators reported higher CPR levels in the He and gasless groups compared to the CO_2 group [66].

Neuroendocrine markers have also been evaluated to compare the effects of stress from laparoscopic and open surgery. Laparoscopic surgery, when compared to open surgery, leads to lower production of cortisol, epinephrine, and norepinephrine in the postoperative period [67, 68].

7 Pneumoperitoneum Complications

Complications can occur either from establishing pneumoperitoneum or its maintenance during a procedure.

Superficial placement of a Veress needle or a trocar can lead to subcutaneous emphysema. This results when CO_2 leaks directly into the subcutaneous or preperitoneal tissue. This is generally a benign, self-limiting complication; however, numerous reports of subcutaneous emphysema leading to hypercarbia exist [69–71]. Because the gas is not contained within the abdominal cavity, it can traverse tissue planes and diffuse into the extrapleural space, mediastinum, or even pericardium. There are descriptions of subcutaneous emphysema causing pneumothorax [72, 73] and pneumopericardium [74, 75]. Small pneumothoraces are generally managed with observation and supportive care, while larger pneumothoraces require decompression and thoracostomy insertion.

Perhaps, the most feared and morbid complication of pneumoperitoneum is a gas embolism. This can result from inadvertent placement of the Veress needle in a vein or into the liver/spleen, wherein gas will infuse directly into the venous circulation. A gas bubble can travel into the right atrium, and from there it can enter the pulmonary circulation. If the bubble sits in the atrium, it can obstruct venous return to the heart, and cardiac output will be compromised. And if the bubble obstructs pulmonary artery flow, pulmonary hypertension and right heart failure can occur. Gas embolism can be identified clinically by observation of a sudden state of hypoxia, hypercarbia, arrhythmia, or hypotension upon insufflation. The patient will also become cyanotic. Capnography and transesophageal echocardiography (TEE) have both been studied as tools to detect gas emboli, with TEE having the highest sensitivity [76–78].

A more theoretical consideration concerning gas emboli is a venous injury during pneumoperitoneum. To test this, O'Sullivan and colleagues made venotomies in pigs undergoing pneumoperitoneum at 10–25 mmHg [78]. They detected gas emboli in 20 of 22 cases. The extent of embolization correlated with a decrease in central venous pressure attributed to blood loss, the duration of the venotomy, and higher intraperitoneal pressure. For significant venous injury during laparoscopic surgery, it is prudent to directly occlude the site of injury and increase intravascular volume.

The treatment of gas embolism involves immediate termination of the pneumoperitoneum, administration of 100% inspired oxygen, and any other resuscitative measures required. The patient should be positioned in the left lateral decubitus position, right side up, and head down. This position will stop the air bubble from transferring into the pulmonary circulation and allows for percutaneous aspiration in the right atrium.

Another complication of pneumoperitoneum is cardiac arrythmia. Bradycardia has been reported with the initiation of abdominal insufflation [79], and may be the result of vagal reflex in response to the stretch of the peritoneum. In a comparison of 100 patients undergoing CO_2 insufflation and 45 patients undergoing N_2O insufflation, the rates of dysrhythmia were 17% and 4%, respectively [80]. The authors attributed the higher rate of dysrhythmia in the CO_2 group (extra-systolic ventricular beats, most commonly) to hypercarbia.

7.1 AIRSEAL® Insufflation Mechanism: A New Generation of Valveless Trocar—How AirSeal® Works

The AirSeal System maintains pressure in two unique ways:

1. Inside the cannula housing of the AirSeal® Access Port, a series of high-pressure nozzles direct gas downward into the cannula until the desired intra-abdominal pressure is achieved. At this point, an equilibrium is reached, creating an invisible, horizontal air barrier inside the cannula housing. As pressure inside the cavity drops (due to a leak or the use of suction), the equilibrium shifts downward allowing more gas to enter the cavity until the set pressure is re-established. Similarly, when pressure in the cavity increases (as it does when external pressure is present and during every ventilation cycle), the equilibrium shifts upward, venting any overpressure almost instantaneously, until the set pressure is again re-established.
2. The iFS measures pressure multiple times per second and responds to changes in pressure by either venting (when an overpressure is present and the cannula cannot respond quickly enough) or by increasing gas flow through to both the 4 holes at the distal end of the cannula and to the jets in the cannula housing when a drop in cavity pressure is sensed.

The AirSeal System continuously clears smoke:

1. A continuous flow circuit is also activated simultaneously evacuating intra-abdominal gas (now containing CO_2 and smoke), filtering it, and recirculating it through the high-pressure nozzles.
2. The smoke evacuation rate can be chosen by the operator. In LOW smoke evacuation mode, gas is evacuated and recirculated at a rate of 3 liters per minute. In HIGH smoke evacuation mode, gas is evacuated and recirculated at a rate of 8 liters per minute (Figs. 1, 2 and 3).

The concept of low-impact laparoscopy (LIL), supported by the European guidelines of Urology, is based on performing the surgery using small-diameter trocars and low insufflation pressures [81]. Previous studies described respiratory and cardiovascular impacts of increased intra-abdominal pressures due to the CO_2 insufflation in laparoscopic procedures. Additionally, the elimination of CO_2 has also been associated with increased postoperative pain and the use of opioids [81]. Therefore, new insufflation systems have been developed to decrease these negative impacts of high intra-abdominal pressure in laparoscopic surgeries.

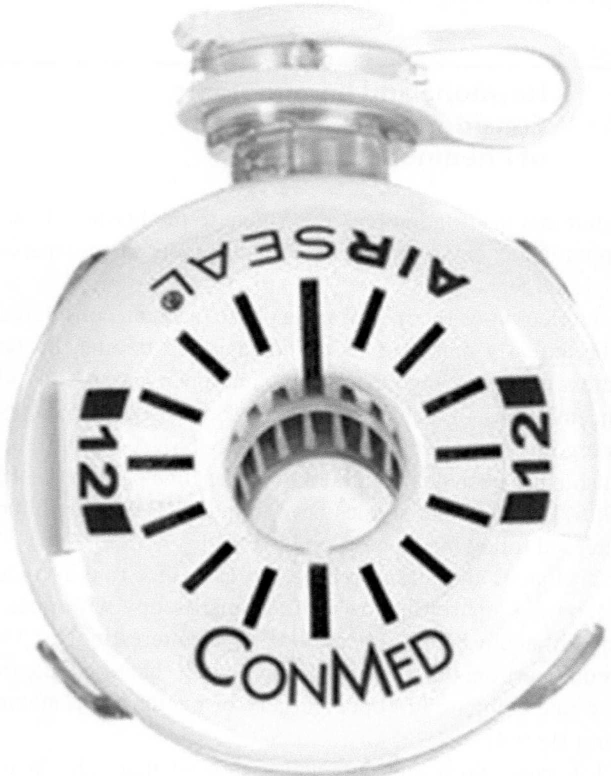

Fig. 1 AIRSEAL® 12 mm cap (available in 8 mm as well) (with permission from Conmed, Largo, FL 33773, USA)

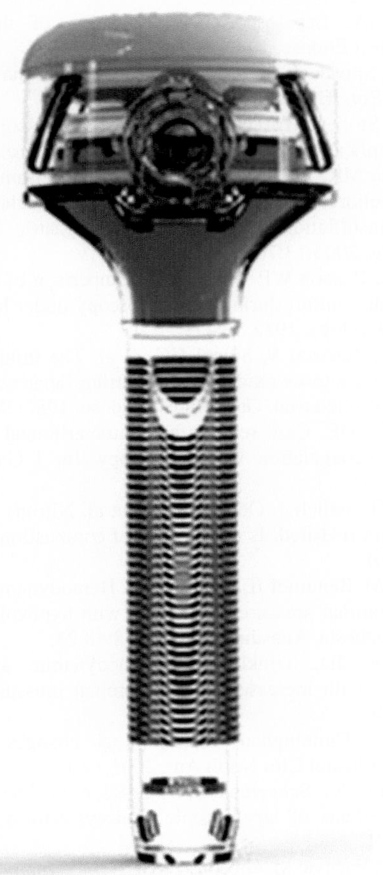

Fig. 2 AIRSEAL® Access port (with permission from Conmed, Largo, FL 33773, USA)

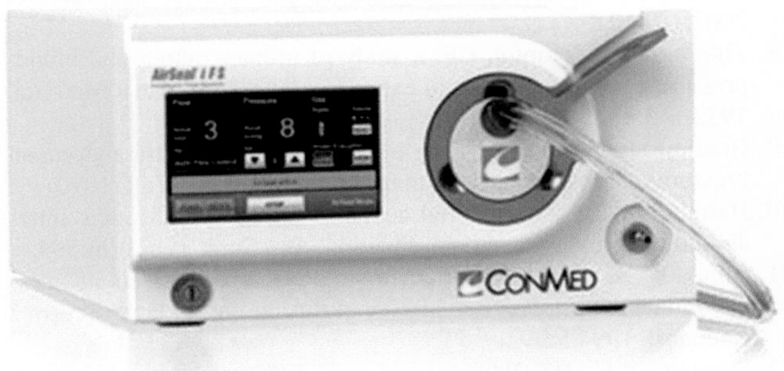

Fig. 3 AIRSEAL® iFS (Intelligent Flow System) (with permission from Conmed, Largo, FL 33773, USA)

The AIRSEAL® Intelligent Flow System (ConMed, New York, USA) is a three-lumen insufflation method with a valveless trocar, which maintains constant intra-abdominal pressure and removes the surgical smoke periodically [82, 83]. Several authors have described in the literature the outcomes of the AIRSEAL® insufflation system compared to the standard CO_2 insufflation (12–15 mmHg) in laparoscopic procedures.

7.1.1 Current Literature Reporting AIRSEAL Use and Outcomes

Intraoperative Performance

Bucur and colleagues, in a study with 56 patients divided into two groups who underwent renal surgery, reported higher blood loss in the AIRSEAL® group compared to the conventional insufflation [84]. On the other hand, several studies reported no significant blood loss and transfusion rates differences between both techniques [82, 85–90].

Different studies assessed the insufflation impact on the surgical field visibility. Madueke-Laveaux et al. reported better surgery visualization when performing cases with the AIRSEAL® [89]. Horstmann and colleagues described no difference in the time spent cleaning the camera in radical prostatectomies [88]. The current literature also has reports of faster operative times associated with the AIRSEAL® use [82, 87, 91].

Postoperative Pain Evaluation and Morphine Analgesia

Some authors had described the impacts of lower pressures on postoperative pain (abdominal or shoulder) [82, 89, 92, 93]. Sroussi and colleagues performed a study enrolling 60 patients who underwent laparoscopic gynecologic surgery comparing the standard intra-abdominal pressure (15 mmHg) with lower pressures (7 mmHg) provided by the AIRSEAL® Intelligent Flow System (ConMed, New York, USA) [93]. The author reported AIRSEAL® benefits to reduce postoperative shoulder pain from four to twenty-four hours after surgery ($p < 0.001$). In addition, patients using this system needed 23.3% less morphine for managing postoperative pain.

Complication Rates

Different authors assessed complication rates at 30 days (using Clavien-Dindo Classification) comparing the AIRSEAL® Intelligent Flow System (ConMed, New York, USA) with the standard CO_2 insufflation [82, 85, 87, 89, 90, 92]. All studies described no differences between both insufflation techniques.

7.1.2 Insufflation Improvements

Since the beginning of the COVID-19 pandemic, the concerns regarding aerosolization of hazards have increased among laparoscopic and robotic surgeons. Some studies described the potential CO_2 leakage and aerosolization associated with the AIRSEAL® system, even with the trocar supplied cap [94]. Therefore, new methods have been tested to improve staff security during the surgery and maintaining the concept of low abdominal pressures in laparoscopic and robotic surgeries.

In this scenario, the recently introduced LEXION (Lexion Medical, MN, USA) system has some modifications compared to the AIRSEAL®. The system also produces a constant intra-abdominal pressure, but instead of using CO_2 gas mixed with air (nitrogen), LEXION (Lexion Medical, MN, USA) provides insufflation using 100% CO_2, which reduces the subcutaneous emphysema, according to the manufacturer. In addition, this system offers ULPA filtration, which filters smaller particles (down to 0.01 micron), eliminating virus and combustion hazards. However, despite the potential advantages of this new system, the literature still lacks comparative studies assessing the advantages of this insufflation mechanism over the standard AIRSEAL®.

7.1.3 Overall Summary and Consideration

Balayssac and colleagues performed a literature review evaluating ten studies from the USA, Europe, and Japan, comparing AIRSEAL® with conventional CO_2 insufflation in laparoscopic surgeries [95]. Four studies were randomized controlled trials (RCT), five were retrospective, and one was prospective non-RCT enrolling a total of 1394 patients (639 AIRSEAL® and 755 CO_2 insufflation). The author concluded that the current literature does not support the benefits of the AIRSEAL® over the conventional CO_2 insufflation in laparoscopic surgeries. However, most studies have less than 100 patients, and most are based on retrospective data analysis with all its inherent risks of bias.

8 Conclusions

With more than five decades of clinical use, laparoscopy has become a foundational component of modern surgery. Carbon dioxide is the most commonly chosen agent for pneumoperitoneum because of its rapid absorption in blood and low combustibility. However, other options for insufflation exist and may be considered for patients with cardiac, pulmonary, and neurologic pathologies that may not tolerate hypercarbia. Pressure effects and gas absorption are well-studied phenomena that promote a variety of physiologic changes in the patient. Understanding the interplay of these physiological changes is vital to patient safety when considering a laparoscopic approach for an operation.

References

1. Wheeless CR. Outpatient laparoscope sterilization under local anesthesia. Obstet Gynecol. 1972;39:767.
2. Dubois F, Icard P, Berthelot G, et al. Coelioscopic cholecystectomy. Preliminary report of 36 cases. Ann Surg. 1990;211:60.
3. Clayman RV, Kavoussi LR, Soper NJ, et al. Laparoscopic nephrectomy: initial case report. J Urol. 1991;146:278.
4. Uhlich GA. Laparoscopy: the question of the proper gas. Gastrointest Endosc. 1982;28:212.
5. Menes T, Spivak H. Laparoscopy: searching for the proper insufflation gas. Surg Endosc. 2000;14:1050.
6. Wolf JS, Stoller ML. The physiology of laparoscopy: basic principles, complications and other considerations. J Urol. 1994;152:294.
7. Brackman MR, Finelli FC, Light T, et al. Helium pneumoperitoneum ameliorates hypercarbia and acidosis associated with carbon dioxide insufflation during laparoscopic gastric bypass in pigs. Obes Surg. 2003;13:768.
8. Sharp JR, Pierson WP, Brady CE. Comparison of CO_2- and N_2O-induced discomfort during peritoneoscopy under local anesthesia. Gastroenterology. 1982;82:453.
9. Minoli G, Terruzzi V, Spinzi GC, et al. The influence of carbon dioxide and nitrous oxide on pain during laparoscopy: a double-blind, controlled trial. Gastrointest Endosc. 1982;28:173.
10. Gunatilake DE. Case report: fatal intraperitoneal explosion during electrocoagulation via laparoscopy. Int J Gynaecol Obstet. 1978;15:353.
11. Hunter JG, Staheli J, Oddsdottir M, et al. Nitrous oxide pneumoperitoneum revisited. Is there a risk of combustion? Surg Endosc. 1995;9:501.
12. Diamant M, Benumof JL, Saidman LJ. Hemodynamics of increased intra-abdominal pressure: interaction with hypovolemia and halothane anesthesia. Anesthesiology. 1978;48:23.
13. Richardson JD, Trinkle JK. Hemodynamic and respiratory alterations with increased intra-abdominal pressure. J Surg Res. 1976;20:401.
14. O'Malley C, Cunningham AJ. Physiologic changes during laparoscopy. Anesthesiol Clin North Am. 2001;19:1.
15. McLaughlin JG, Scheeres DE, Dean RJ, et al. The adverse hemodynamic effects of laparoscopic cholecystectomy. Surg Endosc. 1995;9:121.
16. Dexter SP, Vucevic M, Gibson J, et al. Hemodynamic consequences of high- and low-pressure capnoperitoneum during laparoscopic cholecystectomy. Surg Endosc. 1999;13:376.
17. Neudecker J, Sauerland S, Neugebauer E, et al. The European Association for Endoscopic Surgery clinical practice guideline on the pneumoperitoneum for laparoscopic surgery. Surg Endosc. 2002;16:1121.
18. Thorington J. Schmidt, CF: a study of urinary output and blood-pressure changes resulting in experimental ascites. Am J Med Sci. 1932;165:880.
19. Bradley SE, Bradley GP. The effect of increased intra-abdominal pressure on renal function in man. J Clin Invest. 1947;26:1010.
20. Harman PK, Kron IL, McLachlan HD, et al. Elevated intra-abdominal pressure and renal function. Ann Surg. 1982;196:594.
21. Chiu AW, Azadzoi KM, Hatzichristou DG, et al. Effects of intra-abdominal pressure on renal tissue perfusion during laparoscopy. J Endourol. 1994;8:99.
22. London ET, Ho HS, Neuhaus AM, et al. Effect of intravascular volume expansion on renal function during prolonged CO_2 pneumoperitoneum. Ann Surg. 2000;231:195.
23. McDougall EM, Monk TG, Wolf JS, et al. The effect of prolonged pneumoperitoneum on renal function in an animal model. J Am Coll Surg. 1996;182:317.
24. Chang DT, Kirsch AJ, Sawczuk IS. Oliguria during laparoscopic surgery. J Endourol. 1994;8:349.
25. Kerbl K, Clayman RV, McDougall EM, et al. Laparoscopic nephrectomy: the Washington university experience. Br J Urol. 1994;73:231.
26. Pérez J, Taurá P, Rueda J, et al. Role of dopamine in renal dysfunction during laparoscopic surgery. Surg Endosc. 2002;16:1297.
27. Koivusalo AM, Kellokumpu I, Ristkari S, et al. Splanchnic and renal deterioration during and after laparoscopic cholecystectomy:

a comparison of the carbon dioxide pneumoperitoneum and the abdominal wall lift method. Anesth Analg. 1997;85:886.
28. Caldwell CB, Ricotta JJ. Changes in visceral blood flow with elevated intraabdominal pressure. J Surg Res. 1987;43:14.
29. Evasovich MR, Clark TC, Horattas MC, et al. Does pneumoperitoneum during laparoscopy increase bacterial translocation? Surg Endosc. 1996;10:1176.
30. Irgau I, Koyfman Y, Tikellis JI. Elective intraoperative intracranial pressure monitoring during laparoscopic cholecystectomy. Arch Surg. 1995;130:1011.
31. Josephs LG, Este-McDonald JR, Birkett DH, et al. Diagnostic laparoscopy increases intracranial pressure. J Trauma. 1994;36:815.
32. Rosenthal RJ, Hiatt JR, Phillips EH, et al. Intracranial pressure. Effects of pneumoperitoneum in a large-animal model. Surg Endosc. 1997;11:376.
33. Fujii Y, Tanaka H, Tsuruoka S, et al. Middle cerebral arterial blood flow velocity increases during laparoscopic cholecystectomy. Anesth Analg. 1994;78:80.
34. Abe K, Hashimoto N, Taniguchi A, et al. Middle cerebral artery blood flow velocity during laparoscopic surgery in head-down position. Surg Laparosc Endosc. 1998;8:1.
35. Schöb OM, Allen DC, Benzel E, et al. A comparison of the pathophysiologic effects of carbon dioxide, nitrous oxide, and helium pneumoperitoneum on intracranial pressure. Am J Surg. 1996;172:248.
36. Este-McDonald JR, Josephs LG, Birkett DH, et al. Changes in intracranial pressure associated with apneumic retractors. Arch Surg. 1995;130:362.
37. Halverson AL, Barrett WL, Iglesias AR, et al. Decreased cerebrospinal fluid absorption during abdominal insufflation. Surg Endosc. 1999;13:797.
38. Ben-Haim M, Rosenthal RJ. Causes of arterial hypertension and splachnic ischemia during acute elevations in intra-abdominal pressure with CO_2 pneumoperitoneum: a complex central nervous system mediated response. Int J Color Dis. 1999;14:227.
39. Motew M, Ivankovich AD, Bieniarz J, et al. Cardiovascular effects and acid-base and blood gas changes during laparoscopy. Am J Obstet Gynecol. 1973;115:1002.
40. Gutt CN, Oniu T, Mehrabi A, et al. Circulatory and respiratory complications of carbon dioxide insufflation. Dig Surg. 2004;21:95.
41. Hardacre JM, Talamini MA. Pulmonary and hemodynamic changes during laparoscopy--are they important? Surgery. 2000;127:241.
42. Schwenk W, Böhm B, Witt C, et al. Pulmonary function following laparoscopic or conventional colorectal resection: a randomized controlled evaluation. Arch Surg. 1999;134:6.
43. Hasukić S, Mesić D, Dizdarević E, et al. Pulmonary function after laparoscopic and open cholecystectomy. Surg Endosc. 2002;16:163.
44. Alexander GD, Brown EM. Physiologic alterations during pelvic laparoscopy. Am J Obstet Gynecol. 1969;105:1078.
45. Montalva M, Das B. Carbon dioxide homeostasis during laparoscopy. South Med J. 1976;69:602.
46. Mullett CE, Viale JP, Sagnard PE, et al. Pulmonary CO_2 elimination during surgical procedures using intra- or extraperitoneal CO_2 insufflation. Anesth Analg. 1993;76:622.
47. PRICE, H. L. Effects of carbon dioxide on the cardiovascular system. Anesthesiology. 1960;21:652.
48. Cullen DJ, Eger EI. Cardiovascular effects of carbon dioxide in man. Anesthesiology. 1974;41:345.
49. Seed RF, Shakespeare TF, Muldoon MJ. Carbon dioxide homeostasis during anaesthesia for laparoscopy. Anaesthesia. 1970;25:223.
50. Farhi LE, Rahn H. Dynamics of changes in carbon dioxide stores. Anesthesiology. 1960;21:604.
51. Wallace DH, Serpell MG, Baxter JN, et al. Randomized trial of different insufflation pressures for laparoscopic cholecystectomy. Br J Surg. 1997;84:455.
52. Williams MD, Murr PC. Laparoscopic insufflation of the abdomen depresses cardiopulmonary function. Surg Endosc. 1993;7:12.
53. Joris JL, Noirot DP, Legrand MJ, et al. Hemodynamic changes during laparoscopic cholecystectomy. Anesth Analg. 1993;76:1067.
54. Kelman GR, Swapp GH, Smith I, et al. Caridac output and arterial blood-gas tension during laparoscopy. Br J Anaesth. 1972;44:1155.
55. Chaudhary D, Verma GR, Gupta R, et al. Comparative evaluation of the inflammatory mediators in patients undergoing laparoscopic versus conventional cholecystectomy. Aust N Z J Surg. 1999;69:369.
56. Cho JM, LaPorta AJ, Clark JR, et al. Response of serum cytokines in patients undergoing laparoscopic cholecystectomy. Surg Endosc. 1994;8:1380.
57. Glaser F, Sannwald GA, Buhr HJ, et al. General stress response to conventional and laparoscopic cholecystectomy. Ann Surg. 1995;221:372.
58. Harmon GD, Senagore AJ, Kilbride MJ, et al. Interleukin-6 response to laparoscopic and open colectomy. Dis Colon Rectum. 1994;37:754.
59. Joris J, Cigarini I, Legrand M, et al. Metabolic and respiratory changes after cholecystectomy performed via laparotomy or laparoscopy. Br J Anaesth. 1992;69:341.
60. Maruszynski M, Pojda Z. Interleukin 6 (IL-6) levels in the monitoring of surgical trauma. A comparison of serum IL-6 concentrations in patients treated by cholecystectomy via laparotomy or laparoscopy. Surg Endosc. 1995;9:882.
61. Leung KL, Lai PB, Ho RL, et al. Systemic cytokine response after laparoscopic-assisted resection of rectosigmoid carcinoma: a prospective randomized trial. Ann Surg. 2000;231:506.
62. Roumen RM, van Meurs PA, Kuypers HH, et al. Serum interleukin-6 and C reactive protein responses in patients after laparoscopic or conventional cholecystectomy. Eur J Surg. 1992;158:541.
63. Hill AD, Banwell PE, Darzi A, et al. Inflammatory markers following laparoscopic and open hernia repair. Surg Endosc. 1995;9:695.
64. Chekan EG, Nataraj C, Clary EM, et al. Intraperitoneal immunity and pneumoperitoneum. Surg Endosc. 1999;13:1135.
65. West MA, Baker J, Bellingham J. Kinetics of decreased LPS-stimulated cytokine release by macrophages exposed to CO_2. J Surg Res. 1996;63:269.
66. Sietses C, von Blomberg ME, Eijsbouts QA, et al. The influence of CO_2 versus helium insufflation or the abdominal wall lifting technique on the systemic immune response. Surg Endosc. 2002;16:525.
67. Karayiannakis AJ, Makri GG, Mantzioka A, et al. Systemic stress response after laparoscopic or open cholecystectomy: a randomized trial. Br J Surg. 1997;84:467.
68. Le Blanc-Louvry I, Coquerel A, Koning E, et al. Operative stress response is reduced after laparoscopic compared to open cholecystectomy: the relationship with postoperative pain and ileus. Dig Dis Sci. 2000;45:1703.
69. Wolf JS, Clayman RV, Monk TG, et al. Carbon dioxide absorption during laparoscopic pelvic operation. J Am Coll Surg. 1995;180:555.
70. Kent RB. Subcutaneous emphysema and hypercarbia following laparoscopic cholecystectomy. Arch Surg. 1991;126:1154.
71. Hall D, Goldstein A, Tynan E, et al. Profound hypercarbia late in the course of laparoscopic cholecystectomy: detection by continuous capnometry. Anesthesiology. 1993;79:173.
72. Murray DP, Rankin RA, Lackey C. Bilateral pneumothoraces complicating peritoneoscopy. Gastrointest Endosc. 1984;30:45.
73. Pascual JB, Baranda MM, Tarrero MT, et al. Subcutaneous emphysema, pneumomediastinum, bilateral pneumothorax and pneumopericardium after laparoscopy. Endoscopy. 1990;22:59.
74. Herrerías JM, Ariza A, Garrido M. An unusual complication of laparoscopy: pneumopericardium. Endoscopy. 1980;12:254.
75. Nicholson RD, Berman ND. Pneumopericardium following laparoscopy. Chest. 1979;76:605.

76. Ostman PL, Pantle-Fisher FH, Faure EA, et al. Circulatory collapse during laparoscopy. J Clin Anesth. 1990;2:129.
77. JERNSTROM, P. Air embolism during peritoneoscopy. Am J Clin Pathol. 1951;21:573.
78. O'Sullivan DC, Micali S, Averch TD, et al. Factors involved in gas embolism after laparoscopic injury to inferior vena cava. J Endourol. 1998;12:149.
79. Carmichael DE. Laparoscopy-cardiac considerations. Fertil Steril. 1971;22:69.
80. Scott DB, Julian DG. Observations on cardiac arrythmias during laparoscopy. Br Med J. 1972;1:411.
81. Neudecker J, Sauerland S, Neugebauer E, et al. The european association for endoscopic surgery clinical practice guide- line on the pneumoperitoneum for laparoscopic surgery. Surg Endosc. 2002;16:1121–43. https://doi.org/10.1007/s00464-001-9166-7.
82. Shahait M, Cockrell R, Yezdani M, et al. Improved out- comes utilizing a valveless-trocar system during robot-assisted radical prostatectomy (RARP). Jsls. 2019; https://doi.org/10.4293/jsls.2018.00085.
83. NeppleKG KD, Bhayani SB. Benchtop evaluation of pressure barrier insufflator and standard insufflator systems. Surg Endosc. 2013;27:333–8. https://doi.org/10.1007/s00464-012-2434-x.
84. Bucur P, Hofmann M, Menhadji A, et al. Comparison of pneumoperitoneum stability between a valveless trocar system and conventional insufflation: a prospective randomized trial. Urology. 2016;94:274–80. https://doi.org/10.1016/j.urology.2016.04.022.
85. Herati AS, Andonian S, Rais-Bahrami S, et al. Use of the valveless trocar system reduces carbon dioxide absorption during. Urology. 2011;77(5):1126–32.
86. Covotta M, Claroni C, Torregiani G, et al. A prospective, randomized, clinical trial on the effects of a valveless trocar on respiratory mechanics during robotic radical cystectomy: a pilot 089 study. Anesth Analg. 2017;124:1794–801. https://doi.org/10.1213/ane.0000000000002027.
87. George AK, Wimhofer R, Viola KV, et al. Utilization of a novel valveless trocar system during robotic-assisted laparoscopic prostatectomy. World J Urol. 2015;33:1695–9. https://doi.org/10.1007/s00345-015-1521-8.
88. Horstmann M, Horton K, Kurz M, et al. Prospective comparison between the AirSeal(R) system valve-less trocar and a standard Versaport plus V2 trocar in robotic-assisted radical prostatectomy. J Endourol. 2013;27:579–82. https://doi.org/10.1089/end.2012.0632.
89. Madueke-Laveaux OS, Advincula A, Grimes CL, et al. Comparison of carbon dioxide absorption rates in gynecologic laparoscopy with a valveless versus standard insufflation system: randomized controlled trial. J Minim Invasive Gynecol. 2020;27:225–34. https://doi.org/10.1016/j.jmig.2019.05.005.
90. Miyano G, Nakamura H, Seo S, et al. Pneumoperitoneum and hemodynamic stability during pediatric laparoscopic appendectomy. J Pediatr Surg. 2016;51:1949–51. https://doi.org/10.1016/j.jpedsurg.2016.09.016.
91. Annino F, Topazio L, Autieri D, et al. Robotic partial nephrectomy performed with Airseal versus a standard CO_2 pressure pneumoperitoneum insufflator: a prospective comparative study. Surg Endosc. 2017;31:1583–90. https://doi.org/10.1007/s00464-016-5144-y.
92. Gurusamy KS, Samraj K, Davidson BR. Low pressure versus standard pressure pneumoperitoneum in laparoscopic cholecystectomy. In: The Cochrane Collaboration, editor. Cochrane database of systematic reviews. Chichester: John Wiley; 2009.
93. Sroussi J, Elies A, Rigouzzo A, et al. Low pressure gynecological laparoscopy (7mmHg) with AirSeal((R)) System versus a standard insufflation (15mmHg): a pilot study in 60 patients. J Gynecol Obstet Hum Reprod. 2017;46:155–8. https://doi.org/10.1016/j.jogoh.2016.09.003.
94. Dalli J, Khan MF, Nolan K, Cahill RA. Laparoscopic pneumoperitoneum escape and contamination during surgery using the Airseal Insufflation System - a video vignette. Colorectal Dis. 2020 Sep;22(9):1029–1030. https://doi.org/10.1111/codi.15255. Epub 2020 Sep 1. PMID: 32644263; PMCID: PMC7362043.
95. Balayssac D, Selvy M, Martelin A, et al. Clinical and organizational impact of the AIRSEAL® insufflation system during laparoscopic surgery: a systematic review. World J Surg. 2021;45:705–18. https://doi.org/10.1007/s00268-020-05869-5.

Patient Positioning, Port Placement, and Docking: Si, Xi, and SP Robots

Raymond J. Leveillee, Oscar Schatloff,
Marcio Covas Moschovas, and Jean V. Joseph

1 Introduction

Intuitive Surgical, founded in 1995 and headquartered in Sunnyvale, California, USA., has been the leading computer-assisted surgical device company (aka "robot") for over two decades. This chapter, written in collaboration with my colleagues Oscar Schatloff, MD, Marcio Moschovas, MD, and Jean Joseph, MD, is based on experts' opinion and covers the last 25 years in development and technological improvements since the introduction of the "standard 3-armed Model" in 1998.

This chapter will focus on relevant clinical applications of the four-arm platforms as we currently utilize in our clinical practices for the performance of Radical Prostatectomy. All images are either ones that we have taken ourselves or are readily accessible on the Internet. Appropriate references will be given when warranted. There may be additional modifications/adaptations that other surgeons have utilized. The intent is not to go through the steps of the operation but merely to render our opinions and current practices. We anticipate that future "robotic" surgeons will read these pages with either awe or amusement.

2 Traditional Docking for Prostatectomy (Multiport Robot)

Patient positioning for Multiport Robotic Prostatectomy between the legs using the Si and the Xi Da Vinci Robot involves optimizing placement of the "surgical cart" close to the perineum to allow maximal reach and permit the bedside assistant to manipulate the penis, Foley catheter, and in some instances, the perineum.

The use of a rectal bougie has all but been abandoned by most surgeons currently. Positioning of the vision cart is dictated by the size of the operating room and the length of the cables for the camera and energy cords [often within 3–5 feet (1.0–1.5 meters) from the operating table].

Patient positioning and port placement are similar for the Da Vinci Xi and Si and will be described below. There are many differences between the two systems. The primary difference is that in the Da Vinci Xi, the camera and all the interchangeable instruments are 8 mm in diameter, while in the Si and previous models, the camera is 12 mm in diameter, allowing for "port hopping" with the Xi, which is especially helpful during initial trocar placement, avoiding the use of a separate 5 mm laparoscopic telescope and camera. The arms of the Xi model are also thinner and lighter, allowing a significant improvement in motion and arm clashing for prostate and pelvic surgery.

3 Patient Positioning

Patients are administered a general endotracheal anesthetic with paralysis and put into leg stirrups to allow space and then placed in a 25 to 30 degree supine Trendelenburg (Head down) position to allow gravity displacement of the small intestines once pneumoperitoneum is created. Placement of anti-embolic stockings and sequential compression devices should be routinely done for pelvic surgery. As the risk of a thromboembolic event is thought to be greatest during surgery, we routinely use 5000 UI of unfractionated heparin subcutaneously after the patient is anesthetized. Previous studies have not shown an increase in intraoperative bleeding nor lymphocele.

In sequence, foam rubber padding is often used to protect pressure points, and an anti-sliding foam or conformable vacuum bean bag is placed on the operating table under the

R. J. Leveillee (✉)
Baptist Health South Florida, Bethesda Hospital, Florida, USA

O. Schatloff
Clinica INDISA, Santiago, Chile

M. C. Moschovas
AdventHealth Global Robotics Institute, Florida, USA

J. V. Joseph
University of Rochester Medical Center, Rochester, NY, USA

P. Wiklund et al. (eds.), *Robotic Urologic Surgery*, https://doi.org/10.1007/978-3-031-00363-9_17

patient. The patient is then wrapped across the chest for extra safety. However, care should be taken not to restrain thoracic expansion. The elbows and wrists are positioned to allow slight flexion, and the arms are tucked at the patient's side. The arms should be kept low at the patient's side to avoid contact with the fourth robotic arm or the 12 mm assistant port.

After correctly positioning the patient, the table is turned into Trendelenburg (Head down) of approximately 15 degrees. Patient safety and stability are checked, including inspecting all pressure points and allowing the anesthesia team to visualize the extent to which the patient will be positioned once the drapes are applied. Attention is made to assure that the neck is not hyperextended, and adjustments are made as necessary.

In sequence, the abdomen and genitals are prepared from xiphoid to perineum. Sterile drapes can include cystoscopy leggings, an under buttocks drape, and a standard laparotomy drape. A 16 or 18 French Foley catheter is inserted and kept in the sterile field. Using a blue silicone catheter can improve the visualization of the urethra at the time of prostatic apex division and vesicourethral anastomosis.

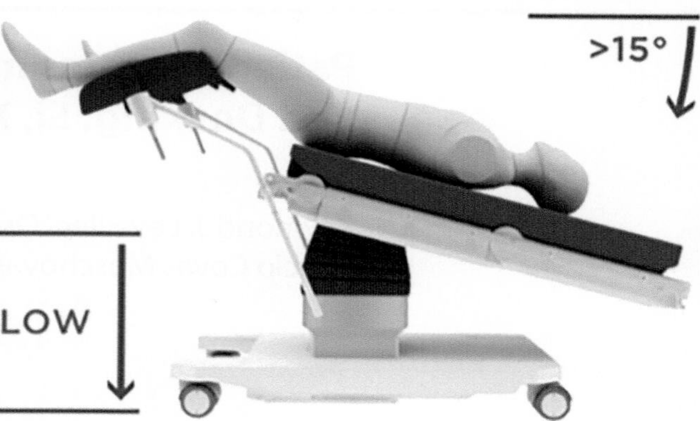

Fig. 1 Diagram illustrating patient positioning with >15 degree Trendelenburg. This is applicable for Davinci S, Si, or Xi. Copyright Intuitive Surgical—reproduced courtesy of the manufacturer)

4 Port Placement (Multiport Robot)

The minimum distance necessary for the arms to move without colliding utilizing the Si is approximately 9 cm. After pneumoperitoneum is created, we recommend placing the 12 mm camera port 2 cm cranial to the umbilicus for better exposure of the cranial part of the pelvis, such as the aortic bifurcation, ureteral crossing, and also for a better view during an extended lymph node dissection. In addition, it allows a higher placement of the robotic arms 1 and 2, to adequately perform the tasks just described. We place the ports in a "W shape." Alternatively a gentle "Rainbow" arc can be used.

After the camera port, we mark a horizontal line 1 cm below the umbilicus and then connect a line from the camera port to the horizontal line a minimum of 9 cm apart. It is better, while entering, to have ports 1 and 2 pointing toward the symphysis pubis in a diagonal direction, so the midpoint between the midline and the iliac crest is usually the optimal place so that a triangle is formed between the camera port and the robotic arms 1 and 2.

We usually place the robotic arm three on the left side of the patient and the 12 mm assistant port on the right side. However, this could be the opposite, according to the surgeon's preference. The 12 mm assistant port is placed at least 9 cm from the robotic arm 1 in a diagonal direction lateral and upwards. The assistant port needs to be placed through the transversus muscles and not through the fascia. Otherwise, it will be too lateral and will collide with the patient's arm and surgical table. This holds true for the third robotic arm on the contralateral side. Finally, we place a 5 mm port below the ribs on the right side for suction, usually on the same vertical line as the right 8 mm port.

The same trocar placement process is performed with the Da Vinci Xi. However, the supraumbilical trocar (camera port) has 8 mm as the other instruments' arms. Another advantage of the Xi with it's overhead, extending and rotational boom is the ability to dock from virtually any angle including the patient's side. This can be especially useful in smaller confined spaces such as older operating rooms. One must remember to make the assistant port on the contralateral side to the docking side. Figures 1, 2, 3, 4, 5, 6, 7 and 8 illustrate the details of port placement with the multiport robot.

5 Single-Port (SP) Robot-Assisted Radical Prostatectomy (RARP)

This century began with the approval of the DaVinci multiport robot-assisted surgery in 2000, ushering in a new era in urologic surgery. While the robot brought forth significant advantages in decreasing surgical invasiveness and easing laparoscopic interventions for surgeons, there has been a relentless pursuit to further decrease the invasiveness of surgeries. From the first standard DaVinci system (Intuitive Surgical, Sunnyvale CA, USA) to the multi-armed platforms (S, Si, and Xi), surgeons have sought ways to decrease the number of ports utilized.

The "single port" (SP) robot was approved by the FDA in 2018, giving surgeons the ability to perform surgery via a single cannula via which all necessary instruments are

PORT PLACEMENT

Measurements should be made AFTER insufflation to 15 mmHg.

> *da Vinci* Camera Port, 12 mm (BLUE); Place port near umbilicus. Place camera port 1-2 cm superior to the umbilicus and make a transverse incision at the midline. Utilizing a transverse incision significantly reduces the risk of incisional hernia.[1, 2]

> *da Vinci* Instrument Arm ① Port, 8 mm (YELLOW); Place 8-10 cm from the camera port on a line to the right anterior iliac spine.

> *da Vinci* Instrument Arm ② Port, 8 mm (GREEN): Place 8-10 cm from the camera port on a line to the left anterior iliac spine.

> *da Vinci* Instrument Arm ① Port, 8 mm (RED): Place on the patient's left side, at least 2-3 cm from the itiac crest and > 8 cm from *da Vinci* Instrument Arm ② Port, just inferior to the camera port.

> Assistant Port #1 (A1), 12 mm (WHITE): During a 3-arm procedure, place the port on the patient's left side, lateral to *da Vinci* instrument arm ②. During a 4-arm procedure, place the port on the patient's right side, lateral to the *da Vinci* instrument arm ① port.

> Assistant Port #2 (A2), 5 mm (**BLACK**): In a 3-arm case, place the port 3-4 cm superior to the camera port and between the camera port and *da vinci* instrument arm ② port. During a 4-arm procedure place the port 3-4 cm superior to the camera port and between the camera port and *da Vinci* instrument arm ① port.

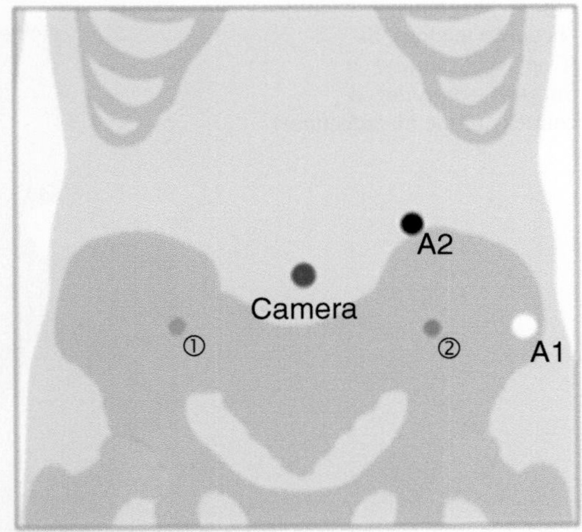

3-ARM SETUP

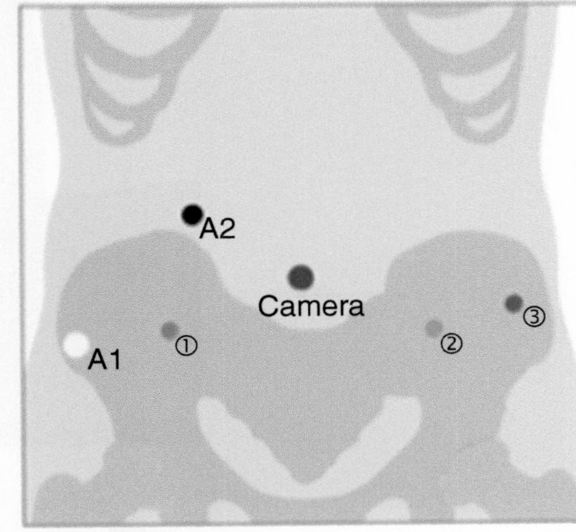

4-ARM SETUP

Fig. 2 Prostatectomy set-up card (3 and 4 arm) Si. (Copyright Intuitive Surgical—reproduced courtesy of the manufacturer)

deployed. Before the arrival of the SP robot, several surgeons had performed single-site surgeries through rearrangement or crossings of the multi-arm robot placed through a single skin incision.

Whether via multiport or single-port robotic surgeries, the adoption of robotic surgery continues to increase. Maneuvering the SP at the surgeon's console mimics the prior robotic systems. Regardless of the approach, proper access, proper patient positioning, and selection remain key. Adequate training and experience of the surgical team are paramount for the success of any new program. In this section, we focus on single-port patient positioning and access for robot-assisted radical prostatectomy.

Radical prostatectomy has been performed with the SP robot using a variety of techniques. These include transperitoneal, extraperitoneal, and perineal. The transperitoneal route can accommodate various techniques, including an anterior or posterior approach and the Retzius sparing.

6 Patient Positioning (SP Robot)

Whether a transperitoneal or an extraperitoneal approach is used, the patients undergoing radical prostatectomy are placed in a supine position. In contrast to the transperitoneal approach, the extraperitoneal access requires less Trendelenburg (less than 10 degrees Trendelenburg for the entire procedure), as illustrated in Fig. 9. The peritoneum serves as a natural barrier keeping all intra-abdominal contents out of the surgical field. Avoiding the peritoneal cavity

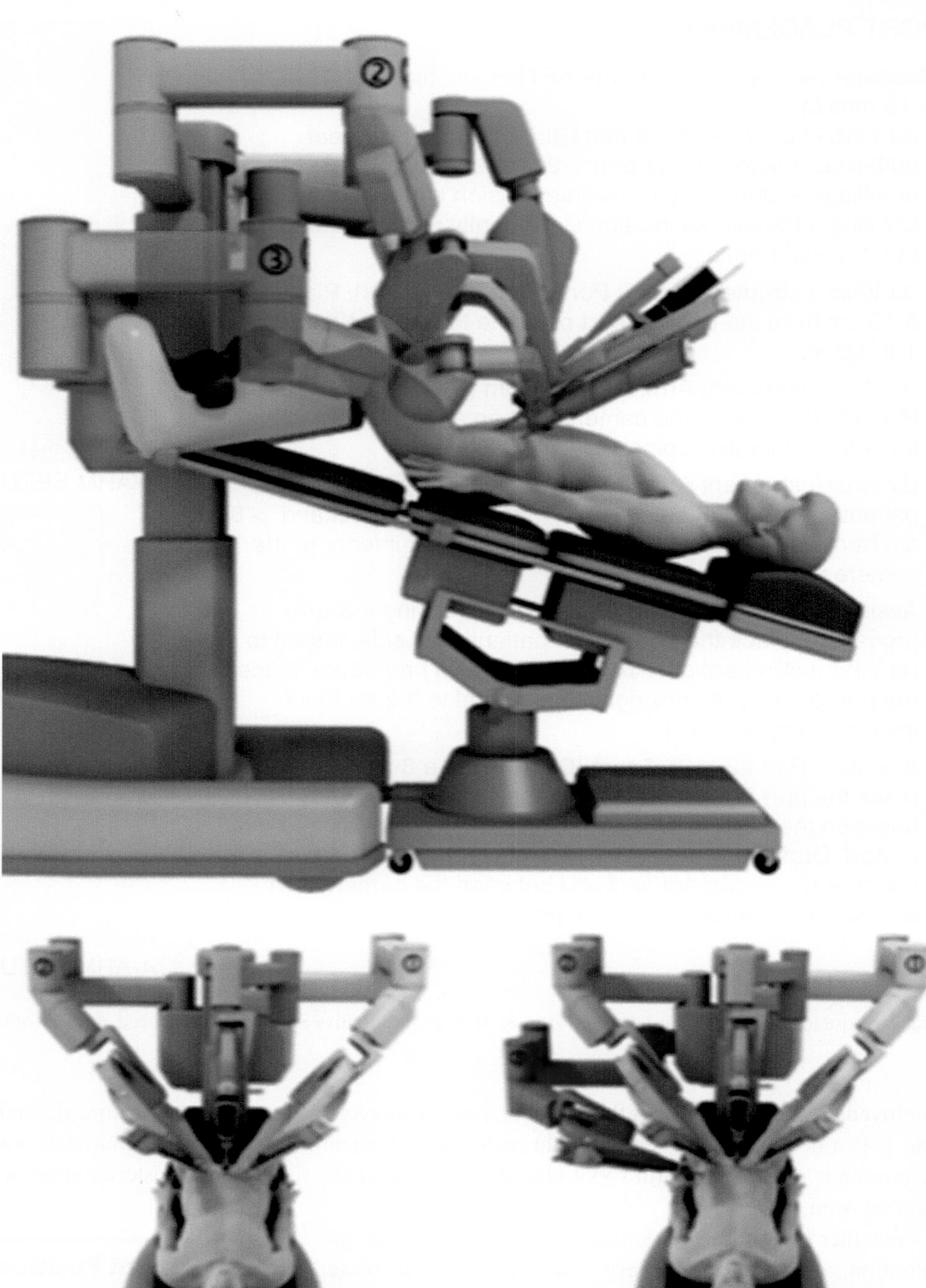

Fig. 3 Diagrams of docking "between the legs, Si." (Copyright Intuitive Surgical—reproduced courtesy of the manufacturer)

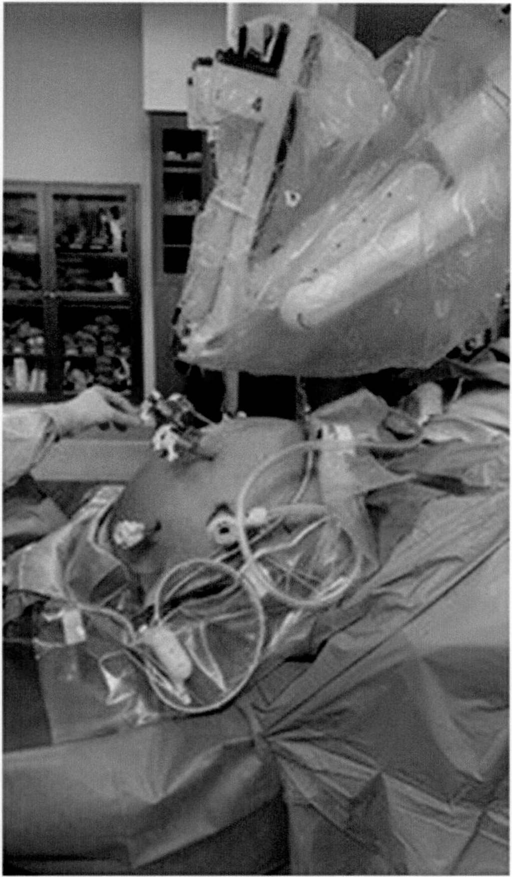

Fig. 4 Traditional docking "between the legs" with the DaVinci Xi. (Photo courtesy R. J. Leveillee, MD, FRCS-G)

provides several advantages, including patients with prior abdominal surgeries, avoiding lysis of adhesions. The abdomen is also left unviolated, easing subsequent abdominal exploration.

7 Da Vinci SP Port Placement

An open Hasson technique is used for the single-port placement. The SP trocar is 2.5 cm in diameter (Fig. 10) and is inserted with a blunt trocar which requires an initial fascial opening. The latter should be kept at less than 2 cm to ensure it stays snug in the fascia. It is an unribbed trocar that can easily slide in and out of the abdominal cavity with motion. Desufflation of the abdomen can cause the abdominal fascia to slide away from the robotic port while the latter stays fixed in space. Intra-Abdominal pressure is routinely kept between 8 and 10 mm Hg.

8 SP Intraperitoneal Access

For a single-port intraperitoneal access, the initial port is best placed cephalad to the umbilicus, usually 20 cm away from the pubis. This facilitates visualization of the necessary landmarks for the bladder take-down step, such as the pubic bone and bilateral vas deferens. The instruments must be deployed about 10 cm away from the tip of the trocar to allow extension of the instrument's elbow and subsequent internal triangulation toward the target organ. Adequate visualization of the medial umbilical ligaments and the urachus is helpful to ensure a good dissection.

9 SP Extraperitoneal Access

A midline 3–4-centimeter incision is made 2–4 cm below the umbilicus (Fig. 11). The fascia is incised in the midline exposing the underlying supravesical fat. A finger can be used to develop the retropubic space bluntly. Given the potential risk of bleeding, we prefer using a balloon dilator to create the extraperitoneal space. With a camera placed inside the balloon, the space is developed under direct vision. Once the epigastric vessels are visualized, the insufflation is discontinued.

There is no need to create additional space laterally even when an additional trocar is used or with a "Plus One" technique (Figs. 12 and 13). This contrasts with the multiport approach where the balloon is inflated maximally to create space laterally for additional robotic arms or assistant trocars. In the early adoption phase of the SP robot, a "Plus One" technique allows the surgeon to benefit from the help of a skilled assistant (Fig. 14). The assistant can retract, use a suction device, or clip as necessary, similar to the standard multiport approach.

Once the retropubic space is developed, the SP trocar can be inserted directly, provided that the fascial opening is less than the trocar site for allowing a tight fit. This approach works for supraumbilical docking. For infraumbilical docking, which is required for the extraperitoneal route, the trocar length and the need for the SP instruments to fully deploy require the trocar entry point to be further away from the fascial opening. In this scenario, we use a GelPOINT (Applied Medical, Rancho Santa Margarita, CA, USA) system to provide the appropriate space for the instrument deployment (Figs. 15 and 16). The SP also has a port access kit that facilitates docking away from the fascial opening. The wound protector is

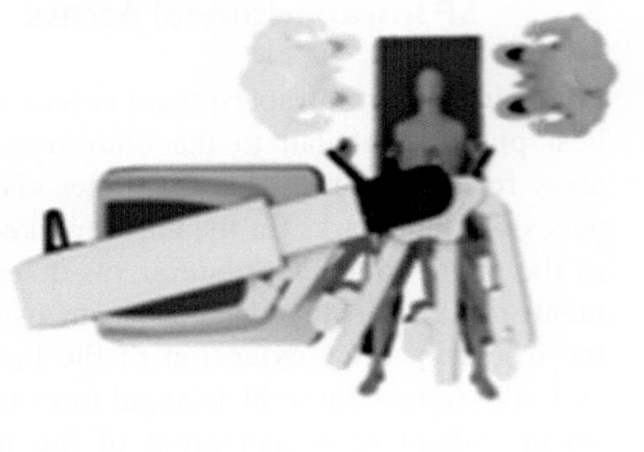

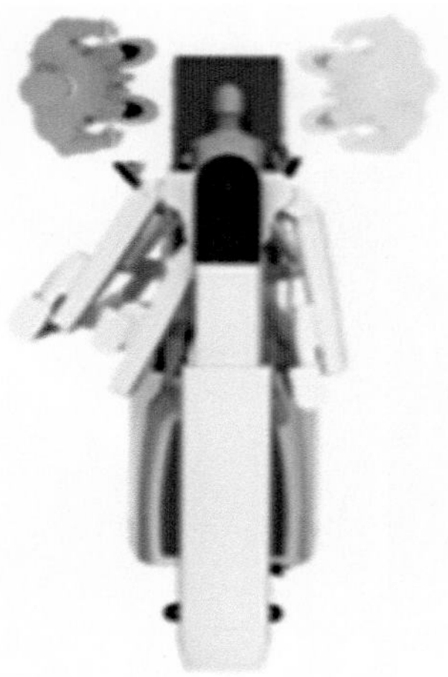

Anatomy	**Anatomy**
Pelvic	Pelvic
Cart Location	**Cart Location**
Patient Right (shown) or Left	Patient Legs
Working Direction	**Working Direction**
Towards Feet	Towards Feet

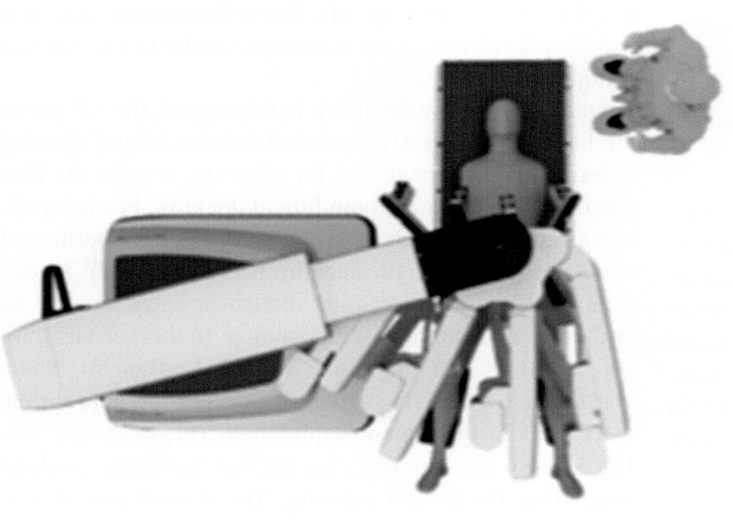

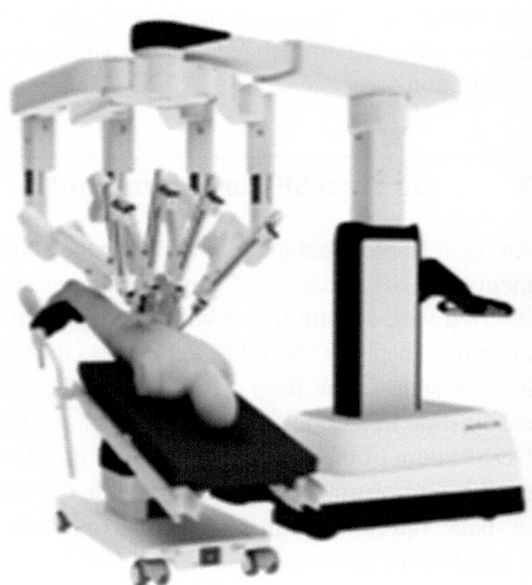

APPROACH 'PATIENT RIGHT' IS SHOWN

Fig. 5 Schematic demonstrating the versatility of the Xi system illustrating the "side docking" approach. (Copyright Intuitive Surgical—reproduced courtesy of the manufacturer)

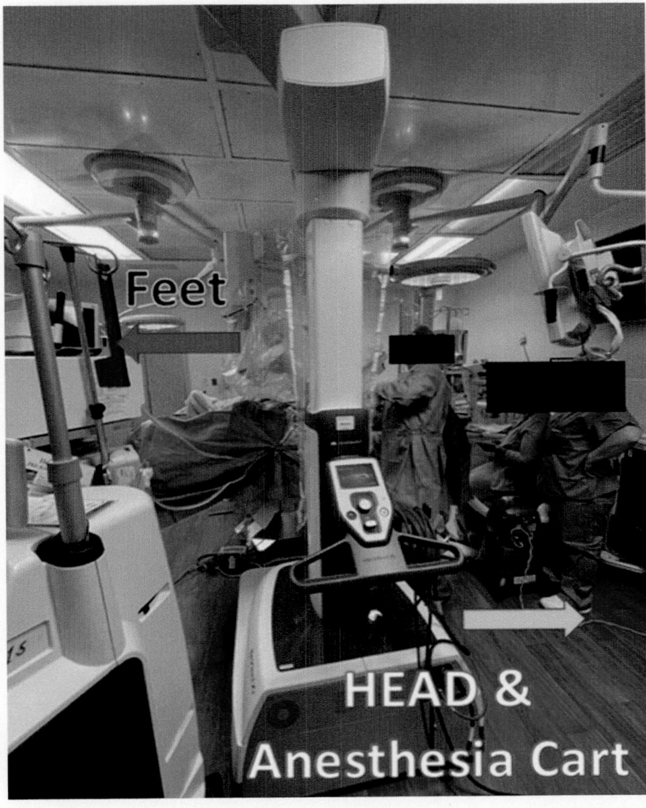

Fig. 6 View of "Side docking" from the patient's left side. Patient feet (red arrow). Patient's head and anesthesia cart (yellow arrow). (Photo courtesy R. J. Leveillee, MD, FRCS-G)

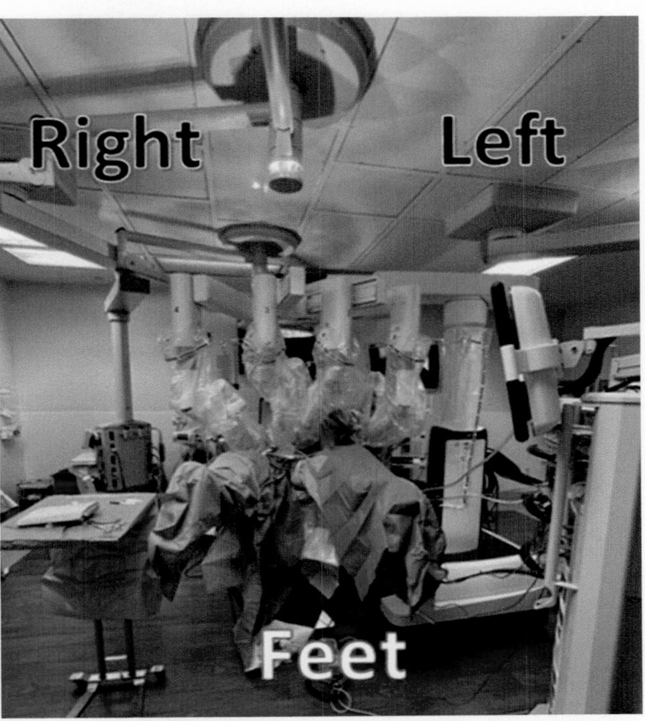

Fig. 7 View of "Side docking" from the patient's feet. Surgical cart is at the patient's left. (Photo courtesy R. J. Leveillee, MD, FRCS-G)

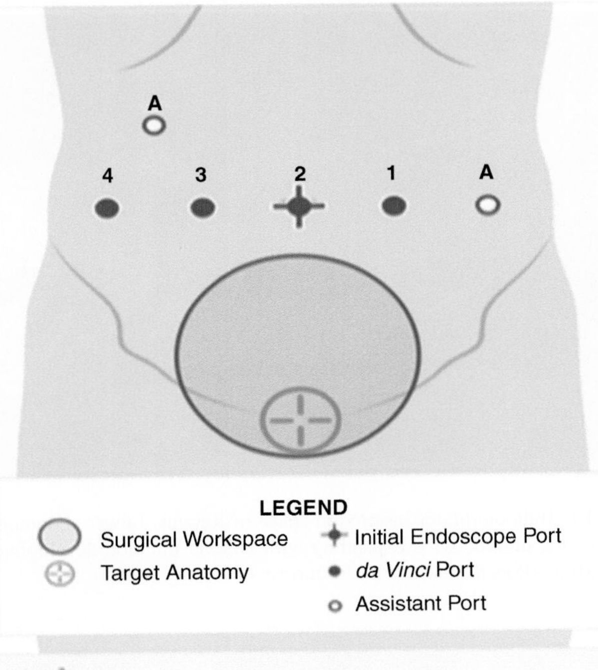

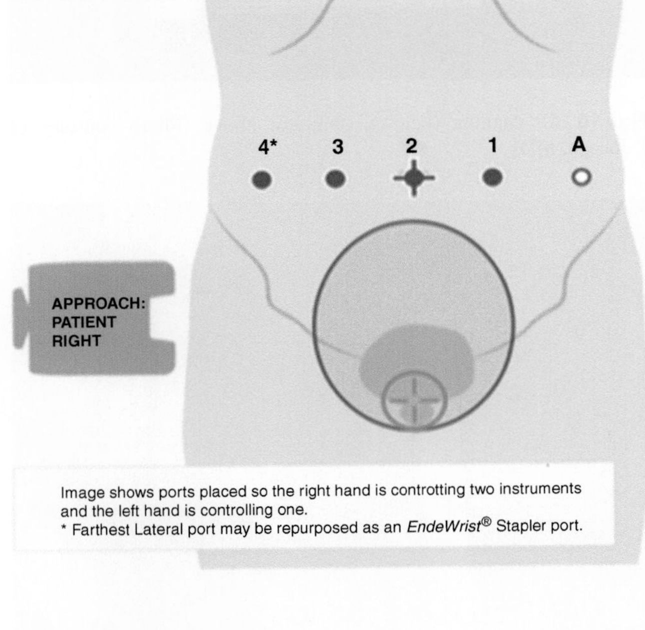

Fig. 8 Schematic demonstrating suggested port placement utilizing the "side docking" approach. For radical prostatectomy (Copyright Intuitive Surgical—reproduced courtesy of the manufacturer)

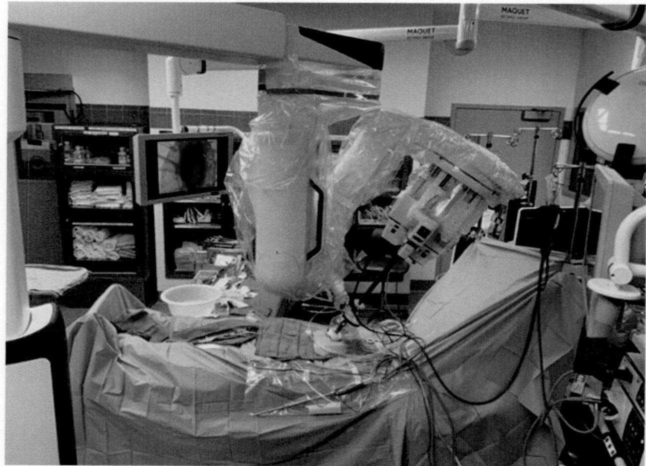

Fig. 9 SP Robot docked. Minimal Trendelenburg positioning (Photo courtesy of J. Joseph, MD)

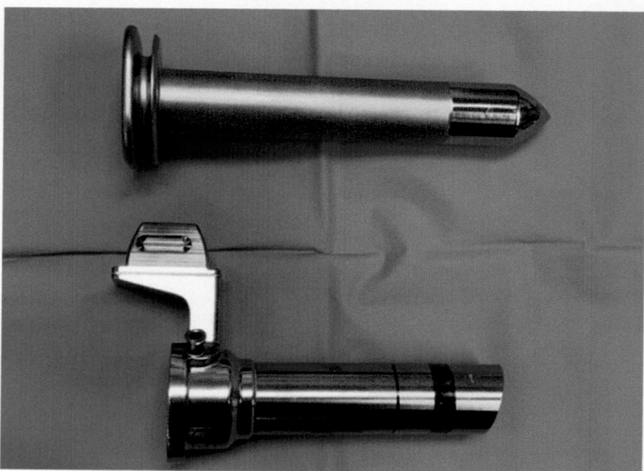

Fig. 10 SP cannula (below), obturator above (Photo courtesy of J. Joseph, MD)

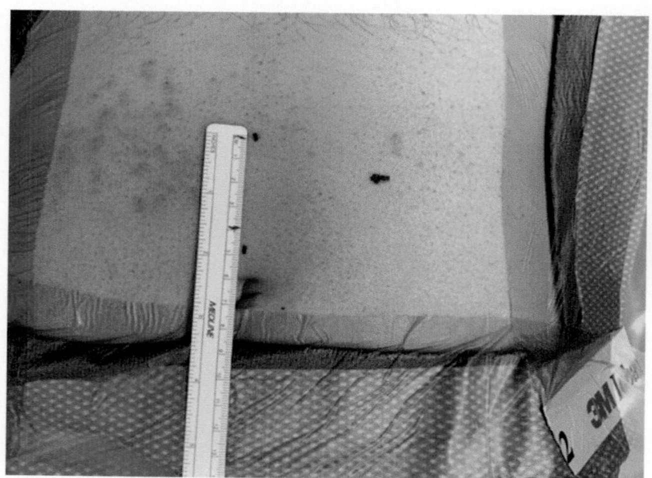

Fig. 11 View of midline (marking) of single-port site, and site of additional trocar for "Plus one" approach, marked in the right lower quadrant (Photo courtesy of J. Joseph, MD)

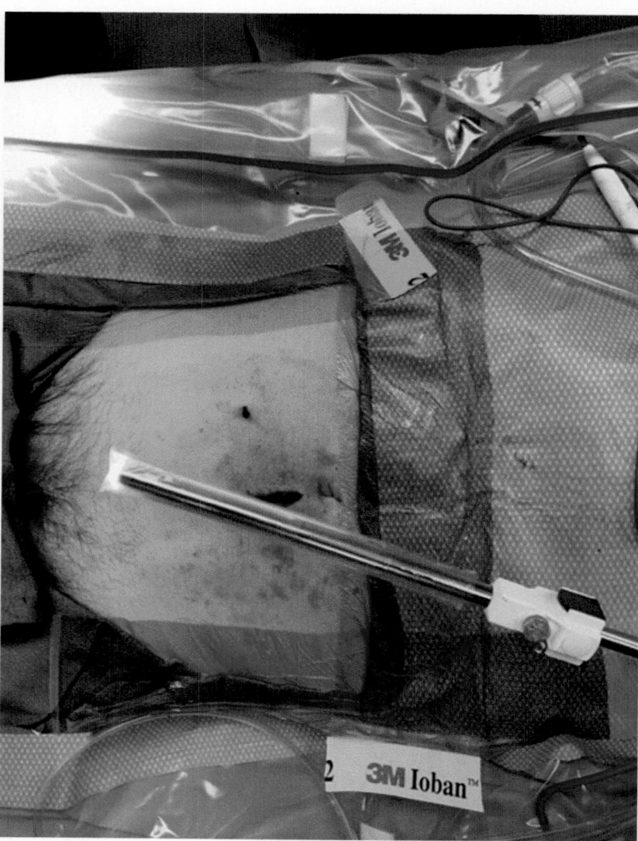

Fig. 12 View of midline single-port incision, with balloon dilator (Photo courtesy of J. Joseph, MD)

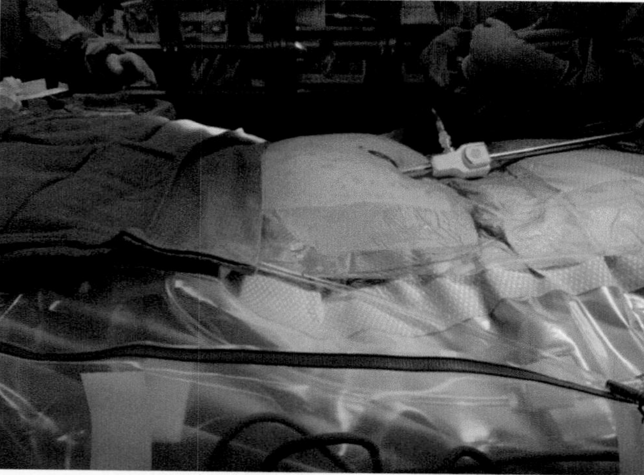

Fig. 13 Balloon dilator inserted in space of Retzius. Lower abdomen (below the umbilicus) is expanding with balloon inflation developing the extraperitoneal space. (Photo courtesy of J. Joseph, MD)

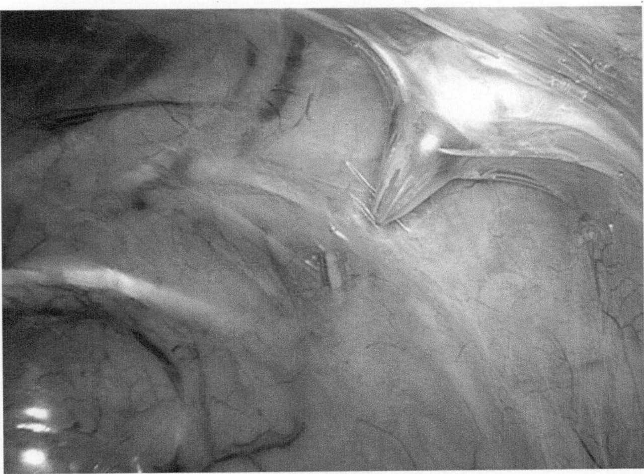

Fig. 14 View of inflated balloon dilator in the space of Retzius. The right epigastric vessels are visualized. The assistant trocar is being inserted in the right lower quadrant, lateral to the epigastric vessels. (Photo courtesy of J. Joseph, MD)

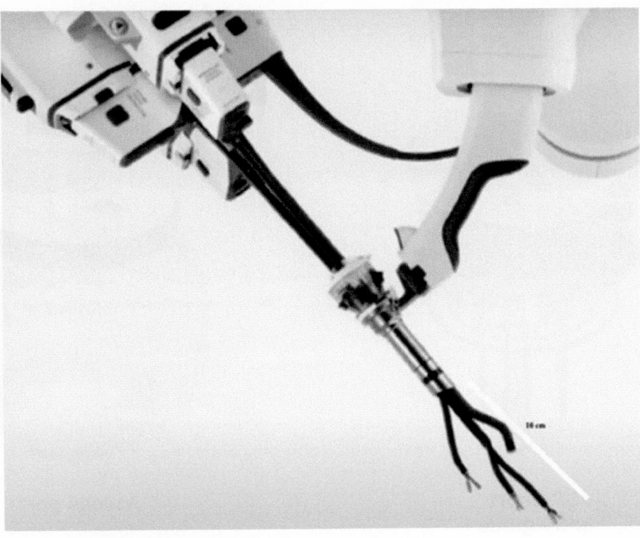

Fig. 16 View of instruments deployed through trocar (Courtesy of Intuitive Surgical, Sunnyvale, CA, USA)

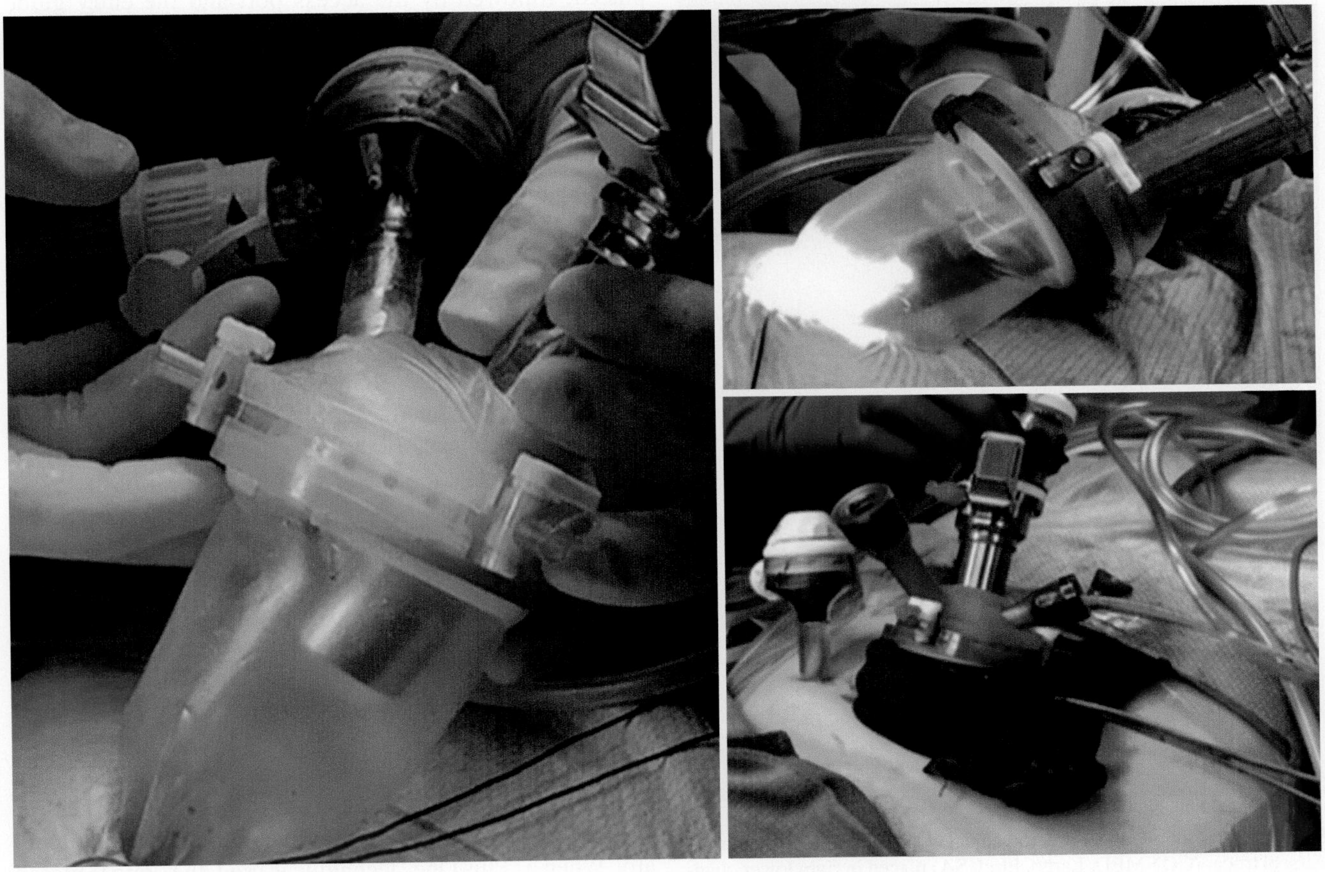

Fig. 15 View of GelPOINT in place with SP port and additional trocar inserted through the gel cap. A wet towel is used to keep gelcap elevated to increase distance from the fascia opening. (Photo courtesy of J. Joseph, MD)

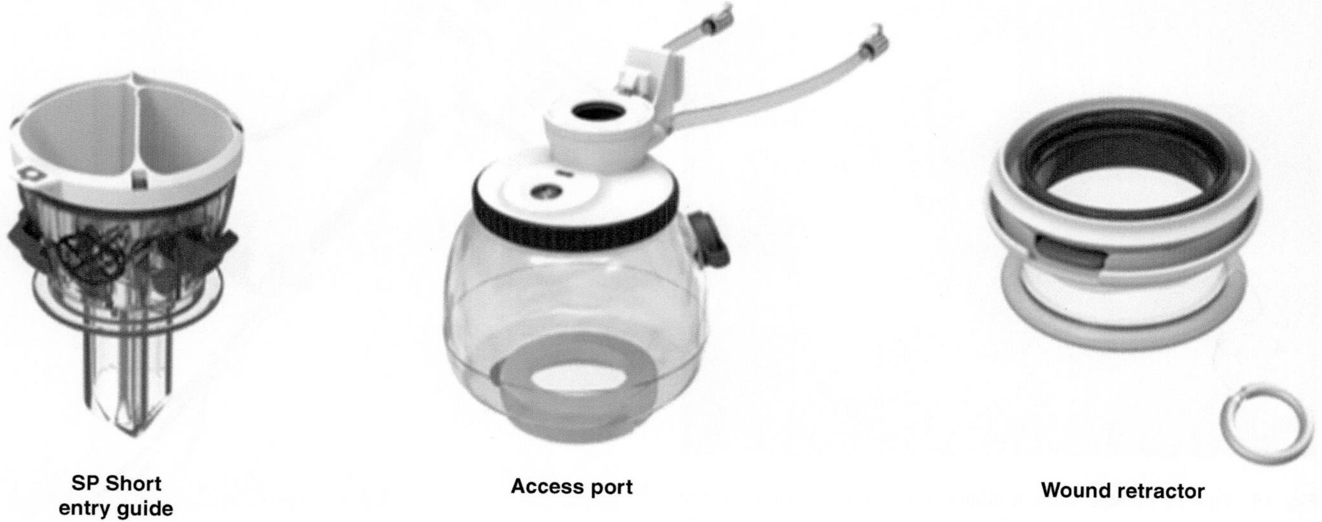

Fig. 17 View of the SP access port and its components. (Courtesy of Intuitive Surgical, Sunnyvale, CA, USA)

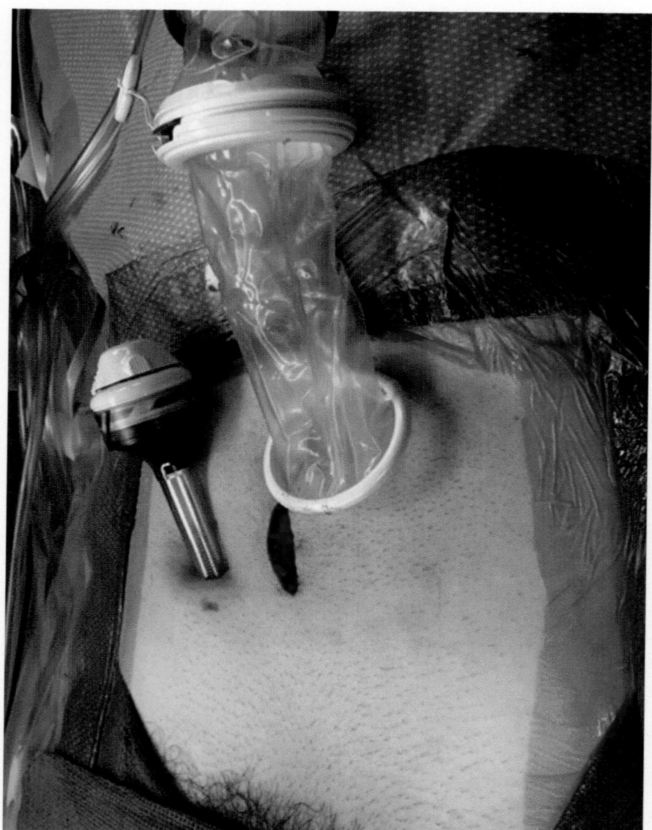

Fig. 18 View of wound retractor adjacent to midline skin opening. Airseal trocar (CONMED, Largo, FL, USA) placed in right lower quadrant (Photo courtesy of J. Joseph, MD)

placed, followed by the access port and the entry guide (Figs. 17 and 18). The metal trocar is not necessary when the entry guide is used, and the robot is directly connected to the latter.

The wound retractor sleeve is rolled inward, coiling all redundant sleeve components into the ring overlying the abdominal wall. Then, the SP access port and guide are connected before docking the robot as illustrated by Figs. 19 and 20. Figure 21 illustrates the final port placement and the robotic docking to SP kit access port.

The SP Kit access port offers several advantages. The clear port allows visualization of the instruments as they pass into the fascial opening. It contains an assistant port that can rotate, allowing entry from multiple directions, including several other accessory ports. With experience, these ports obviate the need for an extra trocar placed via a separate opening. The specimen can be placed in the "bowl" of the SP access port. This is advantageous in the extraperitoneal space where actual spacing can be limiting (Fig. 22). Removing the specimen from the operative field facilitates anastomosis (Fig. 23). The robot can also be quickly undocked to examine the specimen and redocked for the lymph node dissection or the completion of the vesicourethral anastomosis.

Upon completion of the procedure, the midline fascia opening is closed. We routinely use a drain regardless of whether the prostatectomy was done intra or extraperitoneally. When a "Plus One" technique is used, the drain is placed in that site (Fig. 24).

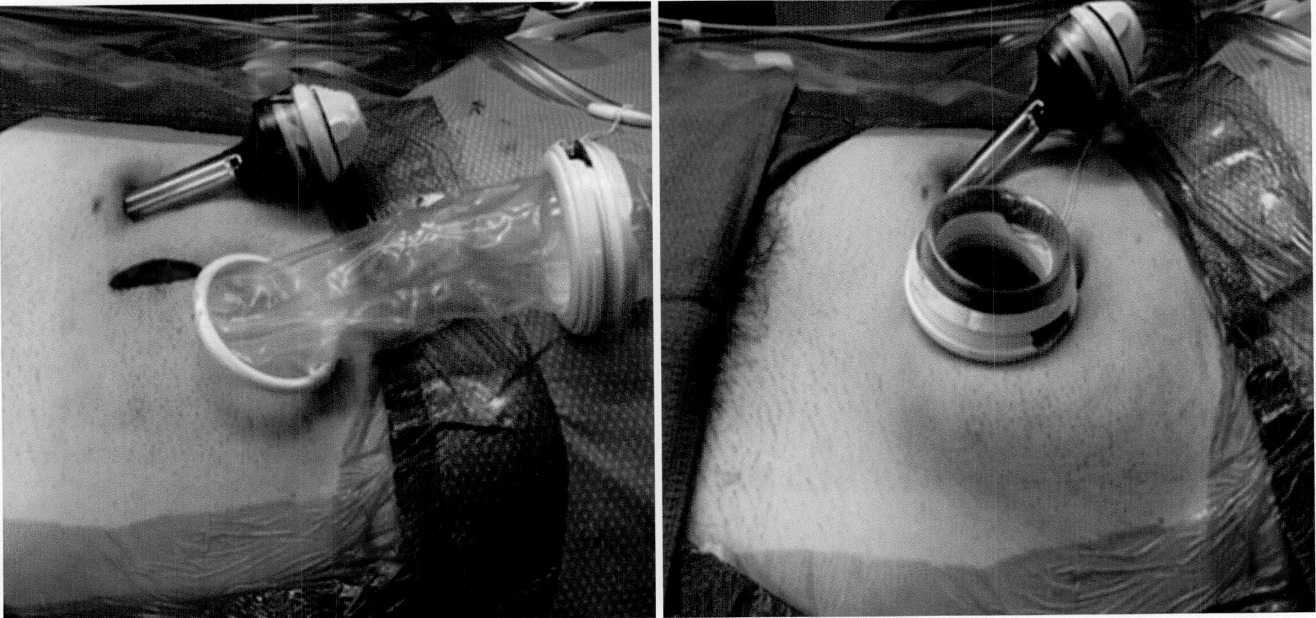

Fig. 19 Wound retractor in place before and after coiling (Photo courtesy of J. Joseph, MD)

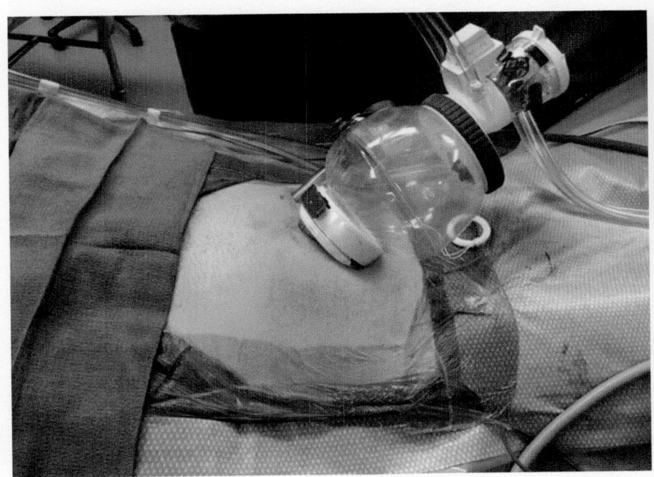

Fig. 20 SP access port and entry guide in place (Photo courtesy of J. Joseph, MD)

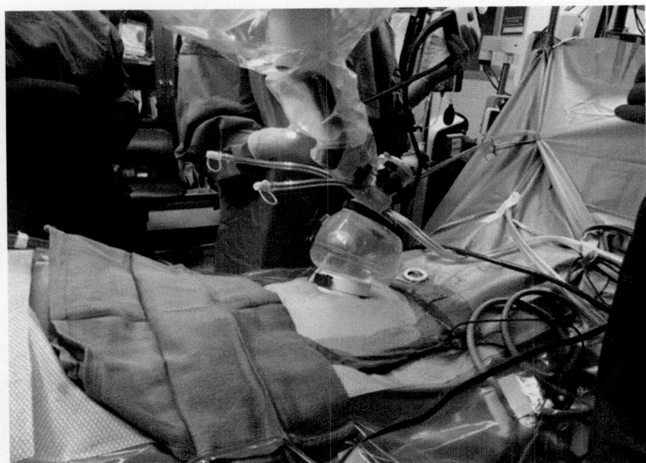

Fig. 21 Close-up view of robot docking using SP kit access port (Photo courtesy of J. Joseph, MD)

10 Conclusion

In this chapter, we have described the details and principles about the trocar placement in patients who underwent radical prostatectomy with the multiport and single-port robotic platforms. After years of experience with robotic surgery, we believe that appropriate patient positioning and port placement are the first step for optimal operative visualization and performance while minimizing the risks of perioperative complications.

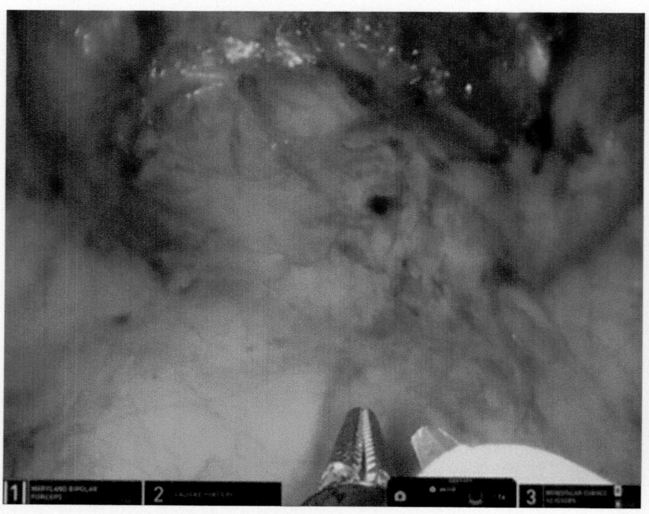

Fig. 22 Retropubic space view after docking (Photo courtesy of J. Joseph, MD)

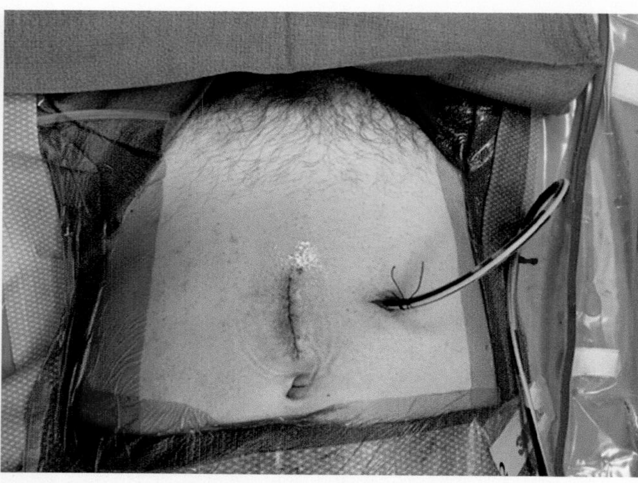

Fig. 24 Postoperative view following prostatectomy. Drain placed in the right lower quadrant (Photo courtesy of J. Joseph, MD)

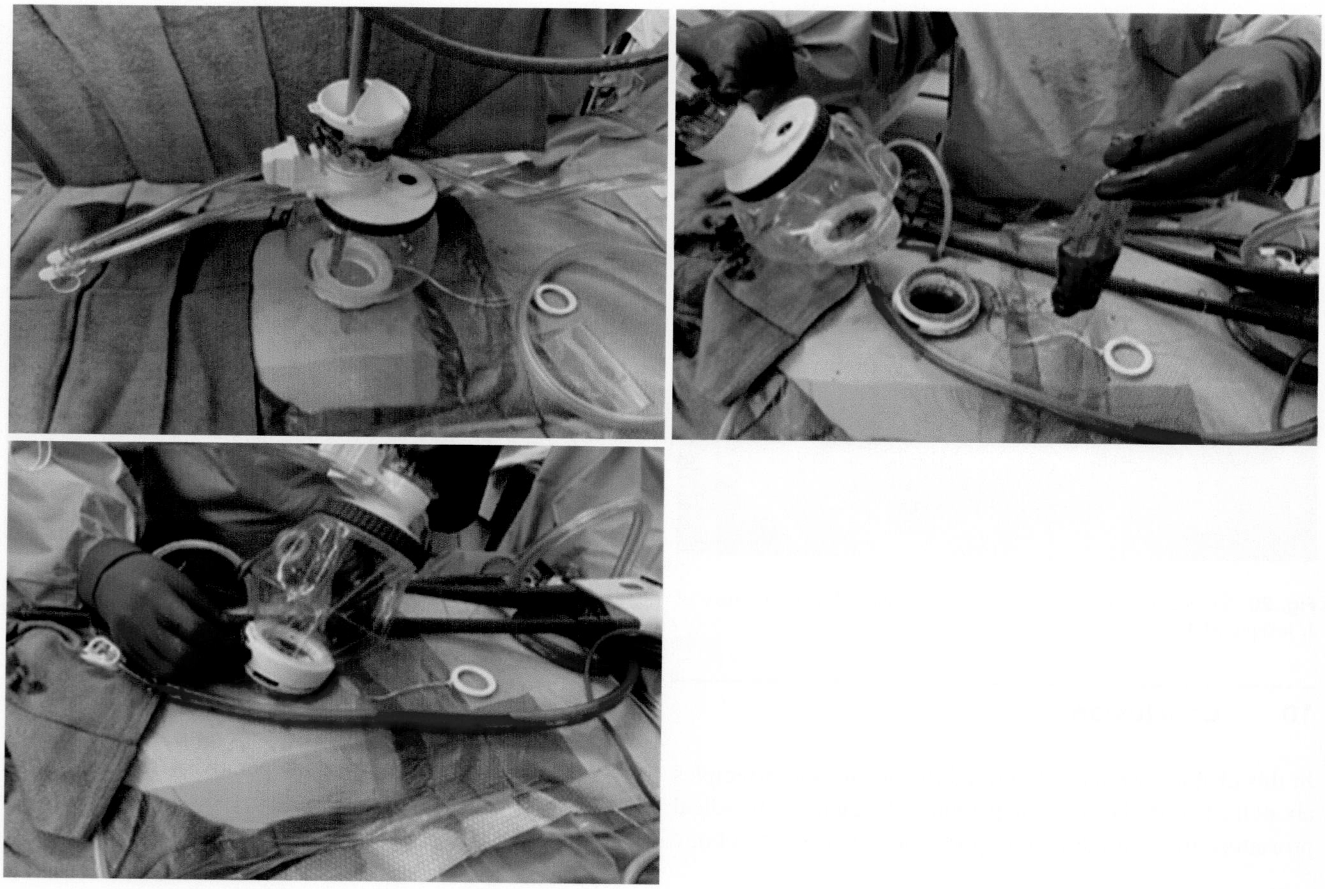

Fig. 23 Transillumination through the access port. The specimen can be visualized (bottom). (Photo courtesy of J. Joseph, MD)

Step-by-Step Approach to Robotic-Assisted Radical Prostatectomy

Marcio Covas Moschovas, Kenneth J. Palmer, Kris Maes, Luísa Alves, and Vipul Patel

1 Introduction

Robotic surgery is constantly evolving since the first procedure was cleared by the FDA (Food and Drug Administration) in 2000. Despite the technological advancements provided by successive generations of the da Vinci Robot, urinary continence, and erectile dysfunction are still unpredictable following robotic-assisted radical prostatectomy (RARP) [1–4]. Recent studies and metanalyses reported incontinence rates ranging from 14% to 31% and erectile dysfunction from 32% to 81% [5, 6]. However, new studies comparing techniques of RARP described improvements in early potency and continence rates after modifying the apical dissection and preserving the lateral prostatic fascia [7].

Among different factors associated with the preservation of functional outcomes following RARP, preoperative SHIM score, degree of nerve sparing, age, pathological stage, and D'Amico class are the most relevant [8]. Excluding the patient's preoperative characteristics, technique with degrees of nerve-sparing is the only factor potentially controlled by the surgeon. In this scenario, the surgical technique is continuously evolving because functional and oncological outcomes still did not reach 100%. In this chapter, we are describing the details of our most recent RARP technique after performing more than 15,000 RARP.

M. C. Moschovas (✉) · V. Patel
AdventHealth Global Robotics Institute, Celebration, USA

University of Central Florida, UCF, Orlando, USA

K. J. Palmer
AdventHealth Global Robotics Institute, Celebration, USA

K. Maes · L. Alves
Hospital da Luz, Lisbon, Portugal

2 Preoperative Routine

For each patient, in our preoperative routine, we consider the age, body mass index (BMI), comorbidities, prostatic-specific antigen (PSA) levels and trends, prostate biopsy report (Gleason /ISUP) [9], and Median Charlson Comorbidity Index age-adjusted. To access the sexual and urinary function, we use the Sexual Health Inventory for Men (SHIM) and American Urologic Association (AUA) symptom score questionnaires before and after the surgery. Before surgery, all patients underwent a complete physical examination and a digital rectal exam (DRE) for cancer staging.

Operative complications are reported according to the modified Clavien–Dindo classification [10]. Continence is defined as the use of no pads and potency as erections firm enough for satisfactory sexual intercourse with or without using PDE-5. Biochemical recurrence was defined as two consecutive prostate-specific antigens (PSA) >0.2 ng/ml.

3 Da Vinci Xi Instruments Setup

- 8 mm Scope
- Monopolar scissors.
- Long Maryland Bipolar.
- Needle drivers.
- Prograsp.

4 Surgical Technique

4.1 Patient Positioning and Trocar Placement

We place the patient in dorsal decubitus with pads in all points of articulations. After general anesthesia and antibiotic prophylaxis, the anesthesia team performs a Transversus abdominis plaine (TAP) block [11].

P. Wiklund et al. (eds.), *Robotic Urologic Surgery*, https://doi.org/10.1007/978-3-031-00363-9_18

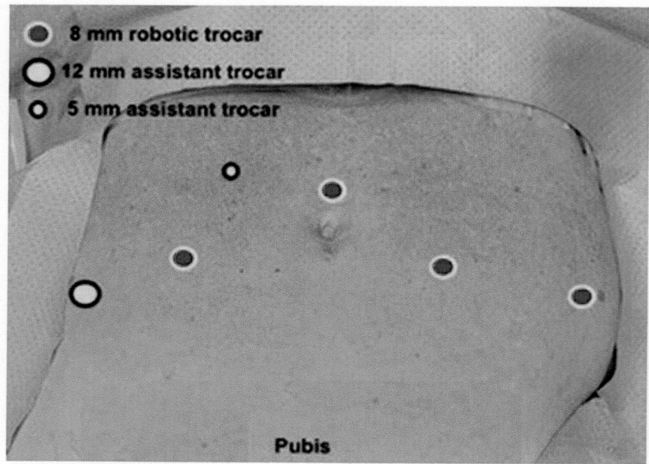

Fig. 1 Trocar placement

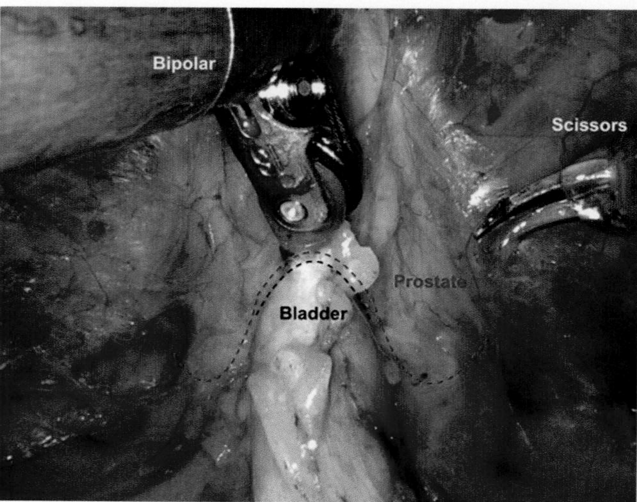

Fig. 2 Anterior bladder neck

After anesthesia, a supraumbilical midline incision is performed and the pneumoperitoneum is achieved with Veress needle. In sequence, we place four robotic trocars and 2 assistant trocars in the conventional position for RARP (Fig. 1). Then, we use an AirSeal® system to provide a constant pneumoperitoneum of 10 mmHg during the procedure. The table is then angled to 26 degrees Trendelenburg position, and the robot is docked on the left side of the patient.

4.2 Retzius Space Access and Bladder Takedown

Instruments used: Scissors (Right arm), Maryland bipolar (Left arm), Prograsp (fourth arm), Scope (30 degrees up or down).

Once the robot is docked, and instruments are placed, the peritoneum is then incised using the bipolar and scissors on the umbilical ligaments to enter Retzius' space extending to the pubic bone up and medially, and the vas deferens laterally, fully exposing the anterior aspect of the prostate. It is crucial to start the Retzius space dissection on the lateral side of both umbilical ligaments.

Once the prostate is accessed, we usually dissect the prostatic fat for skeletonizing the puboprostatic ligaments for optimal apex and dorsal vein complex (DVC) visualization.

4.3 Anterior Bladder Neck Incision

Instruments used: Scissors (Right arm), Maryland bipolar (Left arm), Prograsp (fourth arm).

The precise location of the bladder neck is identified by using the double pinch maneuver and pulling on the catheter repeatedly. In some cases, there is a deviation of the catheter toward one side, which indicates the presence of a possible median lobe or, less frequently, a ureterocele. Once identified, the bladder neck is horizontally incised with scissors and bipolar (applying traction) in a downward direction until reaching the Foley catheter (Fig. 2), which will then be used as upward traction for delineating and approaching the posterior bladder neck.

Some technique variations are described in the literature during this step because some centers, such as Hospital da Luz (Portugal), tend to preserve the bladder neck when anatomically possible [4]. In our technique, we open the BN performing the reconstruction before the anastomosis.

4.4 Posterior Bladder Neck and Seminal Vesicle Dissection

Instruments used: *Scissors (Right arm), Maryland bipolar (Left arm), Prograsp (fourth arm).*

Using the catheter as upward traction (with fourth Prograsp), the plane between the bladder neck and the prostate is dissected until reaching the seminal vesicles. Special care is taken during this step to flatten the lateral aspects of the bladder before entering the posterior dissection. This ensures ample exposure and adequate bladder neck width circumferentially, allowing for a subsequent watertight anastomosis. It is crucial to check the ureteral orifices (UOs) location and anatomy before proceeding to the posterior dissection (Fig. 3). It is necessary to identify the musculofascial plate correctly during the dissection, avoiding the wrong dissection into prostatic tissue. Vertical muscle fibers (retrotrigonal fibromuscular layer) are key landmarks in posterior bladder dissection. A horizontal incision of this tissue will expose fatty tissue until the seminal vesicle space.

Once reached, the seminal vesicles are ligated at the tip using hem-o-loc clips and traction provided by the fourth arm. Upon their release, the SVs are used as upward traction to enter the posterior plane through Denonvilliers' fascia and dissect the rectum of the prostate. It is crucial to minimize the energy use in this step, especially during the seminal vesicle tip, to avoid damaging the posterior neural fibers.

4.5 Denonvilliers' Fascia (DF) and Posterior Neurovascular Bundle (NVB) Preservation

Instruments used: Scissors (Right arm), Maryland bipolar (Left arm), Prograsp (fourth arm), Scope (30 up).

The DF comprises multiple layers of connective tissue created of the fusion between the posterior prostatic fascia and the seminal vesical fascia presenting an enormous interpatient variability in terms of tension and thickness [12]. Laterally, it ends in the neurovascular bundles at the prostatic pedicles.

After incising the posterior fascia, the camera is toggled from 30 degrees down to 30 degrees up. The dissection of this plane encompasses entering in between (Fig. 4a) the layers of DF (pearly white plane). Once we reached and dissected this avascular plane, we start preserving the NVB by accessing the prostatic fascia from 5 to 1 o'clock on the right side and 7 to 11 o'clock on the left side (Fig. 4b). During this step, we use the prostatic vasculature (prostatic artery) as landmarks to guide the nerve-sparing degrees of preservation [13, 14]. The degrees of nerve-sparing vary according to the tumor Grade, tumor location, and Neural bundle anatomy.

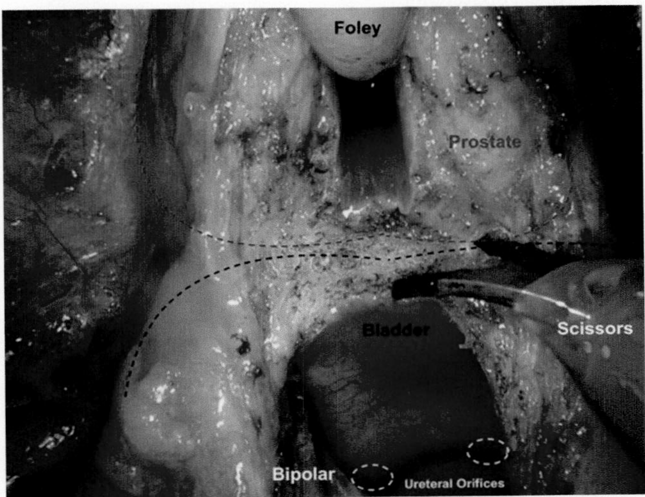

Fig. 3 Posterior bladder neck and ureteral orifices

4.6 Retrograde Neurovascular Preservation

Instruments used: Scissors (Right arm), Maryland bipolar (Left arm), Prograsp (fourth arm), Scope (30 down).

Upon completing the posterior plane, the endopelvic fascia (EF) is opened medially, next to the prostate, to complete a retrograde nerve spare while preserving the lateral aspect of EF. After communicating the lateral with the posterior plane, the nerve preservation is performed with an athermal dissection and by using hem-o-lock clips for vascular control of the prostatic pedicles bilaterally.

Our recent modification described the preservation of the lateral prostatic fascia in selected cases to improve neural preservation and increase early potency rates (Fig. 5) [7]. The Endopelvic fascia is attached to the pelvic fascia diaphragm and tendinous arch covering the levator muscle fibers. Its anterior reflection forms the puboprostatic ligaments. Sharp and blunt dissections during endopelvic fascia incision and release of levator fibers from the

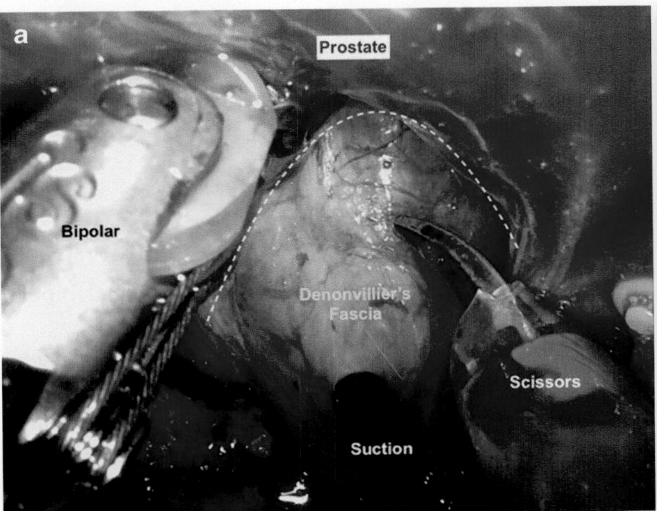

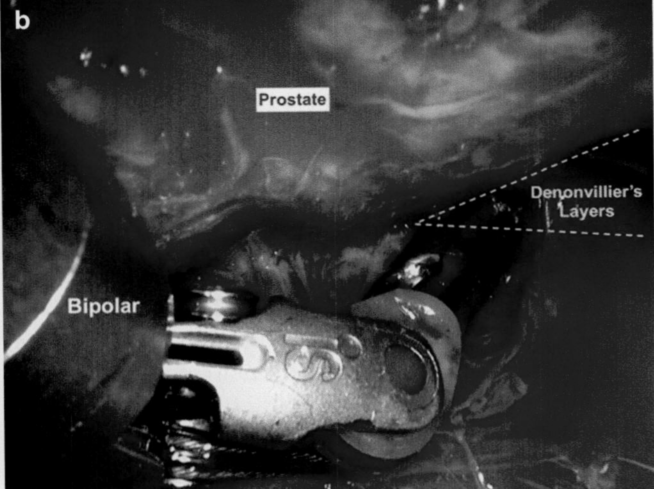

Fig. 4 (**a**) Dissection plane between DF. (**b**) Posterior Nerve-sparing

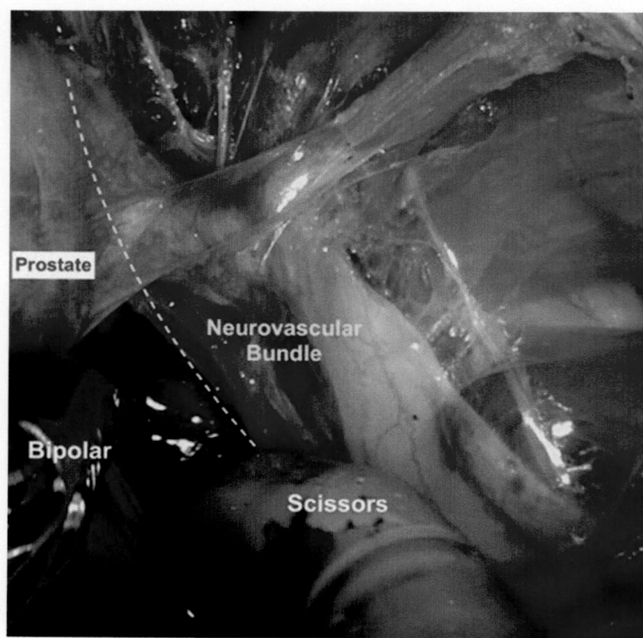

Fig. 5 Retrograde Nerve-sparing dissection

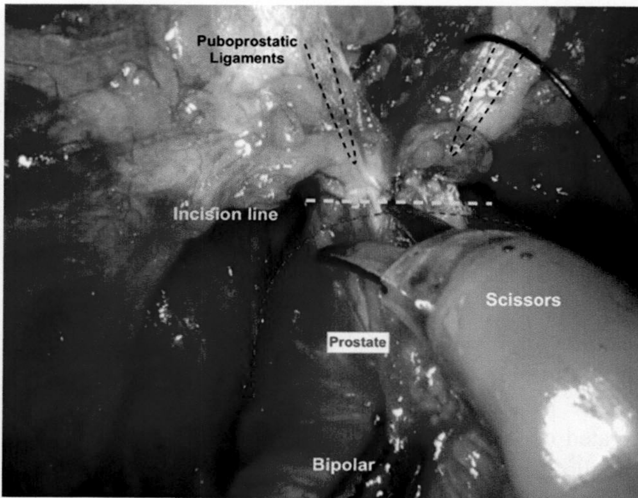

Fig. 6 Apical dissection

prostatic apex could injure the levator muscle, which has crucial importance for continence [15, 16]. Additionally, endopelvic fascia is closely related to the neurovascular bundles, which emerge from the pelvic plexus and run laterally to the bladder neck and on the anterolateral aspect of the prostate [3].

4.7 Apical Dissection and DVC Control

Instruments used: Scissors (Right arm), Maryland bipolar (Left arm), Prograsp (fourth arm).

The apical dissection, another modification of our technique [7], is performed from the base toward the urethra, underneath the puboprostatic ligaments, preserving the maximum amount of periurethral tissue and urethral length (Minimal apical dissection) (Fig. 6). The urethral sphincter is a complex structure distal to the prostate apex and in a close relationship but functionally independent from the muscular pelvic floor. Some challenges in this step regard the variation in apical anatomy and the absence of a clear transition between the prostate capsule and urethra. The correct apical dissection has implications in functional and oncological outcomes [4, 7, 17].

After approaching the urethra, the Prograsp pulls the prostate downward (performing traction), and the DVC is closed with a running suture (Quill® 2.0) while the abdominal pressure is maintained at 6–8 mmHg. After controlling the DVC, we return the pressure to 10 mmHg.

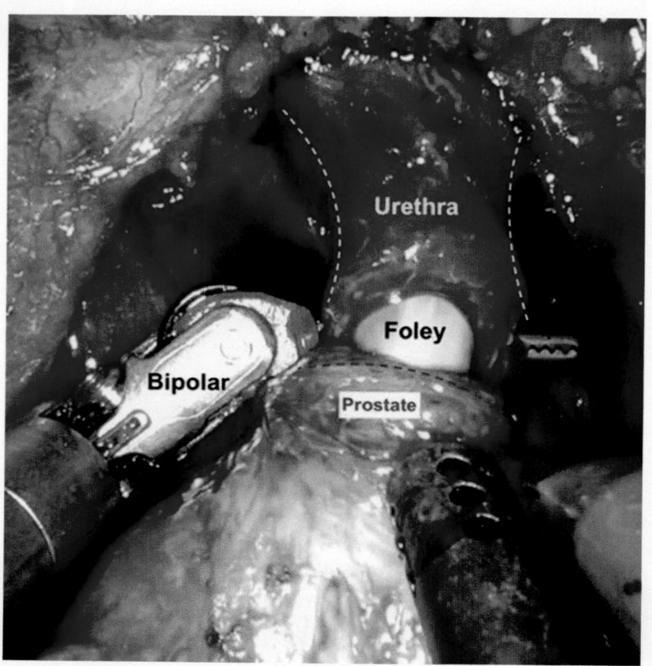

Fig. 7 Urethra division

4.8 Urethra Division

Instruments used: Scissors (Right arm), Maryland bipolar (Left arm), Prograsp (fourth arm).

The urethra is divided with cold scissors, avoiding cautery energy, especially when reaching the mucosa, while ensuring maximum length and periurethral tissue preservation (Fig. 7). During this step, we maintain the Prograsp, applying downward traction on the prostate.

4.9 Bladder Neck and Posterior Reconstruction

Instruments used: Needle drivers (Right and Left arm), Prograsp (fourth arm).

The bladder neck reconstruction is performed by plicating the lateral aspects of the bladder wall with a barbed suture (Quill® 2.0) and running it medially and back laterally (to the place of origin) until the bladder neck and urethra diameters are matched. An essential part of this step is verifying that the ureteral orifices (UOs) are preserved and distant from the edge of the bladder neck.

The posterior reconstruction is performed with Rocco's technique in two planes by approaching the cut edge of Denonvilliers' fascia to the rhabdosphincter (first plane) and then the posterior lip of the bladder neck to the posterior lip of the urethra (second plane) [18]. This step is performed with a single barbed suture (Quill® 2.0) with a loop at the end.

4.10 Anastomosis

Performed as a modified van Velthoven with a bidirectional running barbed suture starting at the 5 o'clock position (using the urethra as reference) and running the posterior aspect of it (clockwise) with one arm until reaching the 10 o'clock position and counterclockwise with the second arm until reaching the same position on the urethral stump where they are tied (Fig. 8) [19]. A new 16 Fr Foley catheter is then inserted and the bladder irrigated with saline solution to clear any clots and confirm a watertight anastomosis.

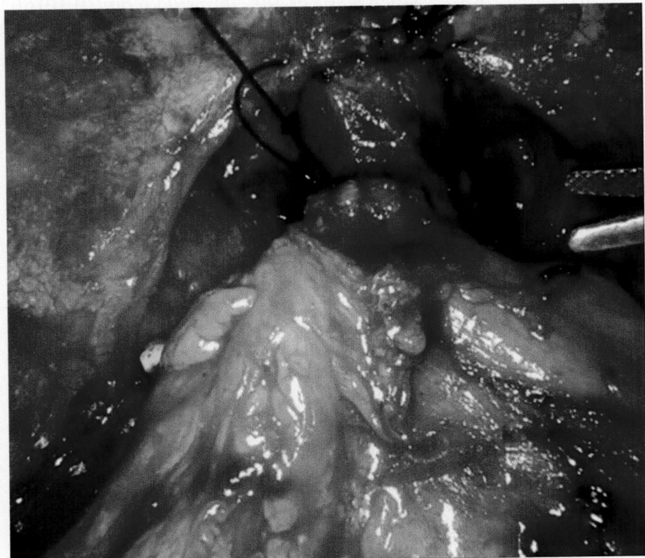

Fig. 8 Anastomosis

After the anastomosis, some centers, such as Hospital da Luz (Portugal), perform the anterior reconstruction, consisting of the re-attachment of the arcus tendinous to the anterior bladder neck through a 2/0 barbed running suture. Attention is taken to avoid piercing any accessory vessels and excessive tightening of the suture. This allows for anterior stabilization of the vesicourethral complex. In addition, after finishing the anastomosis, the peritoneum is closed with a 2/0 barbed running suture.

4.11 Lymphadenectomy

When performing the lymphadenectomy, we remove the standard template anteromedial to the external iliac vein and around the obturator nerve and vessels [20]. In our technique, we use Hem-o-lock® clips on the superior and inferior edges of the lymph node template.

5 Postoperative Routine

In our routine, no abdominal drain is placed at the end of the surgery. The postoperative analgesia is performed with non-opioid medication. The patients are stimulated to ambulate soon after anesthesia recovery, and patients with favorable recovery and clinical conditions are discharged on the same day of surgery.

After discharge, all patients return on the fifth postoperative day to remove the foley catheter and receive the final pathology report. Then, the next appointments are scheduled for six weeks, 3, 6, 9, and 12 months after surgery. During these appointments, we evaluated PSA, SHIM, and AUA scores.

6 RARP Technique Variations

Surgical techniques for RARP are not uniform among the different centers worldwide. However, the common concept to optimize functional and oncological outcomes lies in minimizing thermal and mechanic injury when approaching the neural bundles associated with apical and endopelvic anatomy preservation.

7 Conclusions

In this chapter, we have described our current step-by-step RARP technique after recent refinements. Potency and continence outcomes following Robotic-assisted radical prostatectomy still challenge surgeons and patients due to its multifactorial etiology. In this scenario, as long as we still do not have one hundred percent of the patients with optimal functional and oncological outcomes, we believe that surgical technique is constantly evolving with refinements and modifications in order to further improve functional results in patients undergoing surgical therapy for prostate cancer.

References

1. Bhat KRS, Moschovas MC, Onol FF, Rogers T, Reddy SS, Corder C, Roof S, Patel VR. Evidence-based evolution of our robot-assisted laparoscopic prostatectomy (RALP) technique through 13,000 cases. J Robot Surg 2020 Oct 10. https://doi.org/10.1007/s11701-020-01157-5. Epub ahead of print.
2. Basourakos SP, Kowalczyk KJ, Moschovas M, Dudley V, Shoag JE, Patel V, Hu JC. Robot-assisted radical prostatectomy maneuvers to attenuate erectile dysfunction: technical description and video compilation. J Endourol 2021 May 20. https://doi.org/10.1089/end.2021.0081. Epub ahead of print.
3. Kumar A, Patel VR, Panaiyadiyan S, Seetharam Bhat KR, Moschovas MC, Nayak B. Nerve-sparing robot-assisted radical prostatectomy: current perspectives. Asian J Urol. 2021 Jan;8(1):2–13. https://doi.org/10.1016/j.ajur.2020.05.012. Epub 2020 Jun 11. PMID: 33569267; PMCID: PMC7859364.
4. Martini A, Falagario UG, Villers A, Dell'Oglio P, Mazzone E, Autorino R, Moschovas MC, Buscarini M, Bravi CA, Briganti A, Sawczyn G, Kaouk J, Menon M, Secco S, Bocciardi AM, Wang G, Zhou X, Porpiglia F, Mottrie A, Patel V, Tewari AK, Montorsi F, Gaston R, Wiklund NP, Hemal AK. Contemporary techniques of prostate dissection for robot-assisted prostatectomy. Eur Urol 2020 Oct;78(4):583–591. https://doi.org/10.1016/j.eururo.2020.07.017. Epub 2020 Aug 1.
5. Ficarra V, Novara G, Rosen RC, et al. Systematic review and meta-analysis of studies reporting urinary continence recovery after robot-assisted radical prostatectomy. Eur Urol. 2012;62:405–17.
6. Ficarra V, Novara G, Ahlering TE, et al. Systematic review and meta- analysis of studies reporting potency rates after robot-assisted radical prostatectomy. Eur Urol. 2012;62:418–30.
7. Covas Moschovas M, Bhat S, Onol FF, Rogers T, Roof S, Mazzone E, Mottrie A, Patel V. Modified apical dissection and lateral prostatic fascia preservation improves early postoperative functional recovery in robotic-assisted laparoscopic radical prostatectomy: results from a propensity score-matched analysis. Eur Urol 2020 Dec;78(6):875–884. https://doi.org/10.1016/j.eururo.2020.05.041. Epub 2020 Jun 24.
8. Bhat KRS, Moschovas MC, Sandri M, Dell'Oglio P, Onol FF, Rogers T, Reddy S, Noel J, Roof S, Sighinolfi MC, Rocco B, Patel VR. A predictive pre- and post-operative nomogram for post-operative potency recovery after robot-assisted radical prostatectomy. J Urol. 2021; https://doi.org/10.1097/JU.0000000000001895.
9. Epstein JI, Egevad L, Amin MB, Delahunt B, Srigley JR, Humphrey PA. The 2014 International Society of Urological Pathology (ISUP) con- sensus conference on Gleason grading of prostatic carcinoma: definition of grading patterns and proposal for a new grading system. Am J Surg Pathol. 2016;40:244–52.
10. Dindo D, Demartines N, Clavien PA. Classification of surgical com- plications: a new proposal with evaluation in a cohort of 6336 patients and results of a survey. Ann Surg. 2004;240:205–13.
11. Rogers T, Bhat KRS, Moschovas M. Use of transversus abdominis plain block to decrease pain score and narcotic use following robotic-assisted laparoscopic radical prostatectomy. J Robot Surg. 2020 Apr 22; https://doi.org/10.1007/s11701-020-01064-9.
12. Muraoka K, Hinata N, Morizane S, Honda M, Sejima T, Murakami G, et al. Site-dependent and interindividual variations in Denonvilliers' fascia: a histological study using donated elderly male cadavers. BMC Urol. 2015 May;15:42.
13. Schatloff O, Chauhan S, Sivaraman A, Kameh D, Palmer KJ, Patel VR. Anatomic grading of nerve sparing during robot-assisted radical prostatectomy. Eur Urol 2012 Apr;61(4):796–802. https://doi.org/10.1016/j.eururo.2011.12.048. Epub 2012 Jan 4.
14. Patel VR, Schatloff O, Chauhan S, et al. The role of the prostatic vasculature as a landmark for nerve sparing during robot-assisted radical prostatec- tomy. Eur Urol. 2012;61(3):571–6.
15. Nishimura M, Utsugi R. Impact of total fascia preservation on early recovery of urinary continence after radical prostatectomy. J Clin Urol. 2018;11(4):293–8.
16. Kwon SY, Lee JN, Kim HT, Kim TH, Kim BW, Choi GS, et al. Endopelvic fascia preservation during robot-assisted laparoscopic radical prostatectomy: does it affect urinary incontinence? Scand J Urol. 2014;48(6):506–12.
17. Walz J, Burnett AL, Costello AJ, Eastham JA, Graefen M, Guillonneau B, Menon M, Montorsi F, Myers RP, Rocco B, Villers A. A critical analysis of the current knowledge of surgical anatomy related to optimization of cancer control and preservation of continence and erection in candidates for radical prostatectomy. Eur Urol 2010 Feb;57(2):179–192. https://doi.org/10.1016/j.eururo.2009.11.009. Epub 2009 Nov 11.
18. Rocco B, Cozzi G, Spinelli MG, Coelho RF, Patel VR, Tewari A, Wiklund P, Graefen M, Mottrie A, Gaboardi F, Gill IS, Montorsi F, Artibani W, Rocco F. Posterior musculofascial reconstruction after radical prostatectomy: a systematic review of the literature. Eur Urol. 2012 Nov;62(5):779–90. https://doi.org/10.1016/j.eururo.2012.05.041.
19. Valero R, Schatloff O, Chauhan S, HwiiKo Y, Sivaraman A, Coelho RF, Palmer KJ, Davila H, Patel VR. Bidirectional barbed suture for bladder neck reconstruction, posterior reconstruction and vesicourethral anastomosis during robot assisted radical prostatectomy. Actas Urol Esp. 2012 Feb;36(2):69–74.
20. Walsh PC. Anatomic radical retropubic prostatectomy. In: Walsh PC, Retik AB, Vaughan Jr ED, Wein AJ, editors. Campbell's urology, Chapter 86, vol. III. 7th ed. Philadelphia, WB Saunders; 1997. p. 2565–88.

Outcomes of RALP: An Evidence-Based Approach

Maria Chiara Sighinolfi, Francesco Montorsi, Ahmed Eissa, and Vipul Patel

1 Introduction

Prostate cancer (PCa) is the third most common malignancy (7.3%) following breast (11.7%) and lung cancers (11.4%), and the eighth most common cause of cancer mortality (3.8%) in 2020. Furthermore, it is the most frequently diagnosed male cancer in 112 countries around the globe [1]. PCa represents a major health burden as it was responsible for 7.1 million disability-adjusted life-years (of which, 88% are years of life lost and 12% are years of life with disability) around the world in 2017 [2]. Radical prostatectomy (RP) is considered the mainstay of surgical treatment for men with localized PCa and life expectancy >10 years [3]. The first description of RP for treatment of PCa dates back to the early 1900s, when Young H [4], reported his experience with open perineal prostatectomy in 75 patients; however, this approach was associated with high morbidity and mortality as it was used in the era before the introduction of antibiotics, balloon catheters and blood transfusion in the medical practice. After approximately 40 years, Millin [5] modified the RP approach to be performed through an abdominal incision, yet it was still associated with severe blood loss from the dorsal venous complex (DVC) as it was not tied [6]. Later on, Walsh introduced several modifications to the retropubic RP technique including the ligation of the DVC and the nerve-sparing RP, which reduced the perioperative complications of this surgery and improved its outcomes [6]. As laparoscopic approaches became popular among surgeons, Raboy et al. [7], reported the first case of laparoscopic radical prostatectomy (LRP), which seemed to be associated with several advantages over the ORP, including less intraoperative blood loss and postoperative pain, and shorter hospitalization [8]; however, the laparoscopic approach was not devoid of drawbacks such as the longer operative time and learning curve, and the two-dimensional vision compared to the open approach [6]. In the early 2000s, robotic surgery was introduced and popularized because of its important advantages including three-dimensional (3D) vision, articulated instruments with seven degrees of freedom, magnified vision, tremors filtration, and shorter learning curve [8]. In this setting, the robotic approach to RP was first introduced in 2001 [9], and since then it gained great acceptance among surgeons and patients; as a consequence, to date, approximately 85% of RPs are performed through robotic-assisted laparoscopic approach in the USA [10, 11].

The present chapter reports the highest scientific evidence (Level 1) on robotic-assisted laparoscopic radical prostatectomy (RALP), by considering randomized controlled trials (RCT) and meta-analysis currently available in literature. A PubMed search was performed including the terms "robotic-assisted radical prostatectomy" OR "robotic-assisted laparoscopic prostatectomy" OR "RALP" OR "RARP" AND "randomized controlled" OR "Meta-analysis."

Articles dealing with the following topics were considered:

1. Comparison of different approaches to Radical Prostatectomy (open, laparoscopic, robotic).
2. Outcomes of RALP in special settings.
3. Techniques of prostate dissection.

M. C. Sighinolfi (✉)
Urology Department, ASST Santi Paolo e Carlo, University of Milan, Milan, Italy

F. Montorsi
Department of Urology and Division of Experimental Oncology, Urological Research Institute (URI), IRCCS San Raffaele Scientific Institute, Milan, Italy

A. Eissa
Urology Department, Faculty of Medicine, Tanta University, Tanta, Egypt

V. Patel
Global Robotics Institute, Florida Hospital-Celebration Health Celebration, University of Central Florida School of Medicine, Orlando, FL, USA

P. Wiklund et al. (eds.), *Robotic Urologic Surgery*, https://doi.org/10.1007/978-3-031-00363-9_19

Novelties and tools complementary to RALP were considered separately, with the inclusion of prospective comparative studies and retrospective matched-paired analysis or cohort studies.

1.1 Different Approaches to Radical Prostatectomy

Although robot-assisted approach is the most common approach for RP, there are still limited first-level evidence in the literature to support the superiority of any of the three approaches (ORP, LRP, and RALP) over the other due to the scarcity of randomized controlled trials comparing different approaches, where most of the available evidence is based on observational prospective or retrospective studies with low methodological quality [10, 12]. Furthermore, most of the systematic reviews and meta-analysis showed inconsistent and non-definitive conclusions [10, 13].

1.2 Evidence from Randomized Controlled Trials (RCTs)

Despite RALP being introduced more than two decades ago, there are scarce RCTs in the literature comparing it to other approaches (laparoscopic and open). This may be attributed to the difficult organization of such trials because the patients have the right to decide the type of surgical approach and the randomization concept may be unacceptable for them given the potential life-impacting consequences of different approaches [12]. To date, there are only six RCTs comparing RALP to ORP or LRP in the literature (Table 1) [11, 19–23], of which two RCTs [11, 22] were just an extended follow-up of already published RCTs [20, 21].

1.2.1 RALP Versus LRP

The first RCT was published in 2011 aiming to compare the oncological and functional outcomes of patients treated with RALP or LRP [19]. In this trial, 128 patients with clinically localized PCa were randomly assigned to undergo either RALP (64 patients) or LRP (64 patients). Interestingly, there was no statistically significant difference between the two approaches for all the outcomes under testing (i.e., operative time, estimated blood loss, transfusion rates, complications, positive surgical margins, biochemical recurrence, and post-operative continence recovery) except for the erectile function at 12-months after surgery, where RALP showed statistically significant superiority over LRP (77% vs 32%, $P < 0.0001$) [19]. Similarly, Porpiglia et al. [20], supported RALP superiority over LRP not only on the erectile function recovery at 12-months (80% vs 54.2%, $P = 0.020$) but also on the rates of continence recovery (95% vs 83.3% at 12-months, $p = 0.04$). Notably, the functional outcomes superiority was maintained over 5-years of follow-up (continence OR = 2.47, $p = 0.021$—potency OR 2.35, $p = 0.028$) [11]. Recently, the early results of the largest RCT comparing RALP (547 patients) and LRP (171 patients) were published, endorsing the superiority of RALP for early functional outcomes recovery (at 3-months follow-up) [23].

1.2.2 RALP Versus ORP

On the other hand, only one RCT compared the outcomes between RALP (163 patients) and ORP (163 patients) showing that the two approaches were comparable in terms of functional and oncological outcomes. Regarding perioperative complication rates, even not reaching statistical significance ($p = 0.05$), postoperative complication rate was lower in RARP vs ORP (4 vs 9%). Moreover, this study reported shorter operative time ($p < 0.0001$), lower estimated blood loss ($p < 0.001$), shorter length of stay ($p < 0.001$), and lower intraoperative adverse event rates for RALP ($p = 0.02$) relative to ORP. Similarly, pain relief at 24 hours and 1 week, as well as lymph nodal yield, were in favor of RALP (both $p < 0.001$) [21]. In a recent update of the RCT, patients were further followed up for 24-months showing that the functional outcomes were still comparable among the two surgical approaches; however, the biochemical recurrence rate was significantly higher in the ORP group (4 vs 13 cases of recurrence, 3 vs 9%) [22]. However, as also remarked by the authors, this data needs to be interpreted with cautions due to the absence of standardization in postoperative management between the two trial groups and the use of additional cancer treatments.

1.3 Evidence from Systematic Reviews and Meta-Analysis

Most of the claims in the current literature about the superiority of RALP over other approaches derive from meta-analyses that are based on prospective non-randomized and retrospective studies that are mostly characterized by a low level of evidence [20, 24]. Between 2010 and 2021, 19 systematic reviews and meta-analyses concerned with the comparison between different surgical approaches to RP were identified (Table 2). Of these, five studies compared RALP vs LRP [10, 12, 13, 26, 33], two compared minimally invasive RP (RALP and LRP) vs ORP [24, 25], five compared RALP vs ORP [17, 27–29, 34], and seven included comparison between all the three approaches [8, 30–32, 35–37]. Noteworthy, the results of these systematic reviews and meta-analyses are not consistent and do not provide sufficient evidence to give strong recommenda-

Table 1 Summary of the randomized controlled trials comparing different approaches to radical prostatectomy

Study	Year	Time period	Intervention	No. of patients	Age	BMI	PSA	GS	Prostate volume	IIEF-5 score	NVBS	LND	OT	EBL	Complications	Cont.	EF	PSM	BCR
Stolzenburg JU, et al. [14]	2021	Nov 2014 – Apr 2019	RALP	547	65	27.2	7.7	5 (0.2%) 6 (34%) 7(47%) 8 (11%) 9 (6.4%) 10 (0.7%)	48	14.4	Bilateral (52%) Unilateral (9.8%)	76%	176	250	15%	54%[$]	18%[$]	19%	NA
			LRP	171	65	27	8.1	5 (0%) 6 (32%) 7 (49%) 8 (13%) 9 (5.3%) 10 (0.6%)	47	15	Bilateral (51%) Unilateral (8.5%)	76%	169	210	21%	46%[$]	6.7%[$]	14%	NA
Coughlin GD, et al. [15]	2018	Aug 2010 – Nov 2014	RALP	163	60.4	NA	7.41	2–6 (18%) 7 (67%) 8–10 (15%)	NA	NA	69%	38%	202	443.7	2%	91.3[$$]	46.9[$$]	15%	3%
			ORP	163	59.6	NA	7.57	2–6 (15%) 7 (68%) 8–10 (17%)	NA	NA	69%	35%	234.3	1338	8%	90.9[$$]	45.7[$$]	10%	9%
Yaxley JW, et al. [16]	2016	Aug 2010 – Nov 2014	RALP	163	60.4	NA	7.41	2–6 (18%) 7 (67%) 8–10 (15%)	NA	NA	69%	38%	202	443.7	2%	82.5[$]	35[$]	15%	NA
			ORP	163	59.6	NA	7.57	2–6 (15%) 7 (68%) 8–10 (17%)	NA	NA	69%	35%	234.3	1338	8%	83.8[$]	38.9[$]	10%	NA

(continued)

Table 1 (continued)

Study	Year	Time period	Intervention	No. of patients	Age	BMI	PSA	GS	Prostate volume	IIEF-5 score	NVBS	LND	OT	EBL	Complications	Cont.	EF	PSM	BCR
Porpiglia F, et al. [13]	2016	Jan 2010 – Jan 2011	RALP	60	63.9	26.2	6.9	2–6 (41.7%) 7 (53.3%) 8–10 (5%)	36.2	20.2	Bilateral (28.3%) Unilateral (30%)	21.6%	147.6	202	Minor (16.7%) Major (0%)	96.5%*	74.3%*	NA	6.7%*
			LRP	60	64.7	26.8	8.3	2–6 (58.3%) 7 (33.3%) 8–10 (2.1%)	37.7	18.9	Bilateral (33.3%) Unilateral (25%)	21.6%	138.1	234.1	Minor (11.7%) Major (0%)	84.5%*	51.4%*	NA	10%*
Porpiglia F, et al. [17]	2013	Jan 2010 – Jan 2011	RALP	60	63.9	26.2	6.9	2–6 (41.7%) 7 (53.3%) 8–10 (5%)	36.2	20.2	Bilateral (28.3%) Unilateral (30%)	21.6%	147.6	202	Minor (16.7%) Major (0%)	80%#	80% **	NA	2% **
			LRP	60	64.7	26.8	8.3	2–6 (58.3%) 7 (33.3%) 8–10 (2.1%)	37.7	18.9	Bilateral (33.3%) Unilateral (25%)	21.6%	138.1	234.1	Minor (11.7%) Major (0%)	61.6%#	54.2% **	NA	7.5% **
Anastasios D, et al. [18]	2011	Oct 2007 – Oct 2008	RALP	64	59.6	25.8	8.9	5 (2%) 6 (86%) 7 (12%)	NA	23.2	96.9%	NA	No signif. Diff.	No signif. Diff.	15%	94%**	77%**	15%	No signif. Diff.
			LRP	64	61.1	26.3	7.4	5 (3%) 6 (75%) 7 (22%)	NA	22.7	95.3%	NA			8%	83%**	32%**	10%	

No. Number, *BMI* Body Mass Index, *NVBS* Neurovascular bundle sparing, *LND* Lymph node dissection, *OT* operative time, *EBL* estimated blood loss, *Cont.* continence, *EF* Erectile function, *PSM* positive surgical margins, *BCR* biochemical recurrence, *NA* not available, *signif. Diff.* significant difference

*At 5 years; #at 3 months; **at 1 year; $at 12 weeks; $$EPIC score at 24-month follow-up

Table 2 Summary of the meta-analyses comparing different approaches to radical prostatectomy

Study	Year	Time period	Database searched	No. of studies	Study type	Interven.	No. of patients	Perioperative outcomes				
								OT	EBL	Trans. rate	Hosp. stay	Cath. time
RALP versus LRP												
Carbonara U, et al. [1]	2021	2002–2021	"MEDLINE"; "EMBASE"; "WOS"	26	RCT (3); Pros. Non-Rand. (9); Retro. Case-control (10); Retro. matched cohort (4)	RALP	6135	−ve	NA	NA	−ve	−ve
						LRP	7617					
Wang T., et al. [5]	2019	2005–2018	"PubMed"; "Ovid"; "ScienceDirect"; "EMBASE"	22	RCT; pros. Non-Rand.; retro. Case control; retro matched cohorts	RALP	5170	NA	−ve	NA	NA	NA
						LRP	2782					
Lee SH, et al. [19]	2017	Up to 2014	"MEDLINE"; "EMBASE"; "Cochrane"; "KoreaMed"; "Kmbase"; "KISS"; "RISS"; "KisTi"	30	RCT (2); Prosp. Non-Rand.; Retro. Cohorts	RALP	4272	+ve (favoring RALP)	NA	+ve (favoring RALP)	+ve (favoring RALP)	NA
						LRP	4507					
Huang X, et al. [23]	2016	Up to 2015	"EMBASE"; "MEDLINE"; "PubMed"; "Cochrane"	24	RCT (2); Prosp. Non-Rand. (7); Retro. (15)	RALP	4114	−ve	+ve (favoring RALP)	+ve (favoring RALP)	−ve	−ve
						LRP	5064					
Allan C, et al. [25]	2016	Up to 2014	"MEDLINE"; "SCOPUS"; "Cochrane"	2	RCT	RALP	124	NA	NA	NA	NA	NA
						LRP	124					
Minimally invasive (RALP/LRP) versus ORP												
Cao L, et al. [6]	2019	NA	"PubMed"; "MEDLINE"; "EMBASE"; "Cochrane"	15	RCT (3); Pros. Non-Rand. (12);	Minimally invasive (RALP/LRP)	5051	+ve (favoring ORP)	+ve (favoring RALP/LRP)	+ve (favoring RALP/LRP)	+ve (favoring RALP/LRP)	−ve
						ORP	3496					
Ilic D, et al. [10]	2017	Up to 2017	"Cochrane"; "MEDLINE"; "EMBASE"	2	RCT (2)	Minimally invasive (RALP/LRP)	223	NA	NA	+ve (favoring RALP/LRP over ORP)	+ve (favoring RALP over ORP)	NA
						ORP	223					
RARP versus ORP												
Seo HJ, et al. [24]	2016	1980–2013	"MEDLINE"; "EMBASE"; "Cochrane"; "KoreaMed"; "RISS4U"; "KISS"; "KISTI"; "KMbase"; "NDSL"	61	Prosp. Non-Rand.; retro.	RALP	NA	+ve (favoring ORP)	+ve (favoring RALP)	+ve (favoring RALP)	NA	NA
						ORP	NA					
Srougi V, et al. [20]	2017	Up to 2016	"PubMed"; "EMBASE"; "SCOPUS"	9	Retro. Cohorts	RALP	13,696	NA	NA	NA	NA	NA
						ORP						

(continued)

Table 2 (continued)

Study	Year	Time period	Database searched	No. of studies	Study type	Interven.	No. of patients	Perioperative outcomes				
								OT	EBL	Trans. rate	Hosp. stay	Cath. time
Wang L, et al. [21]	2017	2010–2016	"PubMed"; "EMBASE"; "Cochrane"	20	Double arm prosp. Non-Rand. Cohort (5); Case series (15)	RALP	19,954	NA	NA	NA	NA	NA
						ORP	938					
Tang Q, et al. [22]	2017	NA	"MEDLINE"; "EMBASE"; "PubMed"; "CNKI"	78	Prosp. (35); retro. (43)	RALP	52,767	+ve (favoring ORP)	+ve (favoring RALP)	+ve (favoring RALP)	+ve (favoring RALP)	+ve (favoring RALP)
						ORP	60,125					
Pan XW, et al. [26]	2015	2009–2013	"PubMed"; "Google scholar"; "WOS"; "EMBASE"	6	Prosp. Non-Rand.	RALP	798	+ve (favoring ORP)	NA	−ve	NA	NA
						ORP	1571					
RARP versus LRP versus ORP												
Du Y, et al. [8]	2018	Up to 2017	"Cochrane"; "MEDLINE"; "EMBASE"; "PubMED"; "CNKI"; "Elsevier"	33	Retro. (8); pros. (25)	RALP	10,864	+ve (favoring RALP over LRP but not ORP)	+ve (favoring RALP over LRP and ORP)	+ve (favoring RALP over LRP and ORP)	NA	NA
						LRP	7905					
						ORP	11,336					
Novara G, et al. [27]	2012[a]	2008–2011	"MEDLINE"; "EMBASE"; "WOS"	12	Case series; RCT; Prosp. Non-Rand.; retro. Cohorts	RALP vs ORP	3166/2928	−ve	+ve (favoring RALP)	+ve (favoring RALP)	NA	NA
				7		RALP vs LRP	567/ 461	−ve	−ve	+ve (favoring RALP)		
Ficarra V, et al. [28]	2012[a]	2008–2011	"MEDLINE"; "EMBASE"; "WOS"	8	Case series; RCT; Prosp. Non-Rand.; retro. Cohorts	RALP vs ORP	1402/1411	NA	NA	NA	NA	NA
				8		RALP vs LRP	567/457					
Novara G, et al. [29]	2012[b]	2008–2011	"MEDLINE"; "EMBASE"; "WOS"	13	Case series; RCT; Prosp. Non-Rand.; retro. Cohorts	RALP vs ORP	NA	NA	NA	NA	NA	NA
				8		RALP vs LRP	NA					
Ficarra V, et al. [30]	2012[b]	2008–2011	"MEDLINE"; "EMBASE"; "WOS"	6	Case series; RCT; Prosp. Non-Rand.; retro. Cohorts	RALP vs ORP	956/943	NA	NA	NA	NA	NA
				4		RALP vs LRP	200/212					
Tewari A, et al. [31]	2012	2002–2010	"PubMed"; "SCOPUS"	400	Case series; RCT; Prosp. Non-Rand.; retro. Cohorts	RALP	62,389	NA	+ve (favoring RALP & LRP over ORP)	+ve (favoring RALP & LRP over ORP)	+ve (favoring RALP & LRP over ORP)	NA
						LRP	57,303					
						ORP	167,184					
Coelho RF, et al. [32]	2010	1994–2009	"MEDLINE"	30	Prosp. & retro. Cohorts	RALP	NA	162.6 min	164.2 ml	1.4%	1.43 days	NA
						LRP		205 min	291.5 ml	3.5%	4.87 days	
						ORP		165 min	951 ml	20.1%	NA	

Study	Year	Comp.	Oncological outcomes		Functional outcomes		Limitations
			PSM	BCR	Continence	Potency	
RALP versus LRP							
Carbonara U, et al. [1]	2021	−ve	−ve	+ve (favoring RALP at 12 mo)	+ve (favoring RALP at 12 mo)	+ve (favoring RALP at 12 mo)	1. Absence of long-term oncological outcomes 2. Time bias (learning curve was not comparable) 3. Most centers almost entirely shifted away from laparoscopy
Wang T., et al. [5]	2019	+ve (favoring RALP)	−ve	NA	+ve (favoring RALP at 12 mo)	NA	1. Lack of long-term follow-up 2-. No assessment of the risk of bias was included in the study 3. Time bias
Lee SH, et al. [19]	2017	+ve (favoring RALP for BNC, organ injury)	−ve	+ve (favoring RALP)	+ve (favoring RALP at 12 mo.)	+ve (favoring RALP at 12 mo.)	1. Absence of long-term oncological follow up 2. Significant heterogeneity 3. Time bias
Huang X, et al. [23]	2016	−ve	−ve	−ve	+ve (favoring RALP at 3-, 6-, & 12-mo.)	+ve (favoring RALP at 3-, 6-, & 12-mo.)	1. Few RCT 2. Heterogeneity 3. Lack of long-term follow-up
Allan C, et al. [25]	2016	NA	−ve	−ve	+ve (favoring RALP)	+ve (favoring RALP)	Limited number of included studies with limited number of patients
Minimally invasive (RALP/LRP) versus ORP							
Cao L, et al. [6]	2019	−ve	−ve	−ve (at 3, 12, and 24 mo.)	−ve (comparing only RALP vs ORP at 12 mo.)	−ve (comparing only RALP vs ORP at 12 mo.)	1. Based mainly on low quality studies (only 2 RCT) 2. Strong evidence of heterogeneity 3. Time bias (learning curve was not comparable)
Ilic D, et al. [10]	2017	Little or no difference favoring RALP	NA	NA	Little or no difference favoring RALP	Little or no difference favoring RALP	1. High-performance bias 2. Only 2 RCT "very small sample size"
RARP versus ORP							
Seo HJ, et al. [24]	2016	+ve (favoring RALP for BNC, organ injury, & pulmonary embolism)	−ve	+ve (favoring RALP)	+ve (favoring RALP at 12 mo.)	+ve (favoring RALP at 12 mo.)	1. High heterogeneity 2. No RCT included 3. Varying surgical skills 4. Relatively short follow-up period in the included studies.
Srougi V, et al. [20]	2017	NA	+ve (favoring RALP)	+ve (favoring RALP)	NA	NA	1. Retrospective 2. Heterogeneity 3. Time bias
Wang L, et al. [21]	2017	NA	NA	+ve (favoring RALP at 5 years)	NA	NA	1. No RCT are included 2. Other cancer controls such as metastasis was not studied

(continued)

Table 2 (continued)

Study	Year	Comp.	Oncological outcomes		Functional outcomes		Limitations
			PSM	BCR	Continence	Potency	
Tang Q, et al. [22]	2017	+ve (favoring RALP)	+ve (favoring RALP)	+ve (favoring RALP)	−ve (at 3- & 12-mo)	+ve (favoring RALP)	1. No RCT 2. High heterogeneity 3. Short follow up in most studies
Pan XW, et al. [26]	2015	NA	−ve	NA	−ve (at 3- & 12 mo.)	+ve (favoring RALP at 3- & 12-mo.)	1. Lack of RCT 2. Lack of complete data 3. Lack of follow up
RARP versus LRP versus ORP							
Du Y, et al. [8]	2018	NA	+ve (favoring RALP over LRP but not ORP)	NA	+ve (favoring RALP over LRP and ORP)	+ve (favoring RALP over LRP and ORP)	1. Different surgical techniques 2. Strong heterogeneity 3. Time bias
Novara G, et al. [27]	2012[a]	−ve	NA	NA	NA	NA	Comparison between different approaches was not the primary aim of the meta-analysis
Ficarra V, et al. [28]	2012[a]	NA −ve	NA	NA	+ve (favoring RALP at 12 mo.)	NA	1. Heterogeneity in continence definition 2. Different experiences of the surgeons
Ficarra V, et al. [28]	2012[a]	NA	NA	NA	+ve (favoring RALP at 12 mo.) +ve (favoring RALP at 12 mo.)	NA	1. Heterogeneity in continence definition 2. Different experiences of the surgeons
Novara G, et al. [29]	2012[b]	NA	−ve −ve	−ve −ve	NA	NA	1. Different levels of surgeons' skills 2. High heterogeneity
Ficarra V, et al. [30]	2012[b]	NA	NA	NA	NA	+ve (favoring RALP at 12 mo.) −ve	1. Different levels of surgeons' skills 2. High heterogeneity
Tewari A, et al. [31]	2012	+ve (favoring RALP as regards total perioperative complications)	+ve (favoring RALP over LRP only)	NA	NA	NA	1. Lack of RCT 2. High heterogeneity 3. Due to large number of patients, statistical significance doesn't mean clinical value
Coelho RF, et al. [32]	2010	10.3%	13.6%	NA	92%*	Bi (93.5%*) Uni (59.9%*)	1. Different surgeons with different experience 2. Time bias 3. Use of weighted means
		10.98%	21.3%		84.4%*	Bi (54%*) Uni (31.1%*)	
		10.3%	24%		79%*	Bi (60.6%*) Uni (43.1%*)	

WOS Web of science, *No.* number, *Interven.* intervention, *OT* operative time, *EBL* estimated blood loss, *Trans. Rate* transfusion rate, *Hosp.* hospital, *Cath.* catheterization, *−ve* no statistically significant difference, *+ve* statistically significant difference, *NA* not available, *Comp.* complications, *PSM* positive surgical margins, *BCR* biochemical recurrence, *RALP* Robotic-assisted laparoscopic radical prostatectomy, *RCT* randomized controlled trial, *Pros. Non-Rand.* prospective non-randomized, *Retro.* retrospective, *LRP* Laparoscopic radical prostatectomy, *ORP* open retropubic radical prostatectomy, *mo* months, *BNC* bladder neck contracture, *min* minutes, *Bi* bilateral nerve sparing, *Uni* unilateral nerve sparing

[a]at 1 year

tions as most of them are characterized by the scarcity of RCT, the lack of long-term follow-up in most of the included studies, evident time bias (where the learning curve for each approach was not comparable), high heterogeneity among the included studies in each meta-analysis (in terms of the definition and measurement of continence and potency, the surgical technique used for surgery, and follow-up period). Furthermore, considering that surgical experience is generally accepted as one of the key indicators of high-quality outcomes after RALP, data derived from high-volume centers with highly experienced robotic surgeons usually shows improved outcomes compared to patients operated in low-volume centers by surgeons with lower experience [30, 38–40]. Yet, some of the data in the included systematic reviews may be derived from studies performed in low-volume centers affecting the overall results of the study.

1.3.1 Minimally Invasive (RALP/LRP) Versus ORP

Cao et al. [24], included 15 articles (two RCTs and 13 prospective non-randomized comparative trials) in their pooled analysis showing that minimally invasive RP was significantly associated with reduced estimated blood loss, transfusion rates, and shorter hospital stay compared to ORP; however, there was no difference regarding oncological and functional outcomes between the different approaches. Similarly, Ilic et al. [25], performed a Cochrane systematic review including two RCT supporting the superiority of minimally invasive RP over ORP regarding transfusion rate (low quality of evidence) and hospital stay (moderate quality of evidence). Furthermore, the authors showed that RALP probably results in little or no difference regarding postoperative urinary and sexual functions (moderate quality of evidence).

1.3.2 RALP Versus ORP

Generally, most of the studies showed that RALP is associated with lower rates of biochemical recurrence at follow-up [17, 27, 28, 34]. On the contrary, two meta-analyses demonstrated that RALP was associated with lower rates of positive surgical margins compared to ORP [27, 34]. Only three studies discussed the functional outcomes after RP, where RALP was significantly associated with improved erectile function recovery compared to ORP at 3-,6-, and 12-months [27–29]. On the other hand, Seo et al. [28] reported superior urinary function recovery for RALP compared to ORP at 12-months after surgery. Furthermore, ORP was associated with significantly shorter operative time and higher estimated blood loss compared to RALP [27–29]; however, RALP was associated with lower overall complication rates, especially bladder neck contracture, organ injury, and pulmonary embolism [27, 28].

1.3.3 RALP Versus LRP

Interestingly, Lee et al. [26] and Huang et al. [13] demonstrated that RALP was associated with lower transfusion rates compared to LRP. Furthermore, RALP was associated with lower perioperative complications, especially bladder neck contracture and organ injury compared to LRP [26, 33]. On the contrary, Huang et al. [13] and Carbonara et al. [10] reported that there was no significant difference between these approaches in terms of perioperative complications. Considering oncological outcomes, all the studies reported no superiority of one approach over the other in terms of positive surgical margins and biochemical recurrence, except for Lee et al. [26] and Carbonara et al. [10], who demonstrated statistically significant lower rate of biochemical recurrence after RALP compared to LRP. Regarding functional outcomes, all the available meta-analyses favored RALP over LRP for both continence and potency rates recovery [10, 12, 13, 26, 33].

1.3.4 RALP Versus LRP Versus ORP

In systematic review which performed a pooled comparison of outcomes of all the approaches, operative time resulted similar in RALP and ORP approaches [8, 30, 31], but it was significantly shorter for RALP compared to LRP [8]. In general, estimated blood loss was significantly lower in minimally invasive RP (RALP/LRP) compared to ORP [37]; within the minimally invasive approaches, Du et al. [8] reported that estimated blood loss was significantly lower in patients undergoing RALP compared to LRP. This was also reflected on the transfusion rates, where RALP was associated with significantly lower transfusion rates compared to both LRP and ORP [8, 31, 37]. Furthermore, most of the studies that assessed the perioperative complications demonstrated that there was no significant difference between the three approaches [30, 31]. On the contrary, Tewari et al. [37] supported the superiority of RALP regarding the overall rate of perioperative complications.

Considering oncological outcomes, Tewari et al. [37] and Du et al. [8] were the only authors that demonstrated a superiority for RALP over LRP (but not ORP) regarding positive surgical margins. Moreover, Novara et al. [35] reported that biochemical recurrence rates were not significantly different between the three approaches. On the contrary, RALP was associated with significantly better functional outcomes over LRP and ORP [8, 30, 32, 36]; however, it is worth mentioning that Ficarra et al. [36] showed that the potency recovery was comparable among patients undergoing RALP and LRP.

1.4 Current Status

In the light of these findings, there are few evidences supporting better functional and, to a lesser extent, better oncological outcomes after RALP compared to LRP and ORP; however, this evidence is not sufficient to draw a definitive conclusion on the superiority of RALP. In these settings, both the European Association of Urology (EAU) and the American Urological Association (AUA) guidelines do not recommend yet one approach over another [3, 41]. However, it should be highlighted that the strength of such recommendation ("no approach over another") moved from "Strong" in 2019 to "Weak" in 2020 and 2021—according to the EAU Guidelines—postulating a possible paradigm shift toward robotic approach.

2 Outcomes of RALP in Special Settings

2.1 High-Risk PCa

The setting of high-risk PCa has been considered with a meta-analysis of studies comparing different surgical approaches and their impact on surgical margin and biochemical recurrence. Srougi et al. [34], performed a systematic review of nine retrospective studies comparing ORP and RALP and found that high-risk patients treated with RALP had the least risk of positive surgical margin (risk difference − 0.004) compared to similar patients submitted to ORP. Similarly, from five studies included in the meta-analysis, the risk of BCR was lower with RALP compared to open interventions (HR 0.72). However, the retrospective and observational nature of most of the studies precluded a strong conclusion [34]. Recently, Mazzone et al. [15] described the feasibility of RALP in locally advanced cases with extracapsular extension at preoperative magnetic resonance imaging (MRI). Here, RALP technique was not associated with an increased rate of postoperative complications after surgery compared to previous RALP series on locally advanced cases [16]. This evidence further supports the feasibility and safety profile of this approach in patients with posterior extracapsular extension at MRI. Notably, the robustness of these results on postoperative complications is supported by the use of standardized methodology provided by the EAU [42]. Indeed, by fulfilling all the suggested criteria, the high reliability of data report on postoperative complications was ensured.

2.2 RALP after Previous Benign Prostatic Hyperplasia Surgery

Beyond the comparison between approaches, a certain level of evidence is reported for the use of RALP in special settings, such as after previous bladder outlet surgery or previous treatments for PCa. Minimally invasive radical prostatectomy (RALP + LRP) after previous bladder outlet surgery of benign prostatic hyperplasia (BPH) has been analyzed through a pooled analysis of studies comparing these cases to those patients who did not undergo previous treatments for BPH. Veccia et al. [18] performed a pooled analysis of 12 comparative studies and concluded that previous BPH surgery is associated to lower odds of nerve-sparing completion, longer operative time, higher rate of bladder neck reconstruction, longer catheterization time, higher complication rate, higher PSM rate, higher BCR, and less potency and continence recovery rates. Of note, when considering RALP vs LRP, the robotic approach seems to offer superior outcomes. More recently, Liao et al. [14], performed a meta-analysis of 13 studies specifically addressing PCa patients after transurethral resection of the prostate (TURP) and found similar outcomes in terms of PSM, bladder neck reconstruction rate, nerve-sparing rate, and overall complication rate, with RALP approach being the one with a significant difference in PSM rate between TURP and non-TURP patients. In summary, literature evidence about RALP after previous surgery for BPH confirm its feasibility but confirm the more challenging nature of the procedure.

2.3 Salvage Prostatectomy

The salvage setting (RALP after the failure of previous active treatment for PCa) has been mainly addressed with retrospective studies, including propensity score-matched analyses. Martinez et al. [43] recently compared open (50 patients) and robotic approaches (26 patients) for the management of post-radiotherapy, brachytherapy, and intensity-modulated radiotherapy (IMRT) failure. The authors found that RALP yielded a lower incontinence rate (9.1% vs 34%) and complete absence of anastomotic stricture (0% vs 8.7%) compared to ORP [43]. Onol et al. [44], addressed the issue of different functional outcomes after RALP based on the type of previous treatment, where the authors compared between post-radiation (94 patients) and post-focal ablation (32 patients) cases, reporting that radiation prior to RALP was associated with inferior functional outcomes whereas focal ablation therapies were associated with higher PSM rate and higher risk of non-organ confined disease at final pathology. These findings were confirmed by the retrospective series of DeGroote et al. on 106 patients [45].

The same group of authors recently published a 1:1 prospective propensity-score matched analysis comparing salvage (n = 135) versus primary RALP and concluded that salvage RALP have similar perioperative outcomes with inferior potency rates; consistently with previous studies, a prior whole gland treatment was associated with a higher risk of urinary incontinence [46].

On the same hand, a prospective single-group interventional study about RALP after previous focal therapies

(RAFT clinical trial) was recently published [47]. With the enrolment of 24 men in roughly 2 years, the authors mainly focused on functional outcomes and reported that 96% of patients had an almost complete continence recovery (0/1 pad) one year after surgery. The EPIC-26 questionnaire prior to salvage RALP and after 3 months found that urinary continence was at least similar to preoperative baseline in 74% of patients. This study concluded that salvage RALP after focal therapy provides good urinary outcomes despite being associated with sexual function impairment [47].

Summarizing evidence from the salvage setting, salvage RALP is technically more challenging compared to the primary settings, but it represents a feasible option in high-volume centers. Patients should be counseled that functional outcomes are inferior to those from primary RALP. Adjustment of surgical technique according to the primary treatment may improve surgical outcomes.

3 Techniques of Prostate Dissection and Literature Evidence

RALP has been addressed with Level 1 evidence in the following fields: (1) Surgical access; (2) Retzius sparing vs conventional approach (3) reconstructive techniques (posterior reconstruction, anterior suspension + posterior reconstruction, advanced reconstruction of vesicourethral support) (4) DVC control and sutures.

3.1 Surgical Access: Extra- Versus Transperitoneal

The surgical access represents a matter of debate in the literature; however, over the last decade, the extraperitoneal access gained more popularity and was presented as a safe alternative to the traditional transperitoneal approach [48]. Furthermore, the extraperitoneal approach has been recently gaining more interest due to the introduction of single-port robotic platforms [49]. Each approach has its own advantages and disadvantages. The transperitoneal approach provides a larger working space facilitating the port insertion [50]; however, it carries the risk of bowel injury, complications related to an intraperitoneal urine leak and peritoneal irritation, and the cardiopulmonary complications resulting from the steep Trendelenburg position (30–45 degrees) and the artificial pneumoperitoneum [50, 51]. On the other hand, supporters of the extraperitoneal approach state that it mirrors the technique of ORP, reduces the risk of intraperitoneal complications, and may represent a safer option for patients with histories of previous abdominal surgery, symptomatic inguinal hernia needing mesh repair, or cardiac disease with inserted drug-eluting stents [50, 52, 53].

Only two prospective randomized trials were compared between the two approaches [54, 55]. The first one was carried out by Capello et al. [55], in 2007, showing no significant difference between both approaches in terms of operative times, blood loss, pathological Gleason Score, specimen weight, complications, and PSM rates. Similarly, Akand et al. [54] supported that both approaches have similar oncological outcomes; however, the extraperitoneal approach was associated with significantly shorter operative and anesthesia times, catheterization time, hospital stay, and time to oral diet. These findings were recently supported by a meta-analysis, including 16 studies for an approximative number of 4000 patients, concluding that the extraperitoneal approach offers shorter operative time, decreased length of hospital stay, and decreased rates of postoperative ileus and inguinal hernia formation [48].

3.2 Bladder Detachment Vs Retzius Sparing Approach

Conventionally, in the classical anterior trans-peritoneal approach, RALP requires the access to the Retzius space, potentially disrupting anatomical structures contributing to the urinary continence mechanism. In 2010, Galfano et al. [56] first described the Retzius-sparing technique (RS-RALP) which starts and proceeds from Douglas space onward: this approach maintains the integrity of the anterior compartment—NVBs, pubourethral or puboprostatic ligaments, Aphrodite's veil, accessory pudendal arteries—and carries the perspective of improved and earlier recovery of continence and erectile function. The first prospective trial from the authors reported over 90% of immediate continence at catheter removal and a 70% rate of erectile function at 1 year [57]. Other added benefits are a likely lower incidence of inguinal hernias and Peyronie's disease, less patient-reported penile shortening, and preservation of an untouched Retzius space for patients in whom future surgery is anticipated in this area [58, 59].

Reflecting the increased interest in this RS-RALP, several studies and six meta-analyses were published in just two years on the comparison between anterior RALP and RS-RALP (2019–2020) [60–65]. Phukan et al. [62] performed a systematic review and meta-analysis including 2 RCTs and 4 non-randomized prospective comparative studies for an overall amount of 638 patients. RS-RALP was associated with better early continence rates ($\leq$ 1 month) (moderate-quality evidence) (RR 1.72, 95% CI 1.27, 2.32, $p = 0.0005$) and at 3 months (low quality evidence) (RR 1.39, 95% CI 1.03, 1.88, $p = 0.03$). Furthermore, RS-RALP did not alter T2 positive margin rates (RR 1.67, 95% CI 0.91, 3.06, $p = 0.10$) and T3 positive margin rates (RR 1.08, 95% CI 0.68, 1.70, $p = 0.75$) (very low-quality evidence). Short-term biochemical free survival appears to be similar between the two approaches. Finally, RS-RALP did not alter overall and major complication rates (low-quality evidence) [62].

Dirie et al. [64] drafted similar conclusions; however, it should be noted that their meta-analysis included low-evidence studies (one RCT, six observational studies, two case reports, one case series, and one descriptive study). Similarly, another meta-analysis included 8 studies (2 RCT, 3 retrospective, 3 prospective) for a total of 1620 patients and concluded that the continence rate following RS-RALP may be significantly improved compared to the classical anterior RALP. Notably, PSM rate, complication rate, operative time, EBL, and postoperative hernia were similar between groups [63].

PSM rate represents the major concern of the RS approach. Checcucci et al. [65] reported in their meta-analysis that RS-RALP was associated with improved continence recovery but it was also associated with an increase in the risk of PSM. These findings were further confirmed in the meta-analysis from Tai et al. [60], which included two RCTs and four observational studies, confirming better continence achievement with RS despite a significantly higher PSM rate (OR 1.68, $p = 0.02$). Specifically, higher PSM rates were reported for the anterior site (OR 4.34, $p = 0.03$) and for the subset of RCT (OR 2.80, $p = 0.007$). The authors stated that the limited view of surgeons performing RS-RALP in the anterior aspect of the prostate may account for a higher PSM rate at this site, whereas the PSM rate was similar in other anatomical regions [60].

Evidence about RS-RALP have been analyzed also in a Cochrane review, that pooled data from 5 unique RCT (two published, one in press, two abstract proceedings) for an overall amount of 571 randomized participants. The analysis confirmed that RS-RALP improves continence rate within one week after catheter removal (RR 1.74) and may increase continence at 3 months (RR1.33). The effects of RS-RALP on potency remain uncertain, whereas RS-RALP may increase PSM (RR1.95) [61].

In conclusion, current evidence suggest that RS approach is feasible and may lead to better and earlier continence recovery. However, beyond PSM, some points of concern persist, such as the challenging nature of the approach—especially in the case of anterior tumors, post-TURP or high-volume prostates or median lobes—and the absence of high-level evidence in high-risk diseases.

3.3 Nerve-Sparing Approaches: Antegrade and Retrograde Release of NVB

Approaches for the preservation of NVBs can be performed from the prostate base to the apex (antegrade) or from the apex to the base (retrograde). In 2013, Ko et al. [66] performed a propensity score-matched analysis to compare the outcomes among patients who received antegrade ($n = 235$) and retrograde ($n = 266$) nerve-sparing surgery. The authors reported a higher potency rate in the retrograde approach at 3-,6-, and 9-months (65% vs 80.8% and 72.1% vs 90.1% and 85.3% vs 92.9%, respectively) with similar PSM rates; thus they concluded that a retrograde NS approach facilitates early recovery of potency [66]. The possible benefit of the retrograde NS approach is the avoidance of misplaced clip on the prostatic pedicle as a result of the earlier identification and release of the NVB from the prostate before ligating the prostatic pedicle; moreover, the earlier release of the NVB while the pedicle is still intact may theoretically reduce the neuropraxia [66].

The anatomic principles of nerve-sparing as described by Walsh [67] have been more recently reviewed with micro-anatomical studies finding a complex neuronal distribution around the prostate, including the anterior surface. This finding raised interest toward the preservation of anatomical structures located anteriorly [68, 69]. De Carvalho et al. [70] reported a prospective, non-controlled case series of 128 patients who underwent RALP with retrograde release of NV and preservation of dorsal venous complex (DVC): the approach yielded 85.9% of immediate continence and 86% of potency one year after surgery. Thus, a retrograde NS approach that includes the preservation of anterior fibers seems to enhance the recovery of functional outcomes.

3.4 Reconstructive Techniques

RALP results in the disruption of peri-prostatic structures and the mechanisms underlying urinary continence. It shortens the urethral length and reduces bladder-outlet resistance; RALP may hinder bladder-neck sphincteric function and changes the structure and function of the urinary sphincteric complex. Considering the impact of surgery on these functions, multiple approaches to surgical reconstruction of the pelvic floor have been suggested [71].

The available evidence from reconstruction techniques after robotic prostatectomy has been summarized and divided into: (1) posterior reconstruction (PR) of the rhabdomyosphincter “Rocco stitch” (2) peri-urethral suspension stitch “Patel stitch”, (3) anterior suspension (AS+PR) plus posterior reconstruction techniques, (4) advanced reconstruction of vesicourethral support (ARVUS), (5) total anatomical reconstruction (TAR) [72]. Beyond these reconstruction techniques, the role of preserving of urethral length and bladder neck preservation have been explored in retrospective or non-randomized prospective trials [73–75]. Noteworthy, only one RCTs assessed the value of complete bladder neck preservation on continence recovery showing that this technique is associated with significantly better continence recovery and improved quality of life even at long-term follow-up without compromising the cancer control [76, 77]. Similarly, only one RCT evaluated the potential benefit of maximal urethral length preservation showing that it is associated with earlier recovery of continence [78].

As far as pelvic floor reconstruction is concerned, RCTs comparing a specific technique vs no-reconstruction are available for PR (4 RCT) [79–82], for AS + PR (4 RCT) [83–86], and for ARVUS (1 RCT) [87]. Regarding TAR, a prospective cohort study on 1008 patients, demonstrated a continence rate of 61%, 58%, 79%, 90%, 94%, and 94% at 24 hours, 1,4,12, 48 weeks after catheter removal [88]. Similarly, Checcucci et al. [89] recently published a systematic review of anatomical reconstruction techniques and pooled data from referral centers with more than 250 patients: overall, they included 2 prospective cohort studies and 9 prospective case series, for an overall amount of 10,117 patients. The authors found that total reconstruction showed higher continence recovery rates, compared to their anterior and posterior reconstruction counterparts at 1, 4, 12, 24, and 52 weeks ($p < 0.001$ at all time-points) [89]. Another meta-analysis involved 32 studies for a sample size of 4697 patients and considered the impact of each pelvic floor reconstruction technique on functional outcomes. Nineteen trials evaluated the efficacy of PR, 7 trials evaluated the efficacy of AS, 4 trials evaluated the efficacy of PR + anterior reconstruction (AR), and 2 trials evaluated the efficacy of PR + AS. Seven of these trials were RCTs [90]. Interestingly, this meta-analysis showed that patients who underwent PR had the lowest rates of urinary incontinence, where the pooled results of patients who had solely PR showed significant improvement of the urinary continence at 1–4, 28–42, 90, 180, and 360 days but not after 7–14 days following catheter removal. The use of AS technique was associated with significant improvement only at 28–42 days, whereas the AR + PR was associated with significant urinary continence at 1–4, 90, and 180 days. Furthermore, pooled data from six trials showed that PR was associated with a lower risk of cystogram leakage after surgery (RR = 0.37; $P = 0.004$) [90].

3.5 DCV Control and Sutures

The quality of apical dissection is important as it can affect continence and erectile function and is likely to impact the PSM rate as well. The division of the dorsal venous complex (DVC) represents a cornerstone of apical dissection. The impact of different techniques for DVC management has been addressed in two RCTs. Antonelli et al. [91] performed a prospective randomized trial to compare standard vs delayed approach to DVC (s-DVC vs d-DVC) during RALP. In s-DVC arm, an early suture of the DVC was performed at the beginning of the procedure then the DVC was cut at the time of apical dissection, while in the d-DVC arm the DVC transaction and suturing was delayed at the end of the prostatectomy, prior to apex dissection.

After the enrollment of 162 cases (81 s-DVC, 81 d-DVC), an interim analysis showed significantly higher EBL and significantly higher PSM rate (21.0 vs 14.8%, $p = 0.323$) in the d-DVC arm, with a statistical significance difference in the group of localized tumors (15.5 vs 3.6%, $p = 0.031$). The authors demonstrated that both approaches are feasible; however, the delayed technique may increase the risk of PSM, especially in organ-confined disease with a reduction of risk of apical involvement [91]. The low risk of apical involvement with d-DVC was further confirmed in a systematic review and meta-analysis (OR = 0.39; 95% CI, 0.22 to 0.71; $p = 0.002$) [92].

The other RCT addressed the impact of different techniques for DVC management on urinary continence. The authors considered the effect of endoscopic stapling, division and suture ligation, and suture ligation with suspension of the DVC on 300 patients randomized to three groups [93]. They concluded that there is no difference regarding the overall continence rates at 3 months. On the contrary, at 15 months follow-up, ligation and suspension provided significant superior continence rates (99%) compared to stapler (88%) ($P = 0.002$) and cut and suture ligation (88%) ($P = 0.002$). Furthermore, the authors demonstrated that potency was not affected by the technique of DVC [93].

Finally, the suture materials for the urethrovescical anastomosis were also discussed in the literature. The introduction of unidirectional barbed absorbable poly-glyconate thread—armed with a surgical needle at one end and a welded-loop end effector at the other—challenged the previous Monocryl monofilament and Vicryl braided suture. A meta-analysis of three RCT, four prospective, and two retrospective trials compared barbed with conventional non-barbed sutures. The study concluded that barbed suture could significantly reduce anastomosis time, operative time, and posterior reconstruction time. However, possible complications deriving from the use of barbed suture (such as intra-op leakage/urethral tear and its management, erosion and bladder neck contracture) have not been addressed [94].

4 Novelties and Complementary Tools to RALP

A modified technique of apical dissection with endopelvic fascia preservation has been recently described by Moschovas et al. [95]. This technique allows to maintain NVB untouched and covered together with the maximal preservation of the apical complex and peri-urethral tissues. The authors performed a propensity score matching with a similar group who underwent conventional RALP (104 patients in each group) and found that the modified technique yielded significantly faster continence (mean 46 vs 70 days) and potency recovery (mean 74 vs 118 days) [95].

The preservation of endopelvic fascia alone has been evaluated in another recent RCT enrolling 158 patients randomized in a 1:1 fashion [96]. The approach failed to provide improvement of urinary continence or sexual functions. Similarly, no significant differences in terms of complications and oncological outcomes.

Another preservation approach recently delivered is the “Hood technique,” which includes the sparing of periurethral anatomic structures in the space of Retzius [97]. In this approach, the detrusor apron, puboprostatic ligament complex, arcus tendinous, endopelvic fascia, and pouch of Douglas remain untouched. With a prospective observational study, the authors reported an early return to continence without negatively compromising PSM rates. However, the exclusion of anterior tumor location may have contributed to the low rate of PSM [97]. In summary, recent literature is moving toward the preservation of the anterior compartment to improve functional recovery after RALP.

In more recent years, several technological improvements have been proposed to enhance the recovery of potency. When a nerve-sparing is performed, the intraoperative control of surgical margins at the NVB adjacent site has been proposed in order to ensure oncological safety; the approach further aims to offer a full intrafascial NS surgery also in cases otherwise not elected to, with the direct effect of widening the indication to a nerve-sparing surgery [98]. A recent trial evaluated the reliability of the NeuroSAFE approach and concluded for a concordance between frozen section and the final section with 100% sensitivity and 99.2% specificity [99]. Similarly, Rocco et al. [100, 101], addressed the issue with the use of digital confocal microscopy to verify intraoperatively the absence of PSM at the NVB site. Since the confocal microscope allows the location of PSM with respect to previously positioned markers, the authors described the feasibility of a wedge secondary resection of the primarily preserved NVB, to avoid its complete disruption while pursuing oncological safety [100].

The use of dehydrated human amnion/chorion membrane (dHACM) allograft to wrap and protect the spared NVB has been proposed by Ogaya-Pinies et al. [102], with a propensity score-matched analysis. By comparing 235 patients who underwent a RALP with dHACM with RALP patients without dHACM (1:3 matching), the authors concluded that the device allows for a faster return to potency, regardless of the degree of NS, without compromising oncological outcomes [102]. However, high costs associated with the use dHACM may be an important limitation for its wide implementation in the context of RALP.

The use of a three-dimensional (3D) augmented reality (AR) system to optimize the identification of PCa location during RALP has also been proposed in 2019 by Porpiglia et al. [103]. In their prospective study comparing patients with and without 3D-AR, the authors found that the superimposition of virtual models allows for a possible reduction in PSM rates with maximization of functional outcomes. Similar findings were recently confirmed by a prospective comparative propensity score analysis comparing patients who had 3D-AR and frozen section to patients who had not [104]. Here, the authors showed that PSM at the level of the index lesion was significantly lower with the use of 3DAR, providing guidance toward a tailored dissection and maximization of functional outcomes.

5 Conclusions

Robotic represents the mostly used approach to RP in countries with a widespread diffusion of robotic platforms. However, to date, evidence from the Literature highlighting a clear superiority of the approach are still limited but seemingly emerging. The current evidence-based approach to RALP literature points out the topics that have been comprehensively analyzed through decades. Some technical refinements and robotic complementary tools deserve further insights through RCT in order to strengthen the scientific and surgical impact of RALP advances.

References

1. Sung H, Ferlay J, Siegel RL, Laversanne M, Soerjomataram I, Jemal A, et al. Global cancer statistics 2020: GLOBOCAN estimates of incidence and mortality worldwide for 36 cancers in 185 countries. CA Cancer J Clin. 2021;71:209–49. https://doi.org/10.3322/caac.21660.
2. Fitzmaurice C, Abate D, Abbasi N, Abbastabar H, Abd-Allah F, Abdel-Rahman O, et al. Global, regional, and National Cancer Incidence, mortality, years of life lost, years lived with disability, and disability-adjusted life-years for 29 cancer groups, 1990 to 2017. JAMA Oncol. 2019;5:1749. https://doi.org/10.1001/jamaoncol.2019.2996.
3. Mottet N, van den Bergh RCN, Briers E, Van den Broeck T, Cumberbatch MG, De Santis M, et al. EAU-EANM-ESTRO-ESUR-SIOG guidelines on prostate Cancer-2020 update. Part 1: screening, diagnosis, and local treatment with curative intent. Eur Urol. 2021;79:243–62. https://doi.org/10.1016/j.eururo.2020.09.042.
4. Young HH. VIII. Conservative perineal prostatectomy: the results of two years' experience and report of seventy-five cases. Ann Surg. 1905;41:549–57.
5. Millin T. Retropubic Prostatectomy. J Urol. 1948;59:267–74. https://doi.org/10.1016/S0022-5347(17)69374-1.
6. Costello AJ. Considering the role of radical prostatectomy in 21st century prostate cancer care. Nat Rev Urol. 2020;17:177–88. https://doi.org/10.1038/s41585-020-0287-y.
7. Raboy A, Ferzli G, Albert P. Initial experience with extraperitoneal endoscopic radical retropubic prostatectomy. Urology. 1997;50:849–53. https://doi.org/10.1016/S0090-4295(97)00485-8.

8. Du Y, Long Q, Guan B, Mu L, Tian J, Jiang Y, et al. Robot-assisted radical prostatectomy is more beneficial for prostate cancer patients: a system review and meta-analysis. Med Sci Monit. 2018;24:272–87. https://doi.org/10.12659/MSM.907092.
9. Binder J, Kramer W. Robotically-assisted laparoscopic radical prostatectomy. BJU Int. 2001;87:408–10. https://doi.org/10.1046/j.1464-410X.2001.00115.x.
10. Carbonara U, Srinath M, Crocerossa F, Ferro M, Cantiello F, Lucarelli G, et al. Robot-assisted radical prostatectomy versus standard laparoscopic radical prostatectomy: an evidence-based analysis of comparative outcomes. World J Urol. 2021; https://doi.org/10.1007/s00345-021-03687-5.
11. Porpiglia F, Fiori C, Bertolo R, Manfredi M, Mele F, Checcucci E, et al. Five-year outcomes for a prospective randomised controlled trial comparing laparoscopic and robot-assisted radical prostatectomy. Eur Urol Focus. 2018;4:80–6. https://doi.org/10.1016/j.euf.2016.11.007.
12. Allan C, Ilic D. Laparoscopic versus robotic-assisted radical prostatectomy for the treatment of localised prostate cancer: a systematic review. Urol Int. 2016;96:373–8. https://doi.org/10.1159/000435861.
13. Huang X, Wang L, Zheng X, Wang X. Comparison of perioperative, functional, and oncologic outcomes between standard laparoscopic and robotic-assisted radical prostatectomy: a systemic review and meta-analysis. Surg Endosc. 2017;31:1045–60. https://doi.org/10.1007/s00464-016-5125-1.
14. Liao H, Duan X, Du Y, Mou X, Hu T, Cai T, et al. Radical prostatectomy after previous transurethral resection of the prostate: oncological, surgical and functional outcomes—a meta-analysis. World J Urol. 2020;38:1919–32. https://doi.org/10.1007/s00345-019-02986-2.
15. Mazzone E, Dell'Oglio P, Rosiello G, Puliatti S, Brook N, Turri F, et al. Technical refinements in Superextended robot-assisted radical prostatectomy for locally advanced prostate cancer patients at multiparametric magnetic resonance imaging. Eur Urol. 2021;80(1):104–12. https://doi.org/10.1016/j.eururo.2020.09.009.
16. Gandaglia G, De Lorenzis E, Novara G, Fossati N, De Groote R, Dovey Z, et al. Robot-assisted radical prostatectomy and extended pelvic lymph node dissection in patients with locally-advanced prostate cancer. Eur Urol. 2017;71:249–56. https://doi.org/10.1016/j.eururo.2016.05.008.
17. Wang L, Wang B, Ai Q, Zhang Y, Lv X, Li H, et al. Long-term cancer control outcomes of robot-assisted radical prostatectomy for prostate cancer treatment: a meta-analysis. Int Urol Nephrol. 2017;49:995–1005. https://doi.org/10.1007/s11255-017-1552-8.
18. Veccia A, Antonelli A, Francavilla S, Porpiglia F, Simeone C, Lima E, et al. Minimally invasive radical prostatectomy after previous bladder outlet surgery: a systematic review and pooled analysis of comparative studies. J Urol. 2019;202:511–7. https://doi.org/10.1097/JU.0000000000000312.
19. Asimakopoulos AD, Pereira Fraga CT, Annino F, Pasqualetti P, Calado AA, Mugnier C. Randomized comparison between laparoscopic and robot-assisted nerve-sparing radical prostatectomy. J Sex Med. 2011;8:1503–12. https://doi.org/10.1111/j.1743-6109.2011.02215.x.
20. Porpiglia F, Morra I, Lucci Chiarissi M, Manfredi M, Mele F, Grande S, et al. Randomised controlled trial comparing laparoscopic and robot-assisted radical prostatectomy. Eur Urol. 2013;63:606–14. https://doi.org/10.1016/j.eururo.2012.07.007.
21. Yaxley JW, Coughlin GD, Chambers SK, Occhipinti S, Samaratunga H, Zajdlewicz L, et al. Robot-assisted laparoscopic prostatectomy versus open radical retropubic prostatectomy: early outcomes from a randomised controlled phase 3 study. Lancet. 2016;388:1057–66. https://doi.org/10.1016/S0140-6736(16)30592-X.
22. Coughlin GD, Yaxley JW, Chambers SK, Occhipinti S, Samaratunga H, Zajdlewicz L, et al. Robot-assisted laparoscopic prostatectomy versus open radical retropubic prostatectomy: 24-month outcomes from a randomised controlled study. Lancet Oncol. 2018;19:1051–60. https://doi.org/10.1016/S1470-2045(18)30357-7.
23. Stolzenburg J-U, Holze S, Neuhaus P, Kyriazis I, Do HM, Dietel A, et al. Robotic-assisted versus laparoscopic surgery: outcomes from the first multicentre, randomised, patient-blinded controlled trial in radical prostatectomy (LAP-01). Eur Urol. 2021;79:750–9. https://doi.org/10.1016/j.eururo.2021.01.030.
24. Cao L, Yang Z, Qi L, Chen M. Robot-assisted and laparoscopic vs open radical prostatectomy in clinically localized prostate cancer: perioperative, functional, and oncological outcomes. Medicine (Baltimore). 2019;98:e15770. https://doi.org/10.1097/MD.0000000000015770.
25. Ilic D, Evans SM, Allan CA, Jung JH, Murphy D, Frydenberg M. Laparoscopic and robot-assisted vs open radical prostatectomy for the treatment of localized prostate cancer : a Cochrane systematic review. BJU Int. 2018;121(6):845–53. https://doi.org/10.1111/bju.14062.
26. Lee SH, Seo HJ, Lee NR, Son SK, Kim DK, Rha KH. Robot-assisted radical prostatectomy has lower biochemical recurrence than laparoscopic radical prostatectomy: systematic review and meta-analysis. Investig Clin Urol. 2017;58:152. https://doi.org/10.4111/icu.2017.58.3.152.
27. Tang K, Jiang K, Chen H, Chen Z, Xu H, Ye Z. Robotic vs . Retropubic radical prostatectomy in prostate cancer: a systematic review and a meta-analysis update. Oncotarget. 2017;8:32237–57. https://doi.org/10.18632/oncotarget.13332.
28. Seo H-J, Lee NR, Son SK, Kim DK, Rha KH, Lee SH. Comparison of robot-assisted radical prostatectomy and open radical prostatectomy outcomes: a systematic review and meta-analysis. Yonsei Med J. 2016;57:1165. https://doi.org/10.3349/ymj.2016.57.5.1165.
29. Pan X, Cui X, Teng J, Zhang D, Wang Z, Qu F, et al. Robot-assisted radical prostatectomy vs. open Retropubic radical prostatectomy for prostate cancer: a systematic review and meta-analysis. Indian J Surg. 2015;77:1326–33. https://doi.org/10.1007/s12262-014-1170-y.
30. Coelho RF, Rocco B, Patel MB, Orvieto MA, Chauhan S, Ficarra V, et al. Retropubic, laparoscopic, and robot-assisted radical prostatectomy: a critical review of outcomes reported by high-volume centers. J Endourol. 2010;24:2003–15. https://doi.org/10.1089/end.2010.0295.
31. Novara G, Ficarra V, Rosen RC, Artibani W, Costello A, Eastham JA, et al. Systematic review and meta-analysis of perioperative outcomes and complications after robot-assisted radical prostatectomy. Eur Urol. 2012;62:431–52. https://doi.org/10.1016/j.eururo.2012.05.044.
32. Ficarra V, Novara G, Rosen RC, Artibani W, Carroll PR, Costello A, et al. Systematic review and meta-analysis of studies reporting urinary continence recovery after robot-assisted radical prostatectomy. Eur Urol. 2012;62:405–17.
33. Wang T, Wang Q, Wang S. A meta-analysis of robot assisted laparoscopic radical prostatectomy versus laparoscopic radical prostatectomy. Open Med. 2019;14:485–90. https://doi.org/10.1515/med-2019-0052.
34. Srougi V, Bessa J, Baghdadi M, Nunes-Silva I, da Costa JB, Garcia-Barreras S, et al. Surgical method influences specimen margins and biochemical recurrence during radical prostatectomy for high-risk prostate cancer: a systematic review and meta-analysis. World J Urol. 2017;35:1481–8. https://doi.org/10.1007/s00345-017-2021-9.
35. Novara G, Ficarra V, Mocellin S, Ahlering TE, Carroll PR, Graefen M, et al. Systematic review and meta-analysis of studies

reporting oncologic outcome after robot-assisted radical prostatectomy. Eur Urol. 2012;62:382–404. https://doi.org/10.1016/j.eururo.2012.05.047.

36. Ficarra V, Novara G, Ahlering TE, Costello A, Eastham JA, Graefen M, et al. Systematic review and meta-analysis of studies reporting potency rates after robot-assisted radical prostatectomy. Eur Urol. 2012;62:418–30. https://doi.org/10.1016/j.eururo.2012.05.046.
37. Tewari A, Sooriakumaran P, Bloch DA, Seshadri-Kreaden U, Hebert AE, Wiklund P. Positive surgical margin and perioperative complication rates of primary surgical treatments for prostate cancer: a systematic review and meta-analysis comparing retropubic, laparoscopic, and robotic prostatectomy. Eur Urol. 2012;62:1–15. https://doi.org/10.1016/j.eururo.2012.02.029.
38. Asimakopoulos AD, Annino F, Mugnier C, Lopez L, Hoepffner JL, Gaston R, et al. Robotic radical prostatectomy: analysis of midterm pathologic and oncologic outcomes: a historical series from a high-volume center. Surg Endosc. 2020; https://doi.org/10.1007/s00464-020-08177-0.
39. Roscigno M, La Croce G, Naspro R, Nicolai M, Manica M, Scarcello M, et al. Extended pelvic lymph node dissection during radical prostatectomy: comparison between initial robotic experience of a high volume open surgeon and his contemporary open series. Minerva Urol Nefrol. 2019; https://doi.org/10.23736/S0393-2249.19.03404-0.
40. Xia L, Sperling CD, Taylor BL, Talwar R, Chelluri RR, Raman JD, et al. Associations between hospital volume and outcomes of robot-assisted radical prostatectomy. J Urol. 2020;203:926–32. https://doi.org/10.1097/JU.0000000000000698.
41. Sanda MG, Cadeddu JA, Kirkby E, Chen RC, Crispino T, Fontanarosa J, et al. Clinically localized prostate cancer: AUA/ASTRO/SUO guideline. Part II: recommended approaches and details of specific care options. J Urol. 2018;199:990–7. https://doi.org/10.1016/j.juro.2018.01.002.
42. Mitropoulos D, Artibani W, Graefen M, Remzi M, Rouprêt M, Truss M. Reporting and grading of complications after urologic surgical procedures: an ad hoc EAU guidelines panel assessment and recommendations. Eur Urol. 2012;61:341–9. https://doi.org/10.1016/j.eururo.2011.10.033.
43. Martinez PF, Romeo A, Tobia I, Isola M, Giudice CR, Villamil WA. Comparing open and robotic salvage radical prostatectomy after radiotherapy: predictors and outcomes. Prostate Int. 2021;9:42–7. https://doi.org/10.1016/j.prnil.2020.07.003.
44. Onol FF, Bhat S, Moschovas M, Rogers T, Ganapathi H, Roof S, et al. Comparison of outcomes of salvage robot-assisted laparoscopic prostatectomy for post-primary radiation vs focal therapy. BJU Int. 2020;125:103–11. https://doi.org/10.1111/bju.14900.
45. De Groote R, Nathan A, De Bleser E, Pavan N, Sridhar A, Kelly J, et al. Techniques and outcomes of salvage robot-assisted radical prostatectomy (sRARP). Eur Urol. 2020;78:885–92. https://doi.org/10.1016/j.eururo.2020.05.003.
46. Nathan A, Fricker M, De Groote R, Arora A, Phuah Y, Flora K, et al. Salvage versus primary robot-assisted radical prostatectomy: a propensity-matched comparative effectiveness study from a high-volume tertiary Centre. Eur Urol Open Sci. 2021;27:43–52. https://doi.org/10.1016/j.euros.2021.03.003.
47. Cathcart P, Ribeiro L, Moore C, Ahmed HU, Leslie T, Arya M, et al. Outcomes of the RAFT trial: robotic surgery after focal therapy. BJU Int. 2021;128(4):504–10. https://doi.org/10.1111/bju.15432.
48. Uy M, Cassim R, Kim J, Hoogenes J, Shayegan B, Matsumoto ED. Extraperitoneal versus transperitoneal approach for robot-assisted radical prostatectomy: a contemporary systematic review and meta-analysis. J Robot Surg. 2021; https://doi.org/10.1007/s11701-021-01245-0.
49. Moschovas MC, Seetharam Bhat KR, Onol FF, Rogers T, Ogaya-Pinies G, Roof S, et al. Single-port technique evolution and current practice in urologic procedures. Asian J Urol. 2021;8:100–4. https://doi.org/10.1016/j.ajur.2020.05.003.
50. Kallidonis P, Rai BP, Qazi H, Ganzer R, Do M, Dietel A, et al. Critical appraisal of literature comparing minimally invasive extraperitoneal and transperitoneal radical prostatectomy: a systematic review and meta-analysis. Arab J Urol. 2017;15:267–79. https://doi.org/10.1016/j.aju.2017.07.003.
51. Lee W, Tang J, Li A, Zhu Y, Ling X, Cang J, et al. Transperitoneal versus extraperitoneal robot-assisted laparoscopic radical prostatectomy on postoperative hepatic and renal function. Gland Surg. 2020;9:759–66. https://doi.org/10.21037/gs-20-533.
52. Horovitz D, Feng C, Messing EM, Joseph JV. Extraperitoneal vs. transperitoneal robot-assisted radical prostatectomy in patients with a history of prior inguinal hernia repair with mesh. J Robot Surg. 2017;11:447–54. https://doi.org/10.1007/s11701-017-0678-0.
53. Horovitz D, Feng C, Messing EM, Joseph JV. Extraperitoneal vs Transperitoneal robot-assisted radical prostatectomy in the setting of prior abdominal or pelvic surgery. J Endourol. 2017;31:366–73. https://doi.org/10.1089/end.2016.0706.
54. Akand M, Erdogru T, Avci E, Ates M. Transperitoneal versus extraperitoneal robot-assisted laparoscopic radical prostatectomy: a prospective single surgeon randomized comparative study. Int J Urol. 2015;22:916–21. https://doi.org/10.1111/iju.12854.
55. Capello SA, Boczko J, Patel HRH, Joseph JV. Randomized comparison of Extraperitoneal and Transperitoneal access for robot-assisted radical prostatectomy. J Endourol. 2007;21:1199–202. https://doi.org/10.1089/end.2007.9906.
56. Galfano A, Ascione A, Grimaldi S, Petralia G, Strada E, Bocciardi AM. A new anatomic approach for robot-assisted laparoscopic prostatectomy: a feasibility study for completely Intrafascial surgery. Eur Urol. 2010;58:457–61. https://doi.org/10.1016/j.eururo.2010.06.008.
57. Galfano A, Di Trapani D, Sozzi F, Strada E, Petralia G, Bramerio M, et al. Beyond the learning curve of the Retzius-sparing approach for robot-assisted laparoscopic radical prostatectomy: oncologic and functional results of the first 200 patients with ≥1 year of follow-up. Eur Urol. 2013;64:974–80. https://doi.org/10.1016/j.eururo.2013.06.046.
58. Kowalczyk KJ, Davis M, O'Neill J, Lee H, Orzel J, Rubin RS, et al. Impact of Retzius-sparing versus standard robotic-assisted radical prostatectomy on penile shortening, Peyronie's disease, and inguinal hernia sequelae. Eur Urol Open Sci. 2020;22:17–22. https://doi.org/10.1016/j.euros.2020.09.004.
59. Chang KD, Abdel Raheem A, Santok GDR, Kim LHC, Lum TGH, Lee SH, et al. Anatomical Retzius-space preservation is associated with lower incidence of postoperative inguinal hernia development after robot-assisted radical prostatectomy. Hernia. 2017;21:555–61. https://doi.org/10.1007/s10029-017-1588-9.
60. Tai T-E, Wu C-C, Kang Y-N, Wu J-C. Effects of Retzius sparing on robot-assisted laparoscopic prostatectomy: a systematic review with meta-analysis. Surg Endosc. 2020;34:4020–9. https://doi.org/10.1007/s00464-019-07190-2.
61. Rosenberg JE, Jung JH, Edgerton Z, Lee H, Lee S, Bakker CJ, et al. Retzius-sparing versus standard robot-assisted laparoscopic prostatectomy for the treatment of clinically localized prostate cancer. BJU Int. 2021;128:12–20. https://doi.org/10.1111/bju.15385.
62. Phukan C, Mclean A, Nambiar A, Mukherjee A, Somani B, Krishnamoorthy R, et al. Retzius sparing robotic assisted radical prostatectomy vs. conventional robotic assisted radical prostatectomy: a systematic review and meta-analysis. World J Urol. 2020;38:1123–34. https://doi.org/10.1007/s00345-019-02798-4.

63. Jiang Y-L, Zheng G-F, Jiang Z-P, Zhen-Li, Zhou X-L, Zhou J, et al. Comparison of Retzius-sparing robot-assisted laparoscopic radical prostatectomy vs standard robot-assisted radical prostatectomy: a meta-analysis. BMC Urol. 2020;20:114. https://doi.org/10.1186/s12894-020-00685-4.
64. Dirie NI, Pokhrel G, Guan W, Mumin MA, Yang J, Masau JF, et al. Is Retzius-sparing robot-assisted radical prostatectomy associated with better functional and oncological outcomes? Literature review and meta-analysis. Asian J Urol. 2019;6:174–82. https://doi.org/10.1016/j.ajur.2018.02.001.
65. Checcucci E, Veccia A, Fiori C, Amparore D, Manfredi M, Di Dio M, et al. Retzius-sparing robot-assisted radical prostatectomy vs the standard approach: a systematic review and analysis of comparative outcomes. BJU Int. 2020;125:8–16. https://doi.org/10.1111/bju.14887.
66. Ko YH, Coelho RF, Sivaraman A, Schatloff O, Chauhan S, Abdul-Muhsin HM, et al. Retrograde versus Antegrade nerve sparing during robot-assisted radical prostatectomy: which is better for achieving early functional recovery? Eur Urol. 2013;63:169–77. https://doi.org/10.1016/j.eururo.2012.09.051.
67. Walsh PC. Anatomic radical prostatectomy: evolution of the surgical technique. J Urol. 1998;160(6 Pt 2):2418–24. https://doi.org/10.1097/00005392-199812020-00010.
68. Walz J, Burnett AL, Costello AJ, Eastham JA, Graefen M, Guillonneau B, et al. A critical analysis of the current knowledge of surgical anatomy related to optimization of cancer control and preservation of continence and erection in candidates for radical prostatectomy. Eur Urol. 2010;57:179–92. https://doi.org/10.1016/j.eururo.2009.11.009.
69. Eichelberg C, Erbersdobler A, Michl U, Schlomm T, Salomon G, Graefen M, et al. Nerve distribution along the prostatic capsule. Eur Urol. 2007;51:105–11. https://doi.org/10.1016/j.eururo.2006.05.038.
70. de Carvalho PA, Barbosa JABA, Guglielmetti GB, Cordeiro MD, Rocco B, Nahas WC, et al. Retrograde release of the neurovascular bundle with preservation of dorsal venous complex during robot-assisted radical prostatectomy: optimizing functional outcomes. Eur Urol. 2020;77:628–35. https://doi.org/10.1016/j.eururo.2018.07.003.
71. Puliatti S, Elsherbiny A, Eissa A, Pirola G, Morini E, Squecco D, et al. Effect of puboprostatic ligament reconstruction on continence recovery after robot-assisted laparoscopic prostatectomy: our initial experience. Minerva Urol Nefrol. 2019; https://doi.org/10.23736/S0393-2249.18.03260-5.
72. Vis AN, van der Poel HG, Ruiter AEC, Hu JC, Tewari AK, Rocco B, et al. Posterior, anterior, and Periurethral surgical reconstruction of urinary continence mechanisms in robot-assisted radical prostatectomy: a description and video compilation of commonly performed surgical techniques. Eur Urol. 2019;76:814–22. https://doi.org/10.1016/j.eururo.2018.11.035.
73. Heo JE, Lee JS, Goh HJ, Jang WS, Choi YD. Urethral realignment with maximal urethral length and bladder neck preservation in robot-assisted radical prostatectomy: urinary continence recovery. PLoS One. 2020;15:e0227744. https://doi.org/10.1371/journal.pone.0227744.
74. Kim JW, Kim DK, Ahn HK, Do JH, Lee JY, Cho KS. Effect of bladder neck preservation on Long-term urinary continence after robot-assisted laparoscopic prostatectomy: a systematic review and meta-analysis. J Clin Med. 2019;8:2068. https://doi.org/10.3390/jcm8122068.
75. Mungovan SF, Sandhu JS, Akin O, Smart NA, Graham PL, Patel MI. Preoperative membranous urethral length measurement and continence recovery following radical prostatectomy: a systematic review and meta-analysis. Eur Urol. 2017;71:368–78. https://doi.org/10.1016/j.eururo.2016.06.023.
76. Nyarangi-Dix JN, Radtke JP, Hadaschik B, Pahernik S, Hohenfellner M. Impact of complete bladder neck preservation on urinary continence, quality of life and surgical margins after radical prostatectomy: a randomized, controlled, single blind trial. J Urol. 2013;189:891–8. https://doi.org/10.1016/j.juro.2012.09.082.
77. Nyarangi-Dix JN, Tichy D, Hatiboglu G, Pahernik S, Tosev G, Hohenfellner M. Complete bladder neck preservation promotes long-term post-prostatectomy continence without compromising midterm oncological outcome: analysis of a randomised controlled cohort. World J Urol. 2018;36:349–55. https://doi.org/10.1007/s00345-017-2134-1.
78. Sfoungaristos S, Kontogiannis S, Perimenis P. Early continence recovery after preservation of maximal urethral length until the level of Verumontanum during radical prostatectomy: primary oncological and functional outcomes after 1 year of follow-up. Biomed Res Int. 2013;2013:1–7. https://doi.org/10.1155/2013/426208.
79. Salazar A, Regis L, Planas J, Celma A, Santamaria A, Trilla E, et al. A randomised controlled trial to assess the benefit of posterior Rhabdosphincter reconstruction in early urinary continence recovery after robot-assisted radical prostatectomy. Eur Urol Oncol. 2021; https://doi.org/10.1016/j.euo.2021.02.005.
80. Ogawa S, Hoshi S, Koguchi T, Hata J, Sato Y, Akaihata H, et al. Three-layer two-step posterior reconstruction using peritoneum during robot-assisted radical prostatectomy to improve recovery of urinary continence: a prospective comparative study. J Endourol. 2017;31:1251–7. https://doi.org/10.1089/end.2017.0410.
81. Sutherland DE, Linder B, Guzman AM, Hong M, Frazier HA, Engel JD, et al. Posterior Rhabdosphincter reconstruction during robotic assisted radical prostatectomy: results from a phase II randomized clinical trial. J Urol. 2011;185:1262–7. https://doi.org/10.1016/j.juro.2010.11.085.
82. Jeong CW, Lee JK, Oh JJ, Lee S, Jeong SJ, Hong SK, et al. Effects of new 1-step posterior reconstruction method on recovery of continence after robot-assisted laparoscopic prostatectomy: results of a prospective, single-blind, parallel group, randomized, controlled trial. J Urol. 2015;193:935–42. https://doi.org/10.1016/j.juro.2014.10.023.
83. Hurtes X, Rouprêt M, Vaessen C, Pereira H, Faivre D'Arcier B, Cormier L, et al. Anterior suspension combined with posterior reconstruction during robot-assisted laparoscopic prostatectomy improves early return of urinary continence: a prospective randomized multicentre trial. BJU Int. 2012;110:875–83. https://doi.org/10.1111/j.1464-410X.2011.10849.x.
84. Menon M, Muhletaler F, Campos M, Peabody JO. Assessment of early continence after reconstruction of the Periprostatic tissues in patients undergoing computer assisted (robotic) prostatectomy: results of a 2 group parallel randomized controlled trial. J Urol. 2008;180:1018–23. https://doi.org/10.1016/j.juro.2008.05.046.
85. Koliakos N, Mottrie A, Buffi N, De Naeyer G, Willemsen P, Fonteyne E. Posterior and anterior fixation of the urethra during robotic prostatectomy improves early continence rates. Scand J Urol Nephrol. 2010;44:5–10. https://doi.org/10.3109/00365590903413627.
86. Sammon JD, Muhletaler F, Peabody JO, Diaz-Insua M, Satyanaryana R, Menon M. Long-term functional urinary outcomes comparing single- vs double-layer Urethrovesical anastomosis: two-year follow-up of a two-group parallel randomized controlled trial. Urology. 2010;76:1102–7. https://doi.org/10.1016/j.urology.2010.05.052.
87. Student V, Vidlar A, Grepl M, Hartmann I, Buresova E, Student V. Advanced reconstruction of Vesicourethral support (ARVUS) during robot-assisted radical prostatectomy: one-year functional outcomes in a two-group randomised controlled trial. Eur Urol. 2017;71:822–30. https://doi.org/10.1016/j.eururo.2016.05.032.

88. Manfredi M, Checcucci E, Fiori C, Garrou D, Aimar R, Amparore D, et al. Total anatomical reconstruction during robot-assisted radical prostatectomy: focus on urinary continence recovery and related complications after 1000 procedures. BJU Int. 2019;124:477–86. https://doi.org/10.1111/bju.14716.
89. Checcucci E, Pecoraro A, de Cillis S, Manfredi M, Amparore D, Aimar R, et al. The importance of anatomical reconstruction for continence recovery after robot assisted radical prostatectomy: a systematic review and pooled analysis from referral centers. Minerva Urol Nephrol. 2021;73:165–77. https://doi.org/10.23736/S0393-2249.20.04146-6.
90. Cui J, Guo H, Li Y, Chen S, Zhu Y, Wang S, et al. Pelvic floor reconstruction after radical prostatectomy: a systematic review and meta-analysis of different surgical techniques. Sci Rep. 2017;7:2737. https://doi.org/10.1038/s41598-017-02991-8.
91. Antonelli A, Palumbo C, Veccia A, Fisogni S, Zamboni S, Furlan M, et al. Standard vs delayed ligature of the dorsal vascular complex during robot-assisted radical prostatectomy: results from a randomized controlled trial. J Robot Surg. 2019;13:253–60. https://doi.org/10.1007/s11701-018-0847-9.
92. Li H, Chen J, Cui Y, Liu P, Yi Z, Zu X. Delayed versus standard ligature of the dorsal venous complex during laparoscopic radical prostatectomy: a systematic review and meta-analysis of comparative studies. Int J Surg. 2019;68:117–25. https://doi.org/10.1016/j.ijsu.2019.06.015.
93. Feng T, Heulitt G, Lee JJ, Liao M, Li H-F, Porter JR. Randomised comparison of techniques for control of the dorsal venous complex during robot-assisted laparoscopic radical prostatectomy. BJU Int. 2020;126:586–94. https://doi.org/10.1111/bju.15133.
94. Li H, Liu C, Zhang H, Xu W, Liu J, Chen Y, et al. The use of unidirectional barbed suture for Urethrovesical anastomosis during robot-assisted radical prostatectomy: a systematic review and meta-analysis of efficacy and safety. PLoS One. 2015;10:e0131167. https://doi.org/10.1371/journal.pone.0131167.
95. Covas Moschovas M, Bhat S, Onol FF, Rogers T, Roof S, Mazzone E, et al. Modified apical dissection and lateral prostatic fascia preservation improves early postoperative functional recovery in robotic-assisted laparoscopic radical prostatectomy: results from a propensity score-matched analysis. Eur Urol. 2020; https://doi.org/10.1016/j.eururo.2020.05.041.
96. Siltari A, Riikonen J, Murtola TJ. Preservation of Endopelvic fascia: effects on postoperative incontinence and sexual function – a randomized clinical trial. J Sex Med. 2021;18:327–38. https://doi.org/10.1016/j.jsxm.2020.11.003.
97. Wagaskar VG, Mittal A, Sobotka S, Ratnani P, Lantz A, Falagario UG, et al. Hood technique for robotic radical prostatectomy—preserving Periurethral anatomical structures in the space of Retzius and sparing the pouch of Douglas, enabling early return of continence without compromising surgical margin rates. Eur Urol. 2021;80:213–21. https://doi.org/10.1016/j.eururo.2020.09.044.
98. Eissa A, Zoeir A, Sighinolfi MC, Puliatti S, Bevilacqua L, Del Prete C, et al. "Real-time" assessment of surgical margins during radical prostatectomy: state-of-the-art. Clin Genitourin Cancer. 2020;18:95–104. https://doi.org/10.1016/j.clgc.2019.07.012.
99. Dinneen E, Haider A, Grierson J, Freeman A, Oxley J, Briggs T, et al. NeuroSAFE frozen section during robot-assisted radical prostatectomy: peri-operative and histopathological outcomes from the NeuroSAFE PROOF feasibility randomized controlled trial. BJU Int. 2021;127:676–86. https://doi.org/10.1111/bju.15256.
100. Rocco B, Sarchi L, Assumma S, Cimadamore A, Montironi R, Reggiani Bonetti L, et al. Digital frozen sections with fluorescence confocal microscopy during robot-assisted radical prostatectomy: surgical technique. Eur Urol. 2021; https://doi.org/10.1016/j.eururo.2021.03.021.
101. Rocco B, Sighinolfi MC, Cimadamore A, Reggiani Bonetti L, Bertoni L, Puliatti S, et al. Digital frozen section of the prostate surface during radical prostatectomy: a novel approach to evaluate surgical margins. BJU Int. 2020;126:336–8. https://doi.org/10.1111/bju.15108.
102. Ogaya-Pinies G, Palayapalam-Ganapathi H, Rogers T, Hernandez-Cardona E, Rocco B, Coelho RF, et al. Can dehydrated human amnion/chorion membrane accelerate the return to potency after a nerve-sparing robotic-assisted radical prostatectomy? Propensity score-matched analysis. J Robot Surg. 2018;12:235–43. https://doi.org/10.1007/s11701-017-0719-8.
103. Porpiglia F, Checcucci E, Amparore D, Manfredi M, Massa F, Piazzolla P, et al. Three-dimensional elastic augmented-reality robot-assisted radical prostatectomy using Hyperaccuracy three-dimensional reconstruction technology: a step further in the identification of capsular involvement. Eur Urol. 2019;76:505–14. https://doi.org/10.1016/j.eururo.2019.03.037.
104. Bianchi L, Chessa F, Angiolini A, Cercenelli L, Lodi S, Bortolani B, et al. The use of augmented reality to guide the intraoperative frozen section during robot-assisted radical prostatectomy. Eur Urol. 2021; https://doi.org/10.1016/j.eururo.2021.06.020.

Techniques to Improve Urinary Continence Outcomes Following Robot-Assisted Radical Prostatectomy

Bernardo Rocco, Alberto Martini, Maria Chiara Sighinolfi, and Young Hwii Ko

1 Introduction

Over time, robot-assisted surgery has become more and more common for the removal of the prostate gland. However, owing to the adjacent anatomical location of the prostate to the neurovascular bundles, responsible for erectile function, and the urethral sphincter complex, radical prostatectomy can be associated with adverse functional outcomes, in terms of erectile function and urinary continence. Among them, post-prostatectomy incontinence (PPI) remains a dominant problem for patients who are reluctant to undergo surgery and tend to choose alternative ways instead. To date, the incidence reported by different surgeons considerably varies, in the range of 8–77%.

Since the late 1980s, with the introduction of radical prostatectomy by an open approach, the depth of the anatomical understanding of the structure surrounding the prostate has improved dramatically. That led to the development of new surgical techniques that were consequently aimed at reducing the incidences of PPI. Recent data on PPI from robot-assisted radical prostatectomy (RARP) looks quite acceptable compared to past reports. Nevertheless, urethrovesical anastomosis is still a demanding procedure requiring a steep learning curve for a novice and this can importantly affect patients' quality of life during the early postoperative period. For both patients and surgeons, in addition to the oncological outcomes, functional recovery especially from PPI is being recognized as an important goal of surgery. Therefore, several surgeons suggested various technical refinements to improve urinary continence outcomes following RARP. To this purpose, in this chapter, we aimed to summarize the results of recent studies and systematic reviews regarding PPI following RARP.

1.1 Causes and Frequency of PPI

The prostate gland surrounds the proximal part of the male urethra and it is adjacent to several anatomical structures involved in maintaining urinary continence and responsible for erectile function. As a result, in cases of resection involving the surrounding area, which is the aim of radical prostatectomy, the more successful the process of resection, the greater the risk of impairing urinary continence due to unintended damage to surrounding structures. Considering the close involvement of periprostatic structures in urinary continence, in most patients, PPI shows a pattern of early occurrence followed by gradual recovery over time. Recovery from PPI is usually evaluated by asking the patient about incontinence pad usage, rather than obtaining objective evidence via a 24-hour pad test. This means that the reported incidence is affected by the duration of the investigation and the types of questions being asked. To date, the incidence reported by different surgeons considerably varies, in the range of 8–77% [1], but this seems to be, in part, due to authors using different definitions. Specifically, up to the early 2000s, the most common definition of recovery from incontinence was using 0 or 1 pad per day postoperatively, and this typically included the use of "security" pads. This led to a large number of patients being classified as having recovered from incontinence very early after surgery; however, major differences in quality of life were observed between patients who still used pads in daily living and those who did not, so this classification was criticized for only making surgeons' outcomes appear more favorable. Indeed, one study found that among 1616 patients who were followed up for a mean of 50.7 months (range, 12–216 months) after open retropubic prostatectomy, 1459 (90.3%) reported experiencing urinary leakage, which clearly shows the enor-

B. Rocco (✉) · M. C. Sighinolfi
Department of Urology, Dipartimento di Scienze della Salute, ASST Santi Paolo e Carlo, University of Milan, Milan, Italy

A. Martini
Department of Urology, Vita-Salute San Raffaele University, Milan, Italy

Y. H. Ko
Department of Urology, College of Medicine, Yeungnam University, Daegu, South Korea

P. Wiklund et al. (eds.), *Robotic Urologic Surgery*, https://doi.org/10.1007/978-3-031-00363-9_20

mous effect of the definition of the prevalence of the condition [2]. With regards to the appropriate definition of PPI, Ahlering et al. divided 500 patients who had undergone RARP into groups with daily pad usage of 0 and 1 and reported a significant difference in quality of life between the groups (1.16 vs. 3.41, $p < 0.0005$), arguing, on this basis, that recovery from PPI should be defined as using 0 pads per day [3]. Likewise, the definitions of survival, continence, and potency (SCP) proposed in 2012 by world-leading surgeons as objective indicators to evaluate the outcomes of radical prostatectomy also consider 0 pad usage to be the standard definition for recovery from PPI [4]. However, different authors are still using their own definitions in studies published since then; thus, some caution is required when interpreting individual studies.

1.2 Anatomical Mechanisms of Male Urinary Continence

Although we still cannot claim to fully understand the mechanisms of urinary continence in males, alongside advances in radical prostatectomy techniques and increased numbers of operations, a large amount of related anatomical knowledge has been accumulated. In the 1980s, on the basis of the classical anatomical theory, the urogenital diaphragm, lying flat below the prostate gland, was thought to be a key structure in urinary continence by acting as the urethral sphincter; however, at the end of the 1990s, human and cadaver studies showed that the structure previously identified as the urogenital diaphragm did not exist [5, 6].

Currently, male urinary continence is understood to be achieved by the combined actions of multiple anatomical structures surrounding the prostate gland [7–10]; below, we summarize the major constituent muscular structures in this urethral sphincter complex and their roles.

1. The smooth muscle sphincter (lissosphincter) consists of two layers (inner longitudinal and outer circular) and is innervated by the autonomous nervous system. It forms a spongy structure below the urethral mucosa, and external contraction completely cuts off the flow of urine.
2. The stratified sphincter (rhabdosphincter; the posterior part forms the median fibrous raphe [MFR] with no muscle layer) is responsible for the slow-twitch, passive control. It forms a cylindrical shape that originates from the prostate apex and attaches to the deep transverse perineal muscles. In the transverse cross-section, the muscle in the stratified sphincter is distributed in an omega shape; posteriorly, there is no muscle, but instead, forming the MFR are dense fibrous tissues. The MFR forms a posterior support complex by connecting to the central tendon posteriorly and Denonvilliers' fascia superiorly.
3. The puboperinealis muscle is responsible for fast-twitch, active control. It forms the medial part of the levator ani muscle. In the coronary view of magnetic resonance imaging, the puboperinealis muscle appears as two teardrop shapes running bilaterally, lateral to the urethra. As it attaches to the perineal body posterior to the urethra, the puboperinealis muscle ultimately forms a structure that supports the urethra [9].

Based on this understanding of the urethral sphincter complex, widespread efforts have been made to mitigate PPI by identifying and preserving this complex during surgery. Conceptually, these techniques can be summarized as the preservation of the internal/external sphincters and reconstruction of anterior/posterior support structures. Figure 1 illustrates the operative view of these key structures, once the prostate gland has been dissected free.

Lissosphincter, rhabdosphincter, median fibrous raphe (MFR), puboperinealis muscle.

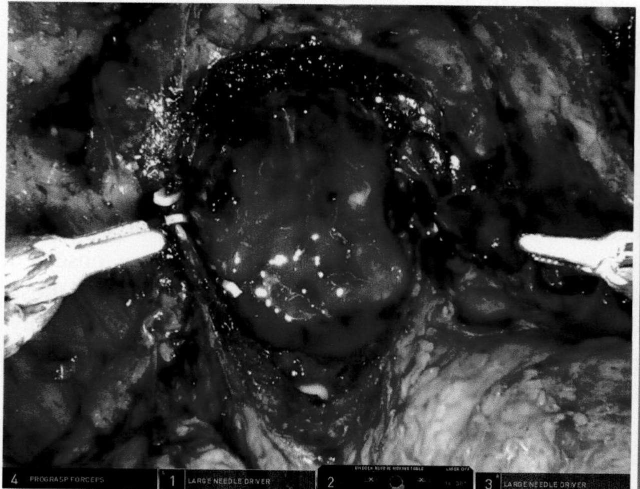

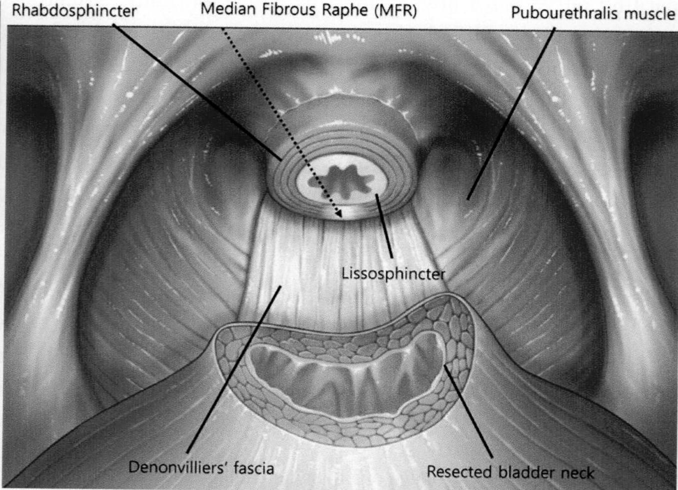

Fig. 1 The key functional structure for continence identified right after the removal of the prostate during RARP

1.3 Correcting PPI Based on Anatomical Understanding: Development of Surgical Techniques and Clinical Outcomes

On the basis of the understanding of the urethral sphincter complex described earlier, widespread efforts have been made to mitigate PPI by identifying and preserving this complex during surgery. Conceptually, these techniques can be summarized as preservation of the internal/external sphincters and reconstruction of anterior/posterior support structures [11].

1.3.1 Preservation of the Bladder Neck

The bladder neck is a structure that includes the intravesical sphincter; in open surgery, broad incision and dissection of the bladder neck is performed to allow complete dissection of the prostate base, followed by suture ligation to restore the original thickness. However, the proximal internal urethral sphincter, previously referred to as the internal sphincter, has been reported to play a role in urinary continence [13]. Many comparative studies have been published where surgical methods aimed at maintaining the bladder neck without any artificial manipulation have been investigated. Friedlander and colleagues reported the largest number of patients recruited (1067 RARP cases). The 791 who underwent bladder neck-sparing surgery showed a significantly shorter time to urinary continence return than the 276 patients who underwent conventional surgery [14]. In a systematic review of 13 studies on this topic, 1130 patients in whom the bladder neck was spared were compared with 1154 control patients and showed a significant improvement in the rate of urinary continence at both 6 and 12 months of follow-up [15]. However, bladder neck sparing is not possible in all the patients, and in patients who have previously undergone endoscopic prostate surgery such as transurethral resection of the prostate or in patients with a medial lobe, proper reconstruction of the bladder neck after resection is essential. In these cases, the bladder neck reconstruction with a transverse plication has been described by Lin et al. in 2009. The technique involves the bilateral plication of the lateral aspect of the bladder, in order to reduce the size of the bladder nack making it matching the size of the membranous urethra [16].

1.3.2 Preservation of the Neurovascular Bundle

From the perspective of classical anatomy, preservation of the neurovascular bundle (NVB) is intended to facilitate early recovery of erectile function rather than to prevent incontinence. However, preservation of the NVB is consistently reported to help recovery from PPI. Ko et al. analyzed 1299 patients operated on by a single surgeon using the same technique and found that recovery from PPI, defined as 0 pad usage within 3 months, was significantly earlier in patients for whom the NVB was even partially spared than in patients with no NVB preservation [17]. A recent systematic review also demonstrated the association between NVB preservation and recovery from PPI [18]; thus, unless NVB preservation is impossible oncologically owing to the presence of aggressive cancer, preservation of the NVB even partially is important to aid recovery from PPI.

1.3.3 Meticulous Apical Dissection

The prostate apex, which is connected to the urethra, communicates immediately with the smooth muscle sphincter and stratified sphincter, so partial dissection of the prostate while sparing these structures is directly related to functional recovery.

1.3.4 Sparing of the External Sphincter

As explained in the discussion of the anatomical structure, the puboperinealis muscle forms a hammock structure that supports the urethra as one aspect of urinary continence. Thus, preservation of the puboperinealis muscle could provide functional benefits in the prevention of PPI. Attached to the lateral part of the prostate apex, this muscle layer should be dissected under careful observation. Takenaka et al. reported that sparing the puboperinealis muscle could reduce the time to recovery from PPI [19].

1.3.5 Posterior Reconstruction and Preservation of Supporting Structures

As anatomical knowledge about the prostate gland increased, the importance of the posterior supporting structures, particularly the posterior support complex, has received greater attention. Posterior reconstruction has become a major milestone in modern prostate surgery; this procedure is also called the Rocco stitch, named after the surgeon who first introduced the concept of reconstructing the posterior structures that are damaged or lost while operating on the prostate [20]. Patel et al. extended this concept to include anterior reconstruction, as the role of the puboprostatic ligament, superior to the prostate apex, is also important in supporting the urethra [21]. Recently, the usefulness of the so-called total anatomical reconstruction has been reported, in which the prostate apex is divided into 5 anatomical units, each of which is reconstructed [22].

Among the suggested techniques to minimize PPI, posterior reconstruction has become a major milestone in modern radical prostatectomy. As a result of prostatectomy, the posterior supportive layers of the bladder and prostate are divided, including Denonvilliers' fascia and its confluence with the posterior rhabdosphincter. Thus, the reconstruction of these supportive structures has been attempted [20]. Several suggested mechanisms for posterior reconstruction include reestablishment of the posterior anatomic support to the bladder and urethra, improving urethral coaptation during voiding, reduced tension at the vesicourethral anastomosis, and increase in the functional length of the striated urethral sphincter complex [23, 24].

Its role in terms of earlier continence recovery has been widely studied across time. While several technical modifications from the original concept should be considered, two initial randomized trials with some technical modifications have found no significant benefits in the earlier regain of continence [25, 26]. Nevertheless, a recent meta-analysis on the published series including the other randomized trial demonstrates that the implementation of posterior reconstruction during radical prostatectomy improves early continence recovery at 3–7, 30, and 90 days after catheter removal, while the continence rate at 180 days was not clinically affected [24, 27]. A recent RCT confirmed a role for an early continence recovery when applying the "no pad usage" definition of continence [28]. A Cochrane review published by Rosemberg et al. in 2021 addressed the effectiveness of posterior reconstruction compared to no posterior reconstruction on early continence recovery after RALP. Authors analyzed 8 unique RCTs, of which 6 were published studies and 2 abstract proceedings. Overall, 963 randomized participants completed the trials. Authors stated that posterior reconstruction may improve urinary continence recovery one week after catheter removal (RR1,25; 95%CI 0.90–1.73) but has little to no effect on urinary continence 3 months after surgery [29]. Another meta-analysis addressed the topic of post-RARP urinary continence by considering all the techniques involved in pelvic floor reconstruction, including anterior suspension, anterior reconstruction, posterior reconstruction, and their combinations [30]. Thirty-two studies were finally included in the meta-analysis, accounting for a total of 4697 patients considered. Authors found that posterior reconstruction is associated with complete urinary continence improval at 1–4, 28–42, 90, 180, and 360 days following catheter removal. Also when considered in combination with other techniques, patients who had posterior reconstruction had the least urinary incontinence [30].

It is also notable that no significant complications related to the posterior reconstruction have been reported so far. The undeniable advantage of posterior reconstruction is that this step reduces the distance between the bladder neck and urethra, thereby facilitating the completion of a tension-free vesicourethral anastomosis, as we illustrated previously. Moreover, the evidence does suggest the incidence of pelvic hematoma may be reduced by performing a posterior reconstruction [31]. In the same context, expending this concept, the usefulness of the so-called total anatomical reconstruction has been suggested, in which the prostate apex is divided into 5 anatomical units, each of which is reconstructed [22].

1.3.6 Urethrovesical Anastomosis: The Surgical Principle

The greatest change and development with the introduction of RARP was, first, that a safe and complete urethrovesical anastomosis became possible as compared to open or laparoscopic approaches, and this change has led to a decrease in the incidence rates of urine leakage and urethral strictures at the urethrovesical anastomosis or bladder neck contracture, which were previously common in the era of non-robotic prostatectomy. Besides posterior reconstruction, though several surgical principles including the preservation of the bladder neck, sparing of the external sphincter, and maximal preservation of the urethral length have been suggested, the secured urethrovesical anastomosis still plays a key role in earlier return to continence.

In the era of robotic surgery, while there are several technical modifications by surgeon's preference, a continuous stitch that distributes tension broadly across multiple points along the bladder neck and urethra utilizing two separate sutures tied together at their ends, which was originally described by van Velthoven et al. [12] became the most typical way. To prevent the suture from slipping thereby maintaining tissue approximation, double-armed barbed sutures are used to accomplish this step. If it is available, two different colors for each suture could be helpful to facilitate visual distinction on each side of the suture. Mucosal eversion sutures at the bladder neck, commonly used during open prostatectomy, are unnecessary when excellent running mucosa-to-mucosa anastomosis is achieved.

1.3.7 Maximal Preservation of the Urethral Length

Ahlering et al. highlighted the remaining length of the urethra after resection of the prostate apex as an important factor in urinary continence [32]. Maintaining urethral length during surgery is essential to facilitate perfect urethrovesical anastomosis, which is one of the most important and demanding aspects of prostatectomy in terms of technical skill. In the dissection of the prostate apex, the final stage of prostatectomy, thorough dissection of the urethra before completely isolating the prostate is crucial to ensure enough urethral length. Meanwhile, unlike other parts of the prostate, the apex is not covered by the prostate capsule, so when cancer develops in this area, the risk of residual cancer after surgery is high. Preserving the length of the urethra can sometimes increase the risk of residual cancer, so when prostate cancer is confirmed to be located in the apex by using histological tests or preoperative imaging, cutting the apex as close to the urethra as possible is recommended.

1.3.8 Watertight Urethrovesical Anastomosis

The greatest change and development with the introduction of RARP was, first, that a safe and complete urethrovesical anastomosis became possible as compared with the previous methods. In the age of open surgery, anastomosis was performed using interrupted stitches in 6 places, but now, by using a continuous stitch, the incidence of leakage has been reduced considerably. This change has led to a decrease in the incidence rates of urethral stricture and bladder neck contracture, which were previously common in the era of open retropubic prostatectomy.

1.3.9 Regenerative Materials

In addition to surgical techniques, another strategy that can be expected to ameliorate PPI is to minimize surgical trauma and to maximize the healing process. Active research has been conducted on techniques such as stem cell injection, but the most successful clinical effort to date was the use of dehydrated human amnion/chorion membrane allograft by Patel et al., reported in 2015. In PPI, defined by the use of safety pads, groups that received the intervention for 1.2 and 1.8 months showed significantly shorter recovery times from incontinence [33], and in a subsequent study on 235 more patients, the use of this material during surgery was reported to have a similar effect of shortening the time to recovery of urinary continence and erectile function [34].

1.3.10 Novel Approaches

A modified technique of apical dissection with endopelvic fascia preservation has been recently described by Moschovas et al. [35]. This technique allows to maintain NVB untouched and covered together with the maximal preservation of the apical complex and peri-urethral tissues. The authors performed a propensity score matching with a similar group who underwent conventional RALP (104 patients in each group) and found that the modified technique yielded significantly faster continence (mean 46 vs 70 days) and potency recovery (mean 74 vs 118 days) [35].

Another preservation approach recently described is the "Hood technique," which includes the sparing of peri-urethral anatomic structures in the space of Retzius [36]. The detrusor apron, puboprostatic ligament complex, arcus tendinous, endopelvic fascia, and pouch of Douglas remain untouched. With a prospective observational study, the authors reported an early return of continence without compromising positive surgical margin rates.

1.3.11 Rehabilitative Approaches: Emphasis on Kegel Exercises

Although the most important factor is to thoroughly apply the aforementioned techniques during surgery and perform the techniques at a high level, exercise can be considered as another important factor that can affect early postoperative recovery from PPI, and Kegel exercises, which can strengthen the urethral sphincter complex, are especially important. In 66 patients who had undergone open retropubic prostatectomy, Park et al. reported statistically significant differences in the extent of PPI, measured by a 24-hour pad test, between a control group and patients who had performed Kegel exercises for 1 hour once a week for 12 weeks [37]. As Kegel exercises can promote considerable recovery from incontinence even when performed sometime after surgery, postoperative patient education and follow-up of exercise levels should not be overlooked in outpatient care after radical prostatectomy.

2 Conclusion

Owing to the increased incidence of prostate cancer due to aging, heightened social interest, and the increase in individuals at high risk of cancer after the modification of the recommendation on the PSA screening since 2012, RARP in the advanced disease is expected to become increasingly common. As this procedure is often performed in elderly patients, postoperative functional recovery will become a more important task in clinical care. As we have seen in this chapter, the incidence of postoperative incontinence has been reduced greatly by focusing on the development of surgical techniques based on anatomical knowledge and advancements in technology. The duration of disease has also decreased considerably since the introduction of robotic surgery.

References

1. Klingler HC, Marberger M. Incontinence after radical prostatectomy: surgical treatment options. Curr Opin Urol. 2006;16:60–4.
2. Peterson AC, Chen Y. Patient reported incontinence after radical prostatectomy is more common than expected and not associated with the nerve sparing technique: results from the Center for Prostate Disease Research (CPDR) database. Neurourol Urodyn. 2012;31:60–3.
3. Liss MA, Osann K, Canvasser N, Chu W, Chang A, Gan J, et al. Continence definition after radical prostatectomy using urinary quality of life: evaluation of patient reported validated questionnaires. J Urol. 2010;183:1464–8.
4. Ficarra V, Sooriakumaran P, Novara G, Schatloff O, Briganti A, Van der Poel H, et al. Systematic review of methods for reporting combined outcomes after radical prostatectomy and proposal of a novel system: the survival, continence, and potency (SCP) classification. Eur Urol. 2012;61:541–8.
5. Kaye KW, Milne N, Creed K, van der Werf B. The 'urogenital diaphragm', external urethral sphincter and radical prostatectomy. Aust N Z J Surg. 1997;67:40–4.
6. Dorschner W, Biesold M, Schmidt F, Stolzenburg JU. The dispute about the external sphincter and the urogenital diaphragm. J Urol. 1999;162:1942–5.
7. Walz J, Burnett AL, Costello AJ, Eastham JA, Graefen M, Guillonneau B, et al. A critical analysis of the current knowledge

of surgical anatomy related to optimization of cancer control and preservation of continence and erection in candidates for radical prostatectomy. Eur Urol. 2010;57:179–92.
8. Walz J, Epstein JI, Ganzer R, Graefen M, Guazzoni G, Kaouk J, et al. A critical analysis of the current knowledge of surgical anatomy of the prostate related to optimisation of cancer control and preservation of continence and erection in candidates for radical prostatectomy: an update. Eur Urol. 2016;70:301–11.
9. Myers RP, Cahill DR, Kay PA, Camp JJ, Devine RM, King BF, et al. Puboperineales: muscular boundaries of the male urogenital hiatus in 3D from magnetic resonance imaging. J Urol. 2000;164:1412–5.
10. Ko YH. Functional recovery after radical prostatectomy for prostate cancer. Yeungnam Univ J Med. 2018 Dec;35(2):141–9.
11. Sridhar AN, Abozaid M, Rajan P, Sooriakumaran P, Shaw G, Nathan S, et al. Surgical techniques to optimize early urinary continence recovery post robot assisted radical prostatectomy for prostate cancer. Curr Urol Rep. 2017;18:71.
12. Van Velthoven RF, Ahlering TE, Peltier A, Skarecky DW, Clayman RV. Technique for laparoscopic running urethrovesical anastomosis:the single knot method. Urology. 2003 Apr;61(4):699–702.
13. Dorschner W, Stolzenburg JU, Neuhaus J. Structure and function of the bladder neck. Adv Anat Embryol Cell Biol 2001;159:III-XII, 1–109.
14. Friedlander DF, Alemozaffar M, Hevelone ND, Lipsitz SR, Hu JC. Stepwise description and outcomes of bladder neck sparing during robot-assisted laparoscopic radical prostatectomy. J Urol. 2012;188:1754–60.
15. Ma X, Tang K, Yang C, Wu G, Xu N, Wang M, et al. Bladder neck preservation improves time to continence after radical prostatectomy: a systematic review and meta-analysis. Oncotarget. 2016;7:67463–75.
16. Lin VC, Coughlin G, Savamedi S, Palmer KJ, Coelho R, Patel V. Modified transverse plication for bladder neck reconstruction during robotic assisted laparoscopic prostatectomy. BJU Int. 2009;104:878–81.
17. Ko YH, Coelho RF, Chauhan S, Sivaraman A, Schatloff O, Cheon J, et al. Factors affecting return of continence 3 months after robot-assisted radical prostatectomy: analysis from a large, prospective data by a single surgeon. J Urol. 2012;187:190–4.
18. Reeves F, Preece P, Kapoor J, Everaerts W, Murphy DG, Corcoran NM, et al. Preservation of the neurovascular bundles is associated with improved time to continence after radical prostatectomy but not long-term continence rates: results of a systematic review and meta-analysis. Eur Urol. 2015;68:692–704.
19. Takenaka A, Tewari AK, Leung RA, Bigelow K, El-Tabey N, Murakami G, et al. Preservation of the puboprostatic collar and puboperineoplasty for early recovery of urinary continence after robotic prostatectomy: anatomic basis and preliminary outcomes. Eur Urol. 2007;51:433–40.
20. Rocco F, Carmignani L, Acquati P, Gadda F, Dell'Orto P, Rocco B, et al. Early continence recovery after open radical prostatectomy with restoration of the posterior aspect of the rhabdosphincter. Eur Urol. 2007;52:376–83.
21. Patel VR, Coelho RF, Palmer KJ, Rocco B. Periurethral suspension stitch during robot-assisted laparoscopic radical prostatectomy: description of the technique and continence outcomes. Eur Urol. 2009;56:472–8.
22. Porpiglia F, Bertolo R, Manfredi M, De Luca S, Checcucci E, Morra I, et al. Total anatomical reconstruction during robot-assisted radical prostatectomy: implications on early recovery of urinary continence. Eur Urol. 2016;69:485–95.
23. Ficarra V, Novara G, Rosen RC, Artibani W, Carroll PR, Costello A, Menon M, Montorsi F, Patel VR, Stolzenburg JU, Van der Poel H, Wilson TG, Zattoni F, Mottrie A. Systematic review and meta-analysis of studies reporting urinary continence recovery after robot-assisted radical prostatectomy. Eur Urol. 2012 Sep;62(3):405–17.
24. Grasso AA, Mistretta FA, Sandri M, Cozzi G, De Lorenzis E, Rosso M, Albo G, Palmisano F, Mottrie A, Haese A, Graefen M, Coelho R, Patel VR, Rocco B. Posterior musculofascial reconstruction after radical prostatectomy: an updated systematic review and a meta-analysis. BJU Int. 2016 Jul;118(1):20–34.
25. Menon M, Muhletaler F, Campos M, Peabody JO. Assessment of early continence after reconstruction of the periprostatic tissues in patients undergoing computer assisted (robotic) prostatectomy: results of a 2 group parallel randomized controlled trial. J Urol. 2008;180:1018–23.
26. Sutherland DE, Linder B, Guzman AM, Hong M, Frazier HA 2nd, Engel JD, Bianco FJ Jr. Posterior rhabdosphincter reconstruction during robotic assisted radical prostatectomy: results from a phase II randomized clinical trial. J Urol. 2011 Apr;185(4):1262–7.
27. Hurtes X, Rouprêt M, Vaessen C, Pereira H, Faivre d'Arcier B, Cormier L, Bruyère F. Anterior suspension combined with posterior reconstruction during robot-assisted laparoscopic prostatectomy improves early return of urinary continence: a prospective randomized multicentre trial. BJU Int. 2012 Sep;110(6):875–83.
28. Salazar A, Regis L, Planas J, Celma A, Santamaria A, Trilla E, Morote J.A Randomised Controlled Trial to Assess the Benefit of PosteriorRhabdosphincter Reconstruction in Early Urinary Continence Recovery after Robot-assisted Radical Prostatectomy. Eur Urol Oncol. 2021 Feb 27:S2588-9311(21)00039-0. https://doi.org/10.1016/j.euo.2021.02.005. Online ahead of print. PMID: 33653674.
29. Rosenberg JE, Jung JH, Lee H, Lee S, Bakker CJ, Dahm P. Posterior musculofascial reconstruction in robotic-assisted laparoscopic prostatectomy for the treatment of clinically localized prostate cancer. Cochrane Database Syst Rev. 2021 Aug 8;8:CD013677. https://doi.org/10.1002/14651858.CD013677.pub2. PMID: 34365635.
30. Cui J, Guo H, Chen S, Zhu Y, Wang S, Wang J, Liu X, WangW HJ, Chen P, Nie S, Yin G, Shi B. Pelvic floor reconstruction after radical prostatectomy: a systematic review and meta-analysis of different surgical techniques. Sci Rep. 2016;7(2737):1–14.
31. Challacombe B, Cathcart P, Roger S. Kirby in chapter 79, Robotic-Assisted Laparoscopic Prostatectomy. In: Hinman's atlas of urologic surgery. 4th ed. Philadelphia, PA: Elsevier; 2019.
32. Borin JF, Skarecky DW, Narula N, Ahlering TE. Impact of urethral stump length on continence and positive surgical margins in robot-assisted laparoscopic prostatectomy. Urology. 2007;70:173–7.
33. Patel VR, Samavedi S, Bates AS, Kumar A, Coelho R, Rocco B, et al. Dehydrated human amnion/chorion membrane allograft nerve wrap around the prostatic neurovascular bundle accelerates early return to continence and potency following robot-assisted radical prostatectomy: propensity score-matched analysis. Eur Urol. 2015;67:977–80.
34. Ogaya-Pinies G, Palayapalam-Ganapathi H, Rogers T, Hernandez-Cardona E, Rocco B, Coelho RF, et al. Can dehydrated human amnion/chorion membrane accelerate the return to potency after a nerve-sparing robotic-assisted radical prostatectomy? Propensity score-matched analysis. J Robot Surg. 2018;12:235–43.
35. Covas Moschovas M, Bhat S, Onol FF, Rogers T, Roof S, Mazzone E, et al. Modified apical dissection and lateral prostatic fascia preservation improves early postoperative functional recovery in robotic-assisted laparoscopic radical prostatectomy: results from

a propensity score–matched analysis. Eur Urol. 2020;78:875–84. https://doi.org/10.1016/j.eururo.2020.05.041.

36. Wagaskar VG, Mittal A, Sobotka S, Ratnani P, Lantz A, Falagario UG, et al. Hood technique for robotic radical prostatectomy—preserving Periurethral anatomical structures in the space of Retzius and sparing the pouch of Douglas, enabling early return of continence without compromising surgical margin rates. Eur Urol. 2021;80:213–21. https://doi.org/10.1016/j.eururo.2020.09.044.
37. Park S, Kim TN, Nam J, Ha H, Shin D, Lee W, Kim M, Chung MK. Recovery of overall excerise ability, quality of life and continence after 12 week combined exercise intervention in elderly patients who underwent radical prostatectomy: a randomized controlled study. Urology. 2012;80:299–305.

Nomograms and RALP Techniques for Management of ECE: Partial Nerve Sparing

Bernardo Rocco, Luca Sarchi, Tommaso Calcagnile, Matthew R. Cooperberg, Zhu Gang, Andrè N. Vis, Simone Assumma, Giorgio Bozzini, and Maria Chiara Sighinolfi

1 Introduction

1.1 Background

Radical prostatectomy (RP) is a trade-off between oncological safety and functional outcomes.

Balancing the risk of positive margins with the goal of improving quality of life is one of the most challenging aspects of performing RP for prostate cancer (PCa). The first described nerve-sparing RP (NSRP) was performed in 1982, and it led to an increase in postoperative sexual function and quality of life [1].

Extracapsular extension (ECE) related to PCa impacts both patient outcomes and surgical technique [2, 3].

ECE reveals the continuous growth of the tumor in non-organ-confined PCa. The presurgical detection of ECE is critical for the disease's appropriate treatment [4, 5].

The persistence of ECE has a negative impact on the choice of surgical preservation of pericapsular structures, particularly the neurovascular bundles (NVB) on the posterolateral side [6].

B. Rocco
Department of Urology, ASST Santi Paolo e Carlo, University of Milan, Milan, Italy

L. Sarchi (✉) · T. Calcagnile · S. Assumma · M. C. Sighinolfi
Department of Urology, Ospedale Policlinico e Nuovo Ospedale Civile S.Agostino Estense Modena, University of Modena and Reggio Emilia, Modena, Italy

M. R. Cooperberg
Department of Urology, University of California San Francisco Medical Center, San Francisco, CA, USA

Z. Gang
Department of Urology, Beijing United Family Hospital and Clinics, Beijing, China

A. N. Vis
VU University Medical Center, Amsterdam, The Netherlands

G. Bozzini
ASST Lariana, Urology Unit, Como, Italy

In case of extrafascial NVB dissection, postoperative functional recovery such as urinary continence [7] and erectile function [8] will likely face an arduous path.

Patient selection is key when planning nerve-sparing (NS) dissection strategy; if patients are properly selected based on tumor location, size, and grade, NS surgery does not impair cancer control [9].

It is established that age and preoperative function might be the most significant factors of postoperative erectile recovery, NS has also been related to better continence results, so it may still be helpful for men with poor sexual function [10].

To date, major urologic guidelines agree on the recommendations to preserve the NVB during RP for organ-confined PCa [11]. However, recent EAU guidelines recommend not to perform NVB preservation when there is a risk of ipsilateral ECE (based on cT stage, ISUP grade, nomogram, multiparametric magnetic resonance imaging) [12].

Historically, PCa clinical staging was related to digital rectal examination (DRE). Nevertheless, the accuracy of preoperative clinical staging based on DRE is limited, with ECE under-staging occurring in 25–30% of instances [13, 14].

Nomograms such as the Partin tables and the Memorial Sloan Kettering Cancer Center nomogram have been described for the prediction of ECE [15, 16].

However, these models do not give insight on ECE's laterality. As ECE is predominantly one-sided (85%), identification of side-specific ECE is critical because in the majority of patients, unilateral NS approach may indeed be feasible [17].

In order to optimize localization of ECE, several side-specific ECE prediction tools have been developed.

The ability to predict a unilateral ECE allows the surgeon to plan a partial preservation of the NVB.

Furthermore, nomograms able to calculate the amount of ECE involving periprostatic layers allow for implementing a partial graduated NS, external to the site involved by malignancy.

P. Wiklund et al. (eds.), *Robotic Urologic Surgery*, https://doi.org/10.1007/978-3-031-00363-9_21

Even if some of these models have been described before the intensive adoption of multiparametric magnetic resonance imaging, and therefore lack of MRI data, they are still able to predict with good accuracy the presence and amount of ECE [17, 18].

In the last few years the use of mpMRI to assist clinical practice, and particularly local staging in prostate cancer, has increased significantly [19].

Though, due to a low per-patient sensitivity of 57 percent for identifying ECE, mpMRI alone has limited efficacy to suggest patient selection for NS [20].

Moreover, the prediction accuracy of ECE by MRI, when integrated with other clinical factors, is not well established yet. The use of mpMRI data in addition to conventional preoperative clinical factors such as biopsy findings and serum prostate-specific antigen (PSA) may help predict adverse postoperative pathology including ECE [21, 22].

Nowadays, the number of available nomograms including a combination of both mpMRI and clinical parameters for the prediction of side-specific ECE is growing.

The goal of this chapter is to provide an overview of all the nomograms able to predict side-specific ECE available for RALP, distinguishing them in clinical nomograms and MRI-included nomograms.

1.2 Anatomical Hints for Partial Nerve Sparing

NVBs run parallel to the prostate's posterolateral margin. Nerves extend as a hammock laterally to the lateral pelvic fascia (LPF) and pararectal fascia junction, posteriorly to the dorsal layer of Denonvilliers' fascia (DF), which constitutes a thick fibrous sheath dividing the prostatic capsule from the rectum. The pelvic fascia has a double layer which separates the levator ani muscle from the prostate [23]. The NVB is not a singular entity but a network of multiple fine dispersed nerves running inside these periprostatic layers.

In order to find a balance between the goal of cancer eradication and functional preservation, Tewari et al. described a risk-stratified approach toward NS according to the patient' s likelihood of ipsilateral ECE. Authors classified 4 different degrees of NVB preservation according to various dissection techniques of specific fascial layers [24] Grade-1 incision inside DF and LPF is just outside the prostatic capsule. This represents the greatest degree of NS possible and is recommended only for patients with minimal risk of extraprostatic extension (EPE). Grade-2 incision through the DF (leaving outer layers on the rectum) and LPF is taken outside the layer of veins of the prostate capsule. This is known as peri-venous plane and preserves most large neural trunks and is used for patients at low risk of EPE.

Grade-3 (partial/incremental NS) incision is taken through the outer compartment of the LPF, excising all layers of DF. This is performed for patients with moderate risk of EPE. Grade-4 (non-NS), in case of high risk of EPE, wide excision of the LPF and DF containing most of the periprostatic neurovascular tissue is performed.

Moreover, Patel et al. described key anatomic landmarks, such as elements of the prostatic vasculature as prostatic and capsular arteries, which allow us to perform a partial NS in a standardized and graded manner. Particularly, a landmark artery, located approximately 2–3 mm outside the capsule, can be used as a visual cue to delineate the extension of the resection of the bundles in case of patients with suspected ECE [25].

Thus, the authors developed a five-point NS score (NSS), which reflects the subtle differences in the amount of nerve preservation needed among individual patients.

As several degrees of partial NS can be obtained, side-specific predictive models were created to guide partial, graded preservation of NVB in patients with low-intermediate or monolateral high risk of ECE.

2 Clinical Nomograms

2.1 Graefen et al. Predictive Tool

Published in March 2001, this study examined a variety of preoperative tumor features, to check if they could predict organ-confined tumor growth for each lobe of the prostate, indicating whether NSRP could be done unilaterally or bilaterally [26].

The authors reported that, until then, selection criteria for NSRP (including DRE, Gleason score in the preoperative biopsy, or intraoperative palpation) were not reliable [27]. A first retrospective analysis on 278 patients – each lobe was evaluated separately since it has its own neurovascular bundle – was published in 1999 [28]. Subsequently, a prospective validation study was performed on 353 consecutive patients, therefore investigating 706 prostate lobes in total.

The retrospective phase included, in both univariate and multivariate regression analyses, nine preoperative tumor features. These characteristics, except for PSA density (PSAD) and serum PSA, were examined separately for each lobe. The statistical analysis was performed to determine, with regard to EPE, the relationship between clinical stage, PSA, PSAD, results of transrectal ultrasound, and systematic sextant biopsy, including a quantitative assessment of cancer in the biopsies with organ-confined tumor growth. The number of positive biopsies on univariate analysis revealed the most useful single parameter able to predict EPE, followed by mm of cancer in the biopsy. On multivariate analysis, only the number of biopsies with high-grade cancer, the number of positive biopsies, and PSA were found to be independent predictors of organ-confined cancer. With a PSA level < 10 ng/ml and no more than 1 biopsy with high-grade cancer in a lobe, organ-confined tumor growth was discovered to be present in 86.1% of cases. The same criteria resulted in an 88.5% incidence of organ-confined prostate cancer on prospective validation. For predicting organ-confined tumor, clinical stage and simple Gleason grade did not provide independent information.

Even if a real nomogram was not introduced, Graefen's tree regression model created and validated objective discrimination rules for selecting patients for NSRP, with an esteem superior to traditional Gleason score derived from the biopsy. This discrimination rule constituted a useful tool for urologists to suggest unilateral or bilateral NSRP.

2.2 Ohori et al. Nomogram

The first real displayed nomogram, mathematical model able to accurately predict the probability of EPE, was developed by Ohori et al. in November 2003 [17] (Fig. 1a and b). The sample consisted in 763 patients, who were subsequently treated with pelvic lymphadenectomy and radical retropubic prostatectomy, with no androgen deprivation therapy or radiotherapy performed in advance. In this population, PCa was diagnosed through systematic needle biopsies from left and right apex, middle, and base.

The area under the ROC curve (AUC) was calculated to estimate the accuracy of predicting the side-specific probability of EPE. PSA (AUC value of 0.627), clinical T stage on each side of the prostate (0.695), and biopsy Gleason sum on each side (0.788) were found to be the most statistically relevant clinical features. Based on the logistic regression model, three nomograms were constructed. Full model included information about the percent positive cores and the percent cancer in the biopsy specimen: its predictive accuracy increased even more than the previous two (AUC 0.806).

Ohori's PTs, especially if considered together with other relevant characteristics as intraoperative findings, are therefore considered the first models that could be applied in clinical practice for discerning the best therapeutic choice between wide dissection versus NSRP.

2.3 Tsuzuki et al. Predictive Tool

Tsuzuki's et al. conducted in 2005 a retrospective study which selected 2660 cases treated with RP – without preoperative adjuvant therapy – at the Johns Hopkins Hospital (Baltimore, Maryland) [29].

3006 prostate lobes were evaluated: 2070 showed organ-confined disease, 620 presented EPE in the neurovascular bundle (NVB) at the posterolateral edge of the gland, and 316 had EPE in a region different from the NVB. Univariate and multivariate logistic regression analyses were performed. On multivariate analysis, PSA (10 or greater versus less than 10), biopsy Gleason score (7 or greater versus 6 or less), DRE (abnormal versus normal), percent of side-specific cores with tumor (greater than 33.3% versus 33.3% or less), and average percent involvement of each positive core (greater than 20% versus 20% or less) resulted in statistically significant independent predictors of NVB penetration. A model was generated, stratifying the variables into high and low risk. If the patient presented 0 or 1 high-risk variable, the probability of EPE in the NVB was less than 10%; on the other hand, the probability was 10% or greater in case of presence of more than 1 high-risk features.

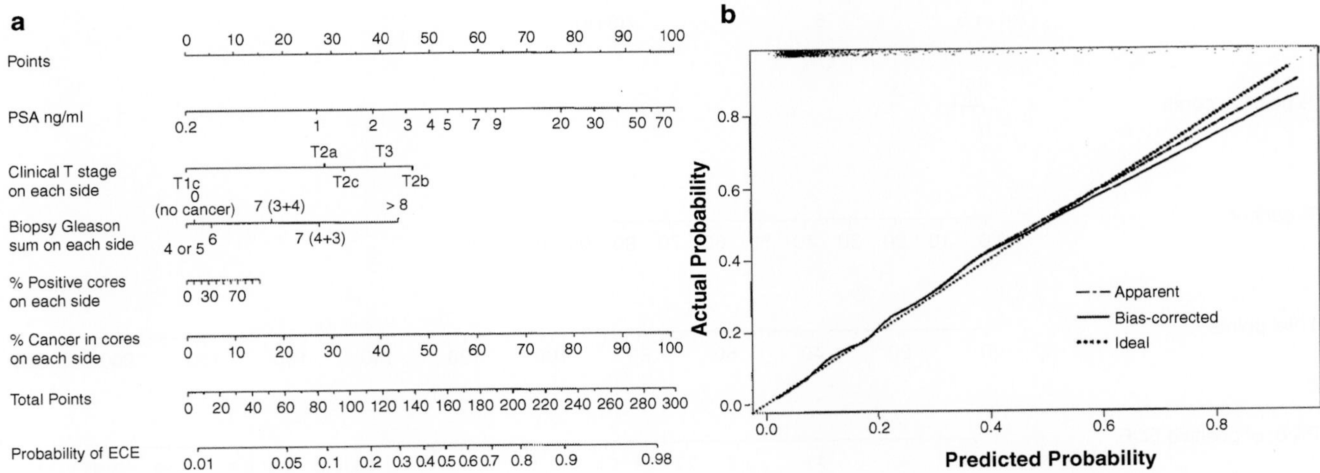

Fig. 1 (**a**) Ohori's nomogram for predicting side-specific EPE. (**b**) calibration of Ohori's nomogram

When applied to the validation set, the PT resulted in a good fit, with an area under the ROC curve of 0.780. Tsuzuki et al. acknowledge as a limitation of the study the absence of assessment of tumor location on biopsy. Nevertheless, it was recognized by the authors that the algorithm introduced in the paper would allow the urologists to predict with 90% or greater accuracy the patients who could be ideal candidates for NSRP.

2.4 Steuber et al. Nomogram

According to Steuber et al., the tree regression model introduced by Graefen et al. lacks quantitative, AUC-based, predictive accuracy estimates, whereas Ohori's nomogram, developed on North American patients, could be barely applied to European men, whose disease characteristics might be different. In 2006, a validated nomogram was therefore generated by analyzing data from 1118 European patients (the 2236 prostate lobes were considered separately to provide side-specific results) [30] (Figs. 2 and 3). Features as pretreatment PSA, clinical stage, biopsy Gleason sum, percent positive cores, and percent cancer in the biopsy specimen were included as predictors in a logistic regression model, which was then used to calibrate a nomogram. EPE was found in 303 out of 1118 RP specimens (27%) and in 385 lobes in total (17%). All the variables included were statistically significant in predicting EPE on multivariate analysis, except the percent of positive biopsy cores.

Based on these findings, Steuber's nomogram is considered a highly accurate method to assist the treatment decision-making process in a European population setting.

2.5 Satake et al. Nomogram

354 patients who underwent radical retropubic prostatectomy and bilateral pelvic lymphadenectomy – with no androgen deprivation therapy or radiotherapy performed before surgery – at Tokyo Medical University (Tokyo, Japan) were enrolled from Satake et al. in a study whose aim was to develop a nomogram able to predict side-specific EPE [31] (Fig. 4a–b).

165 out of 708 prostate lobes (23%) showed EPE. Whereas on univariate logistic regression analysis all the variables were significant in predicting EPE, on multivariate study only clinical stage ($P = 0.039$), Gleason sum ($P = 0.005$), and maximum percent of cancer had statistically significant fea-

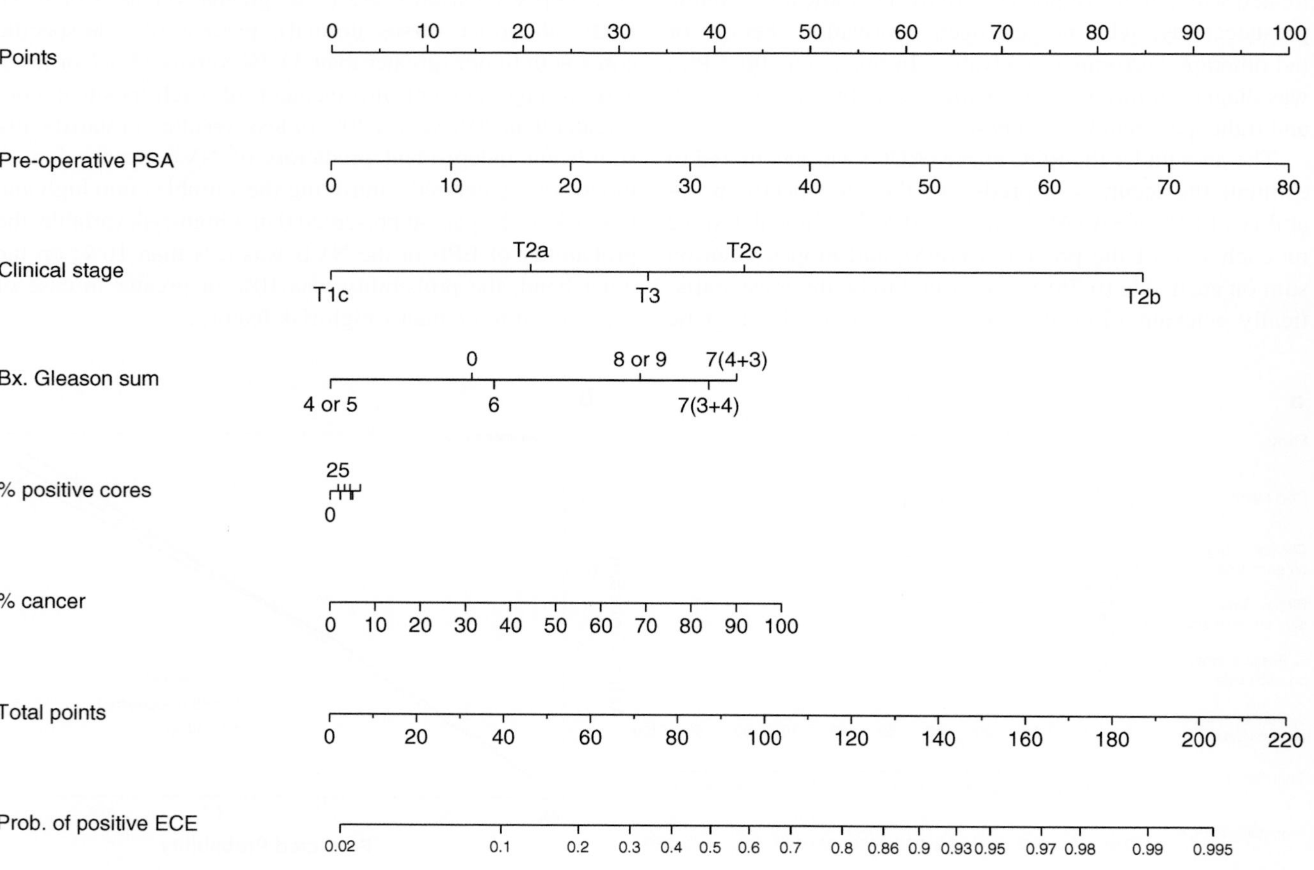

Fig. 2 Steuber nomogram

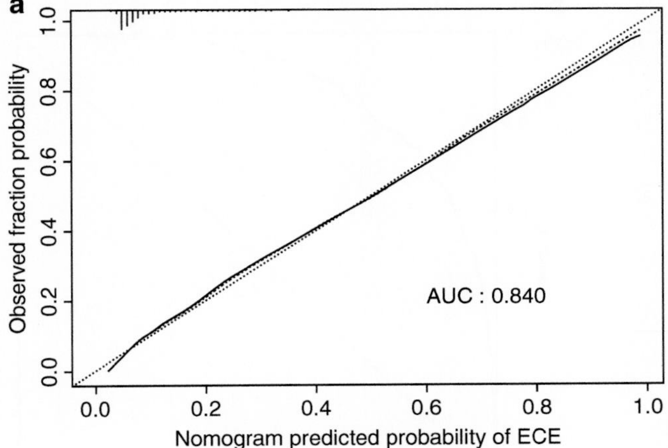

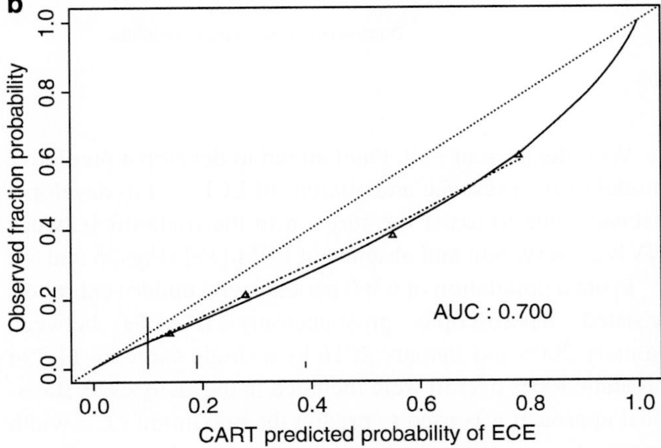

Fig. 3 (**a**) Steuber nomogram calibration plot. (**b**) regression tree analysis. Calibration (CART) plot

tures. An ROC analysis was conducted to examine, separately and in combination, the predictive values of every clinical and pathological feature of interest. Serum PSA had an AUC of 0.624, clinical stage of 0.627, and biopsy Gleason sum on each side of 0.747. AUC increased to 0.773 when the three characteristics were combined; therefore, this was considered as the standard model. The AUC of the standard model did not substantially differ from 0.791 of maximum percent of cancer alone, but it considerably improved (0.799) when maximum percent of cancer on each side was included. A nomogram was later constructed and calibrated, based on the logistic regression analysis.

Because the percent of positive cores was not significant in multivariable logistic regression analysis and provided no more information over the standard plus maximum percent of cancer in ROC analysis, this nomogram only included the standard model and maximum percent of cancer.

A limitation of the study was constituted by the small sample of patients enrolled, which was not enough to make the nomogram as a definitive tool. Nevertheless, it was considered by the authors able to provide an accurate judgment about whether to resect or preserve NVBs.

2.6 Sayyid et al. Nomogram

A nomogram to help surgeons in better selecting patients for an NS versus non-NS approach was developed by Sayyid et al. in 2016 [32] (Fig. 5a–b). Overall, 753 patients – accounting for 1506 evaluable lobes – treated with RP at University Health Network (UHN) were enrolled in the study. Patients whose biopsy lacked side-specific data or

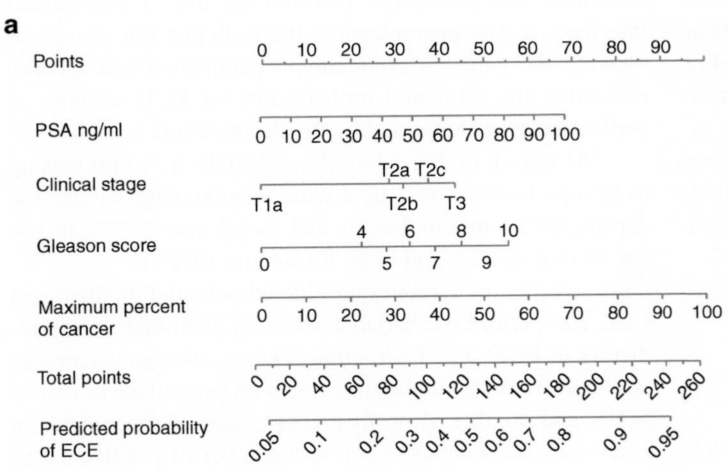

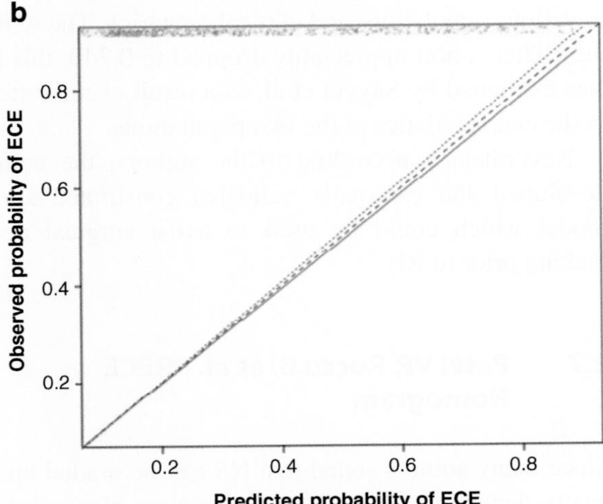

Fig. 4 (**a**) Satake's nomogram. (**b**) calibration of Satake's nomogram

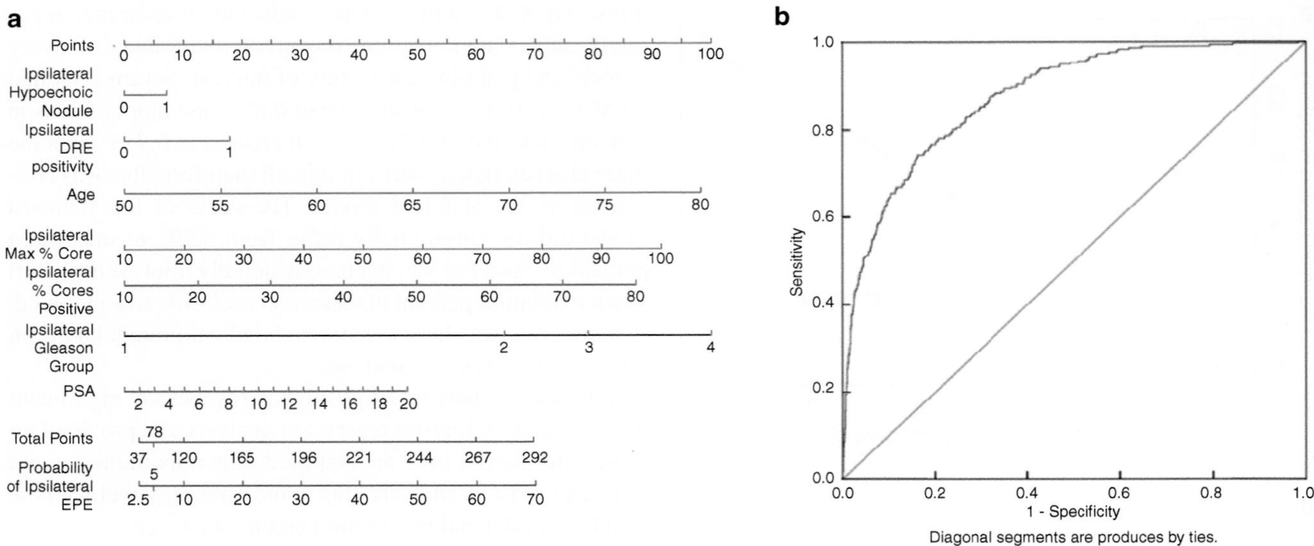

Fig. 5 (**a**) Sayyid's nomogram. (**b**) Sayyid's development cohort ROC curve

missing outcome, as well as those with anterior predominant tumors (hence distant from the NVB), were excluded.

In this developmental cohort, the overall rate of EPE was 19.8% of all the prostate lobes. Age, PSA, percentage of positive cores, highest core involvement, and Gleason score remained significant predictors of EPE risk in both univariate and multivariate analyses ($p < 0.01$). DRE ($p = 0.10$) and the presence of hypoechoic nodule on TRUS ($p = 0.49$) was no longer predictive of EPE risk on multivariate analysis. Based on the logistic regression model, a nomogram was constructed, showing an AUC of 0.880 (Fig. 3a and b).

Similarly, 311 men – 622 sides – from Ottawa Hospital Research Institute (OHRI) were enrolled for the external validation of the model, which confirmed its generalizability to various populations and clinical scenarios. The AUC from the OHRI cohort appreciably dropped to 0.740: this finding was explained by Sayyid et al. as a result of the differences in the characteristics of the two populations.

Nevertheless, according to the authors, the nomogram developed and externally validated constituted a reliable model which could be used to assist surgical decision-making prior to RP.

2.7 Patel VP, Rocco B. et al. PRECE Nomogram

Since many authors stated that NS can be graded up to five levels, depending on the fascial dissection plan on each side of the prostate, the knowledge of the presence and extent of ECE before surgery would help surgeons to tailor the amount of NS [25–31, 33].

With the present tool, Patel aimed to develop a predictive model of the presence and amount of ECE and to develop a decision rule to assist the surgeon in the trade-off between NVB preservation and absence of PSM [18] (Figs. 6 and 7).

From a population of 6360 patients who underwent robot-assisted laparoscopic prostatectomy (RALP) between January 2008 and January 2016 by a single surgeon, 11,794 prostatic lobes overall were included in the analysis. A statistical approach was used to predict the maximum ECE width using clinicopathological parameters. For the presence of ECE and ECE widths of >1, >2, >3, and > 4 mm, five multivariable logistic models were constructed.

A five-zone decision rule, with a lower and a higher threshold, was presented. Through the use of a graphical interface, it was guaranteed to the urologist the chance of viewing the patient's pretreatment parameters and a curve indicating the estimated probabilities for ECE amount, as well as the areas identified by the decision rule.

1351 out of 11,794 lobes showed ECE; its width was up to 15 mm. In 498 cases, the disease was extended beyond the capsule for >1 mm (4.2%), in 261 for >2 mm (2.2%), in 148 for >3 mm (1.3%), and in 99 for >4 mm (0.8%).

A selection of variables considered potential predictors of ECE was performed. Variable selection identified seven predictors of ECE: age, PSA, clinical stage, average percentage of cancer, ratio of number of cores with percentage of cancer >60% and number of positive cores, ratio of the number of cores with Gleason score > 6 and number of positive cores, and rate of positive cores. ROC curves of the regression analysis and their AUCs showed good predictive performances of the models: AUC was 0.810 for ECE, and 0.84, 0.85, 0.88, and 0.90 for ECE width of >1, >2, >3, and > 4 mm, respectively.

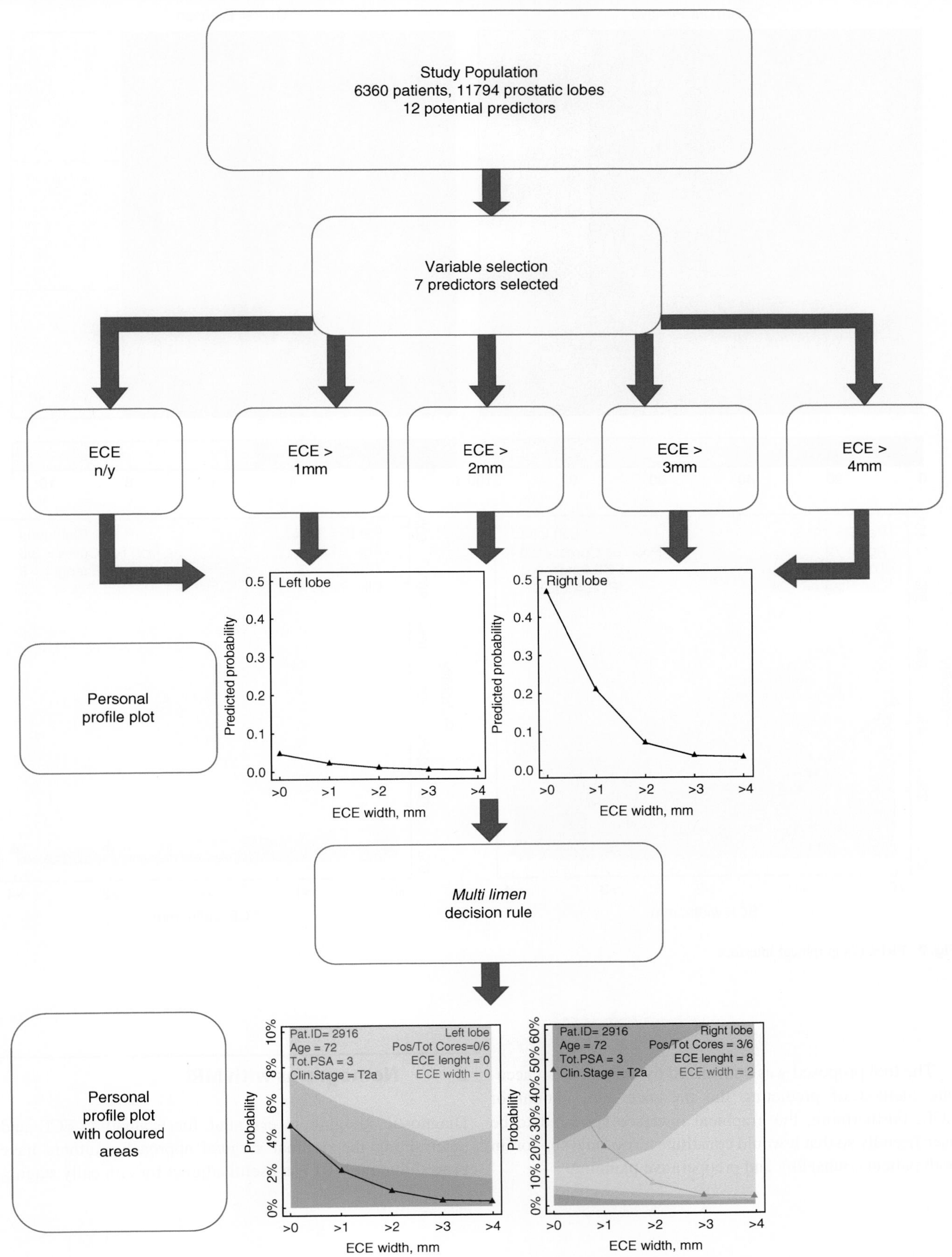

Fig. 6 PRECE's prediction algorithm

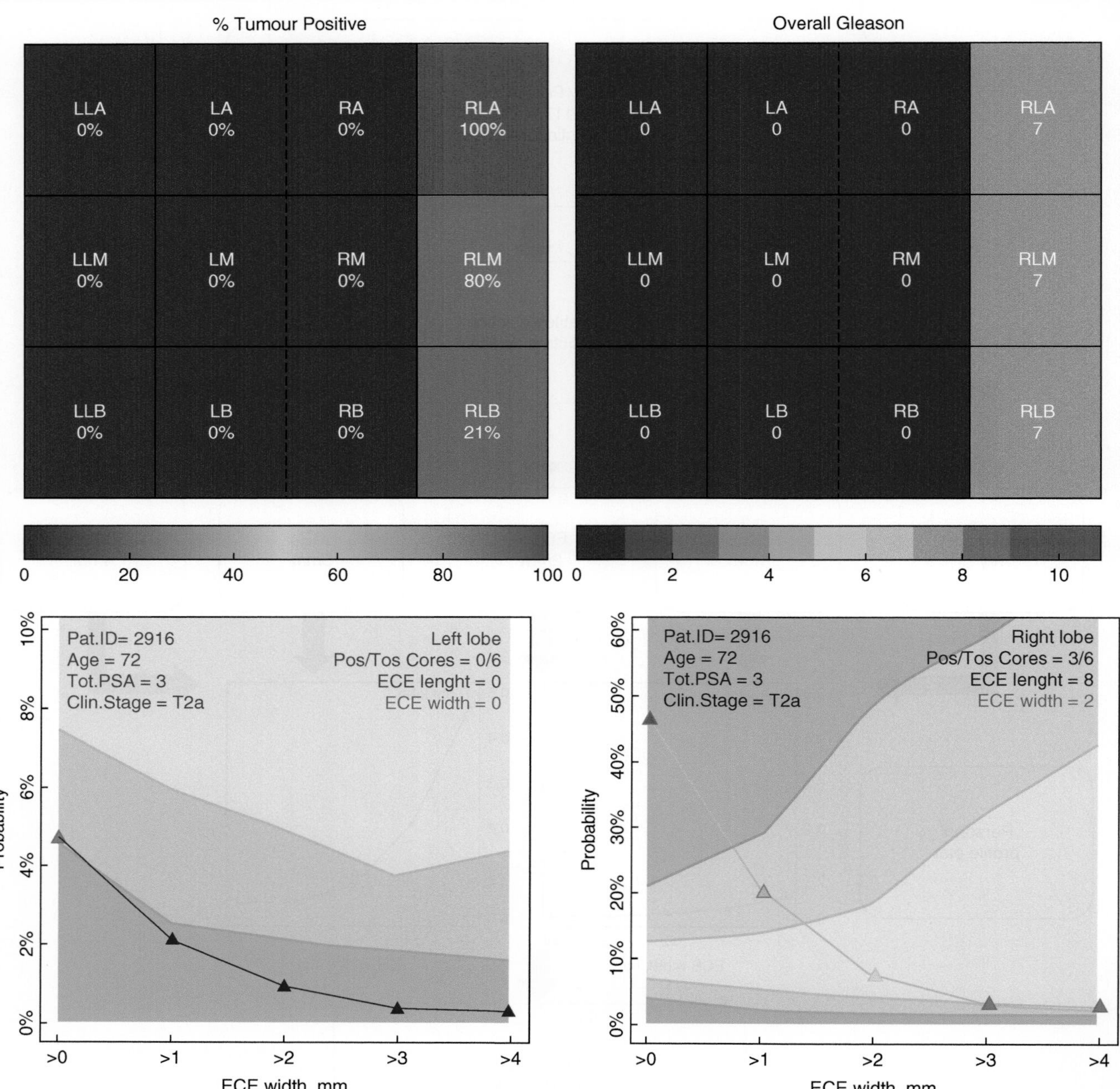

Fig. 7 PRECE's graphical interface

The tool proposed was considered by authors as an accurate method of predicting the presence and amount of ECE. Furthermore, the graphical interface appeared to be user-friendly so that it would constitute an optimal support in both patient counseling and preoperative planning.

3 Nomograms with MRI

Diagnostic imaging is essential for evaluating ECE and determining the optimal surgical approach. Authors have proved that mpMRI is a useful adjunct for clinically staging

PCa, as radiologic data improved accuracy of preexisting clinical nomograms for prediction of pathologic ECE [34].

ECE, which is traditionally diagnosed using T2-weighted imaging, can be confidently predicted with mpMRI (T2-WI). Unfortunately, there is still a wide range of sensitivity and specificity based exclusively on MRI data for ECE, with reports ranging from 30% to 70.7% sensitivity and 73.9–100% specificity, respectively [34].

As a result of these concerns, the necessity to combine radiological and clinical data to increase the predictivity of the risk of ECE arose, prompting the development of several nomograms.

3.1 Giganti et al. Nomogram

Interestingly, one of the first side-specific nomograms was developed by an experienced uro-radiology group, in 2015 [35]. The goal of this study was to develop and verify a nomogram that could predict ECE by combining diffusion-weighted imaging (DWI) data with other imaging and clinical characteristics (Fig. 8).

Authors focused on the importance of evaluating specific phases of mpMRI, in particular on apparent diffusion coefficient (ADC). As DWI provides a significant and clearly visible contrast of tumor site (increased signal intensity) with low ADC values, adding DWI to T2-WI protocol improves sensitivity and specificity to predict ECE. Additionally, tumor ADC—as well as the ratio between pathological and normal ADC—correlates inversely with Gleason grade, implying that they can be considered as ECE predictors [36].

The Giganti nomogram was generated from a population of 70 men affected by PCa, who underwent 1.5 T mpMRI study using an endorectal coil and subsequently treated with RP at a single center. After RP 23 out of 70 patients (33%) showed ECE. Based on T2-WI, 18 out of 70 patients (26%) were diagnosed with ECE. In all, 13 out of 23 patients (57%) were correctly staged with ECE at mpMRI.

The variables considered on the graphic model are normal and pathological ADC, lesion volume, Gleason score, and ECE on T2-WI. The nomogram has been externally validated by another institution on 31 patients; results from the external validation showed an overall accuracy of 81% and a sensitivity, specificity, positive predictive value, and negative predictive value of 65%, 100%, 100%, and 70%, respectively.

The most interesting finding of this study is the significant, increased sensitivity (88%) of this nomogram to detect ECE when DWI is included.

Limitations of the study are represented by the restricted number of patients and the retrospective nature of the study itself.

3.2 Chen et al. Nomogram

In 2016, a group of Chinese researchers described a side-specific ECE nomogram based on a population of 353 Chinese men affected by PCa and treated by RP [37].

All patients underwent preoperative mpMRI using a 1.5 T (113 of 353 patients) or 3.0 T (240 of 353 patients) without an endorectal coil. The authors integrated clinical informa-

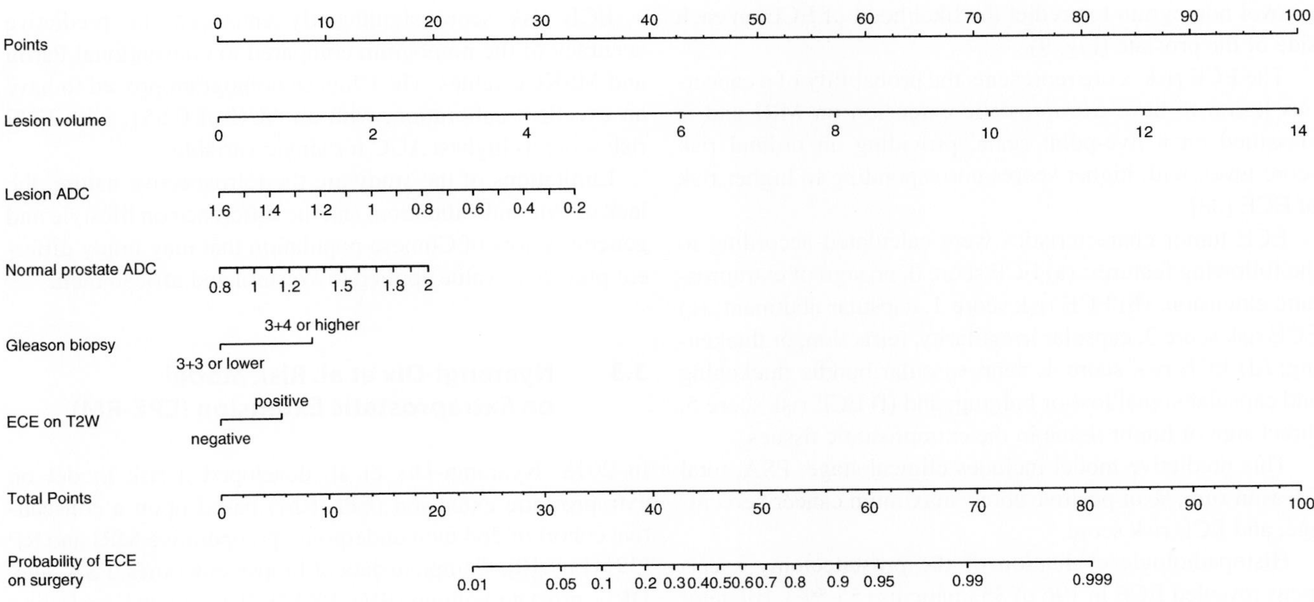

Fig. 8 Giganti nomogram

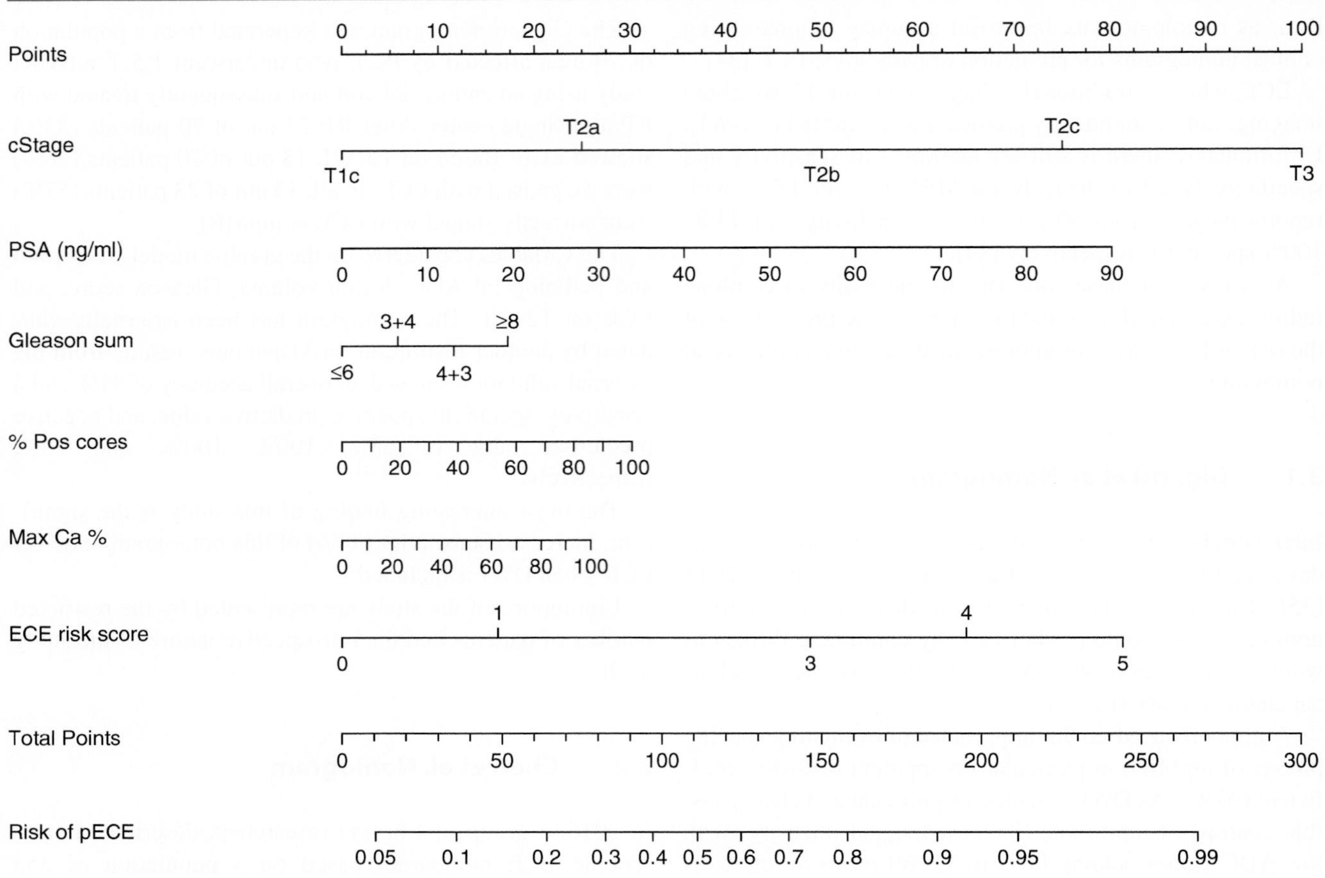

Fig. 9 The Chen nomogram predicting SS probability of ECE

tion from the Partin tables and the MSKCC nomogram with the ECE risk score, obtained from mpMRI data, to construct a novel nomogram to predict the likelihood of ECE on each side of the prostate (Fig. 9).

The ECE risk score represents the probability of a cancerous lesion to have extraprostatic extension on MRI and is classified on a five-point scale, providing an ordinal risk score level, with higher scores corresponding to higher risk of ECE [38].

ECE tumor characteristics were calculated according to the following features: (a) ECE score 0, no sign of extraprostatic extension; (b) ECE risk score 1, capsular abutment; (c) ECE risk score 3, capsular irregularity, retraction, or thickening; (d) ECE risk score 4, neurovascular bundle thickening and capsular signal loss or bulging; and (f) ECE risk score 5, direct sign of tumor tissue in the extraprostatic tissues.

This predictive model includes clinical stage, PSA, total Gleason sum, % of positive cores, maximum cancer percentage, and ECE risk score.

Histopathologic evaluation of the prostatectomy specimens revealed ECE in 196 of 353 patients (55.5%). Bilateral ECE was reported in 49 patients (13.9%), while unilateral left and right ECE was recorded in 87 (24.6%) and 60 (17.0%) patients, respectively. Lobe-specific ECE was present in 245 of 706 prostate lobes (34.7%).

ECE risk score significantly enhanced the predictive accuracy of the nomogram compared to conventional Partin and MSKCC tables. The Chinese nomogram proved to have an excellent calibration, with an AUC of 0.851, with ECE risk score as highest AUC for single variable.

Limitations of the study are the retrospective nature, the lack of external validation, and the difference on lifestyle and genetic factors of Chinese population that may imply different predictive value applied to Western and african men.

3.3 Nyarangi-Dix et al. Risk Model on Extraprostatic Extension (EPE-RM)

In 2018, Nyarangi-Dix et al. developed a risk model on extraprostatic extension (EPE-RM) based upon a consecutive cohort of 264 men undergoing preoperative MRI and RP [39] (Fig. 10). Complete data of biopsy outcomes, PSA, age, DRE, prostate volume (PV), PSAD, RP outcome, including T stage, EPE, and tumor volume (TV) were retrospectively analyzed. In addition, data on PI-RADSv2.0 of every lesion

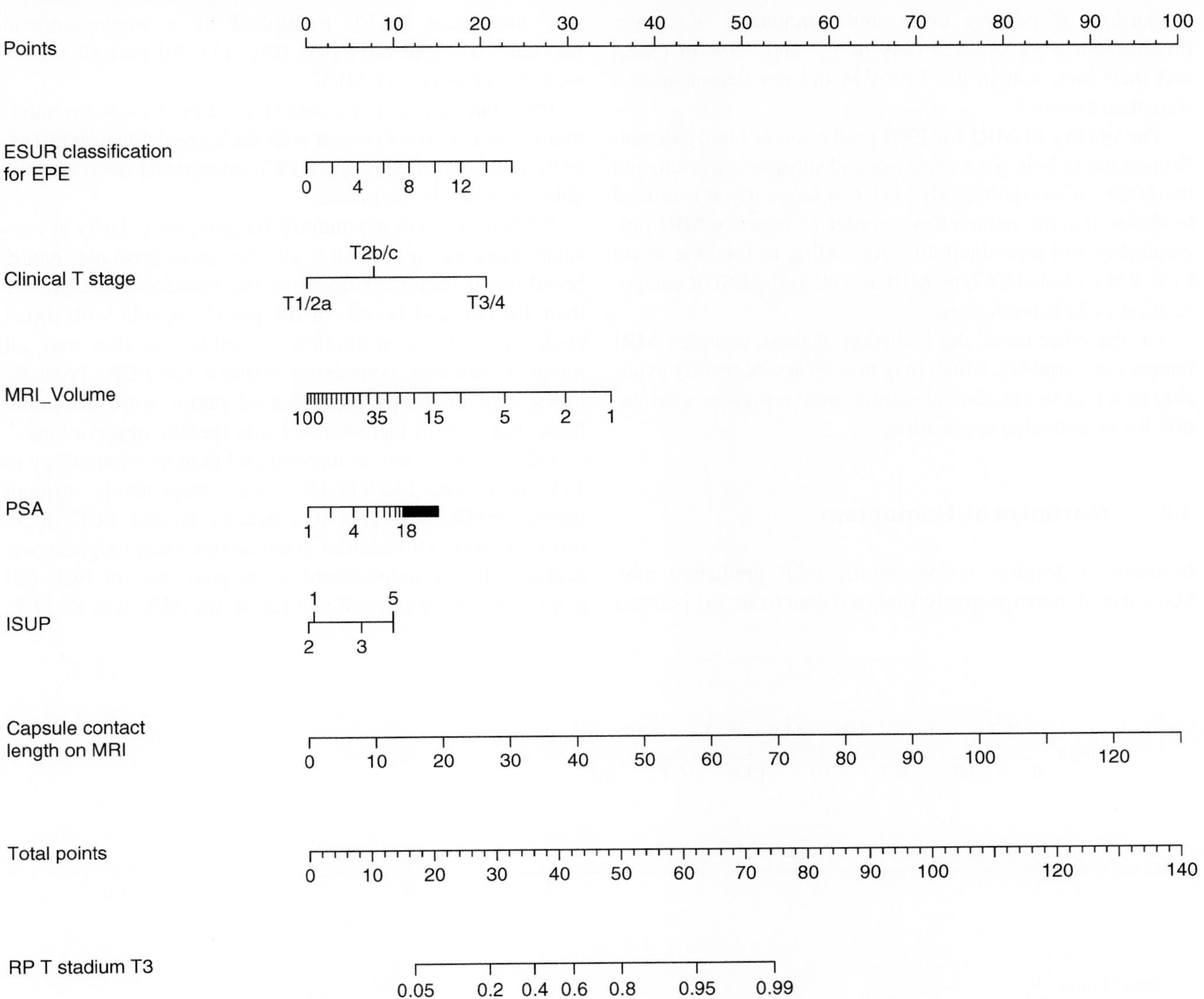

Fig. 10 EPE-RM nomogram

detected by radiologists (in particular, the index lesion), ESUR classification, capsule contact length (CCL), TV and diameter of the lesion on MRI, and localization (side/hemisphere) were collected [39, 40]. These samples served for EPE-RM tool development, generation of a clinical model with MRI, internal validation, and comparisons with ESUR classification, cT, the Steuber, and MSKCC nomograms.

All MRI images were acquired according to the ESUR guidelines with 3Tesla scanners.

Final pathological results showed EPE in the RP specimen on 48% of the patients and 41% of prostate hemispheres overall.

The EPE-RM includes the following parameters: cT stage, PSA, ISUP grade in biopsy, MRI lesion volume, ESUR classification, and capsule contact length [41]. On the multivariate logistical regression analysis for the prediction of EPE, ISUP grade, PV on MRI, ESUR classification, PSA level, cT, and CCL were considered relevant. Conversely, inclusion of the lesion diameter, core involvement in %, percentage of positive cores, and PI-RADSv2.0 in the EPE-RM did not improve discrimination of the model.

EPE-RM, full model, and novel clinical model + MRI reached almost identical AUCs (0.86, 0.86, and 0.85, respectively), all being higher compared with the ESUR classification for EPE (0.81), cT (0.66), the published Steuber (0.70), and MSKCC (0.73) nomograms.

Several comments are discussed in this study: ISUP grade was a significant contributor to regression analysis. This is in contrast to the MSKCC and Steuber nomograms, using Gleason score. The proportion of positive cores and tumorous core involvement in % are often incorporated to predict the potential tumor extension and EPE; in this cohort, both proportion of positive cores and percentage of cancer involvement were selected only in 7% and 7.7% of cases, and their inclusion in the EPE-RM did not demonstrate a statistical benefit.

The quality of MRI for EPE prediction is highly dependent on the radiologist's expertise and subspecialization, and therefore varies significantly [42]. Consequently, it is crucial to define specific parameters in order to improve MRI predictability and reproducibility. According to this, the novel EPE-RM included CCL on MRI as well as the ESUR categorization as EPE predictors.

On the other hand, the inclusion of these complex MRI features as variables, which may not always be readily available in a real-world clinical setting, may represent a limitation for an extended application.

3.4 Martini et al. Nomogram

In order to develop a side-specific ECE predictive tool, Martini et al. retrospectively analyzed data from 561 patients who underwent RARP performed by a single surgeon between 2014 and 2015 [43] (Fig. 11). All patients underwent 3 T preoperative MRI.

PSA, Gleason biopsy grade (1 vs. 2 vs. 3 vs. 4–5), maximum % of core involvement with the highest Gleason (50 vs. >50), and confirmed positive ECE on mpMRI were all variables included in the model.

NVB invasion or asymmetry, bulging, irregularity of capsular margins, obliteration of the recto-prostatic angle, broad-based tumor abutment of the pseudocapsule greater than 1.0 cm, and breach of the pseudocapsule with direct evidence of tumor infiltration or bladder invasion were all imaging elements considered positive for ECE. Prostatic lobes with no biopsy-documented tumor were excluded; thus, study cohort included 829 side-specific observations.

ECE was reported on mpMRI and final histopathology in 115 (14%) and 142 (17.1%) cases, respectively. Among these, mpMRI was able to correctly predict ECE in 57 (40.1%) cases. All variables in the model, except highest percentage of core involvement, were predictors of ECE (all $p \leq 0.006$). After internal validation, the AUC was 82.11%.

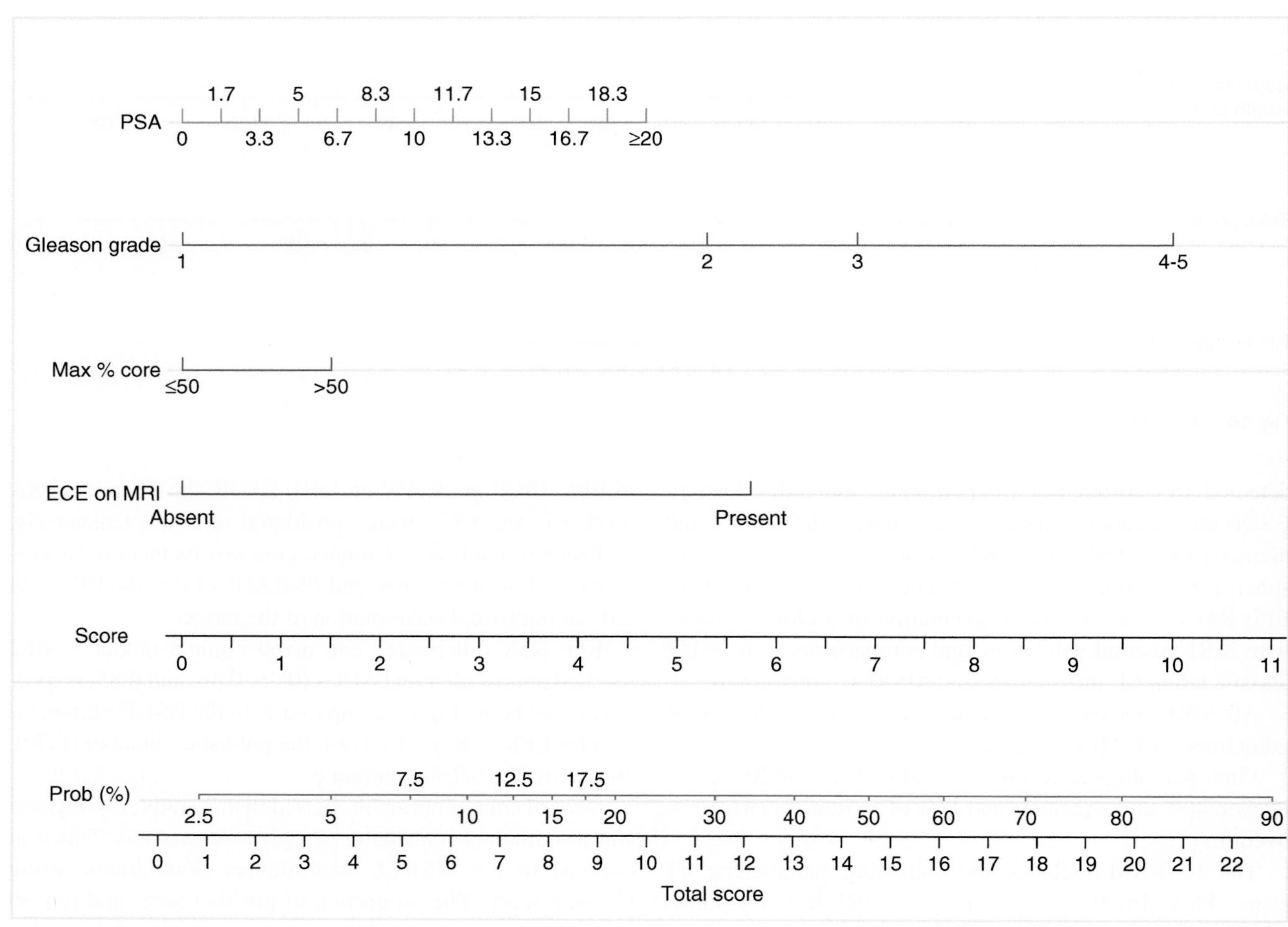

Fig. 11 Martini nomogram to predict side-specific ECE

When compared to relying on just mpMRI prediction of ECE, the model showed better calibration and increased clinical risk prediction.

The Martini model was externally verified by Sighinolfi et al. [44]. At the 20% cutoff, this external validation study revealed moderate to low discriminative performance (AUC 0.68), with sensitivity and specificity of 53.6% and 77.1%, respectively. Thus, when externally validated, this predictive tool revealed a poor calibration with tendency toward underestimation of ECE.

3.5 Soeterik et al. Nomogram

The authors made a retrospective analysis of 1870 consecutive men affected by PCa who underwent RALP from 2014 to 2018 at three different national centers [45].

PSAD, highest ipsilateral ISUP biopsy grade, ipsilateral percentage of positive cores, and side-specific clinical stage determined by DRE and mpMRI were included in four multivariable logistic regression models. The staging data from DRE and mpMRI were divided into 3 subclasses: nonpalpable disease (T1), organ-confined nodal disease (T2), and ECE (T3) about DRE findings. Non-visible lesions (T1), organ-confined lesions (T2), and lesions with ECE about the mpMRI data (T3).

Microscopic bladder neck infiltration (the presence of a tumor between thick smooth muscle bundles in the absence of benign prostate glands) and seminal vesicle involvement were not considered ECE.

Four models were built: model 1 considered PSAD, DRE, ISUP grade, and percentage of positive cores. Model 2 involved PSAD, MRI findings, and ISUP grade. Model 3 involved PSAD, MRI, DRE, and ISUP grade. Model 4 included all previous five predictors. Each patient's right and left prostatic lobes were considered as separate cases.

Overall, 887 men were included in the development cohort, 513 in validation subcohort 1, and 470 in validation subcohort 2. The rates of ECE prevalence on prostatic lobes of these samples were, respectively, 458/1774 (26%), 225/1026 (21%), and 148/940 (16%). PSAD, DRE, mpMRI staging, ISUP grades 3–5, and percentage of positive cores were all found to significantly predict ECE on multivariable analyses. The greatest AUC was obtained by Model 4, which included all available predictors (AUC; 0.82). The other three models had AUCs ranging from 0.80 to 0.81.

In terms of AUC, calibration, and net benefit, the three nomograms based on clinical information associated with mpMRI staging data (models 2, 3, and 4) outperformed the nomogram without mpMRI staging data (model 1). In terms of agreement between predicted and observed probabilities, however, model 2 outperformed both models 3 and 4. As a result, this nomogram should be the favorite tool for predicting side-specific EPE risk. Interestingly, it was also the most simple model in terms of calibration, as it only has three predictor variables (PSAD, highest ISUP grade, and mpMRI staging). This predictive model is freely accessible online at the website https://www.evidencio.com/models/show/2142 (Fig. 12).

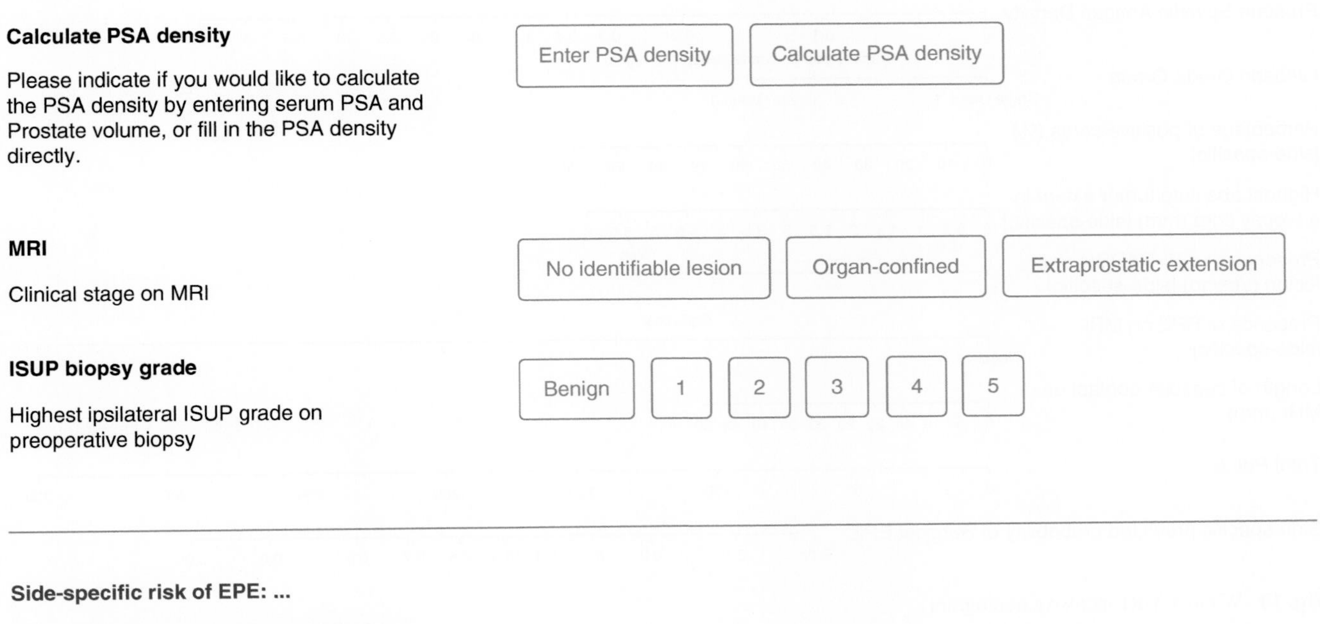

Fig. 12 Soeterik online EPE predictive model

Though the study has some advantages, such as a high number of cases and external validation in two different patient cohorts, it does have few drawbacks that must be addressed. To begin with, the majority of clinical data came from daily clinical practice, and no central histopathological or radiological evaluation was performed. Furthermore, the number of prostatic lobes with one or more incomplete covariates (27%) must be considered as a limit. Finally, both model construction and external validation were carried out by the same research group.

3.6 Wibmer et al. MRI-Inclusive Nomogram

In 2021, ten institutions from the USA and Europe collaborated to develop an international, multicenter nomogram for side-specific prediction of EPE of PCa based on clinical, histological, and radiologic MRI based data [46] (Fig. 13).

Overall, 840 men from these institutions were consecutively enrolled to undergo RP after MRI.

The novel generated nomogram involved the following parameters: age, PSAD, side-specific biopsy results (Gleason grade group, percent positive cores, tumor extent), and side-specific MRI features (presence of a PI-RADS 4 or 5 lesion, level of suspicion for EPE, length of capsular contact).

Imaging was evaluated according to previously published ESUR criteria; the interpreting radiologist scored the likelihood of EPE on a 5-point Likert scale separately for the left and right sides of the gland.

This predictive model showed excellent performance, as AUC ranked at 0.828.

Moreover, the accuracy of the MRI-inclusive nomogram created by the authors was compared to existing models for EPE prediction, based on clinical and biopsy data but lacking radiologic data, such as the MSKCC "Pre-Radical Prostatectomy" nomogram, the updated Partin tables, a validated multi-institutional model from the Belgian Cancer Registry, and the side-specific Steuber nomogram [15, 30, 47, 48].

Authors' findings revealed that MRI-inclusive model significantly outperformed any of the benchmarked statistical models in terms of accuracy of EPE prediction ($p < 0.001$ for all).

Furthermore, the authors claim the importance of the application of their novel nomogram in case of patients with ambiguous MRI findings and/or patients with low/intermediate risk characteristics, in order to evaluate more carefully the likelihood of ECE and partial NS decision.

On the other hand, the nomogram may thus give only limited additional information in high-risk subjects with evident EPE on MRI.

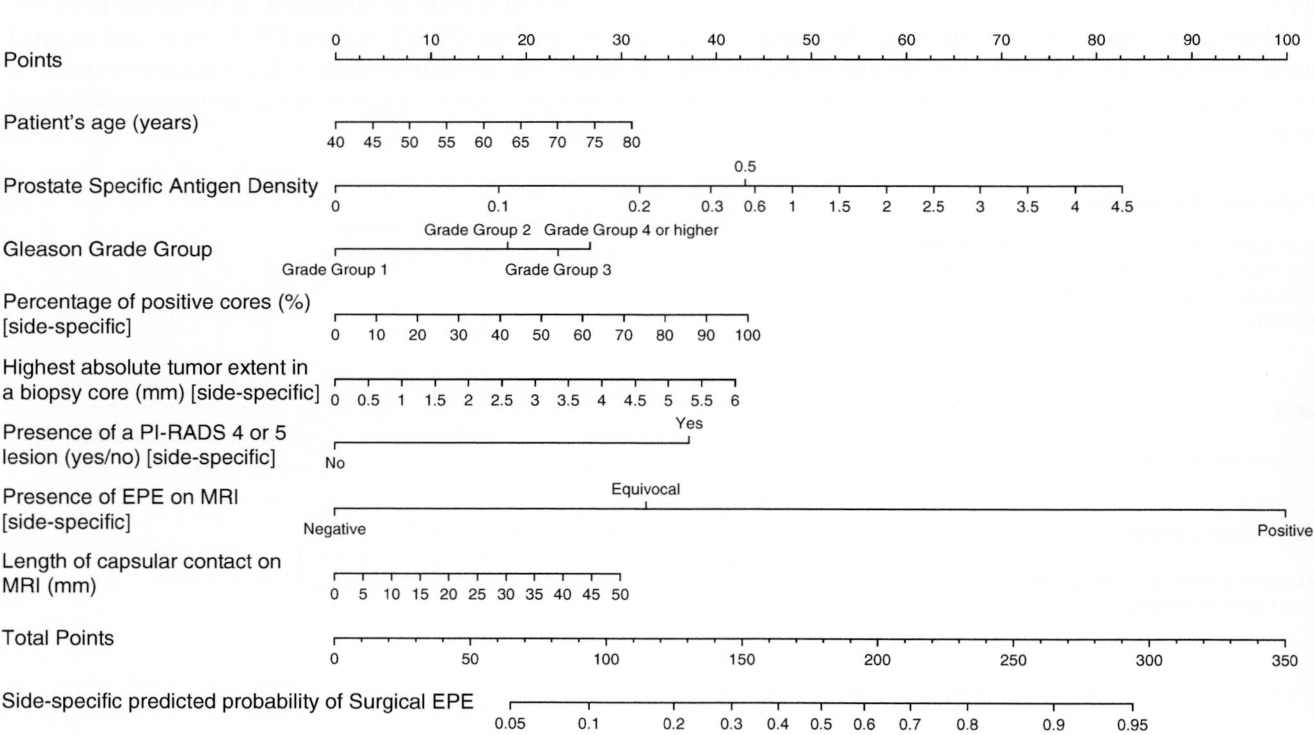

Fig. 13 Wibmer MRI-inclusive nomogram

4 Conclusions

Although MRI has been found to improve PCa preoperative staging, it may not be sufficient alone to properly assess the amount of ECE. When MRI information is integrated into predictive models as nomograms, ECE extension can be predicted more accurately. The application of these statistical tools in clinical practice, especially if combined with intraoperative surgical margins control, can ensure a tailored-graded NS approach and increase functional outcomes without compromising oncological radicality.

References

1. Walsh PC. The discovery of the cavernous nerves and development of nerve sparing radical retropubic prostatectomy. J Urol. 2007 May;177(5):1632–5. https://doi.org/10.1016/j.juro.2007.01.012.
2. Mikel Hubanks J, Boorjian SA, Frank I, et al. The presence of extracapsular extension is associated with an increased risk of death from prostate cancer after radical prostatectomy for patients with seminal vesicle invasion and negative lymph nodes. Urol Oncol. 2014;32:26.e21–7.
3. Partin AW, Borland RN, Epstein JI, Brendler CB. Influence of wide excision of the neurovascular bundle(s) on prognosis in men with clinically localized prostate cancer with established capsular penetration. J Urol. 1993;150:142–6. discussion 146-148
4. Yuh B, Artibani W, Heidenreich A, et al. The role of robot-assisted radical prostatectomy and pelvic lymph node dissection in the management of high-risk prostate cancer: a systematic review. Eur Urol. 2014;65:918–27.
5. Gandaglia G, De Lorenzis E, Novara G, et al. Robot-assisted radical prostatectomy and extended pelvic lymph node dissection in patients with locally-advanced prostate cancer. Eur Urol. 2017;71:249–56.
6. Walz J, Epstein JI, Ganzer R, et al. A critical analysis of the current knowledge of surgical anatomy of the prostate related to optimisation of cancer control and preservation of continence and erection in candidates for radical prostatectomy: an update. Eur Urol. 2016;70:301–11.
7. Michl U, Tennstedt P, Feldmeier L, et al. Nerve-sparing surgery technique, not the preservation of the neurovascular bundles, leads to improved long-term continence rates after radical prostatectomy. Eur Urol. 2016;69:584–9.
8. Nguyen LN, Head L, Witiuk K, et al. The risks and benefits of cavernous neurovascular bundle sparing during radical prostatectomy: a systematic review and meta-analysis. J Urol. 2017;198:760–9.
9. Catalona WJ, Bigg SW. Nerve-sparing radical prostatectomy: evaluation of results after 250 patients. J Urol 1990 Mar;143(3):538–543. https://doi.org/10.1016/s0022-5347(17)40013-9. discussion 544
10. Avulova S, Zhao Z, Lee D, Huang LC, Koyama T, Hoffman KE, Conwill RM, Wu XC, Chen V, Cooperberg MR, Goodman M, Greenfield S, Hamilton AS, Hashibe M, Paddock LE, Stroup A, Resnick MJ, Penson DF, Barocas DA. The effect of nerve sparing status on sexual and urinary function: 3-year results from the CEASAR study. J Urol. 2018 May;199(5):1202–1209. https://doi.org/10.1016/j.juro.2017.12.037. Epub 2017 Dec 16. Erratum in: J Urol. 2018 Aug;200(2):458. PMID: 29253578.
11. Sanda MG, Ronald CC, Crispino T, et al. Clinically Localized Prostate Cancer: AUA/ASTRO/SUO Guideline http://www.auanet.org/guidelines/clinically-localized-prostate-cancer-new-(aua/astro/suo-guideline-2017)
12. EAU Guidelines. Edn. presented at the EAU Annual Congress Milan 2021. isbn 978-94-92671-13-4.
13. Cooperberg MR, Lubeck DP, Mehta SS, Carroll PR, CaPsure. Time trends in clinical risk stratification for prostate cancer: implications for outcomes (data from CaPSURE). J Urol. 2003;170(6 Pt 2):S21–5.
14. Han M, Partin AW, Piantadosi S, et al. Era specific biochemical recurrence-free survival following radical prostatectomy for clinically localized prostate cancer. J Urol. 2001;166:416–9.
15. Memorial Sloan Kettering Cancer Center. Pre-radical prostatectomy tool to predict probability of extraprostatic extension in prostate cancer patients. www.mskcc.org/nomograms/prostate/pre_op.
16. Tosoian JJ, Chappidi M, Feng Z, et al. Prediction of pathological stage based on clinical stage, serum prostate-specific antigen, and biopsy Gleason score: Partin tables in the contemporary era. BJU Int. 2017;119:676–83.
17. Ohori M, Kattan MW, Koh H, et al. Predicting the presence and side of extracapsular extension: a nomogram for staging prostate cancer. J Urol. 2004;171:1844–9.
18. Patel VR, Sandri M, Grasso AAC, et al. A novel tool for predicting extracapsular extension during graded partial nerve sparing in radical prostatectomy. BJU Int. 2018;121:373–82.
19. Caglic I, Kovac V, Barrett T. Multiparametric MRI—local staging of prostate cancer and beyond. Radiol Oncol. 2019;53:159–70.
20. de Rooij M, Hamoen EH, Witjes JA, Barentsz JO, Rovers MM. Accuracy of magnetic resonance imaging for local staging of prostate cancer: a diagnostic meta-analysis. Eur Urol. 2016;70:233–45.
21. Rayn KN, Bloom JB, Gold SA, et al. Added value of multiparametric magnetic resonance imaging to clinical nomograms for predicting adverse pathology in prostate cancer. J Urol. 2018;200:1041–7.
22. Gandaglia G, Ploussard G, Valerio M, et al. The key combined value of multiparametric magnetic resonance imaging, and magnetic resonance imaging-targeted and concomitant systematic biopsies for the prediction of adverse pathological features in prostate cancer patients undergoing radical prostatectomy. Eur Urol. 2020;77:733–41.
23. Costello AJ, Brooks M, Cole OJ. Anatomical studies of the neurovascular bundle and cavernosal nerves. BJU Int. 2004 Nov;94(7):1071–6. https://doi.org/10.1111/j.1464-410X.2004.05106.x.
24. Tewari AK, Srivastava A, Huang MW, Robinson BD, Shevchuk MM, Durand M, Sooriakumaran P, Grover S, Yadav R, Mishra N, Mohan S, Brooks DC, Shaikh N, Khanna A, Leung R. Anatomical grades of nerve sparing: a risk-stratified approach to neural-hammock sparing during robot-assisted radical prostatectomy (RARP). BJU Int. 2011 Sep;108(6 Pt 2):984–92. https://doi.org/10.1111/j.1464-410X.2011.10565.x.
25. Schatloff O, Chauhan S, Sivaraman A, Kameh D, Palmer KJ, Patel VR. Anatomic grading of nerve sparing during robot-assisted radical prostatectomy. Eur Urol 2012 Apr;61(4):796–802. https://doi.org/10.1016/j.eururo.2011.12.048. Epub 2012 Jan 4.
26. Graefen M, Haese A, Pichlmeier U, Hammerer PG, Noldus J, Butz K, Erbersdobler A, Henke RP, Michl U, Fernandez S, Huland HJ A validated strategy for side specific prediction of organ confined prostate cancer: a tool to select for nerve sparing radical prostatectomy. Urol. 2001 Mar;165(3):857–63. PMID: 11176486.
27. O'Dowd GJ, Veltri RW, Orozco R, et al. Update on the appropriate staging evaluation for newly diagnosed prostate cancer. J Urol. 1997;158:687.
28. Graefen M, Noldus J, Pichlmeier U et al. Preoperative prediction of organ-confined (pT2) tumor growth to indicate a bilateral nerve-sparing radical prostatectomy (NSRP). J Urol. 1999;161(Suppl):208, abstract 925

29. Tsuzuki T, Hernandez DJ, Aydin H, Trock B, Walsh PC, Epstein JI. Prediction of extraprostatic extension in the neuro- vascular bundle based on prostate needle biopsy pathology, serum prostate specific antigen and digital rectal examination. J Urol. 2005;173:450–3.
30. Steuber T, Graefen M, Haese A, et al. Validation of a nomogram for prediction of side specific extracapsular extension at radical prostatectomy. J Urol. 2006;175:939–944. discussion 944.
31. Satake N, Ohori M, Yu C, et al. Development and internal validation of a nomogram predicting extracapsular extension in radical prostatectomy specimens. Int J Urol. 2010;17:267–72.
32. Sayyid R, Perlis N, Ahmad A, et al. Development and external validation of a biopsy-derived nomogram to predict risk of ipsilateral extraprostatic extension. BJU Int. 2017;120:76–82.
33. Patel VR, Schatloff O, Chauhan S, et al. The role of the prostatic vasculature as a landmark for nerve sparing during robot assisted radical prostatectomy. Eur Urol. 2012;61:571–6.
34. Feng TS, Sharif-Afshar AR, Wu J, Li Q, Luthringer D, Saouaf R, Kim HL. Multiparametric MRI improves accuracy of clinical nomograms for predicting extracapsular extension of prostate cancer. Urology. 2015 Aug;86(2):332–7. https://doi.org/10.1016/j.urology.2015.06.003.
35. Giganti F, Coppola A, Ambrosi A, Ravelli S, Esposito A, Freschi M, Briganti A, Scattoni V, Salonia A, Gallina A, Dehò F, Cardone G, Balconi G, Gaboardi F, Montorsi F, Maschio AD, De Cobelli F. Apparent diffusion coefficient in the evaluation of side-specific extracapsular extension in prostate cancer: development and external validation of a nomogram of clinical use. Urol Oncol. 2016 Jul;34(7):291.e9–291.e17. https://doi.org/10.1016/j.urolonc.2016.02.015. Epub 2016 Mar 15. PMID: 26992933.
36. De Cobelli F, Ravelli S, Esposito A, Giganti F, Gallina A, Montorsi F, Del Maschio A. Apparent diffusion coefficient value and ratio as noninvasive potential biomarkers to predict prostate cancer grading: comparison with prostate biopsy and radical prostatectomy specimen. AJR Am J Roentgenol 2015 Mar;204(3):550–557. https://doi.org/10.2214/AJR.14.13146. PMID: 25714284.
37. Chen Y, Yu W, Fan Y, Zhou L, Yang Y, Wang H, Jiang Y, Wang X, Wu S, Jin J. Development and comparison of a Chinese nomogram adding multi-parametric MRI information for predicting extracapsular extension of prostate cancer. Oncotarget. 2017 Mar 28;8(13):22095–22103. https://doi.org/10.18632/oncotarget.11559. PMID: 27564265; PMCID: PMC5400649.
38. Boesen L, Chabanova E, Løgager V, Balslev I, Mikines K, Thomsen HS. Prostate cancer staging with extracapsular extension risk scoring using multiparametric MRI: a correlation with histopathology. Eur Radiol 2015 Jun;25(6):1776–1785. https://doi.org/10.1007/s00330-014-3543-9. Epub 2014 Dec 11. PMID: 25504428.
39. Nyarangi-Dix J, Wiesenfarth M, Bonekamp D, Hitthaler B, Schütz V, Dieffenbacher S, Mueller-Wolf M, Roth W, Stenzinger A, Duensing S, Roethke M, Teber D, Schlemmer HP, Hohenfellner M, Radtke JP. Combined clinical parameters and multiparametric magnetic resonance imaging for the prediction of extraprostatic disease-a risk model for patient-tailored risk stratification when planning radical prostatectomy. Eur Urol Focus. 2020 Nov 15;6(6):1205-1212. https://doi.org/10.1016/j.euf.2018.11.004. Epub 2018 Nov 23. PMID: 30477971.
40. Weinreb JC, Barentsz JO, Choyke PL, Cornud F, Haider MA, Macura KJ, Margolis D, Schnall MD, Shtern F, Tempany CM, Thoeny HC, Verma S. PI-RADS prostate imaging - reporting and data system: 2015, version 2. Eur Urol. 2016 Jan;69(1):16–40. https://doi.org/10.1016/j.eururo.2015.08.052.
41. Barentsz JO, Richenberg J, Clements R, Choyke P, Verma S, Villeirs G, Rouviere O, Logager V, Fütterer JJ, European Society of Urogenital Radiology. ESUR prostate MR guidelines 2012. Eur Radiol. 2012 Apr;22(4):746–57. https://doi.org/10.1007/s00330-011-2377-y.
42. Wibmer A, Vargas HA, Donahue TF, Zheng J, Moskowitz C, Eastham J, Sala E, Hricak H. Diagnosis of extracapsular extension of prostate cancer on prostate MRI: impact of second-opinion readings by subspecialized genitourinary oncologic radiologists. AJR Am J Roentgenol 2015 Jul;205(1):W73–W78. https://doi.org/10.2214/AJR.14.13600. PMID: 26102421.
43. Martini A, Gupta A, Lewis SC, Cumarasamy S, Haines KG 3rd, Briganti A, Montorsi F, Tewari AK. Development and internal validation of a side-specific, multiparametric magnetic resonance imaging-based nomogram for the prediction of extracapsular extension of prostate cancer. BJU Int. 2018 Dec;122(6):1025–33. https://doi.org/10.1111/bju.14353.
44. Sighinolfi MC, Sandri M, Torricelli P, Ligabue G, Fiocchi F, Scialpi M, Eissa A, Reggiani Bonetti L, Puliatti S, Bianchi G, Rocco B. External validation of a novel side-specific, multiparametric magnetic resonance imaging-based nomogram for the prediction of extracapsular extension of prostate cancer: preliminary outcomes on a series diagnosed with multiparametric magnetic resonance imaging-targeted plus systematic saturation biopsy. BJU Int. 2019 Aug;124(2):192–4. https://doi.org/10.1111/bju.14665.
45. Soeterik TFW, van Melick HHE, Dijksman LM, Küsters-Vandevelde H, Stomps S, Schoots IG, Biesma DH, Witjes JA, van Basten JA. Development and external validation of a novel nomogram to predict side-specific extraprostatic extension in patients with prostate cancer undergoing radical prostatectomy. Eur Urol Oncol. 2020 Sep 21:S2588-9311(20)30133-4. https://doi.org/10.1016/j.euo.2020.08.008. Epub ahead of print. PMID: 32972895.
46. Wibmer AG, Kattan MW, Alessandrino F, Baur ADJ, Boesen L, Franco FB, Bonekamp D, Campa R, Cash H, Catalá V, Crouzet S, Dinnoo S, Eastham J, Fennessy FM, Ghabili K, Hohenfellner M, Levi AW, Ji X, Løgager V, Margolis DJ, Moldovan PC, Panebianco V, Penzkofer T, Puech P, Radtke JP, Rouvière O, Schlemmer HP, Sprenkle PC, Tempany CM, Vilanova JC, Weinreb J, Hricak H, Shukla-Dave A. International multi-site initiative to develop an MRI-inclusive nomogram for side-specific prediction of extraprostatic extension of prostate cancer. Cancers (Basel). 2021 May 27;13(11):2627. https://doi.org/10.3390/cancers13112627.
47. Eifler JB, Feng Z, Lin BM, Partin MT, Humphreys EB, Han M, Epstein JI, Walsh PC, Trock BJ, Partin AW. An updated prostate cancer staging nomogram (Partin tables) based on cases from 2006 to 2011. BJU Int. 2013 Jan;111(1):22–9. https://doi.org/10.1111/j.1464-410X.2012.11324.x. Epub 2012 Jul 26. Erratum in: BJU Int. 2013 Mar;111(3):524. PMID: 22834909; PMCID: PMC3876476.
48. Tosco L, De Coster G, Roumeguère T, Everaerts W, Quackels T, Dekuyper P, Van Cleynenbreugel B, Van Damme N, Van Eycken E, Ameye F, et al. Development and external validation of nomograms to predict adverse pathological characteristics after robotic prostatectomy: results of a prospective, multi-institutional, nationwide series. Eur Urol Oncol. 2018;1:338–45.

Intraoperative Evaluation and Management of High-Risk Prostate Cancer during Robot-Assisted Radical Prostatectomy

Ahmet Urkmez and John W. Davis

1 Introduction

It has been predicted that high-risk prostate cancer (HRPC) accounts for between 20% and 35% of newly diagnosed patients of localized disease, and approximately 10% of contemporary patients present with locally advanced disease [1–3]. Men with HRPC are at an increased risk of PSA failure, developing metastases, need for adjuvant treatment, and death from prostate cancer (PC) [4, 5]. The PIVOT (Prostate Cancer Intervention Versus Observation Trial) study showed a significantly lower rate of PC-specific death in men with HRPC undergoing surgery compared with observation (9.1% vs 17.5%) as well as a significant decrease in bone metastases at 10- and 12-year follow-up, while PC-specific mortality was not significantly lower in the radical prostatectomy (RP) group among men with low- or intermediate-risk PC [6]. Moreover, SPCG-4 (Scandinavian Prostate Cancer Group) trial demonstrated overall survival advantage with RP over watchful waiting (all-cause mortality, 46.1% vs 52.7%, RR, 0.75; 95% CI, 0.61 to 0.92%) [7]. The risk of death from PC and biochemical recurrence (BCR) after surgery in patients with HRPC was found to be 11.5 and 3.3 times higher, respectively, than in patients with low-risk PC [8].

2 Definition of High-Risk Prostate Cancer

In 1998, D'Amico et al. first suggested a three-group risk stratification system based on preoperative serum PSA level, clinical T stage, and biopsy Gleason score to predict BCR following RP and radiation therapy (RT) [9]. HRPC was defined as having any of the following features: serum PSA ≥ 20 ng/mL, Gleason score ≥ 8, or clinical stage T2c or higher. However, the definition of HRPC covers a very heterogenous population which consequently resulted in wide variability in outcomes [10, 11]. Therefore, the National Comprehensive Cancer Network (NCCN) guidelines suggest subdividing this group to separate patients thought to have the worst prognosis into the very high-risk category [11]. On the other hand, the American Urological Association (AUA) and the European Association of Urology (EAU) guidelines panels did not recommend substratifying HRPC patients into high risk and very high risk because of the similarity in treatment options and lack of clinical utility for substratifying these patients. They alternatively classify clinical T3 or higher disease as locally advanced PC [4, 5]. The EAU guidelines also suggest including preoperative clinal lymph node positivity into this subgroup [5]. Most commonly used definition of locally advanced PC is clinically ≥ T3 disease with any serum PSA and any Gleason score [12].

3 Treatment Options for High-Risk Prostate Cancer

Treatment of HRPC is a subject of constant discussion due to poor prognosis seen in this group. Historically, RARP was not offered to patients with HRPC because of the anticipation of poor oncological and functional outcomes. However, many recent studies proved that RARP in these patients provides at least comparable oncological control with acceptable perioperative complications [13–16]. Even though some of the patients who underwent RARP may require adjuvant treatments (radiotherapy and/or hormonotherapy) in case of BCR, RT and/or hormonotherapy and their toxic effects can be avoided or at least deferred to a later period in a significant number of patients [17]. Besides, when surgery is selected as the first treatment modality, salvage RT is available in case of recurrence. The reverse is also feasible, but salvage RP after RT is a challenging surgery which yields higher rates of complications [18, 19].

A. Urkmez · J. W. Davis (✉)
Department of Urology, MD Anderson Cancer Center, Houston, TX, USA

P. Wiklund et al. (eds.), *Robotic Urologic Surgery*, https://doi.org/10.1007/978-3-031-00363-9_22

Another crucial benefit of RARP with extended lymph node dissection (ePLND) in patients with HRPC or locally advanced disease includes the opportunity to assess the surgical specimen. Because accurate staging in advanced disease is an important determinant of future management strategy [12], both upstaging and downstaging may occur after surgery because clinical staging based on digital rectal examination is subjective and may be discordant between examiners [20, 21]. Another concern is the possibility of upgrading and downgrading. Lavery et al. reported a downgrading rate of 37% (Gleason score 8–10 to Gleason score ≤ 7) and an upgrading rate of 28% (Gleason score 7 to Gleason score 8–9) in patients with HRPC [22]. Additionally, a downgrading rate of 20% and an upgrading rate of 9 to 27% have been reported for locally advanced PC [23, 24].

Today, there is still no consensus regarding the optimal treatment of men with HRPC; definitive therapy options for localized or locally advanced disease include RT with androgen deprivation therapy (ADT) or RP with ePLND, which may be part of multimodal treatment [5]. A recent systematic review comparing RP versus RT and ADT in men with localized HRPC showed that RT without specification of ADT was associated with worse overall (HR 1.65; CI, 1.42–1.91, $p < 0.0001$) and cancer-specific mortality (HR 1.90; CI, 1.61–2.23, $p < 0.0001$). Even though the magnitude of these associations was decreased in the comparison of RT with ADT versus RP relative to the comparison of RT versus RP, a benefit for both overall and cancer-specific mortality in favor of RP was still observed [25].

4 Timing of Surgery

Since there is no gold standard treatment for patients with HRPC, many patients need time to make their decisions and often ask for a second or third opinions, which consequently may cause a significant delay in treatment. Other potential occasions for delayed treatment include patients' anxiety, treatment of comorbidities before surgery, limited surgical capacity, and long waiting lists for some hospitals as well as unprecedented situations as in COVID-19 outbreak [26]. A recent multicenter study from Canada reported that more than 90 days of surgical waiting time (time from biopsy to surgery) was associated with a higher risk of BCR in patients with HRPC [27]. On the contrary, another recent study from Germany observed that a surgical waiting time of >3 and < 6 months compared to ≤3 months does not worsen any of the pathological outcome variables (e.g., pT stage, grading, surgical margin positivity, lymph node involvement, lymphovascular invasion, perineural invasion) nor decrease the chance of nerve-sparing surgery in patients with HRPC [26].

5 The Role of Preoperative Multiparametric MRI

Multiparametric magnetic resonance imaging (mpMRI) is increasingly being utilized in the management of PC, notably in diagnosis and risk stratification, but also in staging and treatment planning [28, 29]. Prediction of adverse pathological features at surgery, in terms of extraprostatic extension (EPE), seminal vesicle invasion (SVI), and node positivity, is of particular interest when assigning the surgical approach. Surgical margin status represents the most important surgery-related oncological outcome of RP and the only factor to be influenced by surgical method and nerve-sparing strategies. Despite the ongoing discussion about the influence of positive surgical margins (PSMs) on long-term outcome, patients with PSMs are at a higher risk of BCR [16, 30, 31]. In HRPC patients, knowledge of the presence and localization of EPE is likely to reduce the number of PSMs since it enables the surgeon to select patients eligible for nerve-sparing procedures [32–34].

Surgeons performing RARP lack tactile sense which may limit the ability to assess the potential involvement of neurovascular bundles. The sensitivity of MRI in predicting EPE tends to increase from low- to high-risk groups (33% vs 80%). In their study, Park et al. reevaluated their nerve-sparing plan during RARP by including mpMRI report, which was initially determined on the basis of the clinical information. After reviewing the mpMRI reports, the surgical plan was changed in 40% of HRPC patients and the change was correct in 89% [35]. Similarly, Kukreja et al. conducted a study to evaluate the added value of mpMRI on presurgical planning of patients with HRPC. Six fellowship-trained urologic oncologists were asked for their surgical planning in regard to degree of nerve sparing and ePLND during RARP, first with only clinical information followed by the addition of mpMRI images and reports. After incorporating mpMRI in decision-making process, 98% of patients had a change in the degree of the planned nerve sparing: wider excision in 32% and increased nerve sparing in 24%. Additionally, lymph node dissection was converted from standard to extended in 17% of patients, and the bladder neck sparing was changed to the appropriate surgical plan in 37% of cases [36]. Moreover, compared to patients who underwent RARP without mpMRI, the overall rate of PSMs was significantly decreased by the use of mpMRI (12.4% vs 24.1%) [37]. In another very recent study including 366 high-risk and very high-risk PC patients who had preoperative mpMRI staging and underwent RP and ePLND, authors reported that in men with HRPC, mpMRI demonstrating no evidence of SVI, EPE, or neurovascular bundle involvement is the most robust independent predictor of organ-confined disease in a multivariate model including other clinical predictors. They also showed that mpMRI adds significantly to model performance in predicting organ-confined disease in men with HRPC [38]. In conclusion, preoperative mpMRI for HRPC appears to have a significant favorable impact on surgical planning and may be the best tool to guide robotic surgeons without haptic feedback to determine the extent of nerve sparing and bladder neck dissection with the potential for decreasing PSMs [35, 36].

6 Technical Aspects of Robot-Assisted Radical Prostatectomy in High-Risk Prostate Cancer

Robot-assisted radical prostatectomy has comparable oncological and functional outcomes in HRPC patients to the traditional open approach with a number of benefits of improved 10x magnification, 3-dimensial (3D) vision, better visualization of tissue planes, precise dissection, and reduced blood loss [14, 18, 39]. However, the lack of tactile feedback in robotic surgery raises concerns about both functional and oncological outcomes after RARP specifically in men with high-risk and locally advanced disease owing to the extracapsular extension of cancer, irregular-bulky borders, and the need for broader dissection in such cases. Therefore, most experts suggest proceeding to perform HRPC cases after acquiring sufficient surgical expertise in low-risk cases [40, 41].

The majority of RARP procedures have been performed via transperitoneal approach owing to the fact that it provides easy access to prostate and offers a large working space which is especially important during the dissection of large-advanced tumors and when ePLND is needed. Six-port transperitoneal approach was used in all of the reported studies in patients with locally advanced PC who underwent RARP [12]. Posterior approach was usually favored to gain a better view of the pelvis. During RARP in HRPC cases, firm seminal vesicles might suggest tumor invasion and requires gentle and careful dissection of tissues in order to prevent PSMs. Besides, in advanced disease, utmost care should be given during the dissection of the plane between the rectum and prostate following incision of Denonvillier's facia. Because anatomical planes might be unclear in such cases due to the extracapsular extension of the tumor and previous ADT, broad dissection might cause rectal injury. Therefore, performing dissections as close as up to the apex between the plane of rectum and prostate facilitates the procedure and prevents rectal injury [42, 43]. Gandaglia et al. described their surgical technique of extrafascial RARP in locally advanced PC which resulted in a large amount of tissue surrounding the prostate specimen. In their technique, the Denonvilliers' fascia was completely dissected free and left on the posterior surface of the seminal vesicles, thus ensuring oncological safety of the procedure. The extrafascial dissection was subsequently carried out laterally to the levator ani fascia. During this approach the neurovascular bundles were clipped and transected below the Denonvillers' fascia [13].

Another crucial step of performing RARP in HRPC patients is dissecting the plane between prostate base and bladder neck. Preoperative mpMRI and virtual 3D printed models could be useful in surgical planning of nerve sparing and bladder neck dissection as well as reducing PSMs in these patients [36, 44]. Intraoperative frozen section analysis during nerve-sparing RARP (nsRARP) in HRPC patients has reduced the rate of PSMs and urinary incontinence [45, 46]. It could also be useful in reducing PSMs during the dissection between bladder neck and prostate base [42]. While dissecting posterior-lateral side of the prostate, visual clues should be considered to reduce the risk of PSMs: color and texture of the tissue, periprostatic veins as a landmark for athermal dissection, and a freely separating bloodless plane showing loose shiny areolar tissue [47].

7 Nerve Sparing Planning/Algorithms

In patients with HRPC, traditionally, nerve sparing was not encouraged because of the anticipation of the increased rate of PSM and BCR after RARP. On the other hand, nsRARP has resulted in better postoperative potency and continence. Therefore, surgeons have the challenge of decreasing the rate of PSM while maintaining the patients' quality of life [40, 48]. Kumar et al. proposed selective nerve sparing in HRPC based on patients' preoperative clinical parameters (clinical stage, positive cores on biopsy) and surgeon's intraoperative judgment (loss of dissection planes, focal bulge of prostate capsule, etc.). Consequently, they reported that complete or partial nsRARP could be performed in 89% of patients with HRPC without compromising the rate of PSM and BCR, and also ensuring better postoperative functional outcomes [40]. Similarly, Lavery et al. suggested using visual clues such as poorly defined or sticky dissection planes, bulging of the prostate capsule, or the appearance of prostate tissue on the preserved neurovascular bundle in selecting patients for nsRARP. Consequently, they were able to perform nsRARP in 73% of patients with HRPC [22]. Punnen et al. compared RARP with open RP in patients with HRPC and reported that RARP patients underwent bilateral nerve sparing more often than open RP patients (54% vs 34%, $p < 0.01$) while PSM rates were comparable in two groups (29% vs 23%, $p = 0.13$) [49]. Shikanov et al. compared extrafascial nsRARP with intrafascial nsRARP and observed a remarkable trend toward lower rate of PSMs in patients with pT3 disease who underwent extrafascial nsRARP compared to intrafascial approach (28% vs 51%). The reduction in PSMs was more prominent in posterolateral and mid-prostate locations [50]. Therefore, extrafascial nsRARP has been suggested over intra- or trans-fascial approach in patients with HRPC to balance oncological safety with preservation of functional outcomes. Besides, surgeons should consider certain preoperative clinical parameters along with intraoperative visual clues to assess the extension and/or invasion of the cancer and to guide selective/individualized nerve sparing since nerve sparing is not "all or none phenomenon" [40].

8 Retzius Sparing in High-Risk Patients

Retzius sparing, also called the Bocciardi approach, provides the maintenance of the normal anatomy as much as possible by preserving supportive structures such as the puboprostatic ligaments, endopelvic fascia, and Santorini plexus [51]. Studies reported excellent postoperative functional outcomes, specifically early return to continence, with this approach. However, these studies mostly include low- and intermediate-risk PC patients [52]. Because Retzius-sparing surgery follows a completely intra- or interfascial plane and requires staying very close to the prostate throughout its mobilization, a concern is raised whether the functional outcomes can be replicated in patients with HRPC without compromising oncological outcomes [53]. A very recent study including 50 men with HRPC (84% of the patients had ≥ pT3 disease) showed that Retzius-sparing RARP was feasible and safe (only 3 patients had Clavien Grade 3 complications related to ePLND; the rest had ≤ Clavien Grade 2 complications) in high-risk and locally advanced PC [54]. Although their PSM rate was seemingly high (43%), it was comparable with other studies on HRPC patients who underwent conventional RARP (16–58%) [12]. Nevertheless, they reported very promising continence (0 or 1 safety liner pad) rates at 3 and 12 months of surgery (82% vs 98%) [54].

9 Extended Pelvic Lymph Node Dissection

Extended pelvic lymph node dissection still represents the most reliable method of detecting lymph node metastases of PC in spite of the recent introduction of Gallium-68 (^{68}Ga)- and Fluorine-18 (^{18}F) prostate-specific membrane antigen (PSMA) positron emission tomography/computed tomography (PET/CT), which provided improved detection of localization of primary or recurrent PC with higher sensitivity and specificity when compared with other imaging modalities [5, 55–57]. The NCCN guidelines for PC treatment recommend performing an ePLND if the nomogram-predicted lymph node metastasis probability is 2% or greater [11], while the EAU guidelines set this cutoff at 5% [5]. Both guidelines suggest following an extended PLND template in patients with HRPC [5, 11]. Despite proven benefits of ePLND in PC staging and consequent guiding of or omitting adjuvant treatment, the therapeutic efficacy of ePLND remains debatable [58–60]. Historically, it was reported that urologists performing RARP were up to five times more prone to omit PLND compared with urologists performing open RP, even in HRPC patients [41, 61]. However, a significantly increased contemporary trend has been observed in the concomitant PLND rate during RARP in patients with intermediate- to high-risk PC likely owing to the increased expertise in robotic surgery [62].

From a technical aspect, ePLND can be performed either before prostatectomy or after prostatectomy and vesicourethral anastomosis. No related oncological or functional outcomes highlight that any of these options as more advantageous than the other. Placing the ports more cranially may help better explore the iliac bifurcation and presacral region during ePLND. Additionally, placement of metal clips instead of hem-o-lock clips at prostate pedicles and in the ePLND site may facilitate targeting of adjuvant RT in case of residual tumor or local recurrence [42]. One of the concerns about performing an ePLND is lymphocele formation. It has been shown that the extent of the PLND is an independent predictor of lymphocele formation [63]. Although various strategies have been proposed to prevent lymphocele development after RARP, randomized controlled trials (RCTs) revealed no significant differences in the rate of symptomatic lymphocele development after RARP with PLND in comparing peritoneal interposition flap with control [64], non-drainage with pelvic drainage [65], titanium clips with bipolar energy [66], TachoSil (a hemostatic sponge) with control [67], and Arista AH (a hemostatic powder) with control [68].

10 Sentinel Node Biopsy and Fluorescence-Supported Lymphography

Studies have shown that 25% of lymphatic landing sites of PC are located outside of the ePLND template owing to the aberrant dissemination pathways [58, 69]. Sentinel node biopsy (SNB) and indocyanine green (ICG)-guided ePLND have been proposed to improve the efficiency of ePLND during RARP [70, 71]. Although SNB appears to increase nodal yield by detecting more affected nodes when combined with ePLND than ePLND alone, it rarely detected positive nodes outside the ePLND template, raising concerns that SNB may not have any additional value over ePLND [72]. A recent RCT showed that ICG-guided ePLND improves the understanding of the lymphatic drainage and detects significantly more lymph nodes with a median number of 25 vs 17 retrieved nodes ($p < 0.001$) [71]. However, due to the reported low sensitivity (44%) in this study, authors suggested combination of ICG guidance with ePLND instead of stand-alone ICG lymph node dissection [71].

11 Complications

A few recent RARP series for HRPC have reported total and major complication rates ranging between 4% and 29% and 0% and 9.1%, respectively [18]. Ham et al. compared the outcomes of RARP performed in organ-confined and locally advanced PC and found no significant differences between two groups in many preoperative features including operation time, estimated blood loss, length of hospital stays, and intraoperative complications [73]. Rogers et al. showed similar recovery period after RARP compared with open RP in the elderly population (≥70-year-old), in which group complications were expected to be higher [74]. Additionally, it has been shown that patients undergoing major urologic surgeries including RARP with ePLND benefited from application of enhanced recovery after surgery (ERAS) protocols such as preoperative counseling, medical optimization, avoidance of fasting and bowel preparation, venous thromboembolism prophylaxis, avoidance of salt and water overload, appropriate antibiotic use, ileus prevention, pain control, early mobilization, and early oral nutrition with avoidance of nasogastric tubes [75].

12 Oncological Outcomes

The avoidance of PSMs during RARP is regarded as the most important surgery-related oncological outcome. Because its presence may signify an indication for adjuvant treatments, such as RT and ADT, which might significantly affect patients' quality of life [16, 76]. RARP currently represents the most commonly performed surgery in men with PC, and several studies have demonstrated significant advantages of RARP compared with open RP regarding blood loss, hospital stays, complication rates, early recovery of urinary incontinence, and erectile dysfunctions [15, 77, 78]. Besides the mentioned benefits of RARP, Suardi et al. showed that RARP was associated with a significantly lower rate of PSMs in HRPC patients compared with open approach (19.7% vs 30.1%, $p < 0.001$), while no significant difference was observed in low- and intermediate-risk patients [16]. However, it should be kept in mind that their analysis was restricted to patients operated on by expert surgeons who have performed a minimum number of 300 procedures per each technique (RARP and open RP) [16]. Current RARP studies in HRPC patients report the BCR rate ranging from 13% to 35% [18]. However, most series lack long-term follow-up.

So far only a few retrospective studies reported oncological outcomes in patients with locally advanced PC. The rates of PSMs in patients with locally advanced PC who underwent RARP ranged from 20% to 60%. BCR rates ranged from 18.5% to 28.6% [12, 13, 21, 73]. Among these studies, Gandaglia et al. reported a relatively lower rate of PSM which might be related to their surgical technique of extrafascial RARP that yields a large amount of tissue surrounding the surgical specimen. Additionally, at 3-year follow-up, two out of three patients were free from BCR as well as 95% of patients were free from clinical recurrence [13].

13 Functional Outcomes

Functional outcomes are major concerns in patients seeking treatment for PC. Surgical techniques, such as nerve-sparing and Retzius-sparing surgery, anterior and posterior reconstruction, and bladder neck preservation approaches, have improved particularly early functional outcomes [4]. A recent study including 764 men with D'Amico HRPC (62% ≥ pT3a) who underwent RARP at two centers in the USA and Europe demonstrated that functional outcomes continue to improve beyond 1 year after RARP. The authors reported urinary incontinence (0 pad or 1 safety liner) and sexual function (SHIM ≥17) recovery rates of 92% and 69%, respectively, at 3-year follow-up of surgery [5]. Along with their report on the oncological safety of RARP in patients with HRPC [6], they suggested that a significant majority of patients with HRCP who underwent RARP can be expected to recover urinary continence and sexual dysfunction without compromising long-term oncological outcomes [5].

References

1. Cooperberg MR, Cowan J, Broering JM, Carroll PR. High-risk prostate cancer in the United States, 1990-2007. World J Urol. 2008 Jun;26(3):211–8. https://doi.org/10.1007/s00345-008-0250-7.
2. Shao YH, Demissie K, Shih W, Mehta AR, Stein MN, Roberts CB, Dipaola RS, Lu-Yao GL. Contemporary risk profile of prostate cancer in the United States. J Natl Cancer Inst. 2009 Sep 16;101(18):1280–3. https://doi.org/10.1093/jnci/djp262.
3. Lowrance WT, Elkin EB, Yee DS, Feifer A, Ehdaie B, Jacks LM, Atoria CL, Zelefsky MJ, Scher HI, Scardino PT, Eastham JA. Locally advanced prostate cancer: a population-based study of treatment patterns. BJU Int. 2012 May;109(9):1309–14. https://doi.org/10.1111/j.1464-410X.2011.10760.x.
4. Sanda MG, Cadeddu JA, Kirkby E, Chen RC, Crispino T, Fontanarosa J, Freedland SJ, Greene K, Klotz LH, Makarov DV, Nelson JB, Rodrigues G, Sandler HM, Taplin ME, Treadwell JR. Clinically localized prostate cancer: AUA/ASTRO/SUO guideline. Part I: risk stratification, shared decision making, and care

options. J Urol. 2018 Mar;199(3):683–90. https://doi.org/10.1016/j.juro.2017.11.095.

5. Mottet N, van den Bergh RCN, Briers E, Van den Broeck T, Cumberbatch MG, De Santis M, et al. EAU-EANM-ESTRO-ESUR-SIOG guidelines on prostate Cancer-2020 update. Part 1: screening, diagnosis, and local treatment with curative intent. Eur Urol. 2021 Feb;79(2):243–62. https://doi.org/10.1016/j.eururo.2020.09.042.
6. Wilt TJ, Brawer MK, Jones KM, Barry MJ, Aronson WJ, Fox S, Gingrich JR, Wei JT, Gilhooly P, Grob BM, Nsouli I, Iyer P, Cartagena R, Snider G, Roehrborn C, Sharifi R, Blank W, Pandya P, Andriole GL, Culkin D, Wheeler T. Prostate cancer intervention versus observation trial (PIVOT) study group. Radical prostatectomy versus observation for localized prostate cancer. N Engl J Med. 2012 Jul 19;367(3):203–13.
7. Bill-Axelson A, Holmberg L, Ruutu M, Garmo H, Stark JR, Busch C, Nordling S, Häggman M, Andersson SO, Bratell S, Spångberg A, Palmgren J, Steineck G, Adami HO, Johansson JE. SPCG-4 investigators. Radical prostatectomy versus watchful waiting in early prostate cancer. N Engl J Med. 2011 May 5;364(18):1708–17. https://doi.org/10.1056/NEJMoa1011967.
8. Boorjian SA, Karnes RJ, Rangel LJ, Bergstralh EJ, Blute ML. Mayo Clinic validation of the D'Amico risk group classification for predicting survival following radical prostatectomy. J Urol 2008 Apr;179(4):1354–1360; discussion 1360-1. https://doi.org/10.1016/j.juro.2007.11.061.
9. D'Amico AV, Whittington R, Malkowicz SB, Schultz D, Blank K, Broderick GA, Tomaszewski JE, Renshaw AA, Kaplan I, Beard CJ, Wein A. Biochemical outcome after radical prostatectomy, external beam radiation therapy, or interstitial radiation therapy for clinically localized prostate cancer. JAMA. 1998 Sep 16;280(11):969–74. https://doi.org/10.1001/jama.280.11.969.
10. Wang Z, Ni Y, Chen J, Sun G, Zhang X, Zhao J, Zhu X, Zhang H, Zhu S, Dai J, Shen P, Zeng H. The efficacy and safety of radical prostatectomy and radiotherapy in high-risk prostate cancer: a systematic review and meta-analysis. World J Surg Oncol. 2020 Feb 24;18(1):42. https://doi.org/10.1186/s12957-020-01824-9.
11. Mohler JL, Antonarakis ES, Armstrong AJ, D'Amico AV, Davis BJ, Dorff T, Eastham JA, Enke CA, Farrington TA, Higano CS, Horwitz EM, Hurwitz M, Ippolito JE, Kane CJ, Kuettel MR, Lang JM, McKenney J, Netto G, Penson DF, Plimack ER, Pow-Sang JM, Pugh TJ, Richey S, Roach M, Rosenfeld S, Schaeffer E, Shabsigh A, Small EJ, Spratt DE, Srinivas S, Tward J, Shead DA, Freedman-Cass DA. Prostate cancer, version 2.2019, NCCN clinical practice guidelines in oncology. J Natl Compr Canc Netw. 2019 May 1;17(5):479–505. https://doi.org/10.6004/jnccn.2019.0023.
12. Saika T, Miura N, Fukumoto T, Yanagihara Y, Miyauchi Y, Kikugawa T. Role of robot-assisted radical prostatectomy in locally advanced prostate cancer. Int J Urol. 2018 Jan;25(1):30–5. https://doi.org/10.1111/iju.13441.
13. Gandaglia G, De Lorenzis E, Novara G, Fossati N, De Groote R, Dovey Z, Suardi N, Montorsi F, Briganti A, Rocco B, Mottrie A. Robot-assisted radical prostatectomy and extended pelvic lymph node dissection in patients with locally-advanced prostate cancer. Eur Urol. 2017 Feb;71(2):249–56. https://doi.org/10.1016/j.eururo.2016.05.008.
14. Abdollah F, Sood A, Sammon JD, Hsu L, Beyer B, Moschini M, Gandaglia G, Rogers CG, Haese A, Montorsi F, Graefen M, Briganti A, Menon M. Long-term cancer control outcomes in patients with clinically high-risk prostate cancer treated with robot-assisted radical prostatectomy: results from a multi-institutional study of 1100 patients. Eur Urol. 2015 Sep;68(3):497–505. https://doi.org/10.1016/j.eururo.2015.06.020.
15. Gandaglia G, Abdollah F, Hu J, Kim S, Briganti A, Sammon JD, Becker A, Roghmann F, Graefen M, Montorsi F, Perrotte P, Karakiewicz PI, Trinh QD, Sun M. Is robot-assisted radical prostatectomy safe in men with high-risk prostate cancer? Assessment of perioperative outcomes, positive surgical margins, and use of additional cancer treatments. J Endourol. 2014 Jul;28(7):784–91. https://doi.org/10.1089/end.2013.0774.
16. Suardi N, Dell'Oglio P, Gallina A, Gandaglia G, Buffi N, Moschini M, Fossati N, Lughezzani G, Karakiewicz PI, Freschi M, Lucianò R, Shariat SF, Guazzoni G, Gaboardi F, Montorsi F, Briganti A. Evaluation of positive surgical margins in patients undergoing robot-assisted and open radical prostatectomy according to preoperative risk groups. Urol Oncol. 2016 Feb;34(2):57.e1–7. https://doi.org/10.1016/j.urolonc.2015.08.019.
17. Parker CC, Clarke NW, Cook AD, Kynaston HG, Petersen PM, Catton C, Cross W, Logue J, Parulekar W, Payne H, Persad R, Pickering H, Saad F, Anderson J, Bahl A, Bottomley D, Brasso K, Chahal R, Cooke PW, Eddy B, Gibbs S, Goh C, Gujral S, Heath C, Henderson A, Jaganathan R, Jakobsen H, James ND, Kanaga Sundaram S, Lees K, Lester J, Lindberg H, Money-Kyrle J, Morris S, O'Sullivan J, Ostler P, Owen L, Patel P, Pope A, Popert R, Raman R, Røder MA, Sayers I, Simms M, Wilson J, Zarkar A, Parmar MKB, Sydes MR. Timing of radiotherapy after radical prostatectomy (RADICALS-RT): a randomised, controlled phase 3 trial. Lancet. 2020 Oct 31;396(10260):1413–21. https://doi.org/10.1016/S0140-6736(20)31553-1.
18. Srougi V, Tourinho-Barbosa RR, Nunes-Silva I, Baghdadi M, Garcia-Barreras S, Rembeyo G, Eiffel SS, Barret E, Rozet F, Galiano M, Sanchez-Salas R, Cathelineau X. The role of robot-assisted radical prostatectomy in high-risk prostate cancer. J Endourol. 2017 Mar;31(3):229–37. https://doi.org/10.1089/end.2016.0659.
19. Chade DC, Eastham J, Graefen M, Hu JC, Karnes RJ, Klotz L, Montorsi F, van Poppel H, Scardino PT, Shariat SF. Cancer control and functional outcomes of salvage radical prostatectomy for radiation-recurrent prostate cancer: a systematic review of the literature. Eur Urol. 2012 May;61(5):961–71. https://doi.org/10.1016/j.eururo.2012.01.022.
20. Connolly SS, Cathcart PJ, Gilmore P, Kerger M, Crowe H, Peters JS, Murphy DG, Costello AJ. Robotic radical prostatectomy as the initial step in multimodal therapy for men with high-risk localised prostate cancer: initial experience of 160 men. BJU Int. 2012 Mar;109(5):752–9. https://doi.org/10.1111/j.1464-410X.2011.10548.x.
21. Casey JT, Meeks JJ, Greco KA, Wu SD, Nadler RB. Outcomes of locally advanced (T3 or greater) prostate cancer in men undergoing robot-assisted laparoscopic prostatectomy. J Endourol. 2009 Sep;23(9):1519–22. https://doi.org/10.1089/end.2009.0388.
22. Lavery HJ, Nabizada-Pace F, Carlucci JR, Brajtbord JS, Samadi DB. Nerve-sparing robotic prostatectomy in preoperatively high-risk patients is safe and efficacious. Urol Oncol. 2012 Jan-Feb;30(1):26–32. https://doi.org/10.1016/j.urolonc.2009.11.023.
23. Xylinas E, Daché A, Rouprêt M. Is radical prostatectomy a viable therapeutic option in clinically locally advanced (cT3) prostate cancer? BJU Int. 2010 Dec;106(11):1596–600. https://doi.org/10.1111/j.1464-410X.2010.09630.x.
24. Mitchell CR, Boorjian SA, Umbreit EC, Rangel LJ, Carlson RE, Karnes RJ. 20-year survival after radical prostatectomy as initial treatment for cT3 prostate cancer. BJU Int. 2012 Dec;110(11):1709–13. https://doi.org/10.1111/j.1464-410X.2012.11372.x.
25. Greenberger BA, Zaorsky NG, Den RB. Comparison of radical prostatectomy versus radiation and androgen deprivation therapy strategies as primary treatment for high-risk localized prostate cancer: a systematic review and meta-analysis. Eur Urol Focus. 2020 Mar 15;6(2):404–18. https://doi.org/10.1016/j.euf.2019.11.007.
26. Engl T, Mandel P, Hoeh B, Preisser F, Wenzel M, Humke C, Welte M, Köllermann J, Wild P, Deuker M, Kluth LA, Roos FC, Chun FKH, Becker A. Impact of "time-from-biopsy-to-prostatectomy" on adverse oncological results in patients with intermediate and high-risk prostate cancer. Front Surg. 2020 Sep 25;7:561853. https://doi.org/10.3389/fsurg.2020.561853.

27. Zanaty M, Alnazari M, Ajib K, Lawson K, Azizi M, Rajih E, Alenizi A, Hueber PA, Tolmier C, Meskawi M, Saad F, Pompe RS, Karakiewicz PI, El-Hakim A, Zorn KC. Does surgical delay for radical prostatectomy affect biochemical recurrence? A retrospective analysis from a Canadian cohort. World J Urol. 2018 Jan;36(1):1–6. https://doi.org/10.1007/s00345-017-2105-6.
28. Ahmed HU, El-Shater Bosaily A, Brown LC, Gabe R, Kaplan R, Parmar MK, Collaco-Moraes Y, Ward K, Hindley RG, Freeman A, Kirkham AP, Oldroyd R, Parker C, Emberton M. PROMIS study group. Diagnostic accuracy of multi-parametric MRI and TRUS biopsy in prostate cancer (PROMIS): a paired validating confirmatory study. Lancet. 2017 Feb 25;389(10071):815–22. https://doi.org/10.1016/S0140-6736(16)32401-1.
29. Kasivisvanathan V, Rannikko AS, Borghi M, Panebianco V, Mynderse LA, Vaarala MH, Briganti A, Budäus L, Hellawell G, Hindley RG, Roobol MJ, Eggener S, Ghei M, Villers A, Bladou F, Villeirs GM, Virdi J, Boxler S, Robert G, Singh PB, Venderink W, Hadaschik BA, Ruffion A, Hu JC, Margolis D, Crouzet S, Klotz L, Taneja SS, Pinto P, Gill I, Allen C, Giganti F, Freeman A, Morris S, Punwani S, Williams NR, Brew-Graves C, Deeks J, Takwoingi Y, Emberton M, Moore CM. PRECISION study group collaborators. MRI-targeted or standard biopsy for prostate-cancer diagnosis. N Engl J Med. 2018 May 10;378(19):1767–77. https://doi.org/10.1056/NEJMoa1801993.
30. Boorjian SA, Karnes RJ, Crispen PL, Carlson RE, Rangel LJ, Bergstralh EJ, Blute ML. The impact of positive surgical margins on mortality following radical prostatectomy during the prostate specific antigen era. J Urol. 2010 Mar;183(3):1003–9. https://doi.org/10.1016/j.juro.2009.11.039.
31. Pfitzenmaier J, Pahernik S, Tremmel T, Haferkamp A, Buse S, Hohenfellner M. Positive surgical margins after radical prostatectomy: do they have an impact on biochemical or clinical progression? BJU Int. 2008 Nov;102(10):1413–8. https://doi.org/10.1111/j.1464-410X.2008.07791.x.
32. McClure TD, Margolis DJ, Reiter RE, et al. Use of MR imaging to determine preservation of the neurovascular bundles at robotic-assisted laparoscopic prostatectomy. Radiology. 2012;262(3):874–83.
33. Hricak H, Wang L, Wei DC, et al. The role of preoperative endorectal magnetic resonance imaging in the decision regarding whether to preserve or resect neurovascular bundles during radical retropubic prostatectomy. Cancer. 2004;100(12):2655–63.
34. Masterson TA, Touijer K. The role of endorectal coil MRI in preoperative staging and decision-making for the treatment of clinically localized prostate cancer. MAGMA. 2008;21(6):371–7.
35. Park BH, Jeon HG, Jeong BC, Seo SI, Lee HM, Choi HY, Jeon SS. Influence of magnetic resonance imaging in the decision to preserve or resect neurovascular bundles at robotic assisted laparoscopic radical prostatectomy. J Urol. 2014 Jul;192(1):82–8. https://doi.org/10.1016/j.juro.2014.01.005.
36. Baack Kukreja J, Bathala TK, Reichard CA, Troncoso P, Delacroix S, Davies B, Eggener S, Smaldone M, Minhaj Siddiqui M, Tollefson M, Chapin BF. Impact of preoperative prostate magnetic resonance imaging on the surgical management of high-risk prostate cancer. Prostate Cancer Prostatic Dis. 2020 Mar;23(1):172–8. https://doi.org/10.1038/s41391-019-0171-0.
37. Schiavina R, Bianchi L, Borghesi M, Dababneh H, Chessa F, Pultrone CV, Angiolini A, Gaudiano C, Porreca A, Fiorentino M, De Groote R, D'Hondt F, De Naeyer G, Mottrie A, Brunocilla E. MRI displays the prostatic cancer anatomy and improves the bundles management before robot-assisted radical prostatectomy. J Endourol. 2018 Apr;32(4):315–21. https://doi.org/10.1089/end.2017.0701.
38. Reichard CA, Kukreja J, Gregg JR, Bathala TK, Achim MF, Wang X, Davis JW, Nguyen QN, Chapin BF. Prediction of organ-confined disease in high- and very-high-risk prostate cancer patients staged with magnetic resonance imaging: implications for clinical trial design. Eur Urol Focus. 2021 Jan;7(1):71–7. https://doi.org/10.1016/j.euf.2019.04.016.
39. Abdollah F, Dalela D, Sood A, Sammon J, Cho R, Nocera L, Diaz M, Jeong W, Peabody JO, Fossati N, Gandaglia G, Briganti A, Montorsi F, Menon M. Functional outcomes of clinically high-risk prostate cancer patients treated with robot-assisted radical prostatectomy: a multi-institutional analysis. Prostate Cancer Prostatic Dis. 2017 Dec;20(4):395–400. https://doi.org/10.1038/pcan.2017.26.
40. Kumar A, Samavedi S, Bates AS, Mouraviev V, Coelho RF, Rocco B, Patel VR. Safety of selective nerve sparing in high risk prostate cancer during robot-assisted radical prostatectomy. J Robot Surg. 2017 Jun;11(2):129–38. https://doi.org/10.1007/s11701-016-0627-3.
41. Canda AE. Re: is robot-assisted radical prostatectomy safe in men with high-risk prostate cancer? Assessment of perioperative outcomes, positive surgical margins, and use of additional cancer treatments. Eur Urol. 2015 Feb;67(2):347. https://doi.org/10.1016/j.eururo.2014.11.017.
42. Stroup SP, Kane CJ. Robotic-assisted laparoscopic prostatectomy for high-risk prostate cancer: technical considerations and review of the literature. ISRN Urol. 2011;2011:201408. https://doi.org/10.5402/2011/201408.
43. Canda AE, Balbay MD. Robotic radical prostatectomy in high-risk prostate cancer: current perspectives. Asian J Androl 2015 Nov-Dec;17(6):908–915; discussion 913. https://doi.org/10.4103/1008-682X.153541.
44. Porpiglia F, Bertolo R, Checcucci E, Amparore D, Autorino R, Dasgupta P, Wiklund P, Tewari A, Liatsikos E, Fiori C. ESUT research group. Development and validation of 3D printed virtual models for robot-assisted radical prostatectomy and partial nephrectomy: urologists' and patients' perception. World J Urol. 2018 Feb;36(2):201–7. https://doi.org/10.1007/s00345-017-2126-1.
45. Mirmilstein G, Rai BP, Gbolahan O, Srirangam V, Narula A, Agarwal S, Lane TM, Vasdev N, Adshead J. The neurovascular structure-adjacent frozen-section examination (NeuroSAFE) approach to nerve sparing in robot-assisted laparoscopic radical prostatectomy in a British setting - a prospective observational comparative study. BJU Int. 2018 Jun;121(6):854–62. https://doi.org/10.1111/bju.14078.
46. Vasdev N, Agarwal S, Rai BP, Soosainathan A, Shaw G, Chang S, Prasad V, Mohan-S G, Adshead JM. Intraoperative frozen section of the prostate reduces the risk of positive margin whilst ensuring nerve sparing in patients with intermediate and high-risk prostate cancer undergoing robotic radical prostatectomy: first reported UK series. Curr Urol. 2016 May;9(2):93–103. https://doi.org/10.1159/000442860.
47. Tewari AK, Patel ND, Leung RA, Yadav R, Vaughan ED, El-Douaihy Y, Tu JJ, Amin MB, Akhtar M, Burns M, Kreaden U, Rubin MA, Takenaka A, Shevchuk MM. Visual cues as a surrogate for tactile feedback during robotic-assisted laparoscopic prostatectomy: posterolateral margin rates in 1340 consecutive patients. BJU Int. 2010 Aug;106(4):528–36. https://doi.org/10.1111/j.1464-410X.2009.09176.x.
48. Yossepowitch O, Briganti A, Eastham JA, Epstein J, Graefen M, Montironi R, Touijer K. Positive surgical margins after radical prostatectomy: a systematic review and contemporary update. Eur Urol. 2014 Feb;65(2):303–13. https://doi.org/10.1016/j.eururo.2013.07.039.
49. Punnen S, Meng MV, Cooperberg MR, Greene KL, Cowan JE, Carroll PR. How does robot-assisted radical prostatectomy (RARP) compare with open surgery in men with high-risk prostate cancer? BJU Int. 2013 Aug;112(4):E314–20. https://doi.org/10.1111/j.1464-410X.2012.11493.x.

50. Shikanov S, Woo J, Al-Ahmadie H, Katz MH, Zagaja GP, Shalhav AL, Zorn KC. Extrafascial versus interfascial nerve-sparing technique for robotic-assisted laparoscopic prostatectomy: comparison of functional outcomes and positive surgical margins characteristics. Urology. 2009 Sep;74(3):611–6. https://doi.org/10.1016/j.urology.2009.01.092.
51. Urkmez A, Ranasinghe W, Davis JW. Surgical techniques to improve continence recovery after robot-assisted radical prostatectomy. Transl Androl Urol. 2020 Dec;9(6):3036–48. https://doi.org/10.21037/tau.2020.03.36.
52. Checcucci E, Veccia A, Fiori C, Amparore D, Manfredi M, Di Dio M, Morra I, Galfano A, Autorino R, Bocciardi AM, Dasgupta P, Porpiglia F. Retzius-sparing robot-assisted radical prostatectomy vs the standard approach: a systematic review and analysis of comparative outcomes. BJU Int. 2020 Jan;125(1):8–16. https://doi.org/10.1111/bju.14887.
53. Stonier T, Simson N, Davis J, Challacombe B. Retzius-sparing robot-assisted radical prostatectomy (RS-RARP) vs standard RARP: it's time for critical appraisal. BJU Int. 2019 Jan;123(1):5–7. https://doi.org/10.1111/bju.14468.
54. Nyarangi-Dix JN, Görtz M, Gradinarov G, Hofer L, Schütz V, Gasch C, Radtke JP, Hohenfellner M. Retzius-sparing robot-assisted laparoscopic radical prostatectomy: functional and early oncologic results in aggressive and locally advanced prostate cancer. BMC Urol. 2019 Nov 12;19(1):113. https://doi.org/10.1186/s12894-019-0550-9.
55. Perera M, Papa N, Roberts M, et al. Gallium-68 prostate-specific membrane antigen positron emission tomography in advanced prostate cancer-updated diagnostic utility, sensitivity, specificity, and distribution of prostate-specific membrane antigen-avid lesions: a systematic review and meta-analysis. Eur Urol. 2020;77:403.
56. Hofman MS, Lawrentschuk N, Francis RJ, et al. Prostate-specific membrane antigen PET-CT in patients with high-risk prostate cancer before curative-intent surgery or radiotherapy (proPSMA): a prospective, randomised, multicentre study. Lancet. 2020;395:1208.
57. Luiting HB, van Leeuwen PJ, Busstra MB, Brabander T, van der Poel HG, Donswijk ML, Vis AN, Emmett L, Stricker PD, Roobol MJ. Use of gallium-68 prostate-specific membrane antigen positron-emission tomography for detecting lymph node metastases in primary and recurrent prostate cancer and location of recurrence after radical prostatectomy: an overview of the current literature. BJU Int. 2020 Feb;125(2):206–14. https://doi.org/10.1111/bju.14944.
58. Fossati N, Willemse PM, Van den Broeck T, van den Bergh RCN, Yuan CY, Briers E, Bellmunt J, Bolla M, Cornford P, De Santis M, MacPepple E, Henry AM, Mason MD, Matveev VB, van der Poel HG, van der Kwast TH, Rouvière O, Schoots IG, Wiegel T, Lam TB, Mottet N, Joniau S. The benefits and harms of different extents of lymph node dissection during radical prostatectomy for prostate cancer: a systematic review. Eur Urol. 2017 Jul;72(1):84–109. https://doi.org/10.1016/j.eururo.2016.12.003.
59. Lestingi JFP, Guglielmetti GB, Trinh QD, Coelho RF, Pontes J Jr, Bastos DA, Cordeiro MD, Sarkis AS, Faraj SF, Mitre AI, Srougi M, Nahas WC. Extended versus limited pelvic lymph node dissection during radical prostatectomy for intermediate- and high-risk prostate cancer: early oncological outcomes from a randomized phase 3 trial. Eur Urol 2020 Dec 5; S0302-2838(20)30941-6. https://doi.org/10.1016/j.eururo.2020.11.040.
60. Preisser F, van den Bergh RCN, Gandaglia G, Ost P, Surcel CI, Sooriakumaran P, Montorsi F, Graefen M, van der Poel H, de la Taille A, Briganti A, Salomon L, Ploussard G, Tilki D, EAU-YAUWP. Effect of extended pelvic lymph node dissection on oncologic outcomes in patients with D'Amico intermediate and high risk prostate cancer treated with radical prostatectomy: a multi-institutional study. J Urol. 2020 Feb;203(2):338–43. https://doi.org/10.1097/JU.0000000000000504.
61. Silberstein JL, Su D, Glickman L, Kent M, Keren-Paz G, Vickers AJ, Coleman JA, Eastham JA, Scardino PT, Laudone VP. A case-mix-adjusted comparison of early oncological outcomes of open and robotic prostatectomy performed by experienced high volume surgeons. BJU Int. 2013 Feb;111(2):206–12. https://doi.org/10.1111/j.1464-410X.2012.11638.x.
62. Xia L, Chen B, Jones A, Talwar R, Chelluri RR, Lee DJ, et al. Contemporary National Trends and variations of pelvic lymph node dissection in patients undergoing robot-assisted radical prostatectomy. Clin Genitourin Cancer 2021 Jan 28; S1558-7673(21)00028-8. https://doi.org/10.1016/j.clgc.2021.01.005.
63. Cacciamani GE, Maas M, Nassiri N, Ortega D, Gill K, Dell'Oglio P, Thalmann GN, Heidenreich A, Eastham JA, Evans CP, Karnes RJ, De Castro Abreu AL, Briganti A, Artibani W, Gill I, Montorsi F. Impact of pelvic lymph node dissection and its extent on perioperative morbidity in patients undergoing radical prostatectomy for prostate cancer: a comprehensive systematic review and meta-analysis. Eur Urol Oncol 2021 Mar 6:S2588-9311(21)00035-3. https://doi.org/10.1016/j.euo.2021.02.001.
64. Bründl J, Lenart S, Stojanoski G, Gilfrich C, Rosenhammer B, Stolzlechner M, Ponholzer A, Dreissig C, Weikert S, Burger M, May M. Peritoneal flap in robot-assisted radical prostatectomy. Dtsch Arztebl Int. 2020 Apr 3;117(14):243–50. https://doi.org/10.3238/arztebl.2020.0243.
65. Chenam A, Yuh B, Zhumkhawala A, Ruel N, Chu W, Lau C, Chan K, Wilson T, Yamzon J. Prospective randomised non-inferiority trial of pelvic drain placement vs no pelvic drain placement after robot-assisted radical prostatectomy. BJU Int. 2018 Mar;121(3):357–64.
66. Grande P, Di Pierro GB, Mordasini L, Ferrari M, Würnschimmel C, Danuser H, Mattei A. Prospective randomized trial comparing titanium clips to bipolar coagulation in sealing lymphatic vessels during pelvic lymph node dissection at the time of robot-assisted radical prostatectomy. Eur Urol. 2017 Feb;71(2):155–8.
67. Buelens S, Van Praet C, Poelaert F, Van Huele A, Decaestecker K, Lumen N. Prospective randomized controlled trial exploring the effect of TachoSil on lymphocele formation after extended pelvic lymph node dissection in prostate cancer. Urology. 2018 Aug;118:134–40.
68. Gilbert DR, Angell J, Abaza R. Evaluation of absorbable hemostatic powder for prevention of lymphoceles following robotic prostatectomy with lymphadenectomy. Urology. 2016 Dec;98:75–80.
69. Mattei A, Fuechsel FG, Bhatta Dhar N, Warncke SH, Thalmann GN, Krause T, Studer UE. The template of the primary lymphatic landing sites of the prostate should be revisited: results of a multimodality mapping study. Eur Urol. 2008 Jan;53(1):118–25. https://doi.org/10.1016/j.eururo.2007.07.035.
70. Mazzone E, Dell'Oglio P, Grivas N, Wit E, Donswijk M, Briganti A, van Leeuwen F, van der Poel H. Diagnostic value, oncological outcomes and safety profile of image-guided surgery technologies during robot-assisted lymph node dissection with sentinel node biopsy for prostate cancer. J Nucl Med. 2021 Feb 5; jnumed.120.259788. https://doi.org/10.2967/jnumed.120.259788.
71. Harke NN, Godes M, Wagner C, Addali M, Fangmeyer B, Urbanova K, Hadaschik B, Witt JH. Fluorescence-supported lymphography and extended pelvic lymph node dissection in robot-assisted radical prostatectomy: a prospective, randomized trial. World J Urol. 2018 Nov;36(11):1817–23. https://doi.org/10.1007/s00345-018-2330-7.
72. Wit EMK, Acar C, Grivas N, Yuan C, Horenblas S, Liedberg F, Valdes Olmos RA, van Leeuwen FWB, van den Berg NS, Winter A, Wawroschek F, Hruby S, Janetschek G, Vidal-Sicart S, MacLennan S, Lam TB, van der Poel HG. Sentinel node procedure in prostate cancer: a systematic review to assess diagnostic accuracy.

Eur Urol. 2017 Apr;71(4):596–605. https://doi.org/10.1016/j.eururo.2016.09.007.

73. Ham WS, Park SY, Rha KH, Kim WT, Choi YD. Robotic radical prostatectomy for patients with locally advanced prostate cancer is feasible: results of a single-institution study. J Laparoendosc Adv Surg Tech A. 2009 Jun;19(3):329–32. https://doi.org/10.1089/lap.2008.0344.
74. Rogers CG, Sammon JD, Sukumar S, Diaz M, Peabody J, Menon M. Robot assisted radical prostatectomy for elderly patients with high risk prostate cancer. Urol Oncol. 2013 Feb;31(2):193–7. https://doi.org/10.1016/j.urolonc.2010.11.018.
75. Rodrigues Pessoa R, Urkmez A, Kukreja N, Baack J. Enhanced recovery after surgery review and urology applications in 2020. BJUI Compass. 2020;1:5–14. https://doi.org/10.1002/bco2.9.
76. Suardi N, Gallina A, Lista G, Gandaglia G, Abdollah F, Capitanio U, Dell'Oglio P, Nini A, Salonia A, Montorsi F, Briganti A. Impact of adjuvant radiation therapy on urinary continence recovery after radical prostatectomy. Eur Urol. 2014 Mar;65(3):546–51. https://doi.org/10.1016/j.eururo.2013.01.027.
77. Ficarra V, Novara G, Rosen RC, Artibani W, Carroll PR, Costello A, Menon M, Montorsi F, Patel VR, Stolzenburg JU, Van der Poel H, Wilson TG, Zattoni F, Mottrie A. Systematic review and meta-analysis of studies reporting urinary continence recovery after robot-assisted radical prostatectomy. Eur Urol. 2012 Sep;62(3):405–17. https://doi.org/10.1016/j.eururo.2012.05.045.
78. Ficarra V, Novara G, Ahlering TE, Costello A, Eastham JA, Graefen M, Guazzoni G, Menon M, Mottrie A, Patel VR, Van der Poel H, Rosen RC, Tewari AK, Wilson TG, Zattoni F, Montorsi F. Systematic review and meta-analysis of studies reporting potency rates after robot-assisted radical prostatectomy. Eur Urol. 2012 Sep;62(3):418–30. https://doi.org/10.1016/j.eururo.2012.05.046.

Management of Challenging Cases during Robot-Assisted Laparoscopic Prostatectomy

Gilberto J. Rodrigues, Peter Sutherland, Vipul Patel, and Rafael F. Coelho

1 Introduction

The first robot-assisted laparoscopic prostatectomy (RALP) emerged in 2000 [1]. Twelve years later, 17 world leaders in prostate cancer and radical prostatectomy brought together in Pasadena, California—the Pasadena Consensus Panel (PCP) [2]—to systematically review available data on RALP and to generate best practice recommendations.

The PCP identified specifically some subgroups of patients who should be treated by experienced surgeons due to the increased difficulties brought by certain scenarios that may require additional dexterity to surpass.

Data from a systematic review showed that 40 RALPs appears to be the minimum to surpass the learning curve and to perform usual cases adequately [3]. However, as surgeons get more confidence with the procedure, there is a natural trend to take on increasingly complex cases [4].

Multiple intra-abdominal adhesions may be present in patients with previous surgery making the creation of pneumoperitoneum more difficult even to start the surgery, as well as the trocars placements and risk to bowel injuries [5]. Previous prostatic surgery may lead to a denser periprostatic dissection plane, resulting in worst rates of nerve-sparing and positive surgical margins (PSM) [6]. Obese patients, presence of median lobe (ML), larger prostates or difficult anatomy may decrease the surgical field increasing the operative time (OT) and the estimated blood loss (EBL) [7–9].

Therefore, in this chapter, we provide some tips and tricks helping to overcome these challenging scenarios and review the surgical outcomes in these subgroups of patients.

G. J. Rodrigues · R. F. Coelho (✉)
University of Sao Paulo, Sao Paulo, SP, Brazil

P. Sutherland
The Royal Adelaide Hospital, Adelaide, SA, Australia

V. Patel
Global Robotic Institute, Florida Hospital, Celebration, FL, USA

2 Challenging Scenarios

2.1 Obese Patients

2.1.1 Tips and Tricks

Particularly in overweight and obese patients, using the usual port placement for RALP as for normal-weight patients, the instruments pass through the abdominal wall at a sharper and more vertical angle and it is frequent to have the distal movements limited by the pubic bones (Fig. 1). This anatomic variation might cause worst visualization of the pelvis, especially to reach properly the apex region of the prostate.

A valuable resource to overcome this situation is to insert the ports at a longer distance from the pubic symphysis making it more cranially. In general, for normal-weight patients, this distance is slightly above the belly button, around 15 cm. For overweight and obese patients, the camera port should be inserted into 15.5 to 18 cm from the pubic bone [10]. The remaining trocars should follow the camera reference and be placed slightly below and in line with the camera port, respecting a minimum distance of 8 cm from each other.

Extra attention must be given during the trocar insertion, always at a perpendicular angle to the abdominal wall so it will pierce the fascia with the correct distance into the abdominal cavity among them, avoiding clashing instrument issues. A tangential insertion will dissect the subcutaneous fat, piercing the fascia in a different location that was previously planned to alter the center point of the trocar creating two wide places of resistance at the skin and fascia, interfering with the instruments' movements.

Initiating the procedure by performing a large periprostatic and perivesical defatting at the bladder neck region in these patients is very helpful to increase the workspace for RALP.

In case the instruments present an inability to reach the surgical field satisfactory, trocars may be advanced into, lower and laterally within the abdominal cavity combining with a decrease in the pneumoperitoneum pressure to 10 mmHg, making the prostatic apex dissection and the vesicourethral anastomosis easier.

P. Wiklund et al. (eds.), *Robotic Urologic Surgery*, https://doi.org/10.1007/978-3-031-00363-9_23

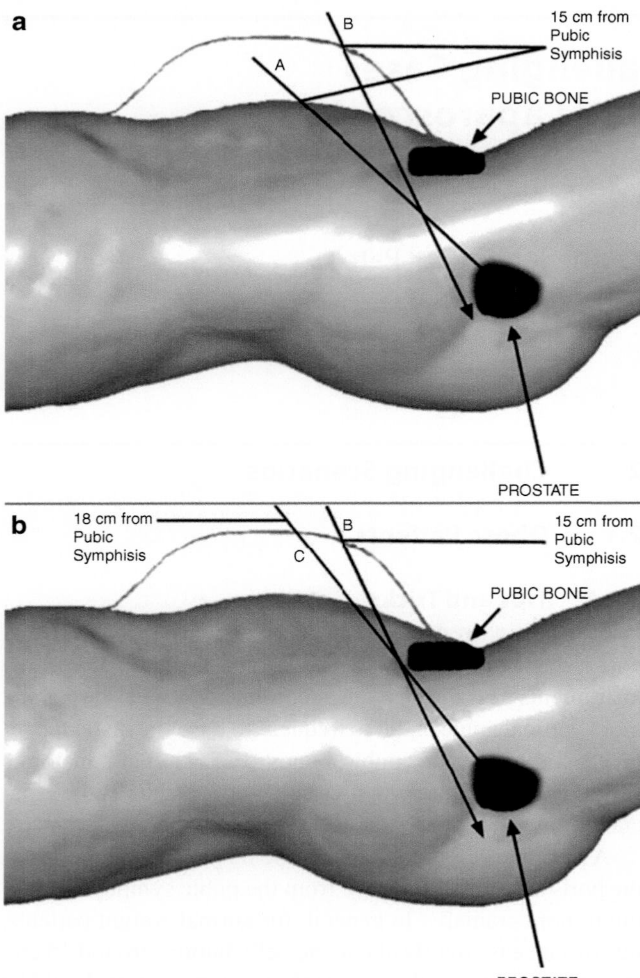

Fig. 1 Schematic model of differences in port placements during a robot-assisted laparoscopic prostatectomy according to patients habitus. (**a**) Instrument trajectory in the presence of a pneumoperitoneum in a normal-weight patient (A) and an obese patient (B) at a distance of 15 cm measured from the pubic symphysis. (**b**) Instrument trajectory in the obese patient in the presence of a pneumo-peritoneum at 15 cm (B) and at 18 cm (C) measured from the pubic symphysis. Pending permission for use: Mikhail, A. A., Stockton, B. R., Orvieto, M. A., Chien, G. W., Gong, E. M., Zorn, K. C., ... Shalhav, A. L. (2006). *Robotic-assisted laparoscopic prostatectomy in overweight and obese patients. Urology, 67(4), 774–779.* https://doi.org/10.1016/j.urology.2005.10

Another maneuver especially useful to get a better visualization of the urethra is a perineal pressure trying to bring the surgical field closer to the instruments. If even though the pubic bone is overriding proper identification of the apex or anastomosis, changing the 30-degree camera lens to 0-degree is an optional resource to achieve a better visualization angle [7].

We routinely perform posterior reconstruction as initially described by Rocco et al. [11] and posteriorly modified by Coelho et al. [12] to get the bladder neck closer to the urethra aiming an anastomosis tension-free and a double posterior layer of running suture to avoid leakage. However, exceptionally in extremely obese patients, due to a very large and fatty bladder, omitting the posterior reconstruction and going straight to the anastomosis is an alternative to get it done easier.

2.1.2 Surgical Outcomes

Surgical outcomes in this challenging scenario had already been described with significant worst functional outcomes at 12 and 24 months regarding potency and continence [13, 14]. Other recurrent findings among series including these patients are mainly longer OT, some higher PSM rates, and complications [14, 15].

Especially in this scenario, higher body mass index (BMI) was already found to be an independent predictive factor (OR: 1.1; 95% CI, 1.0–1.3; $p = 0.0119$) for apical PSM [16]. It was also proved to be an independent predictor of Clavien-Dindo grade 3 complications, increasing chances by 18.4% for each unit rise [17]. Still, results from a national inpatient sample comparing different approaches to radical prostatectomy (53,626 RALPs vs 35,757 open prostatectomies) showed that obesity predisposed to higher rates of perioperative complications in both arms—OR 1.6–1.8 and 1.3–2.8—besides increasing costs in 740$ and 312$, respectively [18].

In a multicenter study from the United Kingdom with 17 institutions and more than 3000 RALPs, although rare, even a serious complication such as lower limb compartment syndrome was observed in nine patients (0.29%) [19]. They identified the main risk factors as: console time longer than 4 hours in 8/9 cases, early learning curve (<20 cases) in 3/9; obesity in 5/9; and peripheral vascular disease in 2/9. One patient was positioned incorrectly.

Another report with 180 consecutives RALP concluded that rhabdomyolysis (creatine kinase >1050 IU/L) occurred in 6.1% of patients with **significant transient decrease in renal function (*p* = 0.007) in 45.5% of them** [20]. **These findings were associated with higher BMI (>25.7; *p* = 0.02) and OT (>188 min; *p* = 0.005).**

In contrast, outcomes from 44 RALPs in morbidly obese patients by a very high-volume surgeon demonstrated that despite technically demanding, it is a safe and feasible procedure [21]. This propensity score-matched analysis showed a significant, but small increase in EBL (**130 ml vs 113 ml; *p* = 0.049) and a more difficult vesicourethral anastomosis (VUA) in these patients (*p* = 0.001). There were similar results in OT, ease of nerve-sparing, transfusion rate, complications, indwelling catheter duration, length of stay (LOS), and pain scores.**

Furthermore, another report from a patient-based model for estimating OT during RALP showed that the main predictor was the surgeon, followed by the BMI [22].

Besides all the complications issues, obesity was found to be a strong predictor (OR = 6.950; $p = 0.002$) of clinically undetected node metastases in intermediate and high-risk prostate cancer patients who underwent RALP associated with extended pelvic lymphadenectomy (ePLND). Also, patients with metabolic syndrome, very prevalent in obese, presented to have higher Gleason grade (≥ 7: 78% vs. 64%, $p < 0.001$) and tumor stage (≥T3 disease: 43% vs. 32%, $p < 0.001$) on final pathology as well were more likely to have upgrading (63% vs. 45%, $P < 0.001$) [23].

Thus, most of the evidence shows so far that a more experienced surgeon is the key to surpassing the challenging scenario of RALP in obese patients and that is not advised to include these patients during the learning curve [7, 14].

Another protective step described for these patients is to promote weight reduction before surgery. During a weight loss program, it was observed that lower weight, fat mass (FM), percent FM, trunk FM, and visceral FM were associated with less surgery-related adverse effects ($r_s = 0.335$ to 0.468, $p < 0.010$) [24]. Still, blood pressure was significantly reduced over the intervention carrying additional protective benefits to surgery.

A narrative review with the main series in this scenario is summarized in Table 1.

Table 1 Narrative review of outcomes from obese with non-obese patients following robot-assisted radical prostatectomy

	N	Study design	Operative time (min)	Estimated blood loss (ml)	Complications	Urinary function	Sexual function	Pathology
Wiltz et al. (2009) [13]	945	Prospective; compare obese patients with normal and overweight	HIGHER	SIMILAR	SIMILAR but higher case abortion due to respiratory-pressure issues	WORSE UB and continence at 12 and 24 months	WORSE SB at 3 months; potency at 12 and 24 months	SIMILAR
Coelho et al. (2010) [16]	876	Prospective; predictive factors for PSM	N/A	N/A	N/A	N/A	N/A	WORSE BMI: Independent predictive factor for apical PSM
Kheterpal et al. (2013) [23]	1051	Retrospective; matched pairs analysis with controls and patients with MS	N/A	N/A	N/A	N/A	N/A	WORSE Gleason grade and pathologic stage
Pridgeon et al. (2013) [19]	3110	Multicenter and retrospective (prevalence of LLCS)	N/A	N/A	N/A	N/A	N/A	N/A
Abdul-Muhsin et al. (2014) [21]	88	Retrospective; propensity score-matched with patients 40 > BMI ≥ 40	SIMILAR but increased difficulty in VUA	HIGHER	SIMILAR	N/A	N/A	SIMILAR
Xu et al. (2015) [14]	6622	Meta-analysis	HIGHER	HIGHER	SIMILAR	WORSE at 1 year	WORSE at 1 year	SIMILAR
Knipper et al. (2019) [18]	53,626	Retrospective	N/A	N/A	HIGHER obesity predicted 5 of 11	N/A	N/A	N/A
Porcaro et al. (2019) [17]	211	Retrospective	N/A	N/A	HIGHER each unit rise in BMI ↑18.4% grade 3 complications	N/A	N/A	N/A
Goßler et al. (2020) [15]	232	Prospective randomized multicenter study	HIGHER (180 vs 160; $p = 0.013$)	N/A	HIGHER (31.4 vs 14.9%; $p = 0.013$)	N/A	N/A	SIMILAR for BMI threshold value of 30 HIGHER for BMI threshold value of 33.7 (34.8 vs 13.4%; $p = 0.013$)
Onagi et al. (2020) [20]	180	Retrospective	N/A	N/A	HIGHER (on multivariate analysis, rhabdomyolysis was significantly associated with BMI > 25.7 kg/m2)	N/A	N/A	N/A

HIGHER or *WORSE* results with statistical significance, *SIMILAR* statistically significance not reached, *N/A* not available, *VUA* vesicourethral anastomosis, *MS* metabolic syndrome, *BMI* body mass index, *PSM* positive surgical margin, *LLCS* lower limb compartment syndrome, *UB* urinary bother, *SB* sexual bother

2.2 Median Lobe

2.2.1 Tips and Tricks

The easier and safer way to not be surprised into a wrong dissection plane due to an ML during the bladder neck dissection is to carefully look at the preoperative images, especially into the sagittal and coronal plane of magnetic resonance of the prostate [25].

The presence of a ML might add some challenges mainly in the surgical step of bladder neck dissection because it may distort the anatomic conformation and carrying difficulty to identify proper surgical planes. A large ML can lead the surgeon to dissect into a wrong plane, causing more bleeding, PSM, or even unintended injuries of the ureteral meatus [26–29]. Trying to overcome these concerns, some tips and tricks have already been described [26, 30].

There are two classical steps to achieve exactly the right plane during the anterior bladder neck dissection. The first is to make a symmetric pressure with the right and left robotic arms at the level of the bladder neck, while pulling the bladder dome cranially with the ProGrasp in the fourth robotic arm, aiming to identify a tent of detrusor fibers over the vesicoprostatic transition (Fig. 2). Next, pushing and pulling the Foley urethral catheter through the prostate boundaries is possible to estimate where the ML is located. If the balloon is laterally shifted during this maneuver, it may be a sign of the presence of a unilateral ML. However, if the Foley balloon does not reach the level of the true visualized bladder neck, it may be a sign of a circumferential or a midline ML.

After precise identification of the vesicoprostatic transition, the next step is to cut the anterior bladder neck with electrocautery and scissor over the detrusor fibers until the identification of the Foley urethral catheter (Fig. 3).

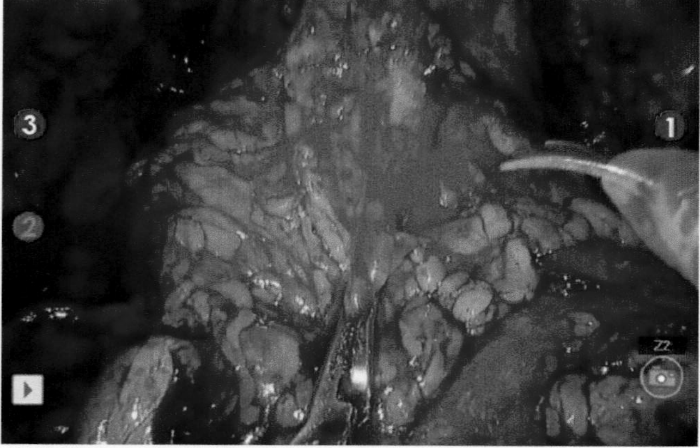

Fig. 2 Identification of a tent over the vesicoprostatic transition while pulling the bladder cranially with the prograsp in the fourth robotic arm. Concomitant to this, pushing and pulling the Foley urethral catheter against the prostate boundaries help proper identification of the bladder neck

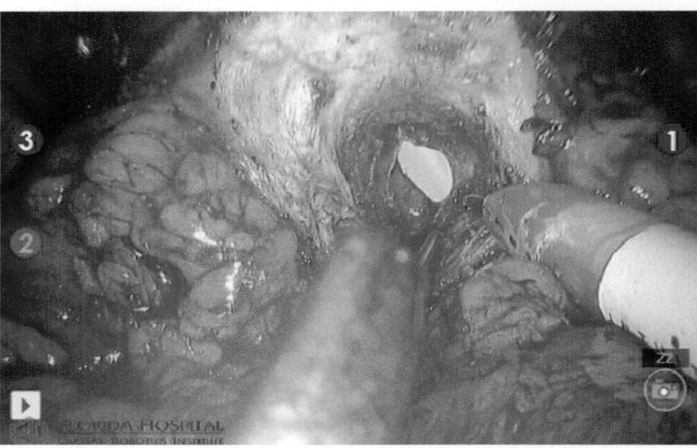

Fig. 3 Using scissor with electrocautery over the detrusor fibers until identification of the Foley urethral catheter

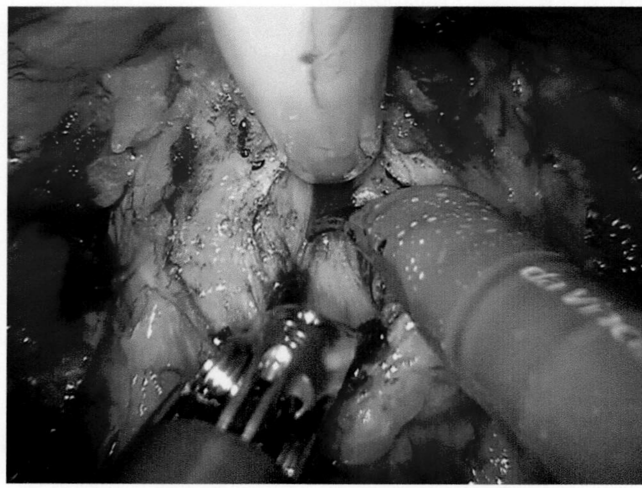

Fig. 4 Usual posterior bladder neck dissection without prominent median lobe: anteriorly traction of Foley urethral catheter with the prograsp into the pubic symphysis combined with a Kocher fixation of its distal extremity

The presence or absence of a bladder drop-off after opening the bladder is another clue for the existence of an ML. In cases without ML, after opening the bladder the posterior bladder neck usually drops downwards into the body of the bladder. While the ML is present, the posterior bladder neck continues straight back without a drop-off.

For a usual posterior bladder neck dissection without a prominent ML, anteriorly traction of Foley urethral catheter with the ProGrasp into the pubic symphysis combined with a Kocher fixation of its distal extremity is usually enough to present an adequate view of the posterior bladder neck (Fig. 4). In cases of a large ML, this region is better exposed retrieving it inside out the bladder applying a continuous traction upwards by the ProGrasp forceps on it (Fig. 5). Another option is to perform a "rescue stitch" on it to pro-

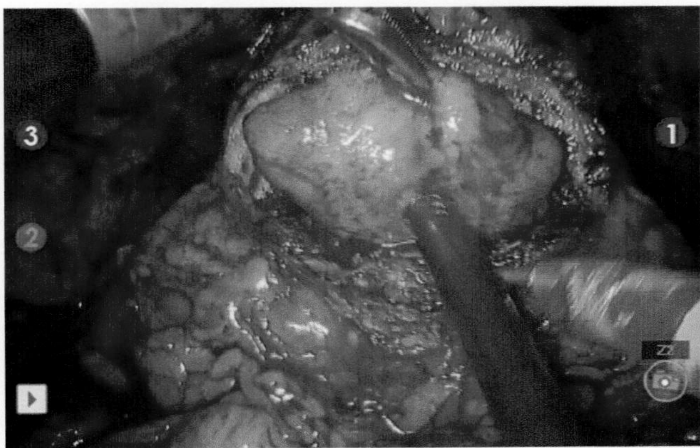

Fig. 5 Retrieving the ML inside out the bladder applying a continuous traction upwards by the prograsp forceps on it

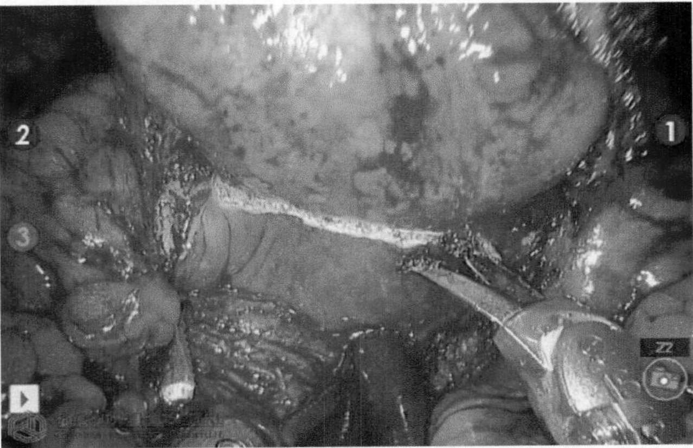

Fig. 6 Maryland bipolar forceps pull the anterior bladder neck cranially; the scissor cuts de posterior bladder neck mucosa respecting the ureteral meatus boundaries

vide a clearer view of the trigonal region to avoid ureteral meatus injuries [30].

After the correct identification of the region to be dissected, the Maryland bipolar forceps pull the anterior bladder neck cranially and the scissor cuts the mucosa over the posterior bladder neck, beginning by the corners and working our way medially and posteriorly, respecting the ureteral meatus boundaries (Fig. 6).

It is frequent to observe a disproportional bigger bladder neck when compared with the diameter of the membranous urethra in a presence of an ML. So, as it occurred in open prostatectomy, bladder neck reconstruction is indicated in this situation. It is an option to perform a tennis-racket or anterior-bladder tube reconstruction as it was performed by the open approach, but due to difficult visualization of the posterior bladder neck in RALP, we prefer to perform a modified bilateral transverse plication as it was described by Lin et al. [31].

In case of iatrogenic meatus injuries or trigone resections, Molinari et al. [26] have already reported an easier fashion way to implant double-pigtail stent during RALP. Preferably after the prostatectomy and posterior plane reconstruction, a guidewire is introduced through the lumen of the Foley urethral catheter by the assistant. After the guidewire is grasped by the robotic arm, it is introduced into the ureteral meatus, the Foley is removed, and the double-pigtail stent is implanted.

2.2.2 Surgical Outcomes

It is already well established that on experienced hands, only the presence of an ML does not affect EBL, PSM, biochemical recurrence (BCR), or complications [8, 32]. When analyzing the OT, an interesting finding was shown by Coelho et al. [8] following 1693 consecutive patients who underwent RALP. Although OT was significantly increased in patients with ML (80 vs 75 minutes, $p < 0.001$), there was no difference in the OT when stratifying this result by prostate weight. Likewise, they did not find any difference in functional outcomes regarding urinary continence between the groups.

Similar findings were recorded by Hamidi et al. [32], but in this series, the presence of ML seems to present a disadvantage in gaining early urinary continence at 1 month following RALP (49.2% and 56.5%, $p = 0.03$) with no major difference from 3 months onwards.

Rajih et al. [33] evaluated several predictor factors for post-prostatectomy urinary incontinence following RALP and found ML did not correlate with delayed continence along 24 months of follow-up. Of note, only prostate size, OT, smoking history, and bladder neck sparing played a role on this outcome.

As well as found by Jenkins et al. [34] in a retrospective review of 345 consecutive RALPs. There were 29 (8%) patients with an ML identified intraoperative. They compared the outcomes of these patients with the 29 consecutive patients without an ML. Patients with ML presented larger prostates (60 vs 23 cm^3; $p = 0.003$) and required reconstruction of the bladder neck more frequently (55 vs 3%; $p < 0.0001$). However, OT, EBL, PSM, final pathological stage, complications and postoperative urinary outcomes were similar between groups.

Still, Alnazari et al. [35] reported no relation between ML and acute urinary retention (AUR) after catheter removal since RALP. Instead, they found a higher rate of AUR for men with catheter removal at Day 4 (4.5% [16/351]) vs. Day 7(0.2% [1/389]) ($p = 0.004$).

Finally, as found in large prostates, Jung et al. [36] showed that patients with ML were less likely to have PSM (16 vs 24.4%; $p = 0.044$). However, in multivariable model, the presence of ML on PSM was not statistically significant (RR 0.97, 95% CI, 0.64–1.47, $p = 0.88$). Despite presenting higher levels of PSA (6.1 vs 5.4; $p = 0.003$), patients with ML had lower Gleason scores (< 7, 58.1% vs 42.1%; $p = 0.012$), lower pathological stages (T2, 87.4% vs 75.4%; $p = 0.024$) and large prostates (64 vs 48 g; $p < 0.0001$), all found to be predictive factors of decreased PSM ($p < 0.01$).

A narrative review with the main series in this scenario is summarized in Table 2.

2.3 Large Prostates

2.3.1 Tips and Tricks

A particular challenge regarding large prostates is exposure and rotation to complete nerve-sparing, reach the apex region, and finishing the prostatectomy itself. Additionally, these patients usually present prostates with a substantial blood supply, posing a risk of major bleeding.

Opening the endopelvic fascia and making early control of the dorsal vein complex may help to reduce vascular flow and bleeding. It is essential a clear visualization of the tissues to avoid getting out of the dissection plane.

During the bladder neck dissection, respecting the contour of the prostate getting all the vesicoprostatic down is advised rather than work in a deep middle hole. The key element for this scenario is a wider exposure, a bloodless field, and reviewing the surgical plane constantly, releasing and pulling the prostate many times as necessary.

2.3.2 Surgical Outcomes

As well as reported by some authors regarding the challenging scenario of RALP in patients with ML, Rajih et al. [33] identified large prostates (≥47 g) as predictors of urinary incontinence following RALP. Besides this, Alenizi et al. [37] showed that prostate volume was also a significant predictor of longer OT not only for individual surgical steps such as dorsal vein complex ligation (OR 1.02), bladder neck division (OR 1.03), pedicle control (OR 1.04), urethral division (OR 1.02) and VUA (OR 1.03) as well for overall OT (1.04).

An inversely proportional outcome of PSM and prostate weight (OR 0.97%; 95% confidence interval [CI] 0.96, 0.99; $P = 0.0003$) was reported by Marchetti et al. [38] from a cohort of 690 men with low-risk prostate cancer who underwent RALP with bilateral nerve-sparing from 2003 to 2009.

Data from a different center with 1168 RALPs by a single surgeon found consistent outcomes of longer OT for prostates ≥75 g and also demonstrated significantly higher EBL in these patients [9]. However, no significant differences were found regarding intraoperative complications and oncologic outcomes (PSM or BCR at 1 year of follow-up).

Coelho et al. [39] reported 1009 consecutive RALPs by a single surgeon and stratified the patients according to prostate weight. They found patients with larger prostate (≥70 g) were older with a median age of 64.9 years ($p < 0.001$), presented higher PSA pretreatment with a median of 6.5 ($p < 0.001$) and had more urinary symptoms (mean AUA-SS

Table 2 Narrative review of outcomes from patients with and without median lobe following robot-assisted radical prostatectomy

	N	Study design	Operative time (min)	Estimated blood loss (ml)	Complications	Urinary function	Sexual function	Pathology
Jenkins et al. 2008 [34]	58	Retrospective	SIMILAR	SIMILAR	SIMILAR	SIMILAR	N/A	SIMILAR
Coelho et al. (2012) [8]	1693	Prospective	HIGHER 80 vs 75; $p < 0{,}001$ But with no difference when stratifying by prostate weight	SIMILAR	SIMILAR	SIMILAR	N/A	SIMILAR only difference in prostate weight, 64 vs 46 g; $p < 0.0001$
Jung et al. 2012 [36]	791	Retrospective	N/A	N/A	N/A	N/A	N/A	BETTER lower PSM, Gleason score and pathological stage
Hamidi et al. (2018) [32]	924	Retrospective	HIGHER (144 vs 136; $p = 0.01$)	SIMILAR	SIMILAR	WORSE at 1 month (49.2% and 56.5%, $p = 0.03$) SIMILAR at 3 months onwards	N/A	SIMILAR
Rajih et al. (2019) [33]	322	Retrospective	N/A	N/A	N/A	SIMILAR	N/A	N/A

HIGHER or WORSE results with statistical significance, *SIMILAR* statistically significance not reached, *N/A* not available, *PSM* positive surgical margin

Table 3 Narrative review of outcomes from patients with and without large prostates following robot-assisted radical prostatectomy

	N	Study design	Operative time (min)	Estimated blood loss (ml)	Complications	Urinary function	Sexual function	Pathology
Marchetti et al. (2011) [38]	690	Retrospective	N/A	N/A	N/A	N/A	N/A	BETTER significant inverse relation between PSM and PV OR 0.97%; 95%CI 0.96, 0.99; $p = 0.0003$
Coelho et al. (2012) [39]	1009	Retrospective	HIGHER 83.3 ± 15.7 $p < 0.001$	HIGHER 129.2 ± 14.6 $p < 0.001$	N/A	SIMILAR	WORSE at 6 weeks 39% were potent $p = 0.01$ SIMILAR at 3 months onwards	BETTER: PSM 7.8%; $p < 0.001$ SIMILAR: Gleason score and pathological stage
Labanaris et al. (2013) [40]	370	Matched pairs analysis	HIGHER 164 vs 144 $p < 0.05$	HIGHER (192 vs 152 $p < 0.05$	Intraoperative: HIGHER 4.8 vs 1.6%; $p < 0.05$ Postoperative: SIMILAR	SIMILAR	WORSE at 12 months 61.9 vs 72.9% $p < 0.05$	BETTER lower PSM, Gleason score, tumor volume and pathological stage
Alenizi et al. (2015) [37]	247	Retrospective	HIGHER (OR.1 0.04)	N/A	N/A	N/A	N/A	N/A
Kim et al. (2019) [9]	1168	Retrospective	HIGHER 61.7 ± 18.3 $p < 0.001$	HIGHER 646 ± 423 $p < 0.001$	SIMILAR	N/A	N/A	SIMILAR: PSM BETTER: Gleason score and pathological stage
Rajih et al. (2019) [33]	322	Retrospective	N/A	N/A	N/A	WORSE PV predicted incontinence along the first 12 months following RALP; $p = 0.02$	N/A	N/A

HIGHER or WORSE results with statistical significance, *SIMILAR* statistical significance not reached, *N/A* not available, *PV* prostate volume, *PSM* positive surgical margin, *RALP* robot-assisted laparoscopic prostatectomy

of 12.8; $p < 0.001$). Despite positive statistic trans operative findings as longer OT (83.3 ± 15.7; $p < 0.001$) and EBL (129.2 ± 14.6; $p < 0.001$), there was only a slightly clinically difference comparing patients with smaller prostate (<30 g) of less than 10 min regarding OT and a few more than 20 ml in terms of EBL. All other perioperative variables were similar among groups of different prostate sizes and the only pathological difference found was lower PSM (7.8%; $p < 0.001$) in larger prostates. Functional outcomes differed significantly in terms of potency rates, patients with larger prostates presented lower early recovery rates at six weeks of the postoperative period (39%; $p < 0.01$), while the intermediate-term results from the third-month postoperative period were similar.

Similar findings were reported by Labanaris et al. [40] in a matched-pairs analysis of 4000 RALPs, comparing 185 men with prostates ≥100 g (large prostates) with individuals whose prostates ≤50 g (smaller prostates) and equivalent clinicopathologic characteristics. Large prostates presented also significant longer OT, need for bladder neck reconstruction, higher EBL, beyond an increase in intraoperative complications rates. There were also less aggressive tumors, PSM and BCR in patients with larger prostates. Despite there being no difference in continence between the groups, it was identified lower-potency rates in patients with larger prostates.

A narrative review with the main series in this scenario is summarized in Table 3.

3 Previous Treatment for Benign Prostatic Hyperplasia

3.1 Tips and Tricks

The scenario of RALP following trans-urethral resection of prostate (TURP) or simple prostatectomy may be even more challenging than ML, due to possible distortions in the anatomy of the bladder neck or to a dense surgical plane harming a clear view and the proper identification of the anatomy.

We believe the best way to achieve the correct plane during the bladder neck dissection in this situation is to quickly enter the bladder in the midline, elevate the prostate and then survey the anatomy from the inside (Fig. 7a). In patients that

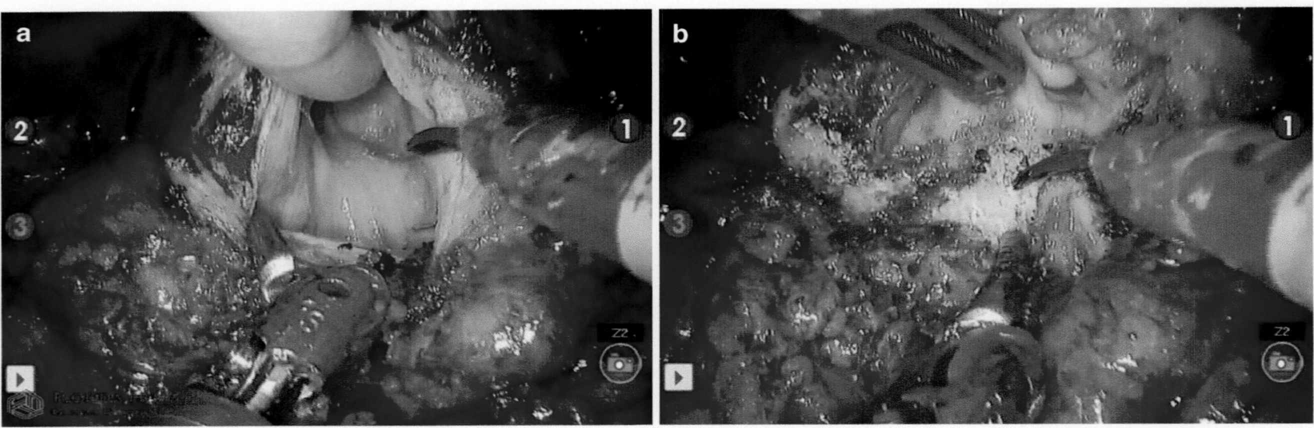

Fig. 7 Anterior bladder open in the midline identifying from inside the bladder distorted prostatic lobes (**a**) and pulling the remaining medium lobe upwards to begin the posterior bladder neck dissection (**b**)

underwent previously a generous TURP, a Foley balloon may lodge inside the prostatic urethra misrepresenting the real location of the bladder neck during a gentle tug on the urethral catheter.

During the posterior bladder neck dissection, the ProGrasp fourth robotic arm pulls upwards the remaining of the ML, while the Maryland bipolar forceps carefully pull cranially the posterior bladder neck (Fig. 7b).

3.2 Surgical Outcomes

Still, in 2008, Hampton et al. [41] analyzed 1768 patients submitted to RALP by six different surgeons, identifying a subgroup of 51 patients that previously underwent TURP surgery as well. Retrospectively compared these two groups and concluded that RALP in post-TURP scenario led to an increase in PSM [35.3% vs 17.6% ($p = 0.015$)], mainly bladder neck margin.

In 2014, a review of RALP following surgery for benign prostate hyperplasia (BPH) recorded contradictory results, while some series reported comparable results to patients without previous prostatic surgeries, others have demonstrated inferior outcomes [6].

Tugcu et al. [42] reported no difference in PSM or BCR in a match-paired analysis of 25 patients with prior surgery for primary bladder outlet obstruction (20 TURP and 5 open prostatectomies). Instead, they observed longer OT, higher EBL as well greater urinary leakage, and anastomotic stricture.

Then, Su et al. [43] reported a cohort of 49 patients who had prior prostatic surgery and compared it with 2644 surgery-naïve patients by a single surgeon. Although observed a greater PSM in patients with prior prostatic surgery around 10%, it wasn't statistically significant ($p = 0.110$). Also, EBL, OT, urinary and sexual functional outcomes were similar. However, bigger rates of weakness of the urinary stream (EPIC #4d) at 12 months were found in the first group ($p = 0.012$).

Similar findings with satisfactory oncological and functional outcomes were reported by Campobasso et al. [44] in 2019, demonstrating that when done by a skilled robotic surgeon, RALP in patients with previous surgery for BPH should be managed as naïve patients when performed by a skilled robotic surgeon. They identified 40 patients from a total of 953 RALPs who also presented a previous surgery for BPH. Only descriptive data was recorded. There was no need for open conversion, neither major intraoperative nor postoperative complications occurred. No blood transfusion was required. Nerve-sparing was performed in all patients and bladder neck reconstruction in 25% of them. The median catheterization time was 5 days [3–14]. Continence rate, defined as usage of 0 or 1 pad/day at 1, 3 and 12 months occurred in 82.5%, 90% and 95%. While PSM was present in 20%, 75% of which was ≥T3.

In contrast, a meta-analysis gathering 13 studies comparing radical prostatectomy (included RALP, open and laparoscopic prostatectomies) in patients with prior BPH surgery with surgery-naïve patients concluded that the first group was found to present significantly higher PSM, need of bladder neck reconstruction, and overall complication rate. While OT, EBL, and 1-year continence rates were comparable between the two groups [45].

Finally, a study from Indiana University described its initial experience of the first 27 patients who underwent RALP with prior history of Holmium Laser Enucleation of the prostate and matched 1:1 with surgery-naïve patients [46]. They found that OT was longer in the first group, as well erection function appeared to be generally poor (despite bilateral nerve-sparing was performed only 11% and the poor initial potency). Also, there were reported higher rates of bladder neck reconstruction, time to continence—while improved with increased experience—and similar low complications rates. While PSM and BCR appeared to be unaffected by previous enucleation.

A narrative review with the main series in this scenario is summarized in Table 4.

3.3 Previous Multiple Prostate Biopsies

3.3.1 Tips and Tricks

The periprostatic inflammation caused due to multiple prostate biopsies is the main concern in this scenario. Although surprisingly variable, increased difficulty can be found especially during the posterior dissection plane above the Denonvilliers fascia and nerve-sparing. Sometimes these tissues are binder to the prostate and harder to dissect.

A general recommendation is to wait at least the first 4 weeks following the last biopsy to perform RALP, or even up to 6 weeks if a prostatitis occurred. Cautiously dissection, trying to keep the field as clean as possible aiming at better identification of structures is highly recommended.

3.3.2 Surgical Outcomes

Since the introduction of prostate cancer screening in the last thirty years, a reduction trend of advanced disease with an increase of low-risk stage was found [47]. The overdiagnosis of these cases led to a challenging scenario of proper identification of candidates who will most benefit from a radical

Table 4 Narrative review of outcomes from patients with and without previous treatment for benign prostatic hyperplasia following robot-assisted radical prostatectomy

	N	Study design	Operative time (min)	Estimated blood loss (ml)	Complications	Urinary function	Sexual function	Pathology
Hampton et al. 2008 [41]	153	Prospective	N/A	N/A	N/A	N/A	N/A	WORSE any PSM: 35.3 vs 17.7% $p = 0.02$ Bladder neck PSM: 13.7 vs 2.0% $p = 0.004$
Su et al. 2015 [43]	2693	Retrospective	SIMILAR	SIMILAR	N/A	SIMILAR (overall) WORSE at 12 months weak stream: 1 vs 0.29% $p = 0.012$	N/A	SIMILAR
Tugcu et al. 2015 [42]	61	Match paired analysis	HIGHER 238 vs 203 $p = 0.028$	HIGHER 187 vs 116 $p = 0.001$	WORSE stricture rate 16 vs 2.8% $p < 0.05$	SIMILAR	SIMILAR	SIMILAR
Liao et al. 2020 [45]	6750	Meta-analysis, including open prostatectomy, laparoscopic prostatectomy and RALP	SIMILAR	SIMILAR	WORSE for overall complication rate OR = 2.09, 95% CI 1.26–3.46, $p = 0.004$, $I^2 = 70\%$ and only for RALP OR = 2.92, 95% CI 1.45–5.90, $p = 0.003$, $I^2 = 0\%$	SIMILAR	N/A	WORSE PSM overall: OR = 1.31, 95% CI 1.09–1.58, $p = 0.004$, $I^2 = 0\%$ PSM only for RALP: OR = 1.71, 95% CI 1.16–2.52, $P = 0.006$, $I^2 = 0\%$
Abedali et al. 2020 [46]	54	Match paired analysis	HIGHER 193.5 vs 164.2 $p < 0.001$	SIMILAR	SIMILAR	0–1 pad/day: SIMILAR 0 pad/day: WORSE 22 vs 74%; $p < 0.001$ WORSE time to continence in months 20 vs 7; $p = 0.007$	SIMILAR	SIMILAR

HIGHER or *WORSE* results with statistical significance, *SIMILAR* statistical significance not reached, *N/A* not available, *PSM* positive surgical margin, *RALP* robot-assisted laparoscopic prostatectomy, *OR* odds ratio, *CI* confidence interval

treatment and who will have an indolent course [48]. Therefore, active surveillance protocols have been developed, including the need for a baseline prostate biopsy with at least an extra follow-up biopsy [49, 50]. Concerns related to multiple biopsies include not only periprocedural complications, such as pain, infection, hematuria and hematospermia, but there are reports suggesting also nerve damage with subsequent erectile dysfunction [51–53].

There are few series correlating outcomes of patients submitted to multiple prostate biopsies and RALP so far. The higher number of transrectal ultrasound-guided prostate biopsy cores were already linked to higher EBL (422 vs 463 ml; $p = 0.003$) and perioperative complications (6.4% vs 8.5%; $p = 0.03$) in RALP. As well as multiple previous prostate biopsies have been shown to decrease postoperative potency rates at 6 months (80% vs 57%; $p = 0.03$) due to local inflammatory process increasing difficulty dissections during neurovascular bundle sparing [54, 55]. No significant impact was found in the postoperative continence for single and multiple biopsies, neither in PSM in both series.

While new series scrutinizing outcomes in this subgroup of patients who underwent RALP are desired, data from the largest open radical prostatectomy series including more than 27,000 patients—of which 4780 (17.3%) were submitted to ≥2 biopsies before surgery—concluded that this subgroup of patients presented higher perioperative blood transfusion rate (12.77 vs 15.50%; $p < 0.0001$), longer LOS (4.6 vs 4.7 days; $p = 0.014$), more need of procedures associated with bladder neck contracture (23.35 vs 27.03%; $p < 0.0001$) and less oncological interventions, such as adjuvant radiation therapy (13.23 vs 10.21%; $p = 0.0001$) or androgen deprivation therapy (4.90 vs 3.41%; $p < 0.0001$) [56]. Readmission rate and 30-day mortality were similar, as well as postoperative functional outcomes of potency and continence.

A narrative review with the main series in this scenario is summarized in Table 5.

3.4 Narrow Pelvis

3.4.1 Tips and Tricks

There are two main challenges to deal with during RALP in this scenario: the intrabdominal limited working space to manipulate the instruments, especially during the apex dissection of the prostate and VUA performance that are limited by the pelvic bones and the clashing instruments externally.

Trying to overcome this, respect a minimum distance of 8 cm among the ports combining with additional maneuvers, such as depressing the fourth arm, elevating and medially rotating the third to prevent them to clash. Constantly adaptations in the robot arms during the surgery may be necessary depending on the site of interest. More experienced surgeons may even perform some steps such as VUA with only one arm in extremally unfavorable cases such as obese patients combined with narrow pelvis.

3.4.2 Surgical Outcomes

The definition of narrow pelvis is not a standard measurement. There are many pelvic dimension references already analyzed, and so far, the best estimation of the working space for robotic arms in the pelvic cavity is the pelvic cavity index (PCI).

Hong et al. [57] developed the PCI multiplying the pelvic inlet by the interspinous distance and dividing it by the pelvic depth. In this series, no pelvic dimensions were associated with increasing OT neither EBL, only PCI approached significance to OT ($p = 0.071$) and only intertuberous distance and interspinous distance approached to EBL ($p = 0.087$ and $= 0.072$, respectively). Only prostate volume had a significant association with OT and EBL, $p = 0.015$ and $p = 0.045$. Again, no pelvic dimension presented any significant effect on PSM or functional outcomes at 6 months following RALP.

Mason et al. [58] proved that patients with larger prostates, narrower and deeper pelvis were predicted to increase

Table 5 Narrative review of outcomes from patients with and without previous multiple prostate biopsy following robot-assisted radical prostatectomy

	N	Study design	Operative time (min)	Estimated blood loss (ml)	Complications	Urinary function	Sexual function	Pathology
Sooriakumaran et al. 2012 [55]	73	Match paired analysis	SIMILAR	SIMILAR	N/A	SIMILAR at 3 and 6 months	WORSE at 6 months 57 vs 80% $p = 0.03$	SIMILAR
Carneiro et al. 2017 [54]	2054, categorized in patients with previous prostate biopsy 12 < cores ≥12	Retrospective	WORSE 146.5 vs 136 $p = 0.01$	WORSE 463 vs 422 $p = 0.003$	WORSE 8.5 vs 6.4% $p = 0.03$	N/A	N/A	SIMILAR

HIGHER or WORSE results with statistical significance, *SIMILAR* statistical significance not reached, *N/A* not available, *PSM* positive surgical margin, *RALP* robot-assisted laparoscopic prostatectomy, *OR* odds ratio, *CI* confidence interval

Table 6 Narrative review of outcomes from patients with and without narrow pelvis following robot-assisted radical prostatectomy

	N	Study design	Operative time (min)	Estimated blood loss (ml)	Complications	Urinary function	Sexual function	Pathology
Hong et al. 2009 [57]	141	Retrospective	SIMILAR	SIMILAR	N/A	SIMILAR	SIMILAR	SIMILAR
Mason et al. 2010 [58]	76	Prospective	Predicted by PV-to-PCI ratio, when >6: 190 vs 166 $p = 0.009$	Predicted by PV-to-PCI ratio, when >6: 201 vs 122 $p = 0.007$	SIMILAR	N/A	N/A	Patients with apical PSM had statistically narrower and deeper pelvises
Yao et al. 2015 [60]	100	Retrospective	Predicted only by PV-to-PCI ratio during the first 50 cases $p = 0.014$, HR 7.12, 95% CI 1.51–12.73	Predicted by PV-to-PCI ratio during the first 50 cases $p = 0.027$, HR 4.12, 95% CI 0.47–7.76	N/A	N/A	N/A	SIMILAR
Chen et al. 2019 [59]	78	Prospective	Associated with PD β: 13.7, $p = 0.039$ as PD increased by 1 cm, surgery time increased by 13.7	SIMILAR	N/A	N/A	N/A	Associated with PCI $p = 0.01$, OR 0.25, 95% CI 0.09–0.72 indicating a lower odd of PSM with a greater PCI (shallow and wide pelvis)

HIGHER or WORSE results with statistical significance, *SIMILAR* statistical significance not reached, *N/A* not available, *PV* prostate volume, *PCI* pelvic cavity index, *PSM* positive surgical margin, *OR* odds ratio, *CI* confidence interval, *PD* pelvic depth

difficulty to RALP. They found a positive relation between prostate volume-to-PCI that could impact OT and EBL significantly. Patients presenting this ratio smaller than 6 had 39% less EBL and 12% shorter OT. Still, an interesting finding regarding PSM was found, patients with apical positive margins presented smaller PCI than those with PSM at other sites (6.53 vs 8.24, $p = 0.0085$).

In a similar way, another report from surgeon automated performance metrics (i.e., camera movement, third-arm swap, energy use, console time) obtained by a systems data recorder (Intuitive Surgical, Sunnyvale, CA, USA) during RALP translated this difficulty into evidence. Analysis from 78 RALPs concluded that narrower and deeper pelvis affected surgeon performance and patient outcomes [59]. On a multivariable linear regression, pelvic depth was found to increase OT, β = 13.5 (95% CI 0.1–26.8; $p = 0.048$). On multivariable logistic regression, PCI was a predictive factor of PSM, odds ratio of 0.25 (95% CI 0.09–0.72; $p = 0.01$), while a wider and shallower pelvis was less likely to result in PSM. Continence recovery was related only to the surgeon's previous experience.

Yao et al. [60] evaluated their RALP learning curve with patient's anatomical dimensions. They found BMI, the prostate anteroposterior diameter, and the prostate volume-to-PCI ratio were all significantly correlated with console time and EBL, on univariate analysis. While on multiple linear regression, only the prostate volume-to-PCI ratio was found to be a significant predictor of console time and EBL. Although with increasing experience, only the first 50 RALPs kept these findings. No positive association was found between anatomical parameters and PSM in this series.

A narrative review with the main series in this scenario is summarized in Table 6.

4 Patients with Previous Abdominal Surgery

4.1 Tips and Tricks

We routinely perform pneumoperitoneum insufflation using the Veress needle through the midline incision where the camera port will be inserted. Patients with previous abdominal surgery may present a variable degree of intraabdominal adhesions that may prevent gas insufflation.

Recently, a comparative study was recorded between patients readmitted to hospital due to adhesion-related surgeries according to laparoscopic or open approach. They found minimally invasive surgeries reduced the incidence of adhesion-related readmissions (1.7% vs 4.3%; $p < 0.0001$) [61].

As well as is in our impression, patients with previous minimally invasive surgery usually do not present major adhesions requiring many adjustments to pneumoperitoneum creation. However, patients with previous larger open access abdominal surgery, especially those who presented inflammatory acute abdomen, can pose a real challenge to the pneumoperitoneum confection.

In our daily clinical practice, we use the three alternatives described by Menon et al. [5] to create the workspace safely, even in this challenging scenario.

The first one is to insert Veress needle on the opposite side from the previous surgical site to insufflate the gas. Following the pneumoperitoneum confection, a possibility is to insert firstly a 5-mm clear tip port to inspect the abdominal cavity, making a minor local trauma and introducing the remaining trocars under direct vision. In case of multiple adhesions, this may avoid major injuries.

The second is to use the Hasson technique, where access to the abdominal cavity is done under direct vision of the fascia and the peritoneum opening.

However, in cases of extensive and thick adhesions when the previous techniques were not enough to perform the pneumoperitoneum properly, a mini midline laparotomy may be done and cautiously adhesiolysis can be carried out. Then, the incision is closed allowing the camera port to pass through it.

Beyond all these surgical modifications to achieve the pneumoperitoneum confection in patients with previous abdominal surgeries, a remarkable evolution of the surgical system was the miniaturization of the previous 12 mm camera size to the newer 8 mm from da Vinci Xi. This mitigated the abdominal trauma and allowed the camera to be inserted through any robotic trocar, allowing intrabdominal visualization in a more versatile way.

4.1.1 Surgical Outcomes

There are few series analyzing outcomes of RALP in patients with prior abdominal or pelvic surgery (PAPS). The two initial series recorded still in 2010 showed feasibility and safety, with no contraindications to RALP in this scenario [5, 62].

In a retrospective review of a prospective database, Ginzburg et al. [62] reported 839 RALPs from 2004 to 2008, embracing 251 (29,9%) patients with PAPS. Interesting to highlight that even the initial cases during the learning curve from all the surgeons were included. Comparing patients with and without PAPS, they found no significant differences in OT (209 vs 204 min; $p = 0.20$), console time (165 vs 163 min; $p = 0.59$), PSM (21.1 vs 27.2%; $p = 0.08$) or incidence of complications (14.3 vs 17.3%; $p = 0.33$).

Analysis from a larger prospective cohort of 3950 consecutive patients submitted to RALP between 2001 and 2008, it was identified 1049 (27%) patients with PAPS [5]. Comparing these two groups of patients, the only positive finding was the increased need for adhesiolysis in patients with PAPS (24 vs 8%; $p < 0.001$). Appendectomy was the most common previous surgery performed (11%) and patients with a previous history of colectomy presented the highest rates of adhesiolysis (72%). There were 5 bowel injuries in 3950 patients, 3 of these patients had PAPS. There were no differences in the preoperative data as BMI (27.8 vs 27.4; $p = 0.2$), PSA baseline (6.1 vs 6.3; $p = 0.07$), clinical stage ($p = 0.71$), as well as in trans-operative findings such as EBL (150 vs 151 ml; $p = 0.79$) and OT (158 vs 155 min; $p = 0.15$).

Still, in a single-surgeon RALP series including 1414 patients, 420 individuals (30%) also presented PAPS [63]. The study found PAPS and the presence of adhesions were associated with increased OT (147 vs 119; $p < 0.001$ and 120 vs 154; $p < 0.001$). In addition, PAPS did not affect the safety either feasibility of RALP, with all patients experiencing comparable perioperative, functional, and oncological outcomes.

Another single-surgeon series reported 339 RALPs from 2008 to 2014, of which 92 (28.4%) had PAPS [64]. They observed no major differences between patients with or without PAPS in terms of mean OT (257 vs 260 min; $p = 0.597$), median lymph node yield (17 vs 16; $p = 0.484$), mean LOS (7.1 vs 7.2; $p = 0.151$), PSM (16.3 vs 12.5%; $p = 0.233$) or complications rates (31.5 vs 26.7%; $p = 0.187$). At a median follow-up of 36 months, neither there were differences in functional (continence in 100 vs 97.9%; $p = 0.329$ and potency 62.2 vs 69.5%; $p = 0.460$) and oncological outcomes (BCR free survival 79.8 vs 78.5%; $p = 0.467$).

Similar findings were reported by a Japanese single-center experience, including 203 RALPs of which 65 (32%) also presented PAPS [65]. Excepting a higher port-insertion time in PAPS patients (22 vs 17 min; $p = 0.01$), there were similar EBL (197 vs 170 ml; $p = 0.29$), catheterization time (7.1 vs 6.8; $p = 0.74$), PSM (26.2 vs 20.2%; $p = 0.32$) and complications rates (12.3 vs 8.7%; $p = 0.42$) between patients with and without history of PAPS. Still, the location of PAPS (above or below the umbilicus) or even if single or multiple surgeries were performed did not affect these outcomes.

Finally, in 2017 Horovitz et al. [66] prospected the role of the extraperitoneal RALP (e-RALP) in patients with PAPS and compared it with transperitoneal RALP (t-RALP) in this setting. They performed a retrospective review of 2927 RALPs and identified 620 (21.18%) patients who were also submitted to PAPS (excluding patients with inguinal hernia repair or unclear surgical histories). Selecting only patients with PAPS, there were 340 patients who underwent e-RALP and 280 t-RALP. Due to the study design and preoperative patient selection, e-RALP patients were younger and healthier and presented lower D'Amico risk. Both approaches were safe to perform surgery, however, on univariate analysis, e-RALP presented lower OT (188.96 vs 197.92 min; $p = 0.003$), extensive lysis of adhesions (0.9 vs 14.3%; $p < 0.0001$), LOS (1.13 vs 1.33 day; $p = 0.003$) and a slightly higher EBL (210.74 vs 190.79; $p = 0.06$). Extraperitoneal approach was also associated with lower rates of gastrointestinal complications (0 vs 3.21%; $p = 0.0007$), overall complications (9.41 vs 15%; $p = 0.03$) and a trend toward lower early postoperative complications (8.53 vs 12.86%; $p = 0.08$).

Table 7 Narrative review of outcomes from patients with and without previous abdominal surgery following robot-assisted radical prostatectomy

	N	Study design	Operative time (min)	Estimated blood loss (ml)	Complications	Urinary function	Sexual function	Pathology
Ginzburg et al. 2010 [62]	839	Prospective	SIMILAR	N/A	SIMILAR	N/A	N/A	SIMILAR
Bernstein et al. 2013 [63]	1414	Prospective	HIGHER 147 vs 119 $p < 0.001$	SIMILAR	SIMILAR	SIMILAR	SIMILAR	SIMILAR
Di Pierro et al. 2016 [64]	339	Prospective	SIMILAR	N/A	SIMILAR	SIMILAR	SIMILAR	SIMILAR
Kishimoto et al. 2016 [65]	203	Retrospective	SIMILAR	SIMILAR	SIMILAR	N/A	N/A	SIMILAR

HIGHER or WORSE results with statistical significance, *SIMILAR* statistical significance not reached, *N/A* not available

A narrative review with the main series in this scenario is summarized in Table 7.

4.2 Renal Transplant Recipients

4.2.1 Tips and Tricks

It is feasible to perform RALP without adapting ports placement. However, inserting them more cephalad and medializing the ipsilateral robot arm, as well putting the assistant port contralateral from transplant graft is a good idea to perform it safer.

As it occurs for previous abdominal surgeries, it is of utmost importance to perform all the ports under direct vision avoiding inadvertent bowel or renal graft injuries.

Besides that, another modification that may prevent ureteral renal graft injury is to perform bladder drop partially, avoiding large dissections ipsilateral to the renal graft. The remaining surgical steps are the same as usual RALP, except for the pelvic lymphadenectomy, which usually is skipped in this scenario or performed only on the contralateral side of the renal graft.

4.2.2 Surgical Outcomes

Initial records of RALP in renal transplant recipients (RTR) consisted of cases and series reports including few patients undergoing surgery from the first decade of the XXI century, since robot-assisted surgery was introduced [67, 68].

Subsequent reports recorded modifications regarding lymphadenectomies templates, port-placement, approach, and reduced insufflation pressure of 10 mmHg aiming to avoid injuries to renal allograft [67, 69–71]. They found satisfactory perioperative, functional, and oncological outcomes encouraging RALP in this scenario.

Even the first case report of a second RTR submitted to RALP was described recently [72]. The first kidney transplant (KT) in the right iliac fossa was performed 20 years ago, patient followed with chronic allograft nephropathy, requiring the second KT (in the left iliac fossa) 8 years ago. The surgical duration was 208 min, and EBL was 50 ml with no intraoperative complications. Until 21 months of follow-up, the patient was continent and biochemical recurrence-free with allograft function preserved.

Then, a better grade of evidence of RALP in this setting was found through a systematic review including 10 articles and 35 RTR [73]. No major technical difficulties precluding the operation were recorded. Technical modifications to the standard technique were described in 10 of the 11 articles specifically including modifications to port placement (54% of patients), development of the space of Retzius (60% of patients), and performance of lymphadenectomy. Graft function did not deteriorate in any patient. Perioperative complication rate was 17.1% (6 of 35 patients), with only one major complication (Clavien ≥3). The rate of PSM was 31.4%. Data on biochemical recurrence revealed a combined rate of 18.1%.

In the last year, the two largest multicenter comparative series so far were reported.

Leonard et al. [74, 75] reported 27 RALPs in RTRs and compared outcomes with patients with similar characteristics except the history of renal transplant. Similar perioperative data was found between groups regarding OT and EBL, respectively, 244 vs 221 min; $p = 0.273$ and 571 vs 543 ml; $p = 0.824$. Hospital stay was shorter in the RTR group (4.4 vs 5.7 days; $p = 0.041$). Similar immediate postoperative complications (29.6 vs 22.2%; $p = 0.279$) were found between groups. Continence rates did not differ between RTR and control group at 3, 6, 12 or 24 months of follow-up (26 vs 26%, 68 vs 57%, 92 vs 82%, 96 vs 85%; $p = 0.186$). As well as at a similar median of follow-up (34.9 vs 47.5 months; $p = 0.052$), there was similar BCR rate (7.4 vs 11.1%; $p = 0.639$). Multivariate analysis showed that a renal graft history was an independent risk factor of shorter BCR-free survival (hazard ratio = 4.291; 95% confidence interval, 2.102–8.761 and $P < 0.001$). Even as the first comparative study on this topic, the low number of men included was the main limitation of this study.

Felber et al. [75] performed an analysis from 5 French referral centers and described the main findings. They retro-

Table 8 Narrative review of outcomes from patients with and without renal transplant recipient following robot-assisted radical prostatectomy

	N	Study design	Operative time (min)	Estimated blood loss (ml)	Complications	Urinary function	Sexual function	Pathology
Zeng et al. 2018 [73]	35	Systematic review	SR: 220 usual RALPs: 180	SR: 383 usual RALPs: 185	17.1%	N/A	N/A	PSM of 31.4%
Léonard et al. 2020 [74]	54	Retrospective multicenter controlled study	SIMILAR	SIMILAR	SIMILAR	SIMILAR	N/A	SIMILAR
Felber et al. 2020 [75]	321	Multicenter with matched pairs analysis	SIMILAR	SIMILAR	HIGHER 51.2 vs 8.2% $p < 0.001$	SIMILAR at 6 months	WORSE at 6 months potency rates of 12.9 vs 31.4% $p = 0.001$	SIMILAR

HIGHER or *WORSE* results with statistical significance, *SIMILAR* Statistical significance not reached, *N/A* not available, *RALPs* robot-assisted laparoscopic prostatectomy

spectively identified between 2008 and 2017 39 RTRs patients who underwent RALP and compared them with 282 matched non-RTR RALP patients (control group). An increased and marginal difference in terms of OT was found (180 × 150 min; $p = 0.0623$) in the RTR group, while similar findings in terms of EBL (150 × 250 mL; $p = 0.1826$) was recorded. RALP was performed safely with no grafts being damaged during surgery. Median LOS was 4 days in RTR patients and 3 days in the control group ($p = 0.0249$). Despite higher rates of postoperative complications in RTR patients (51.2% vs 8.2%; $p < 0.0001$), most of them were minor (41%) according to Clavien–Dindo classification. Pathological tumoral staging and PSM were comparable between groups ($p = 0.77$ and $p = 0.65$). However, ISUP grade was mostly 1 and 2 in RTR patients, while for the control group it was 1, 2, and 3 ($p = 0.0308$), probably due to higher screening rates at this population and earlier diagnosis. At 6 months of follow-up, no major differences were found in terms of recurrence (7.7 vs 8.5%; $p = 0.84$). Erectile function was normal in 12.9% of RTR patients, while it was preserved in 31.4% of the control group ($p = 0.001$). At this same time since RALP, continence was similar between groups (68.8 vs 65.0%; $p = 0.71$) and at one year of follow-up, no patient had a significant preoperative to postoperative change in renal function ($p = 0.07$).

A narrative review with the main series in this scenario is summarized in Table 8.

5 Conclusion

Challenging cases are better managed by high-volume surgeons since the increased difficulty presented in these scenarios requires extra dexterity to surpass them. Surgical outcomes are variable among surgeons and are mainly related to a learning curve. Technique modifications are often required.

The key to achieving proficiency in RALP is a judicious patient selection during the first cases and facing progressively more complex cases in a presence of a more experienced surgeon to guarantee similar favorable results.

References

1. Binder J, Kramer W. Robotically-assisted laparoscopic radical prostatectomy. BJU Int. 2001 Mar;87(4):408–10.
2. Montorsi F, Wilson TG, Rosen RC, Ahlering TE, Artibani W, Carroll PR, et al. Best practices in robot-assisted radical prostatectomy: recommendations of the Pasadena consensus panel. Eur Urol. 2012 Sep;62(3):368–81.
3. Abboudi H, Khan MS, Guru KA, Froghi S, de Win G, Van Poppel H, et al. Learning curves for urological procedures: a systematic review. BJU Int. 2014 Oct;114(4):617–29.
4. Goldstraw MA, Challacombe BJ, Patil K, Amoroso P, Dasgupta P, Kirby RS. Overcoming the challenges of robot-assisted radical prostatectomy. Prostate Cancer Prostatic Dis. 2012 Mar;15(1):1–7.
5. Siddiqui SA, Krane LS, Bhandari A, Patel MN, Rogers CG, Stricker H, et al. The impact of previous inguinal or abdominal surgery on outcomes after robotic radical prostatectomy. Urology. 2010 May;75(5):1079–82.
6. Acar O, Esen T. Robotic radical prostatectomy in patients with previous prostate surgery and radiotherapy. Prostate Cancer. 2014;2014:367675.
7. Samavedi S, Abdul-Muhsin H, Pigilam S, Sivaraman A, Patel VR. Handling difficult anastomosis. Tips and tricks in obese patients and narrow pelvis. Indian J Urol. 2014 Oct;30(4):418–22.
8. Coelho RF, Chauhan S, Guglielmetti GB, Orvieto MA, Sivaraman A, Palmer KJ, et al. Does the presence of median lobe affect outcomes of robot-assisted laparoscopic radical prostatectomy? J Endourol. 2012 Mar;26(3):264–70.
9. Kim MS, Jang WS, Chung DY, Koh DH, Lee JS, Goh HJ, et al. Effect of prostate gland weight on the surgical and oncological outcomes of extraperitoneal robot-assisted radical prostatectomy. BMC Urol. 2019 Jan 3;19(1):1.
10. Mikhail AA, Stockton BR, Orvieto MA, Chien GW, Gong EM, Zorn KC, et al. Robotic-assisted laparoscopic prostatectomy in overweight and obese patients. Urology. 2006 Apr 1;67(4):774–9.
11. Spinelli MG, Cozzi G, Grasso A, Talso M, Varisco D, Abed El Rahman D, et al. Ralp and Rocco stitch: original technique. Urologia. 2011 Oct;78(Suppl 18):35–8.
12. Coelho RF, Chauhan S, Orvieto MA, Sivaraman A, Palmer KJ, Coughlin G, et al. Influence of modified posterior reconstruction of the rhabdosphincter on early recovery of continence and anastomotic leakage rates after robot-assisted radical prostatectomy. Eur Urol. 2011 Jan;59(1):72–80.

13. Wiltz AL, Shikanov S, Eggener SE, Katz MH, Thong AE, Steinberg GD, et al. Robotic radical prostatectomy in overweight and obese patients: oncological and validated-functional outcomes. Urology. 2009 Feb;73(2):316–22.
14. Xu T, Wang X, Xia L, Zhang X, Qin L, Zhong S, et al. Robot-assisted prostatectomy in obese patients: how influential is obesity on operative outcomes? J Endourol. 2015 Feb;29(2):198–208.
15. Goßler C, May M, Rosenhammer B, Breyer J, Stojanoski G, Weikert S, et al. Obesity leads to a higher rate of positive surgical margins in the context of robot-assisted radical prostatectomy. Results of a prospective multicenter study. Cent European J Urol. 2020;73(4):457–65.
16. Coelho RF, Chauhan S, Orvieto MA, Palmer KJ, Rocco B, Patel VR. Predictive factors for positive surgical margins and their locations after robot-assisted laparoscopic radical prostatectomy. Eur Urol. 2010 Jun;57(6):1022–9.
17. Porcaro AB, Sebben M, Tafuri A, de Luyk N, Corsi P, Processali T, et al. Body mass index is an independent predictor of Clavien-Dindo grade 3 complications in patients undergoing robot assisted radical prostatectomy with extensive pelvic lymph node dissection. J Robot Surg. 2019 Feb;13(1):83–9.
18. Knipper S, Mazzone E, Mistretta FA, Palumbo C, Tian Z, Briganti A, et al. Impact of obesity on perioperative outcomes at robotic-assisted and open radical prostatectomy: results from the National Inpatient Sample. Urology. 2019 Nov;133:135–44.
19. Pridgeon S, Bishop CV, Adshead J. Lower limb compartment syndrome as a complication of robot-assisted radical prostatectomy: the UK experience. BJU Int. 2013 Aug;112(4):485–8.
20. Onagi A, Haga N, Tanji R, Honda R, Matsuoka K, Hoshi S, et al. Transient renal dysfunction due to rhabdomyolysis after robot-assisted radical prostatectomy. Int Urol Nephrol. 2020 Oct;52(10):1877–84.
21. Abdul-Muhsin H, Giedelman C, Samavedi S, Schatloff O, Coelho R, Rocco B, et al. Perioperative and early oncological outcomes after robot-assisted radical prostatectomy (RARP) in morbidly obese patients: a propensity score-matched study. BJU Int. 2014 Jan;113(1):84–91.
22. Huben NB, Hussein AA, May PR, Whittum M, Krasowski C, Ahmed YE, et al. Development of a patient-based model for estimating operative times for robot-assisted radical prostatectomy. J Endourol. 2018 Aug;32(8):730–6.
23. Kheterpal E, Sammon JD, Diaz M, Bhandari A, Trinh Q-D, Pokala N, et al. Effect of metabolic syndrome on pathologic features of prostate cancer. Urol Oncol. 2013 Oct;31(7):1054–9.
24. Wilson RL, Shannon T, Calton E, Galvão DA, Taaffe DR, Hart NH, et al. Efficacy of a weight loss program prior to robot assisted radical prostatectomy in overweight and obese men with prostate cancer. Surg Oncol. 2020 Dec;35:182–8.
25. Wasserman NF, Spilseth B, Golzarian J, Metzger GJ. Use of MRI for lobar classification of benign prostatic hyperplasia: potential phenotypic biomarkers for research on treatment strategies. AJR Am J Roentgenol. 2015 Sep;205(3):564–71.
26. Molinari A, Simonelli G, De Concilio B, Porcaro AB, Del Biondo D, Zeccolini G, et al. Is ureteral stent placement by the transurethral approach during robot-assisted radical prostatectomy an effective option to preoperative technique? J Endourol. 2014 Aug;28(8):896–8.
27. Meeks JJ, Zhao L, Greco KA, Macejko A, Nadler RB. Impact of prostate median lobe anatomy on robotic-assisted laparoscopic prostatectomy. Urology. 2009 Feb;73(2):323–7.
28. Huang AC, Kowalczyk KJ, Hevelone ND, Lipsitz SR, Yu H, Plaster BA, et al. The impact of prostate size, median lobe, and prior benign prostatic hyperplasia intervention on robot-assisted laparoscopic prostatectomy: technique and outcomes. Eur Urol. 2011 Apr;59(4):595–603.
29. Jeong CW, Lee S, Oh JJ, Lee BK, Lee JK, Jeong SJ, et al. Quantification of median lobe protrusion and its impact on the base surgical margin status during robot-assisted laparoscopic prostatectomy. World J Urol. 2014 Apr;32(2):419–23.
30. de Castro Abreu AL, Chopra S, Berger AK, Leslie S, Desai MM, Gill IS, et al. Management of large median and lateral intravesical lobes during robot-assisted radical prostatectomy. J Endourol. 2013 Nov;27(11):1389–92.
31. Lin VC, Coughlin G, Savamedi S, Palmer KJ, Coelho RF, Patel VR. Modified transverse plication for bladder neck reconstruction during robotic-assisted laparoscopic prostatectomy. BJU Int. 2009 Sep;104(6):878–81.
32. Hamidi N, Atmaca AF, Canda AE, Keske M, Gok B, Koc E, et al. Does presence of a median lobe affect perioperative complications, oncological outcomes and urinary continence following robotic-assisted radical prostatectomy? Urol J. 2018 Sep 26;15(5):248–55.
33. Rajih E, Meskawi M, Alenizi AM, Zorn KC, Alnazari M, Zanaty M, et al. Perioperative predictors for post-prostatectomy urinary incontinence in prostate cancer patients following robotic-assisted radical prostatectomy: long-term results of a Canadian prospective cohort. Can Urol Assoc J. 2019 May;13(5):E125–31.
34. Jenkins LC, Nogueira M, Wilding GE, Tan W, Kim HL, Mohler JL, et al. Median lobe in robot-assisted radical prostatectomy: evaluation and management. Urology. 2008 May;71(5):810–3.
35. Alnazari M, Zanaty M, Ajib K, El-Hakim A, Zorn KC. The risk of urinary retention following robot-assisted radical prostatectomy and its impact on early continence outcomes. Can Urol Assoc J. 2018 Mar;12(3):E121–5.
36. Jung H, Ngor E, Slezak JM, Chang A, Chien GW. Impact of median lobe anatomy: does its presence affect surgical margin rates during robot-assisted laparoscopic prostatectomy? J Endourol. 2012 May;26(5):457–60.
37. Alenizi AM, Valdivieso R, Rajih E, Meskawi M, Toarta C, Bienz M, et al. Factors predicting prolonged operative time for individual surgical steps of robot-assisted radical prostatectomy (RARP): a single surgeon's experience. Can Urol Assoc J. 2015 Aug;9(7–8):E417–22.
38. Marchetti PE, Shikanov S, Razmaria AA, Zagaja GP, Shalhav AL. Impact of prostate weight on probability of positive surgical margins in patients with low-risk prostate cancer after robotic-assisted laparoscopic radical prostatectomy. Urology. 2011 Mar;77(3):677–81.
39. Coelho R, Chauhan S, Sivaraman A, Palmer K, Orvieto M, Patel V. Does prostate weight affect perioperative, oncologic and early continence outcomes after robotic-assisted laparoscopic radical prostatectomy by an experienced surgeon? SES AUA Annual Meeting. 2012 Mar 21;Poster #63.
40. Labanaris AP, Zugor V, Witt JH. Robot-assisted radical prostatectomy in patients with a pathologic prostate specimen weight ≥100 grams versus ≤50 grams: surgical, oncologic and short-term functional outcomes. Urol Int. 2013;90(1):24–30.
41. Hampton L, Nelson RA, Satterthwaite R, Wilson T, Crocitto L. Patients with prior TURP undergoing robot-assisted laparoscopic radical prostatectomy have higher positive surgical margin rates. J Robot Surg. 2008 Dec;2(4):213–6.
42. Tugcu V, Atar A, Sahin S, Kargi T, Gokhan Seker K, IlkerComez Y, et al. Robot-assisted radical prostatectomy after previous prostate surgery. JSLS. 2015 Dec;19(4):e2015.00080.
43. Su Y-K, Katz BF, Sehgal SS, Yu S-JS SY-C, Lightfoot A, et al. Does previous transurethral prostate surgery affect oncologic and continence outcomes after RARP? J Robot Surg. 2015 Dec;9(4):291–7.
44. Campobasso D, Fiori C, Amparore D, Checcucci E, Garrou D, Manfredi M, et al. Total anatomical reconstruction during robot-assisted radical prostatectomy in patients with previous prostate surgery. Minerva Urol Nefrol. 2019 Dec;71(6):605–11.

45. Liao H, Duan X, Du Y, Mou X, Hu T, Cai T, et al. Radical prostatectomy after previous transurethral resection of the prostate: oncological, surgical and functional outcomes-a meta-analysis. World J Urol. 2020 Aug;38(8):1919–32.
46. Abedali ZA, Calaway AC, Large T, Koch MO, Lingeman JE, Boris RS. Robot-assisted radical prostatectomy in patients with a history of holmium laser enucleation of the prostate: the Indiana University experience. J Endourol. 2020 Feb;34(2):163–8.
47. Loeb S, Bjurlin MA, Nicholson J, Tammela TL, Penson DF, Carter HB, et al. Overdiagnosis and overtreatment of prostate cancer. Eur Urol. 2014 Jun;65(6):1046–55.
48. Klotz L. Active surveillance for prostate cancer: patient selection and management. Curr Oncol. 2010 Sep;17(Suppl 2):S11–7.
49. Mottet N, Cornford P, van den Bergh R, Briers E, De Santis M, Fanti S, et al. EAU guidelines: prostate cancer. Uroweb [Internet]. [cited 2020 Aug 29]; Available from: https://uroweb.org/guideline/prostate-cancer/
50. Sanda MG, Chen RC, Crispino T, Freedland S, Greene K, Klotz L, et al. Prostate cancer: clinically localized guideline - American urological association. [cited 2021 May 3]; Available from: https://www.auanet.org/guidelines/guidelines/prostate-cancer-clinically-localized-guideline
51. Bokhorst LP, Lepistö I, Kakehi Y, Bangma CH, Pickles T, Valdagni R, et al. Complications after prostate biopsies in men on active surveillance and its effects on receiving further biopsies in the prostate cancer research international: active surveillance (PRIAS) study. BJU Int. 2016;118(3):366–71.
52. Fujita K, Landis P, McNeil BK, Pavlovich CP. Serial prostate biopsies are associated with an increased risk of erectile dysfunction in men with prostate cancer on active surveillance. J Urol. 2009 Dec;182(6):2664–9.
53. Zisman A, Leibovici D, Kleinmann J, Siegel YI, Lindner A. The impact of prostate biopsy on patient Well-being: a prospective study of pain, anxiety and erectile dysfunction. J Urol. 2001 Feb;165(2):445–54.
54. Carneiro A, Sivaraman A, Sanchez-Salas R, Nunes-Silva I, Baghdadi M, Srougi V, et al. Higher number of transrectal ultrasound guided prostate biopsy cores is associated with higher blood loss and perioperative complications in robot assisted radical prostatectomy. Actas Urol Esp. 2017 Apr;41(3):155–61.
55. Sooriakumaran P, Calaway A, Sagalovich D, Roy S, Srivastava A, Joneja J, et al. The impact of multiple biopsies on outcomes of nerve-sparing robotic-assisted radical prostatectomy. Int J Impot Res. 2012 Aug;24(4):161–4.
56. Olvera-Posada D, Welk B, McClure JA, Winick-Ng J, Izawa JI, Pautler SE. The impact of multiple prostate biopsies on risk for major complications following radical prostatectomy: a population-based cohort study. Urology. 2017 Aug;106:125–32.
57. Hong SK, Lee ST, Kim SS, Min KE, Hwang IS, Kim M, et al. Effect of bony pelvic dimensions measured by preoperative magnetic resonance imaging on performing robot-assisted laparoscopic prostatectomy. BJU Int. 2009 Sep;104(5):664–8.
58. Mason BM, Hakimi AA, Faleck D, Chernyak V, Rozenblitt A, Ghavamian R. The role of preoperative endo-rectal coil magnetic resonance imaging in predicting surgical difficulty for robotic prostatectomy. Urology. 2010 Nov;76(5):1130–5.
59. Chen J, Chu T, Ghodoussipour S, Bowman S, Patel H, King K, et al. Effect of surgeon experience and bony pelvic dimensions on surgical performance and patient outcomes in robot-assisted radical prostatectomy. BJU Int. 2019 Nov;124(5):828–35.
60. Akihisa Yao, Hideto Iwamoto, Toshihiko Masago, Shuichi Morizane, Masashi Honda, Takehiro Sejima, et al. Anatomical dimensions using preoperative magnetic resonance imaging: impact on the learning curve of robot-assisted laparoscopic prostatectomy. Int J Urol: Official journal of the Japanese Urological Association [Internet]. 2015 Jan [cited 2021 Mar 25];22(1):74-9. Available from: https://pubmed.ncbi.nlm.nih.gov/25212691/
61. Krielen P, Stommel MWJ, Pargmae P, Bouvy ND, Bakkum EA, Ellis H, et al. Adhesion-related readmissions after open and laparoscopic surgery: a retrospective cohort study (SCAR update). Lancet. 2020 Jan 4;395(10217):33–41.
62. Ginzburg S, Hu F, Staff I, Tortora J, Champagne A, Salner A, et al. Does prior abdominal surgery influence outcomes or complications of robotic-assisted laparoscopic radical prostatectomy? Urology. 2010 Nov;76(5):1125–9.
63. Bernstein AN, Lavery HJ, Hobbs AR, Chin E, Samadi DB. Robot-assisted laparoscopic prostatectomy and previous surgical history: a multidisciplinary approach. J Robot Surg. 2013 Jun;7(2):143–51.
64. Di Pierro GB, Grande P, Mordasini L, Danuser H, Mattei A. Robot-assisted radical prostatectomy in the setting of previous abdominal surgery: Perioperative results, oncological and functional outcomes, and complications in a single surgeon's series. Int J Surg. 2016 Dec;36(Pt A):170–6.
65. Kishimoto N, Takao T, Yamamichi G, Okusa T, Taniguchi A, Tsutahara K, et al. Impact of prior abdominal surgery on the outcomes after robotic - assisted laparoscopic radical prostatectomy: single center experience. Int Braz J Urol. 2016 Oct;42(5):918–24.
66. Horovitz D, Feng C, Messing EM, Joseph JV. Extraperitoneal vs. transperitoneal robot-assisted radical prostatectomy in patients with a history of prior inguinal hernia repair with mesh. J Robot Surg. 2017 Dec;11(4):447–54.
67. Smith DL, Jellison FC, Heldt JP, Tenggardjaja C, Bowman RJ, Jin DH, et al. Robot-assisted radical prostatectomy in patients with previous renal transplantation. J Endourol. 2011 Oct;25(10):1643–7.
68. Polcari AJ, Allen JC, Nunez-Nateras R, Mmeje CO, Andrews PE, Milner JE, et al. Multicenter experience with robot-assisted radical prostatectomy in renal transplant recipients. Urology. 2012 Dec;80(6):1267–72.
69. Ghazi A, Erturk E, Joseph JV. Modifications to facilitate extraperitoneal robot-assisted radical prostatectomy post kidney transplant. JSLS. 2012 Jun;16(2):314–9.
70. Fang Y, Chen Z, Juan L, Feng Z, Cao J, Zhou B, et al. Robot-assisted radical prostatectomy in a post-kidney transplant patient: an initial case report in China. Transplant Proc. 2018 Dec;50(10):3978–83.
71. Mistretta FA, Galfano A, Di Trapani E, Di Trapani D, Russo A, Secco S, et al. Robot assisted radical prostatectomy in kidney transplant recipients: surgical, oncological and functional outcomes of two different robotic approaches. Int Braz J Urol. 2019 Apr;45(2):262–72.
72. Minami K, Harada H, Sasaki H, Higuchi H, Tanaka H. Robot-assisted radical prostatectomy in a second kidney transplant recipient. J Endourol Case Rep. 2020;6(4):540–3.
73. Zeng J, Christiansen A, Pooli A, Qiu F, LaGrange CA. Safety and clinical outcomes of robot-assisted radical prostatectomy in kidney transplant patients: a systematic review. J Endourol. 2018 Oct;32(10):935–43.
74. Léonard G, Pradère B, Monléon L, Boutin J-M, Branchereau J, Karam G, et al. Oncological and postoperative outcomes of robot-assisted laparoscopic radical prostatectomy in renal transplant recipients: a multicenter and comparative study. Transplant Proc. 2020 Apr;52(3):850–6.
75. Felber M, Drouin SJ, Grande P, Vaessen C, Parra J, Barrou B, et al. Morbidity, perioperative outcomes and complications of robot-assisted radical prostatectomy in kidney transplant patients: A French multicentre study. Urol Oncol. 2020 Jun;38(6):599.e15–21.

Da Vinci SP Radical Prostatectomy

Marcio Covas Moschovas, Mahmoud Abou Zeinab, Jihad Kaouk, and Vipul Patel

1 Introduction

Robotic surgical technique has been improving since the first procedure in the USA was cleared by the FDA (Food and Drug Administration) in 2000. Since then, this technology has expanded worldwide, and currently Robotic-assisted Radical Prostatectomy (RARP) is the standard surgical treatment for localized prostate cancer in the USA [1]. During this time, five successive models of robotic platforms have been described and efficiently used. The first models (S, Si, Xi, and X) had independent trocars to house each instrument and a rigid scope. In 2018, the FDA cleared a new platform, named da Vinci SP (SP), exclusively built for single port surgery [2, 3]. This novel robot has only one trocar, in which three instruments and one flexible scope are placed at the same time (Fig. 1).

The first urologic surgery performed with the SP was described by Kaouk et al. In this study, 11 of the 19 patients involved underwent radical prostatectomy with transperitoneal access. The author described successful procedures without intraoperative complications [4]. Since then, different centers have also reported SP use in several urologic procedures, with radical prostatectomy being the most common surgery performed with this platform [3]. In this scenario, our chapter will describe details of the SP approach to radical prostatectomy, sharing the experience of pioneers and referral centers using this new robot in the urology field.

M. C. Moschovas (✉)
AdventHealth Global Robotics Institute, Celebration, USA

M. A. Zeinab · J. Kaouk
Cleveland Clinic, Cleveland, OH, USA

V. Patel
AdventHealth Global Robotics Institute, Celebration, USA

University of Central Florida, UCF, Orlando, USA

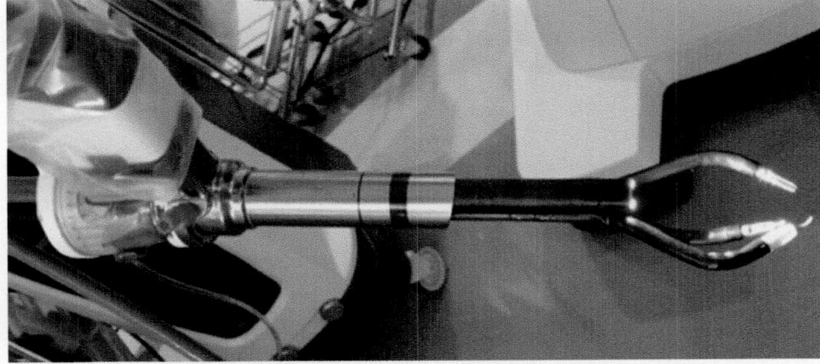

Fig. 1 SP instruments

2 *Da Vinci* SP Modifications and Challenges

2.1 Trocar Placement Differences

Different techniques have been described for the SP-RARP trocar placement [5–7]. In the extraperitoneal approach, the SP trocar is usually attached to a GelPOINT using the floating trocar technique [7, 8]. Other authors have described the transperitoneal approach, placing the robotic trocar in the midline above the umbilicus (Fig. 2) using Hasson's technique, and a 12-mm assistant trocar in the right lower quadrant (SP plus one) [5, 6, 9]. Each SP instrument has two different articulation points (elbow and shoulder-like), and the appropriate working angles and rotations are achieved when these instruments are entirely deployed from the trocar. Therefore, the correct trocar placement is crucial for attaining the optimal triangulation and working distance from the surgical site. Placing the trocar too close to the prostate, with a distance lower than 15 cm from the pubis, inhibits the appropriate instrument triangulation, increasing internal clashing and restricting the scope movement. This is one of the reasons for using the floating trocar on extraperitoneal SP-RARP, because even with an infraumbilical incision, the trocar position (outside of the body) still provides the optimal working distance.

P. Wiklund et al. (eds.), *Robotic Urologic Surgery*, https://doi.org/10.1007/978-3-031-00363-9_24

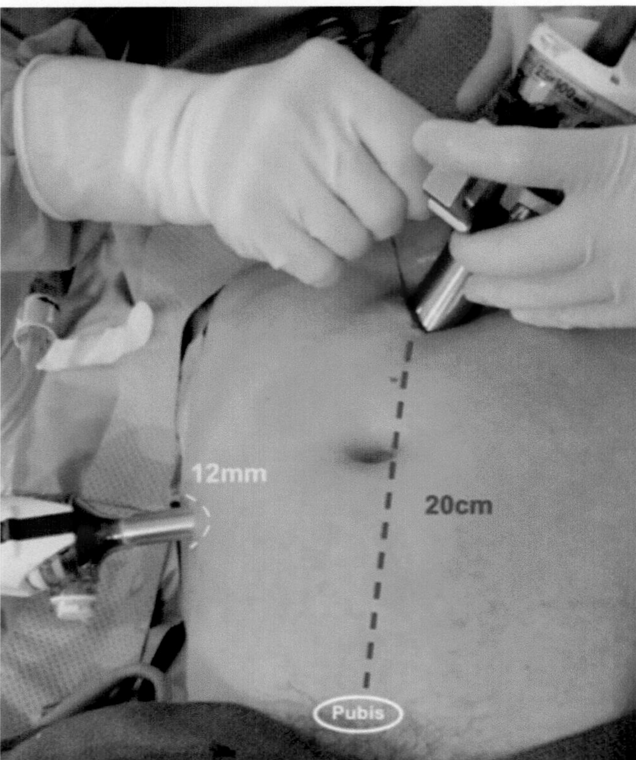

Fig. 2 Transperitoneal technique (SP plus one)

2.2 Different Scope Angles and Working Distances

The SP also presents modifications in the working distance and scope angles that demand a new learning curve. Even with the appropriate trocar placement and instrument triangulation, the working distance differs from the previous multiport console. While the Xi robot enables a close view during the surgery, the SP demands a wider distance (similar to the laparoscopy) because all arms are working simultaneously with constant repositioning to avoid clashing and movement restrictions. The flexible scope has different settings necessary for each surgery step to achieve appropriate angulation and movement [5]. One extra pedal, named the relocation pedal, is responsible for guiding the scope and all instruments to work in a different quadrant (Fig. 3). During this maneuver, all instruments must be located at the center of the screen under visualization to avoid unexpected lesions outside the operative field. This pedal is often used during the lymphadenectomy to guide the robot to the left or right pelvic side. However, this relocation process often adds extra minutes to the total operative time because it usually happens slowly.

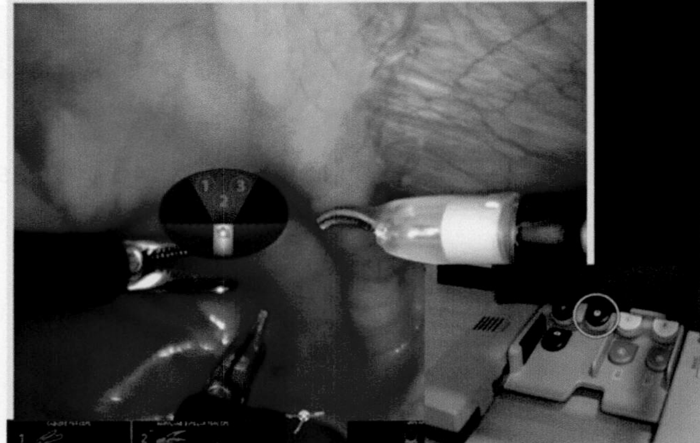

Fig. 3 Relocation pedal

2.3 Traction and Capacity of Dissection

While the multiport Xi console has four 8-mm working ports, the SP has reduced the instrument thickness to 6 mm to enable surgery with a single trocar. However, this modification impacts the capacity of gripping, traction, and dissection of this robot. During our study period in the lab, we realized that cases with a higher need for traction during surgery might not be ideal candidates for SP-RARP [5, 6]. The delicate instrument tip and lack of rigid arms reduced the optimal gripping and traction during surgery. Therefore, to minimize the learning curve challenges, overcome instrument limitations, and maintain the surgical outcomes, some authors have described selection criteria for SP-RARP candidates. The SP selection criteria are not mandatory, because other centers are presenting satisfactory outcomes without selecting patients [10–13].

3 SP-RARP Literature Summary and Outcomes

Table 1 summarizes the current studies reporting SP-RARP outcomes. Not all articles reporting procedures in cadavers or animals were included in our summary. Five different accesses have been described with this platform (extraperitoneal, transperitoneal, Retzius sparing, transperineal, and transvesical). The intraoperative complication rates range from 0 to 5%, with bowel serosal injury being the most common complication. The postoperative complications range from 0 to 45%, with reports ranging from Clavien 1 to Clavien 4B. Total operative time ranges from 114 to 343 minutes, and console time from 80 to 210 minutes. Blood loss ranges from 50 to 750 ml. Positive surgical margins range from 0 to 65.4%.

Table 1 Current series reporting outcomes of SR Radical Prostatectomy

Author	Year	N. of cases	Access	Intraoperative complication rates	Postoperative complication rates (Clavien)	Operative time (min)	Console Time (min)	Blood loss (ml)	Positive margins (%)
Kaouk et al. [4]	2014	11	TPR	None		239		350	18%
Kaouk et al. [10]	2019	3	TPR	None	None	180-300		50-100	33%
Chi-Fai Ng et al. [11]	2019	20	TPR	None	25% (Clavien 1 and 2)	208		296	55%
Deepak A et al. [12]	2019	49	TPR or Retzius	None	8.1% (Clavien 1)	161		200	28%
Kaouk et al. [14]	2019	10	RTP	None	None	197		50-400	50%
Doobs et al. [13]	2019	10	TPR	None	None	234	189	20-150	20%
Kaouk et al. [10]	2019	5	TPR	None	25% (Clavien 2)	180-330		50-750	20%
Doobs et al. [15]	2019	24	TPR	1 Bowel serosal injury	45% (Clavien 1 to 4B)	191-343		75	
Kaouk et al. [7]	2019	46 52	TPR EPT	None None	15% (Clavien1 and 2) 11% (Clavien1 and 2)	201		117	27%
Covas Moschovas et al. [5]	2020	26	TPR	None	None	121	85	50	11%
Kaouk et al. [8]	2020	8 52	TPR EPT	None	None	106-281		50-200	30%
Valero R et al. [16]	2020	1	TPR	None	None	256	108	100	0
Kim et al. [17]	2020	20	TPR	None	None	200-255	165-210	155-300	35%
Jones R et al. [18]	2020	23	TPR	None	26%	236		50	39%
Wilson et al. [19]	2020	60	EPT	None	18% (Clavien 3a)	198		179	23%
Covas Moschovas et al. [6]	2021	50	TPR	None	None	118	80	50	14%
Lenfant et al. [20]	2020	100	EPT	None	16% (Clavien 1-3a)	195		199	24%
Abaza R et al. [21]	2021	59	TPR	NA	NA	NA	NA	NA	NA
Covas Moschovas et al. [22]	2021	71	TPR	None	None	114	80	55	17%
Talamini et al. [23]	2021	20	TPR	1 Bowel serosal injury	20% (Clavien 1-4B)	225	191	20-250	45%
Lenfant et al. [24]	2021	26	RPP	None	50% (Clavien1-3A)	255	NA	100	65.4%
Kaouk et al. [25]	2021	20	TVC	None	None	199	119	135	15%

TNP Transperitoneal, *EPT* Extraperitoneal, *RPP* Radical Perineal Prostatectomy, *NA* non-available data, *TVC* Transvesical

4 SP Radical Prostatectomy: Dr. Patel's Step-by-Step Technique

Our SP-RARP technique follows the same concepts and steps adopted in our conventional multiport RARP [26–29]. The patient undergoes surgery in dorsal decubitus with pad protection in all articulations and contacts with the operative table. After general anesthesia, all patients undergo bilateral transversus abdominis plane (TAP) block [30]. In our technique, we do not place an abdominal drain at the end of the procedure.

4.1 Trocar Placement (Single Port Plus One)

A supraumbilical incision (3 cm) is performed in the midline, at least 20 cm away from the pubis, to place the SP multichannel port with Hasson's technique [9]. In sequence, an extra 12 mm trocar is placed in the right lower quadrant for tableside assistant use. In our experience, the additional trocar was crucial to maintain our established RARP technique, avoiding excessive cautery use on the pedicles. The assistant performs suction and hemostatic clipping, which benefits the patient with operative time reduction.

After placing the trocar, we perform the pneumoperitoneum with the AirSeal system until 8 to 10 mmHg, and then the table is angled in 26 degrees Trendelenburg position.

4.2 Bladder Dropping and Anterior Bladder Neck Dissection

The robotic instruments follow the order: Cadiere–Bipolar–Scissors (Cadiere on the left side, Bipolar at 6 o'clock position, and Scissors on the right side). When dropping the bladder, the pubic bone and vas deferens are landmarks to guide the Retzius space dissection until the anterior bladder neck access. The Cadiere Forceps, placed on the left side, grasp the tissue while the bipolar and scissors perform the dissection. In this step, the relocation pedal is often used to target the robot to different surgical sites. The anterior bladder neck is then opened with scissors, while the Cadiere applies downward contra traction on the bladder (Fig. 4).

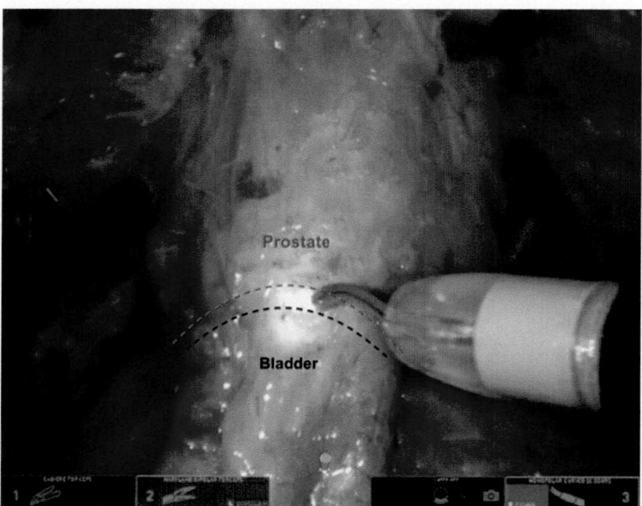

Fig. 4 Anterior bladder neck

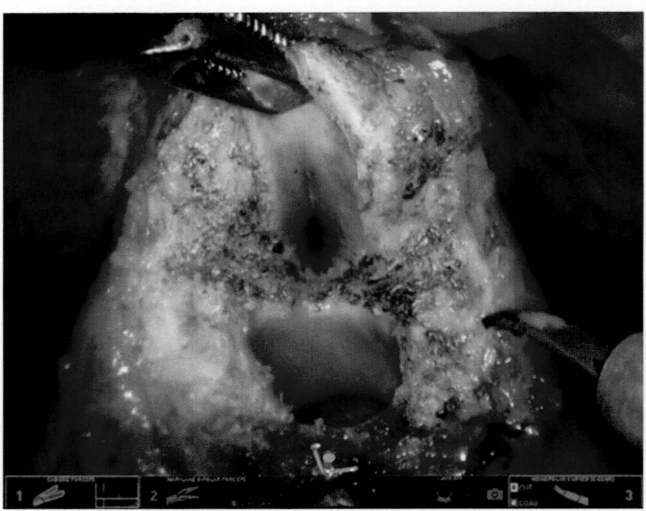

Fig. 5 Posterior bladder neck

4.3 Posterior Bladder Neck Dissection and Seminal Vesicles Approach

After opening the anterior bladder neck, the Foley catheter is lifted and maintained by the Cadiere toward the pubic bone. In sequence, the posterior dissection is performed until the seminal vesicles (SV) plane (Fig. 5). The bipolar applies traction on the bladder neck, while the scissors dissect until reaching the posterior transverse fibers, which separates the posterior bladder wall from the SVs. Then, the vas deferens and SVs are dissected and clipped with Hem-o-lock clips. During this step, we avoid using excessive cautery to minimize prostatic nerve injury. The SP approach to the posterior bladder neck and SVs is more challenging than the Xi robot, especially in prostates with large median lobes, due to the more delicate instruments with less traction capacity and blunt tip scissors.

4.4 Nerve Sparing (Posterior Access and Lateral Dissection)

In our experience, the most challenging step of the SP-RARP is the posterior dissection and nerve sparing (NS), because even with a flexible scope, the angulation used to visualize the posterolateral prostate (between the Denonvilliers layers) is not as good as the Xi, with the scope toggled 30 degrees up. The posterior dissection is performed between the Denonvilliers fascia layers while the prostate is lifted by the seminal vesicles (Fig. 6). In sequence, we deflect the SP scope until visualizing the posterolateral prostate anatomy. The neurovascular bundle and prostatic fascia are then spared

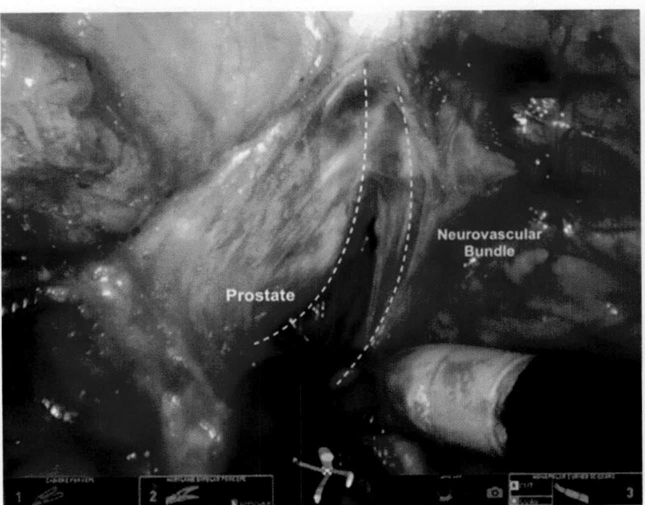

Fig. 6 Nerve sparing

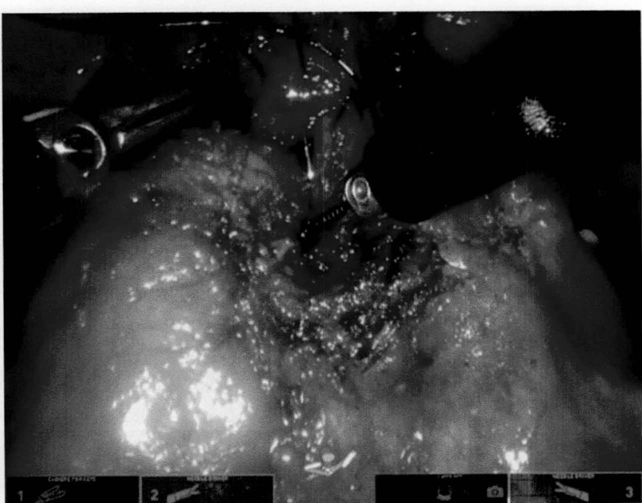

Fig. 7 Anastomosis

bilaterally from the 5 and 7 o'clock positions to the 1 and 11 o'clock positions. Afterward, we open the endopelvic fascia, preserving the lateral prostatic fascia, and perform the lateral neural bundle retrograde dissection. Then, the prostatic arterial pedicles are ligated with Hem-o-lock clips.

4.5 Minimal Apical Dissection and DVC Control

We perform a minimal apical dissection underneath the puboprostatic ligaments, preserving the maximum amount of periurethral tissue, urethra length, and anterior apical attachments to the prostate. Then, the DVC control is performed with a 2-0 running suture (Quill) while the pneumoperitoneum is on 6–8 mmHg. Lowering the intra-abdominal pressure facilitates the identification of bleeding vessels.

4.6 Posterior Reconstruction and Anastomosis

We divide the urethra with scissors avoiding cautery energy, minimizing thermal injury of the urethra mucosa. After the urethra division, we perform a posterior reconstruction with Rocco's technique [31] using a 2-0 Quill, followed by the anastomosis (Fig. 7) performed with a 2-0 bidirectional Quill suture [32].

4.7 Lymphadenectomy

We usually remove the standard template anteromedial to the external iliac vein and around the obturator nerve and vessels [33]. The extremities of the lymph node template are clipped with Hem-o-lock. The instrument configuration follows the same position as the beginning of the surgery (Cadiere–Bipolar–Scissors). In this step, the relocation pedal is often used to guide the robot to the left and right pelvic lymphadenectomy. The Cadiere is used for maintaining the tissue traction, while the bipolar and scissors perform the hemostasis and dissection.

4.8 Postoperative Care and Follow-Up

In the postoperative period, patients complete a questionnaire every six hours, rating their current abdominal pain on a 0–10 scale (0 being no pain, 10 being the most intense pain). Based on the patient's pain score, they are administered non-opiate analgesia if needed. We report postoperative complications according to the modified Clavien–Dindo system classification [34]. Following catheter removal, on the fifth day, patients have postoperative appointments at 6 weeks, and 3, 6, 9, and 12 months after surgery to evaluate the Prostate Specific Antigen (PSA), Sexual Health Inventory for Men (SHIM) score, and American Urological Association (AUA) questionnaires.

5 Extraperitoneal Approach to SP Radical Prostatectomy

In our practice, we offer the SP-RARP using the extraperitoneal approach to patients who have similar indications for the traditional multiport transperitoneal radical prostatectomy (14, 35). Over 200 SP-RARP extraperitoneal cases were performed in our institution. Patients with previous

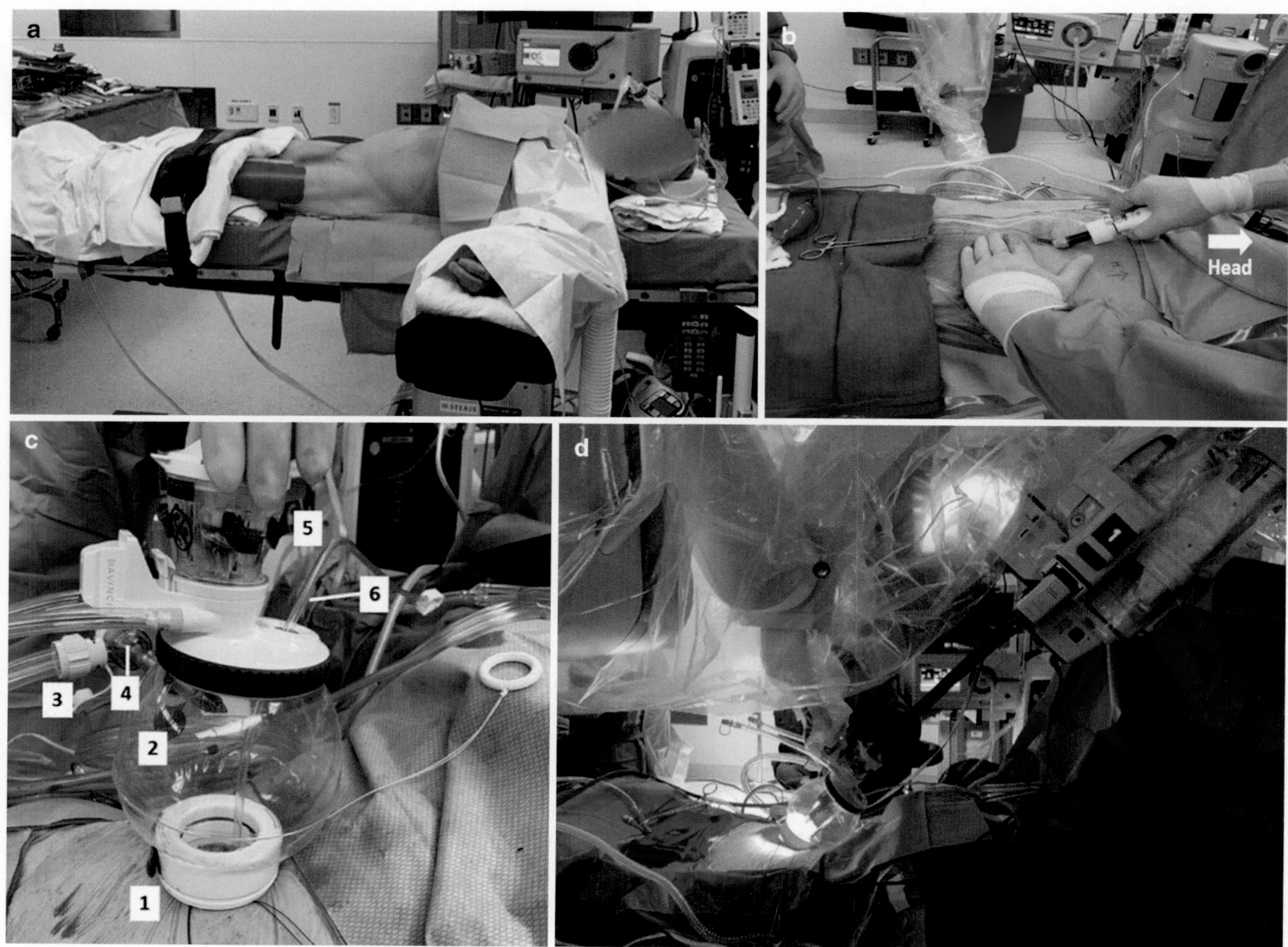

Fig. 8 (**a**) Patient flat positioning in extraperitoneal and transvesical SP-RARP. (**b**) Development of extraperitoneal space. (**c**) The da Vinci Access Port. (1) Wound retractor. (2) Access port. (3) AirSeal. (4) 12-mm assistant port. (5) 25-mm multichannel cannula. (6) ROSI suction device. (**d**) Extraperitoneal SP-RARP Robot docking and instrument insertions

intra-abdominal surgeries and bowel adhesions can particularly benefit from this approach. Patients are positioned in the supine position (Fig. 8a), allowing patients who are unable to tolerate the peritoneal insufflation or Trendelenburg positioning due to significant respiratory disease and glaucoma, to be well suited for the extraperitoneal approach.

5.1 Extraperitoneal Access and SP Docking

Using a 3–3.5 cm infraumbilical incision, a blunt finger dissection is performed between the rectus muscles to partially develop the Retzius space under the pubic bone. We do not go beyond the posterior rectus fascia to avoid entry of the peritoneum. We then introduce the kidney-shaped balloon dilator (Spacemaker™ balloon, Covidien, Dublin, Ireland) below the pubic bone to develop the extraperitoneal space (Fig. 8b).

Similar to the "floating dock" technique described earlier in this chapter [36], we currently use the new da Vinci Access Port (Intuitive Surgical, California, United States) in our SP-RARP (Fig. 8c). The inner ring of the wound retractor is placed into the developed extraperitoneal space. We roll the wound retractor rolling ring and insert the access port. Next, the 25-mm SP multichannel port, 12-mm AirSeal (CONMED, Largo, FL) assistant port, and a ROSI (Remotely Operated Suction Irrigation, Vascular Technology Inc., Nashua, NH) flexible suction device are individually inserted through the access port and insufflate the extraperitoneal space to a pressure of 12 mmHg (Fig. 8d). We do not require any additional port in our SP-RARP procedures. The ROSI device is activated by a foot pedal by the bedside assistant but is entirely controlled by the console surgeon. It allows for both suctioning and retraction during the procedure.

5.2 Postoperative Care and Follow-Up

Foley catheter is removed 6 days postoperative. Patients' follow-up is similar to the one stated earlier.

5.3 Outcomes

Our experience with the extraperitoneal SP-RARP has been widely positive [7, 14, 19, 20]. In comparison to the SP transperitoneal approach, the extraperitoneal approach resulted in shorter operative time, significant reduction of postoperative pain and narcotic use, and shorter hospital stay (4.3 vs 25.7 hours) [7]. Similar results were observed when comparing the SP extraperitoneal to the standard multiport RARP [20]. There was no difference in rates of positive surgical margins, 12 months' biochemical recurrence rate, or 12 months' functional outcomes between the extraperitoneal SP-RARP and the standard transperitoneal multiport RARP [20] (Table 1).

6 Perineal Approach to SP Radical Prostatectomy

SP-RARP using the perineal approach was developed to take advantage of the purpose-built SP platform that presents an excellent narrow profile and allows for procedures in narrow working spaces. In our practice, we offer the perineal approach to patients who are not otherwise candidates for the traditional retropubic robotic approaches [24]. Patients with extensive prior abdominal or pelvic surgeries such as total proctocolectomy and J-pouch, previous pelvic radiotherapy, or kidney transplants are offered the perineal approach to avoid working in a hostile abdomen.

Patients are positioned in a high lithotomy position with a 15-degree Trendelenburg, and arms are tucked (Fig. 9a).

6.1 Perineal Access and SP Docking

At the begining of the surgery, a foley catheter is placed in the bladder, and a modified sterile glove is placed and sutured into the rectum to permit checking the rectum without sterility breaking. Next, an inverted 3 cm semilunar incision is made in the midline between the ischial tuberosities (Fig. 9b). After incision of the central tendon, the rectourethralis and levator ani muscles are dissected, and a subcutaneous space is developed. Suspension sutures are placed to lift the subcutaneous flap. Using the same technique of "Air docking" described earlier, the SP robot is docked (Fig. 9c). ROSI suction tubing is inserted into the GelPOINT. Initially, robotic scissors (right), Cadiere graspers (left), and Maryland bipolar (down) are used.

6.2 Posterior Seminal Vesicles and vas Deferens Dissection

After exposing the levator ani muscle fibers, the Denovilliers are identified and incised, developing the posterior plane toward the base of the prostate. At this point, the seminal vesicles and vas deferens are identified and dissected. The seminal vesicles' blood supply is controlled using a robotic clip applier.

6.3 Vascular Pedicle and Nerve Sparing

The tip of the seminal vesicle is retracted medially to expose the vascular pedicle and neurovascular bundles. The pedicles are sequentially clipped using the robotic clip applier. Once completed, the release of the neurovascular bundle continues apically using sharp dissection, avoiding the use of electrocautery.

6.4 Apical and Bladder Neck Dissection

Next, the urethral-prostatic junction is defined, and the membranous urethra is sharply divided starting from the posterior urethral plate. Care is needed during this step since it is a common site for positive surgical margins. The dissection continues anterolaterally until the bladder is reached. Using the Foley balloon as a guide, the anterior bladder neck is opened and the dissection proceeds in a circumferential fashion and the prostate is freed from the last attachment. The robot is undocked to remove the specimen.

6.5 Pelvic Lymph Node Dissection and Vesicourethral Anastomosis

In the perineal approach, lymph node dissection is performed in a caudal-to-cranial direction, as opposed to the conventional lymph node dissection. The obturator nerve and vein are identified first, and the dissection proceeds anterolateral to expose and dissect the obturator and external iliac lymph nodes (Fig. 9d). The vesicourethral anastomosis is completed using two 4–0 barbed running sutures in a water-tight fashion. Since the anastomosis is above the camera in the perineal approach, the anastomosis begins anteriorly and proceeds posteriorly (Fig. 9e). A pelvic drain is not placed in most of our cases.

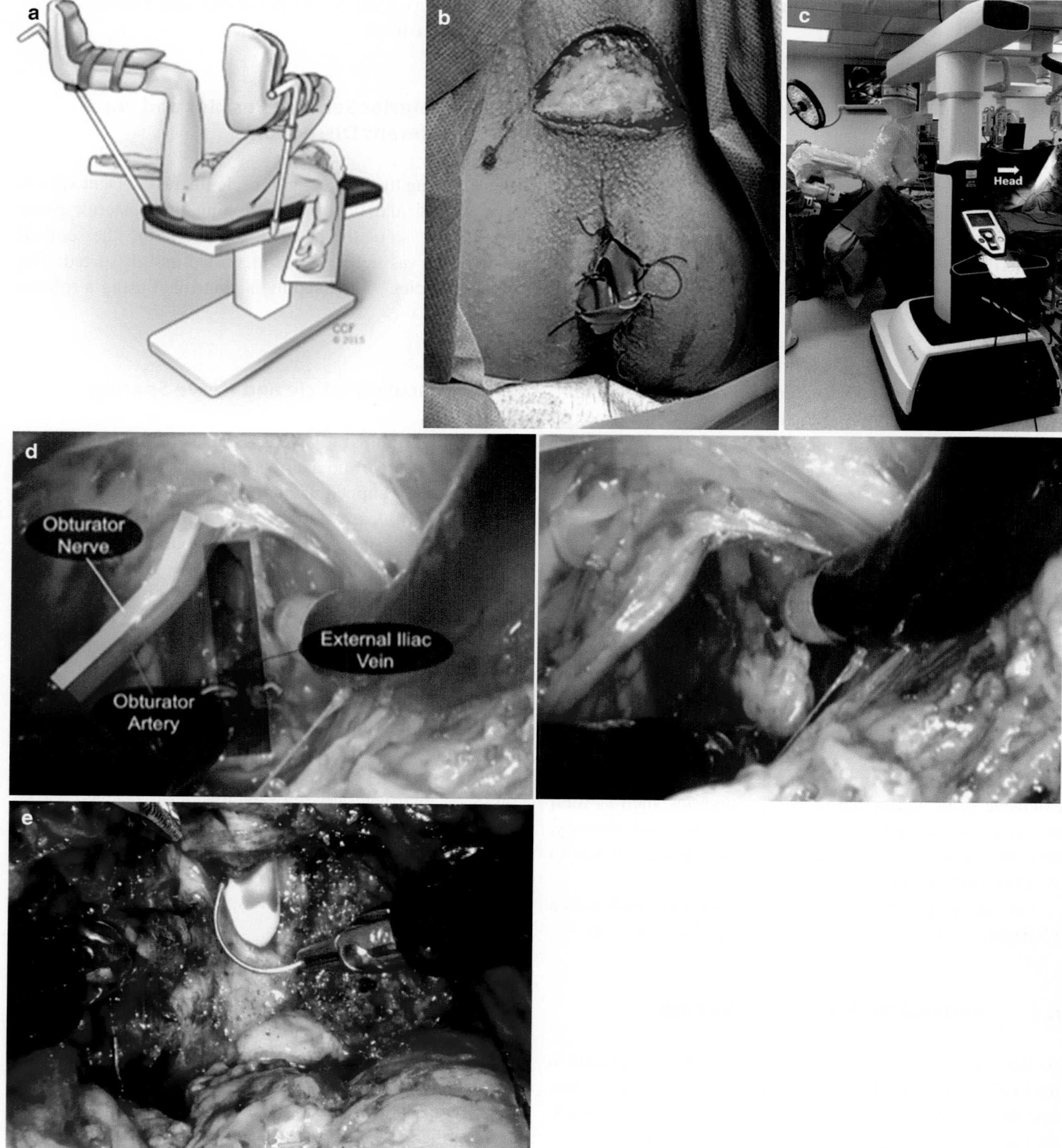

Fig. 9 (**a**) Lithotomy position for perineal SP-RARP. (**b**) Semilunar perineal incision. (**c**) Perineal SP-RARP Robot docking. (**d**) Perineal SP-RARP left lymph node dissection. (**e**) Perineal SP-RARP vesicourethral anastomosis

6.6 Postoperative Care and Follow-Up

Foley catheter is generally removed at postoperative day 7, with a similar follow-up plan to the transperitoneal and extraperitoneal approach.

6.7 Outcomes

Outcomes of the SP-RARP using the perineal approach are presented in Table 1. The perineal approach is an alternative therapeutic option for patients who are poor candidates for other approaches. Compared to the multiport platform, the perineal SP-RARP patients have a shorter hospital stay, higher early continence rates due to the Retzius-sparing approach, faster sexual recovery, and equivalent oncologic outcomes [24, 37, 38].

7 Transvesical Approach to SP Radical Prostatectomy

The narrow profile of the "purpose-built" SP robot allows for many approaches in RARP. After we built the experience with the SP-RARP using the extraperitoneal approach, and the SP transvesical simple prostatectomy [39], we developed the SP-RARP using the transvesical approach [25]. Using this approach, we aim to further improve the patients' perioperative and functional outcomes.

Initially, we offered the transvesical approach to patients with a hostile transperitoneal and/or extraperitoneal space. After the promising data, we expanded our selection to patients with clinically localized, low- and intermediate-risk prostate cancer, according to the guidelines.

The patients are positioned in a supine position, without the need for a Trendelenburg maneuver (Fig. 8a).

7.1 Transvesical Access and SP Docking

A 20 F Foley catheter is inserted into the bladder. A 3–3.5 cm suprapubic midline incision is made, two fingerbreadths above the pubic symphysis. After the rectus fascia is incised, the bladder is identified using a saline distention via the Foley catheter. Four stay sutures are placed on the bladder and a 2 cm cystotomy incision is made (Fig. 10a).

The inner ring of the da Vinci Access Port (Intuitive Surgical, California, United States) is placed directly into the bladder. We roll the wound retractor rolling ring and insert the access port. Next, the 25-mm SP multichannel port, 12-mm AirSeal (CONMED, Largo, FL) assistant port, and a ROSI (Remotely Operated Suction Irrigation, Vascular Technology Inc., Nashua, NH) flexible suction device are individually inserted through the access port (Fig. 8c). The bladder is insufflated to a pressure of 12 mmHg. The camera is inserted at the 12 o'clock position, Monopolar scissors (right), Cadiere forceps (left), and Maryland bipolar forceps (6 o'clock).

7.2 Bladder Neck, vas Deferens, and Seminal Vesicles Dissection

After the identification of the ureteral orifices and maintaining a safe distance, a semilunar incision is made (Fig. 10b), and the dissection extends laterally beyond the detrusor to identify the vas deferens and seminal vesicles. The vas deferens are transected and used as a retractor to expose the seminal vesicles. The tip artery of the seminal vesicles is clipped using robotic Weck clips (Fig. 10c).

7.3 Anterior Dissection

After completing the posterior dissection, the bladder neck is incised anteriorly and the detrusor is incised to reach the endopelvic fascia. After the incision of the endopelvic fascia and the puboprostatic ligaments, the dissection proceeds anteriorly to reach the dorsal venous complex (DVC). A monofilament barbed suture (V-Loc) is used to suture the DVC. Next, the membranous urethra is identified and transected athermally.

7.4 Vascular Pedicle and Nerve Sparing

Using medial traction on the Seminal vesicles, the vascular pedicles are exposed and ligated using the robotic Weck clips (Fig. 10d). Next, the lateral prostatic fascia is incised for better pedicle end identification, and the neurovascular bundle sparing is performed. The prostate is moved into the bladder after freeing it from its attachments.

7.5 Lymph Node Dissection and Vesicourethral Anastomosis

Limited lymph node dissection is performed on patients with over 7% probability of lymph node metastasis according to the Briganti nomogram [40]. Traction is provided laterally on the bladder neck to expose the pelvic sidewall. The obturator nerve is identified using blunt dissection, and lymph node dissection is performed bilaterally (Fig. 10e). Next, a posterior reconstruction with 3–0 V-Loc monofilament barbed suture is performed to reduce the tension on the anas-

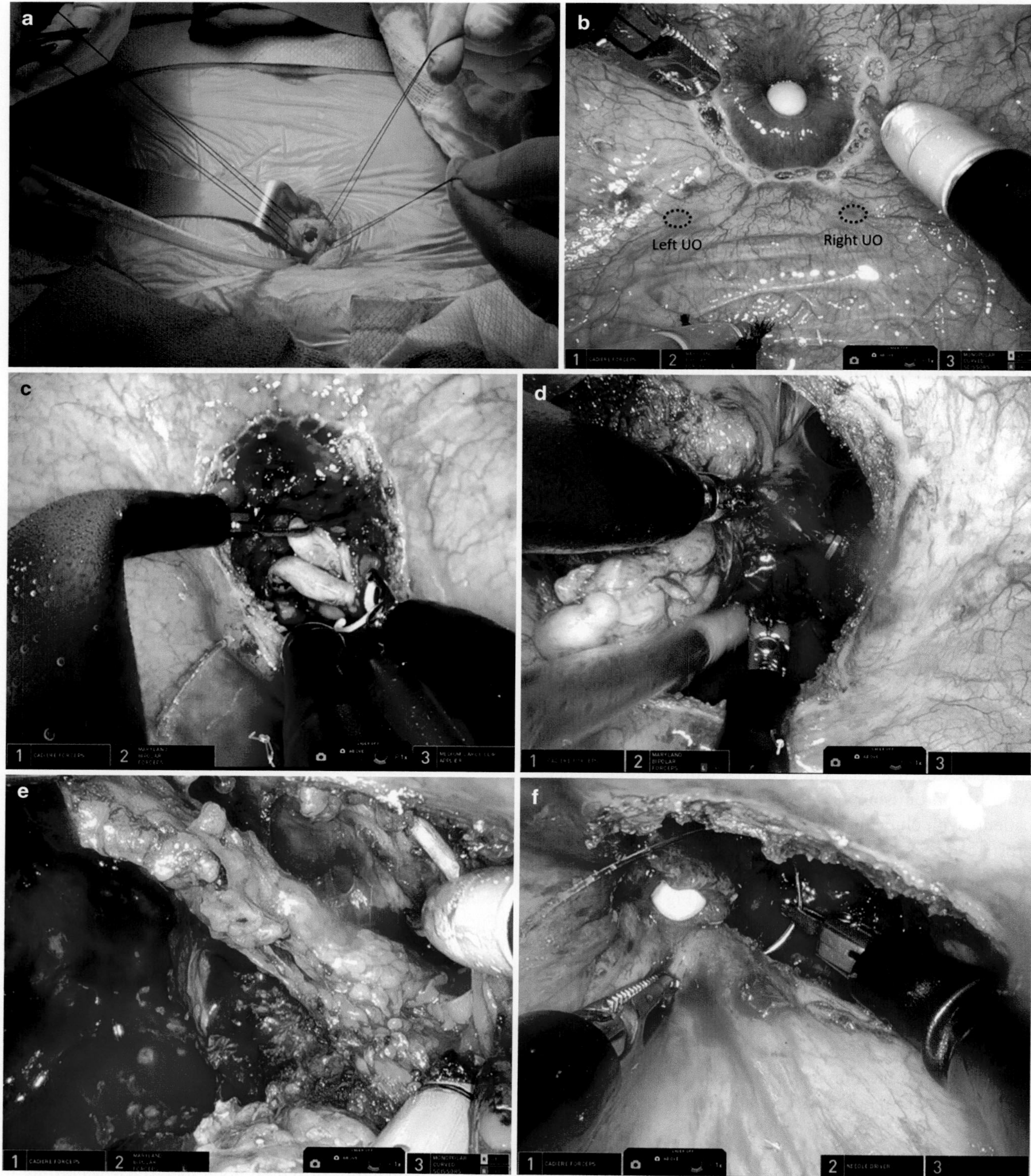

Fig. 10 (**a**) A 3.5 cm midline suprapubic incision. 2 cm cystotomy with four stay sutures on the bladder. (**b**) Figure illustrating the semilunar incision around the prostate, the left and right ureteral orifices (UO) in transvesical RARP. (**c**) Clipping of the tip artery of the right seminal vesicle using a robotic Weck clip in transvesical RARP. Note the left ureteral orifice draining. (**d**) Transvesical RARP clipping of the right vascular pedicle of the prostate. (**e**) Transvesical RARP right lymph node dissection. (**f**) Vesicourethral anastomosis in transvesical RARP

tomosis. Bladder insufflation pressure is dropped to 5 mmHg and the anastomosis is completed (Fig. 10f).

7.6 Postoperative Care and Follow-Up

Patients have similar postoperative care to that discussed earlier. Foley catheter is removed on the third day postoperatively, and patients are followed weekly through a phone call discussing pain control and continence rates, including the number of pads used. Patients have postoperative appointments at 6 weeks, and 3, 6, 9, and 12 months after surgery to evaluate the Prostate Specific Antigen (PSA), Sexual Health Inventory for Men (SHIM) score, and American Urological Association (AUA) questionnaires.

7.7 Outcomes

The outcomes of the Transvesical SP-RARP are presented in Table 1. Early results of this approach are promising in terms of minimal opioid analgesics use, same day discharge, low complication rate, and high rate of immediate urine control after the surgery, without any oncological compromise.

8 Comparative Outcomes between SP and Multiport Robots

It is crucial to emphasize that before comparing the outcomes between the SP and multiport robots, a careful analysis of the current SP data must be performed. All studies reviewed are retrospective series with less than 150 patients, due to the SP learning curve. Only a few studies compared the intraoperative performance and short-term outcomes between both robots (head-to-head) in patients who underwent radical prostatectomy [8, 22, 23]. Prospective comparative data and long-term outcomes are still unknown.

9 Conclusion

The SP technology is promising, but the current studies describing the outcomes for SP radical prostatectomy have only recently appeared in the literature. The available data describes a feasible and safe approach with acceptable perioperative and short-term outcomes. Some articles report benefits in terms of early discharge, pain scores, and perineal approach in patients with previous abdominal surgeries. However, all SP studies are based on retrospective data, which carries inherent risks of bias. Better-designed studies with long-term follow-up are still awaited.

References

1. Martini A, Falagario UG, Villers A, Dell'Oglio P et al. Contemporary techniques of prostate dissection for robot-assisted prostatectomy. Eur Urol. 2020 Oct;78(4):583–591. https://doi.org/10.1016/j.eururo.2020.07.017. Epub 2020 Aug 1.
2. Moschovas MC, Seetharam Bhat KR, Onol FF, Rogers T, Ogaya-Pinies G, Roof S, Patel VR. Single-port technique evolution and current practice in urologic procedures. Asian J Urol. 2021 Jan;8(1):100–104. https://doi.org/10.1016/j.ajur.2020.05.003. Epub 2020 May 22. PMID: 33569276; PMCID: PMC7859361.
3. Covas Moschovas M, Bhat S, Rogers T, Thiel D, Onol F, Roof S, Sighinolfi MC, Rocco B, Patel V. Applications of the da Vinci single port (SP) robotic platform in urology: a systematic literature review. Minerva Urol Nephrol. 2021 Feb;73(1):6–16. https://doi.org/10.23736/S0393-2249.20.03899-0. Epub 2020 Sep 29.
4. Kaouk JH, Haber GP, Autorino R, Crouzet S, Ouzzane A, Flamand V, Villers A. A novel robotic system for single-port urologic surgery: first clinical investigation. Eur Urol. 2014 Dec;66(6): 1033–1043. https://doi.org/10.1016/j.eururo.2014.06.039. Epub 2014 Jul 17.
5. Covas Moschovas M, Bhat S, Rogers T, Onol F, Roof S, Mazzone E, Mottrie A, Patel V. Technical modifications necessary to implement the da vinci single-port robotic system. Eur Urol. 2020 Sep;78(3):415–423. https://doi.org/10.1016/j.eururo.2020.01.005. Epub 2020 Jan 17.
6. Covas Moschovas M, Bhat S, Onol F, Rogers T, Patel V. Early outcomes of single-port robot-assisted radical prostatectomy: lessons learned from the learning-curve experience. BJU Int. 2021 Jan;127(1):114–121. https://doi.org/10.1111/bju.15158. Epub 2020 Aug 2.
7. Kaouk J, Aminsharifi A, Wilson CA, Sawczyn G, Garisto J, Francavilla S, Abern M, Crivellaro S. Extraperitoneal versus transperitoneal single-port robotic radical prostatectomy: a comparative analysis of perioperative outcomes. J Urol. 2020 Jun;203(6):1135–40. https://doi.org/10.1097/JU.0000000000000700.
8. Kaouk J, Aminsharifi A, Sawczyn G et al. Single-port robotic urological surgery using purpose-built single-port surgical system: single-institutional experience with the first 100 cases. Urology. 2020 Mar 3. pii: S0090-4295(20)30224-7. https://doi.org/10.1016/j.urology.2019.11.086
9. Hasson HM. A modified instrument and method for laparoscopy. Am J Obstet Gynecol. 1971 Jul 15;110(6):886–7. https://doi.org/10.1016/0002-9378(71)90593-x.
10. Kaouk J, Garisto J, Bertolo R. Robotic urologic surgical interventions performed with the single port dedicated platform: first clinical investigation. Eur Urol. 2019 Apr;75(4):684–691. https://doi.org/10.1016/j.eururo.2018.11.044. Epub 2018 Dec 3.
11. Ng CF, Teoh JY, Chiu PK, Yee CH, Chan CK, Hou SS, Kaouk J, Chan ES. Robot-assisted single-port radical prostatectomy: a phase 1 clinical study. Int J Urol. 2019 Sep;26(9):878–883. https://doi.org/10.1111/iju.14044. Epub 2019 Jun 30.
12. Agarwal DK, Sharma V, Toussi A, Viers BR, Tollefson MK, Gettman MT, Frank I. Initial experience with da vinci single-port robot-assisted radical prostatectomies. Eur Urol. 2020 Mar;77(3):373–379. https://doi.org/10.1016/j.eururo.2019.04.001. Epub 2019 Apr 19.
13. Dobbs RW, Halgrimson WR, Talamini S, Vigneswaran HT, Wilson JO, Crivellaro S. Single-port robotic surgery: the next generation of minimally invasive urology. World J Urol. 2020 Apr;38(4):897–905. https://doi.org/10.1007/s00345-019-02898-1. Epub 2019 Aug 28.
14. Kaouk J, Valero R, Sawczyn G, Garisto J. Extraperitoneal single-port robot-assisted radical prostatectomy: initial experience and

description of technique. BJU Int. 2020;125(1):182–9. https://doi.org/10.1111/bju.14885.

15. Dobbs RW, Halgrimson WR, Talamini S, et al. Single-port robotic surgery: the next generation of minimally invasive urology. World J Urol. 2020;38:897–905. https://doi.org/10.1007/s00345-019-02898-1.
16. Valero R, Sawczyn G, Garisto J, Yau R, Kaouk J. Multiquadrant combined robotic radical prostatectomy and left partial nephrectomy: a combined procedure by a single approach. Actas Urol Esp. 2020 Mar;44(2):119–124. English, Spanish. https://doi.org/10.1016/j.acuro.2019.06.004. Epub 2019 Dec 18.
17. Kim KH, Song W, Yoon H, Lee DH. Single-port robot-assisted radical prostatectomy with the da Vinci SP system: a single surgeon's experience. Investig Clin Urol. 2020;61(2):173–9. https://doi.org/10.4111/icu.2020.61.2.173.
18. Jones R, Dobbs RW, Halgrimson WR, Vigneswaran HT, Madueke I, Wilson J, Abern MR, Crivellaro S. Single port robotic radical prostatectomy with the da Vinci SP platform: a step by step approach. Can J Urol. 2020 Jun;27(3):10263–9.
19. Wilson CA, Aminsharifi A, Sawczyn G, Garisto JD, Yau R, Eltemamy M, Kim S, Lenfant L, Kaouk J. Outpatient extraperitoneal single-port robotic radical prostatectomy. Urology. 2020 Oct;144:142–146. https://doi.org/10.1016/j.urology.2020.06.029. Epub 2020 Jun 30.
20. Lenfant L, Sawczyn G, Aminsharifi A, Kim S, Wilson CA, Beksac AT, et al. Pure single-site robot-assisted radical prostatectomy using single-port versus multiport robotic radical prostatectomy: a single-institution comparative study. Eur Urol Focus. 2021;7(5):964–72. https://doi.org/10.1016/j.euf.2020.10.006.
21. Abaza R, Murphy C, Bsatee A, Brown DH Jr, Martinez O. Single-port robotic surgery allows same-day discharge in majority of cases. Urology. 2021 Feb;148:159–165. https://doi.org/10.1016/j.urology.2020.08.092. Epub 2020 Nov 17.
22. Moschovas MC, Bhat S, Sandri M, Rogers T, Onol F, Mazzone E, Roof S, Mottrie A, Patel V. Comparing the approach to radical prostatectomy using the multiport da Vinci Xi and da Vinci SP Robots: a propensity score analysis of perioperative outcomes. Eur Urol. 2021 Mar;79(3):393–404. https://doi.org/10.1016/j.eururo.2020.11.042. Epub 2020 Dec 24.
23. Talamini S, Halgrimson WR, Dobbs RW, Morana C, Crivellaro S. Single port robotic radical prostatectomy versus multiport robotic radical prostatectomy: a human factor analysis during the initial learning curve. Int J Med Robot. 2021 Apr;17(2):e2209. https://doi.org/10.1002/rcs.2209. Epub 2020 Dec 29.
24. Lenfant L, Garisto J, Sawczyn G, Wilson CA, Aminsharifi A, Kim S, Schwen Z, Bertolo R, Kaouk J. Robot-assisted radical prostatectomy using single-port perineal approach: technique and single-surgeon matched-paired comparative outcomes. Eur Urol. 2021 Mar;79(3):384–392. https://doi.org/10.1016/j.eururo.2020.12.013. Epub 2020 Dec 21.
25. Kaouk J, Beksac AT, Zeinab MA, Duncan A, Schwen ZR, Eltemamy M. Single port transvesical robotic radical prostatectomy: initial clinical experience and description of technique. Urology. 2021;155:130–7.
26. Covas Moschovas M, Bhat S, Onol FF, Rogers T, Roof S, Mazzone E, Mottrie A, Patel V. Modified apical dissection and lateral prostatic fascia preservation improves early postoperative functional recovery in robotic-assisted laparoscopic radical prostatectomy: results from a propensity score-matched analysis. Eur Urol. 2020 Dec;78(6):875–884. https://doi.org/10.1016/j.eururo.2020.05.041. Epub 2020 Jun 24.
27. Rocha MFH, Picanço Neto JM, Filgueira PHO, Coelho RF, Moschovas MC, Patel V. Robotic-assisted radical prostatectomy with preceptor's assistance: the training experience and outcomes in South America. J Robot Surg. 2021 Mar 24. https://doi.org/10.1007/s11701-021-01233-4. Epub ahead of print.
28. Kumar A, Patel VR, Panaiyadiyan S, Seetharam Bhat KR, Moschovas MC, Nayak B. Nerve-sparing robot-assisted radical prostatectomy: Current perspectives. Asian J Urol. 2021 Jan;8(1):2–13. https://doi.org/10.1016/j.ajur.2020.05.012. Epub 2020 Jun 11. PMID: 33569267; PMCID: PMC7859364.
29. Bhat KRS, Moschovas MC, Onol FF, Rogers T, Reddy SS, Corder C, Roof S, Patel VR. Evidence-based evolution of our robot-assisted laparoscopic prostatectomy (RALP) technique through 13,000 cases. J Robot Surg. 2020 Oct 10. https://doi.org/10.1007/s11701-020-01157-5. Epub ahead of print.
30. Rogers T, Bhat KRS, Moschovas M. Use of transversus abdominis plain block to decrease pain score and narcotic use following robotic-assisted laparoscopic radical prostatectomy. J Robot Surg. 2020 Apr 22; https://doi.org/10.1007/s11701-020-01064-9.
31. Rocco B, Cozzi G, Spinelli MG, Coelho RF, Patel VR, Tewari A, Wiklund P, Graefen M, Mottrie A, Gaboardi F, Gill IS, Montorsi F, Artibani W, Rocco F. Posterior musculofascial reconstruction after radical prostatectomy: a systematic review of the literature. Eur Urol. 2012 Nov;62(5):779–90. https://doi.org/10.1016/j.eururo.2012.05.041.
32. Valero R, Schatloff O, Chauhan S, HwiiKo Y, Sivaraman A, Coelho RF, Palmer KJ, Davila H, Patel VR. Bidirectional barbed suture for bladder neck reconstruction, posterior reconstruction and vesicourethral anastomosis during robot assisted radical prostatectomy. Actas Urol Esp. 2012 Feb;36(2):69–74.
33. Walsh PC. Anatomic radical retropubic prostatectomy. In: Walsh PC, Retik AB, Vaughan Jr ED, Wein AJ, editors. Campbell's urology, Chapter 86, vol. III. 7th ed. WB Saunders: Philadelphia; 1997. p. 2565–88.
34. Dindo D, Demartines N, Clavien PA. Classification of surgical complications: a new proposal with evaluation in a cohort of 6336 patients and results of a survey. Ann Surg. 2004;240(2):205–13.
35. Schaeffer E, Srinivas S, Antonarakis ES, Armstrong AJ, Bekelman JE, Cheng H, et al. NCCN guidelines insights: prostate cancer, version 1.2021. J Natl Compr Canc Netw. 2021;19(2):134–43.
36. Lenfant L, Kim S, Aminsharifi A, Sawczyn G, Kaouk J. Floating docking technique: a simple modification to improve the working space of the instruments during single-port robotic surgery. World J Urol. 2021;39(4):1299–305.
37. Tuğcu V, Akça O, Şimşek A, Yiğitbaşı İ, Şahin S, Yenice MG, et al. Robotic-assisted perineal versus transperitoneal radical prostatectomy: a matched-pair analysis. Turk J Urol. 2019;45(4):265–72.
38. Akca O, Zargar H, Kaouk JH. Robotic surgery revives radical perineal prostatectomy. Eur Urol. 2015;68(2):340–1.
39. Kaouk J, Sawczyn G, Wilson C, Aminsharifi A, Fareed K, Garisto J, et al. Single-port percutaneous transvesical simple prostatectomy using the sp robotic system: initial clinical experience. Urology. 2020;141:173–7.
40. Gandaglia G, Ploussard G, Valerio M, Mattei A, Fiori C, Fossati N, et al. A novel nomogram to identify candidates for extended pelvic lymph node dissection among patients with clinically localized prostate cancer diagnosed with magnetic resonance imaging-targeted and systematic biopsies. Eur Urol. 2019;75(3):506–14.

Textbook of Robotic Urologic Surgery: Retzius-Sparing Robot-Assisted Radical Prostatectomy

Stefano Tappero, Mattia Longoni, Paolo Dell'Oglio, Koon Ho Rha, Antonio Galfano, and Aldo Massimo Bocciardi

1 Background and Technical Rationale

Robot-assisted radical prostatectomy (RARP) is the gold standard for surgical removal of the prostate according to the European Association of Urology (EAU) and the American Urological Association (AUA) guidelines [1]. Since its first appearance in the early 2000s, RARP has undergone an incredible technical evolution, and several approaches were perfectionated in order to optimize the functional outcomes without affecting the oncological efficacy.

Retzius-sparing (RS) RARP was devised by Aldo Massimo Bocciardi at Cà Granda Niguarda Hospital in Milan in 2010, and since then more than 2000 cases have been operated by the Niguarda staff and several thousands in many centers throughout the world [2].

RS-RARP, as the Montsouris approach [3], begins with the incision of the retrovesical pouch, carrying out the subsequent whole prostatectomy through the Douglas space, avoiding bladder detachment, thereby minimizing surgical trauma and preserving normal pelvic anatomy maximally.

The main strength points of RS-RARP are the rapidity of execution, the low complication rates, and the remarkable functional results, certainly due to the anatomical respect of the surrounding structures, in particular the Santorini plexus, the pubo-prostatic ligaments, and the endopelvic fascia [4, 5].

This posterior approach has been standardized for all stages of prostate cancer as first-line or salvage treatment, achieving to be included among the treatment surgical options for prostate cancer by the EAU 2020 guidelines.

S. Tappero (✉) · M. Longoni · P. Dell'Oglio · A. Galfano
A. M. Bocciardi
Urology Unit, Niguarda Hospital, Milan, Italy

K. H. Rha
Department of Urology, Yonsei University, Seoul, South Korea

2 Surgical Technique

2.1 Patient Positioning and Port Placement

Proper patient positioning is of utmost importance. A 25 to 30 degrees Trendelenburg position yields an easy access to the pelvis for robotic arms and displaces the bowels cranially. Patient's arms are fixed along the body. A patient support and non-slipping surfaces prevent the sliding of the patient towards the head of the table while appropriate devices avoid the traction of the brachial plexus.

The Da Vinci robot can be front-docked with legs spread with the Si system, or side-docked with both the Si and Xi.

In non-operated patients, a Veress needle is inserted to induce the pneumoperitoneum, whereas a standard Hasson technique is used in patients with suspect of adhesions. Figure 1 depicts port placement: main operative arms are accommodated through 8-mm trocars with the monopolar scissors on the right and the bipolar Maryland on the lateral left arm. The grasper (usually a Cadiere forceps) is kept in

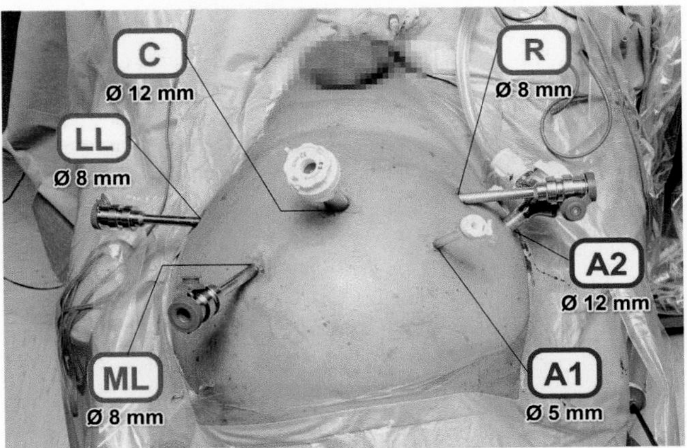

Fig. 1 Port placement. *C* camera, *R* right robotic arm carrying monopolar scissors/large needle driver, *ML* medial left robotic arm carrying the Cadiere forceps, *LL* lateral left robotic arm carrying the Maryland, *A1* left assistant arm, *A2* right assistant arm

P. Wiklund et al. (eds.), *Robotic Urologic Surgery*, https://doi.org/10.1007/978-3-031-00363-9_25

the medial left arm, making mostly upwards and downwards tractions. The latero-umbilical 12-mm trocar is for the 30° lens camera, placed downwards during the initial steps and upwards after the dissection of the seminal vesicles. A 12-mm and a 5-mm table-side assistant ports are placed on the right side. For the initial port placement, the intraabdominal pressure can be raised to 20 mmHg and then reduced to 12–15 mmHg in order to lower the chance of bowel injuries.

2.2 Pansadoro Stitch

In order to expand the surgical field and to reduce the risk of bowel damage, after freeing adhesions of the sigma and left colon, a stay suture with an Ethilon 2-0 straight needle, coming from the 5-mm assistant port and making tension on the epiploic appendices, helps retracting the colon backwards and straightens the rectum (Fig. 2).

2.3 Seminal Vesicles Approach and Transabdominal Stitches

To further increase the surgical field, we strongly recommend placing two transabdominal suprapubic stitches that lift and support the bladder and retract the seminal vesicles.

The grasper lifts up the peritoneum covering the bladder and a peritoneotomy at the anterior surface of the Douglas space is performed; the vas deferens are identified and transected, always bearing in mind that the distal ureter is behind (Fig. 3). The seminal vesicles are carefully dissected until the prostatic base is identified. Two transabdominal prepubic Ethilon 2-0 stitches are positioned laterally at the level of the deferens incision in order to stably lift the bladder and improve the space in the surgical field (Fig. 4).

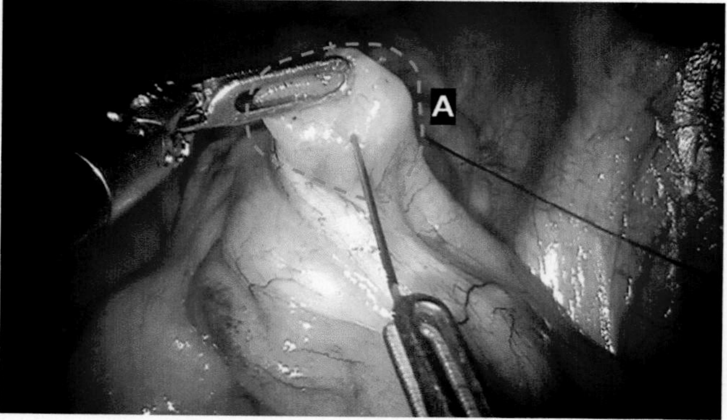

Fig. 2 Pansadoro stich. *A* epiploic appendix

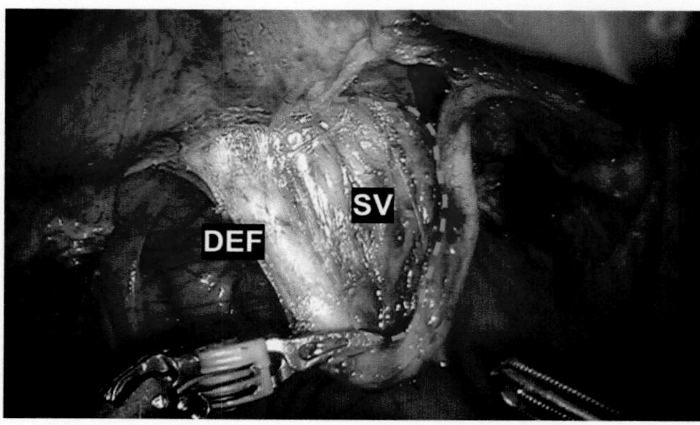

Fig. 3 Dissection of the seminal vesicles. *DEF* vas deferens, *SV* seminal vesicle

2.4 Posterior Prostate Dissection

With a 30° upwards scope, the nerve-sparing level has to be chosen according to the oncological safety and functional needs. The deferenses are lifted upwards by the Cadiere grasper, and the Denonvillier's fascia is separated by the postero-lateral surface of the prostate in an antegrade direction, approximating to the prostatic capsule in order to reach an inter- or intrafascial plane.

A good strategy for finding the desired plane is to start the incision of the Denonvillier's fascia from the midline where less vessels are present, and the plane is clearer (Fig. 5). The grasper traction is moved towards left or right in order to improve lateral exposition and to allow blunt dissection of the lateral aspects of the prostate. In case of adherences, palpable disease or doubts, the surgeon can choose to follow wider dissection planes. After dissection of the prostatic pedicles, laterally to the prostate, a dissection with clips is carried out until the levator ani muscle is identified.

2.5 Anterior Prostate and Bladder Neck Dissection and Removal of the Prostate

The prostate is pushed downwards by the grasper, and the vesicoprostatic junction is identified. The bladder neck is approached starting from its dorsal surface, where a layer represented by the vesicoprostatic muscle covers the circular muscle fibers of the bladder. These fibers can be bluntly dissected and laterally separated from the prostate as far as possible before opening the bladder neck (Fig. 6).

Carefully surrounding the anterior surface of the bladder neck with the bipolar Maryland forceps, the surgeon increases the width of the field and improves the visibility of this structure that otherwise would be hidden. Two quickly absorbable 3-0 stay stitches at 6 and 12 o'clock in the bladder neck help fixing the mucosa and easily recognizing both starting and

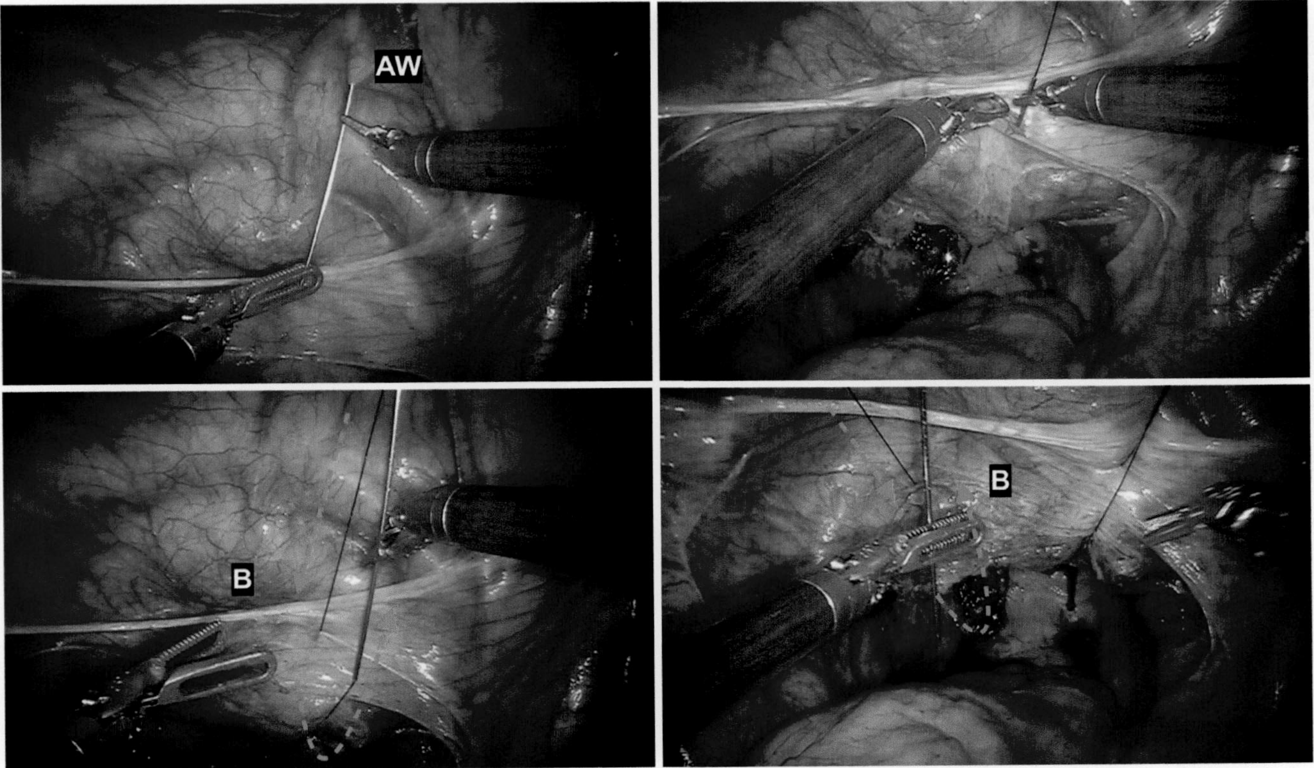

Fig. 4 Transabdominal stiches positioning. *AW* abdominal wall, *B* bladder

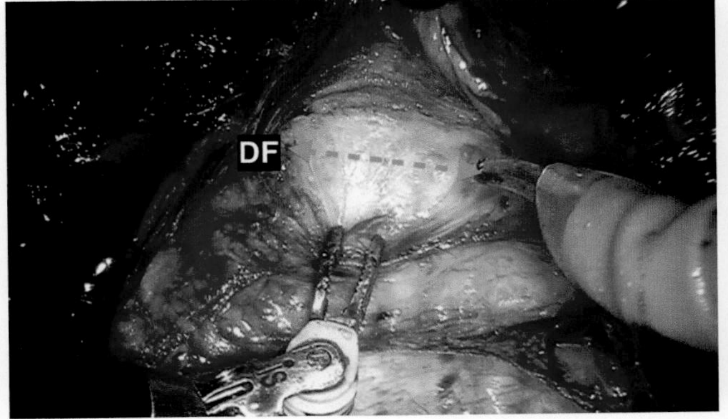

Fig. 5 Incision of the Denonvillier's fascia. *DF* Denonvillier's fascia

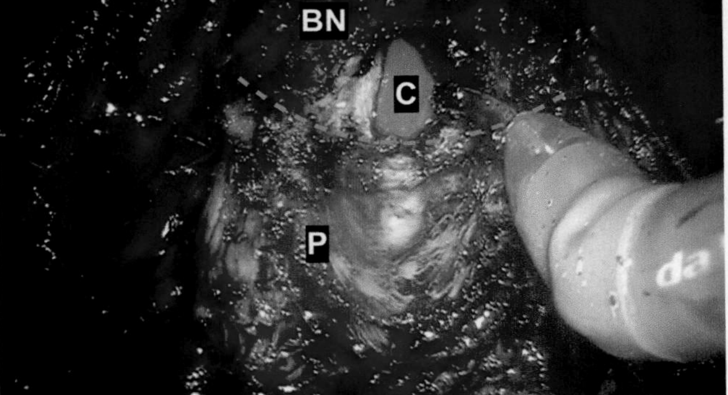

Fig. 6 Bladder neck dissection. *P* prostate, *C* vesical catheter, *BN* bladder neck

ending points of the anastomosis, especially useful in case of small bladder neck.

The anterior surface of the prostate is bluntly isolated from the Santorini plexus without any incision.

In case of dorsal plexus bleeding irrigation with saline water or with glycine solution, instead of suction, allows improved vision. In case of locally advanced anterior prostate cancer, the Santorini plexus can be partially or completely resected. The apex is isolated, and the urethra is incised (Fig. 7). The prostate is positioned into an endobag.

2.6 Vesico-Urethral Anastomosis and Suprapubic Tube Placement

A standard van Velthoven modified anastomosis, starting from 12 o'clock, is the commonly adopted technique at our center (Fig. 8). Using two separated 3-0 barbed stitches, the suture starts from the 12 o'clock position up to the left anterior lateral quarter. The right half circle of the suture is carried out up to 6 o'clock, and the last posterior left quarter is then completed from 9 to 6 o'clock.

To check the water tightness of the anastomosis the bladder is filled with 250–300 cc saline. At this point, the transurethral catheter is removed, and a suprapubic tube is placed by the assistant under direct vision. Since its introduction in our daily practice, this maneuver has been encountered favor for it improves patient's comfort, reduces the probability of involuntary tractions on the anastomosis and does not correlates with higher complication rates when compared to transurethral catheterization. Major contraindications are bladder cancer history and non-watertight anastomosis.

3 The Niguarda Experience

3.1 Perioperative Outcomes

Niguarda Hospital recently turned eleven years of experience in RS-RARP with more than 2000 procedures carried out by nine surgeons, each one on his personal learning curve. The mean prostatectomy console time of the entire equìpe settled at 103 minutes with a mean blood loss rounding 230 ml and, therefore, almost no need for intra-operative transfusions. Major intra-operative complications were principally due to trocar port placement, lysis of adhesions and lymph adenectomy while few directly related to the prostatectomy (Table 1).

Table 2 reports all the 30-d complications recorded in our single institutional series according to the Clavien Dindo classification and the EAU standardized complications reporting system.

Only one procedure was converted to open prostatectomy due to severe respiratory insufficiency.

In the second post-operative day 83.8% of patients were discharged while 5.2% stayed in hospital more than 7 days.

3.2 Oncological Outcomes

When we stratified the entire population according to EAU risk categorization, we found 34.6% of low risk, 44.8% of intermediate risk and 20.6% of high risk and locally advanced PCa patients.

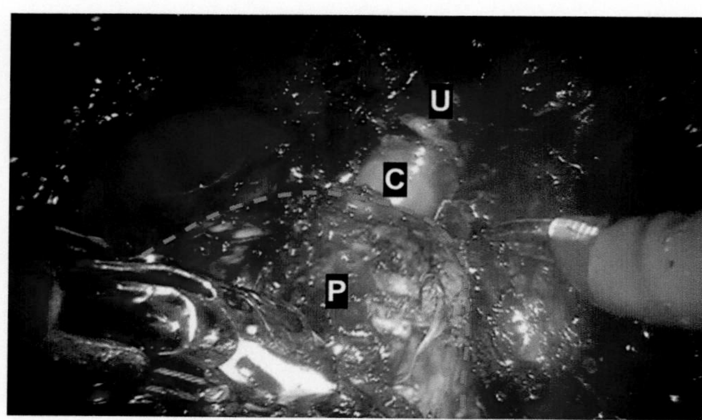

Fig. 7 Final dissection of the prostate apex. *P* prostate, *C* vesical catheter, *U* urethra

Table 1 Intraoperative complications of patients with complete intraoperative data

OVERALL COMPLICATIONS (n = 34–1,8%)			
SURGICAL STEP	TYPE OF COMPLICATION	n	%
Trocar positioning	Injury of the epigastric artery	8	0.4
	Partial lesion of small intestine	1	0.06
Lysis of adhesions	Partial lesion of the colon	2	0.1
	Partial lesion of small intestine	1	0.06
Prostatectomy	Rectal injury	1	0.06
Lymph nodes dissection	Injury of the right external iliac vein	2	0.1
	Injury of the left external iliac vein	1	0.06
	Injury of the left internal iliac artery	2	0.1
	Injury of the left internal iliac vein	1	0.06
	Injury of the right gluteal vein	1	0.06
	Partial injury of the right ureter	4	0.2
	Partial injury of the left ureter	2	0.1
	Complete dissection of the left obturator nerve	1	0.06
	Injury of the bladder nearby right ureteral orifice	2	0.1
	Injury of the bladder below the bladder neck	5	0.3

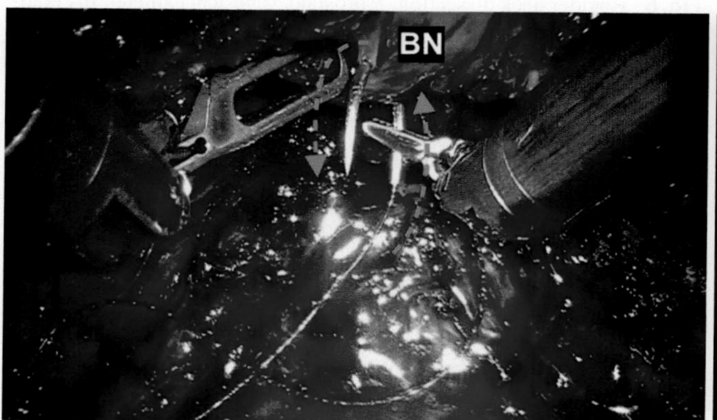

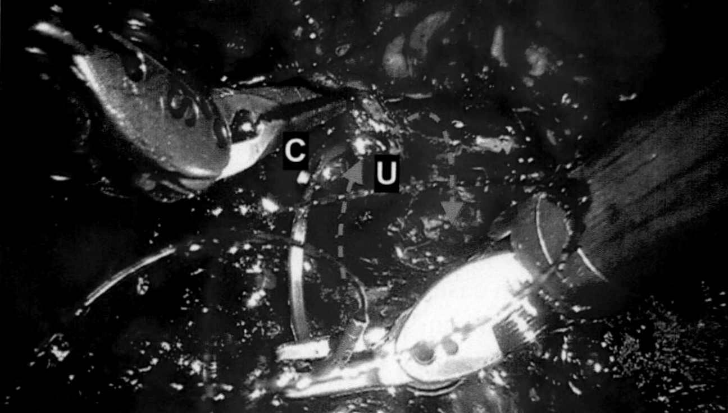

Fig. 8 Vesico-urethral anastomosis. *BN* bladder neck, *C* vesical catheter, *U* urethra

Table 2 Postoperative complications of patients with complete 30-d from surgery data

OVERALL COMPLICATIONS (n = 177 on 141 patients – 9.3%)			
CATEGORY	TYPE OF COMPLICATION	n	%
Clavien Dindo II	Urinary tract infection requiring ABT	26	1.4
	TEP	7	0.4
	DVT	21	1.1
	Post-operative transfusions	33	1.7
Clavien Dindo IIIa	Lymphocele treated with percutaneous drainage	53	2.8
	Acute urinary retention requiring bladder catheterization	29	1.5
Clavien Dindo IIIb	Abdominal hematoma treated with explorative laparotomy and revision of the ureterovesical anastomosis	1	0.01
	Videolaparoscopic removal of needle fragment in pelvic area	1	0.01
	Surgical correction of laparocele	12	0.6
Clavien Dindo V	Death caused by massive pulmonary embolism <30-d from RS-RARP	1	0.01

Overall positive surgical margins (PSM) rate was 26.8%, ranging from 15.2% in pT2 patients to 42.8% in pT3a-b patients. In 76% of cases, PSMs were associated with an ISUP grade tumor ≥3 and the prostate apex resulted as the most common PSM site (26.6%).

Focusing on the high-risk PCa patients, PSM rate raised at 28.8%, with almost the 33% being represented by focal PSMs. Through 47 months of follow-up, 27.7% and 25.9% of these high-risk patients, respectively, needed for adjuvant and salvage treatment.

Overall biochemical disease-free survival (BDFS) was 83.4%, moving from 94.6% in low risk to 64.7% in high-risk PCa patients.

3.3 Urinary Continence Recovery

A recent systematic review of the current literature recognized the SR-RARP superiority, when compared to the standard approach, in terms of urinary continence recovery (UCR) at 1, 3, 6 and 12 months from surgery [6], where continence is meant as no need for safety pad or the use of one 24 hours dry safety pad.

In our complete series, at 7 days from surgery the catheter was removed in around 78% of patients with an acute urinary retention rate of 1.6%.

Functional results obviously depended on the oncological reproducibility of an anatomically nerve sparing surgery. The Pasadena Consensus Conference recommendations in defining full-, partial-, and non-nerve-sparing procedures were taken into account for every single procedure [7].

Stratifying the cohort of patients according to the EAU oncological class of risk, immediate UCR rates settled at 92, 90 and 71% for low, intermediate and high-risk PCa patients, slightly increasing when only considering <65 years old men (95, 94 and 75% respectively). At 12 months of follow-up almost 98% of low and intermediate-risk patients could be considered fully continent and so for the 85% of the high-risk PCa patients.

When we considered the patients according to the exploited nerve-sparing technique, we found a 93, 79 and 70% of immediate UCR rate for full-, partial- and non-nerve-sparing RS-RARP patients, rising at 98, 90 and 82% at 12 months from surgery, respectively.

3.4 Erectile Function Recovery

At a median follow-up of 47 months, 47.7% of our complete series patients were potent, of whom 40% spontaneously.

Identifying the <65 years-old preoperatively potent patients undergoing full intrafascial nerve-sparing RS-RARP, a sexual intercourse within 30 days from surgery was recorded in almost one out of two men. At twelve months, the 79% of this selected population achieved a complete EF recovery.

4 State of Art of the Posterior Approach around the World

At the beginning of 2021, it was performed a well-detailed resume of the oncological and functional outcomes of several published RS-RARP series performed throughout the world, ranging from 30 to more than 600 patients (Table 3) [8].

Turning eleven years since its first description RS-RARP is now spreading worldwide, and it is noteworthy that the current Literature amounts more than 80 articles disguising about this technique, emphasizing its technical feasibility, oncological safety and functional reliability.

Table 3 Results of the *Bocciardi Approach* around the World

Author, year	Country	Patients (n)	Follow up	BDFS (%)	PSM (%)	UCR (%)	EF (%)
Lim et al. 2014 [9]	South Korea	50	4 weeks	NR	14	1-mo: 70	NA
Dalela et al. 2017 [10]	USA	60	3 months	91	11.7	2-mo: 88	NA
Sayyid et al. 2017 [11]	USA	100	12 months	NR	≤T2 16.7 >T3 47.1	12-mo mean n. PPD: 1.5	NA
Chang et al. 2018 [12]	Taiwan	30	12 months	86.7	23.3	12-mo: 100	NA
Eden et al. 2018 [13]	UK	40	4 weeks	NR	T2: 16.7 T3: 31.8	4-w: 90	NA
Menon et al. 2018 [14]	USA	60	12 months	83.8	Focal: 13.3 Non-focal: 11.7	12-mo: 98.3	12-mo: 86.5
Asimakopoulos et al. 2019 [15]	Italy	45	6 months	91.4	T2: 19 T3: 41.2	6-mo: 90.5	NA
Lee et al. 2020 [16]	South Korea	609	6 months	NR	T2: 11 T3: 36	6-mo: 90.5	NA
Egan et al. 2020 [17]	USA	70	12 months	87,1	Focal: 27.1 Non-focal: 7.1	12-mo: 97.6	12-mo: 65,7
Umari et al. 2021 [18]	UK, Italy	282	12 months	98,6	15.6	Immediate: 70.4	Immediate: 13.2

BDFS Biochemical disease-free survival, *PSM* positive surgical margins, *UCR* urinary continence recovery, *EF* erectile function, *PPD* pads per-day

References

1. European Association of Urology. Oncology Guidelines. Treatment: Prostate Cancer; 2020.
2. Galfano A, et al. A new anatomic approach for robot-assisted laparoscopic prostatectomy: a feasibility study for completely intrafascial surgery. Eur Urol. 2010 Sep;58(3):457–61.
3. Guillonneau B, et al. Laparoscopic radical prostatectomy: the Montsouris technique. J Urol. 2000 Jun;163(6):1643–9.
4. Walsh PC, et al. Impotence following radical prostatectomy: insight into etiology and prevention. J Urol. 1982 Sep;128(3):492–7.
5. Walz J, et al. A critical analysis of the current knowledge of surgical anatomy related to optimization of cancer control and preservation of continence and erection in candidates for radical prostatectomy. Eur Urol. 2010 Feb;57(2):179–92.
6. Checcucci E, et al. Retzius-sparing robot-assisted radical prostatectomy vs the standard approach: a systematic review and analysis of comparative outcomes. BJU Int. 2020 Jan;125(1):8–16.
7. Montorsi F, Wilson TG, Rosen RC, Ahlering TE, Artibani W, Carroll PR, et al. Best practices in robot-assisted radical prostatectomy: recommendations of the Pasadena consensus panel. Eur Urol. 2012 Sep;62(3):368–81.
8. Davis M, et al. Retzius-sparing robot-assisted robotic prostatectomy: past, present, and future. Urol Clin North Am. 2021 Feb;48(1):11–23.
9. Lim SK, et al. Retzius-sparing robot-assisted laparoscopic radical prostatectomy: combining the best of retropubic and perineal approaches. BJU Int. 2014 Aug;114(2):236–44.
10. Dalela D, et al. A pragmatic randomized controlled trial examining the impact of the Retzius-sparing approach on early urinary continence recovery after robot-assisted radical prostatectomy. Eur Urol. 2017 Nov;72(5):677–85.
11. Sayyd RK, et al. Retzius-sparing robotic-assisted laparoscopic radical prostatectomy: a safe surgical technique with superior continence outcomes. J Endourol. 2017 Dec;31(12):1244–50.
12. Chang LW, et al. Retzius-sparing robotic-assisted radical prostatectomy associated with less bladder neck descent and better early continence outcome. Anticancer Res. 2018 Jan;38(1):345–51.
13. Eden CG, et al. Urinary continence four weeks following Retzius-sparing robotic radical prostatectomy: The UK experience. J Clin Urol. 2018;11(1):15–20.
14. Menon M, et al. Functional recovery, oncologic outcomes and postoperative complications after robot-assisted radical prostatectomy: an evidence-based analysis comparing the Retzius sparing and standard approaches. J Urol. 2018 May;199(5):1210–7.
15. Asimakopoulos AD, et al. Retzius-sparing versus standard robot-assisted radical prostatectomy: a prospective randomized comparison on immediate continence rates. Surg Endosc. 2019 Jul;33(7):2187–96.
16. Lee J, et al. Retzius sparing robot-assisted radical prostatectomy conveys early regain of continence over conventional robot-assisted radical prostatectomy: a propensity score matched analysis of 1,863 patients. J Urol. 2020 Jan;203(1):137–44.
17. Egan J. et al. Retzius-sparing robot-assisted radical prostatectomy leads to durable improvement in urinary function and quality of life versus standard robot-assisted radical prostatectomy without compromise on oncologic efficacy: single-surgeon series and step-by-step guide. Eur Urol. 2020 Jun 11; Ahead of print.
18. Umari P, et al. Retzius sparing versus standard robot-assisted radical prostatectomy: a comparative prospective study of nearly 500 patients. J Urol. 2021 Mar;205(3):780–90.

Extraperitoneal Robot-Assisted Radical Prostatectomy

Pratik M. S. Gurung,
Vinodh-Kumar-Adithyaa Arthanareeswaran,
Jens-Uwe Stolzenburg, and Jean V. Joseph

1 Introduction

Prostate cancer is the most common solid malignancy in the United States (US) and most western countries [1, 2]. The definitive surgical extirpation for the majority of localized prostate cancer cases, in eligible men, involves radical prostatectomy (RP), with or without pelvic lymph node dissection (PLND), dependent on clinical risk parameters [3, 4]. Although "open" RP and laparoscopic RP are still performed worldwide, the introduction of robot-assisted radical prostatectomy (RARP), about 20 years ago in Europe and the US, and its subsequent rapid adoption worldwide, has meant that RARP is currently considered the standard of care in most developed countries [5–9].

With respect to RARP, there are a multitude of techniques described in the literature [10]. However, based on the method of abdominal/pelvic access to the prostate, RARP can be broadly classified into either transperitoneal (T-RARP) or extraperitoneal (E-RARP) approaches. T-RARP is by far the most commonly performed technique. E-RARP is a less commonly used technique, owing to its perceived technical difficulty and potentially longer learning curve. The extraperitoneal (EP) approach, however, has its merits, particularly in cases where intraperitoneal access may be problematic [10, 11].

Both T-RARP and E-RARP can be performed using either the conventional multi-port (MP) robotic system or the more recent single-port (SP) robotic system [12–14]. With respect to E-RARP, it is felt that the SP system may lend itself particularly well, with purported advantages in terms of better cosmesis, less post-operative analgesic and opioid requirements, and shorter duration of hospital stay [15, 16].

Herein, we will summarize the history of the endoscopic extraperitoneal (EP) approach to radical prostatectomy touching on the salient points of its evolution in the laparoscopic era and subsequent transition into robotics utilizing the multi-port (mp) robotic platform in the last few decades, and more recently, over the last few years, its application using the single-port (sp) robotic platform.

P. M. S. Gurung
Department of Urology, University of Rochester Medical Center, Rochester, NY, USA

Department of Urology, Om Hospital and Research Center, Kathmandu, Nepal

V.-K.-A. Arthanareeswaran · J. U. Stolzenburg
Department of Urology, University of Leipzig, Leipzig, Germany

J.-U. Joseph (✉)
Department of Urology, University of Rochester Medical Center, Rochester, NY, USA

2 History of Radical Prostatectomy with Focus on the Extraperitoneal Approach

2.1 The Beginnings of Radical Prostatectomy

The beginnings of radical prostatectomy date back to the nineteenth century and were based on the experience of partial or complete enucleation of the prostate for prostatic hyperplasia [17]. At that time, prostate cancer had a poor prognosis due to lack of curative treatment options. In 1867, the surgeon Billroth, in Vienna, reported two radical prostatectomies performed through a perineal approach [18]. This was followed in 1883 by Leisring (student of Langenbeck) with the first radical prostatectomy without vesiculectomy. However, the patient survived the procedure only for a short time [19]. The prostatectomy procedure did not achieve a breakthrough until the beginning of the twentieth century when Young (1905) and Proust (1901) described perineal prostatectomy for the treatment of prostate cancer and introduced it into clinical practice [20, 21]. Young additionally removed seminal vesicles, both distal vas deferens and the bladder neck. A decisive advancement in 1945 was the introduction of the retropubic approach to the prostate favored by Millin, which also allowed simultaneous lymphadenectomy [22].

P. Wiklund et al. (eds.), *Robotic Urologic Surgery*, https://doi.org/10.1007/978-3-031-00363-9_26

A general problem with these surgical methods was the extensive intraoperative blood loss, possibly as a result of the lack of understanding of periprostatic anatomy and the high incidence of locally advanced, as opposed to curable organ-confined, tumors at the time. In the early stages, v. Frisch reported up to 30% operative deaths [23]. Removal of the prostatic urethra was initially thought to be the cause of long-term complications such as incontinence and impotence. Only one publication by Wildbolz in 1927 showed the importance of muscular structures on the pelvic floor for continence [24].

2.2 The Anatomically Appropriate Nerve-Sparing Radical Prostatectomy

In the 1980s and 1990s, there was an increase in radical prostatectomies. With the determination and increasing use of prostate specific antigen (PSA) as a serum tumor marker, early stages of prostate cancer were diagnosed more frequently. Further development of the surgical techniques was done by Walsh, who had been intensively involved in radical prostatectomy since the 1970s. Walsh noticed the lack of understanding of many surgeons regarding periprostatic anatomy. This resulted in dissection that was not very true to the anatomy. Little attention was paid to the course of blood vessels and nerves and the sphincter muscle, resulting in a high rate of complications (high blood loss, incontinence, impotence, etc.). Reiner and Walsh described targeted ligation of the dorsal penile vein and Santorini plexus to limit blood loss [25]. Building on the observations of a patient who reported a spontaneous erection 3 months after radical prostatectomy, he began studying the anatomic basis. Walsh met Pieter Donker, a urologist with interest in anatomy, at a conference in Leiden in 1981. During joint anatomical studies, they found that the nerves for erection ran in a dorsolateral vascular nerve bundle outside the prostatic capsule [26]. Walsh applied this finding to his surgical technique and was the first to describe the so-called anatomically nerve-sparing radical prostatectomy in 1983 [27]. By ligating the dorsal venous plexus, intraoperative blood loss decreased, sparing of the external sphincter achieved better continence, and subtle dissection of the vascular nerve bundles ultimately resulted in improved preservation of erectile function [28].

2.3 The Onset of Laparoscopic Prostatectomy

Following introduction of laparoscopic techniques into surgery through the first cholecystectomy, the first laparoscopic operations were extended to urology (varicocele resection, pelvic lymphadenectomy, nephrectomy). Schüssler was the first to report laparoscopic radical prostatectomy in 1991. He operated on a total of nine patients from September 1991 to May 1995 using this method with an average operation time of 580 min and concluded that laparoscopic radical prostatectomy, although feasible, offered no advantages over open surgery [29]. While Schüssler performed prostatectomy in only nine patients laparoscopically in a period of 44 months, a French research group from Bordeaux, led by Richard Gaston, developed a standardized technique of laparoscopic transperitoneal radical prostatectomy (LRPE) in 1998 and introduced it into clinical practice in a very short time. Based on this technique, a research group from Paris, led by Guillonneau and Vallancien, published a first series of 28 LRPE in 1998 [30]. Guillonneau and Vallancien showed that laparoscopic radical prostatectomy could be performed by an experienced team with acceptable operating times. The average operation time was 270 min, and they continuously improved the technique, which is now known as the "Montsouris technique." The oncologic and functional results were comparable to the conventional method [31]. In Germany, the first robot-assisted laparoscopic prostatectomy using the da Vinci system was performed in 2001 by Binder and Kramer from Frankfurt [6]. In 2001, Abbou et al., in France, reported their first case of RARP [5]. At a similar time, in the US, Menon et al. were performing a significant number of RARP cases, transperitoneally, and were describing their technique and outcomes of T-RARP in a series of 50 patients in 2002 [32].

2.4 The Development of Endoscopic Extraperitoneal Radical Prostatectomy

For the first time, Raboy performed a laparoscopic radical prostatectomy in a patient in 1997 using a primarily extraperitoneal (rather than transperitoneal) approach [33]. Further development and standardization of the extraperitoneal technique was performed by Bollens et al. and Stolzenburg et al. [34, 35] Bollens et al. reported the results of 50 patients in 2001. The average operative time was 317 min with four operators. The oncologic and functional outcomes were comparable to laparoscopic and open procedures [34]. Thus, a procedure was developed that combined the advantages of laparoscopy (less invasiveness, less morbidity, faster convalescence, minimal blood loss, good intraoperative vision) with the experience of classic open retropubic prostatectomy. Intraperitoneal complications (bowel injury, intraperitoneal bleeding, intraperitoneal urine leakage) was thereby avoided. Stolzenburg demonstrated the feasibility of the method in 20 patients in 2002. With an average operative time of 170 min, no intraoperative or early post-operative complications occurred [35]. With growing experience and standardization of surgical technique, Stolzenburg established this as the endoscopic extraperitoneal radical prostatectomy (EERPE) technique [36].

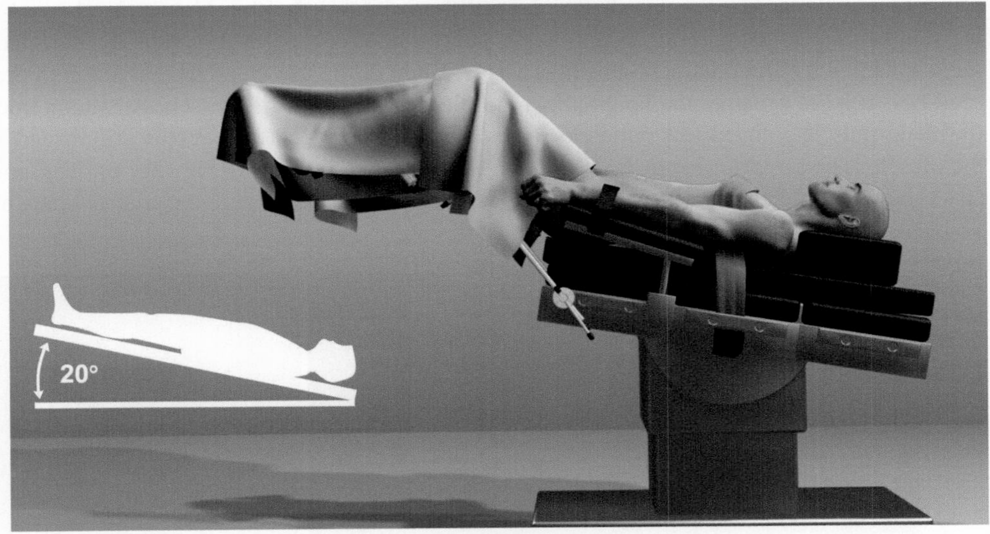

Fig. 1 This diagrammatic image demonstrates the patient positioned with a 20° head down tilt

The focus for improvement of this surgical technique continued on the protection of the so-called vascular nerve bundle. Studies by Kiyoshima show that the neurovascular bundles run dorsolateral to the prostate in only 48% of cases, and in 52% of cases the neurovascular structures are on the lateral side of the prostate [37]. With strictly ventral incision of the periprostatic fascia, preservation of the endopelvic fascia and puboprostatic ligaments, the laterally located nervous structures could be spared [35]. Around the same time, two surgeons presented this technique: described by Menon (Dec 2005) as preservation of the "veil of Aphrodite" and by Stolzenburg (Jan 2006) as "intrafascial nerve-sparing" technique, and both techniques reported significant improvements in early continence and potency outcomes [38, 39].

The robot-assisted approach to radical prostatectomy was adopted initially in centers with significant experience in non-robotic laparoscopic RP or open RP [40]. The interest in robotic prostatectomy has increased exponentially over the years. The technique of robotic prostatectomy is standardized using either a transperitoneal or an extraperitoneal approach [32, 41, 42]. The first patient blinded randomized trial, in Germany, involving 782 patients comparing LRPE and robot-assisted RP was conducted by Stolzenburg et al. [43] The study involved patients who underwent both extraperitoneal and transperitoneal RP. Significantly better earlier return to continence was achieved in the robot-assisted group.

3 Endoscopic Extraperitoneal Approach Adapted to Robot-Assisted Radical Prostatectomy: Emphasis on Port Placement

Endoscopic Extraperitoneal Radical Prostatectomy (EERPE) provides access to the prostate without entering the peritoneal cavity [44, 45]. This may minimize the bowel-related complications that occur with transperitoneal approach [46–48]. Nevertheless, the decision between a transperitoneal or extraperitoneal access to robot-assisted prostatectomy is based on the surgeon's preference and patient status. Today, we predominantly see the indication for extraperitoneal access in patients where we perform nerve-sparing prostatectomy without PLND.

3.1 Patient Positioning

The patient is placed in a classical Trendelenburg position—for the so-called side docking, or in a dorsal supine position with the legs slightly abducted to allow the positioning of the robot between them. A 10–20° head down tilt is sufficient (Fig. 1) for performing the procedure since the bowel does not interfere as in the transperitoneal approach where a 30° head down tilt is often used. The patient is secured on the table with a chest belt and ankle straps. Caution should be made not to exert too much tension and the belt should serve only to stabilize the patient. Both arms of the patient are placed close to the patient's body.

3.2 Development of the Extraperitoneal Space and Insertion of Trocar 1 (Optic Trocar)

The first step of the procedure is to create a preperitoneal space and placement of the first trocar. A 15-mm infraumbilical incision is made 1 cm below and lateral to the right of the umbilicus (right paraumbilical incision, J-US, University of Leipzig; left paraumbilical incision, JVJ, University of Rochester). It is preferred not to go in the midline in order to avoid the linea alba adhesions and inadvertent entry into the peritoneal cavity. A blunt dissection is performed up to the anterior rectus sheath. A small horizontal incision is made in the anterior rectus sheath and this opening is enlarged by blunt dissection using scissors. Blunt dissection is used to separate the longitudinal muscle fibers of the rectus muscle. Langenbeck retractors are used to separate the muscle. The posterior rectus fascia is then exposed. The space between the rectus muscle and the posterior rectus sheath is bluntly developed by finger dissection in the direction of the preperitoneal space. Care should be taken not to use vigorous dissection in order to avoid damage to the epigastric vessels. A balloon trocar is introduced superior to the posterior rectus sheath and insufflated under direct visual control (Fig. 2b, c). The posterior rectus sheath is absent inferior to the arcuate line which leads to creation of the pre-

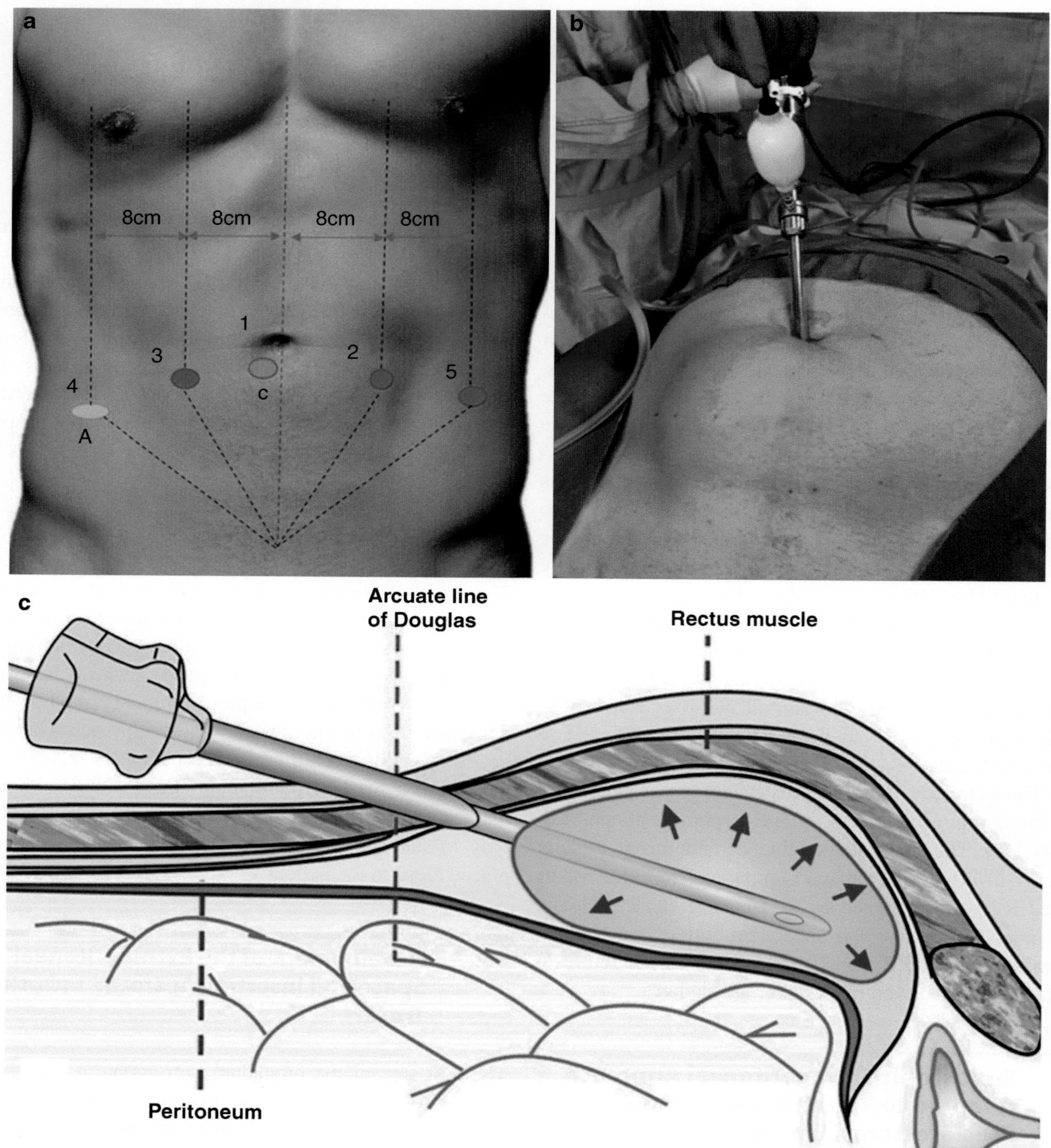

Fig. 2 (**a**) This schematic drawing summarizes the position of all the trocars with the sequence of placement 1–5. The imaginary lines are helpful for orientation (umbilicus, pararectal line, anterior superior iliac spine with 8-cm distance between the lines). A—assistant trocar, C—camera trocar. (**b**) A balloon-optic trocar is introduced superior to the posterior rectus sheath and insufflated under direct visual control. (**c**) The layers of the abdominal wall are shown. After identifying the posterior rectus sheath, the space between the rectus muscle and the posterior rectus sheath is bluntly developed by finger dissection in the direction of the preperitoneal space

peritoneal space. The epigastric vessels are seen ventrally, compressed by the inflated balloon. The pubic arch becomes visible toward the end of the dissection. The balloon trocar is removed and stay sutures are then placed on either end of the anterior rectus sheath incision. A Hasson type balloon—optic port is introduced and fixed (trocar number 1) for the camera (Fig. 2c). We normally use a 30° camera facing downward, which can be easily rotated upward to see the ventral structures. Alternatively, a 0° camera can be used.

3.3 Insertion of the Remaining Trocars

3.3.1 Placement of Trocar 2

After insufflation with CO2 (12-mmHg), an 8-mm trocar (trocar number 2) is positioned 4 fingertips left and lateral to the midline as high as possible. Conventional laparoscopic instruments are used for the gradual extension of the extraperitoneal space to both sides in an attempt to create more space for the insertion of the lateral right and left trocars. Alternatively, the finger can be used with careful sweeping moves to develop this space and the trocar can be inserted using the guidance of the index finger (Fig. 3a).

3.3.2 Placement of Trocar 3

An 8-mm trocar (trocar number 4, arm-1) is placed in the right pararectal line (on the same theoretical line from the spine to the umbilicus) taking care to avoid injury of the epigastric vessels. Injury to the epigastric vessels can be caused during insertion of the fourth trocar (pararectal line, right iliac fossa). For this reason, it is the most dangerous trocar for bleeding. Injury to the epigastric vessels can be avoided by careful inspection of the abdominal wall with the camera before trocar insertion. The third trocar position can be varied medially or laterally aiming to avoid epigastric vessel injury. Alternatively, the index finger dissection technique can be used to place this trocar (Fig. 3b).

3.3.3 Placement of Trocar 4

A 12-mm assisting trocar (trocar number 3) is then positioned two fingers medial and superior to the right anterior superior iliac spine. This line is used as a guide, but the port is ideally placed superior to this. It will vary slightly from patient to patient, but it should be placed as superior as the free edge of peritoneum allows. Trocar 2 must be used to further develop the extraperitoneal space using blunt dissection. This port is used by the bedside assistant for suction. Furthermore, clips as well as needles are inserted and extracted through this trocar.

3.3.4 Placement of Trocar 5

For port placement, the left iliac fossa/left preperitoneal space is dissected through one of the other trocars. An 8-mm trocar (trocar number 5, arm-3) is placed approximately three fingers' breadth medial to and superior to the left anterior superior iliac spine (just above a hypothetical line from the anterior superior iliac spine to the umbilicus). It is important to avoid placement too distally from or too close to the iliac spine, because this can cause problems during apical dissection and anastomosis. The insertion of this arm in the extraperitoneal approach is cumbersome since the caudal positioning of the trocars limits the space for robotic arm movements.

3.4 Docking of the Robot and Insertion of the Instruments

The next step is to dock the robot. The robot is navigated either to the foot of the bed between the patients abducted legs or to the left side of the patient (side docking) and this is what we (J-US, Leipzig) prefer (easier, no limitations, faster). Firstly, the camera port is docked. The camera cable is then clipped in place prior to docking the right-sided ports. This allows for the camera cable to be brought between the camera port and arm-1. The left-sided ports (arms 2 and 3) are docked by the surgeon standing on the patients left, while arm-1 on the right is docked by the bedside assistant. It is important to note that after docking the robotic arms to the trocar, traction can be exerted to the abdominal wall broadening the operative field and gaining space among the trocars. When placing the arms in their final position, a final check should be made to make sure that there is no compression of any body parts. It is important to avoid any injury to the abdominal skin or the legs of the patient due to compression by any of the robotic arms. Thus, all arms should be carefully docked, and the range of movement should be checked.

4 Instrument Use for E-RARP

4.1 Multi-Port (E-RARP-Mp)

The senior author's experience with over 4000 cases since 2003, in a high-volume tertiary cancer referral academic center (JVJ, Rochester), has been previously reported. The technique is broadly similar and the outcomes favorably comparable to those of other experienced centers performing E-RARP using the MP robotic system [41, 42, 49–51].

4.1.1 Access

We have developed a reproducible method to access the extraperitoneal (EP) space (JVJ, Rochester). The patient is placed in the supine position with the arms tucked. A beanbag is used to prevent patient movement when placed in the

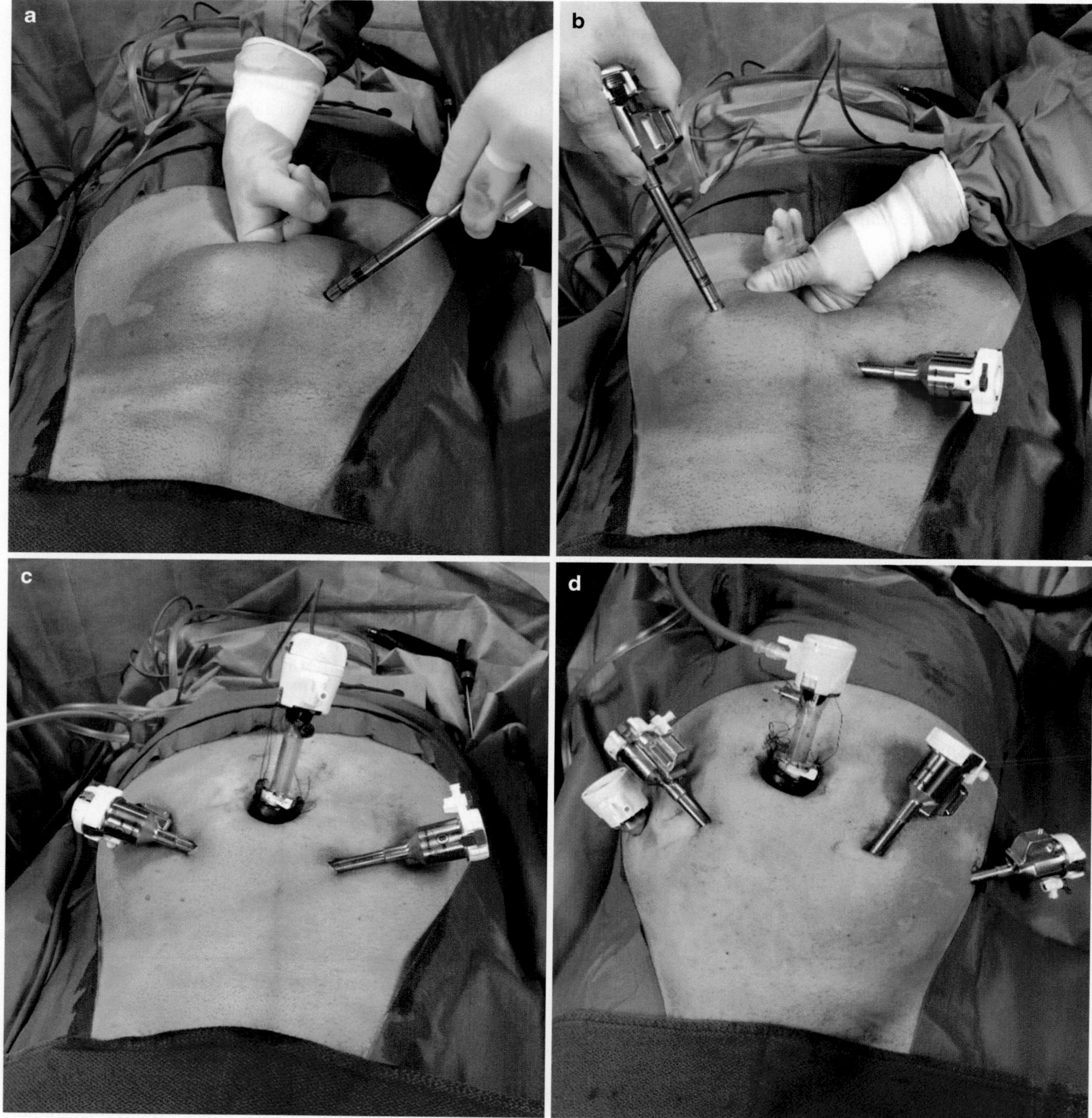

Fig. 3 Port placement for endoscopic extraperitoneal radical prostatectomy (**a**) Placement of da Vinci trocar left side guided by finger dissection (**b**) Placement of da Vinci trocar right side (**c**) camera trocar in place (**d**) All trocars in place

Trendelenburg position. All pressure points are padded. A Foley catheter is placed in a sterile manner after prepping and draping. We use a 3-cm left-sided paraumbilical incision which is carried down to the level of the anterior rectus sheath (Fig. 4a, b). A 1-cm incision is made in the anterior rectus sheath exposing the left belly of the rectus muscle. The latter is swept exposing the posterior rectus sheath. A balloon dilator (Covidien, Dublin, Ireland) is passed beneath the muscle parallel to the posterior rectus sheath, in a caudal direction, accessing the space of Retzius (Fig. 4c). The balloon is manually inflated, gradually expanding the EP space of Retzius. A 0-degree laparoscopic camera, placed inside the balloon dilator, allows direct visualization of the space creation process. The epigastric vessels can be visualized

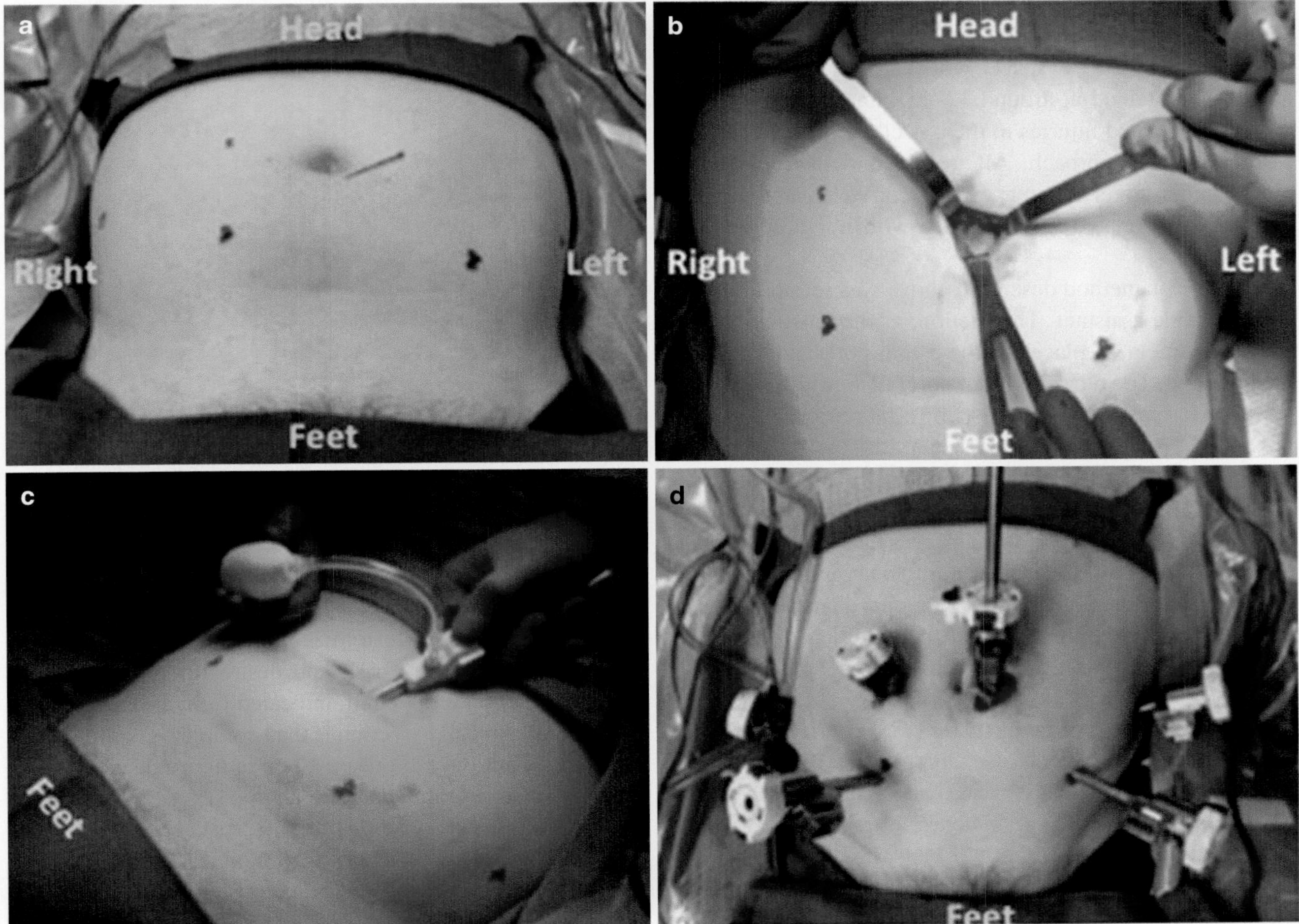

Fig. 4 Extraperitoneal (EP) access and development of EP space. (**a**) Diagrammatic representation of initial access incision in the left paraumbilical area. (**b**) Cut-down entry ("Hasson") into the EP space under vision. (**c**) Laparoscopic camera within balloon dilator and insufflation of balloon dilator in the EP space by manual pump. (**d**) Photo illustrating the final port sites before docking of the robot

anteriorly from their connection with the external iliac vessels. Tearing of the tributaries of the epigastric vessels beneath the muscle can occur at times but is generally of no consequence. Once the space is adequately created, the balloon dilator is withdrawn and replaced by a blunt-ended trocar (Ethicon) via which the space is insufflated. With the scope withdrawn into the trocar to avoid soilage, the tip of the trocar is used to further develop the extraperitoneal space laterally. Additional space creation is obligatory when using a multi-port robot, given the required distance between the robotic arms. When a single-port (SP) robot is used, however, no additional space creation is necessary, which will be discussed later in this chapter.

For placement of additional ports, the inferior epigastric vessels on the anterior abdominal wall can be easily appreciated and avoided. We often place a long 22-gauge hypodermic needle at the proposed site of trocar insertion to help identify the course of the trocar and, thereby, avoid a potential injury to the epigastric vasculature. When using the multi-port Xi da Vinci robot, we routinely place a total of six trocars. Four 8-mm da Vinci ports are used for robot docking (2 about 10-cm lateral and caudal to the umbilicus on either side, and a third placed 5-cm cephalad to the left anterior superior iliac spine) and two by the assistant (5-mm placed 5-cm to the right of the umbilicus, and a 12-mm port placed 5-cm cephalad to the right anterior superior iliac spine) in configuration delineated (Fig. 4d). Prior to robot docking, the paraumbilical initial access trocar used for additional space creation must be replaced by another trocar compatible with da Vinci docking. While a regular 8-mm trocar can be used, we prefer using a 12-mm da Vinci stapler cannula at that site, given the opening in the rectus sheath. The latter is often enlarged with the space creation as the trocar is oriented in multiple directions. We have found it useful to place a purse string suture in the anterior rectus sheath to maintain the required insufflation (Fig. 4d).

Due to the EP nature of the surgical field thus developed, mild Trendelenburg (around 10–15 degrees) is usually more than sufficient. The peritoneum serves as a natural barrier keeping the bowels out of the operative field. Pneumo-insufflation of the EP space, with carbon dioxide, is adequately maintained at around 12–15 mm of mercury (Hg). Access associated injuries to the bowel are avoided with the extraperitoneal approach. All trocars and instruments are placed under direct vision at every step. We have not experienced access related viscus injury with our described EP approach [49].

The access method described above was set up for a left-sided bedside assistant. The suction, as the most commonly used instrument, is placed in the 5-mm port, and used with the left hand. The other assistant port (12-mm) is used by the assistant for passage of sutures, clips, fat retrieval, specimen bag, etc. For a right-handed assistant, the assistant port can be placed in the left lower quadrant, allowing appropriate handling of the necessary instruments, based on the assistant's dexterity. Extraperitoneal access can also be obtained in the midline. We, however, prefer the paraumbilical access with visualization of the consistent rectus anatomy. Entering the linea alba in the midline near the umbilicus may lead to inadvertent entry into the peritoneal cavity.

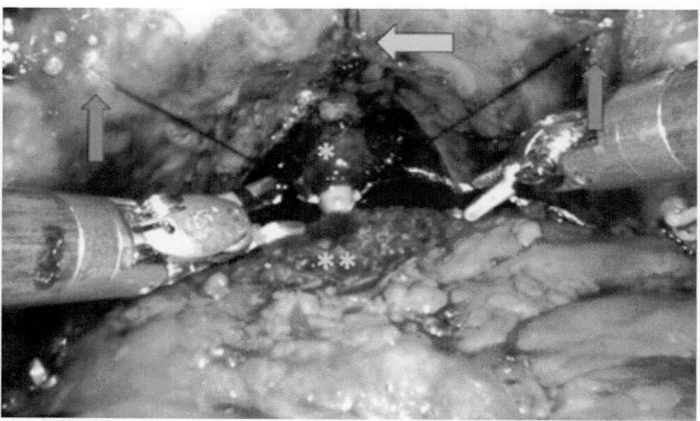

Fig. 5 Anterior suspension after posterior reconstruction. Blue arrows point to the barbed-wire sutures, used in the posterior reconstruction, being hitched bilaterally to the periosteum of the pelvic brim. Yellow arrow points to the barbed-wire suture, which had been used initially for dorsal venous complex (DVC) control, being hitched to the periosteum of the symphysis pubis in the midline anteriorly. This facilitates the anastomosis between the urethra (*) and the bladder (**)

4.1.2 Radical Prostatectomy With or Without Pelvic Lymph Node Dissection (PLND)

As described previously, once adequate EP access is obtained, the prostate is approached anteriorly for a radical prostatectomy, with or without PLND, as indicated clinically [41, 42]. With a few modifications, this approach is similar to the transperitoneal access at this point. The bladder take-down step, necessary with the transperitoneal approach, is not necessary when using the EP technique. The bladder is dissected from the anterior abdominal wall with the initial balloon dilation step. In most patients, the endopelvic fascia is visualized through the balloon dilator. Upon docking, there is quick access to the prostate or lymph node fossa. The prostatectomy begins promptly with incising the endopelvic fascia freeing the prostate from its lateral attachments. The apical dissection leads to visualization of the dorsal venous complex (DVC) which is ligated by a barbed-wire suture. The author's preference is to anchor this suture anteriorly to the pubic symphysis (Fig. 5). Provided there are no issues with high grade/stage lesions in the vicinity of the prostatic base, bladder neck dissection is then performed as anatomically as possible in order to optimally preserve the bladder neck detrusor muscle. Next, release of the vasa and seminal vesicles posteriorly are performed as athermally as possible, depending on the level of neurovascular bundle (NVB) preservation required.

Posterior dissection, anterior to the Denonvillier's fascial space, is continued in the apical direction followed by control of the lateral vascular pedicles. Again, the degree of NVB preservation is customized, on either side, as per the index patient's clinical risk and desire for preservation of erectile function if not contraindicated from a cancer control standpoint. Apical dissection is then completed carefully and athermally not only to preserve pelvic floor muscle but also to avoid inadvertent damage to any preserved NVB distally near the apex. After completing the prostatectomy, bilateral PLND is performed, dictated by clinical indication. The author's preference is to perform a posterior reconstruction, with a double-ended barbed-wire suture, so as to approximate the posterior urethra to the bladder neck in the posterior plane. We routinely use these sutures to perform an "anterior suspension" by hitching the two ends of the barbed-wire suture with Weck clips onto Poupart's ligaments about 5-cm on either side of the midline (Fig. 5). The urethro-vesical anastomosis is carried out using two 3-0 Vicryl sutures, on RB-1 needles, in a semi-continuous fashion. Our practice is to routinely leave a 16-French Jackson-Pratt (JP) drain in the pelvis with the aim of removing it prior to the patient's discharge from hospital the following day. The anterior rectus sheath defect, from the initial incision for access is closed. No additional port or peritoneal closure is necessary. Skin incisions are closed in a subcuticular fashion (Fig. 6). No routine lab/blood tests are ordered post-operatively, unless clinically indicated.

4.1.3 Post-Operative Care and Follow-Up

The patient is reviewed in the outpatient clinic at 1 week to remove the urethral catheter and to discuss the final histopathology dependent on which further follow-up schedules are customized. All data pertaining to pre-operative clinical information, intraoperative details, and post-operative out-

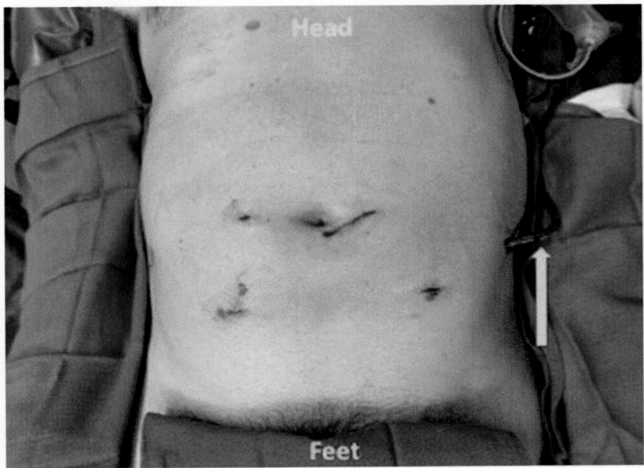

Fig. 6 Wound and skin closure appearance. Yellow arrow points at J-P drain

comes, including oncological and functional results, are maintained in a prospective database with dedicated data managers.

4.2 Single-Port E-RARP

The technical steps relevant to conduct E-RARP using the single-port (SP) robotic system and the various instruments commonly utilized during those steps are summarized in the section below entitled "the single-port promise."

5 Complications of the Extraperitoneal Approach

Surgical complications can be broadly classified into "early" and "late" or "minor" and "major" based largely on the timing and severity, respectively, of post-operative adverse events [52, 53]. In order to reduce the undercapture of complications and to improve standardization of reporting, efforts have been made to include procedure-specific (surgical) as well as general (medical or non-surgical) complications [52, 54]. Furthermore, in recent years, there have also been efforts to include intraoperative adverse events, inclusive of anesthetic events, in order to comprehensively capture and standardize the reporting of all complications relevant to a given surgical case [55–57]. Attempts to standardize the reporting of complications specific to radical prostatectomy, and, in particular, robot-assisted radical prostatectomy (RARP) have meant that data relevant to RARP are more consistently reported in the literature and that meaningful comparisons may be possible between reported series from different institutions [58–62].

With respect to E-RARP, although there are no validated reporting systems specific to the extraperitoneal (EP) approach to robotic radical prostatectomy, there are a number of series in the literature which have attempted to characterize and report complications specific to E-RARP based on their institutional experience [49, 50]. Others have attempted to compare the outcomes, including complications, between E-RARP and T-RARP (transperitoneal RARP) [51, 63–67]. Similarly, others have compared the outcomes of E-RARP and EP laparoscopic radical prostatectomy [68–70]. Evidence on the nuances of the endoscopic approach to EP radical prostatectomy, which includes technical difficulties and specific complications, can also be gleaned from large series of laparoscopic EP radical prostatectomy [44, 71]. The cumulated evidence from these studies enables us to formulate a picture of the profile of complications that may occur from undergoing E-RARP.

5.1 Intraoperative Complications

Firstly, in terms of intraoperative complications, E-RARP seems to have a favorably comparable profile when evaluated against T-RARP, laparoscopic EP radical prostatectomy or open EP radical prostatectomy [49]. The overall intraoperative complication rate seems to be around 0.27% to 0.8% (see Table 1) [49, 72]. This compares to 0.08% to 1.8% for the other aforementioned EP approaches [49]. Specifically, in the series of 1503 E-RARP cases with a median follow-up of 28.9 months, reported in 2013 by Ghazi et al., there was 1 case (0.07%) of intraoperative rectal injury and 3 cases (0.2%) of inadvertent clipping of the obturator nerve, which

Table 1 Comparison characteristics and intraoperative complications of large T-RARP and E-RARP series; adapted from [11, 49]

Study	Coelho et al. 2010 [60]	Agarwal et al. 2011 [62]	Ghazi et al. 2013 [49]	Ploussard et al. 2014 [72]
Approach	T-RARP	T-RARP	E-RARP	E-RARP
Country	US	US	US	France
Cases (*n*)	2500	3317	1503	792
Follow-up (days)	30	30–356	90–1800	570
Intraoperative complications				
Overall %	0.08	1.8	0.27	0.8
Rectal injury %	0.08	N/A	0.07	0.3
Nerve injury %	N/A	N/A	0.2	0.1
Epigastric vessel injury %	N/A	N/A	N/A	0.3
Conversion %	0.08	0.03	0.07	N/A

E-RARP Extraperitoneal robot-assisted radical prostatectomy, *T-RARP* Transperitoneal robot-assisted radical prostatectomy, *US* United States, *N/A* Not applicable/available

were treated intraoperatively with double-layer sutured repair and removal of clip, respectively [49]. With respect to rectal injuries, in a large series comparing E-RARP ($n = 1009$) and laparoscopic EP radical prostatectomy ($n = 1377$), there were 3 (0.3%) and 11 (0.8%) incidences of rectal injuries, respectively [72]. In that comparative study by Poussard et al., both groups had 1 case each of "neurapraxia." [72] In addition, epigastric vessel injuries were found in three cases of E-RARP and four cases of laparoscopic EP radical prostatectomy (**see** Table 1) [72]. Apart from rectal injury, intraoperative bowel (small or large bowel) injury rates appear to be negligible, ranging from 0% to 0.15%, with E-RARP [49, 72]. This seems to be a plausibly advantageous scenario with E-RARP due to the procedure being performed in the EP space, away from potentially intervening loops of bowel which may be overtly or inadvertently injured. The findings are congruent with observations from laparoscopic EP radical prostatectomy series, where intraoperative bowel injury rates were also very low, ranging from 0.1% to 0.8% [44, 71].

On account of the perceived technical difficulty, and associated learning curve, with securing and developing good access in the EP space, one would expect there to be notable instances of the need for intraoperative "conversion" to other modalities, such as to T-RARP, laparoscopic or open radical prostatectomy. However, reported rates of such conversions are surprisingly low. In the study by Ghazi et al., there was 1 case (0.07%) that required conversion to laparoscopic radical prostatectomy on account of robotic malfunction [49]. This compares to conversion rates ranging from 0.03% to 0.48% for T-RARP (see Table 1). It is interesting to note that failed access in itself, with respect to securing and developing the EP space to allow the E-RARP case to proceed, is rare and that conversion to T-RARP or open conversion due to such failed access, is rarely encountered in experienced hands [44, 49, 72].

5.2 Post-Operative and Late Complications

In terms of the severity of complications, as stratified by reported Clavien-Dindo (C-D) grades, the profiles for E-RARP seem comparable to T-RARP, laparoscopic EP radical prostatectomy, and open EP prostatectomy [44, 49, 71, 72]. Specifically, for E-RARP, the overall complications range from approximately 5.1% to 8.45% and this compares to an overall complication rate ranging from 5.08% to 9.8% for T-RARP (see Table 2). The minor (C-D I and II) and major (C-D III-V) complication rates are also comparable between E-RARP and T-RARP (see Table 2).

When scrutinizing the profile of post-operative complications, a few observations stand out as potentially significant in terms of differences between E-RARP and T-RARP. Firstly, the lymphocele rate appears to be higher in E-RARP (see Table 2) and this observation is consistent with findings from laparoscopic EP radical prostatectomy series [44, 71]. This finding may be explained by the fact that, with the EP approach, whether robotic or laparoscopic, any lymph leak subsequent to pelvic lymph node dissection (PLND) would likely be entrapped within the EP space leading to the likelihood of significant lymph collections declaring themselves clinically through symptoms (e.g., pelvic pain, infection, ileus, urinary symptoms on catheter removal, etc.) [73]. In contrast, in the transperitoneal approach, it is theorized that symptomatic lymphocele collections are less likely because the lymph fluid dissipates into the relatively vast intraperitoneal compartment and gets reabsorbed transperitoneally. This has formed the basis for advocating techniques, such as peritoneal fenestration, pleating, flap fixation and interposition, during laparoscopic or robotic radical prostatectomy [74–77]. However, a prospective study investigating the efficacy of peritoneal fixation, during RARP, did not demonstrate a significant reduction in either asymptomatic or

Table 2 Comparison of peri-operative and delayed complications of large T-RARP and E-RARP series; adapted from [11, 49]

Study	Coelho et al. 2010 [60]	Agarwal et al. 2011 [62]	Ghazi et al. 2013 [49]	Ploussard et al. 2014 [72]
Post-operative complications	T-RARP	T-RARP	E-RARP	E-RARP
Overall %	5.08	9.8	8.45	5.1
Minor (C-D I & II)	4.04	7.3	6.99	4.9
Major (C-D III to V)	0.96	3.8	3.06	0.30
Blood transfusion %	0.48	2.1	1.0	2.8
Readmission %	3.5	3.5	3.65	N/A
Lymphocele (adjusted) %	0.80	0.97	3.31	0.90
PLND %	44.5	84.3	44.0	46.1
Ileus %	0.72	0.60	0.06	0.01
Hernia %	0.16	0.21	0	N/A
Bowel injury %	0	0.3	0.06	0.01
Bowel obstruction %	0.08	0.15	0.13	N/A
Urinary retention %	0.53	0.39	0.70	N/A
BNC %	0.12	0.66	1.34	0.50
Anastomotic leak %	1.4	1.17	1.2	2.3
Thromboembolic (DVT, PE) %	0.32	0.27	0.80	0.20
Cardiac %	0.20	0.18	0.30	0.30
Ocular %	N/A	3.8	0.50	N/A

E-RARP Extraperitoneal robot-assisted radical prostatectomy, *T-RARP* Transperitoneal robot-assisted radical prostatectomy, *US* United States, *C-D* Clavien-Dindo, *PLND* Pelvic lymph node dissection, *BNC* Bladder neck contracture, *DVT* Deep vein thrombosis, *PE* Pulmonary embolism, *N/A* Not applicable/available

symptomatic lymphoceles [78]. To add clarity on this issue, there is a larger, better-powered study which is ongoing and is randomizing RARP cases to peritoneal fixation or no fixation [79]. Furthermore, in contradiction to some studies suggesting higher lymphocele rates with the E-RARP approach, there are others comparing E-RARP and T-RARP, which have not demonstrated significant differences [64, 80, 81].

Secondly, the incidence of bowel-related complications, such as bowel injury, ileus, obstruction, and hernia, appears to be lower with the EP approach (see Table 2) [11, 49, 72, 73]. Again, the plausible explanation for this appears to be the fact that the EP approach negates the need to be in the intraperitoneal compartment and, as such, inadvertent contact of bowel with surgical instruments intraoperatively or contact irritation with exposure to urine, blood or lymph fluid, is minimized [82]. Similarly, as all the ports are placed in the EP space, the risk of bowel herniation through such port sites may be mitigated by the EP approach. In fact, in one of the largest series of E-RARP with a median follow-up of 28 months, no instances of post-operative bowel hernia were encountered [49].

Anastomotic complications with E-RARP, whether anastomotic leak in the early post-operative period or anastomotic stricture (bladder neck contracture, BNC) presenting in a late/delayed fashion, appear to be relatively low and comparable to T-RARP series (see Table 2). Specifically, bladder neck contracture (BNC) rates range from 0.5% to 1.34% in E-RARP series and this compares to 0.12% to 0.66% in T-RARP series (see Table 2).

Significant non-surgical (medical) complications, such as myocardial infarctions and thromboembolic events, appear to be relatively infrequent and comparable between E-RARP and T-RARP series (see Table 2). At first glance, it might appear that ocular complications may be lower in the E-RARP (0.5%) cases than in the T-RARP cases (3.8%) (see Table 2). This has led to the suggestion that factors during E-RARP, such as the less steep Trendelenburg required and the lower intraperitoneal diffusion of carbon dioxide, may have a protective effect [49]. However, this needs to be corroborated by other larger studies.

6 Pros and Cons of the Extraperitoneal Technique

Compelling evidence, from randomized studies as well as from large comparative studies, suggests that E-RARP has favorably similar outcomes when compared to T-RARP [42, 63, 64]. In other words, operative parameters, complications, as well as clinical outcomes such as oncological and functional outcomes are not significantly different with either the EP or transperitoneal approaches to RARP. Table 3 summarizes the important pros and cons of E-RARP.

Table 3 Pros and cons of E-RARP

Technique	Pros	Cons
E-RARP	No entry into the peritoneal compartment required	Relatively contraindicated in those with obliterated EP space, for instance due to prior bilateral inguinal hernial mesh repair
	Less risk of bowel-related complications	Relatively contraindicated in those with severe COPD
	Less need for deep Trendelenburg. Therefore, may be advantageous in severely obese patients and those with significant comorbidities	Perceived to be more technically demanding due to unfamiliarity with EP access and EP space development
	May be advantageous when embarking on the recent single-port system	Less working space available in the EP compartment when compared to the intraperitoneal compartment. This issue may be more pronounced in smaller patients

COPD Chronic obstructive pulmonary disease, *E-RARP* Extraperitoneal robotic assisted radical prostatectomy

6.1 Pros: Special Circumstances and Favorable Indications

6.1.1 Previous Abdominal Surgeries

The EP approach is most advantageous when dense intraabdominal adhesions, from previous surgeries, are known or expected. As alluded to above, by virtue of being completely in the EP compartment throughout the procedure, the risk of inadvertently injuring the bowel during access, for placement of ports, and while mobilizing, retracting, and performing adhesiolysis, is significantly minimized. Even in the absence of overt bowel trauma, through inadvertent enterotomies, the need for significant bowel handling for retraction or mobilization or through adhesiolysis may be associated with an ileus which can lengthen the hospital stay and overall recovery. We have not found any prior abdominal surgeries to be limiting in our experience [66]. Even when a low midline incision is present, the space can be developed, but requires incision of the scarred linea alba. In patients with prior major abdominal surgeries, the EP approach likely expedites the procedure, and, thereby, likely impacts favorably on the patient's recovery. A major advantage of the EP approach is the avoidance of creation of intraabdominal adhesions, which can complicate future abdominal interventions.

6.1.2 Concurrent Inguinal Hernia Repair

Inguinal hernia can be detected pre-operatively in a significant proportion of men embarking on radical prostatectomy [83]. Furthermore, symptomatic post-operative inguinal hernia can complicate radical prostatectomy in around 12% to 16% of men [84]. Specifically, with respect to the incidence of inguinal hernia after RARP, a recent systematic review and meta-analysis has estimated the rate to be around 7.9% (95% confidence interval (CI): 5.0% to 10.9%) of which 81.9% were of the indirect type (95% CI: 75.3% to 88.4%) [85]. Although mesh repair of any pre-operatively screened or intraoperatively detected inguinal hernia can be repaired either transperitoneally or in a total EP (TEP) fashion, it is felt that the TEP repair may be advantageous by virtue of avoiding direct contact of mesh with bowel [86, 87]. In the study by Qazi et al., there were no hernia recurrences in 12 patients undergoing E-RARP combined with TEP when followed up for 12 months [86]. In the study by Ludwig et al., there were no hernia recurrences in 11 patients undergoing E-RARP combined with TEP when followed up for a mean duration of 33 months [87]. Even though the two studies mentioned are relatively small, our groups' own anecdotal experience is that recurrence of hernia is indeed rare following mesh repair at the time of E-RARP (JVJ, University of Rochester). This is congruent with the findings of a systematic review of inguinal hernia repair performed concurrently with laparoscopic or robotic radical prostatectomy [88]. Qazi et al. reported no C-D complications in the 12 patients and recorded that unilateral TEP added an average of 12 additional minutes to RARP [86]. Similarly, Ludwig et al., when comparing E-RARP plus TEP versus a matched cohort of laparoscopic EP radical prostatectomy plus TEP, found no significant differences in complications, apart from a case of anterior mesh seroma in the E-RARP group [87]. They found that unilateral TEP and bilateral TEP added, on average, 32 min and 80 min to the E-RARP [87].

6.1.3 Obese Patients

RARP in obese patients may be challenging for a number of reasons. Longer ports may be required to negotiate the abdominal wall girth and optimize the instrumentation angles, quite often within a restricted pelvic field, which can make the whole procedure more challenging. Additionally, steep Trendelenburg may be required to optimize the pelvic operative field. Obese patients quite often have multiple cardiovascular comorbidities and, as such, may not be ideal candidates, from a physiological perspective, for prolonged periods of steep Trendelenburg. Furthermore, they may also have considerable fat and soft tissues around the neck, which make them unfavorable candidates for prolonged periods of ventilation in steep Trendelenburg. Therefore, RARP performed through the EP approach, which requires considerably less Trendelenburg, may be ideally advantageous in significantly obese patients [82, 89].

6.2 Cons: Limitations and Relative Contraindications

6.2.1 Prior Bilateral Inguinal Hernia Repair

In patients in whom the EP space is obliterated, on account of prior operations in that field, it may be more sensible to opt to perform RARP transperitoneally. Patients who have had inguinal hernia repair with mesh previously, particularly if bilateral, fall into this category where E-RARP may be relatively contraindicated owing to the scarred EP space from the dense inflammatory reaction or adhesion created by the mesh. One could theoretically adopt the strategy of attempting E-RARP with a view to "conversion" to T-RARP, if difficulties were encountered; however, port positions would not be optimized to subsequently proceed with T-RARP. It is our preference to immediately proceed with T-RARP in patients with previous bilateral EP mesh inguinal hernia repair.

A corollary of this situation, from a converse standpoint, is when inguinal hernia is known pre-operatively or is encountered intraoperatively and, hence, mesh repair is desirable. The EP approach (E-RARP) does not pose any technical issues when mesh repair of inguinal hernia, whether unilateral or bilateral, is required. Similarly, based on the senior author's (JVJ, University of Rochester) recent and relatively limited experience (>100 cases) of E-RARP using the single-port (SP) system, mesh repair of inguinal hernia is also relatively straightforward using the SP system.

6.2.2 Severe Respiratory Disease

In those with severe chronic respiratory disease (COPD), there is noteworthy evidence, from a randomized study, that performing E-RARP, compared to a transperitoneal approach, may be clinically more risky in terms of less favorable measured respiratory parameters, such as arterial concentration of carbon dioxide (PaCO2) [90]. It is postulated that elevation of PaCO2 may be the result of excess absorption of insufflated CO2 via the disrupted microvascular and lymphatics of the EP surface resulting from development of the EP space [91]. Although significant cardiovascular issues are rarely documented, largely due to vigilant ventilation by the anesthetist intraoperatively to offset any elevation of PaCO2 or alterations in arterial pH, it is nonetheless a significant clinical consideration when considering E-RARP in those with significant COPD. That said, non-surgical management options (surveillance, radiotherapy, etc.) may be more preferable in those with severe comorbidities such as severe COPD. Increased intraabdominal pressure causes diaphragmatic splinting which can impair ventilation in the patient with respiratory compromise.

6.2.3 Extended Lymphadenectomy

As far as pelvic lymph node dissection (PLND) for RARP is concerned, executing this within the field of the standard template, as recommended by international guidelines, is not technically more challenging with the EP approach. "Extended" or "super-extended" lymphadenectomy, incorporating presacral nodes or a more proximal nodal dissection from the common iliac bifurcation, is not recommended for localized prostate cancer. Furthermore, the need for PLND in those with low- or favorable intermediate-risk disease is questionable, and, as such, E-RARP is not technically less advantageous in the vast majority of patients requiring RARP, with or without PLND. We routinely use a zero-degree scope for all prostatectomies. When cephalad dissection is desired for more proximal nodal dissection, a 30 degree-down camera angle may facilitate visualization.

6.2.4 "Non-standard" RARP

"Salvage" radical prostatectomy may be indicated in carefully selected cases of localized prostate cancer which have recurred following prior non-surgical radical interventions, such as radiotherapy, brachytherapy, or HIFU (high-intensity focused ultrasound), which had been delivered with curative intent. However, there is paucity of data on "salvage" RARP performed with the EP technique. Some reports, with limited case numbers and follow-up, suggest that salvage EP *laparoscopic* prostatectomy has similar safety and efficacy to salvage transperitoneal *laparoscopic* prostatectomy and, by inference, similar outcomes to salvage "open" prostatectomy [92]. It is our preference to perform salvage RARP transperitoneally. This is not for the prostatectomy portion, but for the significantly higher risk of lymphocele associated with removal of previously irradiated nodal tissue. There is also paucity of data on single-port (SP) salvage E-RARP. As such, definitive conclusions should not be drawn on the relative merits of salvage E-RARP whether in the context of single-port or multi-port systems.

7 Tips and Tricks

Case Selection

- Avoid E-RARP in patients with severe respiratory compromise, such as significant COPD, due to a higher risk of complications in such cases.
- As per international uro-oncological guidelines, seek alternative management options (for instance, watchful waiting) when patients, though chronologically young, have severe medical comorbidities that would likely complicate surgical intervention. In addition, technically "successful" surgeries may still prove to be futile in the short-to-medium term due to the competing risks for mortality in patients with significant comorbidities.

Access and Development of the EP Space

- Opt for T-RARP (instead of E-RARP) when there is pre-operative evidence of prior bilateral mesh inguinal hernia repair.
- In contrast, E-RARP may be advantageous in cases where the patient is obese or has had prior abdominal surgery.
- Make the initial access incision lateral to the umbilicus (left side is the author's preference, JVJ), rather than in the midline, due to the more consistently appreciable rectus muscle anatomy in the paramedian space and, in contrast, a higher risk of going through-and-through into the intraperitoneal compartment via the linea alba when attempting access in the midline.
- During space creation for additional robotic ports or for assistant ports, it is important to not sweep too vigorously when expanding the EP space in the cephalad direction because the peritoneal layer can be inadvertently torn with consequent entry into the intraperitoneal space.
- Make use of a long 22-gauge hypodermic needle at the proposed site of trocar insertion to help identify the course of the trocar and, thereby, avoid a potential injury to the epigastric vasculature.
- In notably obese patients, make use of longer ports.

E-RARP

- Due to the extraperitoneal nature of the surgical field, mild Trendelenburg (around 10–15 degrees) is usually more than sufficient.
- Make note of any inguinal hernia which could complicate RARP post-operatively. Reduce any hernia and perform a mesh repair with either a total extraperitoneal (TEP) method or a transperitoneal mesh repair method, whichever method one is most familiar with and has good outcomes in one's hands. Depending on one's experience with hernia repair or institutional/national guidelines, it may be necessary to enlist the help of a general surgeon specializing in such hernia surgeries.
- Provided there are no issues with high grade/stage lesions in the vicinity of the prostatic base, perform bladder neck dissection as anatomically as possible in order to optimally preserve the bladder neck detrusor muscle.
- The author's practice is to customize the degree of neurovascular bundle (NVB) preservation, on either side, as per the index patient's clinical risk and desire for preservation of erectile function, if not contraindicated from a cancer control standpoint. Damage to the NVB can occur any-

where along the NVB tract, proximal (prostate base) to distal (prostate apex), and in the author's experience, it is particularly more liable to occur during apical dissection. Careful athermal dissection and avoidance of excessive or prolonged traction are important.

- The author's preference is to utilize anterior suspension, augmented with posterior reconstruction, to optimize the vesicourethral anastomosis step so as to reduce anastomotic urine leaks and achieve earlier zero-pad continence (Fig. 5). However, a multitude of studies have demonstrated conflicting results, with these adjunctive technical maneuvers, with respect to advantages in terms of significantly improved functional outcomes in the longer run.

PLND

- The author's routine practice is to perform, as clinically indicated, a "standard template" for PLND. Performing "extended" and "super-extended" PLND during E-RARP is technically not feasible and, more importantly, the evidence for such extended templates during radical prostatectomy is contentious.
- The author's preference is to utilize meticulous, systematic Weck clip ligation, combined with bipolar diathermy as required, in order to reduce the incidence of symptomatic lymphoceles. In addition, in recent years, the author has also adopted peritoneal fenestration and fixation, as adjunctive techniques, to further minimize the occurrence of symptomatic lymphoceles.

Closure

- The anterior rectus sheath defect, from the initial incision for access, must be closed. This is important to prevent bowel hernia. Similarly, the fascial layer of any assistant port 12-mm or larger needs to be closed. However, no additional port or peritoneal closure is necessary.

Post-operative Care and Follow-up

- Routine lab tests are not required prior to discharge (usually the following day), unless clinically indicated.
- A Jackson-Pratt (JP) drain, which is left in the EP space at the end of the procedure, is removed prior to discharge.
- A 16-Fr Foley urethral catheter, which is placed to protect the anastomosis, is usually removed at 7–10 days upon outpatient review in the clinic with the histopathology report at hand.

8 The Single-Port (SP) Promise

In recent years, the single-port (SP) platform has been applied to a multitude of urological procedures and robotic single-port radical prostatectomy (RARP-sp) has been one of the most common procedures [12–14, 93, 94]. The SP platform seems to be particularly well suited technically when utilizing the EP approach for RARP [15, 95]. Specifically, as opposed to some limitation of space within the EP compartment during multi-port E-RARP, the available EP space seems comfortably adequate when performing E-RARP with the SP system. Additionally, the flexible nature of the camera, offering a wide range of views from unconventional angles, provides tangible technical benefits during certain aspects of critical steps such as NVB preservation, apical dissection, bladder neck dissection, and PLND. Similarly, the angled retraction and swapping of instruments also add technical benefits, which the surgeon can, with increasing experience, fine-tune to their taste. Such features can also enable the surgeon to almost perform the entirety of the procedure "solo," although our advice is to make use of an experienced bedside assistant in the learning phase. Furthermore, with respect to safety, efficacy, and early outcomes, the E-RARP-sp approach appears to be delivering added benefits, compared to multi-port RARP, including same-day outpatient surgery with minimal to no opiate use, excellent pain control, and better cosmesis with fewer, smaller surgical scars [14, 95]. Although highly promising, it should be noted that the currently reported studies on E-RARP-sp are few, with relatively small numbers and short follow-up, and, as such, more studies with larger numbers, longer follow-up, and detailed documentation of complications and outcomes are evidently warranted.

8.1 Access

The EP approach is advantageous when using the SP robotic system. The space creation has been the main factor limiting the adoption of the extraperitoneal route. The use of the MP robot requires a greater space to provide adequate instrument distancing. Additional space creation is necessary laterally, which increases the risk of creating a peritoneal rent, which can reduce the operative space, impacting the overall surgery. When using the SP, there is no need to create any space beyond what is provided by the balloon dilator. Our institution has been among the early adopters of the SP robotic system (JVJ, University of Rochester). Our transition from MP to SP radical prostatectomy has been seamless. As a leading institution accustomed to the EP approach, we anticipated the SP would simplify the access stage. As noted earlier, when using the SP, the space created by the balloon dilator is sufficient for deployment of the SP robotic arms. As with any new technology, there is an associated learning curve. The latter is rather associated with the use of the SP than the space creation, which is now easier. Lateral dissection for MP use, which can be complicated with peritoneotomy, is no longer necessary.

Our method of access for SP is very similar to MP except for a few minor modifications for the SP system. We begin the procedure with a 4–5 cm incision about 5 cm below the umbilicus, the linea alba is incised exposing the perivesical fat (Fig. 7). A balloon dilator is used to create the EP space under direct vision. The noted landmarks include the pubic symphysis caudally and the inferior epigastric vessels on either side are visualized through the balloon dilator. Although the SP cannula is only 2.7 cm, we prefer to have about a 4 cm fascial opening to allow passage of accessory instruments adjacent to the single port. We routinely use a GelPoint Mini Advanced access platform (Applied Medical, CA, US), via which the SP is inserted along with a 5- and 10-mm cannula (Fig. 8a, b). A 5-mm suction tubing is inserted through the GelPoint and kept accessible in the operative field. The 10-mm port is used by the assistant for passage of sutures and the specimen retrieval bag. These additional ports, placed through the GelPoint access, are advanced concurrently into the operative space via the single port of the SP robot. Either accessory port can be used for insufflation for which the AirSeal (ConMed, NY, US) is used. Our preference is to work at a low pressure of 6–10 mm Hg, which is generally enough to provide adequate visualization. Next, the GelPoint is positioned snugly beneath the fascia to maintain adequate pressure in the EP space, prior to docking of the SP robot (Fig. 9). Although we routinely perform the entire procedure through this SP, we often use "SP plus one" approach, where an additional 12-mm port is placed in the right lower quadrant just medial to the umbilical area. This port is used by the assistant and can help expedite the procedure. We often insert this trocar while the balloon is inflated in the EP space. Insertion can be done under direct vision, taking advantage of the countertraction provided by the balloon dilator. Delay associated with clip placement, when the robotic arm clip applier is used by the surgeon himself/herself, can be avoided. The time-saving advantages are most notable during a pelvic lymphadenectomy where clips are used to control the large lymphatics. Incorporating these modifications and optimizing the use of the available expertise, from an experienced bedside assistant, make the whole procedure significantly more efficient, particularly in the very initial phases of the SP learning curve.

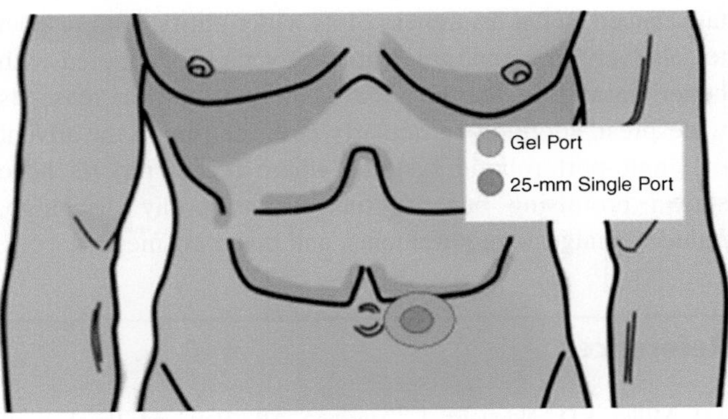

Fig. 7 Diagrammatic representation of planned port positions for single-port extraperitoneal RARP

8.2 Operative Procedure and Post-Operative Care

The technical steps of the RARP and PLND are exactly the same as for the multi-port procedure (EP-RARP-mp), as described above. Due to the different configuration of the robotic arms and the camera in the SP compared to the conventional MP system, optimal use of the robotic arms and camera requires practice. As alluded to above, although the whole procedure can be performed through the single access by utilizing the GelPort platform for further ports, the 5-mm assistant port and AirSeal port, combined with taking advantage of the expertise of an experienced bedside assistant, is highly recommended. To complete the radical prostatectomy, similar to the MP approach, we use da Vinci scissors, Maryland bipolar, and a Cadiere forceps for retraction. The latter is placed at the six o'clock position to allow retraction of the prostate on either side. It is also useful in retracting the

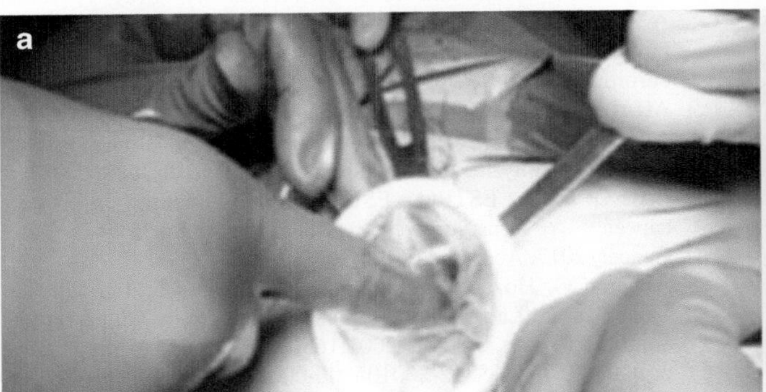

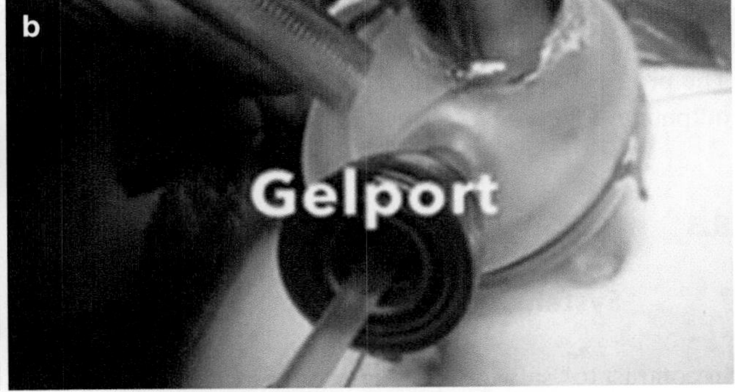

Fig. 8 Gel Port placement. (**a**) Placement of diaphragm of Gel Port within the access wound ensuring a snug fit with the lower/inner lip of the diaphragm. (**b**) Fitting of Gel Port onto upper/outside lip of the diaphragm

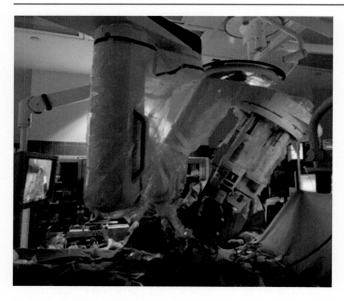

Fig. 9 Single port da Vinci robot after docking

bladder cephalad. Once the bladder is transected, we prefer rotating the entire SP system 180 degrees, placing the Cadiere forceps at the 12 o'clock position and the camera at six o'clock. The scissor and bipolar forceps are reconfigured on either sided based on the surgeon's dexterity. Placing the forceps at the 12 o'clock position allows adequate retraction of the seminal vesicles anteriorly. The posterior prostate dissection and neurovascular bundle (NVB) dissection are facilitated with adequate retraction from the anteriorly located fourth arm or forceps. For the apical dissection and subsequent vesicourethral anastomosis, it is preferable to return the camera to the 12 o'clock location, where the Cadiere forceps can be used to facilitate cephalad dissection as necessary.

The SP consumes a greater amount of time which can be associated with the learning curve. The decreased range of motion, known with the SP robot, secondary to the absence of wristed motion at the instrument tip is associated with increased anastomotic time. With increased experience, we expect this to no longer impact our operative time. At the end of the procedure, the fascial layers of the single-port access site are closed. If an assistant port was used, or a PLND was performed, a drain can be placed in the assistant's port site. The protocol for the immediate post-operative and eventual outpatient follow-up is also similar to that for the MP method.

8.3 Robotic "Simple" Extraperitoneal Prostatectomy with the Single-Port (SP) System

In contrast to "salvage" prostatectomy where there is paucity of studies illustrating the safety and efficacy of E-RARP, there is certainly ample evidence in support of robotic "simple" prostatectomy, for symptomatic benign prostatic hyperplasia (BPH), performed robotically in an EP fashion using multi-port (MP) systems [96–98]. Additionally, with respect to use of the single-port (SP) system for robotic EP simple prostatectomy, there are emerging data, with somewhat limited case numbers and follow-up, which testify to their safety and efficacy [99].

With respect to use of the SP system for "simple" prostatectomy, we prefer to customize it to the clinical situation whereby complex cases, for instance requiring concomitant bladder diverticulectomy, or stone removal, are performed with a transvesical approach (JVJ, University of Rochester) [100]. We routinely use the EP approach for simple prostatectomy, using the MP platform, adopting the Millin technique. The use of the SP in this setting is beyond the scope of this chapter. As noted earlier, our experience with SP transvesical approach for simple prostatectomy is expanding.

9 Conclusions

Extraperitoneal robot-assisted radical prostatectomy, performed with either the multi-port or single-port system, has a significant role in the surgical treatment of localized prostate cancer. Better awareness of its wider utility, with respect to relatively rare contraindications for its use, coupled with better training in learning the technique, may increase its widespread adoption particularly in the setting of the advent of single-port robotic systems where recent reports have shown promising benefits such as same-day discharge, reduced analgesic requirements, and better cosmesis.

References

1. Miller KD, Nogueira L, Mariotto AB, Rowland JH, Yabroff KR, Alfano CM, et al. Cancer treatment and survivorship statistics, 2019. CA Cancer J Clin. 2019;69(5):363–85. https://doi.org/10.3322/caac.21565.
2. Culp MB, Soerjomataram I, Efstathiou JA, Bray F, Jemal A. Recent global patterns in prostate cancer incidence and mortality rates. Eur Urol. 2020;77(1):38–52. https://doi.org/10.1016/j.eururo.2019.08.005.
3. AUA: clinically localized prostate cancer: AUA/ASTRO/SUO guideline. 2017. http://www.auanet.org/guidelines/prostate-cancer-clinically-localized-guideline. Accessed 06 Jul 2021.
4. EAU G: EAU - ESTRO - ESUR - SIOG guidelines on prostate cancer. https://uroweb.org/wp-content/uploads/09-Prostate-Cancer_2017. Accessed 06 Jul 2021.
5. Abbou CC, Hoznek A, Salomon L, Olsson LE, Lobontiu A, Saint F, et al. Laparoscopic radical prostatectomy with a remote controlled robot. J Urol. 2001;165(6 Pt 1):1964–6. https://doi.org/10.1097/00005392-200106000-00027.
6. Binder J, Kramer W. Robotically-assisted laparoscopic radical prostatectomy. BJU Int. 2001;87(4):408–10. https://doi.org/10.1046/j.1464-410x.2001.00115.x.

7. Menon M, Shrivastava A, Tewari A, Sarle R, Hemal A, Peabody JO, et al. Laparoscopic and robot assisted radical prostatectomy: establishment of a structured program and preliminary analysis of outcomes. J Urol. 2002;168(3):945–9. https://doi.org/10.1097/01.ju.0000023660.10494.7d.
8. Cole AP, Trinh QD, Sood A, Menon M. The rise of robotic surgery in the new millennium. J Urol. 2017;197(2s):S213–s5. https://doi.org/10.1016/j.juro.2016.11.030.
9. Costello AJ. Considering the role of radical prostatectomy in 21st century prostate cancer care. Nat Rev Urol. 2020;17(3):177–88. https://doi.org/10.1038/s41585-020-0287-y.
10. Liu S, Hemal A. Techniques of robotic radical prostatectomy for the management of prostate cancer: which one, when and why. Transl Androl Urol. 2020;9(2):906–18. https://doi.org/10.21037/tau.2019.09.13.
11. Semerjian A, Pavlovich CP. Extraperitoneal robot-assisted radical prostatectomy: indications, technique and outcomes. Curr Urol Rep. 2017;18(6):42. https://doi.org/10.1007/s11934-017-0689-4.
12. Kaouk JH, Haber GP, Autorino R, Crouzet S, Ouzzane A, Flamand V, et al. A novel robotic system for single-port urologic surgery: first clinical investigation. Eur Urol. 2014;66(6):1033–43. https://doi.org/10.1016/j.eururo.2014.06.039.
13. Lai A, Dobbs RW, Talamini S, Halgrimson WR, Wilson JO, Vigneswaran HT, et al. Single port robotic radical prostatectomy: a systematic review. Transl Androl Urol. 2020;9(2):898–905. https://doi.org/10.21037/tau.2019.11.05.
14. Checcucci E, De Cillis S, Pecoraro A, Peretti D, Volpi G, Amparore D, et al. Single-port robot-assisted radical prostatectomy: a systematic review and pooled analysis of the preliminary experiences. BJU Int. 2020;126(1):55–64. https://doi.org/10.1111/bju.15069.
15. Kaouk J, Aminsharifi A, Wilson CA, Sawczyn G, Garisto J, Francavilla S, et al. Extraperitoneal versus transperitoneal single port robotic radical prostatectomy: a comparative analysis of perioperative outcomes. J Urol. 2020;203(6):1135–40. https://doi.org/10.1097/ju.0000000000000700.
16. Huang MM, Schwen ZR, Biles MJ, Alam R, Gabrielson AT, Patel HD, et al. A comparative analysis of surgical scar cosmesis based on operative approach for radical prostatectomy. J Endourol. 2020; https://doi.org/10.1089/end.2020.0649.
17. Deutschland. Arbeitsgemeinschaft Bevölkerungsbezogener Krebsregister 2004.
18. Nöske HD, Breitwieser P. Zur Geschichte der Prostatachirurgie. Münch Med Wschr. 1973;115(25):1194–8.
19. Leisrink A, Ahlsberg A. Tumor prostatae; Totale Exstirpation der Prostata. Arch Klin Chir. 1882;28:578–80.
20. Proust R. Technique de la prostatectomie perineal. Ass Franc d'Urol. 1901;5:361.
21. Young HH. The early diagnosis and radical cure of carcinoma of the prostate: being a study of 40 cases and presentations of radical operation which was carried out in 4 cases. Johns Hopkins Hosp Bull. 1905;16:315.
22. Millin T. Retropubic prostatectomy: a new extravesicle technique. Lancet (London). 1945;2:693.
23. von Frisch AZO. Handbuch der Urologie. Berlin, Heidelberg, New York: Springer; 1906. p. 867–91.
24. Budäus LH, Wirth MP, Wolff JM, Bartsch G, Noldus J, Huland H. Prostatakarzinom: gestern – heute – morgen. Urologe (Sonderheft). 2006;45:122–6.
25. Reiner WGWP. An anatomical approach to the surgical management of the dorsal vein and Santorini's plexus during radical retropubic prostatectomy. J Urol. 1979;121:198–200.
26. Walsh PC, Worthington JF. Dr. Patrick Walsh's guide to surviving prostate cancer. 2nd ed. New York: Warner Wellness; 2007.
27. Walsh PCLH, Eggleston JC. Radial prostatectomy with preservation of sexual function: anatomical and pathological considerations. Prostate. 1983;4:473–85.
28. Quinlan DM, Epstein JI, Carter BS, Walsh PC. Sexual function following radical prostatectomy: influence of preservation of neurovascular bundles. J Urol. 1991;145(5):998–1002. https://doi.org/10.1016/s0022-5347(17)38512-9.
29. Schuessler WW, Schulam PG, Clayman RV, Kavoussi LR. Laparoscopic radical prostatectomy: initial short-term experience. Urology. 1997;50(6):854–7. https://doi.org/10.1016/s0090-4295(97)00543-8.
30. Guillonneau B, Cathelineau X, Barret E, Rozet F, Vallancien G. Laparoscopic radical prostatectomy. Preliminary evaluation after 28 interventions. Presse Med. 1998;27(31):1570–4.
31. Guillonneau B, Vallancien G. Laparoscopic radical prostatectomy: the Montsouris experience. J Urol. 2000;163(2):418–22. https://doi.org/10.1016/s0022-5347(05)67890-1.
32. Menon M, Tewari A, Baize B, Guillonneau B, Vallancien G. Prospective comparison of radical retropubic prostatectomy and robot-assisted anatomic prostatectomy: the Vattikuti Urology Institute experience. Urology. 2002;60(5):864–8. https://doi.org/10.1016/s0090-4295(02)01881-2.
33. Raboy A, Ferzli G, Albert P. Initial experience with extraperitoneal endoscopic radical retropubic prostatectomy. Urology. 1997;50(6):849–53. https://doi.org/10.1016/s0090-4295(97)00485-8.
34. Bollens R, Vanden Bossche M, Roumeguere T, Damoun A, Ekane S, Hoffmann P, et al. Extraperitoneal laparoscopic radical prostatectomy. Results after 50 cases. Eur Urol. 2001;40(1):65–9. https://doi.org/10.1159/000049750.
35. Stolzenburg JU, Do M, Pfeiffer H, König F, Aedtner B, Dorschner W. The endoscopic extraperitoneal radical prostatectomy (EERPE): technique and initial experience. World J Urol. 2002;20(1):48–55. https://doi.org/10.1007/s00345-002-0265-4.
36. Stolzenburg JU, Rabenalt R, Do M, Ho K, Dorschner W, Waldkirch E, et al. Endoscopic extraperitoneal radical prostatectomy: oncological and functional results after 700 procedures. J Urol. 2005;174(4 Pt 1):1271–5; discussion 5. https://doi.org/10.1097/01.ju.0000173940.49015.4a.
37. Kiyoshima K, Yokomizo A, Yoshida T, Tomita K, Yonemasu H, Nakamura M, et al. Anatomical features of periprostatic tissue and its surroundings: a histological analysis of 79 radical retropubic prostatectomy specimens. Jpn J Clin Oncol. 2004;34(8):463–8. https://doi.org/10.1093/jjco/hyh078.
38. Menon M, Kaul S, Bhandari A, Shrivastava A, Tewari A, Hemal A. Potency following robotic radical prostatectomy: a questionnaire based analysis of outcomes after conventional nerve sparing and prostatic fascia sparing techniques. J Urol. 2005;174(6):2291–6; discussion 6. https://doi.org/10.1097/01.ju.0000181825.54480.eb.
39. Stolzenburg JU, Rabenalt R, Tannapfel A, Liatsikos EN. Intrafascial nerve-sparing endoscopic extraperitoneal radical prostatectomy. Urology. 2006;67(1):17–21. https://doi.org/10.1016/j.urology.2005.09.052.
40. Menon M, Tewari A. Robotic radical prostatectomy and the Vattikuti Urology Institute technique: an interim analysis of results and technical points. Urology. 2003;61(4 Suppl 1):15–20. https://doi.org/10.1016/s0090-4295(03)00116-x.
41. Joseph JV, Rosenbaum R, Madeb R, Erturk E, Patel HR. Robotic extraperitoneal radical prostatectomy: an alternative approach. J Urol. 2006;175(3 Pt 1):945–50; discussion 51. https://doi.org/10.1016/s0022-5347(05)00340-x.
42. Capello SA, Boczko J, Patel HR, Joseph JV. Randomized comparison of extraperitoneal and transperitoneal access for robot-assisted radical prostatectomy. J Endourol. 2007;21(10):1199–202. https://doi.org/10.1089/end.2007.9906.
43. Stolzenburg JU, Holze S, Neuhaus P, Kyriazis I, Do HM, Dietel A, et al. Robotic-assisted versus laparoscopic surgery: outcomes from the first multicentre, randomised, patient-blinded controlled trial

in radical prostatectomy (LAP-01). Eur Urol. 2021;79(6):750–9. https://doi.org/10.1016/j.eururo.2021.01.030.

44. Stolzenburg JU, Kallidonis P, Minh D, Dietel A, Häfner T, Dimitriou D, et al. Endoscopic extraperitoneal radical prostatectomy: evolution of the technique and experience with 2400 cases. J Endourol. 2009;23(9):1467–72. https://doi.org/10.1089/end.2009.0336.
45. Stolzenburg JU, Liatsikos EN, Rabenalt R, Do M, Sakelaropoulos G, Horn LC, et al. Nerve sparing endoscopic extraperitoneal radical prostatectomy--effect of puboprostatic ligament preservation on early continence and positive margins. Eur Urol. 2006;49(1):103–11; discussion 11–2. https://doi.org/10.1016/j.eururo.2005.10.002.
46. Atug F, Castle EP, Woods M, Srivastav SK, Thomas R, Davis R. Transperitoneal versus extraperitoneal robotic-assisted radical prostatectomy: is one better than the other? Urology. 2006;68(5):1077–81. https://doi.org/10.1016/j.urology.2006.07.008.
47. Stolzenburg J-U, Gettman MT, Liatsikos EN. Endoscopic extraperitoneal radical prostatectomy: laparoscopic and robot-assisted surgery. Springer; 2007.
48. Hung CF, Yang CK, Cheng CL, Ou YC. Bowel complication during robotic-assisted laparoscopic radical prostatectomy. Anticancer Res. 2011;31(10):3497–501.
49. Ghazi A, Scosyrev E, Patel H, Messing EM, Joseph JV. Complications associated with extraperitoneal robot-assisted radical prostatectomy using the standardized Martin classification. Urology. 2013;81(2):324–31. https://doi.org/10.1016/j.urology.2012.07.106.
50. Ploussard G, Salomon L, Parier B, Abbou CC, de la Taille A. Extraperitoneal robot-assisted laparoscopic radical prostatectomy: a single-center experience beyond the learning curve. World J Urol. 2013;31(3):447–53. https://doi.org/10.1007/s00345-012-1014-y.
51. Horovitz D, Feng C, Messing EM, Joseph JV. Extraperitoneal vs. transperitoneal robot-assisted radical prostatectomy in patients with a history of prior inguinal hernia repair with mesh. J Robot Surg. 2017;11(4):447–54. https://doi.org/10.1007/s11701-017-0678-0.
52. Martin RC 2nd, Brennan MF, Jaques DP. Quality of complication reporting in the surgical literature. Ann Surg. 2002;235(6):803–13. https://doi.org/10.1097/00000658-200206000-00007.
53. Dindo D, Demartines N, Clavien PA. Classification of surgical complications: a new proposal with evaluation in a cohort of 6336 patients and results of a survey. Ann Surg. 2004;240(2):205–13. https://doi.org/10.1097/01.sla.0000133083.54934.ae.
54. Donat SM. Standards for surgical complication reporting in urologic oncology: time for a change. Urology. 2007;69(2):221–5. https://doi.org/10.1016/j.urology.2006.09.056.
55. Kaafarani HM, Mavros MN, Hwabejire J, Fagenholz P, Yeh DD, Demoya M, et al. Derivation and validation of a novel severity classification for intraoperative adverse events. J Am Coll Surg. 2014;218(6):1120–8. https://doi.org/10.1016/j.jamcollsurg.2013.12.060.
56. Jung JJ, Elfassy J, Jüni P, Grantcharov T. Adverse events in the operating room: definitions, prevalence, and characteristics. A systematic review. World J Surg. 2019;43(10):2379–92. https://doi.org/10.1007/s00268-019-05048-1.
57. Dell-Kuster S, Gomes NV, Gawria L, Aghlmandi S, Aduse-Poku M, Bissett I, et al. Prospective validation of classification of intraoperative adverse events (ClassIntra): international, multicentre cohort study. BMJ (Clin Res Ed). 2020;370:m2917. https://doi.org/10.1136/bmj.m2917.
58. Hu JC, Nelson RA, Wilson TG, Kawachi MH, Ramin SA, Lau C, et al. Perioperative complications of laparoscopic and robotic assisted laparoscopic radical prostatectomy. J Urol. 2006;175(2):541–6; discussion 6. https://doi.org/10.1016/s0022-5347(05)00156-4.
59. Fischer B, Engel N, Fehr JL, John H. Complications of robotic assisted radical prostatectomy. World J Urol. 2008;26(6):595–602. https://doi.org/10.1007/s00345-008-0287-7.
60. Coelho RF, Palmer KJ, Rocco B, Moniz RR, Chauhan S, Orvieto MA, et al. Early complication rates in a single-surgeon series of 2500 robotic-assisted radical prostatectomies: report applying a standardized grading system. Eur Urol. 2010;57(6):945–52. https://doi.org/10.1016/j.eururo.2010.02.001.
61. Novara G, Ficarra V, D'Elia C, Secco S, Cavalleri S, Artibani W. Prospective evaluation with standardised criteria for postoperative complications after robotic-assisted laparoscopic radical prostatectomy. Eur Urol. 2010;57(3):363–70. https://doi.org/10.1016/j.eururo.2009.11.032.
62. Agarwal PK, Sammon J, Bhandari A, Dabaja A, Diaz M, Dusik-Fenton S, et al. Safety profile of robot-assisted radical prostatectomy: a standardized report of complications in 3317 patients. Eur Urol. 2011;59(5):684–98. https://doi.org/10.1016/j.eururo.2011.01.045.
63. Lee JY, Diaz RR, Cho KS, Choi YD. Meta-analysis of transperitoneal versus extraperitoneal robot-assisted radical prostatectomy for prostate cancer. J Laparoendosc Adv Surg Tech A. 2013;23(11):919–25. https://doi.org/10.1089/lap.2013.0265.
64. Akand M, Erdogru T, Avci E, Ates M. Transperitoneal versus extraperitoneal robot-assisted laparoscopic radical prostatectomy: a prospective single surgeon randomized comparative study. Int J Urol. 2015;22(10):916–21. https://doi.org/10.1111/iju.12854.
65. Kurokawa S, Umemoto Y, Mizuno K, Okada A, Nakane A, Nishio H, et al. New steps of robot-assisted radical prostatectomy using the extraperitoneal approach: a propensity-score matched comparison between extraperitoneal and transperitoneal approach in Japanese patients. BMC Urol. 2017;17(1):106. https://doi.org/10.1186/s12894-017-0298-z.
66. Horovitz D, Feng C, Messing EM, Joseph JV. Extraperitoneal vs transperitoneal robot-assisted radical prostatectomy in the setting of prior abdominal or pelvic surgery. J Endourol. 2017;31(4):366–73. https://doi.org/10.1089/end.2016.0706.
67. Ragavan N, Dholakia K, Ramesh M, Stolzenburg JU. Extraperitoneal vs. transperitoneal robot-assisted laparoscopic radical prostatectomy-analysis of perioperative outcomes, a single surgeon's experience. J Robot Surg. 2019;13(2):275–81. https://doi.org/10.1007/s11701-018-0850-1.
68. Joseph JV, Vicente I, Madeb R, Erturk E, Patel HR. Robot-assisted vs pure laparoscopic radical prostatectomy: are there any differences? BJU Int. 2005;96(1):39–42. https://doi.org/10.1111/j.1464-410X.2005.05563.x.
69. Rozet F, Jaffe J, Braud G, Harmon J, Cathelineau X, Barret E, et al. A direct comparison of robotic assisted versus pure laparoscopic radical prostatectomy: a single institution experience. J Urol. 2007;178(2):478–82. https://doi.org/10.1016/j.juro.2007.03.111.
70. Wang K, Zhuang Q, Xu R, Lu H, Song G, Wang J, et al. Transperitoneal versus extraperitoneal approach in laparoscopic radical prostatectomy: a meta-analysis. Medicine. 2018;97(29):e11176. https://doi.org/10.1097/md.0000000000011176.
71. Verze P, Scuzzarella S, Martina GR, Giummelli P, Cantoni F, Mirone V. Long-term oncological and functional results of extraperitoneal laparoscopic radical prostatectomy: one surgical team's experience on 1,600 consecutive cases. World J Urol. 2013;31(3):529–34. https://doi.org/10.1007/s00345-013-1052-0.
72. Ploussard G, de la Taille A, Moulin M, Vordos D, Hoznek A, Abbou CC, et al. Comparisons of the perioperative, functional, and oncologic outcomes after robot-assisted versus pure extraperitoneal laparoscopic radical prostatectomy. Eur Urol. 2014;65(3):610–9. https://doi.org/10.1016/j.eururo.2012.11.049.

73. Stolzenburg JU, Andrikopoulos O, Kallidonis P, Kyriazis I, Do M, Liatsikos E. Evolution of endoscopic extraperitoneal radical prostatectomy (EERPE): technique and outcome. Asian J Androl. 2012;14(2):278–84. https://doi.org/10.1038/aja.2011.53.
74. Stolzenburg JU, Wasserscheid J, Rabenalt R, Do M, Schwalenberg T, McNeill A, et al. Reduction in incidence of lymphocele following extraperitoneal radical prostatectomy and pelvic lymph node dissection by bilateral peritoneal fenestration. World J Urol. 2008;26(6):581–6. https://doi.org/10.1007/s00345-008-0327-3.
75. Dal Moro F, Zattoni F. P.L.E.A.T.-preventing lymphocele ensuring absorption transperitoneally: a robotic technique. Urology. 2017;110:244–7. https://doi.org/10.1016/j.urology.2017.05.031.
76. Stolzenburg JU, Arthanareeswaran VKA, Dietel A, Franz T, Liatsikos E, Kyriazis I, et al. Four-point peritoneal flap fixation in preventing lymphocele formation following radical prostatectomy. Eur Urol Oncol. 2018;1(5):443–8. https://doi.org/10.1016/j.euo.2018.03.004.
77. Lee M, Lee Z, Eun DD. Utilization of a peritoneal interposition flap to prevent symptomatic lymphoceles after robotic radical prostatectomy and bilateral pelvic lymph node dissection. J Endourol. 2020;34(8):821–7. https://doi.org/10.1089/end.2020.0073.
78. Bründl J, Lenart S, Stojanoski G, Gilfrich C, Rosenhammer B, Stolzlechner M, et al. Peritoneal flap in robot-assisted radical prostatectomy. Dtsch Arztebl Int. 2020;117(14):243–50. https://doi.org/10.3238/arztebl.2020.0243.
79. Neuberger M, Kowalewski KF, Simon V, Wessels F, Siegel F, Worst TS, et al. Peritoneal flap for lymphocele prophylaxis following robotic-assisted laparoscopic radical prostatectomy with pelvic lymph node dissection: study protocol and trial update for the randomized controlled PELYCAN study. Trials. 2021;22(1):236. https://doi.org/10.1186/s13063-021-05168-x.
80. Horovitz D, Lu X, Feng C, Messing EM, Joseph JV. Rate of symptomatic lymphocele formation after extraperitoneal vs transperitoneal robot-assisted radical prostatectomy and bilateral pelvic lymphadenectomy. J Endourol. 2017;31(10):1037–43. https://doi.org/10.1089/end.2017.0153.
81. Motterle G, Morlacco A, Zanovello N, Ahmed ME, Zattoni F, Karnes RJ, et al. Surgical strategies for lymphocele prevention in minimally invasive radical prostatectomy and lymph node dissection: a systematic review. J Endourol. 2020;34(2):113–20. https://doi.org/10.1089/end.2019.0716.
82. Boczko J, Madeb R, Golijanin D, Erturk E, Mathe M, Patel HR, et al. Robot-assisted radical prostatectomy in obese patients. Can J Urol. 2006;13(4):3169–73.
83. Nielsen ME, Walsh PC. Systematic detection and repair of subclinical inguinal hernias at radical retropubic prostatectomy. Urology. 2005;66(5):1034–7. https://doi.org/10.1016/j.urology.2005.05.028.
84. Stranne J, Hugosson J, Lodding P. Post-radical retropubic prostatectomy inguinal hernia: an analysis of risk factors with special reference to preoperative inguinal hernia morbidity and pelvic lymph node dissection. J Urol. 2006;176(5):2072–6. https://doi.org/10.1016/j.juro.2006.07.007.
85. Alder R, Zetner D, Rosenberg J. Incidence of inguinal hernia after radical prostatectomy: a systematic review and meta-analysis. J Urol. 2020;203(2):265–74. https://doi.org/10.1097/ju.0000000000000313.
86. Qazi HA, Rai BP, Do M, Rewhorn M, Häfner T, Liatsikos E, et al. Robot-assisted laparoscopic total extraperitoneal hernia repair during prostatectomy: technique and initial experience. Central Eur J Urol. 2015;68(2):240–4. https://doi.org/10.5173/ceju.2015.562.
87. Ludwig WW, Sopko NA, Azoury SC, Dhanasopon A, Mettee L, Dwarakanath A, et al. Inguinal hernia repair during extraperitoneal robot-assisted laparoscopic radical prostatectomy. J Endourol. 2016;30(2):208–11. https://doi.org/10.1089/end.2015.0393.
88. Fernando H, Garcia C, Hossack T, Ahmadi N, Thanigasalam R, Gillatt D, et al. Incidence, predictive factors and preventive measures for inguinal hernia following robotic and laparoscopic radical prostatectomy: a systematic review. J Urol. 2019;201(6):1072–9. https://doi.org/10.1097/ju.0000000000000133.
89. Agrawal V, Feng C, Joseph J. Outcomes of extraperitoneal robot-assisted radical prostatectomy in the morbidly obese: a propensity score-matched study. J Endourol. 2015;29(6):677–82. https://doi.org/10.1089/end.2014.0661.
90. Dal Moro F, Crestani A, Valotto C, Guttilla A, Soncin R, Mangano A, et al. Anesthesiologic effects of transperitoneal versus extraperitoneal approach during robot-assisted radical prostatectomy: results of a prospective randomized study. Int Braz J Urol. 2015;41(3):466–72. https://doi.org/10.1590/s1677-5538.Ibju.2014.0199.
91. Glascock JM, Winfield HN, Lund GO, Donovan JF, Ping ST, Griffiths DL. Carbon dioxide homeostasis during transperitoneal or extraperitoneal laparoscopic pelvic lymphadenectomy: a real-time intraoperative comparison. J Endourol. 1996;10(4):319–23. https://doi.org/10.1089/end.1996.10.319.
92. Liatsikos E, Bynens B, Rabenalt R, Kallidonis P, Do M, Stolzenburg JU. Treatment of patients after failed high intensity focused ultrasound and radiotherapy for localized prostate cancer: salvage laparoscopic extraperitoneal radical prostatectomy. J Endourol. 2008;22(10):2295–8. https://doi.org/10.1089/end.2008.9713.
93. Dobbs RW, Halgrimson WR, Madueke I, Vigneswaran HT, Wilson JO, Crivellaro S. Single-port robot-assisted laparoscopic radical prostatectomy: initial experience and technique with the da Vinci(®) SP platform. BJU Int. 2019;124(6):1022–7. https://doi.org/10.1111/bju.14864.
94. Covas Moschovas M, Bhat S, Onol F, Rogers T, Patel V. Early outcomes of single-port robot-assisted radical prostatectomy: lessons learned from the learning-curve experience. BJU Int. 2021;127(1):114–21. https://doi.org/10.1111/bju.15158.
95. Wilson CA, Aminsharifi A, Sawczyn G, Garisto JD, Yau R, Eltemamy M, et al. Outpatient extraperitoneal single-port robotic radical prostatectomy. Urology. 2020;144:142–6. https://doi.org/10.1016/j.urology.2020.06.029.
96. Stolzenburg JU, Kallidonis P, Kyriazis I, Kotsiris D, Ntasiotis P, Liatsikos EN. Robot-assisted simple prostatectomy by an extraperitoneal approach. J Endourol. 2018;32(S1):S39–43. https://doi.org/10.1089/end.2017.0714.
97. Wang P, Xia D, Ye S, Kong D, Qin J, Jing T, et al. Robotic-assisted urethra-sparing simple prostatectomy via an extraperitoneal approach. Urology. 2018;119:85–90. https://doi.org/10.1016/j.urology.2018.06.005.
98. Gurung PM, Mithal P, Lu DD, Ghazi AE, Joseph JV. Robot-assisted simple prostatectomy: illustration of a simplified extraperitoneal transcapsular technique. Videourology (New Rochelle). 2019;33(6) https://doi.org/10.1089/vid.2019.0032.
99. Steinberg RL, Passoni N, Garbens A, Johnson BA, Gahan JC. Initial experience with extraperitoneal robotic-assisted simple prostatectomy using the da Vinci SP surgical system. J Robot Surg. 2020;14(4):601–7. https://doi.org/10.1007/s11701-019-01029-7.
100. Gurung PM, Witthaus M, Campbell T, Rashid HH, Ghazi AE, Wu G, et al. Transvesical versus transabdominal - which is the best approach to bladder diverticulectomy using the single port robotic system? Urology. 2020;142:248. https://doi.org/10.1016/j.urology.2020.05.018.

Lymphadenectomy in Prostate Cancer: Technique and Outcomes

Jean Felipe Prodocimo Lestingi, Rafael Sanchez Salas, Kunihiko Yoshioka, and Rafael Ferreira Coelho

1 Introduction

Prostate cancer (PCa) is currently the most common non-cutaneous malignancy and the second leading cause of cancer death in men in Western countries. With the advent of prostate-specific antigen (PSA) and screening programs, although cases of confined organ tumors are currently more frequent, about 10–20% of patients have locally advanced disease or lymph node metastases at the time of diagnosis [1].

The PCa can spread both via the hematogenous route, the axial skeleton being the preferred site of metastases, and via the lymphatic way, represented mainly by the drainage of the pelvic lymph nodes [2]. Despite recent advances in imaging techniques, there are still difficulties in assessing lymph node involvement. The sensitivity of Computed Tomography and Magnetic Resonance in detecting lymph node metastases is close to 35% insufficient [3, 4]. The Positron Emission Tomography (PET) [68Ga] prostate-specific membrane antigen (PSMA) in the setting of primary staging also is controversial, given the paucity of data [5].

Lymphadenectomy, or lymph node dissection (LND), has become part of radical prostatectomy (RP) since the operation became popular in the 1980s by Walsh [6]. The goal of any anatomical lymphadenectomy in patients with high-risk human cancers of any type is to identify microscopic lymph node metastases to improve locoregional staging and facilitate discussions regarding the need for adjuvant systemic therapy and improve long-term oncological outcomes [7].

The actual therapeutic role of LND during RP for the management of PCa remains controversial in terms of oncological impact. Reports suggest that LND improves pathological staging and that extending the pelvic LND (PLND) template may increase its staging accuracy [8]. Nevertheless, the oncological benefit of the procedure is still unclear. Recently, two Randomized Controlled Trials (RCT) comparing extended vs. limited PLND in intermediate- and high-risk PCa patients demonstrated no Biochemical Recurrence differences in a short follow-up [9, 10]. A recent systematic review revealed that performing PLND during RP failed to improve oncological outcomes, including survival [11]. Although, it is generally accepted that extended PLND provides essential information for staging and prognosis.

Furthermore, complications are a significant concern related to the procedure. PLND may be associated with an increased risk of adverse events, morbidity, length of stay, and healthcare costs, mainly related to significant lymphoceles [11]. However, the assertion that more extensive PLND leads to higher complication rates has not always been confirmed [12, 13].

This chapter will review indications, techniques, and results of extended pelvic lymphadenectomy (ePLND) in the surgical treatment of PCa patients.

1.1 Current Guideline Recommendations for Extended PLND in Prostate Cancer

The American Urological Association (AUA) / American Society for Radiation Oncology (ASTRO) / Society of Urologic Oncology (SUO) guidelines reserve the LND for patients with PCa at higher risk for LNI, high-risk or unfavorable intermediate-risk. Still, they do not indicate the extent of the dissection. They also emphasize the importance

J. F. P. Lestingi
Instituto do Cancer do Estado de Sao Paulo – Hospital das Clinicas – Faculdade de Medicina – Universidade de Sao Paulo – ICESP HCFMUSP, São Paulo, Brazil

R. S. Salas
Department of Surgery, Division of Urology, McGill University, Montréal, Canada

K. Yoshioka
Department of Urology, Tokyo Medical University, Tokyo, Japan

R. F. Coelho (✉)
Coordinator of Urology – Instituto do Cancer do Estado de Sao Paulo – Hospital das Clinicas – Faculdade de Medicina – Universidade de Sao Paulo – ICESP HCFMUSP, São Paulo, Brazil

P. Wiklund et al. (eds.), *Robotic Urologic Surgery*, https://doi.org/10.1007/978-3-031-00363-9_27

of guiding patients about LND complications, including lymphocele and its treatment [14].

The European Association of Urology (EAU), European Association of Nuclear Medicine (EANM), European Society for Radiotherapy and Oncology (ESTRO), European Society of Urogenital Radiology (ESUR), and International Society of Geriatric Oncology (SIOG) recommendations indicate the LND for PCa patients with locally advanced, high-risk, and intermediate-risk disease whose LNI estimate is greater than 5% in the preoperative nomograms. In patients where LND is indicated, it should be extended. The recommended extended template dissects the regions bilaterally: obturator, external iliac, and internal iliac. Although, if updated versions of preoperative nomograms are used, including multiparametric Magnetic Resonance Image findings and Target Biopsy results, more patients may spare from an unnecessary PLND (using a threshold of 7%) [15].

The National Comprehensive Cancer Network (NCCN) suggests that an extended PLND is preferred when PLND is performed and recommended for patients whose predicated probability of nodal metastases by nomograms is ≥2%. According to NCCN recommendation, an extended PLND includes removing all node-bearing tissue from an area bound by the external iliac vein anteriorly, the pelvic sidewall laterally, the bladder wall medially, the floor of the pelvis posteriorly, Cooper's ligament distally, and the internal iliac artery proximally. Besides that, PLND can be performed using an open, laparoscopic, or robotic technique [16].

The individual risk of finding positive LNs can be estimated using externally validated preoperative nomograms. Tools currently for identifying ePLND candidates are based on clinical parameters and showed excellent predictive accuracy on internal and external validation [17–20]. The variables included in models predicting lymph node invasion, guidelines, indications, and recommendations to perform PLND are summarized in Table 1.

Table 1 Guidelines, indications, and recommendations to perform pelvic lymph node dissection in prostate cancer

Guideline	Indications to perform PLND	Clinical variables considered	Recommended PLND
AUA / ASTRO / SUO	High-risk	PSA	Do not specify the template
	Unfavorable intermediate-risk	Clinical stage	
		ISUP grade group	
EAU / EANM / ESTRO / ESUR / SIOG	Intermediate-risk according to nomograms	PSA	Extended
	Probability of LNM > 5% (2012 Briganti nomogram)	Clinical stage (mpMRI[a])	
	Probability of LNM > 7% (2018 Gandaglia nomogram)[a]	Primary Gleason grade	
		Secondary Gleason grade	
	High-risk	Positive cores %	
		Maximum lesion diameter at mpMRI[a]	
	Locally advanced	Biopsy Gleason grade group at MRI-targeted biopsy[a]	
		Percentage of cores with clinically significant PCa at systematic biopsy[a]	
NCCN	Probability of nodal metastases by nomogram is ≥2%	Preoperative PSA	Extended
	MSKCC nomogram	Primary biopsy Gleason grade	
		Secondary biopsy Gleason grade	
		Clinical tumor stage	
		Negative biopsy cores	
		Positive biopsy cores	

ASTRO American Society for Radiation Oncology, *AUA* American urological association, *EAU* European Association of Urology, *EANM* European Association of Nuclear Medicine (EANM), *ESTRO* European Society for Radiotherapy and Oncology, *ESUR* European Society of Urogenital Radiology, *LNM* Lymph node metastases, *mpMRI* Multiparametric magnetic resonance imaging, *MSKCC* Memorial Sloan cancer Kettering center, *NCCN* National Comprehensive Cancer Network, *PCa* Prostate cancer, *PLND* Pelvic lymph node dissection, *PSA* Prostate specific antigen, *SIOG* International Society of Geriatric Oncology, *SUO* Society of Urologic Oncology

[a]Exclusive variables

2 Lymphadenectomy and Staging of Prostate Cancer: Templates and Patterns of Lymph Node Involvement

There was a lot of misunderstanding about nomenclature and LND templates. To standardize the extent of this dissection, the reference expert panel from the EAU Prostate Cancer Guideline Panel the following types of LND as follows (Fig. 1):

- ***Limited lymphadenectomy***: obturator lymph nodes.
- ***Standard lymphadenectomy***: obturator and external iliac lymph nodes.

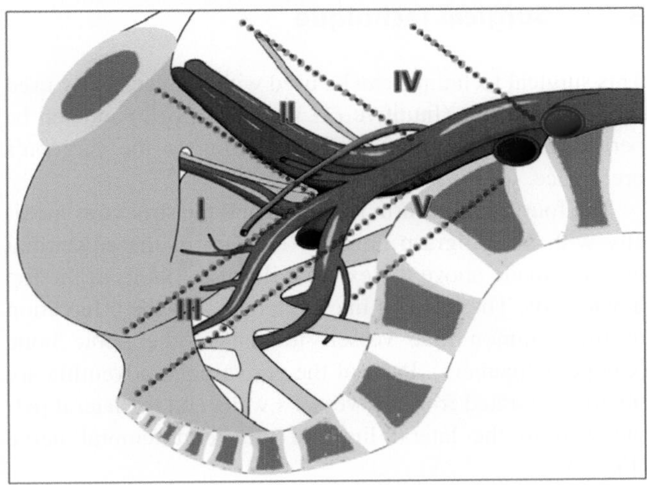

Fig. 1 Anatomical areas for the definition of the extent of dissection. I = obturator nodes; II = external iliac nodes; III = internal iliac nodes; IV = common iliac notes; V = presacral nodes

- ***Extended lymphadenectomy***: obturator lymph nodes, external iliac, and internal iliac.
- ***Super-extended lymphadenectomy***: obturator lymph nodes, external iliac, internal iliac, common iliac, and presacral [11, 21].

The dissection limits of the ePLND template include:

- ***Cranial***: crossing of the ureter over the common iliac vessels.
- ***Caudal***: deep circumflex vein and femoral canal.
- ***Lateral***: genital femoral nerve.
- ***Medial***: perivesical fat [11, 21].

The PCa does not follow a predetermined and constant pattern of nodal dissemination, and about 50% of these lymph node metastases are located along the internal iliac artery [3]. Retrospective series showed that the rate of pelvic lymph nodes invaded in patients with PCA is directly proportional to the extent of LND. The more lymph nodes dissected, the greater the number of affected lymph nodes, denoting the importance of performing ePLND [12, 22–25].

However, studies have indicated that resection of at least 20 lymph nodes is necessary for the PCa staging to be adequate, similar to that demonstrated in the Bladder Cancer LND [26]. Figure 2 illustrates the distribution of positive node patients by dissection area for extended PLND cases with at least one positive lymph node in a recently published trial [9]. Interestingly, almost two-thirds of patients with positive nodes had metastases at the internal iliac area.

A mapping study published by Briganti and colleagues included 19 patients with high-risk PCa (sharing at least two

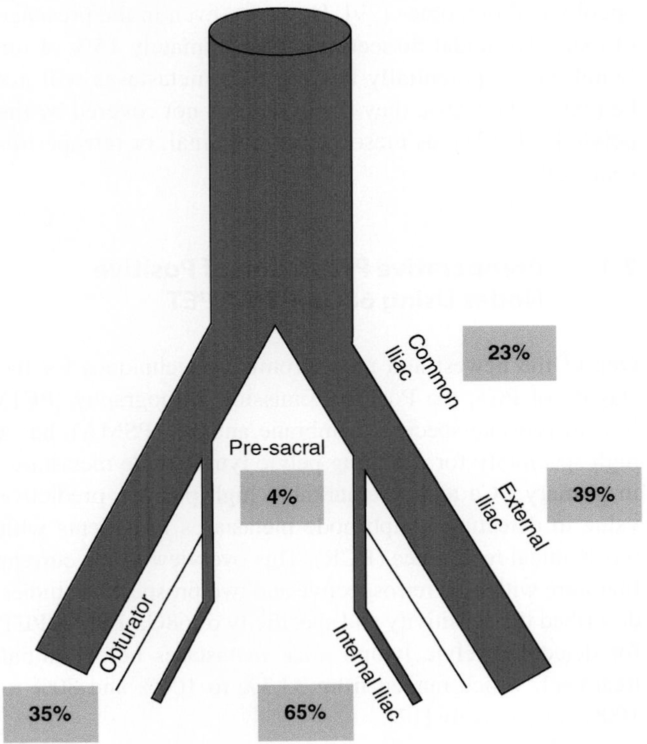

Fig. 2 Distribution of node-positive patients (N1) undergoing extended pelvic lymph node dissection per region [9]

out of the three following parameters: PSA >20 ng/ml, cT3, biopsy Gleason score ≥ 8). All patients were treated with RP and removal of the obturator, hypogastric, external iliac, presacral, common iliac, para-aortal/para-caval, and inter-aortocaval lymph nodes. Only patients with positive common iliac lymph nodes had positive retroperitoneal lymph nodes, demonstrating an ascending pathway for metastatic PCa cells [27].

Another mapping study by Joniau et al. with 74 localized PCa patients and a lymph node involvement risk of ≥10% but ≤35% (Partin tables) or a cT3 tumor provided fundamental insight into the pattern of lymphatic spread. After intraprostatic technetium-99 m nano colloid injection, surgery was performed with a sentinel node procedure and a super-extended LND followed by RP. The predominant site for lymphatic metastases was the internal iliac region. Extended PLND correctly staged the majority of positive lymph nodes patients, but 13% of the positive lymph nodes would have been missed [28].

Extended PLND significantly increases the yield of both total lymph nodes and lymph node metastases independent of the risk classification of PCa. Lymph node metastases will be detected in about 5–6%, 20–25%, and 30–40% of low-, intermediate-, and high-risk PCa, respectively [23].

In high-volume referral centers, the open, laparoscopic, or robotic LND techniques are feasible and have similar oncological outcomes [29]. However, even in the presence of extensive nodal dissections, approximately 15% of the lymph nodes potentially bearing PCa metastases will not be removed because they are in regions not covered by the pelvic LND [21], as mesorectum, inguinal, or retroperitoneal [30].

2.1 Preoperative Prediction of Positive Nodes Using 68Ga-PSMA PET

One of the newest and most promising techniques for the staging of PCa, the Positron Emission Tomography (PET) [68Ga] prostate-specific membrane antigen (PSMA), has a high specificity for detecting pelvic lymph node metastases in primary PCa and a remarkably high positive predictive value in detecting lymph node metastases in patients with biochemical recurrence (BCR). This overview of the current literature with nine retrospective and two prospective studies described the sensitivity and specificity of 68Ga-PSMA PET for detecting pelvic lymph node metastases before initial treatment, which ranged from 33.3% to 100% and 80% to 100%, respectively [17].

Another recent review and meta-analysis included 37 articles and 4790 patients. The results highlighted the excellent sensitivity and specificity of 68Ga-PSMA PET in advanced prostate cancer. Specifically, on a per-patient analysis, the sensitivity and specificity of 68Ga-PSMA PET were 77% and 97%, respectively, following pelvic lymph node dissection at the time of RP. Sensitivity and specificity were 75% and 99% on a per-lesion analysis, respectively [5].

The US Food and Drug Administration (FDA) has recently approved Gallium 68 PSMA-11 as the first drug for PET imaging of PSMA positive lesions in men with PCa. However, one prospective multicenter single-arm open-label phase 3 imaging trial that supported the FDA decision showed a sensitivity of 0.4, also a low sensitivity in evaluating lymph node involvement. From December 2015 to August 2019, 633 intermediate to high-risk PCa patients underwent one 68Ga-PSMA-11 PET for primary staging, and 277/633 (44%) subsequently underwent RP and PLND. The median initial PSA was 11.1 [0.04–147]. Seventy five/two hundred and seventy-seven patients (27%) had N1 disease per histopathology. Sensitivity, specificity, positive predictive value and negative predictive value for N1 detection was 0.40 [0.34, 0.46], 0.95 [0.92, 0.97], 0.75 [0.70, 0.80], 0.81 [0.76, 0.85], respectively. Higher PSAs and larger node sizes correlated with increased sensitivity [18].

Therefore, PET [68Ga] PSMA cannot replace pelvic LND to exclude lymph node metastases: LND is still the gold standard for lymph node staging [5, 17].

3 Surgical Technique

This surgical technique can be used with both currently used robotic platforms (Intuitive *Da Vinci Xi* or *Si*©) and can be performed before or after RP according to the surgeon's preference.

The fourth robotic arm is used to pull the structures medially with the Prograsp Forceps. Incision of the adventitial fascia is made above the external iliac vessels from the top downwards. The incision line stretches from the bifurcation of the common iliac vessels to contact the pubic bone (Cooper's ligament). Parts of the perivascular adventitia are bluntly separated from the vessel's walls and the lateral pelvic wall to the lateral limit of the genitofemoral nerve (Fig. 3).

Slight shifting of the dissected conglomerate to cranial helps to identify the obturator nerve. Furthermore, preparation is strictly along and above the obturator nerve up to the meeting point with the internal iliac artery. The packet is ligated to occlude lymphatic leakage and prevent lymphocele (Fig. 4).

The dissection proceeds caudally to the femoral canal and the deep circumflex vein; the end next to Cooper's ligament is clipped. Sequentially, the tissue along the internal iliac vessels is dissected to skeletonize the obturator nerve (Fig. 5); the back next to the common iliac vessels is clipped.

The ureter, which ascends with the peritoneum, is identified and hitched. The crossing of the ureter at the bifurcation of the common iliac artery marks the caudal end of the dissection (Fig. 6). The bilateral tissue has been released from the extended template and can be extracted safely as a whole using an endo bag.

The Marcille's triangle or fossa is a pelvic anatomical region limited by the fifth lumbar vertebra medially, from the inner edge of the large muscle psoas laterally, from the upper edge of the wing, and the sacrum below. Lymph nodes of this anatomical region are related to the prostate lymphatic system, and some authors discuss Marcille's lymphadenectomy when planning an ePLND in high-risk PCa. Porcaro et al. analyzed 221 patients who underwent ePLND and robotic-assisted RP: Marcille's lymph node involvement was found in 5 (2.3%) patients. However, this involvement was associated with multiple lymph node metastases in other template locations in high-risk PCa patients [19].

The pelvic plexus and the erectile nerves are at risk in standard dissection during the medial dissection in the area of the internal iliac artery and towards the bladder wall. During ePLND, the nerves are also at risk at their origin in the presacral area and medial to the common iliac vessels. Decreased erectile function in patients with a more extended yield of lymph nodes relative to patients with a lower yield or

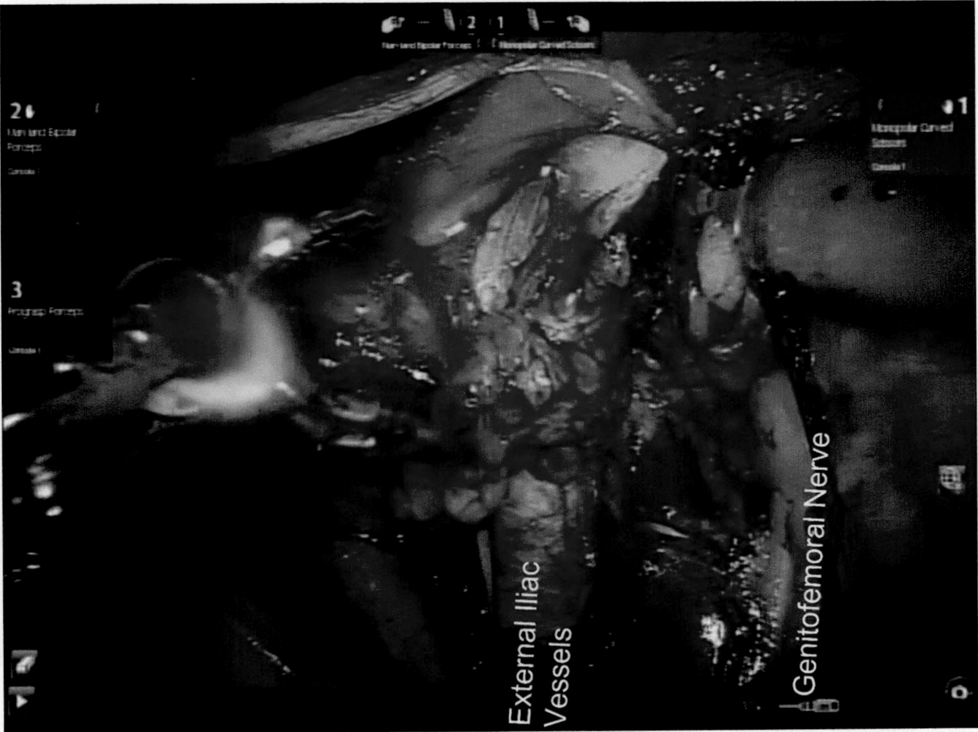

Fig. 3 Extended pelvic lymph node dissection surgical step (right side). Blunt lymphatic dissection anteriorly to the external iliac artery, from common iliac cranially to Cooper's ligament caudally

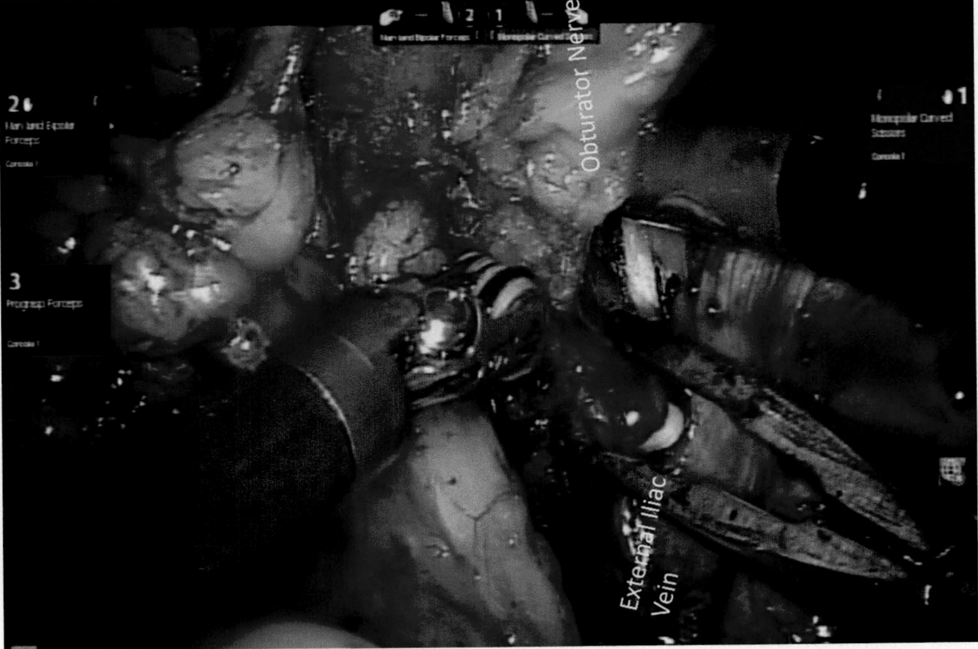

Fig. 4 Extended pelvic lymph node dissection surgical step (right side). Ligation of lymph nodal tissue cranially to the obturator nerve

no lymph node dissection has been demonstrated [20, 31]. Others could not find any influence from the extent of PLND on erectile function [32]. Nevertheless, from an anatomic point of view, ePLND occurs near or inside the pelvic plexus and thus can lead to injury of erectile nerves [33].

Lymphocele is the most common complication after PLND. Over the years, various techniques have been introduced to prevent lymphocele, but no conclusion can be drawn regarding the superiority of one technique over another. In this prospective study, 220 patients undergoing

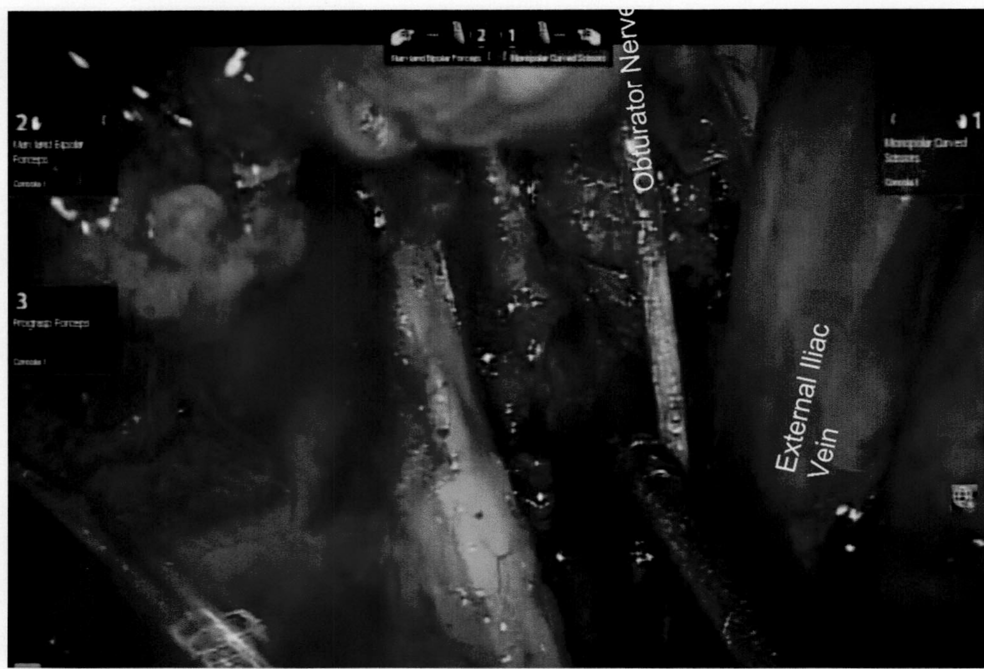

Fig. 5 Extended pelvic lymph node dissection surgical step (right side). Skeletonization of the obturator nerve

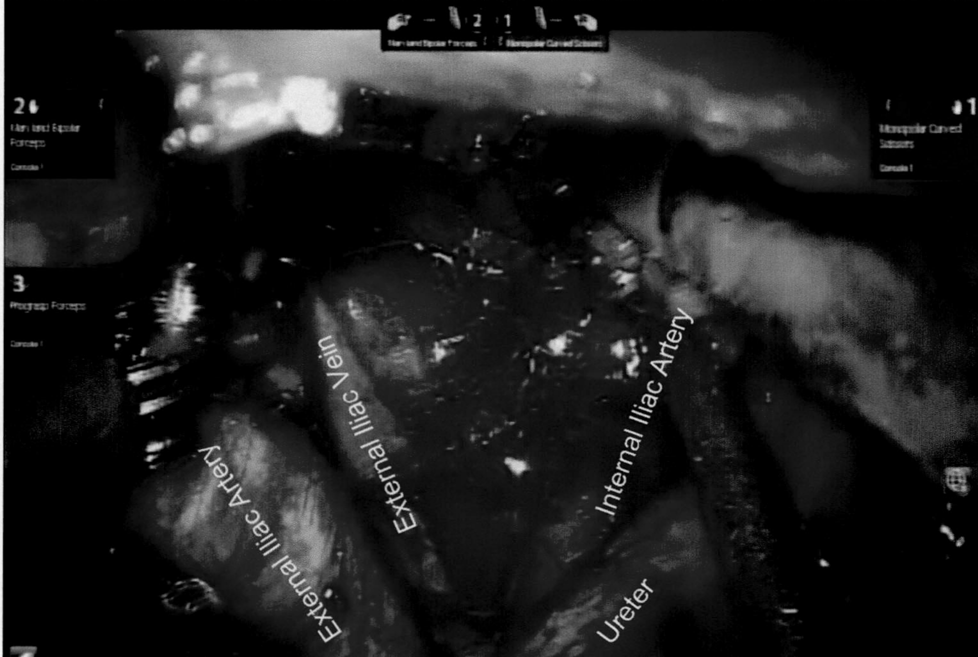

Fig. 6 Extended pelvic lymph node dissection surgical step (left side). The cranial limit of the template is the crossing of the ureter at the bifurcation of the common iliac artery

robot-assisted RP between 2012 and 2015 were randomized to receive titanium clips (group A, $n = 110$) or bipolar coagulation (group B, $n = 110$) to seal lymphatic vessels during ePLND. There were no statistically significant differences between groups A and B regarding overall lymphocele incidence (47% vs. 48%; difference − 0.91%, 95% confidence interval [CI] -2.6 to 0.7; $p = 0.9$) and the rate of clinically significant lymphocele [5% vs. 4%; difference 0.75%, 95% CI, 0.1–3.2; $p = 0.7$]. The two groups were comparable regarding mean (±SD) lymphocele volume (30 ± 32 vs. 35 ± 39 ml; $p = 0.6$), lymphocele location (unilateral, 37% vs. 35%, $p = 0.7$; bilateral, 13% vs. 14%, $p = 0.9$), and time to lymphocele diagnosis (95% vs. 98% on a postoperative day 10; $p = 0.5$) [34].

4 Perioperative Outcomes and Complications

There is much discussion in the literature about what the LND extension model should be. Such doubts are due to the uncertain benefit of LND in therapeutic terms and the potential increase in complications as the dissection limit increases.

The pelvic lymph node dissection is a challenging procedure that is time-consuming and carries a greater risk of surgical complications, with rates ranging from 2 to 51% [8]. One of the most extensive series with 963 patients that compared adverse events of the types of LND showed 19.8% of complications in the extended LND vs. 8.2% in the limited one ($p < 0.001$); when analyzed individually, only the lymphocele was significantly higher in patients undergoing extensive dissection (10.3% vs. 4.6%, respectively; $p = 0.02$) [13]. On the other hand, Bader et al. found only 2.1% of complications needed to prolong the length of hospital stay in patients undergoing ePLND [22].

Similarly, Fossati et al. compared LND vs. no-LND (20 retrospective studies) and compared the extended dissection vs. limited (3 prospective and 15 retrospective studies). LND and extended dissection were associated with significantly worse intra- and postoperative non-oncological outcomes, such as bleeding, lymphocele, and increased surgical time. The retrospective nature of most studies and the lack of standardized definitions for the extension of the LND are the main limitations of its conclusions [11].

The baseline characteristics of the principal comparative studies evaluating non-oncological outcomes are summarized in Table 2 [11, 12, 35]. Overall, 18 studies compared no PLND vs. any form of PLND, while 14 studies compared lPLND/sPLND vs. ePLND/sePLND. The non-oncological results are summarized in Table 3 [11, 12, 35].

4.1 Intraoperative and Perioperative Outcomes

Data were obtained from 16 retrospective studies regarding operative time, blood loss, and postoperative complications [36–51]. In the main, PLND was associated with a significantly higher risk of lymphocele in most studies that addressed the outcome.

In an RCT, 123 patients were randomized to ePLND on the right hemipelvis vs. lPLND on the left hemipelvis. Complications including lymphocele (3% vs. 1%) and lower extremity edema (3% vs. 2%) occurred more commonly on the side subjected to ePLND compared to lPLND [52]. When considering data from nine retrospective studies, conflicting results were observed. Three studies showed significantly higher intraoperative and postoperative complications in the ePLND group than lPLND/sPLND [53–55], while four studies did not find significant differences [56–59]. Similarly, the lymphocele rate was significantly higher in the ePLND group in four studies [53, 54, 60, 61], while no significant differences were observed in three others [56–58].

In another RCT, the rates of grade 2 and grade 3 complications were comparable between the limited (7.3%) and extended PLND groups (6.4%) [10].

4.2 Functional Outcomes

Three retrospective studies did not find any significant differences between PLND and no PLND regarding erectile function recovery [OR 0.95, 95% CI 0.63–1.43, $p = 0.8$ [32]; and HR 0.9; $p = 0.8$ [62]; $p = 0.48$ [59]].

One retrospective comparative study did not find any significant differences regarding urinary continence (HR 1.07, 95% CI 0.87–1.31; $p = 0.5$) and erectile function recovery (HR 1.11, 95% CI 0.75–1.63; $p = 0.6$) between ePLND and lPLND [63].

There were no differences in the International Index of Erectile Function scores in an RCT between ePLND and lPLND [10].

Extending the LND template beyond the ePLND template may cause at least a significant delay in recovery of urinary continence, maybe due to bladder denervation. Seikkula et al. demonstrated in a cohort of 172 PCa patients who underwent RP and PLND that patients undergoing super-extended PLND have a lower chance of regaining urinary continence [hazard ratio (HR) 0.59, 95% CI 0.39–0.90, $p = 0.026$]. Age at the surgery also had a significant influence on continence [64].

Nevertheless, some academic studies have suggested robot-assisted RP superiority over pure laparoscopic or open RP in operative and functional outcomes. Several reviews and meta-analyses of the literature recently highlighted the potential benefit of robot-assisted RP regarding the functional outcomes without hindering oncologic control. Few controlled trials with small cohorts have compared pure laparoscopic radical prostatectomy and robot-assisted RP, suggesting better early functional outcomes using robotic assistance. However, the level of evidence remains weak given the lack of randomized controlled trials and the number of factors (surgeon experience, disease staging, nerve-sparing techniques) that need to be considered [65].

Table 2 Baseline characteristics for studies addressing non-oncological outcomes

Study	Surgical	Treatment	N	Follow-up (mo)	Age (year)	PSA (ng/ml)	Biopsy Gleason score	Clinical T stage	Pathologic T stage	Pathologic Gleason score	Surgical margin	Number of lymph nodes dissected	Number of positive lymph nodes	Outcomes
No PLND versus any PLND														
Ostby-Deglum 2015	Robotic: 100%	No PLND	609	3.0	63	NR	NR	NR	NR	NR	NR	NR	NR	Insufficient
				[0.5–6.1]	[42–78]									Erection
Violette 2015	Robotic: 100%	No PLND	392	NR	60 (7)	6.9 (3)	6: 58.9% ($n = 231$)	NR	NR	NR	NR	NR	NR	OT
							7: 41.1% ($n = 161$)							
Tyritzis 2015	Open: 24%	No PLND	2997	NR	63.5	6.6 [0.1–20.0]	≤6: 58.1% ($n = 1732$)	T1: 65.5% ($n = 1914$)	T2: 77.2% ($n = 2266$)	≤7: 96.2% ($n = 2846$)	NR	NR	NR	DVT
	Robotic: 76%				[37.2–75.0]		3 + 4: 33.9% ($n = 1011$)	T2: 33.2% ($n = 969$)	T3: 22.6% ($n = 662$)	≥8: 3.8% ($n = 113$)				
							4 + 3: 6.1% ($n = 182$)	T3: 1.3% ($n = 38$)	T4: 0.2% ($n = 6$)					
							≥8: 1.8% ($n = 54$)							
		PLND	547		64.8	9.4 [0.7–20.0]	≤6: 13% ($n = 71$)	T1: 35.1% ($n = 187$)	T2: 48% ($n = 258$)	≤7: 78.8% ($n = 423$)				
					[42.3–75.0]		3 + 4: 31.3% ($n = 171$)	T2: 52.2% ($n = 278$)	T3: 50.5% ($n = 271$)	≥8: 21.2% ($n = 114$)				
							4 + 3: 28.9% ($n = 158$)	T3: 12.8% ($n = 68$)	T4: 1.5% ($n = 8$)					
							≥8: 26.7% ($n = 146$)							
Boehm 2015	Open: 95%	No PLND	4884	NR	64 (59–67)	NR	≤6: 29.2% ($n = 3412$)	NR	pT2: 70% ($n = 8172$)	NR	NR	NR	NR	Blood
	Robotic: 5%	PLND	6810				3 + 4: 53.8% ($n = 6303$)		pT3a: 20% ($n = 2327$)					Transfusion
							4 + 3: 13.0% ($n = 1529$)		≥pT3b: 10% ($n = 1223$)					
							≥8: 3.8 ($n = 443$)							

Liss 2013	Robotic: 100%	No PLND	207	NR	61 (6.9)	4.9 (4.0–6.5)	≤6: 93.5% (*n* = 188)	T1: 78.3% (*n* = 162)	T1: 92.3% (*n* = 191)	NR	NR	NA	NA	OT, eBL,
							7: 4.5% (*n* = 9)	T2: 21.7% (*n* = 45)	T2: 6.8% (*n* = 14)					Transfusion
							≥8: 2% (*n* = 4)	T3: 0% (*n* = 0)	T3: 1% (*n* = 2)					Rate, LoS,
														Complication rate,
														Lymphocele rate
		sPLND	231		63 (6.8)	6.1 (4.4–9.2)	≤6: 58.9% (*n* = 136)	T1: 58.9% (*n* = 136)	T1: 72.7% (*n* = 168)			18 [12–25]	0.3% (*n* = 13)	
							7: 39.4% (*n* = 91)	T2: 39.4% (*n* = 91)	T2: 26.4% (*n* = 61)					
							≥8: 1.7% (*n* = 4)	T3: 1.7% (*n* = 4)	T3: 0.9% (*n* = 2)					
		ePLND	54		61 (7.2)	8.5 (5.5–13.5)	≤6: 27.8% (*n* = 15)	T1: 27.8% (*n* = 15)	T1: 42.6% (*n* = 23)			20 (16–28)	2% (*n* = 24)	
							7: 68.5% (*n* = 37)	T2: 68.5% (*n* = 37)	T2: 55.6% (*n* = 30)					
							≥8: 3.7% (*n* = 2)	T3: 3.7% (*n* = 2)	T3: 1.9% (*n* = 1)					
van der Poel 2012	Robotic: 100%	No PLND	464	NR	60.7 (6.2)	NR	< 7: 90.5% (*n* = 420)	T1: 36.4% (*n* = 169)	T0: 1.5% (*n* = 7)	<7: 65.7% (*n* = 305)	NR	0	NA	Lymphocele, DVT,
							7: 8.6% (*n* = 40)	T2: 61.4% (*n* = 285)	T2: 84.5% (*n* = 392)	7: 29.1% (*n* = 135)				Clavien grade,
							>7: 0.7% (*n* = 4)	T3: 2.2% (*n* = 10)	T3: 11.0% (*n* = 51)	>7: 5.2% (*n* = 24)				Hematoma, ileus,
									T4: 3.0% (*n* = 14)					Anastomosis dehiscence
		sPLND	440		62.5 (5.8)	47.9 (23.2)	<7: 25.9% (*n* = 114)	T1: 34.1% (*n* = 150)	T0: 0.2% (*n* = 1)	<7: 65.7% (*n* = 305)		14 [11–19]	8.4% (*n* = 37)	
							7: 54.1% (*n* = 238)	T2: 59.3% (*n* = 261)	T2: 59.8% (*n* = 263)	7: 29.1% (*n* = 135)				
							>7: 20% (*n* = 88)	T3: 20.7 (*n* = 91)	T3: 34.3% (*n* = 151)	>7: 5.2% (*n* = 24)				

(continued)

Table 2 (continued)

Study	Surgical	Treatment	*N*	Follow-up (mo)	Age (year)	PSA (ng/ml)	Biopsy Gleason score	Clinical T stage	Pathologic T stage	Pathologic Gleason score	Surgical margin	Number of lymph nodes dissected	Number of positive lymph nodes	Outcomes
									T4: 5.7% (*n* = 25)					
Schmitges 2012	Open: 93%	No PLND	36,699	NR	61.7 (7.2)	NR	NR	NR	NR	NR	NR	NR	Nx: 56.8% (*n* = 20,862)	DVT
	Minimally												N0–1: 43.2% (*n* = 15,837)	
	Invasive: 7%													
Schmitges 2012	Open: 93%	No PLND	20,862	NR	NR	NR	NR	NR	NR	NR	NR	NR	NR	LoS, hospital charges,
	Minimally													Rectal lacteration rate
	Invasive: 7%													
Gandaglia	Open: 100%	No PLND	161	33.2	62.6	5.43	5: 14.9% (*n* = 24)	T1c: 75.9% (*n* = 122)	T2: 96.3% (*n* = 155)	2–6: 59% (*n* = 95)	NR	0	NR	Erectile function
					(47.8–77.8)	(IQR: 0.25–10)	6: 85.1% (*n* = 137)	T2a: 24.1% (*n* = 39)	T3a: 3.7% (*n* = 6)	7: 41% (*n* = 66)				Recovery rate
									T3b: 0% (*n* = 0)	8–10: 0% (*n* = 0)				
		ePLND	235		62.3	6	5: 23% (*n* = 54)	T1c: 62% (*n* = 147)	T2: 79.1% (*n* = 186)	2–6: 46% (*n* = 108)		20 [1–40]		
					(40.5–78.9)	(IQR: 0.57–10)	6: 77% (*n* = 181)	T2a: 38% (*n* = 88)	T3a: 15.3% (*n* = 36)	7: 48.9% (*n* = 115)				
									T3b: 5.5% (*n* = 13)	8–10: 5.1% (*n* = 12)				
Schmitges 2012	Open: 100%	No PLND	580	NR	64	6.3 (R: 0.5–93)	6: 44.2% (*n* = 637)	T1: 85.4% (*n* = 1230)	T2: 70.2% (*n* = 1011)	6: 28.9% (*n* = 417)	NR	NR	Nx: 40.2% (*n* = 579)	RBC, transfusion,
					(R: 37–77)		7: 35.6% (*n* = 513)	T2: 14.1% (*n* = 203)	T3: 29.8% (*n* = 430)	7: 66.7% (*n* = 961)			N0: 54.7% (*n* = 788)	Prolonged drainage,
							≥8: 8.8% (*n* = 127)	T3: 0.6% (*n* = 8)		8: 4.4% (*n* = 63)			N1–2: 5.1% (*n* = 74)	Lymphocele
Touijer 2011	Lap: 100%	lPND	174	NR	NR	7 [5–11]	<7: 14%	T1: 61%	NR	NR	NR	9 [6–13]	4.5%	OT,
							7: 71%	T2a: 14%						Postoperative

							8–10: 15%	>T2b: 24%						Complications
		sPLND	595			6 [5–9]	<7: 11%	T1: 57%				13 [9–18]	14.3%	
							7: 72%	T2a: 18%						
							8–10: 14%	>T2b: 24%						
		No PLND	202			NR	NR	NR				NA	NA	
Yong 2011	Robotic: 100%	No PLND	182	NR	NR	NR	NR	NR	NR	NR	NR	NR	NR	OT
Eifler 2011	Lap: 100%	No PLND	302	>3	57.7 (6.7)	4.8 (NR)	7: 15.6% (*n* = 47)	NR	NR	NR	NR	0	0	OT, VTE
Khoder 2011	Retro: 89.8%	No PLND	8	NR										Lymphocele
	EERPE: 6.5%													
	Perineal: 3.8%													
Lin 2011	Lap: 100%	No PLND	120	33.9	NR	NR	NR	NR	NR	NR	NR	NR	NR	Inguinal hernia
Hruza 2010	Lap: 100%	No PLND	761	50	63.8 (6.15)	7.6 [IQR: 5.3–11.5]	NR	<T3a: 70.2% (*n* = 1486)	T2: 57.4% (*n* = 1261)	4–5: 10.8% (*n* = 229)	R0: 76.6%	NR	NA	Complication rate
				[IQR: 26–72]					T3a: 26.5% (*n* = 588)	6: 31.8% (*n* = 676)	(*n* = 1683)			
									T3b: 11.8% (*n* = 260)	7: 48.1% (*n* = 1020)				
									T4: 4% (*n* = 89)	8–10: 9.3% (*n* = 197)				
		PLND	1438										1.9% (*n* = 41)	
Zorn 2009	Robotic: 100%	No PLND	859	NR	59.2	5.5	6: 81% (*n* = 696)	cT1c: 71% (*n* = 618)	NR	6: 69.3% (*n* = 595)	NR	NA	NA	OT, eBL, blood
					(R: 40–77)	(R: 0.06–32)	7: 19% (*n* = 163)	cT2a–cT2b: 29% (*n* = 241)		7: 28.8% (*n* = 247)				Transfusions, LoS,
										8–10: 1.9% (*n* = 17)				Postoperative

(continued)

Table 2 (continued)

Study	Surgical	Treatment	N	Follow-up (mo)	Age (year)	PSA (ng/ml)	Biopsy Gleason score	Clinical T stage	Pathologic T stage	Pathologic Gleason score	Surgical margin	Number of lymph nodes dissected	Number of positive lymph nodes	Outcomes
														Complications,
														Symptomatic
														Lymphocele
		PLND	296		61.0	9.0 (R: 0–89-52)	6: 17% (*n* = 52)	cT1c: 61% (*n* = 180)		6: 16.2% (*n* = 48)		12.5 (IQR: 7–16)	7.8% (*n* = 23)	
					(R: 44–85)		7: 62% (*n* = 182)	cT2a–cT2b: 38% (*n* = 112)		7: 67.9% (*n* = 201)				
							8–10: 21% (*n* = 62)	cT3: 1% (*n* = 4)		8–10: 15.9% (*n* = 47)				
Stolzenburg 2005	EERPE: 100%	No PLND	700	17.3	63.4	10.7	NR	NR	T2a: 12.7 (*n* = 89)	4: 11% (*n* = 77)	R1: 19.7%	NR	NR	OT
				(R: 3–39)	(R: 42–77)	(R: 1.4–82)			T2b: 7.7% (*n* = 54)	5: 19.3% (*n* = 135)	(*n* = 138)			
									T2c: 35% (*n* = 245)	6: 23% (*n* = 161)				
									T3a: 32.7 (*n* = 229)	7: 35.4% (*n* = 248)				
									T3b: 11.2 (*n* = 79)	8: 8.3% (*n* = 58)				
									T4: 0.6 (*n* = 4)	9: 2.4% (*n* = 17)				
										10: 0.6% (*n* = 4)				
Limited/standard PLND versus (super) extended PLND														
Hatzichristodoulou 2015	Open: 100%	ePLND	262	48	64.9 (7.5)	8.3 (6.3)	6: 0% (*n* = 0)	≤T1c: 57.3% (*n* = 150)	pT2: 76.3% (*n* = 200)	6: 40.1% (*n* = 105)	NR	20.4 (9.7)	NR	Continence recovery rate
				[R: 24–84]			7: 88.6% (*n* = 232)	>T1c: 42.7% (*n* = 112)	pT3a: 13% (*n* = 34)	7: 47.7% (*n* = 125)				(12 mo), spontaneous EF
							8: 8.0% (*n* = 21)		pT3b: 9.9% (*n* = 26)	8–10: 12.2% (*n* = 32)				Recovery (12 mo),
							9: 3.4% (*n* = 9)		pT4: 0.8% (*n* = 2)					Trifecta rates (2-year)

		lPLND	198		64.6 (7.8)	9.9 (7.8)	6: 100% ($n = 198$)	≤T1c: 74.7% ($n = 148$)	pT2: 80.8% ($n = 160$)	6: 44.9% ($n = 89$)		4.7 (4)		
							7: 0% ($n = 0$)	>T1c: 25.3% ($n = 50$)	pT3a: 13.6% ($n = 27$)	7: 50.6% ($n = 100$)				
							8: 0% ($n = 0$)		pT3b: 5.6% ($n = 11$)	8–10: 4.5% ($n = 9$)				
							9: 0% ($n = 0$)		pT4: 0% ($n = 0$)					
Kim 2013	Robotic: 100%	sPLND	294	36	65	8.4	≤6: 33.4% ($n = 98$)	T1: 66.3% ($n = 195$)	T2: 62.2% ($n = 183$)	NR	NR	12 [R: 9–16]	3.4% ($n = 10$)	Complication rate,
					[R: 60–69]	[R: 5.3–37.7]	7: 48.3% ($n = 142$)	T2: 21.4% ($n = 63$)	T3a: 28.6% ($n = 84$)					Lymphocele, lymphedema,
							≥8: 18.3% ($n = 54$)	T3: 12.3% ($n = 36$)	T3b: 9.2% ($n = 27$)					Neuropraxia
		ePLND	170		66	10.4	≤6: 17.7% ($n = 30$)	T1: 45.9% ($n = 78$)	T2: 56.5% ($n = 96$)			21 [R: 16–25]	13.5% ($n = 23$)	
					[R: 62–70]	[R: 6.6–16.1]	7: 39.4% ($n = 67$)	T2: 41.2% ($n = 70$)	T3a: 28.8% ($n = 49$)					
							≥8: 42.9% ($n = 73$)	T3: 12.9% ($n = 22$)	T3b: 14.7% ($n = 25$)					
Hoshi 2015	Open: 100%	sPLND	599	40 [R: 1–261]	NR	NR	NR	NR	NR	NR	NR	NR	High risk: 7.1% ($n = 13$)	eBL, lymphocele,
													Int risk: 0.6% ($n = 1$)	Intra- and postoperative
													Low risk: 0% ($n = 0$)	Complications
		Semi-ePLND	131										High risk: 20% ($n = 12$)	
													Int risk: 3.3% ($n = 1$)	
													Low risk: 0% ($n = 0$)	

(continued)

Table 2 (continued)

Study	Surgical	Treatment	N	Follow-up (mo)	Age (year)	PSA (ng/ml)	Biopsy Gleason score	Clinical T stage	Pathologic T stage	Pathologic Gleason score	Surgical margin	Number of lymph nodes dissected	Number of positive lymph nodes	Outcomes
Jung 2012	Robotic: 100%	sPLND	155	24	66	8.7	<7: 32.3% (n = 50)	≤T2: 43.9% (n = 68)	T2: 51.6% (n = 80)	<7: 23.9% (n = 37)	R1: 37.4%	15	5.2%	OT, PLND time,
				[IQR: 15–34]	[IQR: 61–70]	[IQR: 5.8–14.3]	7: 33.5% (n = 52)	T3: 56.1% (n = 87)	T3a: 38.1% (n = 59)	7: 50.9% (n = 79)	(n = 58)	[IQR: 11–19]	(n = 8)	eBL, LoS, PLND related
							>7: 34.2% (n = 53)		T3b: 9.0% (n = 14)	>7: 25.2% (n = 39)				Complications
									T4: 1.3% (n = 2)					
		ePLND	45	13	67	15.5	<7: 11.1% (n = 5)	≤T2: 28.9% (n = 13)	T2: 35.6% (n = 16)	<7: 6.7% (n = 3)	R1: 55.6%	24	22.2%	
				[IQR: 10–17]	[IQR: 63–72]	[IQR: 7.6–24.6]	7: 28.9% (n = 13)	T3: 71.1% (n = 32)	T3a: 53.3% (n = 24)	7: 42.2% (n = 19)	(n = 25)	[IQR: 18–28]	(n = 10)	
							>7: 60% (n = 27)		T3b: 8.9% (n = 4)	>7: 51.1% (n = 23)				
									T4: 2.2%% (n = 1)					
Yuh 2013	Robotic: 100%	lPLND	204	NR	64	5.9	6: 6.4% (n = 13)	T1: 72.1% (n = 147)	T2a/b: 7.4% (n = 15)	NR	NR	7 (IQR 5–9)	3.9% (n = 8)	eBL, OT, DVT
					[IQR: 58–70]	[IQR: 4.4–9.1]	3 + 4: 54.9% (n = 112)	T2:27.4% (n = 56)	T2c: 57.8% (n = 118)					Complication rate,
							4 + 3: 22.1% (n = 45)	T3: 0.5% (n = 1)	T3a: 23.5% (n = 48)					Lymphocele,
							8: 12.2% (n = 25)		T3b: 11.3% (n = 923)					Discharge at day 1
							9: 4.4% (n = 9)							
		ePLND	202		64	5.5	6: 5.9% (n = 12)	T1: 68.8% (n = 139)	T2a/b: 12.4% (n = 25)			21.5 (IQR: 17–27)	11.9% (n = 24)	

					[IQR: 58–69]	[IQR: 4.2–8.3]	3 + 4: 59.9% (n = 112)	T2:30.2% (n = 61)	T2c: 60.7% (n = 122)					
							4 + 3: 19.8% (n = 40)	T3: 1% (n = 2)	T3a: 16.8% (n = 34)					
							8: 11.4% (n = 23)		T3b: 10.4% (n = 21)					
							9: 3.0% (n = 6)							
Eden 2010	Lap: 100%	sPLND	311	NR	63	11	7 [4–10]	T1: 32.8% (n = 102)	NR	NR	NR	6.1 [2–8]	NR	Transfusion rate, eBL,
					[43–76]	[2–20]		T2: 63% (n = 196)						OT, LoS, complication
								T3: 4.2% (n = 13)						Rate
		ePLND	121		63	8	7 [6–10]	T1: 33.1% (n = 40)				17.5 [2–23]		
					[43–74]	[1–15]		T2: 57% (n = 174)						
								T3: 9.9% (n = 12)						
Naselli 2010	NR	lPLND	98	≥6 mo	NR	6.43	NR	NR	<T3: 74.5% (n = 73)	≤6: 46.9% (n = 46)	NR	6 [R: 2–14]	N1: 1% (n = 2)	Lymphocele,
						[R: 1.95–65]			T3a: 22.4% (n = 22)	7: 46.9% (n = 46)				Reintervention
									T3b: 8.2% (n = 8)	8–10: 6.1% (n = 6)				
		ePLND	249			7.22			<T3: 67.5% (n = 168)	≤6: 36.9% (n = 92)		16 [R: 10–67]	N1: 11.7% (n = 29)	
						[R: 2.2–98]			T3a: 30.1% (n = 75)	7: 50.6% (n = 126)				
									T3b: 15.7% (n = 39)	8–10: 12.5% (n = 31)				

(continued)

Table 2 (continued)

Study	Surgical	Treatment	*N*	Follow-up (mo)	Age (year)	PSA (ng/ml)	Biopsy Gleason score	Clinical T stage	Pathologic T stage	Pathologic Gleason score	Surgical margin	Number of lymph nodes dissected	Number of positive lymph nodes	Outcomes
Lindberg 2009	NR	lPLND	64	NR	64 (NR)	NR	NR	NR	NR	NR	NR	7 [R: 3–18]	N1: 6% (*n* = 4)	eBL, OT, lymphocele,
														DVT, PE, hematoma,
														Wound infections, sepsis,
														Complication rate
		ePLND	108		64 (NR)							17 [R: 5–40]	N1: 20% (*n* = 22)	
Musch 2008	Open: 100%	lPLND	867	NR	65 (6)	4.1–10: 8% (*n* = 111)	2–6: 65.7% (*n* = 907)	T1: 41.9% (*n* = 578)	T2: 48.3% (*n* = 666)	2–6: 51.8% (*n* = 715)	R: 31.5%	NR	N +: n = 148	Lymphocele,
						10.1–20: 25.4% (*n* = 350)	7: 12.4% (*n* = 171)	T2: 50% (*n* = 690)	T3a: 28.3% (*n* = 391)	7: 26.1% (*n* = 360)	(*n* = 435)			Reintervention
						>20: 13.1% (*n* = 181)	8–10: 17.4% (*n* = 240)	T3: 6.9% (*n* = 95)	T3b: 15.7% (*n* = 217)	8–10: 20.6% (*n* = 284)				
									T4: 5.9% (*n* = 82)					
		ePLND	434											
Klevecka 2007	Open: 100%	lPLND	740	NR	65 (6)	<2.6: 4.9% (*n* = 49)	2–4: 21.8% (*n* = 218)	T1a/b: 3.4% (*n* = 34)	T2a: 7.8% (*n* = 78)	NR	R1: 32.7% (*n* = 327)	NR	10.9% (*n* = 109)	Lymphocele,
						2.6–4.0: 3.6% (*n* = 36)	5–6: 42.2% (*n* = 422)	T1c: 32.7% (*n* = 327)	T2b: 20.5% (*n* = 205)					DVT, PE,
						4.1–10.0: 49.5% (*n* = 495)	7–10: 21.0% (*n* = 210)	T2: 56.8% (*n* = 568)	T2c: 18.9 (*n* = 189)					Reintervention,
						10.1–20.0: 26.6% (*n* = 266)		cT3: 7.1% (*n* = 71)	T3a: 28.8 (*n* = 288)					Postoperative bleeding,
						≥20.1: 15.4% (*n* = 154)			T3b: 17.5% (*n* = 175)					Secondary
									T4: 6.5% (*n* = 65)					Wound healing

		ePLND	236											
Clark 2003	Open: 100%	lPLND	123	NR	61	<10: 84.6% ($n = 104$)	≤6: 67.5% ($n = 83$)	T1c: 72% ($n = 88$)	NR	NR	NR	NR	2.4% ($n = 3$)	Lymphocele, leg edema,
					(R: 45–75)		7: 20.3% ($n = 25$)	T2a: 21% ($n = 26$)						DVT, pelvic abscess,
							8–10: 12.2% ($n = 15$)	T2b: 5.7% ($n = 7$)						Ureteral injury, overall
								T3: 1.3% ($n = 2$)						Unilateral complication
		ePLND	123											
Heidenreich 2002	Open: 100%	sPLND	100	NR	63.5	14.9	5.2 (2.6)	T1c: 10% ($n = 10$)	3.5 (R: 1–4)	NR	NR	11 (R: 6–19)	12% ($n = 12$)	eBL, OT, rectal lesions,
					(R: 49–72)	(R: 1.6–109)		T2: 65% ($n = 65$)						Lymphocele, DVT, PE,
								T3: 25% ($n = 25$)						Obturator nerve lesion
		ePLND	103	NR	61.8	15.9	4.6 (2.3)	T1c: 8.7% ($n = 9$)	3.6 (R: 1–4)	NR	NR	28 (R: 21–42)	26.2% ($n = 27$)	
					(R: 51–71)	(R: 1.2–129)		T2: 59% ($n = 61$)						
								T3: 32% ($n = 33$)						
Mistretta 2017	Robotic: 100%	sPLND	109	32	66.3	12.1	6: 15.6% ($n = 17$)	T1: 45.9% ($n = 50$)	T2a-b: 15.7% ($n = 17$)	6: 15% ($n = 16$)	R1: 21.1%	11	12.8%	eBL, OT, LoS,
				(R: 6–72)	(IQR: 63–71)	(IQR: 4.9–12.9)	3 + 4: 37.6% ($n = 41$)	T2: 50.5% ($n = 55$)	T2c: 50% ($n = 55$)	3 + 4: 41.1% ($n = 44$)	($n = 109$)	[IQR: 7–17]	($n = 14$)	Intraoperative complications,
				($n = 184$)			4 + 3: 22.9% ($n = 25$)	T3: 3.7% ($n = 4$)	T3a: 21.3% ($n = 23$)	4 + 3: 24.3% ($n = 28$)				Postoperative complications,
							8: 15.6% ($n = 17$)		T3b: 13% ($n = 14$)	8: 8.4% ($n = 9$)				Postoperative sexual function
							9: 8.3% ($n = 9$)			9: 11.2% ($n = 12$)				
	Robotic: 100%	ePLND	75		66	13.2	6: 20% ($n = 15$)	T1:37.3% ($n = 28$)	T2a-b: 4% ($n = 3$)	6: 8.2% ($n = 6$)	R1: 33.3%	21	29.3%	

(continued)

Table 2 (continued)

Study	Surgical	Treatment	*N*	Follow-up (mo)	Age (year)	PSA (ng/ml)	Biopsy Gleason score	Clinical T stage	Pathologic T stage	Pathologic Gleason score	Surgical margin	Number of lymph nodes dissected	Number of positive lymph nodes	Outcomes
					(IQR: 59–70)	(IQR: 6.2–17.4)	3 + 4: 32% (*n* = 24)	T2: 50.7% (*n* = 38)	T2c: 48% (*n* = 36)	3 + 4: 47.9% (*n* = 35)	(*n* = 75)	[IQR: 16–29]	(*n* = 22)	
							4 + 3: 18.7% (*n* = 14)	T3: 12% (*n* = 9)	T3a: 26.7% (*n* = 20)	4 + 3: 13.7% (*n* = 12)				
							8: 21.3% (*n* = 16)		T3b: 21.3% (*n* = 16)	8: 11% (*n* = 8)				
							9: 8% (*n* = 6)			9: 19.2% (*n* = 14)				
Touijer 2021	Open	lPLND	700	37.2	62	5.9	6: 10% (*n* = 72)	T1c: 61% (*n* = 400)	T3a: 54% (*n* = 375)	6: 5.9% (*n* = 40)	NR	12 (IQR: 8–17)	11.6% (*n* = 81)	Postoperative complications,
RCT	Lap			(IQR: 18–60)	(IQR: 57–67)	(IQR: 4.3–8.6)	3 + 4: 52% (*n* = 362)	T2a,b,c: 29.4% (*n* = 206)	T3b: 12% (*n* = 85)	3 + 4: 58% (*n* = 399)				Erectile function recovery
	Robotic						4 + 3: 19% (*n* = 135)	T3a,b: 7% (*n* = 49)		4 + 3: 23% (*n* = 160)				
							≥8: 18% (*n* = 129)			≥8: 12% (*n* = 84)				
		ePLND	740		63	5.7	6: 9.4% (*n* = 69)	T1c: 61% (*n* = 418)	T3a: 49% (*n* = 364)	6: 7.3% (*n* = 53)		14 (IQR: 10–20)	13.5% (*n* = 100)	
					(IQR: 57–67)	(IQR: 4.2–8.2)	3 + 4: 52% (*n* = 383)	T2a,b,c: 31.5% (*n* = 233)	T3b: 12% (*n* = 89)	3 + 4: 53% (*n* = 385)				
							4 + 3: 17% (*n* = 125)	T3a,b: 5.3% (*n* = 39)		4 + 3: 24% (*n* = 173)				
							≥8: 22% (*n* = 160)			≥8: 16% (*n* = 118)				

DVT deep venous thromboembolism, *eBL* estimated blood loss, *EERPE* endoscopic extraperitoneal radical prostatectomy, *ePLND* extended PLND, *IQR* interquartile range, *lap* laparoscopic, *LoS* length of hospital stay, *lPLND* limited PLND, *NA* not available, *NR* not reported, *OT* operating time, *PE* pulmonary embolism, *PLND* pelvic lymph node dissection, *RCT* randomized controlled trial, *R* range, *sPLND* standard PLND, *VTE* venous thromboembolism. Data for categorical variables are reported as frequency (proportion). Data for continuous variables are reported as either median [range or IQR] or mean (range or IQR)

Table 3 Results from studies addressing non-oncologic outcomes

Study	Subpopulation	Intervention	Comparator		Outcomes measured	*N at baseline*			*Outcome results*			Reported	Notes
	(if applicable)	(Int)	(Com)			Int	Com		Int		Com	*p* values	
No PLND vs any PLND													
Ostby-Deglum 2015	NA	PLND		No PLND	Insuficient erection	169	440		Univariate analysis: OR 0.95			0.82	
									[95% CI: 0.63–1.43]				
Violette 2015	NA	PLND		No PLND	OT	392			Univariate analysis: OR 1.94			Uni: 0.03	
									[95% CI: 1.09–3.47]			Multi: 0.13	
									MVA: OR 1.65 [95% CI: 0.86–3.17]				
Boehm 2015	NA	PLND		No PLND	Blood transfusion rate	6810	4884		11.4%		9.7%	0.0036	
									RR: 1.18 (95% CI: 1.05–1.32)			NR	
Tyritzis 2015	NA	PLND		No PLND	DVT	547	2997		2.9% ($n = 15$)		0.3% ($n = 10$)	NR	
									Age-adjusted RR: 7.80				
									(95%CI: 3.51–17.30)				
					PE				1.3% ($n = 7$)		0.2% ($n = 6$)		
									Age-adjusted RR: 6.29				
									(95%CI: 2.11–18.73)				
Liss 2013	NA	ePLND	sPLND	No PLND	OT (min)	54	231	207	186	182	176	0.211	
					Blood loss (ml)				150 [100–200]	100 [100–200]	100 [100–200]	0.322	
					Blood transfusion rate				1.9% ($n = 1$)	0.9% ($n = 2$)	2.4% ($n = 5$)	0.436	
					LoS (d)				1.1	1.3	1.6	NR	
					Complication rate				16.7% ($n = 9$)	18.2% ($n = 42$)	13.5% ($n = 28$)	0.412	
					Lymphocele rate (no surgery)				5.6% ($n = 3$)	2.2% ($n = 5$)	0% ($n = 0$)	0.011	
					Lymphocele rate (surgery)				0% ($n = 0$)	3% ($n = 7$)	0% ($n = 0$)	0.018	
van der Poel 2012	NA	sPLND		No PLND	Lymphocele rate	440	464		1.5% ($n = 7$)		0% ($n = 0$)	NR	
					DVT				1.5% ($n = 7$)		0% ($n = 0$)	NR	

(continued)

Table 3 (continued)

Study	Subpopulation	Intervention	Comparator		Outcomes measured	*N at baseline*			*Outcome results*		Reported	Notes
	(if applicable)	(Int)	(Com)			Int	Com		Int	Com	*p* values	
					Clavien grading				1: 6.1% ($n = 27$)	1: 5.0% ($n = 23$)	0.147	
									2: 5.7% ($n = 25$)	2: 4.3% ($n = 20$)		
									3: 2.0% ($n = 9$)	3: 1.7% ($n = 8$)		
									4: 0.2% ($n = 1$)	4: 0% ($n = 0$)		
					Hematoma				3.5% ($n = 15$)	2.1% ($n = 10$)	NR	
					Ileus				0.3% ($n = 1$)	0.2% ($n = 1$)	NR	
					Anastomosis dehiscence				1.1% ($n = 4$)	0.2% ($n = 1$)	NR	
Schmitges 2012	NA	PLND		No PLND	DVT	36,699			MVA: OR: 1.07 (95% CI: 0.67–1.69)	0.78		
									(corrected for: ASC, year of			
									Surgery, age, race, CCI, PLND,			
									Surgical approach)			
Schmitges 2012	NA	PLND		No PLND	LoS >3 d	15,837	20,862		OR 1.50 (95% CI: 1.26–1.78)		ADJ: <0.001	
					Hospital charges >37,621 dollars				OR 0.84 (95% CI: 0.59–1.19)		ADJ: 0.31	
					Rectal lacerations				0.7% ($n = 105$)	0.8% ($n = 159$)	UnADJ: 0.27 ADJ: 0.1	
Gandaglia 2012	NA	ePLND		No PLND E	Erectile function recovery rate	235	161		43.8% ($n = 103$) (1-year)	39.4% ($n = 63$) (1-year)	NR	
									49.7% ($n = 117$) (2-year)	46.6% ($n = 75$) (2-year)		
									Unadjusted HR: 0.8		0.3	
									Adjusted HR: 0.9		0.8	
Schmitges 2012	NA	ePLND	lPLND	No PLND	Transfusion rate (ref = no PLND)	69	792	580	Limited: OR: 1.33 (95% CI: 0.79–2.34)		0.29	
									Extended: OR: 2.04 (95% CI: 0.76–5.51)		0.16	
					Prolonged drainage (ref = no PLND)				Limited: OR: 2.81 (95% CI: 1.32–5.95)		0.007	

									Extended: OR: 3.38 (95% CI: 1.09–10.45)			0.035	
					Pelvic lymphocele (ref = no PLND)				Limited: OR: 12.60 (95% CI: 5.00–31.98)			<0.001	
									Extended: OR: 17.24 (95% CI: 5.37–55.39)			<0.001	
Touijer 2011	NA	ePLND	Lplnd	No PLND	OT (min)	595	174	202	240 [205–270]	210 [180–240]	180 [170–219]	<0.001	
					DVT				1.7% ($n = 10$)	1.1% ($n = 2$)	1.0% ($n = 2$)	1	
					PE				1.3% ($n = 8$)	0.6% ($n = 1$)	0.5% ($n = 1$)	0.5	
					Ureteral injury				0.3% ($n = 2$)	0% ($n = 0$)	0.5% ($n = 1$)	0.7	
					Clavien grading				1: 8.2% ($n = 49$)	1: 4.6% ($n = 8$)	1: 0% ($n = 0$)	0.3	
									2: 3% ($n = 18$)	2: 1.7% ($n = 3$)	2: 1.5% ($n = 3$)		
									3: 4.5% ($n = 27$)	3: 4% ($n = 7$)	3: 0.5% ($n = 1$)		
									4: 0% ($n = 0$)	4: 0% ($n = 0$)	4: 0% ($n = 0$)		
									5: 0% ($n = 0$)	5: 0% ($n = 0$)	5: 0% ($n = 0$)		
									None: 84% ($n = 501$)	None: 90% ($n = 156$)	None: 90% ($n = 156$)		
					Lymphocele rate				5.9% ($n = 35$)	5.2% ($n = 9$)	0% ($n = 0$)	0.9	
					Drainage (ml)				320 [195–540]	235 [140–400]	165 [110–250]	<0.001	
Yong 2011	NA	PLND		No PLND	OT	341	182		OR: 0.66 (95% CI: 0.37–1.18)			0.159	
Eifler 2011	NA	PLND		No PLND	OT (min)	468	302		195		207	0.0008	
					DVT				1.5% ($n = 7$)		0% ($n = 0$)	0.047	
Khoder 2011	NA	PLND		No PLND	Lymphocele rate	1078	85		MVA: OR: 2.6 (95% CI: 1.3–4.9)			0.004	
Lin 2011, retrospective	NA	PLND		No PLND	Inguinal hernia incidence	170	120		HR: 1.02 (95% CI: 0.38–2.75)			0.851	

(continued)

Table 3 (continued)

Study	Subpopulation (if applicable)	Intervention (Int)	Comparator (Com)	Outcomes measured	N at baseline Int	N at baseline Com	Outcome results Int	Outcome results Com	Reported p values	Notes
Hruza 2010	NA	PLND	No PLND	Complication rate	1438	761	MVA: OR: 1.077 (95% CI: 0.834–1.390)		0.570	
Zorn 2009	NA	PLND	No PLND	OT (min)	296	859	224 (R: 160–320)	216 (R: 120–330)	0.09	
				Blood loss (ml)			206 (R: 50–750)	229 (R: 50–700)	0.14	
				Blood transfusion rate			3% ($n = 9$)	1.7% ($n = 15$)	0.4	
				LoS (d)			1.32 (R: 1–5)	1.24 (R: 1–4)	0.4	
				Postoperative complications			9% ($n = 27$)	7% ($n = 63$)	0.8	
				Pelvic lymphocele			2% ($n = 6$)	0% ($n = 0$)	0.9	
				FFS (low)			82%	81%	0.83	
				FFS (intermediate)			63%	71%	0.21	
				FFS (high)			48%	42%	0.45	
Stolzenburg 2005	NA	PLND	No PLND	OT (min)	700		170	115	NR	
Limited/standard PLND vs (super)-extended PLND										
Hatzichristodoulou 2015	NA	ePLND	lPLND	Continence recovery rate (12 mo)	262	198	89.7%	93.4%	0.204	
							MVA: 1.07 [0.87–1.31]		0.508	
							(corrected for age at surgery, preoperative			
							IIEF-5 score, iPSA, pGS, pT, prostate volume)			
				Spontaneous EF recovery (12 mo)			40.4%	47.5%	0.534	
							MVA: 1.11 [0.75–1.63]		0.600	
							(corrected for age at surgery, preoperative			
							IIEF-5 score, iPSA, pGS, pT, prostate volume)			
				Trifecta rates (2-year)			44.1%	47.5%	0.451	
Hoshi 2015	NA	Semi-ePLND	sPLND	Blood loss (ml)	131	599	NR	NR	NS	
				Lymphoceles			0% ($n = 0$)	0% ($n = 0$)	NS	

					Intra- and postoperative complications				0% ($n = 0$)		0% ($n = 0$)	NS	
Kim 2013	NA	ePLND		sPLND	Complication rate	170	294		11.8% ($n = 20$)		2.4% ($n = 7$)	<0.001	
					Lymphocele				2.4% ($n = 4$)		0.3% ($n = 4$)	0.043	
					Lymphedema				8.8% ($n = 15$)		1.4% ($n = 4$)	<0.001	
					Neuropraxia				0.6% ($n = 1$)		0.7% ($n = 2$)	0.905	
Yuh 2013	NA	ePLND		lPLND	Blood loss (ml)	202	204		200 [IQR 150–250]		200 [IQR 150–250]	0.7	
					OT				3 [IQR 2.9–3.3]		2.8 [IQR 2.7–3.2]	<0.001	
					Complication rate				22.8% ($n = 46$)		21.6% ($n = 44$)	0.8	
					Lymphocele				2.5% ($n = 5$)		2.9% ($n = 6$)	NR	
					DVT 1%				($n = 2$) 2.9%		($n = 6$)	NR	
					Major complications				MVA OR: 0.60 (95% CI: 0.25–1.46)			0.3	
					Discharge at day 1				74.8% ($n = 151$)		85.3% ($n = 174$)	0.004	
					Lymphocele plus DVT				NR			0.3	
Jung 2012	NA	ePLND		sPLND	OT (min)	45	155		190 [IQR: 165–211]		196 [IQR: 180–224]	0.027	
					PLND time (min)				26 [IQR: 20–35]		47 [IQR: 36–58]	<0.001	
					Blood loss (ml)				250 [IQR: 150–400]		200 [IQR: 100–300]	0.088	
					LoS (d)				4 [IQR: 3–7]		4 [IQR: 3–7]	0.998	
					PLND-related complications				3.2% ($n = 5$)		2.2% ($n = 1$)	1	
Eden 2010	NA	ePLND		sPLND	Transfusion rate	121	311		2.5% ($n = 3$)		0.8% ($n = 2$)	0.27	
					Blood loss (ml)				200 [10–800]		200 [10–1300]	0.13	
					OT (min)				206.5 [99–331]		180 [117–537]	<0.001	

(continued)

Table 3 (continued)

Study	Subpopulation (if applicable)	Intervention (Int)	Comparator (Com)	Outcomes measured	N at baseline Int	N at baseline Com	Outcome results Int	Outcome results Com	Reported p values	Notes
				LoS (d)			3 [2–4]	3 [2–5]	0.77	
				Complication rate			8.3% ($n = 10$)	3.6% ($n = 9$)	0.10	
Naselli 2010	NA	ePLND	lPLND	Symptomatic lymphocele	249	98	9.6% ($n = 24$)	2% ($n = 2$)	0.028	
							RR: 4.723			
				DVT 1.6%			($n = 4$) 0%	($n = 0$)	NR	
Lindberg 2009	NA	ePLND	lPLND	Blood loss (ml)	108	64	700 [NR]	1100 [NR]	NR	
				OT difference			421 min (ePLND vs lPLND)			
				Lymphocele 1			7.6% ($n = 19$)	9.4% ($n = 6$)		
				DVT			0.9% ($n = 1$)	1.5% ($n = 1$)		
				PE			4.6% ($n = 5$)	1.5% ($n = 1$)		
				Hematoma			1.9% ($n = 2$)	0% ($n = 0$)		
				Wound infections			3.7% ($n = 4$)	0% ($n = 0$)		
				Sepsis			1.9% ($n = 2$)	0% ($n = 0$)		
				Complication rate			30.6% ($n = 33$)	12.5% ($n = 8$)	0.007	
Musch 2008	NA	ePLND	lPLND	Lymphocele	434	867	HR: 2.88 [95% CI: 1.735–4.773]		<0.0001	MVA corrected
										For age, BMI, ASA
				Reintervention			HR: 2.37 [95% CI: 1.494–3.750]		<0.0001	
Klevecka 2007	NA	ePLND	lPLND	Lymphocele	236	740	8.1% ($n = 19$)	2.8% ($n = 21$)	<0.001	Univariate
										Analysis only
				DVT			1.3% ($n = 3$)	1.4% ($n = 10$)	0.93	
				PE			0.9% ($n = 2$)	0.8% ($n = 6$)	0.96	
				Reintervention			10.2% ($n = 24$)	3.1% ($n = 23$)	<0.0001	
				Postoperative bleeding			3.4% ($n = 8$)	1.6% ($n = 12$)	0.10	
				Secondary wound healing			2.1% ($n = 5$)	2.2% ($n = 16$)	0.97	

Clark 2003	NA	ePLND		lPLND	Lymphocele	123	123		3.3% ($n = 4$) (3/4 at side of extended)			NR	Pts randomized
													To one side limited,
													One side extended
					Leg edema				4.1% ($n = 5$) (3/5 at side of extended)				
					DVT				1.6% ($n = 2$) (2/2 at side of extended)				
					Pelvic abscess				0.8% ($n = 1$) (1/1 at side of extended)				
					Ureteral injury				0.8% ($n = 1$) (1/1 at side of extended)				
					Overall unilateral complication rate				75% of total complications on			0.08	
									Side of extended dissection				
Heidenreich 2002	NA	ePLND		sPLND	Blood loss (mL)	103	100		650 (R: 200–1950)		590 (R: 150–2100)	NR	
					OT (min)				179 (R: 140–235)		125 (R: 85–150)	<0.03	
					Rectal lesions				1.1% ($n = 1$)		1% ($n = 1$)	NR	
					Lymphocele				10.6% ($n = 9$)		6% ($n = 6$)	NR	
					DVT				4.2% ($n = 4$)		6% ($n = 6$)	NR	
					PE				2.1% ($n = 2$)		2% ($n = 2$)	NR	
					Obturator nerve lesion				1.1% ($n = 1$)		2% ($n = 2$)	NR	
Mistretta 2017	NA	ePLND		sPLND	OT (min)	75	109		240.4 (IQR: 210–300)		270 (IQR: 215–300)	0.27	
					Blood loss (mL)				150 (IQR: 150–400)		300 (IQR: 150–500)	0.11	
					Intraoperative complications				3.5% ($n = 8$)		8.2% ($n = 12$)	0.2	
					LoS				4 (IQR: 3–6)		3 (IQR: 2–5)	0.07	
					Perioperative complications				30.6% ($n = 34$)		25.3% ($n = 19$)	0.51	
					Anastomotic leak				15.6% ($n = 17$)		12% ($n = 9$)	NR	
					Blood transfusion				1.8% ($n = 2$)		0	NR	

(continued)

Table 3 (continued)

Study	Subpopulation (if applicable)	Intervention (Int)	Comparator (Com)	Outcomes measured	N at baseline Int	N at baseline Com	Outcome results Int	Outcome results Com	Reported p values	Notes
				Lymphocele			6.4% ($n = 7$)	9,3% ($n = 7$)	NR	
				Hematomas			7.3% ($n = 8$)	4% ($n = 3$)	NR	
				Erectile dysfunction			88.3% ($n = 66$)	83% ($n = 90$)	0.48	
Touijer 2021	NA	ePLND	lPLND	Post-operative complication rate	740	400	The rates of grade 2 and grade 3 complications were comparable		NR	
RCT							Between the limited (7.3%) and extended PLND groups (6.4%)			
				Erectile function recovery			In all analyses, the 95% CI excluded a > 1 point reduction in international index of		NR	
							Erectile function scores for the extended template group		NR	

DVT deep venous thromboembolism, *ePLND* extended PLND, *HR* hazard ratio, *EIIF* international index of erectile function, *lPLND* limited PLND, *LRP* laparoscopic surgery, *LoS* length of hospital stay, *MVA* multivariate analysis, *NA* not applicable, *NR* not reported, *OT* operating time, *OR* odds ratio, *PE* pulmonary embolism, *pGS* pathologic Gleason score, *PLND* pelvic lymph node dissection, *PRIAS* prostate cancer research international active surveillance, *PSA* prostate-specific antigen, *RARP* robot-assisted radical prostatectomy, *RCT* randomized clinical trial, *RR* relative risk, *sPLND* standard PLND

5 Oncological Outcomes

The oncological benefit of ePLND is controversial due to the existence of disparate results in the literature.

Furthermore, it should be acknowledged that the positive association between PLND extent and cancer outcome in node-negative patients might be based on a misinterpretation of these data caused by the Will Rogers phenomenon that limits all retrospective studies [66]. Suppose the number of removed negative lymph nodes is investigated as a prognosticator. In that case, patients treated with ePLND have a higher likelihood of being node-negative without overlooked metastases. Suppose a patient has a positive node in an area covered by an extended dissection but not by a limited dissection. In that case, this patient is excluded from the analyses in the group of ePLND patients (as he is node-positive, and only node-negative patients are left in the calculations) but is included in the group with a limited dissection. This means that different groups are compared at a particular disease stage, and the other disease stages can explain the benefit of the group with an extended dissection. In other words, after a limited dissection, the likelihood of overlooked metastases is higher. These missed positive nodes, instead of the removal of negative nodes, influence the prognosis. Similar results can be achieved when considering only patients with positive nodes. Indeed, in patients in whom many nodes are removed, the incidence of finding positive nodes would be high. The outcome of these patients would be relatively good because many patients would have only small-volume metastatic disease. At the same time, when comparing node-positive patients between a series with ePLND or limited PLND, the patients with positive nodes would again have a much better outcome in the series with ePLND because they would contain the patients who had a small nodal disease [8].

It is believed that the advantage, even in negative cases, is due to the resection of micro-metastases. Pagliarulo et al. reexamined 3914 negative lymph nodes in 274 pT3 patients and found that 13.3% of the 180 patients initially defined as pN0 harbored hidden metastases at immunohistochemistry. These patients had worse survival rates than those genuinely negative lymph nodes and had results comparable to patients who had initially been diagnosed as positive lymph nodes [67].

The baseline characteristics of the principal comparative studies evaluating oncological outcomes are summarized in Table 4 [11, 68]. Overall, 16 studies compared no pelvic lymph node dissection (PLND) vs. any form of PLND, whereas 14 studies compared limited PLND (lPLND) or standard PLND (sPLND) vs. extended PLND (ePLND) or super-extended PLND (sePLND). The oncological results are summarized in Table 5 [11, 68] and will be described in more detail below according to biochemical recurrence, distant metastases, cancer-specific survival, overall survival, and RCT.

5.1 Impact of Extended PLND on Biochemical Recurrence

Biochemical recurrence was evaluated in 21 studies, of which five involved lPLND, three sPLND, nine ePLND, and seven undefined PLND [9, 10, 38, 39, 53, 56, 63, 69–81]. Of these, 16 did not find any statistically significant difference between the two groups [9, 10, 53, 56, 59, 63, 70–78, 80]. This negative finding was also applied to the various subgroups of patients (e.g., low-risk disease [72]; also pT2, pT3, or pT2 R0 disease [73]. Therefore, there were no differences in BCR when comparing types of PLND with each other.

Counterintuitive findings were observed in two different retrospective studies regarding the impact of PLND compared to no PLND on BCR [38, 39]. Specifically, Boehm et al. evaluated a cohort of 11,127 patients, including 6810 pN0 patients and 4884 pNx patients treated with radical prostatectomy between 1992 and 2011 [38]. Through multivariable Cox regression analysis, pNx was associated with a lower risk of BCR compared to pN0 (HR 0.81; 95% confidence interval (CI) 0.72–0.9; $p < 0.05$). Despite multivariable analysis, the significant baseline differences between the two groups may explain the higher risk of recurrence among pN0 patients. Furthermore, the extent of PLND was not reported. Conversely, Liss et al. analyzed a cohort of 492 patients treated with robotic-assisted radical prostatectomy between 2007 and 2011 [39]; 54 received ePLND, 231 received sPLND, and 207 did not receive any PLND. At a median follow-up of approximately 1 year, BCR was significantly different among the three groups: 30% vs. 15% vs. 3.4%, respectively ($p < 0.001$). However, when ePLND was compared to sPLND in high-risk patients only, no significant differences were observed ($p = 0.294$). Therefore these two studies showing negative BCR results in the ePLND groups must be due to biases.

EPLND did not provide a better biochemical outcome in two comparative retrospective studies [53, 56]. Allaf et al. showed a statistically significant benefit of ePLND over limited/standard PLND, but only in specific subgroups of patients: pN1 patients with <15% of retrieved nodes affected (43% vs. 10%; $p = 0.01$) [81]. However, counterintuitive findings were observed in a retrospective study in which ePLND was associated with a higher risk of 7-year BCR than lPLND in pT2 patients only (5% vs. 0%; $p = 0.01$) [63]. This result may reflect the selection bias of the study because surgeons tended to perform more extensive nodal dissection in higher risk patients.

Table 4 Baseline characteristics for studies addressing oncological outcomes

Study	Surgical	Treatment	*N*	Follow-up (mo)	Age (year)	PSA (ng/ml)	Biopsy Gleason score	Clinical T stage	Pathologic T stage	Pathologic Gleason score	Surgical margin	Number of lymph nodes dissected	Number of positive lymph nodes	Outcomes
No PLND versus any PLND														
Karl 2015	Open: 87%	No PLND	608	48 [NR]	64.9	<4: 8% (*n* = 43)	NR	NR	pT3a: 100%	≤6: 14% (*n* = 77)	R1: 100%	NR	NR	BRFS
	Lap: 8%				[R: 42–78)	4–9.9: 53% (*n* = 282)				3 + 4: 56% (*n* = 301)				
	Robotic: 2%					10–19.9: 27% (*n* = 142)				4 + 3: 21% (*n* = 112)				
	Perineal: 3%					≥20: 12% (*n* = 64)				8: 9% (*n* = 46)				
Gandaglia 2015	NR	No PLND	1710	40 (32.2)	64	5.4	NR	T1c: 91.2% (*n* = 1560)	NR	NR	NR	NR	NR	BCR
					[IQR: 59–68]	[IQR: 4.2–6.8]		T2: 8.8% (*n* = 150)						
Koo 2015	Open: 29%	No PLND	327	NR	NR	NR	NR	NR	NR	NR	NR	NR	NR	BRFS
	Robotic: 71%	PLND	403											
Boehm 2015	Open: 95%	No PLND	4884	NR	64 (59–67)	NR	≤6: 29.2% (*n* = 3412)	NR	pT2: 70% (*n* = 8172)	NR	NR	NR	NR	BFFS
	Robotic: 5%	PLND	6810				3 + 4: 53.8% (*n* = 6303)		pT3a: 20% (*n* = 2327)					MFS
							4 + 3: 13.0% (*n* = 1529)		≥pT3b: 10% (*n* = 1223)					CSS
							≥8: 3.8 (*n* = 443)							
Liss 2013	Robotic: 100%	No PLND	207	NR	61 (6.9)	4.9 (4.0–6.5)	≤6: 93.5% (*n* = 188)	T1: 78.3% (*n* = 162)	T1: 92.3% (*n* = 191)	NR	NR	NA	NA	BFFS
							7: 4.5% (*n* = 9)	T2: 21.7% (*n* = 45)	T2: 6.8% (*n* = 14)					
							≥8: 2% (*n* = 4)	T3: 0% (*n* = 0)	T3: 1% (*n* = 2)					
		sPLND	231		63 (6.8)	6.1 (4.4–9.2)	≤6: 58.9% (*n* = 136)	T1: 58.9% (*n* = 136)	T1: 72.7% (*n* = 168)			18 [12–25]	0.3% (*n* = 13)	
							7: 39.4% (*n* = 91)	T2: 39.4% (*n* = 91)	T2: 26.4% (*n* = 61)					
							≥8: 1.7% (*n* = 4)	T3: 1.7% (*n* = 4)	T3: 0.9% (*n* = 2)					

		ePLND	54		61 (7.2)	8.5 (5.5–13.5)	≤6: 27.8% (*n* = 15)	T1: 27.8% (*n* = 15)	T1: 42.6% (*n* = 23)			20 (16–28)	2% (*n* = 24)	
							7: 68.5% (*n* = 37)	T2: 68.5% (*n* = 37)	T2: 55.6% (*n* = 30)					
							≥8: 3.7% (*n* = 2)	T3: 3.7% (*n* = 2)	T3: 1.9% (*n* = 1)					
Mitsuzuka 2013	Open: 100%	No PLND	75	NR	63 [NR]	5.9 (NR)	≤6: 45.3% (*n* = 34)	T1c: 90.7% (*n* = 68)		NR	NR	NR	NA	BFFS
							7: 48% (*n* = 36)	T2a: 9.3% (*n* = 9)						MFS
							≥8: 6.7% (*n* = 5)							CSS, OS
		PLND	147		67 [NR}	6.4 (NR)	≤6: 28.6% (*n* = 42)	T1c: 70.1% (*n* = 103)					0.7% (*n* = 1)	
							7: 61.2% (*n* = 90)	T2a: 29.9% (*n* = 44)						
							≥8: 10.2% (*n* = 15)							
Masuda 2013	Single-port	No PLND	379	49.8 (NR)	65.8 (NR)	8.4 (NR)	NR	NR	T3a: 32.5% (*n* = 123)	NR	R1: 25.3% (*n* = 96)	NR	NR	BFFS
	Surgery: 100%								T3b: 4.0% (*n* = 15)					
	(MIES-RP)													
Daimon 2012	Lap: 100%	No PLND	54	69.4 [NR]	65.2 (NR)	6.37 (NR)	NR	NR	NR	NR	NR	NR	NR	BFFS
		Limited	85		54.8 (NR)	6.48 (NR)	NR							
Ost 2012	NR	No PLND	46	60 [6–136]	NR	NR	NR	NR	NR	NR	NR	0	NR	BFFS
		ePLND	179											LFFS
Ku 2011	Open: 88%	No PLND	88	37	66.9 (6.0)	15.8 (15.9)	<7: 11.4% (*n* = 10)	<T2c = 86.4% (*n* = 76)	NR	<7: 9.1% (*n* = 8)	R0: 54.5%	NR	NR	BF
	Lap: 2.5%						7: 13.6% (*n* = 12)	T2c: 13.6% (*n* = 12)		7: 54.4% (*n* = 48)	(*n* = 48)			
	Robotic: 9.5%						8: 48.9% (*n* = 43)			8: 12.5% (*n* = 11)	R +: 45%			
							9: 23.9% (*n* = 21)			9: 22.7% (*n* = 20)	(*n* = 40)			
							10: 2.3% (*n* = 2)			10: 1.1% (*n* = 1)				

(continued)

Table 4 (continued)

Study	Surgical	Treatment	*N*	Follow-up (mo)	Age (year)	PSA (ng/ml)	Biopsy Gleason score	Clinical T stage	Pathologic T stage	Pathologic Gleason score	Surgical margin	Number of lymph nodes dissected	Number of positive lymph nodes	Outcomes
		PLND	111		65.3 (6.9)	21.5 (35.9)	<7: 11.7% (*n* = 13)	<T2c: 89.2% (*n* = 99)		<7: 2.7% (*n* = 3)	R0: 54.1%			
							7: 19.8% (*n* = 22)	T2c: 10.8% (*n* = 12)		7: 66.7% (*n* = 74)	(*n* = 60)			
							8: 42.3% (*n* = 47)			8: 10.8% (*n* = 12)	R +: 45.9%			
							9: 24.3% (*n* = 27)			9: 19.8% (*n* = 22)	(*n* = 51)			
							10: 1.8% (*n* = 2)			10: 0% (*n* = 0)				
Porter 2010	Open: 43%	No PLND	410	139	NR	NR	NR	NR	NR	NR	NR	NR	NR	PCSM
	Perineal: 57%	PLND	342											
Weight 2008	Open: 100%	No PLND	196	88 [NR]	>65: 74%	4: 15% (*n* = 30)	NR	NR	T3a: 45% (*n* = 23)	≤6: 60% (*n* = 117)	NR	NA	NA	BFFS
					(*n* = 146)	4–10: 85% (*n* = 166)			T3b: 2% (*n* = 1)	7: 40% (*n* = 79)				
		PLND	140	94.5 [NR]	>65: 76%	4: 19% (*n* = 19)			T3a: 48% (*n* = 34)	≤6: 54% (*n* = 76)		9 [IQR: 5–13]	NR	
					(*n* = 107)	4–10: 86% (*n* = 121)			T3b: 5% (*n* = 4)	7: 46% (*n* = 64)				
Berglund 2007	NR	No PLND	732	31.9 (40.5)	<65: 74%	<4: 22% (*n* = 155)	2–4: 4% (*n* = 29)	T1: 60% (*n* = 416)	NR	NR	NR	NA	NA	FFS: Free
					(n = 540)	4.1–10: 68% (*n* = 472)	5–6: 81% (*n* = 583)	T2: 39% (*n* = 268)						From BF or
						10.1–20: 7% (*n* = 48)	7: 14% (*n* = 100)	T3: 1% (*n* = 7)						Free from
						>20: 2% (*n* = 16)	8–10: 1% (*n* = 4)	T4: 0% (*n* = 0)						2nd treatment
		lPLND	3961	49.5 (30.4)	< 65: 67%	<4: 14% (*n* = 514)	Gl2–4: 7% (*n* = 278)	T1: 42% (*n* = 1612)				5.8 (5.4)	NR	
					(*n* = 2659)	4.1–10: 64% (*n* = 2372)	Gl5–6: 62% (*n* = 2347)	T2: 56% (*n* = 2123)						
						10.1–20: 16% (*n* = 599)	Gl7: 24% (*n* = 916)	T3: 2% (*n* = 82)						

						>20: 6% ($n = 217$)	Gl8–10: 7% ($n = 254$)	T4: 0% ($n = 2$)						
Bhatta-Dhar 2004	NR	No PLND	196	NR	<65: 74%	≤4: 15% ($n = 30$)	NR	T1–T2a: 95% ($n = 186$)	T3a: 23% ($n = 45$)	≤6: 60% ($n = 117$)	NR	NA	NA	BFFS
					($n = 146$)	4–10: 85% ($n = 166$)		T2b–T2c: 5% ($n = 10$)	T3b: 1% ($n = 2$)	≥7: 40% ($n = 79$)				
		PLND	140		<65: 76%	≤4: 14% ($n = 19$)		T1–T2a: 95% ($n = 133$)	T3a: 34% ($n = 48$)	≤6: 54% ($n = 76$)		NR	NR	
					($n = 107$)	4–10: 86% ($n = 121$)		T2b–T2c: 5% ($n = 7$)	T3b: 4% ($n = 5$)	≥7: 46% ($n = 64$)				
Fergany 2000	Open: 100%	No PLND	203	38	≤65: 74%	≤4: 15% ($n = 31$)	≤6: 100% ($n = 203$)	≤cT1–T2a: 95%	pT3a: 23% ($n = 47$)	≤6: 61% ($n = 123$)	NR	NR	NA	BFFS
				(R: 1–141)	(n = 150)			($n = 193$)	pT3b: 1% ($n = 2$)					
		PLND	372		≤65: 72%	≤4: 24% ($n = 88$)	≤6: 100% ($n = 372$)	≤cT1–T2a: 88%	pT3a: 41% ($n = 153$)	≤6: 60% ($n = 223$)			2% ($n = 6$)	
					(n = 267)			($n = 327$)	pT3b: 4% ($n = 14$)					
Preisser 2020	Open	No PLND	707	60.7	63.6	7.5 (5.5–10.3)	6: 53.6% ($n = 379$)	cT1: 42.1% ($n = 298$)	pT2: 64.9% ($n = 459$)	NR	R1: 29.8%			BFFS
	Lap				(59.1–68.2)		7: 40.9% ($n = 289$)	cT2: 52.5% ($n = 371$)	pT3a: 22.9% ($n = 162$)		($n = 211$)			MFS
	Robotic						≥8: 5.5% ($n = 39$)	cT3: 5.4% ($n = 38$)	≥pT3b: 12.2% ($n = 86$)					CSS
		PLND	9035	30.5	65.5	8.7 (5.8–14.0)	6: 6.1% ($n = 551$)	cT1: 53.7% ($n = 4854$)	pT2: 43.7% ($n = 3951$)	NR	R1: 27.8%	14 (IQR: 8–21)	19% ($n = 1714$)	
					60.2–69.8)		7: 58.8% ($n = 5317$)	cT2: 41.4% ($n = 3736$)	pT3a: 30.2% ($n = 2727$)		(n = 2512)			
							≥8: 35.1% ($n = 3167$)	cT3: 4.9% ($n = 445$)	≥pT3b: 26.1% ($n = 2357$)					

(continued)

Table 4 (continued)

Study	Surgical	Treatment	*N*	Follow-up (mo)	Age (year)	PSA (ng/ml)	Biopsy Gleason score	Clinical T stage	Pathologic T stage	Pathologic Gleason score	Surgical margin	Number of lymph nodes dissected	Number of positive lymph nodes	Outcomes
Limited/standard PLND versus (super) extended PLND														
Hatzichristodoulou 2015	Open: 100%	ePLND	262	48	64.9 (7.5)	8.3 (6.3)	6: 0% (*n* = 0)	≤T1c: 57.3% (*n* = 150)	pT2: 76.3% (*n* = 200)	6: 40.1% (*n* = 105)	NR	20.4 (9.7)	NR	BFFS
				[R: 24–84]			7: 88.6% (*n* = 232)	>T1c: 42.7% (*n* = 112)	pT3a: 13% (*n* = 34)	7: 47.7% (*n* = 125)				
							8: 8.0% (n = 21)		pT3b: 9.9% (*n* = 26)	8–10: 12.2% (*n* = 32)				
							9: 3.4% (*n* = 9)		pT4: 0.8% (*n* = 2)					
		lPLND	198		64.6 (7.8)	9.9 (7.8)	6: 100% (*n* = 198)	≤T1c: 74.7% (*n* = 148)	pT2: 80.8% (*n* = 160)	6: 44.9% (*n* = 89)		4.7 (4)		
							7: 0% (*n* = 0)	>T1c: 25.3% (*n* = 50)	pT3a: 13.6% (*n* = 27)	7: 50.6% (*n* = 100)				
							8: 0% (*n* = 0)		pT3b: 5.6% (*n* = 11)	8–10: 4.5% (*n* = 9)				
							9: 0% (*n* = 0)		pT4: 0% (*n* = 0)					
Kim 2013	Robotic: 100%	sPLND	294	36	65	8.4	≤6: 33.4% (*n* = 98)	T1: 66.3% (*n* = 195)	T2: 62.2% (*n* = 183)	NR	NR	12 [R: 9–16]	3.4% (*n* = 10)	BFFS
					[R: 60–69]	[R: 5.3–37.7]	7: 48.3% (*n* = 142)	T2: 21.4% (*n* = 63)	T3a: 28.6% (*n* = 84)					
							≥8: 18.3% (*n* = 54)	T3: 12.3% (*n* = 36)	T3b: 9.2% (*n* = 27)					
		ePLND	170		66	10.4	≤6: 17.7% (*n* = 30)	T1: 45.9% (*n* = 78)	T2: 56.5% (*n* = 96)			21 [R: 16–25]	13.5% (*n* = 23)	
					[R: 62–70]	[R: 6.6–16.1]	7: 39.4% (*n* = 67)	T2: 41.2% (*n* = 70)	T3a: 28.8% (*n* = 49)					
							≥8: 42.9% (*n* = 73)	T3: 12.9% (*n* = 22)	T3b: 14.7% (*n* = 25)					
Jung 2012	Robotic: 100%	sPLND	155	24	66	8.7	<7: 32.3% (*n* = 50)	≤T2: 43.9% (*n* = 68)	T2: 51.6% (*n* = 80)	<7: 23.9% (*n* = 37)	R1: 37.4%	15	5.2%	BFFS
				[IQR: 15–34]	[IQR: 61–70]	[IQR: 5.8–14.3]	7: 33.5% (*n* = 52)	T3: 56.1% (*n* = 87)	T3a: 38.1% (*n* = 59)	7: 50.9% (*n* = 79)	(*n* = 58)	[IQR: 11–19]	(*n* = 8)	

							>7: 34.2% (*n* = 53)		T3b: 9.0% (*n* = 14)	>7: 25.2% (*n* = 39)				
									T4: 1.3% (*n* = 2)					
		ePLND	45	13	67	15.5	<7: 11.1% (*n* = 5)	≤T2: 28.9% (*n* = 13)	T2: 35.6% (*n* = 16)	<7: 6.7% (*n* = 3)	R1: 55.6%	24	22.2%	
				[IQR: 10–17]	[IQR: 63–72]	[IQR: 7.6–24.6]	7: 28.9% (*n* = 13)	T3: 71.1% (*n* = 32)	T3a: 53.3% (*n* = 24)	7: 42.2% (*n* = 19)	(*n* = 25)	[IQR: 18–28]	(*n* = 10)	
							>7: 60% (*n* = 27)		T3b: 8.9% (*n* = 4)	>7: 51.1% (*n* = 23)				
									T4: 2.2%% (*n* = 1)					
Allaf 2004	Open: 100%	lPLND	1865	93.6 (NR)	57.9	7.2 (NR)	NR	NR	≥T3a: 32% (*n* = 597)	≤6: 64.2% (*n* = 1198)	R1: 9.2%	8.9 (NR)	1.2% (*n* = 22)	BFFS
					(R: 35–74)					7: 30.8% (*n* = 575)	(*n* = 172)			
										8–10: 4.8% (*n* = 90)				
		ePLND	2135	94.8 (NR)	56.7	7.1 (NR)			≥T3a: 32.2% (*n* = 688)	≤6: 67% (*n* = 1431)	R1: 8.4%	11.6 (NR)	3.3% (*n* = 71)	
					(R: 33–74)					7: 28.6% (*n* = 610)	(*n* = 179)			
										8–10: 3.8% (*n* = 82)				
Mistretta 2017	Robotic: 100%	sPLND	109	32	66.3	12.1	6: 15.6% (*n* = 17)	T1: 45.9% (*n* = 50)	T2a-b: 15.7% (*n* = 17)	6: 15% (*n* = 16)	R1: 21.1%	11	12.8%	BCR
				(R: 6–72)	(IQR: 63–71)	(IQR: 4.9–12.9)	3 + 4: 37.6% (*n* = 41)	T2: 50.5% (*n* = 55)	T2c: 50% (*n* = 55)	3 + 4: 41.1% (*n* = 44)	(*n* = 109)	[IQR: 7–17]	(*n* = 14)	Adjuvant
				(*n* = 184)			4 + 3: 22.9% (*n* = 25)	T3: 3.7% (*n* = 4)	T3a: 21.3% (*n* = 23)	4 + 3: 24.3% (*n* = 28)				Therapy
							8: 15.6% (*n* = 17)		T3b: 13% (*n* = 14)	8: 8.4% (*n* = 9)				

(continued)

Table 4 (continued)

Study	Surgical	Treatment	*N*	Follow-up (mo)	Age (year)	PSA (ng/ml)	Biopsy Gleason score	Clinical T stage	Pathologic T stage	Pathologic Gleason score	Surgical margin	Number of lymph nodes dissected	Number of positive lymph nodes	Outcomes
							9: 8.3% (*n* = 9)			9: 11.2% (*n* = 12)				
	Robotic: 100%	ePLND	75		66	13.2	6: 20% (*n* = 15)	T1:37.3% (*n* = 28)	T2a-b: 4% (*n* = 3)	6: 8.2% (*n* = 6)	R1: 33.3%	21	29.3%	
					(IQR: 59–70)	(IQR: 6.2–17.4)	3 + 4: 32% (*n* = 24)	T2: 50.7% (*n* = 38)	T2c: 48% (*n* = 36)	3 + 4: 47.9% (*n* = 35)	(*n* = 75)	[IQR: 16–29]	(*n* = 22)	
							4 + 3: 18.7% (*n* = 14)	T3: 12% (*n* = 9)	T3a: 26.7% (*n* = 20)	4 + 3: 13.7% (*n* = 12)				
							8: 21.3% (*n* = 16)		T3b: 21.3% (*n* = 16)	8: 11% (*n* = 8)				
							9: 8% (*n* = 6)			9: 19.2% (*n* = 14)				
Lestingi 2020	Open: 100%	ePLND	150	55	63.4	10.5	6: 37% (*n* = 55)	T1: 57% (*n* = 82)	T0: 0	6: 2.7% (*n* = 4)	44% (*n* = 65)	17 (IQR: 13–24)	17% (*n* = 25)	BFFS
RCT				(IQR: 35.9–64.3)	(59.1–67)	(IQR: 6.5–17)	3 + 4: 42% (*n* = 63)	T2: 21% (*n* = 31)	T2: 41% (*n* = 61)	3 + 4: 55% (*n* = 83)				MFS
							4 + 3: 12% (*n* = 18)	T3: 22% (*n* = 32)	T3a: 45% (*n* = 67)	4 + 3: 30% (*n* = 45)				CSS
							4 + 4: 5.4% (*n* = 8)		T3b: 14% (*n* = 21)	8: 1.3% (*n* = 2)				
							4 + 5: 3.4% (*n* = 5)		T4: 0.7% (*n* = 1)	9, 10: 11% (*n* = 16)				
		lPLND	150	54.1	63	10.4	6: 36% (*n* = 54)	T1: 52% (*n* = 76)	T0: 0.7% (*n* = 1)	6: 4% (*n* = 6)	37% (n = 55)	3 (IQR: 2–5)	3.4% (*n* = 5)	
				(IQR: 37–61.5)	(58.8–67.3)	(IQR: 6.9–13.9)	3 + 4: 38% (*n* = 57)	T2: 23% (*n* = 33)	T2: 38% (*n* = 57)	3 + 4: 49% (*n* = 73)				
							4 + 3: 13% (*n* = 19)	T3: 25% (*n* = 37)	T3a: 43% (*n* = 64)	4 + 3: 31% (*n* = 46)				
							4 + 4: 8.7% (*n* = 13)		T3b: 18% (*n* = 27)	8: 0.7% (*n* = 1)				
							4 + 5: 4% (*n* = 6)		T4: 0.7% (*n* = 1)	9, 10: 15% (*n* = 23)				

Touijer 2021	Open	lPLND	700	37.2	62	5.9	6: 10% (*n* = 72)	T1c: 61% (*n* = 400)	T3a: 54% (*n* = 375)	6: 5.9% (*n* = 40)	NR	12 (IQR: 8–17)	11.6% (*n* = 81)	BFFS
RCT	Lap			(IQR: 18–60)	(IQR: 57–67)	(IQR: 4.3–8.6)	3 + 4: 52% (*n* = 362)	T2a,b,c: 29.4% (*n* = 206)	T3b: 12% (*n* = 85)	3 + 4: 58% (*n* = 399)				
	Robotic						4 + 3: 19% (*n* = 135)	T3a,b: 7% (*n* = 49)		4 + 3: 23% (*n* = 160)				
							≥8: 18% (*n* = 129)			≥8: 12% (*n* = 84)				
		ePLND	740		63	5.7	6: 9.4% (*n* = 69)	T1c: 61% (*n* = 418)	T3a: 49% (*n* = 364)	6: 7.3% (*n* = 53)		14 (IQR: 10–20)	13.5% (*n* = 100)	
					(IQR: 57–67)	(IQR: 4.2–8.2)	3 + 4: 52% (*n* = 383)	T2a,b,c: 31.5% (*n* = 233)	T3b: 12% (*n* = 89)	3 + 4: 53% (*n* = 385)				
							4 + 3: 17% (*n* = 125)	T3a,b: 5.3% (*n* = 39)		4 + 3: 24% (*n* = 173)				
							≥8: 22% (*n* = 160)			≥8: 16% (*n* = 118)				

BCR biochemical recurrence, *BF* biochemical failure, *BFFS* BF-free survival, *CSS* cancer-specific survival, *ePLND* extended PLND, *IQR* interquartile range, *lap* laparoscopic, *LFFS* local failure-free survival, *lPLND* limited PLND, *MFS* metastases-free survival, *MIESRP* minimum incision endoscopic radical prostatectomy, *NA* not available, *NR* not reported, *OS* overall survival, *PCSM* prostate cancer–specific mortality, *PSA* prostate-specific antigen, *PLND* pelvic lymph node dissection, *R* range, *RCT* randomized clinical trial, *sPLND* standard PLND

Data for categorical variables are reported as frequency (proportion). Data for continuous variables are reported as either median [range or IQR] or mean (range)

Table 5 Results from studies addressing oncologic outcomes

Study	Subgroup if applicable	Intervention (Int)	Comparator (Comp)		Outcome(s)	Int (n)	Comp (n)		Intervention: Outcome	Comparator: Outcome		p value	Comment
No PLND versus any PLND													
Karl 2015	NA	PLND		No PLND	BFFS	357	179		Univariate analysis: HR: 1.69 [1.25–2.29] MVA: HR: 1.29 [0.94–1.78]			Univariate analysis: 0.001 MVA: 0.12	–
Gandaglia 2015	Patients eligible for active surveillance according to PRIAS	PLND		No PLND	BCR	381	1329		MVA: HR: 0.72 [95% CI: 0.37–1.38]			0.3	MVA corrected for: Age, iPSA, PSM, pT, pGS, pN status
Koo 2015	PSM + and undetectable PSA <6 wk	PLND		No PLND	BFFS	403	327		Univariate analysis: 1.099 [95% CI: 0.564–2.141]			0.08	–
Boehm 2015	NA	PLND		No PLND	BFFS	6810	4884		HR: 0.81 (95% CI: 0.72–0.9)			<0.05	pNx versus pN0 (pN + excluded)
					MFS				HR: 0.62 (95% CI: 0.41–0.92)			<0.05	
					OS				HR: 0.92 (95% CI: 0.74–1.14)			0.46	
Liss 2013	NA	ePLND	sPLND	No PLND	BFFS	54	231	207	29.6% ($n = 16$)	14.7% ($n = 34$)	3.4% ($n = 7$)	<0.001	–
Mitsuzuka 2013	Low risk disease	PLND		No PLND	MFS	147	75		100%		100%	NR	Median follow- up PLND: 60 mo no PLND: 26 mo
					CSS				100%		100%	NR	
					OS				98.6% ($n = 145$)		98.7% ($n = 74$)	NR	
					BFFS		NR		NR			0.65	
Masuda 2013	pT2–3 N0/x	PLND		No PLND	BFFS	187	202		MVA total cohort: HR: 1.26 (95% CI: 0.70–2.30)			0.45	Excluded N1
									pT2 disease: HR: 1.00 (95% CI: 0.43–2.26)			1.0	
									pT3 disease: HR: 1.86 (95% CI: 0.75–5.28)			0.19	
									pT2 R0 disease: HR: 0.50 (95% CI: 0.18–1.35)			0.17	

Daimon 2012	NA	lPLND	No PLND	BFFS (5-year)	85	54	90.1% ($n = 77$)	82.4% ($n = 44$)	0.28	
				BFFS (7-year)			88.3% ($n = 75$)	82.4% ($n = 44$)	0.28	
Ost	NA	ePLND	No PLND	BFFS (7-year)	179	46	84%	83%	NR	
							HR: 0.8 [95% CI: 0.2–2.6]		UnADJ: 0.96 ADJ: 0.69	
				LFFS (7-year)			87%	88%	NR	
							HR: 0.09 [95% CI: 0.01–0.6]		UnADJ: 0.35	
									ADJ: 0.009	
Ku 2011	NA	PLND	No PLND	BF	111	88	33.3% ($n = 37$)	35.2% ($n = 31$)	0.36	
Porter 2010	NA	PLND	No PLND	PCSM	342	410	RR: 0.7 (95% CI: 0.2–2.4)		0.6	
Weight 2008	NA	PLND	No PLND	BFFS	140	196	84% (10-year)	88% (10-year)	0.33	
Berglund 2007	NA	lPLND	No PLND	FFS (overall)	3961	732	74%	70%	0.11	
				FFS (low)			82%	81%	0.83	
				FFS(intermediate)			63%	71%	0.21	
				FFS (high)			48%	42%	0.45	
Bhatta-Dhar 2004	NA	PLND	No PLND	BFFS	140	196	86% (6-year)	88% (6-year)	0.28	
Fergany 2000	NA	PLND	No PLND	BFFS	372	203	91% (4-year)	97% (4-year)	0.16	
							MVA: "Not significant"		0.24	
Preisser 2020	NA	PLND	No PLND	BFFS	707	9035	60.4%	65.6%	0.07	2:1 propensity score matching, balanced for PSA, pathologic tumor stage, primary pathologic Gleason and surgical margin status
				MFS			87%	90%	0.06	
				PCSM			95.2%	96.4%	0.2	
Limited/standard PLND versus (super) extended PLND										
Hatzichristodoulou 2015	NA	ePLND	lPLND	BFFS (7-year)	262	198	pT2 94.8% pT3 81.2%	pT2 100% pT3 94.7%	pT2: 0.011 pT3: 0.3	–
Kim 2013	NA	sPLND	ePLND	BFFS (3-year)	170	294	72.7%	79.8%	0.05	(BFFS: Propensity score–matched cohort: $p = 0.497$)
Jung 2012	NA	sPLND	ePLND	BFFS	155	45	77.9%	64.4%	NS	
Allaf 2004	pN+	ePLND	lPLND	BFFS (5-year)	2135	1865	34.4%	16.5%	0.04	
	pN+ (<15% of Retrieved nodes Affected)						42.9%	10%	0.01	

(continued)

Table 5 (continued)

Study	Subgroup if applicable	Intervention (Int)	Comparator (Comp)	Outcome(s)	Int (n)	Comp (n)	Intervention: Outcome	Comparator: Outcome	*p* value	Comment
Mistretta 2017	NA	ePLND	sPLND	BCR	75	109	9.3%	16%	0.32	
Lestingi 2020	ISUP GG 3–5	ePLND	lPLND	BFFS (5-year)	150	150	HR: 0.91 (95% CI 0.63–1.32)		0.6	
RCT										
Touijer 2021	NA	ePLND	lPLND	BFFS	740	700	HR: 1.04 (95% CI 0.93–1.15)		0.5	
RCT										

BCR biochemical recurrence, *BF* biochemical failure, *BFFS* biochemical failure-free survival, *bGS* biopsy Gleason score, *CSS* cancer-specific survival, *eBL* estimated blood loss, *ePLND* extended PLND, *FFS* failure-free survival, *GS* Gleason score, *HR* hazard ratio, *iPSA* initial PSA, *ISUP* international society urological pathology Gleason grade; *lPLND* limited PLND, *IPTW* inverse probability-of-treatment weighting, *LFFS* local failure-free survival, *MFS* metastases-free survival, *MVA* multivariate analysis, *NA* not applicable, *NR* not reported, *OS* overall survival, *PCSM* prostate cancer-specific mortality, *PE* pulmonary embolism, *pGS* pathologic Gleason score, *PLND* pelvic lymph node dissection, *pN+* lymph node positive, *PSM* positive surgical margin, *RCT* randomized clinical trial, *sPLND* standard PLND

5.2 Extended PLND and the Risk of Distant Metastases

Distant metastasis following RP was evaluated in two retrospective studies that reported conflicting results [38, 72]. Mitsuzuka et al. analyzed a series of 222 low-risk patients. They found metastasis-free survival (MFS) of 100% in both sPLND and no-PLND groups at a median follow-up of 60 and 26 mo, respectively [72]. Conversely, the already mentioned study by Boehm et al. found that no PLND was associated with a lower risk of distant metastasis on multivariable analysis (HR 0.62; 95% CI 0.41–0.92; $p < 0.05$) [38]. Baseline differences among pNx and pN0 patients and selection bias may explain these MFS findings.

5.3 Extended PLND and Cancer-Specific and Overall Mortality

Cancer-specific and overall mortality were analyzed in four studies. Of these, PLND was standard in one study [72], while its extent was not reported in the other three studies [38, 80, 82]. Mean follow-up ranged from 30.5 mo [80] to 11 year [82]. None of these studies demonstrated statistically significant differences in cancer-specific mortality [72, 80, 82] or overall mortality [38, 72] between PLND and no PLND.

In a multi-institutional database of 9742 patients (whose probability of lymph node invasion according to the Briganti nomogram was greater than 5%) submitted to RP from 2000 to 2017 with or without PLND, a median of 14 lymph nodes (IQR 8–21) were removed in the PLND cohort and 1714 of these cases (19.0%) harbored lymph node metastasis. After propensity score matching the biochemical recurrence-free, metastasis-free, and cancer-specific mortality-free survival rates were 60.4% vs. 65.6% ($p = 0.07$), 87.0% vs. 90.0% ($p = 0.06$) and 95.2% vs. 96.4% ($p = 0.2$) for pelvic lymph node dissection vs. no pelvic lymph node dissection 120 months after radical prostatectomy. Multivariable Cox regression models adjusted for postoperative and preoperative tumor characteristics revealed that PLND performed at RP was no independent predictor of biochemical recurrence, metastasis, or cancer-specific mortality (all $p \geq 0.1$) [80].

5.4 Randomized Controlled Trials (RCTs)

As already commented, patients undergoing an ePLND are more likely to be correctly staged as pN0 or pN1, making retrospective observational comparisons of oncological results between limited vs. extended dissection problematic (Will Rogers phenomenon) [66].

To fill this knowledge gap, the first phase III randomized controlled trial (RCT) to investigate the therapeutic role of ePLND compared to lPLND in patients with intermediate- and high-risk localized PCa undergoing RP was recently published. Three hundred patients were randomized and treated at a single institution (Instituto do Cancer do Estado de Sao Paulo, Hospital das Clinicas, Faculdade de Medicina da Universidade de Sao Paulo, ICESP-HCFMUSP, Brazil) between May 2012 and December 2016 (1:1; 150 lPLND [obturator nodes bilaterally]; and 150 ePLND [obturator, external iliac, internal iliac, common iliac, and presacral nodes bilaterally]). By showing five times more lymph node metastases in extended dissection, this trial confirmed that ePLND provides better pathological staging, while differences in early oncological outcomes were not demonstrated. The median BRFS was 61.4 mo in the lPLND group and not reached in the ePLND group (hazard ratio [HR] 0.91, 95% CI 0.63–1.32; $p = 0.6$) (Fig. 7a). Median MFS was not

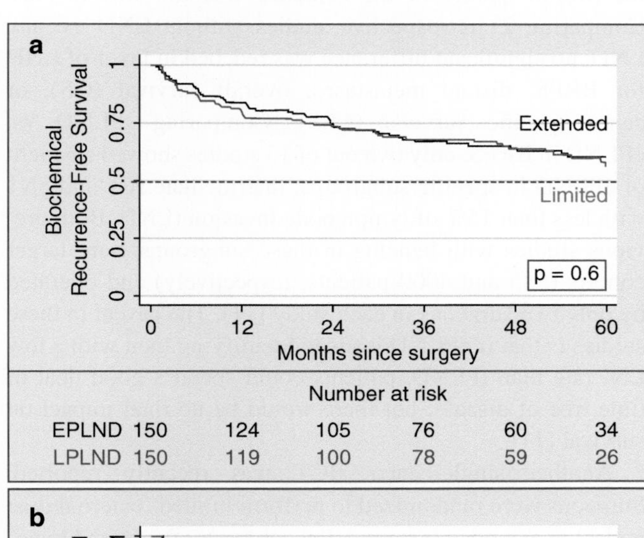

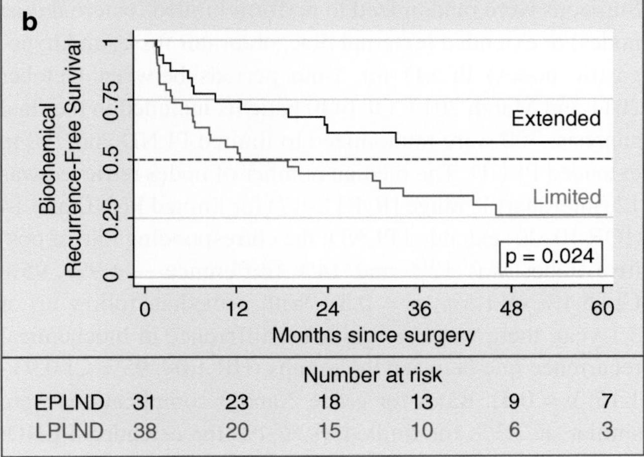

Fig. 7 Kaplan-Meier estimates of biochemical recurrence-free (BRF) survival in the intention-to-treat analysis according to limited (LPLND) or extended pelvic lymph node dissection (EPLND) in (**a**) the overall cohort and (**b**) the subgroup with preoperative biopsy International Society of Urological Pathology grades 3–5 [9]

reached in either group (HR 0.57, 95% CI 0.17–1.8; $p = 0.3$). CSS data were not available because no patient died from PCa before the cut-off date. In an exploratory subgroup analysis, patients with preoperative biopsy International Society of Urological Pathology (ISUP) grade groups 3–5 who were allocated to ePLND had better BRFS (HR 0.33, 95% CI 0.14–0.74, interaction $p = 0.007$) (Fig. 7b) [23]. Therefore, this RCT confirmed that ePLND provides better pathological staging, while differences in early oncological outcomes were not demonstrated. Subgroup analysis suggests a potential BCRFS benefit in patients diagnosed with ISUP grade groups 3–5; however, these findings should be considered hypothesis-generating. Further RCTs with larger cohorts and longer follow-up are necessary to better define the role of ePLND during RP [9].

The oncological results of this RCT were similar to those of the most significant systematic review on the topic (66 studies, 275,269 patients). Fossati et al. demonstrated that the overall quality of the evidence was low due to bias. Comparing 21 retrospective studies without LND vs. any LND, no significant difference was reached in favor of LND for BRFS, distant metastases, overall survival (OS), or cancer-specific survival (CSS). Comparing lPLND vs. ePLND in BRFS, only two out of 13 studies showed a benefit of ePLND in specific subgroups: intermediate risk and pN1 with less than 15% of lymph node invasion (LNI). Both previous studies with benefits in these subgroups were larger cohorts (585 and 4000 patients, respectively) and operated by only two surgeons in each study [11]. The caveat in these studies is that if ePLND leads to identifying men with a low LNI rate than lPLND, patients could spend a good deal of time free of disease, but there would be no final impact on survival [11].

Another single-center RCT was recently reported. Surgeons were randomized to perform limited (external iliac nodes) or extended (external iliac, obturator fossa, and hypogastric nodes) PLND for 3-mo periods between October 2011 and March 2017. Of 1440 patients included in the final analysis, 700 were randomized to limited PLND and 740 to extended PLND. The median number of nodes retrieved was 12 (interquartile range [IQR] 8–17) for limited PLND and 14 (IQR 10–20) extended PLND; the corresponding rate of positive nodes was 12% and 14% (difference − 1.9%, 95% CI -5.4% to 1.5%; $p = 0.3$). With a median follow-up of 3.1 year, there was no significant difference in biochemical recurrence rate between the groups (HR 1.04, 95% CI 0.93–1.15; $p = 0.5$). Rates for grade 2 and 3 complications were similar at 7.3% for limited vs. 6.4% for extended PLND; there were no grade 4 or 5 complications [10]. As the differences between the groups are minimal, a bias has likely occurred by the surgeon. Therefore, extended PLND did not improve freedom from biochemical recurrence over limited PLND for clinically localized prostate cancer men. However, there were smaller than expected differences in the nodal count and the rate of positive nodes between the two templates. Moreover, in the trial by Touijer et al., the number of removed lymph nodes was similar for the limited and extended PLND templates (median 12 vs. 14). Thus, it is not possible to conclude that BCR-free survival is similar in the "limited" vs. "extended" PLND arms because it seems both groups were extended.

A randomized trial comparing PLND to no node dissection is warranted. An RCT has recently started recruiting in Switzerland (NCT03921996) comparing ePLND vs. no PLND during RP for intermediate- and high-risk PCa. Results from clinical trials such as the German SEAL trial (AP 77/13) are also awaited, randomizing a total of 950 patients with intermediate- or high-risk PCa to improve 10-year survival from 83% with lPLND to 88% with ePLND.

5.5 Potential Benefits of Extended PLND in Prostate Cancer

It is also worth mentioning that not all patients with positive lymph nodes have the same risk of progression and death. In a multicenter series of 703 patients with multimodal treatment, those with two or fewer positive lymph nodes had a significantly better result on 15 year-CSS compared to patients with more than two positive lymph nodes (84% vs. 62%, $p < 0.001$). After accounting for all the other predictors, patients with more than two positive nodes had a 1.9-fold higher risk of dying for prostate cancer than patients with two or fewer positive nodes [83].

Another consecutive series of 122 node-positive patients with negative preoperative staging examinations, no neoadjuvant hormonal or Radiotherapy, and who underwent extended PLND (≥10 lymph nodes in the surgical specimen) followed by RP without immediate androgen deprivation therapy (ADT) had similar results. In patients with ≤ two or ≥ three positive nodes removed, median cancer-specific survival at 10 year was 78.6% and 33.4%, respectively ($p < 0.001$). Therefore, there is a direct benefit of PLND for patients with up to two positive lymph nodes, whose oncological evolution is similar to patients with pN0 [84].

Preisser et al. within the Surveillance, Epidemiology and End Results (SEER) database (2004–2014), identified 28,147 patients with D'Amico intermediate- (67.3%) or high-risk (32.7%) characteristics who underwent RP with PLND, without evidence of LNI. Continuously coded removed lymph node count achieved independent predictor status (HR: 0.955, $P = 0.01$), where each additional removed lymph node reduced CSM risk by 4.5% [85].

Recently, Sood et al. analyzed 311,061 PCa patients undergoing RP between 2004 and 2015 on the National Cancer Database (NCDB), and 49,470 (15.9%) patients underwent an ePLND. The median number of lymph nodes removed in patients undergoing none/limited PLND vs. ePLND were 2 and 14, respectively ($P < 0.001$). With a 54-mo median follow-up, they also demonstrated an independent direct benefit of PLND in OS if the risk of LNI is greater than 20% [86].

Another benefit of LND, this time indirect, is to select the patient for adjuvant treatments better. Messing et al. demonstrated that early androgen deprivation therapy (ADT) benefited patients with nodal metastases submitted to RP and LND, compared to those who received treatment later [87].

Abdollah et al. showed benefited from adjuvant Radiotherapy in two groups of patients: (1) patients with positive lymph node (PLN) count ≤2, Gleason score 7 to 10, pT3b/pT4 stage, or positive surgical margins (HR: 0.30; $P = 0.002$); and (2) patients with PLN count of 3 to 4 (HR: 0.21; $P = 0.02$), regardless of other tumor characteristics [88].

Abdollah et al. also examined data of 315 pN1 PCa patients treated with RP and ePLND between 2000 and 2012 at one tertiary care center. All patients received adjuvant hormonal therapy with or without adjuvant Radiotherapy. The number of removed lymph nodes (RLN) independently predicted lower Cancer-Specific Mortality (CSM) rate (HR: 0.93; $p = 0.02$). The most informative cutoff for the number of RLNs was 14. At 10 year, the CSM-free survival rates were significantly higher for patients with ≥14 RLNs compared to their counterparts with <14 RLNs ($p = 0.04$) [89].

Fossati et al. also performed a multi-institutional review of men with a rising PSA after RP treated with salvage radiation therapy (sRT). On multivariable analysis, the risk of BCR after sRT was inversely associated with the number of nodes resected at RP (hazards ratio [HR]: 0.98; 95% CI: 0.96–0.99; $p = 0.049$). The increased extent of dissection was also independently associated with a decreased risk of clinical recurrence after sRT (HR: 0.97; 95%CI: 0.94–0.99; $p = 0.042$). These data support the importance of an extensive LND at surgery and may be used in prognosis assessment when sRT is considered [90].

More recently, Touijer et al., in a retrospective and multicenter cohort of 1338 patients with positive lymph nodes (27% with more than ten years of follow-up), demonstrated that those submitted to Radiotherapy and ADT had better OS and CSS when compared to patients with observation or isolated ADT [91]. Nevertheless, LND is the best option available to determine lymph node metastases and, therefore, the best option to select patients for adjuvant treatments.

6 Salvage Lymphadenectomy

The aims of metastasis-directed therapy in patients with node-only recurrence would optimize locoregional control, limit the risk of distant progression, avoid immediate ADT, and potentially improve cancer-specific survival. In addition, recent developments in PCa recurrence PET/CT imaging have improved the detection of clinical recurrence even at a low PSA level. They could guide node-directed salvage therapy at an early stage of biochemical recurrence [92].

Salvage lymphadenectomy (SLND) is a treatment option offered in high-volume centers by experienced surgeons for patients with BCR post RP. The series of SLND with better oncological outcomes occurs in patients with restricted criteria: PSA < 4 ng/mL, Gleason ≤7 (ISUP 1–3), exclusively low-lymph node disease volume limited to the pelvis proven by PET PSMA. Good disease-free survival could also be anticipated by considering the number of positive nodes during SLND, PSA decrease after surgery, and absence of confirmed extrapelvic positive nodes at the final pathology. Thus, patients with pure pelvic involvement and favorable pathology features may be the ideal candidates for node-directed salvage strategies without a systematic adjuvant approach [92]. These manuscripts showed 9–22% (mean 15%) of patients free of BCR in five years [93, 94]. This benefit may be due to removing lymph nodes guided by imaging tests in patients with positive nodes better selected in the preoperative period.

However, pathological data from SLND studies suggested that only a tiny proportion of patients have lymph node metastases limited to the positive spots. Therefore, any nodal salvage treatment should not be directed only to the suspicious lymph nodes at imaging but also to contiguous nodal areas [95].

The available data suggest that SLND can delay clinical progression and postpone hormonal therapy in almost one-third of the patients, although most will have BCR. An accurate and attentive preoperative patient selection may help improve these outcomes. The most frequent complication after SLND was lymphorrhea (15.3%), followed by fever (14.5%) and ileus (11.2%). It is noteworthy that all examined cohorts originated from retrospective single-institution series, with limited sample size and short follow-up. Consequently, the current findings cannot be generalized and warrant further investigation in future prospective trials [94].

In a recent systematic review and meta-analysis with 27 SLND series, prostate-specific membrane antigen or choline positron emission tomography/computed tomography was the reference detection technique. SLND was performed by open or laparoscopic approach with <10% of grade 3 or more complication rate. Mean follow-up was 29.4 mo. Complete biochemical response after SLND was achieved in

13–79.5% of cases (mean 44.3%). The 2- and 5-year biochemical progression-free survival rates ranged from 23% to 64% and from 6% to 31%, respectively. Five-year overall survival was approximately 84%. The main drawbacks limiting the interpretation of the effectiveness of SLND were the retrospective design of single-center series, heterogeneity between series in terms of adjuvant treatment, endpoints, definitions of progression and study population, and the absence of long-term follow-up. The selection bias is of significant concern in this setting, especially since a control group (standard of care) lacks all except one series. Accumulated data suggest that SLND is a safe metastasis-directed therapy option in nodal recurrence after primary treatment. However, a high level of evidence is still missing to draw any clinically meaningful conclusion about the oncological impact of SLND on long-term endpoints [92].

Similarly, Bravi et al. recently demonstrated in a study that included 189 patients who experienced PSA rise and nodal-only recurrence after RP and underwent SLND at 11 tertiary referral centers between 2002 and 2011. Lymph node recurrence was documented by positron emission tomography/computed tomography (PET/CT) scan using either 11C-choline or 68Ga prostate-specific membrane antigen ligand. A third of men treated with SLND for PET-detected nodal recurrence of PCa died long term, with PCa being the leading cause of death. Salvage LND alone was associated with durable long-term outcomes in a minority of men who significantly benefited from additional treatments after surgery. Taken together, all these data argue against the use of metastasis-directed therapy alone for patients with node-only recurrent PCa. These men should instead be considered at high risk of systemic dissemination already at the time of sLND. Therefore, in general, SLND only helps postpone the introduction of ADT and should be used only as an integral part of multimodal treatment [96].

7 Conclusions

Limited lymphadenectomy significantly underestimates the actual incidence of lymph node metastasis and should no longer be performed for staging.

Extended lymphadenectomy is currently the gold standard in lymph node staging. It should be reserved for patients at higher risk of lymph node invasion:

1. Intermediate-risk patients with a chance of lymph node invasion greater than 5% (Briganti's nomogram) or greater than 7% (if MRI and target biopsy information are used).
2. High-risk.
3. Locally advanced.
4. ISUP Gleason Grade 3–5 in the biopsy.

The oncological role of extended lymphadenectomy is not defined. It can help patients directly (up to two positive lymph nodes), indirectly (select for adjuvant treatments), or may be beneficial in patients with ISUP in biopsy 3–5.

Extended lymph node dissection is also associated with significantly worse intra- and postoperative non-oncological outcomes, such as bleeding, lymphocele, and increased surgical time.

The oncological role of salvage lymphadenectomy also is not clear.

References

1. Siegel RL, Miller KD, Fuchs HE, Jemal A. Cancer statistics, 2021. CA Cancer J Clin. 2021;71(1):7–33.
2. McLaughlin AP, Saltzstein SL, McCullough DL, Gittes RF. Prostatic carcinoma: incidence and location of unsuspected lymphatic metastases. J Urol. 1976;115(1):89–94.
3. Wolf JS, Cher M, Dall'era M, Presti JC, Hricak H, Carroll PR. The use and accuracy of cross-sectional imaging and fine needle aspiration cytology for detection of pelvic lymph node metastases before radical prostatectomy. J Urol. 1995;153(3 Pt 2):993–9.
4. Katz S, Rosen M. MR imaging and MR spectroscopy in prostate cancer management. Radiol Clin N Am. 2006;44(5):723–34. viii
5. Perera M, Papa N, Roberts M, Williams M, Udovicich C, Vela I, et al. Gallium-68 prostate-specific membrane antigen positron emission tomography in advanced prostate cancer-updated diagnostic utility, sensitivity, specificity, and distribution of prostate-specific membrane antigen-avid lesions: a systematic review and meta-analysis. Eur Urol. 2020;77(4):403–17.
6. Hyndman ME, Mullins JK, Pavlovich CP. Pelvic node dissection in prostate cancer: extended, limited, or not at all? Curr Opin Urol. 2010;20(3):211–7.
7. Heidenreich A. Still unanswered: the role of extended pelvic lymphadenectomy in improving oncological outcomes in prostate cancer. Eur Urol. 2021;79(5):605–6.
8. Briganti A, Blute ML, Eastham JH, Graefen M, Heidenreich A, Karnes JR, et al. Pelvic lymph node dissection in prostate cancer. Eur Urol. 2009;55(6):1251–65.
9. Lestingi JFP, Guglielmetti GB, Trinh QD, Coelho RF, Pontes J, Bastos DA, et al. Extended versus limited pelvic lymph node dissection during radical prostatectomy for intermediate- and high-risk prostate cancer: early oncological outcomes from a randomized phase 3 trial. Eur Urol. 2021;79(5):595–604.
10. Touijer KA, Sjoberg DD, Benfante N, Laudone VP, Ehdaie B, Eastham JA, et al. Limited versus extended pelvic lymph node dissection for prostate cancer: a randomized clinical trial. Eur Urol Oncol. 2021;4(4):532–9.
11. Fossati N, Willemse PM, Van den Broeck T, van den Bergh RCN, Yuan CY, Briers E, et al. The benefits and harms of different extents of lymph node dissection during radical prostatectomy for prostate cancer: a systematic review. Eur Urol. 2017;72(1):84–109.
12. Heidenreich A, Varga Z, Von Knobloch R. Extended pelvic lymphadenectomy in patients undergoing radical prostatectomy: high incidence of lymph node metastasis. J Urol. 2002;167(4):1681–6.
13. Briganti A, Chun FK, Salonia A, Suardi N, Gallina A, Da Pozzo LF, et al. Complications and other surgical outcomes associated with extended pelvic lymphadenectomy in men with localized prostate cancer. Eur Urol. 2006;50(5):1006–13.
14. Sanda MG, Cadeddu JA, Kirkby E, Chen RC, Crispino T, Fontanarosa J, et al. Clinically localized prostate cancer: AUA/

ASTRO/SUO Guideline. Part I: risk stratification, shared decision making, and care options. J Urol. 2018;199(3):683–90.

15. Mottet N, van den Bergh RCN, Briers E, Van den Broeck T, Cumberbatch MG, De Santis M, et al. EAU-EANM-ESTRO-ESUR-SIOG guidelines on prostate Cancer-2020 update. Part 1: screening, diagnosis, and local treatment with curative intent. Eur Urol. 2021;79(2):243–62.
16. Mohler JL, Antonarakis ES, Armstrong AJ, D'Amico AV, Davis BJ, Dorff T, et al. Prostate cancer, version 2.2019, NCCN clinical practice guidelines in oncology. J Natl Compr Cancer Netw. 2019;17(5):479–505.
17. Luiting HB, van Leeuwen PJ, Busstra MB, Brabander T, van der Poel HG, Donswijk ML, et al. Use of gallium-68 prostate-specific membrane antigen positron-emission tomography for detecting lymph node metastases in primary and recurrent prostate cancer and location of recurrence after radical prostatectomy: an overview of the current literature. BJU Int. 2020;125(2):206–14.
18. Hope TA, Armstrong WR, Murthy V, Lawhn Heath C, Behr S, Barbato F, et al. Accuracy of 68Ga-PSMA-11 for pelvic nodal metastasis detection prior to radical prostatectomy and pelvic lymph node dissection: a multicenter prospective phase III imaging study. J Clin Oncol. 2020;38(15_suppl):5502.
19. Porcaro AB, Cacciamani GE, Sebben M, Tafuri A, Processali T, Rizzetto R, et al. Lymph nodes invasion of Marcille's fossa associates with high metastatic load in prostate cancer patients undergoing extended pelvic lymph node dissection: the role of "Marcillectomy". Urol Int. 2019;103(1):25–32.
20. Sagalovich D, Calaway A, Srivastava A, Sooriakumaran P, Tewari AK. Assessment of required nodal yield in a high risk cohort undergoing extended pelvic lymphadenectomy in robotic-assisted radical prostatectomy and its impact on functional outcomes. BJU Int. 2013;111(1):85–94.
21. Mattei A, Fuechsel FG, Bhatta Dhar N, Warncke SH, Thalmann GN, Krause T, et al. The template of the primary lymphatic landing sites of the prostate should be revisited: results of a multimodality mapping study. Eur Urol. 2008;53(1):118–25.
22. Bader P, Burkhard FC, Markwalder R, Studer UE. Is a limited lymph node dissection an adequate staging procedure for prostate cancer? J Urol. 2002;168(2):514–8. discussion 8
23. Heidenreich A, Ohlmann CH, Polyakov S. Anatomical extent of pelvic lymphadenectomy in patients undergoing radical prostatectomy. Eur Urol. 2007;52(1):29–37.
24. Touijer K, Rabbani F, Otero JR, Secin FP, Eastham JA, Scardino PT, et al. Standard versus limited pelvic lymph node dissection for prostate cancer in patients with a predicted probability of nodal metastasis greater than 1%. J Urol. 2007;178(1):120–4.
25. Stone NN, Stock RG, Unger P. Laparoscopic pelvic lymph node dissection for prostate cancer: comparison of the extended and modified techniques. J Urol. 1997;158(5):1891–4.
26. Briganti A, Chun FK, Salonia A, Gallina A, Zanni G, Scattoni V, et al. Critical assessment of ideal nodal yield at pelvic lymphadenectomy to accurately diagnose prostate cancer nodal metastasis in patients undergoing radical retropubic prostatectomy. Urology. 2007;69(1):147–51.
27. Briganti A, Suardi N, Capogrosso P, Passoni N, Freschi M, di Trapani E, et al. Lymphatic spread of nodal metastases in high-risk prostate cancer: the ascending pathway from the pelvis to the retroperitoneum. Prostate. 2012;72(2):186–92.
28. Joniau S, Van den Bergh L, Lerut E, Deroose CM, Haustermans K, Oyen R, et al. Mapping of pelvic lymph node metastases in prostate cancer. Eur Urol. 2013;63(3):450–8.
29. Prasad SM, Shalhav AL. Comparative effectiveness of minimally invasive versus open lymphadenectomy in urological cancers. Curr Opin Urol. 2013;23(1):57–64.
30. Barbosa FG, Queiroz MA, Nunes RF, Viana PCC, Marin JFG, Cerri GG, et al. Revisiting prostate cancer recurrence with PSMA PET: atlas of typical and atypical patterns of spread. Radiographics. 2019;39(1):186–212.
31. van der Poel HG, Tillier C, de Blok W, van Muilekom E. Extended nodal dissection reduces sexual function recovery after robot-assisted laparoscopic prostatectomy. J Endourol. 2012;26(9):1192–8.
32. Gandaglia G, Suardi N, Gallina A, Abdollah F, Capitanio U, Salonia A, et al. Extended pelvic lymph node dissection does not affect erectile function recovery in patients treated with bilateral nerve-sparing radical prostatectomy. J Sex Med. 2012;9(8):2187–94.
33. Walz J, Epstein JI, Ganzer R, Graefen M, Guazzoni G, Kaouk J, et al. A critical analysis of the current knowledge of surgical anatomy of the prostate related to optimisation of cancer control and preservation of continence and erection in candidates for radical prostatectomy: an update. Eur Urol. 2016;70(2):301–11.
34. Grande P, Di Pierro GB, Mordasini L, Ferrari M, Würnschimmel C, Danuser H, et al. Prospective randomized trial comparing titanium clips to bipolar coagulation in sealing lymphatic vessels during pelvic lymph node dissection at the time of robot-assisted radical prostatectomy. Eur Urol. 2017;71(2):155–8.
35. Eden CG, Arora A, Rouse P. Extended vs standard pelvic lymphadenectomy during laparoscopic radical prostatectomy for intermediate- and high-risk prostate cancer. BJU Int. 2010;106(4):537–42.
36. Tyritzis SI, Wallerstedt A, Steineck G, Nyberg T, Hugosson J, Bjartell A, et al. Thromboembolic complications in 3,544 patients undergoing radical prostatectomy with or without lymph node dissection. J Urol. 2015;193(1):117–25.
37. Schmitges J, Trinh QD, Jonas L, Budäus L, Larbig R, Schlomm T, et al. Influence of low-molecular-weight heparin dosage on red blood cell transfusion, lymphocele rate and drainage duration after open radical prostatectomy. Eur J Surg Oncol. 2012;38(11):1082–8.
38. Boehm K, Beyer B, Tennstedt P, Schiffmann J, Budaeus L, Haese A, et al. No impact of blood transfusion on oncological outcome after radical prostatectomy in patients with prostate cancer. World J Urol. 2015;33(6):801–6.
39. Liss MA, Palazzi K, Stroup SP, Jabaji R, Raheem OA, Kane CJ. Outcomes and complications of pelvic lymph node dissection during robotic-assisted radical prostatectomy. World J Urol. 2013;31(3):481–8.
40. Violette PD, Mikhail D, Pond GR, Pautler SE. Independent predictors of prolonged operative time during robotic-assisted radical prostatectomy. J Robot Surg. 2015;9(2):117–23.
41. van der Poel HG, de Blok W, Tillier C, van Muilekom E. Robot-assisted laparoscopic prostatectomy: nodal dissection results during the first 440 cases by two surgeons. J Endourol. 2012;26(12):1618–24.
42. Schmitges J, Trinh QD, Sun M, Abdollah F, Bianchi M, Budäus L, et al. Venous thromboembolism after radical prostatectomy: the effect of surgical caseload. BJU Int. 2012;110(6):828–33.
43. Schmitges J, Trinh QD, Sun M, Abdollah F, Bianchi M, Budäus L, et al. Annual prostatectomy volume is related to rectal laceration rate after radical prostatectomy. Urology. 2012;79(4):796–803.
44. Touijer K, Fuenzalida RP, Rabbani F, Paparel P, Nogueira L, Cronin AM, et al. Extending the indications and anatomical limits of pelvic lymph node dissection for prostate cancer: improved staging or increased morbidity? BJU Int. 2011;108(3):372–7.
45. Yong DZ, Tsivian M, Zilberman DE, Ferrandino MN, Mouraviev V, Albala DM. Predictors of prolonged operative time during robot-assisted laparoscopic radical prostatectomy. BJU Int. 2011;107(2):280–2.
46. Eifler JB, Levinson AW, Hyndman ME, Trock BJ, Pavlovich CP. Pelvic lymph node dissection is associated with symptomatic venous thromboembolism risk during laparoscopic radical prostatectomy. J Urol. 2011;185(5):1661–5.
47. Khoder WY, Trottmann M, Buchner A, Stuber A, Hoffmann S, Stief CG, et al. Risk factors for pelvic lymphoceles post-radical prostatectomy. Int J Urol. 2011;18(9):638–43.

48. Lin BM, Hyndman ME, Steele KE, Feng Z, Trock BJ, Schweitzer MA, et al. Incidence and risk factors for inguinal and incisional hernia after laparoscopic radical prostatectomy. Urology. 2011;77(4):957–62.
49. Hruza M, Weiss HO, Pini G, Goezen AS, Schulze M, Teber D, et al. Complications in 2200 consecutive laparoscopic radical prostatectomies: standardised evaluation and analysis of learning curves. Eur Urol. 2010;58(5):733–41.
50. Stolzenburg JU, Rabenalt R, Do M, Ho K, Dorschner W, Waldkirch E, et al. Endoscopic extraperitoneal radical prostatectomy: oncological and functional results after 700 procedures. J Urol. 2005;174(4 Pt 1):1271–5. discussion 5
51. Zorn KC, Katz MH, Bernstein A, Shikanov SA, Brendler CB, Zagaja GP, et al. Pelvic lymphadenectomy during robot-assisted radical prostatectomy: assessing nodal yield, perioperative outcomes, and complications. Urology. 2009;74(2):296–302.
52. Clark T, Parekh DJ, Cookson MS, Chang SS, Smith ER, Wells N, et al. Randomized prospective evaluation of extended versus limited lymph node dissection in patients with clinically localized prostate cancer. J Urol. 2003;169(1):145–7. discussion 7–8
53. Kim KH, Lim SK, Kim HY, Shin TY, Lee JY, Choi YD, et al. Extended vs standard lymph node dissection in robot-assisted radical prostatectomy for intermediate- or high-risk prostate cancer: a propensity-score-matching analysis. BJU Int. 2013;112(2):216–23.
54. Naselli A, Andreatta R, Introini C, Fontana V, Puppo P. Predictors of symptomatic lymphocele after lymph node excision and radical prostatectomy. Urology. 2010;75(3):630–5.
55. Lindberg C, Davidsson T, Gudjónsson S, Hilmarsson R, Liedberg F, Bratt O. Extended pelvic lymphadenectomy for prostate cancer: will the previously reported benefits be reproduced in hospitals with lower surgical volumes? Scand J Urol Nephrol. 2009;43(6):437–41.
56. Jung JH, Seo JW, Lim MS, Lee JW, Chung BH, Hong SJ, et al. Extended pelvic lymph node dissection including internal iliac packet should be performed during robot-assisted laparoscopic radical prostatectomy for high-risk prostate cancer. J Laparoendosc Adv Surg Tech A. 2012;22(8):785–90.
57. Hoshi S, Hayashi N, Kurota Y, Hoshi K, Muto A, Sugano O, et al. Comparison of semi-extended and standard lymph node dissection in radical prostatectomy: a single-institute experience. Mol Clin Oncol. 2015;3(5):1085–7.
58. Yuh BE, Ruel NH, Mejia R, Novara G, Wilson TG. Standardized comparison of robot-assisted limited and extended pelvic lymphadenectomy for prostate cancer. BJU Int. 2013;112(1):81–8.
59. Mistretta FA, Boeri L, Grasso AA, Lo Russo V, Albo G, DE Lorenzis E, et al. Extended versus standard pelvic lymphadenectomy during robot-assisted radical prostatectomy: the role of extended template as an independent predictor of lymph node invasion with comparable morbidity burden. Minerva Urol Nefrol. 2017;69(5):475–85.
60. Musch M, Klevecka V, Roggenbuck U, Kroepfl D. Complications of pelvic lymphadenectomy in 1,380 patients undergoing radical retropubic prostatectomy between 1993 and 2006. J Urol. 2008;179(3):923–8. discussion 8–9
61. Klevecka V, Burmester L, Musch M, Roggenbuck U, Kroepfl D. Intraoperative and early postoperative complications of radical retropubic prostatectomy. Urol Int. 2007;79(3):217–25.
62. Østby-Deglum M, Brennhovd B, Axcrona K, Fosså SD, Dahl AA. A comparative study of erectile function and use of erectile aids in high-risk prostate cancer patients after robot-assisted laparoscopic prostatectomy. Scand J Urol. 2015;49(6):433–9.
63. Hatzichristodoulou G, Wagenpfeil S, Wagenpfeil G, Maurer T, Horn T, Herkommer K, et al. Extended versus limited pelvic lymph node dissection during bilateral nerve-sparing radical prostatectomy and its effect on continence and erectile function recovery: long-term results and trifecta rates of a comparative analysis. World J Urol. 2016;34(6):811–20.
64. Seikkula H, Janssen P, Tutolo M, Tosco L, Battaglia A, Moris L, et al. Comparison of functional outcome after extended versus super-extended pelvic lymph node dissection during radical prostatectomy in high-risk localized prostate cancer. Front Oncol. 2017;7:280.
65. Ploussard G. Robotic surgery in urology: facts and reality. What are the real advantages of robotic approaches for prostate cancer patients? Curr Opin Urol. 2018;28(2):153–8.
66. Gofrit ON, Zorn KC, Steinberg GD, Zagaja GP, Shalhav AL. The will Rogers phenomenon in urological oncology. J Urol. 2008;179(1):28–33.
67. Pagliarulo V, Hawes D, Brands FH, Groshen S, Cai J, Stein JP, et al. Detection of occult lymph node metastases in locally advanced node-negative prostate cancer. J Clin Oncol. 2006;24(18):2735–42.
68. Berglund RK, Sadetsky N, DuChane J, Carroll PR, Klein EA. Limited pelvic lymph node dissection at the time of radical prostatectomy does not affect 5-year failure rates for low, intermediate and high risk prostate cancer: results from CaPSURE. J Urol. 2007;177(2):526–9. discussion 9-30
69. Karl A, Buchner A, Tympner C, Kirchner T, Ganswindt U, Belka C, et al. Risk and timing of biochemical recurrence in pT3aN0/Nx prostate cancer with positive surgical margin - a multicenter study. Radiother Oncol. 2015;116(1):119–24.
70. Gandaglia G, Ploussard G, Isbarn H, Suardi N, De Visschere PJ, Futterer JJ, et al. What is the optimal definition of misclassification in patients with very low-risk prostate cancer eligible for active surveillance? Results from a multi-institutional series. Urol Oncol. 2015;33(4):164.e1–9.
71. Koo KC, Tuliao P, Komninos C, Choi YD, Chung BH, Hong SJ, et al. Prognostic impact of time to undetectable prostate-specific antigen in patients with positive surgical margins following radical prostatectomy. Ann Surg Oncol. 2015;22(2):693–700.
72. Mitsuzuka K, Koie T, Narita S, Kaiho Y, Yoneyama T, Kawamura S, et al. Is pelvic lymph node dissection required at radical prostatectomy for low-risk prostate cancer? Int J Urol. 2013;20(11):1092–6.
73. Masuda H, Fukushima H, Kawakami S, Numao N, Fujii Y, Saito K, et al. Impact of advanced age on biochemical recurrence after radical prostatectomy in Japanese men according to pathological stage. Jpn J Clin Oncol. 2013;43(4):410–6.
74. Daimon T, Miyajima A, Maeda T, Hattori S, Yasumizu Y, Hasegawa M, et al. Does pelvic lymph node dissection improve the biochemical relapse-free survival in low-risk prostate cancer patients treated by laparoscopic radical prostatectomy? J Endourol. 2012;26(9):1199–202.
75. Ost P, Cozzarini C, De Meerleer G, Fiorino C, De Potter B, Briganti A, et al. High-dose adjuvant radiotherapy after radical prostatectomy with or without androgen deprivation therapy. Int J Radiat Oncol Biol Phys. 2012;83(3):960–5.
76. Ku JH, Jeong CW, Park YH, Cho MC, Kwak C, Kim HH. Biochemical recurrence after radical prostatectomy with or without pelvic lymphadenectomy in Korean men with high-risk prostate cancer. Jpn J Clin Oncol. 2011;41(5):656–62.
77. Weight CJ, Reuther AM, Gunn PW, Zippe CR, Dhar NB, Klein EA. Limited pelvic lymph node dissection does not improve biochemical relapse-free survival at 10 years after radical prostatectomy in patients with low-risk prostate cancer. Urology. 2008;71(1):141–5.
78. Bhatta-Dhar N, Reuther AM, Zippe C, Klein EA. No difference in six-year biochemical failure rates with or without pelvic lymph node dissection during radical prostatectomy in low-risk patients with localized prostate cancer. Urology. 2004;63(3):528–31.
79. Fergany A, Kupelian PA, Levin HS, Zippe CD, Reddy C, Klein EA. No difference in biochemical failure rates with or without pelvic lymph node dissection during radical prostatectomy in low-risk patients. Urology. 2000;56(1):92–5.

80. Preisser F, van den Bergh RCN, Gandaglia G, Ost P, Surcel CI, Sooriakumaran P, et al. Effect of extended pelvic lymph node dissection on oncologic outcomes in patients with D'Amico intermediate and high risk prostate cancer treated with radical prostatectomy: a multi-institutional study. J Urol. 2020;203(2):338–43.
81. Allaf ME, Palapattu GS, Trock BJ, Carter HB, Walsh PC. Anatomical extent of lymph node dissection: impact on men with clinically localized prostate cancer. J Urol. 2004;172(5 Pt 1):1840–4.
82. Porter CR, Suardi N, Capitanio U, Hutterer GC, Kodama K, Gibbons RP, et al. A nomogram predicting prostate cancer-specific mortality after radical prostatectomy. Urol Int. 2010;84(2):132–40.
83. Briganti A, Karnes JR, Da Pozzo LF, Cozzarini C, Gallina A, Suardi N, et al. Two positive nodes represent a significant cut-off value for cancer specific survival in patients with node positive prostate cancer. A new proposal based on a two-institution experience on 703 consecutive N+ patients treated with radical prostatectomy, extended pelvic lymph node dissection and adjuvant therapy. Eur Urol. 2009;55(2):261–70.
84. Schumacher MC, Burkhard FC, Thalmann GN, Fleischmann A, Studer UE. Good outcome for patients with few lymph node metastases after radical retropubic prostatectomy. Eur Urol. 2008;54(2):344–52.
85. Preisser F, Bandini M, Marchioni M, Nazzani S, Tian Z, Pompe RS, et al. Extent of lymph node dissection improves survival in prostate cancer patients treated with radical prostatectomy without lymph node invasion. Prostate. 2018;78(6):469–75.
86. Sood A, Keeley J, Palma-Zamora I, Dalela D, Arora S, Peabody JO, et al. Extended pelvic lymph-node dissection is independently associated with improved overall survival in patients with prostate cancer at high-risk of lymph-node invasion. BJU Int. 2020;125(6):756–8.
87. Messing EM, Manola J, Yao J, Kiernan M, Crawford D, Wilding G, et al. Immediate versus deferred androgen deprivation treatment in patients with node-positive prostate cancer after radical prostatectomy and pelvic lymphadenectomy. Lancet Oncol. 2006;7(6):472–9.
88. Abdollah F, Karnes RJ, Suardi N, Cozzarini C, Gandaglia G, Fossati N, et al. Impact of adjuvant radiotherapy on survival of patients with node-positive prostate cancer. J Clin Oncol. 2014;32(35):3939–47.
89. Abdollah F, Gandaglia G, Suardi N, Capitanio U, Salonia A, Nini A, et al. More extensive pelvic lymph node dissection improves survival in patients with node-positive prostate cancer. Eur Urol. 2015;67(2):212–9.
90. Fossati N, Parker WP, Karnes RJ, Colicchia M, Bossi A, Seisen T, et al. More extensive lymph node dissection at radical prostatectomy is associated with improved outcomes with salvage radiotherapy for rising prostate-specific antigen after surgery: a long-term, multi-institutional analysis. Eur Urol. 2018;74(2):134–7.
91. Touijer KA, Karnes RJ, Passoni N, Sjoberg DD, Assel M, Fossati N, et al. Survival outcomes of men with lymph node-positive prostate cancer after radical prostatectomy: a comparative analysis of different postoperative management strategies. Eur Urol. 2018;73(6):890–6.
92. Ploussard G, Gandaglia G, Borgmann H, de Visschere P, Heidegger I, Kretschmer A, et al. Salvage lymph node dissection for nodal recurrent prostate cancer: a systematic review. Eur Urol. 2019;76(4):493–504.
93. Ploussard G, Almeras C, Briganti A, Giannarini G, Hennequin C, Ost P, et al. Management of Node Only Recurrence after primary local treatment for prostate cancer: a systematic review of the literature. J Urol. 2015;194(4):983–8.
94. Abdollah F, Briganti A, Montorsi F, Stenzl A, Stief C, Tombal B, et al. Contemporary role of salvage lymphadenectomy in patients with recurrence following radical prostatectomy. Eur Urol. 2015;67(5):839–49.
95. Passoni NM, Suardi N, Abdollah F, Picchio M, Giovacchini G, Messa C, et al. Utility of [11C]choline PET/CT in guiding lesion-targeted salvage therapies in patients with prostate cancer recurrence localized to a single lymph node at imaging: results from a pathologically validated series. Urol Oncol. 2014;32(1):38.e9–16.
96. Bravi CA, Fossati N, Gandaglia G, Suardi N, Mazzone E, Robesti D, et al. Long-term outcomes of salvage lymph node dissection for nodal recurrence of prostate cancer after radical prostatectomy: not as good as previously thought. Eur Urol. 2020;78(5):661–9.

Robotic-Assisted Salvage Radical Prostatectomy

Senthil Nathan, Christoph Würnschimmel, Arjun Nathan, Markus Graefen, and Vipul Patel

1 Introduction

This chapter aims to describe the history, early reports, guidelines, and current state-of-the-art techniques for salvage robot-assisted radical prostatectomy (sRARP). Evolution of techniques from open to the robotic platform and feasibility trials are described. An exhaustive commentary on patient selection and modifications recommended for sRARP based on primary treatment is quoted. Comparisons between primary RARP and sRARP in propensity matched studies are discussed to evaluate the need and justification of this challenging procedure. Current reports on the oncological and functional outcomes of sRARP are reported with recommendations for future work. Comparative analysis of salvage treatments following prostate sparing treatment is discussed. Finally the the need for training and progression in this extremely challenging surgery is discussed with recommendations for training and requisite surgical expertise.

2 History of Salvage Radical Prostatectomy

In the early years, radiotherapy to the prostate gland with or without adjuvant hormone therapy was the main alternate treatment to radical prostatectomy. When biochemical or clinical local recurrence was diagnosed salvage prostatectomy was contemplated with trepidation. The role of salvage radical prostatectomy following radiation treatment remained controversial due to its extreme surgical complexity, increased complications, and inferior outcomes to primary prostatectomy. Radiation oncologists, to date remain skeptical about advising salvage surgery to their patients and non-experienced urologists tend to shy away from the challenge. Therefore, the most common salvage treatment after failed primary therapy for prostate cancer was androgen deprivation therapy, rarely different modalities of adjuvant or salvage irradiation, and very rarely salvage radical prostatectomy [1–6]. Carson et al. were the first to report on a small series of salvage radical prostatectomy following external beam radiation treatment [7]. This, with other similar studies of open salvage radical prostatectomy in that period, reported poor functional outcomes and high complication rates that were attributed to the complexity of surgery in a previously irradiated field [8–10]. These historical cohorts reported high rates of urinary incontinence, anastomotic strictures, and rectal injury rates that exceeded 15% [11, 12]. With these high perioperative complications, bad functional outcomes, and unknown oncological benefits, salvage radical prostatectomy was not favored by the urological surgeons. This is evidenced from the "Cancer of the Prostate Strategic Urologic Research Endeavor" (CaPSURE) database, where only 2% of radical prostatectomy cases were salvage after failed primary external beam radiotherapy [13, 14].

With the advent of anatomical dissection of the prostate and more refined surgical techniques [15–17], the outcomes of primary radical prostatectomy significantly improved. Urologists became comfortable to expand their surgical expertise in the challenging minefield of salvage surgery. Accordingly, a large series reported by Bonet et al. reported an overall complication rate of 2.3–8.1% which was better than historical literature [18]. With the introduction of the robotic platform in salvage radical prostatectomy, improvement in functional and oncological outcomes was reported while complication rates decreased progressively [5, 19–23]. Currently, with the increased use of innovative prostate sparing therapies such as high intensity focused ultrasound treatment of the prostate, focal cryoablation, focal brachy-

S. Nathan (✉)
University College of London Hospitals NHS Foundation Trust, London, UK

C. Würnschimmel · M. Graefen
University Hospital Hamburg-Eppendorf, Hamburg, Germany

A. Nathan
Division of Surgery and Interventional Sciences, University College of London, London, UK

V. Patel
Global Robotics Institute, Celebration, FL, USA

P. Wiklund et al. (eds.), *Robotic Urologic Surgery*, https://doi.org/10.1007/978-3-031-00363-9_28

therapy, and electroporation of the prostate, the local recurrence rates of prostate cancer have increased leading to increased rates of salvage prostatectomy. Studies have reported the successful use of salvage prostatectectomy in these cases with the procedure now accepted as a feasible operation with comparable outcomes to primary surgery in specialized centers [24, 25].

3 Background

The indication for salvage radical prostatectomy is ambiguous, as agreement on failure following radiation and focal therapies is debated. Radiotherapy failure, is defined as per the ASTRO definition of three serial rises of the prostate-specific antigen, or a rise above 0.2 ng/mL from the nadir [26]. A similar definition does not exist after focal treatments and instead a combination of biochemical failure, imaging, and histology is used. The European Association of Urology (EAU) guidelines for salvage radical prostatectomy advocates strict patient selection based on recommendations from Chade et al., who performed a systematic review and meta-analysis of the literature on open salvage radical prostatectomy [20]. This guideline, with no Level 1 evidence, recommends low co-morbidity profiles and good life expectancy (10 years or more), a prostate-specific antigen value of <10 ng/mL prior to primary therapy, initial biopsy grade of 2/3 or lower (based on the International Society of Urologic Pathology criteria) maximum T2b stage, and no nodal or metastatic disease. Based on the above criteria, Chade et al. showed a significant difference in biochemical recurrence rates following salvage prostatectomy in men who were encompassed within the guidelines compared to those who had more advanced disease [20]. It was evidenced that five- and ten-year biochemical recurrence free survival rates in guideline-encompassed patients versus patients with more advanced disease ranged between 47–82% and 28–53%, respectively. However, ten-year cancer-specific survival and overall survival rates ranged between 70–83% and 53–89%, respectively, in the guideline-encompassed patients [20]. Mandel et al. showed that by adhering to the EAU guidelines, salvage radical prostatectomy was associated with significantly improved oncological outcomes compared to patients who did not fit within these criteria. The five-year biochemical recurrence free rates were 73.9 vs 11.6% between patients who matched with the selection criteria vs patients who did not match the criteria [23]. These findings led to careful consideration of patient selection and who should be offered a sRARP. Further studies showed that early referral of failed cases after focal or whole-gland therapy should be advocated for better oncological and functional outcomes as advised by Nathan et al. [27].

4 Current Status: sRARP

With the introduction of the robotic platform, sRARP has been repeatedly demonstrated to be a safe and feasible procedure. Furthermore, it has been shown to have acceptable oncological and functional outcomes with low perioperative morbidity when performed in high-volume surgeons. Numerous individual studies and meta-analyses have shown that sRARP is safe, feasible with comparable medium-term oncological outcomes. Furthermore, the perioperative complications are same as open surgery with a majority showing better functional outcomes [5, 27–35]. Indeed, compared to the traditional open approach, the novel robotic approach combines the advantage of better vision, improved dexterity and tissue handling which allows very complex prostate anatomy to be safely operated upon [36]. The advantages brought forward by the adoption of the robotic technique in salvage radical prostatectomy have already demonstrated reduced rates of anastomotic stricture, blood loss, hospital stay and improved continence outcomes compared to the open approach [34]. Reports of nerve-sparing techniques, followed by very favorable functional outcomes and low complication rates after sRARP are near similar to primary radical prostatectomy in single institutional studies [18, 25]. Further studies have shown that all outcomes including oncological after salvage radical prostatectomy following focal therapies are favorable against whole-gland primary treatment. sRARP following focal therapies, such as high intensity focused ultrasound treatment of the prostate or cryotherapy, has better outcomes compared to whole-gland treatments such as external beam radiotherapy, high- or low-dose brachytherapy [37–40]. Furthermore, unlike in post-external beam radiation, prostate cancer recurrence after focal therapy can be treated with further focal treatment or salvage external beam radiation besides salvage radical prostatectomy. In this regard, several small studies have shown biochemical recurrence free rates after salvage radiotherapy following focal therapy that were similar to values reported for salvage radical prostatectomy [41–43]. Nathan et al. performed the first comparative effectiveness study in a single institution with a large series of 200 patients to demonstrate the efficacy of salvage radiation versus surgery in local recurrence of prostate cancer following high intensity focal ultrasound treatment or cryotherapy. They compared salvage radiotherapy to salvage radical prostatectomy and showed similar oncological outcomes for men with intermediate-risk disease but potentially superior oncological outcomes for men who had salvage radiotherapy with high-risk disease. However, salvage radiotherapy was associated with a high adverse effect profile and interestingly had similar levels of continence at 2 years [44]. Finally, the inclusion of these novel primary focal therapy options further increases the spectrum of patients eligible for salvage radical prostatectomy. Based on current evidence, salvage radical prostatectomy, and specifically, the robotic approach, should be regarded as a feasible standard alternative for locally recurrent prostate cancer after primary whole or focal therapy. Literature recommends it should be performed only by high-volume experienced robotic surgeons in high-volume centers.

4.1 Salvage Lymph Node Dissection

Dissection and excision of the regional lymph nodes during sRARP can be challenging and potentially morbid. Lymph node dissection in primary RARP remains controversial with no benefit in cancer-specific survival and this remains the case for salvage lymphadenectomy. However, it offers the chance to stage the disease better to initiate early adjuvant treatment. During salvage radical prostatectomy, lymphadenectomy offers a staging surplus, providing an advantage in cancer control and in some cases delays time to systemic therapy [45–48]. Indeed, when depending only on conventional staging methods, the majority of lymph node metastases would be missed, due to their relative miniature [49]. In recent years, with the introduction of molecular imaging and specifically, prostate-specific membrane antigen (PSMA) positron emission tomography, the rates of underdiagnosis of lymph node metastasis have decreased, yet still a considerable amount of micro-metastases may be missed [50]. Thus, lymph node dissection during salvage therapy is regarded as a staging procedure, which is not feasible with any of the other salvage treatments. However, the curative effect of lymph node dissection and the effect of the extent of lymph node dissection (limited, extended, super-extended) are not fully understood, neither in the primary nor in the salvage setting [45, 51–54]. For example, Bravi et al. claimed that no survival advantage in terms of oncological outcomes could be demonstrated by salvage lymph node dissection in a recent multi-institutional analysis [55]. However, this analysis was predominantly based on high-risk locally advanced disease which will not be offered salvage surgery in contemporary practice. Furthermore, with the advent of PSMA positron emission tomography in the recurrent setting, patient selection will be greatly influenced for salvage lymph node dissection in contemporary patients. The advantage of this novel imaging technique, and eventually the combination with intraoperative guidance during salvage lymph node dissection by means of gamma probes ("radioguided surgery"), both in the open and in the robotic setting [56–61], may lead to a much more patient tailored approach. Finally, the potential advantages of lymph node dissection need to be weighed against higher rates of surgical complications (i.e., lymphocele, lymphedema, infection, injury of iliac vessels, injury of the obturator nerve, and thrombosis). These complications are higher in the salvage setting compared to primary lymphadenectomy due to tissue alterations that were induced following primary therapy [62, 63].

The following sections will provide an overview of the current standards of robotic salvage radical prostatectomy and pelvic lymph node dissection that aim to reduce the morbidity and complications, while increasing functional and oncological outcomes.

5 Preoperative Considerations

Patient selection is the main cornerstone to improve outcomes for salvage radical prostatectomy. The EAU advocates the following parameters as most important for clinical decision-making:

- life expectancy over 10 years, no comorbidities,
- clinical T stage ≤2 at initial prostate cancer diagnosis,
- prostate-specific antigen value <10 ng/mL at initial prostate cancer diagnosis,
- initial biopsy grade ≤2/3 (International Society of Urologic Pathology criteria),
- no lymph node involvement,
- no evidence of metastatic disease.

However, one needs to remember that this advocacy is based on retrospective open surgery data with historical Gleason grading and when imaging was not a standard preoperative requirement. Until a new guideline is advocated, this is the best fit advise. When these baseline criteria for a successful salvage radical prostatectomy are fulfilled, further assessments and considerations appear worthwhile in order to increase the chances for favorable outcomes. Contemporary evidence suggests that a wider group of patients may benefit from salvage radical prostatectomy.

Patient Advise should encompass a realistic scenario on the expected functional and oncological outcomes for the patient. Eligible candidates for salvage radical prostatectomy need to be informed explicitly about the inherent risk of postoperative erectile dysfunction and incontinence. Furthermore, depending on the type and quality of the previous radiation therapy, the risk of rectal injuries, higher rates of anastomotic leakage and/or stricture as well as fistula formation, and higher chance for bleeding and infection should be clearly explained.

Preoperative Assessment should include staging by magnetic resonance imaging, in order to evaluate the local disease extent, tissue fibrosis, and adherent anatomical structures and also to provide a roadmap for surgical planning. Indeed, different primary prostate cancer therapies (external beam radiotherapy, high-dose rate, low-dose rate brachytherapy) trigger different magnitudes of tissue fibrosis, in different zones [19, 64, 65]. When there is infiltration of the rectum by the cancer there is a direct relationship in incidence of rectal injury and fistula formation both a after primary and salvage radical prostatectomy [66]. In these locally advanced patients informed consent should always include the potential need for a colostomy. In rare cases of suspected tumor extension into the urinary bladder and/or the ureteric orifices, a preoperative cystoscopy might be indicated. In these cases informed consent should always include the possibility for cystoprostatectomy or ureteric re-implantation. When performing magnetic resonance imaging, some authors advocate that multiparametric magnetic resonance imaging can be replaced by biparametric magnetic resonance imaging in order to detect local recurrence [67]. Finally, as mentioned above, molecular imaging by the means of PSMA positron emission tomography may be considered for eligible patients prior to salvage radical prostatectomy [50]. Indeed, findings from PSMA scans can support clinical decision and surgical planning, especially with regard to assessing the extent of lymph node invasion and the need for a potential multimodal approach [57, 68].

6 Surgical Techniques of Salvage Robotic Assisted Radical Prostatectomy

The technique of sRARP with or without pelvic lymph node dissection generally resembles the approach to primary robotic radical prostatectomy. Most published experience on sRARP relies on the six-port technique using the da Vinci Surgical System (Intuitive Surgical, Sunnyvale, CA, USA) and the proven instrumentation for this surgery is a combination of monopolar scissors, bipolar Maryland forceps, and a ProGrasp forceps, additionally aided by the bed-side surgeon, who uses an atraumatic grasper and a suction unit [22, 27]. The procedure can be carried out using only a 0°binocular scope, but in some cases with impaired visibility, especially in the posterior planes, a 30° binocular scope may be of use.

The commonly used surgical approach for robotic salvage prostatectomy is the "anterior" approach, rather than the "posterior" approach, although both ways are feasible and largely depend on surgeon's experience and preference. Theoretically, the posterior approach facilitates access to the compartments that are usually heavily affected by prior radiation therapies, such as the area around the seminal vesicles. Early mobilization of these structures is facilitated by the posterior approach and is preferred by some. However, sometimes severe adherence is encountered around the rectum and prostatic apex, which cannot be reached easily using the posterior approach. If technically and oncologically feasible, in well-selected patients with preserved functionality regarding erection and continence, a bilateral, athermal nerve-sparing procedure may be performed as in the primary radical prostatectomy. However, lateral adhesions can lead to wrong plane dissection and, therefore, this should only be attempted by experienced surgeons. An extended lymph node dissection is advised in order to increase the staging benefit. The template should encompass nodal tissue along the external and internal iliac vessels, parts of the common iliac vessels up to the ureteric crossing and the obturator fossa [52, 69, 70]. Nevertheless, surgical technique and planning greatly depends on the varying tissue alterations induced by different primary treatment modalities and most likely some individual adjustments in surgical techniques need to be considered in order to yield the most favorable functional and oncological results [27, 71].

6.1 Varied Surgical Technique Based on Primary Prostate Cancer Treatment

For patients after *external beam radiotherapy*, excessive bleeding needs to be expected due to neo-vascularization, especially in the bladder-neck region. The distinction between the lateral margin of the prostate and the levator ani muscle including the sphincter active area maybe indistinguishable due to the effects of radiotherapy. This leads to cutting the endopelvic fascia in the wrong place leading to muscle damage and troublesome bleeding. The whole salvage procedure needs sharp dissection, especially in the posterior part around the seminal vesicles and the posterior Denonvilliers' fascia and the rectum. The seminal vesicles may be sticky, partly due to the concomitantly prescribed androgen deprivation therapy and partly due to radiation effects. They may sometimes need to be excised independently and frequently piece by piece. It is crucial to attempt dissecting the concomitant vasa of the seminal vesicles in order to reach the tips of the seminal vesicles and also to control potential major bleeding in this area.

The prostate is usually adhered to the rectum which should be released with sharp dissection rather than blunt retraction which will tear the rectum. In the apical region, the rectum needs to be separated carefully avoiding thermal injury with sharp dissection. Thermal injury in this area may go unnoticed during the procedure leading to fistula formation. It is prudent to always do a rectal leak test following the excision of the prostate. If rectal injury is suspected, an assistant should perform a rectal examination under visual control by the console surgeon. Injury is confirmed if the gloved finger is visible or there is blood visible on the glove. Alternatively, the "air-distension" technique can be applied.

This method relies on using a rectal catheter that insufflates and distends the rectum with air. The bed-side surgeon fills the perirectal region with irrigation fluid and any signs of air bubbles within the fluid are indicative of rectal injury. Finally, another option might be the use of a proctoscope that illuminates the rectum and transillumination through rectum tissue can be observed in areas where tissue thinning or injury has occurred. This technique will even show just serosal tear without breach to the mucosa. For this option, the robotic endoscope light needs to be reduced to a minimum in order to observe the transillumination.

The anastomosis should ideally be performed using a polydioxanone suture (for example, 3-0 PDS) using Van Velthoven technique [72], by approaching the mucosal ends of the bladder outlet and the urethra. PDS is recommended as it takes 3 months to dissolve in contrast to the usually used monocryl suture which dissolves in 2–3 weeks frequently before healing has occurred in irradiated tissues. Ischemic damage should be avoided by using minimal number of throws for the anastomosis. Apart from keeping the transurethral catheter in place for a longer period of time (approximately 10–14 days), assessment of leakage by the means of cystography should be routine. Catheters with adequate drainage and lower potential for blockage (double hole catheters, 18 Fr) should be used.

Following proton beam therapy extensive adhesions are noted between the lateral surface of the prostate and the levator ani and other structures. It is safe to start in the midline and dissect laterally. Extreme care is needed in large glands adherent to the vascular structures.

After *brachytherapy*, the apex of the prostate is adhered to the sphincter and careful dissection is warranted to prevent damage. Migrated brachytherapy seeds can be disconcerting, and they should be carefully removed. Excessive traction will fracture the prostate along the seed-lines.

After *high intensity focused ultrasound* treatment of the prostate, midline adherence to the rectum is to be expected. Usually, in contrast to external beam radiotherapy, the lateral dissection, including nerve-sparing procedures, is mostly feasible without major difficulty. Following focal treatment dissection should commence primarily from the untreated side, in order to identify the anatomical landmarks [15, 22]. The approach should rely on a "latero-medial direction" with the pedicles dissected first, and sharp dissection of the prostate from the adherent rectum in the midline last. A common occurrence after high intensity focused ultrasound is the development of non-fibrosed cavities and surgeons should avoid entering these. Similar cavities, however, with fibrosis, are encountered after cryotherapy of the prostate [27, 73].

After *electroporation of the prostate*, the gland is irregular with unequal lobes and cavities. Furthermore, after electroporation, the prostatic tissue tends to become more fragile and sticky, especially in the apical part. Therefore, careful application of tension, for example, when handling the urethral catheter, is advised in order to avoid prostate rupture [27].

7 Complications

With regard to improved surgical techniques, and the influence of robotic surgery in salvage radical prostatectomy, the largest and most contemporary comparison on functional outcomes and morbidity after open versus robotic salvage radical prostatectomy was performed by Gontero et al. in 2019 [34]. Their multi-institutional analysis was based on data derived from 18 centers between years 2000 and 2016, on 186 versus 209 patients treated with open and robotic salvage radical prostatectomy, respectively. Gontero et al. reported higher rates of any Clavien–Dindo complication in the open group (19.4 vs 11.0%), as well as higher rates of anastomotic and/or urethral strictures (16.6 vs 7.6%, respectively, for open versus robotic) and renal failure (3.0 vs 0%, respectively, for open versus robotic). Conversely, anastomotic leakage was recorded more frequently in the robotic group (8.9 versus 18.6% for open versus robotic, respectively). Encouragingly, as opposed to more historic series, rectal injuries were low in both open and robotic surgery, but significantly lower in the robotic approach (3.0 vs 0.5% for open versus robotic, respectively). Finally, an important advantage of robotic surgery with regard to morbidity was also low blood loss during surgery (mean 222 mL versus 715 mL), which also translated into higher postoperative blood transfusion rates, however without statistical significance (6.5 vs 2.8% for open versus robotic, respectively, $p = 0.09$). Nathan et al. in a single-center large series of 155 patients showed that when controlling for confounders via propsenity matching, perioperative outcomes and complications for sRARP and primary radical prostatectomy were the same [24].

A recent systematic review by Driscoll et al. reported on 288 patients treated with the open approach versus 207 patients treated with the robotic approach. Their results were derived from data of 31 studies between 1980 and 2018 [32]. Here, acknowledging obvious differences between more historical (open) and more contemporary patients (robotic), Driscoll et al. concluded that the open technique did not exhibit drastically higher rates of complications (38.2 versus 33.8% for open versus robotic, respectively), which contradicts the above study by Gontero et al., but it needs to be mentioned that the severity of complications was higher in the open approach. For example, of all complications, 73.6% Clavien Grade III occurred in the open approach, and also a 5.5% death rate was reported, while the majority of complications in the robotic approach were Grade I complications (47.1%), with no mortality. Therefore, this comparison is flawed and the comment about lower rates of significant complications in the robotic approach remains valid.

8 Functional Outcomes

Functional outcomes after salvage radical prostatectomy have steadily improved in the recent years, due to a combination of several factors. First, the introduction of robotic surgery and improved surgical techniques; second, better patient selection and third, a larger variety and improved quality of primary prostate cancer treatment options that are less destructive, which facilitates salvage surgery.

8.1 Continence and Erectile Function

Regarding preservation of continence, in the analysis by Gontero et al., the robotic approach yielded higher full continence rates at 12 months (63.9 vs 49.2%, $p = 0.055$), which was significant in multivariable analyses (Odds ratio 0.4, $p = 0.02$). Nevertheless, in the overall cohort of open and robotic approaches, severe incontinence after 12 months was still considerably high (24.6%). Regarding preservation of erectile function, Gontero et al. recorded higher rates of nerve sparing in the robotic groups (8.3 vs 19.8% for open versus robotic, respectively). However, the reported data on erectile function was less robust. Generally, unlike in primary radical prostatectomy, patients after salvage radical prostatectomy still need to expect relatively high rates of postoperative erectile dysfunction. Nevertheless, Gontero et al. reported a rate of 8.1% for preserved spontaneous erection after surgery (also by the means of phosphodiesterase-inhibitors), and 15.6% of patients who were potent prior to salvage radical prostatectomy also had preserved erectile function after surgery [34].

8.2 The Influence of Primary Therapy on Functional Outcomes

With regard to the different baseline conditions of patients based on different primary therapies, a recent and contemporary multi-institutional study was performed on 185 patients who received salvage radical prostatectomy following focal therapy versus external beam radiotherapy or brachytherapy [74]. The latter had significantly worse continence at 12 months after salvage radical prostatectomy (49% pad-free vs 83% pad-free, respectively). However, patients following focal therapy exhibited more favorable tumor stages and grade, which limits the outcomes of the study. Nevertheless, the variety of novel primary treatment options needs to be considered when interpreting functional outcomes after salvage radical prostatectomy. Indeed, similar findings were also reported by a high-volume single institution, who examined 185 patients who received robotic salvage radical prostatectomy between 2012 and 2018 after various different primary treatment approaches, such as high intensity focused ultrasound, external beam radiotherapy, seed brachytherapy, cryotherapy, or electroporation/Nanoknife [27]. After 2 years, full continence (no pad use) was reported in 35% versus 58% of treated patients after "whole gland radiation" versus "focal treatment," respectively.

9 Oncological Outcomes

Since the first reports on historical cohorts in the early 80s [7], the oncological outcomes of salvage radical prostatectomy remained unclear, mainly due to very heterogenous tumor and patient profiles and small sample sizes. Recently, a multi-institutional retrospective study on contemporary patients treated with salvage radical prostatectomy addressed this knowledge gap. In this study by Marra et al., 18 institutions reported on overall 414 patients treated with salvage radical prostatectomy between 2000 and 2018, with the endpoint variables of biochemical recurrence, cancer-specific survival, and overall survival [21]. Of these patients, 63.5% received salvage radical prostatectomy after external beam radiotherapy and the majority exhibited a biopsy Gleason score (≤7 in 55.5%), and 93.3% exhibited organ-confined disease (≤cT2) prior to salvage radical prostatectomy. Furthermore, median age and prostate-specific antigen prior to salvage surgery were 66 years and 4.2 ng/mL, respectively. 52.2% received open surgery and 47.8% received robotic surgery, and overall, 84.3% underwent extended or standard lymphadenectomy.

Despite the relatively favorable preoperative tumor characteristics, the postoperative tumor characteristics were predominantly aggressive, as evidenced by the International Society of Urologic Pathology grades of at least 4 in roughly 40% and grades of 5 in 28%. Also, positive lymph nodes were exhibited in 16% and positive surgical margins in roughly 30%. With a median follow-up of 36 months, five-year biochemical recurrence free survival, cancer-specific survival, and overall survival were 56.7, 97.7, and 92.1%, respectively. These rates appear encouraging, despite the aggressive tumor grades. The findings by Marra et al. are even more profound when compared to a more historical study by Chade et al. (treatment years 1985–2009), where lower five-year biochemical recurrence free survival rates were reported (48%) [75]. Chade et al. also provided ten-year biochemical recurrence free, metastasis-free, and cancer-specific mortality-free survival rates. These rates were 37, 77, and 83%, respectively. Chade et al. concluded that patients with low prostate-specific antigen and low Gleason score in the biopsy prior to salvage radical prostatectomy benefit most from surgery, which is in concordance with the European Association of Urology guidelines [6, 23].

Finally, neither Marra et al., nor Chade et al., can ultimately answer the question regarding the true oncological benefit of salvage radical prostatectomy, when compared to alternative salvage treatments, such as androgen deprivation therapy alone. Post radiation salvage hormonal treatment cannot be compared to surgery as it is not curative and castrate resistance can develop in the medium term. In this regard, no prospective randomized trial is feasible to assess efficacy. Furthermore, it has to be considered that patients who underwent salvage radical prostatectomy in these retrospective series may still have more favorable selection criteria and a better overall health status compared to patients who only received androgen deprivation therapy, or even more important, may be influenced by lead-time bias. Therefore, the necessity of large prospective randomized trials investigating the true oncological effect of salvage radical prostatectomy needs to be established, as performed so successfully with salvage radiotherapy [1, 2, 76]. Local control by salvage radical prostatectomy may prove beneficial in patients with very high-risk disease, or with limited nodal or even distant metastasis similar to radiotherapy as shown in the STAMPEDE trial [77]. Indeed, for limited nodal recurrence after primary radical prostatectomy, novel approaches relying on "radioguided surgery" are being implemented more frequently specifically for salvage nodal dissection purpose in experimental settings [58, 59, 78, 79]. In this regard, radioguided salvage lymph node dissection might also be a future key element for the treatment of advanced prostate cancer and therefore may play a role in the salvage radical prostatectomy procedure; however, future study results need to be awaited in order to draw more definitive conclusions.

10 Conclusion

Salvage radical prostatectomy has been proven to be a technically feasible procedure, with comparable cancer outcomes to primary surgery. With the introduction of the robotic platform, the technique has been refined to deliver a feasible procedure with acceptable cancer and quality outcomes. Quality outcomes are significantly better after salvage surgery for focal treatments compared to whole-gland ablations. Nevertheless, surgeon experience is an important factor for safe outcomes especially for this very demanding and challenging surgery.

With increasing focal ablative treatments for localized prostate cancer, robotic salvage radical prostatectomy procedures are expected to increase. Similarly, post radiation salvage surgery is expected to rise as quality outcomes improve with the robotic platform. Surgery for oligometastatic disease (TROMBONE [80]) and consolidation surgery (ATLANTA, NCT03763253) for local control are being studied and may increase the need for urologists to be accomplished in this complex surgery.

References

1. Kneebone A, Fraser-Browne C, Duchesne GM, Fisher R, Frydenberg M, Herschtal A, et al. Adjuvant radiotherapy versus early salvage radiotherapy following radical prostatectomy (TROG 08.03/ANZUP RAVES): a randomised, controlled, phase 3, non-inferiority trial. Lancet Oncol. 2020;21:1331–40. https://doi.org/10.1016/S1470-2045(20)30456-3.
2. Parker CC, Clarke NW, Cook AD, Kynaston HG, Petersen PM, Catton C, et al. Timing of radiotherapy after radical prostatectomy (RADICALS-RT): a randomised, controlled phase 3 trial. Lancet. 2020; https://doi.org/10.1016/S0140-6736(20)31553-1.
3. Hackman G, Taari K, Tammela TL, Matikainen M, Kouri M, Joensuu T, et al. Randomised trial of adjuvant radiotherapy following radical prostatectomy versus radical prostatectomy alone in prostate cancer patients with positive margins or extracapsular extension. Eur Urol. 2019;76:586–95. https://doi.org/10.1016/j.eururo.2019.07.001.
4. Agarwal PK, Sadetsky N, Konety BR, Resnick MI, Carroll PR. Treatment failure after primary and salvage therapy for prostate cancer. Cancer. 2008;112:307–14. https://doi.org/10.1002/cncr.23161.
5. Valle LF, Lehrer EJ, Markovic D, Elashoff D, Levin-Epstein R, Karnes RJ, et al. A systematic review and meta-analysis of local salvage therapies after radiotherapy for prostate cancer (MASTER). Eur Urol. 2020; https://doi.org/10.1016/j.eururo.2020.11.010.
6. Mottet N, van den Bergh RCN, Briers E, Cornford P, De Santis M, Fanti S, et al. EAU - ESTRO - ESUR - SIOG guidelines on prostate cancer 2020. Eur. Assoc. Urol. Guidel. 2020 Ed., vol. presented. Arnhem, The Netherlands: European Association of Urology Guidelines Office; 2020.
7. Carson CC, Zincke H, Utz DC, Cupps RE, Farrow GM. Radical prostatectomy after radiotherapy for prostatic cancer. J Urol. 1980;124:237–9. https://doi.org/10.1016/S0022-5347(17)55384-7.
8. Moul JW, Paulson DF. The role of radical surgery in the management of radiation recurrent and large volume prostate cancer. Cancer. 1991;68:1265–71. https://doi.org/10.1002/1097-0142(19910915)68:6<1265::AID-CNCR2820680615>3.0.CO;2-G.
9. Link P, Freiha FS. Radical prostatectomy after definitive radiation therapy for prostate cancer. Urology. 1991;37:189–92. https://doi.org/10.1016/0090-4295(91)80282-C.
10. Neerhut GJ, Wheeler T, Cantini M, Scardino PT. Salvage radical prostatectomy for radiorecurrent adenocarcinoma of the prostate. J Urol. 1988;140:544–8. https://doi.org/10.1016/S0022-5347(17)41714-9.

11. Chen BT, Wood DP. Salvage prostatectomy in patients who have failed radiation therapy or cryotherapy as primary treatment for prostate cancer. Urology. 2003;62:69–78. https://doi.org/10.1016/j.urology.2003.09.001.
12. Rogers E, Ohori M, Kassabian VS, Wheeler TM, Scardino PT. Salvage radical prostatectomy: outcome measured by serum prostate specific antigen levels. J Urol. 1995;153:104–10. https://doi.org/10.1097/00005392-199501000-00037.
13. Lubeck DP, Litwin MS, Henning JM, Stier DM, Mazonson P, Fisk R, et al. The capsure database: a methodology for clinical practice and research in prostate cancer. Urology. 1996;48:773–7. https://doi.org/10.1016/S0090-4295(96)00226-9.
14. Grossfeld GD, Li Y-P, Lubeck DP, Broering JM, Mehta SS, Carroll PR. Predictors of secondary cancer treatment in patients receiving local therapy for prostate cancer: data from cancer of the prostate strategic urologic research endeavor. J Urol. 2002;168:530–5.
15. Patel VR, Schatloff O, Chauhan S, Sivaraman A, Valero R, Coelho RF, et al. The role of the prostatic vasculature as a landmark for nerve sparing during robot-assisted radical prostatectomy. Eur Urol. 2012;61:571–6. https://doi.org/10.1016/j.eururo.2011.12.047.
16. Schlomm T, Heinzer H, Steuber T, Salomon G, Engel O, Michl U, et al. Full functional-length urethral sphincter preservation during radical prostatectomy. Eur Urol. 2011;60:320–9. https://doi.org/10.1016/j.eururo.2011.02.040.
17. Budäus L, Isbarn H, Schlomm T, Heinzer H, Haese A, Steuber T, et al. Current technique of open intrafascial nerve-sparing retropubic prostatectomy. Eur Urol. 2009;56:317–24. https://doi.org/10.1016/j.eururo.2009.05.044.
18. Bonet X, Ogaya-Pinies G, Woodlief T, Hernandez-Cardona E, Ganapathi H, Rogers T, et al. Nerve-sparing in salvage robot-assisted prostatectomy: surgical technique, oncological and functional outcomes at a single high-volume institution. BJU Int. 2018;122:837–44. https://doi.org/10.1111/bju.14517.
19. Heidenreich A, Richter S, Thüer D, Pfister D. Prognostic parameters, complications, and oncologic and functional outcome of salvage radical prostatectomy for locally recurrent prostate cancer after 21st-century radiotherapy. Eur Urol. 2010;57:437–45. https://doi.org/10.1016/j.eururo.2009.02.041.
20. Chade DC, Eastham J, Graefen M, Hu JC, Karnes RJ, Klotz L, et al. Cancer control and functional outcomes of salvage radical prostatectomy for radiation-recurrent prostate cancer: a systematic review of the literature. Eur Urol. 2012;61:961–71. https://doi.org/10.1016/j.eururo.2012.01.022.
21. Marra G, Karnes RJ, Calleris G, Oderda M, Alessio P, Palazzetti A, et al. Oncological outcomes of salvage radical prostatectomy for recurrent prostate cancer in the contemporary era: a multicenter retrospective study. Urol Oncol Semin Orig Investig. 2021; https://doi.org/10.1016/j.urolonc.2020.11.002.
22. Ogaya-Pinies G, Linares-Espinos E, Hernandez-Cardona E, Jenson C, Cathelineau X, Sanchez-Salas R, et al. Salvage robotic-assisted radical prostatectomy: oncologic and functional outcomes from two high-volume institutions. World J Urol. 2019;37:1499–505. https://doi.org/10.1007/s00345-018-2406-4.
23. Mandel P, Steuber T, Ahyai S, Kriegmair M, Schiffmann J, Boehm K, et al. Salvage radical prostatectomy for recurrent prostate cancer: verification of European Association of Urology guideline criteria. BJU Int. 2016;117:55–61. https://doi.org/10.1111/bju.13103.
24. Nathan A, Fricker M, De Groote R, Arora A, Phuah Y, Flora K, et al. Salvage versus primary robot-assisted radical prostatectomy: a propensity-matched comparative effectiveness study from a high-volume tertiary centre. Eur Urol Open Sci. 2021;27:43–52. https://doi.org/10.1016/j.euros.2021.03.003.
25. Bates AS, Samavedi S, Kumar A, Mouraviev V, Rocco B, Coelho R, et al. Salvage robot assisted radical prostatectomy: a propensity matched study of perioperative, oncological and functional outcomes. Eur J Surg Oncol. 2015;41:1540–6. https://doi.org/10.1016/j.ejso.2015.06.002.
26. Abramowitz MC, Li T, Buyyounouski MK, Ross E, Uzzo RG, Pollack A, et al. The Phoenix definition of biochemical failure predicts for overall survival in patients with prostate cancer. Cancer. 2008;112:55–60. https://doi.org/10.1002/cncr.23139.
27. De Groote R, Nathan A, De Bleser E, Pavan N, Sridhar A, Kelly J, et al. Techniques and outcomes of salvage robot-assisted radical prostatectomy (sRARP). Eur Urol. 2020;78:885–92. https://doi.org/10.1016/j.eururo.2020.05.003.
28. Smith J, Kaffenberger S. Salvage robotic radical prostatectomy. Indian J Urol. 2014;30:429. https://doi.org/10.4103/0970-1591.142074.
29. Eandi JA, Link BA, Nelson RA, Josephson DY, Lau C, Kawachi MH, et al. Robotic assisted laparoscopic salvage prostatectomy for radiation resistant prostate cancer. J Urol. 2010;183:133–7. https://doi.org/10.1016/j.juro.2009.08.134.
30. Dell'Oglio P, Mottrie A, Mazzone E. Robot-assisted radical prostatectomy vs. open radical prostatectomy. Curr Opin Urol. 2020;30:73–8. https://doi.org/10.1097/MOU.0000000000000688.
31. Mantica G, Chierigo F, Suardi N, Gomez Rivas J, Kasivisvanathan V, Papalia R, et al. Minimally invasive strategies for the treatment of prostate cancer recurrence after radiation therapy: a systematic review. Minerva Urol Nefrol. 2020;72:563–78. https://doi.org/10.23736/S0393-2249.20.03783-2.
32. Driscoll K, Goonewardene SS, Challacombe B. Systematic review of open, laparoscopic and robotic salvage radical prostatectomy. In: Salvage therapy for prostate cancer. Cham: Springer; 2021. p. 1–19. https://doi.org/10.1007/978-3-030-57181-8_1.
33. Martinez PF, Romeo A, Tobia I, Isola M, Giudice CR, Villamil WA. Comparing open and robotic salvage radical prostatectomy after radiotherapy: predictors and outcomes. Prostate Int. 2021;9:42–7. https://doi.org/10.1016/j.prnil.2020.07.003.
34. Gontero P, Marra G, Alessio P, Filippini C, Oderda M, Munoz F, et al. Salvage radical prostatectomy for recurrent prostate cancer: morbidity and functional outcomes from a large multicenter series of open versus robotic approaches. J Urol. 2019;202:725–31. https://doi.org/10.1097/JU.0000000000000327.
35. Matei DV, Ferro M, Jereczek-Fossa BA, Renne G, Crisan N, Bottero D, et al. Salvage radical prostatectomy after external beam radiation therapy: a systematic review of current approaches. Urol Int. 2015;94:373–82. https://doi.org/10.1159/000371893.
36. Coughlin GD, Yaxley JW, Chambers SK, Occhipinti S, Samaratunga H, Zajdlewicz L, et al. Robot-assisted laparoscopic prostatectomy versus open radical retropubic prostatectomy: 24-month outcomes from a randomised controlled study. Lancet Oncol. 2018;19:1051–60. https://doi.org/10.1016/S1470-2045(18)30357-7.
37. Herrera-Caceres JO, Nason GJ, Salgado-Sanmamed N, Goldberg H, Woon DTS, Chandrasekar T, et al. Salvage radical prostatectomy following focal therapy: functional and oncological outcomes. BJU Int. 2020;125:525–30. https://doi.org/10.1111/bju.14976.
38. Lawrentschuk N, Finelli A, Van der Kwast TH, Ryan P, Bolton DM, Fleshner NE, et al. Salvage radical prostatectomy following primary high intensity focused ultrasound for treatment of prostate cancer. J Urol. 2011;185:862–8. https://doi.org/10.1016/j.juro.2010.10.080.
39. Nunes-Silva I, Barret E, Srougi V, Baghdadi M, Capogrosso P, Garcia-Barreras S, et al. Effect of prior focal therapy on perioperative, oncologic and functional outcomes of salvage robotic assisted radical prostatectomy. J Urol. 2017;198:1069–76. https://doi.org/10.1016/j.juro.2017.05.071.
40. Marconi L, Stonier T, Tourinho-Barbosa R, Moore C, Ahmed HU, Cathelineau X, et al. Robot-assisted radical prostatectomy after focal therapy: oncological, functional outcomes and predictors of recurrence. Eur Urol. 2019;76:27–30. https://doi.org/10.1016/j.eururo.2019.03.007.
41. Riviere J, Bernhard J-C, Robert G, Wallerand H, Deti E, Maurice-Tison S, et al. Salvage radiotherapy after high-intensity focussed ultrasound for recurrent localised prostate

cancer. Eur Urol. 2010;58:567–73. https://doi.org/10.1016/j.eururo.2010.06.003.

42. Munoz F, Guarneri A, Botticella A, Gabriele P, Moretto F, Panaia R, et al. Salvage external beam radiotherapy for recurrent prostate adenocarcinoma after high-intensity focused ultrasound as primary treatment. Urol Int. 2013;90:288–93. https://doi.org/10.1159/000345631.
43. Marra G, Valerio M, Emberton M, Heidenreich A, Crook JM, Bossi A, et al. Salvage local treatments after focal therapy for prostate cancer. Eur Urol Oncol. 2019;2:526–38. https://doi.org/10.1016/j.euo.2019.03.008.
44. Nathan A, Ng A, Mitra A, Davda R, Sooriakumaran P, Patel S, et al. Comparative effectiveness analyses of salvage prostatectomy and salvage radiotherapy outcomes following focal or whole-gland ablative therapy (high intensity focused ultrasound (HIFU), cryotherapy or electroporation) for localised prostate cancer. Clin Oncol. https://doi.org/10.1016/j.clon.2021.10.012.
45. Wenzel M, Würnschimmel C, Nocera L, Collà Ruvolo C, Tian Z, Shariat SF, et al. The effect of lymph node dissection on cancer-specific survival in salvage radical prostatectomy patients. Prostate. 2021;81:339–46. https://doi.org/10.1002/pros.24112.
46. Ploussard G, Gandaglia G, Borgmann H, de Visschere P, Heidegger I, Kretschmer A, et al. Salvage lymph node dissection for nodal recurrent prostate cancer: a systematic review. Eur Urol. 2018; https://doi.org/10.1016/j.eururo.2018.10.041.
47. Ploussard G, Almeras C, Briganti A, Giannarini G, Hennequin C, Ost P, et al. Management of node only recurrence after primary local treatment for prostate cancer: a systematic review of the literature. J Urol. 2015;194:983–8. https://doi.org/10.1016/j.juro.2015.04.103.
48. Ploussard G, Gandaglia G, Borgmann H, de Visschere P, Heidegger I, Kretschmer A, et al. Salvage lymph node dissection for nodal recurrent prostate cancer: a systematic review. Eur Urol. 2019;76:493–504. https://doi.org/10.1016/j.eururo.2018.10.041.
49. Passoni NM, Fajkovic H, Xylinas E, Kluth L, Seitz C, Robinson BD, et al. Prognosis of patients with pelvic lymph node (LN) metastasis after radical prostatectomy: value of extranodal extension and size of the largest LN metastasis. BJU Int. 2014;114:503–10. https://doi.org/10.1111/bju.12342.
50. Pfister D, Haidl F, Nestler T, Verburg F, Schmidt M, Wittersheim M, et al. 68 Ga-PSMA-PET/CT helps to select patients for salvage radical prostatectomy with local recurrence after primary radiotherapy for prostate cancer. BJU Int. 2020;126:679–83. https://doi.org/10.1111/bju.15135.
51. Lestingi JFP, Guglielmetti GB, Trinh Q-D, Coelho RF, Pontes J, Bastos DA, et al. Extended versus limited pelvic lymph node dissection during radical prostatectomy for intermediate- and high-risk prostate cancer: early oncological outcomes from a randomized phase 3 trial. Eur Urol. 2021;79:595–604. https://doi.org/10.1016/j.eururo.2020.11.040.
52. Mattei A, Würnschimmel C, Baumeister P, Hyseni A, Afferi L, Moschini M, et al. Standardized and simplified robot-assisted superextended pelvic lymph node dissection for prostate cancer: the Monoblock technique. Eur Urol. 2020;78:424–31. https://doi.org/10.1016/j.eururo.2020.03.032.
53. Gandaglia G, Zaffuto E, Fossati N, Bandini M, Suardi N, Mazzone E, et al. Identifying candidates for super-extended staging pelvic lymph node dissection among patients with high-risk prostate cancer. BJU Int. 2018;121:421–7. https://doi.org/10.1111/bju.14066.
54. Suardi N, Gandaglia G, Gallina A, Di Trapani E, Scattoni V, Vizziello D, et al. Long-term outcomes of salvage lymph node dissection for clinically recurrent prostate cancer: results of a single-institution series with a minimum follow-up of 5 years. Eur Urol. 2015;67:299–309. https://doi.org/10.1016/j.eururo.2014.02.011.
55. Bravi CA, Fossati N, Gandaglia G, Suardi N, Mazzone E, Robesti D, et al. Long-term outcomes of salvage lymph node dissection for nodal recurrence of prostate cancer after radical prostatectomy: not as good as previously thought. Eur Urol. 2020;78:661–9. https://doi.org/10.1016/j.eururo.2020.06.043.
56. Würnschimmel C, Wenzel M, Maurer T, Valdés Olmos RA, Vidal-Sicart S. Contemporary update of SPECT tracers and novelties in radioguided surgery: a perspective based on urology. Q J Nucl Med Mol Imaging. 2021; https://doi.org/10.23736/S1824-4785.21.03345-8.
57. Amiel T, Würnschimmel C, Heck M, Horn T, Nguyen N, Budäus L, et al. Regional lymph node metastasis on PSMA PET correlates with decreased BCR-free and therapy-free survival after radical prostatectomy: a retrospective single-center single-arm observational study. J Urol. 2021; https://doi.org/10.1097/JU.0000000000001596.
58. Würnschimmel C, Maurer T. Salvage-lymphadenektomie beim prostatakarzinomrezidiv. Urologe. 2020; https://doi.org/10.1007/s00120-020-01327-1.
59. Maurer T, Robu S, Schottelius M, Schwamborn K, Rauscher I, van den Berg NS, et al. 99mTechnetium-based prostate-specific membrane antigen–radioguided surgery in recurrent prostate cancer. Eur Urol. 2019;75:659–66. https://doi.org/10.1016/j.eururo.2018.03.013.
60. Dell'Oglio P, Meershoek P, Maurer T, Wit EMK, van Leeuwen PJ, van der Poel HG, et al. A DROP-IN gamma probe for robot-assisted radioguided surgery of lymph nodes during radical prostatectomy. Eur Urol. 2021;79:124–32. https://doi.org/10.1016/j.eururo.2020.10.031.
61. Montorsi F, Gandaglia G, Fossati N, Suardi N, Pultrone C, De Groote R, et al. Robot-assisted salvage lymph node dissection for clinically recurrent prostate cancer. Eur Urol. 2017;72:432–8. https://doi.org/10.1016/j.eururo.2016.08.051.
62. Briganti A, Chun FK-H, Salonia A, Suardi N, Gallina A, Da Pozzo LF, et al. Complications and other surgical outcomes associated with extended pelvic lymphadenectomy in men with localized prostate cancer. Eur Urol. 2006;50:1006–13. https://doi.org/10.1016/j.eururo.2006.08.015.
63. Fossati N, Willemse P-PM, Van den Broeck T, van den Bergh RCN, Yuan CY, Briers E, et al. The benefits and harms of different extents of lymph node dissection during radical prostatectomy for prostate cancer: a systematic review. Eur Urol. 2017;72:84–109. https://doi.org/10.1016/j.eururo.2016.12.003.
64. Pfister D, Kokx R, Hartmann F, Heidenreich A. Salvage radical prostatectomy after local radiotherapy in prostate cancer. Curr Opin Urol. 2021;31:194–8. https://doi.org/10.1097/MOU.0000000000000873.
65. Rocco B, Cozzi G, Spinelli MG, Grasso A, Varisco D, Coelho RF, et al. Current status of salvage robot-assisted laparoscopic prostatectomy for radiorecurrent prostate cancer. Curr Urol Rep. 2012;13:195–201. https://doi.org/10.1007/s11934-012-0245-1.
66. Mandel P, Linnemannstöns A, Chun F, Schlomm T, Pompe R, Budäus L, et al. Incidence, risk factors, management, and complications of rectal injuries during radical prostatectomy. Eur Urol Focus. 2018;4:554–7. https://doi.org/10.1016/j.euf.2017.01.008.
67. Barchetti F, Panebianco V. Multiparametric MRI for recurrent prostate cancer post radical prostatectomy and postradiation therapy. Biomed Res Int. 2014;2014:1–23. https://doi.org/10.1155/2014/316272.
68. Maurer T, Eiber M, Schwaiger M, Gschwend JE. Current use of PSMA–PET in prostate cancer management. Nat Rev Urol. 2016;13:226–35. https://doi.org/10.1038/nrurol.2016.26.
69. Gandaglia G, Ploussard G, Valerio M, Mattei A, Fiori C, Fossati N, et al. A novel nomogram to identify candidates for extended pelvic lymph node dissection among patients with clinically localized prostate cancer diagnosed with magnetic resonance imaging-targeted and systematic biopsies. Eur Urol. 2019;75:506–14. https://doi.org/10.1016/j.eururo.2018.10.012.

70. Mattei A, Fuechsel FG, Bhatta Dhar N, Warncke SH, Thalmann GN, Krause T, et al. The template of the primary lymphatic landing sites of the prostate should be revisited: results of a multimodality mapping study. Eur Urol. 2008;53:118–25. https://doi.org/10.1016/j.eururo.2007.07.035.
71. Liu S, Hemal A. Techniques of robotic radical prostatectomy for the management of prostate cancer: which one, when and why. Transl Androl Urol. 2020;9:906–18. https://doi.org/10.21037/tau.2019.09.13.
72. Van Velthoven RF, Ahlering TE, Peltier A, Skarecky DW, Clayman RV. Technique for laparoscopic running urethrovesical anastomosis:the single knot method. Urology. 2003;61:699–702. https://doi.org/10.1016/S0090-4295(02)02543-8.
73. Ghafoor S, Becker AS, Stocker D, Barth BK, Eberli D, Donati OF, et al. Magnetic resonance imaging of the prostate after focal therapy with high-intensity focused ultrasound. Abdom Radiol. 2020;45:3882–95. https://doi.org/10.1007/s00261-020-02577-5.
74. Ribeiro L, Stonier T, Stroman L, Tourinho-Barbosa R, Alghazo O, Winkler M, et al. Is the toxicity of salvage prostatectomy related to the primary prostate cancer therapy received? J Urol. 2021;205:791–9. https://doi.org/10.1097/JU.0000000000001382.
75. Chade DC, Shariat SF, Cronin AM, Savage CJ, Karnes RJ, Blute ML, et al. Salvage radical prostatectomy for radiation-recurrent prostate cancer: a multi-institutional collaboration. Eur Urol. 2011;60:205–10. https://doi.org/10.1016/j.eururo.2011.03.011.
76. Bolla M, van Poppel H, Tombal B, Vekemans K, Da Pozzo L, de Reijke TM, et al. Postoperative radiotherapy after radical prostatectomy for high-risk prostate cancer: long-term results of a randomised controlled trial (EORTC trial 22911). Lancet. 2012;380:2018–27. https://doi.org/10.1016/S0140-6736(12)61253-7.
77. Parker CC, James ND, Brawley CD, Clarke NW, Hoyle AP, Ali A, et al. Radiotherapy to the primary tumour for newly diagnosed, metastatic prostate cancer (STAMPEDE): a randomised controlled phase 3 trial. Lancet. 2018;392:2353–66. https://doi.org/10.1016/S0140-6736(18)32486-3.
78. Knipper S, Tilki D, Mansholt J, Berliner C, Bernreuther C, Steuber T, et al. Metastases-yield and prostate-specific antigen kinetics following salvage lymph node dissection for prostate cancer: a comparison between conventional surgical approach and prostate-specific membrane antigen-radioguided surgery. Eur Urol Focus. 2018; https://doi.org/10.1016/j.euf.2018.09.014.
79. Horn T, Krönke M, Rauscher I, Haller B, Robu S, Wester H-J, et al. Single lesion on prostate-specific membrane antigen-ligand positron emission tomography and low prostate-specific antigen are prognostic factors for a favorable biochemical response to prostate-specific membrane antigen-targeted radioguided surgery in recurrent prostate cancer. Eur Urol. 2019;76:517–23. https://doi.org/10.1016/j.eururo.2019.03.045.
80. Sooriakumaran P. Testing radical prostatectomy in men with prostate cancer and oligometastases to the bone: a randomized controlled feasibility trial. BJU Int. 2017;120:E8–E20. https://doi.org/10.1111/bju.13925.

Histological Evaluations of RADICAL Prostatectomy Specimens

Bernardo Rocco, Alessia Cimadamore, Haiman Aider, Maria Chiara Sighinolfi, and Alexander Haese

1 Introduction

Histological evaluation of RADICAL prostatectomy specimens (RALP) provides essential information on prognostic features for further decision-making. Several factors have to be considered, including the histopathological type, grade, pTNM, and surgical margin status. The presence of lymphovascular invasion and intraductal carcinoma/cribriform architecture is an added feature to be reported as well, together with the location of the dominant tumor; the quantification of tumor burden is still considered optional, but advisable (volume of dominant lesion/percentage of prostate involved).

Beyond the setting of final histopathological analysis on the whole specimen, frozen section analysis of ex vivo prostate has been described too, to guide further steps of radical prostatectomy toward a more conservative (nerve sparing) or wider dissection plane. The chapter will cover the topic of final histopathological analysis together with frozen section modalities and outcomes.

Supplementary Information The online version contains supplementary material available at [https://doi.org/10.1007/978-3-031-00363-9_29].

B. Rocco (✉) · M. C. Sighinolfi
ASST Santi Paolo e Carlo, University of Milan, Milan, Italy

A. Cimadamore
Polytechnic University of the Marche Hospital, Ancona, Italy

H. Aider
University College London Hospitals, NHS, London, UK

A. Haese
Martini Clinic Prostate Cancer Center, University Clinic Eppendorf, Hamburg, Germany

2 Handling and Processing of RALP Specimen in the Regular Setting

The handling of radical prostatectomy specimens is of paramount importance for the accurate assessment of the histopathological parameters and consequent management of the patient. The prostate specimen needs to be handled with great care and according to standardized protocols. Some details of handling and cutting need to be performed according to established procedures, whereas other parts can vary among laboratories also depending on the facilities, costs, and preference of the pathologist.

2.1 Specimen Transportation

As other surgical specimen, the prostate specimen should be sent to the laboratory immediately after surgery in a jar filled with buffered 4–10% formaldehyde solution or a fresh tissue without any fixative solution. The latter procedure offers the possibility to perform intraoperative frozen section evaluation, harvest fresh tissue for research purpose (i.e., bio banking), particular tests preferably conducted on fresh tissue such as hormonal assays and molecular analysis. Right after, the specimen should be immerged in formalin for at least 10 times the prostate volume (at least 500 mL). Presence of proteolytic enzymes in prostatic secretion make the organ more sensitive to autolysis. Compared to an open surgery, robotic prostatectomy (RALP) is characterized by a prolonged warm ischemia. However, in the study of Best et al., no evidence of DNA/RNA and protein degradation was reported in RALP [1]. Formalin has been estimated to penetrate tissue at a speed of approximately 2.4 mm per 24 h. Considering that a prostate gland may have a diameter of 3–7 cm, full penetration of formalin would take several days. Several strategies can be used to enhance formalin fixation such as formalin injection inside the prostatic parenchyma before immersion.

P. Wiklund et al. (eds.), *Robotic Urologic Surgery*, https://doi.org/10.1007/978-3-031-00363-9_29

2.2 Specimen Weight and Dimensions

After fixation, the prostate gland should be weighted and measured in the three dimensions: apex-base, left-right, anterior-posterior diameters. The weight of the specimen is not significant for the pathological examinations, and it is recommended to remove seminal vesicle and vas deferens before weighing and measuring. The diameters of the specimen can be correlated with the weight estimated at preoperative radiological examinations [2].

2.3 Inking the Surface

Surgical margins evaluation is an essential information for the correct management of the patient. To insure an accurate margin assessment the integrity of the specimen is fundamental and is greatly facilitated by inking the specimen. One up to four different colors can be used. The use of different colors helps in the identification of left- and right-side, or anterior- and posterior-side in the case of four colors. The adhesion of the ink can be improved by dipping the prostate in 5% acetic acid. However, side identification can be performed also cutting a specific side of the gland during sampling.

2.4 Slicing the Prostate

The International Society of Urological Pathology (ISUP) Consensus Conference on Handling and Staging of Radical Prostatectomy Specimens provided specific guidelines for the most accurate method to slide the specimen [3].

Since the apex is a common location for positive margins, careful examination is required. The apex should be sliced with the modified cone method by cutting the apical slice in a sagittal way, in order to evaluate the maximum margin surface [4, 5].

The prostate gland then is sliced at 3–4 mm. The base of the prostate should be cut by a modified cone method with sagittal sectioning at a 3-mm interval similar to the apex. A useful tip when cutting the base is to include the basal portion of the seminal vesicle and the transition to the prostate in order to evaluate a seminal vesicle invasion [6]. Sampling of the junction of the seminal vesicles with the prostate is mandatory. Embedding of the entire seminal vesicle and vas deferens is not mandatory, but at least the basal portion should be analyzed microscopically (Fig. 1).

2.5 Partial or Total Embedding of the Radical Prostatectomy Specimen

Prostate cancer is often multifocal with 80–85% arising from the peripheral zone, 10–15% from the transition zone, and 5–10% from the central zone [7]. Compared to other organs, prostate cancer is underestimated and often not visible macroscopically. The safest and most accurate method to avoid undersampling is to submit the entire prostatic tissue for histological examination. Still, about 10% of European laboratories used partial embedding following

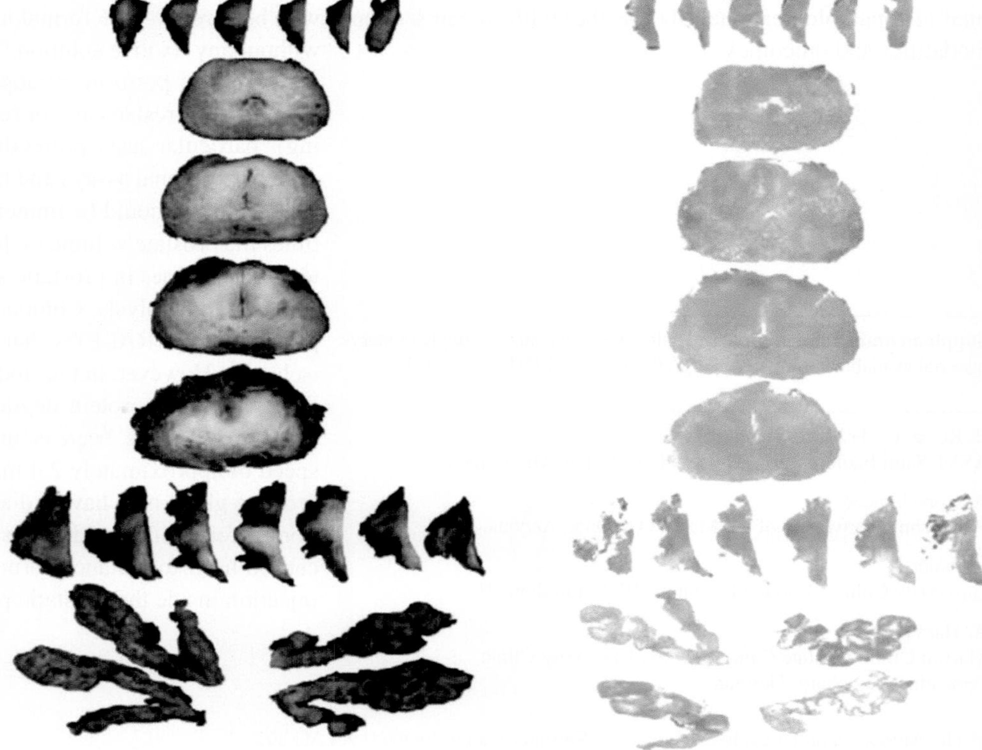

Fig. 1 Sampling of prostatectomy specimen with whole amount sections. The apex and the base are slided with the cone method. On the left, the fixed specimen is inked and cutted. On the right, the same specimen after processing and staining with H&E

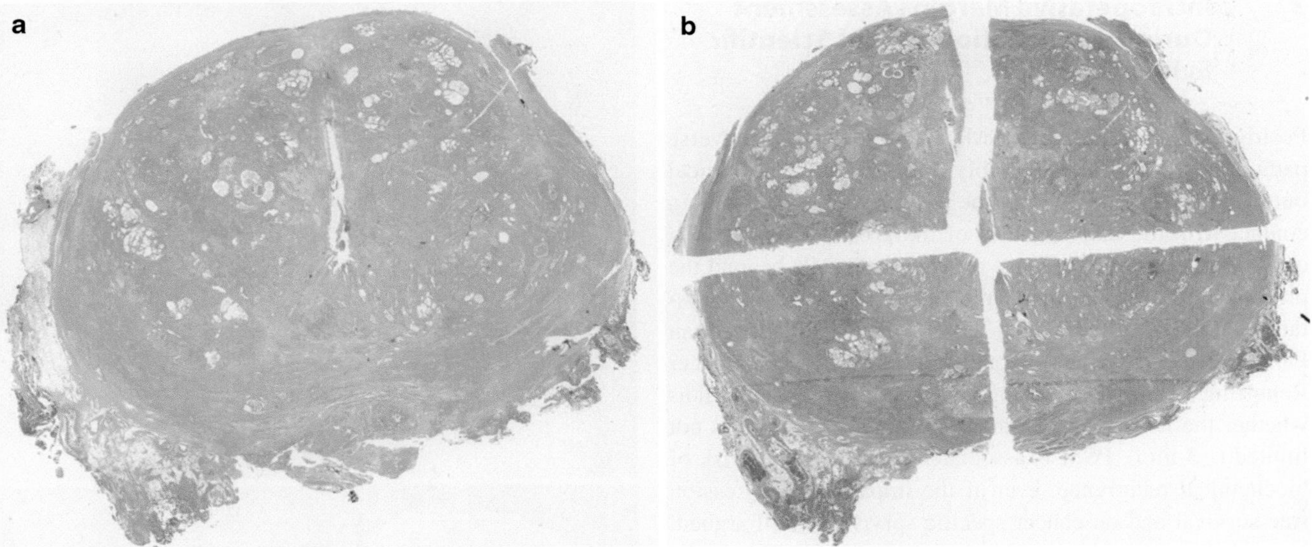

Fig. 2 (**a**) Whole-mount section of a prostate included in a large format cassette. (**b**) Prostate sectioned according to the traditional method in four quadrants, each one included in standard cassette

rigorous criteria for orientation of the specimen [8]. The protocol for partial embedding should include every posterior quadrant and a mid-anterior section on each side. If cancer was found in the anterior sections, additional sections needed to be embedded from the ipsilateral anterior portion of the prostate [9]. However, when partial sampling is adopted some features with diagnostic and, above all, prognostic importance either can be missed such as small cancers ≤3 mm in diameter, extraprostatic extension, especially when focal, presence of positive SMs, and tumor volume evaluation.

2.6 Use of Whole-Mount Versus Standard Sections

Section of prostate gland after slicing can be embedded in standard cassettes or in macrocassettes to obtain whole-mount section. The choice between the two methods depends on the laboratory equipment, technicians' expertise, and pathologist's preference [10–12]. Large format histology has the advantage that the overall appearance of the gland is sampled in one slide, not appreciable when sampling is done with small slides. Considering the pathologist workload with the whole-mount technique vs. standard sections, nine to 14 blocks per slide versus 18–76 blocks per slide are examined with the time to examine the slides being around 30 min and 1 h, respectively. When the whole-mount technique is applied, correlation with digital rectal examination (DRE), transrectal ultrasound (TRUS), mpMRI, surgical operation, and biopsy findings can be straightforward [13]. The joint evaluation of the histological whole-mount sections of RP specimens by the urologist and pathologist can produce much more clinical and prognostic information than that contained in the histopathology report (Fig. 2) [14].

2.7 Digital Versus Light Microscopy Examination

Traditionally, the histopathological examination has been performed using light microscopy. Developments in whole slide imaging and software advances have led to the implementation of digital pathology and virtual microscopy. Interchangeability of light and virtual microscopy by estimation of the intra-observer and inter-observer agreement has been evaluated. Good intra- and inter-observer agreement was achieved for assessment of primary and secondary Gleason pattern, Gleason Grade Groups, extraprostatic extension, and margin status [15–17].

Digital produces data similar to light microscopy with the advantage of more accurate measurements obtained with digital evaluation. Digital images also facilitate remote microscopic diagnosis, allows pathologists to share pathology slides with other pathologist and clinicians using a digital workflow, and provides facile access for remote sign-out. Moreover, digital slides can also be used to perform image analysis and implement artificial intelligence based network.

3 Intraoperative Margins Assessment During RALP: Rationale and Scientific Evidences

Positive surgical margin (PSM) is considered an adverse pathological feature possibly impairing oncological outcomes. PSM is defined as the presence of cancer cells in contact with the inked surface of the prostate specimen. It can be related to the presence of neoplastic cells beyond the prostate capsule (extracapsular extension) or to the intraprostatic surgical dissection. The College of American Pathologists and International Consortium for Cancer Reporting suggested reporting location of a PSM, as well as whether the margin involvement is limited (<3 mm) vs not limited (≥3 mm). PSM is associated to an increased risk of biochemical recurrence, even if the impact on progression free survival and on cancer-specific survival is still argued. Nevertheless, the intra-operative assessment of PSM can be useful to correct the dissection plane by performing a wider removal of tissue [18].

Several methods to assess surgical margin status have been proposed. A review article from Sighinolfi et al. summarizes the intraoperative sampling methods for frozen section analysis and divided them into the following approaches [18]: (1) systematic (analysis of the whole postero-lateral aspect of the prostate specimen); (2) MRI-guided (biopsies from suspicious areas, retrieved by the surgeon in a cognitive way); (3) random biopsies from soft peri-prostatic tissues, in case of uncertain origin (neoplastic/non-neoplastic). Herein, we provide insights on the systematic approach to prostate surface, which could be performed either with conventional frozen section (NeuroSAFE approach) or digital confocal microscopy [18].

3.1 The NeuroSAFE Approach: Handling and Processing of RALP Specimen

Surgical access and procedure: At the beginning of the procedure, through a supraumbilical incision, the 8-mm camera trocar is placed through an Alexis (Applied Medical, Rancho Santa Margarita, CA) wound retractor with laparoscopic cap that attaches to the wound protector/retractor to maintain pneumoperitoneum (Fig. 3a–c).

The NeuroSAFE nerve-sparing robotic prostatectomy is carried out using a transperitoneal antegrade descending approach.

After nerve-sparing prostate dissection and urethral division, the specimen is harvested into an Endocatch bag and then advanced under the Alexis port. The laparoscopic cap of the Alexis port is then detached from the self-retaining Alexis wound protector/retractor such as allowing easy access to the specimen in the Endocatch bag. From there, the surgeon receives the specimen for further processing. After specimen is retrieved, the laparoscopic cap is reattached and pneumoperitonium is re-established. The robotic arms are re-docked to proceed with anatomic reconstruction of the bladder neck and the urethra.

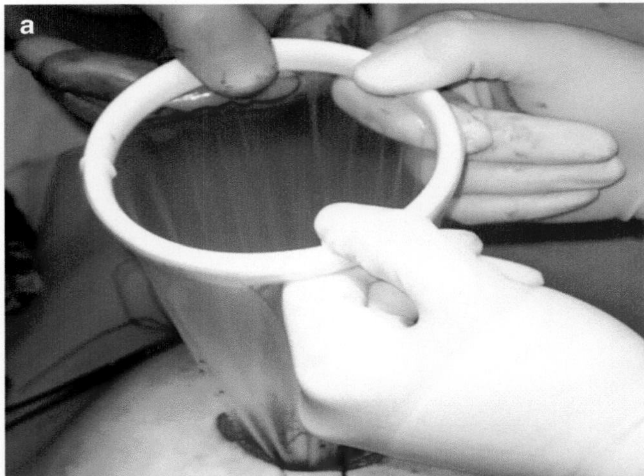

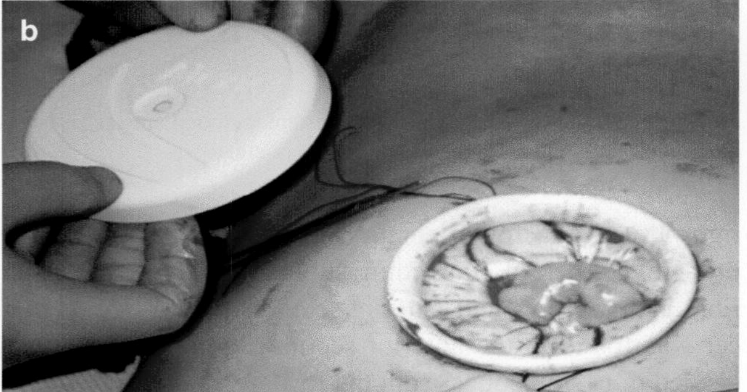

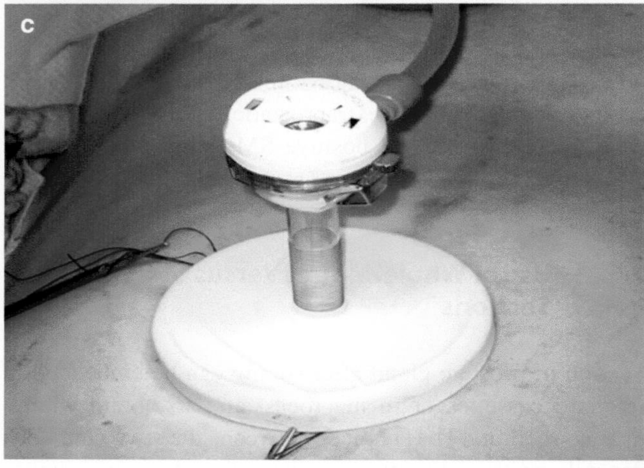

Fig. 3 (**a**–**c**) Alexis port for easy intraoperative harvesting of the specimen

3.2 NeuroSAFE Frozen Section Analysis

Simultaneously to the re-establishment of the pneumoperitoneum, the neurovascular structure-adjacent prostatic tissue is dissected as a wedge of tissue reaching from the apex to the base of the prostate on both sides. The inner and outer surface of the specimen is inked with different colors. The specimen is sent to the Department of Pathology and processed as described. In short, the postero-lateral prostatic margins are dissected and examined in its entirety. Inner (false) margins on both sides are inked with yellow formalin resistant ink while the right and left true surgical (outer) margins are marked with green and blue formalin resistant ink, respectively. The apex is daubed with red ink to assist in anatomical orientation and also to distinguish the apical margin in cases where the same is sent. The specimens are examined for the presence or absence of surgical margins (SM) by a dedicated genitourinary pathology team. A PSM is reported if at least one tumor gland has contact with the inked SM and instigates a secondary neurovascular resection. Histologic recognition of tumor cells in the secondarily resected tissue is defined as EPE.

While the procedure continues with, e.g., lymph node dissection, hemostasis, dorsal double layer reconstruction (Rocco-Stitch), and anastomosis.

3.3 Processing of the Prostate Specimen for NeuroSAFE Frozen Section Analysis [2, 3]

The inked left and right sides of the prostate are sent to the Department of Pathology. There, each side is sectioned at 2–3 mm intervals, from the apex to the base. This results depending on the size of the prostate in 8 (in small prostates) to up to 20 (in large prostates even more) sections per side.

Each section is numbered with 1 starting at the apex. The sections are subsequently stained using standard frozen section protocols. After staining, the dedicated genitourinary pathologist assesses each individual section for tumor contact to either green or blue ink. In experienced hands, with adequate logistics, and staff, the result for the frozen section reaches the surgeon within 35–45 min after the prostate has been harvested.

In case of a negative surgical margin, the procedure can be finished as scheduled.

Management of positive surgical margins: In case of a positive surgical margin, the management depends on the extent of this margin. The pathologist does not only report positive or negative margin, but also location, size, and Gleason Grade of the margin.

In case of singular, small positive margins at one or maximum two sections, the surgeon is able to go back to the affected side. If, for example, the pathologist reports a singular positive margin in section 7 out of 14 on one side with a Gleason Grade 3 touching the ink, the surgeon can locate the corresponding area of the neurovascular bundle and will do a partial resection. If however a large positive margin either expressed by tumor touching the ink in several consecutive or separated sections, the entire neurovascular bundle will be removed [19].

3.4 Results, Internal and External Validation of the NeuroSAFE Frozen Section Analysis

Initial experience with the NeuroSAFE was published in 2006 where NeuroSAFE was applied to palpable disease only [20]. We then described the routine use of the NeuroSAFE technique in 11,069 men who underwent open or RALP in our institution and its impact on nerve-sparing frequency, surgical margin status, and biochemical recurrence (BCR). Positive margins were detected in 25% of NeuroSAFE RPs, leading to a secondary resection of the ipsilateral neurovascular tissue. Secondary resection resulted in conversion to a definitive negative SM (NSM) status in 1180 (86%) patients. In NeuroSAFE RPs, frequency of NS was significantly higher in pT2: (99% vs 92%); pT3a: (94% vs 72%) or pT3b: 88% vs 40%.

Positive margin rates were significantly lower (all stages: 15% vs 22%; pT2: 7% vs 12%; pT3a: 21% vs 32%; $p < 0.0001$) than in the matched non-NeuroSAFE RPs. As for the oncological outcome NeuroSAFE had no negative impact on BCR (pT2, $p = 0.06$; pT3a, $p = 0.17$, pT3b, $p = 0.99$), and BCR-free survival of patients with conversion to NSM did not differ significantly from patients with primarily NSM (pT2, $p = 0.16$; pT3, $p = 0.26$). The accuracy of our NeuroSAFE approach was 97% with a false-negative rate of 2.5% [21].

Subsequently, we validated this approach for the robot-assisted approach and could replicate the findings with both a significant decrease in positive surgical margins and an increase in the rate of nerve-sparing across all pathologic stages [22].

The NeuroSAFE approach has been extensively both, in open and robot-assisted radical prostatectomy validated across multiple institutions [21–28]. Supplementary Table 1 lists the results of published studies.

Beyond that, a randomized controlled trial (NeuroSAFE Proof) has been initiated. After an initial feasibility study demonstrated safety, reproducibility, and excellent histopathological concordance of the NeuroSAFE technique in the NeuroSAFE PROOF trial, which has led to the opening of the NeuroSAFE PROOF randomized controlled trial in the UK [29, 30].

Beyond the simple decrease in positive surgical margin rates and the increase in nerve-sparing observed, a positive effect on improved postsurgical erectile function using the NeuroSAFE approach has been noted [23, 31]. This beneficial effect can be attributed to the fact, that nerve-sparing can be more extensive by approaching the prostatic capsule in a fashion of an intrafascial technique.

Points of consideration: When establishing a NeuroSAFE-Frozen section program, close cooperation with the Department of Pathology is mandatory. Both urologic surgeons and pathologists must agree on a high time priority of the frozen section, as the waiting time must not detrimentally affect OR-time. This limits the usability of NeuroSAFE (as frozen section analysis in general) to hospitals with either an on-site or at least a close-by pathologist.

Similarly, agreement on labeling of the specimen must be ensured. To a very large extent, additional manpower and hardware, in particular on the pathologists side is required, which is, in the absence of reimbursement for such a labor-intense task often a financial challenge. Finally, high-throughput NeuroSAFE frozen sections (in our institution up to 12 prostates, equal to up to 24 prostate specimens, each sliced in up to 20 sections) require a dedicated and trained pathologist. Given the relevance of a missed positive margin for the management of the patient, the expertise of the pathologist cannot be underestimated.

Despite all these challenges, a major advantage is that no specific technology has to be acquired, as frozen section is a routine procedure. Based from our experience, multiple pathologists have visited our institution, and were able to establish a NeuroSAFE program, showing that the transfer of knowledge is possible.

A further limitation is that—given the fact that NeuroSAFE examines tissue blocks at 3 mm intervals—positive margins occur when located exactly between the cuts done for the frozen section, hence are missed during NeuroSAFE assessment hence resulting in a false-negative interpretation. By their very small nature, though, these are usually very small and therefore are probably of a lesser clinical importance. Van der Slot et al. reported 89.4% of such margins to be smaller than 1 mm, 5.3% between 1 and 2 mm, 1% between 2 and 3 mm. No positive margin larger than 3 mm was noted. This is in line with our unpublished evaluation.

As per today, with more than 15 years and 25,000 NeuroSAFE based radical prostatectomies at our institution, the results regarding nerve-sparing rate, decrease in positive margin rate, improved potency, and the oncological safety are remarkably consistent over time. With multiple external validation studies showing the reproducibility of the NeuroSAFE technique, and a randomized trial comparing NeuroSAFE vs Non-NeuroSAFE approach, this surgical technique can be considered as the gold standard in intraoperative margin assessment of clinically localized prostate cancer.

4 Handling and Processing of RALP Specimen with the Confocal Microscope

4.1 Confocal Microscopy Applied to Prostatic Tissue

Fluorescent confocal microscopy (FCM) is an innovative imaging technique that provides microscopical digital picture directly from fresh specimen without any tissue processing. The FCM platform combines two different lasers that enable tissue examination according to fluorescence (488 nm) and reflectance (785 nm) modalities [32]. Fluorescence mode relies on the use of fluorochromes, such as Acridine Orange that specifically binds nucleic acids enhancing the nuclei visualization. The reflectance mode, on the other hand, is based on the natural differences in refractive indices of subcellular structures within the tissues. The digital image in gray-scale pixel is then converted into a digitally stained image with Hematoxylin Eosin fashion, in which nuclei appear purple and collagen and cytoplasm appear pink [32, 33].

The digital image can be shared with a remote pathologist in short time after specimen removal. Compared to frozen tissue section, FCM technique does not need any technical expertise, cryostat, microscope, and the physical presence of the pathologist. The FCM procedure do not alter the original tissue; the specimen can then be processed according to the standard procedures for subsequent histopathological examination and ancillary studies such as immunohistochemistry [34].

The pathological aspect of FCM-obtained digital images is similar to H&E section and pathognomonic criteria for PCa diagnosis are evident such as infiltrative gland architecture, lack of basal cell layer and nuclear atypia with evident nucleoli. Indeed, when FCM technique was applied for the first time in the interpretation of prostate biopsies the agreement between FCM and conventional H&E was 91% with K Cohen coefficient 0.75. Two prospective studies then validated the ability of FCM to interpret in a real-time fashion prostate tissue cores. In the study of Rocco et al. Four hundred and twenty seven cores were processed with FCM and subsequently with standard procedure. All images from FCM digital biopsy and the corresponding H&E digitized slides were presented to 4 pathologists with different experience in a random fashion. The diagnostic agreement between FCM and H&E for detection of neoplastic glands was almost perfect ($K = 0.84$) with a 95.1% of correct diagnoses obtained (range 93.9–96.2%) [35].

Similar results were also obtained by Marenco et al. in different setting. A total of 182 cores from 65 ROI at mpMRI were taken and analyzed with FCM by a single pathologist. Then, HE analysis was performed and HE images were interpreted by a second pathologist, blinded to FCM results. The agreement between FCM and HE of 0.81 and 0.69 at biopsy core and ROI level, with high positive predictive value (85% vs. 83.78%) and negative predictive value (95.1% vs. 85.71%) too, respectively [36].

4.2 Ex Vivo Fluorescence Confocal Microscopy Applied to Surgical Margins During RALP

The intraoperatory microscopical assessment of surgical margin is the most common way to control surgical dissection even if the actual role of frozen section in reducing positive SM is still debated [37, 38]. In the setting of RALP, the application of FCM technique demonstrated to be a promising tool. FCM demonstrated to be adequate in identifying periprostatic soft tissues such as connective, muscular, and fatty components and was able to detect prostate tissue persisting in the periprostatic environment. FCM was then applied for the en face analysis of the prostatic surface, to assess for surgical margin status [39, 40].

FCM procedure is reported in Fig. 4a–c. After orientation of the specimen, the apex is sectioned tangentially to the prostate gland. The prostate specimen is then rotated to expose its right posterolateral margin. Use of a mark (clip) previously positioned on the NVB at the beginning of the NS step (or other lateral dissection performed) and on the corresponding part of the prostate surface helps to identify the proximal and distal boundaries of the lateral shavings. A superficial thin cut is performed tangentially, from the cranial to the distal mark. The whole procedure is then performed on the contralateral left aspect. Occasionally, longitudinal slices were divided into two or three parts to fit the 2.5 cm × 2.5 cm scanning area, depending on prostate volume.

The fresh tissue is then immersed in acridine orange solution for 30 s, then washed in saline solution. The so stained sample is then placed between two glass slides sealed with silicon glue and then positioned onto the FCM stage for image acquisition [26].

The speed for acquisition of digital images on the screen strictly depends on the size of the area to be scanned and may require up to 4–5 min per sample. Once the first digi-

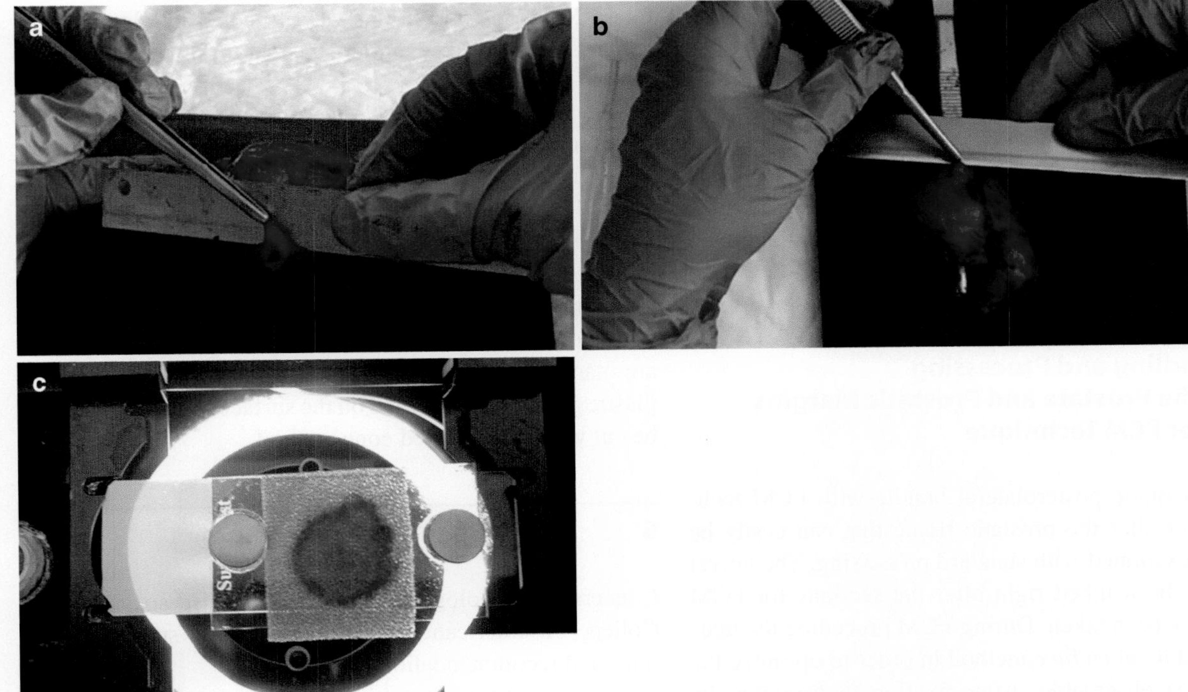

Fig. 4 (**a**) After orientation of the specimen, the apex is sectioned tangentially to the prostate gland. (**b**) The prostate specimen is then rotated to expose its right posterolateral margin. A superficial thin cut is performed tangentially, from the cranial to the distal previously positioned mark. The whole procedure is performed on the contralateral left aspect. (**c**) The stained sample is placed between two glass slides sealed with silicon glue and then positioned onto the FCM stage for image acquisition

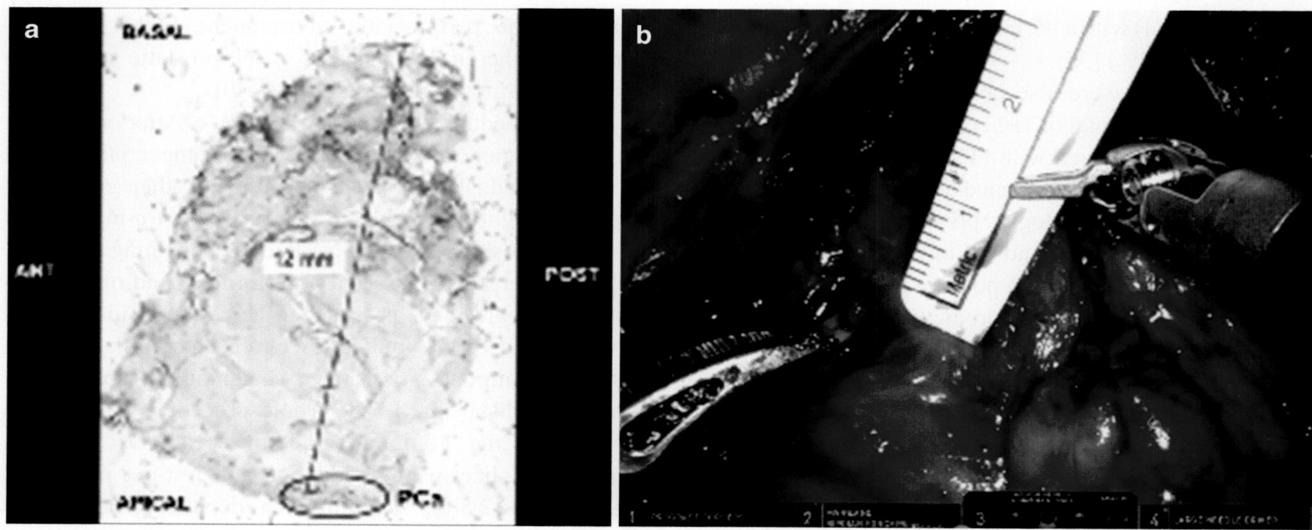

Fig. 5 (**a**) The en face analysis of flat specimens allows measurement of the distance between the cancerous glands and the clip. (**b**) By introducing a ruler within the robotic field, the same length can be tracked on the spared NVB as the distance (mm) from the mark, with an opportunity to achieve a secondary focal wedge resection

tal image (for the apex) is available, the screen can be shared with a remote pathologist. The process for acquisition of digital images from further samples can proceed simultaneously.

In the case of PSM in the NS area, a secondary resection of the bundle is recommended. The en face analysis of flat specimens using the technique allows measurement of the distance between the cancerous glands and the clip (Fig. 5a). By introducing a ruler within the robotic field, the same length can be tracked on the spared NVB as the distance (mm) from the mark, with an opportunity to achieve a secondary focal wedge resection (Fig. 5b). Tissue from the secondary resection undergoes a second FCM evaluation, with efforts to maintain the specimen orientation for evaluation of the outer part.

4.3 Handling and Processing of the Prostate and Prostatic Margins After FCM Technique

Processing prostatic posterolateral bundle with FCM technique does not alter the prostatic tissue that can easily be oriented and examined with standard processing. The lateral surfaces have been inked right after the sections for FCM procedure have been taken. During FCM procedure the margin is oriented in an *en face* method in order to optimize the maximum area observable. After fixation in formalin the same tissue can be oriented and cut in order to see the margin transversally instead of longitudinally and measure the distance of the neoplastic glands from the prostate margin. Margin status can so be assessed and positive linear length measured. The prostatic gland can be processed normally. The shaved area of the prostate is identifiable by the different ink used to recognize the false margin created after cutting for FCM processing. In this way if neoplastic glands are in contact with this inked margin, the margin should not be considered as positive.

After application of FCM technique, the prostate specimen undergoes the conventional processing, including formalin fixation (immersion in 10% neutral buffered formalin for 24-h) and paraffin embedded. After acquisition of all the digital images, the apex and the posterolateral margins samples are sent separately to the laboratory inside biocassettes, maintaining the orientation and providing the pathologist with a description of the material. Shaved prostate surfaces are marked so that they are not considered as PSMs if neoplastic glands are identified on the surface. The apex can then be cut with the modified cone method.

5 RALP Specimen Reporting

Concerning pathological reporting of RALP specimen, the College of American Pathologists provided specific guidelines and recommendation (Table 1).

Histologic type is a required element along with the Grade Group/Gleason score. The most frequent histotypes of PCa

Table 1 College of american pathologists reporting guidelines for radical prostatectomy

Prostate size[a]
Histologic type
Histologic grade
– Primary pattern
– Secondary pattern
– Tertiary pattern
– Gleason score
– Grade group
– Percentage Gleason patterns 4 and 5 (for Gleason score ≥ 7)[a]
Intraductal carcinoma[a]
Tumor quantification
– Percentage of prostate involved by tumor and/or
– Greatest dimension (mm)
Additional dimensions (mm)[a]
Extraprostatic extension
– Focal or nonfocal (if present)
Urinary bladder neck invasion
Seminal vesicle invasion
Margins
– Limited (<3 mm) or non-limited (≥3 mm)
– Linear length of positive margins[a]
– Focality (unifocal or multifocal)[a]
– Location(s) of positive margin
– Margin positivity at area of extraprostatic extension[a]
– Gleason pattern at positive margin[a]
Treatment effect on carcinoma (only required if applicable)
– Lymphovascular invasion[a]
– Perineural invasion[a]
Regional lymph nodes
– Number involved/number examined
– Site of involved lymph nodes[a]
– Size of largest metastatic deposit (mm)[a]
– Size of largest lymph node involved (cm)[a]
– Extranodal extension[a]

[a] Data elements not required for accreditation purposes

is acinar PCa. Variants like ductal carcinoma of the prostate, small cell carcinoma, adenosquamous carcinoma, and sarcomatoid carcinoma are described and are frequently associated with poor prognosis compared to conventional carcinoma. Grade Group/Gleason score is mandatory since are prognostic factor for biochemical recurrence and prostate cancer-specific mortality [41, 42]. Percentage of Gleason pattern 4 and 5 should be reported if applicable as well as the presence of intraductal carcinoma (IDC). Gleason score should be assigned to the dominant nodule(s), if present [43]. In some cases, a dominant nodule is not identified and the grading is based on all carcinomatous areas. Where more than one tumor nodule is clearly identified, the Gleason scores of individual tumors can be reported separately, or, at the very least, a Gleason score of the dominant or most significant lesion (highest Gleason score or pT category, if not the largest) should be recorded.

If three patterns are present, record the most predominant and second most common patterns; the tertiary pattern should be recorded if higher than the primary and secondary patterns but it is not incorporated into the Gleason score if <5% [44]. If the tertiary pattern 5 comprises >5% of the tumor, some pathologists incorporate it into the Gleason score as a secondary pattern.

In case of pretreatment with neoadjuvant or antiandrogen therapy Gleason score should not be assigned.

The percentage of prostate involved by the tumor is a required element by the CAP guidelines and can be performed with multiple methods such as eyeball estimation, use of a grid system, image analysis, measuring the proportion of blocks with tumor, measuring the greatest tumor dimension. However, even though it has been reported that tumor volume predicts pathological stage, biochemical recurrence, and risk of metastasis, it is not an independent predictor of outcome [30, 32, 34, 45–47].

PT2 stage is defined as tumor confined beneath the prostate confines. Subgrouping into T2a,b, and c has been overcome by the current classification because no data exists to allow correlation of pT2 stage with survival in PCa.

PT3 stage is defined as tumors with extension beyond the gland's border represented by a condensed fibromuscular layer of prostatic stroma—"capsule"—better represented in the posterolateral parts of the gland. pT3a is determined by presence of extraprostatic extension (EPE), whereas pT3b by the presence of seminal vesicles invasion (SVI) with or without extracapsular invasion. EPE can be recognizable by the observation of prostatic glands in the periprostatic adipose tissue, or as neoplastic gland within the loose connective tissue and/or perineural spaces of the neurovascular bundles or as tumor nodule that bulges beyond the prostatic border. It is a required element and should be specified if it is focal or non-focal. "Focal" EPE is defined when few neoplastic glands are present outside the prostatic boundaries, or tumor occupying <1 HPF in no more than two sections. The assessment of EPE is particularly challenging in the anterior part of the gland because as described by McNeal the anterior fibromuscular stroma does not have a defined capsule [47]. Both the apex and anterior prostate contain skeletal muscle and this is not a useful indicator of extraprostatic extension.

The presence of extraprostatic extension is associated with an increased risk of biochemical recurrence, distant metastases, and cancer-specific survival.

Bladder neck invasion is staged as pT3a. The practical approach to assess bladder neck invasion is the presence of prostatic adenocarcinoma in thick smooth muscle bundles in the absence of benign prostatic glands. If benign prostatic glands are present, then this should not be considered bladder neck invasion, even if the block comes from the bladder neck region [48, 49].

Seminal vesicle invasion is defined as prostatic tumors infiltrating the SV wall. Invasion of the seminal vesicle(s) indicates a worse prognosis than extraprostatic extension [50, 51]. PT4 is defined when PCa invades adjacent structures (i.e., external sphincter, rectum, bladder, elevator muscle, pelvic wall).

Surgical margins status should be reported and indicated as R1 (residual microscopic disease). By definition, cancer glands must reach ink for the margin to be considered positive. It has been shown that when cancer is close to the margin but not at ink, the risk of recurrence is similar to that of other cases of organ confined cancer [52]. As previously stated, linear length of positive margin should be reported and defined as "limited" if the positive margin measures <3 mm or "non-limited" if it is more or equal to 3 mm. Focality—"unifocal" vs. "multifocal"—and location of the positive margin are also important, especially if intraprostatic or extraprostatic. Presence of benign prostate glands at surgical margin is also a useful parameter for the clinician during PSA monitoring. Gleason pattern at positive margin should be reported since it has been demonstrated to be an independent predictor of biochemical recurrence [53, 54].

6 Conclusions

Histopathological evaluation of prostatectomy specimen provides useful information to tailor post-surgical strategy and to predict patient's prognosis. The intraoperative control of surgical margins is likely to reduce PSM rate; further validation studies are required to standardize the systematic approach and to spread these novel techniques complementary to RALP.

References

1. Best S, Sawers Y, Fu VX, Almassi N, Huang W, Jarrard DF. Integrity of prostatic tissue for molecular analysis after robotic-assisted laparoscopic and open prostatectomy. Urology. 2007;70(2):328–32. https://doi.org/10.1016/j.urology.2007.04.005.
2. Samaratunga H, Montironi R, True L, et al. International society of urological pathology (ISUP) consensus conference on handling and staging of radical prostatectomy specimens. Working group 1: specimen handling. Mod Pathol. 2011;24(1):6–15. https://doi.org/10.1038/modpathol.2010.178.
3. Egevad L, Srigley JR, Delahunt B. International society of urological pathology (ISUP) consensus conference on handling and staging of radical prostatectomy specimens: rationale and organization. Mod Pathol. 2011;24(1):1–5. https://doi.org/10.1038/modpathol.2010.159.
4. Tan PH, Cheng L, Srigley JR, et al. International society of urological pathology (ISUP) consensus conference on handling and staging of radical prostatectomy specimens. Working group 5: surgical margins. Mod Pathol. 2011;24(1):48–57. https://doi.org/10.1038/modpathol.2010.155.
5. Smith JA, Chan RC, Chang SS, et al. A comparison of the incidence and location of positive surgical margins in robotic assisted laparoscopic radical prostatectomy and open retropubic radical prostatectomy. J Urol. 2007;178(6):2385–90. https://doi.org/10.1016/j.juro.2007.08.008.
6. Samaratunga H, Samaratunga D, Perry-Keene J, Adamson M, Yaxley J, Delahunt B. Distal seminal vesicle invasion by prostate adenocarcinoma does not occur in isolation of proximal seminal vesicle invasion or lymphovascular infiltration. Pathology. 2010;42(4):330–3. https://doi.org/10.3109/00313021003767330.
7. Andreoiu M, Cheng L. Multifocal prostate cancer: biologic, prognostic, and therapeutic implications. Hum Pathol. 2010;41(6):781–93. https://doi.org/10.1016/j.humpath.2010.02.011.
8. Egevad L, Algaba F, Berney DM, et al. Handling and reporting of radical prostatectomy specimens in Europe: a web-based survey by the European Network of Uropathology (ENUP). Histopathology. 2008;53(3):333–9. https://doi.org/10.1111/j.1365-2559.2008.03102.x.
9. Sehdev AES, Pan CC, Epstein JI. Comparative analysis of sampling methods for grossing radical prostatectomy specimens performed for nonpalpable (Stage T1c) prostatic adenocarcinoma. Hum Pathol. 2001;32(5):494–9. https://doi.org/10.1053/hupa.2001.24322.
10. Cimadamore A, Cheng L, Lopez-Beltran A, et al. Added clinical value of whole-mount histopathology of radical prostatectomy specimens: a collaborative review. Eur Urol Oncol. 2020; https://doi.org/10.1016/j.euo.2020.08.003.
11. Montironi R, Lopez Beltran A, Mazzucchelli R, Cheng L, Scarpelli M. Handling of radical prostatectomy specimens: total embedding with large-format histology. Int J Breast Cancer. 2012;2012:1–6. https://doi.org/10.1155/2012/932784.
12. Montironi R, Lopez-Beltran A, Scarpelli M, Mazzucchelli R, Cheng L. Handling of radical prostatectomy specimens: total embedding with whole mounts, with special reference to the Ancona experience. Histopathology. 2011;59(5):1006–10. https://doi.org/10.1111/j.1365-2559.2011.03908.x.
13. Montironi R, Scarpelli M, Galosi AB, et al. Total submission of lymphadenectomy tissues removed during radical prostatectomy for prostate cancer: possible clinical significance of large-format histology. Hum Pathol. 2014;45(10):2059–62. https://doi.org/10.1016/j.humpath.2014.06.023.
14. Montironi R, Cheng L, Lopez-Beltran A, et al. Joint appraisal of the radical prostatectomy specimen by the urologist and the uropathologist: together, we can do it better. Eur Urol. 2009;56(6):951–5. https://doi.org/10.1016/j.eururo.2009.08.016.
15. Zelic R, Giunchi F, Lianas L, et al. Interchangeability of light and virtual microscopy for histopathological evaluation of prostate cancer. Sci Rep. 2021;11(1) https://doi.org/10.1038/s41598-021-82911-z.
16. Volavšek M, Henriques V, Blanca A, et al. Digital versus light microscopy assessment of extraprostatic extension in radical prostatectomy samples. Virchows Arch. 2019;475(6) https://doi.org/10.1007/s00428-019-02666-x.
17. Volavšek M, Blanca A, Montironi R, et al. Digital versus light microscopy assessment of surgical margin status after radical prostatectomy. Virchows Arch. 2018;472(3):451–60. https://doi.org/10.1007/s00428-018-2296-2.
18. Sighinolfi MC, Eissa A, Spandri V. Positive surgical margin during radical prostatectomy: overview of sampling methods and techniques for the secondary resection of the neurovascolar bundles. BJU Int. 2020;125:656–63.
19. NeuroSAFE Martini-Klinik. https://www.youtube.com/watch?v=rD3BMjyESqo&t=5s.
20. Eichelberg C, Erbersdobler A, Haese A, Schlomm T, Chun FK, Currlin E, Walz J, Steuber T, Graefen M, Huland H. Frozen section for the management of intraoperatively detected palpable tumor lesions during nerve-sparing scheduled radical prostatectomy. Eur Urol. 2006;49(6):1011–6; discussion 1016–8.

21. Schlomm T, Tennstedt P, Huxhold C, et al. Neurovascular structure-adjacent frozen-section examination (NeuroSAFE) increases nerve-sparing frequency and reduces positive surgical margins in open and robot-assisted laparoscopic radical prostatectomy: experience after 11,069 consecutive patients. Eur Urol. 2012;62:333–40.
22. Beyer B, Schlomm T, Tennstedt P, et al. A feasible and time-efficient adaptation of NeuroSAFE for da Vinci robot-assisted radical prostatectomy. Eur Urol. 2014;66:138–44.
23. Mirmilstein G, Rai BP, Gbolahan O, et al. The neurovascular structure-adjacent frozen-section examination (NeuroSAFE) approach to nerve sparing in robot-assisted laparoscopic radical prostatectomy in a British setting – a prospective observational comparative study. BJU Int. 2018;121:854–62.
24. Preisser F, Theissen L, Wild P, et al. Implementation of intraoperative frozen section during radical prostatectomy: short-term results from a German tertiary-care center. Eur Urol Focus. 2019; https://doi.org/10.1016/j.euf.2019.03.007.
25. Vasdev N, Agarwal S, Rai BP, et al. Intraoperative frozen section of the prostate reduces the risk of positive margin whilst ensuring nerve sparing in patients with intermediate and high-risk prostate cancer undergoing robotic radical prostatectomy: first reported UK series. Curr Urol. 2016;9:93–103.
26. van der Slot MA, den Bakker MA, Klaver S, Kliffen M, Busstra MB, Rietbergen JBW, Gan M, Hamoen KE, Budel LM, Goemaere NNT, Bangma CH, Helleman J, Roobol MJ, van Leenders GJLH. Intraoperative assessment and reporting of radical prostatectomy specimens to guide nerve-sparing surgery in prostate cancer patients (NeuroSAFE). Histopathology. 2020;77(4):539–47.
27. von Bodman C, Brock M, Roghmann F, Byers A, Löppenberg B, Braun K, Pastor J, Sommerer F, Noldus J, Palisaar RJ. Intraoperative frozen section of the prostate decreases positive margin rate while ensuring nerve sparing procedure during radical prostatectomy. J Urol. 2013;190(2):515–20.
28. Hatzichristodoulou G, Wagenpfeil S, Weirich G, Autenrieth M, Maurer T, Thalgott M, Horn T, Heck M, Herkommer K, Gschwend JE, Kübler H. Intraoperative frozen section monitoring during nerve-sparing radical prostatectomy: evaluation of partial secondary resection of neurovascular bundles and its effect on oncologic and functional outcome. World J Urol. 2016;34(2):229–36.
29. Dinneen E, Haider A, Allen C, Freeman A, Briggs T, Nathan S, Brew-Graves C, Grierson J, Williams NR, Persad R, Oakley N, Adshead JM, Huland H, Haese A, Shaw G. NeuroSAFE robot-assisted laparoscopic prostatectomy versus standard robot-assisted laparoscopic prostatectomy for men with localised prostate cancer (NeuroSAFE PROOF): protocol for a randomised controlled feasibility study. BMJ Open. 2019;9(6):e028132.
30. Dinneen E, Haider A, Grierson J, Freeman A, Oxley J, Briggs T, Nathan S, Williams NR, Brew-Graves C, Persad R, Aning J, Jameson C, Ratynska M, Ben-Salha I, Ball R, Clow R, Allen C, Heffernan-Ho D, Kelly J, Shaw G. NeuroSAFE frozen section during robot-assisted radical prostatectomy: peri-operative and histopathological outcomes from the NeuroSAFE PROOF feasibility randomized controlled trial. BJU Int. 2021;127(6):676–86.
31. Fosså SD, Beyer B, Dahl AA, Aas K, Eri LM, Kvan E, Falk RS, Graefen M, Huland H, Berge V. Improved patient-reported functional outcomes after nerve-sparing radical prostatectomy by using NeuroSAFE technique. Scand J Urol. 2019;53(6):385–91.
32. Rocco B, Cimadamore A, Sarchi L, et al. Current and future perspectives of digital microscopy with fluorescence confocal microscope for prostate tissue interpretation: a narrative review. Transl Androl Urol. 2021;10(3):1569–80. https://doi.org/10.21037/tau-20-1237.
33. MAVIG. Datasheet VivaScope® 2500M-G4 [Internet]. 2018. https://www.vivascope.de/wp-content/uploads/2019/06/DS_VS-2500M-G4_287_0219-ohne-Mohs.pdf
34. Bertoni L, Puliatti S, Reggiani Bonetti L, et al. Ex vivo fluorescence confocal microscopy: prostatic and periprostatic tissues atlas and evaluation of the learning curve. Virchows Arch. 2020;476(4):511–20. https://doi.org/10.1007/s00428-019-02738-y.
35. Rocco B, Sighinolfi MC, Sandri M, et al. Digital biopsy with fluorescence confocal microscope for effective real-time diagnosis of prostate cancer: a prospective, comparative study. Eur Urol Oncol. 2020; https://doi.org/10.1016/j.euo.2020.08.009.
36. Marenco J, Calatrava A, Casanova J, et al. Evaluation of fluorescent confocal microscopy for intraoperative analysis of prostate biopsy cores. Eur Urol Focus. 2020; https://doi.org/10.1016/j.euf.2020.08.013.
37. Dinneen EP, Van Der Slot M, Adasonla K, et al. Intraoperative frozen section for margin evaluation during radical prostatectomy: a systematic review. Eur Urol Focus. 2020;6(4):664–73. https://doi.org/10.1016/j.euf.2019.11.009.
38. Eissa A, Zoeir A, Sighinolfi MC, et al. "Real-time" assessment of surgical margins during radical prostatectomy: state-of-the-art. Clin Genitourin Cancer. 2020;18(2):95–104. https://doi.org/10.1016/j.clgc.2019.07.012.
39. Rocco B, Sighinolfi MC, Cimadamore A, et al. Digital frozen section of the prostate surface during radical prostatectomy: a novel approach to evaluate surgical margins. BJU Int. 2020;126(3):336–8. https://doi.org/10.1111/bju.15108.
40. Rocco B, Sarchi L, Assumma S, et al. Digital frozen sections with fluorescence confocal microscopy during robot-assisted radical prostatectomy: surgical technique. Eur Urol. 2021; https://doi.org/10.1016/j.eururo.2021.03.021.
41. Savdie R, Horvath LG, Benito RP, et al. High Gleason grade carcinoma at a positive surgical margin predicts biochemical failure after radical prostatectomy and may guide adjuvant radiotherapy. BJU Int. 2012;109(12):1794–800. https://doi.org/10.1111/j.1464-410X.2011.10572.x.
42. Epstein JI, Egevad L, Amin MB, Delahunt B, Srigley JR, Humphrey PA. The 2014 international society of urological pathology (ISUP) consensus conference on Gleason grading of prostatic carcinoma definition of grading patterns and proposal for a new grading system. Am J Surg Pathol. 2016;40(2):244–52. https://doi.org/10.1097/PAS.0000000000000530.
43. Pierorazio PM, Walsh PC, Partin AW, Epstein JI. Prognostic Gleason grade grouping: data based on the modified Gleason scoring system. BJU Int. 2013;111(5):753–60. https://doi.org/10.1111/j.1464-410X.2012.11611.x.
44. Humphrey PA, Vollmer RT. Intraglandular tumor extent and prognosis in prostatic carcinoma: application of a grid method to prostatectomy specimens. Hum Pathol. 1990;21(8):799–804. https://doi.org/10.1016/0046-8177(90)90048-A.
45. Stamey TA, McNeal JE, Yemoto CM, Sigal BM, Johnstone IM. Biological determinants of cancer progression in men with prostate cancer. J Am Med Assoc. 1999;281(15):1395–400. https://doi.org/10.1001/jama.281.15.1395.
46. Salomon L, Levrel O, Anastasiadis AG, et al. Prognostic significance of tumor volume after radical prostatectomy: a multivariate analysis of pathological prognostic factors. Eur Urol. 2003;43(1):39–44. https://doi.org/10.1016/S0302-2838(02)00493-1.
47. McNeal JE. The zonal anatomy of the prostate. Prostate. 1981;2(1):35–49. https://doi.org/10.1002/pros.2990020105.
48. Magi-Galluzzi C, Evans AJ, Delahunt B, et al. International society of urological pathology (ISUP) consensus conference on handling and staging of radical prostatectomy specimens. Working group 3: extraprostatic extension, lymphovascular invasion and locally advanced disease. Mod Pathol. 2011;24(1):26–38. https://doi.org/10.1038/modpathol.2010.158.
49. Osunkoya AO, Grignon DJ. Practical issues and pitfalls in staging tumors of the genitourinary tract. Semin Diagn

Pathol. 2012;29(3):154–66. https://doi.org/10.1053/j.semdp.2011.10.001.
50. Tefilli MV, Gheiler EL, Tiguert R, et al. Prognostic indicators in patients with seminal vesicle involvement following radical prostatectomy for clinically localized prostate cancer. J Urol. 1998;160(3 Pt 1):802–6. https://doi.org/10.1097/00005392-199809010-00047.
51. Epstein JI, Partin AW, Potter SR, Walsh PC. Adenocarcinoma of the prostate invading the seminal vesicle: prognostic stratification based on pathologic parameters. Urology. 2000;56(2):283–8. https://doi.org/10.1016/S0090-4295(00)00640-3.
52. Epstein JI, Sauvageot J. Do close but negative margins in radical prostatectomy specimens increase the risk of postoperative progression? J Urol. 1997;157(1):241–3. https://doi.org/10.1016/S0022-5347(01)65336-9.
53. Fleshner NE, Evans A, Chadwick K, Lawrentschuk N, Zlotta A. Clinical significance of the positive surgical margin based upon location, grade, and stage. Urol Oncol Semin Orig Investig. 2010;28(2):197–204. https://doi.org/10.1016/j.urolonc.2009.08.015.
54. Patel AA, Chen MH, Renshaw AA, D'Amico AV. PSA failure following definitive treatment of prostate cancer having biopsy Gleason score 7 with tertiary grade 5. J Am Med Assoc. 2007;298(13):1533–8. https://doi.org/10.1001/jama.298.13.1533.

Management of Extracapsular Extension and Positive Surgical Margins Following Robot-Assisted, Laparoscopic Radical Prostatectomy

Scott A. Greenberg, Hao G. Nguyen, and Peter R. Carroll

1 Introduction

The widespread implementation of prostate specific antigen (PSA) screening for prostate cancer in the late-1980s led to more men diagnosed with clinically localized disease [1, 2]. In contemporary practice, approximately 77% of the estimated 248,530 annual prostate cancer diagnoses in the United States present as clinically localized disease and are eligible for several potentially curative therapies including external beam radiotherapy, brachytherapy, cryotherapy, and emerging partial gland treatment modalities [3, 4]. With that said, the radical prostatectomy (RP) continues to be a common standard for the definitive treatment of clinically localized prostate cancer. Compared to conservative management, RP is associated with improved oncologic outcomes including progression-free survival, metastasis-free survival, cancer-specific survival, and overall survival in selected men with intermediate and high-risk disease [5].

Following the first published report of RP with robotic assistance in 2000, use of the surgical robot to perform robot-assisted laparoscopic prostatectomy (RALP) increased rapidly with a majority of RPs performed by RALP in the United States by 2008 [6, 7]. By 2013, over 85% of RPs were performed with robot assistance [8]. Currently, utilization of the surgical robot to perform RPs is associated with less intraoperative blood loss, fewer transfusions, shorter hospital stays and appears to be cost effective at 1 year following surgery with fewer additional treatments and days of missed work [9–12].

With regard to oncologic benefits, RALP has conflicting outcomes in the literature when compared to open radical prostatectomy (ORP). Positive surgical margins (PSMs), an independent predictor of biochemical failure, have been found by several series to occur less frequently in RALP cases [7, 10, 13, 14]. However, other series—including a 2012 systematic review as well as a contemporary CaPSURE publication containing more than 1800 men—found no significant difference in PSM rates between the different surgical modalities [15, 16]. Furthermore, RALP and ORP have similar outcomes with respect to cancer-specific and overall survival, which questions the clinical significance of any theoretical difference in PSM rates between modalities [12].

During robotic surgery's infancy, the incidents of PSMs were up to 59% in small cohorts of men treated by RALP [17]. Now, PSM rates range from 6.5 to 32% [18]. This reduction in PSMs is likely multifactorial but at least partially attributable to a "learning curve"—the period for which inexperience results in a surgeon finding procedures more difficult, with longer operative times, lower efficacy, and potentially higher complication rates [19]. For a urologist's RALP learning curve to plateau, studies have quoted the need to perform anywhere from 50 to 1600 cases to achieve an acceptable PSM rate [19]. With that said, even for those who have plateaued on their learning curve, patient selection is a critical determinant for PSM risk. Men diagnosed with pT2 disease have a reported incidents of PSMs between 7.3 and 17.4% [20, 21] while those found to have extracapsular extension (ECE; T3a disease) may have up to a 59% risk of PSMs on final pathology [22]. Such statistics should not dissuade surgeons from operating on those with higher-risk disease, as this patient population may benefit most from surgery [23]. In these high-risk patients, surgeons may consider altering their surgical approach to minimize the risk of PSMs.

Despite the suboptimal surgical and oncologic outcome PSMs represents, the patient's clinical prognosis is not invariably affected [18]. As covered later in this chapter, PSMs are independently associated with biochemical recurrence (BCR), local recurrence, and decreased prostate cancer-specific survival [24]. However, a very significant fraction of men found to have PSMs will remain BCR-free on extended follow-up [25]. Nevertheless, remaining BCR-free does not preclude men from significant psychological distress on postoperative follow-up as those with PSMs are

S. A. Greenberg (✉) · H. G. Nguyen · P. R. Carroll
Department of Urology, UCSF – Helen Diller Family Comprehensive Cancer Center, University of California, San Francisco, San Francisco, CA, USA

P. Wiklund et al. (eds.), *Robotic Urologic Surgery*, https://doi.org/10.1007/978-3-031-00363-9_30

more fearful of poor oncologic outcomes than their negative surgical margin counterparts [26].

This chapter will review the definition, risk factors, and natural history of both ECE and PSMs as well as the available treatment (or non-treatment) options for such patients after RALP.

2 Definition and Location of Extracapsular Extension

Extracapsular extension, used interchangeably with the term "extraprostatic extension," is defined as "an extension of tumor into periprostatic soft tissue" and is stage T3a in the American Joint Commission on Cancer (AJCC) version 8 (Fig. 1) [27, 28]. This pathologic diagnosis is almost exclusively made on RP final pathology with only 0.2–0.6% of positive biopsies found to have ECE [29]. For those diagnosed with ECE on prostate biopsy, poorer oncologic outcomes after RP have been reported. A 2019 publication of 83 men diagnosed with ECE on prostate biopsy found ECE present on final pathology for 98% with 59% experiencing PSMs, 45% with seminal vesicle invasion, and 37% with lymph node involvement [29]. At 3 years, 48% of men with ECE on prostate biopsy were BCR-free and almost 25% had developed metastatic disease.

The most common location for ECE on RP pathology is the mid-posterolateral gland with tracking of the tumor along perineural spaces [28, 30]. Other common locations include the mid-posterior and posterior base of the prostate [30]. Although the location of ECE is commonly included in pathology reports, there has been no evidence that *location* of ECE carries prognostic value or relevance for adjuvant therapy after RP [28].

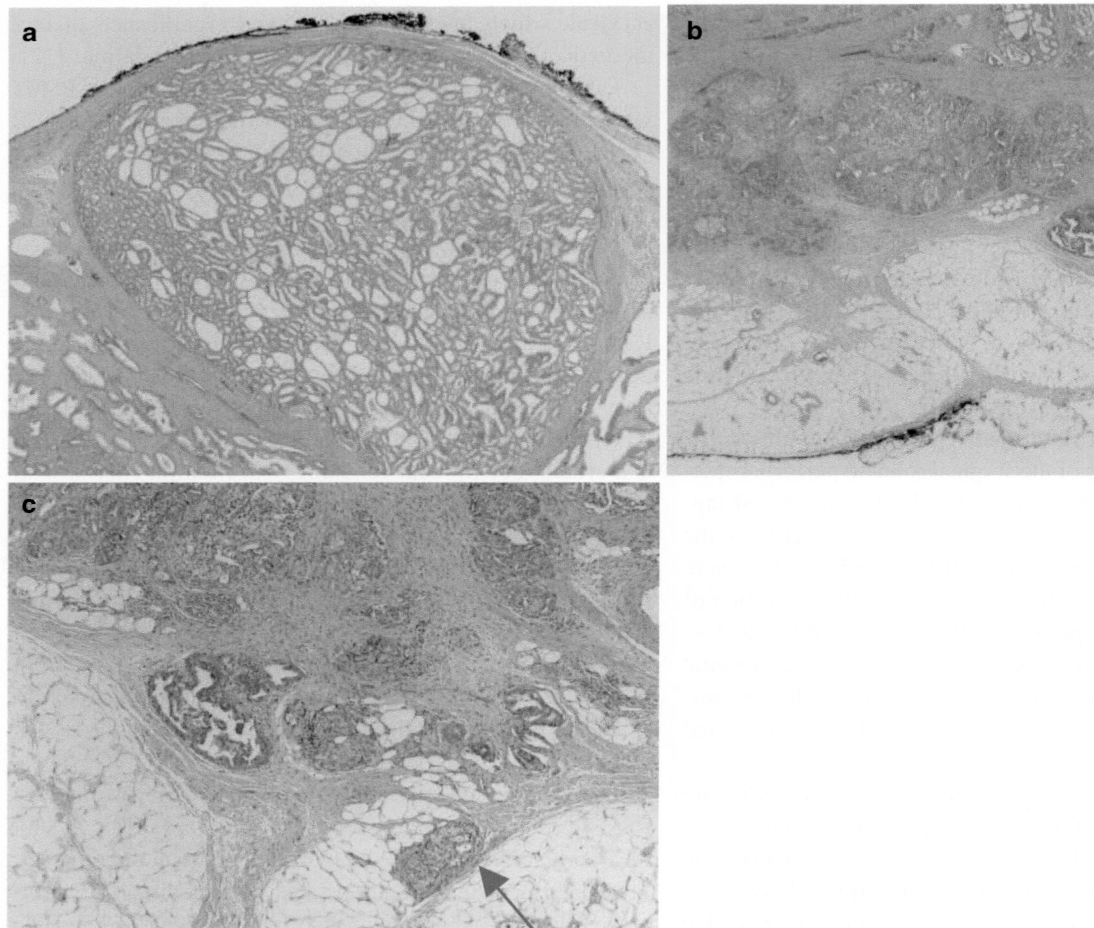

Fig. 1 (**a**) Tumor approaching the prostatic capsule (×20 magnification). (**b**) Extracapsular extension, arrow marking tumor beyond prostatic capsule into periprostatic fat (×20 magnification). (**c**) Extracapsular extension, arrow marking tumor beyond prostatic capsule into periprostatic fat (×40 magnification). Images provided by Dr. Jeffry Simko. Department of Pathology and the Helen Diller Family Comprehensive Cancer Center, University of California San Francisco

3 Risk Factors and Prediction of Extracapsular Extension

Rates of ECE vary widely in literature depending on clinicopathologic characteristics of the evaluated cohort but range from 17 to 50% in studies that include all risk groups [31, 32]. For men with Gleason score 6 prostate cancer on RP, ECE is incredibly rare—under 0.3% [33]. Historically, the preoperative risk of ECE on RP has been estimated with tools such as the Memorial Sloan Kettering Cancer Center (MSKCC) nomogram and the Partin tables [34]. These risk stratification tools utilize clinical characteristics such as stage, preoperative PSA, age, biopsy Gleason score, and percentage of positive biopsy cores to evaluate the likelihood of ECE—as well as organ-confined disease, seminal vesicle invasion (SVI), and lymph node involvement [35, 36]. However, the MSKCC nomogram and Partin tables were created prior to the widespread adoption of prostate imaging with multiparametric magnetic resonance imaging (mpMRI) and thus do not employ prognostic information from this contemporary tool.

mpMRI utilizes a scoring system known as "PI-RADS" (Prostate Imaging—Reporting and Data System) to score imaged lesions from 1 to 5 based on the likelihood of clinically significant prostate cancer with 1 "highly unlikely" and 5 "highly likely" [37]. PI-RADS score has been demonstrated to be a significant predictor of adverse pathology at RP and multiple guidelines recommend implementation of mpMRI prior to entering active surveillance for clinically localized prostate cancer [38]. By adding "grade group at MRI-targeted biopsy" as a clinical variable to preoperative PSA, maximum diameter of mpMRI index lesion, and presence of clinically significant prostate cancer, Gandaglia et al. created a new nomogram that demonstrated improved risk stratification for both ECE and SVI when compared to the MSKCC nomogram and the Partin tables [34]. Adding mpMRI findings to risk stratification models has been found to improve ECE predictive accuracy, compared to the MSKCC nomogram and the Partin tables, in several other studies as well [39, 40].

In addition to improving nomogram risk stratification, mpMRI also has a high specificity for ECE. mpMRI subjective findings such as capsular contact or bulging; irregular or angulated prostatic margin adjacent to the tumor; obliteration of the rectoprostatic angle; or asymmetry or thickening of the neurovascular bundle have been used by radiologist to predict the presence of ECE (Fig. 2). Studies have found mpMRI ECE specificity to range from 87 to 92% with corresponding high negative predictive values [40]. However, ECE sensitivity and positive predictive value are less robust with sensitivity calculated to be 35–58% in the same studies. It is important to note that the reading radiologist interpreting prostate mpMRI is a key factor in the assessment of ECE. One study found genitourinary radiologists at a single high volume tertiary care center had poor agreement with the ECE assessment by outside radiologists on referral mpMRIs (30% of cases; $\kappa = 0.35$) [41]. The differing second-opinion reports by the specialized radiologists were correct in 86% of the histopathologic results and demonstrated a much higher sensitivity (66% vs. 24%; $p < 0.01$) but similar specificity (87% vs. 93%; $p = 0.3$).

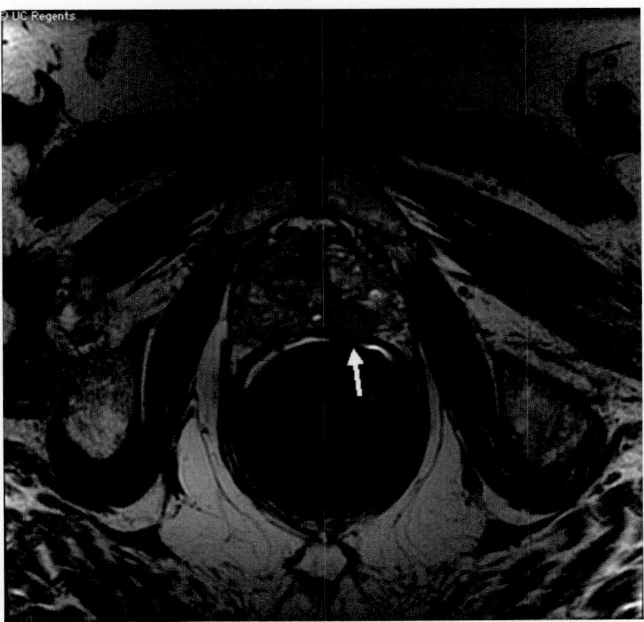

Fig. 2 Axial T2-weighted Magnetic Resonance Image (MRI) of extracapsular extension. Arrow indicates prostate cancer extension through the capsule and invasion into Denonvilliers' fascia. Images provided by Dr. Ron Zagoria. Department of Radiology and Biomedical Imaging, University of California San Francisco

For surgeons, assessing the risk for ECE is important for operative decision making and prognostication in patients who elect to undergo RP. Prostate cancer is often multifocal in nature and the largest tumor focus is the lesion most likely to contribute to ECE—as well as PSM—on surgical pathology [37]. Additionally, the length of the tumor in contact with the prostate capsule, as determined on preoperative mpMRI, is associated with likelihood of ECE on RP pathology. In one study, tumor contact length on MRI outperformed targeted-biopsy cancer core involvement and the Partin tables in accurately predicting microscopic ECE [42]. Finally, while the anatomic extent of ECE is often modest with 90% of cases within 4 mm of the prostate capsule, ECE > 1 mm predicts the risk of recurrence [43, 44].

ECE is an important clinicopathologic characteristic to be taken into consideration for clinical decision making, operative planning, and prognosis. However, after RP, one needs to be careful to not conflate the pathologic diagnosis of ECE and PSMs—related but distinct entities.

4 Definition, Causes, and Location of Positive Surgical Margins

A positive surgical margin is defined as "A tumor extending to the inked surface of the prostatectomy specimen that the surgeon has cut across" [45]. There are three circumstances which can lead to a PSM pathologic diagnosis: (1) the tumor tissue invades the prostatic capsule to reach the external, inked surface, (2) extracapsular extension is present and the tumor is incised, and (3) the surgeon incises the prostatic capsule or parenchyma and reaches tumor tissue that was actually confined within the prostate—referred to as "capsular incision" (Fig. 3) [18]. The risk of progression is similar for PSMs caused by either capsular incision or focal ECE. However, individuals with PSMs caused by capsular incision have a significantly higher recurrence rate than patients with focal ECE but without PSMs [46].

Due to anatomic considerations of the prostate in the pelvis—specifically the close contact of the prostate capsule with the rectum, bladder, external urinary sphincter, and neurovascular bundles—it can be difficult for the surgeon to perform a *wide* surgical resection; possibly accounting for the high incidents of PSMs after RP compared to other oncologic surgical procedures [47]. As previously stated, the incidence of PSMs in RALP cases is between 6.5 and 32% with increasing risk of PSMs associated with increasing pathologic T-stage. A 2012 systematic review and meta-analysis of RALP studies including at least 100 cases by Novara et al. found pathologic T2 cases experienced PSMs 4–23% (mean 9%), pT3 29–50% (37%), and pT4 40–75% (50%) [16]. With regard to location, the same study found PSMs at the apex in 5%, posterolateral in 2.6%, bladder neck in 1.6%, anterior in 0.6%, and in a multifocal distribution in 2.2% of cases. The increased risk of an apical PSMs may result from dividing the urethra in a straight, perpendicular plane causing inadvertent incision into prostates where the urethra enters proximal and anterior to the apex [18, 48]. Further complicating resection of apical tumors is the need to avoid over-dissecting the urethra and periurethral muscles to improve recovery of urinary continence postoperatively [48].

In addition to the surgical challenges the prostatic apex poses, there are obstacles in the dissection of the posterolateral margins, posterior margin, and bladder neck as well. Preservation of the neurovascular bundle (NVB) is of the utmost importance for preservation of erectile function but even experienced surgeons may have difficulty obtaining negative margins on the posterolateral aspect of the prostate if bulky or high-risk tumors lie in close proximity to the NVB [48]. Denonvilliers' fascia on the posterior of the prostate is also commonly involved with extraprostatic tumor extension and it has been recommended to remove this fascia en bloc with the RP specimen while acknowledging the potential to injure nerves originating from the NVB running between the anterior rectal wall and the prostate [48–50]. Finally, on systematic review, bladder neck-sparing surgery—an increasingly common procedure designed to aid the early return of urinary continence after RP—may increase the risk of PSMs compared to patients without bladder neck-sparing surgery (4.9% vs. 1.9%) [51]. There are, however, conflicting reports from earlier studies, including patients predominantly treated by ORP, that did not find increased risk of PSMs in patients undergoing bladder neck-sparing surgery [52].

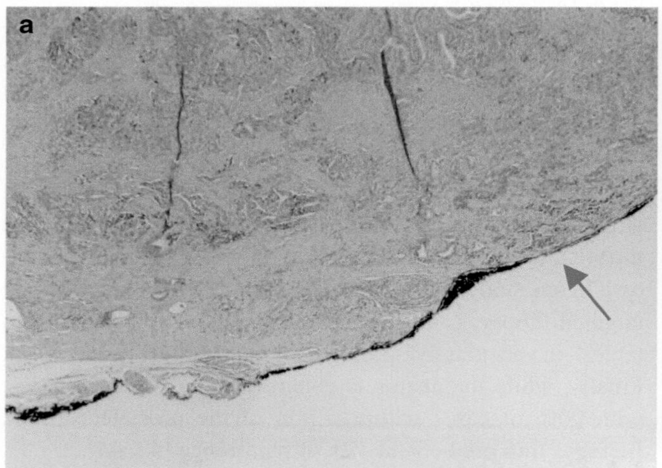

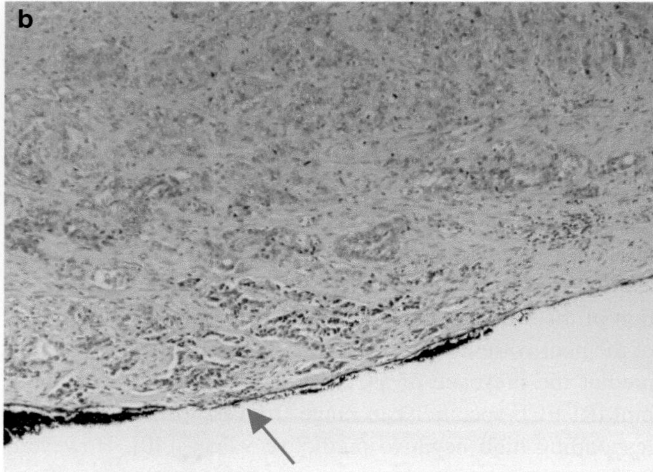

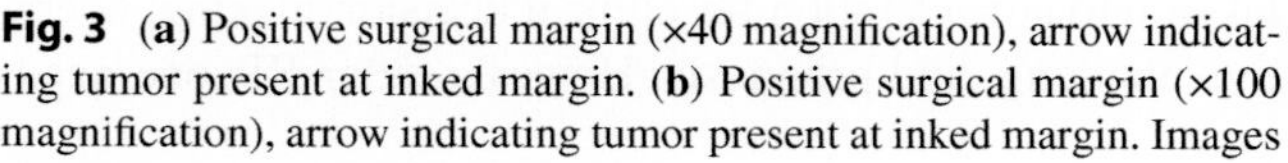
Fig. 3 (**a**) Positive surgical margin (×40 magnification), arrow indicating tumor present at inked margin. (**b**) Positive surgical margin (×100 magnification), arrow indicating tumor present at inked margin. Images provided by Dr. Jeffry Simko. Department of Pathology and the Helen Diller Family Comprehensive Cancer Center, University of California San Francisco

5 Risk Factors and Prediction of Positive Surgical Margins

As described in the previous section of this chapter, the risk of PSMs increases as the pathologic T-stage increases. From a 2012 systematic review and meta-analysis of studies including >100 RALP cases, the mean PSM rate for pT2 tumors was 9% (4–23%), increasing to 37% (29–50%) for pT3 tumors and 50% (40–75%) for pT4 [16]. In addition to pathologic T-stage, multiple studies have sought to identify the association of PSMs with clinical and pathologic factors, surgical approach, and surgeon experience.

Clinical factors including clinical T-stage, prostate volume, PSA, PSA density, biopsy Gleason score, percent biopsy positive, BMI, and even case order have been associated with increased risk of PSMs [18, 22, 53, 54]. With that said, there is great heterogeneity within the literature regarding these proposed clinical factors and their association with PSMs. For example, at least one study found higher BMI to be protective of focal PSMs (odds ratio [OR] 0.94) [53], three found no association with PSMs [22, 54, 55], and one found an association between higher BMI and PSMs [56]. Prostate volume also has divergent findings with Ficarra et al. finding smaller prostates to be protective of PSMs (HR 0.42) and Patel et al. demonstrating increased size as protective (OR 0.98) [22, 56]. Conflicting findings such as these have led most authors to conclude that patient factors which increase surgical difficulty likely have an insignificant impact on the PSM rate [18]. Furthermore, other clinical variables, such as preoperative PSA, have been found to have inconsistent risk of PSMs as well. Zhang et al. found preoperative PSA to be associated with risk of PSMs, yet at least two other studies found no association [22, 53, 54]. Considering the discrepancies in the surgical literature, it is difficult to draw meaningful conclusions regarding the clinical factors which have strong associations with PSMs.

Pathologic factors, on the other hand, have a clearer association with the increased risk of PSMs. The presence of higher pathologic Gleason score, perineural invasion, lymph node involvement, ECE, and SVI have been demonstrated to increase the risk for PSMs on RP [18, 22, 53, 54]. Ficarra et al. found pathologic Gleason scores ≥8 (HR 6.9), perineural invasion (HR 3.4), and ≥pT3 (HR 11.9) all associated with PSMs and concluded that "pathological extension of the primary tumor [is] the most relevant predictor of [PSM]" [22]. Similarly, Zhang et al. found pathologic Gleason score ≥7 (OR 2.5), ≥pT3 (OR 3.9), lymph node involvement (OR 3.1), ECE (OR 4.4), and SVI (OR 4.2) as independent predictors of PSMs [54]. Finally, Porcaro et al. found ECE (OR 2.7) and SVI (OR 2.9) associated with PSMs but, interestingly, failed to find an association with lymph node involvement [53].

When considering the association of tumor location and risk of PSMs the apex is the most common location of PSMs on RP (29–38%) with the posterolateral aspect of the prostate often considered the second most common with about 22% [16, 57]. Interestingly, it is this posterolateral margin, in which the NVBs run, that is associated with increased risk of PSMs in pT2 disease and can prove to be a barrier to surgeons—unwilling to compromise oncologic safety—from providing more aggressive nerve-sparing approaches [58–60]. To improve rates of nerve-sparing RP, while maintaining oncologic principles, intraoperative frozen-section analysis of the surgical margins overlying the NVBs has been proposed to provide surgeons immediate oncologic feedback. To perform this intraoperative evaluation, the NeuroSAFE (neurovascular structure-adjacent frozen-section examination) technique was developed.

The NeuroSAFE protocol calls for immediate removal of the RP specimen once the apex is transected and sending an extracorporeally dissected and inked wedge of neurovascular structure-adjacent prostate for immediate pathologic assessment [61]. The surgeon regains insufflation and continues with a pelvic lymph node dissection as the pathologic specimens are being analyzed. If there is a positive surgical margin identified, a secondary resection of the NVB and Denonvilliers fascia is performed [61]. Using this technique at the Martini clinic, rates of nerve-sparing have risen from 81 to 97% across all stages with PSM rates declining from 22–24% to 15–16% [59]. In a recent study of 157 men treated without and 120 with NeuroSAFE, the PSM rates were 17.8% and 9.2%, respectively, with improved potency at 12 months in the NeuroSAFE group—despite the NeuroSAFE cohort containing more high-risk pathologic features [59]. Our experience at UCSF has also found intraoperative assessment of surgical margins allows for a greater likelihood of nerve preservation in higher-risk cases that would otherwise be considered for wide excision. It should be noted, however, that undergoing additional resection for positive margins often yields no residual tumor in the additionally resected tissue.

Another emerging technology is the use of intraoperative imaging to better identify (and resect) the extent of malignancy to reduce the likelihood of PSMs. UCSF is completing a Phase 1, single-site, interventional clinical trial evaluating the safety and efficacy of IS-002 intravenous (IV) injection (a novel PSMA fluorophore) for fluorescent identification of positive cancer margins and metastatic lymph nodes during RALP using the da Vinci® X/Xi Surgical System with Firefly® Fluorescent Imaging (Fig. 4) [62]. Results to date are quite encouraging and a phase 2 trial is planned. Such technology, if found to be of value, could be widely disseminated given the florescent imaging capability and widespread distribution of the Intuitive DaVinci Xi platform

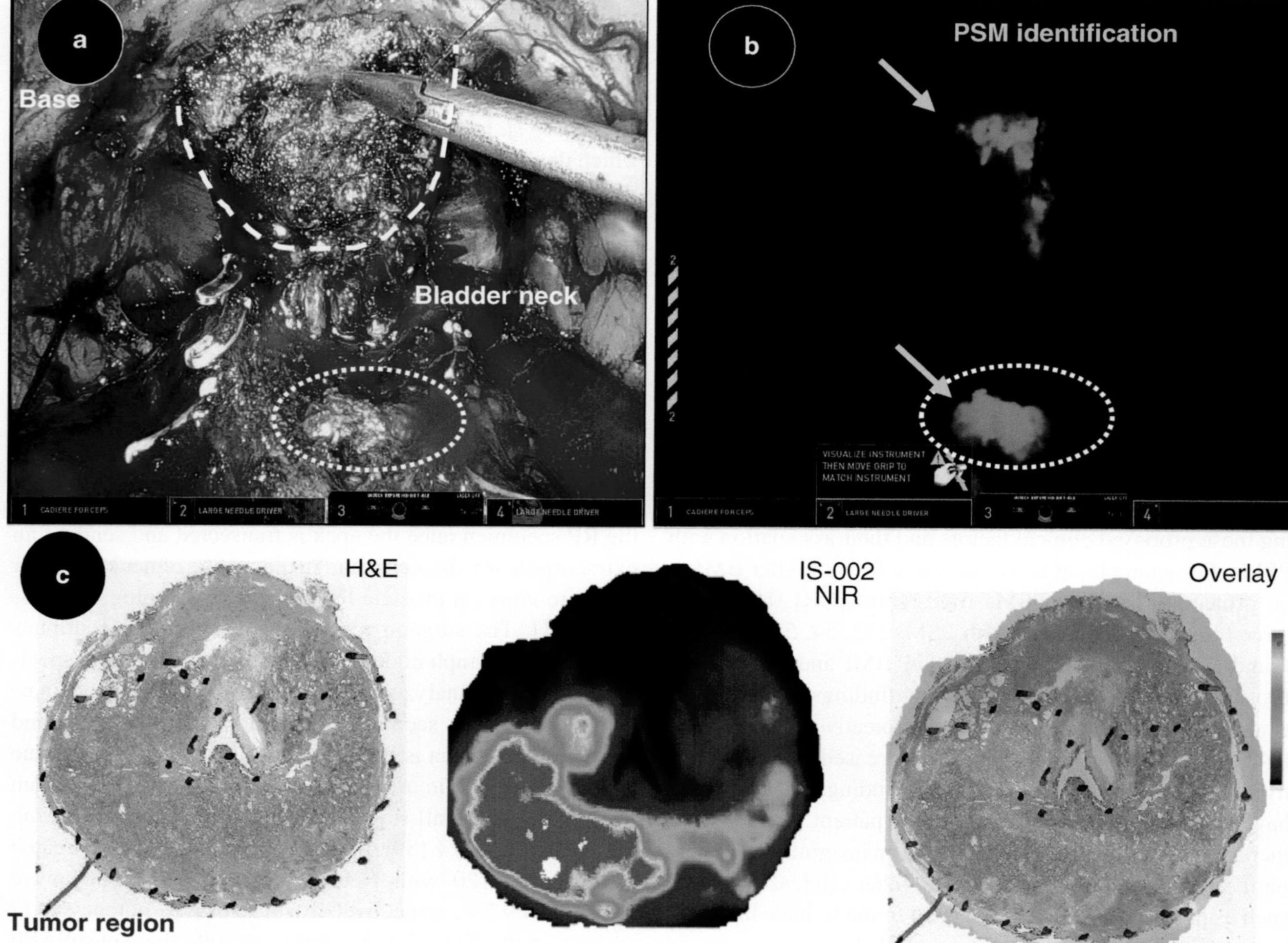

Fig. 4 (**a**) Robot-assisted laparoscopic prostatectomy (RALP) performed with the endoscope plus using the da Vinci® X/Xi Surgical System. White light intraoperative image after transection of prostate base (white dotted line) from bladder neck (white dotted circle). (**b**) Same intraoperative image using Sensitive Firefly with IS-002 intravenous injection ~24 h prior to surgery for fluorescent identification of positive cancer margins. Yellow arrows indicate IS-002 fluorescence. (**c**) (Left image) Pathologic specimen stained with hematoxylin and eosin (H&E) under white light with tumor outlined with dotted line. (Middle image) Same pathologic specimen under near-infrared spectrum light from patient treated with IS-002 intravenous injection prior to RALP. (Right image) Overlay of white and near-infrared spectrum light images demonstrating correlation between IS-002 molecule targeting and tumor location. Images provided by Dr. Hao Nguyen. Department of Urology, UCSF—Helen Diller Family Comprehensive Cancer Center, University of California San Francisco

[63]. Other, similar agents and techniques are being developed and/or refined [64–66].

In addition to clinical and pathologic characteristics, surgeon experience serves as an additional risk factor for PSMs. As mentioned in the introduction, surgeons experience a "learning curve" when learning to perform a procedure. The learning curve—defined as the period for which inexperience results in a surgeon finding procedures more difficult, with longer operative times, lower efficacy, and potentially higher complication rates—for an acceptable rate of PSMs while performing RALP has been quoted anywhere between 50 and 1600 cases; although most studies quote ≤200 [19]. A recent retrospective study including more than 2200 patients treated by surgeons performing their initial RALP surgeries at a single institution found greater experience was associated with lower probability of PSMs [67]. The risk of PSMs after ten cases was 15.3% and after 250 cases was 6.7%. Furthermore, for ≥T3 disease, the probability of PSMs decreased from 41.5 to 21.1% between the 10th and 250th RALP performed. A related finding by Porcaro et al. was that RALP by a high-volume surgeon (>500 career RALPs), compared to low-volume surgeons (>50 career RALPs), at a single high-volume center was protective of PSMs on multivariate analysis [53].

When different RP modalities are compared (ORP, laparoscopic radical prostatectomy, RALP), the risk of PSMs for patients undergoing RALP has conflicting findings in the literature. Multiple studies have found RALP to have less risk of PSMs than ORP. In 2003 Tewari et al. published one of the first comparisons of ORP and RALP techniques and found PSMs more frequent in ORP (23%) compared to RALP (9%) in the 300 men included [10]. More contemporary studies have found similar results. Using SEER data, Hu et al. demonstrated improved PSM rates after RALP versus ORP in >13,000 men (OR 0.7) and Basiri et al. found ORP to have an increased risk of PSMs compared to RALP (OR 1.18) on a systematic analysis of 104 publications including >227,000 men [7, 13]. In 2012, Tewari et al. again evaluated PSMs across RP modalities in a meta-analysis of 400 studies and found RALP superior to ORP and laparoscopic RP on unadjusted analysis but, on propensity-adjusted estimates, only laparoscopic RP had higher PSM rates than RALP [14]. Similarly, several other studies of large cohorts have found no difference in risk. Herlemann et al. evaluated almost 1900 men in the CAPSURE database and found similar PSM rates between RALP and ORP in both pT2 and pT3 patients while Novara et al. found no significant difference in PSM rates between RALP and ORP in the full cohort of 6419 men and the pT2 subgroup [15, 16]. The conflicting results from these comparison studies do not allow for a strong argument for one modality over another. With that said, RALP appears very unlikely to increase the risk of PSMs compared to other RP surgical modalities.

Finally, RALP approach has been reported to affect PSM outcomes. There are many different approaches in addition to the classic transperitoneal RALP approach including extraperitoneal, transvesical, and Retzius-sparing. Extraperitoneal and transperitoneal approaches appear to demonstrate similar outcomes but Retzius-sparing has been found in some studies to have increased risk of PSMs [68]. In a 2019 systematic review including 451 patients, Checcucci et al. found standard RALP to have a lower likelihood of PSMs than Retzius-sparing RALP (15.2% vs. 24%) [69]. However, as Retzius-sparing is a relatively new RALP approach for many surgeons, there is suspicion that the difference in PSM rates could be confounded by a learning curve [68]. Indeed, a new comparative prospective study of three high-volume RALP surgeons—one who performed transperitoneal RALPs, one who performed Retzius-sparing RALPs, and one who performed both—found no difference in PSM rates between approaches [70]. Such results, however, are subject to patient selection.

From the data presented here, it is more likely that the pathologic characteristics of tumor and surgeon experience, rather than the surgical modality or approach, influence the risk of PSMs on RALP.

6 Natural History of Patients with Positive Surgical Margins and Extracapsular Extension

It is well established that PSMs are associated with an increased risk of detectable serum PSA after RP—commonly referred to as a biochemical recurrence (BCR) [18, 71, 72]. By current American Urologic Association guidelines, BCR is defined as two consecutive increases in PSA ≥0.2 ng/ml at least 8 weeks after surgery; although some historic and non-US based studies have used other thresholds (ex. PSA greater than 0.1 or 0.4 ng/ml after RP, or an initial post-RP PSA >0.2) [73]. BCR is often studied as a surrogate endpoint for oncologic outcomes in surgically treated prostate cancer patients due to the long natural history of localized disease [74]. Poor oncologic outcomes including reduced local recurrence-free survival, distant metastasis-free survival, and prostate cancer-specific survival are associated with the development of BCR [18, 75–78].

The hazard ratio (HR) for BCR after RP with PSMs, compared to patients with negative margins, ranges from 0.87 to 5.0 in individual studies with a vast majority calculating a HR >1 [18, 73]. A meta-analysis by Zhang et al. found the multivariate pooled HR of BCR in the setting of PSMs from 41 high-quality studies to be 1.35 (95% CI 1.27–1.43; $p < 0.001$) [73]. Furthermore, several studies have found PSM length >3.0 mm (HR 1.9–2.5) and multifocal PSMs (HR 2.2–3.4) further increase the risk of developing a BCR [79–83].

Despite the risk of BCR in the setting of PSMs, it is also important to recognize a very significant proportion of patients diagnosed with PSMs do not experience BCR and a significant percentage of men who experience BCR will not further experience disease progression. In the open era, progression to BCR was found in 27% of men at 6 years, 40% at 7 years, and 54% of men at 10 years in the setting of PSMs [71, 84, 85]. In patients treated by RALP with PSMs, BCR has been found in 6% of men at 1 year, 11% at 4 years, and 29% at 6 years [22, 77, 86]. With regard to further progression (i.e., local recurrence or metastasis), Pound et al. found 37% of men experienced disease progression in the first 5 years after a BCR diagnosis and only 24% of the men progressed within 15 years of BCR diagnosis in a study by Boorjian et al. [87, 88] Clearly, other clinical variables such as time-to-BCR, PSA doubling time (PSADT), pathologic Gleason score, and pathologic stage also play an important role in progression risk stratification of RP patients in addition to PSMs [72, 76, 89, 90].

Similar oncologic outcomes have also been found in men diagnosed with ECE on RP. BCR, decreased cancer-specific survival, and decreased overall survival have all been associated with pathologic ECE [39, 91]. In the open RP era, approximately half of the men diagnosed with ECE on RP experience prostate cancer progression at 10 years and were found to be at a seven times relative risk for death from prostate cancer compared to men with organ-confined disease [92, 93]. A recent meta-analysis including 28 articles from 2004 to 2018 by Jiang et al. found a pooled HR of 1.3 (95% CI 1.2–1.4) for the risk of BCR in the setting of ECE—compared to organ-confined disease—on multivariate analysis [94]. Eggener et al. found ECE on RP to have a 2.9–10% 15-year prostate cancer-specific mortality risk, however, when calculating "competing cause mortality" discovered the risk of competing causes to be 6.6–27% [95]. Thus, while ECE is associated with BCR, it is important to recognize many men with prostate cancer also have competing comorbidities that may have a greater risk to their overall survival.

The extent of ECE appears to further drive risk of poor oncologic outcomes. ECE can be subcategorized as "focal," "established," or "non-focal"/"multifocal" with multiple studies demonstrating disparate outcomes between the groups. In over 15,500 men treated with RP between 1982 and 2012, Jeong et al. identified 27% of men to have ECE—of which 44% had focal ECE and 56% with non-focal ECE [96]. In the generated multivariable model, compared to organ-confined disease, focal ECE carried a BCR HR of 2.3 and non-focal ECE's HR was 3.2. Comparing the risk of BCR between non-focal and focal ECE, there was also a statistically significant difference between groups (non-focal ECE HR 1.4). However, for prostate cancer-specific survival and overall survival, there was no statistically significant difference between focal and non-focal ECE cohorts. Other studies have quoted the rates of 10-year progression-free survival as 67–69% for focal ECE, 36–58% for established ECE, and 29% for multifocal ECE; with established and multifocal ECE HRs for progression 3.1 and 3.5, respectively [97]. The significantly different risk between ECE subgroups has led some experts to recommend further subcategorizing pT3a disease into pT3aF (focal) and pT3aNF (non-focal) to better identify men at higher risk of recurrence and consider them for additional therapy [96].

7 Management of Extracapsular Extension and Positive Surgical Margins

For men diagnosed with ECE or PSMs on RP, current guidelines from the National Comprehensive Cancer Network (NCCN) recommend management with either observation or external beam radiation therapy with or without androgen depravation [98]. Several studies have established that adjuvant radiation therapy in high-risk prostate cancer patients (ECE, PSMs, or SVI) improves BCR-free survival and local recurrence-free survival compared to observation alone [99–101]. However, the studies failed to demonstrate meaningful improvements in metastasis-free survival or overall survival. In addition, late adverse effects such as proctitis, rectal bleeding, urethral strictures, and total urinary incontinence were significantly more common in the radiation treatment arms of these studies.

The improved cancer progression outcomes associated with adjuvant radiation, in conjunction with increased adverse events without demonstrating a survival advantage, has led to somewhat conflicting recommendations from different medical societies. The American Urologic Association's "Adjuvant and Salvage Radiotherapy After Prostatectomy" guidelines state "patients should be counseled that high-quality evidence indicates that use of adjuvant radiotherapy in patients with adverse pathology reduces the risk of biochemical recurrence, local recurrence, and clinical progression" [102]. Yet the European Society of Medical Oncology guidelines indicate that providers should "not offer immediate postoperative radiotherapy after radical prostatectomy" [103]. For the past three decades, observation has been the most frequently employed adjuvant modality and continues to be utilized at an increasing rate [104]. Using the CAPSURE database to compare patients with adverse features treated by RP between 1990 and 1994 and those treated between 2005 and 2017, Balakrishnan et al. found a decrease in adjuvant external beam radiation therapy from 10.1 to 2.6% while observation increased from 51.3 to 88.0% over that time period [104].

Recently, three prospective randomized, controlled phase III trials were published comparing adjuvant radiotherapy to observation with early salvage radiotherapy following RP in men with undetectable PSA but high risk of progression. The RAVES trial (TROG 08.03) randomly assigned 333 men to adjuvant radiotherapy or observation with salvage radiotherapy once a PSA recurrence ≥0.2 ng/ml was detected with the primary endpoint being freedom from BCR [105]. GETUG-AFU 17 enrolled 424 men and randomized them to adjuvant radiotherapy or observation with salvage radiotherapy (PSA recurrence defined as ≥0.2 ng/ml) with the primary endpoint being event-free survival (PSA >0.4 ng/ml after radiotherapy, clinical progression, death) [106]. Finally, RADICALS-RT randomized 697 men to adjuvant radiotherapy and 699 to observation with salvage radiotherapy (PSA recurrence ≥0.1 ng/ml) with the primary outcome being freedom from distant metastases [107]. The three studies had median follow-up of 6.1, 6.3, and 4.9 years, respectively.

Comparing adjuvant radiotherapy and observation with salvage radiotherapy cohorts, the RAVES trial found similar 5-year freedom from BCR (86% adjuvant vs 87% salvage; $p = 0.15$), GETUG-AFU 17 found similar 5-year event-free survival (92% adjuvant vs 90% salvage; p = 0.42), and RADICALS-RT did not sufficiently mature for the outcome of freedom from distant metastases [105–107]. However, the secondary outcomes for RADICALS-RT included BCR-free survival (85% adjuvant vs 88% salvage; p = 0.56) and freedom from non-protocol hormone therapy (93% adjuvant vs 92% salvage; p = 0.53) which were both similar between cohorts. All three studies reported a statistically significant increase in adverse events in the adjuvant radiotherapy cohort compared to the observation with salvage radiotherapy cohort: grade 2 or worse genitourinary toxicity, grade 2 or worse late erectile dysfunction, and grade 3/4 urethral strictures. All three trials concluded that the results do not support the use of adjuvant radiotherapy after RP in patients with pathologic high-risk features [105–107]. The RADICAL-RT authors further concluded that observation with early salvage radiotherapy should be the current standard of care [107].

The results of these studies should be interpreted carefully, however, as the majority of men enrolled in the trials had relatively favorable pathologic findings. In patients with adverse pathologic features (high PSA, high Gleason score, seminal vesicle invasion, or node positivity) there is evidence that adjuvant therapy should be considered [108]. Indeed, a recent analysis in men with pN1 or pathologic Gleason score 8–10 and pT3/T4 disease after RP with undetectable PSA, adjuvant radiation was associated with significantly lower all-cause mortality compared to those undergoing early salvage radiotherapy [109]. Together, these studies suggest that early, adjuvant radiation may improve survival in high-risk patients.

8 Conclusion

ECE and PSMs portend adverse oncologic outcomes for RP patients. Men with PSMs on RP have a 35% greater risk of experiencing a BCR than their counterparts with negative margins. Those with ECE have a 30–70% chance of experiencing disease progression within 10 years, depending on the extent. There is a great heterogeneity, however, in the clinical courses experienced by patients with these poor prognostic findings. Additional risk factors such as time-to-BCR, PSA doubling time (PSADT), pathologic Gleason score, and pathologic stage, as well as the patient's life expectancy, likely contribute to the variable progression and cancer-specific survival observed in these patients.

Despite the unfavorable prognosis, in the setting of undetectable disease after RP, there appears to be no survival advantage from adjuvant radiotherapy for all patients with ECE or PSMs. Adjuvant radiotherapy puts men at greater risk for radiation-associated adverse events including urethral stricture, erectile dysfunction, and other genitourinary toxicities. However, men with high-risk features (i.e., pT3/4, Gleason score 8–10) may benefit from adjuvant rather than early salvage therapy. Randomized trials in this cohort would be of great value.

References

1. Catalona WJ, Smith DS, Ratliff TL, et al. Detection of organ-confined prostate cancer is increased through prostate-specific antigen-based screening. JAMA. 1993;270:948.
2. Shieh Y, Eklund M, Sawaya GF, et al. Population-based screening for cancer: hope and hype. Nat Rev Clin Oncol. 2016;13:550.
3. Pinsky PF, Prorok PC, Kramer BS. Prostate cancer screening—a perspective on the current state of the evidence. N Engl J Med. 2017;376:1285.
4. Siegel DA, O'Neil ME, Richards TB, et al. Prostate cancer incidence and survival, by stage and race/ethnicity—United States, 2001-2017. MMWR Morb Mortal Wkly Rep. 2020;69:1473.
5. Vernooij RW, Lancee M, Cleves A, et al. Radical prostatectomy versus deferred treatment for localised prostate cancer. Cochrane Database Syst Rev. 2020;6:CD006590.
6. Abbou CC, Hoznek A, Salomon L, et al. [Remote laparoscopic radical prostatectomy carried out with a robot. Report of a case]. Prog Urol. 2000;10:520.
7. Hu JC, Gandaglia G, Karakiewicz PI, et al. Comparative effectiveness of robot-assisted versus open radical prostatectomy cancer control. Eur Urol. 2014;66:666.
8. Leow JJ, Chang SL, Meyer CP, et al. Robot-assisted versus open radical prostatectomy: a contemporary analysis of an all-payer discharge database. Eur Urol. 2016;70:837.
9. Okhawere KE, Shih IF, Lee SH, et al. Comparison of 1-year health care costs and use associated with open vs robotic-assisted radical prostatectomy. JAMA Netw Open. 2021;4:e212265.
10. Tewari A, Srivasatava A, Menon M, et al. A prospective comparison of radical retropubic and robot-assisted prostatectomy: experience in one institution. BJU Int. 2003;92:205.
11. Trinh QD, Sammon J, Sun M, et al. Perioperative outcomes of robot-assisted radical prostatectomy compared with open radical prostatectomy: results from the nationwide inpatient sample. Eur Urol. 2012;61:679.
12. Hu JC, O'Malley P, Chughtai B, et al. Comparative effectiveness of cancer control and survival after robot-assisted versus open radical prostatectomy. J Urol. 2017;197:115.
13. Basiri A, de la Rosette JJ, Tabatabaei S, et al. Comparison of retropubic, laparoscopic and robotic radical prostatectomy: who is the winner? World J Urol. 2018;36:609.
14. Tewari A, Sooriakumaran P, Bloch DA, et al. Positive surgical margin and perioperative complication rates of primary surgical treatments for prostate cancer: a systematic review and meta-analysis comparing retropubic, laparoscopic, and robotic prostatectomy. Eur Urol. 2012;62:1.
15. Herlemann A, Cowan JE, Carroll PR, et al. Community-based outcomes of open versus robot-assisted radical prostatectomy. Eur Urol. 2018;73:215.
16. Novara G, Ficarra V, Mocellin S, et al. Systematic review and meta-analysis of studies reporting oncologic outcome after robot-assisted radical prostatectomy. Eur Urol. 2012;62:382.
17. Ficarra V, Cavalleri S, Novara G, et al. Evidence from robot-assisted laparoscopic radical prostatectomy: a systematic review. Eur Urol. 2007;51:45.
18. Yossepowitch O, Briganti A, Eastham JA, et al. Positive surgical margins after radical prostatectomy: a systematic review and contemporary update. Eur Urol. 2014;65:303.

19. Abboudi H, Khan MS, Guru KA, et al. Learning curves for urological procedures: a systematic review. BJU Int. 2014;114:617.
20. Adili AF, Di Giovanni J, Kolesar E, et al. Positive surgical margin rates during the robot-assisted laparoscopic radical prostatectomy learning curve of an experienced laparoscopic surgeon. Can Urol Assoc J. 2017;11:E409.
21. Asimakopoulos AD, Annino F, Mugnier C, et al. Robotic radical prostatectomy: analysis of midterm pathologic and oncologic outcomes: a historical series from a high-volume center. Surg Endosc. 2021;35(12):6731–45.
22. Ficarra V, Novara G, Secco S, et al. Predictors of positive surgical margins after laparoscopic robot assisted radical prostatectomy. J Urol. 2009;182:2682.
23. Cooperberg MR, Vickers AJ, Broering JM, et al. Comparative risk-adjusted mortality outcomes after primary surgery, radiotherapy, or androgen-deprivation therapy for localized prostate cancer. Cancer. 2010;116:5226.
24. Zhang B, Zhou J, Wu S, et al. The impact of surgical margin status on prostate cancer-specific mortality after radical prostatectomy: a systematic review and meta-analysis. Clin Transl Oncol. 2020;22:2087.
25. Nielsen ME. How bad are positive margins after radical prostatectomy and how are they best managed? J Urol. 2009;182:1257.
26. Hong YM, Hu JC, Paciorek AT, et al. Impact of radical prostatectomy positive surgical margins on fear of cancer recurrence: results from CaPSURE. Urol Oncol. 2010;28:268.
27. Maubon T, Branger N, Bastide C, et al. Impact of the extent of extraprostatic extension defined by Epstein's method in patients with negative surgical margins and negative lymph node invasion. Prostate Cancer Prostatic Dis. 2016;19:317.
28. Magi-Galluzzi C, Evans AJ, Delahunt B, et al. International Society of Urological Pathology (ISUP) consensus conference on handling and staging of radical prostatectomy specimens. Working Group 3: extraprostatic extension, lymphovascular invasion and locally advanced disease. Mod Pathol. 2011;24:26.
29. Faisal FA, Tosoian JJ, Han M, et al. Clinical, pathological and oncologic findings of radical prostatectomy with extraprostatic extension diagnosed on preoperative prostate biopsy. J Urol. 2019;201:937.
30. Johnson MT, Ramsey ML, Ebel JJ, et al. Do robotic prostatectomy positive surgical margins occur in the same location as extraprostatic extension? World J Urol. 2014;32:761.
31. Gupta R, O'Connell R, Haynes AM, et al. Extraprostatic extension (EPE) of prostatic carcinoma: is its proximity to the surgical margin or Gleason score important? BJU Int. 2015;116:343.
32. Rosen MA, Goldstone L, Lapin S, et al. Frequency and location of extracapsular extension and positive surgical margins in radical prostatectomy specimens. J Urol. 1992;148:331.
33. Anderson BB, Oberlin DT, Razmaria AA, et al. Extraprostatic extension is extremely rare for contemporary gleason score 6 prostate cancer. Eur Urol. 2017;72:455.
34. Gandaglia G, Ploussard G, Valerio M, et al. The key combined value of multiparametric magnetic resonance imaging, and magnetic resonance imaging-targeted and concomitant systematic biopsies for the prediction of adverse pathological features in prostate cancer patients undergoing radical prostatectomy. Eur Urol. 2020;77:733.
35. Eifler JB, Feng Z, Lin BM, et al. An updated prostate cancer staging nomogram (Partin tables) based on cases from 2006 to 2011. BJU Int. 2013;111:22.
36. Memorial Sloan Kettering Cancer Center. Pre-radical prostatectomy.
37. Weinreb JC, Barentsz JO, Choyke PL, et al. PI-RADS prostate imaging—reporting and data system: 2015, version 2. Eur Urol. 2016;69:16.
38. Bjornebo L, Olsson H, Nordstrom T, et al. Predictors of adverse pathology on radical prostatectomy specimen in men initially enrolled in active surveillance for low-risk prostate cancer. World J Urol. 2021;39(6):1797–804.
39. Feng TS, Sharif-Afshar AR, Smith SC, et al. Multiparametric magnetic resonance imaging localizes established extracapsular extension of prostate cancer. Urol Oncol. 2015;33:109 e15.
40. Jansen BHE, Nieuwenhuijzen JA, Oprea-Lager DE, et al. Adding multiparametric MRI to the MSKCC and Partin nomograms for primary prostate cancer: improving local tumor staging? Urol Oncol. 2019;37:181 e1.
41. Wibmer A, Vargas HA, Donahue TF, et al. Diagnosis of extracapsular extension of prostate cancer on prostate MRI: impact of second-opinion readings by subspecialized genitourinary oncologic radiologists. AJR Am J Roentgenol. 2015;205:W73.
42. Baco E, Rud E, Vlatkovic L, et al. Predictive value of magnetic resonance imaging determined tumor contact length for extracapsular extension of prostate cancer. J Urol. 2015;193:466.
43. Kir G, Arikan EA, Seneldir H, et al. Determining the cut-off values of tumor diameter, degree of extraprostatic extension, and extent of surgical margin positivity with regard to biochemical recurrence of prostate cancer after radical prostatectomy. Ann Diagn Pathol. 2020;44:151431.
44. Sohayda C, Kupelian PA, Levin HS, et al. Extent of extracapsular extension in localized prostate cancer. Urology. 2000;55:382.
45. Epstein JI, Amin M, Boccon-Gibod L, et al. Prognostic factors and reporting of prostate carcinoma in radical prostatectomy and pelvic lymphadenectomy specimens. Scand J Urol Nephrol Suppl. 2005;34.
46. Chuang AY, Epstein JI. Positive surgical margins in areas of capsular incision in otherwise organ-confined disease at radical prostatectomy: histologic features and pitfalls. Am J Surg Pathol. 2008;32:1201.
47. Orosco RK, Tapia VJ, Califano JA, et al. Positive surgical margins in the 10 most common solid cancers. Sci Rep. 2018;8:5686.
48. Yossepowitch O, Bjartell A, Eastham JA, et al. Positive surgical margins in radical prostatectomy: outlining the problem and its long-term consequences. Eur Urol. 2009;55:87.
49. Costello AJ, Brooks M, Cole OJ. Anatomical studies of the neurovascular bundle and cavernosal nerves. BJU Int. 2004;94:1071.
50. Villers A, McNeal JE, Freiha FS, et al. Invasion of Denonvilliers' fascia in radical prostatectomy specimens. J Urol. 1993;149:793.
51. Bellangino M, Verrill C, Leslie T, et al. Systematic review of studies reporting positive surgical margins after bladder neck sparing radical prostatectomy. Curr Urol Rep. 2017;18:99.
52. Smolski M, Esler RC, Turo R, et al. Bladder neck sparing in radical prostatectomy. Indian J Urol. 2013;29:338.
53. Porcaro AB, Sebben M, Corsi P, et al. Risk factors of positive surgical margins after robot-assisted radical prostatectomy in high-volume center: results in 732 cases. J Robot Surg. 2020;14:167.
54. Zhang L, Zhao H, Wu B, et al. Predictive factors for positive surgical margins in patients with prostate cancer after radical prostatectomy: a systematic review and meta-analysis. Front Oncol. 2020;10:539592.
55. Marchetti PE, Shikanov S, Razmaria AA, et al. Impact of prostate weight on probability of positive surgical margins in patients with low-risk prostate cancer after robotic-assisted laparoscopic radical prostatectomy. Urology. 2011;77:677.
56. Patel VR, Coelho RF, Rocco B, et al. Positive surgical margins after robotic assisted radical prostatectomy: a multi-institutional study. J Urol. 2011;186:511.
57. Wadhwa H, Terris MK, Aronson WJ, et al. Long-term oncological outcomes of apical positive surgical margins at radical prostatectomy in the Shared Equal Access Regional Cancer Hospital cohort. Prostate Cancer Prostatic Dis. 2016;19:423.

58. Marcq G, Michelet A, Hannink G, et al. Risk of biochemical recurrence based on extent and location of positive surgical margins after robot-assisted laparoscopic radical prostatectomy. BMC Cancer. 2018;18:1291.
59. Mirmilstein G, Rai BP, Gbolahan O, et al. The neurovascular structure-adjacent frozen-section examination (NeuroSAFE) approach to nerve sparing in robot-assisted laparoscopic radical prostatectomy in a British setting—a prospective observational comparative study. BJU Int. 2018;121:854.
60. Preston MA, Breau RH, Lantz AG, et al. The association between nerve sparing and a positive surgical margin during radical prostatectomy. Urol Oncol. 2015;33:18 e1.
61. Beyer B, Schlomm T, Tennstedt P, et al. A feasible and time-efficient adaptation of NeuroSAFE for da Vinci robot-assisted radical prostatectomy. Eur Urol. 2014;66:138.
62. Carroll PR. A phase 1 study of IS-002 injection in patients undergoing robotic prostatectomy. 2020.
63. https://www.intuitive.com/en-us. 2021.
64. Derks YHW, Lowik D, Sedelaar JPM, et al. PSMA-targeting agents for radio- and fluorescence-guided prostate cancer surgery. Theranostics. 2019;9:6824.
65. Maurer T, Robu S, Schottelius M, et al. (99m)Technetium-based prostate-specific membrane antigen-radioguided surgery in recurrent prostate cancer. Eur Urol. 2019;75:659.
66. Olde Heuvel J, de Wit-van der Veen BJ, van der Poel HG, et al. (68)Ga-PSMA Cerenkov luminescence imaging in primary prostate cancer: first-in-man series. Eur J Nucl Med Mol Imaging. 2020;47:2624.
67. Bravi CA, Tin A, Vertosick E, et al. The impact of experience on the risk of surgical margins and biochemical recurrence after robot-assisted radical prostatectomy: a learning curve study. J Urol. 2019;202:108.
68. Martini A, Falagario UG, Villers A, et al. Contemporary techniques of prostate dissection for robot-assisted prostatectomy. Eur Urol. 2020;78:583.
69. Checcucci E, Veccia A, Fiori C, et al. Retzius-sparing robot-assisted radical prostatectomy vs the standard approach: a systematic review and analysis of comparative outcomes. BJU Int. 2020;125:8.
70. Umari P, Eden C, Cahill D, et al. Retzius-sparing versus standard robot-assisted radical prostatectomy: a comparative prospective study of nearly 500 patients. J Urol. 2021;205:780.
71. Stephenson AJ, Wood DP, Kattan MW, et al. Location, extent and number of positive surgical margins do not improve accuracy of predicting prostate cancer recurrence after radical prostatectomy. J Urol. 2009;182:1357.
72. Swindle P, Eastham JA, Ohori M, et al. Do margins matter? The prognostic significance of positive surgical margins in radical prostatectomy specimens. J Urol. 2008;179:S47.
73. Zhang L, Wu B, Zha Z, et al. Positive surgical margin is associated with biochemical recurrence risk following radical prostatectomy: a meta-analysis from high-quality retrospective cohort studies. World J Surg Oncol. 2018;16:124.
74. Gharzai LA, Jiang R, Wallington D, et al. Intermediate clinical endpoints for surrogacy in localised prostate cancer: an aggregate meta-analysis. Lancet Oncol. 2021;22:402.
75. Van den Broeck T, van den Bergh RCN, Briers E, et al. Biochemical recurrence in prostate cancer: the European Association of Urology Prostate Cancer Guidelines Panel recommendations. Eur Urol Focus. 2020;6:231.
76. Freedland SJ, Humphreys EB, Mangold LA, et al. Risk of prostate cancer-specific mortality following biochemical recurrence after radical prostatectomy. JAMA. 2005;294:433.
77. Sachdeva A, Veeratterapillay R, Voysey A, et al. Positive surgical margins and biochemical recurrence following minimally-invasive radical prostatectomy—an analysis of outcomes from a UK tertiary referral centre. BMC Urol. 2017;17:91.
78. Pfitzenmaier J, Pahernik S, Tremmel T, et al. Positive surgical margins after radical prostatectomy: do they have an impact on biochemical or clinical progression? BJU Int. 2008;102:1413.
79. Dev HS, Wiklund P, Patel V, et al. Surgical margin length and location affect recurrence rates after robotic prostatectomy. Urol Oncol. 2015;33:109 e7.
80. Keller EX, Bachofner J, Britschgi AJ, et al. Prognostic value of unifocal and multifocal positive surgical margins in a large series of robot-assisted radical prostatectomy for prostate cancer. World J Urol. 2019;37:1837.
81. Preisser F, Coxilha G, Heinze A, et al. Impact of positive surgical margin length and Gleason grade at the margin on biochemical recurrence in patients with organ-confined prostate cancer. Prostate. 2019;79:1832.
82. Servoll E, Vlatkovic L, Saeter T, et al. The length of a positive surgical margin is of prognostic significance in patients with clinically localized prostate cancer treated with radical prostatectomy. Urol Int. 2014;93:289.
83. Sofer M, Hamilton-Nelson KL, Civantos F, et al. Positive surgical margins after radical retropubic prostatectomy: the influence of site and number on progression. J Urol. 2002;167:2453.
84. Chalfin HJ, Dinizo M, Trock BJ, et al. Impact of surgical margin status on prostate-cancer-specific mortality. BJU Int. 2012;110:1684.
85. Mauermann J, Fradet V, Lacombe L, et al. The impact of solitary and multiple positive surgical margins on hard clinical end points in 1712 adjuvant treatment-naive pT2-4 N0 radical prostatectomy patients. Eur Urol. 2013;64:19.
86. Sooriakumaran P, Srivastava A, Shariat SF, et al. A multinational, multi-institutional study comparing positive surgical margin rates among 22393 open, laparoscopic, and robot-assisted radical prostatectomy patients. Eur Urol. 2014;66:450.
87. Boorjian SA, Thompson RH, Tollefson MK, et al. Long-term risk of clinical progression after biochemical recurrence following radical prostatectomy: the impact of time from surgery to recurrence. Eur Urol. 2011;59:893.
88. Pound CR, Partin AW, Eisenberger MA, et al. Natural history of progression after PSA elevation following radical prostatectomy. JAMA. 1999;281:1591.
89. Artibani W, Porcaro AB, De Marco V, et al. Management of biochemical recurrence after primary curative treatment for prostate cancer: a review. Urol Int. 2018;100:251.
90. Simmons MN, Stephenson AJ, Klein EA. Natural history of biochemical recurrence after radical prostatectomy: risk assessment for secondary therapy. Eur Urol. 2007;51:1175.
91. Ball MW, Partin AW, Epstein JI. Extent of extraprostatic extension independently influences biochemical recurrence-free survival: evidence for further pT3 subclassification. Urology. 2015;85:161.
92. Bill-Axelson A, Holmberg L, Ruutu M, et al. Radical prostatectomy versus watchful waiting in early prostate cancer. N Engl J Med. 2011;364:1708.
93. Epstein JI, Partin AW, Sauvageot J, et al. Prediction of progression following radical prostatectomy. A multivariate analysis of 721 men with long-term follow-up. Am J Surg Pathol. 1996;20:286.
94. Jiang W, Zhang L, Wu B, et al. Prognostic roles of extraprostatic extension in evaluating biochemical recurrence after radical prostatectomies: PRISMA-compliant systematic review and meta-analysis. Int J Clin Exp Med. 2019;12(5):4550–62. https://e-entury.us/web/journal_search.php?journal=ijcem&q=prognostic%20roles%20of%20extraprostatic%20extension. https://e-century.us/files/ijcem/12/5/ijcem0090957.pdf.
95. Eggener SE, Scardino PT, Walsh PC, et al. Predicting 15-year prostate cancer specific mortality after radical prostatectomy. J Urol. 2011;185:869.

96. Jeong BC, Chalfin HJ, Lee SB, et al. The relationship between the extent of extraprostatic extension and survival following radical prostatectomy. Eur Urol. 2015;67:342.
97. Farchoukh L, Laframboise WA, Nelson JB, et al. Multifocal extraprostatic extension of prostate cancer. Am J Clin Pathol. 2020;153:548.
98. Schaeffer E, Srinivas S, Antonarakis ES, et al. NCCN guidelines insights: prostate cancer, version 1.2021. J Natl Compr Canc Netw. 2021;19:134.
99. Bolla M, van Poppel H, Tombal B, et al. Postoperative radiotherapy after radical prostatectomy for high-risk prostate cancer: long-term results of a randomised controlled trial (EORTC trial 22911). Lancet. 2012;380:2018.
100. Thompson IM Jr, Tangen CM, Paradelo J, et al. Adjuvant radiotherapy for pathologically advanced prostate cancer: a randomized clinical trial. JAMA. 2006;296:2329.
101. Wiegel T, Bartkowiak D, Bottke D, et al. Adjuvant radiotherapy versus wait-and-see after radical prostatectomy: 10-year follow-up of the ARO 96-02/AUO AP 09/95 trial. Eur Urol. 2014;66:243.
102. Pisansky TM, Thompson IM, Valicenti RK, et al. Adjuvant and salvage radiotherapy after prostatectomy: ASTRO/AUA guideline amendment 2018-2019. J Urol. 2019;202:533.
103. NICE Guidance - Prostate cancer: diagnosis and management: (c) NICE (2019) Prostate cancer: diagnosis and management. BJU Int. 2019;124:9.
104. Balakrishnan AS, Zhao S, Cowan JE, et al. Trends and predictors of adjuvant therapy for adverse features following radical prostatectomy: an analysis from cancer of the prostate strategic urologic research endeavor. Urology. 2019;131:157.
105. Kneebone A, Fraser-Browne C, Duchesne GM, et al. Adjuvant radiotherapy versus early salvage radiotherapy following radical prostatectomy (TROG 08.03/ANZUP RAVES): a randomised, controlled, phase 3, non-inferiority trial. Lancet Oncol. 2020;21:1331.
106. Sargos P, Chabaud S, Latorzeff I, et al. Adjuvant radiotherapy versus early salvage radiotherapy plus short-term androgen deprivation therapy in men with localised prostate cancer after radical prostatectomy (GETUG-AFU 17): a randomised, phase 3 trial. Lancet Oncol. 2020;21:1341.
107. Parker CC, Clarke NW, Cook AD, et al. Timing of radiotherapy after radical prostatectomy (RADICALS-RT): a randomised, controlled phase 3 trial. Lancet. 2020;396:1413.
108. Sachdev S, Carroll P, Sandler H, et al. Assessment of post-prostatectomy radiotherapy as adjuvant or salvage therapy in patients with prostate cancer: a systematic review. JAMA Oncol. 2020;6:1793.
109. Tilki D, Chen M-H, Wu J, et al. Adjuvant versus early salvage radiation therapy for men at high risk for recurrence following radical prostatectomy for prostate cancer and the risk of death. J Clin Oncol. 2021;39(20):2284–93.

Managing Postoperative Complications After Robot-Assisted Radical Prostatectomy

Aldo Brassetti, Flavia Proietti, David Bouchier-Hayes, and Vito Pansadoro

1 Rectourethral Fistula

Rectourethral fistula (RUF) is a connection between the lower urinary tract and the distal part of the rectum. It was first described by Jones in 1858, although an earlier reference to a colovesical fistula is attributed to Rufus of Ephesus in 200 AD [1].

1.1 Incidence and Etiology

RUFs can be congenital or acquired. The first ones, usually related to imperforate anus, represent a small subset of this pathology and are managed by pediatric surgeons. Most of acquired RUFs are iatrogenic, resulting from prostate/bowel surgery or ablative treatments complications [1]; less commonly, fistulae can be a consequence of a trauma [2], Fournier' gangrene [3], or Crohn's disease [4].

The vast majority of RUFs are related to prostate cancer (PCa) treatment, and a 0.53–9% fistulization rate was observed after radical prostatectomy (RP) [5, 6], 0–6% after external beam radiotherapy (EBRT) [7], 0.4–8.8% after brachytherapy (BT) [8, 9], and 0.4–3% after cryotherapy and high-intensity focused ultrasound [10, 11]. Interestingly, while in the 1990s most of RUFs resulted from complications of prostate surgery, to date up to 52% of patients with a fistula has received radiation [12], often as a second-line treatment for biochemical recurrence. In contrast to primary treatment, in fact, salvage EBRT/BT could increase RUF incidence rate from 0.6 to 3% [13].

Considering that surgery still represents the most common treatment option in patients with a resectable tumor, most of the observed RUFs occur after prostatectomy and are often secondary to an unrecognized rectal injury (RI) during the operation [1]. According to a recent population-based study on 614,294 patients who underwent RP, perforation occurred in 2900 cases (0.5%) with a 26% decline from 2003–2006 to 2009–2012 ($p < 0.01$). Multivariable analysis identified concurrent benign prostatic hyperplasia (OR, 2.33; 95% CI, 1.16–4.69; p 0.02) and metastatic cancer (OR, 2.31; 95% CI, 1.53–3.5; $p < 0.01$) as predictors of RI, while robotic approach (OR, 0.38; 95% CI, 0.29–0.50; $p < 0.01$), high-volume hospital (OR, 0.58; 95% CI, 0.46–0.72; $p < 0.01$), and obesity (OR, 0.56; 95%CI, 0.34–0.93; p 0.02) reduced the risk [14]. Post-RP RUFs are commonly found in close proximity of the urethrovesical anastomosis: experts in the field observed that most of these fistulae are not actually located through the anastomosis but rather at the "tennis racket handle" between the ureters, where a foreign body (usually a hemostatic clip) migrated causing fibrosis and fistulization [13]. Prior radiation and/or ablative therapies increase the risk of fistula, in a dose-dependent manner, and decrease the likelihood of its spontaneous closure as a result of ischemia and fibrosis they induced [12]. Moreover, these therapies also complicate the repair surgery due to the lack of laxity and the avascularity of the surrounding tissues [7].

1.2 Diagnosis and Evaluation

RUF diagnosis is clinical, and an appropriate medical interview is imperative. Pneumaturia is the most common sign (67–85%) followed by urine leakage through the rectum during micturition (40–100%) and fecaluria (39–65%), which is also the most specific. Other common findings are recurrent urinary tract infections (73 %), abdominal pain (22 %), and dysuria (14.6%) [15]. An acute presentation (0–3 weeks from hospital discharge) is common in post-RP cases, while

A. Brassetti (✉)
Fondazione Vincenzo Pansadoro, Rome, Italy

IRCCS "Regina Elena" National Cancer Institute, Rome, Italy

F. Proietti · V. Pansadoro
Fondazione Vincenzo Pansadoro, Rome, Italy

D. Bouchier-Hayes
Galway Clinic, Galway, Ireland

P. Wiklund et al. (eds.), *Robotic Urologic Surgery*, https://doi.org/10.1007/978-3-031-00363-9_31

a delayed onset of symptoms (>14 weeks from treatment) is more common in irradiated patients.

Digital rectal examination allows identification of the fistula and direct size estimation: usually post-surgical RUFs are small and barely palpable, while those post-EBRT are larger.

Radiologic evaluation (CT scan, magnetic resonance imaging, voiding cystourethrogram, retrograde urethrography) and endoscopic procedures (cystoscopy, proctoscopy) help in delineating the anatomy and selecting the appropriate treatment strategies (Fig. 1).

1.3 Classification

The use of a standardized classification for RUFs would allow both selection of the optimal treatment for each patient and comparison of outcomes among different series. An attempt was done by Prof. Anthony Mundy, who distinguished between direct and cavitating fistulae merely on the basis of their morphological features [13]. Hanna et al. suggested to classify RUFs according to their distance from the rectal sphincter (<2 cm vs. >2 cm) as distal ones could better benefit from a transperineal approach rather that transsphincteric surgery. More clinically relevant was the classification proposed by Montorsi et al. (Table 1) who differentiated RUFs on the basis of their size and etiology. In fact, the diameter of the fistulae causes symptom burden (as smaller ones usually present with pneumaturia and are not associated with fecaluria and recurrent UTI) [7], while the vascularization of the surrounding tissues, which primarily depends on their degree of irradiation, affects chances to heal (99% success rate after RUFs repair when no prior non-surgical treatment has been administered vs. 87% for fistulas caused by treatment with energy ablation as either primary or adjuvant) [16].

1.4 Management

Although over 40 techniques have been described which all share the basic principles for urinary fistula surgical repair (Table 2), there is no consensus on the optimal approach,

Table 1 Classification of rectourethral fistulas after primary treatment of prostate cancer based on size and etiology

Stage	Size	Grade	Etiology
I	<1.5 cm	0	Surgical accidental rectal injury with no prior radiotherapy
II	>1.5 cm	1	Primary or adjuvant prostate cancer treatment modality that uses physical agents
III	Any diameter with urethral sphincter damage	2	Salvage prostatectomy or prostatic ablation

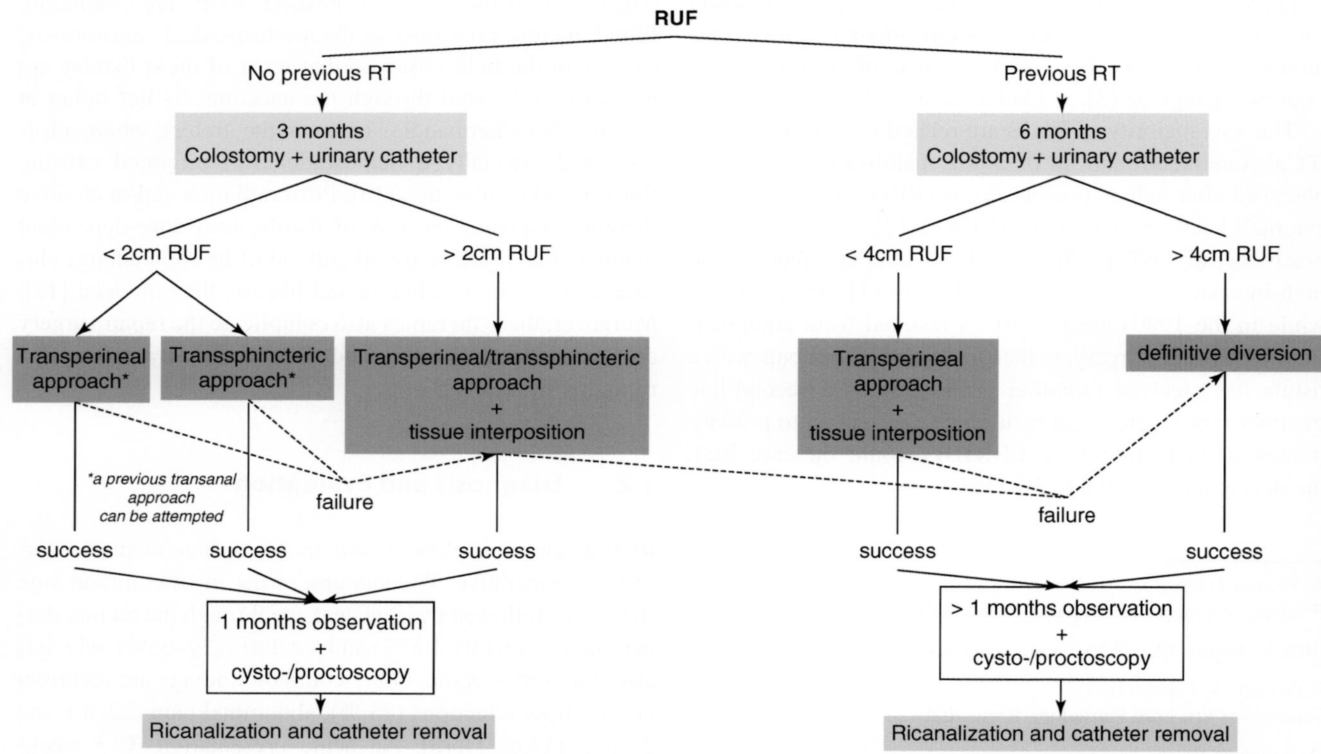

Fig. 1 Suggested algorithm to guide treatment selection in patients with RUFs

Table 2 Common principles of urinary fistulae surgical repair

Adequate exposure of the fistulous tract
Good hemostasis and minimal use of electrocautery
Well-vascularized, healthy tissue for repair
Multiple layer closure
Watertight closure of each layer
Tension-free, non-overlapping suture lines
Adequate urinary drainage after repair
Prevention of infection and nutritional optimization

whereby the vast majority of currently available studies consist of single-institution experiences, small case series, or case reports. Moreover, no comparative series with long-term follow-up are currently available to identify the best approach for patients with RUFs after PCa treatment.

1.4.1 Conservative Management

It has been suggested that a RUF might close spontaneously, but it only occurred within 6 weeks from PCa surgery, before the track had epithelialized [17]. Otherwise, there is no report of an established fistula closing spontaneously and permanently, and no suggestion at all that a post-irradiation one would do so [18–20].

In the early post-RP period, in order to control symptoms, an indwelling catheter and a colostomy may be necessary, especially in patients with extravasation of urine and fecal leakage: as the flow gradient is from the urinary tract to the rectum, the catheter is more likely to be helpful than fecal diversion [13]. As a matter of fact, most patients with RUF, whether post-surgical or post-irradiation, receive a colostomy either in the hope that this might promote a spontaneous healing or otherwise to "prepare" the subsequent repair. The decision to perform a temporary colostomy/ileostomy is not standardized, and some groups base this decision on clinical facts: for patients only suffering from pneumaturia or urine leakage through the anus, resolution through a low-residue diet is first attempted, while those experiencing fecaluria or sepsis are considered for colostomy straightaway [13, 17, 18].

In recent years, new approaches using sealant or fibrin glue [21] have emerged. In 2001, Bardari et al. reported the use of cyanoacrylate glue for the treatment of a post-RP fistula [22]. Similarly, Bhandari et al. further resorted to the same approach to heal a neobladder fistula after radical cystoprostatectomy [23]. These reports of favorable outcomes are however anecdotal, and further cases are necessary to validate those results.

1.4.2 Transanal Approaches

The Latzko Procedure

First conceived in 1914 for the treatment of vesicovaginal or enterovaginal fistulae, the transanal Latzko technique was used by Noldus et al. in 1997 to repair RUFs occurred after radical retropubic prostatectomy [24]. Although it provides poor visibility and limited instruments maneuverability, it is simple, does not require fistulous tract excision, and may be repeated as many times as necessary. It is indicated for small proximal fistulae.

The patient is placed in the lithotomy position, and cystoscopy is performed to localize the fistula. A 5F ureteral catheter is placed through the fistula endoscopically, and the area of the fistula at the site of the rectum is exposed with an anal retractor. Trendelenburg position may improve the visualization of the anterior rectal wall. A solution containing adrenalin (1:20,000) is injected around the fistulous opening to facilitate dissection and decrease bleeding. A circular area of rectal mucosa is incised for 1.0–1.5 cm from the fistulous opening. The rectal mucosa is denuded in four quadrants (Fig. 2a). No rectal mucosa is allowed to remain between the edges of the incision and the fistulous opening. The ureteral catheter is removed, and the fistula is closed with two layers of separate side-by-side 3-0 absorbable sutures (Fig. 2b, c). The margins of the rectal wound are similarly closed thereafter. A transurethral Foley catheter is placed in the bladder.

Endorectal Wall Advancement Flap

The use of transanal flaps in the management of fistulas involving the rectum was first published by Jones et al. in 1987 [25] and further popularized by Dreznik for the treatment of RUFs [26]. The technique is simple and safe, does not require a colostomy, and avoids any division of the sphincteric mechanism. It is indicated for proximal fistulae.

The operation is performed in the prone jack-knife position with the table flexed at the level of the hip joint. A self-retaining Parks' self-retaining anal retractor is inserted, to expose the anterior rectal wall. A local injection of diluted adrenalin (1:20,000) may decrease bleeding and ease dissection. The fistulous tract is excised to leave a transverse defect of 1–2 cm in the anterior rectal wall. A longitudinal incision is made in the rectum from each lateral edge of the defect for 3–4 cm proximally, and an intersphincteric sharp dissection is performed so that a U-shaped rectal flap can be obtained (Fig. 3a). The defect in the urethra is closed using 3-0 absorbable interrupted sutures (Fig. 3b). The rectal flap is then advanced over the fistula and sutured to the rectal wall with interrupted 2-0 braided sutures ensuring the absence of tension (Fig. 3c). Three weeks later, the urinary catheter is removed.

To overcome the inherent limitations of poor visibility and limited instrument maneuverability that characterize transanal approaches, the resort to endoscopic microsurgery (TEM-TAMIS) has also been proposed, with different treatments of the fistulous tract, urethral orifice, and rectal opening: experiences in this field are limited to small series and case reports [27–30].

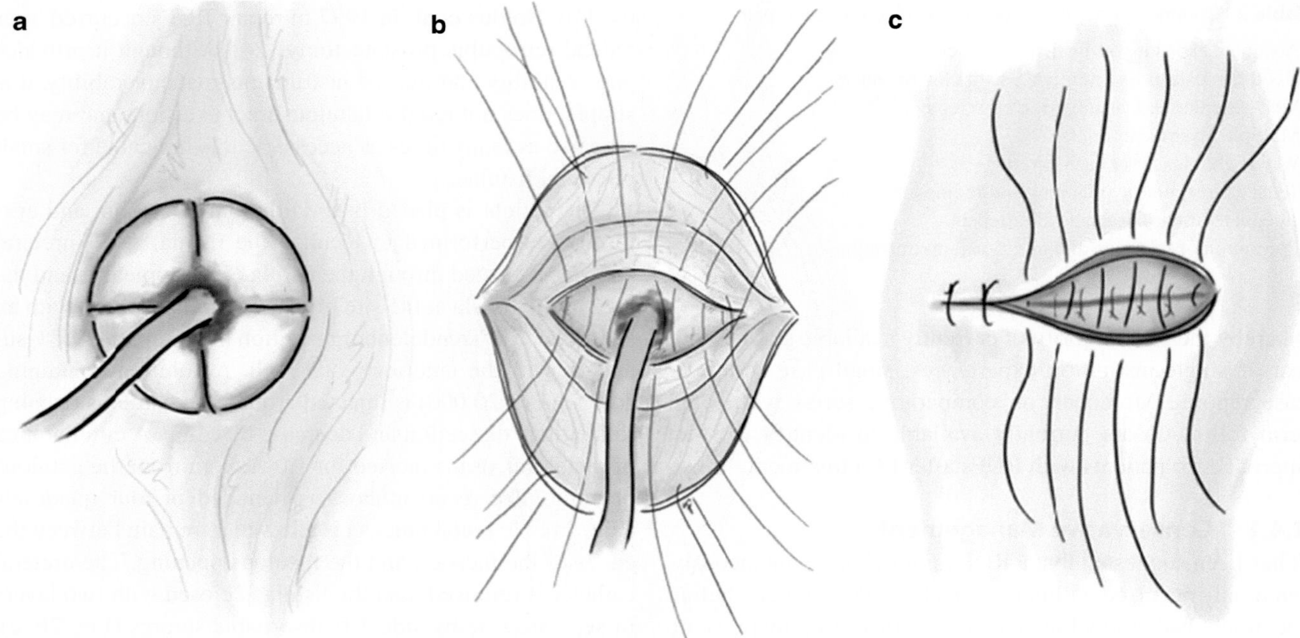

Fig. 2 A circular area of rectal mucosa is incised for 1.0–1.5 cm from the fistulous opening, and the rectal mucosa is denuded in four quadrants (**a**). The ureteral catheter is removed, and the fistula is closed with two layers of separate side-by-side 3-0 absorbable sutures (**b**). The margins of the rectal wound are similarly closed thereafter (**c**)

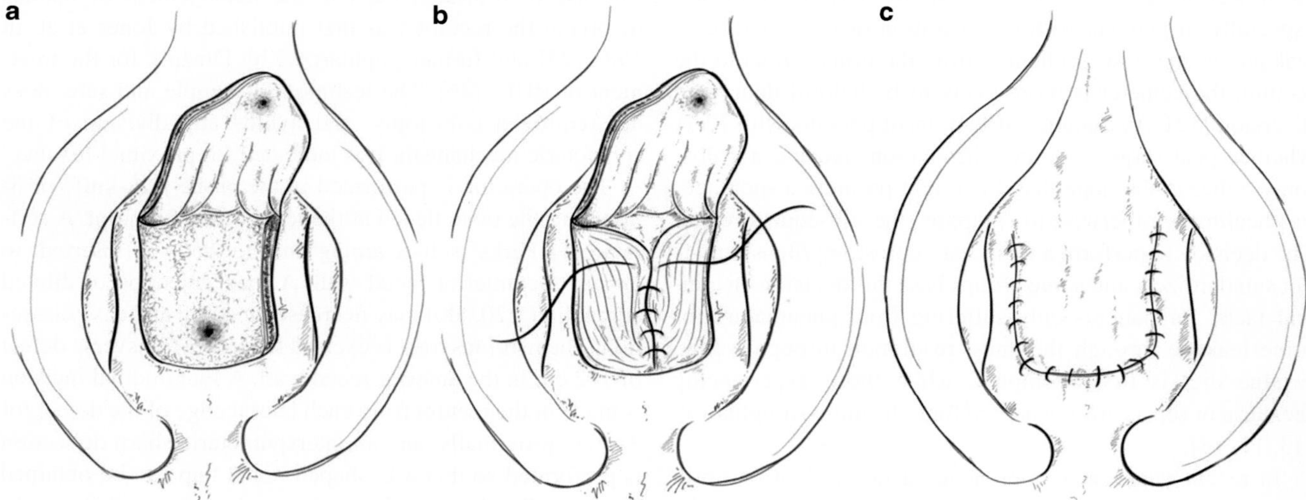

Fig. 3 Approximately 1 cm far from the fistulous tract, a U-shaped incision of the anterior rectal wall is performed, and an intersphincteric sharp dissection is carried on until a flap is obtained (**a**). The defect at the level of the urinary tract is closed using 3-0 absorbable interrupted sutures (**b**). The fistulous tract is resected from the rectal flap which is then advanced over the fistula and sutured to the rectal wall with interrupted 2-0 braided sutures (**c**)

1.4.3 Transperineal Repair

First described by H.H. Young in 1926, the transperineal approach for the treatment of RUFs was popularized by Goodwin in the 1950s. The technique is popular among urologists as they are familiar with this surgical route to the prostate gland. It provides a good exposure of the fistula and allows for tissue interposition between the rectum and the urinary tract. Its success rate ranges between 78 and 100%, with one or several interventions [31, 32].

The patient is placed in a lithotomy position, and a transurethral catheter is inserted. A wide inverted-U-shaped perineal incision is made outside the anus (2 cm far from its

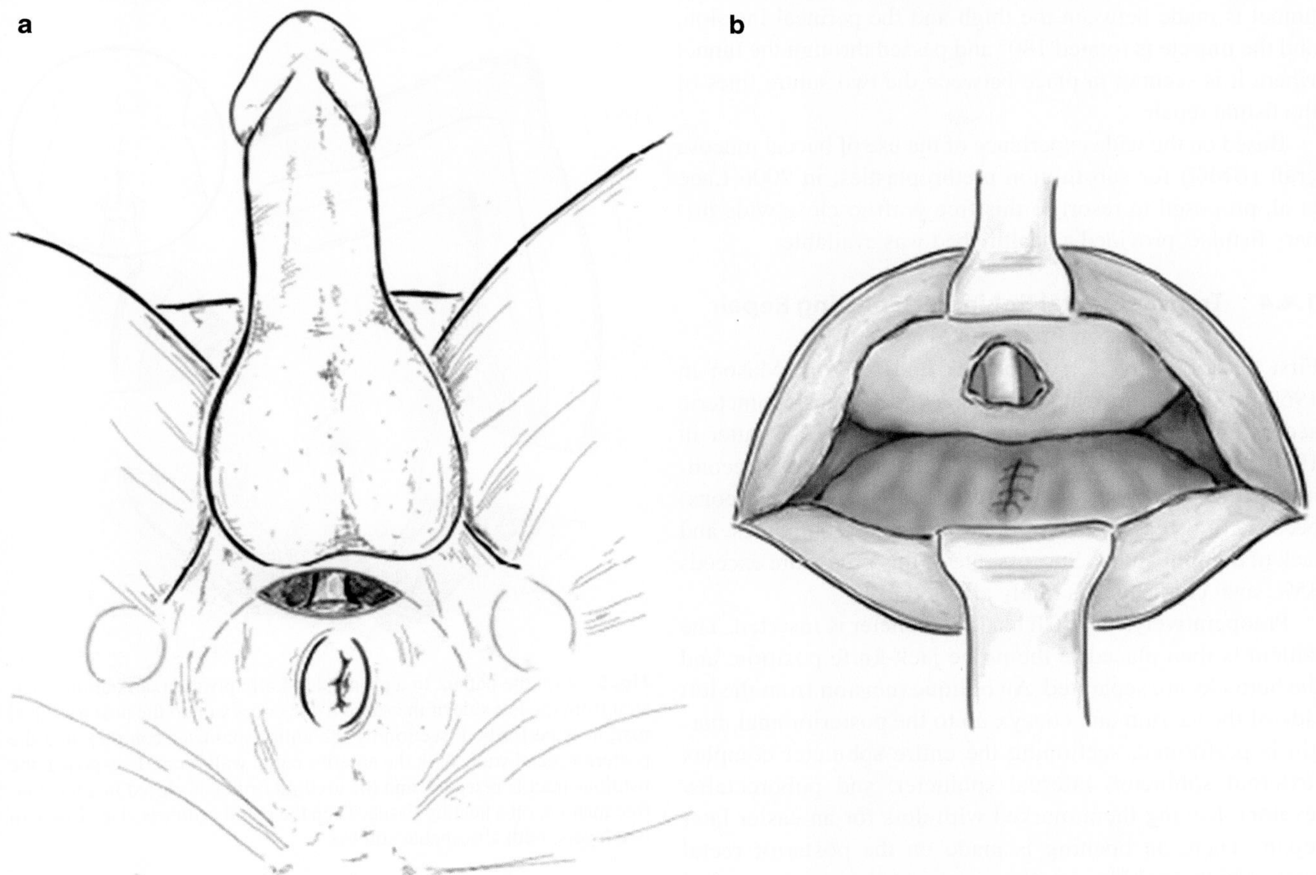

Fig. 4 With the patient in a lithotomy position, a wide inverted-U-shaped perineal incision is made outside the anus and inside the ischial tuberosities (**a**). With blunt dissection, the two ischiorectal fossae are developed. The central tendon of the perineum is transected, and the anterior rectal wall exposed. The fistulous tract is carefully identified and excised: the urethral and rectal orifices are released and sutured in two planes, forming a right angle between them (**b**)

verge) and inside the ischial tuberosities (Fig. 4a). The subcutaneous tissue is divided, and a fingertip is used to bluntly develop the two ischiorectal fossae. The central tendon of the perineum is transected, and the anterior rectal wall exposed. The scarring between the urethra, the bladder, and the anterior rectal wall is dissected sharply until the fistulous tract is identified and completely excised. The preoperative endoscopic placement of a Pollack catheter through the fistula may help in identifying it during surgery. Both the urethral and rectal orifices are released and sutured in two planes, forming a right angle between them (Fig. 4b). Lane first proposed implanting a buccal mucosa patch to close wide fistulas, ensuring a healthy and epithelized tissue [12]. Adequate separation of the urinary tract from the rectum by the interposition of either the levator ani muscle or other transposition flaps [33] (with the gracilis [31], dartos [34], and gluteal muscles [35]) is advised, especially in the setting of post-radiation fibrosis, large/multiple fistulas, or other risk factors for failure of primary repair [33] (Fig. 1). A perineal drainage is left in place. The bladder catheter should not be removed before 14–60 days. To restore intestinal continuity, a mean accepted period is 3 months.

In 1979, Ryan first used the gracilis muscle for the treatment of three urinary fistulae: since then the technique has been replicated by many authors with high healing rates (83–95%), although the published series are very limited [31, 32]. Spiegel et al. also proposed an endoscopic approach to harvest the flap [36].

With the patient in a lithotomy position, an 8-cm longitudinal incision is made on the medial thigh, starting at the estimated location of the vascular pedicle (which can be identified on the anterior boarder of the muscle with the help of Doppler). A small counter incision is made distally over the site of insertion of the muscle just below the medial condyle of the tibia. The muscle is lifted off the belly of the underlying adductor magnus with cautery and blunt dissection. The distal tendinous insertion is transected, and the muscle is pulled through the proximal incision. Then, a tunnel is made between the thigh and the perineal incision, and the muscle is rotated 180° and passed through the tunnel where it is secured in place between the two suture lines of the fistula repair.

Based on the wide experience of the use of buccal mucosa graft (BMG) for substitution urethroplasties, in 2006 Lane et al. proposed to resort to this free graft to close wide urinary fistulae, provided a healthy bed was available.

1.4.4 Transanorectal Sphincter-Splitting Repair (York Mason Procedure)

First described by F.R. Kilpatrick and A. York Mason in 1969 [37] with a parasacral-coccygeal trans-sphincteric access, the technique was further modified by the latter in 1970 [38]. With small variations this approach is recommended by numerous authors (especially general surgeons) because of its ease, accessibility, satisfactory outcomes, and lack of complications. Success rate of this procedure exceeds 85%; anal continence is rarely affected [39].

Preoperatively, an 18Ch bladder catheter is inserted. The patient is then placed in the prone jack-knife position, and the buttocks are separated. An oblique incision from the left side of the sacrum and coccyx up to the posterior anal margin is performed, sectioning the entire sphincter complex (external sphincter, internal sphincter, and puborectalis/levator), leaving them marked with dots for an easier later repair. Then, an opening is made on the posterior rectal wall, which enables a perfect view of the anterior rectal aspect with its fistulous orifice. The entire fistulous tract is resected, including the rectal wall, the urethral wall, and the surrounding tissues, thus enabling the correct suture of healthy tissues. There is no consensus regarding the need for urethral orifice closure (unless it is achieved in a tension-free manner and on healthy tissue), while the rectal orifice should be closed in two planes (submucosa and muscle in the first, everted mucosa in the second) both with absorbable stitches (Fig. 5). The urethral and rectal sutures should not overlap: occasionally, a rectal advancement flap is required [2]. The final step is the closure of the posterior rectal wall and sphincter and subcutaneous and skin reconstruction, leaving a suction drainage at the subcutaneous level for 24–48 h. The bladder catheter should remain placed for 6–8 weeks. With respect to the need of a fecal diversion, even though most authors recommend it, the possibility of omitting it is also accepted in cases of small fistulae, without extensive fibrosis, and in the absence of uncontrolled systemic infection, sepsis, or abscess [39]. If a colostomy is made, the closure will take place between 2 and 3 months after the procedure. Prior to restoring the intestinal continuity, the complete closure of the fistula should be confirmed by cystoscopy, retrograde cystourethrogram, rectoscopy, and even opaque enema, to confirm there is no communication.

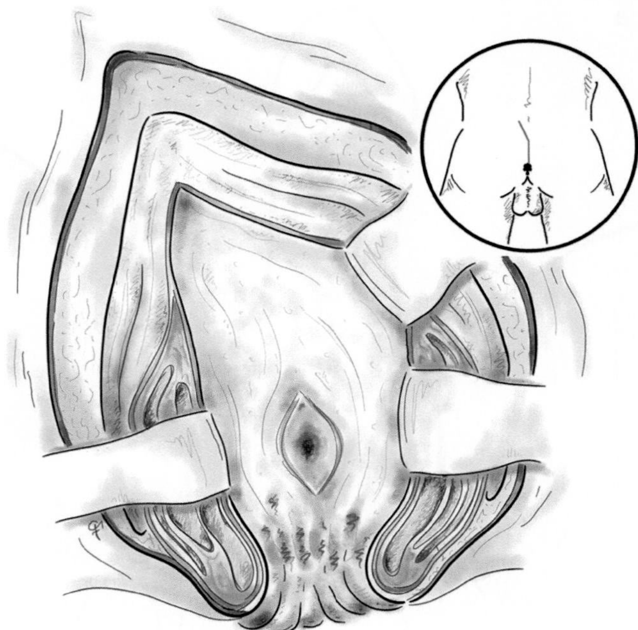

Fig. 5 With the patient in a prone jack-knife position, an oblique incision from the left side of the sacrum and coccyx up to the posterior anal margin is performed, sectioning the entire sphincter complex and the posterior rectal wall. With the anterior rectal wall properly exposed, the fistulous tract is resected, and the urethral orifice is closed in a tension-free manner, on a healthy tissue. Then the rectal orifice is also closed, in two layers, with absorbable stitches

1.4.5 Transabdominal

This has been for decades the less commonly used approach. Although it provides access to both the omentum and peritoneum so that pedunculated and free flap for interposition could be obtained, open surgery via a violated abdominal cavity implies greater morbidity and, more importantly, poor exposure of the deep pelvis. In recent years, a renewed interest toward this route was observed thanks to minimally invasive techniques. Using a laparoscopic approach, Sotelo et al. treated three patients with simple RUF [40], while Bollens successfully treated a 5-cm-wide recto-vesical fistula [41]. Similarly, other authors recently shared their experiences with the use of a robot-assisted approach in this field [42, 43].

1.4.6 Urinary Diversion

In certain extremely complex cases, a permanent urinary and/or fecal diversion and even pelvic exenteration may be needed [7, 12, 18].

2 Lymphocele

The word "lymph" derives from the Roman deity of fresh water, *Lympha*. First termed as lymphocyst by Mori in 1955 [44], lymphocele (LY) is a collection of lymphatic fluid surrounded by a fibrotic wall that lacks epithelial lining.

2.1 Incidence and Etiology

The pathophysiology of LY formation is largely speculative: during lymph node dissection (LND), leaking fluid from unsealed lymph channels may collect in the pelvis being further walled off from the peritoneal cavity, confined into a pseudocyst with a hard fibrous capsule. If lymphadenectomy is not performed, the risk of LYs is negligible [45].

Their true incidence has not been defined yet, as most are asymptomatic. Orvieto et al. routinely performed postoperative CT scans at 6 and 12 weeks after surgery in 76 men that underwent robot-assisted radical prostatectomy (RARP) with pelvic LND (PNLD): 51% of patients developed LYs, and 15% of which were symptomatic [46].

Various authors investigated possible risk factors for LY formation, but results were inconclusive. Capitanio et al. highlighted that lymph node yield during PLND was an independent predictor, and, for every node removed additional to a threshold of 20, the risk increased by 5% [47]. Conversely, Khoder et al. found no correlation between the number of excised lymph nodes and the rate of LY [48]. Interestingly, Liss [45] provided evidence that also the actual extent of PLND does not predict the risk of LY formation, and, in a longitudinal study on patients that underwent RARP with extended ($n = 202$) or standard PLND ($n = 204$), no differences in the rate of radiologic (22% vs. 23%) and symptomatic LYs (3% vs. 2.5%) were observed [49].

Another potential risk factor for LY formation is performing an extraperitoneal vs. a transperitoneal prostatectomy. In fact, it is thought that the latter approach promotes reabsorption of the lymphatic fluid by the peritoneum. So far, there have been no prospective randomized trials attempting to verify this hypothesis, and few supporting evidences arise from retrospective analyses [50, 51]. Interestingly, Stolzenburg et al. observed a significant reduction in incidence of LY following extraperitoneal radical prostatectomy (RP) and PLND by bilateral peritoneal fenestration, compared to conventional technique (radiologic LYs, 6% vs. 32%; $p < 0.001$; symptomatic LYs, 0% vs. 14%; $p < 0.001$) [52].

Since lymph also contains coagulative factors as plasma, the use of perioperative heparin (to prevent deep vein thrombosis [DVT] and pulmonary embolism [PE]) could prolong the closure of the afferent lymphatic channels injured during LND. However, this theoretical correlation is still controversial: Tomic et al. observed a sevenfold greater incidence of LY formation in patients that received heparin [53], while other studies failed to prove the same [54]. Overall, the potential for life-threatening thromboembolic events should overweight the possible increased risk of LYs with perioperative low-molecular-weight heparin.

2.2 Clinical Spectrum

Although most LYs occur asymptomatically, up to 15% can become symptomatic [46] because of superinfection (causing fever and/or sepsis) or compression on adjacent structures (potentially resulting in abdominal discomfort, venous drainage impairment, lower limb edema, DVT/PE). While thromboembolic events after RARP with PLND are rare (<1%), LY infection occurs in a non-negligible percentage of cases (3%), and Gram-positive cocci represent the most common (73%) causative organisms [55], probably coming from skin flora. Although codified antibiotic regimens are not available yet, patients with infected LYs should be treated for about 4–6 weeks, similar to abdominal abscess, and Gram-positive coverage is a reasonable empiric therapy choice; in case of sepsis, anti-*Pseudomonas* and anti-anaerobes agents such as piperacillin/tazobactam or cefepime plus metronidazole should be considered [55].

2.3 Management

2.3.1 Potential Preventative Strategies

Various strategies to prevent LY formation have been explored over the years. Leaving a drain longer to divert lymphorrhea sounds intuitive; however, a randomized study demonstrated no statistically significant difference in the incidence of LY (asymptomatic and symptomatic) between patients that had their drain in place for 1 day, 7 days, or no drainage at all [51]. These results were further confirmed by Chenam et al., in a robotic series [56]. Similarly, Gotto et al. found that the number of pelvic drains does not predict the risk of symptomatic LYs after RP with LND [57]. Probably, pelvic drainage adds little value to prevent this complication, and most of the studies failed to prove its role as tubes were removed quite early, considering that most lymph collections are diagnosed 3 weeks after surgery [58].

It is commonly believed that a meticulous ligation of the afferent lymphatic channels minimizes lymphorrhea. Few authors identified monopolar energy as the worst sealing technique, followed by bipolar and ultrasonic energy, while clips appeared as the most effective option [46, 59].

On the contrary, a Swiss prospective randomized trial failed to prove any difference between the use of clips and electrical coagulation during RARP with PLND in terms of overall (47% vs. 48%; $p = 0.9$) and symptomatic (5% vs. 4%; $p = 0.7$) LY rates [60]. Indeed, the major limitation of that study was the application of titanium clips only at the femoral canal; as such, Devis and colleagues reported an <1% incidence of LY after extensive clipping during PLND [61].

Fibrant and hemostatic sealants (such as Floseal [62], Tachosil [63], Arista AH [64], Vivostat [65]) have been proposed as adjuvant measures to mitigate lymphorrhea, but definitive evidence in their favor still lacks.

The transperitoneal approach to prostatectomy has been associated to a reduced risk of LYs [50, 51]. In case the extraperitoneal route is chosen instead, making large fenestration in the peritoneum at the end of the procedure may prevent lymph from collecting in a closed space [52].

In 2012, at the Lahey Institute of Urology, the *peritoneal interposition flap* was conceived: after transperitoneal RP with PLND, the visceral serosa covering the bladder is folded on its lateral aspects and sutured there to prevent the organ from adhering to and walling off the LND bed while allowing continuous egress of lymphatic fluid into the peritoneal cavity. Its efficacy was proved in a non-randomized study, where the LY rate in the Lahey-stitch group was 0% vs. 11.6% in the control group [66]. This technique was slightly modified by Dal Moro [67] and Stolzemburg [68], who provided evidence that peritoneum reconfigurations (Fig. 6) significantly reduce the risk of pelvic lymph collections. Results from randomized controlled studies (NCT03567525) are awaited.

2.3.2 Treatment Options

Once considered the treatment of choice, surgical evacuation with fenestration or marsupialization (either via laparotomy or laparoscopy) is nowadays outdone by a wide range of radiologic interventions. At present, the gold standard treatment option is percutaneous catheter drainage; sclerotherapy with chemical agents can improve its efficacy by triggering a chemical reaction that obliterates the lymph vessels and cavity preventing further leakage. As little data exist, consensus is lacking on the best sclerosing agent, its dosage, and the length of administration. Ethanol, povidone-iodine, and tetracyclines are frequently used, as these are affordable, easily available and generally well tolerated.

Other LY treatment options include percutaneous fine needle aspiration and embolization during lymphangiography (in which *N*-butyl cyanoacrylate glue is directly injected into lymph nodes or lymph vessels to treat downstream leaks). According to a recent systematic review, lymph aspiration provided the lowest success rate (0.341; 95% CI, 0.185–0.542), followed by percutaneous catheter placement (0.612; 95% CI, 0.490–0.722). When sclerotherapy was added, efficacy increased up to 0.890 (95% CI, 0.781–0.948) for delayed addition and 0.872 (95% CI, 0.710–0.949) for instantaneous addition. The embolization group showed the highest success rate (0.922; 95% CI, 0.731–0.981). Complication rate was the highest after percutaneous catheter drainage, while lymph node embolization appeared as the safest approach. However, further prospective research with correction for predisposing and aggravating factors, and focus on differentiation between primary and secondary treatments, is required to ultimately determine the optimal treatment modality for symptomatic postoperative pelvic LYs [69].

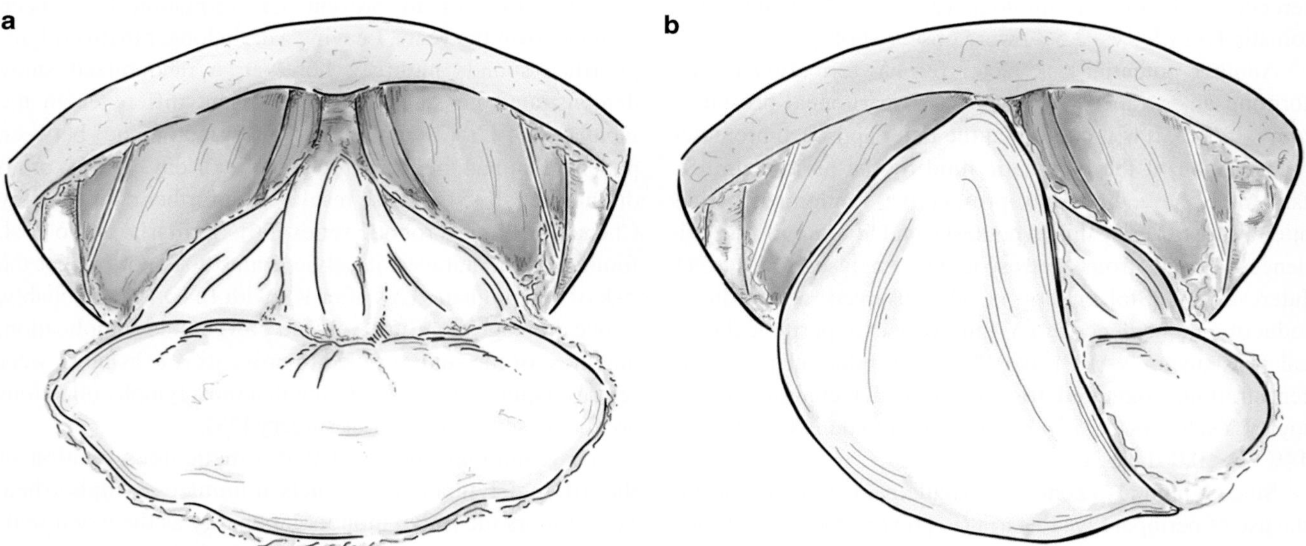

Fig. 6 The concept of *peritoneal advancement flap* requires that the visceral serosa covering the bladder is exposed to the iliac vessels and obturator fossae. To achieve this, the peritoneum-lined aspects of the taken-down bladder (**a**) are sutured to the anterior and lateral pelvic sidewalls (**b**)

3 Vesico-urethral Anastomotic Stenosis

Bladder neck contracture (BNC), also termed as vesico-urethral anastomotic stenosis (VUAS), is a potential complication after radical prostatectomy (RP) which presents as scar tissue obstructing the bladder outlet.

3.1 Incidence and Etiology

Its true incidence is unknown as there are no available studies routinely assessing urethral patency after surgery: thus, only patients complaining for postoperative voiding symptoms have been eventually diagnosed with BNC. Interestingly, the rate has declined over the years as it was 2.6–7.5% after open RP (ORP) vs. 0–2.1% in the robot-assisted era [70, 71].

The underlying molecular mechanisms are poorly understood: in the physiological wound healing process, fibrogenesis is tightly regulated and leads to successful tissue repair. If the fragile balance between cytokines, growth factors, mesenchymal cells, and extracellular matrix is deregulated, excessive scar tissue formation may happen. It is thought that an association between peripheral vascular disease and BNC exists: in fact, current cigarette smoking is its strongest independent predictor, followed by coronary artery disease, hypertension, and diabetes [72]. Similarly, men undergoing adjuvant radiotherapy showed a twofold increased risk of VUAS [73] compared to prostatectomy alone. The type of suture used for the anastomosis and the duration of catheterization do not affect contracture incidence, while an increased number of sutures/takes does [70, 72].

3.2 Clinical Presentation and Diagnosis

Most symptoms occur within 6–12 months from RP: obstructed urine flow, recurrent infections, retention, and occasionally urinary incontinence are strongly suggestive of BNC [74].

According to international guidelines, the workup should start with a medical interview, and baseline continence status should be assessed. Urinalysis with culture should be included to rule out other etiologies that may mimic stenosis; prostate-specific antigen test should be performed to exclude cancer recurrence. Uroflowmetry and post-void residual urine measurement could be considered to objectify symptoms. Cystoscopy is helpful to confirm clinical suspicion of BNC, and it is crucial to identify stenotic involvement of the external sphincter. Also retrograde urography with voiding cystogram could provide valuable information about the status of anterior and posterior urethra [75]: it is usually reserved for cases in which complete cystourethroscopy cannot be performed for multiple strictures, complete urethral obliteration, and patients unwilling to undergo a procedure in an ambulatory setting [76].

3.3 Management

3.3.1 Dilation

Interruption of the stenotic bladder neck is the central premise of endourologic procedures for VUAS. However, according to SIU/ICUD consultation on urethral strictures, dilation is indicated in early postoperative stenoses (<6 months) [76]. The endoscopic placement of a guidewire and the use of co-axial sounds or balloon dilators will reduce the risk of false passage creation or disruption of a fresh anastomosis. Up to 59% success rate has been reported for these approaches; very few evidences, however, support favorable long-term outcomes [77, 78].

3.3.2 Direct Vision Internal Urethrotomy (DVIU)

For strictures that fail initial dilation or occur >6 weeks after RP, a low-energy urethrotomy is recommended [76, 79]. There is low-level evidence supporting a certain superiority of holmium laser over cold-knife incision [80]. The original technique was proposed by Dalkin in 1996: two deep incisions at 4 and 8 o'clock positions are performed with a cold-knife urethrotome, down to the bleeding tissue, from the proximal area of the contracture to its distal extent. Pinpoint coagulation is only used in case of major arterial bleeding. At the end of the procedure, a 20–22 Ch urethral catheter is left in place for 72 h [81]. A *triradial* technique was further proposed by Vanni et al. [82]: however, aggressive incisions at 6 and 12 o'clock positions are strongly discouraged because of the risk of rectal injury and urosymphyseal fistulation, respectively [83]. DVIU for obliterative VUAS is not advised because of the limited success rate and the considerable risk of perforation [84]. De novo urinary incontinence was observed in 0–10% of cases; interestingly, a non-negligible (20–52%) share of patients with pre-existing leakage experienced improvements after surgery [85, 86]. Patency after the first urethrotomy ranges between 25 and 80% [85, 86]; repetitive endoluminal treatments can be attempted to stabilize recalcitrant strictures [79], but ultimately 6–10% of patients will require permanent urinary diversion [87]. Intralesional injections of different drugs were also attempted to treat recurrent BNCs: after corticosteroid injections the success rate was 50–100% [88, 89] and 58–79% after mitomycin C [90, 91]. With this regard, however, Redshaw et al. also reported osteitis pubis, bladder neck necrosis, and rectourethral fistula in few patients which had the latter drug injected [90].

The role of intermittent self-catheterization in reducing recurrence after surgery has not been established yet: we recommend *self-hydropneumatic dilations* for a couple of weeks after DVIU, which is achieved by means of intermittent compressions of penile urethra during micturition.

3.3.3 Transurethral Electrosurgical Incision/Resection (TUR)

It has been used when dilation and DVIU have failed. The greater risk of incontinence (14–50%) should be considered against the likelihood of long-term urethral patency (40%) [84, 89, 92].

3.3.4 ReDo Vesico-urethral Anastomosis and Y-V Plasty

All endoscopic therapies inherit the risk of recurrence: in these patients further attempts should be avoided, and surgical reconstruction of the vesico-urethral anastomosis (VUA) discussed. Temporary suprapubic cystostomy drainage will allow planning for reconstruction. Patient age, previous surgery or radiation, cancer stage, and life expectancy must be assessed before intervention. The primary goal should be urethral patency, with many men requiring an artificial urinary sphincter (after 3–6 months, at least) [76, 79].

Different techniques (abdominal retropubic, transperineal, combined) and approaches (open [93, 94], robotic [95–97]) have been proposed. With this regard, the introduction of the SP-DaVinci platform may offer significant advantages allowing the surgeon to operate in extremely narrow spaces [96].

In patients with adequate bladder function and in the absence of periurethral pathology (necrosis, calcifications, fistulas), the retropubic/abdominal route should be preferred [76, 79]: if an extensive urethral mobilization can be avoided, preservation of continence is possible. In these cases, the bladder neck is approached anteriorly by developing the space of Retzius. The dissection is then carried inferiorly, beneath the pubic symphysis, to the area of the bladder neck. At this point, either a urethral catheter or flexible cystoscope may be placed to identify the location and distal extent of stenosis. The bladder can be opened anteriorly at the bladder neck to help localize the proximal extent of the scar, which is excised completely using electrocautery and sharp dissection. Once the bladder neck is circumferentially freed, the VUA is re-sewn. Alternatively Y-V plasty of the bladder neck can be performed: this avoids dissection of the stenotic urethra posteriorly and any potential rectal complications. A longitudinal incision through the anterior aspect of the scar is performed, and then an inverted-V incision is made on the anterior aspect of the bladder wall, at the level of the bladder neck. The apex of the V-shaped bladder flap is advanced into the distal aspect of the scar incision (Fig. 7). Patency rates vary between 83 and 100%, with 14–45 months of follow-up. De novo incontinence rate ranges from 0 to 14% [94–97].

The transperineal approach inherits the advantages of operating in an unspoiled surgical field and allows for an easier mobilization of the urethra; incontinence, however, is unavoidable. The patient is placed in an exaggerate lithotomy position. A transperineal inverted-U-shaped incision is performed, and the urethra is dissected under digital rectal examination. A complete exposition of the anastomotic area is obtained, and the scar is excised until healthy tissue is reached. Wide mobilization of both the urethra and bladder should be obtained to guarantee a tension-free anastomosis. The urethra is spatulated dorsally, and the reanastomosis is sutured under direct vision control [93]. To increase visualization of anatomical structures, the use of a robotic camera has been recently proposed [98]. Patency rate up to 90% was reported [93, 98].

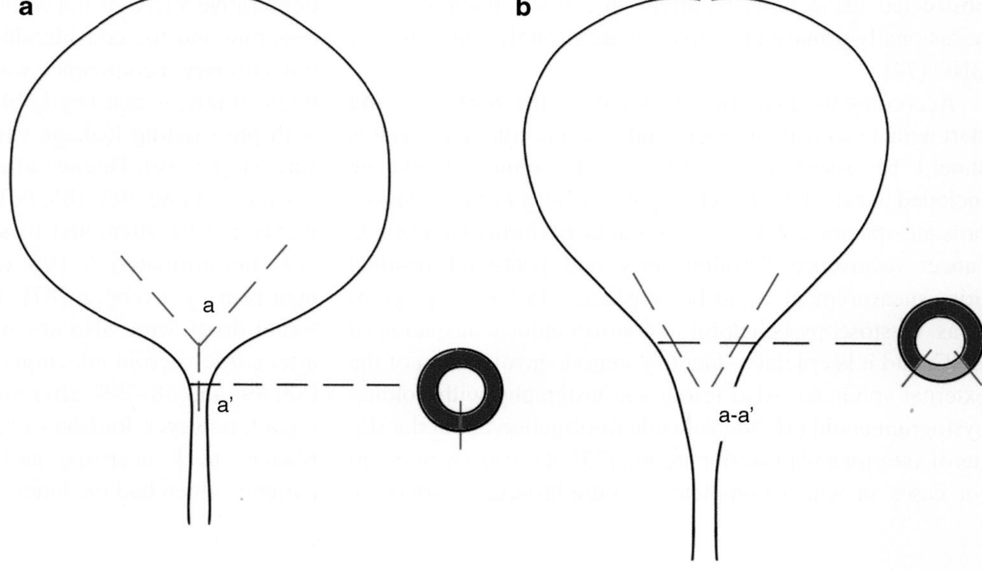

Fig. 7 Y-V plasty of the bladder neck. A longitudinal section through the anterior aspect of the scar is performed, together with an inverted-V incision of the bladder neck (**a**). The apex *a* of the advancement flap is then sutured to the most caudal point *a′* of the incised scar (**b**)

3.3.5 Stents

Several semi-/permanent metallic stents have been used in the setting of VUAS [99, 100]. Their use is currently discouraged by international guidelines [79] because of their limited efficacy and challenges with migration, tissue regrowth, or intrusion.

4 Well Leg Compartment Syndrome

Compartment syndrome is an uncommon complication of robot-assisted radical prostatectomy due to the increased pressure in the muscles of the lower extremities which leads to hypoperfusion of the tissues and necrosis.

4.1 Incidence and Etiology

Compartment syndrome is a rare complication after robot-assisted radical prostatectomy (RARP). The underlying cause of compartment syndrome is the increase in pressure in the muscle compartments surrounded by inelastic fascia when swelling or edema occurs, leading to an eventual increase in pressure in the compartment above perfusion pressure, leading to disruption of oxygenated blood flow and subsequent tissue necrosis [101]. Outcomes can be devastating and include loss of motor function, foot drop, permanent disability and restriction of mobility, lower limb amputation, renal failure from rhabdomyolysis, and death.

It is an uncommon condition in RARP, with an incidence of 0.29%, but that equates to three cases per thousand [102], so it is possible that most moderate- to high-volume surgeons may come across it once in their career, and the potential adverse outcomes are so severe that it must be taken very seriously as a condition. Lower limb compartment syndrome (LLCS) is often related to the use of the lithotomy position, with pressure being put on the calf muscles by the weight of the leg being suspended in stirrups of various designs. The use of Trendelenburg positioning can also contribute to LLCS in the setting of RARP [101]. Predisposing factors [102] include:

1. Extended time in lithotomy. It is traditionally felt that lithotomy duration of over 4 h increases the risk of LLCS, but it can occur in cases that last less than an hour.
2. Blood loss/hypovolemia
3. Hypotension
4. Obesity
5. Muscular, tight calves
6. Smoking
7. Peripheral vascular disease
8. Compression of iliac vessels such as during lymphadenectomy

The underlying pathophysiology that occurs is a rise of the internal compartment pressure to above 30 mmHg, although it can occur at lower pressures. The normal pressure is 0–10 mmHg. A rise in pressure causes a rise in compartmental pressure, leading to venous occlusion causing a rise in intracompartmental pressure to above mean arterial pressure with subsequent ischemia, as mentioned [102].

4.2 Clinical Presentation

LLCS usually manifests itself in the first few hours after injury but may present later. Pain is usually the first major complaint, with the pain being out of proportion to the injury. Pain is usually significantly increased on passive stretching. The tissue may also feel tense and "woody." The traditional conglomeration of symptoms is described under the "the five Ps," those being pain, pulselessness, paresthesia, pallor, and paralysis [101]. However, these may be late signs, and pain should be considered a cardinal sign, although this may be confused with the pain from deep vein thrombosis and may be masked by epidural analgesia use. There may paresthesia or loss of sensation in the first interdigital web space in the foot. The diagnosis is a clinical one, but measurement of intracompartmental pressures is a useful adjunct. This can be done by using either a transducer-tipped catheter or by a conventional fluid-filled system. There is no universal agreement on the precise intracompartmental pressure at which intervention should be considered. The decision to operate should be made in conjunction with clinical findings although a value of >30 mmHg usually shows that surgical decompression is needed. Alternatively, one can use the perfusion pressure of the compartment, or compartment delta pressure, which is the diastolic pressure minus the intracompartmental pressure. If this is less than 30 mmHg, then there is an imminent risk of anoxia and ischemia, and intervention is required [103]. Serial creatine kinase levels may be helpful, especially if they are increasing in a serial manner as sequentially elevated levels occur with increasing muscle damage [104]. Renal function should also be serially assessed as renal impairment may occur secondary to rhabdomyolysis [105].

4.3 Surgical Management

The procedure of choice for LLCS is urgent fasciotomy of the compartments of the below-knee compartments to allow the release of pressure. This should be done as soon as possible and usually requires the intervention of orthopedic, trauma, plastic, or general surgery depending on what expertise is available. It is vital to open the anterior compartment as this is the one most commonly affected, but more extensive fasciotomy with opening of the other compartments is often needed. Any necrotic tissue should be excised, and the compartments closed loosely. Repeat inspections of the muscle bellies under anesthesia are usually needed, and skin grafts are often employed to close the resultant defect [103].

Compartment syndrome is a surgical emergency that is rare and unexpected in urology, which puts an onus on the clinician to suspect it in any patient complaining of severe pain in the lower limb following RARP, which is not a procedure associated with lower limb pain usually. The risk is lowered by reduced operative time and keeping the legs in a flat position, as opposed to using stirrups and the lithotomy position. There is no significant association of the use of mechanical thromboprophylaxis, lithotomy position, and compartment syndrome [106]. The diagnosis is a clinical diagnosis, and once the possibility of LLCS has been raised, it is appropriate to get urgent specialist advice and proceed quickly to fasciotomy, as if LLCS is present, there will be ongoing muscle tissue destruction, with potentially catastrophic resultant outcomes.

References

1. Ramírez-Martín D, Jara-Rascón J, Renedo-Villar T, Hernández-Fernández C, Lledó-García E. Rectourethral fistula management. Curr Urol Rep. 2016;17:1–6.
2. Al-Ali M, Kashmoula D, Saoud IJ. Experience with 30 posttraumatic rectourethral fistulas: presentation of posterior transsphincteric anterior rectal wall advancement. J Urol. 1997;158:421–4.
3. Ruiz-Lopez M, Mera S, Gonzalez-Poveda I, Becerra R, Carrasco J, Toval JA, et al. Fournier's gangrene: a complication of surgical glue treatment for a rectourethral fistula in a patient with human immunodeficiency virus infection. Color Dis. 2012;14 https://doi.org/10.1111/j.1463-1318.2011.02822.x.
4. Hébuterne X, Filippi J, Al-Jaouni R, Schneider S. Nutritional consequences and nutrition therapy in Crohn's disease. Gastroentérologie Clin Biol. 2009;33(Suppl):3. https://doi.org/10.1016/s0399-8320(09)73159-8.
5. Thomas C, Jones J, Jäger W, Hampel C, Thüroff JW, Gillitzer R. Incidence, clinical symptoms and management of rectourethral fistulas after radical prostatectomy. J Urol. 2010;183:608–12.
6. Elliott SP, McAninch JW, Chi T, Doyle SM, Master VA. Management of severe urethral complications of prostate cancer therapy. J Urol. 2006;176:2508–13.
7. Chrouser KL, Leibovich BC, Sweat SD, Larson DW, Davis BJ, Tran NV, et al. Urinary fistulas following external radiation or permanent brachytherapy for the treatment of prostate cancer. J Urol. 2005;173:1953–7.
8. Shah SA, Cima RR, Benoit E, Breen EL, Bleday R. Rectal complications after prostate brachytherapy. Dis Colon Rectum. 2004;47:1487–92.
9. Shakespeare D, Mitchell DM, Carey BM, Finan P, Henry AM, Ash D, et al. Recto-urethral fistula following brachytherapy for localized prostate cancer. Color Dis. 2007;9:328–31.
10. Netsch C, Bach T, Gross E, Gross AJ. Rectourethral fistula after high-intensity focused ultrasound therapy for prostate cancer and its surgical management. Urology. 2011;77:999–1004.
11. Badalament RA, Bahn DK, Kim H, Kumar A, Bahn JM, Lee F. Patient-reported complications after cryoablation therapy for prostate cancer. Urology. 1999;54:295–300.
12. Lane BR, Stein DE, Remzi FH, Strong SA, Fazio VW, Angermeier KW. Management of radiotherapy induced rectourethral fistula. J Urol. 2006;175:1382–8.
13. Mundy AR, Andrich DE. Urorectal fistulae following the treatment of prostate cancer. BJU Int. 2011;107:1298–303.
14. Barashi NS, Pearce SM, Cohen AJ, Pariser JJ, Packiam VT, Eggener SE. Incidence, risk factors, and outcomes for rectal injury during radical prostatectomy: a population-based study. Eur Urol Oncol. 2018;1:501–6.
15. Beatty JD, Witherow R. Diagnostic lessons learnt from a series of enterovesical fistulae [2]. Color Dis. 2005;7:196.
16. Harris CR, McAninch JW, Mundy AR, Zinman LN, Jordan GH, Andrich D, et al. Rectourethral fistulas secondary to prostate cancer treatment: management and outcomes from a multi-institutional combined experience. J Urol. 2017;197:191–4.
17. Goodwin WE, Turner RD, Winter CC. Rectourinary fistula: principles of management and a technique of surgical closure. J Urol. 1958;80:246–54.
18. Nyam DCNK, Pemberton JH. Management of iatrogenic rectourethral fistula. Dis Colon Rectum. 1999;42:994–7.
19. Garofalo TE, Delaney CP, Jones SM, Remzi FH, Fazio VW. Rectal advancement flap repair of rectourethral fistula: a 20-year experience. Dis Colon Rectum. 2003;46:762–9.
20. Dafnis G. Transsphincteric repair of rectourethral fistulas: 15 years of experience with the York Mason approach. Int J Urol. 2018;25:290–6.
21. Verriello V, Altomare M, Masiello G, Curatolo C, Balacco G, Altomare DF. Treatment of post-prostatectomy rectourethral fistula with fibrin sealant (Quixil™) injection: a novel application. Tech Coloproctol. 2010;14:341–3.
22. Bardari F, D'Urso L, Muto G. Conservative treatment of iatrogenic urinary fistulas: the value of cyanoacrylic glue. Urology. 2001;58:1046–8.
23. Bhandari Y, Khandkar A, Chaudhary A, Srimali P, Desai D, Srinivas V. Post-radical prostatectomy rectourethral fistula: endosopic management. Urol Int. 2008;81:474–6.
24. Noldus J, Fernandez S, Huland H. Rectourinary fistula repair using the Latzko technique. J Urol. 1999;161:1518–20.
25. Jones IT, Fazio VW, Jagelman DG. The use of transanal rectal advancement flaps in the management of fistulas involving the anorectum. Dis Colon Rectum. 1987;30:919–23.
26. Dreznik Z, Alper D, Vishne TH, Ramadan E. Rectal flap advancement—a simple and effective approach for the treatment of rectourethral fistula. Color Dis. 2003;5:53–5.
27. Nicita G, Villari D, Caroassai Grisanti S, Marzocco M, Li Marzi V, Martini A. Minimally invasive transanal repair of rectourethral fistulas. Eur Urol. 2017;71:133–8.
28. Atallah S, Albert M, deBeche-Adams T, Larach S. Transanal minimally invasive surgery (TAMIS): applications beyond local excision. Tech Coloproctol. 2013;17:239–43.
29. Pigalarga R, Patel NM, Rezac C. Transanal endoscopic microsurgery-assisted rectal advancement flap is a viable option for iatrogenic rectourethral fistula repair: a case report. Tech Coloproctol. 2011;15:209–11.
30. Andrews EJ, Royce P, Farmer KC. Transanal endoscopic microsurgery repair of rectourethral fistula after high-intensity focused ultrasound ablation of prostate cancer. Color Dis. 2011;13:342–3.
31. Ryan JA, Beebe HG, Gibbons RP. Gracilis muscle flap for closure of rectourethral fistula. J Urol. 1979;122:124–5.
32. Ghoniem G, Elmissiry M, Weiss E, Langford C, Abdelwahab H, Wexner S. Transperineal repair of complex rectourethral fistula using gracilis muscle flap interposition-can urinary and bowel functions be preserved? J Urol. 2008;179:1882–6.
33. Margules AC, Rovner ES. The use of tissue flaps in the management of urinary tract fistulas. Curr Urol Rep. 2019;20 https://doi.org/10.1007/s11934-019-0892-6.

34. Yamazaki Y, Yago R, Toma H. Dartos flap interposition in the surgical repair of rectourethral fistulas. Int J Urol. 2001;8:564–7.
35. Krand O, Unal E. Management of enema tip-induced rectourethral fistula with gluteus maximus flap: report of a case. Tech Coloproctol. 2008;12:131–3.
36. Spiegel JH, Lee C, Trabulsy PP, Coughlin RR. Endoscopic harvest of the gracilis muscle flap. Ann Plast Surg. 1998;41:384–9.
37. Kilpatrick FR, Mason AY. Post-operative recto-prostatic fistula. Br J Urol. 1969;41:649–54.
38. Mason AY. Surgical access to the rectum—a transsphincteric exposure. Proc R Soc Med. 1970;63(Suppl):91–4.
39. Kasraeian A, Rozet F, Cathelineau X, Barret E, Galiano M, Vallancien G. Modified York-Mason technique for repair of iatrogenic rectourinary fistula: the Montsouris experience. J Urol. 2009;181:1178–83.
40. Sotelo R, Garcia A, Yaime H, Rodríguez E, Dubois R, De Andrade R, et al. Laparoscopic rectovesical fistula repair. J Endourol. 2005;19:603–6.
41. Bollens R. 5 cm Vesicorectal fistula post radical prostatectomy. https://www.youtube.com/watch?v=iXmlb6famCE&t=9396s&ab_channel=RenaudBollens. Accessed 4 May 2021.
42. Sotelo R, de Andrade R, Carmona O, Astigueta J, Velasquez A, Trujillo G, et al. Robotic repair of rectovesical fistula resulting from open radical prostatectomy. Urology. 2008;72:1344–6.
43. Linder B, Frank I, Dozois E, Elliott D. V405 robotic transvesical rectourethral fistula repair following a robotic radical prostatectomy. J Urol. 2013;189:e164–5.
44. Mori N. Clinical and experimental studies on the so-called lymphocyst which develops after radical hysterectomy in cancer of the uterine cervix. J Jpn Obstet Gynecol Soc. 1955;2:178–203.
45. Liss MA, Palazzi K, Stroup SP, Jabaji R, Raheem OA, Kane CJ. Outcomes and complications of pelvic lymph node dissection during robotic-assisted radical prostatectomy. World J Urol. 2013;31:481–8.
46. Orvieto MA, Coelho RF, Chauhan S, Palmer KJ, Rocco B, Patel VR. Incidence of lymphoceles after robot-assisted pelvic lymph node dissection. BJU Int. 2011;108:1185–9.
47. Capitanio U, Pellucchi F, Gallina A, Briganti A, Suardi N, Salonia A, et al. How can we predict lymphorrhoea and clinically significant lymphocoeles after radical prostatectomy and pelvic lymphadenectomy? Clinical implications. BJU Int. 2011;107:1095–101.
48. Khoder WY, Trottmann M, Buchner A, Stuber A, Hoffmann S, Stief CG, et al. Risk factors for pelvic lymphoceles post-radical prostatectomy. Int J Urol. 2011;18:638–43.
49. Yuh BE, Ruel NH, Mejia R, Novara G, Wilson TG. Standardized comparison of robot-assisted limited and extended pelvic lymphadenectomy for prostate cancer. BJU Int. 2013;112:81–8.
50. Kowalczyk KJ, Levy JM, Caplan CF, Lipsitz SR, Yu HY, Gu X, et al. Temporal national trends of minimally invasive and retropubic radical prostatectomy outcomes from 2003 to 2007: results from the 100% medicare sample. Eur Urol. 2012;61:803–9.
51. Danuser H, Di Pierro GB, Stucki P, Mattei A. Extended pelvic lymphadenectomy and various radical prostatectomy techniques: is pelvic drainage necessary? BJU Int. 2013;111:963–9.
52. Stolzenburg JU, Wasserscheid J, Rabenalt R, Do M, Schwalenberg T, McNeill A, et al. Reduction in incidence of lymphocele following extraperitoneal radical prostatectomy and pelvic lymph node dissection by bilateral peritoneal fenestration. World J Urol. 2008;26:581–6.
53. Tomic R, Granfors T, Sjödin JG, Öhberg L. Lymph leakage after staging pelvic lymphadenectomy for prostatic carcinoma with and without heparin prophylaxis. Scand J Urol Nephrol. 1994;28:273–5.
54. Sieber PR, Rommel M, Agusta VE, Breslin JA, Harpster LE, Huffnagle HW, et al. Is heparin contraindicated in pelvic lymphadenectomy and radical prostatectomy? J Urol. 1997;158:869–71.
55. Yamamoto S, Ikeda M, Kanno Y, Okamoto K, Okugawa S, Moriya K. Microbiological analysis of infectious lymphocele: case series and literature review. J Infect Chemother. 2021;27:172–8.
56. Chenam A, Yuh B, Zhumkhawala A, Ruel N, Chu W, Lau C, et al. Prospective randomised non-inferiority trial of pelvic drain placement vs no pelvic drain placement after robot-assisted radical prostatectomy. BJU Int. 2018;121:357–64.
57. Gotto GT, Yunis LH, Guillonneau B, Touijer K, Eastham JA, Scardino PT, et al. Predictors of symptomatic lymphocele after radical prostatectomy and bilateral pelvic lymph node dissection. Int J Urol. 2011;18:291–6.
58. Canes D, Cohen MS, Tuerk IA. Laparoscopic radical prostatectomy: omitting a pelvic drain. Int Braz J Urol. 2008;34:151–8.
59. Box GN, Lee HJ, Abraham JB, Deane LA, Elchico ER, Abdelshehid CA, et al. Comparative study of in vivo lymphatic sealing capability of the porcine thoracic duct using laparoscopic dissection devices. J Urol. 2009;181:387–91.
60. Grande P, Di Pierro GB, Mordasini L, Ferrari M, Würnschimmel C, Danuser H, et al. Prospective randomized trial comparing titanium clips to bipolar coagulation in sealing lymphatic vessels during pelvic lymph node dissection at the time of robot-assisted radical prostatectomy. Eur Urol. 2017;71:155–8.
61. Davis JW, Shah JB, Achim M. Robot-assisted extended pelvic lymph node dissection (PLND) at the time of radical prostatectomy (RP): a video-based illustration of technique, results, and unmet patient selection needs. BJU Int. 2011;108:993–8.
62. Waldert M, Remzi M, Klatte T, Klingler HC. Floseal reduces the incidence of lymphoceles after lymphadenectomies in laparoscopic and robot-assisted extraperitoneal radical prostatectomy. J Endourol. 2011;25:969–73.
63. Simonato A, Varca V, Esposito M, Venzano F, Carmignani G. The use of a surgical patch in the prevention of lymphoceles after extraperitoneal pelvic lymphadenectomy for prostate cancer: a randomized prospective pilot study. J Urol. 2009;182:2285–90.
64. Gilbert DR, Angell J, Abaza R. Evaluation of absorbable hemostatic powder for prevention of lymphoceles following robotic prostatectomy with lymphadenectomy. Urology. 2016;98:75–80.
65. Garayev A, Aytaç Ö, Tavukcu HH, Atug F. Effect of autologous fibrin glue on lymphatic drainage and lymphocele formation in extended bilateral pelvic lymphadenectomy in robot-assisted radical prostatectomy. J Endourol. 2019;33:761–6.
66. Lebeis C, Canes D, Sorcini A, Moinzadeh A. Novel technique prevents lymphoceles after transperitoneal robotic-assisted pelvic lymph node dissection: peritoneal flap interposition. Urology. 2015;85:1505–9.
67. Dal Moro F, Zattoni F. P.L.E.A.T.—preventing lymphocele ensuring absorption transperitoneally: a robotic technique. Urology. 2017;110:244–7.
68. Stolzenburg JU, Arthanareeswaran VKA, Dietel A, Franz T, Liatsikos E, Kyriazis I, et al. Four-point peritoneal flap fixation in preventing lymphocele formation following radical prostatectomy. Eur Urol Oncol. 2018;1:443–8.
69. ten Hove AS, Tjiong MY, Zijlstra IAJ. Treatment of symptomatic postoperative pelvic lymphoceles: a systematic review. Eur J Radiol. 2021;134 https://doi.org/10.1016/j.ejrad.2020.109459.
70. Modig KK, Godtman RA, Bjartell A, Carlsson S, Haglind E, Hugosson J, et al. Vesicourethral anastomotic stenosis after open or robot-assisted laparoscopic retropubic prostatectomy—results from the laparoscopic prostatectomy robot open trial. Eur Urol Focus. 2021;7:317–24.
71. Wang R, Wood DP, Hollenbeck BK, Li AY, He C, Montie JE, et al. Risk factors and quality of life for post-prostatectomy vesicourethral anastomotic stenoses. Urology. 2012;79:449–57.
72. Borboroglu PG, Sands JP, Roberts JL, Amling CL. Risk factors for vesicourethral anastomotic stricture after radical prostatectomy. Urology. 2000;56:96–100.

73. Sowerby RJ, Gani J, Yim H, Radomski SB, Catton C. Long-term complications in men who have early or late radiotherapy after radical prostatectomy. J Can Urol Assoc. 2014;8:253–8.
74. Parihar JS, Ha Y-S, Kim IY. Bladder neck contracture-incidence and management following contemporary robot assisted radical prostatectomy technique. Prostate Int. 2014;2:12–8.
75. Campos-Juanatey F, Osman NI, Greenwell T, Martins FE, Riechardt S, Waterloos M, et al. European Association of Urology guidelines on urethral stricture disease (part 2): diagnosis, perioperative management, and follow-up in males. Eur Urol. 2021; https://doi.org/10.1016/j.eururo.2021.05.032.
76. Herschorn S, Elliott S, Coburn M, Wessells H, Zinman L. SIU/ICUD consultation on urethral strictures: posterior urethral stenosis after treatment of prostate cancer. Urology. 2014;83 https://doi.org/10.1016/j.urology.2013.08.036.
77. Ramchandani P, Banner MP, Berlin JW, Dannenbaum MS, Wein AJ. Vesicourethral anastomotic strictures after radical prostatectomy: efficacy of transurethral balloon dilation. Radiology. 1994;193:345–9.
78. Herschorn S, Carrington E. S-shaped coaxial dilators for male urethral strictures. Urology. 2007;69:1199–201.
79. Lumen N, Campos-Juanatey F, Greenwell T, Martins FE, Osman NI, Riechardt S, et al. European Association of Urology guidelines on urethral stricture disease (part 1): management of male urethral stricture disease. Eur Urol. 2021; https://doi.org/10.1016/j.eururo.2021.05.022.
80. Labossiere JR, Cheung D, Rourke K. Endoscopic treatment of vesicourethral stenosis after radical prostatectomy: outcomes and predictors of success. J Urol. 2016;195:1495–500.
81. Dalkin BL. Endoscopic evaluation and treatment of anastomotic strictures after radical retropubic prostatectomy. J Urol. 1996;155:206–8.
82. Vanni AJ, Zinman LN, Buckley JC. Radial urethrotomy and intralesional mitomycin C for the management of recurrent bladder neck contractures. J Urol. 2011;186:156–60.
83. Shapiro DD, Goodspeed DC, Bushman W. Urosymphyseal fistulas resulting from endoscopic treatment of radiation-induced posterior urethral strictures. Urology. 2018;114:207–11.
84. Barratt R, Chan G, La Rocca R, Dimitropoulos K, Martins FE, Campos-Juanatey F, et al. Free graft augmentation urethroplasty for bulbar urethral strictures: which technique is best? A systematic review. Eur Urol. 2021;80 https://doi.org/10.1016/j.eururo.2021.03.026.
85. Lagerveld BW, Laguna MP, Debruyne FMJ, De La Rosette JJMCH. Holmium:YAG laser for treatment of strictures of vesicourethral anastomosis after radical prostatectomy. J. Endourol. 2005;19:497–501.
86. Giannarini G, Manassero F, Mogorovich A, Valent F, De Maria M, Pistolesi D, et al. Cold-knife incision of anastomotic strictures after radical retropubic prostatectomy with bladder neck preservation: efficacy and impact on urinary continence status. Eur Urol. 2008;54:647–56.
87. Brede C, Angermeier K, Wood H. Continence outcomes after treatment of recalcitrant postprostatectomy bladder neck contracture and review of the literature. Urology. 2014;83:648–52.
88. Eltahawy E, Gur U, Virasoro R, Schlossberg SM, Jordan GH. Management of recurrent anastomotic stenosis following radical prostatectomy using holmium laser and steroid injection. BJU Int. 2008;102:796–8.
89. Kravchick S, Lobik L, Peled R, Cytron S. Transrectal ultrasonography-guided injection of long-acting steroids in the treatment of recurrent/resistant anastomotic stenosis after radical prostatectomy. J Endourol. 2013;27:875–9.
90. Redshaw JD, Broghammer JA, Smith TG, Voelzke BB, Erickson BA, McClung CD, et al. Intralesional injection of mitomycin C at transurethral incision of bladder neck contracture may offer limited benefit: TURNS Study Group. J Urol. 2015;193:587–92.
91. Sourial MW, Richard PO, Bettez M, Jundi M, Tu LM. Mitomycin-C and urethral dilatation: a safe, effective, and minimally invasive procedure for recurrent vesicourethral anastomotic stenoses. Urol Oncol Semin Orig Investig. 2017;35(672):e15–672.e19.
92. Kranz J, Reiss PC, Salomon G, Steffens J, Fisch M, Rosenbaum CM. Differences in recurrence rate and de novo incontinence after endoscopic treatment of vesicourethral stenosis and bladder neck stenosis. Front Surg. 2017;4 https://doi.org/10.3389/fsurg.2017.00044.
93. Schuettfort VM, Dahlem R, Kluth L, Pfalzgraf D, Rosenbaum C, Ludwig T, et al. Transperineal reanastomosis for treatment of highly recurrent anastomotic strictures after radical retropubic prostatectomy: extended follow-up. World J Urol. 2017;35:1885–90.
94. Pfalzgraf D, Beuke M, Isbarn H, Reiss CP, Meyer-Moldenhauer WH, Dahlem R, et al. Open retropubic reanastomosis for highly recurrent and complex bladder neck stenosis. J Urol. 2011;186:1944–7.
95. Granieri MA, Weinberg AC, Sun JY, Stifelman MD, Zhao LC. Robotic Y-V plasty for recalcitrant bladder neck contracture. Urology. 2018;117:163–5.
96. Boswell TC, Hebert KJ, Tollefson MK, Viers BR. Robotic urethral reconstruction: redefining the paradigm of posterior urethroplasty. Transl Androl Urol. 2020;9:121–31.
97. Kirshenbaum EJ, Zhao LC, Myers JB, Elliott SP, Vanni AJ, Baradaran N, et al. Patency and incontinence rates after robotic bladder neck reconstruction for vesicourethral anastomotic stenosis and recalcitrant bladder neck contractures: the Trauma and Urologic Reconstructive Network of Surgeons Experience. Urology. 2018;118:227–33.
98. Şimşek A, Danacıoğlu YO, Arıkan Y, Özdemir O, Yenice MG, Atar FA, et al. Perineoscopic vesicourethral reconstruction: a novel surgical technique for anastomotic stricture following radical prostatectomy. Turk J Urol. 2021;47:51–7.
99. Nathan A, Mazzon G, Pavan N, De Groote R, Sridhar A, Nathan S. Management of intractable bladder neck strictures following radical prostatectomy using the Memokath®045 stent. J Robot Surg. 2020;14:621–5.
100. Elliott DS, Boone TB, Chancellor M. Combined stent and artificial urinary sphincter for management of severe recurrent bladder neck contracture and stress incontinence after prostatectomy: a long-term evaluation. J Urol. 2001;165:413–5.
101. Simms MS, Terry TR. Well leg compartment syndrome after pelvic and perineal surgery in the lithotomy position. Postgrad Med J. 2005;81:534–6.
102. Pridgeon S, Bishop CV, Adshead J. Lower limb compartment syndrome as a complication of robot-assisted radical prostatectomy: the UK experience. BJU Int. 2013;112:485–8.
103. Tillinghast C, Gary J. Compartment syndrome of the lower extremity. In: Mauffrey C, Hak DJ, Martin III MP, editors. Compartment syndrome: a guide to diagnosis and management. Cham: Springer; 2019. p. 67–81.
104. Nilsson A, Alkner B, Wetterlöv P, Wetterstad S, Palm L, Schilcher J. Low compartment pressure and myoglobin levels in tibial fractures with suspected acute compartment syndrome. BMC Musculoskelet Disord. 2019;20 https://doi.org/10.1186/S12891-018-2394-Y.
105. Zutt R, van der Kooi AJ, Linthorst GE, Wanders RJA, de Visser M. Rhabdomyolysis: review of the literature. Neuromuscul Disord. 2014;24:651–9.
106. Gelder C, McCallum AL, Macfarlane AJR, Anderson JH. A systematic review of mechanical thromboprophylaxis in the lithotomy position. Surgeon. 2018;16:365–71.

Penile Rehabilitation After Robot-Assisted Laparoscopic Radical Prostatectomy

Kristina Buscaino, Rafael Carrion, Jeff Brady, and Lawrence S. Hakim

1 Introduction

Erectile dysfunction (ED) after robot-assisted laparoscopic radical prostatectomy (RALRP) ranges from 20 to 90% [1–3]. As there are increasingly rising survival rates in younger and sexually active men undergoing RALRP, the number of men suffering from ED after their surgery will continue to rise [4]. This may ultimately affect the patient's quality of life, self-esteem, and overall sexual health [4, 5]. Although nerve-sparing techniques may not prevent ED in every patient [4], utilizing the robotic approach often leads to a faster recovery and may ensure better erectile function (EF) outcomes compared to the open or laparoscopic approach [6–8]. It has also been demonstrated that in some cases, it may take up to 2 years for erectile function to return even after a successful nerve-sparing surgery is performed [4, 9, 10].

2 Risk Factors for Post-RALRP ED

The likelihood of recovery of erectile function is often multifactorial. Numerous predictors have been mentioned in the literature including utilizing the nerve-sparing technique, patient's age, degree of pre-operative erectile function, existing comorbidities, intraoperative complications, and cancer stage or grade [5].

The neurovascular bundle (NVB) was first identified and described during radical retropubic prostatectomy by Walsh and Donker [11]. As the NVB travels posterolateral to the prostate, injury to the NVB may vary [6, 7, 12]. Tumor stage may act as a predictor of surgical complexity [13] and ability to perform nerve-sparing RALRP. Therefore, surgical details should always be reported, especially to specify the degree of nerve sparing, in order to better predict post-operative erectile function [14]. Neurovascular injury may include reversible neuropraxia caused by excessive retraction, ischemic and/or thermal damage and local inflammatory effects [15], or complete transection. The resulting nerve injury leads to the loss of neural connections to the corpora cavernosa and its neuroregulatory functions [5].

It has been reported that return of erectile function is inversely correlated with age. Men younger than 60 years of age may have faster return and recovery due to greater neuroplasticity [16–18]. Rabbani et al. reported that for patients aged ≤60, 60–65, and ≥65, EF recovery after prostatectomy is 70%, 45%, and 30%, respectively [19]. Another study demonstrated that men in their 40s undergoing RALRP had a much greater chance of returning to their baseline EF as compared to their 70-year-old counterparts [20].

Knowing the patient's baseline erectile function prior to RALRP is important as it assists with predicting post-operative EF recovery [13]. Up to 48% of patients who undergo RALRP may have a suboptimal EF prior to surgery [21, 22]. Pre-operative EF assessment should be done prior to cancer diagnosis if possible. If obtained after cancer diagnosis and/or prior to surgery, it may affect the patient's libido and overall sexual activity, underestimating their baseline EF [23, 24]. In addition, depression and decreased libido are common in these patients due to cancer-related psychological stress [25].

Studies have demonstrated that having two or more vascular comorbidities, such as diabetes, hypertension, and hyperlipidemia, decreases the success rate of penile rehabilitation due to endothelial dysfunction [26]. Diabetic men with hyperglycemia have impaired nitric oxide synthase (NOS), which reduces NOS and endothelial-mediated smooth muscle relaxation [27–29] and causes structural changes to the corpora cavernosa [30]. Hyperlipidemia decreases cavernosal endothelial cells [31] and impairs eNOS function and

K. Buscaino · R. Carrion
University of South Florida, Tampa, FL, USA

J. Brady
Department of Urology, AdventHealth Medical Group, AdventHealth Physician Network, Orlando, FL, USA

L. S. Hakim (✉)
Department of Urology, Cleveland Clinic Florida, Weston, FL, USA

P. Wiklund et al. (eds.), *Robotic Urologic Surgery*, https://doi.org/10.1007/978-3-031-00363-9_32

endothelium relaxation [31–36]. Hypertension may damage endothelial lining and smooth muscle and causes thinning of tunica albuginea and increased collage deposition [30, 37–40].

3 Penile Rehabilitation

The goal of penile rehabilitation is to decrease and prevent cavernosal tissue damage during the timeframe of neural recovery [4]. It is based on three important concepts: (1) cavernosal oxygenation, (2) endothelial protection, and (3) cavernosal nerve regeneration [4, 46]. There is an important balance between low cavernosal oxygenation (flaccid penis) and high cavernosal oxygenation (erect penis), with pO2 of 35–40 mmHg and pO2 70–100 mmHg, respectively [41]. Cavernosal oxygen levels affect multiple factors that are released. Low cavernosal pO2 will increase the release of fibrogenic cytokines, whereas normal or high cavernosal pO2 will upregulate prostanoids and cyclic adenosine monophosphase (cAMP) [4]. Prostanoids counteract the production of fibrogenic cytokines [4]. If flaccidity remains constant, fibrogenic cytokine production will continue, leading to cavernosal smooth muscle fibrosis [4]. Endothelial NOS lines cavernosal sinusoids and plays an important role in maintaining erections [42]. Endothelial dysfunction is affected by vascular compromise, including diabetes mellitus, hypercholesterolemia, hypertension, and aging [30, 43], as discussed above. Cavernosal nerve injury will ultimately lead to hypoxic conditions within the corpora, causing increased release of fibrogenic cytokines and endothelial apoptosis [44–46]. Transforming growth factor β1 (TGF-β1) production from penile hypoxia will worsen collagen accumulation and fibrosis [41]. Normally, cAMP and prostaglandin E1 (PGE1) prevent TGF-β1 collagen synthesis; however, both are inhibited with low pO2 [47]. TGF-β1 will also increase endothelin-1 production, causing constriction of the penile smooth muscle [47].

It is important to consider starting penile rehabilitation early, as the later it is started, the more likely venous leak will occur due to worsening corporal fibrosis [4]. It has been shown on corporal biopsies that lower smooth muscle content is associated with a higher flow-to-maintain value during cavernosometry, which confirms cavernosal tissue fibrosis resulting in venous leakage [48]. Venous leakage after radical prostatectomy has been found to be time dependent. In animal studies, after cavernosal nerve damage, peak neuropraxia-induced apoptosis was at day 3, with decreased smooth muscle-to-collagen ratio by day 30 and venous leak at day 45 [49]. In patients who have undergone radical prostatectomy, venous leak was noted at 30% and 50% at 8 and 12 months, respectively [50]. If penile duplex Doppler is performed and venous leakage is seen, there is a lower likelihood of return of spontaneous erections and a poor response to phophodiesterase type 5 inhibitors (PDE5-Is) may be expected [50]. Only 8% of patients diagnosed with venous leakage had recovery of spontaneous erections that were firm enough for intercourse [50].

Various regimens have been suggested as part of a post-RALRP penile rehabilitation program. These may include monotherapy or combination of oral PDE5-Is, intracavernosal injections (ICI), intraurethral alprostadil, penile vacuum erection devices (VED), and/or penile vibratory stimulation (PVS). Studies have suggested that penile rehabilitation results in better post-operative EF in comparison to placebo or no treatment [25].

PDE5-Is are typically considered the first-line therapy, but response is dependent on cavernous nerve function [5] and eNOS [26], making preservation of the NVB imperative to maximize PDE5-I efficacy [26]. The more nerve tissue that is preserved correlates with better spontaneous EF and response to PDE5-Is [51–53]. PDE5-Is induce cavernosal oxygenation even in the flaccid state and protect endothelial tissue [4]. There is no randomized data that shows which specific PDE5-I agent is more superior or when to start therapy [5]. Numerous studies have demonstrated that cavernosal nerve-injured animals treated with PDE5-Is have preservation of EF due to decreased smooth muscle loss and increased preservation of endothelial factor staining [54–56]. Earlier onset of PDE5-I rehabilitation improves EF and has demonstrated better results in younger men with high pre-operative IIEF [57, 58]. When starting penile rehabilitation within 6 months after nerve-sparing radical prostatectomy, patients had an increased likelihood of return of spontaneous erections and/or erections with sildenafil 2 years post-operatively [58].

ICI may also be utilized if patients have a poor response, cannot tolerate, or have a contraindication to PDE5-I usage. The efficacy is independent of cavernous injury, unlike PDE5-Is. The most common formulations are alprostadil (PGE1), bimix (papaverine, phentolamine), and trimix (papaverine, phentolamine, and alprostadil). Each component acts on different erectile mechanisms [5]. Papaverine is a non-specific PDE-I that increases cavernosal cAMP and cGMP. Phentolamine is an alpha-blocker that induces smooth muscle relaxation. Alprostadil is PGE1 which increases cavernosal cAMP. These mechanisms ultimately increase cavernosal oxygenation and increase blood flow to the corpora. In 1977, Montorsi et al. was the first to investigate penile rehabilitation using alprostadil ICI to increase recovery time of spontaneous erections [59]. Thirty patients were randomized and received either no injections or intracavernosal alprostadil injections three times a week for 12 weeks after prostatectomy. The study demonstrated that 67% of the men in the alprostadil ICI group had recovered erections that allowed for intercourse without medical assistance versus only 20% in the control group [59]. By adding ICI to PDE5-Is, improved rates of spontaneous erections and response to PDE5-Is have been demonstrated 18 months post-operatively [60].

Intraurethral alprostadil is a urethral suppository that delivers PGE1, increasing cAMP within the erectile tissue indirectly [61–63]. This mechanism bypasses the cavernosal nerve and is independent of cavernosal nerve injury. As the mode of effect is via urethra, the most common side effect is urethral burning and penile pain. There has been no clinical data that demonstrates a significant difference in return of EF [61]. Intraurethral alprostadil may improve erections in patients with ED, but studies are limited after RALRP.

The function of a vacuum erection device (VED) is to provide negative pressure, drawing blood into both the intra- and extra-corporal spaces of the penis and distending the corporal sinusoids [64]. In rat models, daily VED demonstrated improved intracavernosal pressure, increased eNOS, and decreased hypoxia-induced factor 1α and TGF-β1 levels and smooth muscle apoptosis [65, 66]. Two randomized studies have looked at the use of VED after radical prostatectomy. Kohler et al. [67] studied early (4 weeks post-operatively) versus delayed treatment group (before intercourse) with or without PDE5-Is. There were significantly higher IIEF scores at 3 and 6 months with the early treatment group; however no significant differences were noted after 1 year. In both groups, spontaneous erections were not adequate for penetration at 1 year. Raina et al. [68] randomized nerve-sparing and non-nerve-sparing radical prostatectomy with daily VED use for 9 months versus no VED use. At 9 months, mean IIEF-5 scores were higher in the treatment group versus the control group. However, return of spontaneous erections between both groups was not significant. Mixed efficacy is demonstrated among studies; however, VED use has been shown to prevent loss of penile length [64]. Therefore, VED may be offered as a supportive measure or in conjunction with other penile rehabilitation modalities [69].

Penile vibratory stimulation (PVS) stimulates the pudendal nerves along the penile shaft. A reflex parasympathetic erection occurs by activating nerve terminal endings, releasing NO, and inhibiting sympathetic fibers [61]. Fode et al. studied the effects of PVS by stimulating the frenulum once daily for 1 week before surgery and again after catheter removal for 6 weeks. IIEF-5 scores were higher with PVS; however they were statistically insignificant compared to the control group without PVS [69].

4 Conclusion

Despite improvement in surgical procedures, loss of erectile function remains a serious concern for men undergoing RALRP. There are a wide range of outcomes reported in the literature with regard to the return of erectile function post-RALRP due to the heterogeneity of risk factors, EF assessment, and penile rehabilitation protocols. While there is no published consensus as to the single best penile rehabilitation strategy, studies have demonstrated improved outcomes in EF with early onset of either monotherapy or combination therapy with PDE5-I oral agents, ICI, intraurethral alprostadil, VED, and PVS. Further studies regarding the ideal starting time, dosing regimens, combinations, and treatment protocols for post-RALRP penile rehabilitation are needed.

References

1. Catalona WJ, Basler JW. Return of erections and urinary continence following nerve sparing radical retropubic prostatectomy. J Urol. 1993;150:905.
2. Jønler M, Messing EM, Rhodes PR, et al. Sequelae of radical prostatectomy. Br J Urol. 1994;74:352.
3. Litwin MS, Flanders SC, Pasta DJ, et al. Sexual function and bother after radical prostatectomy or radiation for prostate cancer: multivariate quality-of-life analysis from CaPSURE. Cancer of the prostate strategic urologic research endeavor. Urology. 1999;54:503–8.
4. Mulhall JP, Morgantaler A. Penile rehabilitation should become the norm for radical prostatectomy patients. J Sex Med. 2007;4:538–43.
5. Chung E, Brock GB. Delayed penile rehabilitation post radical prostatectomy. J Sex Med. 2010;7:3233–6.
6. Salonia A, Adaikan G, Buvat J, et al. Sexual rehabilitation after treatment for prostate cancer-Part 1: recommendations from the Fourth International Consultation for Sexual Medicine (ICSM 2015). J Sex Med. 2017;14:285–96.
7. Walz J, Epstein JI, Ganzer R, et al. A critical analysis of the current knowledge of surgical anatomy of the prostate related to optimisation of cancer control and preservation of continence and erection in candidates for radical prostatectomy: an update. Eur Urol. 2016;70:301–11.
8. Ficarra V, Novara G, Ahlering TE, et al. Optimal timing to evaluate prediagnostic baseline erectile function in patients undergoing robot-assisted radical prostatectomy. J Sex Med. 2012;9:602–7.
9. Lee JK, Assel M, Thong AE, et al. Unexpected long-term improvements in urinary and erectile function in a large cohort of men with self-reported outcomes following radical prostatectomy. Eur Urol. 2015;68:899–905.
10. Mandel P, Preisser F, Graefen M, et al. High chance of late recovery of urinary and erectile function beyond 12 months after radical prostatectomy. Eur Urol. 2017;71:848–50.
11. Walsh PC, Donker PJ. Impotence following radical prostatectomy: insight into etiology and prevention. J Urol. 1982;128:492–7.
12. Pederzoli F, Campbell JD, Matsui H, et al. Surgical factors associated with male and female sexual dysfunction after radical cystectomy: what do we know and how can we improve outcomes? Sex Med Rev. 2018;6:469–81.
13. Capogrosso P, Pozzo EP, Celentano V, et al. Erectile recovery after radical pelvic surgery: methodological challenges and recommendations for data reporting. J Sex Med. 2020;17:7–16.
14. Capogrosso P, Vertosik EA, Benfante NE, et al. Are we improving erectile function recovery after radical prostatectomy? Analysis of patients treated over the last decade. Eur Urol. 2018;75:221–8.
15. Burnett AL. Rational for cavernous nerve restorative therapy to preserve erectile function after radical prostatectomy. Urology. 2003;61:491–7.
16. Quinlan DM, Epstein JI, Carter BS, et al. Sexual function following radical prostatectomy: Influence of preservation of neurovascular bundles. J Urol. 1991;145:998–1002.

17. Flanigan KM, Lauria G, Griffin JW, et al. Age-related biology and diseases of muscle and nerve. Neurol Clin. 1998;16:659–69.
18. Burnett AL. Strategies to promote recovery of cavernous nerve function after radical prostatectomy. World J Urol. 2003;20:337–42.
19. Rabbani F, Stampleton AM, Kattan MW, et al. Factors predicting recovery of erections after radical prostatectomy. J Urol. 2000;164:1929–34.
20. Kundu SD, Roehl KA, Eggener SE, et al. Potency, continence and complications in 3,477 consecutive radical retropubic prostatectomies. J Urol. 2004;172:2227–31.
21. Salomon G, Isbarn H, Budaeus L, et al. Importance of baseline potency rate assessment of men diagnosed with clinically localized prostate cancer prior to radical prostatectomy. J Sex Med. 2009;6:498–504.
22. Salonia A, Zanni G, Gallina A, et al. Baseline potency in candidates for bilateral nerve-sparing radical retropubic prostatectomy. Eur URol. 2006;50:336–65.
23. Salonia A, Gallina A, Briganti A, et al. Remembered International Index of Erectile Function domain scores are not accurate in assessing preoperative potency in candidates for bilateral nerve-sparing radical retropubic prostatectomy. J Sex Med. 2008;5:677–83.
24. Kim DS, Chung YG, Kim DJ, et al. Optimal timing to evaluate prediagnostic baseline erectile function in patients undergoing robot-assisted radical prostatectomy. J Sex Med. 2012;9:602–7.
25. Salonia A, Adaikan G, Buvat J, et al. Sexual rehabilitation after treatment for prostate cancer-Part 2: recommendations from the Fourth International Consultation for Sexual Medicine (ICSM 2015). J Sex Med. 2017;14:297–315.
26. Muller A, Parker M, Waters BW, et al. Penile rehabilitation following radical prostatectomy: predicting success. J Sex Med. 2009;6:2806–12.
27. Saenz de Tejada I, Goldstein I, Azadzoi K, Krane RJ, Cohen RA. Impaired neurogenic and endothelium-mediated relaxation of penile smooth muscle from diabetic men with impotence. N Engl J Med. 1989;320:1025–30.
28. Cellek S, Foxwell NA, Moncada S. Two phases of nitrergic neuropathy in streptozotocin-induced diabetic rats. Diabetes. 2003;52:2353–62.
29. Podlasek CA, Zelner DJ, Bervig TR, Gonzalez CM, McKenna KE, MeVary KT. Characterization and localization of nitric oxide synthase isoforms in the BB/WOR diabetic rat. J Urol. 2001;166:746–55.
30. Musicki B, Burnett AL. eNOS function and dysfunction in the penis. Exp Biol Med (Maywood). 2006;231(2):154–65. https://doi.org/10.1177/153537020623100205. PMID: 16446491
31. Kim JH, Klyachkin ML, Svendsen E, Davies MG, Hagen PO, Carson CC 3rd. Experimental hypercholesterolemia in rabbits induces cavemosal atherosclerosis with endothelial and smooth muscle cell dysfunction. J Urol. 1994;151:198–205.
32. Kim SC, Kim IK, Seo KK, Baek KJ, Lee MY. Involvement of superoxide radical in the impaired endothelium-dependent relaxation of cavernous smooth muscle in hypercholesterolemic rabbits. Urol Res. 1997;25:341–6.
33. Kim SC. Hyperlipidemia and erectile dysfunction. Asian J Androl. 2000;2:161–6.
34. Azadzoi KM, Saenz de Tejada I. Hypercholesterolemia impairs endothelium-dependent relaxation of rabbit corpus cavernosum smooth muscle. J Urol. 1991;146:238–40.
35. Behr-Roussel D, Bernabe J, Compagnie S, Rupin A, Verbeuren TJ, Alexandre L, Giuliano F. Distinct mechanisms implicated in atherosclerosis-induced erectile dysfunction in rabbits. Atherosclerosis. 2002;162:355–62.
36. Seo KK, Yun HY, Kim H, Kim SC. Involvement of endothelial nitric oxide synthase in the impaired endothelium-dependent relaxation of cavernous smooth muscle in hypercholesterolemic rabbit. J Androl. 1999;20:298–306.
37. Toblli JE, Stella I, Inerra F, Ferder L, Zeller F, Mazza ON. Morphological changes in cavernous tissue in spontaneously hypertensive rats. Am J Hypertens. 2000;13:686–92.
38. Jiang R, Chen JH, Jin J, Shen W, Li QM. Ultrastructural comparison of penile cavernous tissue between hypertensive and normotensive rats. Int J Impot Res. 2005;17(5):417–23.
39. Behr-Roussel D, Gorny D, Mevel K, Compagnie S, Kern P, Sivan V, Bernabe J, Bedigian MP, Alexandre L, Giuliano F. Erectile dysfunction: an early marker for hypertension? A longitudinal study in spontaneously hypertensive rats. Am J Physiol Regul Integr Comp Physiol. 2005;288:R276–83.
40. Okabe H, Hale TM, Kumon H, Heaton JP, Adams MA. The penis is not protected-in hypertension there are vascular changes in the penis which are similar to those in other vascular beds. Int J Impot Res. 1999;11:133–40.
41. Moreland RB. Is there a role of hypoxemia in penile fibrosis: a viewpoint presented to the Society for the Study of Impotence. Int J Impot Res. 1998;10:113.
42. Burnett AL. Nitric oxide in the penis: physiology and pathology. J Urol. 1997;157:320.
43. Jackson G. The cardiac urologist. Int J Clinc Pract. 2007;61:181.
44. Carrier S, Zvara P, Nunes L, et al. Regeneration of nitric oxide synthase-containing nerves after cavernous nerve neurotomy in the rat. J Urol. 1995;153:1722.
45. Leungwattanakij S, Bivalacqua TJ, Usta MF, et al. Cavernous neurotomy causes hypoxia and fibrosis in rat corpus cavernosum. J Androl. 2003;24:239.
46. User HM, Hairston JH, Zelner DJ, et al. Penile weight and cell subtype specific changes in a post-radical prostatectomy model for erectile dysfunction. J Urol. 2003;169:1175.
47. Mullerad M, Donohue JF, Li PS, et al. Functional sequelae of cavernous nerve injury in the rat: is there model dependency? J Sex Med. 2006;3:77–83.
48. Nehra A, Azadzoi KM, Moreland RB, et al. Cavernosal expandability is an erectile tissue mechanical property which predicts trabecular histology in an animal model of vasculogenic erectile dysfunction. J Urol. 1998;159:2229.
49. Ferrini MG, Kowanecz I, Sanchez S, et al. Fibrosis and loss of small muscle in the corpora cavernosa precede corporal veno-occlusive dysfunction (CVOD) induced by experimental cavernosal nerve damage in the rat. J Sex Med. 2009;6:415–28.
50. Mulhall JP, Slovick R, Hotaling J, et al. Erectile dysfunction after radical prostatectomy: hemodynamic profiles and their correlation with the recovery of erectile function. J Urol. 2002;167(3):1371–5.
51. Fulton D, Gratton JP, McCabe TJ, Fontana J, Fujio Y, Walsh K, Franke TF, Papapetropoulos A, We S. Regulation of endothelium-derived nitric oxide production by the protein kinase Akt. Nature. 1999;399:597–601.
52. Michell BJ, Chen Z, Tiganis T, Stapleton D, Katsis F, Power DA, Sim AT, Kemp BE. Coordinated control of endothelial nitric-oxide synthase phosphorylation by protein kinase C and cAMP-dependent protein kinase. J Biol Chem. 2001;276:17625–8.
53. Fleming I, Fisslthaler B, Dimmeler S, Kemp BE, Busse R. Phosphorylation of Thr(495) regulates Ca(2+)/calmodulin-dependent endothelial nitric oxide synthase activity. Circ Res. 2001;88:E68–75.
54. Ferrini MG, Davila HH, Kovanecz I, et al. Vardenafil prevents fibrosis and loss of corporal smooth muscle that occurs after bilateral cavernosal nerve resection in the rat. Urology. 2006;68:429.
55. Donohue JF, Mullerad M, Kobylarz K, et al. The functional and structural consequences of cavernous nerve injury in the rat model are ameliorated by sildenafil citrate. J Urol. 2005:173–285.
56. Vignozzi L, Filippi S, Morelli A, et al. Effect of chronic tadalafil administration on penile hypoxia induced by cavernous neurotomy in the rate. J Sex Med. 2006;3:419–31.

57. Hatzimouratidis K, Burnett AL, Hatzichristou D, McCullough AR, Montorsi F, Mulhall JP. Phosphodiesterase type-5 inhibitors in postprostatectomy erectile dysfunction: a critical analysis of the basic science rational and clinical application. Eur Urol. 2009;55:334–47.
58. Mulhall JP, Parker M, Waters BW, Flanigan R. The timing of penile rehabilitation after bilateral nerve-sparing radical prostatectomy affects the recovery of erectile function. BJU Int. 2009;105:37–41.
59. Montorsi F, Guazzoni G, Strambi LF, Da Pozzo LF, Nava L, Barbieri L, Rigatti P, Pizzini G, Miani A. Recovery of spontaneous erectile function after nerve sparing radical retropubic prostatectomy with and without early intracavernous injections of alprostadil: results of a prospective, randomised trial. J Urol. 1997;158:1408–10.
60. Mulhall J, Land S, Parker M, Waters WB, Flanigan RC. The use of an erectogenic pharmacotherapy regimen following radical prostatectomy improves recovery of spontaneous erectile function. J Sex Med. 2005;2:532–40. Discussion 540–2.
61. Clavell-Hernandez J, Wang R. Penile rehabilitation following prostate cancer treatment: review of current literature. Asian J Androl. 2015;17(6):916–22; discussion 921. https://doi.org/10.4103/1008-682X.150838. PMID: 25851656; PMCID: PMC4814961.
62. Alba F, Wang R. Current status of penile rehabilitation after radical prostatectomy. CML Urol. 2010;16:93–101.
63. McCullough AR, Hellstrom WG, Wang R, Lepor H, Wagner KR, et al. Recovery of erectile function after nerve sparing radical prostatectomy and penile rehabilitation with nightly intraurethral alprostadil versus sildenafil citrate. J Urol. 2010;183:2451–6.
64. Qian SQ, Gao L, Wei Q, Yuan J. Vacuum therapy in penile rehabilitation after radical prostatectomy: review of hemodynamic and antihypoxic evidence. Asian J Androl. 2016;18(3):446–51. https://doi.org/10.4103/1008-682X.159716. PMID: 26289397; PMCID: PMC4854102.
65. Yuan J, Westney OL, Wang R. Design and application of a new rat-specific vacuum erectile device for penile rehabilitation research. J Sex Med. 2009;6:3247–53.
66. Yuan J, Lin H, Li P, Zhang R, Luo A, et al. Molecular mechanisms of vacuum therapy in penile rehabilitation: a novel animal study. Eur Urol. 2010;58:773–80.
67. Kohler TS, Pedro R, Hendlin K, Utz W, Ugarte R, Reddy P, et al. A pilot study on the early use of the vacuum erection device after radical retropubic prostatectomy. BJU Int. 2007;100:858–62. https://doi.org/10.1111/j.1464-410X.2007.07161.x.
68. Raina R, Agarwal A, Ausmundson S, Lakin M, Nandipati KC, Montague DK, Mansour D, Zippe CD. Early use of vacuum constriction device following radical prostatectomy facilitates early sexual activity and potentially earlier return of erectile function. Int J Impot Res. 2006;18:77–81.
69. Nicolai M, Urkmez A, Sarikaya S, Fode M, Falcone M, Albersen M, Gul M, Hatzichristodoulou G, Capogrosso P, Russo GI. Penile rehabilitation and treatment options for erectile dysfunction following radical prostatectomy and radiotherapy: a systematic review. Front Surg. 2021;8:636974. https://doi.org/10.3389/fsurg.2021.636974. PMID: 33738297; PMCID: PMC7961076

Part III

Kidney, Adrenals, and Ureter

Renal Anatomy, Physiology, and Its Clinical Relevance to Renal Surgery

Ruben De Groote, Chandru Sundaram, and Pieter De Backer

1 Introduction to Renal Anatomy and Its History

Due to its complexity, renal anatomy has a long-standing research history with a specific focus on renal vascularization, as it is crucial to surgical hemostasis. Renal vascular segments were first recognized in the middle of the eighteenth century by Hunter and Bertin [1, 2]. Hyrtl [3] confirmed the compartmentalization hypothesis in 1882 and noted that, due to the renal artery's branching nature with blind endings, the kidney is particularly sensitive to ischemia as compared to other organs. In 1901, Brödel [4] described surgical planes of renal division to avoid blood loss, which he had defined through the production of human renal casts.

The next major breakthrough in renal vascularization was published in 1954 by Graves [5]. He described the first renal artery classification, proposing a renal division into five commonly found segments, based on the corresponding five extrarenal divisions of the renal artery (Fig. 1). This division can be considered a gold standard up to present, although the following research showed the renal vascularization to have a high degree of variation without a "one-size-fits-all" formula.

Due to advancements in the availability and power of different imaging systems, researchers continue to gain more insights into normal and aberrant renal anatomy, and it remains an active topic of study. Our knowledge vastly expands due to the increase in urological, interventional radiological, vascular, and renal transplantation surgeries, all of which require profound knowledge of the vascular tree and renal anomalies [7, 8]. Shifting from open to robotic surgery further facilitates this research.

Another consequence of the advancements in imaging is a rise in the incidence of renal tumors during the last decades [9]. Due to the often accompanying early diagnosis, the majority of these lesions are found at the clinical T1 stage, with distant metastases being present in up to 12% at the time of diagnosis [10], making most of them amenable for partial nephrectomy (chapter "RAPN"). Since minimally invasive approaches have become a viable alternative for open partial nephrectomy [11], a strong focus on the integration of the patient-specific renal anatomy into these technical environments is observed during recent years (chapter "Current Imaging Modalities and Virtual Models for Renal Tumors"). Traditionally, partial nephrectomy was performed open with full hilar clamping and cold ischemia. As such, the relevance of renal vasculature and its anomalies was not readily apparent. The advent of laparoscopic and robotic approaches with their warm ischemia approach and concomitant possible renal ischemic damage required a shift in this approach. Improved ability to dissect and identify vessels and the concern of warm ischemia caused surgeons to shift toward selective clamping or off-clamp tumor resections. As such, knowledge of the patient-specific anatomy and implications for selective clamping has found their way into clinical routine.

A detailed understanding of the patient's anatomy facilitates pre-operative planning as well as peri-operative technique and allows for optimization of functional and oncological surgical outcome.

In this chapter, we describe the embryology, physiology, and surgical anatomy of kidneys and adrenals in order to provide a holistic approach to pre-operative robotic renal surgery planning. A strong emphasis is put on the detection and treatment of vascular anomalies in order to facilitate dissection of atypical vasculature. We also describe practicalities in anticipating and overcoming these difficulties.

R. De Groote (✉)
ORSI Academy, Melle, Belgium

Department of Urology, OLV, Aalst, Belgium

C. Sundaram
Indiana University School of Medicine, Indianapolis, IN, USA

P. De Backer
ORSI Academy, Melle, Belgium

Department of Urology, Ghent University Hospital, Ghent, Belgium

P. Wiklund et al. (eds.), *Robotic Urologic Surgery*, https://doi.org/10.1007/978-3-031-00363-9_33

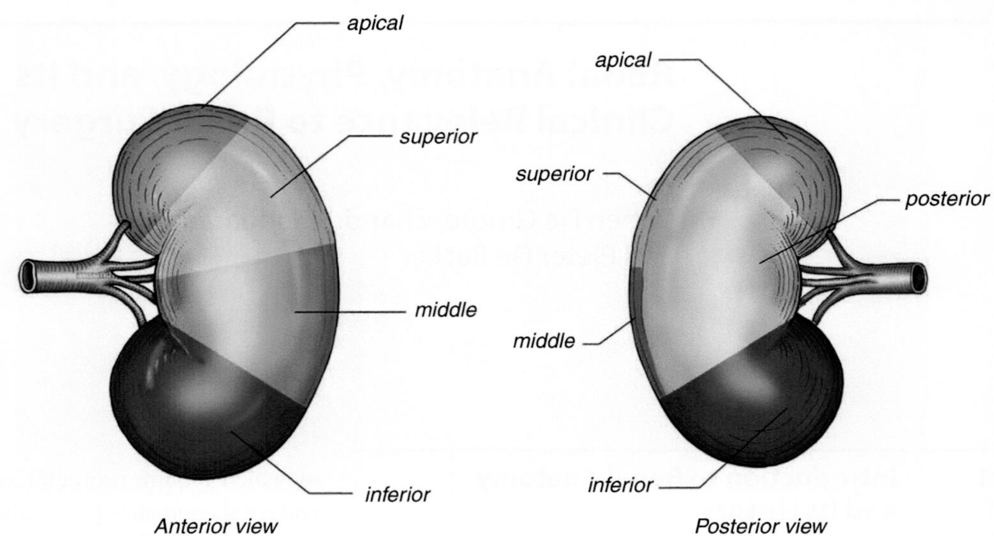

Fig. 1 Segmental division following extrarenal arterial branching as described by Graves [6]. The apical part encompasses the superior pole, the superior part encompasses the remainder of the anteromedial portion of the superior pole, the inferior part occupies the lower pole, the middle part occupies the remaining anteromedial part, and the posterior zone includes the posterior renal part between the apical and inferior segments

2 Renal Physiology

Renal function can be categorized in three main categories:

- Firstly, an excretory function, in which metabolic waste products are excreted toward the urine.
- Secondly, an endocrine function that controls red blood cell production by bone marrow and activates vitamin D.
- Thirdly, a homeostatic role in controlling blood pressure, tissue osmolality, electrolyte and water balance, and plasma pH.

Both excretory and homeostatic properties are carried out through a complex process of filtration, reabsorption, secretion, and excretion.

Renal anatomy and its functions are closely linked. The medial surface of the kidney consists of a hilum through which the renal artery, vein, lymphatics, renal nerves, and ureter access the inner part of the kidney. On sectioning, the kidney parenchyma consists of two main regions: the cortex, seen as a pale outer region, and the medulla, which is the darker inner region. The medulla typically consists of 8–18 conical regions called renal pyramids. Each pyramid is separated by renal cortex; these septa of surrounding cortical tissue are called the columns of Bertin. The base of each medullary pyramid lies at the cortex-medullary border, and the apex ends at so-called papilla, which merges with the pyelum through a minor calyx, the start of the collecting system. These minor calyces fuse into two or three major calyces, which subsequently form the renal pelvis, draining into the ureter. The calyceal walls, pelvis, and ureters are lined with smooth muscles that can propel urine forward by peristalsis. The cortex and medulla form the functional part of the kidney and consist of about 1.3 million nephrons. A corticopapillary osmotic gradient is in place, with a renal cortex osmolality (300 mOsm/kg), being close to plasma osmolality, and a high inner medulla osmolality (1200 mOsm/kg). This osmotic gradient is essential for normal renal function as it allows to recover virtually all of the daily filtered water, which is approximately 180 l.

The cortex contains approximately 85% of the nephrons, and the other 15% are so-called juxta-medullary nephrons. The nephron is the functional kidney unit and consists of a renal corpuscle which is the initial filtering component and a renal tubule which processes and finally carries away the filtered urine.

The renal corpuscle of the juxta-medullary nephron is situated at the border of the medulla but still in the cortex, and their proximal convoluted tubule and the associated loop of Henle occur deeper in the medulla than the cortical nephron. It is to be noted that the juxta-medullary nephrons are the most functional of all nephrons, as they have the capacity to hyperconcentrate urine. This is due to their long loops of Henle reaching deep into the hyperosmolar inner medulla. Their tubuli are the only ones surrounded by vasa recta. The vasa rectum is a long looping vascular structure around the tubular loop, able to generate a hyperosmolar gradient and generate hyperconcentration. As such, the renal pyramids, consisting mainly of the tubuli and vasa recta of juxta-medullary nephrons, can be considered the primary functional unit of the kidney. The juxta-medullary nephron is often depicted when explaining the function of the kidney. Each kidney filters approximately 1 l of blood per minute. This high filtration rate has two major advantages. Firstly, circulating toxins can be cleared from the circulation in as little as 30 min. Secondly, the kidney is only selective on what it recovers from the large filtrate volume, so any substance that is not reabsorbed is automatically secreted without further due.

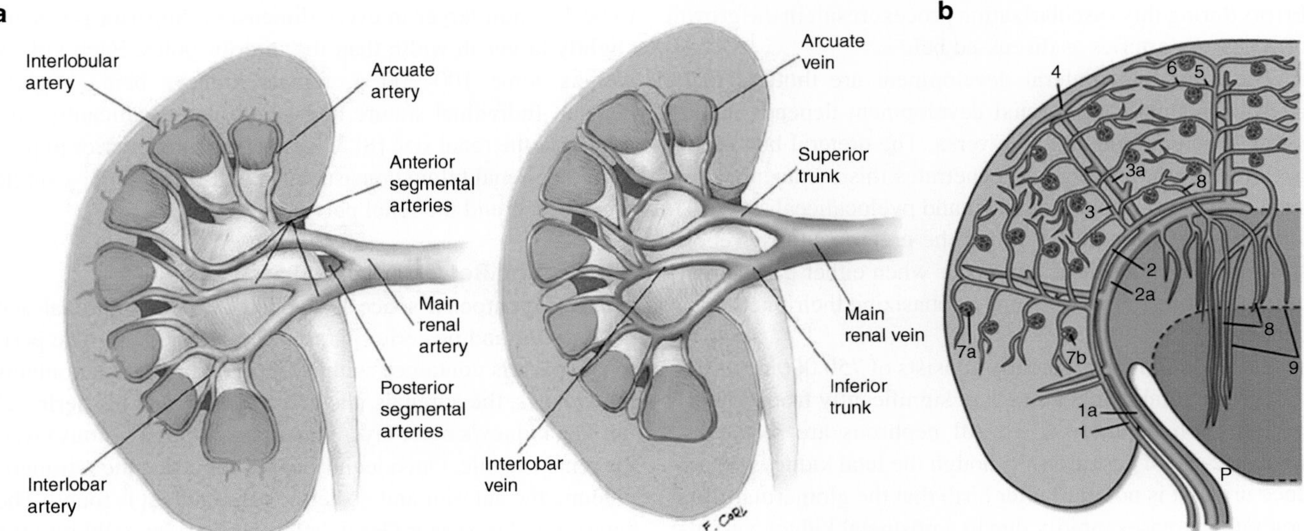

Fig. 2 Vascular system of the kidney. (**a**) Macrovascular network of the kidney. Derived from [12]. (**b**) Microvascular network. (1) Interlobar arteries; (1a) interlobar vein. (2) Arcuate arteries; (2a) arcuate veins. (3) Cortical radial or interlobular arteries; (3a) interlobular veins. (4) Stellate vein. (5) Afferent arterioles. (6) Efferent arterioles. (7a, 7b) Glomerular capillary networks. (8) Descending vasa recta. (9) Ascending vasa recta. Derived from [13]

As depicted in Fig. 2, the vascular supply of the kidney forms a complex network. The renal artery splits into segmental arteries as discussed thoroughly in Sect. 4. These segmental arteries subsequently divide into interlobar arteries which enter the parenchyma at the level of the renal sinus and subsequently travel toward the cortex in the Bertin columns. As such, they extend along the boundary of each renal lobe, explaining their name. These interlobar arteries subsequently branch in right angles to arcuate arteries, found at the corticomedullary border. From these arcuate arteries, cortical radial arteries or interlobular arteries arise in a 90-degree angle and oriented radially as their name suggests. From there on, the arterioles provide oxygen-rich blood to renal corpusculi, tubuli, and vasa recta. Compared to other organs, there is relatively little branching until the capillary region of the vasculature is reached, resulting in higher capillary bed pressures, necessary to sustain the high filtration rate.

Two main factors contribute to the renal sensitivity in hypoperfusion.

Firstly, as stated above, the medullary region is crucial in renal function yet receives only 10% of the arterial blood supply. This is explained by the cortex having a high energy demand of sodium/potassium ATPase, responsible for 99% of the filtration reabsorption into the blood [14]. The lower medullary perfusion however implies that during restricted oxygen delivery such as trauma/crush/arterial clamping, this important functional part becomes anoxic, and renal failure can follow. We also note that it is exactly this lower medullary perfusion rate which contributes the medullary region to be hyperosmolar, as compared to the medullary cortex.

Secondly, the renal branches are non-anastomotic [15]. Even though the arcuate arteries may illicit similarities to arcuate artery in the human feet, the renal arterial system is terminal. This is also clearly noted in renal infarction, with typical triangular defects.

Venous blood drains through a similar cascade of venules, interlobular veins, arcuate veins, interlobar veins, and eventually the renal vein. In contrast to the arterial system, this system is non-terminal, with several anastomoses inside the kidney but also with veins in the perinephric fat, through a subcapsular plexus of stellate veins.

3 Embryology

The renal organogenesis starts at the level of the three germ leaves. More specifically, the kidneys originate from the intermediate mesoderm. Nephrogenesis starts in the 4th week of gestation. In utero, renal development is characterized by three subsequent phases, pronephros, mesonephros, and metanephros, which is the precursor of the final kidney [16].

At week 6, the metanephros ascends from the pelvis toward its final lumbar position where it meets the adrenal gland. While the kidneys are still in the pelvis, they are supplied by the median sacral artery and internal and external iliac vessels. In normal organogenesis, these arteries atrophy and newly cranial arteries are formed as the kidneys' ascent. As such, the kidneys generate arteries along their path, making new cranial arteries, while lower caudal arteries atrophy.

Errors during this vascularization process result in the growth of accessory arteries as discussed below.

The renal and ureteral development are thought to be interdependent: normal renal development depends upon a normal ureteral bud and vice versa. The ureteral bud undergoes orderly branching and penetrates this metanephros, as such forming the collecting duct and pyelocaliceal system. It will also elongate, thus forming the ureter. Autopsy reports show that renal agenesis can occur when either parenchyma or ureteral bud fail to develop, emphasizing their interdependence [17].

Each adult kidney typically consists of 750,000 nephrons, though the total number can vary significantly from 250,000 to 2 million nephrons [18]. All nephrons are formed by weeks 32–36 of gestation. Although the fetal kidneys do produce urine, it is not until after birth that the glomerular filtration rate increases rapidly due to a postnatal kidney vascular resistance drop and accompanying increased renal perfusion. Nephron maturation also continues postnatally.

4 Surgical Renal Anatomy

4.1 Renal Anatomical Relationships

4.1.1 Renal Topology

The position of the right kidney is 1–2 cm lower than the left kidney due to the liver, positioned above. Both kidneys are positioned retroperitoneally and rest with their posterior upper third against the diaphragm, covered by the 12th rib. The left kidney is also covered by the 11th rib. Their longitudinal axes parallel the oblique and inclined psoas muscle, on which their posterior medial two thirds rest, while the lateral posterior two thirds is bordered by the quadratus lumborum. Both muscles are separated from the kidney by Gerota's fascia, a layer of posterior pararenal fat and the transversus abdominis fascia [19]. Due to the conical psoas muscle shape, the superior poles are more inclined toward posterior and medial in comparison to the inferior poles.

Anteriorly, the kidneys are lined by the left and right colon with their mesentery on the respective sides. The right kidney is bordered by the liver and attached to it by the hepatorenal ligament. Its renal hilum is overlayed by the descending part of the duodenum and the pancreatic head. The left kidney is superiorly bordered by the pancreatic tail and splenic hilum, in which the inferior mesenteric vein fuses. The posterior gastric wall can also overly the left kidney. It is attached to the spleen by the splenorenal ligaments, and care should be taken in applying excessive downward pressure on the left kidney to avoid splenic capsular lesions.

Mean renal length is estimated at approximately 11.1 cm, with a thickness of 3.3 cm. The superior width is found to be 1.1 cm wider than the inferior pole. The left kidney is found to be 1–3 mm larger in every dimension. Superior poles are slightly larger in width than the inferior poles. Each kidney weighs some 100–200 g, female kidneys being slightly heavier. Individual stature and length are significantly correlated to the renal size [8]. Classically, from anterior to posterior, the renal hilum consists of a single renal vein, a single renal artery, and the renal pelvis.

4.1.2 The Retroperitoneal Space

The retroperitoneal space is divided into the perirenal and the anterior and posterior pararenal space (Fig. 3). The perirenal space is contained within Gerota's fascia and contains the kidneys, the adrenals, the great vessels, and the perirenal fat. The kidney's outer layer consists of a tough fibrous layer, the renal capsule. Outside the Gerota but inside the retroperitoneum, the anterior and posterior pararenal fat is found. The anterior and posterior Gerota's fasciae fuse laterally into the lateroconal fascia, which subsequently fuses with the peritoneum lateral to the colon, as such forming the white line of Toldt. Superiorly, Gerota's fascia attaches to the diaphragmatic crura, while inferiorly, no fusion occurs, as such leaving a potential open space.

4.1.3 The Adrenal Glands

The adrenal glands are paired structures, located on the medial upper kidney pole within Gerota's fascia. They are surrounded by adipose and connective tissue, forming a pseudocapsule which facilitates dissection. The right adrenal gland is positioned lower than the left adrenal gland, in concordance with relative position of the right kidney as compared to the left kidney. It is positioned between the liver and the diaphragm, just right to the IVC, with the duodenum covering it anteromedially. The left adrenal lies more medial than its contralateral equivalent. In contrast to the right adrenal vein which drains directly in the IVC, the lower left adrenal drains into the midpoint of the left renal vein. This explains its more medial position and why it is more easily drawn down with the left kidney itself. The superior left adrenal drains into the inferior phrenic vein. Similarly to the upper left kidney pole, the left adrenal's anterior and upper aspects are also related to the pancreatic tail and splenic vessels, as well as the stomach. Bilateral arterial adrenal supply is identical and threefold: inferior branches from the ipsilateral renal artery, middle branches directly from the abdominal aorta, and superior branches from the inferior phrenic arteries (Fig. 4).

4.1.4 Variations

Horseshoe kidneys are one of the most commonly found renal fusion anomalies with a reported frequency of 1 in 500 patients and a male preponderance (2:1) [22]. In a horseshoe kidney, both kidneys are connected by an isthmus, most often at the level of the lower pole. The isthmus is found

Anterior Gerota's fascia
Anterolateral abdominal muscles
Psoas major muscle
IVC
Aorta
Kidney
Peritoneum
Perirenal fat
Lateroconal fascia
Posterior Gerota's fascia (Zuckerkandl fascia)
Transversalis fascia
Pararenal fat
Quadratus lumborum muscle

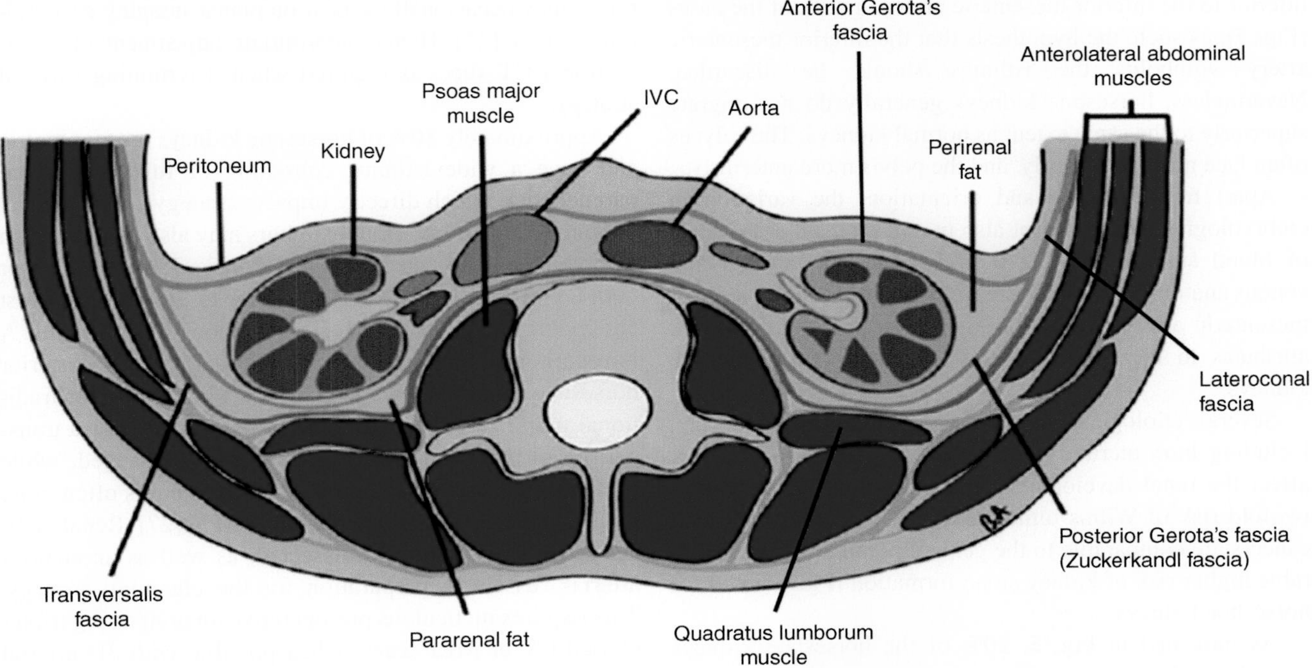

Fig. 3 Retroperitoneal organization. Adapted from [20]

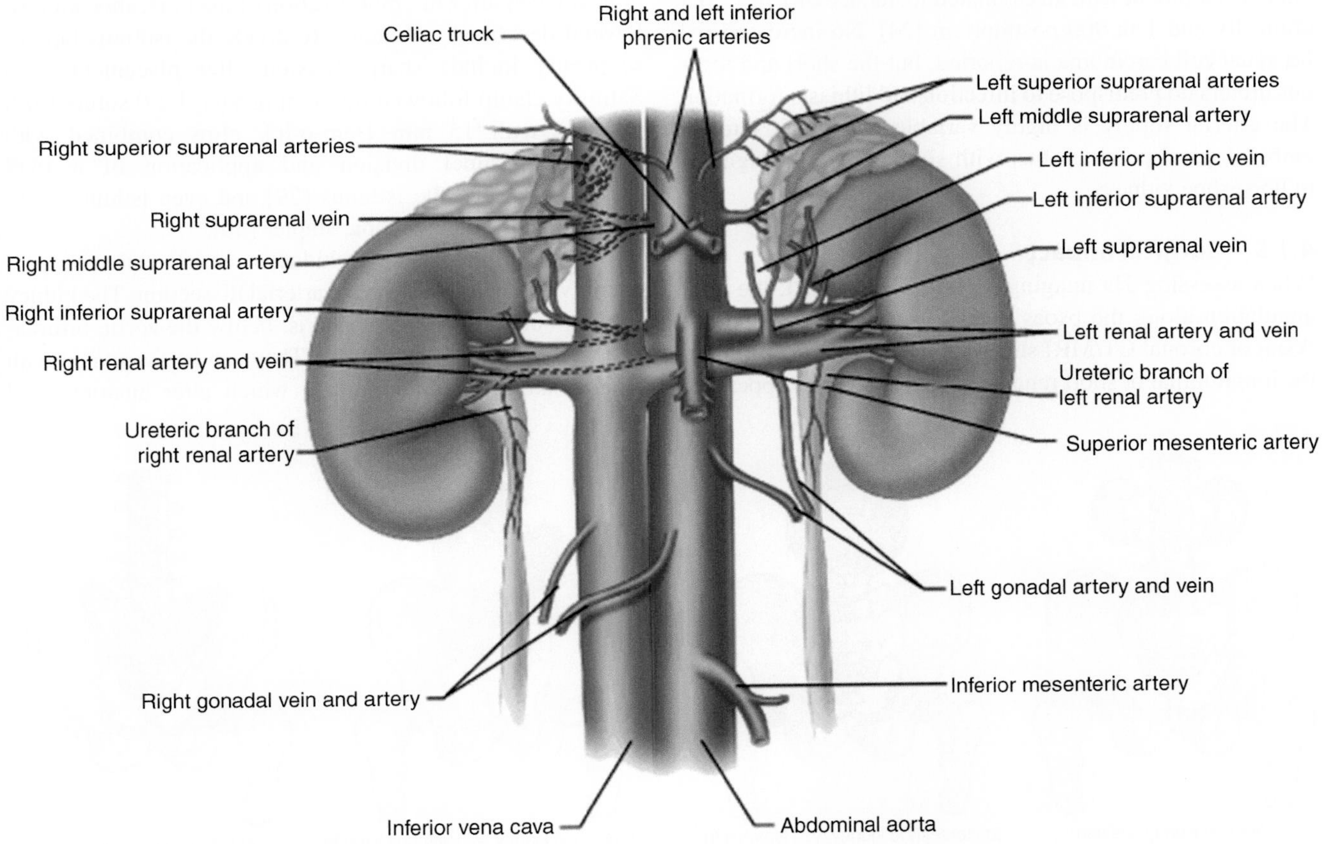

Celiac truck
Right and left inferior phrenic arteries
Left superior suprarenal arteries
Left middle suprarenal artery
Left inferior phrenic vein
Left inferior suprarenal artery
Left suprarenal vein
Left renal artery and vein
Ureteric branch of left renal artery
Superior mesenteric artery
Right superior suprarenal arteries
Right suprarenal vein
Right middle suprarenal artery
Right inferior suprarenal artery
Right renal artery and vein
Ureteric branch of right renal artery
Left gonadal artery and vein
Inferior mesenteric artery
Right gonadal vein and artery
Inferior vena cava
Abdominal aorta

Fig. 4 Renal and adrenal vascularization overview. Derived from [21]

inferior to the inferior mesenteric artery in 40% of the cases (Fig. 5); as such, the hypothesis that the inferior mesenteric artery withholds the isthmus should be discarded. Nevertheless, horseshoe kidneys generally do not migrate superiorly to the same extent as normal kidneys. The calyces often face more posteriorly, and the pelvis more anteriorly.

Apart from location and orientation, the variation in embryological development also manifests itself at the level of blood supply, showing a highly variable arterial and venous anatomy. Arteries arise from any of the aorta, inferior mesenteric artery, iliac vessels, or even sacral artery. This attributes to the complex surgical anatomy of horseshoe kidneys.

Several etiological factors are thought to contribute, including intra-uterine, genetic, and structural factors that affect the renal development and migration. Apart from a twofold risk of Wilms tumor [23], rates of other renal cell cancers are comparable to the general population. A comparable higher risk of kidney stone formation is also noted for horseshoe kidneys.

As indicated in Fig. 5, 20% of the horseshoe kidneys never leave the pelvis.

When unfused, non-ascending of pelvic kidneys forms another frequent finding of migrational errors during embryonal development with an estimated incidence of 1 in 12,000 clinically and 1 in 900 postmortem [24]. No increased risk for renal cell carcinoma is reported, but the short and tortuous ureters do predispose to infection and lithiasis formation. The arterial supply is highly variable and confers to the embryological pelvic status, with similar arterial origins as in horseshoe kidneys.

4.1.5 Surgical Impact

When assessing 2D imaging such as CT or MRI, the renal angulation along the psoas muscle becomes very relevant. Axial or coronal CT/MRI slices are not aligned according to the longitudinal or short renal axis, and as such an upper pole tumor may occasionally appear on planar imaging as a mid-renal tumor [25]. Hence, appropriate adjustment of cross-sectional CT slices is required when determining surgical strategy.

Approximately 80% of horseshoe kidneys are symmetric and have a wide isthmus consisting of functional renal parenchyma, which directly impacts strategy during partial or heminephrectomy. Double ureters may also be present on or both sides (6%) in horseshoe kidneys [26], and one or both ureters can rarely travel posterior to the isthmus. Most commonly the great vessels lie posterior to the isthmus. A retroperitoneal approach might be essential in posterior horseshoe tumors as the anatomy does not allow for traditional mobilization and flipping of the kidney. For a transperitoneal approach, patient position is unchanged, while port placement needs to be individualized but is often more medial and caudal than in classical RAPN [27]. Renal pedicle needs to be carefully dissected, as well as anomalous arterial vessels in preparation for the clamping strategy. This requires meticulous pre-operative imaging using triple-phased CT or MRI scans, when possible with 3D arterial reconstruction. Tumor dissection can be challenging as the kidney is still supplied by the other half through the isthmus. When heminephrectomy is required, the isthmus needs to be divided after full mobilization of the horseshoe kidney. Several described techniques to divide the isthmus laparoscopically include sharp division after placement of a Satinsky clamp followed by running Vicryl 2-0 suture [28], clipping with 15 mm Hem-o-lok clips combined with Harmonic scalpel division and application of a PDS Endoloop around the isthmus [29] and even isthmus transection using a laparoscopic stapler [30].

Similarly, ectopic pelvic kidneys require extensive pre-operative imaging and precise arterial dissection. The kidney is often buried deep in the pelvis, below the aortic bifurcation, and hidden by the sacrum. They can be associated with other anatomical abnormalities which alter anatomy and

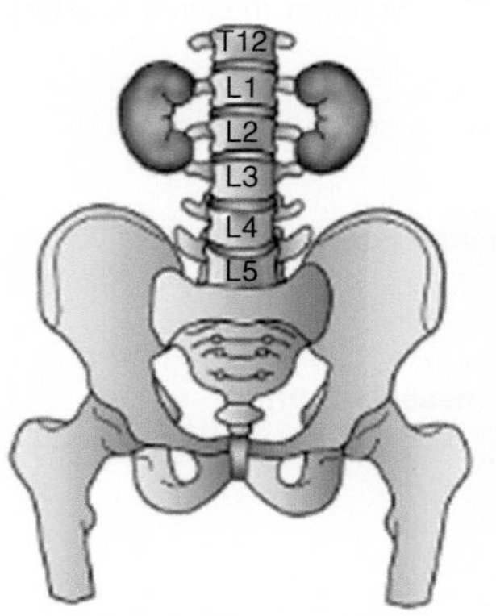

1) Normal kidney position.

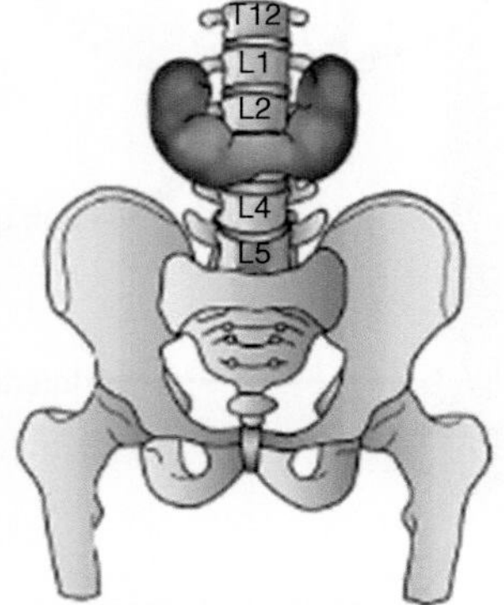

2) Horseshoe kidney with isthmus in normal position of lower poles (40%).

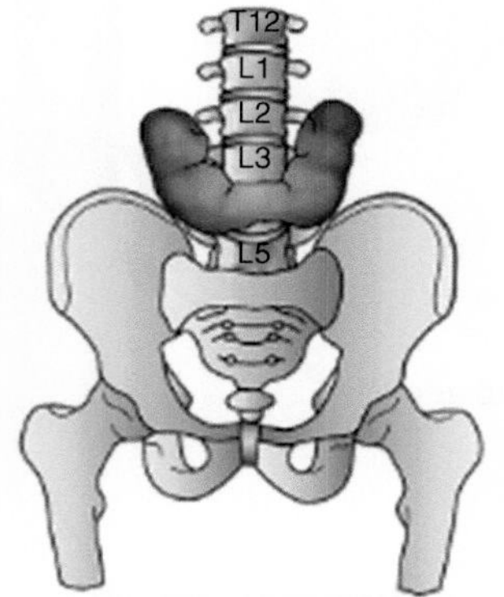

3) Horseshoe kidney with isthmus lying at L4 below inferior mesenteric artery (40%).

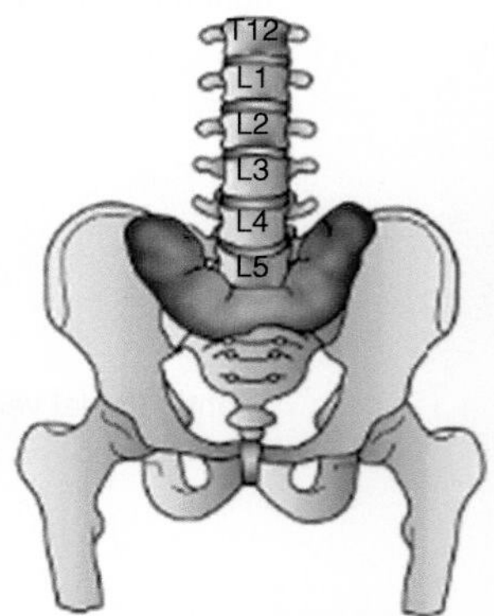

4) Horseshoe kidney with isthmus inthe pelvis (20%).

Fig. 5 Position-distribution of inferiorly fused horseshoe kidneys as compared to the normal position. Horseshoe kidneys fused at the lower pole account for 90% of all horseshoe kidneys, and 20% of these horseshoe kidneys never leave the pelvis. Derived from [22]

complicate access. Just as horseshoe kidneys, these procedures should be left in the hands of experienced robotic surgeons [27].

Regarding renal topology, several renal anatomical relationships need to be appreciated during kidney mobilization and renal surgery. Due to the vicinity of the pancreatic tail near the left renal hilum, one should always be aware of the possibility of pancreatic tail lesions during RAPN or left nephrectomy. Unlike splenic injuries, which are easily recognized pre-operatively due to extensive bleeding, pancreatic lesions tend to be recognized in the post-operative period when pancreatic fistula's or peripancreatic collections become apparent. As these complications require re-interventions in the majority of cases and have a considerable mortality rate, pancreatic lesions during renal surgery account for one of the most significant complications. Care should be given to the pancreas tail during descending colon mobilization in left-sided renal surgery during which wide exposure and a meticulous surgical technique are key [31].

The close relationship between the left kidney and the spleen demands carefulness during upper pole mobilization of the left kidney. Iatrogenic injury to the spleen is not an uncommon complication. Left nephrectomy has been reported as the second most common cause of iatrogenic splenectomy with a reported incidence between 1.3 and 24%. Moreover, iatrogenic splenectomy is associated with significant morbidity and mortality. With the advent of hemostatic agents, smaller splenic injuries could be managed conservatively. As mobilization of the splenic flexure of the colon most often is not deemed necessary for a good exposure, this could prevent iatrogenic splenic capsule laceration and splenic vessel damage [32–34].

Left-sided kidney exposure demands mobilization of the descending colon along the paracolic gutter (i.e., Toldt's fascia). During right-sided renal surgery, it is deemed necessary by many surgeons to completely mobilize the ascending colon along Toldt's fascia. However, the splenic flexure lies at a higher level compared with the hepatic flexure, as it is held on to the diaphragm by a peritoneal fold, the phrenicocolic ligament on which the spleen sits. Therefore, a full ascending colon might not be necessary in the majority of cases. An alternative technique is to start the right hilar dissection at the level of the fat-free region of the inferior caval vein under the liver border and to follow it more caudally until the renal vein is met. A minimal mobilization of hepatic colic flexure and duodenum is only necessary [35].

4.2 Arterial System

4.2.1 Normal Anatomy

In general, each kidney has one single renal artery which finds its origin on the abdominal aorta slightly below the superior mesenteric artery. It is bilaterally positioned posterior to the renal vein. However, in approximately one in three patients, the renal artery is located anterior to the renal vein [25].

Due to the lowered position of the right kidney and the left-sided aortic origin, the right renal artery has a longer and downward course, traversing behind the inferior vena cava (IVC). The left renal artery however typically arises somewhat lower on the abdominal aorta, as such having a horizontal orientation toward to the superiorly positioned left kidney.

The renal artery typically gives rise to an anterior and posterior trunk, which subsequently subdivides into four to five segmental arteries which supply a corresponding segmental parenchymal part (Fig. 6). The anterior trunk is con-

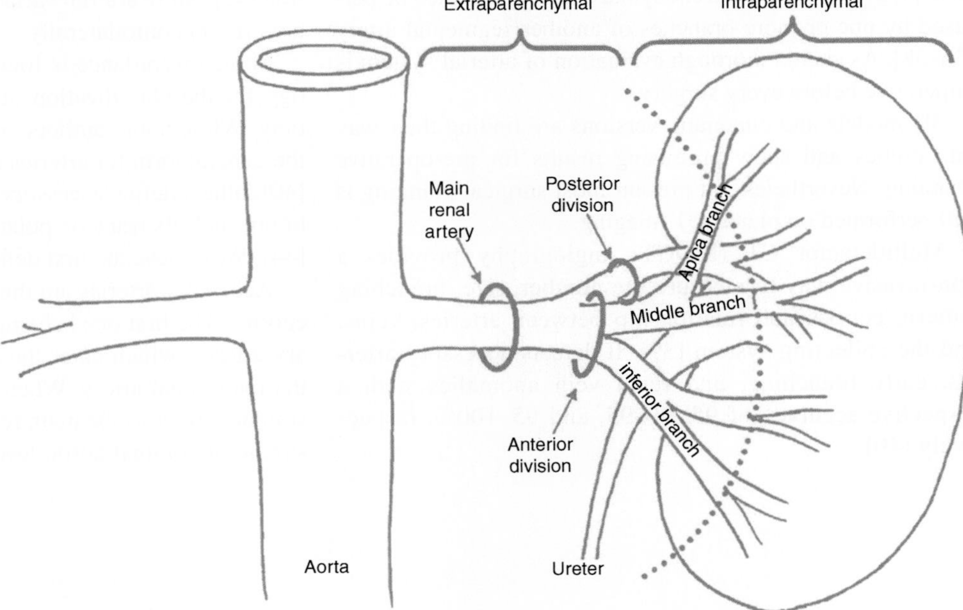

Fig. 6 Classical extrarenal anatomic division of the renal artery into five segmental arteries: an anterior trunk giving rise to an apical, upper, middle, and lower segmental artery and a posterior trunk perfusing the posterior segment. Derived from [25]

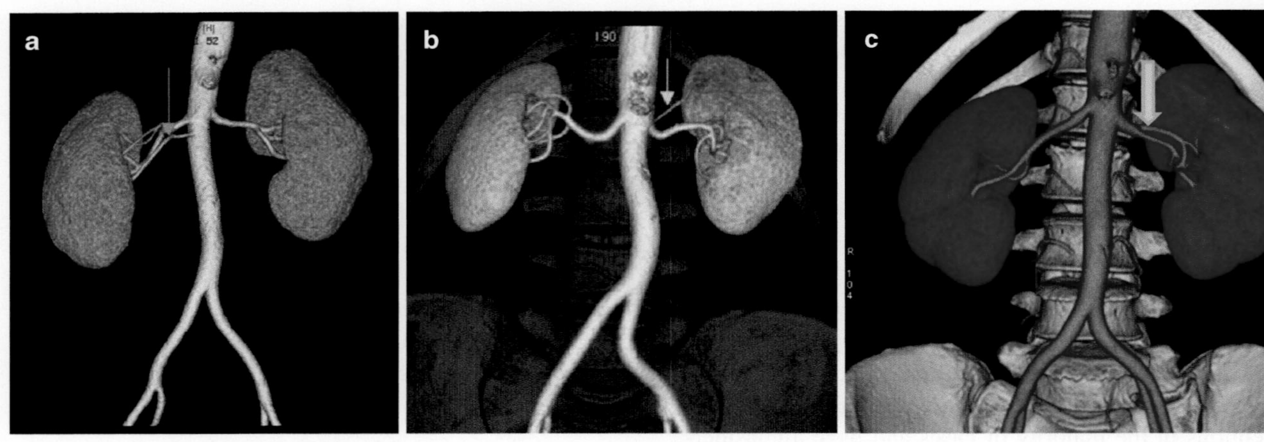

Fig. 7 Cinematic renders of supernumerary renal artery categories. Pictures adapted from [45]. (**a**) Accessory hilar renal artery on the right side, as indicated by the blue arrow. The artery has its origin in the abdominal aorta and enters at the level of the renal hilum. (**b**) Accessory polar artery on the right side as indicated by the yellow arrow. The artery has its origin in the abdominal artery and enters the kidney outside the renal hilum. (**c**) Early arterial branching on the left side, as indicated by the yellow arrow. The artery has its origin in the renal artery itself, within 1.5 cm of the arterial ostium

sidered dominant in perfusion, carrying approximately 75% of the renal blood supply [25]. The anterior-posterior division gives rise to an avascular frontal plane, along the so-called line of Brödel as defined in 1901, passing through the row of minor posterior calyces, which is currently however less used in surgical planning.

The corresponding perfusion zones for these segmental arteries, as defined by Graves in 1954, can be seen in Fig. 1. Subsequent division of segmental arteries up onto the interlobular level is discussed in Sect. 2.

Graves' classification is considered the gold standard for the classification of the arterial renal system. Nevertheless, a high variability is present both at the level of the main renal artery and its segmental arteries. Several studies estimate the percentage deviating from Graves' classification around 40% [1, 2, 36]. Single parenchymal segment can also be perfused by one or more branches of another segmental artery [36–38]. As such a thorough evaluation of arterial system is imperative before every surgery.

3D models and cinematic versions are finding their way into clinics and show promising results for pre-operative planning. Nevertheless, at present most surgical planning is still performed on planar CT imaging.

Multidetector CT (MDCT) angiography provides a non-invasive way to measure the number, size, branching pattern, course, and relationship between arteries, veins, and the collecting system [39]. It detects accessory arteries, early branching, and renal vein anomalies with a respective accuracy of 95, 90–95, and 95–100%, respectively [40].

4.2.2 Renal Artery Variations

As mentioned above, the renal vasculature has consistent patterns, but it can still be very subject to variation (Fig. 7). One reason for this variation is the renal ascent in utero in which arteries are subsequently generated and atrophied. As such, supernumerary or accessory renal arteries are found up to 25–30% of the population, while the other two thirds are estimated to have a classical single renal artery [2, 41, 42]. As such, the presence of these multiple or accessory renal arteries is the most common anatomic variation [43]. Up to five accessory arteries have been reported.

Accessory arteries originate most commonly from the abdominal aorta, supplying the inferior pole [40]. Accessory or multiple renal arteries are more common on the right side [25] and can be present bilaterally in 10–15% of the population [42]. More arterial variation is also seen when anomalies are present contralaterally.

Some discordance is found in literature on the terminology for the classification of anomalous arterial renal anatomy. While some authors consider accessory arteries to be the general term for arteries not following a classical pattern [40], others define accessory arteries as arteries reaching the hilum and aberrant or polar arteries as the other category [44]. We choose the first definition.

Accessory arteries are thus subdivided into two main categories. The first one is being the hilar arteries, supernumerary arteries which enter the kidney at the hilum along with the main renal artery. When a hilar accessory artery is of a similar caliber as the main renal artery and originates from a similar abdominal aortic level, it is sometimes named "second main renal artery." The second category is formed by polar arteries which enter the kidney directly from the capsule outside the hilum. Both groups usually originate from the abdominal aorta or iliac arteries. Rarely, both categories of accessory arteries may also arise from the lower thoracic aorta and lumbar or mesenteric arteries.

Both groups are not to be confused with the so-called prehilar or early arterial branching, in which the first renal arterial branch arises within 1.5 cm of the renal artery ostium, with an estimated prevalence of 12% of the population [44]. Early arterial branching is also more objectivated on the right side [45–47].

4.2.3 Surgical Impact

Several studies have shown that both parenchymal segments [31] and tumors are often perfused by several segmental arteries [2, 37, 38]. This means that segmental clamping will often be insufficient to reach satisfactory tumor ischemia. These crossing vessels are most frequently found between the middle, inferior, and superior segments. As such, tumors at the posterior segment have a smaller risk of collateral blood supply from anterior segmental arteries. Bloodless resection after selective clamping is expected to follow [36]. This can be considered a present equivalent to the avascular plane as defined by Brödel.

Evenly important is that the renal arterial system is terminal. As stated above, this makes the parenchyma very sensitive to ischemic damage.

As such, both aspects have a direct impact on the clamping strategy.

We refer to chapter "Hilar Dissection: Selective Clamping and Early Unclamping Techniques for Clamping Strategies."

Concerning the variant anatomy on the right-hand side, a surgeon needs to be aware renal artery typically originates posterior to the IVC, but early bifurcation or accessory artery can result in the part of the right renal artery being anterior to the IVC, therefore accruing the risk of damaging the IVC [47].

4.3 Venous System

4.3.1 Normal Anatomy

As discussed in the arterial section, the right renal artery generally crosses the inferior vena cava posteriorly. This relative position is most often maintained upon the renal hilum, where the renal vein usually lies anterior to the renal artery. Due to the IVC's rather right-sided position, the left renal vein is almost three times longer than the right renal vein [20]. Unlike the right renal vein, the left renal vein receives several tributaries before joining the IVC: the left adrenal vein superiorly, the left gonadal vein inferiorly, and a lumbar vein posteriorly. It reaches the IVC more cranially and anterolaterally as compared to the right renal vein. Direct confluence of gonadal or adrenal veins into the right renal vein is seen in only 7 and 30% of cases, respectively. The renal vein's position can vary up to 1–2 cm cranio-caudally with respect to the artery.

Up until the level of the segmental branches, the venous anatomy correlates with the arterial system. These segmental branches next coalescence in two to five venous trunks which will eventually the renal vein.

In contrast to the arterial supply, the venous system has plenty of intra- and extrarenal anastomotic vessels. They anastomose at the level of the sinus (first order), pyramids (second order), and marginal veins (third order) [48]. The veins are also in relation to interlobar, arciform, and stellate veins. As noted earlier, the venous drainage indeed also communicates with veins inside the perinephric fat via a subcapsular venous plexus of stellate veins.

We discuss the anomalies on CT angiography. The venous anatomy is readily to be appreciated on the arterial phase. However, some large venous tributaries might require additional evaluation of nephrographic phase images [49, 50].

4.3.2 Renal Vein Anomalies

In contrast to the high arterial variation, venous anatomy is less variable.

The most commonly encountered venous variation is the presence of multiple renal veins, encountered in 15–30% of patients [42]. Multiple renal veins are more present on the right side [44], most probably due to the short distance to the IVC. The left renal vein is nearly always singular. Two left gonadal veins can be observed in 15% of patients, and the gonadal vein can become very large on the left side, being diagnosed a prominent gonadal vein which is 5 mm or larger (Fig. 8). In 59–88% of patients, the retroperitoneal veins (lumbar, ascending lumbar, and hemiazygos veins) drain into the left renal vein.

Figure 9 provides an overview of the most common left renal vein anomalies and peculiarities.

The most common anomaly of the left renal venous system is the circumaortic renal vein, seen in up to 17% of the population (Fig. 9b) [42, 44]. Here, the left renal vein splits into an anterior and posterior part that encircles the abdominal aorta. The retro-aortic component can vary in size. The adrenal vein typically joins the anterior part, while the gonadal vein typically joins the posterior vein. The posterior component often joins the aorta at a more caudal level, which also explains its relation to the gonadal vein.

More rare is a complete retro-aortic renal vein, seen in 2–3% of patients. Here, the single left renal vein courses posterior to the aorta before draining into the IVC (Fig. 9C).

Less common variants include a late venous confluence, in which the venous branch coalescences within 1.5 cm of the anastomosis of the renal vein with the IVC. As such, it is the venous analogy of early arterial branching.

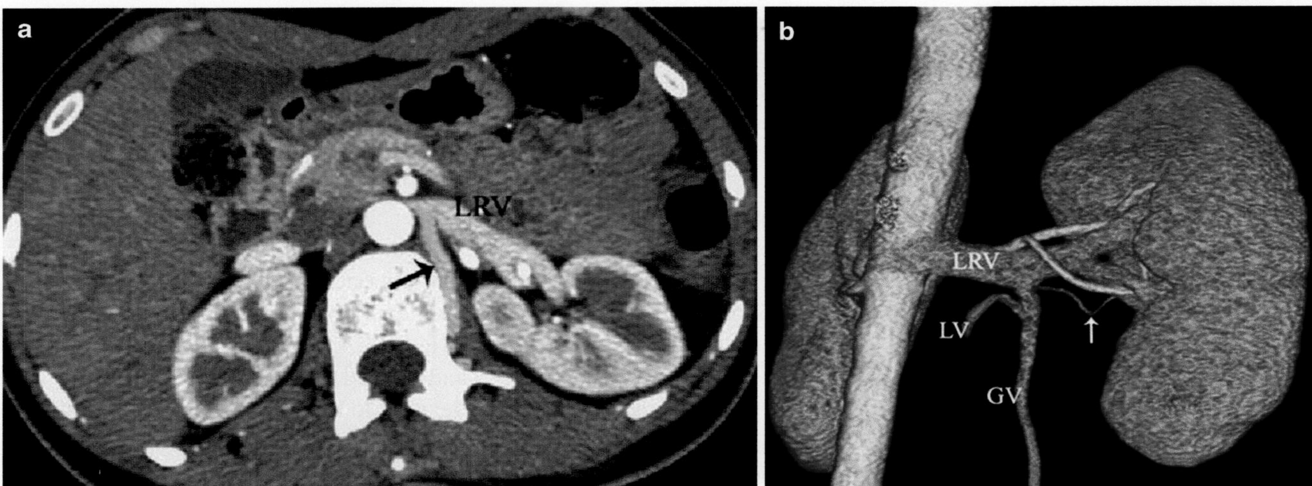

Fig. 8 Prominent gonadal and retroperitoneal veins. (**a**) Large lumbar vein draining into the left renal vein (LRV), as indicated by the black arrow [42]. (**b**) Cinematic render showing a prominent left gonadal vein (GV), draining into the left renal vein (LRV), as well as a lumbar vein (LV) and small renal venous branch (arrow) draining into the left gonadal vein

Right-sided late venous confluence is very poorly described, as almost every right-sided venous drainage happens within 1.5 cm of the renal vein ostium due to the short venous length.

4.3.3 Surgical Impact

As discussed earlier, the renal venous system is not terminal but widely collateral. This implies that segmental branches can be occluded without hampering venous outflow or without subsequent renal damage.

MDCT allows for pre-operative detection of minor venous variants such as lumbar or gonadal veins. This may facilitate dissection in partial and radical nephrectomy and help avoid hemorrhagic complications.

If an IVC thrombus is present, both collateral venous circulation and drainage of the retroperitoneal veins will be hampered, causing them to dilate and further increasing the risk of hemorrhagic complications.

4.4 Renal Collecting System and the Ureter

4.4.1 Renal Papillae, Calyces, and Pelvis

The renal papillae are the tip of a medullary pyramid and constitute the first gross structure of the renal collecting system (Fig. 10). Typically, each kidney has 7–9 papillae, but this number is variable, ranging from 4 to 18. Each of these papillae is cupped by a minor calyx. At the upper and lower poles, compound calyces are often encountered. These compound calyces are the result of renal pyramid fusion and because of their anatomy dare more likely to allow reflux into the renal parenchyma.

After cupping an individual papilla, each minor calyx narrows to an infundibulum. Just as there is frequent variation in the number of calyces, the diameter and length of the infundibula vary greatly. Infundibula combine to form two or three major calyceal branches. These are frequently termed the upper, middle, and lower pole calyces, and these calyces in turn combine to form the renal pelvis. The renal pelvis itself can vary greatly in size, ranging from a small intrarenal pelvis to a large predominantly extrarenal pelvis. Eventually the pelvis narrows to form the ureteropelvic junction, marking the beginning of the ureter.

4.4.2 Ureter

The key to many urologic procedures is an understanding of ureteral anatomic relationships. The ureter begins at the ureteropelvic junction, which lies posterior to the renal artery and vein. It then progresses inferiorly along the anterior edge of the psoas muscle. Anteriorly, the right ureter is related to the ascending colon, cecum, colonic mesentery, and appendix. The left ureter is closely related to the descending and sigmoid colon and their accompanying mesenteries. Approximately a third of the way to the bladder, the ureter is crossed anteriorly by the gonadal vessels. As it enters the pelvis, the ureter crosses anterior to the iliac vessels. This crossover point is usually at the bifurcation of the common iliac into the internal and external iliac arteries, thus making this a useful landmark for pelvic procedures [53, 54].

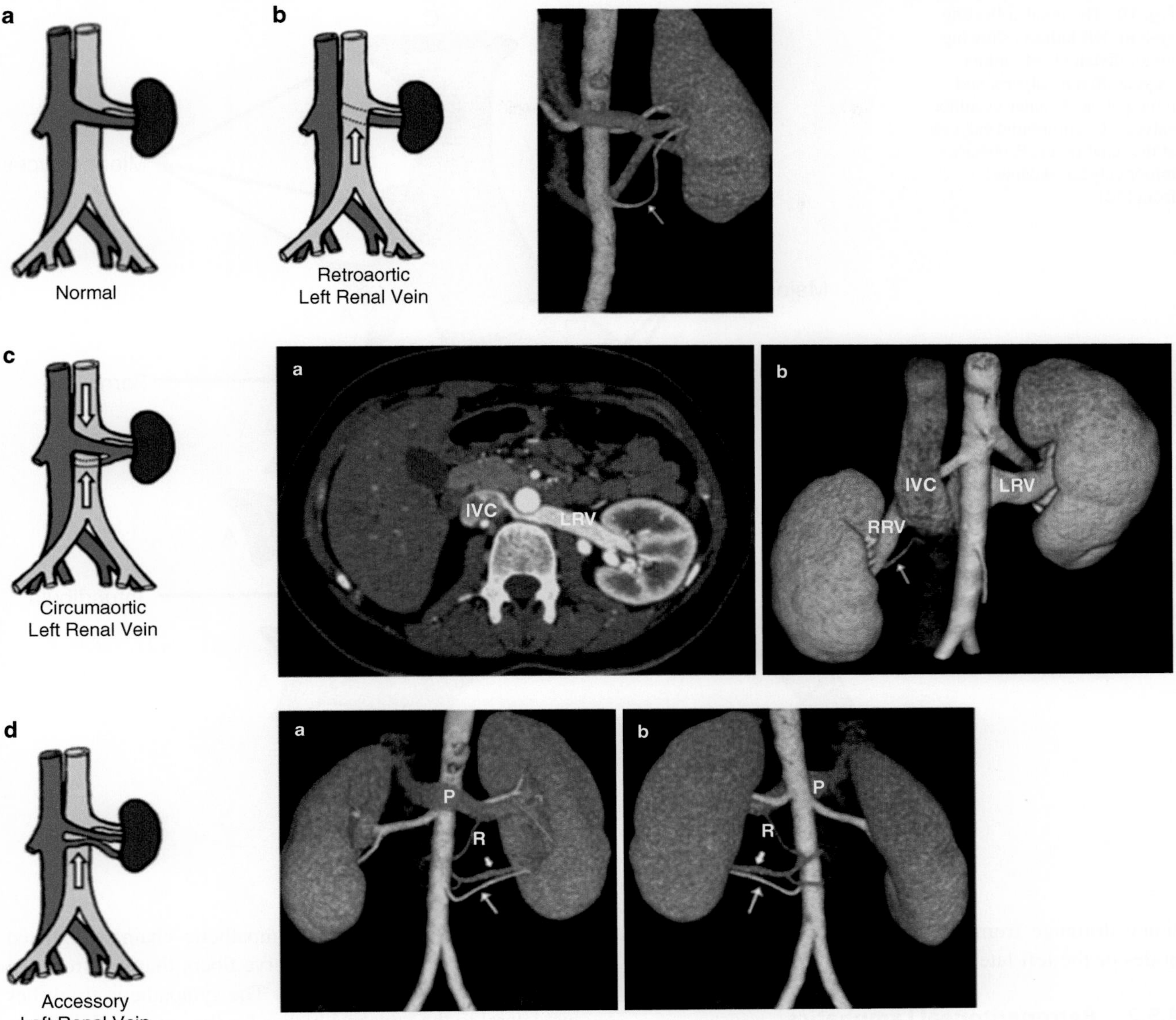

Fig. 9 An overview of the congenital left renal vein and IVC anomalies. Adapted from [42, 51]. (**a**) Normal anatomical situation. (**b**) Circumaortic left renal vein. Cinematic render shows how the posterior vein is more caudally oriented. We also note the accessory hilar artery. (**c**) Retro-aortic left renal vein (LRV). Note the second small right renal vein (arrow) (RRV, right renal vein; IVC, inferior vena cava). (**d**) Accessory second renal vein (short arrow), with a small retro-aortic component, and a polar artery (long arrow)

4.5 Lymphatics, Retroperitoneal Nodes and Sympathetic Ganglia

4.5.1 Renal Lymphatics

The renal lymphatics largely follow blood vessels through the columns of Bertin and then form large lymphatic trunks within the renal sinus. As these lymphatics exit the hilum, branches from the renal capsule, perinephric tissues, renal pelvis, and upper ureter drain into these lymphatics. They then empty into lymph nodes associated with the renal vein near the renal hilum. From here, the lymphatic drainage between the two kidneys differs between sides. On the left, primary lymphatic drainage is into the left lateral para-aortic lymph nodes including nodes anterior and posterior to the aorta between the inferior mesenteric artery and the diaphragm. Occasionally, there will be additional drainage from the left kidney into the retrocrural nodes or directly into the thoracic duct above the diaphragm. On the right, drainage is into the right interaortocaval and right paracaval lymph nodes, including nodes located anterior and posterior to the vena cava, from the common iliac vessels to the diaphragm. Occasionally, there will be addi-

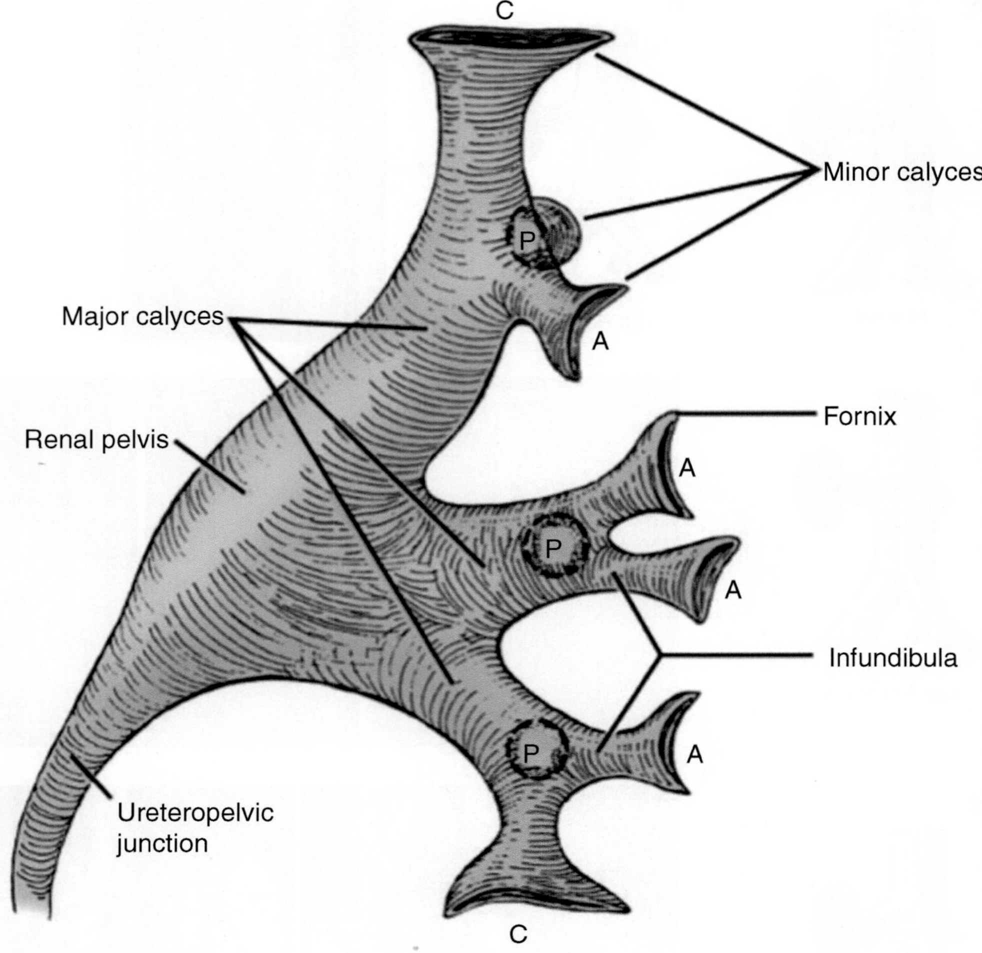

Fig. 10 The renal collecting system (left kidney) showing major divisions into minor calyces, major calyces, and renal pelvis. A, anterior minor calyces; C, compound calyces at the renal poles; P, posterior minor calyces. Adapted from [52]

tional drainage from the right kidney into the retrocrural nodes or the left lateral para-aortic lymph nodes.

4.5.2 Retroperitoneal Lymphatics

The retroperitoneal lymphatics form a very rich and extensive chain. As a general rule, lymphatics follow the arteries, and named lymph nodes are found at the root of the arteries. Retroperitoneal nodes of the abdomen comprise the inferior diaphragmatic nodes and the lumbar nodes. The latter are classified as left lumbar (aortic), intermediate lumbar (interaorticovenous), and right lumbar (caval). These nodes surround the aorta and the inferior vena cava. Around the aorta lie the para-aortic nodes, preaortic nodes (including celiac, superior mesenteric, and inferior mesenteric nodes collecting lymph from the splanchna supplied by the homonymous arteries), and retro-aortic nodes. Similarly, around the vena cava lie the paracaval, precaval, and retrocaval nodes. Pelvic nodes include the common iliac, external and internal iliac, obturator, and sacral nodes.

The sympathetic trunks (sympathetic chain, gangliated cord) are a paired bundle of nerve fibers that run from the base of the skull to the coccyx. The sympathetic trunk lies just lateral to the vertebral bodies for the entire length of the vertebral column. During renal surgery it is very rare that these structures are encountered [55, 56].

4.5.3 Surgical Impact

The role of performing lymphadenectomy during renal surgery is still controversial. There is no consensus on the fact whether retroperitoneal lymph node dissection should be part of renal oncological surgery. Data suggest that lymph node dissection is not associated with improved oncologic outcomes among patients at high risk who undergo radical nephrectomy for M0 renal cell carcinoma. If deemed necessary, a meticulous surgical technique with the use of surgical clips and hemostatic agents might be beneficial to lower peri-operative complications [57, 58].

References

1. Mishra GP, Bhatnagar S, Singh B. Anatomical variations of upper segmental renal artery and clinical significance. J Clin Diagn Res. 2015;9(8):AC01–3.
2. Borojeni S, Borojeni A, Panayotopoulos P, Bouvier A, Aubé C, Azzouzi AR, et al. Study of renal and kidney tumor vascularization using data from preoperative three-dimensional arteriography prior to partial nephrectomy. Eur Urol Focus. 2020;6(1):112–21.
3. Hyrtl J. Handbuch der topographischen Anatomie. Wien; 1982.
4. Brödel M. The intrinsic blood-vessels of the kidney and their significance in nephrotomy. Bull Johns Hopkins Hosp. 1901;12(10)
5. Graves F. The anatomy of the intrarenal arteries and its application to segmental resection of the kidney. Br J Surg. 1954;42(1722):132–9.
6. Weld KJ, Bhayani SB, Belani J, Ames CD, Hruby G, Landman J. Extrarenal vascular anatomy of kidney: Assessment of variations and their relevance to partial nephrectomy. Urology. 2005;66(5):985–9.
7. Sampaio FJB, Passos MARF. Renal arteries: anatomic study for surgical and radiological practice. Surg Radiol Anat. 1992;14(2):113–7.
8. Sampaio FJB. Renal anatomy: endourologic considerations. In: Minimally invasive surgery of the kidney: a problem-oriented approach. Philadelphia, PA: W.B. Saunders; 2000. p. 585–607.
9. Capitanio U, Bensalah K, Bex A, Boorjian SA, Bray F, Coleman J, et al. Epidemiology of renal cell carcinoma. Vol. 75, European urology. Elsevier; 2019. p. 74–84.
10. Siegel RL, Miller KD, Jemal A. Cancer statistics, 2018. CA Cancer J Clin. 2018;68(1):7–30.
11. EAU Guidelines. Edn. presented at the EAU Annual Congress Milan 2021. EAU Guidelines Office, Arnhem, The Netherlands. 2021. http://uroweb.org/guidelines/compilations-of-all-guidelines/.
12. Urban BA, Ratner LE, Fishman EK. Three-dimensional volume-rendered CT angiography of the renal arteries and veins: normal anatomy, variants, and clinical applications 1 learning objectives for test 2 CME feature. RadioGraphics. 2001;21:373–86.
13. Koeppen BM, Stanton BA. Chapter 32: Elements of renal function. In: Berne & Levy physiology. Elsevier Health Sciences; 2009.
14. Johns EJ, Ahmeda AF. Renal circulation. In: Reference module in biomedical sciences. 2014. Available from: https://doi.org/10.1016/B978-0-12-801238-3.00200-2
15. Breshears MA, Confer AW. The urinary system. Pathol Basis Vet Dis Expert Consult. 2017;617–81.e1.
16. Upadhyay KK, Silverstein DM. Renal development: a complex process dependent on inductive interaction. Curr Pediatr Rev. 2014;10(2):107–14.
17. Shapiro E, Goldfarb DA, Ritchey ML. The congenital and acquired solitary kidney. Rev Urol [Internet]. 2003;5(1):2–8.
18. Schreuder MF, Nauta J. Prenatal programming of nephron number and blood pressure. Kidney Int [Internet]. 2007;72:265–8. Available from: http://www.kidney-international.org
19. Smith J, Howards S, Preminger G, Dmochowski R. Hinman's atlas of urologic surgery, vol. 49. 4th ed. Philadelphia, PA: Elsevier; 2019. 1008 p
20. Karam IM, Oliver A, Hubert J. Surgical anatomy of kidneys and adrenals. In: John H, Wiklund P, editors. Robotic urology [Internet]. Cham: Springer; 2018. p. 63–70. Available from: https://doi.org/10.1007/978-3-319-65864-3_4
21. Furst J, Kurra S. Adrenal physiology. In: Surgical endocrinopathies. 2015. p. 187–95.
22. Taghavi K, Kirkpatrick J, Mirjalili SA. The horseshoe kidney: Surgical anatomy and embryology. J Pediatr Urol [Internet]. 2016;12(5):275–80. Available from: https://doi.org/10.1016/j.jpurol.2016.04.033
23. Neville H, Ritchey ML, Shamberger RC, Haase G, Perlman S, Yoshioka T. The occurrence of Wilms tumor in horseshoe kidneys: A report from the National Wilms Tumor Study Group (NWTSG). J Pediatr Surg. 2002;37(8):1134–7.
24. Khougali HS, Alawad OAMA, Farkas N, Ahmed MMM, Abuagla AM. Bilateral pelvic kidneys with upper pole fusion and malrotation: a case report and review of the literature. J Med Case Rep [Internet]. 2021;15(1):1–6. Available from: https://doi.org/10.1186/s13256-021-02761-1
25. Klatte T, Ficarra V, Gratzke C, Kaouk J, Kutikov A, Macchi V, et al. A literature review of renal surgical anatomy and surgical strategies for partial nephrectomy. Eur Urol [Internet]. 2015;68(6):980–92. Available from: https://doi.org/10.1016/j.eururo.2015.04.010
26. Glodny B, Petersen J, Hofmann KJ, Schenk C, Herwig R, Trieb T, et al. Kidney fusion anomalies revisited: clinical and radiological analysis of 209 cases of crossed fused ectopia and horseshoe kidney. BJU Int. 2009;103(2):224–35.
27. Raison N, Doeuk N, Malthouse T, Kasivisvanathan V, Lam W, Challacombe B. Challenging situations in partial nephrectomy. Int J Surg [Internet]. 2016;36:568–73. Available from: https://doi.org/10.1016/j.ijsu.2016.05.070
28. Rebouças RB, Monteiro RC, Souza TN, Barbosa PF, Pereira GG, Britto CA. Pure laparoscopic radical heminephrectomy for a large renal-cell carcinoma in a horseshoe kidney. Int Braz J Urol. 2013;39(4):604.
29. Khan A, Myatt A, Palit V, Biyani CS, Urol D. Laparoscopic heminephrectomy of a horseshoe kidney. J Soc Laparoendosc Surg. 2011;15(3):415–20.
30. Rogers CG. Robotic nephrectomy for kidney cancer in a horseshoe kidney with renal vein tumor thrombus: novel technique for thrombectomy. J Endourol. 2008;22(8):1563.
31. Horesh N, Abu-Ghanem Y, Erlich T, Rosin D, Gutman M, Zilberman DE, et al. Management of pancreatic injuries following nephrectomy. Isr Med Assoc J. 2020;22(4):244–8.
32. Wang JK, Tollefson MK, Kim SP, Boorjian SA, Leibovich BC, Lohse CM, et al. Iatrogenic splenectomy during nephrectomy for renal tumors. Int J Urol Off J Jpn Urol Assoc. 2013;20(9):896–902.
33. Tan K, Lewis GR, Chahal R, Browning AJ, Sundaram SK, Weston PMT, et al. Iatrogenic splenectomy during left nephrectomy: a single-institution experience of eight years. Urol Int. 2011;87(1):59–63.
34. Fonouni H, Kashfi A, Majlesara A, Stahlheber O, Konstantinidis L, Gharabaghi N, et al. Hemostatic efficiency of modern topical sealants: Comparative evaluation after liver resection and splenic laceration in a swine model. J Biomed Mater Res B Appl Biomater. 2018;106(3):1307–16.
35. Jacob S. Human anatomy. 1st ed. New York: Elsevier; 2007.
36. Macchi V, Crestani A, Porzionato A, Sfriso MM, Morra A, Rossanese M, et al. Anatomical study of renal arterial vasculature and its potential impact on partial nephrectomy. BJU Int. 2017;120(1):83–91.
37. Shao P, Tang L, Li P, Xu Y, Qin C, Cao Q, et al. Precise segmental renal artery clamping under the guidance of dual-source computed tomography angiography during laparoscopic partial nephrectomy. Eur Urol. 2012;62(6):1001–8.
38. Bjurlin MA, Gan M, McClintock TR, Volpe A, Borofsky MS, Mottrie A, et al. Near-infrared fluorescence imaging: Emerging applications in robotic upper urinary tract surgery. Eur Urol [Internet]. 2014;65(4):793–801. Available from: https://doi.org/10.1016/j.eururo.2013.09.023
39. Sauer B, Flocquet M, Batch T, Blum A, Hubert J. Vascular renal anatomy and the ureteropelvic junction: Preoperative multidetec-

tor CT scanning with split-bolus injection as a predictor of laparoscopic findings. J Endourol. 2008;22(1):13–7.
40. Türkvatan A, Akıncı S, Yıldız Ş, Ölçer T, Cumhur T. Multidetector computed tomography for preoperative evaluation of vascular anatomy in living renal donors. Surg Radiol Anat. 2009;31(4):227–35.
41. Özkan U, Oğuzkurt L, Tercan F, Kizilkiliç O, Koç Z, Koca N. Renal artery origins and variations: Angiographic evaluation of 855 consecutive patients. Diagn Interv Radiol. 2006;12(4):183–6.
42. Türkvatan A, Özdemir M, Cumhur T, Ölçer T. Multidetector CT angiography of renal vasculature: Normal anatomy and variants. Eur Radiol. 2009;19(1):236–44.
43. Wein AJ. Campbell-Walsh urology. 9th ed. Philadelphia, PA: Elsevier; 2007. 3323 p
44. Kumar S, Neyaz Z, Gupta A. The utility of 64 channel multidetector CT angiography for evaluating the renal vascular anatomy and possible variations: A pictorial essay. Korean J Radiol. 2010;11(3):346–54.
45. Munnusamy K. Variations in branching pattern of renal artery in kidney donors using CT angiography. J Clin Diagn Res [Internet]. 2016 [cited 14 June 2021]. Available from: http://jcdr.net/article_fulltext.asp?issn=0973-709x&year=2016&volume=10&issue=3&page=AC01&issn=0973-709x&id=7342
46. Famurewa OC, Asaleye CM, Ibitoye BO, Ayoola OO, Aderibigbe AS, Badmus TA. Variations of renal vascular anatomy in a Nigerian population: A computerized tomography study. Niger J Clin Pract. 2018;21(7):840–6.
47. de Mello Júnior CF, Araujo Neto SA, de Carvalho Junior AM, Rebouças RB, Negromonte GRP, de Oliveira CD. Multidetector computed tomography angiography of the renal arteries: normal anatomy and its variations. Radiol Bras. 2016;49(3):190–5.
48. Sampaio FJ, Aragão AH. Anatomical relationship between the renal venous arrangement and the kidney collecting system. J Urol [Internet]. 1990;144(5):1089–93. Available from: http://europepmc.org/abstract/MED/2231877
49. Raman SS, Pojchamarnwiputh S, Muangsomboon K, Schulam PG, Gritsch HA, Lu DSK. Surgically relevant normal and variant renal parenchymal and vascular anatomy in preoperative 16-MDCT evaluation of potential laparoscopic renal donors. Am J Roentgenol. 2007;188(1):105–14.
50. Holden A, Smith A, Dukes P, Pilmore H, Yasutomi M. Assessment of 100 live potential renal donors for laparoscopic nephrectomy with multi-detector row helical CT. Radiology. 2005;237(3):973–80.
51. Truty MJ, Bower TC. Congenital anomalies of the inferior vena cava and left renal vein: implications during open abdominal aortic aneurysm reconstruction. Ann Vasc Surg. 2007;21(2):186–97.
52. Wein AJ. Campbell-Walsh urology. 10th ed. Philadelphia, PA: Elsevier; 2011.
53. Elkoushy M, Andonian S. Campbell-Walsh urology: surgical, radiographic, and endoscopic anatomy of the kidney and ureter. 2015. p. 967–77.
54. Anderson JK, Cadeddu J. surgical anatomy of the retroperitoneum, adrenals, kidneys, and ureters. Abdominal Key [Internet]. [cited 10 Aug 2021]. Available from: https://abdominalkey.com/surgical-anatomy-of-the-retroperitoneum-adrenals-kidneys-and-ureters/
55. Mirilas P, Skandalakis JE. Surgical anatomy of the retroperitoneal spaces, Part III: Retroperitoneal blood vessels and lymphatics. Am Surg. 2010;76(2):139–44.
56. Baniel J, Foster RS, Donohue JP. Surgical anatomy of the lumbar vessels: implications for retroperitoneal surgery. J Urol. 1995;153(5):1422–5.
57. Gershman B, Thompson RH, Moreira DM, Boorjian SA, Lohse CM, Costello BA, et al. Lymph node dissection is not associated with improved survival among patients undergoing cytoreductive nephrectomy for metastatic renal cell carcinoma: a propensity score based analysis. J Urol. 2017;197(3 Pt 1):574–9.
58. Gershman B, Thompson RH, Boorjian SA, Larcher A, Capitanio U, Montorsi F, et al. Radical nephrectomy with or without lymph node dissection for high risk nonmetastatic renal cell carcinoma: a multi-institutional analysis. J Urol. 2018;199(5):1143–8.

Training and Challenges to Perform Robot-Assisted Renal Surgeries

Stefano Puliatti, Pietro Piazza, Rui Farinha, Thomas Raju, and Anthony G. Gallagher

1 Introduction

Over the last two centuries, medical training has been based on the Halstedian "see one, do one, teach one" model [1], consisting of observing, performing, and then teaching others as part of the learning process. The introduction of new rules limiting work shifts, increasing paperwork, and concerns about neophytes operating on patients [2] have shown the need for a paradigm shift in surgical training. Halsted's methodology has been proven to be flawed, as trainees need more than mere observation to be able to perform a procedure and teach it to other trainees.

Historically, surgeons have learned how to perform surgeries on live patients and, despite having completed their training, may still find themselves at the initial phases of the learning curve for certain techniques and procedures [3]. This finding is of the utmost importance, considering that several studies on perioperative morbidity following minimally invasive procedures have shown that the majority of complications occur in the early part of the learning curve [4]. Surgical training should focus on providing an optimal setting in which skills can be developed following a specific, structured, and validated process; furthermore, trainers should evaluate whether a trainee has reached a specified proficiency level of performance before dismissing or allowing them to move to the next step. Nowadays, standard courses do not rely on structured teaching methodology and do not include an end-of-course objective assessment of the acquired skills. Learning new procedures should be grounded on validated approaches, such as proficiency-based progression training, and include a cognitive understanding of the procedure itself. Trainees should be aware of what they should and, more importantly, what they should not do when performing the procedure [5]. Procedures should be learned and practiced, until the quantitatively defined proficiency benchmark is demonstrated, in a laboratory setting or through simulation training, improving patient safety [6]. Only when proficiency is demonstrated with established benchmarks, trainees should proceed to perform the procedure in a real-life setting, moving from an exposure-based to a proficiency-based assessment. Without this paradigm shift, it is unlikely that an adequate quality of skills will be achieved.

2 The Role of Robot-Assisted Procedures in Renal Surgery

Over the last years, the role of robot-assisted procedures in renal diseases' treatment has drastically increased. Several studies have proven the benefits of robot-assisted surgery (RAS) for most of the diseases over traditional techniques. Partial nephrectomy is one of the most challenging urologic surgeries, requiring careful handling of the renal parenchyma and rapidity in the excision to reduce the loss of renal function. Technical and technological improvements associated

S. Puliatti (✉)
University of Modena and Reggio Emilia, Modena, Italy

Department of Urology, Onze-Lieve-Vrouwziekenhuis, Aalst, Belgium

ORSI Academy, Melle, Belgium

P. Piazza
Department of Urology, Onze-Lieve-Vrouwziekenhuis, Aalst, Belgium

Division of Urology, IRCCS Azienda Ospedaliero-Universitaria di Bologna, Bologna, Italy

Università degli Studi di Bologna, Bologna, Italy

R. Farinha
Department of Urology, Onze-Lieve-Vrouwziekenhuis, Aalst, Belgium

ORSI Academy, Melle, Belgium

T. Raju
Department of Urology, Tulane University School of Medicine, New Orleans, LA, USA

A. G. Gallagher
Faculty of Life and Health Sciences, Ulster University, Northern Ireland, UK

P. Wiklund et al. (eds.), *Robotic Urologic Surgery*, https://doi.org/10.1007/978-3-031-00363-9_34

with robotic system can help in maximizing renal function preservation after partial nephrectomies. The use of intraoperative ultrasound can help identify and define tumor's border, locate hilar structure, and evaluate renal ischemia after renal artery clamping [7]. By allowing a better determination of the vascularization of the kidney and renal tumor, fluorescence imaging, through Firefly technology, can assist in its identification, guide selective ischemia, and provide real-time guidance during resection and assessment of tumor margins [8]. Finally, surgical navigation systems that synchronize real-time endoscopic images with virtual reality 3D models might help improve the quality of the surgical procedure [9]. The combined use of these technologies can also improve the access and selection of the best clamping technique. Considering that clamping the renal pedicle has a direct impact on the warm ischemia time and, therefore, on kidney function preservation, RAS can assist the surgeon in significantly reducing ischemia-related renal injury [10]. The increased dexterity associated with Endowrist technology can finally impact functional outcomes of RA partial nephrectomy allowing surgeons to perform more selective resection and more accurate hemostasis, even in case of complex tumor, totally intrarenal, while still maintaining high standard of oncological safety [11].

Treatment of pyelo-ureteral junction disease (PUJD) via RAS has also quickly gained consensus due to comparable outcomes with laparoscopic surgery while being associated with a shorter learning curve and reduced operative time, mostly due to the reduced difficulty of the reconstructive step [12]. Moreover, due to the intrinsic risk of failure of the procedure, the use of RAS has grown, thanks to its safety and ease to approach scarred anastomotic tissue in a minimally invasive way [13].

Living-donor nephrectomy and kidney transplantation are two of the most challenging surgical procedures. Being conducted in healthy volunteers, living-donor nephrectomies need to guarantee the safety of the donor. Moreover, a good vascular dissection is of utmost to obtain enough vessel length and to minimize warm ischemia time during transplantation. Robot-assisted procedures have shown to ease this complex task [14]. Robotic kidney transplantation is rapidly gaining consensus, showing encouraging results [15], mostly due to increased dexterity offered by the use of wristed robotic instruments [16]. However, robot-assisted transplantation has shown to require a structured training in order to surpass the steep learning curve associated with the procedure.

3 Training Curricula for Renal Surgery

No guidelines on training for robot-assisted renal surgery (RARS) are currently available. As previously stated, to reduce the exposure of patients to possible risks, the introduction of structured, standardized, validated, and effective curricula is mandatory. A series of validated and non-validated robotic curriculum have been developed for robotic training, either based on simulation (FSRS, fundamental skills of robotic surgery [17]; proficiency-based robotic curriculum [18]; BSTC, basic skill training curriculum [4]) or structured curricula (ERUS curriculum for partial nephrectomy) [19]. However, all these curricula lack an objective assessment of trainees' performances. Trainees, despite their previous expertise, should exhibit a quantitatively defined performance standard before advancing along the curriculum's steps and therefore being allowed to use the robotic system on actual patients. Proficiency-based progression (PBP) training has been proven to help trainees achieve better performances in clinical setting when compared to trainees trained with traditional methods [20]. PBP is based on metrics derived from the experience of experts, and, after validation, these are used to set benchmarks which trainees must demonstrate before progressing [6]. This approach assures the skill level of trainees at the completion of the training path and helps systematize performance levels in robotic surgery [21].

4 Proficiency-Based Progression Training

Skills needed to perform robot-assisted renal surgery (RARS) should be acquired in an organized, sequential, and structured fashion. Proficiency-based progression (PBP) training had been successfully applied in the development of several surgical skills [22, 23] and, recently, has been used as the method of choice for the construction of robot-assisted radical prostatectomy curriculum [24]. According to PBP methodology, a specific procedure is subdivided in several phases. All phases are then divided in discrete procedural steps. For each step, errors and critical errors are identified. All the steps are performed in a certain order identified by a panel of experts. Subsequently, these metrics are analyzed through a modified Delphi panel [21]. The Delphi consensus-approved metrics constitute the core of the curriculum. PBP-based curricula are divided into a theoretical, pre-clinical, and clinical part. These phases will be discussed in detail in the following subsections.

In order to progress along the curriculum, a certain benchmark has to be demonstrated for each step. Benchmarks are based on the standard performance of experts who have completed the same assessment. Thus, at the end of the process, trainees must demonstrate theoretical and practical skills comparable with experienced surgeons. Moreover, assessment allows trainers to acquire data about trainees' involvement and average skill. This could provide trainers valuable information on the quality and appropriateness of the contents and on which aspect a certain trainee has to improve before reattempting the assessment. Of note, mindlessly repeating the same action does not assure the improvement of performances. Repeated practice may lead to replicating the same mistakes over and over, without learning from them. To avoid this training loophole, PBP methodology has introduced the use of deliberate practice. Thanks to deliberate practice, a constant formative feedback on their performance through the whole training process [25] is provided. Thanks to PBP, trainees can get a precise overview on their errors. As the complexity of the procedural skills increases, the risk of not performing the procedure correctly drastically increases. Deliberate practice focuses on reinforcing small steps toward the final goal rather than reinforcing only the final outcome, leading to major retention and better acquisition of performance characteristics.

Finally, participants will practice the skill in the most effective way, shortening the progression along the learning curve and assuring the retention of technical skill. In case of failure, trainees will not need to retake the entire course. They will only have to demonstrate proficiency.

4.1 Curriculum's Pre-clinical Phase

The pre-clinical phase should start with an e-learning module. Interactive, web-based media have shown to improve surgical skills and reduce error rates and operative time [26]. The ability to subdivide contents to ease their assimilation, interactivity to maintain a consistently high level of attention, and personalization of the learning experience allow participants to create their own learning plan. Each lecture should contain a combination of text and videos on each step, explaining and showing both errors and the successful completion of the step according to the metrics, other than the metrics itself. At the end of the theoretical part of the course, students should be assessed through an interactive questionnaire. The score obtained at the end of this test must be high enough to reach the pre-set benchmarks. A final assessment is mandatory before accessing to skills laboratories. One of the main problems of skills laboratories is that the level of skills taught in a particular course is tied to the level of the trainee with the lowest level of preparation. e-Learning and the correct use of assessment could be important tools able to raise the level of the trainees to a point where minimal time is wasted teaching unprepared trainee's theoretical concepts they should already possess. This practical approach guarantees that time in the skills lab is used efficiently.

The e-learning module should be followed by technical training on the robotic platform. According to the indication of the ORSI Consensus Meeting on European Robotic Training (OCERT) [21], the technical training should be performed by specialists from the company producing the robot and should focus on all the technical aspects of the robotic platform, including safety features and how to manage system errors and emergency situations. Technical training is followed by a baseline assessment of trainee's starting surgical skills.

Regardless of the outcomes of this assessment, the trainee will undergo a skill development module, in which the basic skills will be developed and reinforced via the use of exercise in a simulated environment.

Surgical simulators have been proven to improve trainee's surgical skills, reduce the learning curve, and shorten the length of the surgical procedures [20]. Ideal simulators should be economic and easy to setup and have a long life span, but their validation as training simulators and the need to define specific metrics for the procedure they want to simulate make their development a challenging task. Currently, different simulators are present on the market that can be used to acquire basic robotic dexterity, suturing, and manipulation skills, as well as perform full surgical cases. The improvements in computing power and software design improvement have been directly linked with development of new surgical simulators [27]. Virtual reality simulators can be both useful for novices and for more expert surgeons, thanks to the possibility of performing full-length real procedures [28]. However, most of these simulators lack realistic tissue responsiveness, are flawed by delays in signal processing, and provide inadequate measurements of surgeon's skills leading to lower cost-effectiveness when compared with other options available on the market [29].

In a dry-laboratory setting, several models can be found, despite most of them not being currently validated for robotic surgical training. Dry-lab models include simulators built from several types of materials, 3D printed models, harvested animal organs, and animal cadavers. Simpler models, built from balloons, porcine ureter, silicone, and thermoplastic elastomers, have been described in robotic renal surgery training, especially for pyeloplasty [30–33]. Three-dimensional printed models have recently grown in popularity. 3D printing allows the production of countless, standardized, and affordable models and therefore the construction of a free-access library of surgical cases. Despite the extraordinary evolution observed in the 3D printing, the price of the equipment (3D printer, 3D printing software, and printing materials) is still high. Moreover, 3D models lack realism in terms of malleability, tear strength, hardness, resistance to cut and needle driving, and simulated vascular blood flow; therefore their use for advanced skills acquisition is still suboptimal [34]. The use of chicken cadavers for training renal RAS-associated skills has been described for pyeloplasty and has been proven to be an easily replicable inexpensive model, despite its longer preparation time. Finally, harvested animal organs such as porcine kidneys, despite their low cost, provide a good model for simulating tissue handling, resection, and suturing [35]. These models provide realistic support for surgical exercises and allow the performance of more than one RAPN in one single kidney [36].

After an initial phase of skill development on virtual and dry-lab simulator, the trainees should be involved in an intensive structured course, providing guided dry-lab simulations, live-case observation of procedures performed by experts, and then proctored hands-on wet lab, allowing familiarization with the main steps of the procedure in a safe setting prior to moving to the clinical phase. Wet laboratories are characterized by the use of higher reality and higher-cost training models [37], such as living anesthetized pigs and the human cadaver. The living anesthetized porcine model is the most commonly animal used for basic and advanced robotic renal surgery training, due to its anatomical similarity to the human [38]. Several papers described the use of porcine training models for training partial nephrectomy, pyeloplasty, and renal transplantation, allowing trainees to develop skills of tissue handling, resection, and intracorporeal suturing in a realistic environment [39, 40]. In spite of some anatomical differences, the researchers were able to develop valid high-fidelity models, with the advantage of cost reduction by allowing bilateral kidney procedures in the same animal model [41] or simulating several crucial steps of renal surgery [42].

Despite the anatomical similarity to the human body and the existence of live tissue perfusion, the small amount of perinephric fat, the intraperitoneal localization of the colon, and the large variations in its renal vascular anatomy make this model incompletely representative.

Being considered the gold standard model for robotic renal surgery training, human cadaver model allows a realistic simulation, also providing anatomical variability and pathological conditions of the vessels and viscera [43]. Using this model, it is possible to train a complete surgery while dealing with tissues reacting similarly to the one encountered in routine clinical setting. However, the need of embalming, storing, and transporting makes it a very expensive training model [44]. Moreover, the risk of transmissible diseases, the absence of blood perfusion, and ethical concerns constitute some drawbacks to its use in a daily setting [45].

After completion of the intensive training and after having proven to have reached a benchmarked proficiency level during the final assessment of the course, trainees should be allowed to proceed to the final phase of the training curriculum.

4.2 Curriculum's Clinical Phase

During this phase, the console activity of the trainee should be monitored by an expert surgeon, providing feedbacks about trainee's progression. The concept of modular proficiency-based progression training, initially developed by Stolzenburg [46], after being successfully applied to robot-assisted radical prostatectomy's curriculum, has been applied to robot-assisted partial nephrectomy training, showing promising results as well as a potential transferability to other renal RAS. According to Stolzenburg's methodology, each surgery is divided into different steps according to a chronological sequence; each step is then ranked according to complexity using a scale ranging from I (easy) to V (complex); and steps with similar complexity are then grouped into modules. Each module will constitute a unit with similar complexity, regardless of their chronological order. Proctors will follow the evolution of the trainees throughout this proficiency-based modular progression, ensuring that the least complex modules are completed before advancing to more complex ones [19]. Once proficiency is achieved in all the established modules, trainees will be allowed to perform a full procedure independently. The renal RAS full case should be recorded and then evaluated by experts, blinded to the identity of the surgeon, according to a procedure-specific evaluation scale, after which the trainee will be considered certified and independent in this specific procedure. Clearly defined and properly validated assessment tools based on objective procedural metrics will allow trainees to progress throughout the learning curve until they will reach clinical proficiency, guaranteeing proper development of surgical skills and helping improve the training program [47].

5 Summary

Robot-assisted renal surgery training is still under definition, and validated robotic curricula are still lacking. The implementation of the proficiency-based progression (PBP) training model can provide an objective and effective tool to help develop skills and create standardized and efficient curricula.

References

1. Hasson HM. Open laparoscopy. Biomed Bull. 1984;5:1–6.
2. Maybury C. The European Working Time Directive: a decade on. Lancet Lond Engl. 2014;384:1562–3. https://doi.org/10.1016/s0140-6736(14)61972-3.
3. Bridges M, Diamond DL. The financial impact of teaching surgical residents in the operating room. Am J Surg. 1999;177:28–32. https://doi.org/10.1016/s0002-9610(98)00289-x.
4. Foell K, Finelli A, Yasufuku K, Bernardini MQ, Waddell TK, Pace KT, et al. Robotic surgery basic skills training: evaluation of a pilot multidisciplinary simulation-based curriculum. Can Urol Assoc J J Assoc Urol Can. 2013;7:430–4. https://doi.org/10.5489/cuaj.222.
5. Gallagher AG. Metric-based simulation training to proficiency in medical education: what it is and how to do it. Ulster Med J. 2012;81:107–13.

6. Gallagher AG, Ritter EM, Champion H, Higgins G, Fried MP, Moses G, et al. Virtual reality simulation for the operating room: proficiency-based training as a paradigm shift in surgical skills training. Ann Surg. 2005;241:364–72. https://doi.org/10.1097/01.sla.0000151982.85062.80.
7. Hyams ES, Kanofsky JA, Stifelman MD. Laparoscopic Doppler technology: applications in laparoscopic pyeloplasty and radical and partial nephrectomy. Urology. 2008;71:952–6. https://doi.org/10.1016/j.urology.2007.11.062.
8. Hekman MCH, Rijpkema M, Langenhuijsen JF, Boerman OC, Oosterwijk E, Mulders PFA. Intraoperative imaging techniques to support complete tumor resection in partial nephrectomy. Eur Urol Focus. 2018;4:960–8. https://doi.org/10.1016/j.euf.2017.04.008.
9. Hughes-Hallett A, Mayer EK, Marcus HJ, Cundy TP, Pratt PJ, Darzi AW, et al. Augmented reality partial nephrectomy: examining the current status and future perspectives. Urology. 2014;83:266–73. https://doi.org/10.1016/j.urology.2013.08.049.
10. Mattevi D, Luciani LG, Mantovani W, Cai T, Chiodini S, Vattovani V, et al. Fluorescence-guided selective arterial clamping during RAPN provides better early functional outcomes based on renal scan compared to standard clamping. J Robot Surg. 2019;13:391–6. https://doi.org/10.1007/s11701-018-0862-x.
11. Buffi NM, Saita A, Lughezzani G, Porter J, Dell'Oglio P, Amparore D, et al. Robot-assisted partial nephrectomy for complex (PADUA score ≥10) tumors: techniques and results from a multicenter experience at four high-volume centers. Eur Urol. 2020;77:95–100. https://doi.org/10.1016/j.eururo.2019.03.006.
12. Buffi NM, Lughezzani G, Fossati N, Lazzeri M, Guazzoni G, Lista G, et al. Robot-assisted, single-site, dismembered pyeloplasty for ureteropelvic junction obstruction with the new da Vinci platform: a stage 2a study. Eur Urol. 2015;67:151–6. https://doi.org/10.1016/j.eururo.2014.03.001.
13. Jacobson DL, Shannon R, Johnson EK, Gong EM, Liu DB, Flink CC, et al. Robot-assisted laparoscopic reoperative repair for failed pyeloplasty in children: an updated series. J Urol. 2019;201:1005–11. https://doi.org/10.1016/j.juro.2018.10.021.
14. Giacomoni A, Di Sandro S, Lauterio A, Concone G, Buscemi V, Rossetti O, et al. Robotic nephrectomy for living donation: surgical technique and literature systematic review. Am J Surg. 2016;211:1135–42. https://doi.org/10.1016/j.amjsurg.2015.08.019.
15. Sood A, Ghosh P, Menon M, Jeong W, Bhandari M, Ahlawat R. Robotic renal transplantation: current status. J Minimal Access Surg. 2015;11:35–9. https://doi.org/10.4103/0972-9941.147683.
16. Lee JY, Alzahrani T, Ordon M. Intra-corporeal robotic renal autotransplantation. Can Urol Assoc J J Assoc Urol Can. 2015;9:E748–9. https://doi.org/10.5489/cuaj.3015.
17. Stegemann AP, Ahmed K, Syed JR, Rehman S, Ghani K, Autorino R, et al. Fundamental skills of robotic surgery: a multi-institutional randomized controlled trial for validation of a simulation-based curriculum. Urology. 2013;81:767–74. https://doi.org/10.1016/j.urology.2012.12.033.
18. Dulan G, Rege RV, Hogg DC, Gilberg-Fisher KM, Arain NA, Tesfay ST, et al. Developing a comprehensive, proficiency-based training program for robotic surgery. Surgery. 2012;152:477–88. https://doi.org/10.1016/j.surg.2012.07.028.
19. Larcher A, De Naeyer G, Turri F, Dell'Oglio P, Capitanio U, Collins JW, et al. The ERUS curriculum for robot-assisted partial nephrectomy: structure definition and pilot clinical validation. Eur Urol. 2019;75:1023–31. https://doi.org/10.1016/j.eururo.2019.02.031.
20. Mazzone E, Puliatti S. A systematic review and meta-analysis on the impact of proficiency-based progression simulation training on performance outcomes. Ann Surg. 2021;274(2):281–9.
21. Vanlander AE, Mazzone E, Collins JW, Mottrie AM, Rogiers XM, van der Poel HG, et al. Orsi Consensus Meeting on European Robotic Training (OCERT): results from the first multispecialty consensus meeting on training in robot-assisted surgery. Eur Urol. 2020;78:713–6. https://doi.org/10.1016/j.eururo.2020.02.003.
22. Angelo RL, Ryu RKN, Pedowitz RA, Beach W, Burns J, Dodds J, et al. A proficiency-based progression training curriculum coupled with a model simulator results in the acquisition of a superior arthroscopic bankart skill set. Arthrosc J Arthrosc Relat Surg. 2015;31:1854–71. https://doi.org/10.1016/j.arthro.2015.07.001.
23. Puliatti S, Mazzone E, Amato M, De Groote R, Mottrie A, Gallagher AG. Development and validation of the objective assessment of robotic suturing and knot tying skills for chicken anastomotic model. Surg Endosc. 2020; https://doi.org/10.1007/s00464-020-07918-5.
24. Satava R, Gallagher AG. Proficiency-based progression process training for fundamentals of robotic surgery curriculum development. Ann Laparosc Endosc Surg. 2020;5:14. https://doi.org/10.21037/ales.2020.02.04.
25. Ericsson KA. Towards a science of the acquisition of expert performance in sports: clarifying the differences between deliberate practice and other types of practice. J Sports Sci. 2020;38:159–76. https://doi.org/10.1080/02640414.2019.1688618.
26. Davis JS, Garcia GD, Wyckoff MM, Alsafran S, Graygo JM, Withum KF, et al. Knowledge and usability of a trauma training system for general surgery residents. Am J Surg. 2013;205:681–4. https://doi.org/10.1016/j.amjsurg.2012.07.037.
27. Hung AJ, Jayaratna IS, Teruya K, Desai MM, Gill IS, Goh AC. Comparative assessment of three standardized robotic surgery training methods. BJU Int. 2013;112:864–71. https://doi.org/10.1111/bju.12045.
28. Hung AJ, Shah SH, Dalag L, Shin D, Gill IS. Development and validation of a novel robotic procedure specific simulation platform: partial nephrectomy. J Urol. 2015;194:520–6. https://doi.org/10.1016/j.juro.2015.02.2949.
29. Simmerman E, Simmerman A, Lassiter R, King R, Ham B, Adam B-L, et al. Feasibility and benefit of incorporating a multimedia cadaver laboratory training program into a didactics curriculum for junior and senior surgical residents. J Surg Educ. 2018;75:1188–94. https://doi.org/10.1016/j.jsurg.2018.03.012.
30. Rod J, Marret J-B, Kohaut J, Aigrain Y, Jais JP, de Vries P, et al. Low-cost training simulator for open dismembered pyeloplasty: development and face validation. J Surg Educ. 2018;75:188–94. https://doi.org/10.1016/j.jsurg.2017.06.010.
31. Raza SJ, Soomroo KQ, Ather MH. "Latex glove" laparoscopic pyeloplasty model: a novel method for simulated training. Urol J. 2011;8:283–6.
32. Timberlake MD, Garbens A, Schlomer BJ, Kavoussi NL, Kern AJM, Peters CA, et al. Design and validation of a low-cost, high-fidelity model for robotic pyeloplasty simulation training. J Pediatr Urol. 2020;16:332–9. https://doi.org/10.1016/j.jpurol.2020.02.003.
33. Lima JCS, Rocha HAL, Mesquita FJC, Araújo DABS, da Silveira RA, Borges GC. Simulated training model of ureteropyelic anastomosis in laparoscopic pyeloplasty. Acta Cir Bras. 2020;35:e351108. https://doi.org/10.1590/ACB351108.
34. Ahmed K, Jawad M, Abboudi M, Gavazzi A, Darzi A, Athanasiou T, et al. Effectiveness of procedural simulation in urology: a systematic review. J Urol. 2011;186:26–34. https://doi.org/10.1016/j.juro.2011.02.2684.
35. Ames CD, Vanlangendonck R, Morrissey K, Venkatesh R, Landman J. Evaluation of surgical models for renal collecting system closure during laparoscopic partial nephrectomy. Urology. 2005;66:451–4. https://doi.org/10.1016/j.urology.2005.03.033.
36. Silberstein JL, Maddox MM, Dorsey P, Feibus A, Thomas R, Lee BR. Physical models of renal malignancies using standard cross-sectional imaging and 3-dimensional printers: a pilot study. Urology. 2014;84:268–72. https://doi.org/10.1016/j.urology.2014.03.042.

37. Liss MA, McDougall EM. Robotic surgical simulation. Cancer J Sudbury Mass. 2013;19:124–9. https://doi.org/10.1097/PPO.0b013e3182885d79.
38. Bestard Vallejo JE, Raventós Busquets CX, Celma Doménech A, Rosal Fontana M, Esteve M, Morote Robles J. [Pig model in experimental renal transplant surgery]. Actas Urol Esp. 2008;32:91–101. https://doi.org/10.1016/s0210-4806(08)73800-2.
39. Fu B, Zhang X, Lang B, Xu K, Zhang J, Ma X, et al. New model for training in laparoscopic dismembered ureteropyeloplasty. J Endourol. 2007;21:1381–5. https://doi.org/10.1089/end.2006.0317.
40. Díaz-Güemes Martín-Portugués I, Hernández-Hurtado L, Usón-Casaús J, Sánchez-Hurtado MA, Sánchez-Margallo FM. Ureteral obstruction swine model through laparoscopy and single port for training on laparoscopic pyeloplasty. Int J Med Sci. 2013;10:1047–52. https://doi.org/10.7150/ijms.6099.
41. Cavallari G, Tsivian M, Bertelli R, Neri F, Faenza A, Nardo B. A new swine training model of hand-assisted donor nephrectomy. Transplant Proc. 2008;40:2035–7. https://doi.org/10.1016/j.transproceed.2008.05.034.
42. Tiong HY, Goh BYS, Chiong E, Tan LGL, Vathsala A. Robotic kidney autotransplantation in a porcine model: a procedure-specific training platform for the simulation of robotic intracorporeal vascular anastomosis. J Robot Surg. 2018;12:693–8. https://doi.org/10.1007/s11701-018-0806-5.
43. Holland JP, Waugh L, Horgan A, Paleri V, Deehan DJ. Cadaveric hands-on training for surgical specialties: is this back to the future for surgical skills development? J Surg Educ. 2011;68:110–6. https://doi.org/10.1016/j.jsurg.2010.10.002.
44. Huri E, Ezer M, Chan E. The novel laparoscopic training 3D model in urology with surgical anatomic remarks: fresh-frozen cadaveric tissue. Turk J Urol. 2016;42:224–9. https://doi.org/10.5152/tud.2016.84770.
45. Minneti M, Baker CJ, Sullivan ME. The development of a novel perfused cadaver model with dynamic vital sign regulation and real-world scenarios to teach surgical skills and error management. J Surg Educ. 2018;75:820–7. https://doi.org/10.1016/j.jsurg.2017.09.020.
46. Stolzenburg J-U, Schwaibold H, Bhanot SM, Rabenalt R, Do M, Truss M, et al. Modular surgical training for endoscopic extraperitoneal radical prostatectomy. BJU Int. 2005;96:1022–7. https://doi.org/10.1111/j.1464-410X.2005.05803.x.
47. Dai JC, Lendvay TS, Sorensen MD. Crowdsourcing in surgical skills acquisition: a developing technology in surgical education. J Grad Med Educ. 2017;9:697–705. https://doi.org/10.4300/JGME-D-17-00322.1.

Current Imaging Modalities and Virtual Models for Kidney Tumors

F. Porpiglia, C. Rogers, P. De Backer, and F. Piramide

1 Introduction

During the last decades, the progressive diffusion and technological improvements of renal tumor imaging have played a pivotal role in changing the natural history of this disease.

The widespread diffusion of ultrasound (US) and computed tomography (CT) scan increased the number of incidentally detected renal tumors. Nowadays it is estimated that up to 66% of small renal masses are incidentally found.

The amount of renal masses detected at an earlier stage and amenable to less invasive or conservative treatment has increased with a subsequent increase in overall and cancer-specific survival [1].

On the other hand, the technological advancement of CT scan and magnetic resonance imaging (MRI) lets clinicians to progressively better characterize the masses and help the surgeon choose the better surgical approach. Moreover, the recent advent of 3D virtual models has furtherly increased surgeons' comprehension of anatomical details with a subsequently more accurate preoperative planning.

In the following chapter, an overview of the current imaging modalities and the new technologies available for the diagnosis and the treatment of renal tumors is presented.

2 Ultrasound (US)

Since its advent in clinical practice, US showed its great potential as a low-cost and less-invasive imaging modality but is able to provide clinicians with a large amount of information in almost every anatomical district. Concerning the urogenital system and focusing in the renal oncological setting, US is worldwide considered a reasonable first-line option to identify and characterize a renal mass [2].

For renal US a standard transabdominal 3–6 MHz convex probe is usually used with the patients in supine or lateral position [3].

Renal masses are typically identified thanks to the deformation of the normal kidney structure. They are usually spherical and causing an alteration of kidney's margins (if not completely endophytic). US mainly distinguishes renal tumors in solid or cystic masses and could provide some preliminary information about their dimension, polar location, and growth pattern.

Solid renal masses could appear as isoechoic, hyperechoic, or hypoechoic with respect to the healthy parenchyma. Despite several studies tried to classify renal tumor histotype according to their US aspect, up to now the echogenicity has shown a poor correlation with tumor subtype except for angiomyolipoma (AML); thanks to its fatty content, this benign tumor usually appears as a hyperechoic solid mass.

Concerning cystic masses, US can be a useful tool for an initial study. In fact, US is able to visualize and describe the aspect of cystic walls, presence of calcifications or septa, and an eventual solid component.

Additional information could be provided by the application of color Doppler. As known, renal cell carcinoma (RCC) is a highly angiogenetic malignancy; the large number of new vessels around the tumor can be easily identified with a color Doppler US. The increased Doppler signal could be very useful especially in case of isoechoic endophytic lesion that could easily be missed if they have a small size [3].

Despite its large field of application and its good performance, US has some limits in renal masses assessment. To overcome these limitations and to expand its indication, contrast-enhanced ultrasound (CEUS) and intraoperative ultrasound have been introduced.

F. Porpiglia (✉) · F. Piramide
Department of Oncology, Division of Urology, University of Turin, Orbassano (Turin), Italy

C. Rogers
Department of Urology, Vattikuti Urology Institute, Detroit, MI, USA

P. De Backer
ORSI Academy, Melle, Belgium

P. Wiklund et al. (eds.), *Robotic Urologic Surgery*, https://doi.org/10.1007/978-3-031-00363-9_35

2.1 Contrast-Enhanced Ultrasound (CEUS)

An important step further in increasing US sensibility and specificity for renal masses has been provided by contrast agents. US is performed after intravenously injection of gas microbubbles (with low diffusion and solubility, as perfluorocarbon or sulfur hexafluoride) surrounded by biocompatible materials. These bubbles, smaller than erythrocytes, could easily arrive in the arterial circulation and here being confined, since they neither diffuse into the interstitial space nor be filtered by the glomeruli.

Therefore, in this technique only two enhancement phases will occur: the cortical and the parenchymal (in which both cortical and medullar portions are vascular) phases.

After the bubbles being insonated, they send a high-intensity transient signal revealing precisely the vascularization of a specific mass or district [4].

Finally, the bubbles are eliminated by the lung and the surrounding shell by the liver which thus also allows to apply this imaging modality in patients with end-stage chronic kidney disease (CKD).

The above characteristics of this technique allow clinicians to better distinguish various renal conditions. For example, thanks to its high sensitivity to vascularization, CEUS could easily distinguish hypovascularized tumors from hemorrhagic cysts (which may not be purely anechoic).

Moreover, CEUS could be very useful in case of pseudotumors (as dromedary hump, prominent column of Bertin, congenic lobulation, etc.) and in other conditions in which there is a deformation of the normal shape of the kidney. Despite tumors usually being correctly identified by conventional US, sometimes it is necessary to perform additional investigations. In these cases, CEUS may reveal the absence of different vascular patterns with respect to the normal parenchyma and consequently exclude the suspect of neoplasm in the major part of the cases (95%) [5]. In the 5% of isoenhancing tumors, the normal US mode usually detects a difference in terms of echogenicity with the surrounding healthy tissue.

One of the other most frequent fields of application of CEUS is surely the characterization of complex renal cysts (Bosniak III–IV, see below). In this setting, thanks to a precise enhancement evaluation, it is possible to correctly differentiate benign from malignant cysts with high sensitivity (100%), high specificity (97%), and a negative predictive value of 100% ($\kappa = 0.95$) [6].

Lastly, CEUS is more commonly adopted for postprocedural follow-up after thermal ablation techniques. The success of the procedure is usually deemed after a few weeks, and the pivotal condition is the absence of enhancement at the lesion's core [7]. In this setting CEUS showed promising results with quite comparable performances of CT scan and MRI (79% of sensitivity and 100% of specificity) [7].

In conclusion, CEUS could represent a very useful tool in a large variety of settings, especially in case of indeterminate results of CT, with the advantages of avoiding radiation exposure and being a less invasive procedure also accessible to CKD patients.

2.2 Intraoperative Ultrasound

Ultrasound has long been used to provide an intraoperative real-time assistance during partial nephrectomy. Since the advent of laparoscopic technique, many companies have produced their own laparoscopic probe for an intraoperative use. At the beginning of the robotic era, the assistant usually handled the probe. However, in recent years, dedicated probes to be manipulated by the surgeon have been developed with an integrated view of the US images on the console screen (Fig. 1) [8].

The intraoperative examination with a dedicated probe allows to better recognize tumor location, borders (especially in case of partially or completely endophytic masses), and its relationship with other anatomical structures (e.g., calices or vessels). Moreover, it could reveal aspects missed by preoperative imaging exams, like multifocal disease or cystic component [8]. As for the preoperative setting, it is possible to apply the Doppler mode and CEUS to the intra-

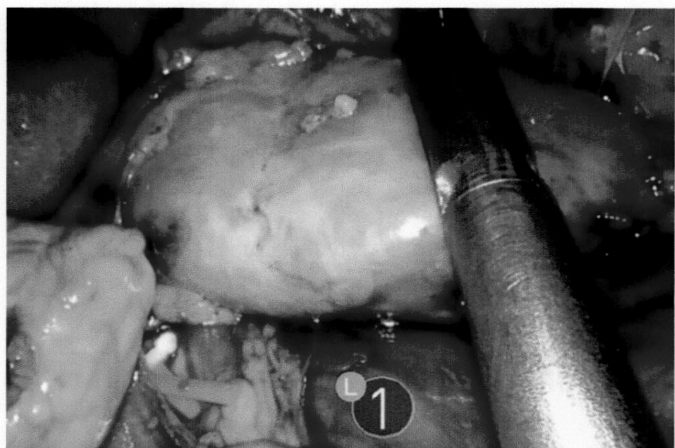

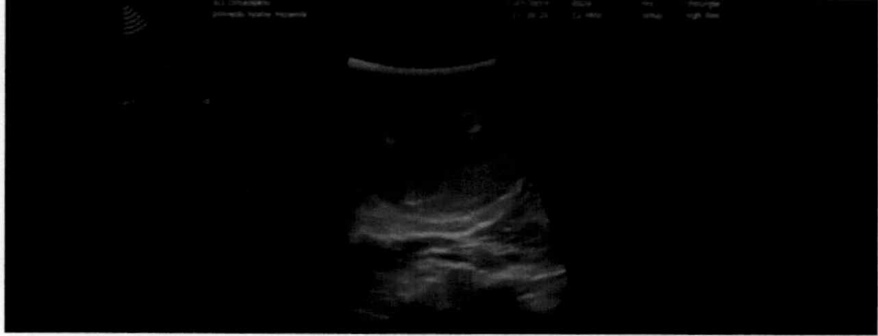

Fig. 1 Intraoperative US application during robot-assisted partial nephrectomy to correctly identify tumor margins and its relationship with intrarenal structures

operative one. In these cases, surgeon could also utilize them to double-check the selective clamping accuracy [9].

All the above applications are usually performed in a static phase of the intervention, typically after hilum identification and kidney's defatting. The knowledge on US application during the resection phase of the procedure is rather limited since it may prolong the ischemia time with important drawbacks.

3 Computed Tomography (CT) Scan

CT scan is widely considered the gold standard imaging modality for an initial characterization and staging of renal masses [1]. This role has been achieved thanks to its high diagnostic yield, its rapid time of execution, and its availability.

An ideal CT scan protocol is performed with a minimum slice thickness of 3 mm combined with multiplanar reconstructions and includes unenhanced images followed by an arterial (corticomedullary) and a parenchymal (nephrographic) phase. Additionally, an excretory phase could be obtained 3–5 min after contrast injection and provide more details about the relationship of the mass with the upper collecting system [10].

Thanks to a precise study of the above phases, with CT scan it is possible to collect a lot of information about the tumor biology and its aggressiveness (e.g., presence of enhancement, irregular margins, necrotic areas, size).

Using the non-enhanced phase only, it is not easy to characterize a renal mass. The presence of calcifications is typical of RCC, whereas the macroscopic presence of fat is more indicative of AML.

Considering also the abovementioned injection phases, it is possible to assess the presence of enhancement, and the diagnostic yield of CT scan rises substantially. The presence of enhancement is defined as a modification in terms of Hounsfield units (HUs) before, and after, contrast administration. A change of at least 15 HUs in the solid tumor parts is considered positive for enhancement and with a high likelihood of malignancy. Moreover, the histological subtypes of RCC have different and typical enhancement patterns which sometimes allow preliminary diagnosis. For example, clear cell RCC (ccRCC) enhances avidly on corticomedullary phase and rapidly washes out during the nephrographic phase (Fig. 2), while papillary tumors show a slow and progressively enhancement more visible during the nephrographic phase (Fig. 3).

More challenging, even for experienced radiologist, is the differentiation between oncocytoma and chromophobe RCC (chRCC). Moreover, to differentiate them from ccRCC is challenging. The typical stellate scar is present in almost one-third of oncocytomas, but it is not considered a pathognomonic feature, since it could be simulated by RCC with central area of necrosis. Oncocytoma and chRCC could vary from homogeneous to heterogeneous pattern and show a hyperenhancement in the corticomedullary phase with progressive or persistent hyperenhancement in the nephrographic phase [11] (Fig. 4).

Concerning the staging of a renal mass, CT scan usually provides reliable information for both local and distant staging. The evaluation includes the lymph nodes, adrenal gland, and renal vein. A venous involvement is usually due to tumor thrombus inside the lumen of the vein, while a direct invasion of the wall is less common, but, in those cases, MRI could provide additional details.

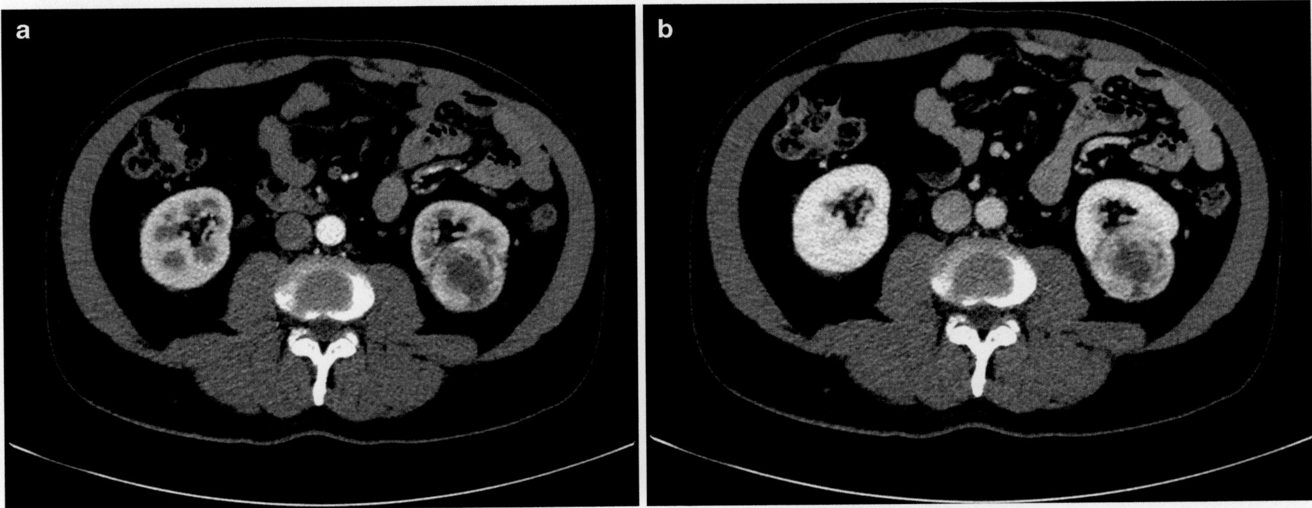

Fig. 2 CT scan appearance of ccRCC. As shown, it has a rapid enhancement during corticomedullary phase (**a**) with rapid washout at nephrographic phases (**b**)

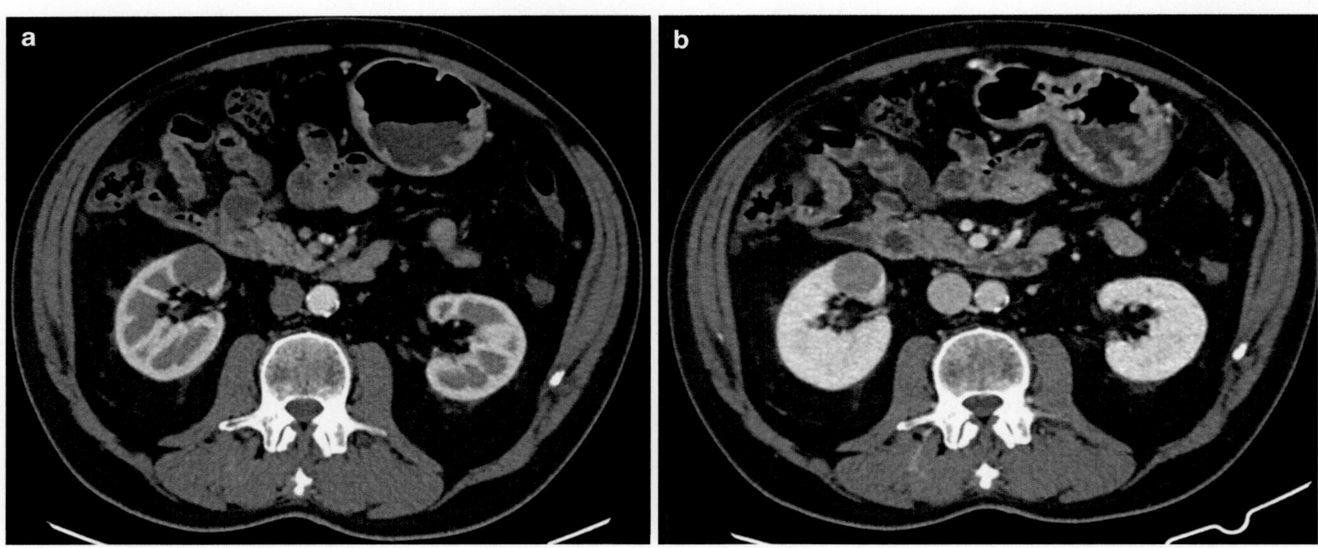

Fig. 3 CT scan appearance of papillary RCC (pRCC) with progressive enhancement as shown in corticomedullary (**a**) and nephrographic phases (**b**)

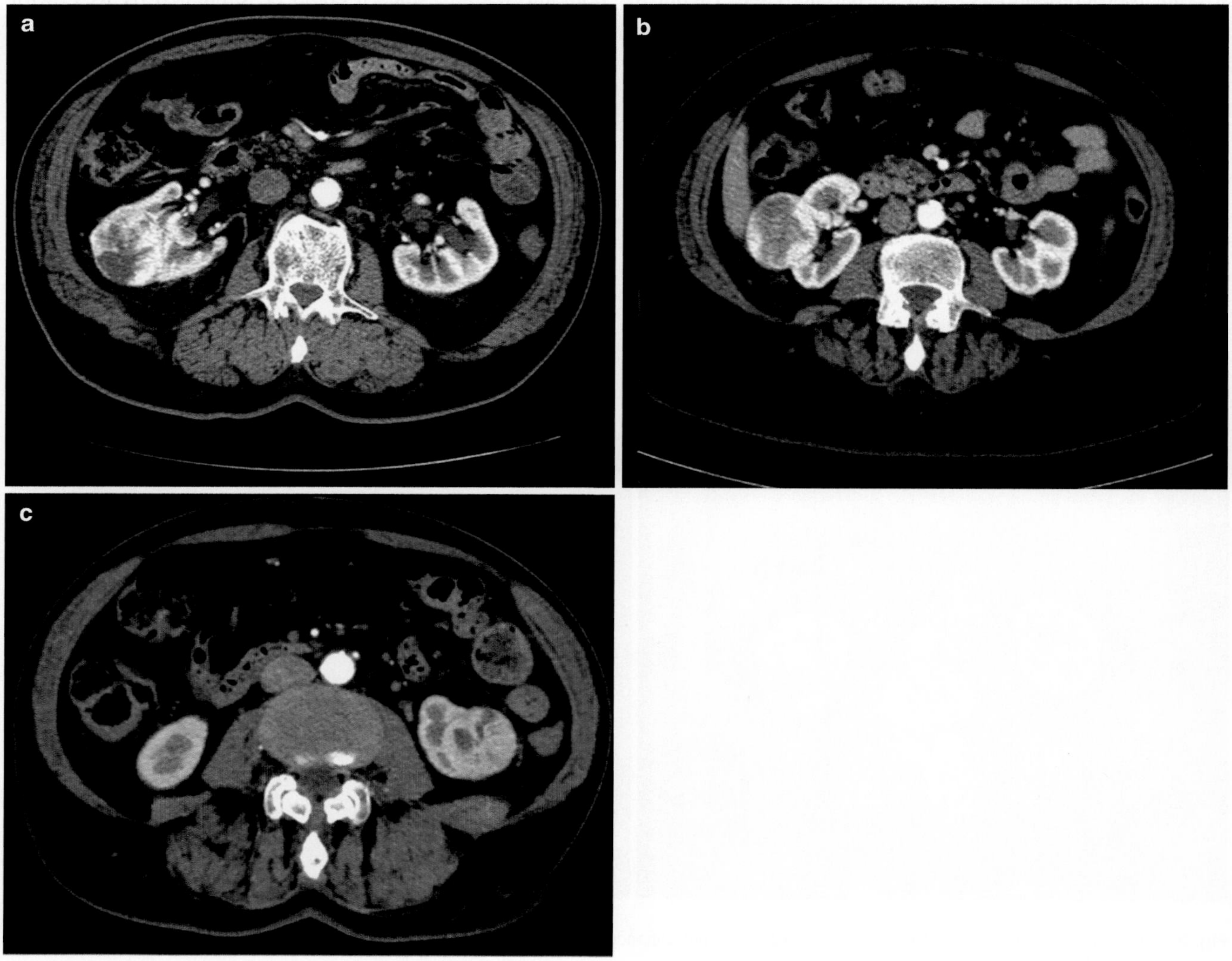

Fig. 4 Example of renal masses with similar radiological aspect: ccRCC (**a**), oncocytoma (**b**), and chRCC (**c**)

Finally, CT scan may also be useful for a preliminary assessment of the function and morphology of the contralateral kidney. On the basis of these features, clinicians can better identify patients eligible to undergo preoperative renal scan to have a more reliable assessment of renal function. According to renal scan results, the surgeon could decide to consider or not to attempt a conservative approach [1].

3.1 Classification of Cystic Masses

The main features analyzed to describe cystic renal masses and to assess their risk of malignancy have been reported for the first time by Bosniak in 1986. This CT-based system has been recently updated and adapted to guarantee also MRI and CEUS application [12] (Table 1). The Bosniak classification system is a simple and reproducible tool, created to categorize cystic renal neoformation and to simplify clinicians' communication. The lesions are classified in five groups correlating with the risk of malignancy and the consequent clinical management. These reasons explain why this system is still widely accepted and employed.

Between the evaluated features, we again find the presence of enhancement. Enhancement could be limited to cystic wall and just perceived (Bosniak II–IIF), or it could be significant and measurable either at the cystic wall, septa, or solid nodules (Bosniak III–IV).

Another important aspect is intralesional homogeneity: it is critical to ensure that the content is homogeneous and that there are no subtle or peripheral heterogeneous elements.

In case of intralesional septa, it is mandatory to establish the number of septa (three being the maximum for Bosniak II), their thickness, and enhancement.

Table 1 Bosniak classification of renal cystic masses

Bosniak category	Characteristics	Management
I	Hairline-thin wall without septa, calcification, or solid components. Same density as water and does not enhance with contrast medium	Benign
II	Benign cyst with few hairline-thin septa or fine calcification	Benign
IIF	More hairline-thin septa. Minimal enhancement of a hairline-thin septum or wall. Minimal thickening of the septa or wall The cyst may contain calcification, which may be nodular and thick, with no contrast enhancement. No enhancing soft tissue elements	Follow-up
III	Indeterminate cystic masses with thickened irregular walls or septa with enhancement	Surgery or active surveillance
IV	Complex cyst containing enhancing soft tissue components	Surgery

Overall, the diagnostic yield of CT scan for Bosniak IIF–III is limited (sensitivity 36% and specificity 76%; $\kappa = 0.11$), and usually it requires additional investigations. In this setting MRI and CEUS showed good performances due to a higher detection of enhancement (MRI, 71% sensitivity and 91% specificity [$\kappa = 0.64$]; CEUS, 100% sensitivity and 97% specificity [$\kappa = 0.95$]) [6].

4 Magnetic Resonance Imaging (MRI)

Despite being widely rated compared to CT scan for renal mass assessment, MRI is mainly adopted as a problem-solving imaging technique in case of indeterminate lesions. Moreover, it is the preferred technique in the case of patient with CT contrast allergy or severe CKD, and it is an opportunity to reduce the X-ray exposure in young patients [1].

A standard multiparametric MRI protocol includes conventional morphological sequences (T2 and T1 weighted—T2W and T1W) and functional ones (chemical shift imaging—CSI; dynamic contrast-enhanced—DCE; diffusion-weighted imaging—DWI; apparent diffusion coefficient—ADC) [13].

T2W sequence is useful especially in detecting and characterizing cystic lesions, whereas in case of solid ones, it could help in identifying the RCC subtypes. T1W gives its best contribution in detecting hemosiderin residuals and macro- or microscopic fat inside a renal mass. Here a well-defined loss of signal due to intralesional macroscopic fat is diagnostic for AML, whereas a more diffused and undefined signal loss remains of uncertain attribution. In fact, it could be representative not only of lipid-poor AML (due to the interposition of fat and other soft tissue within the same voxel) but also of ccRCC (due to intracellular fat).

The possibility of MRI to reproduce multiple soft tissue contrast allows to potentially differentiate RCC subtypes. For example, an intermediate to high signal intensity on T2W with hyperenhancement after contrast injection has been described as suggestive of ccRCC. Moreover, in case of concomitant microscopic fat, the likelihood of finding a ccRCC at renal biopsy or surgery is relevant. Following these concepts, Johnson et al. reported a new algorithm to facilitate ccRCC diagnosis in MRI [14]. This new tool named "clear cell likelihood score" (ccLS) classifies a renal mass in five levels according to the risk of being a ccRCC, ranging from "very likely" to "very unlikely." The diagnostic yield of this score was prospectively assessed in 57 patients with small renal masses. Its high diagnostic rate was further confirmed in a large retrospective cohort of 434 patients. ccLS score reached a positive predicted value of 93% for ccLS5 and 78% for ccLS4, with a sensitivity and specificity of 91% and 56%, respectively. ccLS was found to be independently predictive of ccRCC at multivariate analysis [15].

In conclusion MRI can be considered a valid alternative to CT scan with comparable diagnostic yield which in some special conditions (e.g., cystic masses) has shown to be even better. Notwithstanding the possibility to be performed also in pregnant, young, or CKD patients, the lower availability of MRI platform throughout the territory, the higher costs, and the scanning time explain why this imaging modality is more utilized in case of indeterminate masses rather than the irst imaging technique.

5 Near-Infrared Fluorescence Guidance with Indocyanine

The progressive trend in adopting nephron-sparing surgery as the referral treatment option for renal tumors has forced urologist to face more and more challenging cases. In order to correctly manage these complex masses, many intraoperative tools have been developed. Among the different intraoperative imaging modalities, near-infrared fluorescence (NIRF) guidance with indocyanine green (ICG) is one of the most common adopted thanks to its large field of applications.

After intravenous injection, the indocyanine molecules are bound by plasma proteins and consequently confined inside the vascular system until they are entirely removed by the hepatic filter. There is no renal filtration, so this technology can be safely used in CKD patients. After adsorbing near-infrared wavelengths of lights, ICG releases slight longer wavelengths detected by the NIRF camera. In the last years, the Firefly® system has been introduced, incorporating the NIRF technology inside the da Vinci camera. With this technology, surgeons have the possibility to rapidly switch from to the near-infrared view by a simple console touch.

Since the ICG advent in robotics, many experiences have been reported exploring its possible applications. Thanks to the aforementioned features, ICG guidance may represent as a valid tool in assessing the success of selective clamping (Fig. 5) prior to incision of the renal parenchyma. Alternatively, ICG could be very useful in a global clamping setting if there is a doubt regarding the presence of misdiagnosed accessory or aberrant renal arteries. In these conditions the use of ICG may be fundamental, since it could confirm or change the urologist's intraoperative strategy.

Moreover, ICG could be very useful in tumor identification and margins demarcation thanks to its hypo-fluorescent appearance as opposed to the highly vascularized healthy parenchyma. This application of ICG is particularly useful in case of partially endophytic renal masses with limited deformation of the kidney's shape, hence improving the precision of surgical resection and the amount of spared healthy tissue.

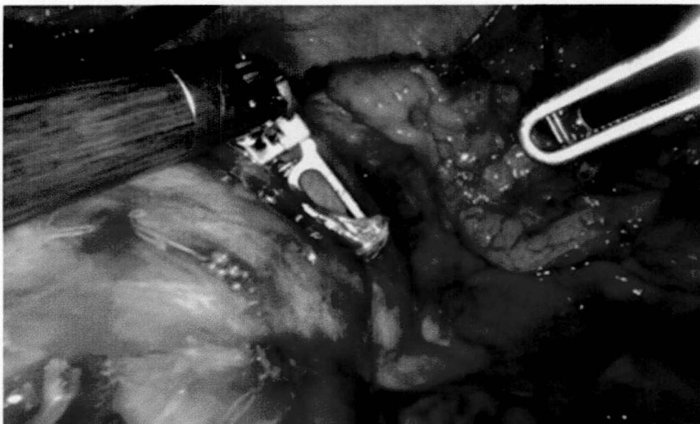

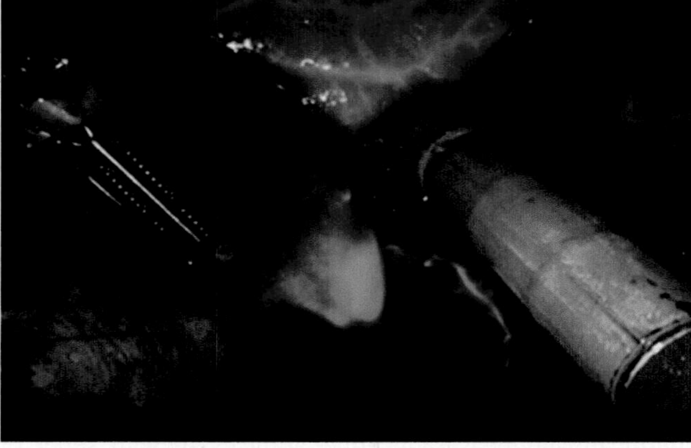

Fig. 5 Intraoperative view during ICG-RAPN: the NIRF vision confirmed the success of the selective clamping with the sparing of the blood supply of the upper pole of the kidney

Lastly, the ICG guidance may be applied to assess the vascularization of the remnant vital parenchyma at the end of the procedure.

All these fields of application have been well described and reported, but usually a few number of patients were included in these studies [16, 17]. Recently, Diana et al. [18] published a multi-institutional analysis including more than 300 patients undergoing ICG-guided robot-assisted partial nephrectomy (RAPN). Besides the abovementioned ICG advantages, the authors also outlined other possible challenging settings of application, such as solitary, horseshoe, or pelvic kidney. In all these anatomical abnormalities, the vascularization is often aberrant and difficult to preoperatively assess with the assistance of the standard 2D imaging. In this retrospective series, ICG was found to be an independent predicting variable of achievement of trifecta (negative surgical margins, warm ischemia time <25 minutes, and no perioperative complications).

Besides the intraoperative surgical advantages of ICG guidance, a recent pooled analysis by Veccia et al. [19] demonstrates higher postoperative eGFR levels of ICG-guided RAPN compared to standard robot-assisted partial nephrectomy (RAPN) and no difference in terms of operative time, blood loss, and perioperative complications.

Notwithstanding the abovementioned advantages of ICG-guided procedures over the standard ones, ICG is prone to some limitations: firstly, it is a one-shot opportunity because once injected the molecule remains in the circulation for several minutes, so it cannot be repeated in case of wrong clamping; secondly, the rate of failed selective clamping (defined as converted procedure to global clamping due to excessive bleeding) is around 20–25% according to the different available data; thirdly, it only provides surface information, and the surgeon has no idea on the perfusion status inside the parenchyma.

6 Virtual Reality and 3D Models

In the current era of precision surgery, the classical surgical principles have been widely revised. A perfect balance between the oncological and the functional outcomes is therefore needed [20]. Image-guided surgery plays a key role in achieving this balance and is enabled by novel technological improvements.

In the last years, 3D models had a widespread diffusion thanks to their very promising clinical applications. A 3D model is a physical or virtual representation of the surface of an object. In medicine, and even more in the surgical setting, they could overcome the limits of the current 2D imaging. In fact, the correct understanding of standard imaging modalities requires a lot of clinical experience linked with a rigorous knowledge of anatomy. Moreover, the subsequent step requires a good mental representation to translate the 2D information in 3D ones.

Therefore, it is easy to understand why 3D models have gained popularity in the daily clinical practice and contributed to the so-called surgery 4.0 [21]. This innovative movement also involved the renal surgical setting where many pioneering experiences have been published and described with the aim of improving the quality of the procedure for both the oncological and the functional aspects. In the following sections, a brief overview of the current 3D model technologies and their application is performed.

6.1 How to Make a 3D Model Reconstruction

The creation of 3D model begins from CT scan or MRI 2D image processing. The "original" 3D models, automatically obtained from DICOM (Digital Imaging and COmmunications in Medicine) viewers, consisted mainly of cinematic volume renders and maximum intensity projections [22], based on angiographic CTs. Despite adding some extra information when compared to classical 2D images, these automatic 3D models were often poor in resolution, lack many details, and cannot be manipulated freely. Therefore, surgeons cannot rely on them to plan surgery. Technological advancements in engineering and strong collaborations between surgeons and engineers lead to more precise models with a higher anatomical accuracy, as such overcoming these limits.

Practically speaking, the process starts with the acquisition of CT scan or MRI images in DICOM format. The image quality and slice thickness (no more than 5 mm) are pivotal since they allow to increase the precision of the reconstruction. Then a preprocessing phase takes place, in which the target organ is analyzed and interested images are selected and adjusted (e.g., image luminosity and contrast). Subsequently, software packages analyze the images and automatically generate the first prediction in a process called "segmentation." Here, the software (semi-)automatically generates a preliminary model which indicates for each pixel in each slice of the CT scan to which part anatomical structure it belongs. In case of renal surgery, this is typically the parenchyma, arteries, veins, pyelocaliceal system, tumor, and when applicable some renal cysts. Whereas this used to be a tedious time-consuming task, artificial intelligence techniques can now speed up this step significantly. At the end of this (semi-)automatic process, the reconstruction is manually refined by an engineer/technician/clinician in order to improve the accuracy of the model. Afterward, the project is saved in .stl (standard triangulation language) format and further modified by the operator using dedicated 3D manipulation software. Finally the virtual 3D model is completed and could be displayed on electronic devices or printed using different 3D printing technologies (Fig. 6).

6.2 3D Model Applications

3D reconstruction can be used in two main applications: printed and displayed on an electronic device (virtual models).

Printed 3D models allow surgeons to handle the model increasing the comprehension of the anatomy and the accuracy of preoperative surgical planning. A recent feasibility study on 3D printed models has been published by Maddox et al. [23]. In this experience, 3D printed models of seven patients were constructed with materials approximating the in vivo tissue on the basis of preoperative CT scan. Surgeons had the possibility to simulate the procedure on the model and thereafter perform the procedure on real patients. Notwithstanding the larger tumor size and complexity of the 3D group, significant lower estimated blood loss was recorded. Finally 3D models have been proposed to facilitate patients' understanding of their disease and communications with clinicians [24, 25]. The need for a 3D printer and the high costs explain the limited diffusion of this technology

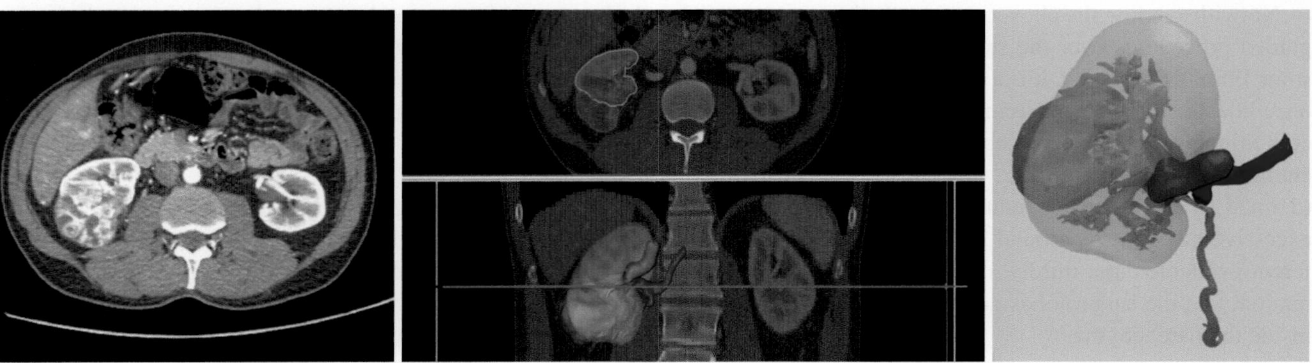

Fig. 6 3D model processing: from CT scan to image segmentation and 3D model visualization

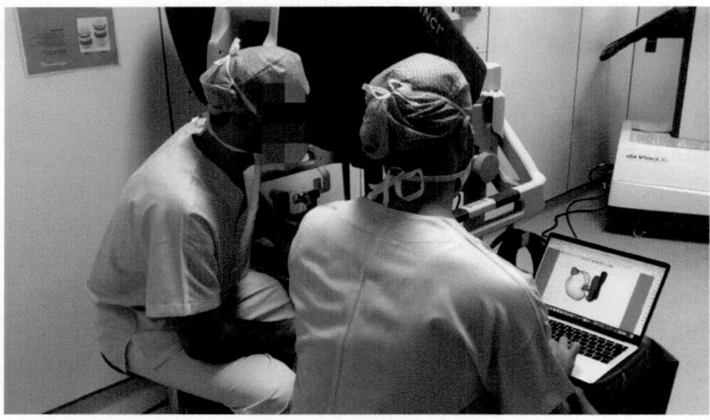

Fig. 7 Visualization of the 3D models during cognitive robotic partial nephrectomy

and mainly reserve it for highly complex cases. However, recent advancement in materials field may furtherly decrease the production costs overcoming this limit.

Conversely, virtual models are seeing a widespread diffusion thanks to their great variety in technological applications. Indeed, virtual 3D models can be variably displayed according to surgeons' needs and available devices:

- **2D screen view** (e.g., PC, tablet, smartphone): In this setting the 3D model is displayed as a navigable file (e.g., 3D pdf (portable document format) or other formats to be opened in 3D viewers), in which the surgeon can pan, zoom, and rotate by using the touch screen or a dedicated joystick or mouse. Moreover, it is possible to modify the model's color or transparency to increase the understanding of anatomical details as necessitated by the operator. Finally, thanks to a dedicated assistant, they could be used on-demand during the surgical procedure (Fig. 7).

  Porpiglia et al. [26] recently investigated the reliability of 3D models using the so-called "hyper-accuracy three-dimensional" (HA3D™) reconstructions to reproduce the patients' anatomy. They compared the perioperative outcomes of RAPN for complex renal tumors when the preoperative planning was performed either with the assistance of HA3D™ or without it (e.g., based on planar CT data only). The surgeon had the possibility to study the 3D models preoperatively, simulating the clamping strategies. Moreover, he could consult the HA3D™ intraoperatively on a tablet manually oriented by a dedicated operator, according to the intraoperative anatomy. Authors managed to perform up to 90% of selective clamping as preoperatively planned vs 60% in the standard group based on CT scan only.

  These preliminary results have been later confirmed by Shirk et al. [27] who conducted a RCT where 3D-assisted RAPN was compared to standard RAPN. The 3D models helped in reducing estimated blood loss, clamp time, and length of hospital stay. While Shirk found a reduced operative time, Michiels et al. [28] found a lengthening of the procedural time but again with overall better surgical outcomes: better trifecta achievement, lower transfusion rates, less major complications, and less conversion to radical nephrectomy. They also report an additional impact on short-term renal function.
- **Virtual reality (VR):** This technology permits the user, using dedicated visors, to interact with a fully virtual environment excluding completely the real one. Virtual surgical simulators based on this technology [e.g., for robotic surgery, dV-Trainer (Mimic, Seattle, WA, USA) and da Vinci Skills Simulator (Intuitive Surgical, Sunnyvale, CA, USA)] are currently used for surgeons' training: thanks to different levels of difficulty, the trainer can improve his/her skills step by step in specific tasks and operations (e.g., partial nephrectomy or radical prostatectomy). In this scenario surgeons will be able to simulate preparatory surgical gestures interacting with the 3D model while planning the more suitable surgical strategy.
- **Mixed reality (MR):** Thanks to the use of dedicated devices (e.g., HoloLens®), it is possible to merge together

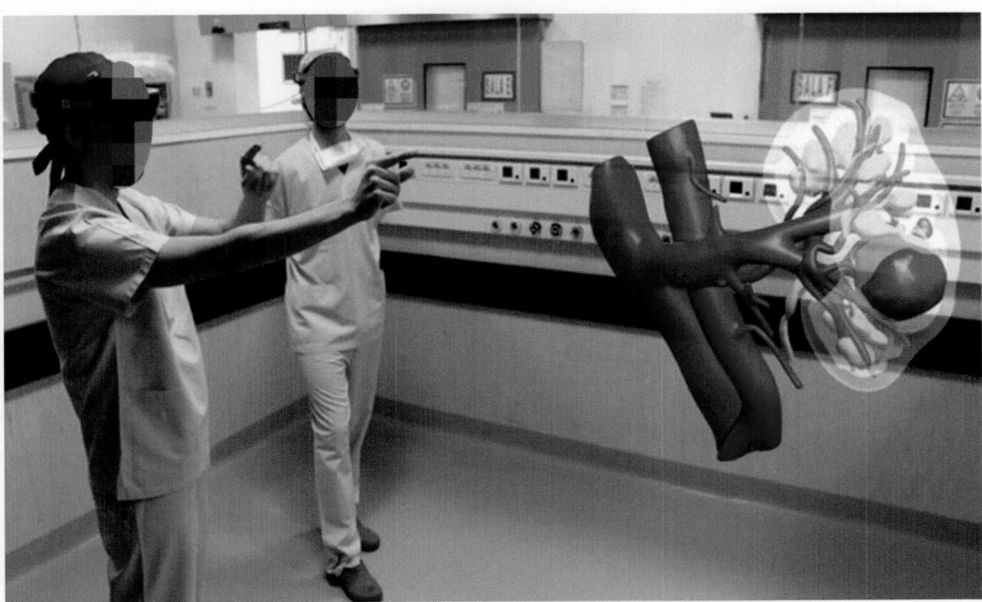

Fig. 8 3D mixed reality visualization of the 3D virtual model for preoperative surgical planning

the virtual and real images. In this way the 3D model can be visualized inside the physical environment, and the operator can interact with the model and view it from different positions in the room (Fig. 8).

Moreover, the superimposed images can be broadcasted, allowing the model to be viewed by a large number of people simultaneously. Thanks to this complete involvement of the operators, this technology is perfectly suited for preoperative planning as shown recently by several authors [29, 30]. In particular Antonelli et al. [29] studied a mixed reality platform using a Windows-based laptop (the zSpace workstation), linked to a stereoscopic screen displaying virtual objects (e.g., 3D virtual kidney model). This specifically designed platform allowed the authors to improve the preoperative planning for partial nephrectomy thanks to the higher-resolution details when compared to standard CT scan.

Similar advantages were described by Checcucci et al. [30] using the HoloLens® device: during an international urological meeting, several surgeons had the possibility to analyze the HA3D™ reconstruction of their case in a MR setting prior to the live surgical procedure and to share their surgical planning with the audience. This technology was rated favorably by the surgeons both for anatomical accuracy (scored 9/10) and surgical planning (8/10) on 1–10 Likert scale. Moreover, its potential in influencing surgeons' planning was investigated: in 64.4% and 44.4% of the cases, surgeons shift toward a more selective clamping and more nephron-sparing technique, respectively, compared to CT scan-based preoperative planning.

– **Augmented reality (AR)**: In this setting the virtual object is overlaid onto the real environment in order to enhance its features. Intraoperative navigation forms an ideal use case for AR: the overlapping of digital and real images may help surgeons in the identification of hidden anatomy features (tumor's location, vascular anatomy).

Despite its very appealing application, few studies in literature have explored the in vivo feasibility of AR. In 2009 an AR stereo-endoscopic RAPN obtained with an intraoperatory tracking system was described by Su et al. [31]. In this preliminary experience, an error of just 1 mm among the superimposed and real images was identified. Another interesting experience was published in 2018: Wake et al. described a new 3D printed and AR model created with Unity® software and adopted during RAPN. AR 3D model application showed to be safe, feasible, and able to influence the surgical planning [32].

A recent comparative prospective study has been reported by Porpiglia et al. [33]. A dedicated software able to merge together the HA3D™ reconstruction with the da Vinci surgical console was developed. With a dedicated software (developed with the Unity® platform), the 3D models were loaded on a dedicated AR platform, where it was possible to precisely reproduce the displacements and elastic modifications of the target organ during the surgery (Fig. 9). The AR platform combined the receiving stream from the endoscopic video of the robotic camera with the 3D model images, and the resulting stream was sent back to the remote console by using the Tile-Pro™. As such, the overlapped 3D model augments the live surgical feed inside the robotic console (Fig. 10).

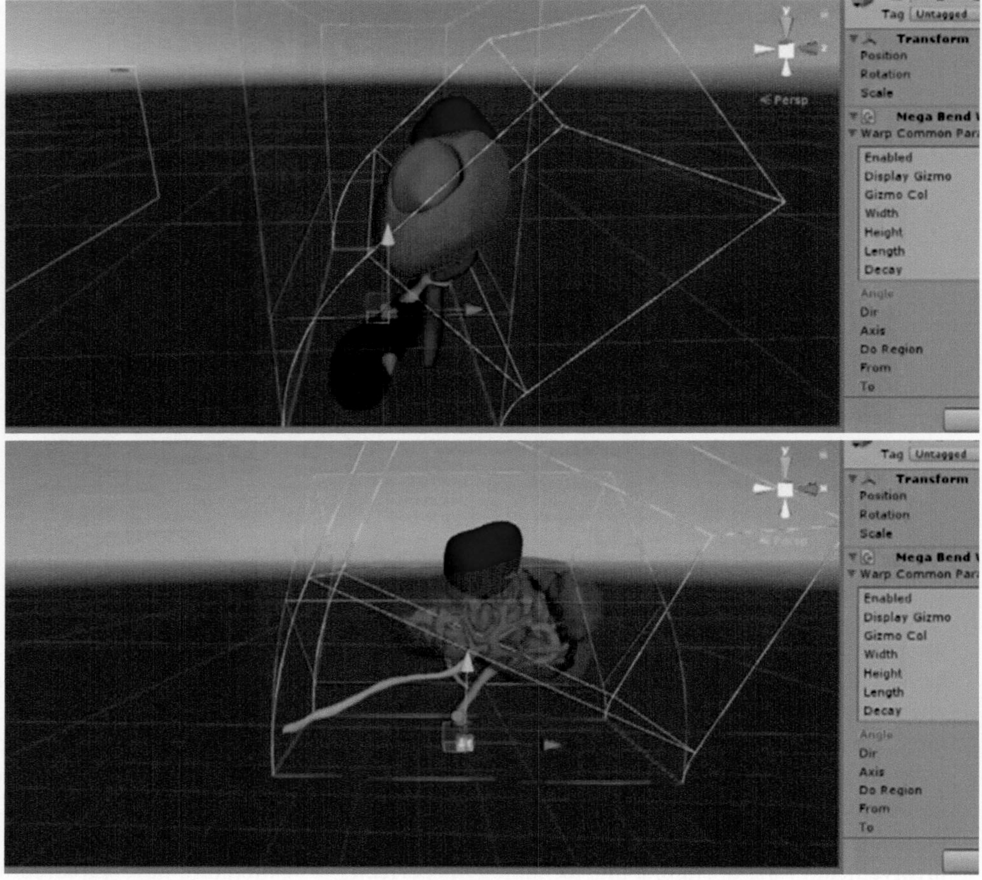

Fig. 9 The 3D elastic augmented reality system: thanks to the application of non-linear parametric deformation, it is possible to approximate the manipulation of the kidney during the intervention

To improve the aid given to the surgeon, it was possible to modify the transparency of the 3D model in order to show the hidden anatomical details of the organ or the tumor's margins. All the above movements of the HA3D™ model were manually performed by an assistant by using a dedicated mouse.

The AR 3D technology was compared with the standard intraoperative US guidance during RAPN performed for complex renal tumors (PADUA score ≥10) [33]. The AR 3D technology provided a more accurate intraoperative guidance than the standard US one, able to identify the position of renal vessels (facilitating the selective clamping procedures) and of endophytic and posterior tumors.

6.3 Future Perspectives

Notwithstanding the high-quality resolution obtained with the HA3D reconstruction, there are still some limitations that need to be addressed.

The higher accuracy of the last 3D models compared to the first generation of 3D automatic reconstructions headed to a new frontier in the field of selective clamping. The possibility to clearly identify the segmental branches of the renal artery might inform surgeons on how to perform super-selective RAPN, with possible benefits in terms of functional outcomes. Here, the perfusion zones per arterial branch are estimated. Notwithstanding promising results of the first preliminary experience, sometimes the preoperative planning failed due to an imprecise estimation of the regions perfused by each branch (10% in one of the most recent series) [26]. This field of application is therefore one of the more interesting that should further be investigated.

In the AR setting, the need for an assistant to constantly manipulate the model in order to maintain the correct overlapping is one of the main limitations of the aforementioned technique. Researchers are now developing strategies to achieve a complete automatic AR procedure. Two main approaches have been proposed to overcome this limit. The first strategy implies the identification of landmarks on the endoscopic vision that could be subsequently detected by the

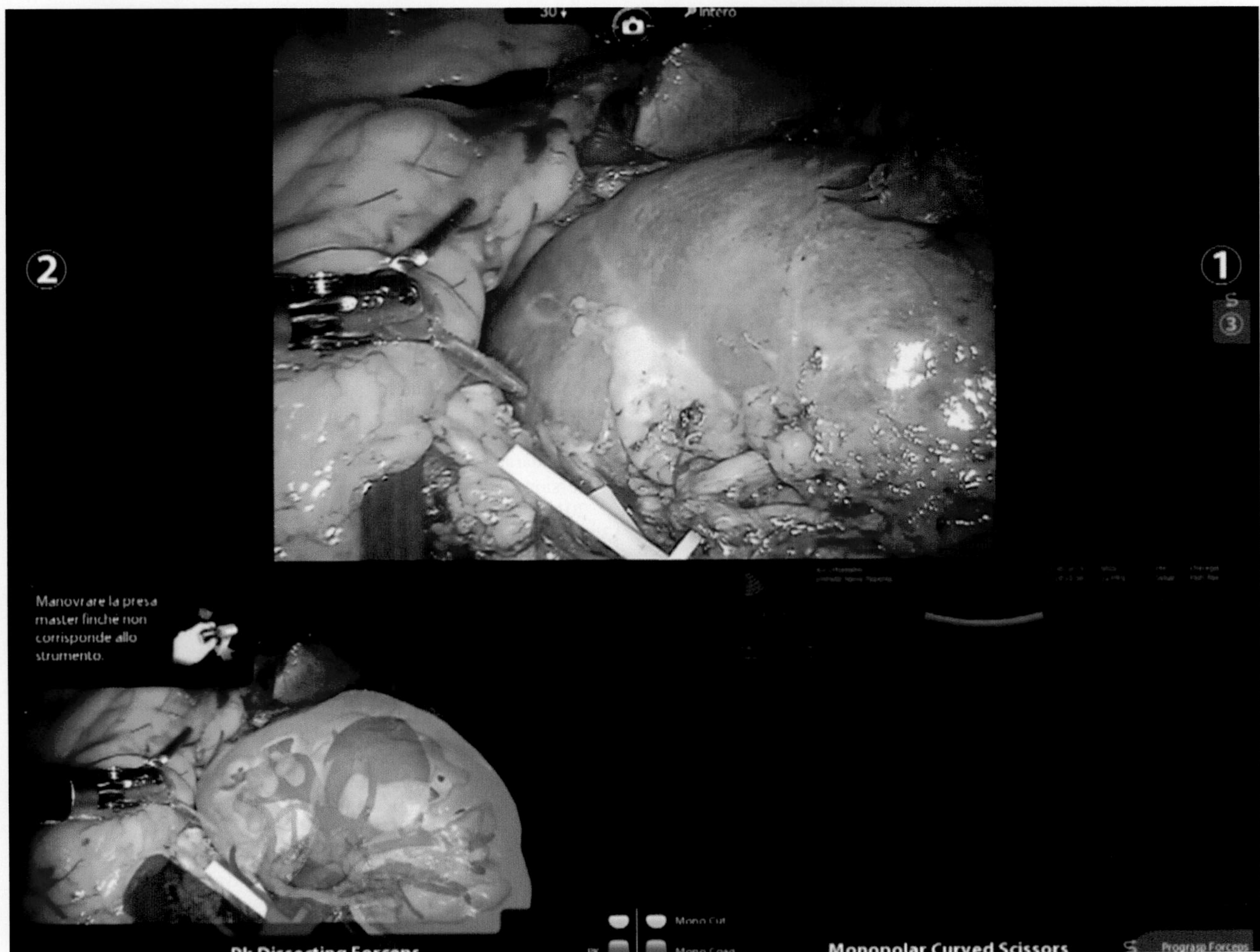

Fig. 10 The view of the da Vinci console camera after activating the Tile-Pro to see the overlapping of the 3D model to the real anatomy. In this case of completely endophytic tumor, this technology provides a precise estimation of tumor's margins and its relationship with the intrarenal structures

AR software [29, 34]. The alternative approach is based on a "markerless" strategy. A preliminary "markerless" experience has been recently reported by Amparore et al. [35]: thanks to a new computer vision algorithm, it has been possible to correctly estimate the position of the target organ on the operative field. To overcome the similarity of colors of the operative field, the "registration" process (e.g., the identification and anchoring of the model) was performed with the assistance of ICG guidance: the boundaries of the kidney, appearing as a bright green arc, are easily identified by the algorithm, and the model is anchored. Then it is possible to switch to standard vision and perform the procedure (Fig. 11).

7 Conclusion

The state of the art in pre- and intraoperative imaging modalities for kidney tumors is rapidly evolving thanks to technological improvements. Built on the standard imaging techniques, new tools in this surgical setting could provide the best-tailored patient-specific treatment. With the help of these new technologies, it is estimated to further increase the number of complex renal masses suitable for nephron-sparing surgery and to reduce the postoperative functional impairment thanks to more conservative resection techniques and more selective clamping procedures.

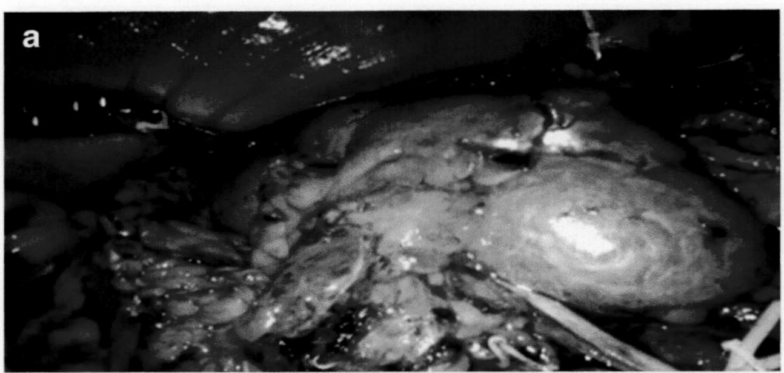

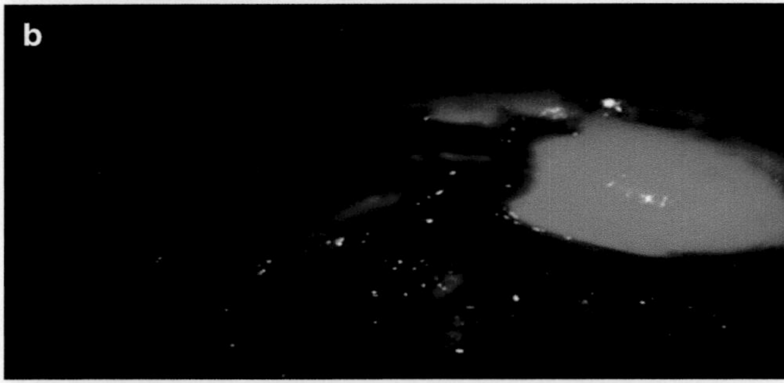

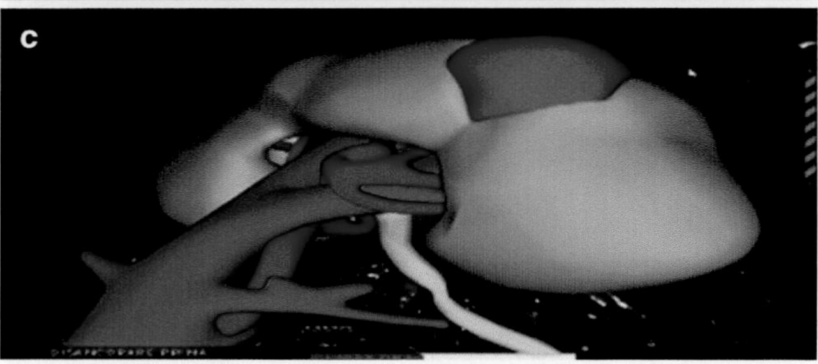

Fig. 11 Automatic overlapping of the 3D model. After kidney surface exposure (**a**), the indocyanine is injected (**b**). Thereafter the software is able to recognize the organ and to overlap the 3D model (**c**)

References

1. Ljungberg B, Albiges L, Abu-Ghanem Y, Bensalah K, Dabestani S, Fernández-Pello S, et al. European Association of Urology Guidelines on Renal Cell Carcinoma: limited update March 2021. Eur Urol [Internet]. 2021;75(5):799–810. Available from: https://linkinghub.elsevier.com/retrieve/pii/S0302283821000075
2. van Oostenbrugge TJ, Fütterer JJ, Mulders PFA. Diagnostic imaging for solid renal tumors: a pictorial review. Kidney Cancer. 2018;2(2):79–93.
3. Rumack C, Wilson S. Diagnostic ultrasound: general adult. 4th ed. Saunders; 2014.
4. Bertolotto M, Bucci S, Valentino M, Currò F, Sachs C, Cova MA. Contrast-enhanced ultrasound for characterizing renal masses. Eur J Radiol [Internet]. 2018;105(May):41–8. Available from: https://doi.org/10.1016/j.ejrad.2018.05.015
5. Bertolotto M, Cicero C, Catalano O, Currò F, Derchi LE. Solid renal tumors isoenhancing to kidneys on contrast-enhanced sonography: differentiation from pseudomasses. J Ultrasound Med. 2018;37(1):233–42.
6. Defortescu G, Cornu JN, Béjar S, Giwerc A, Gobet F, Werquin C, et al. Diagnostic performance of contrast-enhanced ultrasonography and magnetic resonance imaging for the assessment of complex renal cysts: a prospective study. Int J Urol. 2017;24(3):184–9.
7. Hoeffel C, Pousset M, Timsit MO, Elie C, Méjean A, Merran S, et al. Radiofrequency ablation of renal tumours: diagnostic accuracy of contrast-enhanced ultrasound for early detection of residual tumour. Eur Radiol. 2010;20(8):1812–21.
8. Hekman MCH, Rijpkema M, Langenhuijsen JF, Boerman OC, Oosterwijk E, Mulders PFA. Intraoperative imaging techniques to support complete tumor resection in partial nephrectomy. Eur Urol Focus [Internet]. 2018;4(6):960–8. Available from: https://doi.org/10.1016/j.euf.2017.04.008
9. Correas JM, Anglicheau D, Joly D, Gennisson JL, Tanter M, Hélénon O. Ultrasound-based imaging methods of the kidney—recent developments. Kidney Int. 2016;90(6):1199–210.
10. Diaz de Leon A, Pedrosa I. Imaging and screening of kidney cancer. Radiol Clin North Am. 2017;55(6):1235–50.
11. Sasaguri K, Takahashi N. CT and MR imaging for solid renal mass characterization. Eur J Radiol [Internet]. 2018;99(Dec 2017):40–54. Available from: https://doi.org/10.1016/j.ejrad.2017.12.008
12. Silverman SG, Pedrosa I, Ellis JH, Hindman NM, Wang ZJ, Chandarana H, et al. Bosniak classification of cystic renal masses, version 2019 : an update proposal and needs assessment. Radiology. 2019;292:26–38.
13. Wang ZJ, Westphalen AC, Zagoria RJ. CT and MRI of small renal masses. Br J Radiol. 2018;91(1087):20180131.
14. Johnson BA, Kim S, Steinberg RL, de Leon AD, Pedrosa I, Cadeddu JA. Diagnostic performance of prospectively assigned clear cell Likelihood scores (ccLS) in small renal masses at multiparametric magnetic resonance imaging. Urol Oncol Semin Orig Invest. 2019;37(12):941–6.
15. Steinberg RL, Rasmussen RG, Johnson BA, Ghandour R, De Leon AD, Xi Y, et al. Prospective performance of clear cell likelihood scores (ccLS) in renal masses evaluated with multiparametric magnetic resonance imaging. Eur Radiol. 2021;31(1):314–24.
16. Krane LS, Manny TB, Hemal AK. Is near infrared fluorescence imaging using indocyanine green dye useful in robotic partial nephrectomy: a prospective comparative study of 94 patients. Urology [Internet]. 2012;80(1):110–8. Available from: https://doi.org/10.1016/j.urology.2012.01.076
17. Bjurlin MA, McClintock TR, Stifelman MD. Near-infrared fluorescence imaging with intraoperative administration of indocyanine green for robotic partial nephrectomy. Curr Urol Rep. 2015;16(4)
18. Diana P, Buffi NM, Lughezzani G, Dell'Oglio P, Mazzone E, Porter J, et al. The role of intraoperative indocyanine green in robot-assisted partial nephrectomy: results from a large, multi-institutional series. Eur Urol. 2020;78(5):743–9.
19. Veccia A, Antonelli A, Hampton LJ, Greco F, Perdonà S, Lima E, et al. Near-infrared fluorescence imaging with indocyanine green in robot-assisted partial nephrectomy: pooled analysis of comparative studies. Eur Urol Focus. 2020;6(3):505–12.
20. Autorino R, Porpiglia F, Dasgupta P, Rassweiler J, Catto JW, Hampton LJ, et al. Precision surgery and genitourinary cancers. Eur J Surg Oncol [Internet]. 2017;43(5):893–908. Available from: https://doi.org/10.1016/j.ejso.2017.02.005
21. Feußner H, Park A. Surgery 4.0: the natural culmination of the industrial revolution? Innov Surg Sci. 2017;2(3):105–8.
22. Fishman EK, Ney DR, Heath DG, Corl FM, Horton KM, Johnson PT. Volume rendering versus maximum intensity projection in CT angiography: what works best, when, and why. Radiographics. 2006;26(3):905–22.
23. Maddox MM, Feibus A, Liu J, Wang J, Thomas R, Silberstein JL. 3D-printed soft-tissue physical models of renal malignancies for individualized surgical simulation: a feasibility study. J Robot Surg. 2018;12(1):27–33.
24. Bernhard JC, Isotani S, Matsugasumi T, Duddalwar V, Hung AJ, Suer E, et al. Personalized 3D printed model of kidney and tumor anatomy: a useful tool for patient education. World J Urol. 2016;34(3):337–45.

25. Porpiglia F, Amparore D, Checcucci E, Autorino R, Manfredi M, Iannizzi G, et al. Current use of three-dimensional model technology in urology: a road map for personalised surgical planning. Eur Urol Focus [Internet]. 2018;4(5):652–6. Available from: https://doi.org/10.1016/j.euf.2018.09.012
26. Porpiglia F, Fiori C, Checcucci E, Amparore D, Bertolo R. Hyperaccuracy three-dimensional reconstruction is able to maximize the efficacy of selective clamping during robot-assisted partial nephrectomy for complex renal masses. Eur Urol [Internet]. 2018;74(5):651–60. Available from: https://doi.org/10.1016/j.eururo.2017.12.027
27. Shirk JD, Thiel DD, Wallen EM, Linehan JM, White WM, Badani KK, et al. Effect of 3-dimensional virtual reality models for surgical planning of robotic-assisted partial nephrectomy on surgical outcomes: a randomized clinical trial. JAMA Netw Open. 2019;2(9):1–11.
28. Michiels C, Khene ZE, Prudhomme T, Boulenger de Hauteclocque A, Cornelis FH, Percot M, et al. 3D-Image guided robotic-assisted partial nephrectomy: a multi-institutional propensity score-matched analysis (UroCCR study 51). World J Urol [Internet]. 2021;0123456789. Available from: https://doi.org/10.1007/s00345-021-03645-1
29. Antonelli A, Veccia A, Palumbo C, Peroni A, Mirabella G, Cozzoli A, et al. Holographic reconstructions for preoperative planning before partial nephrectomy: a head-to-head comparison with standard CT scan. Urol Int. 2019;102(2):212–7.
30. Checcucci E, Amparore D, Pecoraro A, Peretti D, Aimar R, De Cillis S, et al. 3D mixed reality holograms for preoperative surgical planning of nephron-sparing surgery: evaluation of surgeons' perception. Minerva Urol Nefrol. 2021;73(3):367–75.
31. Su LM, Vagvolgyi BP, Agarwal R, Reiley CE, Taylor RH, Hager GD. Augmented reality during robot-assisted laparoscopic partial nephrectomy: toward real-time 3D-CT to stereoscopic video registration. Urology [Internet]. 2009;73(4):896–900. Available from: https://doi.org/10.1016/j.urology.2008.11.040
32. Wake N, Bjurlin MA, Rostami P, Chandarana H, Huang WC. Three-dimensional printing and augmented reality: enhanced precision for robotic assisted partial nephrectomy. Urology [Internet]. 2018;116:227–8. Available from: https://doi.org/10.1016/j.urology.2017.12.038
33. Porpiglia F, Checcucci E, Amparore D, Piramide F, Volpi G, Granato S, et al. Three-dimensional augmented reality robot-assisted partial nephrectomy in case of complex tumours (PADUA ≥10): a new intraoperative tool overcoming the ultrasound guidance. Eur Urol [Internet]. 2020;78(2):229–38. Available from: https://doi.org/10.1016/j.eururo.2019.11.024
34. Nosrati MS, Abugharbieh R, Peyrat JM, Abinahed J, Al-Alao O, Al-Ansari A, et al. Simultaneous multi-structure segmentation and 3D nonrigid pose estimation in image-guided robotic surgery. IEEE Trans Med Imaging. 2016;35(1):1–12.
35. Amparore D, Checcucci E, Piazzolla P, Piramide F, De Cillis S, Piana A, et al. Indocyanine green drives computer vision based 3D augmented reality robot assisted partial nephrectomy: the beginning of "automatic" overlapping era. Urology. 2022;19:S0090-4295(22)00029-2. https://doi.org/10.1016/j.urology.2021.10.053. Epub ahead of print. PMID: 35063460.

Patient Positioning for Renal Surgery

Louis Saada, Nikhil Sapre, and Benjamin J. Challacombe

1 Standard Position for a Transperitoneal Approach

Before positioning the patient, it is important to ensure that they are catheterised and have the necessary deep vein thrombosis prophylaxis in place. Ideally intermittent pneumatic compression devices should be used. One must also ensure that the anaesthetic team are satisfied with vascular access and pressure point padding and have applied any necessary monitoring apparatus.

The patient should then be placed in a 60° lateral decubitus (flank) position with the contralateral side down. Full back supports, along with 10 cm tapes at the level of the pelvis and the chest, can be used to secure the torso. The table is flexed slightly to open the space between the 12th rib and the iliac crest, allowing for better access to the ipsilateral kidney. To achieve this, the patient should be positioned with their umbilicus at the level of the table break. Before breaking the table, it is important to check that the shoulders, spine and hip are aligned. This will ensure the patient stays centrally placed on the table once flexed.

The dependent leg should be flexed at the hip and knee and placed on a supportive jelly pad. The non-dependent leg should sit in a straight position on top with a pillow in between the legs. A tape can then be applied to secure the legs. The arms should be flexed at the shoulders and elbows, away from the torso. The arms should rest on padding in a 'sleeping baby' position or the dependent one in a gutter, and an axillary roll may be placed. The head should be supported on pillows, keeping it in line with the spine. A warming blanket can then be placed over the patient before draping.

L. Saada · N. Sapre · B. J. Challacombe (✉)
The Urology Centre, Guy's and St Thomas' Hospitals, London, UK

2 Variation for a Retroperitoneal Approach

A retroperitoneal approach requires a slight adjustment to the above positioning to allow for the greater degree of posterolateral access required. To facilitate this, the patient must be placed in the full lateral decubitus position. Care must be taken when securing the patient in this position. Robotic arms can clash with bulky full back supports, so rolled blankets or pillows should be used instead. These can be positioned on both sides of the patient for extra security, and straps should be placed over the top as standard.

When using the retroperitoneal approach, all attempts must be made to create sufficient space for port site placement in the flank. This can be one of the major challenges of this approach. In contrast to the partial table flex used for the transperitoneal approach, fully flexing the table can help create this space for this retroperitoneal access. To achieve enough flexion, it is essential to position the patient with the space between their 12th rib and iliac crest directly over the table break.

The rest of the positioning should proceed as standard. Adjustments may need to be made to support the limbs and head with the greater degree of rotation used in this position.

3 Difficulties with Positioning

For obese patients, or those with larger hips, difficulties can arise with inferior robotic arms clashing with the iliac crest or overlying soft tissue. One way to address this is to further flex the table, bringing the hip down and out of the way. Alternatively, the patient can be moved caudally down the table before it is broken.

For patients with poor spinal flexibility, adopting the lateral decubitus position with a flexed table can be challenging. Applying further pressure or traction to achieve the desired positioning can be dangerous. Instead this issue

P. Wiklund et al. (eds.), *Robotic Urologic Surgery*, https://doi.org/10.1007/978-3-031-00363-9_36

should be considered and discussed during pre-operative planning, and measures put into place to avoid unnecessary table flexion. For example, it may be possible to perform the operation with a transperitoneal approach where a lesser degree of table flexion is required.

4 Positioning-Related Complications

There are a number of complications that can arise from poor patient positioning. These tend to be the result of excessive pressure onto soft tissue structures and bony promontories. While taking the time to appropriately position patients for surgery has made these complications rare, they can still occur regardless.

One of the most common groups of positioning-related complications is peripheral nerve injuries. The most commonly damaged nerves are the ulnar nerve, the common peroneal nerve and the nerves of the brachial plexus [1]. These are all potentially at risk in the lateral decubitus position, and specific measures should be taken to prevent them.

Ulnar nerve injuries are typically the result of pressure on the nerve as it passes through the cubital tunnel. In the lateral decubitus position, these injuries can result from the lack of padding underneath the dependent arm but could also be caused by positioning the patient with excessive elbow flexion [2]. These injuries can also be the result of incorrect placement of blood pressure monitoring cuffs over the cubital fossa.

Common peroneal nerve injuries are more classically associated with the lithotomy position but can also be seen in the lateral decubitus position. They tend to occur as a result of excessive pressure on the nerve as it traverses the fibular head and can be avoided with sufficient padding of this area.

Brachial plexus injuries occur more frequently in other patient positions but can occur in the lateral decubitus position when the patient's arms are flexed up and away from their neutral position. This can result in the plexus being compressed between the chest wall and the unpadded operating table. The use of axillary rolls can prevent these injuries.

Positioning-related injuries to the skin can also occur in the form of decubitus pressure ulcers [3]. Like peripheral nerve injuries, these are seen when appropriate measures to apply padding and support are not taken. This can result in regions of the soft tissue being exposed to prolonged periods of pressure. Any shearing forces generated from incorrectly restrained patients slipping on the table can exacerbate these pressure injuries, increasing the severity of the resulting ulcers.

5 Port Placement

The optimal placement of ports is influenced by several factors including the robotic platform used, the surgical approach and the position of the tumour.

5.1 The Influence of Robotic Platform on Port Placement

The two major robotic platforms we will discuss are the Da Vinci Si and the Da Vinci Xi [Intuitive Surgical Inc., USA]. Both platforms allow for one camera arm and three instrument arms. However, the updated Xi platform brought with it significantly more flexibility. The arms have a greater degree of movement and a longer reach and can be placed much closer together. The platform also has a rotating boom from which the arms originate, allowing for simpler docking and facilitating multi-quadrant surgery. This flexibility allows for simpler port placement, without the need to triangulate positions or worry about spacing to the same degree as with the Si platform.

The Da Vinci range also includes the X platform sitting between the Si and the Xi models. This platform performs much like the Si but with upgraded optics and thinner arms. While the Da Vinci X can bring some greater flexibility with its upgraded arms when compared to the Si system, its lack of rotating boom means it does not match the performance of the Xi platform.

In practical terms, using the Xi platform can allow for easier port placement in more challenging situations where space may be limited by body habitus or previous surgical sites. While such cases may still be possible with the Si and X platforms, the lack of flexibility may mean sacrifices have to be made with less room for the fourth arm or assistant ports.

5.2 Port Placement for the Transperitoneal Approach

For both platforms, port placement starts with insertion of the camera port and establishing a pneumoperitoneum. Initial access can be achieved using the Veress needle or open Hasson technique. The Veress needle technique is a blind entry technique using a needle with a dull spring-loaded stylet that advances upon entry into the peritoneal cavity, protecting the viscera. The Hasson technique, often considered safer, involves a cut-down through the layers of the abdominal wall with direct vision. The peritoneum is then elevated with a pair of haemostats and excised in a controlled manner. Once the camera port has been positioned, it can be used to insert the remaining ports under direct vision.

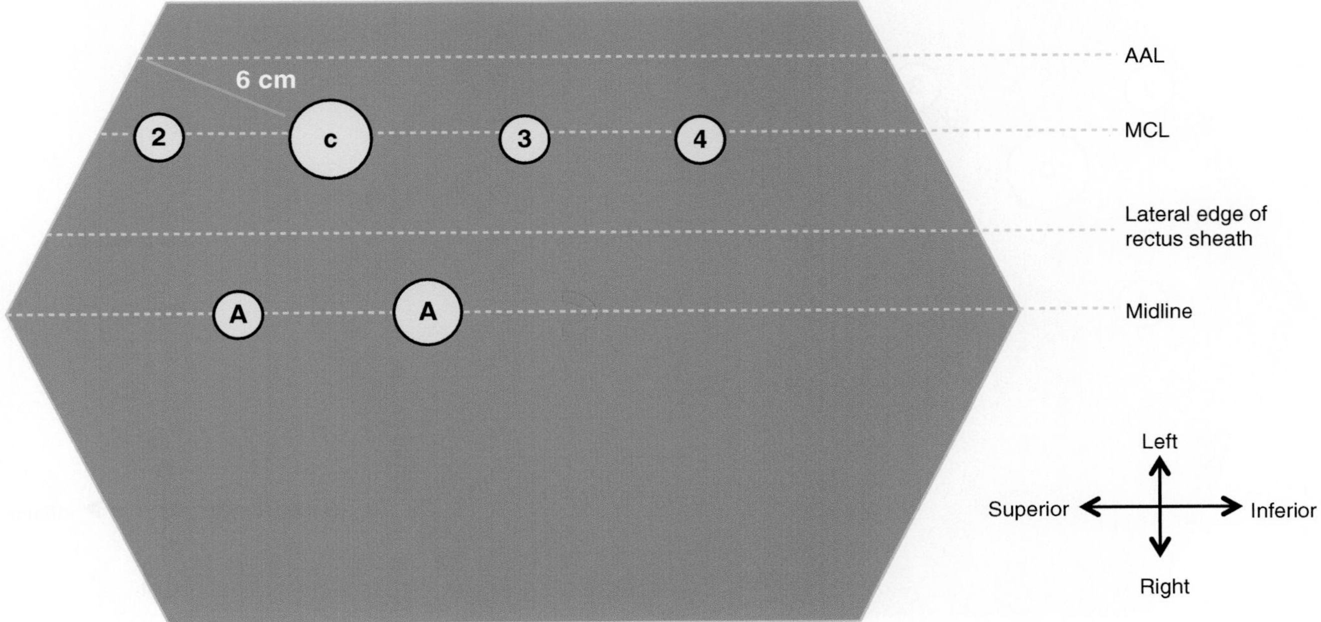

Fig. 1 Port placement for a transperitoneal approach to the left kidney with the Xi platform. *AAL* anterior axillary line, *MCL* medial clavicular line, *C* camera port, *A* assistant port, the remaining ports are numberedmm assistant port for suction

Port placement is simple when using the Xi platform (see Fig. 1). The camera port is placed in the mid-clavicular line 6 cm infero-medial to the costal margin. The remaining three robotic ports will then also be positioned directly in the mid-clavicular line: one cephalad and the other two caudally. A 12-mm assistant port can be placed around 6 cm superior to the umbilicus, with a further 5 mm assistant port for suction 6 cm superior to that if required.

For the Si platform, the instruments, and therefore port sites, need to be triangulated to a greater degree and spaced 6–8 cm apart. There are two main approaches to this, characterised by the position of the camera in relation to the second and third arms. The decision between the two can be influenced by the position of the tumour but tends to be determined by the surgeon's personal experience and preference.

For the medial camera trocar arrangement (see Fig. 2), the camera port will be placed 6 cm infero-medial to the costal margin near the lateral edge of the rectus sheath. The second and third ports can then be triangulated out laterally. One will be placed around 6 cm supero-lateral (near the costal margin) and the other 6 cm infero-lateral. Two assistant ports can be triangulated medially from the camera port, sitting supero-medially and infero-medially near the midline. A fourth arm port can be placed 6 cm inferior to the inferior robotic arm port. The medial camera trocar arrangement provides a 'front-on' working view that can be useful when approaching hilar or anterior renal masses.

For the lateral camera trocar arrangement (see Fig. 3), the camera is instead placed more laterally in the mid-clavicular or anterior axillary line. The second and third ports are then placed medially at the lateral edge of the rectus sheath. As above, it is important to ensure that the ports are placed at least 6 cm apart. Similarly, the fourth arm can be placed inferiorly in line with the camera port or in line with the other two arm ports. The lateral camera trocar arrangement provides a 'top-down' working view that can be useful when approaching lateral or posterior masses.

Depending on surgeon preference, an additional small sup-xiphoid port can be added for right-sided operations for the insertion of a liver retractor. This is less relevant when the fourth arm is available but may still be included.

5.3 Port Placement for the Retroperitoneal Approach

For both platforms, port placement starts with insertion of the camera port just above the iliac crest in the mid-axillary line. Initially a kidney-shaped balloon dilator is used to create space in the retroperitoneum. The ports are then placed sequentially under direct vision with a pledget often being used to increase the retroperitoneal space and push the peritoneum away.

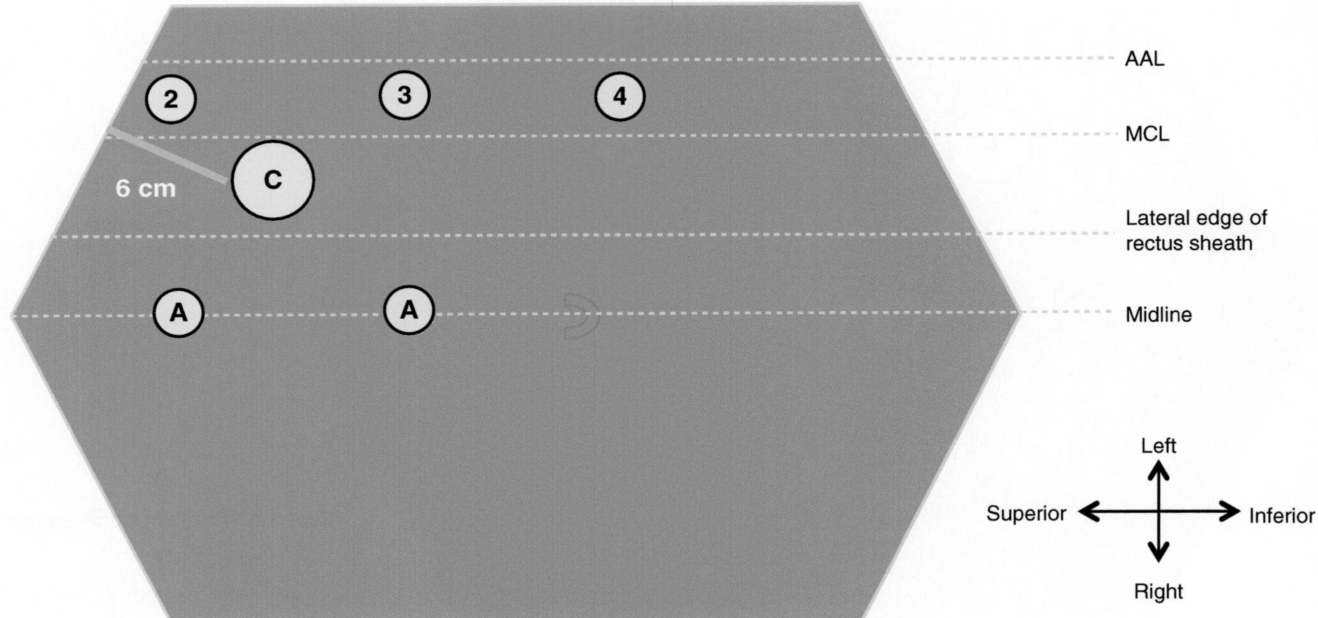

Fig. 2 The medial camera trocar arrangement of port placement for the transperitoneal approach to the Left kidney with the Si platform. *AAL* anterior axillary line, *MCL* medial clavicular line, *C* camera port, *A* assistant port, the remaining ports are numbered

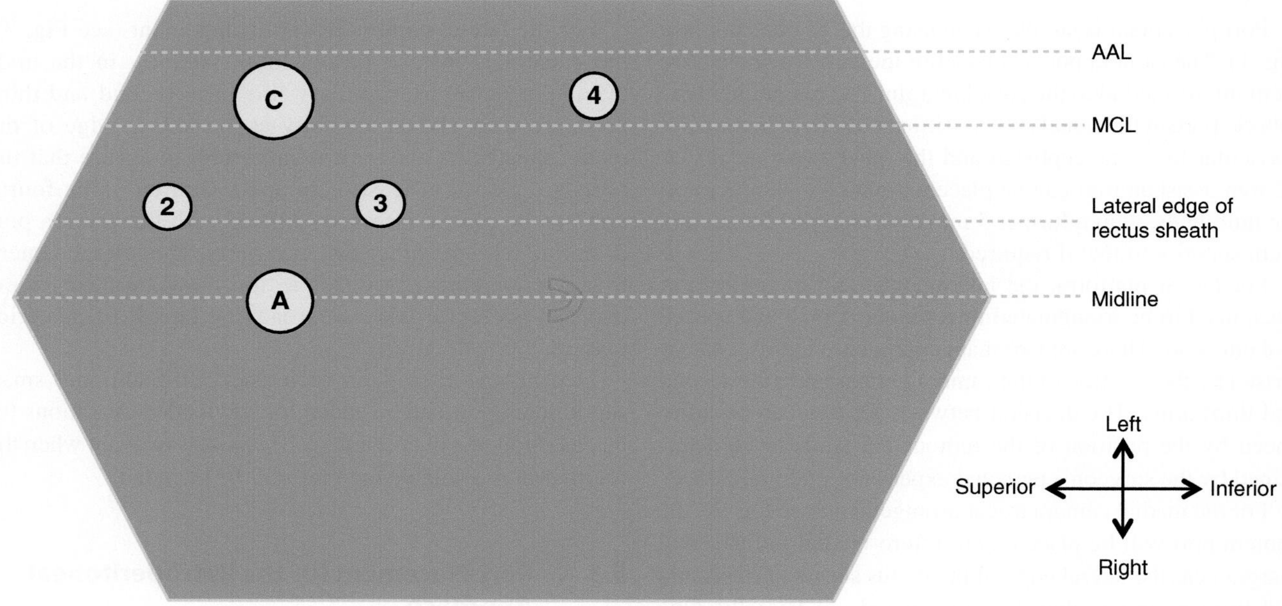

Fig. 3 The lateral camera trocar arrangement of port placement for the transperitoneal approach to the Left kidney with the Si platform. *AAL* anterior axillary line, *MCL* medial clavicular line, *C* camera port, *A* assistant port, the remaining ports are numbered

For the Xi platform (see Fig. 4), the lateral and medial ports can be placed in the posterior and anterior axillary lines, respectively. Without the concern about arm clashing and poor flexibility that are encountered in the Si platform, the ports do not need to be triangulated superiorly and can therefore be placed along one slightly curved line running in the axial plane. The fourth arm can be placed 6 cm medial to the medial third arm rather than placing it more inferiorly. The assistant port, however, should be placed off this line, 6–8 cm medial and inferior to the camera port in a position just superior to the anterior superior iliac spine.

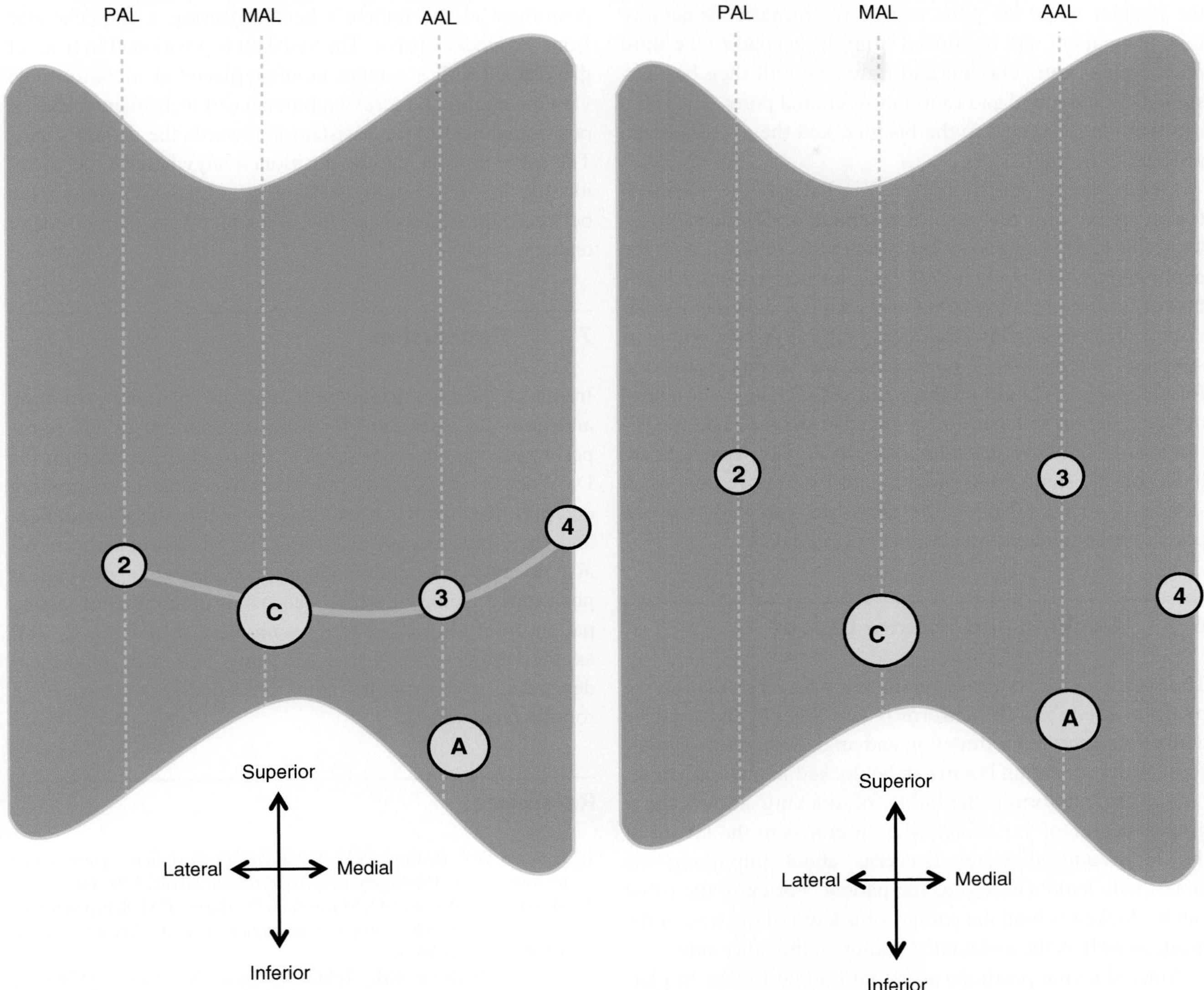

Fig. 4 Port placement for the retroperitoneal approach to the Right kidney with the Xi platform. *PAL* posterior axillary line, *MAL* medial axillary line, *AAL* anterior axillary line, *C* camera port, *A* assistant port, the remaining ports are numbered

Fig. 5 Port placement for the transperitoneal approach to the Right kidney with the Si platform. *AAL* anterior axillary line, *MCL* medial clavicular line, *C* camera port, *A* assistant port, the remaining ports are numbered

For the Si platform (see Fig. 5), the second robotic port should be triangulated out into a position 6–8 cm superior and lateral to the camera port, in the posterior axillary line. Next, the third robotic port should be inserted into a position 6–8 cm superior and medial to the camera port, in the anterior axillary line. The assistant port can be placed in a position around 6–8 cm inferior and medial to the camera port, sitting just superior to the anterior superior iliac spine. If space allows, the fourth arm port can be added 6–8 cm inferior and medial to the third arm or put on the other side of the camera port towards Arm 2.

Adjustments to standard positions can be made depending on the tumour location. For example, to reach the upper pole lesions, the ports can be placed more cranially, while lower pole tumours may require ports to be shifted caudally.

5.4 Port Placement for a Transperitoneal Nephroureterectomy

The Xi platform has been specifically designed to perform multi-quadrant surgery without the need for the complex port positions and adjustments that were required for the Si platform. With its improved reach and flexibility, it can easily target both the kidney and the bladder without the need for repositioning, making it the ideal platform for a robotic nephroureterectomy. Standard transperitoneal nephrectomy port sites can be used when performing a transperitoneal nephroureterectomy using the Xi platform. The only adjustment necessary comes when switching from the kidney to the bladder when the ports can be reallocated. To achieve this, the camera will be moved from the second to the third most cranial port. The left and right arm will then be reassigned to the second and fourth most cranial ports. The robot can then be retargeted to the bladder, and the operation can proceed as normal.

Before the introduction of the Xi platform, the transperitoneal nephroureterectomy represented a significant challenge for robotic surgeons. Initial attempts to reach both the nephrectomy and bladder cuff excision sites required insertion of further port sites, robot re-docking and patient repositioning. However, with experience, several groups proposed solutions where simply reassigning the second, third and fourth arm ports could produce sufficient changes in angles of triangulation and therefore avoided re-docking and repositioning [4–7]. In essence these patterns of port placement are based on the standard Si patterns outlined above, but when switching to the bladder, the arms are swapped between ports to triangulate down towards the pelvis.

6 Docking and Theatre Layout

The docking process varies significantly based on the robotic platform used. The Si platform is less flexible and must be docked in a particular direction and angle, while the Xi platform with its rotating boom can be docked in any direction.

The Xi platform's flexibility of docking allows for a greater degree of variability when it comes to the layout of the room and alleviates concerns about impinging the anaesthetic team's access to the patient. For ease, the robot can be docked behind the patient's back out of the way of the head, as well as the assistant standing on the other side.

Since docking positions are more limited for the Si platform, one must be more careful when planning theatre layout. For transperitoneal approaches the robot will be docked just behind the patient's head, and for retroperitoneal cases, it will be docked directly above the patient's head. This can potentially impact on the access the anaesthetic team has to the patient's airway. Measures must be taken to ensure this is not significantly impaired. Similarly, care must be taken when positioning anaesthetic equipment and raising drapes at the head end as these could potentially clash with the working robotic arms.

Once plans for docking are established, the rest of the room layout can be determined. The anaesthetist will be positioned at the patient's head, ensuring a safe distance from any docked robot. The assistant is positioned in front of the patient with a camera monitor placed at a comfortable viewing angle. The scrub technician and instrument table are positioned next to the assistant at towards the patient's legs. The robot console can be positioned anywhere in the room, ideally in a position facilitating clear communication between the surgeon and the other members of the theatre team.

7 Conclusion

In this chapter we discussed the optimal patient positioning and port site placement for both transperitoneal and retroperitoneal robotic renal surgical approaches across both the Da Vinci Si and X/Xi robotic platforms. Correct positioning and port placement can facilitate entry into the surgical field and therefore successful completion of the operation. We also reviewed the complications associated with poor patient positioning, some of which can result in significant lasting patient morbidity. Familiarity with these principles, as well as the ability to adjust positioning and port placement depending on particular situations, underpins success in robotic renal surgery.

References

1. Hewson DW, Bedforth NM, Hardman JG. Peripheral nerve injury arising in anaesthesia practice. Anaesthesia. 2018;73:51–60.
2. Warner MA, Warner DO, Matsumoto JY, Harper CM, Schroeder DR, Maxson PM. Ulnar neuropathy in surgical patients. Anesthesiology. 1999 Jan;90(1):54–9.
3. Tourinho-Barbosa RR, Tobias-Machado M, Castro-Alfaro A, Ogaya-Pinies G, Cathelineau X, Sanchez-Salas R. Complications in robotic urological surgeries and how to avoid them: A systematic review. Arab J Urol [Internet]. 2018;16(3):285–92.
4. Eun D, Bhandari A, Boris R, Rogers C, Bhandari M, Menon M. Concurrent upper and lower urinary tract robotic surgery: strategies for success. BJU Int. 2007 Nov;100(5):1121–5.
5. Lee Z, Cadillo-Chavez R, Lee DI, Llukani E, Eun D. The technique of single stage pure robotic nephroureterectomy. J Endourol. 2013 Feb;27(2):189–95.
6. Badani KK, Rothberg MB, Bergman A, Silva MV, Shapiro EY, Nieder A, et al. Robot-assisted nephroureterectomy and bladder cuff excision without patient or robot repositioning: description of modified port placement and technique. J Laparoendosc Adv Surg Tech [Internet]. 2014;24(9):647–50.
7. Teo XL, Lim SK. Robot-assisted nephroureterectomy: current perspectives. Robot Surg. 2016:37–48.

Port Placement for Robotic Renal Surgery

Christophe Vaessen, Elisabeth Grobet-Jeandin, Jens-Uwe Stolzenburg, Vinodh-Kumar-Adithyaa Arthanareeswaran, and James Porter

1 Introduction

Nephrectomy was the first urological surgical procedure performed by laparoscopy in 1991 [1]. Since year 2000, the da Vinci® surgical system (Intuitive Surgical Inc., Sunnyvale, CA, USA) has revolutionized the management of renal tumors with tremendous technological advancement [2]. After two decades of experience, robot-assisted laparoscopic partial or radical nephrectomy is now part of the surgical armamentarium for the treatment of renal cancer [3] and can be considered equivalent to open surgery in terms of cancer control and preservation of renal function [4].

Under the influence of laparoscopy, the transperitoneal approach has long been the most widely used for robot-assisted kidney surgery. This approach allows to work in a space with well-known anatomical landmarks in a large space allowing to distance the trocars from each other and to avoid external robotic arm clashing [5]. However, posterior renal tumors require complete mobilization and medial rotation of the kidney [6]. The retroperitoneal approach provides direct access to the renal hilum and posterior tumors. It has been shown to decrease operative times and narcotic need and permit quicker return of bowel function [6]. Furthermore, surgical outcomes of retroperitoneal are comparable to transperitoneal approach [7]. Therefore, the retroperitoneal approach is becoming increasingly important in robot-assisted kidney surgery, particularly for posterior or lateral renal tumors. This chapter provides various configurations of port placement for renal surgery.

2 General Objectives and Rules for Port Placement

Beyond the skills of the surgeon and of his dedicated surgical team, the key to a successful robot-assisted intervention is the correct positioning of the patient and proper placement of the trocars [8]. The main objectives of a proper positioning of the trocars are as follows [9]:

- Optimize access to the target organ and to adjacent structures.
- Avoid any patients' body injury which could occur due to the bulky nature of the robot (e.g., head trauma, leg or arm compression).
- Avoid external robotic arm clashing and internal instrument collision.
- Minimize intraoperative range-of-motion limits.
- Assure easy access for the bedside assistant.
- Use the fewest ports necessary to minimize cosmetic impact.

For transperitoneal or retroperitoneal renal surgery, 8-mm da Vinci® surgical system trocars (Intuitive Surgical Inc., Sunnyvale, CA, USA) should be chosen. This bladeless trocar should be inserted respecting the upper black line which indicates the level of the skin and the lower black line which determines the level of the peritoneum (see Fig. 1). The tap of the ports must always be positioned on the side opposite to the patient to avoid skin injuries. It is suggested to place each of these trocars 8 cm apart to reduce conflict between arms or instruments.

C. Vaessen (✉)
Sorbonne University, GRC 5, Predictive Onco-Urology, APHP, Pitié-Salpêtrière Hôpital, Urology, Paris, France

E. Grobet-Jeandin
Sorbonne University, GRC 5, Predictive Onco-Urology, APHP, Pitié-Salpêtrière Hôpital, Urology, Paris, France

Division of Urology, Geneva University Hospitals, Geneva, Switzerland

J.-U. Stolzenburg · V.-K.-A. Arthanareeswaran
Department of Urology, University of Leipzig, Leipzig, Germany

J. Porter
Swedish Urology Group, Seattle, WA, USA

P. Wiklund et al. (eds.), *Robotic Urologic Surgery*, https://doi.org/10.1007/978-3-031-00363-9_37

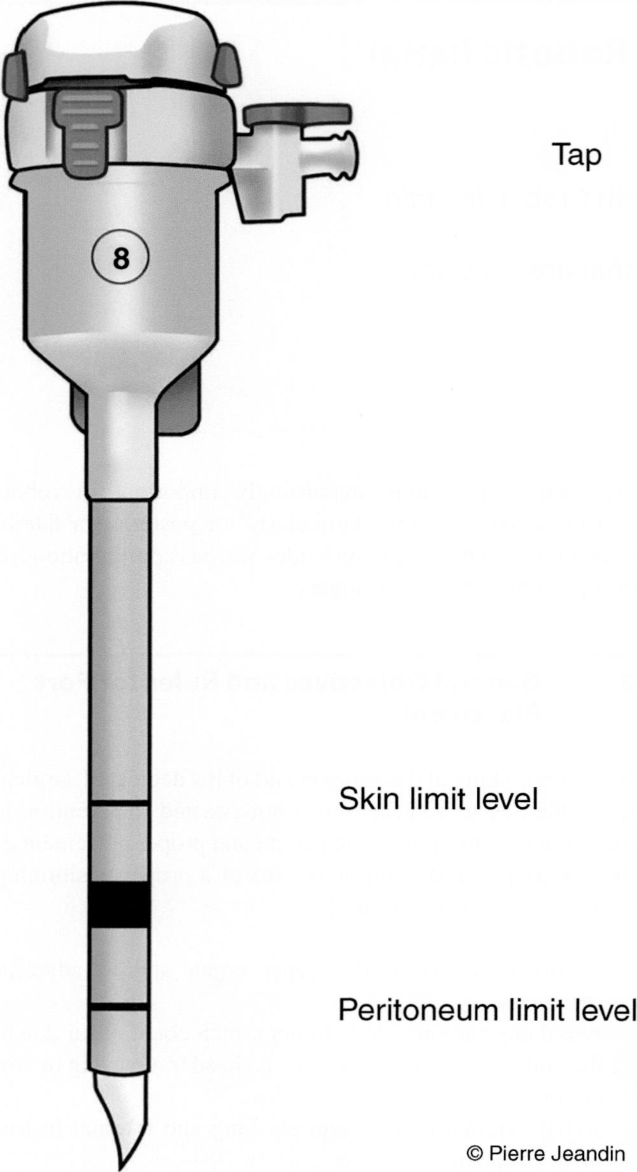

Fig. 1 da Vinci Xi 8-mm bladeless optical obturator (standard)

3 Port Placement for Transperitoneal Robotic Partial Nephrectomy

J. Stolzenburg and V. Arthanareeswaran

Although there are different possibilities, we describe the trocar placement that we use in our department [10–16].

3.1 Step 1: Patient Positioning

The induction of anesthesia is performed in supine position. A urinary catheter is inserted. The patient is now turned to the lateral position, and the urinary bag is placed either at the top or bottom end of the bed for access by the anesthetist. The legs are separated and protected with either pillows or a specially designed foam or rubber device between them. This relieves any weight on pressure points. All other bony points, including shoulders and hips, are protected by the rubber or foam mat. The head and neck are supported with either pillows or a rubber head ring in order to maintain them in a neutral position.

3.2 Step 2: Flexion of the Table

A patient with right-sided renal tumor is positioned in the left lateral position at an angle of 110° to the horizontal. The table is flexed at the level of the umbilicus by approximately 10–15° (Fig. 2). The patient is positioned on the table toward the edge of the table facing the surgeons. This prevents interference of the robotic instruments with the table during the procedure. The patient's arms are slightly flexed at the elbow, and the arm boards are positioned approximately 90–110° toward the head. The arm above should be positioned as low as possible. They are both supported appropriately with arm rests, and all bony and nerve pressure points are well padded. The arms are secured in the rests with Velcro strapping, leaving both forearms and antecubital fossae available to the

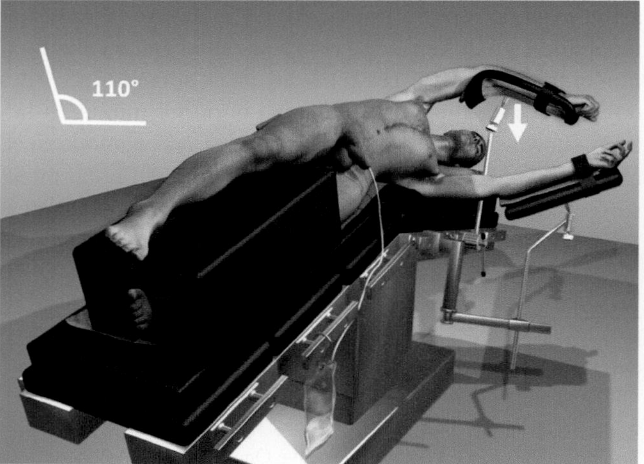

Fig. 2 Patient positioning

anesthetist at all stages. Both the anesthetist and the surgeon should finally check the position of the arms together to make sure that there is no interference with instrument movements during the procedure.

3.3 Step 3: Fixation of the Patient

The patient's thoracic and lumbar areas are supported in the lateral position with table attachments which are well padded and which must be securely fixed to the table because the patient is rotated posteriorly. The patient is firmly supported with Velcro tapes across both forearms and secured with a wide-diameter belt at the level of the pelvis. A blanket is used to cover the patient to assist maintenance of body temperature. It must also be noted that sequential compressing stockings should be fitted to all patients prior to surgery.

3.4 Step 4: Marking the Anatomical Landmarks

The trocar placements are done using a number of imaginary lines guided by anatomical landmarks on the patient. For transperitoneal access, the most important lines are midline, para-rectal line, mid-clavicular line, anterior axillary line, midaxillary line, and posterior axillary line (Fig. 3a). These anatomical landmarks are bounded by the subcostal margin superiorly and the iliac crest inferiorly.

3.5 Step 5: Marking "Imaginary" Vertical Lines

Next a vertical line is marked at the level of the umbilicus that is perpendicular to the direction of the operating kidney and da Vinci instrument. Two lines are drawn on either side, parallel to this vertical line, so that the distance between each is 6 to 8 cm.

3.6 Step 6: da Vinci X and Xi Port Placement

The port placement in da Vinci X and Xi robotic platform is in a linear fashion as shown in Fig. 3b, c. The four da Vinci trocars are usually placed in the intersection of the vertical lines and the mid-clavicular line. This can vary between the para-rectal line and the anterior axillary line based on the patient size (more laterally in obese/larger patient and medially in slim/smaller patient). A 12-cm assistant port is placed as shown in Fig. 3a at the level of para-rectal line. Some groups prefer to place this port at the same line but cranially to the umbilicus. We prefer to place the Alexis port (green) at this position which allows easy removal of the specimen for frozen section or faster specimen removal.

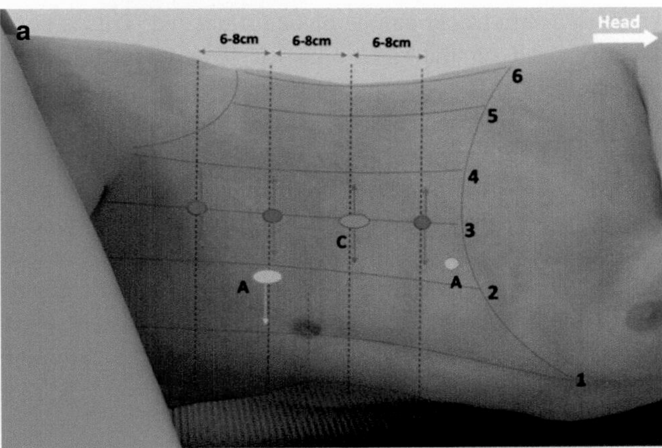

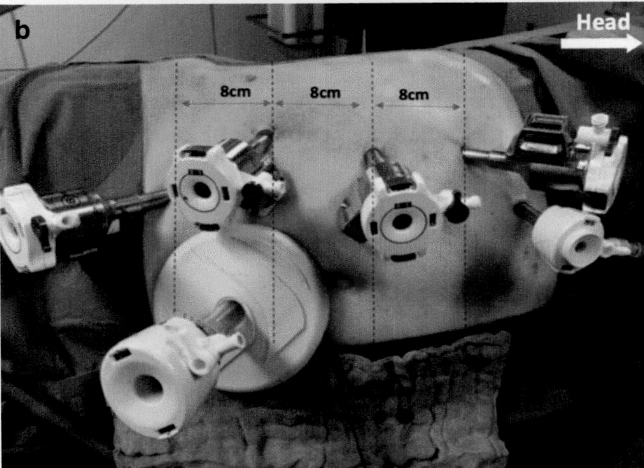

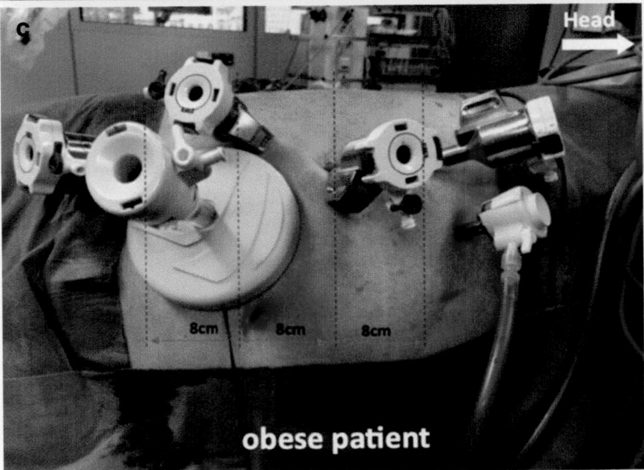

Fig. 3 (**a**) da Vinci Xi trocar placement in the right side: 1 = midline, 2 = para-rectal line, 3 = mid-clavicular line, 4 = anterior axillary line, 5 = midaxillary line, and 6 = posterior axillary line. A, 5-mm assistant trocar predominantly for liver retraction on the right side; C, camera trocar. (**b**) Thin patient with Alexis assistant port with 12-mm assistant trocar in the midline. (**c**) Obese patient with Alexis assistant port in paramedian position

An extra 5-mm trocar can be placed if needed. This is consistently used on the right side for liver retraction. The placement of this additional 5-mm assisting port depends on the surgeon's preference and tumor complexity. In patients who are relatively thin and short, the 12-cm assistant trocar or Alexis port can be placed in the midline (Fig. 3b). All ports (apart from the first port) are placed under direct visual control. We normally use a 30° camera facing downward, which can be easily rotated upward to visualize the ventral structures. A 0° optic can also be used depending on the preference of the surgeon and location of the tumor.

3.7 Step 6: (b) da Vinci Si Port Placement

The port placement in da Vinci Si is different compared to Xi as shown in Fig. 4. The camera trocar is placed at the lever of intersection of the third vertical line and the para-rectal line as it is done if the da Vinci Xi is used. The da Vinci trocars for da Vinci Si are placed in a triangular fashion as shown in Fig. 4 to avoid collision of the da Vinci arms and instruments. A 12-cm assistant port is placed on the intersection of the second vertical line and para-rectal line. This trocar is used for the insertion of large-bore instruments such as staplers, clip applicators, and endobags. Alternatively, an Alexis port can be additionally used as described previously. Care should be taken to minimize collision between the robotic and assistant's instruments. For right-sided surgery, an additional 5-mm trocar is often used under the xiphoid for liver retraction and facilitating upper pole exposure. The robotic working trocars should be carefully inserted under direct visual control (like always!) to avoid collision between the robotic arms.

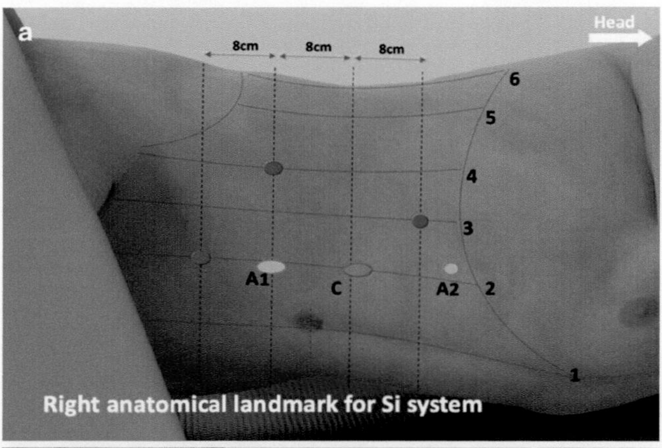

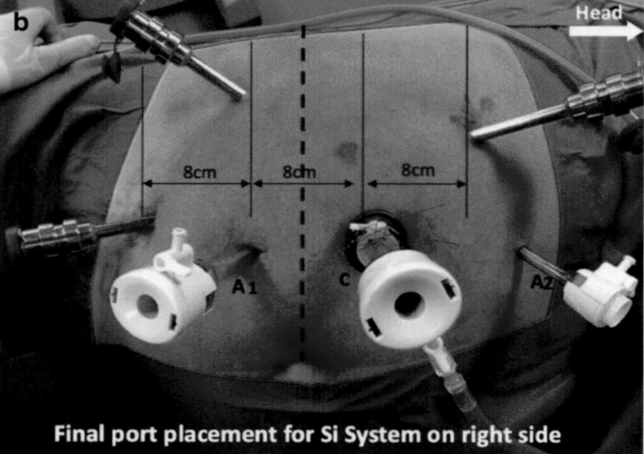

Fig. 4 daVinci Si trocar placement. Right side: 1 = midline, 2 = pararectal line, 3 = mid-clavicular line, 4 = anterior axillary line, 5 = midaxillary line, and 6 = posterior axillary line. A1, assistant trocar; A2, assistant trocar for liver retraction on right side; C, camera trocar

4 Port Placement for Retroperitoneal Robotic Partial Nephrectomy

J. Porter

The early experience with robotic renal surgery was an extension of laparoscopic surgery, and, therefore, most procedures were performed via the transperitoneal approach. Given that the robotic arms were quite large, the increased space afforded by the transperitoneal approach allowed for adequate range of motion of the robotic arms and decreased external conflict. This leads to the transperitoneal approach becoming the standard technique for robotic nephron-sparing surgery (NSS). However, posterior renal masses can be difficult to remove using the transperitoneal technique and are more directly accessed with the retroperitoneal approach. The application of the robot to the retroperitoneal space for renal surgery has gained in popularity, and the technique has become standardized and reproduced by several groups [5, 17]. As the technique to gain access to the retroperitoneum has become more standardized, concerns regarding space limitations and disorientation are no longer barriers to adoption [18–29].

4.1 Positioning

For the retroperitoneal approach, patients are placed in a complete, full flank position to facilitate access and increase the space between the 12th rib and iliac crest. A gel roll is used as the axillary support, and the arms are extended 90 degrees with the lower arm resting on an arm rest. Pillows are placed between the arms and legs with tape securing them from moving. Prior to flexing the bed, the position of the patient is then checked ensuring that the patient is in full flank and the shoulder and hip are inline. The bed is then maximally flexed without raising the kidney rest. The patient is then secured to the table with wide adhesive tape (Fig. 5).

4.2 Access

The iliac crest, 11th rib, and 12th rib are marked out. An incision is made just above the iliac crest directly in the midaxillary line (Fig. 6). Tissues are divided with cautery until the external oblique fascia is reached. This is incised, and finger dissection is utilized to bluntly gain access into the retroperitoneum. A 10-mm kidney-shaped balloon dilator (Fig. 7) is inserted into the space and inflated under direct vision using a 10-mm laparoscope or the robotic endoscope with a 30-degree lens. Ideally, the balloon is placed between the posterior body wall and the kidney which is still surrounded by Gerota's fascia.

As the balloon inflates, the kidney will be pushed anteriorly if the balloon has been placed properly. The psoas muscle will become visible along with the gonadal vessels, the ureter, and the edge of the peritoneum as it is mobilized off of the transversus abdominis muscle anteriorly. The other key landmark is the posterior layer of Gerota's fascia, which will be pushed off the psoas muscle by the balloon dilator. After the balloon has been fully inflated, it is removed, and a camera port is inserted through the midaxillary incision. For the da Vinci Si, a 12-mm Hasson balloon port is used for the robotic endoscope, and for the da Vinci Xi, the 8-mm port through a Hasson cone (Fig. 8).

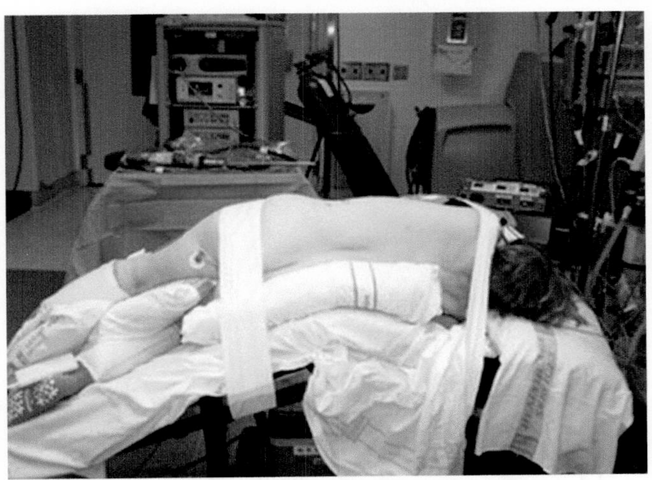

Fig. 5 Patient positioning

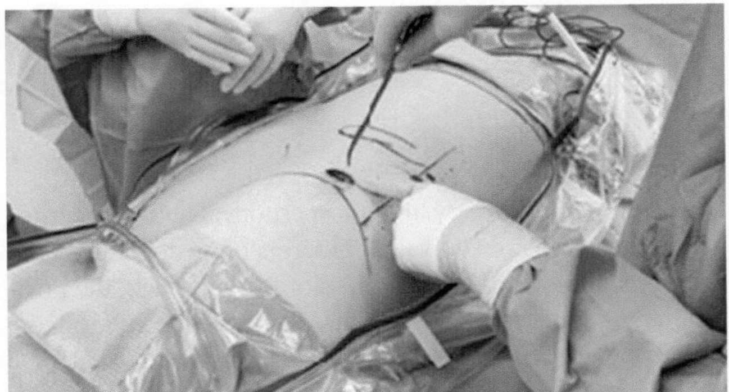

Fig. 6 First trocar incision

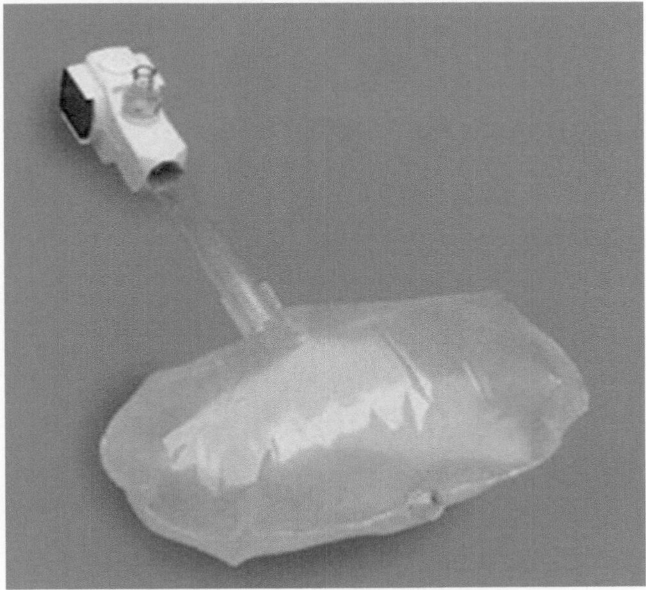

Fig. 7 Balloon dilator

4.3 Port Placement

For the da Vinci Si system, three robotic ports are placed in a "V" configuration with the point of the V being the camera port (Fig. 9). The camera port is placed in the midaxillary line 1 to 2 cm above the iliac crest. The posterior port is placed 7 to 8 cm from the camera port and just below the 12th rib in the posterior axillary line. The anterior port is placed 7 to 8 cm from the camera in the anterior axillary line. The assistant port is placed near the anterior superior iliac spine and is 8 cm inferior to the anterior port.

For the da Vinci Xi, we use four robotic ports with the addition of a fourth arm port for retraction (Fig. 10). After placing the camera port and posterior port in the posterior axillary line, a blunt laparoscopic instrument is passed through the posterior port to gently push the peritoneal reflection off of the transversus abdominis muscle to create more space anteriorly for the two additional robotic ports and the 12-mm assistant port. This dissection is best done using the 30-degree up lens, and care is taken to avoid inad-

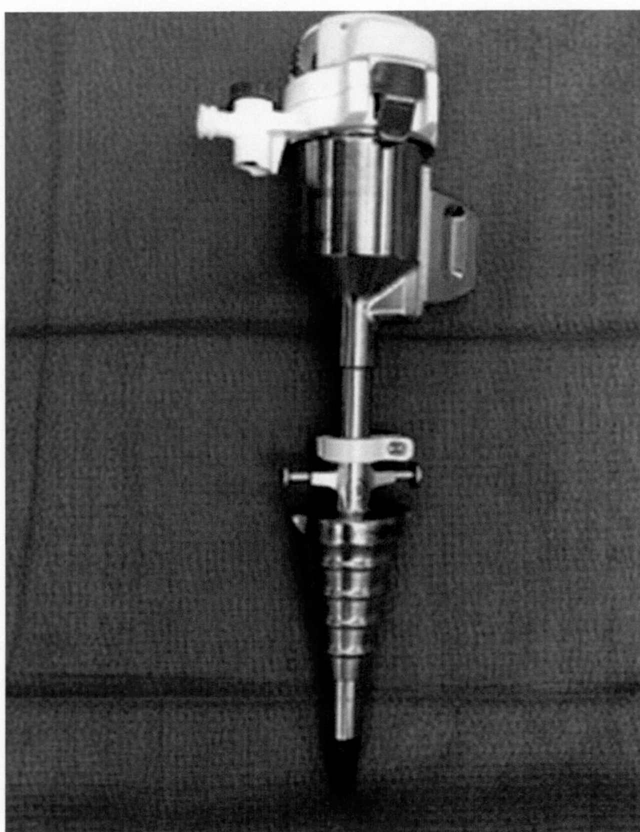

Fig. 8 Hasson cone

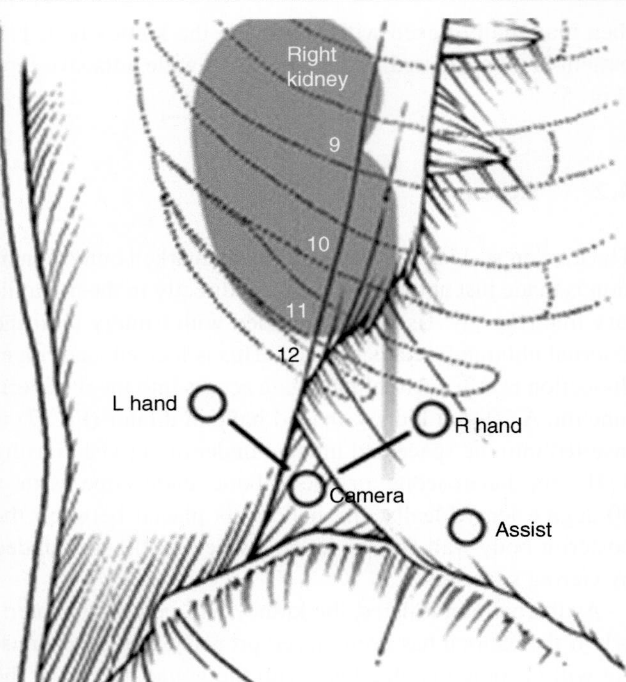

Fig. 9 da Vinci Si port positioning

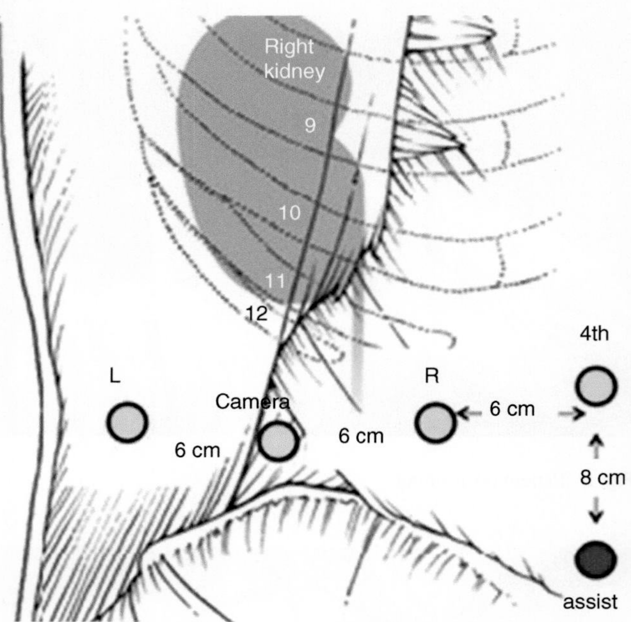

Fig. 10 da Vinci Xi port positioning

vertent entry into the peritoneum during mobilization. The ports are placed in an arc configuration with the distance between ports being 5–6 cm. The 12-mm assistant port is usually a valveless high-flow insufflation port such as the AirSeal device (CONMED) and is placed near the anterior superior iliac spine and is 8 cm inferior to the anterior port.

4.4 Docking

Using the da Vinci Si, the robot is docked directly over the patient's head parallel to the spine.

Using the da Vinci Xi with a rotating boom, the robot can be brought in at several different locations and the tower rotated to align with the trocars. We routinely dock posteriorly over the hip at a 45-degree angle.

5 Conclusion

Proper positioning of the trocars is a key to success in renal robot-assisted surgery. A good port placement allows an optimized access to the kidney and the tumor, avoids patient's injury, and minimizes intraoperative range-of-motion limits. For renal robotic surgery, the transperitoneal and retroperitoneal approach seem equivalent in terms of postoperative and oncological outcomes. Regardless of the approach, the positioning of the trocars for kidney surgery depends on the robotic device (Si, X, or Xi da Vinci® surgical system), the patient's morphology, the location of the tumor, and the preferences of the surgeon.

References

1. Clayman RV, Kavoussi LR, Soper NJ, Dierks SM, Merety KS, Darcy MD, et al. Laparoscopic nephrectomy. N Engl J Med. 1991;324(19):1370–1.
2. Kallingal GJS, Swain S, Darwiche F, Punnen S, Manoharan M, Gonzalgo ML, et al. Robotic partial nephrectomy with the Da Vinci Xi. Adv Urol. 2016;2016:9675095.
3. Mikhail D, Sarcona J, Mekhail M, Richstone L. Urologic robotic surgery. Surg Clin N Am. 2020;100(2):361–78.
4. Durand X, Molimard B, Bayoud Y. Néphrectomie partielle par voie laparoscopique robot-assistée transpéritonéale. EMC – Techniques chirurgicales – Urologie. 2014;7(4):1–5.
5. Mittakanti HR, Heulitt G, Li H-F, Porter JR. Transperitoneal vs. retroperitoneal robotic partial nephrectomy: a matched-paired analysis. World J Urol. 2020;38(5):1093–9.
6. Patel M, Porter J. Robotic retroperitoneal partial nephrectomy. World J Urol. 2013;31(6):1377–82.
7. M P, J P. Robotic retroperitoneal surgery: a contemporary review. Current opinion in urology [Internet]. janv 2013 [cité 18 juin 2021];23(1). Disponible sur: https://pubmed.ncbi.nlm.nih.gov/23159992/
8. Hemal AK, Goldberg H. NARUS 2019: port placement principles for Xi and Si robots. 3rd Annual North American Robotic Urology Symposium (NARUS). 2019.
9. Pathak RA, Patel M, Hemal AK. Comprehensive approach to port placement templates for robot-assisted laparoscopic urologic surgeries. J Endourol. 2017;31(12):1269–76.
10. Ljungberg B, Hanbury DC, Kuczyk MA, Merseburger AS, Mulders PFA, Patard J-J, et al. Renal cell carcinoma guideline. Eur Urol. 2007;51(6):1502–10.
11. Aron M, Gill IS. Minimally invasive nephron-sparing surgery (MINSS) for renal tumours part I: laparoscopic partial nephrectomy. Eur Urol 2007;51(2):337–46; discussion 46–47.
12. Singh I. Robot-assisted laparoscopic partial nephrectomy: current review of the technique and literature. J Minim Access Surg. 2009;5(4):87–92.
13. Atalla MA, Dovey Z, Kavoussi LR. Laparoscopic versus robotic pyeloplasty: man versus machine. Expert Rev Med Devices. 2010;7(1):27–34.
14. Casale P, Lughezzani G, Buffi N, Larcher A, Porter J, Mottrie A, et al. Evolution of robot-assisted partial nephrectomy: techniques and outcomes from the transatlantic robotic nephron-sparing surgery study group. Eur Urol. 2019;76(2):222–7.
15. Stolzenburg J-U, Türk IA, Liatsikos EN, éditeurs. Laparoscopic and robot-assisted surgery in urology: Atlas of standard procedures. Berlin: Springer; 2011.
16. Benway BM, Bhayani SB, Rogers CG, Porter JR, Buffi NM, Figenshau RS, et al. Robot-assisted partial nephrectomy: an international experience. Eur Urol. 2010;57(5):815–20.
17. Sammon JD, Karakiewicz PI, Sun M, Ravi P, Ghani KR, Jeong W, et al. Robot-assisted vs. laparoscopic partial nephrectomy: utilization rates and perioperative outcomes. Int Braz J Urol. 2013;39(3):377–86.
18. Wright JL, Porter JR. Laparoscopic partial nephrectomy: comparison of transperitoneal and retroperitoneal approaches. J Urol. 2005;174(3):841–5.
19. Hu JC, Treat E, Filson CP, McLaren I, Xiong S, Stepanian S, et al. Technique and outcomes of robot-assisted retroperitoneoscopic partial nephrectomy: a multicenter study. Eur Urol. 2014;66(3):542–9.
20. Xia L, Zhang X, Wang X, Xu T, Qin L, Zhang X, et al. Transperitoneal versus retroperitoneal robot-assisted partial nephrectomy: a systematic review and meta-analysis. Int J Surg. 2016;30:109–15.
21. Kim EH, Larson JA, Potretzke AM, Hulsey NK, Bhayani SB, Figenshau RS. Retroperitoneal robot-assisted partial nephrectomy for posterior renal masses is associated with earlier hospital discharge: a single-institution retrospective comparison. J Endourol. 2015;29(10):1137–42.
22. Choo SH, Lee SY, Sung HH, Jeon HG, Jeong BC, Jeon SS, et al. Transperitoneal versus retroperitoneal robotic partial nephrectomy: matched-pair comparisons by nephrometry scores. World J Urol. 2014;32(6):1523–9.
23. Hughes-Hallett A, Patki P, Patel N, Barber NJ, Sullivan M, Thilagarajah R. Robot-assisted partial nephrectomy: a comparison of the transperitoneal and retroperitoneal approaches. J Endourol. 2013;27(7):869–74.
24. Maurice MJ, Kaouk JH, Ramirez D, Bhayani SB, Allaf ME, Rogers CG, et al. Robotic partial nephrectomy for posterior tumors through a retroperitoneal approach offers decreased length of stay compared with the transperitoneal approach: a propensity-matched analysis. J Endourol. 2017;31(2):158–62.
25. Tanaka K, Shigemura K, Furukawa J, Ishimura T, Muramaki M, Miyake H, et al. Comparison of the transperitoneal and retroperitoneal approach in robot-assisted partial nephrectomy in an initial case series in Japan. J Endourol. 2013;27(11):1384–8.
26. Huang WC, Levey AS, Serio AM, Snyder M, Vickers AJ, Raj GV, et al. Chronic kidney disease after nephrectomy in patients with renal cortical tumours: a retrospective cohort study. Lancet Oncol. 2006;7(9):735–40.
27. Kim SP, Murad MH, Thompson RH, Boorjian SA, Weight CJ, Han LC, et al. Comparative effectiveness for survival and renal function of partial and radical nephrectomy for localized renal tumors: a systematic review and meta-analysis. J Urol. 2012.
28. Fan X, Xu K, Lin T, Liu H, Yin Z, Dong W, et al. Comparison of transperitoneal and retroperitoneal laparoscopic nephrectomy for renal cell carcinoma: a systematic review and meta-analysis. BJU Int. 2013;111(4):611–21.
29. Xia L, Talwar R, Taylor BL, Shin MH, Berger IB, Sperling CD, et al. National trends and disparities of minimally invasive surgery for localized renal cancer, 2010 to 2015. Urol Oncol. 2019;37(3):182.e17–27.

Early Unclamping, Selective, Superselective, and Unclamped Robotic Partial Nephrectomy

Andrew B. Chen, Giovanni E. Cacciamani, and Mihir M. Desai

1 Introduction

Kidney cancer is the third most common urologic malignancy, of which the vast majority are renal cell carcinoma [1]. The increase in access to axial imaging has been associated with a similar increase in the diagnosis of clinically localized small renal masses [2, 3]. Partial nephrectomy (PN) is considered the prioritized management of the majority of T1a and select T1b renal tumors when intervention is indicated with favorable oncologic outcomes and minimization of the risk of chronic kidney disease (CKD) or CKD progression [4]. Over the past two decades, there has been a rapid uptake of minimally invasive approaches such as laparoscopic and robotic approaches to performing PN. The advent of robotic surgery has led to improvements in perioperative outcomes with lower conversion rate to radical nephrectomy, shorter length of hospital stay, and shorter warm ischemia time (WIT) when comparing the robotic approach to the laparoscopic approach [5].

Main renal artery clamping remains the most common technique of vascular control during PN, allowing for tumor resection and reconstruction of the renal remnant in a bloodless field, and it comes at the cost of variable warm ischemia. The adverse impact of warm ischemic clamping is controversial and as such beyond the scope of this writing [6]. Overall, the goal of partial nephrectomy is to achieve an oncologically complete tumor resection with the minimum impact on renal function while avoiding complications. This principle would inherently require the ischemic clamping and amount of normal parenchyma excised to be the minimum. Various techniques have evolved to minimize ischemia time from main artery clamping as well as the impact of global renal ischemia including early unclamping, selective clamping, superselective clamping, and unclamped partial nephrectomy.

2 Terminology

There is a lack of standardized terminology to define the various techniques that employ less than global renal ischemia during PN.

2.1 Selective Clamping

This technique is defined as isolation and clamping of a single or multiple first-order segmental renal artery branches that cover the tumor. While selective clamping avoids global renal ischemia, there is typically a variable amount of collateral ischemia to the renal remnant.

2.2 Superselective Clamping

This refers to further renal vascular microdissection within the renal sinus with clamping of tertiary or higher-order arterial branches [7]. Only tumoral/peritumoral blood flow is eliminated by anatomic microdissection and tumor-specific devascularization [8]. Additionally, the access to higher-order tumor-specific branches may also require radial nephrotomies at the renal sinus margin.

2.3 Unclamped Partial Nephrectomy

Unclamped partial nephrectomy refers to no vascular control and performing either a minimum margin tumor excision (also referred to as enucleo-resection) or an actual enucleation staying on the tumor pseudocapsule. It must be mentioned that the latter does generate concerns about oncologic adequacy and has not been universally embraced outside a few centers.

A. B. Chen · G. E. Cacciamani · M. M. Desai (✉)
USC Institute of Urology, Los Angeles, CA, USA

P. Wiklund et al. (eds.), *Robotic Urologic Surgery*, https://doi.org/10.1007/978-3-031-00363-9_38

2.4 Zero-ischemia

At our institution, zero-ischemia refers to superselective clamping that provides tumor-specific devascularization or elimination of all vascular clamping and tumor excision with a minimal margin adjacent to the tumor capsular edge [9]. Essentially, we have used this term to refer to elimination of collateral ischemia, and the technical nuances are detailed in this chapter.

3 Patient Selection

Patient selection is critical for performing zero-ischemia partial nephrectomy. Tumor factors predominantly dictate the feasibility and safety of achieving tumor-specific devascularization or minimal margin enucleo-resection. Typically hilar and polar tumors have a predictable vascular supply that is easy to identify and control during resection and are ideal for this technique (Fig. 1). In contrast, broad-based lateral tumors have multiple sources of vascularity and a broad-based attachment to the renal parenchyma that entails a more difficult resection with a higher blood loss (Fig. 2). Tumor contact surface area (CSA) is an important measure of the degree of attachment of the tumor to the renal parenchyma, and a greater CSA may be a clinically important measure to assess safety of performing unclamped partial nephrectomy [10]. Radiographic assessment of the "stickiness" of the peri-nephric fat is also an important factor that influences the ease of intra-hilar dissection as patients with unfavorable fat may not be suitable for zero-ischemia partial nephrectomy. Finally, one must always balance the technical feasibility of performing superselective clamping or unclamped partial nephrectomy with the need for nephron sparing. Patients with normal baseline renal function should only be offered these techniques if tumor factors are highly favorable.

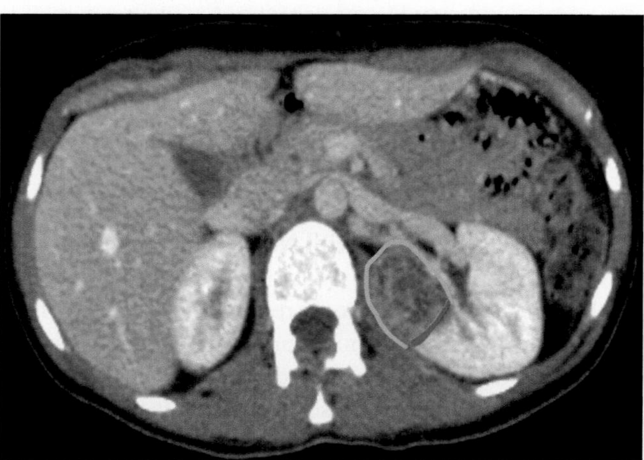

Fig. 1 CT image of favorable tumor for zero-ischemia PN. The tumor is hilar, and the majority of the circumference abuts the peri-nephric fat or hilar fat and structures (green line), while only a small portion is attached to the renal parenchyma (red line)

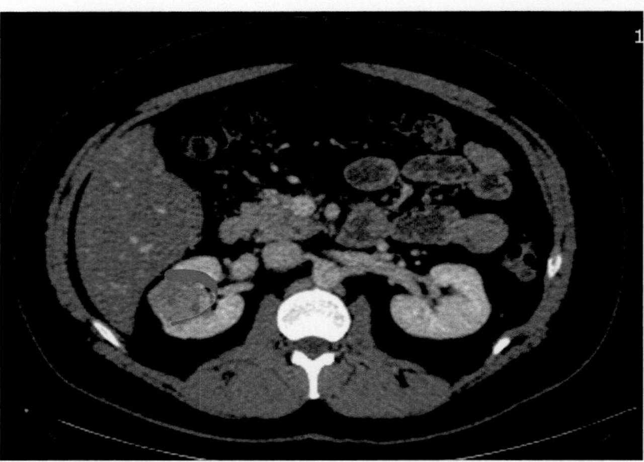

Fig. 2 CT image of unfavorable tumor for zero-ischemia PN. This tumor has a broad attachment to the parenchyma (red line) and an unpredictable vascular supply

4 Preoperative Imaging

Precise evaluation of renal vasculature and tumor anatomy is essential to performing zero-ischemia partial nephrectomy. To this end, we perform multi-phasic CT of the kidneys with 0.5 mm thickness to assess tertiary and quaternary branches of renal vasculature as well as measure the contact surface area of the tumor to renal parenchyma [10] (Fig. 3). While detailed 3D model rendering can be performed by most radiologists, easy-to-use commercial applications are now developed that provide the surgeon with detailed views of the tumor and relationship with renal vasculature and collection system anatomy [11].

5 Surgical Technique

Preoperative preparation: At our institution, enhanced recovery after surgery (ERAS) protocols is employed. Patients also receive a combination of oral non-narcotic pain medications including gabapentin, acetaminophen, and celecoxib, with dose adjustments made for age or comorbidities. A broad-spectrum antibiotic (first-generation cephalosporin) is administered intravenously as well. In addition to sequential compression devices (SCDs), patients will receive 5000 units of subcutaneous heparin upon induction of anesthesia. An orogastric tube is placed intraoperatively and removed at the conclusion of the procedure.

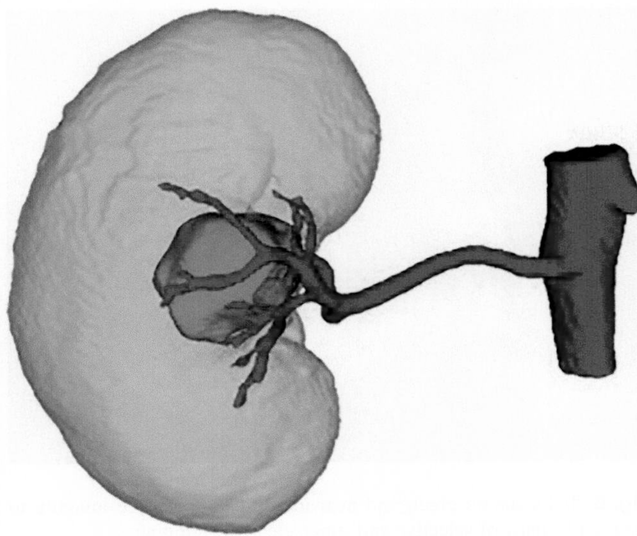

Fig. 3 Preoperative 3D modeling using thin-slice CT imaging to help identify tumor and vascular anatomy. Thin-slice (0.5 mm) multi-phase CT with segmentation and reconstruction provides the essential roadmap for tumor resection during superselective clamping

6 Patient Positioning and Trocar Placement

The patient is positioned in a 60-degree flank position. A warming blanket is applied to the upper body just above the rib line. An alcohol-based prep is used to prep the entirety of the abdomen. Initial access into the abdominal cavity is obtained in the lower lateral quadrant. Pneumoperitoneum is established to a pressure of 15 mmHg. The ports are then placed in a five- to six-port configuration with four 8-mm ports, which include the left and right arm, camera, and fourth arm. Bipolar fenestrated forceps are placed in the left arm. A monopolar scissors is placed in the right, and Prograsp forceps are used for the fourth arm. The 12-mm AirSeal continuous insufflation port is placed between the camera and the caudal arm, and a 5-mm subxiphoid port is placed for liver retraction if the mass is in the right kidney. If necessary, another 5-mm assistant port can be triangulated between the cephalad arm and the camera. The da Vinci Xi Surgical System (Intuitive Surgical) is then brought in and docked in the usual fashion.

7 Hilar Dissection

Gerota's fascia of the kidney is exposed by medializing the colon. The duodenum is Kocherized if working on the right kidney, and mobilization of the spleen is performed if working on the left. We then mobilize the ureter and gonadal vein laterally off the psoas muscle and trace these structures cephalad to identify the main renal artery and vein. We recommend renal hilar dissection in all patients where superselective clamping or unclamped partial nephrectomy is being considered. This provides a safety net in case of excessive bleeding during the procedure. It is important to perform the least amount of hilar dissection to perform expeditious and safe clamping.

8 Kidney Mobilization

The location of the tumor determines the amount of kidney mobilization required. Anterior hilar tumors in the interpolar and lower pole locations require minimal mobilization. However, a 180-degree rotation of the kidney may be necessary for posterior hilar lesions, thus requiring significant kidney mobilization including upper pole dissection of the kidney from the adrenal gland.

9 Color Doppler Ultrasound

Once the mass is localized, a drop-in US probe is placed through the 12-mm AirSeal and used to delineate the margins of the tumor. We then score the proposed parenchymal margins with electrocautery.

10 Selective and Superselective Clamping

Once parenchymal margins of resection of the hilar or polar tumor are scored, dissection proceeds toward the section of the renal sinus enclosed in the proposed area of resection. Segmental arteries and veins are identified and mobilized inside the renal sinus. Based on the preoperative knowledge of the tumor vascularity, the tertiary and quaternary branches are identified. Branches that are thought to be directly supplying the tumor are clipped and divided. The robotic Hem-o-lok applicator is particularly useful as the Endowrist provides optimal angles in securing these third- and fourth-level branches inside the renal sinus. Branches that are supplying the immediate peritumoral parenchyma are temporarily occluded using micro-bulldog clamps (Fig. 4). Several techniques can be employed to assess the adequacy of peritumor vascular control during selective and superselective clamping. Color Doppler may be helpful in assessing the immediate tumor and peritumor vascularity but requires significant surgeon experience with this technique (Fig. 5). A more rapid and easy-to-determine method is the use of indocyanine green and visualization using near-infrared imaging

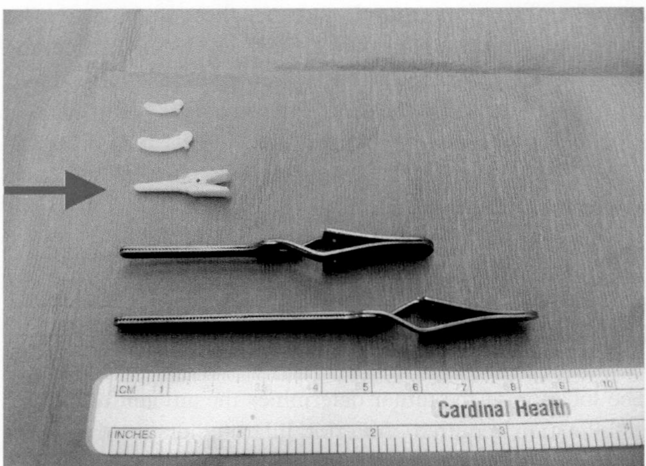

Fig. 4 Photograph of micro-bulldog clamp used during superselective clamping

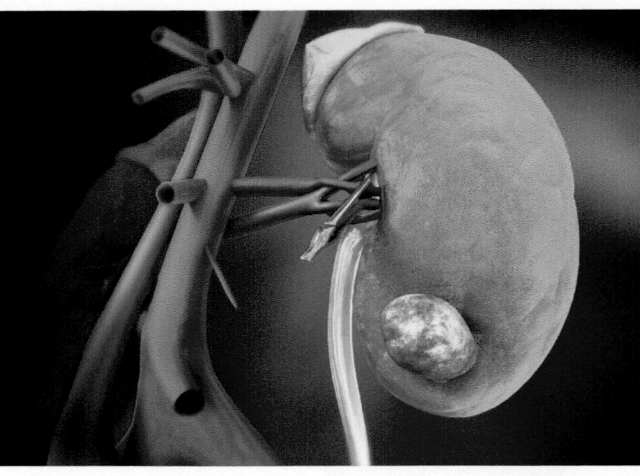

Fig. 6 Indocyanine green and near-infrared fluorescence imaging to assess adequacy of selective and superselective clamping

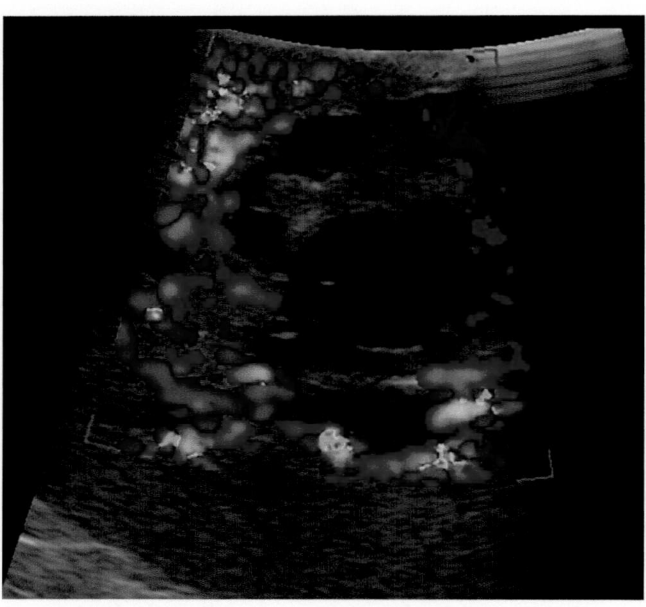

Fig. 5 Color Doppler to assess peritumor vascularity during superselective clamping. The series of photographs shows a progressive reduction in peritumor vascularity with superselective occlusion of sub-segmental vessels

(Fig. 6). Once the renal sinus dissection is complete, the portion of the tumor circumference within the renal sinus would have already been mobilized, and the remaining part attached to the parenchyma is carefully separated keeping a minimum margin similar to the completely unclamped technique described below. Vascular supply encountered during this phase can be cauterized or suture ligated using 4–0 polyglactin 910 figure-of-8 sutures.

11 Unclamped Partial Nephrectomy: Minimal Margin Resection or Enucleo-resection

A nephrotomy is created along the scored margins with monopolar robotic shears. The incision is then deepened circumferentially to prevent over-dissection in one location. This is best achieved by gradual opening of the blunt-tipped fenestrated grasper to split the renal parenchyma with occasional strategic use of electrocautery for parenchymal/cortical vessels. The cortical incision is taken all the way to the renal sinus fat. The tumor should be carefully retracted away from the PN bed to facilitate dissection. Throughout this dissection, the bedside assistant will provide critical visualization through suction and transient compression of specific bleeding vessels. Once the central sinus is reached, intra-renal vessels supplying the tumor can be isolated and taken with Hem-o-lok clips or sutures. Thus, the tumor is then excised using a combination of cold cutting and monopolar.

12 Hemostasis and Kidney Reconstruction

The majority of hemostasis is performed during the tumor enucleo-resection. After resection of tumor, any collecting system injury is closed with 3–0 polyglactin 910 sutures on an SH-1 needle. Any bleeders in the resection bed are sutured with point-specific 3-0 polyglactin 910 sutures on an SH-1 needle with care to avoid incorporation of hilar vessels and the pelvi-calyceal system. The parenchymal edge is repaired with a pledgeted CTX 1 or CT-1 number 1 polyglactin 910 suture. After thorough inspection of hemostasis, biological hemostatic agent is layered on the resection bed and covered with a sheet of Surgicel. Gerota's fascia is reconstructed to cover the PN defect.

13 Early Unclamping

Early unclamping refers to the technique of PN performed under full hilar clamping where the vascular occlusion clamps are removed after the inner medullary closure but prior to any capsular renorrhaphy. The primary objective of early unclamping is not reduction of ischemia time but rather the ability to identify and suture any bleeding vessel missed by the inner medullary suture. Subsequently, capsular renorrhaphy may or may not be necessary based on the surgeon assessment of the security of closure.

14 Extraction of the Specimen and Closure of Port Sites

A Blake drain is placed in the peri-nephric space through one of the robotic ports and secured to the skin. The tumor is placed in an EndoCatch bag and extracted via the assistant port site. The fascia of all port sites larger than 8 mm is closed using the Carter-Thomason port closure system and number 1 polyglactin 910 sutures. The skin is then closed with 4–0 poliglecaprone 25 sutures, and Dermabond is applied. We extract and bivalve the inked specimen to confirm grossly negative margins before completing laparoscopic exit and final closure.

15 Post-Operative Care

The patient is then extubated at the conclusion of the procedure, and the orogastric tube is removed. Post-operative ERAS protocols are followed which include several non-narcotic analgesic medications, gastrointestinal and DVT prophylaxis, early clear liquid diet, and early ambulation. Body fluid analysis of creatinine from drain fluid is performed during hospitalization.

16 Outcomes of Superselective and Unclamped PN

A comprehensive meta-analysis of various hilar control techniques demonstrated that while the off-clamp group had higher estimated blood loss (WMD = 47.83, $p < 0.001$), renal function outcomes were superior in regard to short-term absolute eGFR (WMD = 16.05, $p = 0.06$), short-term percentage change in eGFR (WMD = 7.02, $p < 0.001$), long-term absolute eGFR (WMD = 6.59, $p = 0.02$), and long-term percentage change in eGFR (WMD = 4.09, $p = 0.005$). Both groups were similar in regard to transfusion rates, open conversion rates, hospital stay, positive margin rates, and post-operative complications [12].

References

1. Siegel RL, Miller KD, Fuchs HE, Jemal A. Cancer statistics, 2021. CA Cancer J Clin. 2021;71(1):7–33.
2. Mathew A, Devesa S, Fraumeni J Jr, Chow W. Global increases in kidney cancer incidence, 1973–1992. Eur J Cancer Prev. 2002;11(2):171–8.
3. Nguyen MM, Gill IS, Ellison LM. The evolving presentation of renal carcinoma in the United States: trends from the surveillance, epidemiology, and end results program. J Urol. 2006;176(6):2397–400.
4. Campbell SC, Clark PE, Chang SS, Karam JA, Souter L, Uzzo RG. Renal mass and localized renal cancer: evaluation, management, and follow-up: AUA guideline part I. J Urol. 2021:https://doi.org/10.1097/JU.0000000000001911.
5. Choi JE, You JH, Kim DK, Rha KH, Lee SH. Comparison of perioperative outcomes between robotic and laparoscopic partial nephrectomy: a systematic review and meta-analysis. Eur Urol. 2015;67(5):891–901.
6. Thompson RH, Lane BR, Lohse CM, et al. Every minute counts when the renal hilum is clamped during partial nephrectomy. Eur Urol. 2010;58(3):340–5.
7. Abreu AL, Gill IS, Desai MM. Zero-ischaemia robotic partial nephrectomy (RPN) for hilar tumours. BJU Int. 2011;108(6b):948–54.
8. Desai MM, de Castro Abreu AL, Leslie S, et al. Robotic partial nephrectomy with superselective versus main artery clamping: a retrospective comparison. Eur Urol. 2014;66(4):713–9.
9. Satkunasivam R, Tsai S, Syan S, et al. Robotic unclamped "minimal-margin" partial nephrectomy: ongoing refinement of the anatomic zero-ischemia concept. Eur Urol. 2015;68(4):705–12.
10. Leslie S, Gill IS, de Castro Abreu AL, et al. Renal tumor contact surface area: a novel parameter for predicting complexity and outcomes of partial nephrectomy. Eur Urol. 2014;66(5):884–93.
11. Cacciamani GE, Okhunov Z, Meneses AD, et al. Impact of three-dimensional printing in urology: state of the art and future perspectives. A systematic review by ESUT-YAUWP Group. Eur Urol. 2019;76(2):209–21.
12. Cacciamani GE, Medina LG, Gill TS, et al. Impact of renal hilar control on outcomes of robotic partial nephrectomy: systematic review and cumulative meta-analysis. Eur Urol Focus. 2019;5(4):619–35.

Tips and Tricks for Kidney Mobilization in Robot-Assisted Renal Surgery

Daniele Cignoli, Ruben De Groote,
Marcio Covas Moschovas, and Alessandro Larcher

1 Robot-Assisted Partial Nephrectomy (RAPN)

1.1 The Use of the Fourth Arm to Elevate the Ureter and the Lower Pole of the Kidney to Access Renal Hilum

Lateral retraction of the kidney is a maneuver aimed at the suspension upward of the kidney to allow the renal hilum to be on stretch and better dissect the different renal vessels [1–3]. Similarly, in an open surgery with a flank incision, surgeons lateralize the kidney during the dissection from the psoas muscle, to better expose the renal hilum. This technique has already been described for laparoscopic partial nephrectomy and can be applied to the context of robot-assisted surgery.

After reflection of the colon, Gerota's fascia is grasped, and the kidney is lifted laterally to help expose the ureter and the gonadal vein. After the identification of the ureter, the psoas muscle is identified medial to the ureter. The ProGrasp or any other instrument installed on the fourth arm is used to elevate the ureter off the psoas muscle, allowing a clear path to the renal hilum (Fig. 1). The hilum is identified by tracing the gonadal vein. On the left, the gonadal is traced directly to its insertion in the renal vein. On the right, the gonadal is traced first to the vena cava and after followed to the renal vein. Once the renal vein is identified, the renal artery is dissected. It is usually behind the vein, and the visualization of its pulsations may help in identifying its location and course. To better perform this step, the fourth arm can be placed under the lower pole of the kidney and used to elevate the kidney away from the great vessels (Fig. 2). This maneuver stretches the renal hilum and allows the creation of a better working space between the great vessels and the kidney. This also stretches any remaining colon-renal attachments that can be taken down sharply.

1.2 Gerota's Opening

The incision of Gerota's fascia is another crucial step of robot-assisted partial nephrectomy. Technically, removing the fat around the tumor is not difficult except in patients with copious adherent perinephric fat. In these cases, this step can be difficult and extensively time-consuming. To open the Gerota's fascia, the fourth arm, the ProGrasp, is used to provide anteromedial kidney retraction to achieve the proper tension on Gerota's fascia. Then, Gerota's fascia is entered using the monopolar scissors, and the incision is carried cranio-caudally. As in laparoscopic surgery, the plane of the psoas muscle should be used for orientation, as the horizon. After the incisions of the Gerota's fascia, "defatting" the kidney adequately allows the correct exposure of the renal tumor. Removal of the adipose tissue should be done preferentially along the renal capsular plane (Fig. 3).

Correct execution of this step allows adequate exposure of the tumor and mobilizes the kidney to achieve a wide surgical field to perform the excision. To better distinguish tumor margins, a drop-in ultrasound probe could be introduced and manipulated by the surgeon.

On behalf of the Junior ERUS/YAU Working Group on Robot-Assisted Surgery of the European Association of Urology.

D. Cignoli · A. Larcher (✉)
Unit of Urology, Division of Experimental Oncology, URI Urological Research Institute, IRCCS San Raffaele Scientific Institute, Vita-Salute San Raffaele University, Milan, Italy

R. De Groote
Department of Urology, Onze Lieve Vrouw Hospital, Aalst, Belgium

ORSI Academy, Melle, Belgium

M. C. Moschovas
AdventHealth Global Robotics Institute, Celebration, FL, USA

P. Wiklund et al. (eds.), *Robotic Urologic Surgery*, https://doi.org/10.1007/978-3-031-00363-9_39

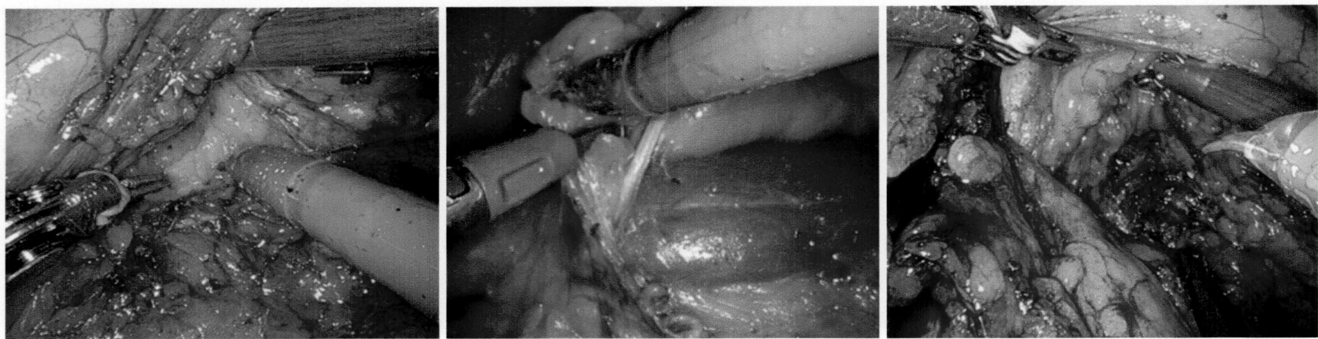

Fig. 1 Fourth arm lifting the ureter and creating the plane between the ureter and psoas muscle

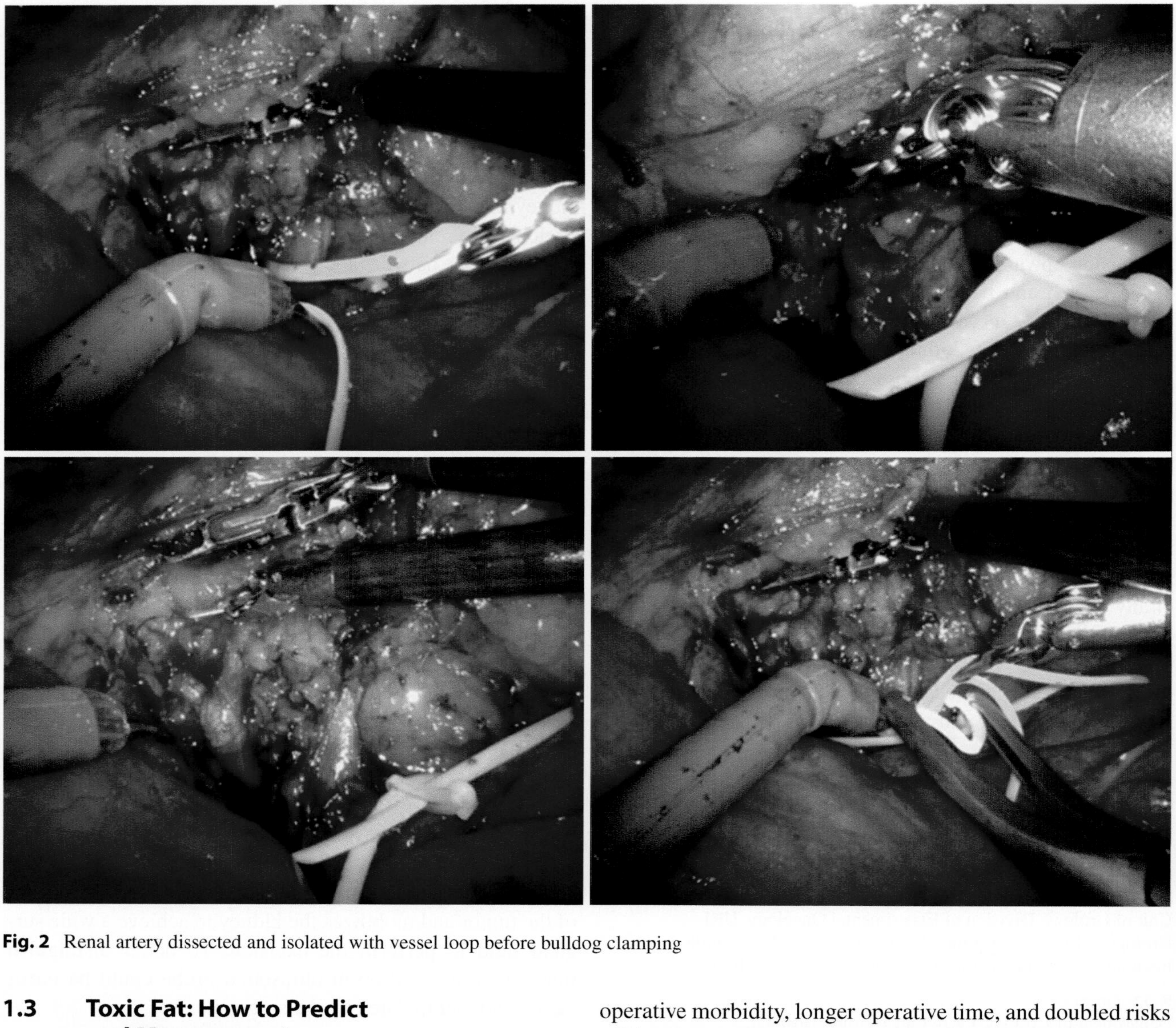

Fig. 2 Renal artery dissected and isolated with vessel loop before bulldog clamping

1.3 Toxic Fat: How to Predict and Management

Toxic fat (TF) is defined as inflammatory perirenal fat adhering to the renal parenchyma that makes kidney dissection very difficult (Fig. 4). TF is linked with increased perioperative morbidity, longer operative time, and doubled risks of bleeding and transfusion [4]. The reason for such increased morbidity is related to the difficult dissection of TF from renal parenchyma, often resulting in kidney decapsulations and increased intraoperative blood loss due to lesions to be inflamed in hyper-vascularized TF as the result of an inflam-

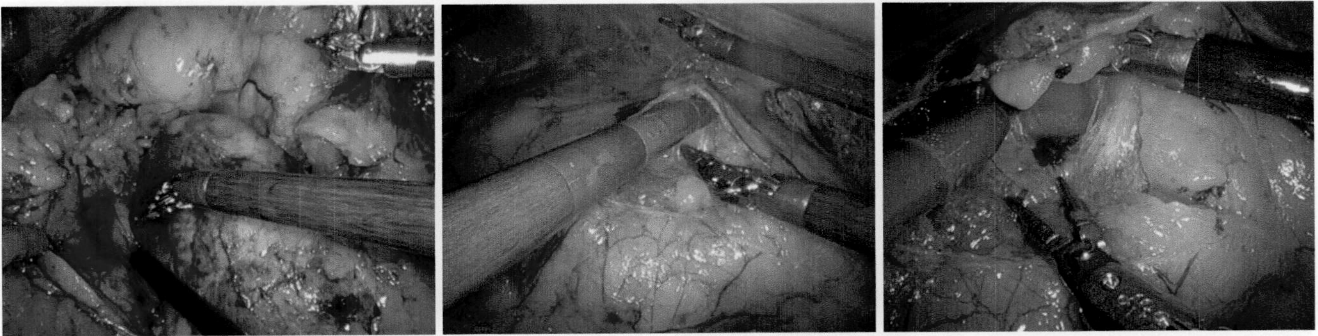

Fig. 3 Gerota's fascia opening and access to the renal tumor

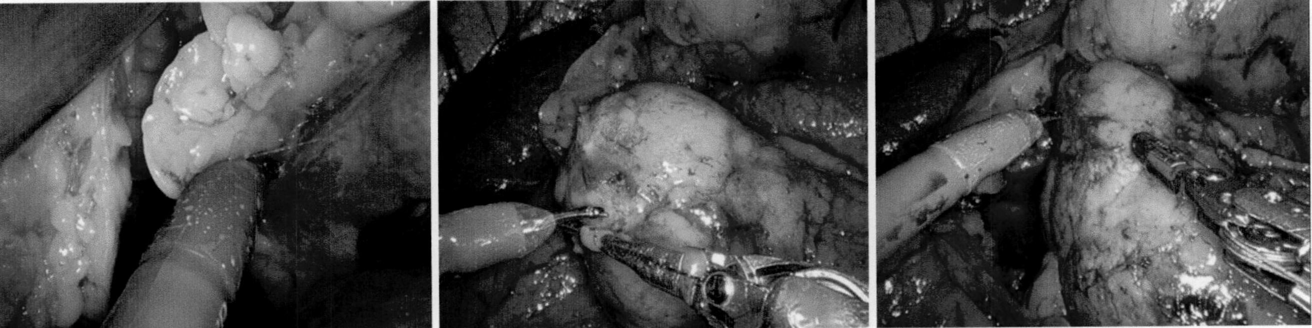

Fig. 4 Right kidney tumor with toxic fat

matory process. The presence of TF is also linked with an increased risk of conversion to radical nephrectomy or to open surgery [4]. Therefore, it is crucial to predict the presence of TF before surgery due to its intraoperative challenging potential. Unfortunately, RENAL and PADUA scores are based on tumor anatomical characteristics and do not consider other factors, as the presence of TF [5]. From a biological standpoint, the pathogenesis of TF is unclear. There are several factors, including fibrosis, autoimmune response, and inflammation. It also seems to be linked with cardiovascular risk factors and BMI, which induce a generalized hyperinflammation [6, 7]. Furthermore, the Mayo Adhesive Probability (MAP) radiological score seems to be the strongest predictor of TF [4, 8]. It could be used in a pre-operative set, to better define the presence or not of TF and program the best surgical approach for the patient.

To surmount this potential obstacle, good training is fundamental. Intraoperative ultrasound identification of tumor margins could be useful to better define where to go to remove the fat around the tumor.

1.4 Complete Renal Flipping to Access the Posterior Face of the Kidney

A challenge in RAPN is the difficult approach to posterior renal masses [9]. RAPN can be performed via either transperitoneal (tRAPN) or retroperitoneal (rRAPN) approach. Available evidence comparing tRAPN vs. rRAPN are discordant and mostly based on studies with small sample sizes [10, 11]; thus, current guidelines do not provide recommendations on the issue [12, 13]. Some authors proposed rRAPN for posterior renal masses, because there is no need for bowel mobilization and more direct access to the posterior aspect of the kidney and renal hilum [14]. Recently, Dell'Oglio et al. [15] compared data from a multi-institutional database of patients undergoing tRAPN vs. rRAPN, with a specific focus on tumor's location. An interaction test analysis revealed no advantages in the tRAPN for anterior tumors or rRAPN for posterior tumors. Moreover, it is important to consider that RAPN is a complex surgical procedure with a relatively long learning curve in which suboptimal surgical outcomes might be achieved [16]. In consequence, the choice of the approach should be driven by the surgeon's expertise [9].

During tRAPN, a maneuver that could be performed to access the posterior face of the kidney is flipping the kidney medially on its vertical axis. An accurate and complete dissection of the entire kidney is necessary to allow such step. A complete flipping of the kidney is achieved either by placing a robotic arm under the lateral border of the kidney or turning it medially (Fig. 5). This maneuver allows better visualization of the posterior renal face and an easy dissection of posterior renal masses.

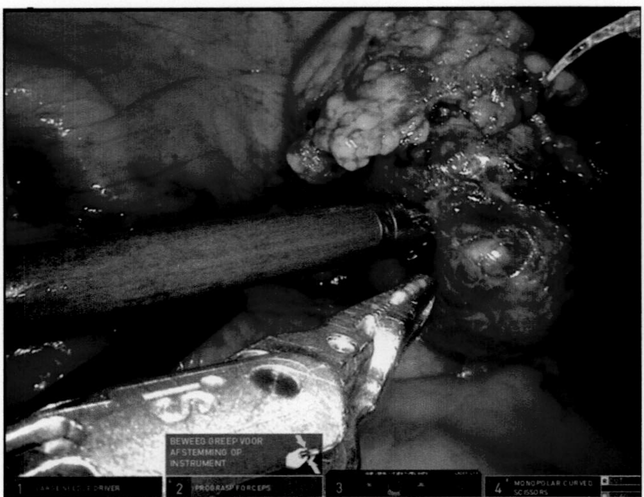

Fig. 5 Kidney release and flipping

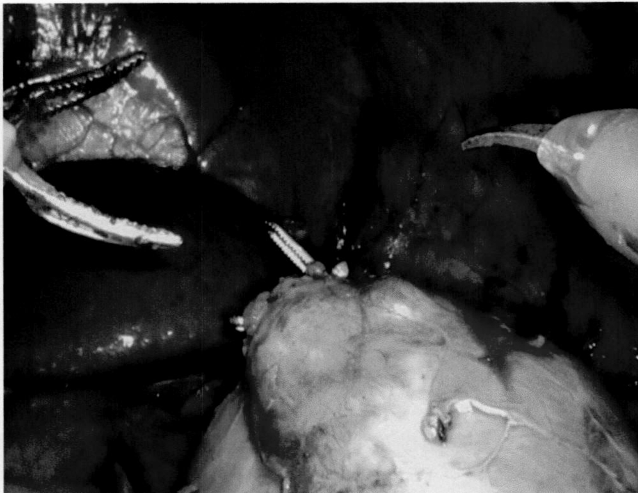

Fig. 6 Robotic arm pushing the lower pole down to present the upper pole renal mass

1.5 Maneuvers to Rotate the Kidney to Access the Upper Pole

RAPN for upper pole renal masses, especially if located posteriorly, can be challenging because of difficult visualization during tumor excision and renorrhaphy. Few studies assess these difficult conditions in the literature, but all of them agree that minimally invasive partial nephrectomy (MIPN) (both laparoscopic and robotic) for upper pole tumors is associated with a high complication rate and blood loss [17, 18]. To solve this problem, some maneuvers have been described to rotate the kidney to better access the upper pole.

One of these maneuvers is to use a robotic arm, usually the fourth, to push down the lower pole of the kidney and to present upper pole renal masses or, in contrast, to elevate the upper pole (Fig. 6). The position of the upper pole can be further improved by placing a gauze or more under the upper pole. This procedure allows a better view and an easy dissection of the mass. Usually, a combination of the two modalities is used, especially in case of four-arm transperitoneal RAPN. For both maneuvers, a previous accurate and complete dissection of the entire kidney is crucial.

Renal transposition is another safe technique that facilitates nephron-sparing transperitoneal laparoscopic resection of difficult-to-reach upper pole tumors [19]. The first step is to dissect all the attachments to the kidney outside of Gerota's fascia. Second, all the adipose tissue superior to the renal hilum must be dissected, including complete separation of the adrenal gland from the upper pole. Third, the ureter must be dissected from the lower pole of the kidney to the renal hilum. These three steps allow a complete kidney rotation around the hilar axis, by rotating the upper pole anteriorly and inferiorly and the lower pole posteriorly and superiorly.

It is noteworthy that renal transposition cannot be performed in patients with multiple renal vessels that don't allow complete rotation. It is recommended to clamp the renal hilum after complete transposition to avoid any risk of trauma to the vessels. In this case, it could be difficult to separately clamp the renal artery after transposition, and en bloc clamping of the entire renal hilum with a bulldog may be necessary [19].

2 Robot-Assisted Radical Nephrectomy (RARN)

2.1 How to Carefully Mobilize a Previously Treated Kidney

Surgical treatment in case of local recurrence after a previous partial nephrectomy or local tumor ablation can be very challenging. In case of re-surgery, the patient is older by definition and has the potential increase of comorbidities. The tumor-specific phenotype should be considered more dangerous, in either a more aggressive residual primary or another independent oncologic event. Finally, the surgical field is not naïve. Previous surgery promotes the formation of adhesions that may distort tissue planes, alter the position of anatomical landmarks, and fix bowel to the anterior abdominal wall, making subsequent trocar position more difficult. Because of the presence of abdominal scars, the position of trocars may be alternative to standard sites and subsequently suboptimal, potentially increasing the risk of conflict of robotic arms or difficult manipulation of instruments by the assistant during the procedure. After trocars are placed, it could be necessary to dissect adhesions before docking the robot, increasing the risk of bleeding and bowel injury. In addition, the distortion of normal anatomy may decrease visibility during the procedure and limit the identification of precise anatomical landmarks. This results in an increased technical complexity of both RAPN and RARN and in an increased risk of intra- or postoperative complications.

Salvage treatment for local recurrence after previous treatment for kidney cancer has been poorly investigated in the literature, and there are few retrospective studies demonstrating the safety of salvage renal surgery [20–24].

A recent multicenter investigation observed that salvage robot-assisted renal surgery includes multiple and heterogeneous clinical and surgical scenarios that could be very challenging and reported significant morbidity with respect to intraoperative complications, despite an acceptable rate of postoperative complication rate in the hands of expert surgeons at high-volume institutions [25].

The first port should preferably be placed away from the scar of previous surgery. Open insertion of the first port or using optical access trocars may prevent bowel injury. Attention must be taken during the dissection of adhesions to avoid the risk of bleeding or bowel injury. A significant experience is key to reduce the risk of intraoperative complications, because of the distortion of anatomical landmarks and the challenges of these procedures. A correct and accurate dissection of the kidney could be useful to better reach the renal hilum and the tumor to dissect (Fig. 7). In the case of the target lesion located in the upper pole, the spleen or liver might be mobilized, depending on the side. Intraoperative ultrasound can be used to locate the tumor, especially in the case of endophytic lesions [25].

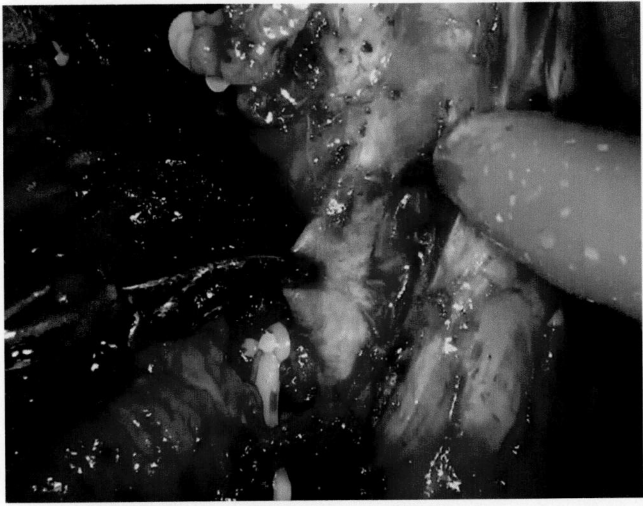

Fig. 7 Accurate dissection of a previously treated kidney

2.2 Difficult Mobilization of Upper Pole in Case of Psoas Muscle Infiltration

Bulky tumors with extensive infiltration of perirenal tissue represent an uncommon and worrisome scenario that can make kidney isolation during RARN extremely difficult. In such circumstances, we advise preferentially avoiding blunt maneuvers and proceed with sharp dissection with the robotic scissors and with generous use of coagulation. Usually, in these episodes, the tumoral invasion leads to a neovascularization state which increases the caliber of the peripheral vessels and potentializes blood loss and surgical challenges.

2.3 Examples of Surgical Plane for Adrenal/Removal Sparing

Recent guidelines recommend not performing ipsilateral adrenalectomy, both in RN and in PN, if there is no clinical evidence of invasion of the adrenal gland [12]. Accordingly, ipsilateral adrenalectomy has no advantage in the absence of clinically evident adrenal involvement [26].

If the latter scenario, dissection can be performed directly along the renal capsule to leave the adrenal gland and the upper pole perinephric fat undisturbed. An adrenal gland violation often leads to venous bleeding. It is important to perform the upper pole dissection prior to detach the kidney laterally to avoid the kidney falling medially and obscure the upper pole and the adrenal fossa. Difficulties with this part of the procedure include dissecting within the correct plane between the adrenal gland and kidney or being unable to reach the upper part of the kidney secondary to a large tumor mass.

In case of tumor extension or metastasis on the right side, the adrenal vein must be divided. Care must be taken as the adrenal vein on the right side drains directly into the inferior vena cava, is of short length, and can easily be avulsed. On both sides, the medial edge of the adrenal gland should be identified, and dissection should proceed superiorly and posteriorly with Gerota's fascia intact since the adrenal gland is within Gerota's fascia (Fig. 8).

Finally, besides vascular lesions, robot-assisted adrenalectomy is associated with hepatic, splenic, and pancreatic lesions due to the close contact between the adrenal and these organs. In these scenarios, it is important to repair the lesion as soon as it is recognized. In some cases, especially in pancreatic injuries, it is crucial to have the general surgery team as a backup [27].

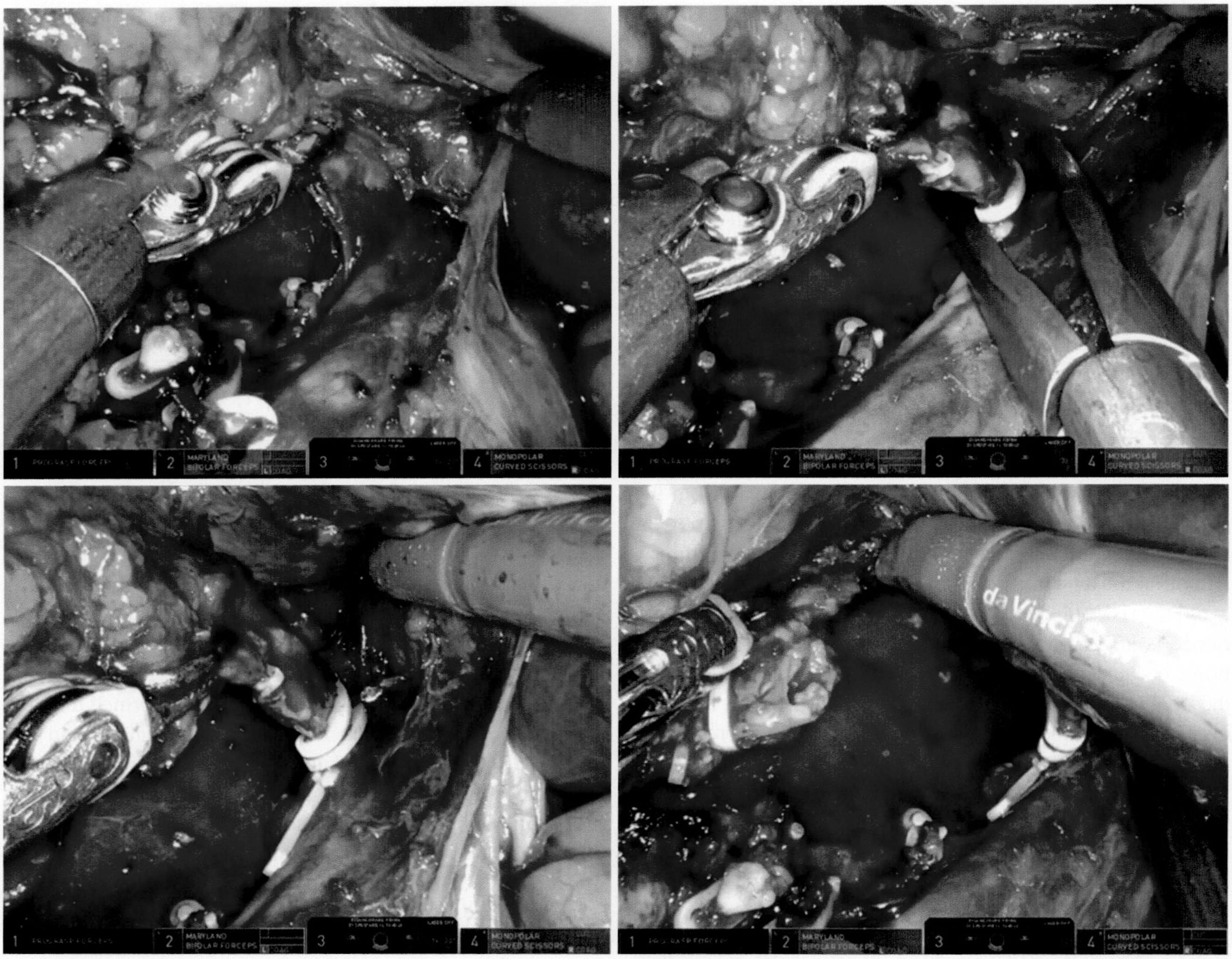

Fig. 8 Dissection of right adrenal gland within the right kidney

2.4 Avoid Diaphragmatic Injury

During upper pole dissection, care should be taken to avoid diaphragmatic injury. This adverse event should be suspected in the presence of increasing ventilatory difficulty or paradoxical diaphragmatic movements intraoperatively. When the upper pole of the kidney is dissected, the movement of the surgeon must phase with the respiratory excursion of the diaphragm, and cautery should be avoided in any case to maximally reduce the risk of diathermal lesion to the diaphragm (Fig. 9).

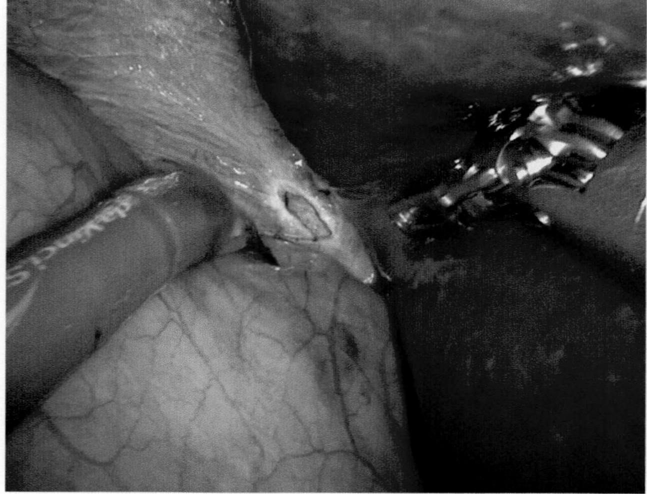

Fig. 9 Diaphragmatic injury during the right kidney dissection

References

1. Kallingal GJS, Swain S, Darwiche F, Punnen S, Manoharan M, Gonzalgo ML, et al. Robotic partial nephrectomy with the Da Vinci Xi. Adv Urol. 2016;2016:9675095.
2. Patel MN, Bhandari M, Menon M, Rogers CG. Robotic-assisted partial nephrectomy: has it come of age? Indian J Urol. 2009;25(4):523–8.
3. Bhayani SB. da Vinci robotic partial nephrectomy for renal cell carcinoma: an atlas of the four-arm technique. J Robot Surg. 2008;1(4):279–85.
4. Khene Z-E, Peyronnet B, Mathieu R, Fardoun T, Verhoest G, Bensalah K. Analysis of the impact of adherent perirenal fat on peri-operative outcomes of robotic partial nephrectomy. World J Urol. 2015;33(11):1801–6.
5. Long J-A, Arnoux V, Fiard G, Autorino R, Descotes J-L, Rambeaud J-J, et al. External validation of the RENAL nephrometry score in renal tumours treated by partial nephrectomy. BJU Int. 2013;111(2):233–9.
6. Macleod LC, Hsi RS, Gore JL, Wright JL, Harper JD. Perinephric fat thickness is an independent predictor of operative complexity during robot-assisted partial nephrectomy. J Endourol. 2014;28(5):587–91.
7. Bylund JR, Qiong H, Crispen PL, Venkatesh R, Strup SE. Association of clinical and radiographic features with perinephric "sticky" fat. J Endourol. 2013;27(3):370–3.
8. Davidiuk AJ, Parker AS, Thomas CS, Leibovich BC, Castle EP, Heckman MG, et al. Mayo adhesive probability score: an accurate image-based scoring system to predict adherent perinephric fat in partial nephrectomy. Eur Urol. 2014;66(6):1165–71.
9. Cignoli D, Fallara G, Larcher A, Rosiello G, Montorsi F, Capitanio U. How to improve outcome in nephron-sparing surgery: the impact of new techniques. Curr Opin Urol. 2021;31(3):255–61.
10. Cacciamani GE, Medina LG, Gill T, Abreu A, Sotelo R, Artibani W, et al. Impact of surgical factors on robotic partial nephrectomy outcomes: comprehensive systematic review and meta-analysis. J Urol. 2018;200(2):258–74.
11. Pavan N, Derweesh I, Hampton LJ, White WM, Porter J, Challacombe BJ, et al. Retroperitoneal robotic partial nephrectomy: systematic review and cumulative analysis of comparative outcomes. J Endourol. 2018;32(7):591–6.
12. EAU Guidelines. Edn. presented at the EAU Annual Congress Milan 2021. ISBN 978-94-92671-13-4.
13. Campbell S, Uzzo RG, Allaf ME, Bass EB, Cadeddu JA, Chang A, et al. Renal mass and localized renal cancer: AUA guideline. J Urol. 2017;198(3):520–9.
14. Arora S, Heulitt G, Menon M, Jeong W, Ahlawat RK, Capitanio U, et al. Retroperitoneal vs transperitoneal robot-assisted partial nephrectomy: comparison in a multi-institutional setting. Urology. 2018;120:131–7.
15. Dell'Oglio P, De Naeyer G, Xiangjun L, Hamilton Z, Capitanio U, Ripa F, et al. The impact of surgical strategy in robot-assisted partial nephrectomy: is it beneficial to treat anterior tumours with transperitoneal access and posterior tumours with retroperitoneal access? Eur Urol Oncol [Internet]. 2019. https://doi.org/10.1016/j.euo.2018.12.010
16. Larcher A, Muttin F, Peyronnet B, De Naeyer G, Khene ZE, Dell'Oglio P, et al. The learning curve for robot-assisted partial nephrectomy: impact of surgical experience on perioperative outcomes. Eur Urol [Internet]. 2019;75(2):253–6. https://doi.org/10.1016/j.eururo.2018.08.042
17. Venkatesh R, Weld K, Ames CD, Figenshau SR, Sundaram CP, Andriole GL, et al. Laparoscopic partial nephrectomy for renal masses: effect of tumor location. Urology. 2006;67(6):1169–1174; discussion 1174.
18. Zorn KC, Gong EM, Mendiola FP, Mikhail AA, Orvieto MA, Gofrit ON, et al. Operative outcomes of upper pole laparoscopic partial nephrectomy: comparison of lower pole laparoscopic and upper pole open partial nephrectomy. Urology. 2007;70(1):28–34.
19. Kaplan JR, Chang P, Percy AG, Wagner AA. Renal transposition during minimally invasive partial nephrectomy: a safe technique for excision of upper pole tumors. J Endourol. 2013;27(9):1096–100.
20. Kriegmair MC, Bertolo R, Karakiewicz PI, Leibovich BC, Ljungberg B, Mir MC, et al. Systematic review of the management of local kidney cancer relapse. Eur Urol Oncol. 2018;1(6):512–23.
21. Jiménez JA, Zhang Z, Zhao J, Abouassaly R, Fergany A, Gong M, et al. Surgical salvage of thermal ablation failures for renal cell carcinoma. J Urol. 2016;195(3):594–600.
22. Gilbert D, Abaza R. Robotic excision of recurrent renal cell carcinomas with laparoscopic ultrasound assistance. Urology. 2015;85(5):1206–10.
23. Autorino R, Khalifeh A, Laydner H, Samarasekera D, Rizkala E, Eyraud R, et al. Repeat robot-assisted partial nephrectomy (RAPN): feasibility and early outcomes. BJU Int. 2013;111(5):767–72.
24. Watson MJ, Sidana A, Diaz AW, Siddiqui MM, Hankins RA, Bratslavsky G, et al. Repeat robotic partial nephrectomy: characteristics, complications, and renal functional outcomes. J Endourol. 2016;30(11):1219–26.
25. Martini A, Turri F, Barod R, Rocco B, Capitanio U, Briganti A, et al. Salvage robot-assisted renal surgery for local recurrence after surgical resection or renal mass ablation: classification, techniques, and clinical outcomes. Eur Urol. 2021.
26. Lane BR, Tiong H-Y, Campbell SC, Fergany AF, Weight CJ, Larson BT, et al. Management of the adrenal gland during partial nephrectomy. J Urol. 2009;181(6):2430–7.
27. Seetharam Bhat KR, Moschovas MC, Onol FF, Rogers T, Roof S, Patel VR, Schatloff O. Robotic renal and adrenal oncologic surgery: a contemporary review. Asian J Urol. 2021;8(1):89–99. https://doi.org/10.1016/j.ajur.2020.05.010. Epub 2020 Jun 3. PMID: 33569275; PMCID: PMC7859360.

Tips and Tricks for Excision of Renal Tumours

C. J. Anderson, D. Aggarwal, A. Mottrie, and C. Vaessen

1 Introduction

Partial nephrectomy is considered the standard of care for T1a and appropriate T1b tumours [1]. Originally robotic partial nephrectomy was performed for accessible, mainly exophytic, tumours with low nephrometry parameters. As experience has matured, excision of more complex tumours has become part of the armamentarium of robotic partial nephrectomy [2, 3]. This chapter discusses the standard approach to tumour excision but also addresses the management of multiple, endophytic, hilar and cystic tumours.

2 Kidney Mobilisation

The colon is reflected along the line of Toldt. The plane between the colonic mesentery and Gerota's fascia is created by blunt and sharp dissection with medial retraction of the colon and gentle lateral pressure applied toward the kidney. The fourth arm can assist by pulling Gerota's fascia anterolaterally. The lower pole is mobilised, and gonadal vein is usually encountered early. This is helpful in locating the ureter. Surgeons differ in their approach to the hilum with some looking for the early signs of waving of the renal vein and commencing skeletonisation of renal vein and artery by dissecting directly onto them. On the left side, it is common to mobilise the lower pole with ureter and gonadal vein and place the fourth arm under the kidney to elevate it. This facilitates access to the high-level vessels. On the right side, initial dissection from the direction of the upper pole to the hilum is commonly practised. However, mobilisation of the lower pole with elevation by the fourth arm is also feasible on that side.

3 Preparing for Excision

Notwithstanding the variety of technical descriptions in the literature, there are generally accepted basic principles regarding the technique of tumour excision.

Preoperatively the surgeon develops a 3D impression of the tumour characteristics by thorough appraisal of the CT or MRI images. This aids in preparation, port placement, approach to mobilising perinephric fat and tumour excision (Figs. 1 and 2).

During the procedure a drop-in ultrasound probe is placed by the assistant into the surgical field to allow the surgeon to specifically identify the tumour contours and facilitate complete tumour excision. The TilePro™ facility integrates the ultrasound images with the console enabling the ultrasound view to be seen simultaneously by the console surgeon [4]

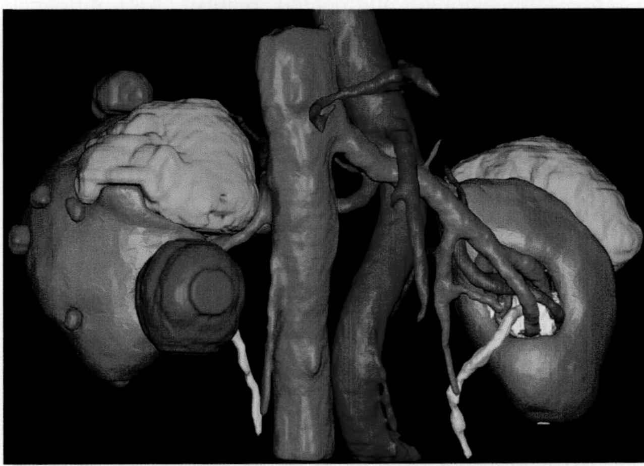

Fig. 1 Three-dimensional reconstruction of bilateral renal tumours (biopsy-confirmed tumour—green)

C. J. Anderson (✉) · D. Aggarwal
St. Georges University Hospital, London, UK

A. Mottrie
Onze Lieve Vrouw Hospital, Aalst, Belgium

ORSI Academy, Melle, Belgium

C. Vaessen
Pitie-salpetriere Academic Hospital, Assistance publique-hopitaux de Paris, Sorbonne Universite, Paris, France

P. Wiklund et al. (eds.), *Robotic Urologic Surgery*, https://doi.org/10.1007/978-3-031-00363-9_40

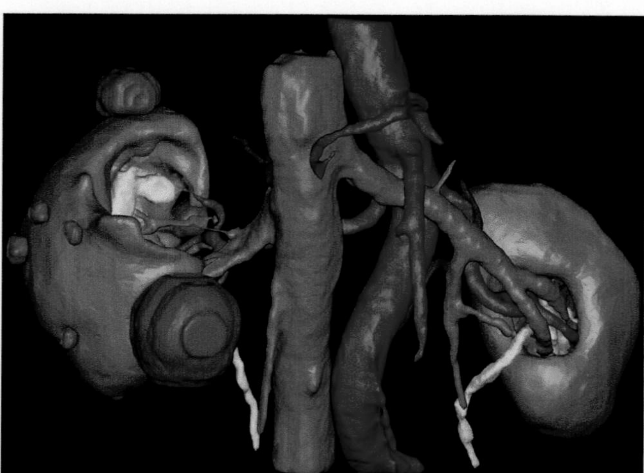

Fig. 2 Subtraction of tumour to determine relationship to the collecting system and vessels

(Fig. 3). Both the fenestrated bipolar or Maryland forceps and the ProGrasp can be used to hold the probe to ensure imaging at all angles is possible. It is sometimes necessary to withdraw the scissors and replace it with the ProGrasp forceps to align more feasibly with the direction that the ultrasound probe has entered the surgical field.

With the assistance of the ultrasound guidance, the anticipated excision boundary around the tumour is scored on the renal capsule using monopolar cautery. After scoring it may be helpful to cut into the cortex circumferentially along the scored area so as to lessen the amount of excision required during the warm ischaemic time. This might cause minor bleeding but does not generally compromise subsequent vision.

Intraoperative ultrasound is not helpful at the time of excision of tumour due to its bulkiness and limited manoeuvrability around the abdomen as well as the fact that it occupies the main assistant port.

Three-dimensional, augmented reality (AR) guidance potentially will be very useful in complex renal tumours. Real-time 3D image display can be viewed on the console using TilePro™ [5, 6]. It has facilitated tumour identification and helped with precise dissection as well as assisted in identifying high-order renal artery branches for selective arterial clamping. This has demonstrated superior perioperative outcomes in comparison to 2D ultrasound guidance. One study showed that the use of 3D AR guidance allowed optimisation of the outcomes of both the extirpative and reconstructive phases of the surgery; US guidance, on the contrary, turned out to be useful only for some outcomes of the extirpative phase [7]. A higher rate of tumour enucleation with a reduced rate of collecting system violation and ischaemia was reported with its use [5].

Other modalities for intraoperative tumour localisation have been evaluated. Near-infrared fluorescent (NIRF) imaging with indocyanine green dye (ICG) has been shown to differentiate tumour from normal surrounding parenchyma. This is because ICG is transported to the proximal tubule of the normal kidney, becomes hyperfluorescent and is not taken up by malignant cells. The tumour therefore remains hypofluorescent. The ICG is injected intravenously at a dose of 5–10 mg. This differentiation is easier to distinguish in more exophytic lesions [8]. However, its effectiveness was not proven in completely endophytic tumours [9].

NIRF is probably more commonly used in selective arterial clamping after skeletonisation of segmental branches and subsequent selective clamping. The normally fused renal parenchyma will fluoresce green with the area containing the tumour remaining dark. In so doing the surgeon can verify whether the correct artery has been clamped. If persistent arterial inflow is suspected, then either additional arterial branches can be sorted or complete clamping can be used (Fig. 4a–b) [10]. One limitation is that one can't inject a second bonus of ICG until the previous one has washed out. Therefore, whatever alternatives in strategy in terms of clamping have to be made without further ICG.

4 Tumour Resection

Tumour excision can be done by enucleoresection which involves excising the tumour with sharp and blunt dissection with a rim of normal parenchyma. Alternatively, a wider wedge resection might be required with more endophytic tumours in which a broader margin of healthy parenchyma is included.

Another option is enucleation where the tumour is shelled out within the natural plane between the pseudo-capsule of the tumour and the healthy parenchyma. This dissection plane represents a less vascularised region. Enucleation has been described as being equivalent to enucleoresection and wedge resection [11] (Fig. 5a–b).

A potential drawback is inadequate resection in cases where the tumour has invaded the pseudo-capsule [11]. However the risk of positive surgical margins (PSM) nevertheless remains low, and enucleation is considered oncologically safe [12]. In a systematic review and meta-analysis comparing wide excision with enucleation, there was no significant difference in PSM, loco-regional or renal recurrence [13].

The fourth arm can be used to stabilise the kidney and help position the kidney at an appropriate angle to assist the dissection. The use of the fourth arm is possible when using Si, X and Xi systems.

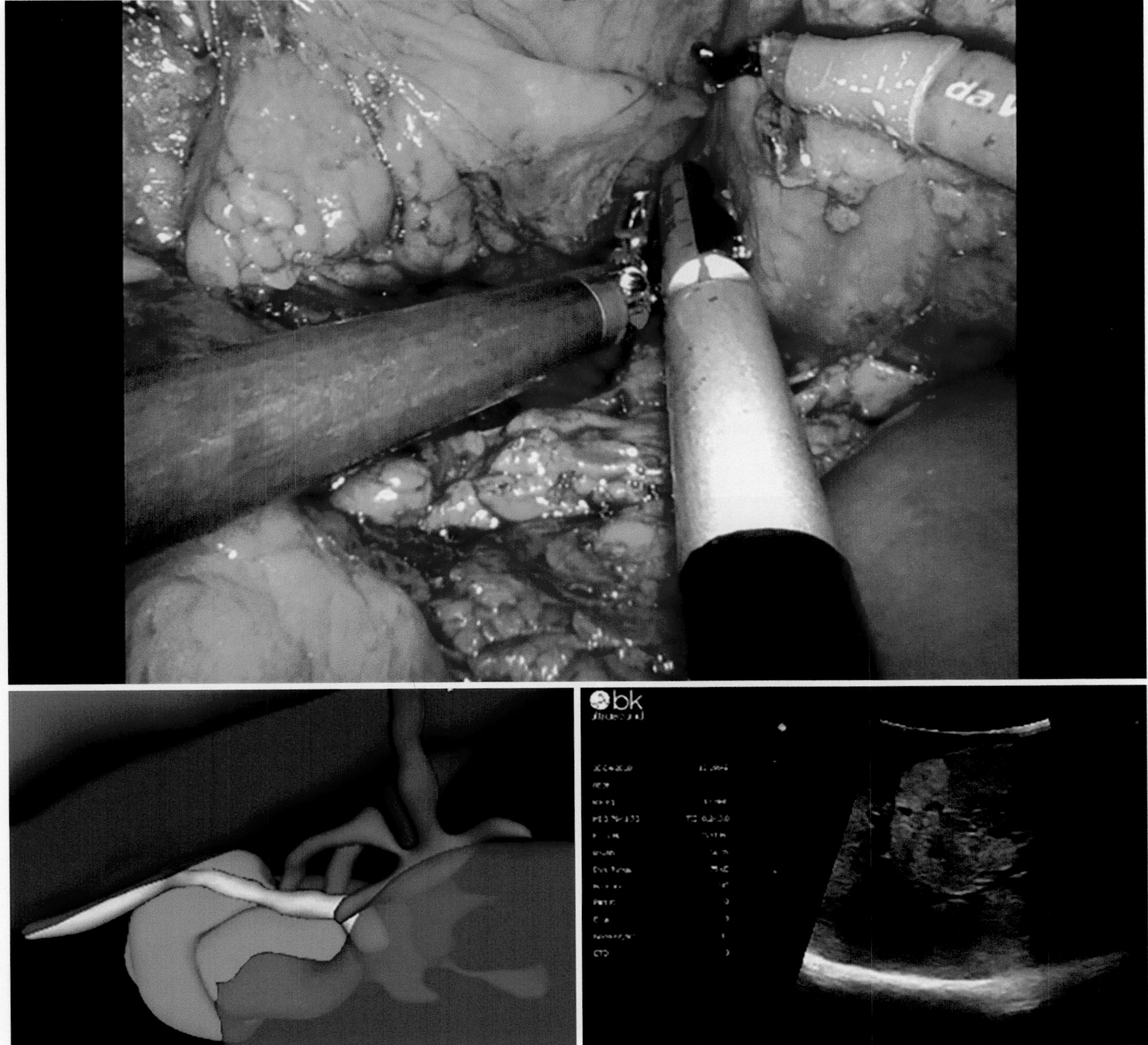

Fig. 3 TilePro™ integration of the ultrasound images and 3D reconstruction with the console view

After initial incision into the parenchyma and subsequent clamping (Scanlan® Reliance Bulldog Clamp), further progress is made along the circumference of the tumour by a combination of blunt and sharp dissection. By opening the fenestrated bipolar or Maryland forceps in the dissection plane, the scissors can be placed between the jaws, thereby facilitating exposure of the narrow surgical field. The assistant uses suction to aid with visibility during the resection, and the suction device might also be useful at certain angles in applying counter traction. Care must be taken to avoid overzealous suction by the assistant to prevent significant movement of the kidney. Sharp dissection is usually used when cutting through renal papilla.

Intraoperative haemorrhage can be prevented in most cases by meticulous dissection. Significant bleeding can also be reduced by temporarily increasing pneumoperitoneum.

In order to minimise bleeding in the tumour bed, an attempt must be made to ligate large intrarenal vessels that become visible during resection of the tumour. To manage localised bleeding into the tumour bed, a figure-of-eight suture (3–0 Vicryl on an SH needle) can be used on bleeding areas. This can also be used to repair any previously identi-

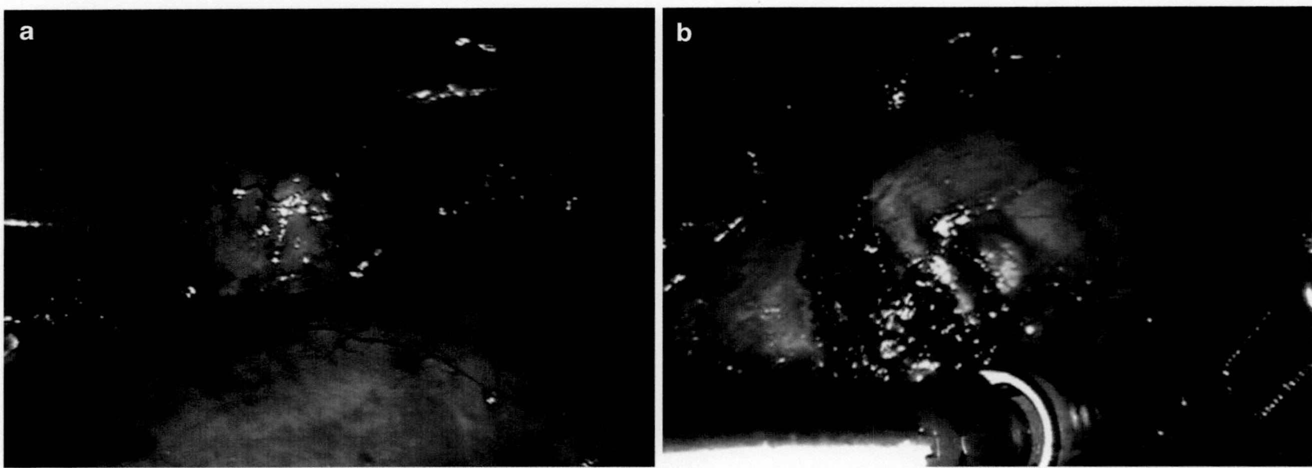

Fig. 4 Near-infrared fluorescent (NIRF) imaging with indocyanine green dye (ICG) showing proper (**a**) or insufficient (**b**) clamping of the region of interest [10]

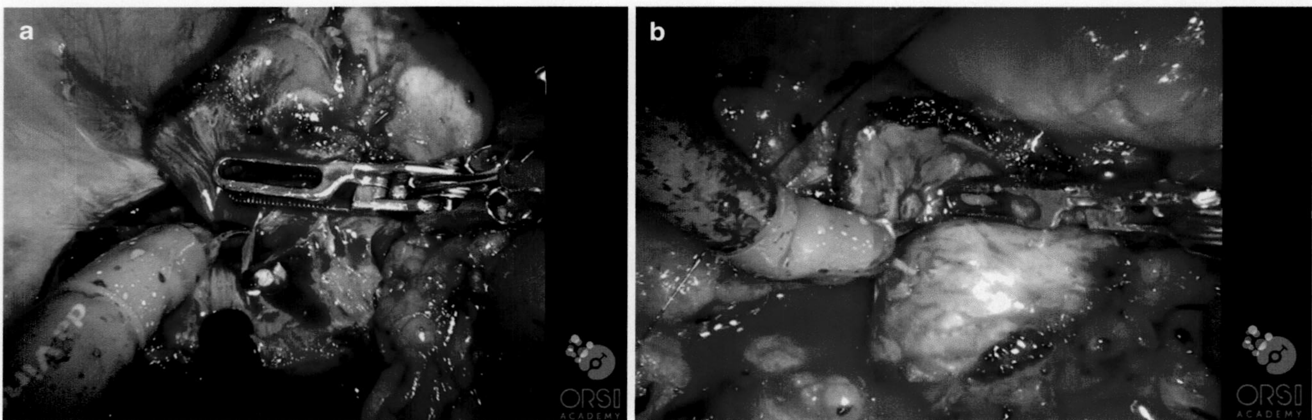

Fig. 5 Tumour resection following an enucloresection (**a**) or enucleation (**b**) plane

fied entry into the collecting system. For diffuse bleeding running V-Loc™ (Medtronic) barbed suture may be utilised.

Currently, a two-layer closure of the renal defect is advocated in most of the studies. Thereby, the first layer is used to close the collecting system and suture medullary vessels, while the second layer is used to approximate renal cortex. Significant calyceal defects may be closed individually. Surgeons differ in their choice of suture material for the first layer and use monofilament or barbed sutures. With a monofilament suture, the suture tension is increased by traction on both ends after completion, as the suture will glide through the tissues. However, barbed sutures are likely to maintain their traction at the time the suture is placed.

After the mini-bulldog clips are removed, a final bolus ICG can be administered to confirm that global perfusion is restored [10].

4.1 Endophytic Tumours

There is a paucity of literature regarding endophytic tumour as it is challenging and performed less frequently than partial nephrectomy for more common tumours. The open surgical approach is still often used despite the availability of minimally invasive surgery (MIS). This is due to perceived advantages of better access to hilar vessels, cold ischaemia, direct compression of the parenchyma and more secure renorrhaphy [4].

Robotic partial nephrectomy for endophytic tumours is considered very challenging, as the surgeon does not have gross tumour visualisation. The difficult manoeuvrability and limited external view may potentially increase the risk of complication and affect overall outcomes.

The most challenging component is tumour identification and to identify the depth of tumour. Overlying fat is dissected off. Intracorporeal ultrasound is used to define edges and depth of tumour. The TilePro™ and multi-image display mode of robotic system allows better integration and localisation of tumour. The Doppler mode may allow localisation of renal hilum anatomy and aberrant vessels.

The renal capsule is scored usually with an attempt to start the dissection plane wider than normal so as to approach the tumour in a more horizontal or shallow trajectory. Resection commences after clamping along the scored margin using monopolar scissors. The left-hand forceps might be used to widen the plane between tumour and healthy parenchyma. The assistant might assist with traction at various angles with the sucker and also remove blood from the operating field to maximise visibility. Super-selective clip ligation of small arterial feeders is optional to control haemorrhage.

An intraoperative frozen section from resected bed area may help in confirming negative surgical margins, and, if found positive, the resection bed can be extended.

Completely endophytic tumours may leave a larger and deeper cavity after resection, which increases difficulty in renorrhaphy. A two-layer closure is highly advocated as already discussed.

4.2 Hilar Tumours

It is helpful for port placement to allow the camera to be deliberately placed directly over the hilum in managing hilar tumours.

A ureteric catheter might be considered if there is significant collecting system breach anticipated, so as to avoid or minimise post-operative urinary leak.

Hilar microdissection is performed medial to lateral to identify specific divisions of the branching arterial tree that might supply the tumour. Hilar fat is removed to improve access to the artery and vein, and robotic mini clamps (Scanlan) are applied to secondary-, tertiary- or quaternary-level branches. If the tumour is completely anterior or posterior to Brodel's line, only the anterior or posterior branches are dissected out.

Intraoperative ultrasound is necessary for tumour delineation for hilar tumours. Scoring is done in an inverted-U shape with the open end being at the hilum. Selective clamping and using ICG might be appropriate depending on the surgeon's preference. With hilar tumours there is often more opportunity to detect arterial vessels feeding directly into the tumour than usual. Therefore, these can be individually ligated where possible [14–16].

If the lesion is hilar and endophytic, the same principles are applied in their resection. As with endophytic tumours, a wider parenchymal margin is made to create a shallow trajectory to the base of the tumour. Tumour excision can be started at the cortical level before clamping in order to minimise ischaemic time. When bleeding starts to obscure, the visual field clamping can be performed. Predominantly blunt dissection is used to avoid cutting into the collecting system or cause vascular injury [17].

Once the tumour has been removed, the collecting system and radially traversing vessels will be seen in the tumour bed. If bleeding vessels require ligation, care must be taken to do this in a radial direction rather than placing sutures perpendicular to the radially traversing vessels. The collecting system is repaired if breached. The tumour bed is left open, or haemostatic agents and sealants may be used according to the surgeon's preference. A hilar suture renorrhaphy method has been described ('V' hilar suture) whereby inner layer sutures are placed in a way to reshape the parenchymal defect [18].

4.3 Cystic Tumours

The frequency of cystic tumours in the nephrectomy/partial nephrectomy published series is 12 to 18% [19, 20]. Studies vary in terms of malignancy in resected cysts: in one study 64.8% for Bosniak III and IV [21] and in another 56% and 74% for Bosniak III and IV, respectively [22]. When comparing the pathology between similar tumour dimensions of cystic and solid tumours, the latter has higher rate of malignancy as well as higher pathological grades [23–25]. Nevertheless, the malignancy rates in complex Bosniak III and IV cystic tumours support the use of nephron-sparing surgery [22, 23].

There are few publications on robotic partial nephrectomy for cystic renal masses. A large multi-institutional retrospective series of cystic tumours showed that robotic partial nephrectomy was associated with less operating time, but all the following parameters were similar to partial nephrectomy for solid lesions. These were blood loss, ischaemic time, post-operative complications, PSM, renal function and pathology [26]. Due to the risk of cystic wall rupture during resection and risk of tumour spillage, handling of cystic masses requires special care and skills. In one study there was a higher rate of rupture in cysts with more complex nephrometry (higher E and N in RENAL classification), Bosniak III cysts and where the surgeon had experience of fewer than 20 cases [27].

In one study data was compared between matched open and cystic partial nephrectomy [22]. There was no difference in perioperative outcomes between each group, and the volume of healthy rim of renal parenchyma resected with the tumours was equivalent. This negated the hypothesis that there might be a tendency to remove more renal parenchyma than necessary to avoid cyst rupture. This is a significant finding as the volume of resected tissue is an important predictor of renal function preservation [28, 29].

It seems therefore that in experienced hands the selection of patients for partial nephrectomy should not be influenced by the fact that lesions are cystic and they should be dealt with in the same way as solid lesions. The experience of the surgeon is paramount, and nephrometry scoring and appropriate patient selection are essential due to the risk of rupture if the cystic mass is mishandled.

During partial nephrectomy for solid lesions, a surgeon can alter the plane of dissection section if the lesion margin is breached. This is not possible with cystic lesions due to the potential for cyst rupture. Meticulous preoperative planning with high-quality imaging is necessary. 3D reconstructions are likely to be extremely beneficial in this group. Judicious use of intraoperative ultrasound is recommended to facilitate knowledge of the exact dimensions and depth of lesion [22]. Preferably, the cortex should be scored with scissors, with the help of intraoperative ultrasound, to determine the exact entrypoint for the subsequequent incision. Thereafter, circumferential incision with a rim of normal parenchyma, is performed in the same way as for solid tumours. Care must be taken not to lever over or compress the cystic tumour. At the end of the procedure, the endoscopic bag extraction must be performed through large-enough incision to avoid rupture.

4.4 Multiple Tumours

The incidence of multifocal lesions is 6 to 25% in the sporadic population [30]. It is obviously higher in hereditary syndromes like von Hippel Lindau syndrome, hereditary papillary renal cancer and Birt-Hogg-Dube syndrome.

Generally hereditary cancers are closely monitored, and surgery is indicated when the tumours reach 3 cm in size [31]. Intervention at this stage is important due to the risk of recurrence requiring repeat intervention and possible need for dialysis if left too late. Renal function preservation is the most important consideration in the motivation for nephron-sparing surgery in these patients. They are keen to avoid dialysis and the complexities of transplant, and reported data supports that renal insufficiency is an independent risk factor for cardiovascular disease, hospitalisation and all-cause mortality brackets [32].

The robotic approach with its magnification, articulation and pneumoperitoneum offers the opportunity for enucleation of multiple tumours with minimal vascular compromise and blood loss, even in endophytic tumours. Due to multiplicity of lesions, excision without a rim of normal parenchyma is preferred [33].

By intervening when lesions are small, surgeons can perform enucleation of tumours with zero ischaemia in appropriate cases. This would be determined by surgeon experience and location and accessibility of the lesions. In so doing hilar dissection is avoided, which might be beneficial in repeat partial nephrectomy and reducing vascular complications [34, 35]. Furthermore by using MIS, and preferably with no hilar dissection, the approach during a re-operation procedure is likely to be less challenging than re-operation after open surgery. These cases are good for the use of sealants, but otherwise the described variety of techniques for renorrhaphy can be utilised.

5 Conclusion

Robotic partial nephrectomy has proven to be oncologically safe and functionally effective and routinely practsced for tumours of low complexity. Endophytic, hilar, multifocal and complex cystic tumours can be a barrier for many surgeons, but as surgeon experience increases, the evidence shows that the robotic approach is feasible for these challenging cases. Meticulous preparation and patient selection, together with judicious use of improving imaging technologies, enable favourable outcomes and afford a minimally invasive option in the management of these cases.

References

1. Ljungberg B, Bensalah K, Canfield S, Dabestani S, Hofmann F, Hora M, et al. EAU guidelines on renal cell carcinoma: 2014 update. Eur Urol. 2015;67(5):913–24.
2. White MA, Haber G-P, Autorino R, Khanna R, Hernandez AV, Forest S, et al. Outcomes of robotic partial nephrectomy for renal masses with nephrometry score of ≥7. Urology. 2011;77(4):809–13.
3. Long J-A, Yakoubi R, Lee B, Guillotreau J, Autorino R, Laydner H, et al. Robotic versus laparoscopic partial nephrectomy for complex tumors: comparison of perioperative outcomes. Eur Urol. 2012;61(6):1257–62.
4. Kim DK, Komninos C, Kim L, Rha KH. Robot-assisted partial nephrectomy for endophytic tumors. Curr Urol Rep. 2015;16(11):76.
5. Furukawa J, Miyake H, Tanaka K, Sugimoto M, Fujisawa M. Console-integrated real-time three-dimensional image overlay navigation for robot-assisted partial nephrectomy with selective arterial clamping: early single-centre experience with 17 cases: Real-time 3D image navigation for robot-assisted partial nephrectomy. Int J Med Robot. 2014;10(4):385–90.
6. Hughes-Hallett A, Pratt P, Mayer E, Martin S, Darzi A, Vale J. Image guidance for all – TilePro display of 3-dimensionally reconstructed images in robotic partial nephrectomy. Urology 2014;84(1):237–242.
7. Porpiglia F, Checcucci E, Amparore D, Piramide F, Volpi G, Granato S, et al. Three-dimensional augmented reality robot-assisted partial nephrectomy in case of complex tumours (PADUA ≥10): a new intraoperative tool overcoming the ultrasound guidance. Eur Urol. 2020;78(2):229–38.

8. Tobis S, Knopf JK, Silvers C, Messing E, Yao J, Rashid H, et al. Robot-assisted and laparoscopic partial nephrectomy with near infrared fluorescence imaging. J Endourol. 2012;26(7):797–802.
9. Hekman MCH, Rijpkema M, Langenhuijsen JF, Boerman OC, Oosterwijk E, Mulders PFA. Intraoperative imaging techniques to support complete tumor resection in partial nephrectomy. Eur Urol Focus. 2018;4(6):960–8.
10. Bjurlin MA, Gan M, McClintock TR, Volpe A, Borofsky MS, Mottrie A, et al. Near-infrared fluorescence imaging: emerging applications in robotic upper urinary tract surgery. Eur Urol. 2014;65(4):793–801.
11. Minervini A, Carini M. Tumor enucleation is appropriate during partial nephrectomy. Eur Urol Focus. 2019;5(6):923–4.
12. Minervini A, Campi R, Di Maida F, Mari A, Montagnani I, Tellini R, et al. Tumor-parenchyma interface and long-term oncologic outcomes after robotic tumor enucleation for sporadic renal cell carcinoma. Urol Oncol. 2018;36(12):527.e1–527.e11.
13. Minervini A, Campi R, Sessa F, Derweesh I, Kaouk JH, Mari A, et al. Positive surgical margins and local recurrence after simple enucleation and standard partial nephrectomy for malignant renal tumors: systematic review of the literature and meta-analysis of prevalence. Minerva Urol Nefrol. 2017;69(6):523–38.
14. Borofsky MS, Gill IS, Hemal AK, Marien TP, Jayaratna I, Krane LS, et al. Near-infrared fluorescence imaging to facilitate super-selective arterial clamping during zero-ischaemia robotic partial nephrectomy: Near-infrared fluorescence imaging in zero ischaemia RPN. BJU Int. 2013;111(4):604–10.
15. Feliciano J, Stifelman M. Robotic retroperitoneal partial nephrectomy: a four-arm approach. JSLS. 2012;16(2):208–11.
16. Dulabon LM, Kaouk JH, Haber G-P, Berkman DS, Rogers CG, Petros F, et al. Multi-institutional analysis of robotic partial nephrectomy for hilar versus nonhilar lesions in 446 consecutive cases. Eur Urol. 2011;59(3):325–30.
17. Arora S, Rogers C. Partial nephrectomy in central renal tumors. J Endourol. 2018;32(S1):S63–7.
18. Khalifeh A, Autorino R, Hillyer SP, Kaouk JH. V-hilar suture renorrhaphy during robotic partial nephrectomy for renal hilar tumors: preliminary outcomes of a novel surgical technique. Urology. 2012;80(2):466–71.
19. Spaliviero M, Herts BR, Magi-Galluzzi C, Xu M, Desai MM, Kaouk JH, et al. Laparoscopic partial nephrectomy for cystic masses. J Urol. 2005;174(2):614–9.
20. Bielsa O, Lloreta J, Gelabert-Mas A. Cystic renal cell carcinoma: pathological features, survival and implications for treatment. Br J Urol. 1998;82(1):16–20.
21. Pinheiro T, Sepulveda F, Natalin RH, Metrebian E, Medina R, Goldman SM, et al. Is it safe and effective to treat complex renal cysts by the laparoscopic approach? J Endourol. 2011;25(3):471–6.
22. Akca O, Zargar H, Autorino R, Brandao LF, Laydner H, Kaouk JH, et al. Robotic partial nephrectomy for cystic renal masses: a comparative analysis of a matched-paired cohort. Urology. 2014;84(1):93–8.
23. Nassir A, Jollimore J, Gupta R, Bell D, Norman R. Multilocular cystic renal cell carcinoma: a series of 12 cases and review of the literature. Urology. 2002;60(3):421–7.
24. You D, Shim M, Jeong IG, Song C, Kim JK, Ro JY, et al. Multilocular cystic renal cell carcinoma: clinicopathological features and preoperative prediction using multiphase computed tomography: multilocular cystic renal cell carcinoma. BJU Int. 2011;108(9):1444–9.
25. Aubert S, Zini L, Delomez J, Biserte J, Lemaitre L, Leroy X. Cystic renal cell carcinomas in adults. Is preoperative recognition of multilocular cystic renal cell carcinoma possible? J Urol. 2005;174(6):2115–9.
26. Novara G, La Falce S, Abaza R, Adshead J, Ahlawat R, Buffi NM, et al. Robot-assisted partial nephrectomy in cystic tumours: analysis of the Vattikuti Global Quality Initiative in Robotic Urologic Surgery (GQI-RUS) database. BJU Int. 2016;117(4):642–7.
27. Chen S-Z, Wu Y-P, Chen S-H, Li X-D, Sun X-L, Huang J-B, et al. Risk factors for intraoperative cyst rupture in partial nephrectomy for cystic renal masses. Asian J Surg. 2021;44(1):80–6.
28. Simmons MN, Hillyer SP, Lee BH, Fergany AF, Kaouk J, Campbell SC. Functional recovery after partial nephrectomy: effects of volume loss and ischemic injury. J Urol. 2012;187(5):1667–73.
29. Mir MC, Campbell RA, Sharma N, Remer EM, Simmons MN, Li J, et al. Parenchymal volume preservation and ischemia during partial nephrectomy: functional and volumetric analysis. Urology. 2013;82(2):263–8.
30. Baltaci S, Orhan D, Soyupek S, Bedük Y, Tulunay O, Gögüs O. Influence of tumor stage, size, grade, vascular involvement, histological cell type and histological pattern on multifocality of renal cell carcinoma. J Urol. 2000;164(1):36–9.
31. Herring JC, Enquist EG, Chernoff A, Linehan WM, Choyke PL, Walther MM. Parenchymal sparing surgery in patients with hereditary renal cell carcinoma: 10-year experience. J Urol. 2001;165(3):777–81.
32. Go AS, Chertow GM, Fan D, McCulloch CE, Hsu C-Y. Chronic kidney disease and the risks of death, cardiovascular events, and hospitalization. N Engl J Med. 2004;351(13):1296–305.
33. Boris R, Proano M, Linehan WM, Pinto PA, Bratslavsky G. Initial experience with robot assisted partial nephrectomy for multiple renal masses. J Urol. 2009;182(4):1280–6.
34. Johnson A, Sudarshan S, Liu J, Linehan WM, Pinto PA, Bratslavsky G. Feasibility and outcomes of repeat partial nephrectomy. J Urol. 2008;180(1):89–93.
35. Bratslavsky G, Liu JJ, Johnson AD, Sudarshan S, Choyke PL, Linehan WM, et al. Salvage partial nephrectomy for hereditary renal cancer: feasibility and outcomes. J Urol. 2008;179(1):67–70.

Renorrhaphy Techniques in Robot-Assisted Partial Nephrectomy

Elio Mazzone, Alexandre Mottrie, and Andrea Minervini

1 Introduction

Recently, in the context of robot-assisted partial nephrectomy (RAPN), the suture technique has been mentioned among the factors influencing the functioning of the residual renal parenchyma. Indeed, reducing the healthy parenchyma incorporated in the renorrhaphy has been proposed to minimize the injury from the reconstructive phase [1, 2]. Based on this concept, to date, there is a consensus suggesting that one of the main predictors of the ultimate renal function is the quantity of the preserved parenchyma after partial nephrectomy: this said, it will result from the healthy parenchyma spared during the resection that does not suffer of ischemia due to the renorrhaphy [3, 4].

The majority of the studies on the impact of renorrhaphy on outcomes were focused on "to suture or not to suture" rather than "single-layer versus double-layer suture," but literature is still lacking about the best practice. The issue is underlined by the fact that, to date, we still lack a standardized report about the optimal suture technique after RAPN. This would be of key importance in increasing the scientific impact of the studies about the renal function after RAPN. Nonetheless, current guidelines do not provide specific recommendations to tailor renorrhaphy technique according to patient- or tumor-related characteristics to maximize parenchymal preservation [5, 6].

E. Mazzone (✉)
Division of Oncology/Unit of Urology, URI, IRCCS Ospedale San Raffaele, Milan, Italy

Vita-Salute San Raffaele University, Milan, Italy

A. Mottrie
Orsi Academy, Melle, Belgium

Department of Urology, OLV, Aalst, Belgium

A. Minervini
Unit of Urological Robotic Surgery and Renal Transplantation, University of Florence, Florence, Italy

Department of Experimental and Clinical Medicine, University of Florence, Florence, Italy

Of note, in order to maximize the amount of healthy residual parenchyma after surgery, minimal-margin resection and minimal renorrhaphy are necessary, since penetration into the renal parenchyma may cause intraparenchymal vessel injuries, leading to increased loss of functional nephrons [7]. In the same direction, current literature suggests that ischemia time and amount of healthy renal parenchyma resected are the main modifiable factors affecting renal function and volume loss after RAPN [8]. Regarding suture, performing single-layer renorrhaphy while omitting cortical renorrhaphy appears to improve postoperative renal function according to very limited data [9]. Lastly, recent studies have demonstrated the feasibility of "sutureless" techniques, which may ideally spare substantial renal parenchyma [10]. However, such evidence is still sparse, and no prospective well-designed studies are currently available to disentangle this issue. In the current chapter, we will outline the available evidence on different techniques for renorrhaphy in RAPN.

2 Main Body of the Chapter

2.1 Surgical Techniques for Renorrhaphy in Robotic Partial Nephrectomy

Before focusing on the main features of renorrhaphy, the first crucial step to achieve maximum parenchyma preservation is represented by the precise excision of the tumor. To obtain an optimal tumor excision, after isolating the hilum, a robotic bulldog clamp is applied to the renal artery to minimize bleeding, and, in selected cases, this is followed by another on the renal vein [11]. The clamping marks the triggering of a stopwatch, to measure warm ischemic time (WIT). The tumor is excised with consideration of surgical margins, with the assistant surgeon ensuring the field is adequately exposed by suctioning away blood. Thereafter, the sliding-clip renorrhaphy principle is applied to close the renal defect, in multiple layers. The traditional approach to renal reconstruction during RAPN is represented by a two-layer closure, first

P. Wiklund et al. (eds.), *Robotic Urologic Surgery*, https://doi.org/10.1007/978-3-031-00363-9_41

described in 2004 [12]. The deep layer of the renorrhaphy is performed with the monofilament 3–0 suture, using a Hem-o-Lock ligating clip already attached at one end. A continuous suture runs through the base of the defect closing any open collecting system and small vessels. If arterial bleeds are detected, these can be sutured individually with additional monofilament sutures to ensure meticulous hemostasis. Once the running suture is applied, a second Hem-o-Lock clip locks the other loose end. Traction is applied to the suture end to snug the clip down against the renal capsule, bringing the renal defect together. Larger defects may require multiple sutures. From a technical point of view, it is important to orient the suture at right angles with respect to the line of the arcuate arteries and to take into account the radial anatomy of the renal lobes and their respective interlobar arteries (Fig. 1) [13]. Early "off-clamp" technique is generally accepted after the deep sliding-clip renorrhaphy is complete, in the order of release of renal vein, followed by the artery, where the vein has been previously clamped. This allows to reduce the WIT, preserving a higher amount of healthy parenchyma. At this stage, hemostasis is adequate to complete the superficial sliding-clip renorrhaphy suture with a larger suture. In this layer, clips are applied at every throw through the renal capsule to further approximate the defect. A second locking clip is then applied above every previous clip on the sliding suture to prevent slipping. During the cortical suture, it is recommended to avoid including the arcuate arteries to preserve the medullar blood supply and to avoid overcompressing the tissue to minimize the ischemic compression of the renal parenchyma (Fig. 2) [13]. The use of adjuncts to hemostasis is not essential but may provide added security and further minimize blood loss. This may be in the form of FloSeal®, Surgicel®, or Evicel®. After completing the renorrhaphy, the hilum and the excision site are carefully inspected following this step, to ensure hemostasis is achieved.

In summary, as described above, robotic renorrhaphy classically consists of a double-layer technique [11] including a medullary suture, often performed in a knotless fashion by using Lapra-Ty (Ethicon, Somerville, New Jersey, USA) or Hem-o-Lock clips, and a cortical suture (running or interrupted) to re-approximate the renal defect, typically performed with sliding-clip technique [14]. Hemostatic agents may be used according to the surgeon's preference to complete hemostasis. To reduce renorrhaphy time, some authors reported the use of self-retaining barbed sutures either for inner-layer renorrhaphy [15–23] or during cortical renorrhaphy [19]. Of note, in their study on unclamped, minimal-margin RAPN, Satkunasivam et al. reported a double-layer, bolsterless, renorrhaphy technique aimed to maximize the preservation of the vascularized healthy renal parenchyma [24].

In case of accidental injury of urinary collecting system (UCS) during tumor resection, several renorrhaphy techniques have been described to close UCS entries during RAPN. In most studies, entries into the UCS (more frequent in case of larger and/or anatomically complex renal masses) were repaired using variable suture materials with either

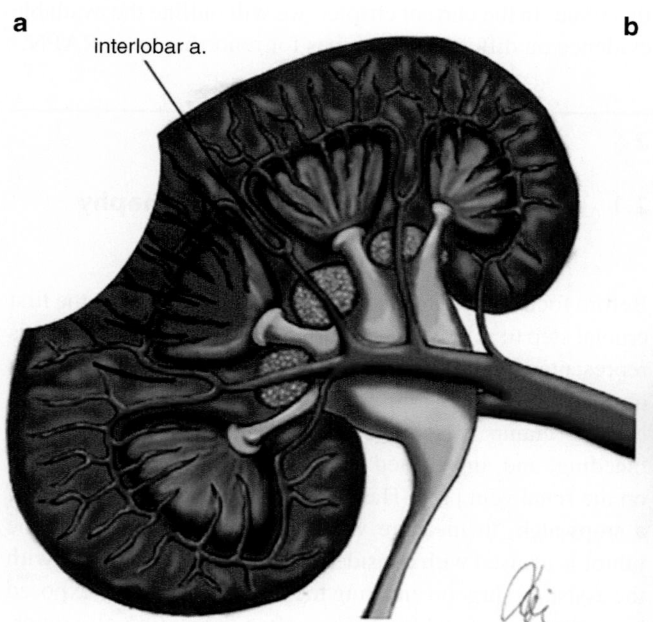

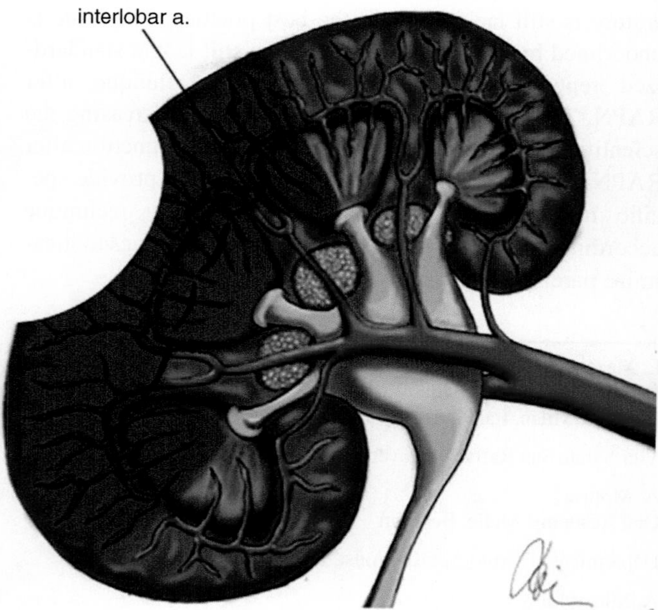

Fig. 1 Suture of the medulla. (**a**) The suture has been performed while taking into account the radial anatomy of the renal lobe (the pyramid) and its respective interlobar arteries. (**b**) Interlobar arteries have been included in the suture. Surrounding renal parenchyma will be devascularized due to the consequent ischemia of the respective arcuate arteries originating from the sutured interlobar arteries [13]

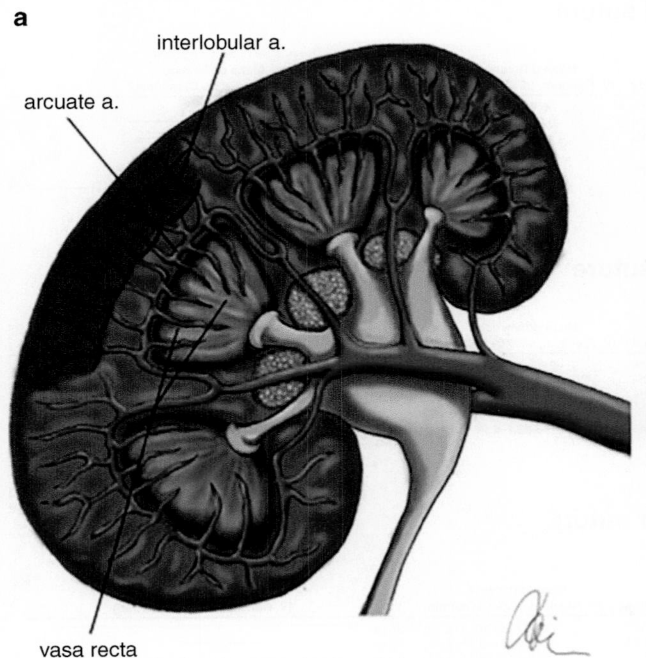

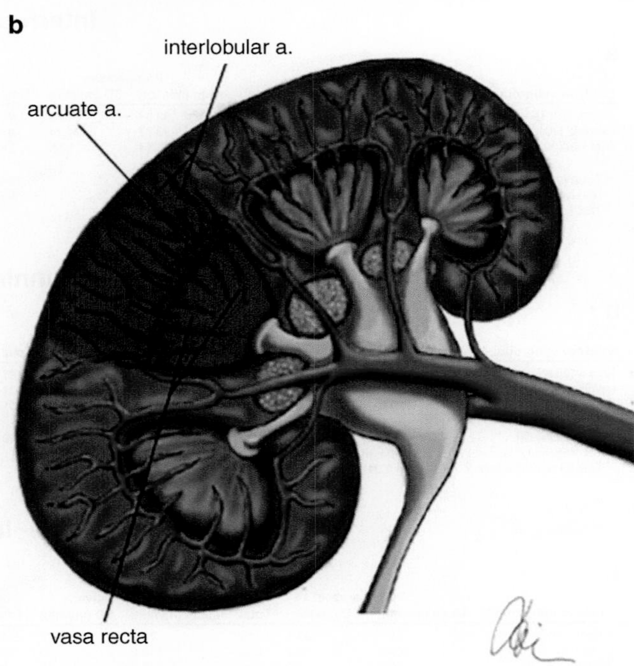

Fig. 2 Suture of the cortex. (**a**) The suture has been performed superficial enough in order to avoid the involvement of the arcuate arteries: the blood supply to the medullar parenchyma by the vasa recta is spared. (**b**) The suture has been deepened with involvement of the arcuate arteries and subsequent ischemia of both the cortical and the medullar parenchyma [13]

selective interrupted sutures or during the running suture performed for inner-layer renorrhaphy. When repairing UCS, it is recommended to stay superficial, avoiding calyx involvement leading to its exclusion [13]. In their study comparing renorrhaphy with and without repair for UCS entries, Desai and co-workers found that UCS repair was associated with significantly longer WIT but no differences in functional outcomes or complications rate. Of note, tumor size was significantly higher in patients requiring UCS repair [25].

Among studies comparing running versus interrupted sutures, four studies reported a dedicated suture of the UCS [15, 16, 26, 27]. The most common suture used was 2–0 or 3–0 polyglactin suture (Vicryl). One study reported the use of 3–0 polydioxanone (PDS) [27]. In the study by Williams et al. [28], omitting the inner-layer suture (and therefore a dedicated UCS closure) and closing the outer layer by sliding-clip renorrhaphy did not result in an increased risk of complications or renal function impairment as compared to double-layer renorrhaphy.

2.2 The Impact of Different Suture Techniques on Outcomes

In a recent systematic review, six studies analyzed the impact of running versus interrupted suture on outcomes [15–18, 21, 26, 29, 30]. The groups under evaluation were comparable in terms of preoperative characteristics, namely, age, body mass index (BMI), and tumor size. A significant advantage in terms of operative time (mean difference −17.12 [95% CI −24.30, −9.94] minutes), WIT (−8.73 [95% CI −12.41, −5.06] minutes), and occurrence of postoperative complications (odds ratio (OR) 0.54 [95% CI 0.32, 0.89]) and transfusions (OR 0.30 [95% CI 0.15, 0.59]) favored running suture. Conversely, no significant differences were found for urinary leakages. No significant differences were found between pre- and postoperative estimated glomerular filtrations (eGFRs) in both patients who received an interrupted suture (mean difference −4.88 ml/min, 95% confidence interval [CI] −11.38; 1.63, $p = 0.14$) and those who received a running suture (−3.42 ml/min, 95% CI −9.96; 3.12, $p = 0.31$) (Fig. 3a–b) [29, 30].

Similarly, studies testing the impact of barbed versus non-barbed sutures on outcomes were analyzed [31–34]. Here, significant advantage in terms of operative time (mean difference −8.80 [95% CI −12.97, −4.64] minutes), WIT (−6.70 [95% CI −7.82, −5.57] minutes), and blood losses (−46.31 [95% CI −55.23, −37.39] mL) favored running suture. No differences were found in postoperative complications, transfusions, and urinary leakages [29, 30].

Lastly, in analyses comparing single- versus double-layer sutures, three studies were considered [8, 28, 35]. Groups were comparable in terms of age and tumor size (cumulative analysis for BMI not performed due to insufficient data). A

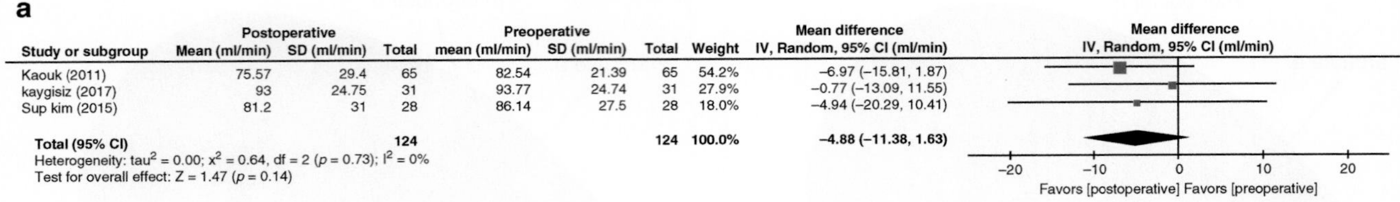

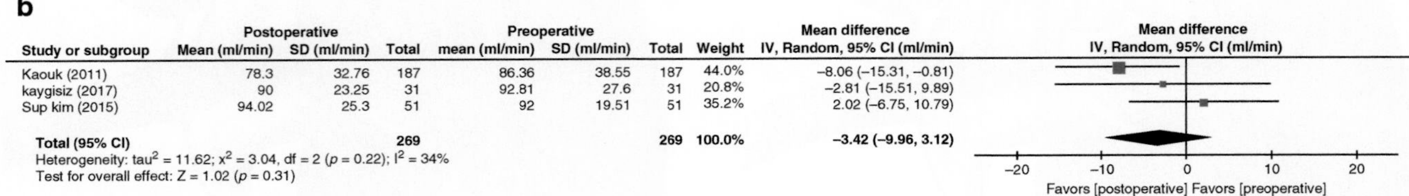

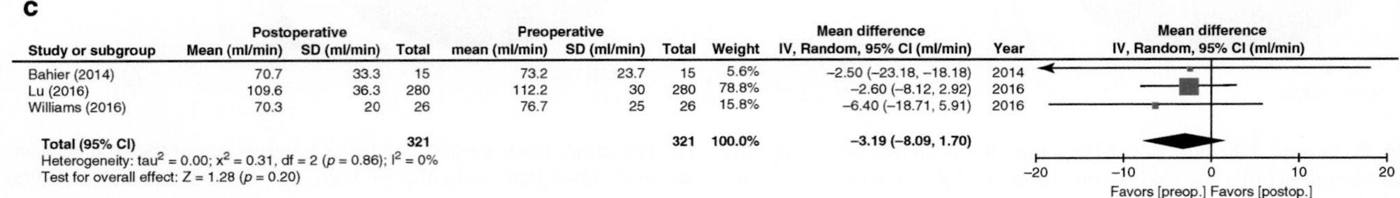

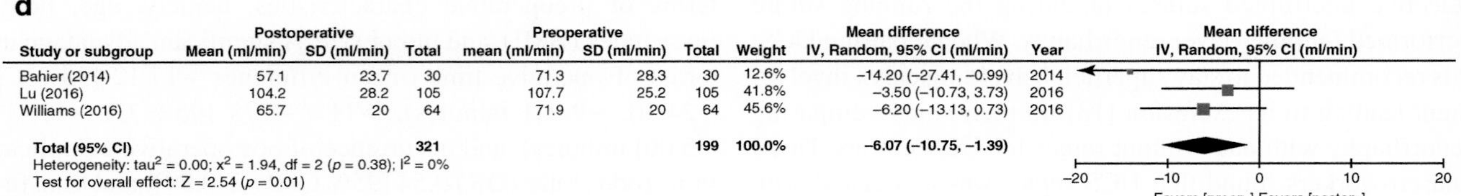

Fig. 3 (**a**) Interrupted suture: pooled analysis of post- versus preoperative estimated glomerular filtration rate (ml/min). (**b**) Running suture: pooled analysis of post-versus preoperative estimated glomerular filtration rate (ml/min). (**c**) Single-layer suture: pooled analysis of post- versus preoperative estimated glomerular filtration rate (ml/min). (**d**) Double-layer suture: pooled analysis of post-versus preoperative estimated glomerular filtration rate (ml/min) [30]. *CI* confidence interval, *IV* interval variable, *SD* standard deviation

significant advantage in terms of operative time (mean difference −11.13 [95% CI −20.14, −2.13] minutes) and WIT (−3.39 [95% CI −4.53, −2.24] minutes) favored single-layer technique. Conversely, no significant differences were found in terms of blood losses, postoperative complications, and urinary leakages. When analyzing eGFR, a benefit in functional outcomes in favor of the single-layer technique (−3.19 ml/min, 95% CI −8.09; 1.70, $p = 0.2$ versus −6.07 ml/min, 95% CI −10.75; −1.39, $p = 0.01$) has been reported (Fig. 3c–d) [29, 30]. In general, according to the available evidence and expert opinions, when a single-layer renorrhaphy is attempted, the cortical rather than the medullary layer should be omitted.

2.3 Feasibility of "Sutureless" RAPN

With the evolution of renorrhaphy techniques, especially during RAPN, the use of surgical bolsters to fill the renal defect after inner-layer renorrhaphy has gradually declined. However, few studies have proposed, in very selected cases, to fully omit inner and/or outer renorrhaphy in case of limited bleeding in order to preserve the maximum amount of safe parenchyma. To achieve this goal, several hemostatic agents have been employed by surgeons to improve hemostasis during RAPN. Overall, the use and type of hemostatic agents were based on the surgeon's preference, and no studies formally compared the differential role of renorrhaphy techniques and hemostatic agents on RAPN outcomes. Moreover, the aim of hemostatic agents (i.e., to improve hemostasis versus to fill the renal defect) was rarely reported in most studies.

Minervini et al. were the first to describe the use of TachoSil (Nycomed, Zurich, Switzerland) without capsular re-approximation in case of wide resection beds or after sutureless hemostasis for small cortical lesions [36]. More recently, Farinha et al. described a novel surgical "sutureless" technique aimed at maximally preserving vital parenchyma. In their classical technique (standard RAPN), inner renorrhaphy was performed with a running 4–0/3–0 suture and outer renorrhaphy with a 1–0 Vicryl running suture. Hem-o-Lok clips were placed on both sides of the thread and tightened to compress the renal parenchyma as needed if cortical bleeding occurs. These parenchymal running suture and renorrhaphy steps were omitted during the novel sutureless RAPN. When no arterial bleeding was observed, no suturing was carried out, and a hemostatic agent (TachoSil, Nycomed GmbH, Zurich, Switzerland, or Veriset, Medtronic, Minneapolis, MN, USA) was applied to the tumor bed. When analyzing outcomes of the novel technique, only one patient (3.4%) in the sutureless RAPN group experienced an intraoperative complication, namely, venous bleeding during hilar dissection. Two sutureless RAPN patients (6.9%) versus four standard RAPN patients (13.8%) experienced 30-day postoperative complications. Of note, at a 6-month follow-up, the median eGFR decrease was −5.6 (interquartile range [IQR], −3.4–8.3) for the sutureless RAPN group versus −9.1% (IQR, −7.3–11) for the standard RAPN group ($p < 0.01$). Finally, only one sutureless RAPN patient (3.4%) versus five standard RAPN patients (17%) experienced postoperative acute kidney injury ($p = 0.2$) [10]. Overall, these findings demonstrate the safety and feasibility of sutureless RAPN. However, this study represents the initial experience of a high-volume surgeon who had already reached the plateau of his learning curve; as such, prospective randomized trials with a larger cohort are needed to further support these observations.

3 Conclusion

The renorrhaphy techniques have evolved over time toward the concept of a nephron-sparing renal reconstruction. Besides achieving hemostasis and closure of the collecting system, the aim of renorrhaphy is to maximize preservation of vascularized parenchyma, which may translate into a benefit of ultimate renal function. Based on the available evidence, single-layer renorrhaphy may favor improved postoperative renal functional outcomes; however, this is based on very limited retrospective studies. On the other hand, the use of "sutureless" techniques in very selected cases might be the optimal choice in the setting of chronic renal insufficiency or solitary kidney, when technically feasible. Overall, surgeon experience and skills remain the key drivers of current reconstruction techniques, which should be tailored to a single clinical scenario.

Acknowledgments Disclosure: The authors declare no conflict of interest.

Financial Disclosures

Elio Mazzone certifies that all conflicts of interest, including specific financial interests and relationships and affiliations relevant to the subject matter or materials discussed in the manuscript (e.g., employment/affiliation, grants or funding, consultancies, honoraria, stock ownership or options, expert testimony, royalties, or patents filed, received or pending), are the following: None.

References

1. Simmons MN, Hillyer SP, Lee BH, et al. Functional recovery after partial nephrectomy: effects of volume loss and ischemic injury. J Urol. 2012;187:1667–73.
2. Minervini A, Campi R, Sessa F, et al. Positive surgical margins and local recurrence after simple enucleation and standard partial nephrectomy for malignant renal tumors: systematic review of the literature and meta-analysis of prevalence. Minerva Urol Nefrol. 2017;69:523–38.
3. Wen D, Jitao W, Chalairat S-O, et al. Devascularized parenchymal mass associated with partial nephrectomy: predictive factors and impact on functional recovery. J Urol. 2017;198:787–94.
4. Bertolo RG, Zargar H, Autorino R, et al. Estimated glomerular filtration rate, renal scan and volumetric assessment of the kidney before and after partial nephrectomy: a review of the current literature. Minerva Urol Nefrol. 2017;69:539–47.
5. Campbell SC, Uzzo RG, Karam JA, et al. Renal mass and localized renal cancer: evaluation, management, and follow-up: AUA guideline: Part II. J Urol. 2021;206:209–18.
6. EAU Guidelines. Edn. presented at the EAU Annual Congress Milan 2021. ISBN 978-94-92671-13-4. 2021.
7. Takagi T, Kondo T, Omae K, et al. Assessment of surgical outcomes of the non-renorrhaphy technique in open partial nephrectomy for ≥T1b renal tumors. Urology. 2015;86:529–33.
8. Bahler CD, Dube HT, Flynn KJ, et al. Feasibility of omitting cortical renorrhaphy during robot-assisted partial nephrectomy: a matched analysis. J Endourol. 2015;29:548–55.
9. Shatagopam K, Bahler CD, Sundaram CP. Renorrhaphy techniques and effect on renal function with robotic partial nephrectomy. World J Urol. 2020;38:1109–12.
10. Farinha R, Rosiello G, Paludo ADO, et al. Selective suturing or sutureless technique in robot-assisted partial nephrectomy: results from a propensity-score matched analysis. Eur Urol Focus. 2021:1–8.
11. Kaouk JH, Khalifeh A, Hillyer S, et al. Robot-assisted laparoscopic partial nephrectomy: step-by-step contemporary technique and surgical outcomes at a single high-volume institution. Eur Urol. 2012;62:553–61.

12. Gettman MT, Blute ML, Chow GK, et al. Robotic-assisted laparoscopic partial nephrectomy: technique and initial clinical experience with Da Vinci robotic system. Urology. 2004;64:914–8.
13. Porpiglia F, Bertolo R, Amparore D, Fiori C. Nephron-sparing suture of renal parenchyma after partial nephrectomy: which technique to go for? Some Best Practices Eur Urol Focus. 2019;5:600–3.
14. Benway BM, Wang AJ, Cabello JM, Bhayani SB. Robotic partial nephrectomy with sliding-clip renorrhaphy: technique and outcomes. Eur Urol. 2009;55:592–9.
15. Baumert H, Ballaro A, Shah N, et al. Reducing warm ischaemia time during laparoscopic partial nephrectomy: a prospective comparison of two renal closure techniques. Eur Urol. 2007;52:1164–9.
16. Canales BK, Lynch AC, Fernandes E, Anderson JK, Ramani AP. Novel technique of knotless hemostatic renal parenchymal suture repair during laparoscopic partial nephrectomy. Urology. 2007;70:358–9.
17. Kawa G, Kinoshita H, Komai Y, et al. Uninterrupted suturing of renal parenchyma in laparoscopic partial nephrectomy decreases renal ischemic time and intraoperative blood loss. Int J Urol Off J Japanese Urol Assoc. 2010;17:382–4.
18. Kaouk JH, Hillyer SP, Autorino R, et al. 252 robotic partial nephrectomies: evolving renorrhaphy technique and surgical outcomes at a single institution. Urology. 2011;78:1338–44.
19. Sukumar S, Rogers CG. Robotic partial nephrectomy: surgical technique. BJU Int. 2011;108:942–7.
20. Seideman C, Park S, Best SL, Cadeddu JA, Olweny EO. Self-retaining barbed suture for parenchymal repair during minimally invasive partial nephrectomy. J Endourol. 2011;25:1245–8.
21. Kim HS, Lee YJ, Ku JH, et al. The clinical application of the sliding loop technique for renorrhaphy during robot-assisted laparoscopic partial nephrectomy: surgical technique and outcomes. Korean J Urol. 2015;56:762–8.
22. Rassweiler JJ, Klein J, Tschada A, Gözen AS. Laparoscopic retroperitoneal partial nephrectomy using an ergonomic chair: demonstration of technique and matched-pair analysis. BJU Int. 2017;119:349–57.
23. Hennessey DB, Wei G, Moon D, et al. Strategies for success: a multi-institutional study on robot-assisted partial nephrectomy for complex renal lesions. BJU Int. 2018;121(Suppl 3):40–7.
24. Satkunasivam R, Tsai S, Syan S, et al. Robotic unclamped "minimal-margin" partial nephrectomy: ongoing refinement of the anatomic zero-ischemia concept. Eur Urol. 2015;68:705–12.
25. Desai MM, Gill IS, Kaouk JH, Matin SF, Novick AC. Laparoscopic partial nephrectomy with suture repair of the pelvicaliceal system. Urology. 2003;61:99–104.
26. Kaygisiz O, Çelen S, Vuruşkan BA, Vuruşkan H. Comparison of two different suture techniques in laparoscopic partial nephrectomy. Int Braz J Urol. 2017;43:863–70.
27. Kim KS, Choi SW, Kim JH, et al. Running-clip renorrhaphy reducing warm ischemic time during laparoscopic partial nephrectomy. J Laparoendosc Adv Surg Tech A. 2015;25:50–4.
28. Williams RD, Snowden C, Frank R, Thiel DD. Has sliding-clip renorrhaphy eliminated the need for collecting system repair during robot-assisted partial nephrectomy? J Endourol. 2017;31:289–94.
29. Bertolo R, Campi R, Klatte T, et al. Suture techniques during laparoscopic and robot-assisted partial nephrectomy: a systematic review and quantitative synthesis of peri-operative outcomes. vol. 123. 2019.
30. Bertolo R, Campi R, Mir MC, et al. Systematic review and pooled analysis of the impact of renorrhaphy techniques on renal functional outcome after partial nephrectomy. Eur Urol Oncol. 2019;2:572–5.
31. Sammon J, Petros F, Sukumar S, et al. Barbed suture for renorrhaphy during robot-assisted partial nephrectomy. J Endourol. 2011;25:529–33.
32. Olweny EO, Park SK, Seideman CA, Best SL, Cadeddu JA. Self-retaining barbed suture for parenchymal repair during laparoscopic partial nephrectomy; initial clinical experience. BJU Int. 2012;109:906–9.
33. Jeon SH, Jung S, Son H-S, Kimm SY, Chung BI. The unidirectional barbed suture for renorrhaphy during laparoscopic partial nephrectomy: Stanford experience. J Laparoendosc Adv Surg Tech A. 2013;23:521–5.
34. Erdem S, Tefik T, Mammadov A, et al. The use of self-retaining barbed suture for inner layer renorrhaphy significantly reduces warm ischemia time in laparoscopic partial nephrectomy: outcomes of a matched-pair analysis. J Endourol. 2013;27:452–8.
35. Lu Q, Zhao X, Ji C, et al. Modified laparoscopic simple enucleation with single-layer suture technique versus standard laparoscopic partial nephrectomy for treating localized renal cell carcinoma. Int Urol Nephrol. 2017;49:239–45.
36. Minervini A, Tuccio A, Masieri L, et al. Endoscopic robot-assisted simple enucleation (ERASE) for clinical T1 renal masses: description of the technique and early postoperative results. Surg Endosc. 2015;29:1241–9.

Robot-Assisted Radical Nephrectomy and Vena Cava Thrombus Management

Gang Zhu, Ronney Abaza, Xu Zhang, and Qingbo Huang

1 Introduction

Laparoscopic radical nephrectomy (LRN) was first performed in 1991 by Clayman [1]. Not more than a decade later, urologists are leading the way in robotic surgeries as it overcomes many technical and ergonomic difficulties associated with conventional laparoscopic procedures. Further, robotic surgery helps surgeons challenge more technically difficult minimally invasive procedures, such as inferior vena cava (IVC) tumor thrombectomy.

Klingler has first reported the robot-assisted radical nephrectomy (RARN) [2]. Since then, there was no stopping debate on the application of robotics in RARN as it was with longer operative times and similar outcomes but a higher cost than LRN. A multi-institutional database study compared RARN and LRN for large renal masses (≥ cT2). Over the study period, there is a trend of the increasing use of RARN (annual increase of 11.75%) over LRN (annual decline of 5.39%). RARN is being performed for more advanced disease, higher histological grade, and higher rate of lymphadenopathy and higher BMI patients. RARN cases were more likely to include lymph node dissection (LND). There were no significant differences in operative times (OT), estimated blood loss (EBL), transfusion rate, length of stay (LOS), conversion rate, intraoperative complications, and postoperative complications between these two groups [3, 4]. RARN has equivalent perioperative complication rate with LRN [5].

On the other hand, with the recognition of oncological outcomes and improvements in instruments and surgical techniques, in particular the robotic surgery, the indication of partial nephrectomy (PN) has been expanded in clinically localized renal cell carcinoma (RCC) [6].

G. Zhu (✉)
Beijing United Family Hospital, Beijing, China

R. Abaza
Central Ohio Urology Group, Columbus, OH, USA

X. Zhang · Q. Huang
Chinese PLA General Hospital, Beijing, China

A systemic review and meta-analysis of comparative studies of PN vs. radical nephrectomy (RN) for cT1b and T2 RCCs found out that the PN group had a lower risk of tumor recurrence, cancer-specific mortality, and all-cause mortality compared to the RN group. For T2 tumors the EBL and risk of complications were higher for PN, but the recurrence rate and cancer-specific mortality were lower for PN [7]. PN even extended its indication in metastatic RCC (mRCC), in which cytoreductive PN was shown to be associated with improved OS in mRCC patients, although this effect was limited to patients with primary tumors <4 cm [8]. In general, the need for RN decreases.

2 Indications and Contraindications

2.1 Indications

RCC patients indicated for open or laparoscopic RN are the potential candidates for RARN. The use of a RARN depends on the availability of robotic platform, surgeon's preference, and shared decision-making.

The robotic platform has expended the indications for RARN to larger masses, locally advanced disease stages, cytoreductive nephrectomy (CN) in mRCC, RN with concurrent lymph node dissection (LND), and/or inferior vena cava (IVC) tumor thrombectomy [9].

RARN is not suggested in patients with T1 tumors for whom a PN is feasible by any approach, including open [6]. RN is the recommended standard treatment option for the curative treatment of large or central renal masses where a PN is not feasible [10].

While systemic therapy is strongly suggested for contemporary treatment in mRCC, CN is still indicated in well-selected patients, such as patients with good general status Eastern Cooperative Oncology Group (ECOG) Performance Status <2), estimated survival times >12 months, no brain metastasis, or three or fewer International Metastatic RCC Database Consortium (IMDC) prognostic factors [10, 11].

P. Wiklund et al. (eds.), *Robotic Urologic Surgery*, https://doi.org/10.1007/978-3-031-00363-9_42

2.2 Contraindications

RN is not indicated in patients with T1 tumors for whom a PN is feasible by any approach, including open.

The absolute contraindication for RARN is diminishing. But the uncorrected coagulopathy, sepsis, and peritonitis are still generally accepted as absolute contraindications.

Other relative rather than absolute contraindications include:

- Bleeding disorders and anticoagulated patients.
- Severe chronic obstructive pulmonary disease (COPD).
- Difficulty body habitus.
- Tumor extends beyond the Gerota's fascia, and perinephric inflammation may increase the chance of conversion to open surgery.
- Previous abdominal adhesions may consider retroperitoneal approach.
- Previous retroperitoneal surgery or percutaneous kidney and surrounding structure procedures may consider transperitoneal approach.
- Extremely large tumors (>15 cm) may be difficult because of limited working space.
- Patient's preference after fully informed consent.

2.3 Lymph Node Dissection (LND)

In patients with T1–T2, clinically negative lymph nodes, and absence of unfavorable clinical and pathologic characteristics, regional LND offers limited staging information and no benefit in terms of decreasing disease recurrence or improving survival.

An extended LND may be potentially beneficial in RCC patients with locally advanced disease (T3–T4) and/or unfavorable clinical and pathologic characteristics, such as high WHO/ISUP (International Society of Urological Pathology) grade, larger tumors, presence of sarcomatoid features, coagulative tumor necrosis, and high risk for regional lymph node involvement [12].

The NCCN Guidelines suggested that regional LND is optional but is recommended for patients with adenopathy on preoperative imaging or palpable/visible adenopathy at the time of surgery [10].

It has been suggested that the lymph nodes from the ipsilateral great vessel and the interaortocaval region be removed from the crus of the diaphragm to the common iliac artery when performing LND for high-risk nodal metastasis RCC cases [13].

Robotic platform has enabled the adoption of LND at RARN [14].

2.4 Adrenalectomy

Do not perform ipsilateral adrenalectomy if there is no clinical evidence of adrenal gland invasion [15].

3 Preoperative Preparation

3.1 Preoperative Evaluation

We need to consider for the general risks of the surgical procedures, including anesthetic risk, bleeding, infection, deep vein thrombosis, wound infection, and other specific risks and evaluate patients properly.

A thorough preoperative assessment is necessary including a deep history and physical examination in evaluation of general conditions, cardio-circulatory, respiratory, endocrine, neuromuscular, hepatic, renal, hematology, obese, obstructive sleep apnea, etc. Laboratory evaluation should focus on renal functional capacity. Blood type and screen are required. In difficult cases, autologous and/or cross-matched blood preparation is suggested.

As the lung is a common site of RCC metastasis, a chest CT is routinely suggested.

Chemical or mechanic prophylaxis of venous thromboembolism (VTE) will be considered depending on the pre- or post-surgery evaluation.

A fully informed consent is essential. The risk is low, but the patient needs to be informed the risk of converting to open surgery.

3.2 Imaging

Diagnostic staging involving a contrast CT or MRI is mandatory prior to the initiation of the surgical procedure. For the concerns over vascular details of the tumor and aberrant vascular structure, a CT angiography (CTA) or three-dimensional (3D) image reconstruction based on contrast CT or MRI is suggested.

The 3D imaging is more precise than 2D imaging in evaluating the surgical complexity of the renal tumor by showing the tumor location in the kidney and relations of tumor with surrounding organs and vessels as shown in Fig. 1. Nowadays, there is an emergence of 3D imaging navigation in robotic surgery. By adjusting the 3D images extracorporeally, the fused 3D images with the real structure will guide surgeons to the vessel, lymph nodes, and other important structures during the surgical procedure. 3D imaging technique had reduced operative time, estimated blood loss, complications, and length of hospital stay. There are more benefits from the 3D imaging in a more challenging case [16–19].

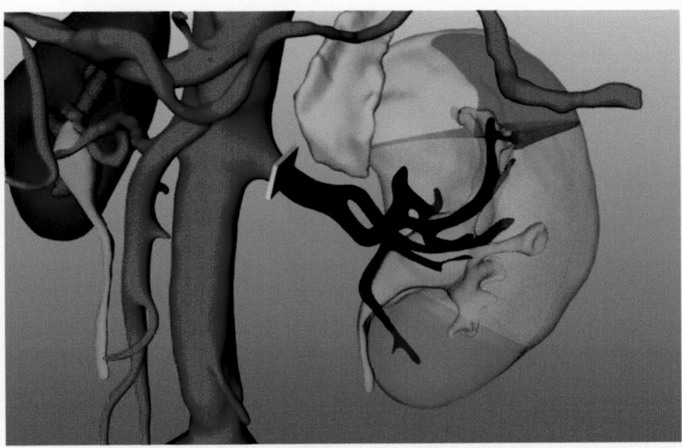

Fig. 1 Holographic 3D image showed the renal artery, its branches, collecting system, ureter, and adrenal gland with simulation of the clamped left renal artery

Depending on the individual cases and procedures, special images including ultrasound, dynamic renal scintigraphy, etc. may be needed.

4 Surgical Technique

As in LRN, both transperitoneal and retroperitoneal approaches are feasible for RARN.

Currently, it's hard to find randomized clinical trials comparing the transperitoneal and retroperitoneal RARN. However, as RARN is a special type of laparoscopic surgery, we use the laparoscopy surgery data as reference.

A retrospective analysis showed that retroperitoneal laparoscopic RN (RLRN) has similar oncological outcomes with transperitoneal laparoscopic RN (TLRN) in patients with the final pathological diagnosis of clear cell RCC [20]. A systemic review that involved 12 studies has assessed TLRN vs. RLRN approaches. The RLRN approach had a shorter time to renal artery control and a lower overall complication rate than TLRN. There were no significant differences between the retroperitoneal and transperitoneal approaches in perioperative and postoperative complications and oncological results. In appropriately selected patients, particularly patients with posteriorly located renal tumors, the retroperitoneal approach may be faster and equally safe compared with the transperitoneal approach [21].

For RARN, the transperitoneal approach has the advantages of a wider working space and more easily identifiable anatomical landmarks. However, it also requires bowel mobilization and adhesiolysis which resulted from previous abdominal surgery. The retroperitoneal approach, on the other hand, allows extra-peritoneal dissection and fast access to the renal hilum while avoiding the need for bowel mobilization. Relative indications for a retroperitoneal approach include a hostile surgical abdomen resulted from previous transperitoneal surgical procedures, peritoneal dialysis, morbid obesity, and pregnancy [22, 23].

4.1 Retroperitoneal RARN

For retroperitoneal RARN, there is a need to develop an adequate working space in the retroperitoneum before trocar placement. The anatomic landmarks are different, particularly for surgeons not using the retroperitoneal approach very often.

In pregnant patients, this approach may minimize peritoneal and uterine stimulation and risk of preterm labor [22]. In morbidly obese patients, this approach may directly access to the renal hilum, avoiding the abdominal apron [23].

Limitations of this approach include the smaller working space and reduced traction and instrument mobility.

4.1.1 Patient Positioning and Port Placement

Generally, a three-port technique is enough for retroperitoneal RARN, while the fourth robotic arm will facilitate the procedure in complex cases. The fourth robotic arm provides the console surgeon more independence from the assistant in retraction, ligation, or clamping of hilar vessels [22, 24].

Similar to laparoscopic retroperitoneal kidney surgery, in retroperitoneal RARN, the patient is placed in a lateral decubitus position with the umbilicus over the break of the operating table. The table is flexed to increase the space between costal margin and iliac crest. Position is secured by placing the posterior thoracic support. The arms are flexed with the shoulder at 90 degree to the chest in armrests. Pressure points should be properly padded, and an axillary roll should be placed in prevention of neuropraxia [25, 26].

A peripheral warming blanket and graduated compression stockings (GCS) or intermittent pneumatic compression (IPC) pump are applied in preventing deep venous thrombosis (DVT) and pulmonary embolism (PE).

A 10–15 degree anterior rotation of the operative table results the abdominal contents and peritoneum drop ventrally and more retroperitoneal working space.

The assistant surgeon stands in front of the patient with suction or laparoscopic fenestrated graspers.

A 12-mm camera port position is 3 cm above the iliac crest. The lateral and medial trocars are placed in the lateral margin of sacrospinalis and anterior axillary line parallel to the camera port. The assistant trocar is placed 2 cm about the iliac crest in the anterior axillary line as shown in Figs. 2 and 3.

A 3-cm horizontal incision is made 3 cm above the iliac crest, and blunt dissection is used to the level of thoracolumbar fascia by artery forceps. An index finger is introduced through the muscle layer to sweep the space and increase the

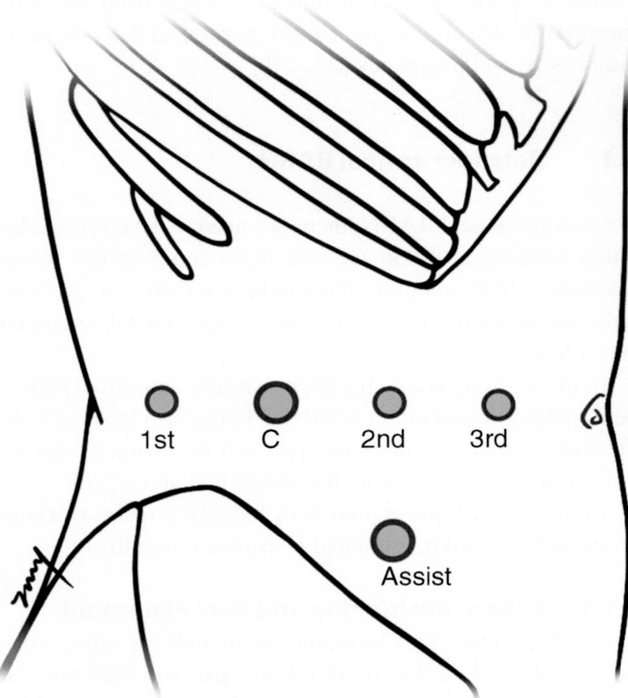

Fig. 2 Retroperitoneal RARN port placement

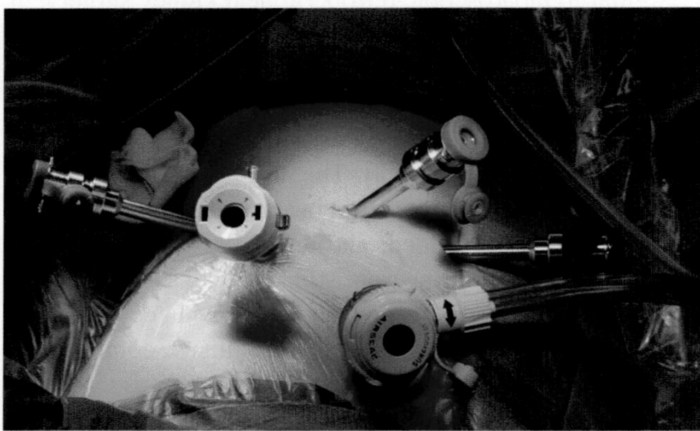

Fig. 3 Retroperitoneal RARN port placement with AirSeal

space for balloon dilation between the psoas muscle lying fascia and Gerota's fascia. Usually the finger can feel the 12th rib tip upward and kidney lower pole downward. A trocar-mounted balloon dilator or a self-made dilator is inserted and distended up to 600–800 ml; the dilation can be monitored by the scope.

After removal of the dilator, 8-mm lateral and medial trocars are placed under direct vision or with finger guidance. Be aware of the sharp injury risk. The third 8-mm robotic arm trocar is optional and is placed in the medial and interior of the field, approximately 8 cm from the anterior axillary line. Our experience found out that even the trocar distance less than 8 cm, there was not a lot of robotic arm collision and interference of the operation. Under direct vision, the peritoneum is swept medially toward the paramedian plane by laparoscopic grasping forceps.

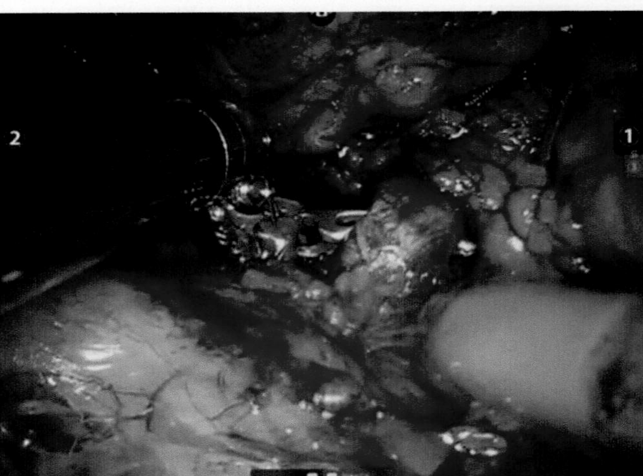

Fig. 4 Dissection of the renal hilum on the right side with fourth-arm ProGrasp forceps retraction

A 12-mm camera trocar was placed, CO_2 pneumoperitoneum is established, and pressure maintained at 12 mmHg.

For da Vinci *Si* system, the robot is docked over the patient head or 45° position to the operative table, for da Vinci *Xi* system, the robot can be docked from back or front [26]. Thirty-degree or zero-degree lens can be used depending on the surgeon's preference.

4.1.2 Kidney Preparation

In most cases, monopolar curved scissors and Maryland bipolar forceps or fenestrated bipolar forceps can do very precise dissection. ProGrasp forceps is often used in the fourth arm for retraction as shown in Fig. 4. Harmonic ACE-curved shears can be used for better bleeding control in large tumor case.

It is important to dissect the fatty tissue between psoas muscle fascia and Gerota's fascia. As it may interfere the surgical procedure, the fatty tissue is better to be freed and moved down to the iliac space. By this maneuver, the operation field will be expanded with clear anatomical landmarks, such as psoas muscle and ipsilateral peritoneal reflection.

After opening the posterolateral Gerota's fascia longitudinally along the kidney, further dissection can be carried along the psoas muscle to expose the ureter, the IVC on the right, and the aorta with pulsations on the left side. With good retraction, the renal hilum is readily accessible for dissection, and the size of the renal mass or kidney is not a significant issue during the hilar dissection.

Once the upper pole is defined, a transversely dissection between the kidney and adrenal gland is carried out within

Gerota's fascia. If an adrenalectomy is indicated, the adrenal vein is identified, clipped, and sectioned, and the whole adrenal gland is with the kidney specimen.

Mobilization of the specimen along avascular planes around Gerota's fascia will further develop and enlarge the retroperitoneal space as the dissection proceeds. The entire procedure can be achieved without a peritoneal opening.

4.1.3 Radical Nephrectomy

RN should remove the whole kidney bearing the tumor with Gerota's fascia incorporating the perinephric fat. The adrenal gland should be spared if there is no clinical evidence of adrenal gland invasion or metastasis.

The dissection is performed external to Gerota's fascia. On both sides, the renal hilum can be accessed directly. Then the renal artery is dissected. The renal artery is secured with two Hem-o-lok clips proximally and one clip distally and sectioned.

On the left side, after sectioning the renal artery, the adrenal vein, gonadal vein, and lumbar vein will be dissected and exposed. These veins and the renal vein can be secured with two Hem-o-lok clips proximally and one clip distally and sectioned.

On the right side, the IVC, gonadal vein, and ureter are exposed, and then the renal vein will be dissected. The gonadal vein can be spared. The renal vein can be secured with two Hem-o-lok clips proximally and one clip distally and sectioned. Caution should be taken in distinguishing the left ureter and lower pole renal artery aberrant branches.

The mobilization of the kidney and Gerota's fascia is from posterior surface to cephalad. The upper pole can be freed as shown in Fig. 5, often with spared adrenal gland. The dissection continues at the anterior aspect between Gerota's fascia and the peritoneum. At this point, the duodenum should be protected by careful dissection between Gerota's fascia and the duodenum. The lower pole is free, and the ureter is Hem-o-lok clip ligated and sectioned as far distally as possible.

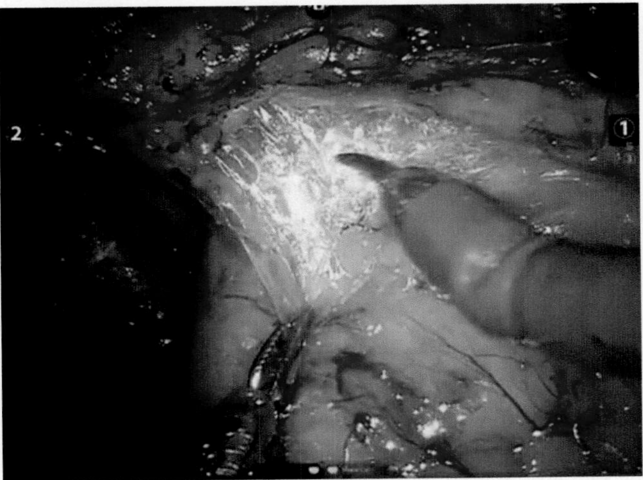

Fig. 5 The dissection at the anterior aspect between Gerota's fascia and the peritoneum and freeing the right upper pole of the kidney

The specimen is placed into a retrieval bag which is inserted through the 12-mm assistant trocar to minimize the risk of direct contact with the tumor.

Lymphadenectomy can then be performed. Lymphatic tissue should be dissected and ligated with clips, bipolar coagulation, or harmonic shears.

The specimen is then retrieved through an iliac incision, which is usually a linked incision between two trocar sites. A free drainage is placed into the retroperitoneal space for 24 hours. The extraction wound is closed in layers. Other trocar sites are closed with intracutaneous absorbable running sutures and dressed.

4.2 Transperitoneal RARN

4.2.1 Patient Positioning

For transperitoneal RARN, patient positioning is similar to what is used for laparoscopic or robotic kidney surgery. The flank position involves the patient lying on their side with the involved kidney side elevated. Positioning should be done carefully to prevent pressure points, particularly for longer procedures.

Flank position for laparoscopic or robotic surgery has been described anywhere from 30 to 90 degrees with some surgeons using 45 or 60 degrees. The use of the full 90 degrees of laterality, though, will provide more gravity retraction of the small bowel after mobilization of the colon, and the duodenum and spleen will remain out of the operative field without deliberate retraction since gravity alone will provide this. This can reduce the number of robotic arms needed or assistant ports for retraction. Flexion of the operative table is not necessary in robotic surgery, and the kidney rest should not be used as it may increase the risk of rhabdomyolysis or other injuries by placing pressure on the spine and perispinal muscles.

4.2.2 Port Placement

The patient side cart should ideally approach the patient from behind the side of the involved kidney, particularly if the da Vinci® *S* or *Si* system (Intuitive Surgical, Inc., Sunnyvale, CA) is used, while the da Vinci® *Xi* robot is more flexible and can approach the bedside from multiple directions. The *Xi* patient side cart can be docked to the bedside from multiple directions since the tower holding the robotic arms can be rotated.

A three-port approach can be used to perform robotic nephrectomy, including a camera port and two ports for robotic instruments. The robotic camera port can be placed at the umbilicus or above or below this level still along the linea alba to avoid muscle puncture. Alternatively, with the *Xi*, the camera port can be placed lateral to the midline, but this will lessen the field of view or ability to back away from the target anatomy for a wider view. The 30-degree down lens is commonly used.

The robotic ports for the left and right robotic arms are placed above and below the camera port location and are taken care of to avoid placing the ports in line with each other so as to prevent arm collisions. For complex procedures or earlier in a surgeon's learning curve, a port can be placed for the fourth arm and/or for the assistant to perform suction or retraction as needed. In right-sided nephrectomies, a liver retractor is optional and may be recommended for less-experienced surgeons. Alternatively, the robotic surgeon can lift the liver and keep it above the shaft of the right arm instrument throughout the dissection without needing a liver retractor port.

4.2.3 Robotic Instruments

RARN is commonly performed with monopolar cautery in the right hand using the hook cautery or cautery scissor and with a bipolar instrument in the left hand. To avoid an addition of an assistant port, clipping of the vessels can be performed by using robotic Hem-o-lok clips or the robotic stapler rather than having the assistant perform this critical step. A minimum of two clips should be placed on the renal artery and vein. If the fourth arm is used, the ProGrasp is usually used for retraction.

4.2.4 Transperitoneal Right RARN

In both right and left transperitoneal RARN, the first step is reflection of the colon. The plane between the colon and Gerota's fascia should be preserved since early entry into Gerota's fascia can be disorienting or worse. After the colon is reflected medially enough to allow gravity to keep it out of the field, the hilum can be approached without needing retraction. The duodenum is next seen as well as the vena cava in thinner patients. Kocherization of the duodenum will then allow identification of the vena cava if not previously seen. The vena cava can then be followed until the take-off of the right renal vein is found.

The kidney can then be lifted away from the underlying psoas plane lateral to the vena cava starting at the level of the lower pole of the kidney and then moved cephalad toward the hilum. The kidney and surrounding Gerota's fascia are lifted laterally to keep the renal vessels on stretch. To allow dissection with two hands, either the fourth-arm instrument or assistant retractor can accomplish this stretch, but alternatively in a three-port approach, a single clip between Gerota's fascia and interior side wall will suspend the kidney equally well (Fig. 6).

The renal vein entry to the vena cava is approached posteriorly to identify the renal artery behind the vein. The renal artery is clipped or stapled first followed by the vein. Again, a minimum of two clips should be left on the artery if not stapling it with the kidney end of the renal artery either clipped as well or cauterized to prevent back bleeding. The renal vein is also clipped leaving two clips in the patient or stapled.

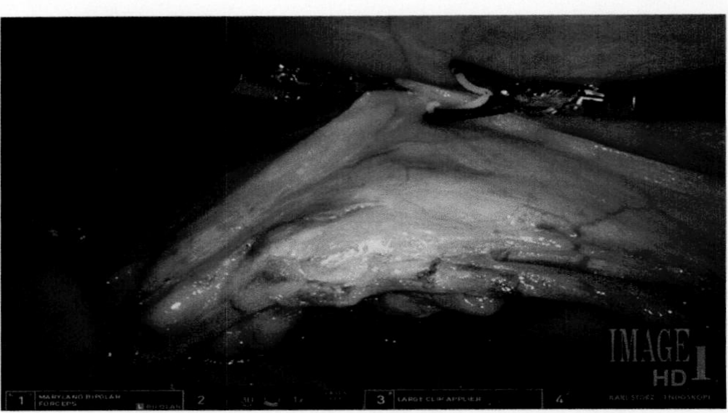

Fig. 6 Placing the left kidney on stretch with a clip to allow hilar dissection

The adrenal gland can be spared in most cases. Vessels between the upper pole of the kidney and adrenal should be carefully controlled with bipolar cautery at a minimum since this can be a common area of postoperative bleeding if not carefully divided.

If the adrenal gland is being removed with the specimen, the adrenal vein must be identified as it enters the vena cava posteriorly and controlled with a clip or bipolar cautery or both. The ureter is then clipped and divided with the lateral attachments taken last so that the specimen does not fall medially during the remainder of the dissection. The specimen is extracted in a bag ideally without cutting the muscle through the linea alba or with a Pfannenstiel incision.

4.2.5 Transperitoneal Left RARN

Left RARN begins the same way as on the right side by reflecting the colon medially. The spleen should be reflected en bloc with the colon as well by continuing the incision of the line of Toldt cranially above the spleen so that the colon and spleen will reflect medially as one unit along with the pancreas. The left kidney within Gerota's fascia is then lifted up from the psoas muscle as on the right to place the hilum on stretch. The psoas plane is followed cephalad until the renal vein is identified. The renal artery is usually found behind the renal vein as on the right. The artery and vein are then controlled with clips or stapling as on the right side. One distinction from the right side is that the artery should not be clipped directly on the aorta as a stump of artery is necessary to prevent the clips from being pushed off the aorta from the blood pressure behind them. The adrenal can be taken or spared, but unlike on the right, the adrenal vein will empty into the left renal vein.

4.3 Postoperative Management

Following multimodal pain control protocols to control and prevent perioperative pain, the postoperative pain is usually well controlled with intravenous or oral narcotics.

As suggested in ERAS protocol [27], mobilization of patient is recommended as early as the patient tolerates. A clear liquid diet can be started the same day of surgery if there was no risk of bowel injury during the procedure and advance to regular diet if the patient can tolerate the day after. Foley catheter can be removed the same day or at day 1 after the surgery. The drainage can be removed at day 1 after the surgery. The patient can be discharged on the first or second postoperative day.

4.4 Complications and Management

As RARN is indicated in more complex cases, the risk of complication is an unavoidable consequence even in experienced hands. To minimize the risk of complications, adequate pre-surgery preparation and pre-surgery imaging are essential.

Generally, RARN had similar intraoperative and postoperative complications as those of LRN [5, 28]. However, Gershman has reported that RARN was associated with lower perioperative morbidity than conventional LRN (20.4 vs. 27.2%, $p < 0.001$) [29].

The potential complications of a RARN have been well described [30]. Access-related complications include abdominal wall hematomas, vascular injuries, and organ injuries. Intraoperatively, liver laceration and pancreas, spleen, and vascular injuries were reported. Transfusion rate was reported of 7.9%. Mechanical failure and bleeding requiring conversion were reported as well. Bowel injury is another potential risky complication [31]. Postoperative complications such as wound dehiscence, wound infection, incisional hernias, prolonged ileus, pneumonia, pulmonary embolism, and atrial fibrillation were reported as well [30].

5 RARN with IVC Thrombectomy

RCC with venous tumor thrombus extending to the IVC has an estimated prevalence of 4–10% [32].Surgically complete resection of tumor thrombus is the only treatment option that offers the potential cure for these patients [33, 34]. Radical nephrectomy with IVC tumor thrombectomy is a technically and physically challenging procedure and has traditionally been performed open approach with high risks of perioperative morbidity and mortality [35]. It has been reported that the perioperative mortality rates range from 3.5 to 9.6% [36–38].

The robotic surgery technology has enabled urologists to perform the RARN with concurrent inferior vena cava (IVC) thrombectomy to reduce perioperative complications including massive blood loss, shorter operating time, and length of hospital stay and overcomes the limitations of a conventional laparoscopic approach [39–41].

In 2011, Abaza reported the first successful robotic IVC thrombectomy [40]. After that, there were several groups who reported their experience and techniques of RARN with IVC thrombectomy from level I to level III IVC thrombus [42–49]. Our team (Zhang Xu and Ma Xin) performed robotic IVC thrombectomy (R-IVCTE) since 2013 and have reported our experience of robotic RN with level I–IV IVC thrombectomy [9, 50–53]. In the section, we describe the detailed techniques of different levels of thrombus mainly based on our techniques.

5.1 Indications and Contraindications

5.1.1 Indications

Robotic RARN and IVC tumor thrombectomy are the treatment options for following RCC with IVC tumor thrombus patients.

RARN and IVC thrombectomy are recommended for RCC with tumor thrombus level I thrombus (thrombus extending ≤2 cm above the renal vein, Mayo classification) and Level II thrombus (thrombus extending >2 cm above the renal vein, but below the hepatic veins). However, only highly selected level III thrombus (thrombus extending hepatic vein, but below the diaphragm) and level IV thrombus (thrombus extending above diaphragm or into the right atrium) could be managed by robotic approach.

It is suggested that the operation of level III–IV thrombus should be completed by a multidisciplinary team, including experts from urology, hepatobiliary surgery, and cardiac surgery if cardiopulmonary bypass (CPB) is needed.

5.1.2 Contraindications

Patient with uncorrected coagulopathy.

Patient who are medically unfit for general anesthesia.

There was a history of abdominal operation and severe abdominal adhesion.

Huge primary tumor or enlarged congestive liver.

5.2 Preoperative Preparation

5.2.1 General Patient Preparation

Preoperative patient preparations are similar as those for transperitoneal robotic surgery, including preoperative skin preparation, bowel preparation, prophylactic antibiotics, etc.

5.2.2 Special Patient Preparation

Low molecular heparin (if indicated) is given to decrease the risk of pulmonary embolism.

Preoperative renal artery embolization on the left side is recommended. For the right side cases, preoperative embolization is helpful in reducing intraoperative bleeding, dissecting IVC and renal vein, and extracting tumor thrombus.

Temporary IVC filter is not recommended due to the risk of thrombogenesis of contralateral renal vein and hepatic vein, which may affect tumor thrombus dissection during the operation.

Preoperative color Doppler ultrasound re-examination for IVC is recommended especially for level II–IV thrombus to ensure the latest status of tumor thrombus.

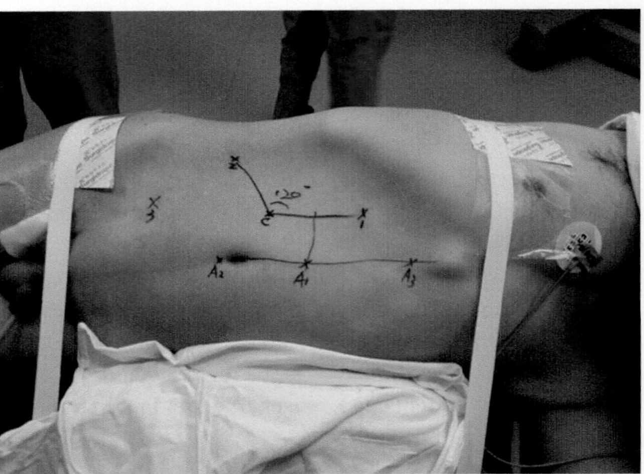

Fig. 7 Patient position and port placement sites

5.3 Step-by-Step Operative Technique

5.3.1 Anesthesia and Patient Position

After general anesthesia and Foley catheter placement, the patient is positioned to 60- to 70-degree left lateral recumbent position with flank extension supported by gel pad. Other than respiration and ECG monitoring, blood pressure monitoring via jugular vein and radial artery are required for all cases. Multichannel venous access should be established, which is helpful for medication and fluid infusion. For right RCC, R-IVCTE and RARN can be both completed through this position. For the left RCC, R-IVCTE can also be completed through this position. After R-IVCTE, left RARN will be performed in 60–70° right lateral decubitus position.

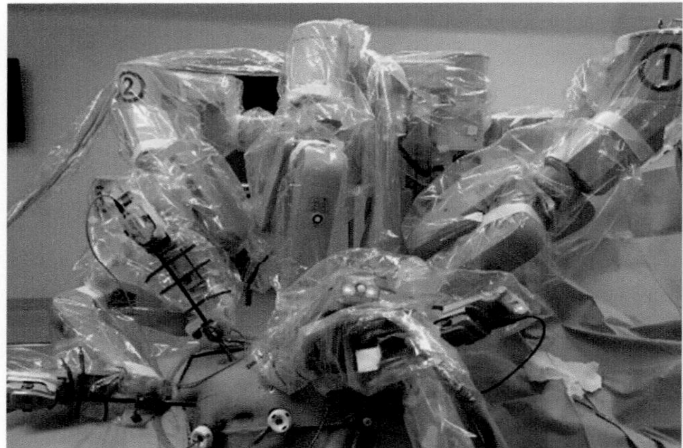

Fig. 8 Port placement and docking

5.3.2 Right RARN and IVC Thrombectomy

Patient Position and Port Placement

The patients were positioned in a 70° left lateral decubitus position (Fig. 7). The first assistant trocar is placed at 6 cm above the umbilicus for the insertion of the suction device. The second assistant trocar is placed at the subumbilical cord for the application of Hem-o-lok clips, and the third assistant trocar is placed near the xiphoid under the costal margin for liver retraction. A monopolar curved scissor, bipolar Maryland clamp, and ProGrasp grasper are inserted as the first, second, and third arms, respectively. All the instruments are placed in to the abdominal cavity under direct vision. During the operation, the instruments on the second and third arm can be exchanged as indicated (Fig. 8).

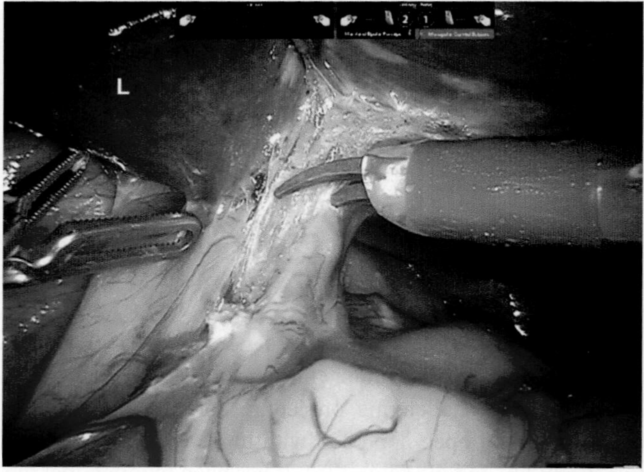

Fig. 9 The hepatocolic ligament is divided (L, liver)

Dissection of Inferior Vena Cava, Left Renal Vein, and Right Renal Vein

The hepatocolic ligament and hepatorenal ligament are divided (Figs. 9 and 10). The liver is retracted upward with a needle holder (Fig. 11), and the retraction is secured by

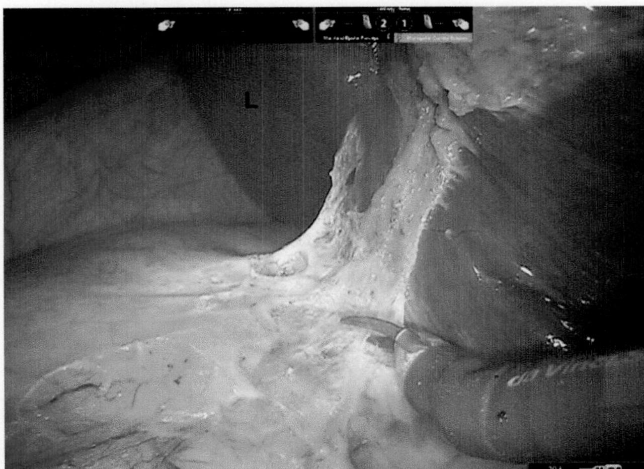

Fig. 10 The hepatorenal ligament is divided (L, liver)

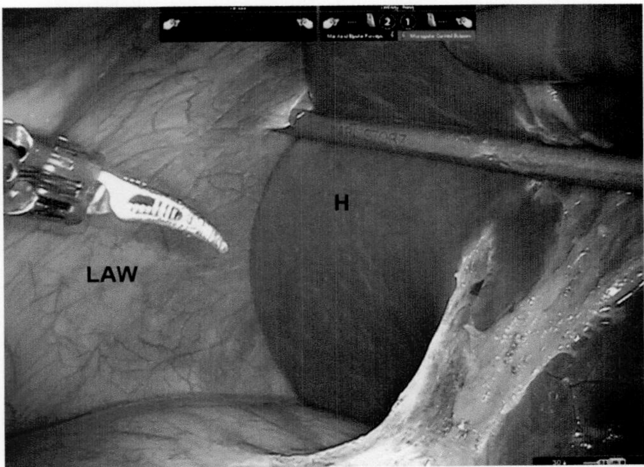

Fig. 11 The liver is retracted upward with a needle holder (L, liver; LAW, lateral abdominal wall)

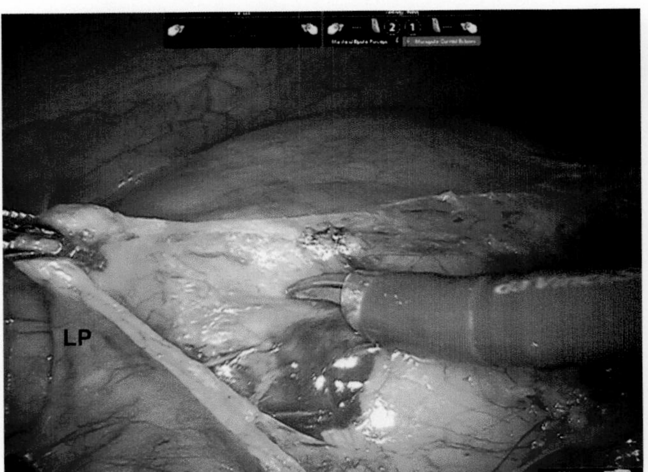

Fig. 12 The peritoneum is incised, and the retroperitoneum space is exposed (LP, lateral peritoneum)

clamping the needle holder at the lateral abdominal wall for exposure of the operating field. The ascending colon is medialized to expose the retroperitoneum space (Fig. 12). The duodenum is mobilized until the IVC is fully exposed (Figs. 13 and 14). The perivascular fascia is dissected to skeletonize the IVC, right renal vein, and left renal vein (Figs. 15 and 16).

Dissection of the IVC at the Thrombus Level, Left Renal Vein, and Part Lumbar Vein

The ventral surface of the IVC is exposed. For level II IVC thrombus, the accessory hepatic vein and right suprarenal vein are clipped and divided for cross-clamping of the IVC (Fig. 17). The left renal vein was dissected circumferentially at the interaortocaval space (Fig. 18). Then the dorsal surface of the IVC is mobilized, and the affected lumbar vein was clipped and divided (Figs. 19 and 20).

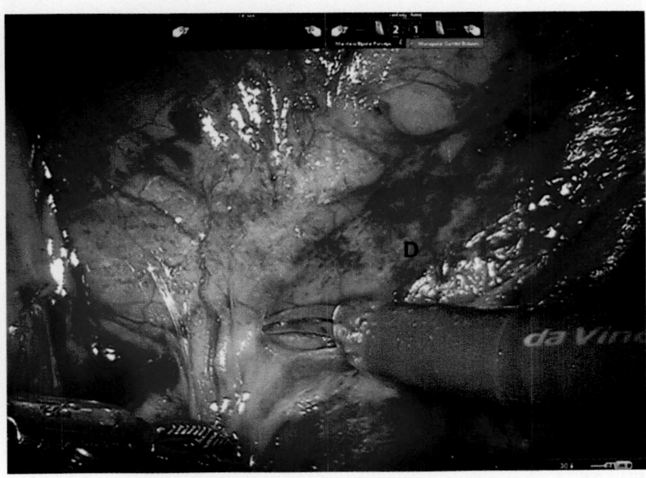

Fig. 13 The duodenum is mobilized medially (D, duodenum)

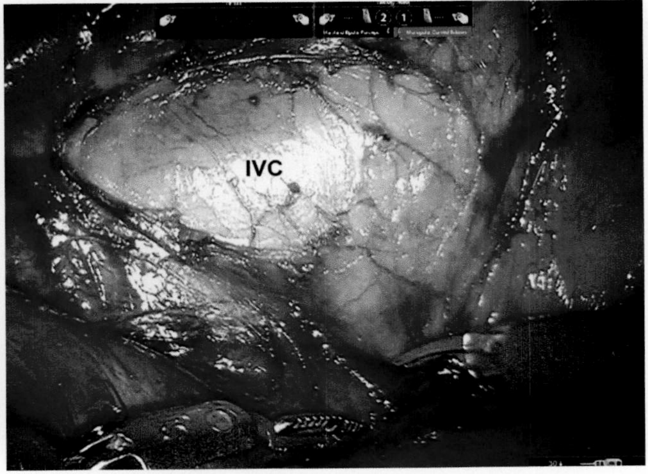

Fig. 14 IVC exposure (IVC, inferior vena cava)

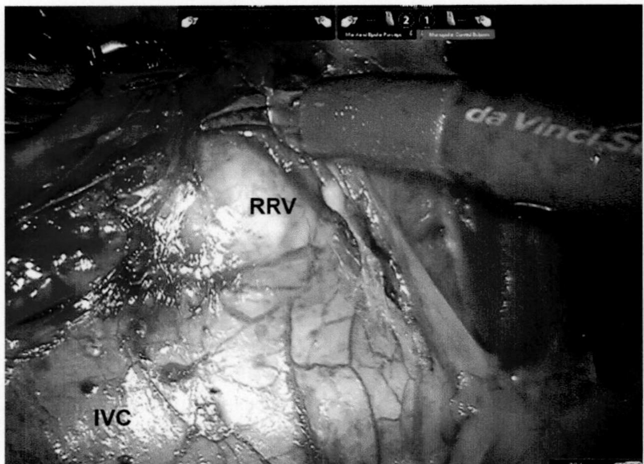

Fig. 15 Right renal vein exposure (IVC, inferior vena cava; RRV, right renal vein)

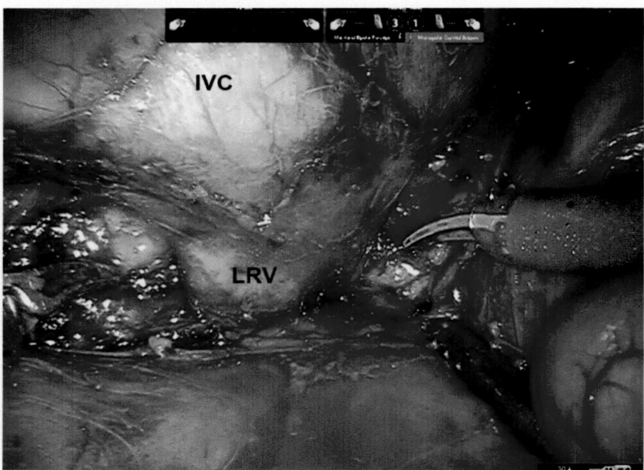

Fig. 16 Left renal vein exposure (IVC, inferior vena cava, LRV, left renal vein)

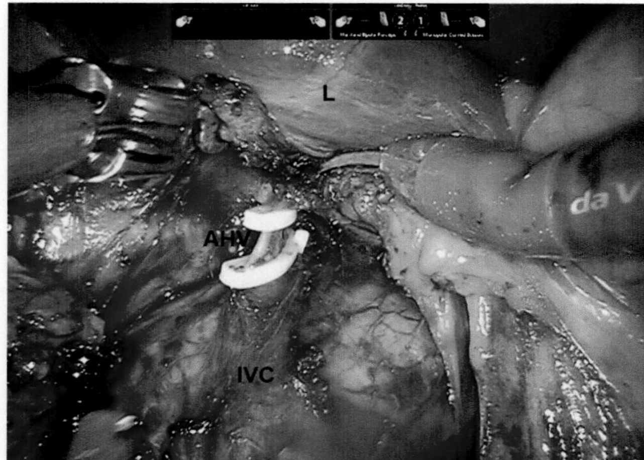

Fig. 17 The accessory hepatic vein is divided and clipped with Hem-o-lok clips (L, liver; AHV, accessory hepatic vein; IVC, inferior vena cava)

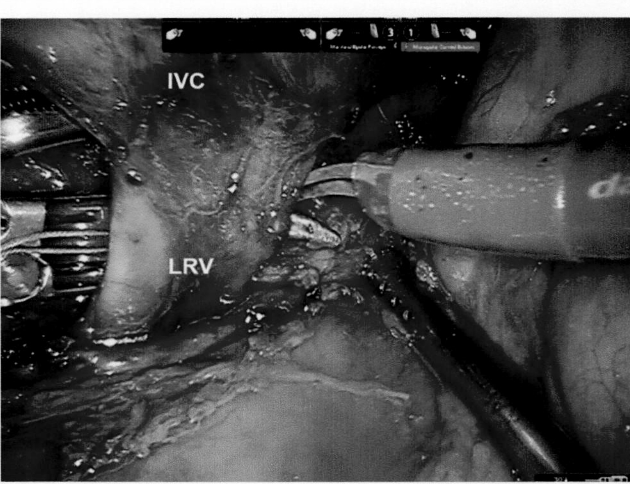

Fig. 18 The left renal vein is isolated (IVC, inferior vena cava; LRV, left renal vein)

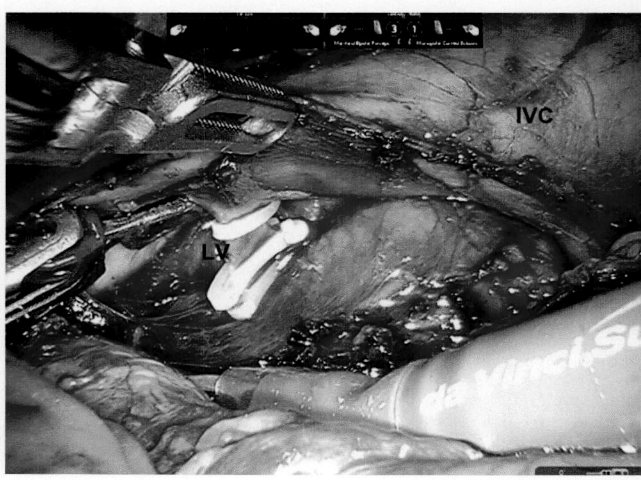

Fig. 19 The lumbar veins are divided and then clipped (IVC, inferior vena cava; LV, lumbar vein)

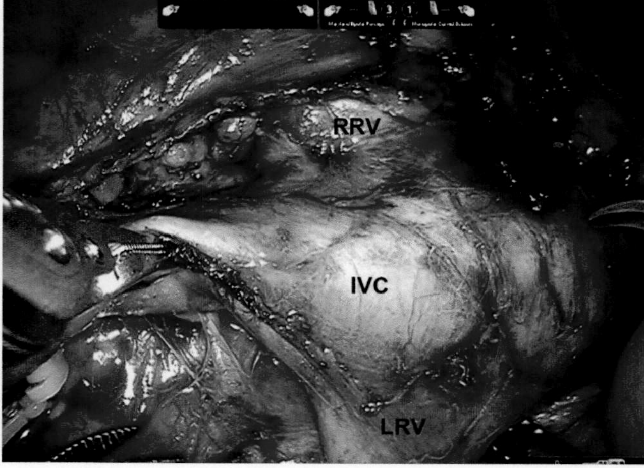

Fig. 20 Complete exposure of the IVC, left renal vein, and right renal vein (IVC, inferior vena cava; LRV, left renal vein; RRV, right renal vein)

Sequential Occlusion of the Distal IVC, Left Renal Vein, and Proximal IVC.

The IVC proximal and distal to the thrombus and the left renal vein are double looped with vessel loop and secured with Hem-o-lok clip for surgeon control (Figs. 21, 22, 23). The distal IVC, left renal vein, and proximal IVC were sequentially occluded (Fig. 24).

5.3.3 Extraction of Thrombus

After the sequential occlusion, the IVC wall is incised, and the thrombus is removed (Figs. 25 and 26). After irrigation of the IVC lumen with heparinized saline, the IVC is closed with 5–0 polypropylene suture (Fig. 27). Occlusion at the proximal IVC, left renal vein, and distal IVC is released in order. Hemostasis is secured. The thrombus is inserted into a specimen bag to avoid tumor dissemination.

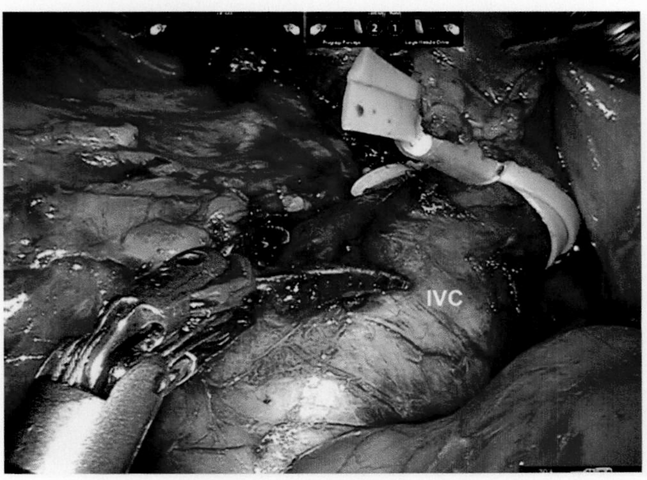

Fig. 23 The vessel loops were wrapped twice around the proximal IVC (IVC, inferior vena cava)

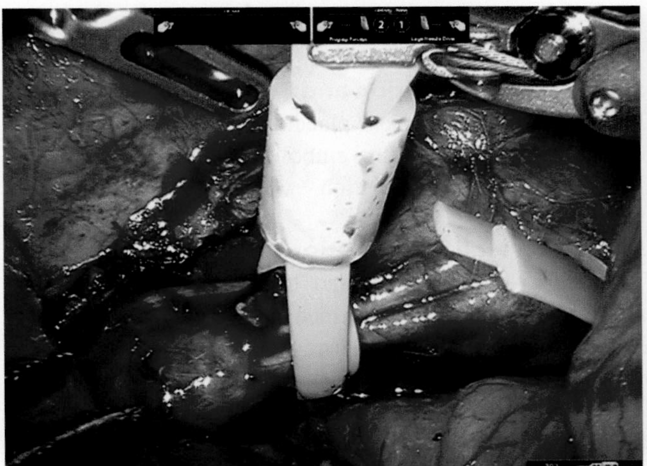

Fig. 21 The vessel loops were wrapped twice around the cephalic IVC

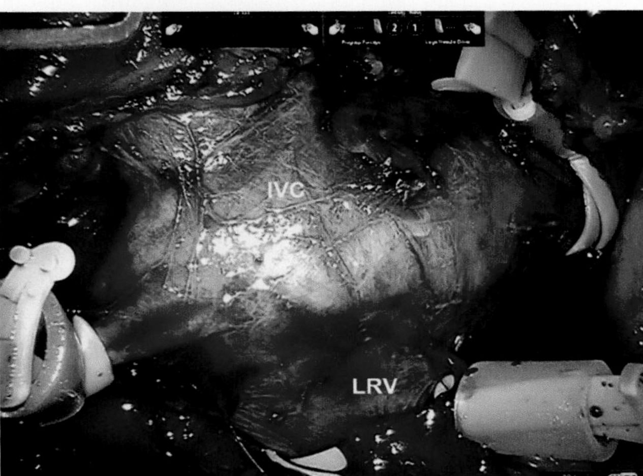

Fig. 24 The caudal IVC, left renal vein, and cephalic IVC were sequentially clamped (IVC, inferior vena cava; LRV, left renal vein)

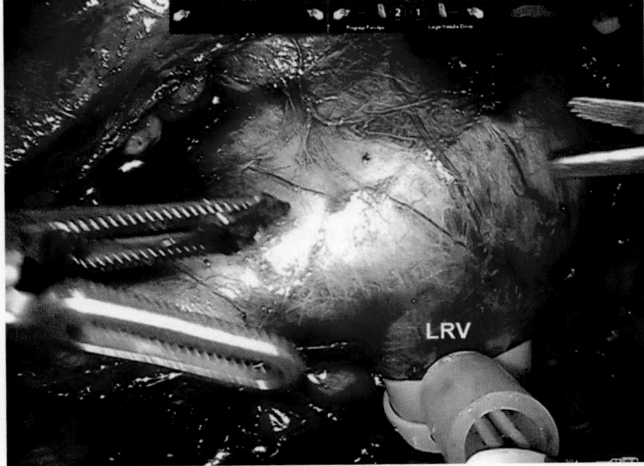

Fig. 22 The vessel loops were wrapped twice around the left renal vein (LRV, left renal vein)

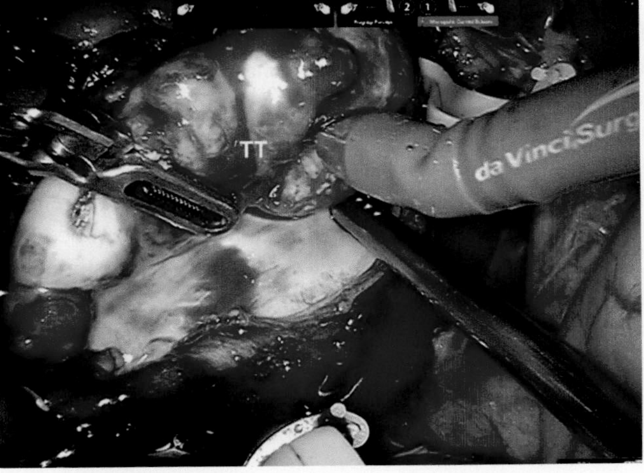

Fig. 25 The IVC thrombus is exposed and excised (TT, tumor thrombus)

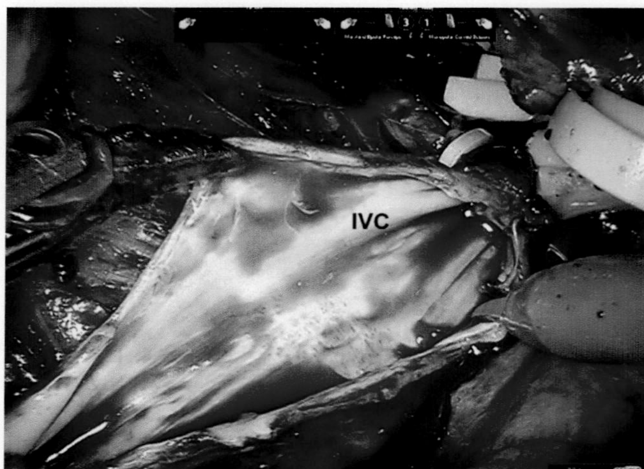

Fig. 26 The IVC thrombus was completely removed (IVC, inferior vena cava)

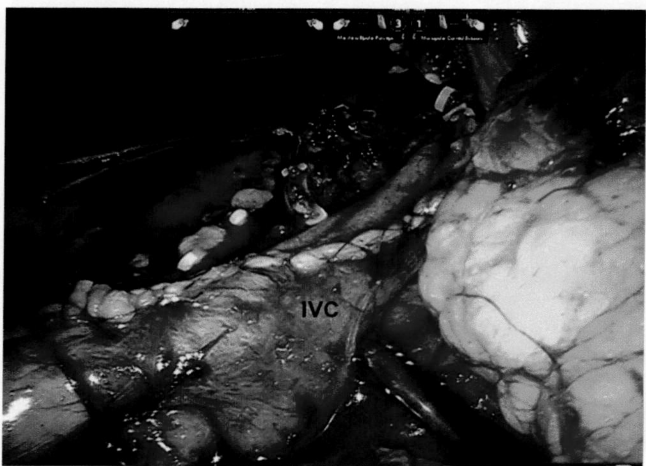

Fig. 27 The IVC is closed by a running suture (IVC, inferior vena cava)

Right Radical Nephrectomy

In the same position, the right renal artery is isolated, clipped with Hem-o-lok clips, and divided (Fig. 28). The right kidney and adrenal gland are mobilized as described in previous section. Right renal artery embolization is recommended 1–2 h before operation. In cases in which renal artery embolization is not performed, a modified technique can be used. The right renal artery is dissected and ligated in the interaortocaval space before IVC clamping. The right kidney is removed together with the IVC thrombus if possible. If they can't be removed together, the right renal vein will be transected with Endo-GIA before clamping the IVC.

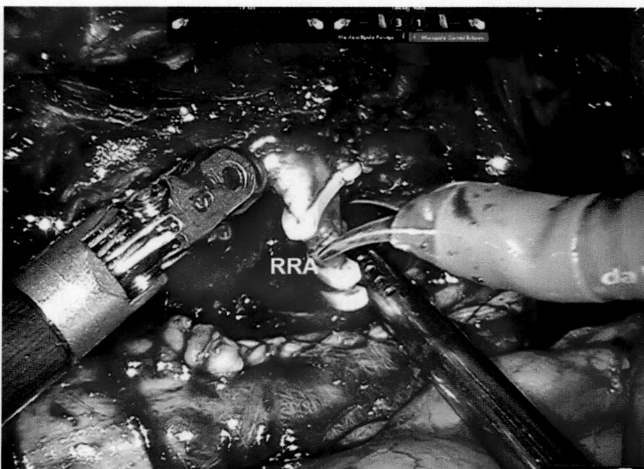

Fig. 28 The right renal artery is clipped with Hem-o-lok clips and then divided (RRA, right renal artery)

5.4 Left RARN and IVC Thrombectomy

5.4.1 Patient Position and Port Placement

Patient position and trocar placement are similar as for the right RCC. Left renal artery embolization must be performed 1–2 hours before the operation.

5.4.2 Dissection of Inferior Vena Cava

The hepatocolic ligament and hepatorenal ligament were incised, and the liver is retracted upward. The ascending colon is medialized. The perirenal fascia is dissected. The duodenum is medialized to expose the IVC (Fig. 29).

5.4.3 Isolation of the Right and Left Renal Veins

The right renal vein (Fig. 30) and left renal vein (Fig. 31) are skeletonized. The left renal vein, including the thrombus, was transected with Endo-GIA (Figs. 32 and 33).

The procedure of IVC tumor thrombus removal was the same as that of the right tumor. After the removal of IVC tumor thrombus, the patient was repositioned in a 70° right lateral decubitus position, and the nephrectomy of the left side was completed.

5.5 Robot-Assisted Level III IVC Thrombectomy: Left Side

5.5.1 Preoperative Preparation

Renal artery embolization on the affected side was conducted 1–2 hours preoperatively for patients with left-sided or right-

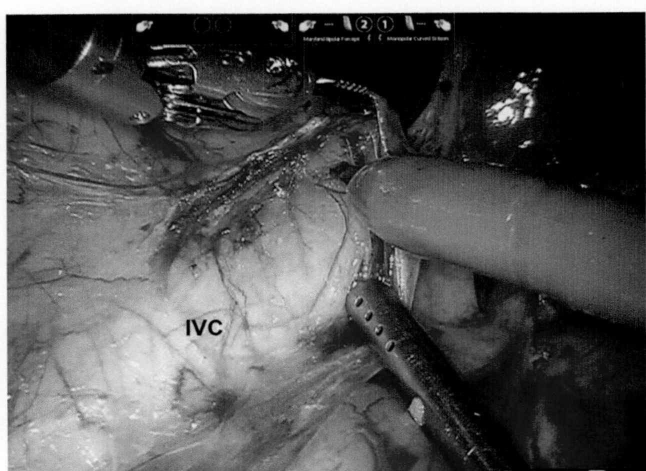

Fig. 29 IVC exposure (IVC, inferior vena cava)

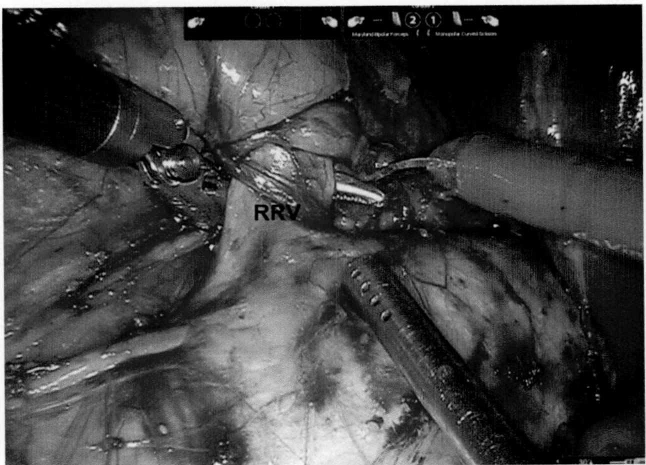

Fig. 30 The right renal vein is dissected (RRV, right renal vein)

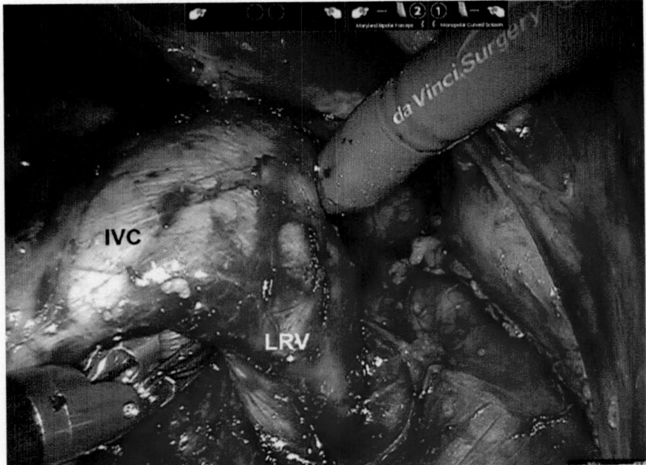

Fig. 31 The left renal vein is dissected (LRV, left renal vein; IVC, inferior vena cava)

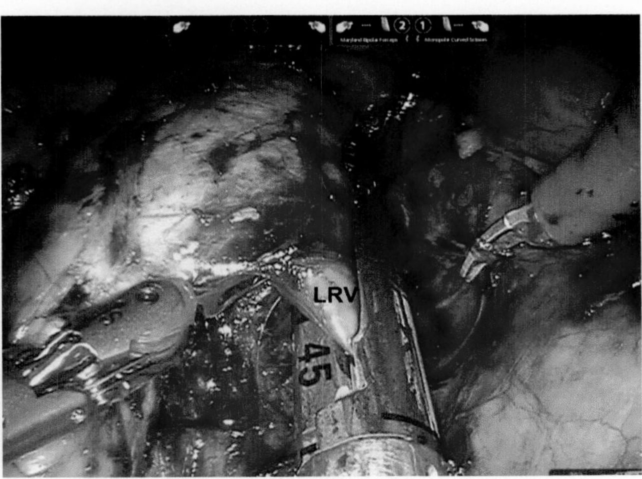

Fig. 32 The left renal vein is transected with Endo-GIA stapler (LRV, left renal vein)

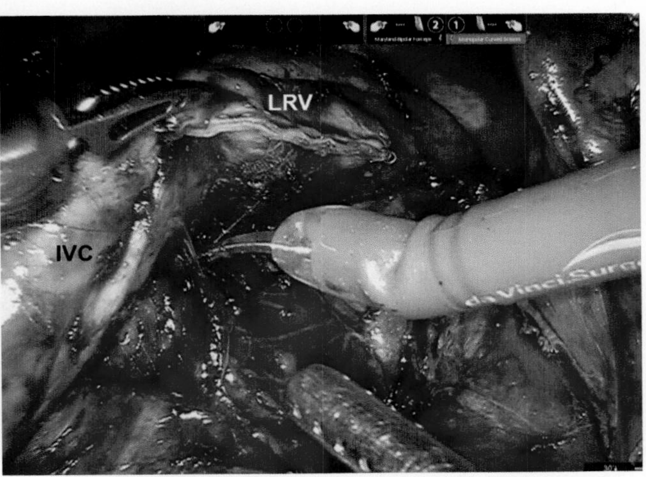

Fig. 33 The left renal vein is divided (LRV, left renal vein; IVC, inferior vena cava)

sided large kidney tumor. Transesophageal ultrasound was prepared for intraoperative monitoring of thrombus extent/tip stability during manipulation.

5.5.2 Patient Position and Trocar Placement

For liver mobilization, the patients were placed in a 30–45° dorsal elevated lithotomy position (Fig. 34a), and the five-port method for trocar placement was deployed (Fig. 34b).

Then the patients were repositioned in a modified left lateral decubitus position with a 70° bump (thrombectomy position, Fig. 34c), and the seven-port method for trocar placement was used (Fig. 34d). Four trocars can be reused (points A1, C, 1, and 2 in Fig. 34b and d).

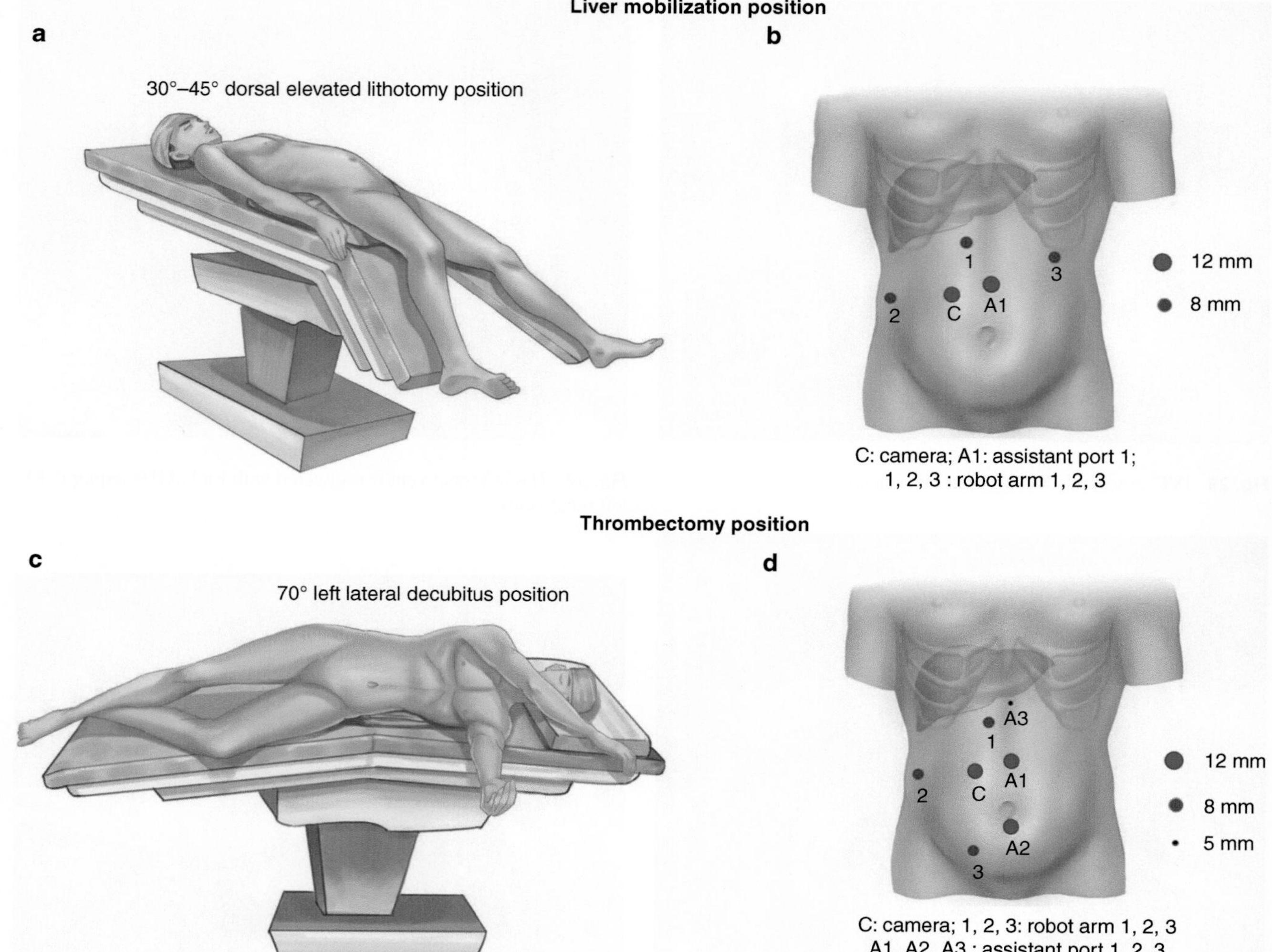

Fig. 34 Liver mobilization position and thrombectomy position

5.5.3 Surgical Strategy

Under the "liver mobilization position," we mobilized both the right and left lobes of the liver to expose retrohepatic IVC and control the suprahepatic infradiaphragmatic IVC. Under the "thrombectomy position," the left thrombus-involved renal vein was stapled by Endo-GIA; the caudal IVC, right renal artery (RRA), right renal veins (RRV), first porta hepatis (FPH), and suprahepatic infradiaphragmatic IVC were sequentially clamped; and the thrombi were removed (Fig. 35).

For the left kidney tumor, the perihepatic ligaments, including the round and falciform ligaments (Fig. 36), the right and left triangular and coronary ligaments, and hepatocolic ligament, were disconnected under the "liver mobilization position" (Figs. 37, 38, 39, 40, 41). Additional SHVs were ligated to fully expose the retrohepatic IVC (Figs. 42 and 43). Both the right and left liver lobes were mobilized off the IVC. A 10-Fr catheter was placed in the suprahepatic and infra-diaphragmatic IVC above the proximal IVC thrombus (Fig. 44). Then, the robotic transabdominal control of the suprahepatic and infra-diaphragmatic IVC would be achieved. After liver mobilization, patients were repositioned in a "thrombectomy position." The tumor-bearing left renal vein (LRV) was dissected circumferentially. Finally, the LRV was stapled (Fig. 45). Subsequently, the caudal IVC, right renal artery (RRA), right renal vein (RRV), first porta hepatis (FPH), and suprahepatic and infra-diaphragmatic IVC were clamped in order (Figs. 46, 47, 48, 49, 50). Finally, the IVC wall was incised, and the tumor thrombus was removed (Figs. 51 and 52).

For the right kidney tumor, the position and placement of trocars for liver mobilization and thrombectomy were the

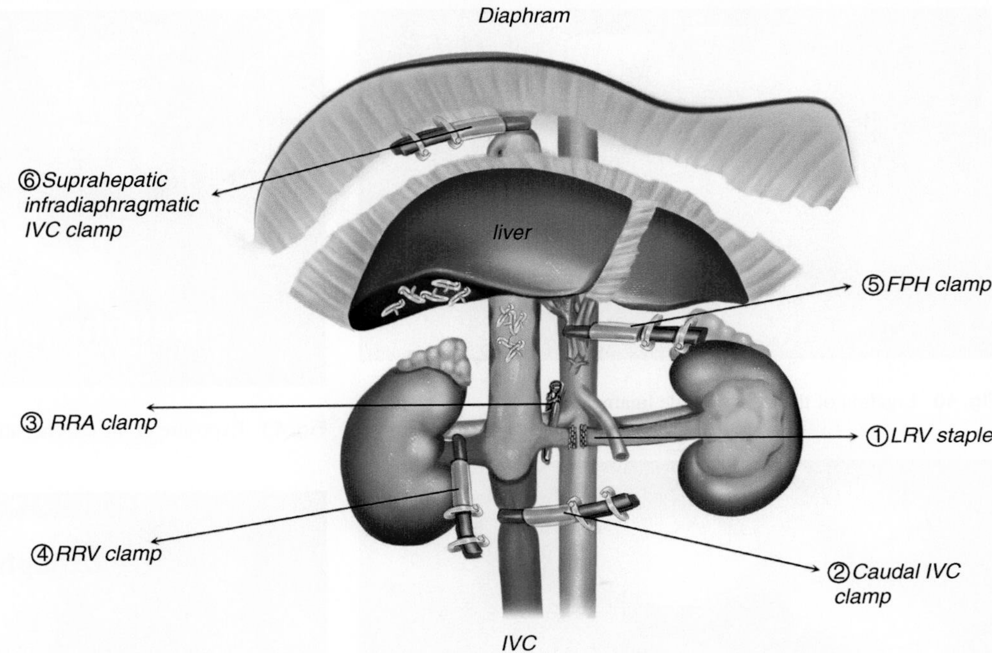

Fig. 35 A surgical strategy diagram for level III thrombus on the left side

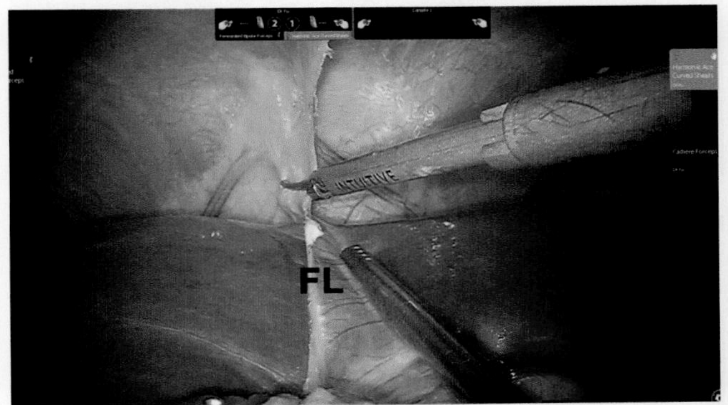

Fig. 36 Ligation of the liver falciform ligament (FL)

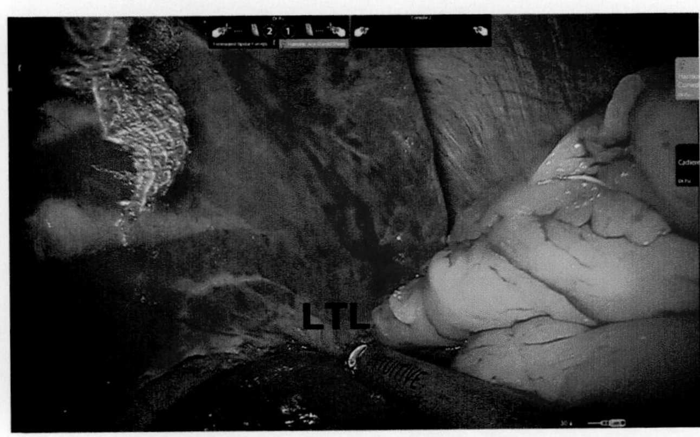

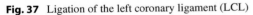

Fig. 38 Ligation of the left triangle ligament (LTL)

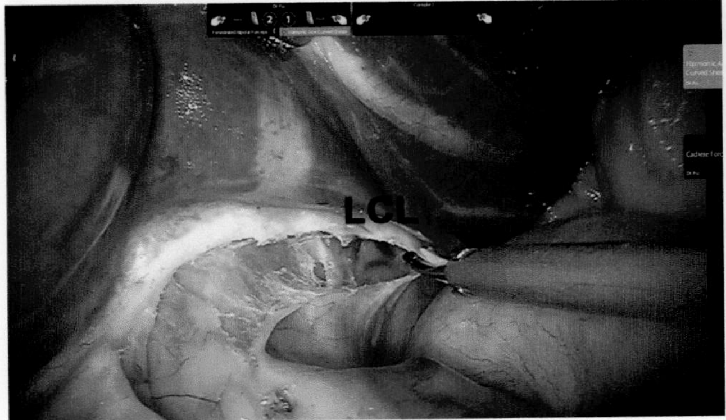

Fig. 37 Ligation of the left coronary ligament (LCL)

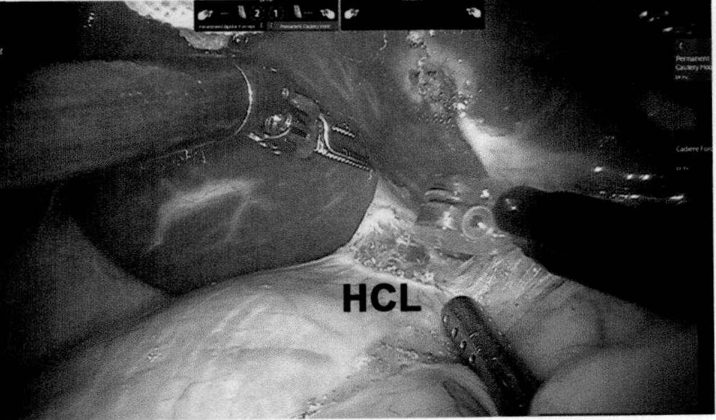

Fig. 39 Ligation of the hepatocolic ligament (HCL)

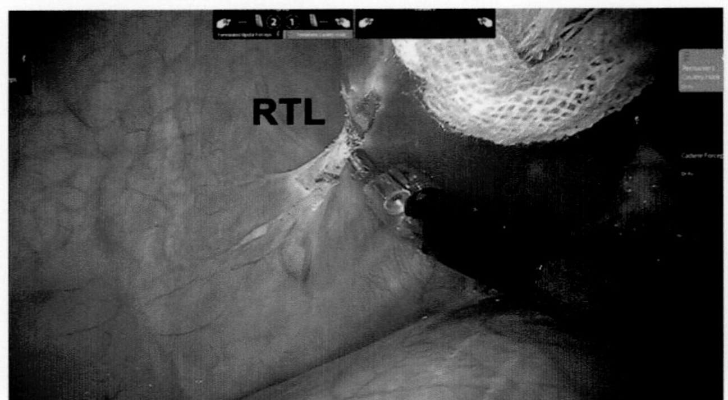

Fig. 40 Ligation of the right triangle ligament (RTL)

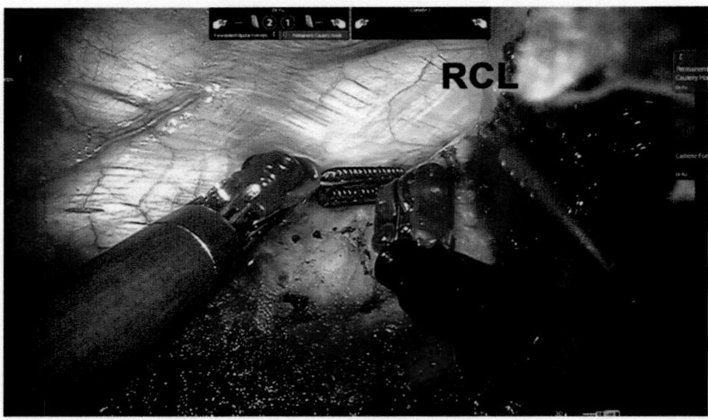

Fig. 41 Ligation of the right coronary ligament (RCL)

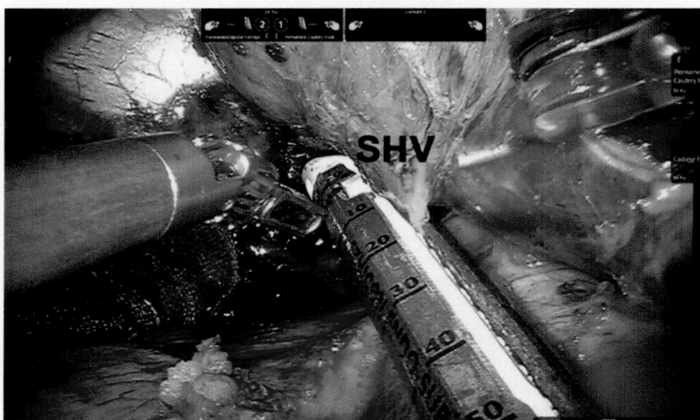

Fig. 42 Transection of the short hepatic vein (SHV)

same as for the left RTs. The steps were similar except for clamping of renal vessels. For the right kidney tumor, we clamped the LRV, while we did not staple the tumor-bearing RRV, and we did not clamp the left renal artery.

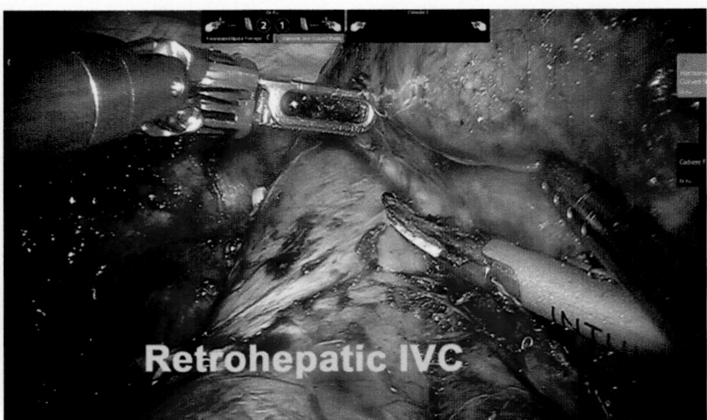

Fig. 43 Exposure of the retrohepatic IVC

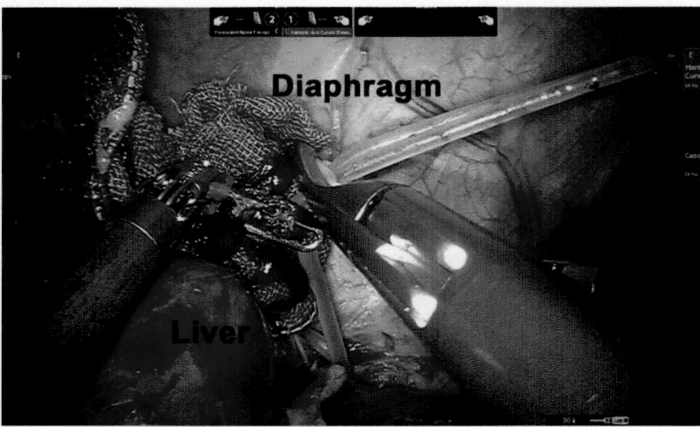

Fig. 44 Placement of suprahepatic infradiaphragmatic IVC tourniquet with a 10-Fr catheter

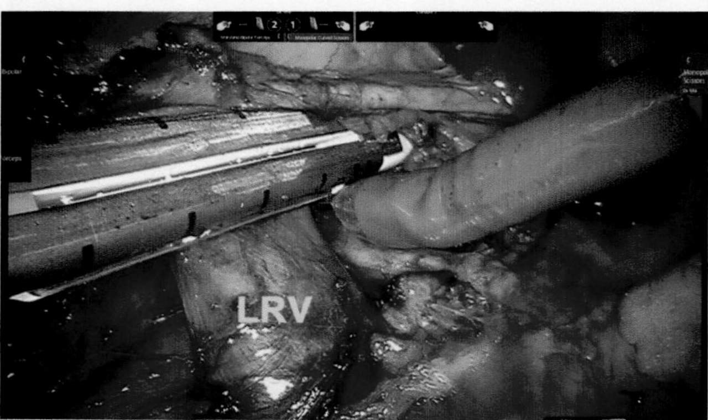

Fig. 45 Transection of the left renal vein (LRV)

In summary, level III RA-IVCT requires liver mobilization and clamping of the FPH and suprahepatic and infradiaphragmatic IVC.

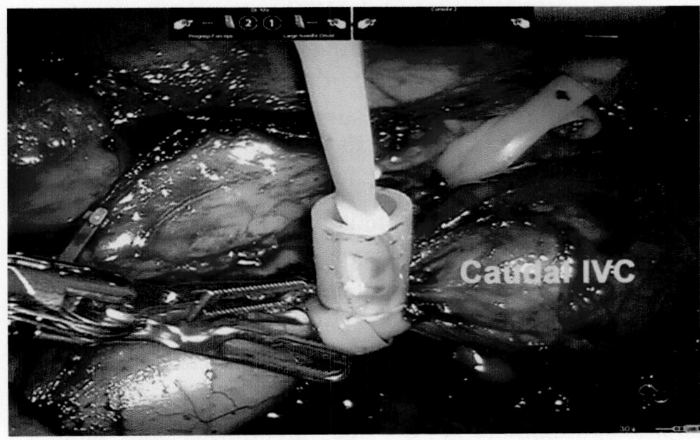

Fig. 46 Clamping of the caudal IVC

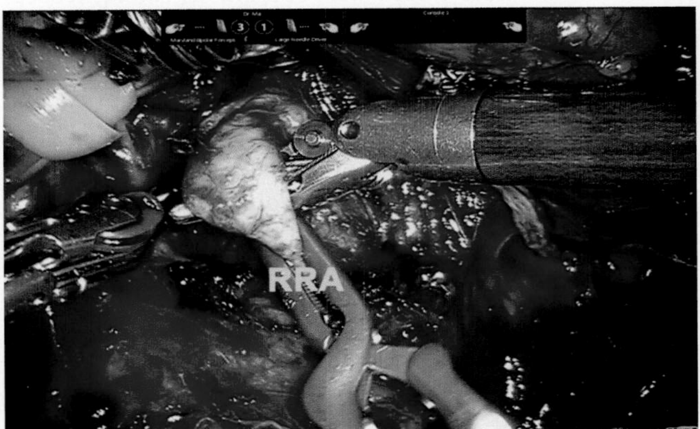

Fig. 47 Clamping of the right renal artery (RRA)

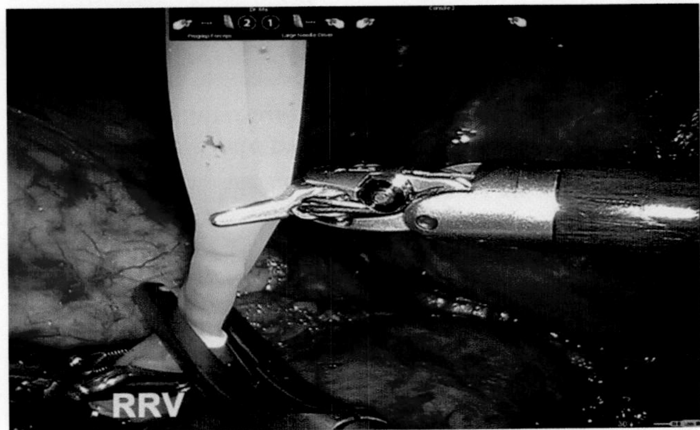

Fig. 48 Clamping of the right renal vein (RRV)

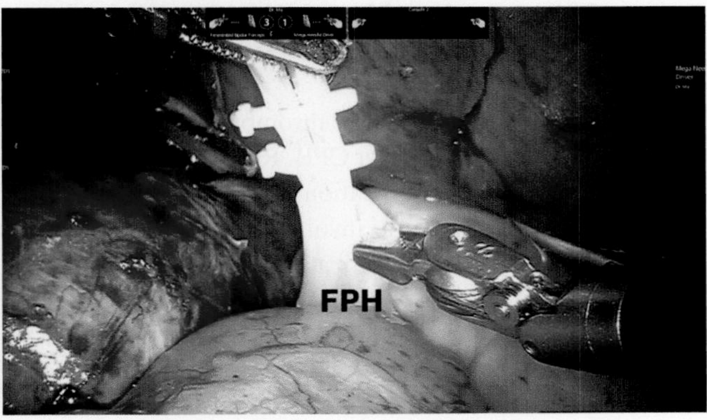

Fig. 49 Clamping of the first porta hepatis (FPH)

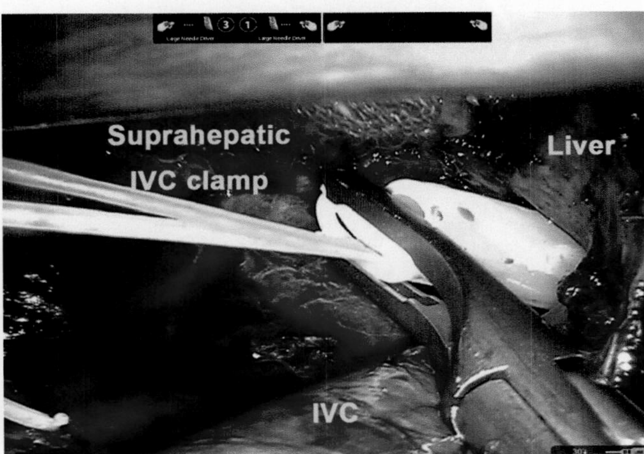

Fig. 50 Clamping of the suprahepatic infradiaphragmatic IVC

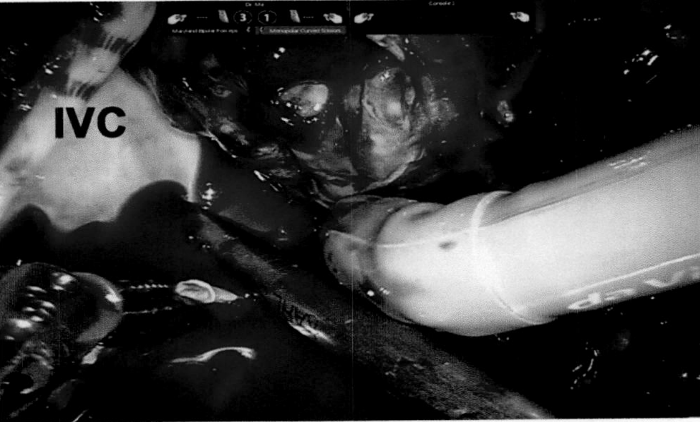

Fig. 51 IVC tumor thrombectomy

5.6 Robot-Assisted Level IV IVC Thrombectomy: Right Side

Patients with level IV tumor thrombus underwent "segmented thrombectomy" under CPB. Routinely, we used two-stage approach (liver mobilization and IVC thrombectomy). SHVs were ligated, and the involved retrohepatic IVC was dissociated. After liver mobilization, the right renal artery was clipped initially with Hem-o-lock interaortocaval. The involved infrahepatic IVC, caudal IVC, left renal vein (LRV), and FPH were mobilized circumferentially. Vessel loops were wrapped twice around the IVC below the tumor thrombus, around the LRV, and around the FPH, prepared for clamping (Fig. 53a).

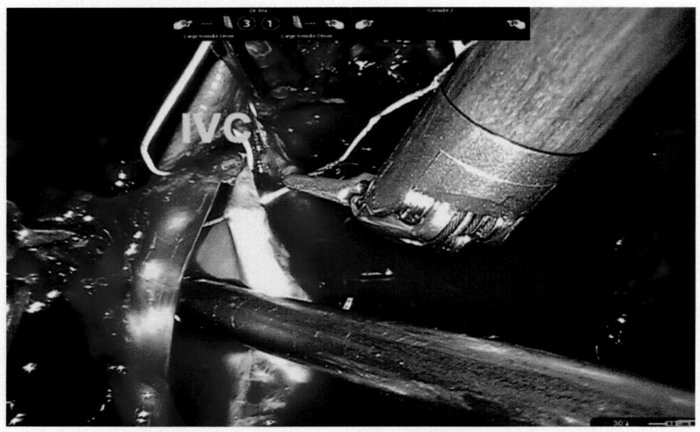

Fig. 52 IVC suture

Firstly, the cardiovascular surgeons established CPB. The right internal jugular vein was cannulated (Fig. 53b). The fifth intercostal small incision of 6 cm was taken to prepare for thoracoscopy-assisted small incision operation (Fig. 53c). Then, the right femoral artery and vein were cannulated (Fig. 53d). After pericardium incision, the superior vena cava (SVC) was mobilized and clamped (Fig. 54). The right atrium was incised (Fig. 55), and the thrombus above the diaphragm was transected and removed (Fig. 56). Then, the supradiaphragmatic IVC was mobilized and clamped (Fig. 57). Subsequently, the LRV, caudal IVC, and FPH were clamped; the IVC was incised, and the IVC thrombus below the diaphragm was transected and removed. Finally, the IVC and the atrium were closed with continuous suture, respectively (Fig. 58). The FPH, LRV, caudal IVC, SVC (Fig. 59), and supradiaphragmatic IVC (Fig. 60) were released in order, and the CPB was stopped. Finally, protamine (3.3 mg/kg) was neutralized, and then blood products, including platelets, plasma, and cryoprecipitate, were replenished according to the assessed bleeding volume.

Taken together, level IV RA-IVCT requires establishment of CPB. Thoracoscopy-assisted thrombectomy was performed for the intra-atrium part of the thrombus under

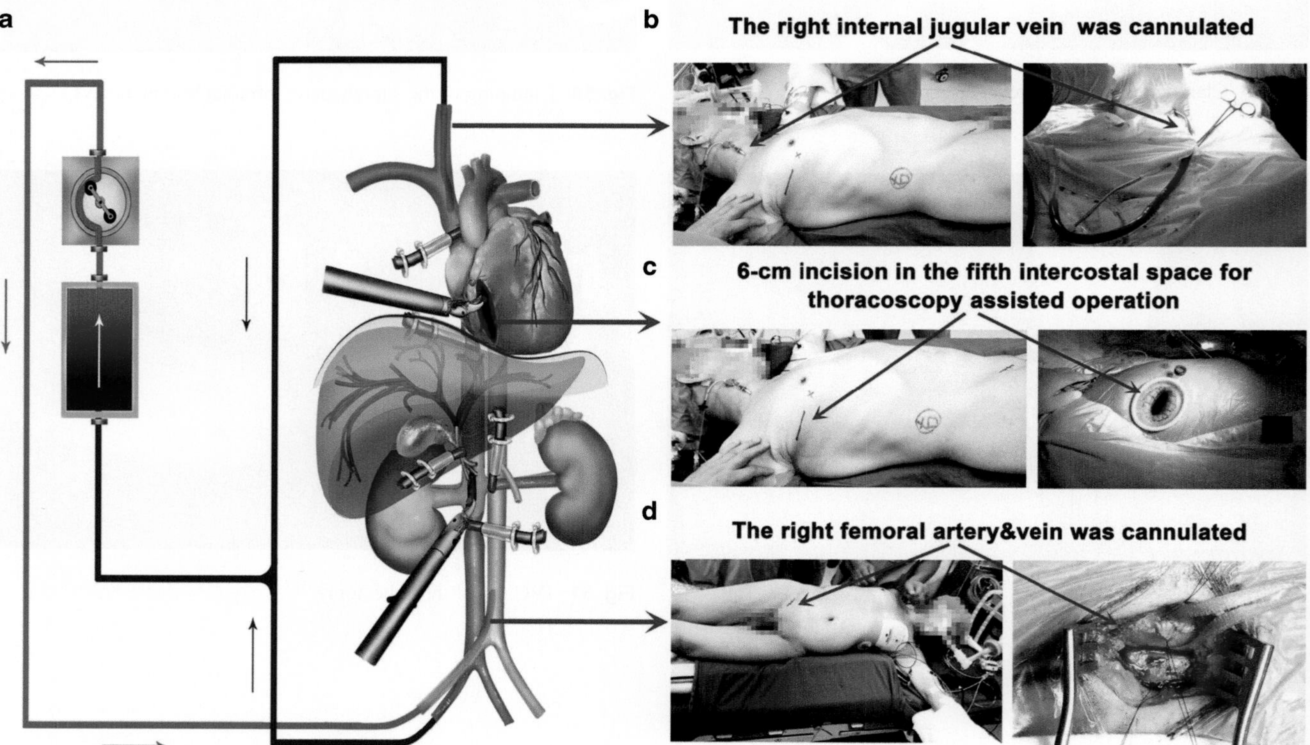

Fig. 53 The establishment of cardiopulmonary bypass

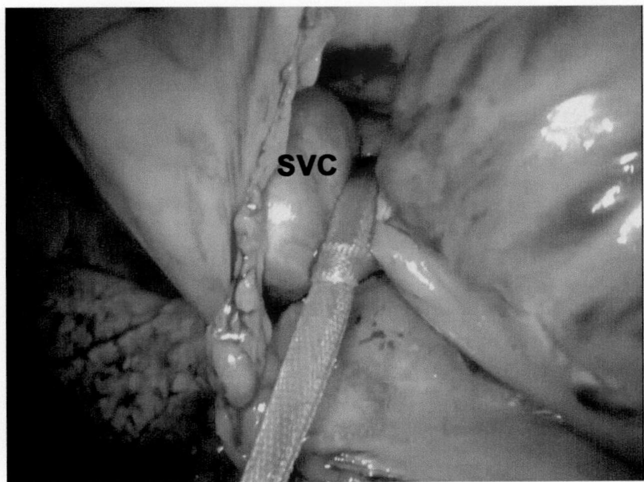

Fig. 54 Clamping of the superior vena cava (SVC)

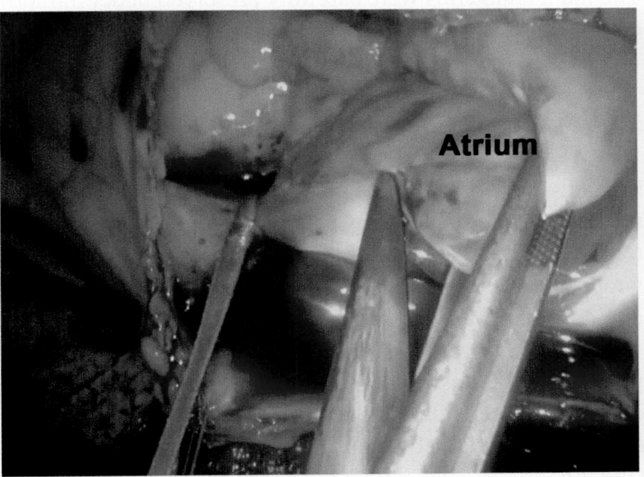

Fig. 55 Incision of the right atrium

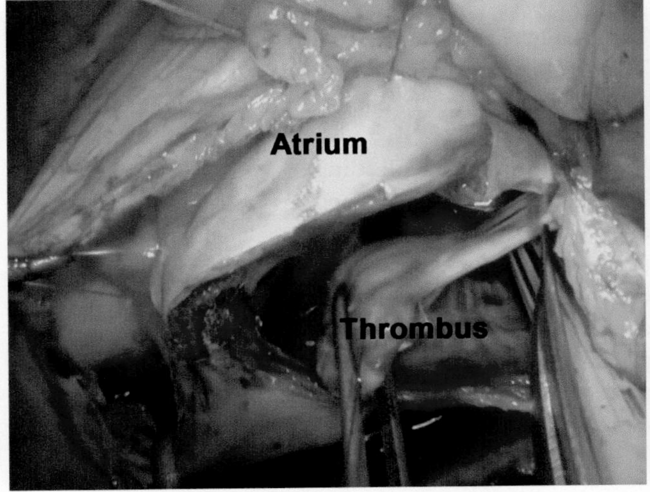

Fig. 56 Removal of the atrium thrombus

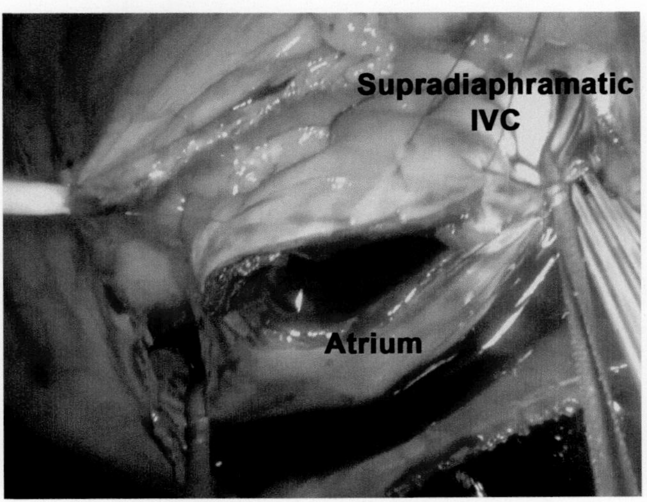

Fig. 57 Clamping of the supradiaphragmatic IVC

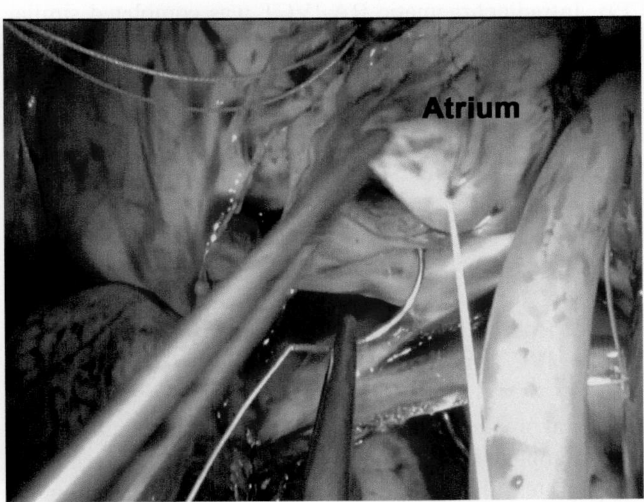

Fig. 58 Suturing of the right atrium

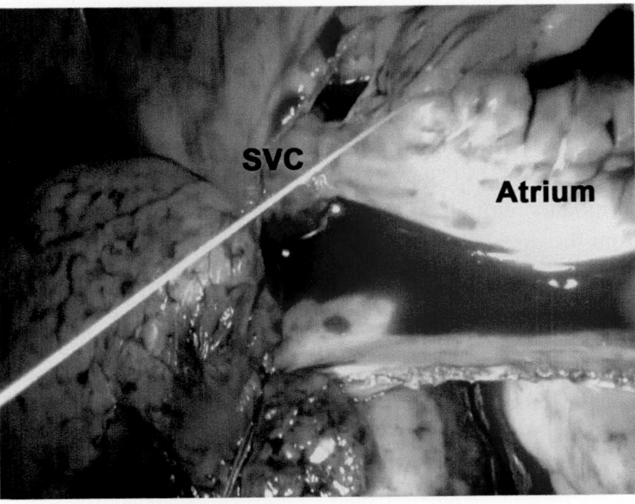

Fig. 59 Release of the superior vena cava (SVC) clamp

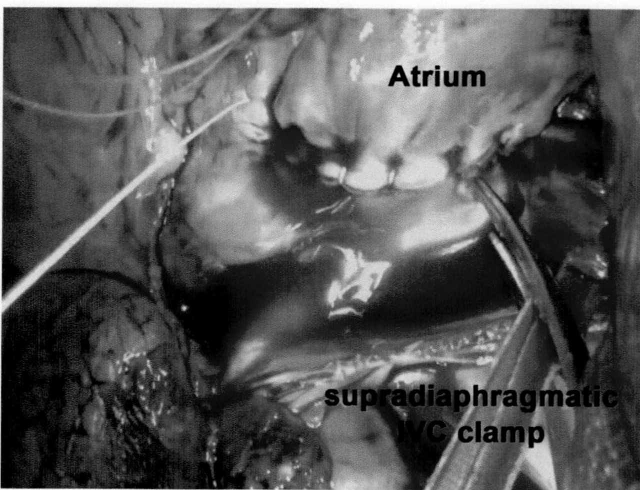

Fig. 60 Release of the supradiaphragmatic IVC clamp

CPB. Infradiaphragmatic RA-IVCT was completed similar as level III RA-IVCT.

The steps of RA-IVCT for left-sided RTs were similar with that for right-sided RTs, except clamping of renal vessels. For left-sided RTs, the tumor-bearing LRV should be stapled, and RRA and RRV should be both clamped, the same as the controlling of infradiaphragmatic IVC in level III.

5.7 Robotic-Assisted Cavectomy for Level II IVC Thrombectomy

In clinical practice, some IVC tumor thrombi are bulky, leading to complete obstruction of the IVC. Collateral circulation compensates in the process of chronic obstruction of IVC. The blood return of the distal IVC mainly flows back to the superior vena cava through the lumbar vein, ascending lumbar vein, azygous vein, and semi-azygous vein system (Fig. 61). At this time, cavectomy of tumor-bearing IVC has little effect on the distal IVC blood return. Furthermore, for tumor thrombus invading the IVC wall, cavectomy including tumor-bearing IVC is more suitable for tumor control [54]. In addition, if there is a long unresectable bland thrombosis in the distal IVC, cavectomy also was used to prevent pulmonary embolism caused by bland thrombus shedding from the distal IVC. For the right renal tumor, the left renal vein can return through its rich branches (gonadal vein, central adrenal vein, ascending lumbar vein, etc.). Therefore, it was safe to perform cavectomy of the tumor-bearing IVC and staple the left renal vein. However, it should be noted that for left renal tumors, due to the lack of natural genus of the right renal vein, the right renal vein return should be restored after it is disconnected, usually through the caudal IVC, the lumbar vein, azygous vein, and semi-azygous vein system from the distal end of inferior vena cava. In addition, in order not to affect the hepatic blood return, cavectomy should be performed below the hepatic vein.

5.8 RAC-IVCT for Right-Sided RCC with IVCT

The surgical strategy for right-sided RCC with IVCT was demonstrated in Fig. 62. The cephalic IVC below the hepatic veins was stapled, leaving a minimal segment of the cava caudal to the hepatic veins, thereby limiting turbulence and potential thrombosis (Fig. 63). Subsequently, the left renal vein was circumferentially dissected, looped, and stapled (Fig. 64). The right renal artery was exposed and ligated in the interaortocaval space. The caudal tumor-bearing IVC was further dissected circumferentially and stapled (Fig. 65). The main collaterals were carefully preserved under intraoperative ultrasound guidance during caudal IVC stapling.

5.9 RAC-IVCT for Left-Sided RCC with IVCT

For left-sided RCC with IVCT, the cephalic IVC and left renal vein were sequentially stapled. The IVC was dissected retrogradely and circumferentially. The vessel loops were wrapped twice around the IVC between the superior border of the right renal vein and inferior border of the left renal vein. The IVC wall was cut 1–2 cm cephalic to the loop; precaution was taken to preserve the orifice of preexisting collaterals. Thereafter, the caudal IVC was reconstructed to ensure the right renal venous return through IVC collaterals (Fig. 66).

5.10 Complications and Management

Tumor Thrombus Detachment

This fatal complication rarely occurs. Once this happens, it can result in pulmonary embolism or myocardial infarction.

Vascular Injury and Bleeding

During the operation, the blood vessels are skeletonized and exposed to the risk of injury. Vascular injury usually happened during dissection of the IVC and renal vein, especially lumbar vein dissection (Fig. 67). Familiarity of the anatomy and gentle dissection are the key components of primary prevention. Once bleeding occurs, gauzes can be placed, and pneumoperitoneum pressure can be increased to tamponade the bleeding. The injured vessel wall can be

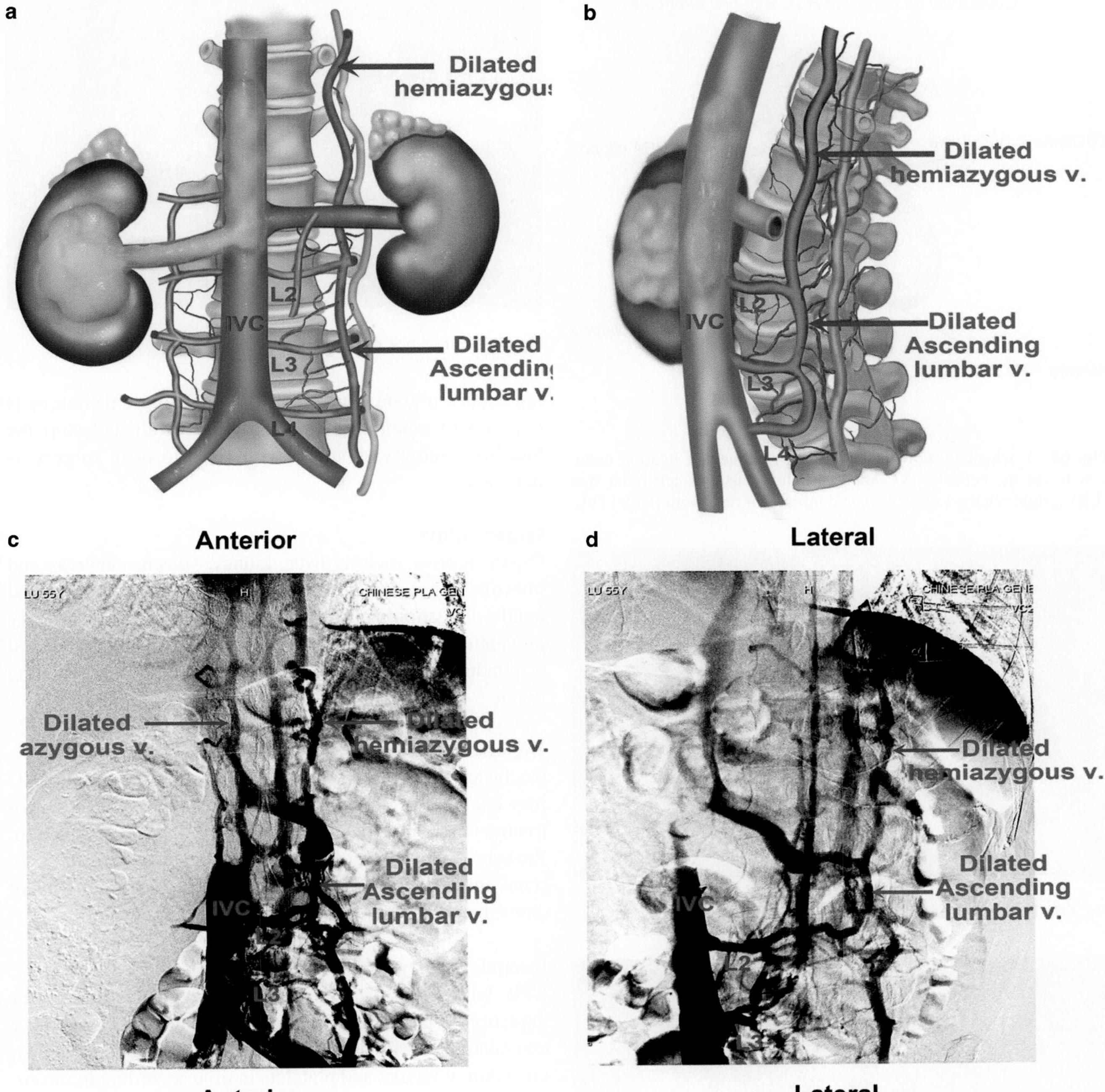

Fig. 61 A schematic drawing and cavography images represents the collateral circulation of a caudal inferior vena cava (IVC) incrementally occluded by a thrombus. (**a**, **b**) A diagram illustrates the collateral circulation through the caudal IVC to the dilated lumbar vein, ascending lumbar vein, and hemiazygos and azygos veins. (**c**, **d**) Cavography images shows the collateral circulation through the caudal IVC to the dilated lumbar vein, ascending lumbar vein, and hemiazygos and azygos veins

repaired continuously with absorbable suture (Fig. 68). IVC looping proximal and distal to the thrombus is associated with the high risk of bleeding as well. IVC tributaries are clipped with Hem-o-lok clips and left in situ; vessel loops might dislodge the Hem-o-lok clips and cause bleeding (Fig. 69). IVC tributaries adjacent to the cross-clamping location should be sutured; Hem-o-lok clips may be dislodged during looping of vessel loops (Fig. 70). Once bleed-

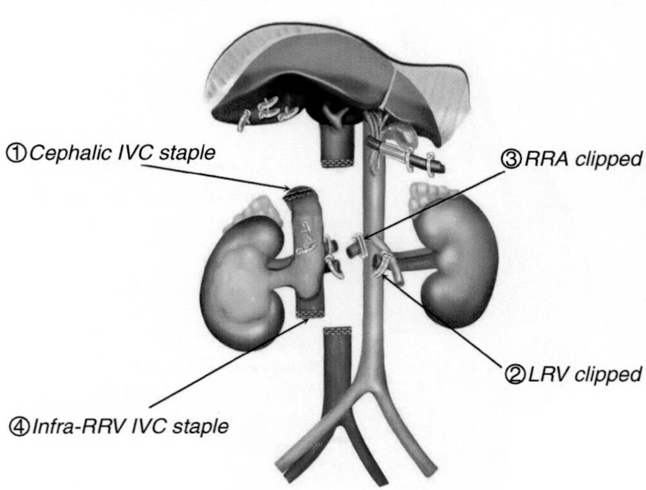

Fig. 62 A schematic drawing represents a sequential ligation order, which was the cephalic IVC above the thrombus end, left renal vein (LRV), right renal artery (RRA), and infra-right renal vein (RRV) IVC

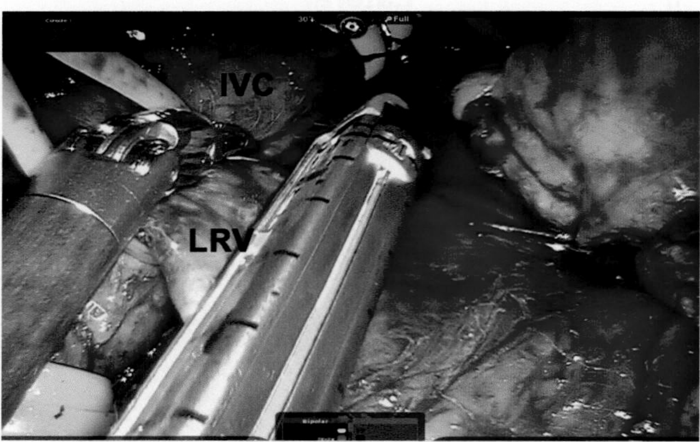

Fig. 64 Transection of the left renal vein (LRV)

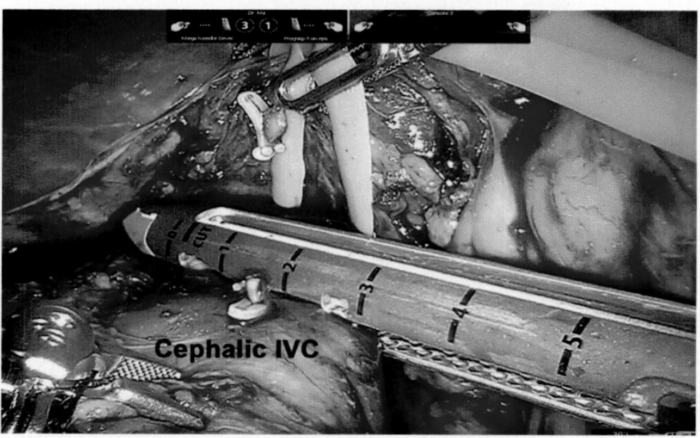

Fig. 63 Transection of the cephalic IVC

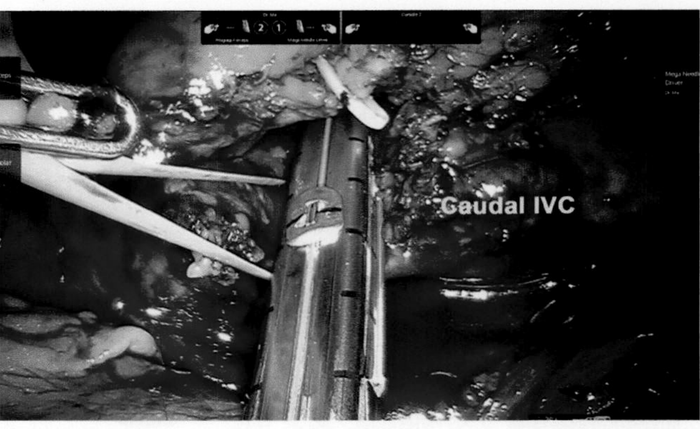

Fig. 65 Transection of the caudal IVC

ing occurs, a good mastering of robotic suture technique is required to repair the damaged vessel wall and stop the bleeding. Surgery should be converted to open surgery as indicated.

Organ Injury

Organ injuries such as liver, kidney, spleen, pancreas and intestinal injury rarely occur. Familiarity of the anatomy and gentle dissection again are the key components of primary prevention. Once organ injury occurs, management should be conducted according to the principle of the corresponding organ.

Hepatic and Renal Dysfunction

Occlusion of the first porta hepatis and suprahepatic IVC may lead to acute hepatic dysfunction, and pharmacological treatment should be taken to protect hepatic function. Prolonged occlusion of the renal hilum may lead to acute renal insufficiency or even acute renal failure. In severe cases, hemodialysis is needed.

Coagulation Dysfunction

CPB with heparinization can lead to coagulation factor depletion, platelet dysfunction, hemodilution, and other coagulation dysfunctions. It is necessary to supplement coagulation factors and platelets in time according to thromboelastogram and coagulation factor detection and timely adjust blood coagulation and heparin.

Edema of Lower Limbs

If cavectomy was chosen in the insufficient establishment of collateral circulation, edema of lower limbs may occur, which could be alleviated by diuresis and elevation of affected limbs. With the establishment of collateral circulation, edema can gradually disappear.

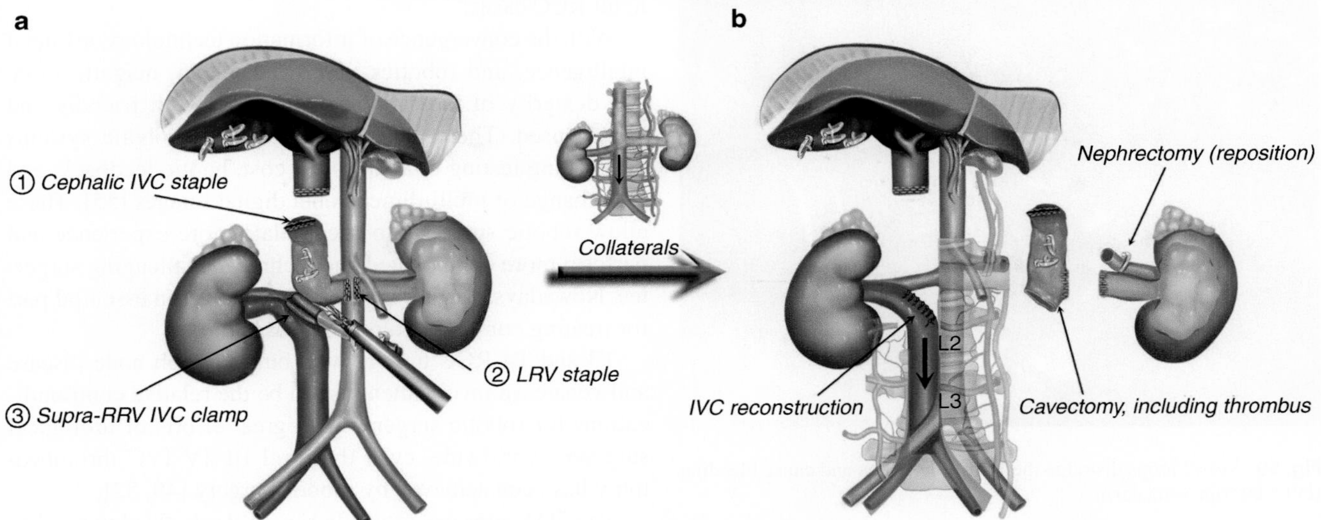

Fig. 66 A schematic drawing represents a sequential ligation order and collateral circulation. After the cephalic IVC and left renal vein (LRV) are stapled, venous return of the right renal vein (RRV) was through the caudal IVC, lumbar vein, lumbar ascending vein, and hemiazygos and azygos vein systems (right). Arrows indicate the direction of venous blood

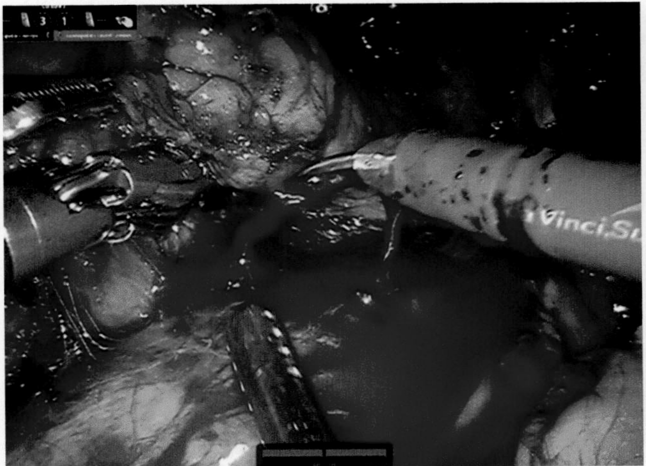

Fig. 67 Bleeding from an injured tributary of the IVC

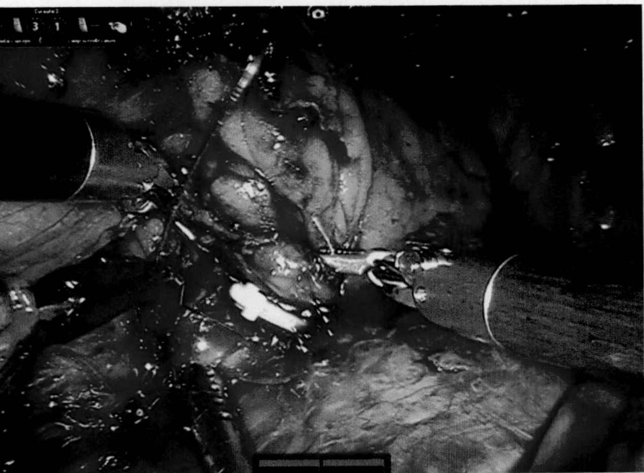

Fig. 68 The IVC defect is closed by a running suture

Surgical Site Infection
Surgical site infection is managed with regular dressing. Colligated drain can be inserted as indicated, to drain the exudate. Antibiotic should be started according to the sensitivity when the patient has fever.

Peritonitis
Peritonitis rarely occurs; however it can occur in patients with primary intraperitoneal infection. Postoperative intraperitoneal collection and hematoma can aggravate the infection. Optimal drainage is crucial in addition to appropriate antibiotic prescription. Intraperitoneal lavage can be performed as indicated.

Pneumonia
It usually occurs in patients with primary lung diseases. Preoperative lung function test and blood gas analysis are important for this kind of patient during preoperative evaluation. Postoperatively, the patient should rest in a 45-degree prompt-up position whenever possible. Chest physiotherapy should be initiated as soon as possible, and the patient is encouraged for early ambulation. Good inhalation and exha-

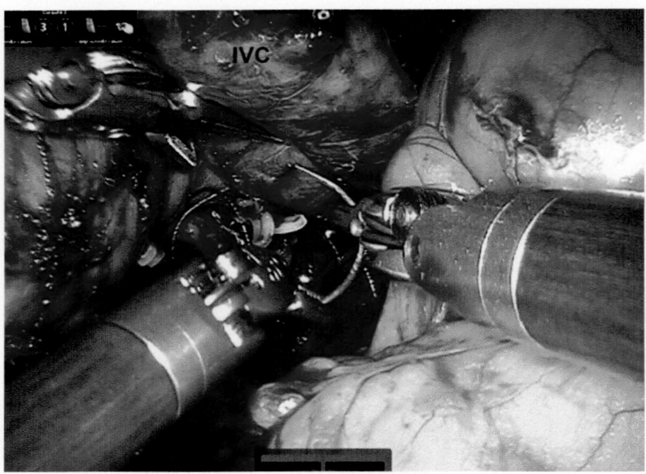

Fig. 69 Vessel loops dislodge the Hem-o-lok clips and cause bleeding (IVC, inferior vena cava)

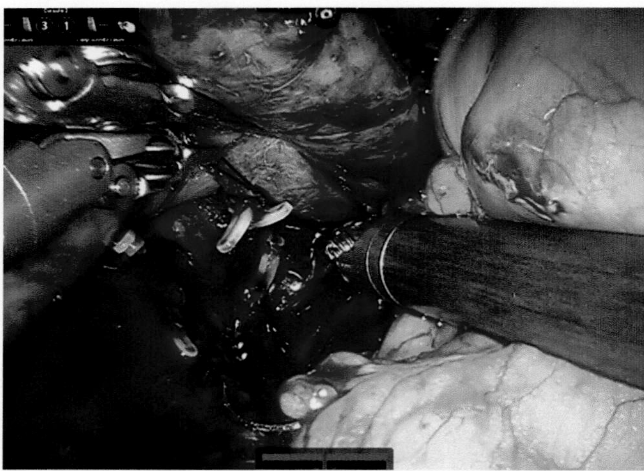

Fig. 70 Preventive suturing to avoid bleeding

lation techniques are emphasized to the patient. The patient needs to be ensured for performing intensive spirometry regularly. If the patient is complicated with pneumonia, chest physician can be consulted.

Other Complications

Other complications include postoperative lymphatic leakage, lower limb deep venous thrombosis, etc.

6 Future Perspectives for RARN and IVC Thrombectomy

Before the advent of robotic surgery, RCC with massive tumors, adjacent organ invasion, and need for lymphadenectomy and IVC tumor thrombectomy were often performed by open surgery. Robotic surgery has been validated to be an alternative to open surgery for the management of these difficult RCC cases.

With the convergence of information technology, artificial intelligence, and robotics, improved vision, magnification, and dexterity of the robotic platform make it friendly and widely used. There are a number of new robotic systems undergoing testing to address the cost, haptic feedback, and interchange of multi-dimensional digital images [55]. These allow robotic surgeons to accumulate more experience and perform more complicated and technical challenging surgeries. Nowadays, robotic surgery has become an essential part for treating complex urologic diseases [56].

T3 and T4 RCC tumors with bulky lymph node disease and vena cava involvement use to be the relative contraindications for robotic surgery. With great efforts of urological surgeons worldwide, even the level III–IV IVC thrombectomy has been achieved by robotic surgery [49, 52].

The FDA approval of the da Vinci SP robotic platform has led to its usage in urologic malignancy treatment. SP robotic system has been used in both retroperitoneal and transperitoneal RARN approved to be a feasible surgical technique in the management of RCC [57].

RARN is a reproducible surgical technique, which will be mastered by more urological surgeons. There is a great potential for development and application of RARN in the future.

References

1. Clayman RV, Kavoussi LR, Soper NJ, Dierks SM, Meretyk S, Darcy MD, et al. Laparoscopic nephrectomy: initial case report. J Urol. 1991;146(2):278–82.
2. Klingler DW, Hemstreet GP, Balaji KC. Feasibility of robotic radical nephrectomy—initial results of single-institution pilot study. Urology. 2005;65(6):1086–9.
3. Anele UA, Marchioni M, Yang B, Simone G, Uzzo RG, Lau C, et al. Robotic versus laparoscopic radical nephrectomy: a large multi-institutional analysis (ROSULA Collaborative Group). World J Urol. 2019;37(11):2439–50.
4. Ashrafi AN, Gill IS. Minimally invasive radical nephrectomy: a contemporary review. Transl Androl Urol. 2020;9(6):3112–22.
5. Li J, Peng L, Cao D, Cheng B, Gou H, Li Y, et al. Comparison of perioperative outcomes of robot-assisted vs. laparoscopic radical nephrectomy: a systematic review and meta-analysis. Front Oncol. 2020;10:551052.
6. Ljungberg B, Albiges L, Abu-Ghanem Y, Bensalah K, Dabestani S, Fernández-Pello S, et al. European association of urology guidelines on renal cell carcinoma: the 2019 update. Eur Urol. 2019;75(5):799–810.
7. Mir MC, Derweesh I, Porpiglia F, Zargar H, Mottrie A, Autorino R. Partial nephrectomy versus radical nephrectomy for clinical T1b and T2 renal tumors: a systematic review and meta-analysis of comparative studies. Eur Urol. 2017;71(4):606–17.
8. Lenis AT, Salmasi AH, Donin NM, Faiena I, Johnson DC, Drakaki A, et al. Trends in usage of cytoreductive partial nephrectomy and effect on overall survival in patients with metastatic renal cell carcinoma. Urol Oncol. 2018;36(2):78.e21–8.

9. Shen D, Du S, Huang Q, Gao Y, Fan Y, Gu L, et al. A modified sequential vascular control strategy in robot-assisted level III–IV inferior vena cava thrombectomy: initial series mimicking the open 'milking' technique principle. BJU Int. 2020;126(4):447–56.
10. Motzer RJ, Jonasch E, Michaelson MD, Nandagopal L, Gore JL, George S, et al. NCCN Guidelines Insights: Kidney Cancer, Version 2.2020. J Natl Compr Canc Netw. 2019;17(11):1278–85.
11. Heng DY, Wells JC, Rini BI, Beuselinck B, Lee JL, Knox JJ, et al. Cytoreductive nephrectomy in patients with synchronous metastases from renal cell carcinoma: results from the International Metastatic Renal Cell Carcinoma Database Consortium. Eur Urol. 2014;66(4):704–10.
12. Blute ML, Leibovich BC, Cheville JC, Lohse CM, Zincke H. A protocol for performing extended lymph node dissection using primary tumor pathological features for patients treated with radical nephrectomy for clear cell renal cell carcinoma. J Urol. 2004;172(2):465–9.
13. Crispen PL, Breau RH, Allmer C, Lohse CM, Cheville JC, Leibovich BC, et al. Lymph node dissection at the time of radical nephrectomy for high-risk clear cell renal cell carcinoma: indications and recommendations for surgical templates. Eur Urol. 2011;59(1):18–23.
14. Abaza R, Lowe G. Feasibility and adequacy of robot-assisted lymphadenectomy for renal-cell carcinoma. J Endourol. 2011;25(7):1155–9.
15. Bekema HJ, MacLennan S, Imamura M, Lam TB, Stewart F, Scott N, et al. Systematic review of adrenalectomy and lymph node dissection in locally advanced renal cell carcinoma. Eur Urol. 2013;64(5):799–810.
16. Porpiglia F, Amparore D, Checcucci E, Manfredi M, Stura I, Migliaretti G, et al. Three-dimensional virtual imaging of renal tumours: a new tool to improve the accuracy of nephrometry scores. BJU Int. 2019;124(6):945–54.
17. Shirk JD, Thiel DD, Wallen EM, Linehan JM, White WM, Badani KK, et al. Effect of 3-dimensional virtual reality models for surgical planning of robotic-assisted partial nephrectomy on surgical outcomes: a randomized clinical trial. JAMA Netw Open. 2019;2(9):e1911598.
18. Zhang K, Zhu G, Li HB, Martinez Portillo FJ, et al. Application of 3D image reconstruction in robotic urological surgery. Chin J Urol. 2018;39(9):690–3.
19. Zhu G, Xing JC, Weng GB, et al. Application of holographic image navigation in urological laparoscopic and robotic surgery. Chin J Urol. 2020;41(2):117–23.
20. Ha US, Hwang TK, Kim YJ, Oh TH, Jeon YS, Lee W, et al. Comparison of oncological outcomes of transperitoneal and retroperitoneal laparoscopic radical nephrectomy for the management of clear-cell renal cell carcinoma: a multi-institutional study. BJU Int. 2011;107(9):1467–72.
21. Fan X, Xu K, Lin T, Liu H, Yin Z, Dong W, et al. Comparison of transperitoneal and retroperitoneal laparoscopic nephrectomy for renal cell carcinoma: a systematic review and meta-analysis. BJU Int. 2013;111(4):611–21.
22. Yin L, Zhang D, Teng J, Xu D. Retroperitoneal laparoscopic radical nephrectomy for renal cell carcinoma during pregnancy. Urol Int. 2013;90(4):487–9.
23. Berglund RK, Gill IS, Babineau D, Desai M, Kaouk JH. A prospective comparison of transperitoneal and retroperitoneal laparoscopic nephrectomy in the extremely obese patient. BJU Int. 2007;99(4):871–4.
24. Jing TLXD, Wang P, et al. Utility of the third arm in robotic-assisted laparoscopic partial nephrectomy for complex renal tumor. Chin J Urol. 2017;38(7):507–10.
25. Caputo PA, Ko O, Patel R, Stein R. Robotic-assisted laparoscopic nephrectomy. J Surg Oncol. 2015;112(7):723–7.
26. Patel M, Porter J. Robotic retroperitoneal surgery: a contemporary review. Curr Opin Urol. 2013;23(1):51–6.
27. Daneshmand S, Ahmadi H, Schuckman AK, Mitra AP, Cai J, Miranda G, et al. Enhanced recovery protocol after radical cystectomy for bladder cancer. J Urol. 2014;192(1):50–5.
28. Crocerossa F, Carbonara U, Cantiello F, Marchioni M, Ditonno P, Mir MC, et al. Robot-assisted radical nephrectomy: a systematic review and meta-analysis of comparative studies. Eur Urol. 2020.
29. Gershman B, Bukavina L, Chen Z, Konety B, Schumache F, Li L, et al. The association of robot-assisted versus pure laparoscopic radical nephrectomy with perioperative outcomes and hospital costs. Eur Urol Focus. 2020;6(2):305–12.
30. Asimakopoulos AD, Miano R, Annino F, Micali S, Spera E, Iorio B, et al. Robotic radical nephrectomy for renal cell carcinoma: a systematic review. BMC Urol. 2014;14:75.
31. Nik-Ahd F, Souders CP, Houman J, Zhao H, Chughtai B, Anger JT. Robotic urologic surgery: trends in food and drug administration-reported adverse events over the last decade. J Endourol. 2019;33(8):649–54.
32. Marshall FF, Dietrick DD, Baumgartner WA, Reitz BA. Surgical management of renal cell carcinoma with intracaval neoplastic extension above the hepatic veins. J Urol. 1988;139(6):1166–72.
33. Skinner DG, Pfister RF, Colvin R. Extension of renal cell carcinoma into the vena cava: the rationale for aggressive surgical management. J Urol. 1972;107(5):711–6.
34. Skinner DG, Vermillion CD, Colvin RB. The surgical management of renal cell carcinoma. J Urol. 1972;107(5):705–10.
35. Blute ML, Leibovich BC, Lohse CM, Cheville JC, Zincke H. The Mayo Clinic experience with surgical management, complications and outcome for patients with renal cell carcinoma and venous tumour thrombus. BJU Int. 2004;94(1):33–41.
36. Ciancio G, Manoharan M, Katkoori D, De Los SR, Soloway MS. Long-term survival in patients undergoing radical nephrectomy and inferior vena cava thrombectomy: single-center experience. Eur Urol. 2010;57(4):667–72.
37. Wagner B, Patard JJ, Méjean A, Bensalah K, Verhoest G, Zigeuner R, et al. Prognostic value of renal vein and inferior vena cava involvement in renal cell carcinoma. Eur Urol. 2009;55(2):452–9.
38. Martínez-Salamanca JI, Huang WC, Millán I, Bertini R, Bianco FJ, Carballido JA, et al. Prognostic impact of the 2009 UICC/AJCC TNM staging system for renal cell carcinoma with venous extension. Eur Urol. 2011;59(1):120–7.
39. Lee JY, Mucksavage P. Robotic radical nephrectomy with vena caval tumor thrombectomy: experience of novice robotic surgeons. Korean J Urol. 2012;53(12):879–82.
40. Abaza R. Initial series of robotic radical nephrectomy with vena caval tumor thrombectomy. Eur Urol. 2011;59(4):652–6.
41. Gu L, Ma X, Gao Y, Li H, Li X, Chen L, et al. Robotic versus open level I–II inferior vena cava thrombectomy: a matched group comparative analysis. J Urol. 2017;198(6):1241–6.
42. Chopra S, Simone G, Metcalfe C, de Castro Abreu AL, Nabhani J, Ferriero M, et al. Robot-assisted level II–III inferior vena cava tumor thrombectomy: step-by-step technique and 1-year outcomes. Eur Urol. 2017;72(2):267–74.
43. Gill IS, Metcalfe C, Abreu A, Duddalwar V, Chopra S, Cunningham M, et al. Robotic level III inferior vena cava tumor thrombectomy: initial series. J Urol. 2015;194(4):929–38.
44. Nelson RJ, Maurice MJ, Kaouk JH. Robotic radical left nephrectomy with inferior vena cava level III thrombectomy. Urology. 2017;107:269.
45. Ramirez D, Maurice MJ, Cohen B, Krishnamurthi V, Haber GP. Robotic level III IVC tumor thrombectomy: duplicating the open approach. Urology. 2016;90:204–7.
46. Bratslavsky G, Cheng JS. Robotic-assisted radical nephrectomy with retrohepatic vena caval tumor thrombectomy (level III)

combined with extended retroperitoneal lymph node dissection. Urology. 2015;86(6):1235–40.
47. Sood A, Jeong W, Barod R, Bahnson E, Kirura P, Abdollah F, et al. Robot-assisted hepatic mobilization and control of suprahepatic infradiaphragmatic inferior vena cava for level 3 vena caval thrombectomy: an IDEAL stage 0 study. J Surg Oncol. 2015;112(7):741–5.
48. Abaza R, Eun DD, Gallucci M, Gill IS, Menon M, Mottrie A, et al. Robotic surgery for renal cell carcinoma with vena caval tumor thrombus. Eur Urol Focus. 2016;2(6):601–7.
49. Murphy C, Abaza R. Complex robotic nephrectomy and inferior vena cava tumor thrombectomy: an evolving landscape. Curr Opin Urol. 2020;30(1):83–9.
50. Wang B, Li H, Ma X, Zhang X, Gu L, Li X, et al. Robot-assisted laparoscopic inferior vena cava thrombectomy: different sides require different techniques. Eur Urol. 2016;69(6):1112–9.
51. Wang B, Li H, Huang Q, Liu K, Fan Y, Peng C, et al. Robot-assisted retrohepatic inferior vena cava thrombectomy: first or second porta hepatis as an important boundary landmark. Eur Urol. 2018;74(4):512–20.
52. Wang B, Huang Q, Liu K, Fan Y, Peng C, Gu L, et al. Robot-assisted level III–IV inferior vena cava thrombectomy: initial series with step-by-step procedures and 1-yr outcomes. Eur Urol. 2020;78(1):77–86.
53. Shi T, Huang Q, Liu K, Du S, Fan Y, Yang L, et al. Robot-assisted cavectomy versus thrombectomy for level II inferior vena cava thrombus: decision-making scheme and multi-institutional analysis. Eur Urol. 2020;78(4):592–602.
54. Rodriguez Faba O, Linares E, Tilki D, Capitanio U, Evans CP, Montorsi F, et al. Impact of microscopic wall invasion of the renal vein or inferior vena cava on cancer-specific survival in patients with renal cell carcinoma and tumor thrombus: a multi-institutional analysis from the international renal cell carcinoma-venous thrombus consortium. Eur Urol Focus. 2018;4(3):435–41.
55. Fan S, Dai X, Yang K, Xiong S, Xiong G, Li Z, et al. Robot-assisted pyeloplasty using a new robotic system, the KangDuo-Surgical Robot-01: a prospective, single-centre, single-arm clinical study. BJU Int. 2021.
56. Mikhail D, Sarcona J, Mekhail M, Richstone L. Urologic robotic surgery. Surg Clin North Am. 2020;100(2):361–78.
57. Fang AM, Saidian A, Magi-Galluzzi C, Nix JW, Rais-Bahrami S. Single-port robotic partial and radical nephrectomies for renal cortical tumors: initial clinical experience. J Robot Surg. 2020;14(5):773–80.

Robotic Renal Transplantation

Pietro Diana, Andrea Gallioli, Karel Decaestecker, Mani Menon, and Alberto Breda

1 Introduction

Kidney transplantation (KT) is considered one of the cornerstones in the treatment of end-stage renal disease (ESRD) since transplanted patients reach superior survival rates and an improved quality of life compared to hemodialysis, and the open kidney transplantation (OKT) is considered the gold standard technique [1]. The first KT was performed by Dr. Joseph Murray (Nobel Prize for Medicine, 1990) in 1953 and is reputed to be revolutionary in the history of surgery. Despite the OKT being the standard approach, in the era of minimally invasive surgery, technical alternatives have been performed targeting an improvement of the surgical outcomes and a reduction of the postoperative complications. In 2009, the first laparoscopic KT (LKT) has been performed [2, 3] followed by the publication in 2013 of the first large LKT series compared to the conventional approach that reported the results from 72 living donor for KT and 145 OKT. Results showed for LKT and OKT a mean operating time of 224 vs 175 min, and the mean rewarming time was 60 vs 30 min ($p = 0.03$). Functional outcomes were comparable in terms of graft and patient survival, with a median follow-up of 22 months. The LKT provided advantages regarding wound infections and analgesic therapy, with a subsequent faster recovery and aesthetic results. However, the procedure resulted to be challenging and needing a solid expertise in laparoscopy to reach acceptable operative times and avoid complications as patients with ESRD have a higher risk to develop respiratory acidosis and hypertension due to the slower elimination of carbon dioxide used for pneumoperitoneum. Obvious limitations of laparoscopic suturing techniques did not allow a widespread adoption of laparoscopic surgery for KT. To overcome the limitations of the laparoscopic approach, robot-assisted kidney transplantation (RAKT) was introduced and is showing promising results as a less invasive alternative to the open approach, with the advantages of the robotic technique such as a shorter learning curve and a high dexterity with enhanced visualization of the surgical field [4–6]. Since the first RAKT in 2010, the surgical technique has been refined and standardized by centers highly experienced in robotic surgery and KT. Few authors compared surgical and functional results with the open approach, showing possible advantages in selected cases, such as obese patients and multiple-vessel graft [7, 8]. Furthermore, a structured program was developed in order to expand RAKT's indication to deceased donors [9].

2 Robot-Assisted Kidney Transplantation (RAKT): Living Donor

2.1 Background

2.1.1 Living-Donor Nephrectomy

About 20% of all KT in Europe are performed using living-donor grafts, while in the USA, the percentage raises up to 40% [10]. Living donors are generally part of the patient's family or emotionally related to the patient, and compared to deceased donor kidney, the use of living-donor graft has reported advantages in graft function and survival, other than reducing the organ waiting list [11]. Furthermore, in

P. Diana
Fundació Puigvert, Department of Urology, Autonomous University of Barcelona, Barcelona, Spain

Department of Urology, Humanitas Clinical and Research Institute IRCCS, Rozzano, Italy

A. Gallioli · A. Breda (✉)
Fundació Puigvert, Department of Urology, Autonomous University of Barcelona, Barcelona, Spain

K. Decaestecker
Department of Urology, Ghent University Hospital, Ghent, Belgium

M. Menon
VCORE – Vattikuti Urology Institute Center for Outcomes Research, Analytics and Evaluation, Henry Ford Hospital, Detroit, MI, USA

P. Wiklund et al. (eds.), *Robotic Urologic Surgery*, https://doi.org/10.1007/978-3-031-00363-9_43

the case of donation from an ABO blood group system-compatible family member, the recipients need a less aggressive immunosuppressive regimens. The left kidney is generally preferred for donation because of a longer renal vein compared to the contralateral one; however, if the renal function differs between the two kidneys, the one with the lower function is employed. Since 1995, the living-donor nephrectomy for graft retrieval is performed through the laparoscopic technique [2] that reported better results in terms of pain control, blood loss, hospital stay, and aesthetic results, compared to the open technique. In 2001, a group at the University of Illinois (Chicago) reported the first series of robot-assisted laparoscopic donor nephrectomies, using the da Vinci Surgical System (Intuitive Surgical, Sunnyvale, CA, USA) [12]. This new approach, despite the feasibility and safety of the technique, reported high costs and no substantial advantages compared to the laparoscopic technique.

2.1.2 Living-Donor Kidney Transplantation

The first RAKT was performed in the USA and reported by Giulianotti et al. [13]. This technique was then replicated and refined by other surgeons. In 2014, Menon et al. described a standardized technique using a transperitoneal approach, guaranteeing regional hypothermia with the Vattikuti-Medanta technique [14, 15]. In Europe, the first two RAKTs were performed in July 2015 by Breda et al. [16]. In 2016, the European Association of Urology (EAU) Robotic Urology Session (ERUS-RAKT) formed a working group in order to report the surgical outcomes and standardize the technique [17, 18]. Today 11 centers joined the ERUS-RAKT working group, reporting more than 300 surgeries with 1 year of follow-up, showing comparable outcomes with OKT as reported in the literature [19].

2.2 Surgical Technique

2.2.1 Living-Donor Nephrectomy

The gold standard approach to perform living-donor nephrectomy is the transperitoneal laparoscopic approach. Considering its functional and operative outcomes, the laparoscopic technique is comparable to the open approach, and it bears the advantages of the minimally invasive approach, maintaining an acceptable cost-benefit compared to the robotic approach.

2.2.2 Bench Table Preparation

After donor nephrectomy, the graft preparation is carried out on the bench table. After nephrectomy, the kidney is positioned in a metallic basin filled with ice slush in order to reduce the graft temperature, and here the reperfusion of the organ is performed with 1 L of cold storage solution (Custodiol®, Celsior®, Institut Georges Lopez-1®). At this point, the vascular dissection, with eventual reconstruction in the case of multiple vessels, takes place [20]. After these steps, according to the preference of the surgeon, the ureter can be pre-stented with a double-J. Once the graft is ready for transplantation, the kidney is packed into a cooling system consisting of a gauze filled with ice slush and subsequently positioned inside the operative field, according to Vattikuti-Medanta technique, in order to provide a low graft temperature during the rewarming time and to protect the kidney from injuries [14]. At the level of the renal hilum, the gauze is opened to form a window in order to access the renal vessels and perform the anastomosis while the graft is kept cool (Fig. 1). As the ice slush melts rapidly, every 15 min, it is added through the GelPOINT® (Applied Medical, Rancho Santa Margherita, CA, USA) via modified Toomey syringes in order to keep the graft temperature below 20 °C until the anastomosis is performed.

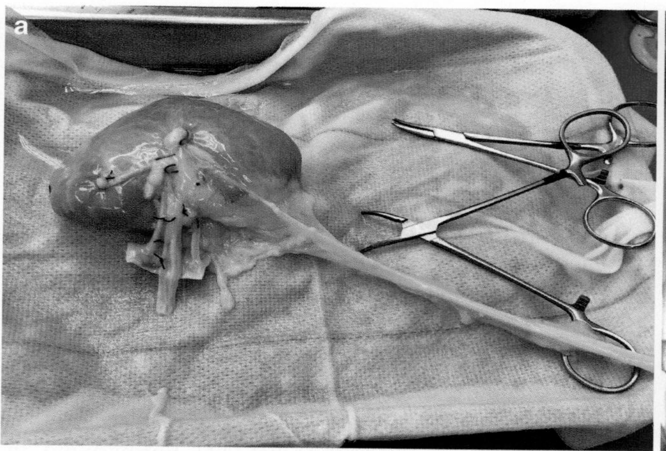

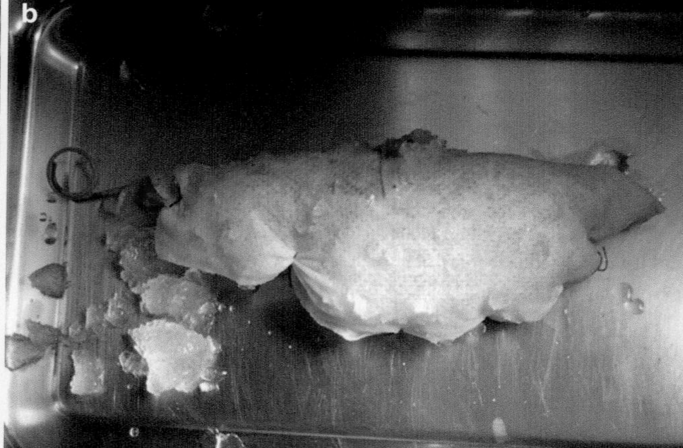

Fig. 1 (**a**) Defatted kidney graft with dissected graft vessels and ureter (**b**) Kidney graft wrapped in gauze filled with ice slush with a central hole for the renal vessels and DJ stent (12 cm, 4.8 French)

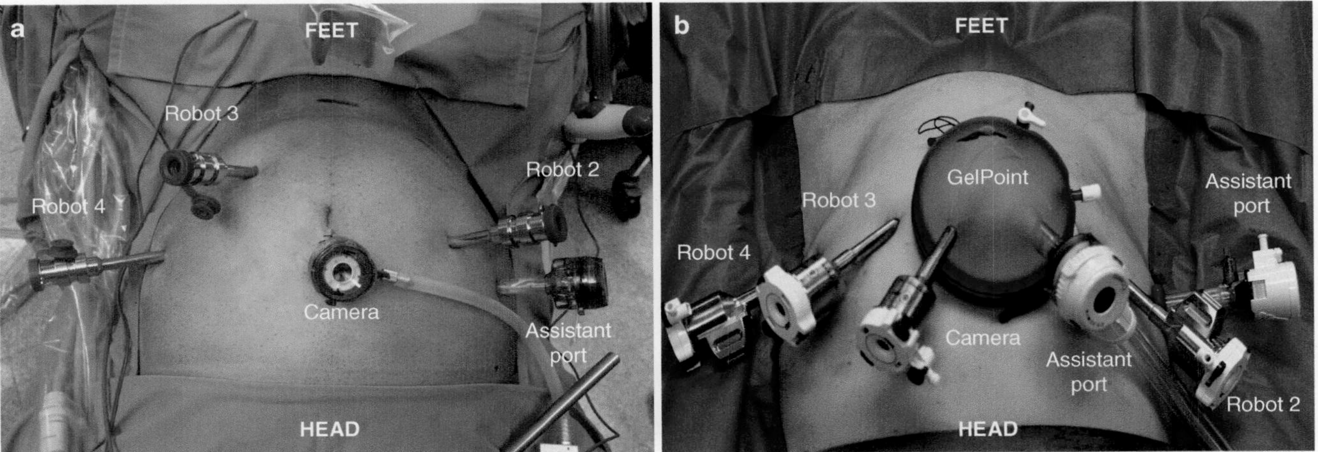

Fig. 2 Port placement in (**a**) Si and X DaVinci systems and (**b**) Xi DaVinci System

2.2.3 Patient and Trocar Positioning

Patient positioning depends on the robotic system employed. The lithotomy position is provided when the DaVinci Si® or X® system is employed, while the dorsal decubitus position is preferred in the case the surgeon uses the DaVinci Xi®. In all cases a 20–30° Trendelenburg is recommended. Firstly, the pneumoperitoneum is created with a 12 mm camera port inserted in the supra-umbilical area. Alternately, the Veress needle puncture, optical trocar access, or the Hasson technique [21] may also be used. Then, three 8 mm robotic ports are placed under vision and docking of robot is performed. If DaVinci Si® is used, the 8 mm port for arm 3 is positioned on the intersection between the line joining the pubis to arm 4 with the umbilicus anterior superior iliac spine line. If RAKT is carried out with Da Vinci Xi®, the robotic ports are placed in line in a simple and reproducible scheme (Fig. 2). In order to introduce the graft in the abdominal cavity and to allow ice slush introducing, a GelPOINT® is positioned, replacing the camera trocar through a 6–8 cm periumbilical incision. The assistant port is placed through the GelPOINT®. Transvaginal access has been proposed as an alternative being a minimally invasive technique in women [22]. In some centers the AirSeal® (Conmed, Utica, NY, USA) system is used to maintain a constant and low pressure at 8 mmHg.

2.2.4 Transplant Bed Preparation

The external iliac vessels are carefully dissected to gain an operative field that allows vascular control, clamping, and arteriotomy/venotomy; a retroperitoneal pouch is created through an incision of the peritoneum in order to allow graft covering after reperfusion (retroperitonealization).

2.2.5 Vascular Anastomosis

For the first step, the anastomotic time is the venous anastomosis between the renal graft vein and the external iliac vein. Two clamps are placed in the external iliac vein to avoid blood loss and a longitudinal venotomy is realized. The end-to-side anastomosis is carried out with a continuous suture using a 6/0 Gore-Tex® CV-6 TTc-9 or THc-12 needle (W.L. Gore and associates Inc., Flagstaff, AZ, USA). A continuous running suture is performed starting from a tight knot at the cranial angle of the posterior wall of the renal vein to the caudal angle, passing the needle in an outside-inside direction. Consequently, the needle is passed in an inside-outside fashion to close the anterior wall of the vein. Before completing the anastomosis, the lumen is flushed with an heparin solution using a 4.8 F ureteric catheter. Finally, a clamp is placed on the graft, vein and the two clamps are removed from the external iliac vein and placed on the external iliac artery.

As soon as the external iliac artery circulation is interrupted, arteriotomy may be realized with a cold linear incision that may be converted to circular incision using a laparoscopic aortic punch. At this point, a continuous suture is performed similar to the venous technique (Fig. 3). The peculiar difference of the arterial anastomosis regards to the first knot at the cranial angle, which is not tightened until the needle has passed through the vessel, otherwise the subsequent needle passage would result to be harder because of the smaller lumen of the artery. When the anastomosis is completed, a clamp is placed on the graft's artery and the external iliac artery clamps are removed. If no signs of bleeding are observed, the graft's vascular clamps are removed, and the reperfusion starts. The evaluation of the kidney's reperfusion is primarily visual, but a Doppler ultrasound might provide an objective evaluation of the flow.

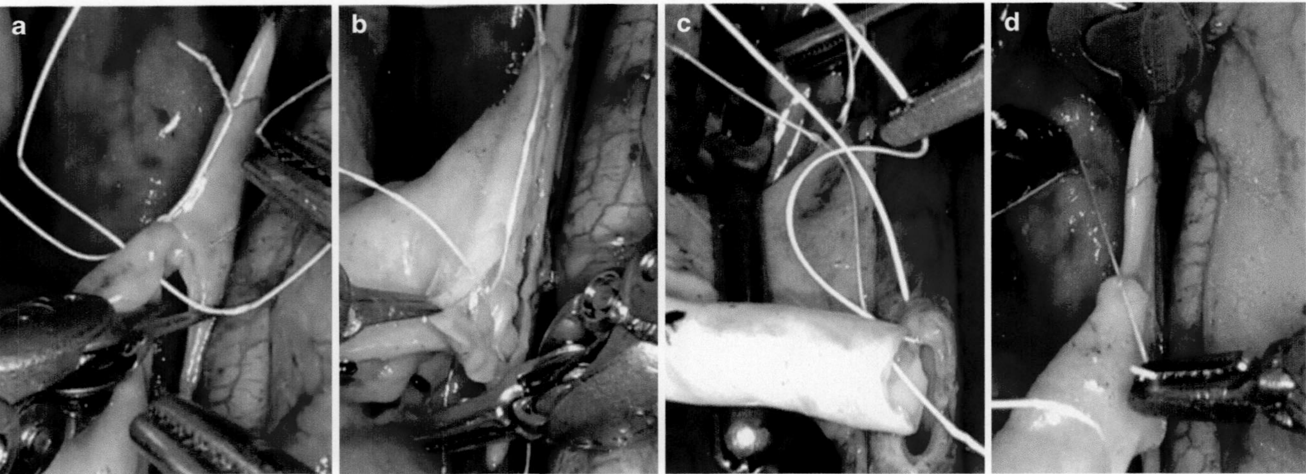

Fig. 3 (**a–b**) Venous anastomosis. (**c–d**) Arterial anastomosis

2.2.6 Ureteroneocystostomy

After reperfusion, ureteroneocystostomy is performed according to the Lich-Gregoir technique using a Monocryl or PDS 5/0 (Ethicoin Inc., Cincinnati, OH, USA) running suture. At this point the retroperitonealization of the graft is performed to avoid complications such as the torsion of the renal pedicle and facilitate eventual graft biopsies. Peritoneal closure is performed with Hem-o-lock® to assure lymph reabsorption from the peritoneum and minimize the risk of lymph collection.

3 Results

The first standardization of the RAKT technique was described by Menon et al., reaching an operative time of 214.1 ± 39.8 min and a rewarming time of 46.6 ± 9.3 min. These results were subsequently in subsequent series showing that a rewarming time below 48 min was correlated with better functional recovery of the kidney 1 month after the operation [17]. The first ERUS-RAKT study showed the results from 147 patients followed for 1 year; positive functional outcomes were reported with a median eGFR of 57.4 mL/min/1.73 m^2 [19]. ERUS-RAKT published consequently another study that compared the first 120 cases of RAKT with the following 171 cases, reporting a statistically significantly shorter total operative time in the second population (p = 0.005). Regarding postoperative complications, 7.5% of patients experienced Clavien-Dindo ≥3 complications, comprehending a 1.7% of delayed graft function (DGF); in 2% of cases, a surgical exploration was required due to active bleeding, and 0.3% of cases underwent transplantectomies performed for acute rejection. Late complications included 3% lymphoceles, 2% ureteric stenosis, and 1% incisional hernias [18]. Few studies from referral centers analyzed the learning curve in RAKT [4, 5]. Gallioli et al. estimated that 35 procedures were associated to a 75% probability to achieve RAKT's trifecta [6]. The comparison between RAKT and OKT was reported in the literature despite the consistent limitations due to the lack of randomized control trials. In the latest retrospective series from Ahlawat et al. [23] with a median follow-up of 2 years, graft postoperative function was comparable to OKT despite a higher operative and rewarming time in the RAKT group. Moreover, the RAKT provided a lower intraoperative estimated blood loss, a reduced use of analgesia, and a decrease incidence of wound infections and symptomatic lymphoceles (Table 1).

4 Complex Surgical Scenarios

4.1 Obese Patient

Obese patients were traditionally considerate a relative contraindication in some countries (BMI > 35 kg/m^2) or at least a strong challenge to KT. A part from the higher technical difficulties, obese patients bear a higher risk of developing wound infections that, in the case of immunocompromised patients, may also lead to graft loss [7].

The first experience of RAKT was reported from the University of Illinois using a 7 cm periumbilical incision and a hand-assisted device. The total surgical time was 223 min and warm ischemia time was 50 min [13]. A subsequent similar series of 28 obese patients (mean BMI 42.6) was published by the same group in 2013, showing higher creatinine at discharge in the robotic group compared to the open group (2.0 vs 1.4 mg/dl) but similar renal function at 6 months (1.5 vs 1.6 mg/dl). Surgical site/wound infection was significantly at a lower rate in the RAKT group compared to the open approach one (28.6% vs 3.6%; p = 0.004) [7].

Table 1 Postoperative outcomes in comparative series of robot-assisted kidney transplantation (RAKT) and open kidney transplantation (OKT)

Author	Surgical approach	Patients (n)	Follow-up (months)	Analgesia (morphine derivatives)	Wound infection	Delayed graft function	Symptomatic lymphocele	Length of hospital stay	Creatinine (last follow-up)	Mortality
Tuğcu (2018)	OKT	40	6	–	3 (7.5)	0	2 (5)	–	0.87 ± 0.73	2 (5)
	RAKT	40	6	–	1 (2.5)	1 (2.5)	0	–	0.95 ± 0.9	0 (0)
Pein (2019)	OKT	21	–	–	0 (0)	1 (4.7)	–	23.5 ± 11.7	145.7 ± 42	0 (0)
	RAKT	21	–	–	0 (0)	0 (0)	–	15 ± 4.1*	182.6 ± 115.9	0 (0)
Maheshwari (2020)	OKT	152	29	3.1 ± 0.45	10 (6.6)	8 (5.2)	2 (1.3)	–	1.1 (0.5–6)	0 (0)
	RAKT	55	27	1.3 ± 0.12*	0 (0)	5 (9.0)	0 (0)	–	1.1 (0.4–7.5)	1 (1.8)
Bansal (2020)	OKT	21	31	3 (2–4)	3 (14.3)	0 (0)	0 (0)	9 (9–9)	1.1 (0.9–1.5)	0 (0)
	RAKT	4	30.5	1.5 (1–2)*	0 (0)	0 (0)	0 (0)	9 (9–11.5)	1.35 (1.08–1.63)	0 (0)
Ahlawat (2020)	OKT	378	23.2	31.2 ± 7.2	15 (4)	9 (2.4)	20 (7)	8 (6–14)	1.2 (1–1.5)	8 (2.1)
	RAKT	126	24.7	20.1 ± 9.5*	0 (0)*	0 (0)	0 (0)*	8 (5–12)	1.2 (1–1.4)	5 (3.9)

*$p < 0.05$

Prudhomme et al. recently compared renal function (eGFR) at 1-year follow-up in the population database of the ERUS-RAKT working group, stratifying the groups according to BMI, and no statistical significant difference between the two groups could be underlined. The median eGFR was 54 (45–60) vs 57 (46–70) vs 63 (49–78) ml/min/1.73 m^2 ($p = 0.5$) in obese (≥30 kg/m^2 BMI), overweight (<30/≥25 kg/m^2 BMI), and non-overweight recipients (<25 kg/m^2 BMI) [24].

4.2 Multiple Vessels

RAKT has been studied, and a few studies have shown its effectiveness also in those setting where the graft is characterized by a complex surgical vascular anatomy that requires reconstruction. The vascular reconstruction may be performed extra, during bench surgery, or intracorporeally with two different techniques. The pantaloon anastomosis provides a latero-lateral anastomosis of the vessel branches. In alternative, an end-to-side anastomosis may be preferred if the branches significantly differ in caliber.

A study from Siena et al. recorded the results from the multi-institutional ERUS-RAKT working group database that compared 21 patients that underwent RAKT from living donors using grafts characterized by a complex vasculature or multiple-vessel grafts (MVGs) to 127 single-vessel ones. The ex vivo vascular reconstruction was carried out on the bench table after living-donor nephrectomy. Total operative time and cold ischemia time were significantly longer in the MVG group ($p = 0.004$ and $p = 0.003$, respectively), but no differences were found for rewarming and anastomotic time. However, at the multivariate analysis, RAKT applied to MVG was not associated with a worse postoperative renal function at 1 month (eGFR <45 ml/min/1.73 m^2) [20]. Another study showed that the number of graft arteries was independently associated with worse GFR at 1 month postoperatively ($p = 0.02$) in obese recipients [24]. In a recent retrospective analysis, 43 MVG patients underwent RAKT were compared with 43 MVG treated with OKT. The pain score, use of analgesic medications, and hospital stay were significantly lower in the robotic group ($p = 0.03$, $p = 0.02$, and $p = 0.05$, respectively), and functional outcomes were comparable between the two populations ($p = 0.9$) [25]. The overall complication rate was similar between the two groups except for wound-related events in favor of the robotic approach ($p = 0.002$).

5 Limitations

5.1 Robot-Assisted Kidney Transplantation: Deceased Donor

Deceased donor grafts are still one of the main limitation in RAKT due to either logistic matter and recipient features. Firstly, the deceased donor KT is performed in an emergency setting usually via an open approach, due to the unpredictable availability of the graft and the expertise needed to perform RAKT. Secondly, the population subjected to KT is at ESRD and under hemodialytic treatment; thus, they bear cardiovascular problems, comprehending the possibility to present with multiple external iliac artery plaques that contraindicate the RAKT. RAKT is contraindicated in these cases because the surgeon lacks the tactile feedback and the choice to position the clamps placement and the portion to perform arteriotomy on the external iliac artery is arbitrary. The first experience in RAKT from deceased donor was carried out at the University of Florence, which developed a dedicated structured program to overcome this limit [9]. Five key phases of RAKT were highlighted, so that each of them was adapted to the emergency setting of a deceased donor's RAKT (Table 2).

The largest cohort of deceased donor RAKT in the literature has been reported by the group of Florence counting 21 patients. When compared to the same technique performed

Table 2 Key phases to perform in deceased donor's RAKT, according to the University of Florence's dedicated protocol

Surgical team	• One experienced surgeon in RAKT. • Two experienced bedside assistants in laparoscopic urologic surgery. • Robotic operating room nursing staff.
Recipient	• Absence of exclusion criteria for RAKT (age < 18 years, contraindications for robotic surgery, multiple previous abdominal surgery, previous transplant). • Absence of severe atheromatic plaques at the level of the iliac vessels.
Robotic operating room	• Setting of a dedicated emergency robotic operating room available during the weekends and at nighttime. • Full availability of the robotic operating room during daytime according to elective surgeries scheduled.
Cold ischemia	• Availability of the operating room with the possibility to start the bench surgery within 16 hours from the beginning of cold storage.
Graft	• Absence of exclusion criteria at bench table, such as in the case of a graft with multiple vessels.

in living donors (LD), surgical outcomes did not significantly differ in the deceased donor's cohort (mean rewarming time was 59 min in LD vs 56 min in DD, $p = 0.4$). In two cases (9.5%), significative postoperative complications (Clavien >2) were recorded, and the other two patients experienced delayed graft function, being on dialysis at the last follow-up. No cases of Clavien-Dindo IV or V were recorded. Moreover, an increasing trend of eGFR from postoperative day 1 to the last follow-up (median of 16 months) was observed, reaching satisfactory graft function and holding all the forementioned advantages of a minimally invasive approach for the patient and all the enhanced movements and visualization for the surgeon [26].

6 Future Perspectives

Since the first experience, the indications for RAKT have been pushed, and obese patients, multiple-vessel grafts, and deceased donors can now be treated by a robotic approach. Some points still remain critical and need to be faced to improve RAKT operative outcomes.

6.1 Intracorporeal Graft Cooling Systems

One of the main critical steps of the KT, especially evident since the robotic approach took over, regards to the rewarming time consisting in the time running from the graft placement into the abdominal cavity of the recipient to graft revascularization, and it is associated with ischemic/reperfusion damage. In order to preserve the graft function during vascular anastomosis, ice slush is commonly used to maintain a low temperature, according to the Vattikuti-Medanta technique described by Menon et al. [15]. In the standard RAKT procedure, graft temperature should be kept below 20 °C before graft revascularization. This regional hypothermia minimizes the potential risk associated with the rewarming time. However, this cooling technique may be suboptimal and the ice slush may affect bowel function [25]. Several cooling devices have been implemented to overcome this limit during the surgical procedure, but due to the scarcity of results and the unavailability on the market, they have not been implemented in the human model. Recently, a cold ischemia device (CID) (Fig. 4) has been described by Territo et al. [27] to maintain a low graft temperature during surgery through the IDEAL phases 0 and 1. In all the preliminary tests of IDEAL phase 0 and in the animal model, the CID was able to maintain a low and constant graft temperature. The IDEAL phase 1 in humans demonstrated feasibility of both OKT and RAKT using the CID, and the graft temperature never exceeded 20 °C (mean temperature: OKT 15.7 °C vs RAKT 18.3 °C).

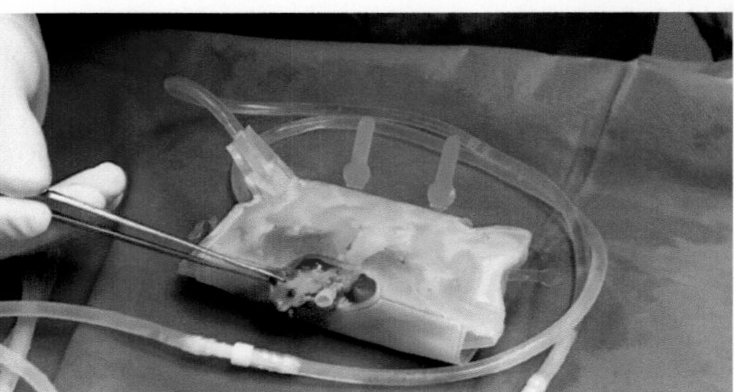

Fig. 4 Cold ischemia device

6.2 Iliac Artery Plaque Tracking

In the majority of cadaveric donor recipients, it is possible to detect multiple arterial plaques of the iliac artery due to advanced renal disease up to ESRD and to the long-term consequences of the hemodialysis to the cardiovascular apparatus. RAKT in these patients is usually contraindicated due to the surgeon's lack of intraoperative haptic feedback that usually guides the surgeon in deciding where to clamp the vessel and perform the arteriotomy. The use of 3D augmented reality technology can overcome this limitation, expanding the indication of RAKT to this new cohort of patients.

6.3 Robot-Assisted Kidney Autotransplantation (RAKAT)

Another novel application of the robotic-assisted renal transplantation is in the field of autotransplantation with RAKAT. The indications to perform a RAKAT are healthy patients with a proximal and/or medium ureteral stricture that can be iatrogenic or functional, in which an in situ reconstruction or an endoscopic approach cannot be performed. Two main techniques have been described, using the DaVinci Si and Xi robotic platform: the extracorporeal and the totally intracorporeal techniques. In the extracorporeal technique, the graft is prepared on the bench table, whereas in the total intracorporeal technique, the kidney is prepared inside the operative field. The transplant technique mimics the standard RAKT steps mentioned before. The largest series of kidney autotransplantation available on literature included seven patients treated with both extracorporeal and totally intracorporeal techniques with no need for open conversion during the procedure [28]. Mean serum postoperative creatinine levels showed a significant improvement. A recent study by Breda et al. was published describing the largest population of patients ($n = 29$) undergoing RAKAT, and they compared the intra-versus extracorporeal approach [29]. They concluded that both e RAKAT = RAKAT represent promising minimally invasive techniques in selected cases with acceptable ischemia time, and, despite a quicker renal function recovery seen in the eRAKAT approach in the short-term, the long-term operative outcomes are comparable [29].

References

1. Collins AJ, Foley RN, Gilbertson DT, Chen S-C. United States Renal Data System public health surveillance of chronic kidney disease and end-stage renal disease. Kidney Int Suppl. (2011). 2015;5(1):2–7. https://doi.org/10.1038/kisup.2015.2.
2. Rosales A, Salvador JT, Urdaneta G, et al. Laparoscopic kidney transplantation. Eur Urol. 2010;57(1):164–7. https://doi.org/10.1016/j.eururo.2009.06.035.
3. Modi P, Pal B, Modi J, et al. Retroperitoneoscopic living-donor nephrectomy and laparoscopic kidney transplantation: experience of initial 72 cases. Transplantation. 2013;95(1):100–5. https://doi.org/10.1097/TP.0b013e3182795bee.
4. Ahlawat RK, Tugcu V, Arora S, et al. Learning curves and timing of surgical trials: robotic kidney transplantation with regional hypothermia. J Endourol. 2018;32(12):1160–5. https://doi.org/10.1089/end.2017.0697.
5. Sood A, Ghani KR, Ahlawat R, et al. Application of the statistical process control method for prospective patient safety monitoring during the learning phase: robotic kidney transplantation with regional hypothermia (IDEAL phase 2a-b). Eur Urol. 2014;66(2):371–8. https://doi.org/10.1016/j.eururo.2014.02.055.
6. Gallioli A, Territo A, Boissier R, et al. Learning curve in robot-assisted kidney transplantation: results from the European Robotic Urological Society Working Group. Eur Urol. 2020;78(2):239–47. https://doi.org/10.1016/j.eururo.2019.12.008.
7. Oberholzer J, Giulianotti P, Danielson KK, et al. Minimally invasive robotic kidney transplantation for obese patients previously denied access to transplantation. Am J Transplant. 2013;13(3):721–8. https://doi.org/10.1111/ajt.12078.
8. Lynch RJ, Ranney DN, Shijie C, Lee DS, Samala N, Englesbe MJ. Obesity, surgical site infection, and outcome following renal transplantation. Ann Surg. 2009;250(6):1014–20. https://doi.org/10.1097/SLA.0b013e3181b4ee9a.
9. Vignolini G, Campi R, Sessa F, et al. Development of a robot-assisted kidney transplantation programme from deceased donors in a referral academic centre: technical nuances and preliminary results. BJU Int. 2019;123(3):474–84. https://doi.org/10.1111/bju.14588.
10. Cohen B, Smits JM, Haase B, Persijn G, Vanrenterghem Y, Frei U. Expanding the donor pool to increase renal transplantation. Nephrol Dial Transplant. 2005;20(1):34–41. https://doi.org/10.1093/ndt/gfh506.
11. Banasik M. Living donor transplantation—the real gift of life. Procurement and the ethical assessment. Ann Transplant. 2006;11(1):4–6.
12. Horgan S, Vanuno D, Benedetti E. Early experience with robotically assisted laparoscopic donor nephrectomy. Surg Laparosc Endosc Percutan Tech. 2002;12(1):64–70. https://doi.org/10.1097/00129689-200202000-00011.
13. Giulianotti P, Gorodner V, Sbrana F, et al. Robotic transabdominal kidney transplantation in a morbidly obese patient. Am J Transplant. 2010;10(6):1478–82. https://doi.org/10.1111/j.1600-6143.2010.03116.x.
14. Menon M, Abaza R, Sood A, et al. Robotic kidney transplantation with regional hypothermia: evolution of a novel procedure utilizing the IDEAL guidelines (IDEAL phase 0 and 1). Eur Urol. 2014;65(5):1001–9. https://doi.org/10.1016/j.eururo.2013.11.011.
15. Menon M, Sood A, Bhandari M, et al. Robotic kidney transplantation with regional hypothermia: a step-by-step description of the Vattikuti Urology Institute-Medanta technique (IDEAL phase 2a). Eur Urol. 2014;65(5):991–1000. https://doi.org/10.1016/j.eururo.2013.12.006.
16. Breda A, Gausa L, Territo A, et al. Robotic-assisted kidney transplantation: our first case. World J Urol. 2016;34(3):443–7. https://doi.org/10.1007/s00345-015-1673-6.
17. Breda A, Territo A, Gausa L, et al. Robot-assisted kidney transplantation: the European experience. Eur Urol. 2018;73(2):273–81. https://doi.org/10.1016/j.eururo.2017.08.028.
18. Musquera M, Peri L, Ajami T, et al. Robot-assisted kidney transplantation: update from the European Robotic Urology Section (ERUS) series. BJU Int. 2021;127(2):222–8. https://doi.org/10.1111/bju.15199.
19. Territo A, Gausa L, Alcaraz A, et al. European experience of robot-assisted kidney transplantation: minimum of 1-year follow-up. BJU Int. 2018;122(2):255–62. https://doi.org/10.1111/bju.14247.
20. Siena G, Campi R, Decaestecker K, et al. Robot-assisted kidney transplantation with regional hypothermia using grafts with multiple vessels after extracorporeal vascular reconstruction: results from the European association of urology robotic urology section working group. Eur Urol Focus. 2018;4(2):175–84. https://doi.org/10.1016/j.euf.2018.07.022.
21. Bianchi G, Martorana E, Ghaith A, et al. Laparoscopic access overview: Is there a safest entry method? Actas Urol Esp. 2016;40(6):386–92. https://doi.org/10.1016/j.acuro.2015.11.011.
22. Doumerc N, Roumiguié M, Rischmann P, Sallusto F. Totally robotic approach with transvaginal insertion for kidney transplantation. Eur Urol. 2015;68(6):1103–4. https://doi.org/10.1016/j.eururo.2015.07.026.
23. Rajesh A, Akshay S, Wooju J, et al. Robotic kidney transplantation with regional hypothermia versus open kidney transplanta-

tion for patients with end stage renal disease: an ideal stage 2B study. J Urol. 2021;205(2):595–602. https://doi.org/10.1097/JU.0000000000001368.

24. Prudhomme T, Beauval JB, Lesourd M, et al. Robotic-assisted kidney transplantation in obese recipients compared to non-obese recipients: the European experience. World J Urol. Published online June 19, 2020. https://doi.org/10.1007/s00345-020-03309-6.
25. Nataraj SA, Zafar FA, Ghosh P, Ahlawat R. Feasibility and functional outcome of robotic assisted kidney transplantation using grafts with multiple vessels: comparison to propensity matched contemporary open kidney transplants cohort. Front Surg. 2020;7:51. https://doi.org/10.3389/fsurg.2020.00051.
26. Vignolini G, Greco I, Sessa F, et al. The university of florence technique for robot-assisted kidney transplantation: 3-year experience. Front Surg. 2020;7:583798. https://doi.org/10.3389/fsurg.2020.583798.
27. Territo A, Piana A, et al. Step-by-step development of a cold ischemia device for open and robotic-assisted renal transplantation. Eur Urol. 2021 May 28;S0302-2838(21)01795-4. https://doi.org/10.1016/j.eururo.2021.05.026.
28. Decaestecker K, Van Parys B, Van Besien J, et al. Robot-assisted kidney autotransplantation: a minimally invasive way to salvage kidneys. Eur Urol Focus. 2018;4(2):198–205. https://doi.org/10.1016/j.euf.2018.07.019.
29. Breda A, Diana P, et al. Intracorporeal versus extracorporeal robot-assisted kidney autotransplantation: experience of the ERUS RAKT Working Group. Eur Urol. 2021. EPub. https://doi.org/10.1016/j.eururo.2021.07.023.

Nephroureterectomy and Bladder Cuff Excision

Ashok K. Hemal, Sumit Saini, David Albala, and Riccardo Autorino

1 Introduction

Upper tract urothelial carcinoma is a relatively uncommon malignancy and accounts for 5–10% of all urothelial carcinomas [1]. Radical nephroureterectomy (RNU) and bladder cuff excision along with template-based lymphadenectomy is now considered the gold standard procedure for all high-risk upper tract urothelial carcinomas [2]. The laparoscopic approach is marred with inferior oncological outcomes despite delivering improved perioperative outcomes in comparison to open approach [3, 4]. With laparoscopic approach, meticulous bladder cuff excision and watertight closure of the cystotomy require intracorporeal suturing which could be the most daunting task even for the most experienced laparoscopic surgeons. The data concerning the robot-assisted approach suggests comparable oncological outcomes to open and laparoscopic approaches while allowing favorable perioperative outcomes in terms of blood loss, length of hospital stay, and complications [5]. The most recent National Cancer Database (NCDB)-based analysis favors a robot-assisted approach over the laparoscopic approach regarding the rates of lymph node dissection/yield and better oncological outcomes [6].

The robotic EndoWrist technology (*da Vinci*), with the three-dimensional visualization and magnification, allows for the performance of this part of the procedure with utmost precision and ease. Also, the evidence is mounting regarding the benefit of template-based lymphadenectomy, even in clinically node-negative patients, where robot-assisted procedure seems to have an edge [2, 6].

One of the challenges of the RNU procedure is the need to address both the upper and lower urinary tract. Indeed, discussion on the best way to manage the bladder cuff fueled the debate in the laparoscopic era [5]. One of the advantages of robot-assisted overstandard laparoscopy for this procedure is that the robotic platform facilitates the "multi-quadrant" approach which is required for ablative and reconstructive components. Initial robotic experience was mainly based on the use of the S® and Si® platforms that would typically require robot re-docking and/or patient repositioning. However, the concept of a "single-stage" approach was then introduced with pioneering work by Hemal et al. and others with the main aim of reducing the operative time while maintaining surgical effectiveness [7, 8]. More recently, the introduction of the da Vinci Xi® Surgical System further facilitated this approach [9, 10].

In this chapter, we aim to describe our technique for robotic-assisted nephroureterectomy with bladder cuff excision and template-based lymphadenectomy in a step-by-step manner with tips and tricks to help surgeons perform this procedure efficiently and with ease.

2 Case Selection and Preparing for Surgery

Regardless of the tumor location, radical nephroureterectomy with bladder cuff excision is the standard management of nonmetastatic, organ-confined, high-risk upper tract urothelial carcinoma. Due to the inferior oncological outcomes

A. K. Hemal
Department of Urology, Comprehensive Cancer Center, Wake Forest Institute for Regenerative Medicine, Robotics Committee, Baptist Medical Center, Robotics and Minimally Invasive Surgery, Atrium Health Wake Forest Baptist & Wake Forest School of Medicine, Winston-Salem, NC, USA

S. Saini (✉)
Department of Urology, Robotics and Minimally Invasive Surgery, Atrium Health Wake Forest Baptist, Winston-Salem, NC, USA
e-mail: ssaini@wakehealth.edu

D. Albala
State University of New York, Downstate Health Sciences University, Urology, Crouse Hospital, Associated Medical Professionals, Syracuse, NY, USA

R. Autorino
Urologic Oncology, Division of Urology, VCU Health, GU Disease Working Group, VCU Massey Cancer Center, Richmond, VA, USA

P. Wiklund et al. (eds.), *Robotic Urologic Surgery*, https://doi.org/10.1007/978-3-031-00363-9_44

in non-organ-confined disease (pT3/T4 +/– bulky lymph nodes), minimally invasive surgery is a contraindication [4, 11]. Other contraindications for robot-assisted procedure include medical conditions including severe cardiopulmonary disease which precludes general anesthesia. Multiple previous abdominal surgeries are also relative contraindication. However, in these cases, a retroperitoneal approach can be adopted.

A thorough history and physical examination is necessary including the review of all the imaging studies. Urethrocystoscopy is also an integral part of the evaluation to rule out concomitant bladder carcinoma. Even when highly suspicious, imaging studies alone are usually not sufficient to proceed with RNU. However, in the case of a poorly functioning kidney, or pyonephrosis or severe hydroureteronephrosis with gross hematuria and periureteral or perinephric stranding, a positive urine cytology can be deemed sufficient to proceed. If there is any doubt, then ureterorenoscopy and guided biopsies should be performed to stage/risk stratify the disease.

Patients on antiplatelets and anticoagulants should be seen by their primary care physician/cardiologists, and appropriate clearances should be sought to either hold the medications or to bridge with heparin in the perioperative period depending upon the patient's cardiovascular condition. Aspirin can be continued throughout the perioperative period and in high-risk cases, we also give heparin.

Informed consent is ideally obtained in the clinic prior to scheduling the surgery. Both usual and unusual risks associated with the procedure and anesthesia, which includes bleeding, infection, damage to adjacent structures (including the bowel, pancreas, spleen, liver), urine leak, hernia formation, testicular pain, renal insufficiency, disease recurrence, myocardial infarction, stroke, deep venous thromboembolism, pulmonary embolism, and very rarely death, should be discussed with the patients. All patients should also be informed regarding the need for conversion to an open procedure with a low threshold in the event of any difficulty (technical/surgical) encountered.

3 Patient Positioning

After induction of anesthesia in the supine position, per urethral catheter is placed (16/18 Fr). The abdomen is shaved from the costal margins till pubic symphysis. The patient is then placed in a full-flank position with the lower leg flexed at the hip and knee joint, with the upper leg fully extended. This provides stability and prevents forward roll in this position. A pillow is placed between the knees, and the table may be flexed to open up the space between the costal margin and the iliac crest. Table flexion is not essential while using Xi in which the table is usually kept flat or if desired, flexion can be done to open the space between the iliac crest and costal cartilage. To prevent the neurovascular bundle injury or compression, an axillary roll is placed under the patient's axilla. The back of the patient is supported by bolsters or bean bags, and Velcro straps are also used to secure the patient both at the chest and hips. The dependent arm is secured on a padded arm board straight out and the nondependent arm is either placed on the Allen's rest with the elbow flexed or kept straight down the side of the patient and secured. Once positioned, all the pressure points must be padded as appropriate.

We currently employ a four-armed transperitoneal robotic technique using the da Vinci Xi with an additional port (12 mm) for the bedside assistant. For right side cases, an additional 5 mm port to accommodate a locking grasper for liver retraction can be used. The scrub technician also stays on the same side next to the bedside assistant for the ease of instrument placement and exchanges.

4 Instrumentation and Equipment

Robotic Equipment

- da Vinci Xi Surgical System (Intuitive Surgical Inc., Sunnyvale, CA),
- Fenestrated bipolar forceps.
- Monopolar curved scissors.
- ProGrasp forceps or tip-up fenestrated grasper.
- Large suture cut needle driver.
- Large needle driver (optional).
- Maryland bipolar forceps (optional).
- Vessel sealer (optional).

Trocars

- 8 mm robotic trocars × 4
- 12 mm AirSeal port (Surgiquest Inc., Milford, CT)
- 5 mm port (optional, for right side cases).

Sutures

- 3-0 barbed V-Loc suture (Covidien, Minneapolis, MN) or 3-0 poliglecaprone suture
- 3-0 polyglactin 910 suture
- 0-polydioxanone (PDS) suture
- 4-0 poliglecaprone suture
- 4-0 silk or nylon suture (for drain).

Laparoscopic Instruments for Bedside Assistant

- Needle driver.
- Blunt grasper.
- Suction irrigator.
- Hem-o-Lok clip applier.
- Endovascular stapler with vascular loads (optional).
- Endo Catch II or bag for specimen retrieval.
- Locking grasper or Allis (optional for right side cases).

5 Surgical Technique

5.1 Step 1: Abdominal Access

Using either the closed (Veress needle) which we do routinely or open-access (Hasson) technique, very infrequently based on the surgeon's preference, pneumoperitoneum is created. While using Hasson's technique for entry into the abdominal cavity, a point in the midline 3–4 cm above the umbilicus is chosen. This could later serve as the 12 mm assistant port (AirSeal, if available). The abdomen is insufflated. Higher pressures up to 15–20 mm Hg could be used at the time of port placement based on the surgeon's preference and then should be brought down to 10–13 mm of Hg.

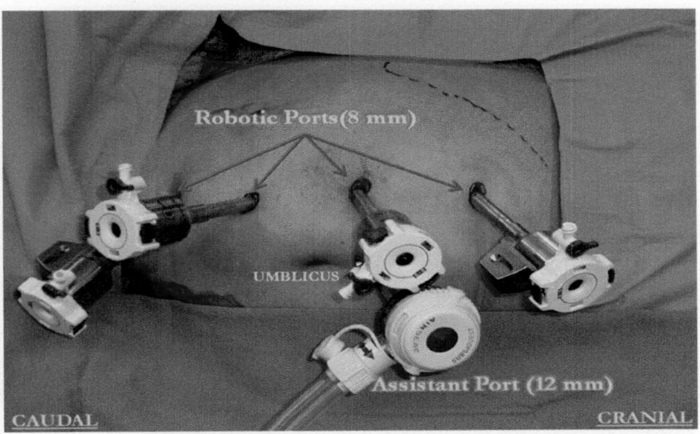

Fig. 2 Depiction of port placement (right RNU-BCE) on a patient

5.2 Step 2: Port Placement and Configuration

Once the pneumoperitoneum is created, the initial intra-abdominal visualization may be done using a 0-degree lens, which could also be utilized for placement of the ports. Port placement is a crucial step but has been simplified over time to almost a standard template for the robotic radical nephroureterectomy with bladder cuff excision, which allows for dissection in both abdomen and the pelvis, without the need for patient repositioning or re-docking of the robot which has been a major advance for this surgery. All ports are 8 mm in size and positioned in a linear/curvilinear fashion (Figs. 1 and 2). The first port is placed just lateral to the rectus muscle, immediately cranial to the level or above the umbilicus as per patient built. The second port is placed in line with the first port, around 2 fingerbreadths inferior to the costal margin. The third port is placed 6–8 cm caudal to the first port and immediately lateral to the rectus muscle. The final/fourth port is placed 6–8 cm caudal to the third either in line with the rest of the three ports or slightly toward the midline. Another 12 mm assistant port (*AirSeal*, if available) is also placed in the midline, around 3–4 cm cranial to the umbilicus. An additional 5 mm port can be placed in the subxiphoid area to accommodate a locking Allis or grasper for liver retraction in right side cases. Once all the ports are in position, the robot is docked perpendicular to the table, over the patient's back.

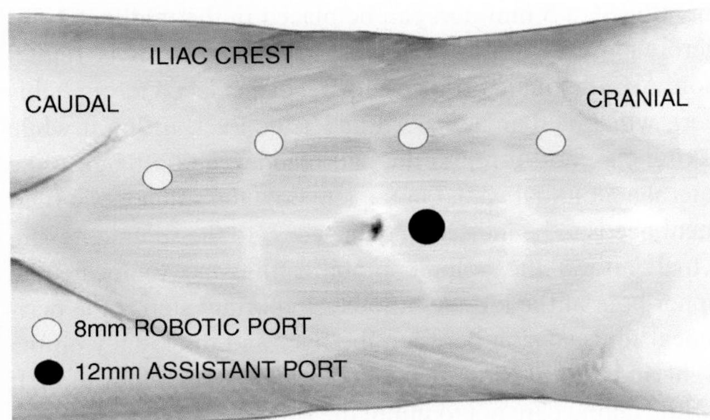

Fig. 1 Illustration for port placement (right RNU-BCE + LND) for the da Vinci Xi platform. The ports can be placed medially/laterally based on the patient's body habitus

The camera hopping and targeting/retargeting feature of Xi allows for the multi-quadrant approach to this surgery as needed. During the abdominal component of the procedure, the camera is positioned in the first port just cranial to the level of the umbilicus, but during the pelvic component, the camera can be hopped to the port placed 6–8 cm caudal to the first port. The arms are then completely disconnected and the ipsilateral ureterovesical junction is targeted. This allows the robotic boom to rotate, reorient, and reposition the robotic arms, to maximize the range of motion and patient clearance.

With all ports and the robotic arms docked in position (Fig. 3), we proceed with the radical nephrectomy portion of the procedure typically with the 30° lens. Under direct vision, robotic instruments are inserted into the cannulas by the bedside assistant into the surgical field. As the camera is positioned through the first port, the instruments placed in position through the second and third ports serve as the right/left working arms based on the side of the surgery. For the right-sided procedure, the second port which is the most cranial port becomes the right working arm, and the third port which is placed 6–8 cm from the camera port serves as the left working arm. This orientation is reversed for the left-sided procedure, where the third port which is 6–8 cm caudal to the camera port becomes the right arm and the most cranial

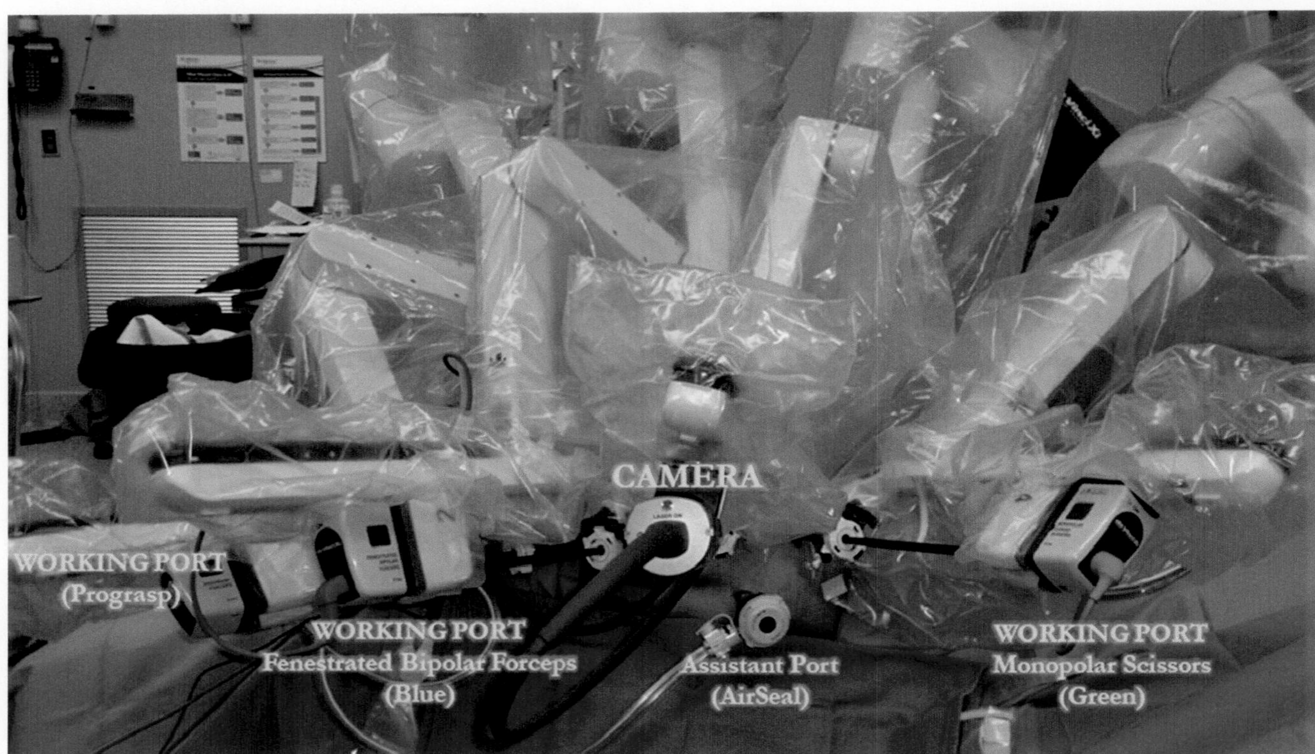

Fig. 3 Ports/robotic arms docked (right RNU-BCE) with instruments in position

or the second port serves as the left arm. Monopolar curved scissors are placed in the right working arm, and the fenestrated bipolar forceps are placed in the left working arm (Fig. 3). The ProGrasp or tip-up fenestrated grasper is placed through the most caudal or the fourth port cannula (Fig. 3). We keep the energy setting of 3 or 5 for both coagulation and cutting depending on the steps of the procedure (e.g., 3 near the hilar structures or for lymphadenectomy or bladder cuff excision) while using the Xi which has an integrated ERBE VIO dV generator.

5.3 Step 3: Colon Mobilization

Upon entering the abdominal cavity, if any adhesions are encountered between the abdominal structures (omentum/mesentery, etc.) and the peritoneum, these are taken down sharply in the avascular plane closest to or at the abdominal wall. The first step while performing the radical nephroureterectomy is colonic mobilization. The colon is mobilized medially by incising the relatively avascular white line of Toldt, using gentle sweeping motions. Mesocolon is swept over the Gerota's fascia without breaching either of these. The color and compactness of the fat allow for the differentiation between the two. Mesocolic fat is bright yellow and more loosely packed, while the perinephric fat is densely packed and pale yellow. The colon is reflected from the hepatic/splenic flexure to the pelvic inlet. This allows adequate exposure of the kidney and proximal ureter.

On the right side, the liver usually obstructs the view of the colon and/or kidney. For better exposure, the right coronary ligament can be incised which helps in retracting the liver to allow access to the Morrison's pouch. As already mentioned, a 5 mm port can be placed in the midline, 2 fingerbreadths away from the xiphoid process for liver retraction. An atraumatic grasper with a lock is placed through this port, which is then advanced under the liver, lifting it while taking care not to injure the gall bladder, and affixed to the lateral abdominal wall. On the left side, the splenocolic ligament needs to be incised to gain access to the splenic flexure which allows the colonic mobilization and to locate the upper pole of the kidney. Another important step is the peritoneal fold incision between the liver and the kidney on the right and the division of the lienorenal ligament on the left (while taking care not to injure the splenic vessels). Based on the surgeon's preference, this step could be done at the time of upper pole mobilization after renal vessel ligation/hilar dissection or at the beginning during colon mobilization.

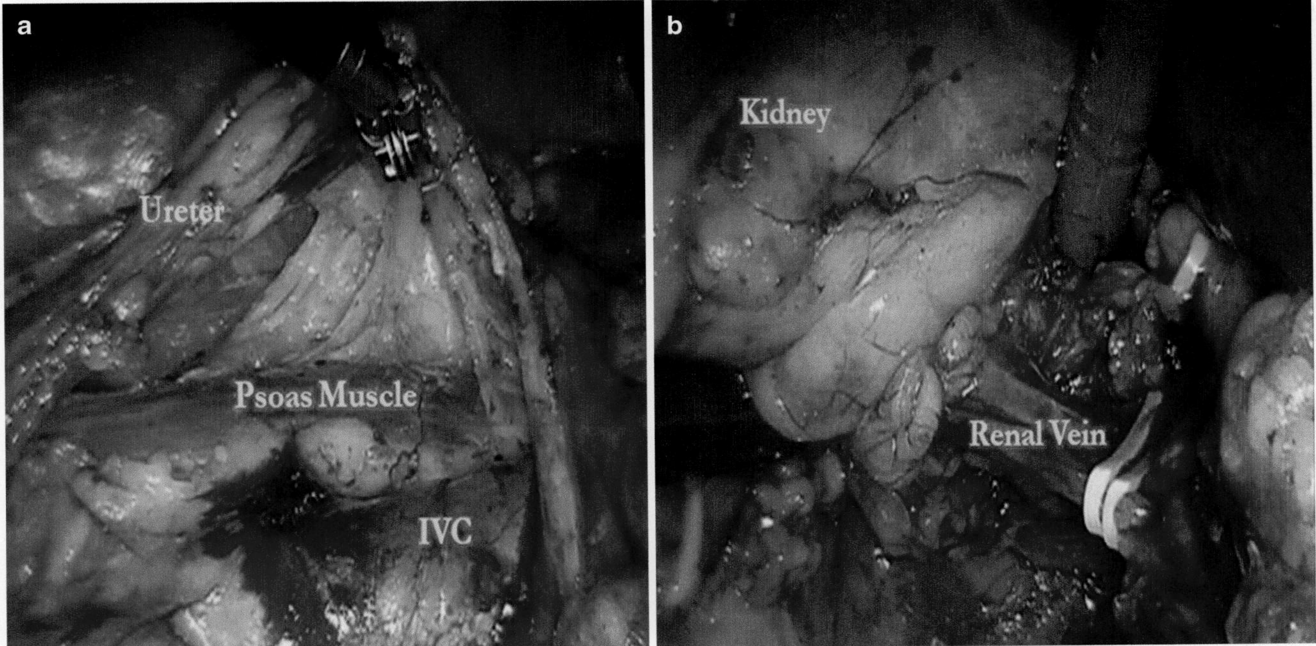

Fig. 4 (**a**) Depiction of lifting the right ureter off the psoas muscle. (**b**) Depiction of Hilar dissection immediately following the renal artery division; renal vein clipped

5.4 Step 4: Dissection of the Ureter and Identification of the Renal Hilum

On the right side, the duodenum is kocherized to expose the inferior vena cava (IVC) which is a necessary step not just for the renal hilar dissection but also for the lymph node dissection. After colonic mobilization, the lower pole of the kidney is identified and lifted with the tip-up grasper (fourth arm). Dissecting further down and medially, the ureter and gonadal vein are identified. They are then traced back to the hilum by gently lifting only the ureter on the right and ureter and gonadal vein together on the left. A window is also created over the psoas muscle, while gently lifting these structures, dissection is continued cranially (Fig. 4a). On the right side, the gonadal vein is traced to its insertion in the IVC, while on the left, it is traced back to its insertion in the left renal vein.

5.5 Step 5: Hilar Dissection

As we proceed cranially, the renal hilum is reached. Fine dissection at the renal hilum can be aided using additional instruments like vessel sealer, Maryland bipolar forceps, or the monopolar hook. Typically, we continue to use the monopolar scissors and the fenestrated bipolar forceps to save the cost and the time required to switch the instruments. Hilar dissection is done with utmost precision to skeletonize the proximal renal artery and renal vein for about 2–3 cm segment, individually. During the dissection, the fourth robotic arm with ProGrasp or tip-up grasper in position aids in continued retraction of the kidney laterally. The assistant can provide additional help in retracting other structures like the colon, duodenum, and IVC on the right side and the colon, pancreas, and spleen on the left side, for unhindered dissection at the renal hilum. Considerable attention must also be given to identify accessory renal vessels, lumbar vessels, adrenal vessels, and early branching of the main renal artery or the renal vein. Preoperative dedicated CT scans such as CT angiogram of the abdomen or the three-dimensional reconstruction is of great importance to identify these structures intraoperatively. Once the renal hilum is dissected, the renal artery is divided first using extra-large Hem-o-Lok clips 3 on the stay side and one distal toward the kidney; if complex dissection, then we apply one clip over the artery and proceed for renal vein dissection and division using extra-large Hem-o-Lok clips 3 on the stay side and one distal toward the kidney (Fig. 4b). Other potential options are suture ligation with 0-silk or using an endovascular stapler. If the stapler is used, we try and place at least one extra-large Hem-o-Lok clip proximally on the renal artery and vein before stapling, to decrease the risk of vascular fistula formation or in event of misfire or any other issue. The bedside assistant should be facile in deploying the stapler and understanding the device.

5.6 Step 6: Adrenal Gland Dissection and Kidney Mobilization

Immediately after the ligation of renal vessels, the ureter is clipped. The clipping of the ureter is done only after the renal vessels have been ligated to prevent the buildup of the urine in the renal pelvis which might obscure the hilar dissection. Ureteral clipping plays an important role in the prevention of any tumor spillage or the shed tumor cells to move along the natural transit of the urine, from the pelvicalyceal system caudally into the ureter and the bladder, especially for tumors in the renal pelvis.

After the ligation of renal vessels and clipping of the ureter, the upper pole of the kidney is mobilized usually with an adrenal sparing technique unless there is evidence of direct tumor involvement into the adrenal, either visually or radiographically. The adrenal glands may have a complex vascular supply, and this should be borne in mind while dissecting the adrenals from the renal capsule. Once the adrenal gland is preserved and the upper polar mobilization is complete (incision of peritoneal folds between the liver and kidney on the right and lienorenal ligament division on the left side, if not done before), the dissection is continued laterally and behind the kidney to divide all the attachments, and the kidney is freed from all around. The dissection is then continued caudally along the ureter toward the true pelvis. Until the bladder cuff excision, the kidney (within the Gerota's fascia) is left in the upper quadrant.

5.7 Step 7: Lymphadenectomy

For the tumors arising from the renal pelvis/ureter, template-based lymphadenectomy is usually performed. EAU guidelines suggest a survival benefit even in clinically and pathologically node-negative patients if template-based lymphadenectomy is performed for all tumors with muscle-invasive disease (>/= T2) [2].

The following templates can be used [12].

- Renal Pelvis/Proximal Ureter
  - Right side: hilar, paracaval, precaval, and retrocaval ± interaortocaval.
  - Left side: hilar, para-aortic, and preaortic ± interaortocaval.
- Mid-ureter
  - Right side: paracaval + interaortocaval + right common iliac.
  - Left side: para-aortic + interaortocaval + left common iliac.
- Distal Ureter (Extended Pelvic Lymphadenectomy)
  - Right side: right pelvic nodes (obturator, internal and external iliac, and common iliac lymph nodes) ± paracaval.
  - Left side: left pelvic nodes (obturator, internal and external iliac, and common iliac lymph nodes) ± para-aortic.

Lymph node dissection is done using blunt and sharp dissection without the use of electrocautery to avoid any inadvertent damage to the major vessels. Each nodal packet is clipped both proximally and distally to avoid/reduce the risk of lymphocele and sent for pathological analysis separately. Vessel-sealing device, if used, is very helpful during this step as it avoids the need to use several clips.

5.8 Step 8: Dissection of the Distal Ureter and Bladder Cuff

As we move caudally into the pelvis, the robotic arms require some adjustments to allow the transition from the abdomen to the pelvic component of the procedure. All the robotic arms are completely removed, and the camera is hopped to the third port (6–8 cm caudal to the first/periumbilical port; see port placement section). Once the camera is switched to this new position, it is then centered/focused on the ipsilateral ureterovesical junction, and the boom is retargeted. This is an inherent automatic feature of Xi which allows for multi-quadrant surgery in the same patient position. The boom rotates and the robotic arms align themselves in the most convenient position allowing maximum range of motion and patient clearance. The instruments of choice (surgeon's preference) are inserted taking into consideration that the right working arm is through the most caudal port and the left working arm is through the port just above the level of the umbilicus (previous camera port). The fourth robotic arm is placed in the most cranial robotic port.

While ureteral dissection is continued caudally (Fig. 5a), the vas deferens in males and the broad ligament in females are encountered. These are then clipped and divided if needed. The medial umbilical ligament is then divided to allow for the rotation of the bladder for easier access to the bladder cuff if needed or else retraction with one arm is sufficient. The coverings of the bladder in the peri-ureteral region are also incised, allowing the visualization of the detrusor muscle fibers. The ureter is then grasped and placed on traction by either using the fourth arm or with the help of the bedside assistant, which assists in the identification of the ureteral insertion into the bladder and clear delineation of ureterovesical junction (Fig. 5b).

5.9 Step 9: Bladder Cuff Excision

We typically use the extra-vesical technique for the bladder cuff excision. At Atrium Health Wake Forest Baptist, we prefer Gemcitabine intra-vesical instillation in the beginning

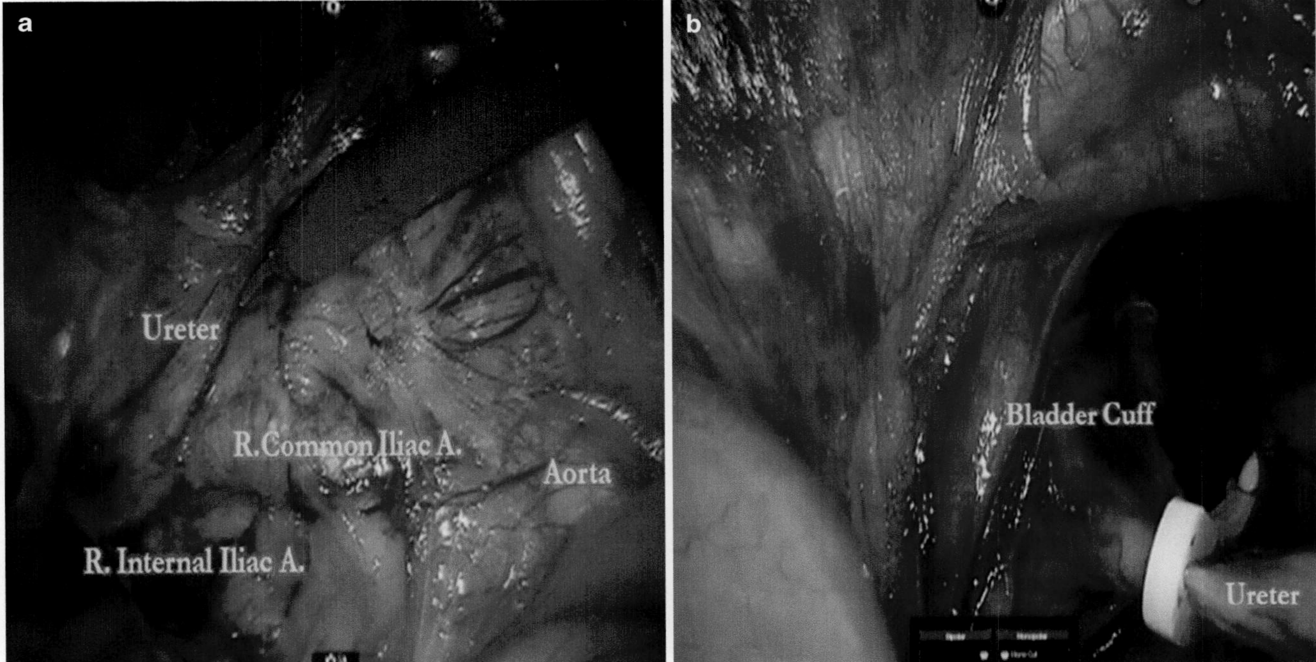

Fig. 5 (a) Dissection continued caudally; lifting the ureter at the level of crossing over the iliac vessels. (b) Depiction of the bladder cuff with the ureter placed on traction

which is left for 60 minutes, and the bladder is emptied prior to excision of bladder cuff to minimize the risk of urine spillage/intravesical chemotherapeutic, into the peritoneal cavity. A full-thickness stay suture using either a 3-0 barbed suture or polyglactin on the lateral aspect of the bladder cuff is placed to prevent the retraction of the bladder mucosa once the bladder cuff is completely excised, using suture cut needle driver in one hand and ProGrasp or bipolar forceps in the other hand. The use of a second needle driver can be avoided to reduce the cost. Monopolar scissors are then used to dissect the bladder cuff with a 1–1.5 cm margin all around the ureterovesical junction. Using sharp dissection/incisions, the bladder lumen is entered, and the bladder cuff is excised. The contralateral ureteral orifice can be visualized once inside the bladder lumen, and caution must be taken to avoid its injury. Once this step is completed, the whole specimen (en bloc) is placed into a specimen bag for extraction later.

5.10 Step 10: Bladder Repair/Cystotomy Closure

Bladder repair is done in layers, with mucosal closure being the first layer. We typically use 3-0 poliglecaprone suture in a continuous fashion for mucosal layer closure. After the complete closure of the first layer, the second full-thickness closure is done using the previously placed 3-0 barbed stay suture, again in the continuous fashion. Otherwise one can run the same stay suture incorporating the mucosa and detrusor and second full-thickness layer. We then check the integrity of the bladder repair by retrograde filling through the Foley catheter, by instilling saline (+/– methylene blue). Insufflation pressure is then reduced to 5 mm Hg, and the hemostasis is confirmed at all the dissection sites (abdomen and pelvis). If easy and peritoneal flap is available, we retroperitonealize.

5.11 Step 11: Retrieval of the Specimen and Closure

We deploy a 15 Fr Jackson Pratt closed suction drain through the most caudal 8 mm port if the specimen is planned to be retrieve through the supraumbilical assistant port (midline) and secure this with the absorbable suture. In most of the cases if not necessary, we do not place the drain, and the specimen is retrieved through the most caudal 8 mm port site (extending incision laterally in transverse direction). All 12 mm ports are required to be closed at the fascial level if not used for specimen retrieval. Subsequent to the specimen removal, the fascia is closed using a 0-polydioxanone suture in a continuous fashion. The robot is un-docked and all

Table 1 Reported outcomes of robotic nephroureterectomy

Reference	Year	No. of cases	Robotic system	LND (%)	>/=pT3 (%)	OT, min	EBL, ml	LOS, days	Overall complication rate, %
Hemal et al. [7]	2011	15	S/Si	20	26.6	183	103	2.7	0
Lim et al. [13]	2013	32	S/Si	34[a]	40.6	250	263	6.2	28
Lee et al. [14]	2013	17	S/Si	80	23.5	161	99	3.0	20
Zargar et al. [8]	2014	31	S/Si	45	45.1	300	200	5.0	19
Ambani et al. [15]	2014	22	S/Si	59	36.4	298	380	3.1	37
Melquist et al. [16]	2016	37	Si	100	19	306	150	5.0	14
Patel et al. [17]	2018	87	S/Si/Xi	S/Si: 54 Xi: 84	S/Si: 33.3 Xi: 41	S/Si: 232 Xi: 184	S/Si: 156 Xi: 122	S/Si: 2.6 Xi: 2.3	S/Si: 17 Xi: 13
De Groote et al. [18]	2019	78 (Si/Xi: 69/9)	Si/Xi	41	29.5	167	124	4.0	24.4
Lee et al. [19]	2019	124	S/Si/Xi	NR	28.22	248.5	200.5	10.3	9.7
Ye et al. [20]	2020	29	Si	NR	20.8	300	100	5.0	NR
Veccia et al. [10]	2021	148	Xi	38.1	30.8	215.5	100	2.0	17.7

Bladder cuff excision was extravesical in all series
NR: not reported
[a] Retroperitoneal lymph node dissection was not performed, only pelvic LND

8 mm ports are removed. These ports do not require fascial closure and typically only the skin closure is needed. Scarpa's fascia is closed with interrupted 4-0 polyglactin suture, and the skin is closed using the 4-0 poliglecaprone (continuous, subcuticular). The port sites are also closed using the same suture.

6 Postoperative Management

Patients are started on a clear liquid diet on postoperative day 0/1 and maintenance intravenous fluids based on the hydration status/urine output. We typically use acetaminophen tablet 1000 mg and ketorolac as the analgesic adjunct. We avoid narcotics and follow care pathways. Patients are also encouraged to ambulate, starting from the evening of the surgery or the postoperative day 1, with assistance. The diet is advanced, as tolerated. Typically, the drain is removed on postoperative day 1, and the patient is discharged or as needed. Per urethral catheter is usually kept for 7 days. Cystogram is not usually required unless there is clinical suspicion of a urine leak.

7 Steps to Avoid Complications

- Empty the bladder before dividing the bladder cuff to prevent spillage of urine. Also, empty chemotherapeutic agent if it is instilled.
- Judicious use of electrocautery to minimize the risk of any inadvertent vascular/bowel injury.
- Use clips or vessel-sealing device at the time of lymphadenectomy to minimize the risk of lymphatic leak/lymphocele.
- Perform a two-layered closure for the cystotomy repair to minimize urine leak.
- Place clips over the artery/vein proximally, before firing endovascular stapler (if employed) to prevent the risk of fistula formation or use extra-large Hem-o-Lok clips, and divide in between to save on cost.
- Carefully dissect the distal ureter in females, to avoid any inadvertent injury due to its proximity to the cervix/vagina, as it may lead to the creation of a vesicovaginal fistula. The bedside assistant may provide some help during this step by placing a swab on sponge stick in the vagina to aid in its identification.

8 Outcomes

An overview of studies reporting on robot-assisted nephroureterectomy for the surgical management of upper tract urothelial carcinoma is provided in Table 1.

9 Discussion

Robot-assisted RNU is a challenging procedure that includes both an extirpative (nephroureterectomy/abdominal component with lymphadenectomy) and a reconstructive (bladder cuff excision and bladder repair/pelvic component) portion. With continued advancements in the robotic surgical systems over time, the surgical technique has evolved as well, and by and large all across the globe, surgeons prefer using Xi robot for this surgery.

While the earlier description of this procedure required the repositioning of the patient and re-docking/repositioning of the robot, the first series with a description of complete robot-assisted RNU and bladder cuff excision without patient repositioning or re-docking of the robot was published in 2011 (using S/Si systems) [7]. With the launch of the robotic system, da Vinci Xi in 2014. the overhead configuration of the robotic arms, features like camera hopping, multi-quadrant access using targeting/retargeting, and patient clearance, further facilitated the surgical procedure. One retrospective analysis compared the two surgical systems where the Xi system was found to have an edge over the S/Si system. Operative times, anesthesia costs, and overall hospitalization costs were found to be significantly lower than the S/Si surgical system while simultaneously allowing for the single docking technique. This analysis suggested improved outcomes with advancing technology [17].

Template-based lymph node dissection has been studied both prospectively and retrospectively. Based upon the side and location of the primary tumor, upper tract urothelial carcinoma has a characteristic pattern of retroperitoneal lymph nodal metastases with a tendency for the involvement of interaortocaval lymph nodes (tumors of the renal pelvis on the right side) and right to left spread [12, 21]. Lymph node dissection (template-based) at the time of radical nephroureterectomy has recently been included in the guidelines secondary to the emerging evidence supporting the survival benefit. In patients with muscle-invasive and locally advanced disease, template-based lymph node dissection demonstrated staging and survival benefits [22]. Even in clinically and pathologically node-negative disease, a definite survival advantage has been demonstrated [23, 24]. It has also been found that the template-based dissection, rather than the lymph node yield, has a greater impact on survival [25].

Surgical approach to the RNU has been found to have an impact on this inclusion of lymph node dissection. Over the years increased utilization of robot-assisted procedures has been demonstrated. With increased adoption, it has also been noted that in clinically node-negative patients who underwent a robot-assisted procedure, there is a higher likelihood of receiving lymph node dissection. At the same time, it was also noted that patients who underwent a robot-assisted procedure have significantly better perioperative morbidity and overall survival [6]. This is a very important finding as the robotic approach allows for meticulous lymph node dissection with ease (three-dimensional visualization, magnification, and EndoWrist technology) which in turn is associated with better survival outcomes and without any antecedent increase in perioperative morbidity.

Following RNU, the rate of bladder recurrence is 22–47% [2]. Postoperative intravesical instillation of mitomycin C, pirarubicin, epirubicin, and gemcitabine has been tried previously to reduce such recurrences. Significant reductions in recurrences have been found in a few randomized prospective trials like ODMIT-C (mitomycin C) and THP Monotherapy Study Group Trial (pirarubicin) [26, 27], although the ideal time for such instillation is not yet clear as various time points after RNU was used in these studies (0–10 days) for the intravesical instillation of chemotherapy. A few retrospective analyses have also evaluated the impact of intraoperative instillation and found significant reductions in bladder recurrences with this approach when compared to postoperative instillation [28, 29]. Although the benefit of maintenance intravesical instillations seems plausible (extrapolating the results/advantage of maintenance intravesical chemotherapy in non-muscle-invasive bladder carcinoma), yet no current evidence supports this hypothesis. A prospective randomized trial evaluated this hypothesis and found some potential delay in recurrences with maintenance intravesical instillations but fails to register significant recurrence-free survival benefit in this regard when compared to single intravesical instillation [30]. Thus, the current guidelines recommend only a single postoperative intravesical chemotherapy instillation to reduce bladder recurrences [2].

There is also an emerging role of perioperative chemotherapy for high-risk upper tract urothelial carcinoma. The current guidelines recommend postoperative/adjuvant chemotherapy [2], as the data regarding its use and benefit is more robust which is primarily derived from a phase III randomized trial using gemcitabine-cisplatin-based chemotherapy. Significant improvement in disease-free survival was seen in patients with muscle-invasive and/or node-positive disease if the chemotherapy is initiated within 90 days [31]. The main criticism for adjuvant chemotherapy is the expected impact of nephroureterectomy on the residual renal function. Due to this, delivering a full dose of cisplatin-based chemotherapy could be challenging following the radical surgery. Neoadjuvant chemotherapy, however, would not have such an impact. Patients are subjected to chemotherapy before losing their renal reserve with an opportunity of pathological downstaging. On the flip side, the disease may progress with possible deterioration of the performance status of the patient (toxicity) which may impact the feasibility of subsequent surgical resection. The data regarding its use is still evolving, and a recent phase II trial (accelerated methotrexate, vinblastine, doxorubicin, and cisplatin in patients with creatinine clearance of more than 50 ml per minute) suggested a 14% complete pathological response with acceptable toxicity [32]. A retrospective analysis also suggested a significant survival advantage (progression-free, cancer-specific, and overall survival) with platinum-based neoadjuvant chemotherapy in locally advanced upper tract urothelial carcinoma [33].

10 Conclusions

Robot-assisted RNU with bladder cuff excision is a safe and feasible procedure that allows for meticulous dissection (lymph node dissection) and intracorporeal suturing (cystotomy closure). The introduction of the Xi system allowed facilitating the implementation of a multi-quadrant single-stage approach, which translated into reduced operative time and favorable perioperative and oncological outcomes.

References

1. Siegel RL, Miller KD, Fuchs HE, Jemal A. Cancer Statistics, 2021. CA Cancer J Clin. 2021;71(1):7–33.
2. Rouprêt M, Babjuk M, Burger M, Capoun O, Cohen D, Compérat EM, Cowan NC, Dominguez-Escrig JL, Gontero P, Hugh Mostafid A, Palou J, Peyronnet B, Seisen T, Soukup V, Sylvester RJ, Rhijn BWGV, Zigeuner R, Shariat SF. European association of urology guidelines on upper urinary tract urothelial carcinoma: 2020 update. Eur Urol. 2021;79(1):62–79.
3. Ni S, Tao W, Chen Q, Liu L, Jiang H, Hu H, Han R, Wang C. Laparoscopic versus open nephroureterectomy for the treatment of upper urinary tract urothelial carcinoma: a systematic review and cumulative analysis of comparative studies. Eur Urol. 2012;61(6):1142–53.
4. Simone G, Papalia R, Guaglianone S, Ferriero M, Leonardo C, Forastiere E, Gallucci M. Laparoscopic versus open nephroureterectomy: perioperative and oncologic outcomes from a randomized prospective study. Eur Urol. 2009;56(3):520–6.
5. Veccia A, Antonelli A, Francavilla S, Simeone C, Guruli G, Zargar H, Perdoná S, Ferro M, Carrieri G, Hampton LJ, Porpiglia F, Autorino R. Robotic versus other nephroureterectomy techniques: a systematic review and meta-analysis of over 87,000 cases. World J Urol. 2020;38(4):845–52.
6. Kenigsberg AP, Smith W, Meng X, Ghandour R, Rapoport L, Bagrodia A, Lotan Y, Woldu SL, Margulis V. Robotic nephroureterectomy *vs* laparoscopic nephroureterectomy: increased utilization, rates of lymphadenectomy, decreased morbidity robotically. J Endourol. 2021;35(3):312–8.
7. Hemal AK, Stansel I, Babbar P, Patel M. Robotic-assisted nephroureterectomy and bladder cuff excision without intraoperative repositioning. Urology. 2011;78(2):357–64.
8. Zargar H, Krishnan J, Autorino R, Akca O, Brandao LF, Laydner H, Samarasekera D, Ko O, Haber GP, Kaouk JH, Stein RJ. Robotic nephroureterectomy: a simplified approach requiring no patient repositioning or robot redocking. Eur Urol. 2014;66(4):769–77.
9. Patel MN, Aboumohamed A, Hemal A. Does transition from the da Vinci Si to Xi robotic platform impact single-docking technique for robot-assisted laparoscopic nephroureterectomy? BJU Int. 2015;116(6):990–4.
10. Veccia A, Carbonara U, Derweesh I, Mehrazin R, Porter J, Abdollah F, Mazzone E, Sundaram CP, Gonzalgo M, Mastroianni R, Ghoreifi A, Cacciamani GE, Patel D, Marcus J, Danno A, Steward J, Bhattu AS, Asghar A, Reese AC, Wu Z, Uzzo RG, Minervini A, Rha KH, Ferro M, Margulis V, Hampton LJ, Simone G, Eun DD, Djaladat H, Mottrie A, Autorino R. Single stage Xi® robotic radical nephroureterectomy for upper tract urothelial carcinoma: surgical technique and outcomes. Minerva Urol Nephrol. 2021 Mar 29.
11. Peyronnet B, Seisen T, Dominguez-Escrig JL, Bruins HM, Yuan CY, Lam T, Maclennan S, N'dow J, Babjuk M, Comperat E, Zigeuner R, Sylvester RJ, Burger M, Mostafid H, van Rhijn BWG, Gontero P, Palou J, Shariat SF, Roupret M. Oncological outcomes of laparoscopic nephroureterectomy versus open radical nephroureterectomy for upper tract urothelial carcinoma: an European association of urology guidelines systematic review. Eur Urol Focus. 2019;5(2):205–23.
12. Matin SF, Sfakianos JP, Espiritu PN, Coleman JA, Spiess PE. Patterns of lymphatic metastases in upper tract urothelial carcinoma and proposed dissection templates. J Urol. 2015;194(6):1567–74.
13. Lim SK, Shin TY, Kim KH, Chung BH, Hong SJ, Choi YD, Rha KH. Intermediate-term outcomes of robot-assisted laparoscopic nephroureterectomy in upper urinary tract urothelial carcinoma. Clin Genitourin Cancer. 2013;11(4):515–21.
14. Lee Z, Cadillo-Chavez R, Lee DI, Llukani E, Eun D. The technique of single stage pure robotic nephroureterectomy. J Endourol. 2013;27(2):189–95.
15. Ambani SN, Weizer AZ, Wolf JS Jr, He C, Miller DC, Montgomery JS. Matched comparison of robotic vs laparoscopic nephroureterectomy: an initial experience. Urology. 2014;83(2):345–9.
16. Melquist JJ, Redrow G, Delacroix S, Park A, Faria EE, Karam JA, Matin SF. Comparison of single-docking robotic-assisted and traditional laparoscopy for retroperitoneal lymph node dissection during nephroureterectomy with bladder cuff excision for upper-tract urothelial carcinoma. Urology. 2016;87:216–23.
17. Patel MN, Hemal AK. Does advancing technology improve outcomes? Comparison of the Da Vinci Standard/S/Si to the Xi robotic platforms during robotic nephroureterectomy. J Endourol. 2018;32(2):133–8.
18. De Groote R, Decaestecker K, Larcher A, Buelens S, De Bleser E, D'Hondt F, Schatteman P, Lumen N, Montorsi F, Mottrie A, De Naeyer G, YAU Robotic and Urothelial Group. Robot-assisted nephroureterectomy for upper tract urothelial carcinoma: results from three high-volume robotic surgery institutions. J Robot Surg. 2020;14(1):211–9.
19. Lee H, Kim HJ, Lee SE, Hong SK, Byun SS. Comparison of oncological and perioperative outcomes of open, laparoscopic, and robotic nephroureterectomy approaches in patients with non-metastatic upper-tract urothelial carcinoma. PLoS One. 2019;14(1):e0210401.
20. Ye H, Feng X, Wang Y, Chen R, Zhang C, Zhang W, Guo F, Wang Z, Fang Y, Wu Z, Yang Q, Yang B, Lü C, Wang L. Single-docking robotic-assisted nephroureterectomy and extravesical bladder cuff excision without intraoperative repositioning: The technique and oncological outcomes. Asian J Surg. 2020;43(10):978–85.
21. Kondo T, Hara I, Takagi T, Kodama Y, Hashimoto Y, Kobayashi H, Iizuka J, Omae K, Yoshida K, Tanabe K. Template-based lymphadenectomy in urothelial carcinoma of the renal pelvis: a prospective study. Int J Urol. 2014;21(5):453–9.
22. Seisen T, Shariat SF, Cussenot O, Peyronnet B, Renard-Penna R, Colin P, Rouprêt M. Contemporary role of lymph node dissection at the time of radical nephroureterectomy for upper tract urothelial carcinoma. World J Urol. 2017;35(4):535–48.
23. Dong F, Xu T, Wang X, Shen Y, Zhang X, Chen S, Zhong S, Zhang M, Ding Q. Lymph node dissection could bring survival benefits to patients diagnosed with clinically node-negative upper urinary tract urothelial cancer: a population-based, propensity score-matched study. Int J Clin Oncol. 2019;24(3):296–305.
24. Lenis AT, Donin NM, Faiena I, Salmasi A, Johnson DC, Drakaki A, Gollapudi K, Blumberg J, Belldegrun A, Pantuck A, Chamie K. Role of surgical approach on lymph node dissection yield and survival in patients with upper tract urothelial carcinoma. Urol Oncol. 2018;36(1):9.e1–9.
25. Kondo T, Hashimoto Y, Kobayashi H, Iizuka J, Nakazawa H, Ito F, Tanabe K. Template-based lymphadenectomy in urothelial carcinoma of the upper urinary tract: impact on patient survival. Int J Urol. 2010;17(10):848–54.
26. O'Brien T, Ray E, Singh R, Coker B, Beard R, British Association of Urological Surgeons Section of Oncology. Prevention of

bladder tumours after nephroureterectomy for primary upper urinary tract urothelial carcinoma: a prospective, multicentre, randomised clinical trial of a single postoperative intravesical dose of mitomycin C (the ODMIT-C Trial). Eur Urol. 2011;60(4):703–10.
27. Ito A, Shintaku I, Satoh M, Ioritani N, Aizawa M, Tochigi T, Kawamura S, Aoki H, Numata I, Takeda A, Namiki S, Namima T, Ikeda Y, Kambe K, Kyan A, Ueno S, Orikasa K, Katoh S, Adachi H, Tokuyama S, Ishidoya S, Yamaguchi T, Arai Y. Prospective randomized phase II trial of a single early intravesical instillation of pirarubicin (THP) in the prevention of bladder recurrence after nephroureterectomy for upper urinary tract urothelial carcinoma: the THP Monotherapy Study Group Trial. J Clin Oncol. 2013;31(11):1422–7.
28. Noennig B, Bozorgmehri S, Terry R, Otto B, Su LM, Crispen PL. Evaluation of intraoperative versus postoperative adjuvant mitomycin c with nephroureterectomy for urothelial carcinoma of the upper urinary tract. Bladder Cancer. 2018;4(4):389–94.
29. Freifeld Y, Ghandour R, Singla N, Woldu S, Bagrodia A, Lotan Y, Rapoport LM, Gazimiev M, Delafuente K, Kulangara R, Robyak H, Petros FG, Raman JD, Matin SF, Margulis V. Intraoperative prophylactic intravesical chemotherapy to reduce bladder recurrence following radical nephroureterectomy. Urol Oncol. 2020;38(9):737.e11–6.
30. Harraz AM, El-Shabrawy M, El-Nahas AR, El-Kappany H, Osman Y. Single versus maintenance intravesical chemotherapy for the prevention of bladder recurrence after radical nephroureterectomy for upper tract urothelial carcinoma: a randomized clinical trial. Clin Genitourin Cancer. 2019;17(6):e1108–15.
31. Birtle A, Johnson M, Chester J, Jones R, Dolling D, Bryan RT, Harris C, Winterbottom A, Blacker A, Catto JWF, Chakraborti P, Donovan JL, Elliott PA, French A, Jagdev S, Jenkins B, Keeley FX Jr, Kockelbergh R, Powles T, Wagstaff J, Wilson C, Todd R, Lewis R, Hall E. Adjuvant chemotherapy in upper tract urothelial carcinoma (the POUT trial): a phase 3, open-label, randomised controlled trial. Lancet. 2020;395(10232):1268–77.
32. Margulis V, Puligandla M, Trabulsi EJ, Plimack ER, Kessler ER, Matin SF, Godoy G, Alva A, Hahn NM, Carducci MA, Hoffman-Censits J, Collaborators. Phase II trial of neoadjuvant systemic chemotherapy followed by extirpative surgery in patients with high grade upper tract urothelial carcinoma. J Urol. 2020;203(4):690–8.
33. Hosogoe S, Hatakeyama S, Kusaka A, Hamano I, Iwamura H, Fujita N, Yamamoto H, Tobisawa Y, Yoneyama T, Yoneyama T, Hashimoto Y, Koie T, Ohyama C. Platinum-based neoadjuvant chemotherapy improves oncological outcomes in patients with locally advanced upper tract urothelial carcinoma. Eur Urol Focus. 2018;4(6):946–53.

Current Status of Robotic-Assisted Pyeloplasty in Adults

Pietro Diana, Simone Scarcella, Raymond J. Leveillee, Geert De Naeyer, and Nicolomaria Buffi

1 Definition and Indications (When to Operate and When to Wait)

Ureteropelvic junction obstruction (UPJO), or pelvic-ureteric junction obstruction, represents the most common cause of antenatal/neonatal hydronephrosis. It is characterized by an impaired flow of urine from the renal pelvis into the proximal upper ureter, due to blockage or obstruction, that can determine an increased back pressure on the kidney parenchyma. If left untreated, a progressive dilatation and distension of the renal pelvis and calyces could occur, leading to interstitial fibrosis, loss of nephrons, reduction of kidney function, and, ultimately renal failure. UPJO affects sporadically 1 per 1000/1500 newborns with a 4:1 male-female ratio: two-thirds of congenital cases is predominantly left-sided with a 10–46% variable incidence of bilateral occurrences; also familiar inheritance has been reported [1]. It can be detected at any time, from uterine development during prenatal ultrasonography to older age; it has been estimated that up to 50% of the patients presenting antenatal hydronephrosis will be diagnosed with UPJO at further radiological evaluations during life [2]. There are multiple possible causes, either transient or physiologic, which can be categorized as intrinsic/extrinsic and congenital/acquired (Table 1).

P. Diana (✉) · N. Buffi
Department of Urology, Humanitas Clinical and Research Institute IRCCS, Rozzano, Italy

S. Scarcella
Department of Urology, Onze Lieve Vrouw Hospital, Aalst, Belgium

Department of Urology, Polytechnic University of Marche Region, University Hospital "Ospedali Riuniti", Ancona, Italy

R. J. Leveillee
Department of Urology, Jackson Memorial Hospital, Miami, FL, USA

G. De Naeyer
Department of Urology, Onze Lieve Vrouw Hospital, Aalst, Belgium

Table 1 Causes of ureteropelvic junction obstruction

	Congenital	Acquired
Intrinsic	– Aperistaltic ureteric segment (replacement of spiral musculature with fibrous tissue). – True ureteral stricture. – Scarring of the ureteric valve. – Ureteric kinking.	– Renal calculi. – Traumatic stricture following instrumentation. – Urothelial neoplasm.
Extrinsic	– Crossing lower pole vessels distorting the UPJ configuration (e.g.,, renal artery, aorta, vena cava, or iliac vessels). – Horseshoe kidney. – Duplex kidney.	– Scarring after surgical instrumentation of the ureter. – Fibroepithelial polyps.

Several theories have been proposed regarding UPJO development, but despite several studies focusing on different lines of investigation including embryological, histological, anatomical, functional, and more recently molecular causes, the exact determinant of UPJO remains unknown [3].

Among possible etiologies, intrinsic causes include the following:

- Ureteric valves scarring due to incomplete ureteral recanalization during development, resulting in stenosis/obstruction.
- Neurogenic/muscular dysfunction at the level of the ureteropelvic junction determining abnormal peristalsis.
- Discontinuity of ureteral smooth muscle, replaced with collagen fibers, determining ureteric hypoplasia with disruption of regular peristalsis.

Extrinsic causes include the following:

- Impaired urine drainage due to high insertion of the ureter in the renal pelvis.
- Abnormal kidney rotation (renal ectopy or hypermobility), causing intermittent obstruction in relation to the ureteric position.

P. Wiklund et al. (eds.), *Robotic Urologic Surgery*, https://doi.org/10.1007/978-3-031-00363-9_45

- Secondary UPJO, determined by prior surgery or stone burden.
- Aberrant, accessory, or early branching renal vessel crossing the lower renal pole and determining ureteral compression and urine flow obstruction; anterior crossing vessels are more common than posterior ones. This occurrence can be the only determinant in ≤40% of cases, while in the remaining ones is concomitant to an intrinsic UPJO cause.
- Congenital renal abnormalities (horseshoe or duplex kidneys).
- Iatrogenic scar formation secondary to ureteric manipulation by previous surgery.
- Fibroepithelial polyps.

All these etiologies lead to an acute obstruction of urine flow from the upper tracts with increased ureteric, renal pelvic, and blood pressures. As consequence of the chronic rising of the ureteric pressure, the renal pelvis starts dilating, and renal blood flow decreases due to efferent arteriole vasoconstriction. In the long term, a decreased overall glomerular filtration rate occurs due to tubular dilation, inflammation, glomerulosclerosis, and fibrosis of the kidney secondary to UPJO [4].

For this reason, it is therefore of vital importance to understand how to early diagnose and treat this condition. Patients affected by UPJO can manifest multiple signs and symptoms and at any age. Of these, the most frequent ones are flank pain, nausea and vomiting, hematuria, recurrent infections progressing to pyelonephritis/pyonephrosis, and palpable mass in the lumbar region. Adults are more likely to present with UPJO secondary to acquired causes, such as kidney stones or previous surgeries, with symptoms of acute renal colic and chronic back pain that can be exacerbated by increased fluid intake and diuretics. Rarely, UPJO remains asymptomatic and is detected incidentally during radiological investigations performed to exclude other diseases [5].

The natural history of UPJO remains not clearly defined, without a widely accepted consensus regarding how to manage patients affected by this condition and when to treat them conservatively or surgically. Some indications for surgical intervention in adult patients with UPJO include the following:

- Obstructive symptoms such as flank pain, hematuria, and recurrent infection nonresponsive to medical therapies.
- Impaired split renal function at MAG3 diuretic renography with at least 40% differential function of the affected renal unit.
- Anterior/posterior diameter of the renal pelvis higher than 20 mm on ultrasonographic scan.
- Concomitant presence of renal calculi on CT scan.
- Hypertension development at a young age.

An effective management is mandatory; it requires early identification of signs and symptoms, prompt diagnosis, and targeted treatment with the aim of improving renal drainage and function. In the absence of these indications, patients can be monitored closely with both radiological and blood sample investigations. Their treatment algorithm has to be tailored according to progression of clinical symptoms and/or worsening of renal function.

2 Preoperative Evaluations

UPJO reduces the normal flow of urine from the renal pelvis to the ureter and if misdiagnosed or left untreated, can significantly affect renal function. In this setting, radiological imaging techniques are of paramount importance in UPJO syndrome diagnosis and treatment planning. The main objectives of radiological imaging techniques for UPJO are to determine the presence and degree of renal obstruction, to assess renal function, and to determine the possible etiology. All patients presenting with UPJO symptoms should be evaluated with a full set of blood exams, including complete blood count, kidney function tests with serum creatinine, eGFR, and BUN. The majority of patients will present high levels of creatinine and decreased eGFR; in the case of concomitant urinary tract infections (UTI), leukocytosis can be detected. A urine sample should always be sent for analysis and cultures, as UTI are commonly seen in these patients.

2.1 Ultrasonography

Ultrasonography (US) is the reference standard methodology used for evaluating the urinary system in patients suspected for hydronephrosis. This technology is characterized by various advantages such as being noninvasive, cost and time saving, easily accessible in most institutions, and repeatable without the need of radiation exposure. The widespread use of abdominal US screening leads to higher detection rates of UPJO in both pediatric and adult populations. Hydronephrosis can be detected as an incidental finding during abdominal US exams performed for other reasons and might reflect an underlying UPJO. Each kidney should routinely be assessed both in transverse and longitudinal planes. Specific ultrasonographic characteristics of UPJO are the presence of multiple dilated calyces of uniform size communicating with the dilated renal pelvis that abrupt narrowing at the level of the UPJ, continuing in a ureter with a regular caliber [6].

US examination provides essential information regarding laterality, kidney size, appearance (such as echogenicity, corticomedullary differentiation, cyst), parenchymal thickness, presence of pelvicalyceal dilatation, and extension of the stenotic tract. US also gives important information about the contralateral kidney, ureter, and bladder. It is mandatory to screen the complete urinary tract system due to the increased incidence of concomitant congenital abnormalities in patients with UPJO such as vesicoureteral reflux, renal duplication, ureterovesical obstruction, and bilateral UPJO. The exams can be completed with the color Doppler mode evaluation that can give additional information identifying the eventual presence of crossing vessels. It represents one of the extrinsic causes of UPJO occurring at older ages compared to intrinsic causes. These vessels usually originate from both the renal artery or the aorta and supply the lower renal pole.

2.2 Computed Tomography

Abdominal contrastenhanced CT scan is the gold standard radiological investigation for the diagnosis of UPJO with a 97% sensitivity and 92% specificity. High-resolution imaging modalities provide detailed anatomical information such as location, orientation, and presence of aberrant vessels regarding the obstruction. Moreover, it can help identify possible underlying causes, such as urinary stones or urothelial tumors, and provide additional 3D reconstruction images of the vascular anatomy. Providing a detailed preoperative knowledge regarding the renal arterial supply is of paramount importance in order to aid treatment decision-making, reducing the occurrence of potential intraoperative complications with improved prognosis [7].

With a resolution thickness of 1 mm, CT technology provides an accurate urinary tract reconstruction in both coronal and sagittal planes with additional 2D/3D reconstructions and volume rendering images allowing the anatomical visualization of both the renal collecting system and vascular structures. Application of CT scan for the evaluation of the urinary tract is called CT urography (CTU), while the study of vascular anatomy is called CT angiography (CTA). CTU examination should always be performed in cases of suspected UPJO because the assessment of the excretory phase is mandatory. A separate non-enhanced phase should be obtained to detect eventual urinary stones that may occur secondary to obstruction. During the contrast enhanced excretory CT scan, the obstructed kidney is characterized by delayed opacifications and excretions of the radiographic contrast agent. The arterial phase CTA is crucial in order to detect eventual crossing vessels, and the multiplanar 3D images reconstruction is essential to properly plan surgical intervention [8].

In conclusion, both CTU and CTA phases provide important information for the anatomy and the function of the urinary tract (renal parenchyma, collecting system, accessory vessel, stone formation, and contrast excretion) with higher acquisition speed, especially in those patients who are unable to undergo MRI or in centers where MRI is not available. However, the grade of collecting system dilatation detected on CT does not always relate to the functional obstruction, and a nuclear medicine scan with an added diuretic phase should be performed to quantify the entity of renal pelvic dilatation.

2.3 Magnetic Resonance Urography

Magnetic resonance urography (MRU) technology, thanks to both technological software and hardware developments, has progressed during the last decade, becoming a reliable alternative in patients who are not evaluable with CT imaging techniques. MRU allows the complete study of both upper and lower urinary tract anatomy, providing detailed information regarding differential renal function and the eventual presence of UPJO, without using radiation [9]. Known disadvantages of this technology are longer operative time, the need of sedation to prevent motion artifacts in noncomplying patients, the use of gadolinium (the risk of nephrogenic systemic fibrosis in patients with low eGFR), and the impossibility to scan patients with metallic prosthesis.

MRU represents a promising alternative to CT scan, being able to assess the entire urinary tract during a single session providing both anatomical and functional information. In addition, it enables the study of the whole ureter course with the eventual identification of ectopic insertions and potential causes of obstructions [10].

2.4 Diuretic Renography

Diuretic renography represents the most effective radiological investigative tool to assess differential renal function for a patient with UPJO, quantifying the degree of obstruction. Moreover, it allows the evaluation of renal plasma clearance compared to CT scan, which is characterized by a superior radiological resolution of the urological tract anatomy. The exam is performed under diuretic stimulation (Furosemide), and whereas a mechanical obstructive hydronephrosis is detected, it will show no downward slope progression of the tracer on renogram, with retention in the collecting system. The radiopharmaceutical agent of choice is Technetium Tc-99 m-MAG3 that has replaced Tc-99 m-DTPA due to a clearer gamma resolution, faster renal clearance, and a lower background activity. Thanks to these advantages, it is possible to compare isotope uptake and renal blood afferent flow in both kidneys measuring differential renal function. O'Reilly et al. [11] was the first one to define and publish renogram curves characterizing Tc-99 m-MAG3 uptake and drainage in both physiological and pathological conditions. The standard time (t½) to excrete 50% of the radionuclide tracer is inferior to 10 min in normal conditions, while a t½ longer than 20 minutes is highly suggestive of an anatomical obstructive condition. Prior to submitting patients to the radiolabelled pharmaceutical agent injection, they should have been properly hydrated with the bladder completely emptied [12]. In conclusion Tc-99 m-MAG3 diuretic renography should always be preferred as pharmacological agent in patients with suspected UPJO and normal renal function, thanks to its safer profile. In the case of chronic renal function impairment, Tc-99 m-DTPA should be used due to a 20% lower rate of renal clearance resulting in less than half of Tc-99 m-MAG3 one.

2.5 Intravenous Pyelography

Intravenous pyelography (IVP) or intravenous urography (IVU) was the gold standard radiological modality to study the urinary tract, but its indications decreased over time due to technological advances. Nowadays, it is rarely used in centers where more advanced imaging methods are limited. Typical findings, characterizing obstructive hydronephrosis, are collecting system dilatation, parenchymal changes during the nephrographic phase and delayed excretion of medium contrast [13]. Some known drawbacks of this technique are insufficient visualization of poorly functioning kidneys due to reduced contrast excretion, impaired image quality in the case of concomitant bowel gas abundance, and contrast nephrotoxicity and hypersensitivity reactions to contrast tracer.

2.6 Preoperative Stenting

Preoperative retrograde JJ stent placement should not be performed routinely. According to different reports within the scientific literature, it can reduce the risk of intraoperative complications, providing an enhanced anatomical delineation and consequent better dissection of the surgical planes around the ureteropelvic junction. Furthermore, it allows the decompression of the obstructed renal pelvis and might hamper the posterior suturing of the anastomosis between the reduced pelvis and the ureter [14]. In opposition, other authors strongly suggested to avoid preoperative ureteral stenting reporting that it reduces both surgeons' ability and surgical vision during the suture of the posterior anastomosis layer, requiring repeated multiple manipulations to keep it distant from the suturing line, with increased risks of ureteral laceration. Moreover, additional complications during JJ stent placement could occur including ureteral perforation or displacement and increased periureteral tissue fixation due to inflammatory reaction [15].

2.7 Preoperative Nephrostomy

In the case of pyonephrosis, it can be mandatory to insert a nephrostomy tube. The pyeloplasty is best done some weeks later, when the inflammatory reaction has been disappeared. The nephrostomy tube can stay in place until the moment of surgery, but can be removed afterward.

3 OR Setting and Patient Positioning

The setting of the operative room for a robotic transperitoneal pyeloplasty is the same as for any transperitoneal robotic procedure with the patient in lateral decubitus positioning. The patient is positioned in a full lateral decubitus positioning with the ventral surface on the edge of the table for a transperitoneal approach. The lower leg is bended, the upper leg is stretched, and a pillow is supporting the upper leg, with flexion of the table of about 30–40 degrees (Fig. 1). To prevent shoulder plexus lesions, a supportive roll is placed under the patient at the tip of the scapula. Mostly a shoulder support is used to prevent the patient from turning down. The arms are drained over the chest. The lower limbs are secured by a tape. In the case of a necessity to use a flexible cystoscope to take out some stones of the pelvis, the possibility of having an additional screen for this scope should be taken into consideration.

3.1 The Port Placement

Depending on surgeons' preference, the procedure can be done with a standard three-arm approach or a four-arm robotic approach. The camera trocar is placed about 3 cm cranial of the umbilicus at the para-rectal line, with an 8 mm

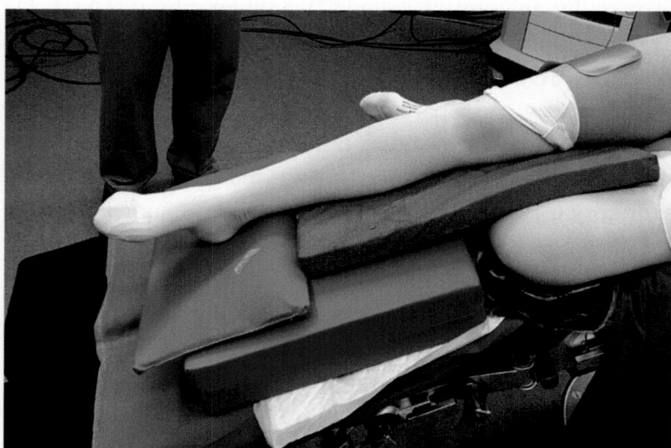

Fig. 1 Extensive padding of all pressure points when positioning the patient in lateral decubitus should prevent nerve entrapment

trocar just below the lower rib and two other 8 cm trocars toward the lower abdomen on one line. An 12 mm assisting port is placed at the level of the umbilicus (see Figs. 2 and 3). When the port placement has been done, the abdomen is inflated by the pneumoperitoneum pressure of about 8 mm of Hg, according to the principals of low pressure laparoscopy.

3.2 Surgical Procedure

As the kidney is located in the retroperitoneum, the conventional steps of bowel mobilization and reclination of the colon is the first step in a robotic pyeloplasty. Care should be taken to identify the correct plane in between the mesocolon and the Gerota's fascia. The reclination of the colon is started at the lower pole of the kidney following up toward the renal pelvis. After identification of the psoas muscle, the ureter is identified. The ureter is then followed toward the lower pole of the kidney where UPJ stenosis can be identified. One should be careful not to damage the gonadal vessels. In the case of a preoperative stent placement, the periureteral inflammation can make these steps more bloody and more difficult. The UPJ is nicely dissected, where the principal of avoiding excessive coagulation on tissues is respected in order to prevent devascularization of the proximal ureter. In the case of an intrinsic UPJO, the dissection is continued toward the inflated or hydronephrotic pelvis. In the case of an extrinsic UPJO with a crossing vessel, the surgeon should be careful not to damage the vessels which could lead to excessive bleeding. After the UPJ has clearly been identified, the next step will be to do a dismembering of the UPJ. One should be careful not to have the ureter to much rotated in order to know which side is medial and which side is lateral. After dismembering, the ureter is best immediately spatulated over about 1 to 2 cm. Next, the pelvis is further opened as well over about 1–2 cm. After it has been checked that the pelvis and the ureter can be brought together without too much traction, the anastomosis can be started. The sutures that are used for the anastomosis can be chosen according to the surgeons' preference (monofilament or poly-filament absorbable sutures). For the size of the suture, mostly a 4/0 to 6/0 suture is chosen. More important is in fact the size of the needle. One can choose for a continuing suturing or interrupted suturing. The anastomosis is started on the posterior side where the posterior anastomosis is made toward the level of the upper pelvis. It is advised that the first knot is a double knot as it will better keep the ureter and pelvis together. After the posterior anastomosis has been made, the JJ stent can be introduced.

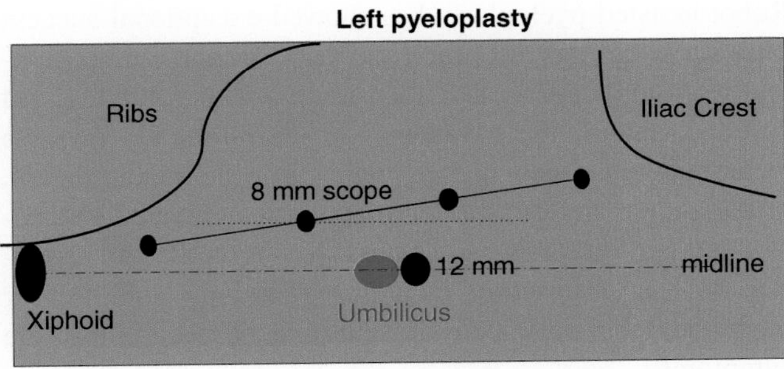

Fig. 2 Schematic presentation of port placement for robotic left-sided pyeloplasty with the da Vinci Xi system

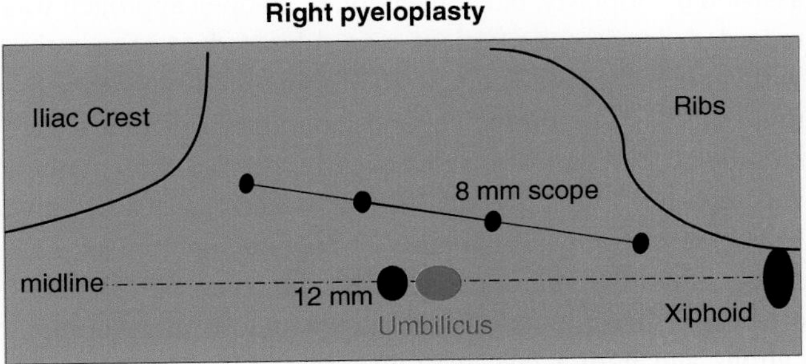

Fig. 3 Schematic presentation of port placement for robotic right-sided pyeloplasty with the da Vinci Xi system

3.3 Ureteral Stenting

The size of the J splint can vary according to the size of the ureter. For normally sized ureters, a conventional 6 Fr double J splint is used. First, the guide wire is introduced by the table assistant. This ca be done through the accessory port or can be done by placing a transcutaneous 13–15 G needle. The tip of the guide wire is introduced in the ureter toward the bladder by the console surgeon. One should check that the guide wire is smoothly going downward the ureter and is not placed submucosally. After it is realized that the guide wire is safely in the bladder, the J splint can be introduced over the guide wire toward the bladder. When the J splint is with its proximal curl in the bladder, the guide wire can be removed, and the upper part of the J splint should be brought into the pelvis. This can sometimes be difficult as the splint might always have the intention to flip out of the pelvis (Fig. 4). This can sometimes be solved by putting a temporary stitch on the pelvis. After the J splint has been brought into the pelvis, the anterior part of the anastomosis can be made, and both anterior and posterior sutures are tied to each other. After the anastomosis has been finished, the Gerota's fascia can be closed with a resorbable suture, but this step is optional. It is advised to put a small drain during the first postoperative day(s).

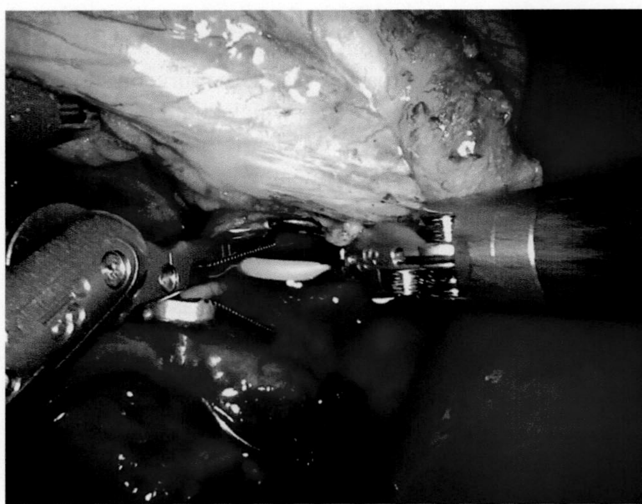

Fig. 4 Putting the splint into the pyelum can sometimes be a challenge

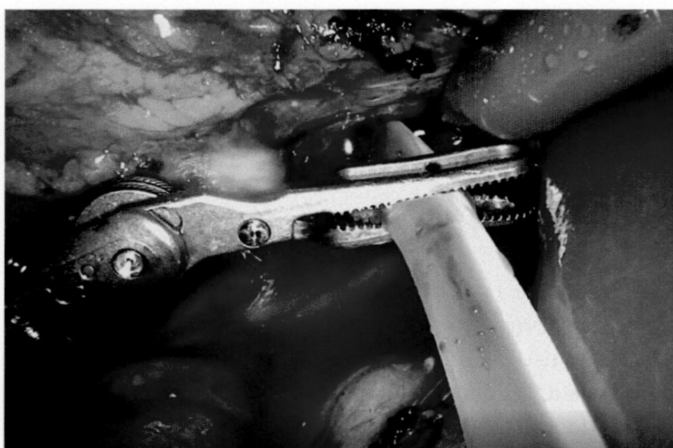

Fig. 5 A silicone tube can be used to rinse the pyelum and flush out the stones

3.4 The Pelvic Stone Treatment

In the case of concomitant pelvic stones, the stones need to be removed. In some cases it is necessary to use a gastric silicone tube to rinse the pelvis and flush out the stones (Fig. 5). One can also use a flexible cystoscope that can be introduced through the accessary port to remove those pelvic stones.

4 Tips and Tricks

In patients with a really hydronephrotic pelvis and a very thin mesocolon, one could take the option to go for a transmesocolic pyeloplasty. In these cases, the mesocolon is opened parallel to the mesenteric vessels at different levels in order to have a good access to the ureter and the UPJ. The different steps of ureteral dismembering and anastomosis are similar. One should not forget to close the mesocolon afterward, because that could otherwise lead to internal herniation.

It is advised not to empty the dilated pelvis too early, because the dissection will be easier to be done with a dilated pelvis instead of an empty pelvis. In some cases where the traction on the anastomosis will be too much, it is sometimes indicated to release the kidney out of the Gerota's fascia and bring the kidney toward a more lower level on the psoas muscle and to do a kind of nephropexy at the psoas muscle.

In some cases a transcutaneous needle can be used to fix the pelvis toward the abdominal wall and better present the area of interest. To check that the J splint is in the bladder, some surgeons have the preference to put a three-way bladder catheter, fill the bladder with a solution of methylene blue, and check that there is reflux of this blue fluid through the splint. When using a flexible cystoscope to extract some stones out of the pelvis, it can be helpful to use an Airseal® system (Conmed, Largo, USA) as this will keep the pneumoperitoneum more constant.

5 Surgical Outcomes

Robot-assisted pyeloplasty has showed exceptional success rates for symptoms resolution and very low peri- and postoperative complications and recurrences. The robot-assisted approach retains the advantages of the minimally invasive technique, but with a higher precision in the manipulation, visualization, and a faster learning curve compared to laparoscopy. Several tools can be employed to verify the resolution of the obstruction including radiology and nuclear medicine, laboratory analysis, and clinical resolution of the symptoms.

Getmann et al. reported the first series of robotic pyeloplasty in 2002 [16] comprehending nine consecutive patients affected by UPJO and treated with transperitoneal robot-assisted pyeloplasty. No conversion to an open approach was recorded despite one patient was subjected to reoperation with an open approach due to the formation of a urinary fistula. Successful radiological and laboratory outcomes were recorded for all patients. Subsequently, a series of 50 patients was reported. Operative success was described as a negative MAG3 renography. The totality of patients reported surgical success, and the authors concluded that robotic pyeloplasty offers short-term functional efficacy with low rate of complications and with a fast learning curve [17]. Mufarrij et al. published a multicentric population of 140 patients affected by either primary of secondary UPJO with a median follow-up of 29 months. Surgical success rate was 96% and obstruction recurrence was seen in about 4% of cases. Overall

Table 2 Summary of studies on robotic pyeloplasty

Authors	Number of patients	Transperitoneal/ retroperitoneal approach	Operative time (min)	Conversion rate (%)	Complication rate (%)	Hospital stay (days)	Follow-up (mo)
Patel (2005)	50	Transperitoneal	122	0	32	1.1	11.7
Olsen (2007)	67	Retroperitoneal	146	1.5	17,9	2	12.1
Schwentner (2007)	92	Transperitoneal	108	0	NA	4.6	39.1
Mufarrij (2008)	140	Transperitoneal	217	0	10	2.1	29
Gupta (2010)	86	Transperitoneal	121	2.3	9.3	2.5	13.6
Etafy (2011)	61	Transperitoneal	335	0	11.4	2	18
Sivaraman (2012)	168	Transperitoneal	134.9	0	6.6	1.5	39
Buffi (2017)	145	Both	120	2.8	8.3	4.7	24

complication rate was 7.1%. Regarding major complication, the double J stent migration was the most common adverse event in the postoperative time, and regarding minor complications, fever was the most commonly reported [18]. Schwentner et al. published in 2007 a large series of 92 patients (80 and 12 patients were affected by primary and secondary UPJO, respectively). The median follow-up was 40 months and the surgical success rate was 96%. In the secondary obstruction patients group failure rate after robotic pyeloplasty was slightly higher [19]. These optimal results were then confirmed by other single and multi-institutional studies exploring also the retroperitoneal approach reporting short- and long-term excellent and reproducible results [17, 19–22]. Summary of the surgical outcome is reported in Table 2.

5.1 Comparative Studies

Autorino et al. published a meta-analysis that demonstrates no statistically significant difference in terms of success and complication rate between minimally invasive and open approach in the adult population; however, minimally invasive approaches provide a shorter hospital stay and a better pain management compared to open surgery [23].

Basatac et al. confirmed the significant decrease in the length of hospital stay, estimated blood loss, earlier drainage removal, and the decrease of the need for painkillers [24]. In terms of success rates, intraoperative complications and conversions, no significant differences were found. Furthermore, a shorter time for robotic surgery has been recorded although they considered exclusively the console time. Hanske et al., when evaluating a large number of patients undergoing minimally invasive vs. open, report a statistically significant difference in the percentage of patients requiring prolonged operation time (<236 min): 29.6% for minimally invasive pyeloplasty vs. 15.3% for open pyeloplasty [25].

5.2 The Role of Robotic System in the Treatment of Recurrent UPJO

The robotic approach is feasible, safe, and effective for treating recurrent obstruction [26]. Secondary minimally invasive pyeloplasty is obviously a more challenging procedure due to the fibrosis and the adhesions formed after the previous surgery. The precise movements with the robotic assistance and the amplified vision provide higher precision, thus, a bloodless dissection, and a higher quality of the suture above all in complex patients.

Thom et al. found that nine secondary robotic procedures done at their center required longer operative time with an increased blood loss and failure rate (22%) [27]. Atug et al. show data from seven patients undergoing redo RP. The outcomes were compared with data from a series of 37 patients that underwent RP for primary ureteropelvic junction obstruction. The mean operative time was 60 min longer in the secondary RP group. However, EBL, hospital stay, and overall success were comparable [28].

Hemal et al. described the outcomes of nine patients (mean age: 16.4 year) treated for secondary UPJO after failure of a previous open pyeloplasty and additional failed endoscopic pyelotomy. All patients were treated robotically and reported clinical resolution of symptoms and no sign of residual obstruction at postoperative renal scan [29].

Data from a series of 20 patients treated for secondary obstruction were published. Redo RP was successful in 94% of cases and the procedure was reported as feasible and safe [30].

6 Novelties and New Technologies

6.1 Single-Site Robot-Assisted Pyeloplasty

Ureteropelvic junction obstruction (UPJO) is a condition that is usually encountered in young patients. As such, the cosmetic results represent a crucial point in this population besides the resolution of the obstruction. For this reason, laparoendoscopic single-site surgery (LESS) has been introduced in this setting with the objective to offer a better cosmetic result limiting the invasiveness of the procedure, offering a limited postoperative pain and a quicker recovery. However, LESS remains a challenging procedure as the instrument triangulation is lacking, requiring solid surgical skills to allow proper laparoscopic suturing that is crucial in the treatment of UPJO beside the reduced visibility and maneuverability associated with the coaxial orientation of instruments [31, 32]. This resulted in longer operative time compared to the open technique, leading the patients with postoperative complications related to anesthesiology and surgical bed positioning. The introduction of the da Vinci Surgical System (Intuitive Surgical, Sunnyvale, CA, USA) brought higher dexterity in suturing and less conflicts between surgical instruments. Robotic laparoendoscopic single site (R-LESS) pyeloplasty has been introduced as a feasible technique in the urologist's armamentarium to overcome the technical problems and satisfy both the surgical requirements and cosmetic results [31, 32]. R-LESS pyeloplasty is performed by positioning a GelPort system through a 2.5–5 cm periumbilical incision through which the SP system trocar is inserted [33–35]. The SP robotic system is docked and the camera and robotic instruments inserted. A first preliminary study on a series of nine patients confirmed the feasibility of this technique with a mean operative time of 166 min, and no intraoperative complications were recorded [31]. Clinical resolution of symptoms and a laboratory renal function recovery were observed and maintained during a short follow-up of 6 months [31]. A follow-up study with a larger population was published by the same group 2 years after confirming both the safety and feasibility of the procedure in a series of 30 patients [32]. In this study, in two cases, a conversion into a classic laparoscopic was necessary, and in three cases, an additional 3 mm trocar was placed [32]. Surgical success was reached in 28 patients (93.3%) at a median follow-up of 13 (range 3–21) months in terms of absence of symptoms and functional recovery both through blood analysis and postoperative imaging. Lenfant et al. published a series of ten patients that underwent an R-LESS pyeloplasty with a mini-Pfannenstiel approach [36]. Mean operative time was 166 minutes (interquartile range [IQR] 146–181) and EBL was minimal. The only complication recorded was a postoperative urinary tract infection treated with antibiotics. Surgical success at 3 months after surgery was 100%. Exclusion criteria for this approach are a body mass index (BMI) >30 kg/m2, previous surgical procedure, an extremely dilated kidney pelvis, and complicated UPJO (presence of kidney stones, pelvic kidney, and horseshoe kidney) [22, 37]. Despite the good aesthetic results and the comparable short-term functional results, functional advantages in the long term are still under investigation.

6.2 The Role of Indocyanine Green in Pyeloplasty

The use of intraureteral injection indocyanine green (ICG) dye and the visualization under near-infrared fluorescence (NIRF) in urological surgery have been extensively employed in highlighting the vasculature and the viable tissue in the real time, permitting the surgeon to perform an ICG-guided procedure [38, 39]. In the setting of ureteral reconstruction, ICG has been employed in both the identification of viable ureteral tissue and stricture margins, in order to avoid to leave fibrotic tissue and increase the possibility to recur as well as to identify the ureter itself if imbedded in a fibrotic surrounding occurring in the case of a redo pyeloplasty or previous radiotherapy [40, 41]. The procedure to perform an ICG-guided procedure in this setting consists in inserting a 6 Fr ureteral catheter into the diseased ureter, and 10 ml ICG solution is injected retrogradely into the ureteral lumen, above and below the level of stricture if possible. Once injected the NIRF vision is activated, and both the ureter and the stricture (as fibrotic tissue loses its transparency) itself can be identified (Fig. 6). ICG can also be injected intravenously (2 to 4 mL of a 2.5 mg/mL solution) in order to highlight the healthy tissue that appears bright green and the fibrotic one darker as less perfused. Several series were published proving that the intraureteral injection of ICG is reproducible, safe, easy to perform, and involves minimal additional costs. All cases were clinically and radiographically successful, and no patient has required a repeat operation for stricture recurrence [40].

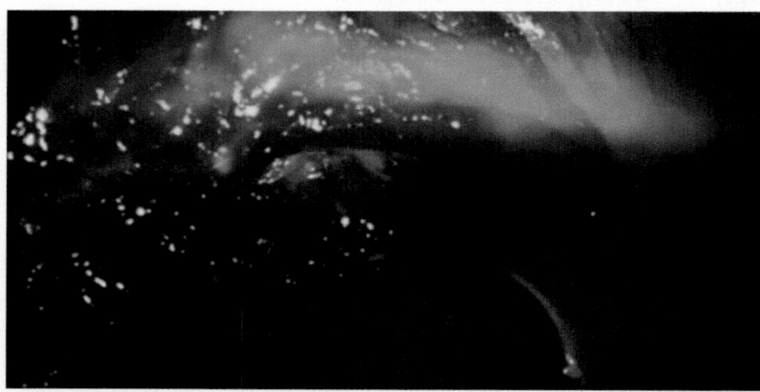

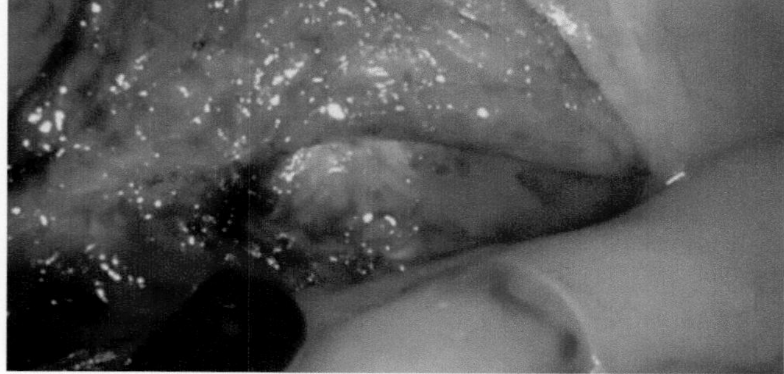

Fig. 6 Intraureteral injection of indocyanine green in a redo pyeloplasty

6.3 Buccal Mucosal Graft in Pyeloplasty

Management of recurrent UPJO has lower success rate compared to primary treatment. Redo pyeloplasty is not always feasible because the surgery could result to be challenging due to the fibrotic surrounding and tissue entrapment that brings to broader resections to find the healthy and well-vascularized ureteral tissue for the anastomosis and resolve the disorder. Buccal mucosal grafts (BMG), already in use for ureteral reconstruction, have been advised in cases of UPJO refractory to surgery and endoscopic treatment [42].

The surgery consists in the identification of the obstruction at the level of the UPJ, a longitudinal dissection of the ureter on the anterior face of the stricture comprehending about 1 cm below and above the stricture to ensure exposure of vascularized tissue. After the positioning of an 8 Fr ureteral stent from the incision itself over the guidewire, a single buccal graft is harvested from the right inner cheek, avoiding to compromise the Stensen's ducts. The graft is adapted as an anterior anastomotic onlay, over the ureteral defect, and sutured with two semicontinuous suture (4–0 Vicryl). The repair and entire surgical fields are wrapped in omentum after assuring that the ureteral anastomosis are watertight with filling of the bladder with 100 cc of methylene blue solution.

Although a handful of cases have been reported, it is a feasible and safe technique. In the two studies, three and two patients were recorded and a complete resolution of symptoms with radiological and biochemical stability over the follow-up with a median of 10 and 7 months in the two studies. No postoperative complications were recorded [43, 44].

References

1. Cohen B, Goldman SM, Kopilnick M, Khurana A V., Salik JO. Ureteropelvic junction obstruction: its occurrence in 3 members of a single family. J Urol. 1978. https://doi.org/10.1016/S0022-5347(17)57175-X.
2. Bultitude MF. Campbell-walsh urology tenth edition. BJU Int. 2012. https://doi.org/10.1111/j.1464-410x.2011.10907.x.
3. Park JM, Bloom DA. The pathophysiology of UPJ obstruction: current concepts. Urol Clin North Am. 1998. https://doi.org/10.1016/S0094-0143(05)70004-5.
4. Lam JS, Breda A, Schulam PG. Ureteropelvic junction obstruction. J Urol. 2007. https://doi.org/10.1016/j.juro.2007.01.056.
5. O'Reilly PH, Brooman PJC, Mak S, et al. The long-term results of Anderson-Hynes pyeloplasty. BJU Int. 2001. https://doi.org/10.1046/j.1464-410X.2001.00108.x.
6. Siegel CL, McDougall EM, Middleton WD, et al. Preoperative assessment of ureteropelvic junction obstruction with endoluminal sonography and helical CT. Am J Roentgenol. 1997. https://doi.org/10.2214/ajr.168.3.9057502.
7. Stabile Ianora AA, Scardapane A, Chiumarullo L, Calbi R, Rotondo A, Angelelli G. Congenital stenosis of ureteropelvic junction: assessment with multislice CT. Radiol Med. 2003.
8. Khaira HS, Platt JF, Cohan RH, Wolf JS, Faerber GJ. Helical computed tomography for identification of crossing vessels in ureteropelvic junction obstruction – Comparison with operative findings. Urology. 2003. https://doi.org/10.1016/S0090-4295(03)00156-0.
9. Silay MS, Spinoit AF, Bogaert G, Hoebeke P, Nijman R, Haid B. Imaging for vesicoureteral reflux and ureteropelvic junction obstruction. Eur Urol Focus. 2016. https://doi.org/10.1016/j.euf.2016.03.015.
10. Zielonko J, Studniarek M, Markuszewski M. MR urography of obstructive uropathy: diagnostic value of the method in selected clinical groups. Eur Radiol. 2003. https://doi.org/10.1007/s00330-002-1550-8.
11. O'Reilly PH, Lawson RS, Shields RA, Testa HJ. Idiopathic hydronephrosis – the diuresis renogram: a new non-invasive method of assessing equivocal pelvioureteral junction obstruction. J Urol. 1979. https://doi.org/10.1016/S0022-5347(17)56703-8.
12. Perez-Brayfield MR, Kirsch AJ, Jones RA, Grattan-Smith JD. A prospective study comparing ultrasound, nuclear scintigraphy and dynamic contrast enhanced magnetic resonance imaging in the evaluation of hydronephrosis. J Urol. 2003. https://doi.org/10.1097/01.ju.0000086775.66329.00.
13. Esmaeili M, Esmaeili M, Ghane F, Alamdaran A. Comparison between diuretic urography (IVP) and diuretic renography for diagnosis of ureteropelvic junction obstruction in children. Iran J Pediatr. 2016. https://doi.org/10.5812/ijp.4293.
14. Mandhani A, Goel S, Bhandari M. Is antegrade stenting superior to retrograde stenting in laparoscopic pyeloplasty? J Urol. 2004. https://doi.org/10.1097/01.ju.0000116546.06765.d1.
15. Papalia R, Simone G, Leonardo C, et al. Retrograde placement of ureteral stent and ureteropelvic anastomosis with two running sutures in transperitoneal laparoscopic pyeloplasty: tips of success in our learning curve. J Endourol. 2009. https://doi.org/10.1089/end.2008.0617.
16. Gettman MT, Neururer R, Bartsch G, Peschel R. Anderson-Hynes dismembered pyeloplasty performed using the da Vinci robotic system. Urology. 2002. https://doi.org/10.1016/S0090-4295(02)01761-2.
17. Patel V. Robotic-assisted laparoscopic dismembered pyeloplasty. Urology. 2005. https://doi.org/10.1016/j.urology.2005.01.053.
18. Mufarrij PW, Woods M, Shah OD, et al. Robotic dismembered pyeloplasty: a 6-year, multi-institutional experience. J Urol. 2008. https://doi.org/10.1016/j.juro.2008.06.024.
19. Schwentner C, Pelzer A, Neururer R, et al. Robotic Anderson-Hynes pyeloplasty: 5-year experience of one centre. BJU Int. 2007. https://doi.org/10.1111/j.1464-410X.2007.07032.x.
20. Sivaraman A, Leveillee RJ, Patel MB, et al. Robot-assisted laparoscopic dismembered pyeloplasty for ureteropelvic junction obstruction: a multi-institutional experience. Urology. 2012. https://doi.org/10.1016/j.urology.2011.10.019.
21. Gupta NP, Nayyar R, Hemal AK, Mukherjee S, Kumar R, Dogra PN. Outcome analysis of robotic pyeloplasty: a large single-centre experience. BJU Int. 2010. https://doi.org/10.1111/j.1464-410X.2009.08983.x.
22. Cestari A, Buffi NM, Lista G, et al. Retroperitoneal and transperitoneal robot-assisted pyeloplasty in adults: techniques and results. Eur Urol. 2010;58(5):711–8. https://doi.org/10.1016/j.eururo.2010.07.020.
23. Autorino R, Eden C, El-Ghoneimi A, et al. Robot-assisted and laparoscopic repair of ureteropelvic junction obstruction: a systematic review and meta-analysis. Eur Urol. 2014. https://doi.org/10.1016/j.eururo.2013.06.053.
24. Başataç C, Boylu U, Önol FF, Gümüş E. Comparison of surgical and functional outcomes of open, laparoscopic and robotic pyeloplasty for the treatment of ureteropelvic junction obstruction. Turk Urol Derg. 2014. https://doi.org/10.5152/tud.2014.06956.

25. Hanske J, Sanchez A, Schmid M, et al. Comparison of 30-day perioperative outcomes in adults undergoing open versus minimally invasive pyeloplasty for ureteropelvic junction obstruction: analysis of 593 patients in a prospective national database. World J Urol. 2015. https://doi.org/10.1007/s00345-015-1586-4.
26. Buffi NM, Lughezzani G, Hurle R, et al. Robot-assisted surgery for benign ureteral strictures: experience and outcomes from four tertiary care institutions. Eur Urol. 2017. https://doi.org/10.1016/j.eururo.2016.07.022.
27. Mei H, Pu J, Yang C, Zhang H, Zheng L, Tong Q. Laparoscopic versus open pyeloplasty for ureteropelvic junction obstruction in children: A systematic review and meta-analysis. J Endourol. 2011. https://doi.org/10.1089/end.2010.0544.
28. Thom MR, Haseebuddin M, Roytman TM, Benway BM, Bhayani SM, Figenshau RS. Robot-assisted pyeloplasty: outcomes for primary and secondary repairs, a single institution experience. Int Braz J Urol. 2012. https://doi.org/10.1590/S1677-55382012000100011.
29. Atug F, Burgess S V., Castle EP, Thomas R. Role of robotics in the management of secondary ureteropelvic junction obstruction. Int J Clin Pract. 2006. https://doi.org/10.1111/j.1368-5031.2006.00701.x.
30. Hemal AK, Mishra S, Mukharjee S, Suryavanshi M. Robot assisted laparoscopic pyeloplasty in patients of ureteropelvic junction obstruction with previously failed open surgical repair. Int J Urol. 2008. https://doi.org/10.1111/j.1442-2042.2008.02091.x.
31. Cestari A, Buffi NM, Lista G, et al. Feasibility and preliminary clinical outcomes of robotic laparoendoscopic single-site (R-LESS) pyeloplasty using a new single-port platform. Eur Urol. 2012. https://doi.org/10.1016/j.eururo.2012.03.041.
32. Buffi NM, Lughezzani G, Fossati N, et al. Robot-assisted, single-site, dismembered pyeloplasty for ureteropelvic junction obstruction with the New da Vinci Platform: a stage 2a study. Eur Urol. 2015. https://doi.org/10.1016/j.eururo.2014.03.001.
33. Lindgren BW, Hagerty J, Meyer T, Cheng EY. Robot-assisted laparoscopic reoperative repair for failed pyeloplasty in children: a safe and highly effective treatment option. J Urol. 2012. https://doi.org/10.1016/j.juro.2012.04.118.
34. Niver BE, Agalliu I, Bareket R, Mufarrij P, Shah O, Stifelman MD. Analysis of robotic-assisted laparoscopic pyleloplasty for primary versus secondary repair in 119 consecutive cases. Urology. 2012. https://doi.org/10.1016/j.urology.2011.10.072.
35. Desai MM, Berger AK, Brandina R, et al. Laparoendoscopic single-site surgery: initial hundred patients. Urology. 2009. https://doi.org/10.1016/j.urology.2009.02.083.
36. Lenfant L, Wilson CA, Sawczyn G, Aminsharifi A, Kim S, Kaouk J. Single-port robot-assisted dismembered pyeloplasty with mini-pfannenstiel or peri-umbilical access: initial experience in a single center. Urology. 2020;143:147–52. https://doi.org/10.1016/j.urology.2020.05.041.
37. Buffi NM, Lughezzani G, Fossati N, et al. Robot-assisted, single-site, dismembered pyeloplasty for ureteropelvic junction obstruction with the New da Vinci Platform: a stage 2a study. Eur Urol. 2015;67(1):151–6. https://doi.org/10.1016/j.eururo.2014.03.001.
38. Diana P, Buffi NM, Lughezzani G, et al. The role of intraoperative indocyanine green in robot-assisted partial nephrectomy: results from a large, multi-institutional series. Eur Urol. 2020. https://doi.org/10.1016/j.eururo.2020.05.040.
39. Pathak RA, Hemal AK. Intraoperative ICG-fluorescence imaging for robotic-assisted urologic surgery: current status and review of literature. Int Urol Nephrol. 2019;51(5):765–71. https://doi.org/10.1007/s11255-019-02126-0.
40. Lee Z, Moore B, Giusto L, Eun DD. Use of indocyanine green during robot-Assisted ureteral reconstructions. Eur Urol. 2015;67(2):291–8. https://doi.org/10.1016/j.eururo.2014.08.057.
41. Lee M, Lee Z, Strauss D, et al. Multi-institutional experience comparing outcomes of adult patients undergoing secondary versus primary robotic pyeloplasty. Urology. 2020;145:275–80. https://doi.org/10.1016/j.urology.2020.07.008.
42. Zhao LC, Weinberg AC, Lee Z, et al. Robotic ureteral reconstruction using buccal mucosa grafts: a multi-institutional experience. Eur Urol. 2018;73(3):419–26. https://doi.org/10.1016/j.eururo.2017.11.015.
43. Ahn JJ, Shapiro ME, Ellison JS, Lendvay TS. Pediatric robot-assisted redo pyeloplasty with buccal mucosa graft: a novel technique. Urology. 2017;101:56–9. https://doi.org/10.1016/j.urology.2016.12.036.
44. Zampini AM, Nelson R, Zhang JJH, Reese J, Angermeier KW, Haber GP. Robotic salvage pyeloplasty with buccal mucosal onlay graft: video demonstration of technique and outcomes. Urology. 2017;110:253–6. https://doi.org/10.1016/j.urology.2017.07.023.

Reconstructive Surgery for Ureteral Strictures: Boari Flap, Psoas Hitch, Buccal Mucosa, and Other Techniques

Nathan Cheng and Michael Stifelman

1 Introduction

Ureteral reconstruction, a field that aims to surgically correct pain, renal dysfunction, and infection risk associated with obstructed urinary flow from the kidney to the bladder, has been expanding with the popularization of robotic techniques. Ischemia, iatrogenic trauma, non-iatrogenic trauma, retroperitoneal fibrosis, radiation, malignancy, or impacted ureteral calculi are all possible etiologies for ureteral stricture formation. The fine dissecting ability, decreased postoperative pain, and use of adjunctive measures to confirm tissue perfusion in robotic reconstruction suggest equivalent, if not better, outcomes than that of traditional open and laparoscopic procedures [1].

1.1 Proximal Ureter

Radiologically, the proximal ureter is defined to be the segment between the renal pelvis and the superior border of the sacroiliac joint. Proximal ureteral blood supply arises medial-to-lateral, mostly from the main renal artery with some contribution from smaller branches directly off the aorta as well as the gonadal artery. The more proximal the ureteral stricture, the more the reconstruction benefits from robust vascularity, as is closer to the main renal artery branches, one of the reasons why pyeloplasty outcomes are excellent. Tracing distally, there are watershed regions of the proximal ureter between plexuses from the renal artery branches, aortic branches, and gonadal artery branches. Thus, surgical principles of proximal ureteral reconstruction state that dissection of the proximal ureter must be precise with care to leave as much adventitia on the ureter as possible and to avoid lateralizing the ureter extensively.

N. Cheng · M. Stifelman (✉)
Hackensack Meridian School of Medicine, Nutley, NJ, USA

Hackensack University Medical Center, Hackensack, NJ, USA

1.2 Mid-Ureter

The mid-ureter is defined to be the segment of the ureter between the superior border of the sacroiliac joint and the inferior border of the sacroiliac joint, or more simply, the pelvic inlet. This segment obtains its vascularity from posterior to anterior originating from the common iliac artery.

1.3 Distal Ureter

The segment between the pelvic inlet and the ureterovesical junction is the distal ureter. Its vascularity originates lateral to medial from branches off of the internal iliac artery and its branches (e.g., superior vesical, uterine, inferior vesical, middle rectal, etc.). Similar to the rest of the ureter, its perfusion from these adventitia plexuses are tenuous, and blood supply to the bladder will almost always be superior to that of the distal ureter; thus, ureteroneocystostomy is the reconstructive technique of choice when managing distal ureteral strictures.

1.4 Identification and Isolation of Strictured Segment

First, the colon should be reflected medially by incising the white line of the Toldt in order to expose the retroperitoneum for strictures in the proximal or mid-ureter. When operating on the right side, Kocherizing the duodenum medially in order to visualize the hilar strictures of the kidney, including the gonadal vessels, is often necessary to aid in the identification of the ureter. In distal ureteral strictures, the ureter can often be identified crossing the bifurcation of the common iliacs into the external and internal after medial retraction of bowel.

There are certain cases, particularly in radiation, malignant, or retroperitoneal fibrosis etiologies, where there may be strong fibrotic or desmoplastic reactions in the retroperi-

P. Wiklund et al. (eds.), *Robotic Urologic Surgery*, https://doi.org/10.1007/978-3-031-00363-9_46

toneum that complicate ureteral identification. Fibrotic rinds may encase the ureter and distort the expected location of the ureter (e.g., retroperitoneal fibrosis medializing the ureter). It is important, in these cases, to identify normal ureter outside of the diseased segment to trace it into unknown territory.

Should anatomic considerations be inadequate in identifying the ureter, there are some adjunctive techniques that may help. Intraoperative ultrasonography with robotic or laparoscopic probes are useful in identifying indwelling ureteral stents or catheters that can be placed cystoscopically or antegrade via nephrostomy access at the time of surgery—there may be some cases of operating on a patient with an indwelling ureteral stent already in place, which will be discussed later to be disadvantageous to reconstructive outcomes. Ureteroscopy is very helpful when performing ureteral reconstruction, as it allows for correlation between the intraluminal status of the ureter with the extraluminal appearance robotically. Most recent robotic console softwares include a near-infrared imaging (NIRF) modality, which enhances the light emanating from the ureteroscope, allowing for identification of the ureter. The use of intraureteral indocyanine green (ICG) is also a useful tool that takes advantage of NIRF. 5 mL of diluted ICG can be instilled intraureterically. ICG binds to the tissues of the ureter and is fluorescent green in the NIRF setting. ICG has also been commonly used intravenously (2 mL) to assess for tissue perfusion (Fig. 1). The disadvantage of intraureteral ICG for ureteral identification is that it precludes one from using intravenous ICG to confirm ureteral perfusion, as it will be illuminated fluorescent green regardless of perfusion status. Thus, if the ureter can be identified without using intraureteral ICG, it may be advantageous to save the ICG to be used intravenously.

Once the ureter is identified, it must be isolated. Sharp dissection over the anterior tissues overlying the ureter should be performed, with judicious electrocautery use. The anterior ureter is generally safe to dissect, but surgeons may choose to hedge toward one side or the other based on the direction of blood supply to the diseased segment location, i.e., anterolaterally in proximal ureter and anteromedially in distal ureter. Circumferential isolation of the ureter is usually performed, but depending on the etiology of stricture, may not be necessary. If the ureteral stricture is secondary to extrinsic compression from extraluminal tissue (e.g., retroperitoneal fibrosis), circumferential isolation must be performed. If an omental wrap is going to be performed (e.g., buccal mucosal ureteroplasty), getting completely around the ureter is often needed. However, there are circumstances when ureteral dissection is difficult and may compromise the adventitia and its vascular plexus and the surgeon is able to reconstruct the ureter without circumferential ureteral transection (e.g., appendiceal bypass or side-to-side reimplantation).

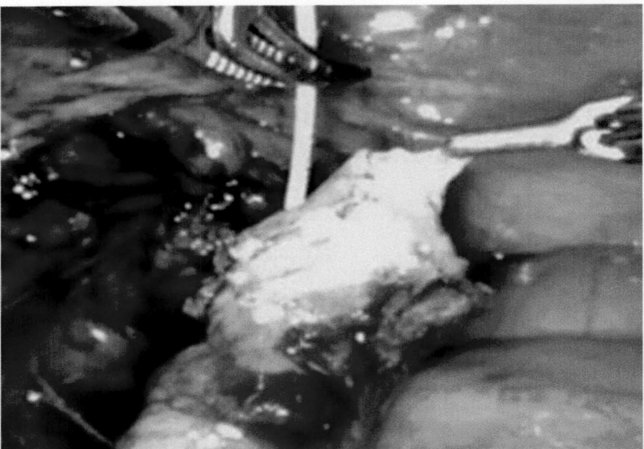

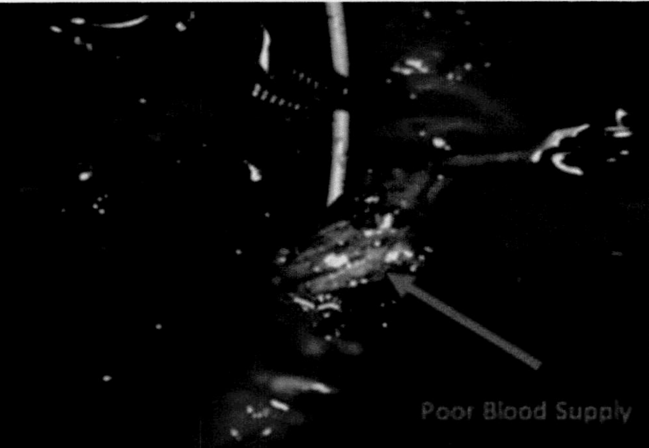

Fig. 1 After transection of a strictured ureteral segment, the use of near-infrared imaging (NIRF) following 2 mL of intravenous indocyanine green shows that the distal extent of the stump is poorly perfused and thus warrants further trimming

Finally and perhaps the most important concept of ureteral identification and dissection is discerning healthy tissue versus unhealthy tissue. Reconstructive surgical principles state to trim or exclude unhealthy tissue until viable ureter is seen, so only healthy ureter is involved in urine passage. Poorly perfused ureter is at risk for scarring and recurrence of stricture—these tissues are generally pale or discolored with minimal to no bleeding when cutting into. If there is any question about viability of tissues, 2 mL intravenous ICG, as mentioned above, is an excellent modality to assess for tissue perfusion.

1.5 Ureteral Rest

The universally accepted urethral reconstructive principle of urethral rest has been translated to upper tract reconstruction as ureteral rest, the absence from ureteral instrumentation or hardware leading up to the operation. It has been proven to be beneficial in ureteral reconstructive outcomes, with patients who had no indwelling ureteral stent or percutaneous nephroureteral tube for at least 4 weeks prior to surgery having 90.7% success versus 77.5% in those without ureteral rest ($p = 0.057$) in a multi-institutional retrospective study of 234 patients [2]. While not yet studied at a histologic level, the hypothesized physiology is tissue recovery with maturation of the stricture, as continued hardware (indwelling ureteral stent or nephroureteral tube) increases ureteral and periureteral tissue inflammation.

2 Ureterolysis

2.1 Retroperitoneal Fibrosis

Ureterolysis is a procedure reserved to manage patients who have ureteral obstruction secondary to extrinsic compression. Causes may include tumor, infection, and, most commonly, retroperitoneal fibrosis (RPF). RPF is a process characterized by fibrosis and chronic retroperitoneal inflammation, usually originating from peri-aortic and other great vessels' adventitia. RPF is a general term, with some of its causes including endovascular stents (e.g., for abdominal aortic aneurysms), spinal hardware, prior retroperitoneal surgery, radiation, medication adverse effects especially that of ergot alkaloids (such as methysergide), and other processes that recruit inflammatory reactions affecting the retroperitoneum. RPF is a broad disease process with multiple etiologies including idiopathic RPF. While rare, with an incidence of 0.1–1.3 cases/100,000 people annually, idiopathic RPF is thought to have an etiology from disease processes on the spectrum of autoimmune disorders such as large vessel vasculitides [3]. A relationship to IgG4 has been described over the past decade, with its pathophysiology hypothesized to be a lymphoplasmacytic, fibrotic, and IgG4+ plasma cell infiltration of various organ systems. It is associated with other autoimmune disorders such as rheumatoid arthritis, ankylosing spondylitis, systemic lupus erythematosus, and, most commonly, thyroiditis.

Ureteral involvement, either bilateral or unilateral, is the most common sequelae of RPF. Although rare, at time of diagnosis of unilateral disease, the contralateral side can be affected gradually between weeks and years [4]. Multiple studies have shown that the risk of contralateral obstruction is low, and thus, bilateral ureterolysis for unilateral disease is not required [5–7]. Classically, the mid- to proximal ureter is affected, extrinsically compressed, and deviated medially.

The etiology of RPF should be determined, if possible, prior to surgical intervention [5, 8–10]. After ruling out secondary causes of RPF and an idiopathic etiology is deemed most likely, glucocorticoid and/or other immunosuppression trials with temporary urinary drainage (e.g., indwelling ureteral stents or nephrostomy tube) have been studied, particularly in mild to moderate ureteral obstruction. The first-line medicinal therapy is prednisone with initial dose of 0.75–1 mg/kg/day and a titration 5–7.5 mg/day within 6–9 months [11]. Immunosuppressive agents such as mycophenolate mofetil and cyclophosphamide may also be considered. Some studies have suggested that tissue diagnosis of the RPF should be performed in order to guide treatment, as lymphoma and other diseases may mimic RPF. Surgical excisional biopsy should be performed at the time of ureterolysis in these scenarios [12].

2.2 Patient Positioning and Trocar Placement

For unilateral operations, patients should be in semilateral decubitus with modified low lithotomy, particularly for urethral access in female patients. All four arms of the da Vinci Xi system are used, with one 5 mm bedside assistant trocar. All trocars except the most inferior should be equidistant away from the vertical midline, approximately 2–3 cm on the ipsilateral side. The inferior-most trocar for retraction should be further medial right at midline, as shown in Fig. 2.

For bilateral operations, the patient is positioned supine with low modified lithotomy. This positioning and trocar placement is almost identical to that of robotic retroperitoneal lymph node dissections, except for the low modified lithotomy, with all ports along the Pfannenstiel line, as seen in Fig. 3.

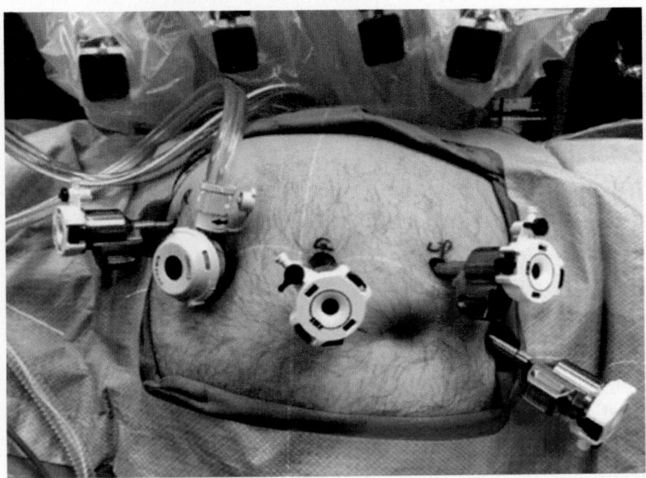

Fig. 2 Robotic trocar placement for left-sided ureterolysis

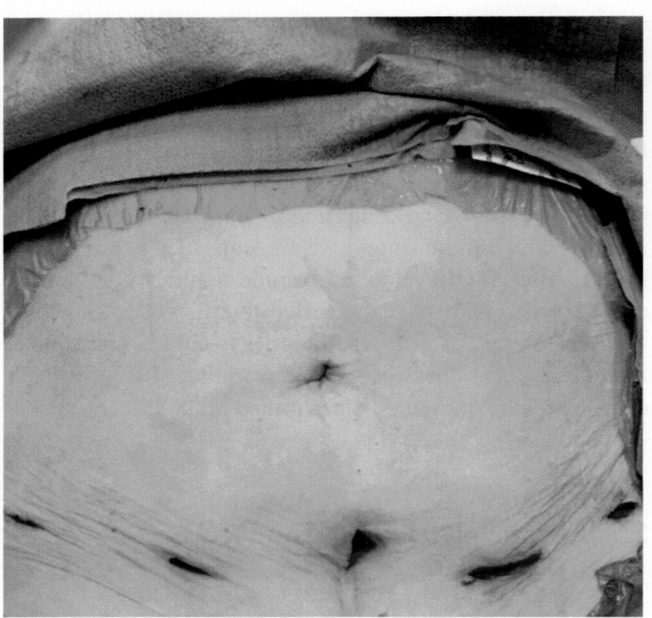

Fig. 3 Robotic trocar placement (post-procedure and with trocars removed) for bilateral ureterolysis

2.3 Technique

Ureterolysis should be done in a systematic fashion by peeling back anterior tissue, then dissecting circumferentially to free the ureter from its posterior fibrosis. The use of a vessel loop after the posterior has been freed is helpful to provide soft traction anteriorly to continue ureterolysis proximally and distally until normal periureteral fat is encountered. Once the correct plane has been established, the fibrotic rind is usually not difficult to peel off of the ureter. Fine dissection using Potts scissors may be helpful.

Biopsy of the periureteral tissues and retroperitoneal mass should be sent off for pathologic evaluation. The ureter should then be assessed for its perfusion, as occasionally, it may be necessary to excise the segment and perform uretero-ureterostomy or other techniques, such as buccal graft ureteroplasty, if there is perfusion compromised to the disease ureteral segment.

Omental wrap is then performed. Healthy omentum encasing the entire length of the ureter is used to prevent recurrence of ureteral obstruction from its surrounding fibrotic tissues. The distal edge of the omentum is bifurcated. Enough should be mobilized to wrap the entire length of the ureter, and if more length is needed, the short gastric vessels can be ligated, freeing the omentum from the stomach. Care must be taken to preserve the left and right gastroepiploic arteries. If there is inadequate omentum, peritonealizing the ureter can be performed, although not preferred. The idea is to anteriorly displace the ureter and keep it out of the fibrotic retroperitoneum by tacking the peritoneal attachments of the colon underneath the ureter to the side wall. This technique does not provide the additional vascularity to the ureter as omental wraps, and thus it is the opinion of the authors to use this technique as a last resort only if the omentum is not accessible.

3 Ureteroneocystostomy (Ureteral Reimplantation)

Distal ureteral strictures may be managed with ureteral reimplantation of healthy ureter proximal to the diseased segment into well-vascularized bladder tissue. Robotic ureteroneocystostomy has been shown to have similar outcomes to open surgery but with the benefits of minimally invasive surgery: decreased postoperative narcotic use and shorter length of stay [13].

3.1 Patient Positioning and Robotic Trocar Placement

Male patients can be positioned supine on the operating room table, whereas female patients may require low/modified lithotomy for urethral access. Urethral access is important for urethral catheter placement to test watertightness as well as ureteroscopy, if necessary.

All four arms of the da Vinci Xi robot are used, in addition to one 5 mm bedside assistant trocar. The camera port should be supraumbilical. The two working arms should be several centimeters lateral to the camera port, with the contralateral working arm being a few centimeters more caudal. The retracting fourth arm trocar, as mentioned above, is contralateral to the disease ureter of concern and even more caudal than the contralateral working arm, so that it is relatively close to the anterior superior iliac spine (ASIS) with enough distance away (usually just a couple centimeters) to not be restricted when moving the arm. The 5 mm assistant trocar should be a few centimeters cephalad to the midway point between the ipsilateral working trocar and camera trocar (Fig. 4). It is recommended that all trocars be placed under direct visualization.

After all robotic trocars are placed, the operating table should be tilted to moderate-to-steep Trendelenburg position to allow for the bowel to fall cephalad.

3.2 Technique

After the strictured distal ureteral segment has been identified, it is traced up proximally until healthy ureter is seen,

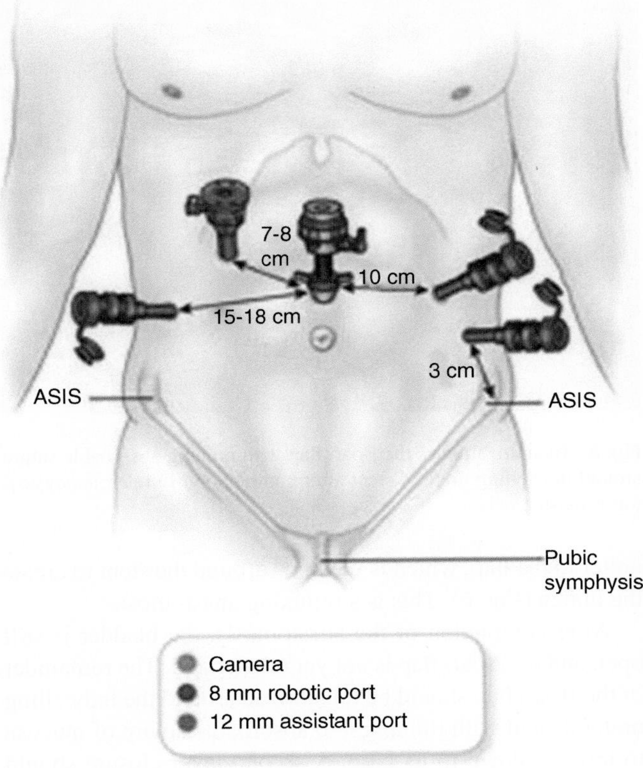

Fig. 4 Robotic trocar placement for right-sided ureteral reimplantation

where the ureter is then transected. The dissection of this transected ureteral stump is generally circumferential in order to give it mobility for reimplantation to the dome of the bladder. Newer techniques have been utilized, as will be discussed later in this chapter, for a non-transecting ureteral reimplantation that minimizes dissection in order to preserve ureteral blood supply. After the transected ureteral stump is mobilized enough to reach to the dome of the bladder, which usually requires mobilization of the anterior aspect of the bladder off of the pelvic and lower abdominal wall, the bladder is filled with approximately 300 mL of normal saline. The ureter is then spatulated approximately 2–3 cm and anastomosed to the cystotomy created about the same size, with attention to have mucosal-to-mucosal apposition. An indwelling ureteral stent should be left prior to completion of the anastomosis. Postoperatively, the Foley catheter is left between 7 and 10 days and the ureteral stent 4 and 6 weeks.

4 Psoas Hitch

The psoas hitch is an adjunctive mobility technique to make up length to facilitate more proximal ureteral reimplantations and also a technique that takes off tension on the anastomosis.

After the space of Retzius is developed and adequate bladder mobility is achieved, an absorbable suture is used to tack the posterolateral aspect of the bladder to the ipsilateral psoas fascia. Either smooth or barbed absorbable sutures may be used. When suturing the psoas fascia, it is important to take the bite longitudinal to the fascial fibers, reducing the risk of catching the genitofemoral nerve, which runs along the anterior surface of the psoas muscle. For strength, the psoas hitch suture can be thrown a few times before tying down.

5 Boari Flap

This technique should be considered for more mobility when it is not possible to create a tension-free ureteroneocystostomy anastomosis, even after bladder mobilization with psoas hitch. This may be seen in mid- to distal ureteral strictures occurring iatrogenically from pelvic radiation, retroperitoneal fibrosis, or other surgical interventions causing scarring. The robotic modality for Boari flaps have shown to have improved outcomes [14]. All patients under consideration for a Boari flap reconstruction should have bladder capacity and compliance tested to be within normal or tolerable limits prior with preoperative cystogram or urodynamics. Patients exhibiting poor capacity and/or compliance may have significant urinary frequency, urgency, and other symptoms secondary to decreased bladder volume, as the effective intraluminal bladder volume is decreased due to the elongated reconfiguration, after Boari flap reconstruction. In addition to these significant quality-of-life measures, patients with preexisting low bladder capacity and/or compliance may have increased filling and/or voiding pressures, predisposing the patient to vesicoureteral reflux, regardless of non-tunneled or tunneled reconstructions. Furthermore, a patient with baseline small bladder volume may not have enough flap tissue to accommodate a tension-free reimplantation anyhow. Thus, patients with preoperative testing showing low capacity and/or compliance should have other types of reconstructive methods that may be better suited to achieve the safest and most patient-favorable outcomes.

5.1 Patient Positioning and Robotic Trocar Placement

Positioning is similar to that of a non-Boari flap ureteral reimplantation.

The trocar placement is also similar to that of unilateral non-Boari flap ureteral reimplantation, with all ports a few centimeters more superior. How proximal the stricture is dictates how much more cephalad the trocars are placed.

5.2 Technique

The Boari flap reconstruction starts after transecting the ureter proximal to the diseased segment, mobilizing the bladder adequately, and completing the psoas hitch. The bladder is first filled with 300–500 mL of normal saline. The shape of the flap is then marked out by scoring over the bladder serosa with electrocautery. If bladder capacity is adequate, a flap length up to 10–15 cm can be developed, with a shape of an inverted "U." The apex of the flap will become the proximal aspect that is anastomosed to the ureter after its construction. In order to minimize the risk of flap ischemia, it is important that the base of the inverted "U," which corresponds to the junction between the bladder and the Boari flap, is wide, often described to be at least 4 cm wide.

The flap is then incised transmurally. Minimal electrocautery may be used for hemostasis, but similar to the principles of ureteral dissection, sharp cutting is preferred in order to retain the bladder's intrinsic vascularity. The apex of the flap is then brought up to the ureteral stump. The posterior aspect of the flap can be tacked to the psoas fascia, if the surgeon decides it is necessary to take off more tension. The ureter should be spatulated posteriorly about 1.5–2.0 cm. After that is done, the posterior plate of the ureter-Boari flap anastomosis is created by absorbable 4–0 suture, taking the apex of the Boari flap to the crotch of the posterior ureteral spatulation (Fig. 5). Once the posterior plate is completed, ensuring adequate mucosa-to-mucosa apposition, an indwelling ureteral stent is placed. The anterior aspect can then be completed with 4–0 absorbable suture by anastomosing the anterior ureter to the flap, which is wrapped around the stent to create the lumen (Fig. 6). This is a refluxing anastomosis.

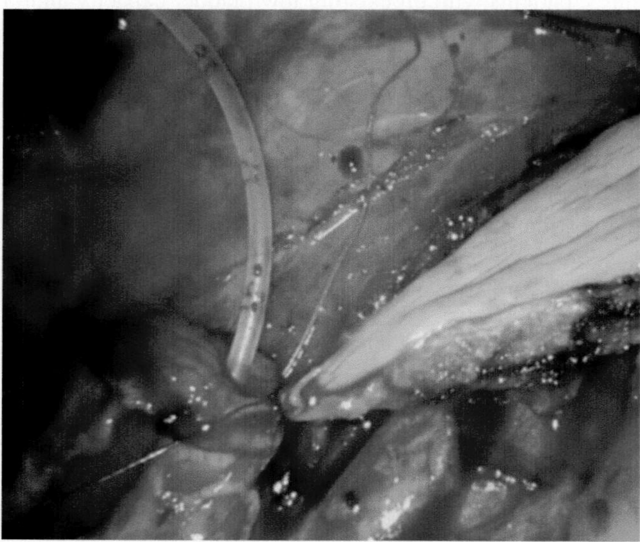

Fig. 5 Posterior anastomosis of the Boari flap (right) to the spatulated ureteral stump (left) with absorbable suture

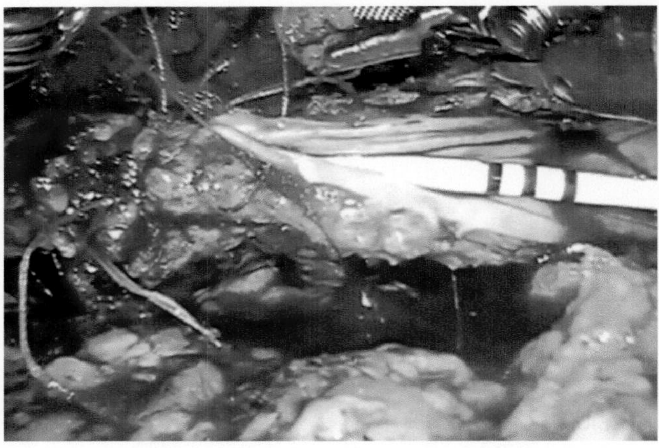

Fig. 6 Tubularization of the Boari flap with running absorbable suture around indwelling ureteral stent after completion of ureteroneocystostomy anastomosis

After completion of the anastomosis, the bladder is still open and the Boari flap is not yet tubularized. The remainder of the Boari flap should be tubularized around the indwelling ureteral stent with running 4–0 absorbable suture of mucosa to mucosa down to its base. A second layer closure should then be performed with 3–0 or 4–0 absorbable suture to reapproximate the detrusor over the newly tubularized flap. The bladder defect can then be repaired in the usual one- or two-layer repair with 3–0 absorbable suture.

After completion of the Boari flap tubularization and cystorrhaphy, the closure should be tested by instilling 300 mL of normal saline via the Foley catheter. Additional sutures may be placed in order to repair leaks.

As with all ureteral anastomoses, a surgical drain should be left. The Foley catheter should be left for 10–14 days and the ureteral stent for 4–6 weeks. A cystogram may be performed to ensure that the bladder has completely healed before removal of the Foley catheter.

6 Non-transecting Side-to-Side Ureteral Reimplantation

As alluded to earlier, there are certain circumstances in which circumferential isolation and transection of the ureter are not needed, and, in fact, may compromise blood supply to the ureter. Non-transecting side-to-side ureteral reimplantations have been become more popular recently [15], a useful tool in a reconstructive urologist's armamentarium for distal ureteral strictures within severely fibrotic tissues, particularly in the setting of prior radiation therapy.

6.1 Patient Positioning and Robotic Trocar Placement

Patient positioning and robotic trocar placement are similar to that of standard ureteral reimplantation. A Foley catheter may be placed either on or off the sterile field: if off the sterile field, a circulating assistant should be available to irrigate the Foley catheter with normal saline. This is used to assist with bladder mobilization as well as testing the ureteroneocystostomy anastomosis.

6.2 Technique

After the distal ureter is identified, the strictured segment is followed up proximally until healthy ureter is seen. Again, there is no rule for circumferentially dissecting out the ureter, particularly over the posterolateral aspect of the adventitia where the blood supply in this segment originates from. A 3–4-cm-long ureterotomy is made over the anterior (or even anteromedial) aspect of the healthy ureter. The strictured segment of the ureter distal to this ureterotomy is left in situ, hence the term non-transecting.

The bladder is then mobilized in order to have the length to reach the ureterotomy created. While dropping the bladder of its anterior attachments to the abdominal wall and pelvis may give enough length, sometimes further mobilization of the bladder of its lateral attachments may be necessary. The same adjunctive techniques of psoas hitch and even Boari flap can be utilized if necessary. After the bladder is adequately mobilized, a transmural cystotomy is made over the posterolateral aspect on the ipsilateral side in order to be anastomosed to the ureterotomy.

The ureterotomy-cystotomy anastomosis is performed first over the medial side to create the posterior plate with 4–0 absorbable suture. After this posterior plate is completed, a double J indwelling ureteral stent with a guidewire straightening out the proximal curl is introduced into the abdominal cavity through the assistant port and placed in a retrograde fashion through the ureterotomy. After the proximal aspect of the stent is in the approximate position, the guidewire is removed, and the distal curl can be placed into the bladder through the cystotomy. Now with the ureteral stent in place, the anterior aspect of the anastomosis can be completed with another 4–0 absorbable suture (Fig. 7).

After the anastomosis is completed, the bladder is filled with at least 200 mL of normal saline in order to test the watertightness of the side-to-side ureteroneocystostomy. Should there be areas of leakage, additional interrupted 4–0 absorbable sutures can be placed, with care not to take bites too deep in order to avoid suturing the indwelling ureteral stent. A pelvic drain is then placed through the most inferior robotic trocar.

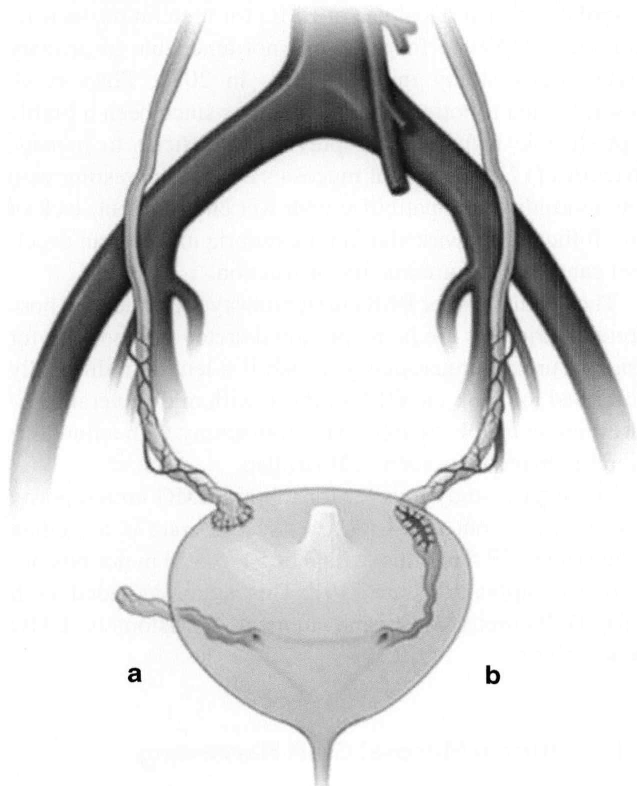

Fig. 7 Illustration of right-sided transecting (**a**) versus left-sided non-transecting side-to-side (**b**) ureteral reimplantation

The drain is usually removed prior to discharge, assuming the output is low and, if not, drain fluid creatinine is consistent with serum creatinine. The Foley catheter remains for approximately 1 week. Some surgeons elect to perform a cystogram to ensure no urine leak prior to removing the Foley catheter. The indwelling ureteral stent is removed in approximately 4 weeks.

6.3 Outcomes

As this is a newly popularized technique, there are not many published studies reporting the outcomes. However, in a recent series of 16 patients across three institutions, all patients had radiographically improved hydronephrosis, and 15 out of 16 (93.8%) patients had improvement in flank pain at a median follow-up time of 12 months [15].

7 Buccal Mucosal Ureteroplasty

Much like the concept of preoperative ureteral rest, buccal mucosal graft (BMG) for urologic reconstruction is a technique borrowed from urethral reconstruction. The first described open surgical use of BMG for ureteral reconstruction was by Naude for strictures not amenable to primary ureteroureterostomy in 1999 [16]. In 2015, Zhao et al. described the robotic technique and has since been a highly reproducible technique for previously difficult to manage strictures [17]. The buccal mucosa's ease of harvesting with low morbidity, compatibility with wet environment, lack of hair follicles, and vascular lamina propria makes it an excellent candidate for ureteral reconstruction.

The candidates for BMG ureteroplasty are patients whose ureteral strictures are in the proximal ureter and too long for primary ureteroureteroplasty, which is a length traditionally described to be >3 cm [18], or those with mid-ureteral strictures not amenable to ureteroneocystostomy with adjunctive mobility maneuvers such as Boari flap.

The largest study thus far for robotic BMG ureteroplasty has shown 47 out of 54 (87.0%) success rate at a median follow-up of 27.5 months, with 3 of 54 (5.6%) major postoperative complication rate [19]. This study included both onlay BMG ureteroplasty and augmented anastomotic BMG ureteroplasty.

7.1 Buccal Mucosal Graft Harvesting

The endotracheal tube should be secured to the side of the mouth ipsilateral to the ureteral pathology to allow for enough space to operate on the dependent cheek. The BMG harvest relies on intraoperative measurement of the ureteral stricture in order to guide the length of graft, so should be done concurrently with the robotic portion of the case if possible. The width of the graft should be about 1.5 cm.

The buccal mucosa is first infiltrated with lidocaine with epinephrine for hydrodissection and then sharply excised off the buccinator muscle. Usually proximal toward the molars and on the upper half of the cheek mucosa, the Stensen's duct, the duct that drains salivary fluid into the mouth from the parotid gland, must be visualized in order to avoid injury. After harvest, it is important to keep note which side of the buccal mucosal graft is the shiny oral epithelium and which side is the more dull submucosa. The graft is prepared on a back table by sharply removing the submucosal tissue and fat to expose the lamina propria, so that the BMG will have an oral epithelium on one side facing the ureteral lumen and lamina propria on the other side in direct contact with the omentum or other vascular tissues. Minimal submucosa tissues and fat on the lamina propria side ensure maximal direct contact of the lamina propria to its perfusion environment to optimize graft take.

After achieving hemostasis, the BMG harvest site can either be left open to heal via secondary intention or closed with absorbable suture. Postoperatively, the patient is allowed to have oral intake of food and fluid immediately, as tolerated. Oral rinses that contain local anesthetic with or without antiseptic agents help with symptomatic relief.

7.2 Onlay Buccal Mucosal Graft Ureteroplasty

Strictures with narrowed ureteral lumen are candidates for the BMG onlay technique [20]. Importantly, patients with complete ureteral obliteration are not candidates for the BMG onlay. A longitudinal ureterotomy is made over the strictured segment until the lumen is exposed. The length of the incision should be made so that there is adequate healthy ureteral tissue over the proximal- and distal-most aspects of the ureterotomy.

The BMG should then be trimmed to the shape of the ureterotomy and then secured over the ureterotomy with absorbable sutures. Midway through the BMG anastomosis, an indwelling ureteral stent should be placed.

7.3 Augmented Anastomotic Buccal Mucosal Graft Ureteroplasty

Strictures with obliterated ureteral lumens must be excised. After excision, the posterior plate of the ureteroplasty is created by anastomosing the proximal and distal transected ureteral stumps with absorbable suture, making sure to confirm this posterior ureteral plate is healthy. Intravenous ICG is useful here. An indwelling ureteral stent is then placed. The anterior tissue of the proximal and distal ureteral stumps should also be confirmed to be healthy; further trimming of tissue may be done, and spatulation can also be performed if lumen is narrowed. The remaining anterior defect is then covered with BMG and secured with absorbable suture similar to the onlay technique (Fig. 8).

7.4 Omental Wrap

An omental, perinephric, or even mesenteric fat flap should be used to supply blood to the BMG as it heals and incorporates into the ureter. The technique for harvesting omentum is discussed previously. For ureteroplasties that were circumferentially dissected, the preferred omental flap technique is passing the pedicle posterior to the ureter, securing it to the psoas fascia posteriorly, and then securing the pedicle around medially to cover the anterior side of the ureter so that the ureter is in contact with a vascular supply circumferentially. It is important that the BMG has maximal contact with the omental wrap, and a useful technique is to directly secure the omentum to the "serosa" of the BMG with absorbable suture. Placing sutures on the omentum should be done carefully

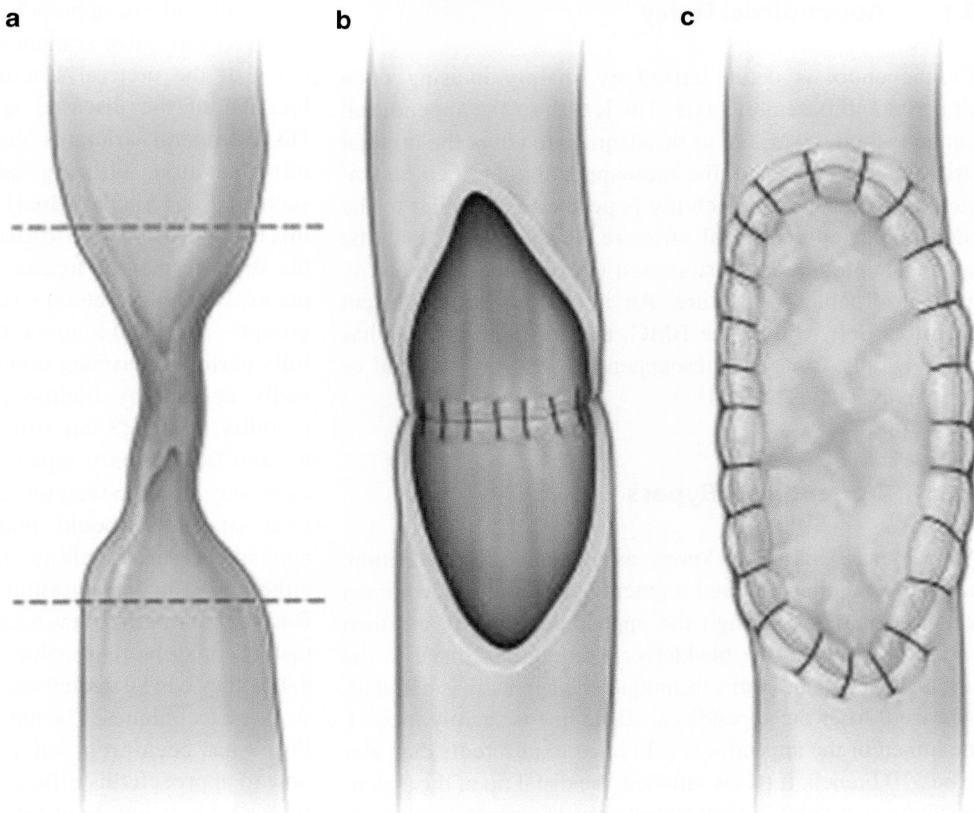

Fig. 8 Illustration of the steps for an augmented anastomotic buccal mucosal graft ureteroplasty, with an obliterated ureteral segment (**a**) transected, the posterior ureteroureteral plate anastomosis (**b**), and the onlay of the buccal mucosal graft over the anterior defect (**c**)

along its longitudinal axis and in an interrupted fashion as to not compromise pedicle perfusion. Intravenous ICG can also be used to confirm omental flap vascularity. For ureteroplasties that were not circumferentially dissected, the omental pedicle is placed over the anterior surface of the ureter, with absorbable suture placed between the omentum and BMG "serosa" to maximize contact and secured laterally.

8 Appendiceal Ureteroplasty

Appendiceal utilization in ureteral reconstruction was described as early as 1912 by Melnikoff with both open and laparoscopic techniques being evaluated in the literature [21–24]. While simple distal ureteral strictures may be corrected with some variation of a ureteroneocystostomy, more complex distal ureteral strictures, mid-, or proximal ureteral strictures may be approached with appendiceal ureteroplasty, if the appendix is present. This is another tool as a substitute to BMG ureteroplasty. The robotic modality for appendiceal ureteroplasty was recently shown to have a 92% success rate in a multi-institutional early retrospective database of 12 patients [25].

Patients are placed in a modified lateral decubitus position with both the genitalia and nephrostomy tube prepped into the field. Similar to the previous reconstructive techniques, females had their legs in modified lithotomy for access to urethra. The bedside assistant trocar should be a 12 mm port in order to accommodate the laparoscopic stapler to divide the appendix from the cecum; however, one can also sharply divide the appendix from the cecum and close the cecal defect with two-layer suture. After the diseased ureteral segment has been isolated, attention is then paid to the appendix.

A window in the mesoappendix is made, with care not to disturb its intrinsic vascularity. The laparoscopic stapler is then used to divide the appendix from the cecum, with care to keep the mesoappendix intact. The staple line on the appendix side is then sharply opened with suctioning of fecal material if present. The appendix may then need to be mobilized in order to reach the region of the ureteral stricture. Intravenous ICG can be used to ensure adequate appendiceal and mesoappendiceal perfusion post-mobilization.

Similar to BMG onlay versus augmented anastomotic BMG ureteroplasty, the use of the appendix depends on whether the stricture lumen is narrowed or obliterated. Obliterated lumens require an appendiceal bypass. Narrowed lumens are managed with appendiceal onlay but can also be managed with appendiceal bypass.

8.1 Appendiceal Onlay

The appendix is detubularized by sharply incising open along its antimesenteric axis. The length of the appendiceal lumen is then made sure to be adequate to cover the ureteral stricture. If inadequate, the mesoappendix can then be stapled across and appendectomy is performed. Similar to the BMG onlay, the ureteral stricture is split open, and the appendiceal onlay is anastomosed to cover the ureterotomy with absorbable 4–0 suture. An indwelling ureteral stent should be left. Unlike the BMG, the appendix already has blood supply from the mesoappendix; thus no, omental or perinephric flap is needed.

8.2 Appendiceal Bypass

Appendiceal bypass, also known as appendiceal interposition, keeps the ureteral strictured segment in situ with a new lumen for urine passage through the appendiceal lumen and then either directly into the bladder or to the ureter distal to the strictured segment. In this technique, the appendix is not detubularized. After the appendiceal staple line is sharply incised, the lumen of the appendix is calibrated to ensure its diameter to be >10 French. If this is satisfied, the distal tip of the appendix (anticecal side) is then sharply cut to expose the lumen. This distal tip of the appendix will be anastomosed to the ureter proximal to the stricture, while the cecal side is anastomosed distal to the stricture (either the bladder or ureter). Both open ends of the appendix are spatulated approximately 2–3 cm in length for anastomosis. An indwelling ureteral stent should be left through the appendiceal lumen and ureter.

9 Technique Summary and Algorithmic Approach

Robotic surgical principles in ureteral reconstruction are the same as those of open surgery, with many concepts extrapolated from urethral reconstruction: minimizing ureteral blood supply disruption, creating tension-free anastomoses, ensuring mucosa-to-mucosa apposition (for the ureter, bladder, or BMG), and, more recently studied, allowing the stricture to mature with ureteral rest. Minimizing ureteral blood supply disruption is a function of both technique and decision-making: dissection of the ureter should be minimized with as much adventitial tissue left on as possible, circumferential dissection should be limited if unnecessary, and ureteral reimplantation is preferred when possible as the bladder's vascularity is superior to the ureter.

An algorithmic approach for these novel tools in our ureteral reconstructive armamentarium based on the characteristics of the ureteral stricture should be used. First, the location of the diseased segment should be considered. Distal ureteral strictures should be repaired with ureteral reimplantation, utilizing adjunctive mobility techniques such as psoas hitch or Boari flap when needed. However, if this is not possible due to characteristics of the bladder, then the stricture may be treated similar to that of the proximal ureter. Proximal ureteral strictures should be placed in two groups—short and long—referring to the ability to successfully perform a primary ureteroureterostomy and not necessarily abiding by traditional 3 cm cutoff, as, based on mobility, some <3 cm strictures may not be amenable to tension-free primary repair. Short proximal ureteral strictures may undergo ureteroureterostomy. Long proximal ureteral strictures should undergo BMG ureteroplasty or appendiceal ureteroplasty. Mid-ureteral strictures can go either way in the algorithm: if the bladder is amenable, Boari flap or perhaps even just a psoas hitch ureteroneocystostomy may be reasonable, and if the bladder is not amenable, they can be treated accordingly with proximal ureteral stricture techniques. The algorithm by Zhao et al. as seen in Fig. 9 has been proposed and is a good guide to deciding how to approach this difficult urologic disease process with such a wide spectrum of severity [1].

10 Single-Port Robotic System

With the increased popularity of single-port robotic systems after the rollout of the da Vinci Single-Port (SP) platform (Intuitive Surgical Inc., Sunnyvale, CA) in 2018, urologic procedures that have been mastered with the previous iterations of the multi-port robotic consoles have now been translated over the this novel device [26]. With the proposed advantages of improved cosmesis (Fig. 10), ability to work in tighter spaces (e.g., deep in the pelvis for the bladder neck or proximal urethral reconstructions), and ease of staying extraperitoneal for certain procedures (e.g., radical prostatectomy), the SP system has been utilized across the country and is being shown to be feasible for operations that have been performed multi-port, including ureteral reconstructions [27, 28]. While there is a learning curve to the SP system and its current limitations including the lack of NIRF, smaller working space, and increased difficulty with tissue retraction, ureteral reconstruction using the SP system has been shown to be safe and effective in early case series [29], with larger studies with longer follow-up data in the works (Figs. 11 and 12).

Location

Distal

Proximal/Mid

<3 cm

Appendix present and amenable?

Reimplantation

Uretero-ureterostomy (at surgeon preference)

No appendix or not amenable

Appendiceal Onlay

+ Psoas hitch

Appendix not amenable?

Buccal Graft

+ Boari flap

Illeal Ureter[a]

Autotransplant

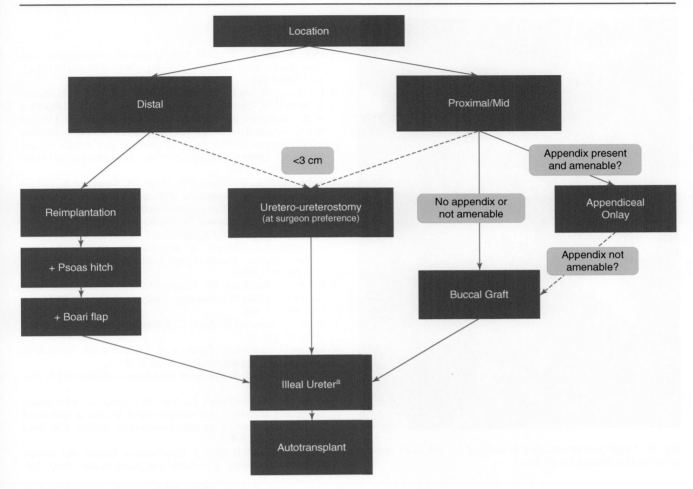

Fig. 9 Ureteral reconstruction algorithm, as proposed by [30]

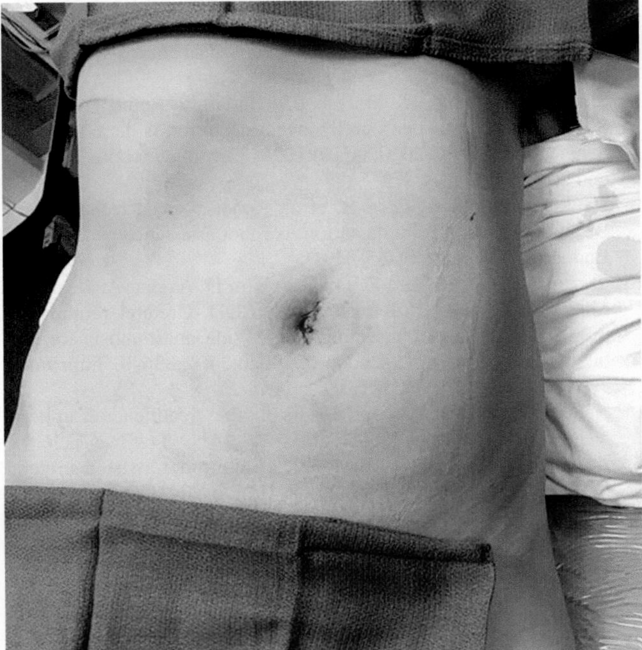

Fig. 10 Periumbilical single-port robotic incision

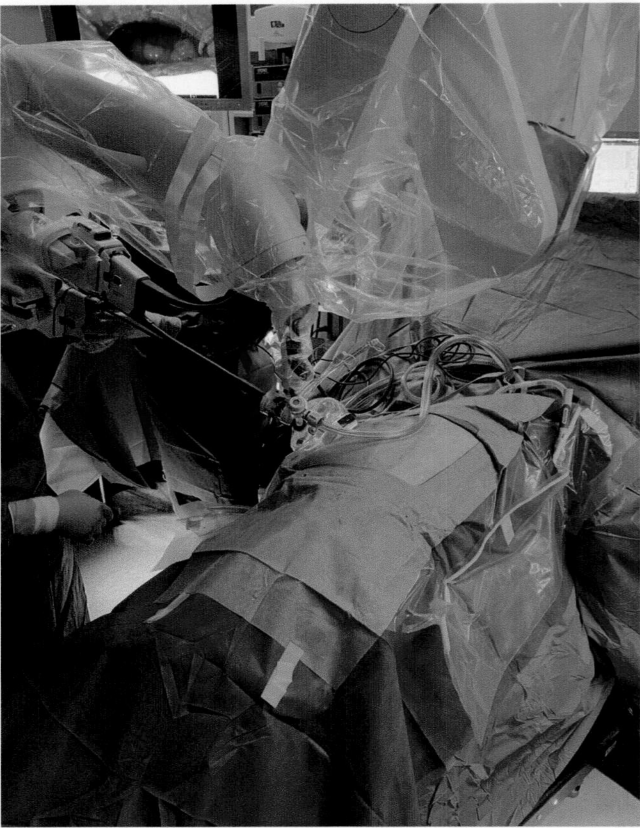

Fig. 11 Single-port robotic system docking for left-sided ureteral reconstruction, intraoperative photo

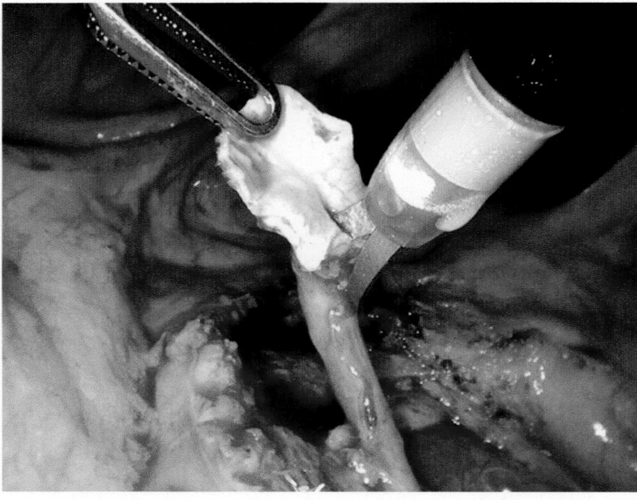

Fig. 12 Intraoperative photo of ureteral spatulation using the single-port robotic system

References

1. Drain A, Jun MS, Zhao LC. Robotic ureteral reconstruction. Urol Clin North Am. 2021;48(1):91–101. https://doi.org/10.1016/j.ucl.2020.09.001.
2. Lee Z, Lee M, Lee R, Koster H, Cheng N, Siev M, Jun M, Munver R, Ahmed M, Zhao LC, Stifelman MD, Eun DD, Collaborative of Reconstructive Robotic Ureteral Surgery (CORRUS). Ureteral rest is associated with improved outcomes in patients undergoing robotic ureteral reconstruction of proximal and middle ureteral strictures. Urology. 2021;152:160–6. https://doi.org/10.1016/j.urology.2021.01.058.
3. Khosroshahi A, Carruthers MN, Stone JH, Shinagare S, Sainani N, Hasserjian RP, Deshpande V. Rethinking Ormond's disease: "idiopathic" retroperitoneal fibrosis in the era of IgG4-related disease. Medicine (Baltimore). 2013;92:82–91.
4. Kermani TA, Crowson CS, Achenbach SJ, Luthra HS. Idiopathic retroperitoneal fibrosis: a retrospective review of clinical presentation, treatment, and outcomes. Mayo Clin Proc. 2011;86:297–303.
5. Baker LR, Mallinson WJ, Gregory MC, et al. Idiopathic retroperitoneal fibrosis. A retrospective analysis of 60 cases. Br J Urol. 1987;60:497–503.
6. Vaglio A, Salvarani C, Buzio C. Retroperitoneal fibrosis. Lancet. 2006;367:241–51.
7. Simone G, Leonardo C, Papalia R, et al. Laparoscopic ureterolysis and omental wrapping. Urology. 2008;72:853–8.
8. Kottra J, Dunnick N. Retroperitoneal fibrosis. Radiol Clin N Am. 1996;34:1259–75.
9. Drieskens O, Blockmans D, Van Den Bruel A, Mortelmans L. Riedel's thyroiditis and retroperitoneal fibrosis in multifocal fibrosclerosis: positron emission tomographic findings. Clin Nucl Med. 2002;27:413–5.
10. Drake M, Nixon P, Crew J. Drug-induced bladder and urinary disorders: incidence, prevention and management. Drug Saf. 1998;19:45–55.
11. Vaglio A, Palmisano A, Alberici F, Maggiore U, Ferretti S, Cobelli R, Ferrozzi F, Corradi D, Salvarani C, Buzio C. Prednisone versus tamoxifen in patients with idiopathic retroperitoneal fibrosis: an open-label randomized controlled trial. Lancet. 2011;378:338–46.
12. Keehn A, Mufarrij P, Stifelman M. Robotic ureterolysis for relief of ureteral obstruction from retroperitoneal fibrosis. Urology. 2010;77(6):1370–4.
13. Skupin PA, Stoffel JT, Malaeb BS, Barboglio-Romo P, Ambani SN. Robotic versus open ureteroneocystostomy: is there a robotic benefit? J Endourol. 2020;34(10):1028–32. https://doi.org/10.1089/end.2019.0715.
14. Do M, Kallidonis P, Qazi H, et al. Robot-assisted technique for Boari flap ureteral reimplantation: is robot assistance beneficial? J Endourol. 2014;28:679–85.
15. Slawin J, Patel NH, Lee Z, Dy GW, Kim D, Asghar A, Koster H, Metro M, Zhao L, Stifelman M, Eun DD. Ureteral reimplantation via robotic nontransecting side-to-side anastomosis for distal ureteral stricture. J Endourol. 2020;34(8):836–9. https://doi.org/10.1089/end.2019.0877.
16. Naude JH. Buccal mucosal grafts in the treatment of ureteric lesions. BJU Int. 1999;83:751.
17. Zhao LC, Yamaguchi Y, Bryk DJ, et al. Robot-assisted ureteral reconstruction using buccal mucosa. Urology. 2015;86:634.

18. Andrade HS, Kaouk JH, Zargar H, et al. Robotic ureteroureterostomy for treatment of a proximal ureteric stricture. Int Braz J Urol. 2016;42:1041–2.
19. Lee Z, Lee M, Koster H, Lee R, Cheng N, Jun M, Slawin J, Zhao LC, Stifelman MD, Eun DD, Collaborative of Reconstructive Robotic Ureteral Surgery (CORRUS). A multi-institutional experience with robotic ureteroplasty with buccal mucosa graft: an updated analysis of intermediate-term outcomes. Urology. 2021 Jan;147:306–10. https://doi.org/10.1016/j.urology.2020.08.003.
20. Lee Z, Waldorf BT, Cho EY, Liu JC, Metro MJ, Eun DD. Robotic ureteroplasty with buccal mucosa graft for the management of complex ureteral strictures. J Urol. 2017;198(6):1430–5. https://doi.org/10.1016/j.juro.2017.06.097.
21. Alcantara-Quispe C, Xavier JM, Atallah S, et al. Laparoscopic left ureteral substitution using the cecal appendix after en-bloc rectosigmoidectomy: a case report and video demonstration. Tech Coloproctol. 2017;21:817–8.
22. Adani GL, Pravisani R, Baccarani U, et al. Extended ureteral stricture corrected with appendiceal replacement in a kidney transplant recipient. Urology. 2015;86:840–3.
23. Melnikoff A. Sur le replacement de l'uretere par anse isolee de l'intestine grele. Rev Clin Urol. 1912;1:601.
24. Duty BD, Kreshover JE, Richstone L, Kavoussi LR. Review of appendiceal onlay flap in the management of complex ureteric strictures in six patients. BJU Int. 2015;115:282–7.
25. Jun MS, Stair S, Xu A, Lee Z, Asghar AM, Strauss D, Stifelman MD, Eun D, Zhao LC, Collaborative of Reconstructive Robotic Ureteral Surgery (CORRUS). A multi-institutional experience with robotic appendiceal ureteroplasty. Urology. 2020 Nov;145:287–91. https://doi.org/10.1016/j.urology.2020.06.062.
26. Dobbs RW, Halgrimson WR, Talamini S, Vigneswaran HT, Wilson JO, Crivellaro S. Single-port robotic surgery: the next generation of minimally invasive urology. World J Urol. 2020;38(4):897–905. https://doi.org/10.1007/s00345-019-02898-1.
27. Steinberg RL, Johnson BA, Cadeddu JA. Ureteral reconstruction using the DaVinci SP robotic platform: an initial case series. J Endourol Case Rep. 2019;5(2):60–3. https://doi.org/10.1089/cren.2018.0115.
28. Kaouk JH, Garisto J, Eltemamy M, Bertolo R. Robot-assisted surgery for benign distal ureteral strictures: step-by-step technique using the SP® surgical system. BJU Int. 2019;123:733–9. https://doi.org/10.1111/bju.14635.
29. Billah MS, Stifelman M, Munver R, Tsui J, Lovallo G, Ahmed M. Single port robotic assisted reconstructive urologic surgery-with the da Vinci SP surgical system. Transl Androl Urol. 2020;9(2):870–8. https://doi.org/10.21037/tau.2020.01.06.
30. Drain A, Jun MS, Zhao LC. Robotic Ureteral Reconstruction. Urol Clin North Am. 2021;48(1):91–101. https://doi.org/10.1016/j.ucl.2020.09.001. Epub 2020 Nov 5. PMID: 33218597.

Robot-Assisted Adrenalectomy Workup and Management

Stefano Puliatti, Pietro Piazza, Declan Murphy, and Erdem Canda

1 Introduction

While their role and identity as individual organs have been neglected until the late nineteenth century, the first surgical adrenalectomy dates back to 1860, when Thornton successfully removed a 9-kg adrenal tumor, along with the ipsilateral kidney, from a 36-year-old woman. Over the past two decades, minimally invasive treatment of adrenal glands has grown in popularity and eventually became the treatment of choice for adrenal neoplasms. Minimally invasive procedures are associated with better cosmetic outcomes, less postoperative pain, and a shorter hospital stay than traditional open procedures [1]. After the first robot-assisted adrenalectomy in 1999 by Piazza et al., several studies comparing the robotic approach with laparoscopy were published [2]. The first randomized clinical trial comparing laparoscopic and robot-assisted adrenalectomy was published in 2004 by Morino et al. and yielded controversial results, mainly due to the surgeons' lack of experience in using the robotic platform [3]. However, subsequent studies supported the safety and feasibility of the technique [4, 5]. In patients with secreting adrenal tumors, the use of robotic technology could help surgeons limit manipulation of the gland, reducing the risk of intraoperative complications. Robotic surgery has also been associated with safer treatment of larger tumors [6], other than in morbidly obese patients [7]. Because of these advantages, despite the lack of a concrete indication from urological guidelines, robotics is now used worldwide as a safe and practical minimally invasive technology for adrenal surgery.

S. Puliatti (✉)
Department of Urology, Onze Lieve Vrouw Hospital, Aalst, Belgium

ORSI Academy, Melle, Belgium

Department of Urology, University of Modena & Reggio Emilia, Modena, Italy

P. Piazza
Department of Urology, Onze Lieve Vrouw Hospital, Aalst, Belgium

ORSI Academy, Melle, Belgium

Division of Urology, IRCCS Azienda Ospedaliero-Universitaria di Bologna, Bologna, Italy

Università degli Studi di Bologna, Bologna, Italy

D. Murphy
Division of Cancer Surgery, Peter MacCallum Cancer Centre, Melbourne, VIC, Australia

Sir Peter MacCallum Division of Oncology, University of Melbourne, Parkville, VIC, Australia

E. Canda
Department of Urology, School of Medicine, Koç University, Istanbul, Turkey

2 Indications for Radical Adrenalectomy

The main indication for adrenalectomy is the treatment of primary or secondary neoplasm of the adrenal gland.

Adrenal neoplasms are discussed in the following sections [8].

2.1 Adrenal Carcinoma

Adrenal carcinoma is a rare neoplasm that affects 0.8–2 people per million annually. It is usually diagnosed in the first or fourth decade of life. It is bilateral in 2–6% of cases, and it is usually associated with an underlying genetic disease (MEN1, Li-Fraumeni syndrome, Lynch syndrome, McCune-Albright syndrome). Although several oncogenes have been identified, their role in tumor pathogenesis is still largely unknown. Adrenal carcinomas are secretory in up to 70% of cases and result in overproduction of adrenal hormones, with associated symptoms depending on the type of hormone produced. The most common secreting molecule is cortisol, causing Cushing's syndrome. In the case of non-secreting carcinoma, the most common symptoms are back pain, nausea, and vomiting.

P. Wiklund et al. (eds.), *Robotic Urologic Surgery*, https://doi.org/10.1007/978-3-031-00363-9_47

Table 1 Weiss criteria for differential diagnosis between adrenal adenoma and carcinoma

Weiss criteria
High nucleolar grade (Furman 3–4)
High mitotic rate (>5 mitosis per field)
Presence of atypical mitosis
Low percentage of clear cells
Altered architecture of tumoral cells
Presence of necrosis
Vascular structure invasion
Sinusoids invasion
Tumoral capsule invasion

On diagnostic imaging, these tumors appear as irregularly shaped masses, with intraparenchymal calcifications and areas of necrosis, and with high density level. Weiss criteria are used for the differential diagnosis between adenoma and carcinoma (Table 1) [9].

Usually, adrenal carcinomas are diagnosed at advanced stages; therefore, 5-year survival rates are low, around 20–40%, with a high recurrence rate (60–80%). Robot-assisted adrenalectomy with regional lymphadenectomy can be safely performed even in locally advanced and metastatic diseases. Although not an absolute contraindication, tumors larger than 12 cm should raise concerns about the possibility of achieving complete oncologic excision with minimally invasive approaches. Invasion of surrounding organs, involvement of vascular tissue, vena cava thrombosis, and widespread metastatic disease are relative contraindications.

2.2 Pheochromocytoma

Pheochromocytoma is a tumor arising from the chromaffin cells of the adrenal medulla. It is a rare tumor with an incidence of 2–8 cases per million inhabitants/year. It is mainly diagnosed in the third, fourth, and fifth decades of life. Historically, it was defined as the 10% tumor: 10% extra-adrenal, 10% familial, 10% bilateral, 10% pediatric, and 10% malignant. Today, this term is no longer used as it has been shown that the extra-adrenal forms account for about 25% and that it is familial in 30–40% of cases. It is often associated with multiple endocrine neoplasia type 2 (MEN 2), von Hippel-Lindau disease, and neurofibromatosis type 1. Symptoms are related to high levels of circulating catecholamines, including headache, palpitations, and sweating; anxiety, fatigue, fever, hyperglycemia, hypertension, and indolent hematuria may also be present. Typical manifestations of pheochromocytomas are the so-called crises, acute manifestations due to a sudden massive release of catecholamines into the bloodstream. These crises usually manifest with anxiety and fear of impending death, dyspnea, epigastric or chest pain, nausea and vomiting, tremor, and palpitations. Pheochromocytoma should be suspected when one or more of the following conditions are present: hyperadrenergic crises, treatment-refractory hypertension, genetic syndromes (MEN type 2, VHL disease, neurofibromatosis type 1), or a family history of pheochromocytoma. The diagnosis is confirmed by the detection of fractionated metanephrines and catecholamines in 24-h urine (positive test if Met >400 microg). Contrast-enhanced computed tomography is used to localize the tumor. The gold standard treatment for pheochromocytomas is surgical excision. To prevent a catecholaminergic "crisis" during surgery, a well-established pharmacological preparation for surgery is required, which will be discussed in the following sections. As this is a benign pathology, surgical excision is curative in most cases, but annual follow-up by urinary catecholamine assay should be performed to exclude delayed occurrence of multiple primary tumors or, in the case of a malignant neoplasm, the occurrence of metastases.

2.3 Metastases

Adrenal glands are a typical location of secondary dissemination for melanoma, lung, kidney, breast, and colon malignancies [10]. In the case of secondary localization to the adrenal glands, the aim of surgery is to enucleate the tumor while preserving as much function as possible, making minimally invasive surgery the best suitable option.

2.4 Benign Tumors

Benign adrenal tumors, which can be classified in secreting and non-secreting, are the most common indication for minimally invasive adrenalectomy [11]. The active metabolite synthesis of these tumors causes clinical manifestations. Cushing's syndrome, Conn's syndrome, and virilization are caused by tumors that produce corticosteroids, aldosterone, or sex steroids, respectively.

The vast majority of benign adrenal neoplasms are non-secreting tumors, with adenoma being the most common histologic type, accounting for 82.4% of all incidentally discovered adrenal lesions. Despite their low level of threat, they are difficult to distinguish from adrenal carcinoma on a computed tomography or MRI scan, posing a challenging differential diagnosis. Taking this into account, the need for resection is determined by the patient's functional status, clinical manifestations, and cancer risk. Tumor size is often used to determine malignancy risk, but the threshold is still controversial. According to Song et al., the risk of malignancy in tumors <4 cm is negligible. The likelihood of malignant tumors increases whit lesions larger than 5 cm, with lesions larger than 8 cm having a 95% chance of being malignant in individuals with a positive history.

Oncocytoma is a rare benign tumor. It is more common in women (2.5:1) and has the same histologic features as renal oncocytoma, but unlike the latter, in most cases, does not show a spoke-wheel appearance at CT and can reach a size of more than 20 cm. Treatment consists of surgical resection.

Myelolipoma is a rare benign neoplasm, with an estimated prevalence of 0.1% in the world population. It is formed by fatty and myelopoietic cells and is usually non-secreting. On CT scans, it appears as a well-circumscribed adrenal lesion with contextual adipose tissue; these specific features allow a fairly simple diagnosis. Treatment is conservative, limiting surgical approach to symptomatic cases.

Ganglioneuroma is a rare benign tumor that can develop in various sites of the body (e.g., retroperitoneum or mediastinum), including the adrenal gland. It is more common in young people, with rapid growth that can cause compressive symptoms. It can secrete Vasoactive Intestinal Peptide (VIP), so it is often associated with diarrhea. Diagnosis is usually histological after surgical removal.

Schwannoma, is a benign tumor arising from cells of the peripheral nervous system and may rarely present as adrenal neoplasm. It is associated with neurofibromatosis type 1 and may present as a malignant tumor in 10% of cases. The treatment of choice is surgical excision.

Adrenal cysts are found incidentally in about 0.1% of autopsies. They can be divided into epithelial cysts, endothelial cysts, and pseudocysts. Pseudocysts are malignant in 7% of cases. Treatment depends on the characteristics of the cyst; however, any therapeutical choice should be weighed with caution given the malignant potential of these neoformations.

2.5 Other Diseases

Infections [12] and persistent Adreno Cortico Tropic Hormone (ACTH)-producing masses caused by Cushing's syndrome [13] are two less common indications for surgical removal of the adrenal glands.

3 Preoperative Imaging

Diagnostic imaging in adrenal gland disease is of paramount importance. The current gold standard procedure is abdominal contrast-enhanced computed tomography (CECT), followed by magnetic resonance imaging. The use of abdominal ultrasonography is limited by the location and size of the adrenal glands.

3.1 Contrast-Enhanced Computed Tomography (CECT)

CECT is the technique of choice for the evaluation of the adrenal glands [14]. Thanks to the difference in density of the adrenal glands with the retroperitoneal fat, tomography allows clear identification of the organs.

The right adrenal gland is shaped like an inverted "Y" and is located immediately posterior to the inferior vena cava (IVC), posterior to the liver, and anterior to the kidney. The left adrenal gland, triangular in shape, is located medial and anterior to the superior pole of the ipsilateral kidney, posterior to the pancreas, and lateral to the aorta.

Density values and enhancement features after contrast administration allow characterization of the lesions and help in differential diagnosis (Table 2). CECT also plays a role in performing adrenal biopsies.

3.2 Magnetic Resonance Imaging (MRI)

MRI is considered as a second level investigation [15]. Its role is limited to the differential diagnosis of adrenal adenomas, preoperative assessment of relationships with adjacent organs, and in patients with impaired renal function.

4 Vascular Anatomy

A comprehensive knowledge of the vascular anatomy of the adrenal glands is essential when performing an adrenalectomy (Fig. 1). Each adrenal gland is irrorated by branches arising

Table 2 CECT scan characteristics of the most common adrenal tumors

	Size	Morphology	Density	Other characteristics
Adenoma	<3 cm >3 cm (usually non producing)	Round shaped	<10 UH (fatty appearance)	Hypotrophic contralateral adrenal
Pheochromocytoma	Variable	Irregular	Uneven (necrosis)	Hypervascularization (marked contrast enhancement)
Primary adrenal carcinoma	Usually quite large (>6 cm)	Irregular, with local invasion	Uneven (necrosis, calcifications, bleeding)	Uneven contrast enhancement; absence of adiposity
Metastases	Variable	Variable	>20 UH Uneven	Rapid and prolonged contrast enhancement; sometimes bilateral

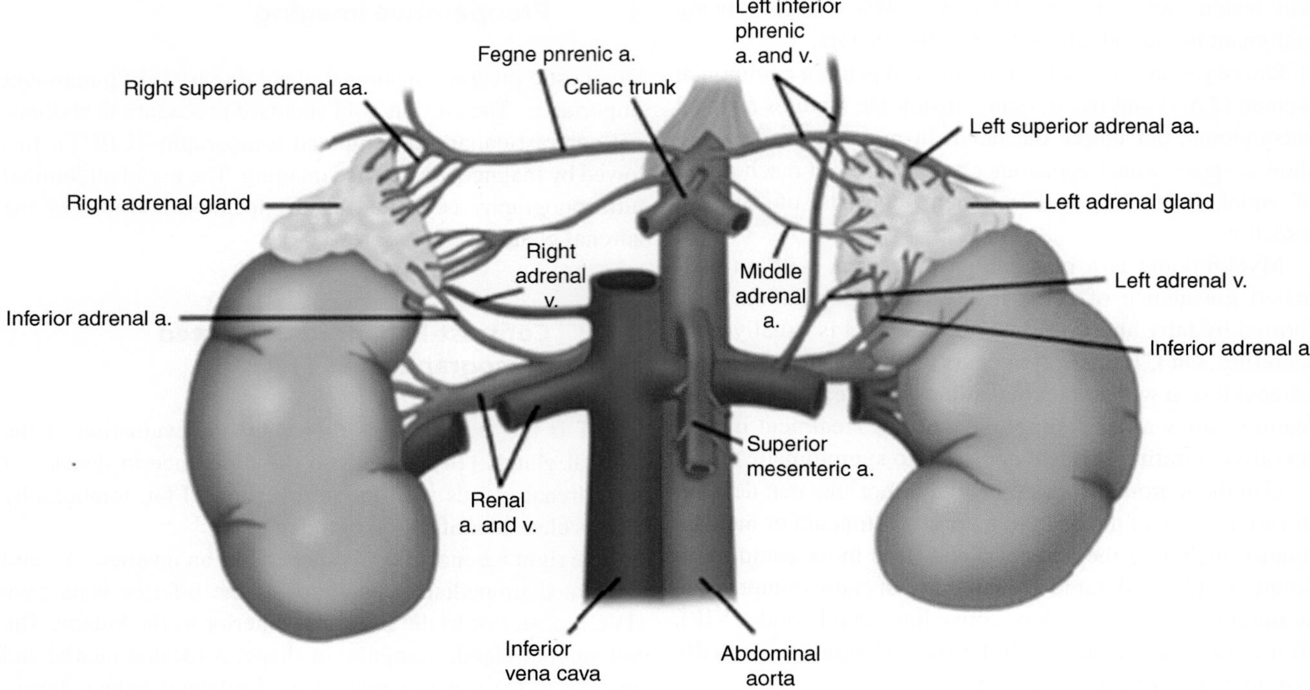

Fig. 1 Adrenal glands vascular supply

from the inferior phrenic artery, the renal artery, and the aorta. These arteries enter the gland along the superior and medial borders, making the inferolateral, posterior, and anterior surfaces of the gland typically avascular. The right adrenal vein originates on the superomedial surface of the gland, runs few millimeters along the anterior surface of the gland, and empties into the inferior vena cava (IVC). The left adrenal vein exits the gland at the inferior border and drains into the left renal vein. Compared to the insertion of the left gonadal vein, the left adrenal vein is found on the opposite side of the vein, slightly more medial. There are typically multiple collateral veins present. These veins are usually easily distinguished from the main adrenal vein because they tend to be more tortuous, have thinner walls, and are usually located below the main adrenal vein.

5 Preoperative Setting

Surgical preparation for adrenal disease is complex and may require specialized endocrinologic, anesthesiologic, and cardiology consultation depending on the metabolic characteristics of the tumor [16].

5.1 Pheochromocytoma

Excessive secretion of catecholamines can lead to tachycardia, sweating, headache, hypertension, arrhythmias, left ventricular dysfunction, and impaired glucose tolerance. Therefore, the following preoperative investigations are recommended: cardiac evaluation, electrocardiogram, echocardiography, and assessment of hypertension induced by the hormone-producing tumors. To achieve adequate hemodynamic and glucose control, administration of sympathetic therapy with drugs blocking alpha-adrenergic receptors (e.g., doxazosin and terazosin) should be started 2 weeks before surgery. During surgery, hypertensive episodes can be anticipated and controlled by intravenous use of nitroglycerin, nicardipine, phentolamine, and nitroprusside. Beta blockers with short half-life are also an appropriate choice. Limited surgical manipulation of the pheochromocytoma is also of utmost importance. In the immediate postoperative period, careful fluid administration and the use of vasopressor medications to control hypotension are required. Correction of electrolyte alterations and hypoglycemia may also be necessary.

5.2 Conn's Syndrome

Primary hyperaldosteronism associated with this syndrome can lead to electrolyte and acid-base imbalances such as hypokalemia, hypomagnesemia, and alkalosis; fluid loss or retention; refractory hypertension; cardiac dysfunction; and arrhythmia. These changes should be treated preoperatively by administration of aldosterone antagonists (e.g., spironolactone) and further monitored postoperatively. Fluids or diuretics should be administered depending on the state of volume saturation. If bilateral manipulation or excision is planned, preoperative cortisol administration may be required, which should be continued for 24 h after surgery; in addition, supplemental therapy with mineral corticoids or glucocorticoids should be administered.

5.3 Cushing's Syndrome

Hypercortisolism can lead to hypertension, diabetes, myopathy, hypokalemia, fluid retention, and cardiac dysfunction. For these reasons, adequate anesthesiologic and cardiopulmonary evaluation preoperatively is recommended. Fluid balance, blood pressure, glucose control, and electrolyte changes must then be carefully evaluated and treated. In patients with cortisol-producing masses, steroids are administered preoperatively because of the contralateral adrenal gland inhibition due to the high cortisol production of the mass.

Hormone replacement therapy is continued for several weeks after surgery to allow the contralateral adrenal gland to normalize. Myopathy and changes in bowel motility can lead to postoperative respiratory problems and "ab ingestis" pneumonia. Respiratory gymnastics should be started as soon as possible after surgery.

6 Patients' Setup

The operation is performed under general endotracheal anesthesia. Before positioning the patient, a urethral indwelling urinary catheter is inserted. The patient is positioned in the flank position with an angle of 45°–60° for a transperitoneal approach or 90° for a retroperitoneal approach. Using the kidney as anatomical landmark and placing it at the level of the table break, moderate table flexion (approximately 15°) is provided to maximize the distance between the costal margin and the iliac crest (Fig. 2). The elbows, wrists, and hands are padded, and the arms are extended in front of the patient with the aid of an upper arm support. Caution must be exercised to avoid hyperextension of the shoulder, which can lead to neuropraxia. The lower leg is flexed, the upper leg is extended, and all lower limbs' pressure points are padded. To keep the patient immobilized throughout the procedure, the patient is tethered to the table with fabric tape and Velcro straps at the level of the iliac crest and knees. All pressure areas are examined, including the head, neck, armpit, arms, hips, knees, and ankles, and more padding is applied as needed. This position is used when closing trocar wounds at the end of the procedure and to convert to an open procedure in the event of an emergency.

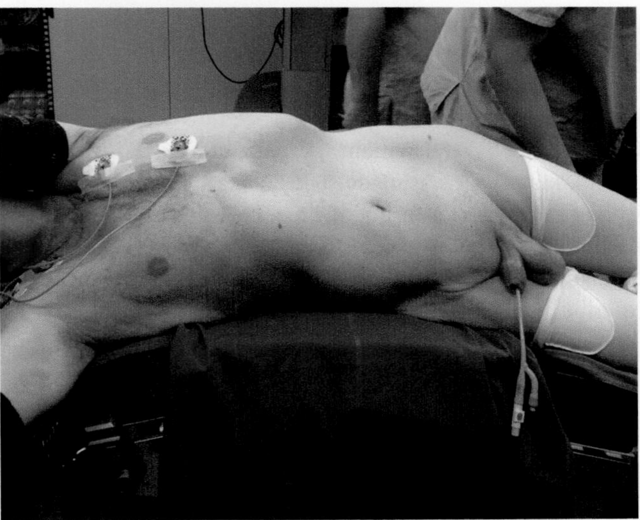

Fig. 2 Patient's positioning for robot-assisted radical adrenalectomy

7 Robot-Assisted Radical Adrenalectomy

Several techniques, such as lateral transabdominal and posterior retroperitoneal, have been described for robot-assisted radical adrenalectomy. None of them has been recognized as favorable and has been associated with significant advantages over the other. The choice for the best approach is still controversial and depends mainly on the surgeon's experience. The lateral transabdominal technique is currently the most popular. This approach is preferable by others because of the larger working space and familiarity with the anatomical structures. This approach also allows the surgeon to perform multiple abdominal surgeries simultaneously [17]. In addition, the transabdominal approach is recommended for morbidly obese patients or patients with large tumors because of its applicability and larger workspace [18]. The main advantage of the posterior approach is the convenient access to the Gerota's space. This approach should be preferred in patients who have previously undergone extensive abdominal surgery or who require bilateral adrenalectomy. However, due to the limited retroperitoneal surgical space, this method is not recommended for large tumors [19].

7.1 Transperitoneal Approach

Trocar Positioning The placement of trocars in robotic surgery depends on the robotic platform used and the surgeon's preference. This section describes the technique used by Prof. A. Mottrie for the robot "Da Vinci Xi." The first trocar to be placed is the 12 mm "Airseal" trocar, a CO2 insufflation system that allows the pressure (set at 8 mmHg according to early recovery after surgery protocols) to be kept constant during the robotic procedure and to minimize CO_2 uptake by the patient. A peri-umbilical incision of approximately 2 cm is made. The planes are digitally opened so that the posterior fascia of the rectus muscles is reached. At this level, the "Airseal" trocar is used to create a small hole in the posterior fascia of the muscles, performing a rotation movement without applying pressure. The hole is digitally enlarged, and the trocar is inserted in the abdominal cavity. The robotic endoscope is inserted, and the correct placement of the trocar in the peritoneal cavity is verified. This trocar is then used by the table assistant for suction, clip placement, and suture insertion. The four 8 mm robotic trocars are then placed 8–10 cm apart. The first trocar is placed two fingers below the costal arch along the paramedian line. The others are placed at the aforementioned distance along a line slightly oblique and lateral to the paramedian line (Fig. 3).

Surgical Steps For left adrenalectomy, the most common approach involves dissection along Toldt's line, medialization of the descending colon, and incision of the splenocolic ligament. The lienorenal ligament is then transected, and the retroperitoneal space is accessed at the level of the inferior border of the pancreas. With adequate and gentle retraction of the spleen and pancreas, the left adrenal vein is exposed. The adrenal vein is then isolated to its origin at the level of the left renal vein. Three metal clips are placed, two proximal to the renal vein and one near the origin of the vein from the adrenal gland, and then transected. The medial edge of the gland is separated from the aortic plane. With gentle traction on the kidney by the table-side assistant, the plane between the upper pole of the kidney and the adrenal gland is dissected. A small amount of fat is left on the adrenal gland to minimize direct manipulation of the gland. Small adrenal arteries are clipped or coagulated as they are identified. Dissection of the left adrenal gland from the upper renal pole is then completed, taking care not to injure superior polar renal vessels. In right adrenalectomy, after transperitoneal entry, the hepatic flexure is mobilized inferiorly, and the liver is retracted superiorly. The second part of the duodenum is then mobilized to expose the inferior vena cava. The following surgical steps resemble the left adrenalectomy.

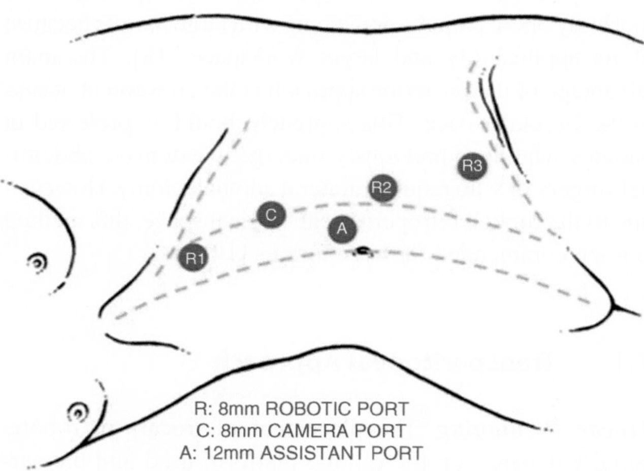

Fig. 3 Trocar positions for robot-assisted transperitoneal adrenalectomy using the Xi system

Closure Once the dissection of the adrenal gland is complete, the surgical specimen is placed in an Endobag and then removed through the 12 mm port. Pneumoperitoneum pressure is then reduced to 5 mmHg to verify adequate hemostasis. After removal of the robotic instruments, the robot is undocked, and the trocars are removed. The 12 mm port is closed according to the anatomical planes.

7.2 Retroperitoneal Approach

Trocar Positioning The 8 mm optic trocar is inserted approximately 1–2 cm inferior to the 12th rib. A finger dissection or balloon trocar may be applied in order to develop the retroperitoneal space. The CO_2 insufflation pressure should be higher than the lateral transabdominal approach at approximately 20 mmHg, in order to properly expand the space. After insufflation, two 8-mm working arms are placed to lateral and medial sides of the optic trocar at a distance of 8–10 cm, in order to avoid instrument collisions.

Surgical steps Anatomic landmarks are difficult to identify. The psoas muscle should be identified through a medial dissection, followed by the retroperitoneal major vessels. Next, the renal hilum should be identified. With a retroperitoneal approach, the artery, posterior to the vein, is identified first. The adrenal vein should be identified and isolated at the level of the inferior medial border of the adrenal gland. The adrenal vein is then closed using a three-clip technique, as described for the transperitoneal approach, and then transected. Dissection of the adrenal gland is then completed, taking care to carefully cauterize the small adrenal arteries that originate directly from the aorta.

Closure The gland is placed in an "Endobag" and then removed. A drain is usually placed. Pneumoperitoneum pressure is then reduced to 5 mmHg to verify adequate hemostasis. After removal of the robotic instruments, the robot is undocked, and the trocars are removed.

8 Postoperative Care

Patients must remain in the hospital overnight. In the recovery room, a diet is established, narcotics are avoided, and deambulation is encouraged. A complete blood count and a basic metabolic assessment are performed the day after surgery. Cushing's syndrome patients are started on high-dose steroids and oral hydrocortisone at discharge. In patients without Cushing's syndrome, oral steroids are not necessary at discharge if the blood glucose level is higher than 10 g/dL. If the patient shows evidence of adrenal insufficiency or the morning cortisol level are lower than 10 g/dL, steroids are administered, and an endocrinology consultation is scheduled. In patients with primary hyperaldosteronism, their aldosterone and renin levels are checked. In patients with pheochromocytoma, catecholamine levels are checked once a month and then once a year [20].

9 Complications

Vascular injury, intestinal injury, liver, and splenic injury are all potential complications associated with this operation. Vascular injury is reported to occur in 0.7–5.4% of cases, while transfusion rates are around 10% [21]. While large vascular injury is immediately noticed, small vessel injury may go unnoticed initially due to the pneumoperitoneum pressure. Therefore, small vascular injuries usually show up during the postoperative period, causing hematomas and, in some cases, hemodynamical instability. Bowel damage is another common complication of minimally invasive adrenalectomy, potentially leading to severe consequences if left untreated. Small bowel is the most frequently injured organ, with duodenal injury having the most serious consequences. The most common type of intestinal injury is thermal injury [22]. When working near the bowel, especially around the duodenum, cautery should be avoided. Adrenalectomy can also potentially cause liver and splenic damage. Instrument insertion or forceful retraction might cause capsular tears. Adequate adhesion lysis before the start of the procedure can help prevent these injuries. To avoid harming any viscera, all trocars and table-side assistant's instruments should be inserted under direct vision. In the following paragraphs, some common surgical and metabolic complications associated with robot-assisted adrenalectomy are reported.

9.1 Intraoperative Complications

Access Related Abdominal wall hemorrhage, cutaneous nerve injury, and endo-abdominal organ injury from Verres needle or trocars insertion.

Hemorrhagic Caused by injury to retroperitoneal large vessels, adrenal vein, lienal or hepatic vessels, and lumbar vessels or by bleeding from the resection bed following partial adrenalectomy.

Ischemic May be caused by erroneous ligation of the superior mesenteric artery or superior mesenteric vein or renal vessels.

Injury to Adjacent Organs Result from incorrect choice of dissection plan or diathermic insult. The organs affected may include the kidneys, pancreas, spleen, and liver.

Hemodynamic Instability Typically encountered in the case of pheochromocytoma.

9.2 Postoperative Complications

Patients with Primary Hyperaldosteronism May experience hypokalemia resulting from a prolonged loss of potassium or hyperkalemia if the contralateral gland does not compensate by adequate secretion of aldosterone.

Patients with Cushing's Syndrome Hypocortisolism due to inadequate replacement therapy, fractures due to osteoporosis, hyperglycemia, inadequate wound healing, and infections.

Patients with Pheochromocytoma Hemodynamic alterations.

General Complications Hemorrhage, pneumothorax, pancreatitis, and intra-abdominal collections.

10 Outcomes

Several studies have supported the safety of robotic adrenalectomy when compared with laparoscopy and open surgery [23]. Despite the existing literature has not yet shown a significant advantage of one technique over the other, robot-assisted procedures appear to have some advantages over other minimally invasive approaches [24]. The conversion rates of robot-assisted and laparoscopic adrenalectomy have been reported to be 0–5% [25] and 1–6% [7], respectively, showing a slight advantage of the robotic over the laparoscopic approach. Although conversion rate is not considered a direct indicator of safety, it may influence outcomes such as pain, hospital stay, and cosmetic effects and therefore should be considered. Other authors showed that robotic surgery was associated with a lower complication rate compared to laparoscopic surgery (3.6% vs. 6.8%) [26]. In terms of blood loss, all current studies showed a significant reduction in blood loss with robotic surgery. In addition, patients treated with robot-assisted adrenalectomy had a statistically lower hospital stay compared to the traditional open procedure [1]. All of these outcomes correlate strongly with the learning curve of robot-assisted adrenalectomy. According to current research, the learning curve cutoff for robot-assisted adrenalectomy is 20 procedures; however, these results are mainly from tertiary institutions and referrable to experienced surgeons [27]. Regarding the oncologic outcomes of these procedures, the current level of evidence is low. However, one of the largest studies, involving 289 patients, suggests that robot-assisted adrenalectomy has comparable oncologic outcomes when compared with open procedures [28]. Further studies with higher level of evidence are needed.

11 Robot-Assisted Partial Adrenalectomy

The diffusion of robotic surgery has also contributed to new interest in partial adrenalectomy, a procedure currently limited to patients with single adrenal gland or with genetic diseases associated with multiple adrenal tumors, such as VHL, neurofibromatosis, or MEN II.

Several studies have demonstrated the safety and feasibility of partial adrenalectomy [29–31]. Partial adrenalectomy may help patients preserve part of the hormone-producing function, reducing the risk of adrenal insufficiency and Addisonian crisis and the morbidity associated with long-term adrenal steroid replacement. To date, few case reports have been published on partial adrenalectomy using a robot-assisted approach [29–31]. The use of intraoperative ultrasonography has significantly changed the way partial adrenalectomy is performed. Ultrasound allows more precise delineation of tumor margins within the adrenal gland [32]. Thanks to the special vascularization of the adrenal gland, which is supplied with blood by various arteries, it is possible to selectively remove the adrenal tumor and spare the remaining parenchyma. In addition, the use of Firefly technology along with indocyanine green (ICG) helps the surgeon to properly identify both the tumor and its vascularization [33].

Patient positioning, trocar placement, and surgical setup are identical to total adrenalectomy as previously described. The same technique is used to access the adrenal gland as in total adrenalectomy. After isolation of the adrenal gland, a flexible ultrasound drop-in probe is inserted through the 12 mm assistant trocar and used to detect the tumor and define its anatomical margins. It is of utmost importance to mobilize only the portion of the adrenal gland affected by the neoplasm in order to preserve the necessary residual vascularity of the gland. After mobilization of the gland, the tumor is resected. After removal, the surgical specimen is placed in an Endobag and then extracted via the 12 mm periumbilical trocar incision. The use of frozen section histological examination is strongly recommended.

12 Conclusions

Robot-assisted approach for adrenalectomy is feasible and safe. Although adrenalectomy is a purely extirpative procedure requiring no further reconstruction, wristed instruments, increased precision, and magnified three-dimensional vision may aid in dissection of large and small vessels and more precise delineation of the tumor lesion during both radical and partial adrenalectomies. These advantages may allow more surgeons, including those with limited laparoscopic experience, to offer their patients an effective and minimally invasive approach to adrenalectomy.

References

1. Heger P, Probst P, Hüttner FJ, Gooßen K, Proctor T, Müller-Stich BP, et al. Evaluation of open and minimally invasive adrenalectomy: a systematic review and network meta-analysis. World J Surg. 2017;41:2746–57. https://doi.org/10.1007/s00268-017-4095-3.
2. Piazza L, Caragliano P, Scardilli M, Sgroi AV, Marino G, Giannone G. Laparoscopic robot-assisted right adrenalectomy and left ovariectomy (case reports). Chir Ital. 1999;51:465–6.
3. Morino M, Benincà G, Giraudo G, Del Genio GM, Rebecchi F, Garrone C. Robot-assisted vs laparoscopic adrenalectomy: a prospective randomized controlled trial. Surg Endosc. 2004;18:1742–6. https://doi.org/10.1007/s00464-004-9046-z.
4. Aliyev S, Karabulut K, Agcaoglu O, Wolf K, Mitchell J, Siperstein A, et al. Robotic versus laparoscopic adrenalectomy for pheochromocytoma. Ann Surg Oncol. 2013;20:4190–4. https://doi.org/10.1245/s10434-013-3134-z.
5. Karabulut K, Agcaoglu O, Aliyev S, Siperstein A, Berber E. Comparison of intraoperative time use and perioperative outcomes for robotic versus laparoscopic adrenalectomy. Surgery. 2012;151:537–42. https://doi.org/10.1016/j.surg.2011.09.047.
6. Brunaud L, Bresler L, Ayav A, Zarnegar R, Raphoz A-L, Levan T, et al. Robotic-assisted adrenalectomy: what advantages compared to lateral transperitoneal laparoscopic adrenalectomy? Am J Surg. 2008;195:433–8. https://doi.org/10.1016/j.amjsurg.2007.04.016.
7. Aksoy E, Taskin HE, Aliyev S, Mitchell J, Siperstein A, Berber E. Robotic versus laparoscopic adrenalectomy in obese patients. Surg Endosc. 2013;27:1233–6. https://doi.org/10.1007/s00464-012-2580-1.
8. Chow G, Blute ML. Chapter 58: Surgery of adrenal glands. In: Campbell-Walsh urology. 10th ed. Philadelphia: Saunders; 2012. p. 1737–52.
9. Weiss LM, Medeiros LJ, Vickery AL. Pathologic features of prognostic significance in adrenocortical carcinoma. Am J Surg Pathol. 1989;13:202–6. https://doi.org/10.1097/00000478-198903000-00004.

10. Sarela AI, Murphy I, Coit DG, Conlon KCP. Metastasis to the adrenal gland: the emerging role of laparoscopic surgery. Ann Surg Oncol. 2003;10:1191–6. https://doi.org/10.1245/aso.2003.04.020.
11. Young WF. Management approaches to adrenal incidentalomas. A view from Rochester, Minnesota. Endocrinol Metab Clin North Am. 2000;29(159–85):x. https://doi.org/10.1016/s0889-8529(05)70122-5.
12. Imisairi AH, Hisham AN. Adrenal tuberculosis: the atypical presentations of eggshell-like calcifications. ANZ J Surg. 2009;79:488–9. https://doi.org/10.1111/j.1445-2197.2009.04953.x.
13. Smith PW, Turza KC, Carter CO, Vance ML, Laws ER, Hanks JB. Bilateral adrenalectomy for refractory Cushing disease: a safe and definitive therapy. J Am Coll Surg. 2009;208:1059–64. https://doi.org/10.1016/j.jamcollsurg.2009.02.054.
14. Boland GWL. Adrenal imaging. Abdom Imaging. 2011;36:472–82. https://doi.org/10.1007/s00261-010-9647-z.
15. Hussain HK, Korobkin M. MR imaging of the adrenal glands. Magn Reson Imaging Clin N Am. 2004;12(515–44):vii. https://doi.org/10.1016/j.mric.2004.03.008.
16. Torricelli FCM, Coelho RF. Adrenalectomy. In: Sotelo R, Arriaga J, Aron M, editors. Complications in robotic urologic surgery. Cham: Springer; 2018. p. 135–9. https://doi.org/10.1007/978-3-319-62277-4_15.
17. Henry JF. Minimally invasive adrenal surgery. Best Pract Res Clin Endocrinol Metab. 2001;15:149–60. https://doi.org/10.1053/beem.2001.0132.
18. Taskin HE, Berber E. Robotic adrenalectomy. Cancer J Sudbury Mass. 2013;19:162–6. https://doi.org/10.1097/PPO.0b013e31828ba0c7.
19. Mercan S, Seven R, Ozarmagan S, Tezelman S. Endoscopic retroperitoneal adrenalectomy. Surgery. 1995;118:1071–5. https://doi.org/10.1016/s0039-6060(05)80116-3.
20. Kahramangil B, Berber E. Robotic adrenalectomy. In: Tsuda S, Kudsi OY, editors. Robotic assisted minimally invasive surgery. Cham: Springer; 2019. p. 109–15. https://doi.org/10.1007/978-3-319-96866-7_13.
21. Permpongkosol S, Link RE, Su L-M, Romero FR, Bagga HS, Pavlovich CP, et al. Complications of 2,775 urological laparoscopic procedures: 1993 to 2005. J Urol. 2007;177:580–5. https://doi.org/10.1016/j.juro.2006.09.031.
22. Bishoff JT, Allaf ME, Kirkels W, Moore RG, Kavoussi LR, Schroder F. Laparoscopic bowel injury: incidence and clinical presentation. J Urol. 1999;161:887–90. https://doi.org/10.1016/s0022-5347(01)61797-x.
23. Brunaud L, Bresler L, Ayav A, Tretou S, Cormier L, Klein M, et al. Advantages of using robotic Da Vinci system for unilateral adrenalectomy: early results. Ann Chir. 2003;128:530–5. https://doi.org/10.1016/s0003-3944(03)00220-7.
24. Brandao LF, Autorino R, Zargar H, Krishnan J, Laydner H, Akca O, et al. Robot-assisted laparoscopic adrenalectomy: step-by-step technique and comparative outcomes. Eur Urol. 2014;66:898–905. https://doi.org/10.1016/j.eururo.2014.04.003.
25. Dickson PV, Alex GC, Grubbs EG, Jimenez C, Lee JE, Perrier ND. Robotic-assisted retroperitoneoscopic adrenalectomy: making a good procedure even better. Am Surg. 2013;79:84–9.
26. Brandao LF, Autorino R, Laydner H, Haber G-P, Ouzaid I, De Sio M, et al. Robotic versus laparoscopic adrenalectomy: a systematic review and meta-analysis. Eur Urol. 2014;65:1154–61. https://doi.org/10.1016/j.eururo.2013.09.021.
27. Rosoff JS, Otto BJ, Del Pizzo JJ. The emerging role of robotics in adrenal surgery. Curr Urol Rep. 2010;11:38–43. https://doi.org/10.1007/s11934-009-0079-7.
28. Mishra K, Maurice MJ, Bukavina L, Abouassaly R. Comparative efficacy of laparoscopic versus robotic adrenalectomy for adrenal malignancy. Urology. 2019;123:146–50. https://doi.org/10.1016/j.urology.2018.08.037.
29. Asher KP, Gupta GN, Boris RS, Pinto PA, Linehan WM, Bratslavsky G. Robot-assisted laparoscopic partial adrenalectomy for pheochromocytoma: the National Cancer Institute technique. Eur Urol. 2011;60:118–24. https://doi.org/10.1016/j.eururo.2011.03.046.
30. Boris RS, Gupta G, Linehan WM, Pinto PA, Bratslavsky G. Robot-assisted laparoscopic partial adrenalectomy: initial experience. Urology. 2011;77:775–80. https://doi.org/10.1016/j.urology.2010.07.501.
31. Gupta NP, Nayyar R, Singh P, Anand A. Robot-assisted adrenal-sparing surgery for pheochromocytoma: initial experience. J Endourol. 2010;24:981–5. https://doi.org/10.1089/end.2009.0351.
32. Barod R, Rogers CG. Robot-assisted total and partial adrenalectomy. In: Su L-M, editor. Atlas of robotic urologic surgery. Cham: Springer; 2017. p. 63–75. https://doi.org/10.1007/978-3-319-45060-5_5.
33. Dip FD, Roy M, Perrins S, Ganga RR, Lo Menzo E, Szomstein S, et al. Technical description and feasibility of laparoscopic adrenal contouring using fluorescence imaging. Surg Endosc. 2015;29:569–74. https://doi.org/10.1007/s00464-014-3699-z.

Single-Port Approach to Kidney Surgery

Alireza Aminsharif, Mahmoud Abou Zeinab, and Jihad Kaouk

1 Introduction

Since 2018, with the adoption of the single-port robotic surgery platform at many institutes, single-site surgery has evolved. Potential benefits of single-port robotic surgery have been shown in recent radical prostatectomy series. Early evidence showed that single-port robotic radical prostatectomy can be associated with less postoperative morbidity, shorter hospital stay, and a quicker recovery compared to conventional approaches [1–4].

Similarly, the specific characteristics of a dedicated system for single-port robotic surgery such as a non-bulky platform, double-arm flexible instruments, and the camera would make it an ideal system for single-site robotic surgery for upper urinary tract pathologies. In this chapter, we describe the potential application of single-port robotic surgery for partial nephrectomy and pyeloplasty as common upper tract surgical procedures. Technical details of single-port retroperitoneal robotic partial nephrectomy and single-port robotic pyeloplasty through Pfannenstiel's abdominal incision will be discussed. As emerging techniques in this field, both approaches can potentially offer a less morbid surgical procedure with a short hospital stay and a rapid convalescence period.

2 Single-Port Retroperitoneal Robotic Partial Nephrectomy

With the da Vinci SP® system, a single robotic arm is docked to a 25 mm multichannel port, and a 12 × 10 mm articulating camera and three 6 mm articulating instruments can be passed through one entry access point. All instruments and the camera have a double articulating design to provide intracorporeal triangulation. Moreover, the system has an extra clutch by which the surgeon can move the camera and working arms as one unit during surgery. With these characteristics, this novel system can be applied for extraperitoneal robotic partial nephrectomy via a single flank incision.

Although several groups attempted to integrate conventional robotic platforms for single-site surgery, several technical issues such as limited working space or external clashing of robotic arms limited the widespread application of single-site robotic surgery using conventional platforms [5, 6].

Maurice et al. were the first who described the feasibility of robotic-assisted single-site surgery for retroperitoneal partial and radical nephrectomy in a cadaveric model [7]. Later on, the clinical application of the SP® platform for partial nephrectomy was reported by Kaouk et al. in three patients [8]. A transperitoneal approach was used in this initial experience with single-port robotic partial nephrectomy. All three procedures were completed as planned without any conversion to multiport robotic or open surgery with a mean operative time of 186 min and warm ischemia time of 25 min. One patient required angioembolization for management of active postoperative bleeding.

Recently, Na et al. compared the performance of a conventional Xi® system versus a dedicated SP® system for doing single-site robotic partial nephrectomy [9]. Docking time was significantly shorter with the SP® platform. Limitation of working space and intracorporeal docking clashing were more evident with the use of the Xi® system, which led to conversion to the conventional multiport robotic procedure in one case. Moreover, with the use of the Xi® system for single-site surgery, the authors had to add an assistant abdominal port away from the site of robot docking; however, with the SP® system, all procedures were completed without any additional abdominal ports [9]. Notably, when the Xi® system is used for single-site surgery, dissection of upper pole tumors was challenging, while with the SP® system, tumor dissection in various locations would

A. Aminsharif
Department of Urology, Pennsylvania State University, Hershey Medical Center, Hershey, PA, USA

M. Abou Zeinab · J. Kaouk (✉)
Glickman Urological & Kidney Institute, Cleveland Clinic Foundation, Cleveland, OH, USA

P. Wiklund et al. (eds.), *Robotic Urologic Surgery*, https://doi.org/10.1007/978-3-031-00363-9_48

be easier [7–9]. In general, the bulky configuration of the multiport system can restrict the movement of arms because of extracorporeal clashing.

Fang et al. reported a series of single-port robotic partial nephrectomy ($n = 13$) with transperitoneal ($n = 6$) and retroperitoneal ($n = 7$) approaches [10]. They placed a separate 5–12 mm AirSeal® (ConMed Corp, Utica, NY, USA) port to facilitate the procedure. All procedures were accomplished with zero ischemia (off-clamp enucleation). The mean tumor size was 3.4 cm, and they were able to approach exophytic or endophytic tumors in various locations (i.e., upper, interpolate, or lower pole) with this platform. The mean operative time was 176 min in this series. The authors reported a case of conversion from single-port retroperitoneal partial nephrectomy to open radical nephrectomy due to significant adhesion in the surgical field caused by previous transperitoneal laparoscopic partial nephrectomy. They had also difficulties in progression and localization of the recurred mass [10].

Similar outcomes were reported by Shukla et al. on a series of 12 patients who underwent single-port robotic partial nephrectomy with a transperitoneal approach (mean tumor size = 3.1 cm). They used an additional 12 mm assistant port, about 7 cm away from the SP® cannula. All procedures were successful with an average operative time of 172 min and warm ischemia time of 25 min. No conversion was reported [11].

3 Single-Port Retroperitoneal Robotic Partial Nephrectomy: Surgical Technique

With this procedure, partial nephrectomy can be accomplished through a small 25 mm incision without any additional ports. The retroperitoneal approach can potentially be associated with a shorter hospital stay and a quicker recovery due to a lower incidence of postoperative ileus [12, 13].

4 Patient Selection

At least in initial experience, the authors recommend excluding patients with complex renal hilum anatomy, previous history on ipsilateral kidney [10], or morbid obesity. Tumors larger than 4 cm (T1a disease) [11], those with high complexity scores, or with high-risk features may not be good candidates in the initial experience.

The procedure is done under general anesthesia, and the patient is placed in a lateral flank position (Fig. 1a). Prophylactic single-dose intravenous antibiotics and subcutaneous heparin can be administered.

5 Access

The docking point should be about an inch above the anterior superior iliac spine over the anterior axillary line. The access point should be ideally ≥10 cm away from the renal hilum [11]. A 2–3 cm incision is made, and with blunt and sharp dissections, the retroperitoneal space will be entered (Fig. 1b). After blunt dissection of the perinephric fat, the psoas sheath will be palpable. The Spacemaker™ (Covidien, Dublin, Ireland) surgical balloon dissection system is placed into the retroperitoneal space over the psoas muscle and guided toward the lower pole of the kidney. Adequate working space can be developed in the retroperitoneum by inflating the balloon with 400 cc of air (Fig. 1c).

6 Port Placement

The GelPOINT Mini System (Applied Medical, Rancho, Santa Margarita, CA) is used for port placement. The wound retractor/protector component (Alexis®) is fixed to the wound by securing its inner ring under the transversalis fascia (Fig. 1d). After insertion of the 25 mm, SP® cannula with a multichannel guide port as well as a 12 mm AirSeal® port into the GelSeal cap, the GelSeal cap is attached to the Alexis® (Fig. 1e). Then the SP® robot is docked to the cannula and insufflation is established (Fig. 1f).

7 Floating Technique (Air Docking)

To increase the working space for robotic instruments, the Alexis® wound retractor must be left unrolled. Therefore, the SP® cannula remains away from the patient's body and maximal working space will be provided for robotic instruments [14].

8 Partial Nephrectomy

After docking, retroperitoneal partial nephrectomy can be followed step by step in standard technique [6–8]. With the retroperitoneal approach, the ureter and renal hilum can be easily seen and dissected by lateral and upward retraction of the lower pole. The renal artery can be approached behind the renal vein. After sharp dissection of the Gerota's fascia, the perinephric fat can be dissected from the kidney to identify the renal mass. Intraoperative ultrasound can be passed through the assistant port and used to identify and circumscribe the margin of resection. The assistant can also pass the laparoscopic bulldog clamp as well as Vicryl sutures through the assistant port.

After clamping of the renal artery, the tumor can be resected by cold scissors. Renorrhaphy will then be started

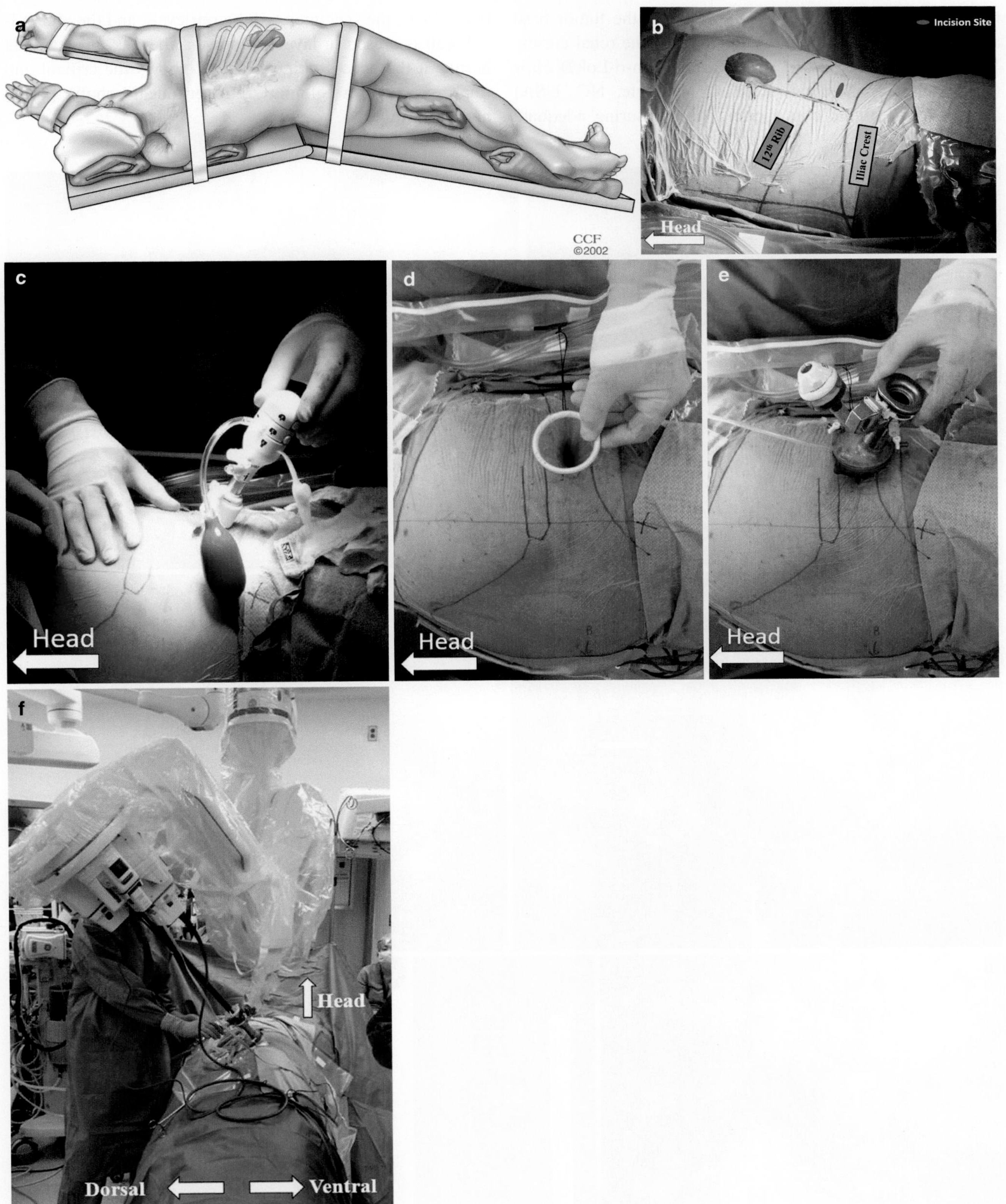

Fig. 1 (**a**) Patient positioned in a flank position. (**b**) The 2–3 cm incision made between the 12th rib and iliac crest. (**c**) Development of retroperitoneal space. (**d**) Placement of Alexis® wound retractor. (**e**) Placement of the GelPOINT Mini System, SP multichannel cannula, and an assistant port. (**f**) SP robot docking and instrument insertion

by running deep Vicryl sutures to oversew the tumor base and superficial interrupted sutures to close the renal cortex. Sutures can be buttressed with 5 mm Hem-o-Lok® clips (Weck, Teleflex Medical, Research Triangle, NC, USA) applied by a robotic clip applier. After ensuring adequate hemostasis, the specimen will be retrieved, and the abdominal wall is closed in layers to prevent the risk of incisional hernia at the access point. Figure 2 shows the critical and final aspects of single-port retroperitoneal robotic partial nephrectomy.

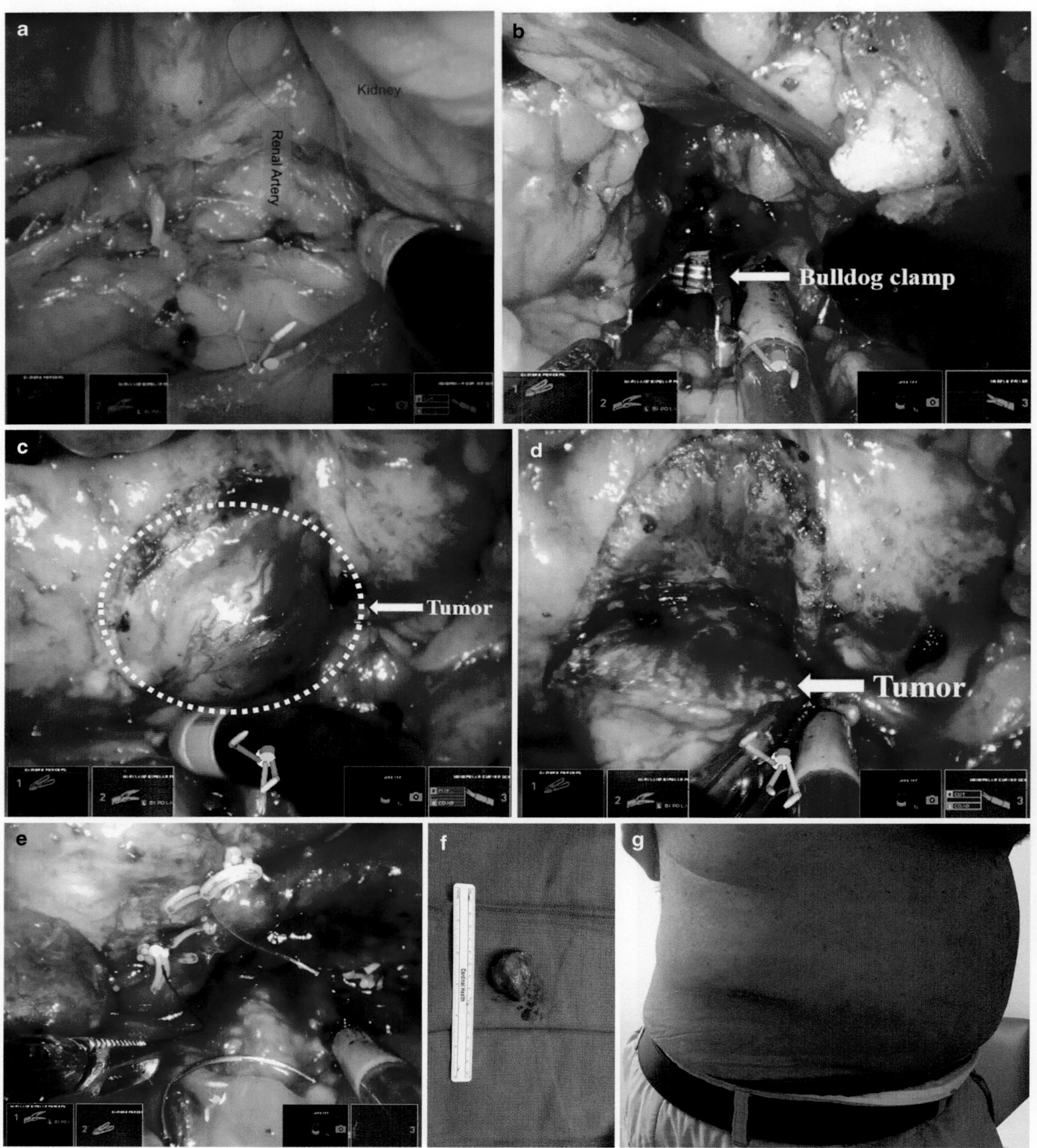

Fig. 2 (**a**) Identification of the renal artery. (**b**) Clamping the renal artery using a bulldog clamp. (**c**) Identification of the tumor. (**d**) Excision of the tumor. (**e**) Renorrhaphy of the tumor base. (**f**) Renal tumor specimen after excision. (**g**) Scar of the incision 6 weeks post-surgery

9 Technical Remarks

With the single-port robotic platform, retroperitoneal partial nephrectomy is feasible without the need for any abdominal port. However, especially in early experience, the addition of an assistant port at the level of umbilicus can be helpful [11]. The multi-quadrant feature of the SP® robotic system and its non-bulky configuration is helpful to approach both anteriorly and posteriorly located tumors via the retroperitoneal access point. The relocation pedal repositions the camera and all instruments as one unit and is very helpful to adjust the position of working instruments with tumor location. Mastery of new SP® camera control ("Cobra" mode) is beneficial to improve visualization during dissection of tumor and suturing of the tumor bed. In general, single-port robotic instruments tend to have weaker grasping strength than their conventional robotic counterparts. Therefore, a standard robotic bulldog clamp cannot be loaded, opened, and applied using one single-port robotic instrument. Usually, two robotic arms should be used to apply or remove the bulldog clamp [15].

10 Single-Port Robotic Pyeloplasty Through a Pfannenstiel Abdominal Incision

After presenting the initial series of robotic pyeloplasty in 2002 [16], there has been an interest in the use of conventional multiport robotic systems for single-site surgery [17, 18]. Despite this initial interest, single-site surgery with multi-arm robotic systems was not widely adopted due to potential difficulties and clashing during suturing. After the initial utilization of the dedicated SP® robot for extirpation surgery, its application was rapidly expanded to reconstructive procedures [19, 20].

Potential benefits of pure single-site pyeloplasty include a shorter hospital stay and a faster recovery [21], reduced postoperative pain, and improved cosmetic results [21, 22]. Recently, we reported our experience with single-port robotic pyeloplasty via a periumbilical or Pfannenstiel abdominal incision [22]. Although access through a periumbilical incision is standard practice [19], we showed that to further improved the cosmetic results and reduce postoperative pain, a mini-Pfannenstiel incision can be used as a potential access point for single-point robotic pyeloplasty [22]. Previously, the advantages of Pfannenstiel incision compared to abdominal incisions in reducing postoperative pain and morbidity have been shown in laparoscopic nephrectomy series [23]. The dedicated characteristics of the SP® robotic platform such as its multi-quadrant feature and its non-bulky configuration would be very helpful for conducting an upper tract surgery through a Pfannenstiel incision especially in the pediatric population.

11 Surgical Technique

It is recommended that the surgical team completes a formal training course before doing pyeloplasty with SP® robotic platform. The SP® platform has double articulating instruments with an intracorporeal triangulation feature. The arm movements with SP® instruments are slightly different from conventional robotic arms. Due to the added elbow joint to the instruments, the wrist function of the instrument is modified, and therefore, suturing and knot tying need practice for skill development [20]. Moreover, the use of single-port robotic surgery should be cautious in patients with previous abdominal surgery especially early in the surgeon's learning curve.

12 Positioning, Pfannenstiel Incision, Access, and Port Placement

The patient is positioned in a lateral flank position with a 20–30° tilt away from the robot (Fig. 3a). The patient is widely prepared and draped from symphysis pubis to the subcostal area. Through a small 2.5 cm transverse incision over the ipsilateral pubic tubercle (Pfannenstiel incision), the rectus fascia is exposed and sharply incised. The rectus muscles are retracted, and the peritoneal cavity will be entered by incising the peritoneum. The inner ring of the Alexis® device (Applied Medical, Rancho, Santa Margarita, CA) is then placed in the peritoneal cavity and is secured under the rectus fascia.

Then the GelSeal cap into which the 25 mm SP® cannula and an assistant port (a 12 mm AirSeal® port) have been placed will be attached to the Alexis® (Fig. 3b). The SP® robot is docked to the cannula, insufflation is established, and the SP® cannula remains away from the patient's body with a floating technique [14].

13 Exposing the Renal Pelvis and Ureteropelvic Junction (UPJ)

Using the relocation pedal, all robotic instruments can be directed toward the kidney. After incising the white line, the colon is reflected radially. On the right side, the duodenum can also be carefully dockerized. The proximal ureter can usually be easily identified, and dissection is carried in the cephalad direction to the UPJ. Crossing vessels can be identified during dissection of UPJ and should be preserved to save maximum renal perfusion. In the case of any bleeding around the UPJ, the use of bipolar energy would be preferred for meticulous hemostasis and minimal collateral damage.

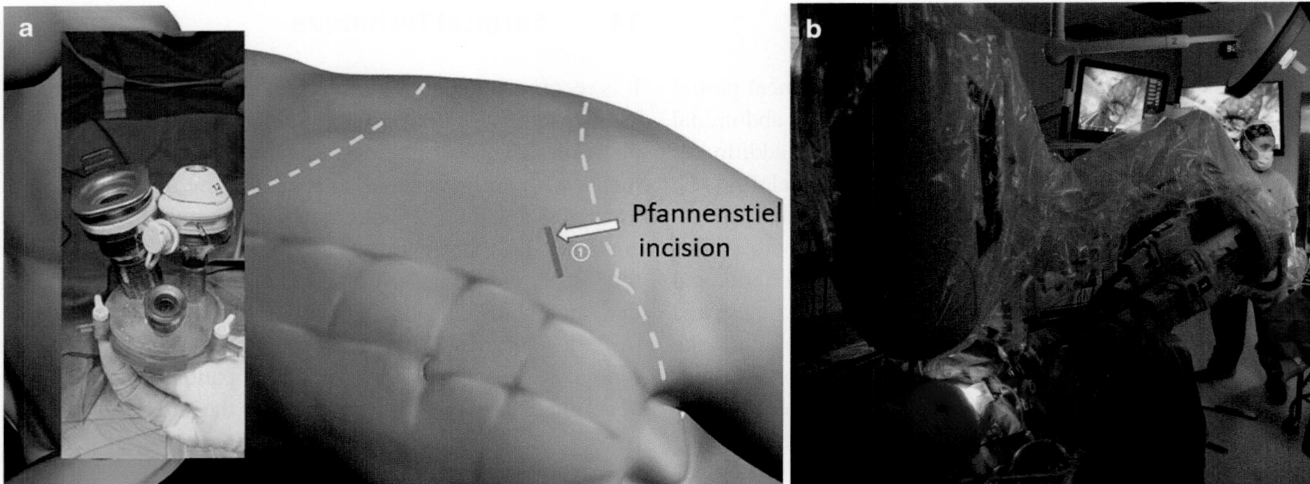

Fig. 3 (**a**) Pfannenstiel skin incision and port orientation. (**b**) SP robot docking using the floating dock technique

14 Dismembered Pyeloplasty

After adequate mobilization of the proximal ureter, UPJ, and renal pelvis, the UPJ is dismembered, and the stenotic segment is excised. The proximal ureter is then spatulated 2 cm laterally, and the ureter is anastomosed to the most dependent part of the renal pelvis with a 4–0 Polyglactin suture. The posterior edge of the ureteropelvic anastomosis is completed with the same suture material in a running fashion. The flexible 3D HD camera and its "Cobra" configuration provide enhanced visualization during suturing. Then a double J can be passed over a guidewire anterogradely. The stent and sutures can be easily advanced through the assistant port. After placement of the double J, the anterior aspect of anastomosis is completed with another 4–0 Polyglactin suture. The renal pelvis is closed at the end of the procedure. External drainage is not typically required; however, a JP drain can be placed through a separate small incision in lower quadrants.

After completion of the procedure, the robot is undocked and the access point should be closed in layers to prevent any incisional hernia. The double J stent will be removed in 4–6 weeks. Figure 4 shows the critical and final aspects of the robotic pyeloplasty through a Pfannenstiel abdominal incision.

15 Conclusion

Single-port robotic surgery is feasible and is being rapidly adopted in the urology community for upper tract urological procedures. The multi-quadrant feature of this platform is very helpful to perform partial nephrectomy through single-site retroperitoneal access, irrespective of the tumor location. The same concept is true to approach the UPJ for pyeloplasty through a Pfannenstiel abdominal incision. Potential limitations with these techniques include limited data and evidence with regard to long-term post-procedural outcomes. The learning curve with single-port robotic surgery and the surgeon-bedside assistant coordination may be challenging during the early phase of implementation of these new systems and procedures.

Several studies on various urological procedures have shown the potential for same-day discharge (i.e., short hospital stay) with the use of single-port robotic surgery. Comparative trials with conventional robotic platforms and cost-analysis studies will be very interesting to determine the cost-effectiveness of these new approaches.

Disclosures Dr. Jihad Kaouk has a consultant agreement with *Intuitive Surgical*.

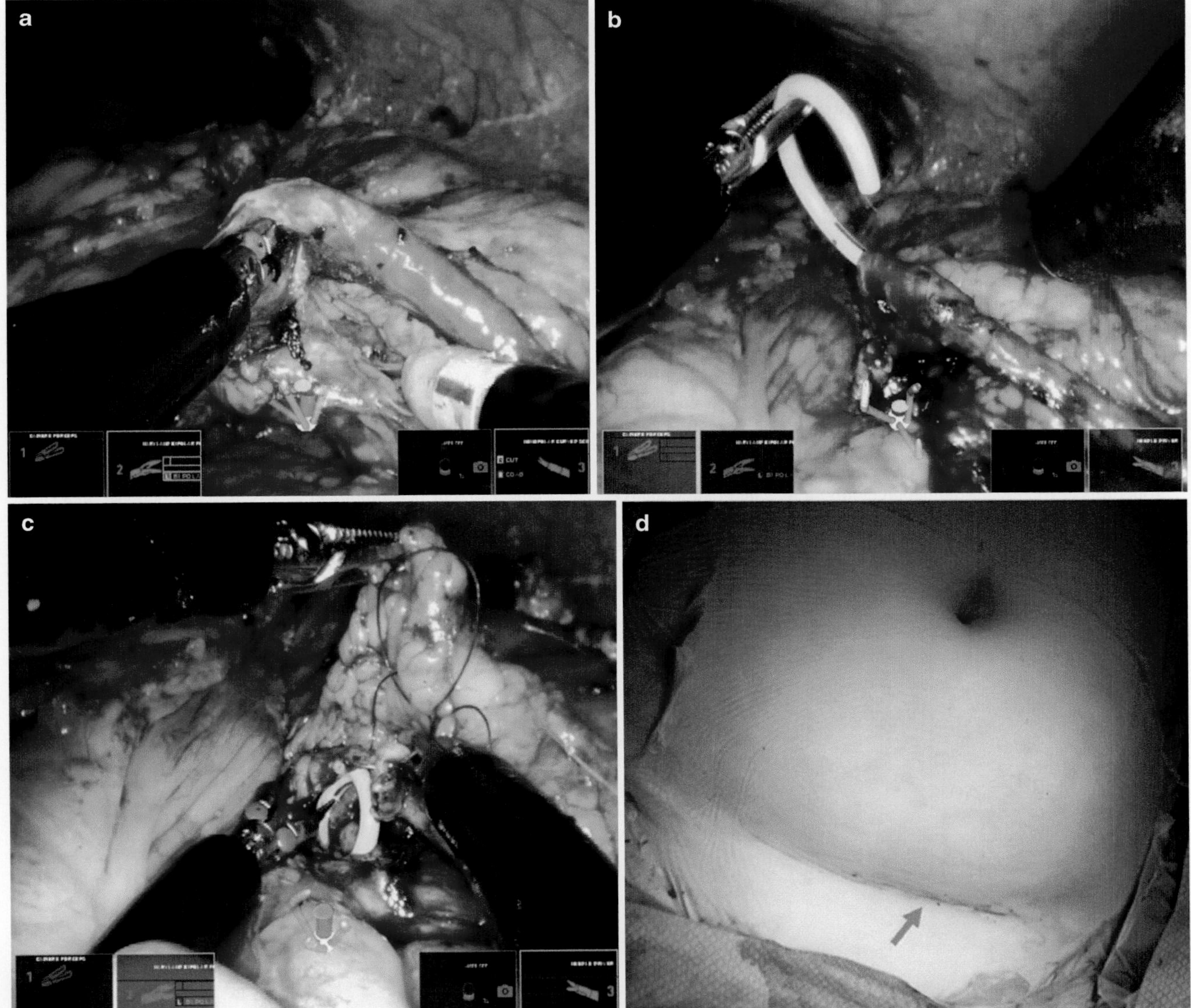

Fig. 4 (**a**) Identification of the proximal ureter. (**b**) Insertion of JJ stent into the ureter. (**c**) Ureteropelvic anastomosis. (**d**) Final incision

References

1. Sathianathen NJ, Lamb AD, Lawrentschuk NL, et al. Changing face of robot-assisted radical prostatectomy in Melbourne over 12 years. ANZ J Surg. 2018;88(3):E200–3.
2. Walsh AL, Dasgupta P. A comparative analysis of single port versus multi-port robotic assisted radical prostatectomy for prostate cancer. Investig Clin Urol. 2020;61(4):335–7.
3. Wilson CA, Aminsharifi A, Sawczyn G, et al. Outpatient Extraperitoneal single-port robotic radical prostatectomy. Urology. 2020;144:142–6.
4. Kaouk J, Aminsharifi A, Wilson CA, et al. Extraperitoneal versus transperitoneal single port robotic radical prostatectomy: a comparative analysis of perioperative outcomes. J Urol. 2020;203(6):1135–40.
5. Nelson RJ, Chavali JSS, Yerram N, Babbar P, Kaouk JH. Current status of robotic single-port surgery. Urol Ann. 2017;9(3):217–22.
6. Bertolo R, Garisto J, Gettman M, Kaouk J. Novel system for robotic single-port surgery: feasibility and state of the art in urology. Eur Urol Focus. 2018;4(5):669–73.
7. Maurice MJ, Ramirez D, Kaouk JH. Robotic laparoendoscopic single-site retroperitoneal renal surgery: initial investi-

gation of a purpose-built single-port surgical system. Eur Urol. 2017;71(4):643–7.

8. Kaouk J, Garisto J, Eltemamy M, Bertolo R. Pure single-site robot-assisted partial nephrectomy using the SP surgical system: initial clinical experience. Urology. 2019;124:282–5.
9. Na JC, Lee HH, Yoon YE, Jang WS, Choi YD, Rha KH, Han WK. True single-site partial nephrectomy using the SP surgical system: feasibility, comparison with the Xi single-site platform, and step-by-step procedure guide. J Endourol. 2020;34(2):169–74.
10. Fang AM, Saidian A, Magi-Galluzzi C, Nix JW, Rais-Bahrami S. Single-port robotic partial and radical nephrectomies for renal cortical tumors: initial clinical experience. J Robot Surg. 2020;14(5):773–80.
11. Shukla D, Small A, Mehrazin R, Palese M. Single-port robotic-assisted partial nephrectomy: initial clinical experience and lessons learned for successful outcomes. J Robot Surg. 2021;15(2):293–8.
12. Xia L, Zhang X, Wang X, Xu T, Qin L, Zhang X, Zhong S, Shen Z. Transperitoneal versus retroperitoneal robot-assisted partial nephrectomy: a systematic review and meta-analysis. Int J Surg. 2016;30:109–15.
13. Mittakanti HR, Heulitt G, Li HF, Porter JR. Transperitoneal vs. retroperitoneal robotic partial nephrectomy: a matched-paired analysis. World J Urol. 2020;38(5):1093–9.
14. Lenfant L, Kim S, Aminsharifi A, Sawczyn G, Kaouk J. Floating docking technique: a simple modification to improve the working space of the instruments during single-port robotic surgery. World J Urol. 2021;39(4):1299–305.
15. Shumaker L, Rais-Bahrami S, Nix J. Renal hilar clamping with a standard robotic bulldog clamp using the single port da Vinci robot. Urology. 2020;145:297.
16. Gettman MT, Neururer R, Bartsch G, Peschel R. Anderson-Hynes dismembered pyeloplasty performed using the da Vinci robotic system. Urology. 2002;60(3):509–13.
17. Desai MM, Rao PP, Aron M, Pascal-Haber G, Desai MR, Mishra S, Kaouk JH, Gill IS. Scarless single-port transumbilical nephrectomy and pyeloplasty: first clinical report. BJU Int. 2008;101(1):83–8.
18. Kaouk JH, Goel RK, Haber GP, Crouzet S, Stein RJ. Robotic single-port transumbilical surgery in humans: initial report. BJU Int. 2009;103(3):366–9.
19. Billah MS, Stifelman M, Munver R, Tsui J, Lovallo G, Ahmed M. Single port robotic assisted reconstructive urologic surgery-with the da Vinci SP surgical system. Transl Androl Urol. 2020;9(2):870–8.
20. Steinberg RL, Johnson BA, Cadeddu JA. Ureteral reconstruction using the da Vinci SP robotic platform: an initial case series. J Endourol Case Rep. 2019;5(2):60–3.
21. Abaza R, Murphy C, Bsatee A, Brown DH Jr, Martinez O. Single-port robotic surgery allows same-day discharge in majority of cases. Urology. 2021;148:159–65.
22. Lenfant L, Wilson CA, Sawczyn G, Aminsharifi A, Kim S, Kaouk J. Single-port robot-assisted dismembered pyeloplasty with mini-Pfannenstiel or peri-umbilical access: initial experience in a single center. Urology. 2020;143:147–52.
23. Binsaleh S, Madbouly K, Matsumoto ED, Kapoor A. A prospective randomized study of Pfannenstiel versus expanded port site incision for intact specimen extraction in laparoscopic radical nephrectomy. J Endourol. 2015;29(8):913–8.

Robotic Single-Port Kidney Surgery: The Chicago Approach

Susan Talamini and Simone Crivellaro

The single-port da Vinci robotic system (SP) offers a unique approach to the treatment of renal masses. Specifically, those tumors located posteriorly and laterally which can be addressed via the retroperitoneal approach are uniquely suited for the single-port robot. The small footprint of the robot makes working within the narrow confines of the retroperitoneum more ergonomic.

1 Introduction

Given the widespread availability of cross-sectional imaging, renal tumors are increasingly diagnosed well before becoming symptomatic [1]. Often, these tumors are diagnosed incidentally and at an earlier stage of the disease [2]. As compared to radical nephrectomy, the benefit of nephron-sparing surgery in order to preserve renal function and reduce the progression of chronic kidney disease (CKD) when feasible for small renal masses has been demonstrated throughout the literature [3–5]. Thus, for the appropriately selected patient, those with cT1a lesions, solitary kidney, bilateral disease, or familial disorders, nephron-sparing surgery has become standard of care [5].

Historically, partial nephrectomy has been managed via open, laparoscopic, and robotic approaches. Considerations such as depth of invasion, size of the mass, and location of the mass (nearness to hilum, anterior or posterior location) have been used to gauge the complexity of the case and select the most appropriate approach [6]. In recent years, the robotic approach has been preferred over laparoscopic and open approaches for the properly selected mass due to decreased clamp times, better visualization, decreased transfusion rates, and a shorter learning curve as compared to laparoscopy [7–11].

The robot-assisted partial nephrectomy (RAPN) has traditionally included transperitoneal (TP-RAPN) and retroperitoneal (RP-RAPN) approaches. Initially performed laparoscopically first by Gill and colleagues in 1994, the retroperitoneal partial nephrectomy is a unique anatomical approach with surgical benefits to the well-selected mass [12]. Lesions located posteriorly or laterally often require a significant amount of mobilization when approaching transperitoneal. In order to reach some posterior lesions, the kidney may need complete medial mobilization and may still pose surgical challenges. The retroperitoneal approach makes these lesions more easily accessible with minimal mobilization. Additionally, avoiding entrance into the peritoneum reduces bowel manipulation, decreasing incidence of ileus and risk of bowel injury, and leads to shorter hospital stays [13, 14]. In patients with a history of previous abdominal surgery, the retroperitoneal approach avoids potential adhesions and scarring. The retroperitoneal approach using the da Vinci multiport (MP-RAPN) system presents the challenges of a multiarmed robotic system working within a very confined space.

Recent advances in robotic surgery have led to the development of the da Vinci single-port robotic platform (Intuitive Surgical, Sunnyvale Ca), which has found unique application in the realm of renal surgery [15, 16].

The SP system is uniquely suited to retroperitoneal partial nephrectomy owing to the narrow profile of the device and flexible, articulated camera. This chapter will review the role of the single-port robot in the approach to the RP-RAPN and address specific technical considerations.

2 Overview and Key Points

The retroperitoneal approach to partial nephrectomy offers the advantage of direct access to the renal hilum, avoidance of the peritoneal space, and decreased postoperative ileus, blood loss, and hospital stay [13, 17, 18]. This approach provides considerable benefit when dealing with a complex abdomen with a history of previous interventions. The decrease in spillage of blood and urine into the intraabdomi-

S. Talamini (✉) · S. Crivellaro
Urology Department, University of Illinois at Chicago, Chicago, IL, USA

P. Wiklund et al. (eds.), *Robotic Urologic Surgery*, https://doi.org/10.1007/978-3-031-00363-9_49

nal cavity and avoidance of bowel manipulation and mobilization may play a role in the reduction of ileus [13].

The appropriate patient selection is crucial for success. A thorough history and physical exam must be performed, including documentation of prior renal surgery or retroperitoneal surgery [10, 19]. The patient must be counseled regarding the risks of the surgery, including the need to convert to a radical nephrectomy if there is a risk of compromise to oncologic outcomes due to anatomical challenges or concern for positive margins and conversion to an open procedure.

When considering renal masses, those lesions which are very posterior or would require significant renal mobilization to reach via a transabdominal approach are well suited to the retroperitoneal technique, whereas anterior or medially located lesions may be better addressed via transabdominal approaches [13]. Patients with a history of previous retroperitoneal surgery, percutaneous nephrostomy or percutaneous nephrolithotomy may represent a contraindication to RP-RAPN [14].

Previously, major drawbacks of the retroperitoneal approach included the limited working space, making laparoscopic surgery challenging in this space. The SP robot is uniquely suited for the small space of the retroperitoneum, and some patients may even be considered for same-day discharge [20].

3 Positioning

The patient is placed on the operating room table in the supine position initially. IV access is obtained, bilateral sequential compression devices applied, and intubation performed. A Foley catheter is placed for maximum decompression of the urinary system. The patient is the placed in lateral decubitus position. We prefer to place gel rolls for lumbar support, and axillary gel roll may be placed as well. No-slip padding on the operating table pads pressure points and allows for table rotation, and the patient is further secured using circumferential tape. The arms are also secured in place in a neutral position and protected using either foam or pillow for padding. The kidney rest may be lifted, or a break in the table may be flexed to aid in opening the space for dissection. Cross-sectional imaging should be displayed in the operating room for review.

4 Access

The narrow operative space for retroperitoneal surgery necessitates careful port placement. The 11th and 12th ribs superiorly and the iliac crest inferiorly are marked out. The anterior and posterior axillary lines are delineated as anterior and posterior margins, and the midaxillary line is used to guide the middle of the port incision. A 3 cm marking is made transversely approximately half the distance between the bottom margin of the 12th rib and the iliac crest (Fig. 1). If the port is placed too inferiorly, the assistant may be restricted by the iliac crest while directing instruments superiorly.

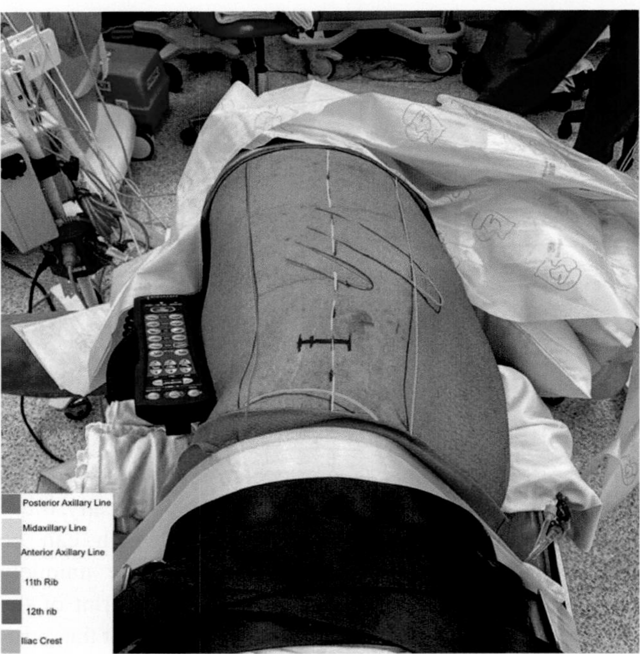

Fig. 1 Patient positioning and anatomical landmarks for port placement

The incision is made sharply, and dissection is carried down to the thoracolumbar fascia which is divided. Once the retroperitoneal space is entered, blunt finger dissection is used to further develop the space posterior to the kidney to allow for placement of the balloon spacemaker. The psoas muscle can be felt posteriorly and the lower pole of the kidney inside Gerota's fascia anteriorly. Typically, the kidney is pushed anteriorly during blunt dissection. Whereas the multiport approach would require extensive dissection to position four trocars, the single port requires much less dissection to allow port placement and therefore minimal with risk of perforating the peritoneum.

A Balloon Dissector Spacemaker™ (Covidien, Dublin, Ireland) trocar is placed into the space, trocar removed, and the balloon inflated. Care must be taken to ensure proper orientation of the balloon, which is oblong and football shaped. This balloon can inadvertently violate the peritoneal space if not oriented correctly. A 0-degree 10 mm laparoscopic camera is placed into the trocar to confirm adequate development of the space, utilizing visualization of the psoas muscle posteriorly as an anatomical landmark. The balloon is deflated, and the device is removed.

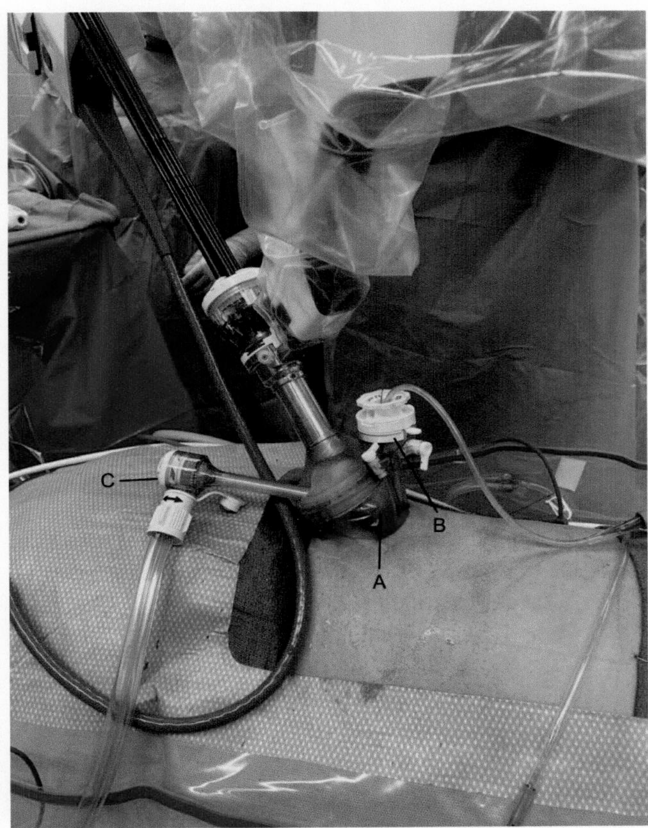

Fig. 2 (A) Floating configuration of Alexis retractor; (B) 12 mm assistant port in side car configuration; (C) 5 mm AirSeal port

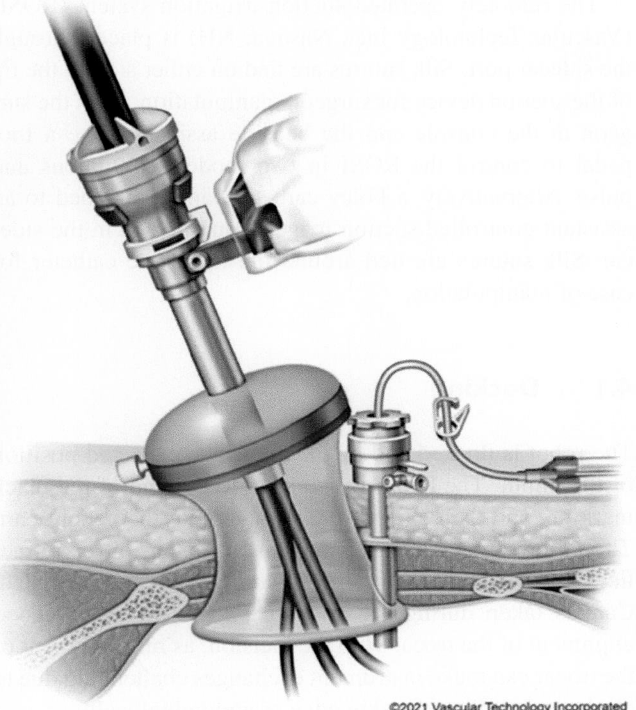

Fig. 3 Floating dock and sidecar technique with GelPOINT Mini

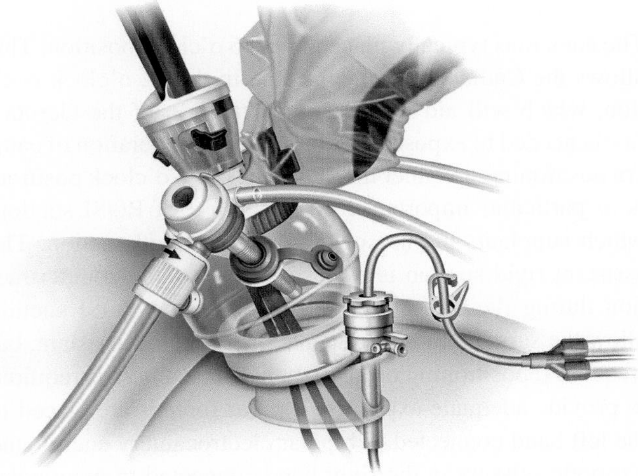

Fig. 4 Floating dock and sidecar technique with SP access port

Multiple techniques have been used for access and port placement. One key concept is the floating dock (Fig. 2). This approach essentially extends the port outside the body using insufflation of the unrolled portion of the Alexis wound protector. The floating dock allows for significantly more working space and greater deflection and angulation of the robot [21, 22].

When using the GelPOINT Mini advanced access platform (Applied Medical, Rancho Santa Margarita, CA), an Alexis wound protector is inserted into the incision, and the ring is rolled downward, leaving some space in the plastic for the floating technique, and a green GelPOINT device is placed over the Alexis. The metal SP trocar is inserted through the gel, and a 5 mm AirSeal (ConMed, Utica, NY) is also inserted through the gel. A 12 mm trocar is placed in the sidecar fashion by using the same skin incision and placing the trocar through a separate fascial incision through the plastic of the Alexis retractor (Fig. 3).

Currently, we favor the use of the SP access port which is a purpose-specific device designed to allow an all-in-one approach to SP surgery (Fig. 4). This device allows for maximum floating ability, and the space within the access port allows for seamless bedside assistance, such as suture exchanges and specimen placement outside of the abdominal cavity which can be extracted later.

An Alexis-type retractor is placed into the incision in the retroperitoneal space, again leaving some space in the plastic to allow for a floating configuration. The SP access port is placed onto the retractor, which includes the robotic trocar and a custom-designed space for placement of the 5 mm AirSeal device for insufflation. A 12 mm trocar is placed in the side car fashion.

The remotely operated suction irrigation system (ROSI) (Vascular Technology Inc., Nashua, NH) is placed through the sidecar port. Silk sutures are tied on either side of the tip of the suction device for surgeon manipulation. Both the surgeon at the console and the bedside assistant have a foot pedal to control the ROSI in two modes, continuous and pulse. Alternatively, a Foley catheter can be attached to an assistant-controlled suction irrigator and placed in the sidecar. Silk sutures are tied around the tip of the catheter for ease of manipulation.

4.1 Docking

The robot is docked and aligned with the expected position of the hilum. The boom is extended to the end of the black marking, and then slightly drawn back into the patient cart. This allows for additional movement, extension or retraction, or "burping" of the trocar during the case if needed. Care is taken during the docking process to ensure good alignment of the trocar with the incision, as misalignment of the trocar can make instrument exchanges challenging due to clashes with either the skin edge or abdominal wall.

4.2 Instruments and Equipment

The camera is typically placed in the 6 o'clock position. This allows the Cadiere instrument to be in the 12 o'clock position, which will aid in the upward traction of the Gerota's fascia needed to expose the hilum. The consideration of camera positioning, in either the 12 o'clock or 6 o'clock position, is of particular importance given the use of ROSI suction, which supplants the use of the assistant rigid suction. The assistant rigid suction is often used to provide countertraction during the dissection. The Cadiere and ROSI suction allow the surgeon more independence from the assistant, but frequent repositioning of instruments and camera is required to provide adequate exposure. Bipolar forceps are placed in the left hand connected to bipolar electrocautery energy and a robotic scissors in the right hand connected to monopolar energy.

The assistant is crucial in the control of the renal hilum with the placement of bulldog laparoscopic clamps (Aesculap, Center Valley, PA), and a selection of clamps may be available including straight and curved clamps, both in short and long varieties.

A Robotic Drop-In ultrasound transducer or laparoscopic ultrasound probe (BK Medical ApS, Herlev, Denmark) can be utilized with Tile Pro to better visualize the lesion. The Drop-In probe is a flexible transducer that can be controlled robotically by the primary surgeon, and again, decreasing reliance on the bedside assistant. Cadiere is the recommended instrument to hold the probe. The laparoscopic probe can be inserted through the 12 mm assistant trocar, however, can be difficult to manipulate given the small operative space.

In consideration of the renorrhaphy, 2–0 and 3–0 Vicryl or V-loc barbed sutures may be used for hemostasis, and laparoscopic Hem-o-Lok clips (Weck Closure Systems, Research Triangle Park, NC, USA) can be placed by the assistant to secure the suture. Robot Hem-o-Lok clips are available for the SP system and can be utilized instead of the laparoscopic clips depending on surgeon preference. When using a sliding clip technique for renorrhaphy, the sutures should be prepared ahead of time on the back bench as ischemia time is affected by any additional preparation needed intraoperatively. Additional suture to consider include 5–0 Prolene prepared with Lapra-Ty clips for repair of vascular injury.

Hemostatic agents to consider may include Surgicel (Ethicon, Raritan NJ), Surgiflo (Ethicon, Raritan NJ), and Floseal (Baxter, Deerfield IL).

5 Surgical Technique

The key operative considerations of the SP-RAPN include patient positioning, access into the retroperitoneal space, robot docking, and familiarity with anatomical landmarks. If any of these points are miscalculated, the case may become increasingly challenging and progress hindered.

After docking considerations are taken into account as mentioned in Sect. 49.4.1, the trocar is positioned and directed toward the expected location of the hilum. Minimal initial dissection is typically needed as the balloon dissector opens the retroperitoneal space bluntly. The psoas muscle can be identified posteriorly and the Gerota's fascia medially. Gerota's is observed for pulsations, and then dissection is directed toward creating a window for isolation and control of the renal hilum. The perirenal fat is lifted upward by the Cadiere, which will provide much of the counter traction during the procedure. Countertraction can be applied with the bipolar forceps, and minimal monopolar energy is needed as dissection is carried out in an avascular plane. Adequate traction and counter traction is crucial during the procedure and as a general rule when using the Single Port robot. Once the hilum is encountered, the renal artery is typically encountered first, considering its posterior location to the renal vein, and dissected circumferentially in order to allow the assistant to place a bulldog clamp without resistance. The consideration of renal vein clamping can be taken in the context of a very centrally located lesion, interpolar lesion, or to prevent CO_2 gas embolism though rare [23–25]. There is evidence to suggest that concurrent renal artery and renal vein clamping do not adversely affect renal function, though data is still conflicting [26–29].

The remainder of the dissection and resection are analogous to the transperitoneal approach with either MP or SP.

Prior to clamping, the dissection is then carried out over the expected location of the mass. Intraoperative ultrasound can be utilized at this time to aide in identification of the lesion. Once accurately identified, the perirenal fat over the lesion is cleared in order to achieve a 1 cm margin. One can proceed with enucleation or wedge resection of the mass based on surgeon preference. Caution should be taken when attempting enucleation of cystic or partially cystic lesions. Risk of entering or perforating a cystic lesion during enucleation increases risk of malignant seeding, and consideration should be given to a wedge resection of these lesions.

Prior to initiating the resection, the parenchyma may be scored circumferentially around the tumor to guide the dissection. Fat overlaying the tumor may be sent to pathology as a separate specimen, if this tissue needs to be removed to aid in the dissection. At this point, if proceeding with a clamped resection, the bedside assistant will place a bulldog clamp around the renal artery and/or vein. The resection can be carried out with sharp dissection cold or with electrocautery. Using energy during the dissection may alter tissue planes, making visualizing the correct plane between the tumor and healthy parenchyma more challenging.

Once resection is complete, monopolar scissors and fenestrated bipolar respectively ay 3 and 9 o'clock are switched with needle drivers. The tumor bed and renorrhaphy can be completed in one or two layers. A deep running stitch can be performed using Vicryl or V-loc suture with a Hem-o-Lok clip placed after a knot on the end of the stitch and double clip placed after completion of the stitch. Interrupted 2–0 Vicryl prepared with Hem-o-Lok clips are placed to bring together the defect and are sequentially tightened gently using the sliding clip technique, with care taken not to tear through the parenchyma by placing undue traction on sutures [30]. Clip is placed ensuring suture in the middle of the clip to avoid tearing of tissue and evenly dispersed parenchymal pressure. Clips should remain outside the parenchyma, as migrated clips into the collecting system or stone formation on clips that have migrated have been reported [31–33]. The insufflation pressure should be dropped down to 8 to assess hemostasis. Needles are typically left on the suture until the defect is completely closed and adequate hemostasis is confirmed.

6 Limitations

We were able to reproduce this technique in a wide variety of patients, with different levels of tumor complexity with renal scores ranging from 4 to 12, BMI ranging from 18 to 55, and in patients with previous renal surgery. It is a reliable, reproducible technique, however associated with some objective limitations. The need of having a good alignment of the platform with the target might pose more challenges when approaching upper pole or lower pole lesions. The camera and the instruments need to be frequently repositioned during the dissection introducing a small learning curve. The strength of the needle drivers does not allow the surgeon to apply the same pressure to the Hem-o-Lok clips when using the sliding clip technique that could be applied with the multiport robot. This necessitates the positioning of multiple sutures to be able to properly close the defect without tearing the tissue. Finally, though the single port has firefly technology capabilities, it has not yet received FDA approval.

7 Conclusions

Overall, the single-port platform offers the opportunity to exploit different approaches than the classic transperitoneal route. Single-port kidney surgery can be easily performed via the retroperitoneal approach, reducing the technical challenges of retroperitoneal surgery encountered via a multiport technique due to the slim profile of the device. The improved technical feasibility will decrease the learning curve associated with this approach, providing benefits to our patients by reducing the invasiveness and morbidity of the procedure, not only due to the single 3 cm incision but through the benefits obtained from avoiding the peritoneal cavity, allowing easy access to the pedicle and decreasing pain and length of hospital stay.

References

1. Zagoria RJ. Imaging of small renal masses: a medical success story. Am J Roentgenol. 2000;175(4):945–55. https://doi.org/10.2214/ajr.175.4.1750945.
2. Gill IS, Aron M, Gervais DA, Jewett MAS. Small renal mass. N Engl J Med. 2010;362(7):624–34. https://doi.org/10.1056/NEJMcp0910041.
3. Uzzo RG, Novick AC. Nephron sparing surgery for renal tumors: indications, techniques and outcomes. J Urol. 2001;166(1):6–18. https://doi.org/10.1016/S0022-5347(05)66066-1.
4. Fergany AF, Hafez KS, Novick AC. Long-term results of nephron sparing surgery for localized renal cell carcinoma: 10-year followup. J Urol. 2000;163(2):442–5. https://doi.org/10.1016/S0022-5347(05)67896-2.
5. Campbell S, Uzzo RG, Allaf ME, et al. Renal mass and localized renal cancer: AUA guideline. J Urol. 2017;198(3):520–9. https://doi.org/10.1016/j.juro.2017.04.100.
6. Kutikov A, Uzzo RG. The R.E.N.A.L. nephrometry score: a comprehensive standardized system for quantitating renal tumor size, location and depth. J Urol. 2009;182(3):844–53. https://doi.org/10.1016/j.juro.2009.05.035.
7. Wang AJ, Bhayani SB. Robotic partial nephrectomy versus laparoscopic partial nephrectomy for renal Cell Carcinoma: single-surgeon analysis of >100 consecutive procedures. Urology. 2009;73(2):306–10. https://doi.org/10.1016/j.urology.2008.09.049.

8. Pierorazio PM, Patel HD, Feng T, Yohannan J, Hyams ES, Allaf ME. Robotic-assisted versus traditional laparoscopic partial nephrectomy: comparison of outcomes and evaluation of learning curve. Urology. 2011;78(4):813–9. https://doi.org/10.1016/j.urology.2011.04.065.
9. Link RE, Bhayani SB, Allaf ME, et al. Exploring the learning curve, pathological outcomes and perioperative morbidity of laparoscopic partial nephrectomy performed for renal mass. J Urol. 2005;173(5):1690–4. https://doi.org/10.1097/01.ju.0000154777.24753.1b.
10. Benway BM, Mottrie A, Bhayani SB. Robot-assisted partial nephrectomy. In: Patel VR, editor. Robotic urologic surgery. Springer: London; 2012. p. 295–302. https://doi.org/10.1007/978-1-84882-800-1_28.
11. Ghani KR, Sukumar S, Sammon JD, Rogers CG, Trinh Q-D, Menon M. Practice patterns and outcomes of open and minimally invasive partial nephrectomy since the introduction of robotic partial nephrectomy: results from the nationwide inpatient sample. J Urol. 2014;191(4):907–13. https://doi.org/10.1016/j.juro.2013.10.099.
12. Gill IS, Delworth MG, Munch LC. Laparoscopic retroperitoneal partial nephrectomy. J Urol. 1994;152:1539–42. https://doi.org/10.1016/S0022-5347(17)32465-5.
13. Wright JL, Porter JR. Laparoscopic partial nephrectomy: comparison of transperitoneal and retroperitoneal approaches. J Urol. 2005;174(3):841–5. https://doi.org/10.1097/01.ju.0000169423.94253.46.
14. Patel M, Porter J. Robotic retroperitoneal partial nephrectomy. World J Urol. 2013;31(6):1377–82. https://doi.org/10.1007/s00345-013-1038-y.
15. Shukla D, Small A, Mehrazin R, Palese M. Single-port robotic-assisted partial nephrectomy: initial clinical experience and lessons learned for successful outcomes. J Robot Surg. 2021;15(2):293–8. https://doi.org/10.1007/s11701-020-01106-2.
16. Kaouk J, Garisto J, Eltemamy M, Bertolo R. Pure single-site robot-assisted partial nephrectomy using the SP surgical system: initial clinical experience. Urology. 2019;124:282–5. https://doi.org/10.1016/j.urology.2018.11.024.
17. Feliciano J, Stifelman M. Robotic retroperitoneal partial nephrectomy: a four-arm approach. JSLS. 2012;16(2):208–11. https://doi.org/10.4293/108680812X13427982376149.
18. Ren T, Liu Y, Zhao X, et al. Transperitoneal approach versus retroperitoneal approach: a meta-analysis of laparoscopic partial nephrectomy for renal cell carcinoma. PLoS One. 2014;9(3):e91978. https://doi.org/10.1371/journal.pone.0091978.
19. Partin AW, Dmochowski RR, Kavoussi LR, Peters CA. Campbell-Walsh-Wein urology. Philadelphia, PA: Elsevier; 2021.
20. Abaza R, Murphy C, Bsatee A, Brown DH, Martinez O. Single-port robotic surgery allows same-day discharge in majority of cases. Urology. 2021;148:159–65. https://doi.org/10.1016/j.urology.2020.08.092.
21. Lenfant L, Kim S, Aminsharifi A, Sawczyn G, Kaouk J. Floating docking technique: a simple modification to improve the working space of the instruments during single-port robotic surgery. World J Urol. 2021;39(4):1299–305. https://doi.org/10.1007/s00345-020-03307-8.
22. Zhao LC. Management of urethral stenosis after treatment for prostate cancer: NYU case of the month, august 2020. Rev Urol. 2020;22(3):133–4.
23. Hou W, Zhong J, Pan B, et al. Paradoxical carbon dioxide embolism during laparoscopic surgery without intracardiac right-to-left shunt: two case reports and a brief review of the literature. J Int Med Res. 2020;48(8):030006052093381. https://doi.org/10.1177/0300060520933816.
24. Li Y, Zhang E, Yuan H. Cerebral carbon dioxide embolism after kidney cancer laparoscopic surgery with full neurological recovery: a case report. Medicine (Baltimore). 2020;99(27):e20986. https://doi.org/10.1097/MD.0000000000020986.
25. Cottin V, Delafosse B, Viale J-P. Gas embolism during laparoscopy: a report of seven cases in patients with previous abdominal surgical history. Surg Endosc. 1996;10(2):166–9. https://doi.org/10.1007/BF00188365.
26. Blum KA, Paulucci DJ, Abaza R, et al. Main renal artery clamping with or without renal vein clamping during robotic partial nephrectomy for clinical T1 renal masses: perioperative and long-term functional outcomes. Urology. 2016;97:118–23. https://doi.org/10.1016/j.urology.2016.08.028.
27. Akpinar C, Suer E, Baklaci U, et al. The effect of renal artery-only or renal artery–vein clamping during partial nephrectomy on short and long-term functional results: is clamping technique important? Int Urol Nephrol. 2021;53(7):1317–23. https://doi.org/10.1007/s11255-021-02812-y.
28. Funahashi Y, Kato M, Yoshino Y, Fujita T, Sassa N, Gotoh M. Comparison of renal ischemic damage during laparoscopic partial nephrectomy with artery-vein and artery-only clamping. J Endourol. 2014;28(3):306–11. https://doi.org/10.1089/end.2013.0446.
29. Cao J, Zhu S, Ye M, et al. Comparison of renal artery *vs* renal artery-vein clamping during partial nephrectomy: a system review and meta-analysis. J Endourol. 2020;34(4):523–30. https://doi.org/10.1089/end.2019.0580.
30. Benway BM, Wang AJ, Cabello JM, Bhayani SB. Robotic partial nephrectomy with sliding-clip renorrhaphy: technique and outcomes. Eur Urol. 2009;55(3):592–9. https://doi.org/10.1016/j.eururo.2008.12.028.
31. Lee Z, Reilly CE, Moore BW, Mydlo JH, Lee DI, Eun DD. Stone formation from nonabsorbable clip migration into the collecting system after robot-assisted partial nephrectomy. Case Rep Urol. 2014;2014:1–3. https://doi.org/10.1155/2014/397427.
32. Park KS, Sim YJ, Jung H. Migration of a Hem-o-Lok clip to the ureter following laparoscopic partial nephrectomy presenting with lower urinary tract symptoms. Int Neurourol J. 2013;17(2):90–2. https://doi.org/10.5213/inj.2013.17.2.90.
33. Shrivastava P, Nayak B, Singh P. Migrated Hem-o-Lok clips in the ureter: a rare cause of recurrent urinary tract infection. BMJ Case Rep. 2017;2017:bcr2016219143. https://doi.org/10.1136/bcr-2016-219143.

Complications in Robot-Assisted Renal Surgery

Marcio Covas Moschovas, Elio Mazzone, and Alexandre Mottrie

1 Introduction

Several authors have described the benefits of robotic surgery to approach renal tumors [1]. In this scenario, in the USA, robot-assisted partial nephrectomy has become the standard surgery for managing renal tumors smaller than 5 cm [2]. Some authors have described renal function preservation of up to 90% in favor of PN versus 70% of the radical nephrectomy group [3]. The finesse provided by robotic technology associates the intraoperative 3D digital image with highly precise instruments, maximizing renal parenchyma preservation and postoperative recovery. However, despite its advantages, robotic surgery is not devoid of complications. In this chapter we describe the management of the most common complications associated with the robotic approach to renal surgery.

2 Intraoperative Complications and Management

2.1 Patient Positioning

The first step to avoid complications in robotic surgery starts with patient positioning. All patients must have pad protection in all articulations and points of body contact with the operative table. In addition, head and face protection is crucial in this process to avoid trauma to the patient's eyes. In some reports, the chances of corneal abrasions in robotic surgery can reach up to 6.5-fold compared to open surgery [4].

In the current literature, several authors have described complications during this initial step of the surgery, being skin lesion, the most common issue reported, and operative time the most important risk factor for nerve injuries [5–7]. Common nerve injuries include brachial nerve plexus due to hyperabduction in kidney surgery, ulnar nerve injury due to elbow compression against the table corner, radial nerve injury due to hand and wrist compression, and femoral nerve injury due to the lithotomy position in radical prostatectomies and cystectomies. For each additional hour of surgery, it is estimated that the nerve injury increases up to 100-fold [8, 9].

Finally, the collision between the robotic arms and the patient's body is another source of skin complications. In these cases, the tableside assistant and anesthesia team must monitor these robotic movements during the surgery and provide an appropriate external arm angulation and trocar burp when required [10].

2.2 Trocar Placement and Bowel Lesion

Appropriate trocar placement is imperative for the success of the robot-assisted surgical procedure. The correct trocar triangulation associated with a standardized technique is crucial to avoid internal lesions and optimize robotic movements during the surgery. In renal surgeries, especially partial nephrectomies, the trocar placement is always adapted according to the type of robot used (S, Si, X, Xi, and SP), patient's size, body habitus, tumor location, and renal anatomy. In addition, the past surgical history is a determinant factor while placing the trocars due to the highest chances of intra-abdominal adhesions, which increases vascular and bowel lesions during the abdominal access. In these cases, the most appropriate trocar placement is performed with Hasson's technique or Palmer's point access [11, 12].

M. C. Moschovas (✉)
AdventHealth Global Robotics Institute, Celebration, FL, USA

ORSI Academy, Melle, Belgium

University of Central Florida, UCF, Orlando, USA

E. Mazzone
ORSI Academy, Melle, Belgium

Division of Oncology/Unit of Urology, URI, IRCCS Ospedale San Raffaele, Milan, Italy

A. Mottrie
ORSI Academy, Melle, Belgium

OLV Hospital, Aalst, Belgium

P. Wiklund et al. (eds.), *Robotic Urologic Surgery*, https://doi.org/10.1007/978-3-031-00363-9_50

Recent studies reported the chances of vascular and bowel lesions in robot-assisted surgeries in up to 0.1% of the cases, being vascular injury the most common complication [13]. However, despite the small likelihood, an adverse and unrecognized injury can cause serious impacts on the patient's health. In this scenario, it is crucial to inspect the whole abdominal with the robotic or laparoscopic scope after placing the first trocar and before proceeding with the next trocars. In the case of any organ damage, the repair must be performed immediately.

Extra attention must be paid to patients with small body habitus and low BMI due to a smaller distance between the skin incision and the aortocaval space, which increases the chances of damaging these structures while placing the Veress needle or the robotic trocar.

Besides the trocar placement, bowel injury can happen while releasing the colon to access the kidney in both sides. Two different types of injury mechanisms are described: mechanical and thermal.

Mechanical injuries are usually associated with retraction and blunt dissection. Due to the lack of tactile feedback, some delicate organs and structures are damaged with inappropriate mechanical manipulation.

In general, robotic instruments provide two types of energy: monopolar and bipolar. Both have potential for thermal lesions of the bowel. Monopolar energy causes more lateral thermal spread and produces higher temperatures than bipolar electrocautery, the Harmonic scalpel, and LigaSure [14]. Thermal injury is usually more extensive than expected, and conservative management can result in acute perforation during the postoperative period. Intraoperative repair is usually the best management. If a bowel repair is required, all bowel edges must be refreshed, and all affected tissue removed before the primary repair [14]. The injured site should be drained, and the patient must be prescribed antibiotic treatment [15].

Unrecognized bowel injuries usually present as sepsis and acute abdominal pain in the postoperative period. Other signs and symptoms are leukopenia or leukocytosis, fever, orifice pain trocar, ileus, nausea, or vomiting. In these scenarios, a CT scan usually supports the diagnosis. In cases of suspicion, a diagnostic laparoscopy should be performed.

Technical refinement is the best way of minimizing complications during trocar placement and bowel manipulation. When using bipolar or monopolar energy, the surgeon must ensure that the instruments are not touching each other and that the arm is not touching the bowel, vessels, or adjacent structures; only the tip of the instrument must be in contact with the bleeding tissue to be cauterized. In addition, the surgeon must avoid manipulating the bowel with tools with delicate tips such as scissors and Maryland.

2.3 Potential Issues with Pneumoperitoneum

Insufflation of CO_2 and pneumoperitoneum pressures during the surgical procedure are always potential factors of complications. In addition, extended operative time is associated with hypercapnia and metabolic acidosis, especially in smokers and patients with chronic obstructive pulmonary disease (COPD). In such cases, some authors have described pneumoperitoneum insufflation with helium gas as an alternative to CO_2 [16–18].

The CO_2 insufflation rate is also important due to the increased risk of embolic events, hypotension, and vagal response. Monitoring the rapid increase of intra-abdominal pressure is crucial, mainly when operating patients with cardiovascular diseases and morbid obesity due to the asystole and ventilation issues during the surgery [6].

2.4 Hepatic, Splenic, and Pancreatic Lesions

Hepatic, splenic, and pancreatic lesions are uncommon events in robot-assisted renal surgery. Some authors have reported up to 0.3% of splenic lesions in left upper urinary tract surgeries while mobilizing the spleen to access the upper pole of the kidney [19]. On the other hand, hepatic lesions are difficult to estimate because minor injuries are not usually reported. Bile duct injuries appear in the right adrenalectomy and partial nephrectomy. In these cases, the general surgery team must be contacted immediately to manage ductal lesions appropriately.

It is estimated that pancreatic injury rates reach up to 0.2% during left kidney surgery. Despite the uncommon event, it has substantial morbidity. The best advice to prevent this complication is a careful dissection of the upper renal pole, between the tail of the pancreas and Gerota's fascia [14]. It is also recommended to have an intraoperative evaluation of the general surgery team when suspecting or recognizing an inadvertent pancreatic lesion.

2.5 Vascular Injury and Management

Controlling the renal hilum and manipulation of large-caliber vessels are common steps of robot-assisted renal surgery. However, being direct branches of the aorta and vena cava, any lesion of the renal artery or vein has deadly potential. In this scenario, preoperative imaging studies, including 3D reconstructions, are crucial for avoiding accidental vascular lesions [20].

In our experience, after dissecting the renal artery and vein, a vessel loop is used to repair these branches and facilitate the manipulation while placing the bulldog clamp (Fig. 1). These repairs are important landmarks to identify the vessels in the case of any accidental vascular lesion and massive bleeding. Placing vessel loops is also an option to minimize the blood loss in large-caliber vessels such as aortic injuries, allowing an appropriate surgical view during the repair (Fig. 2).

The bedside assistant has a fundamental role during these episodes of vascular injuries. The assistant must associate an efficient suction with compression of the bleeding source

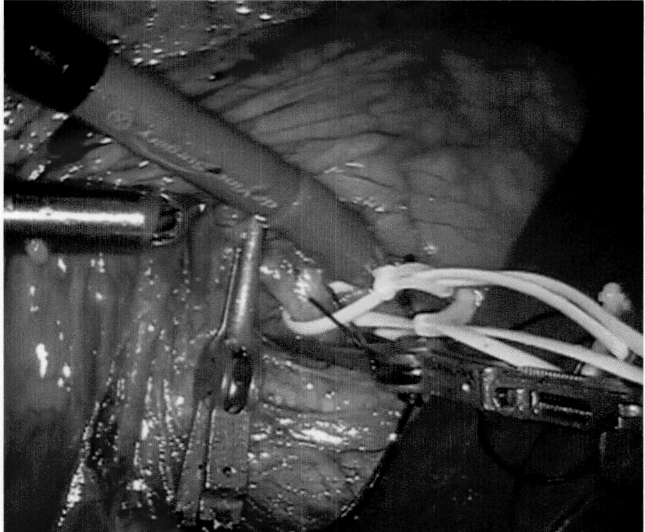

Fig. 1 Renal artery repaired by vessel loops

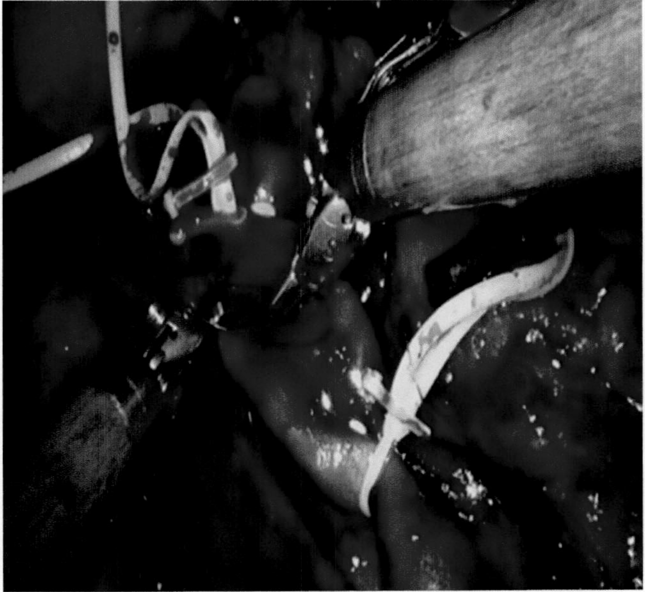

Fig. 2 Aorta injury. Vessel loops repairing the edges of the lesion to decrease blood loss and improve visualization

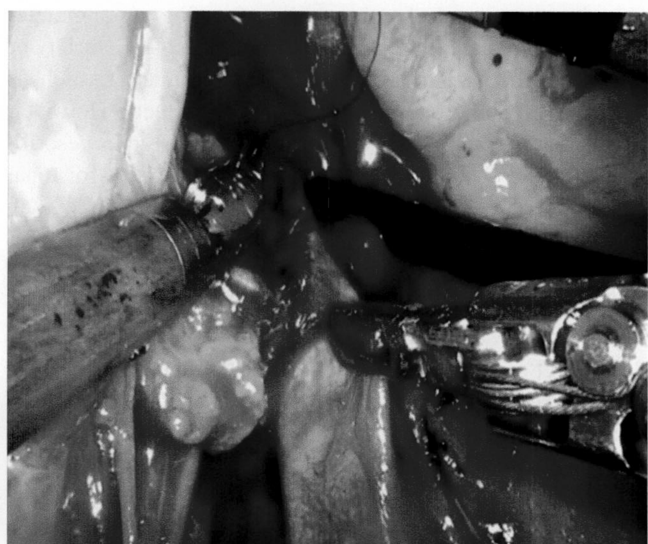

Fig. 3 Bedside assistant associating pressure and suction to improve the operative view while decreasing blood loss

(Fig. 3). Performing the blood suction without applying local compression increases the blood loss and, in the case of massive bleeding, will not properly clean the surgical site for identifying and repairing the lesion. The assistant can also use other resources to help the robotic surgeon, such as introducing a compress through the 12 mm port for improving the compression surface, placing a new trocar to work with both hands, or using additional bulldog clamps to decrease the active bleeding while the surgeon repairs the lesion.

Sliding Hem-o-Lok clips is another situation that usually leads to massive bleeding, especially when only one clip is placed in large-caliber vessels. For this reason, we usually apply two clips on the renal artery or direct branches of the aorta. In addition, the assistant must have extra caution when using the suction over a clamped artery because the tip of the suction device can displace or slide the clip, causing substantial bleeding.

Finally, some patients present a hemorrhagic state after unclamping the renal artery and vein due to a medullar or cortical vessel that was not controlled during the renorrhaphy. In our technique, all sutures used in the renorrhaphy have Hem-o-Lok clips on their tips. In these episodes of parenchymal bleeding after unclamping, the first step is the suture tightening by sliding the Hem-o-Lok of the suture. However, sometimes, the suture adjustment is not enough to stop the bleeding. In such cases, we usually release the suture and apply new stitches to the bleeding site.

2.5.1 Hemostatic Agent's Role in Bleeding Episodes

Several groups have reported the role of hemostatic agents in robot-assisted renal surgery for the final hemostasis and for reducing the warm ischemia when performing tumor enucleation without clamping the renal artery [21–24]. A variety of brands and materials are available in the market, such as hemostatic patches, foam, and powder products. However, the current literature still lacks well-designed studies describing which hemostatic agent is the most appropriate for renal surgery.

In our experience, hemostatic patches such as TachoSil are effective for minimizing renal sutures in enucleations of small and peripheral tumors (Fig. 4). The patch is placed on the tumor bed, and the robotic arm performs a local pressure with a wet gauze over the patch. After 5 min of pressure, the gauze is removed, and the hemostasis is checked with low-pressure insufflation (Fig. 5). These patches can also be used in the hemostasis of hepatic and splenic inadvertent lesions.

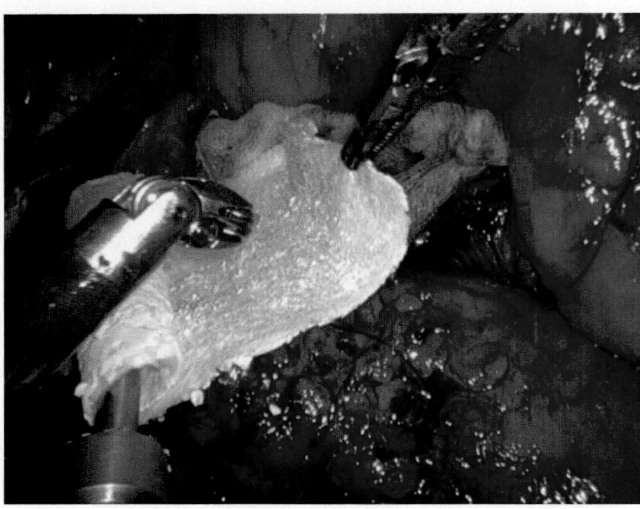

Fig. 4 Hemostatic patch before application

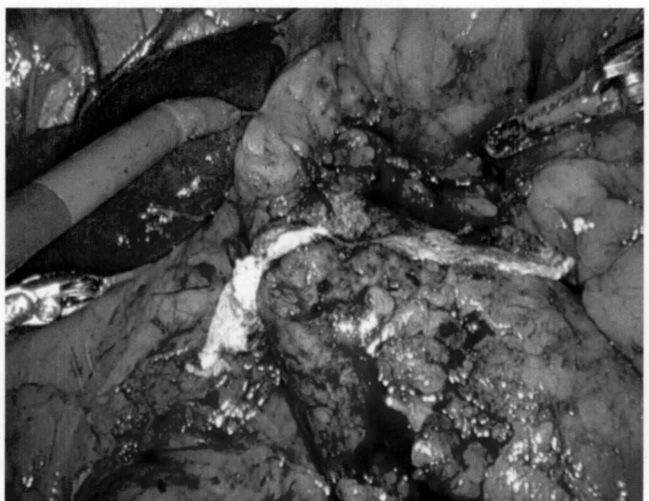

Fig. 5 Hemostatic patch after 5 min

2.6 Instrument Malfunction and Material Issues

Some studies in the literature described up to 4.6% of issues associated with the materials used in robot-assisted surgery, including software-related, mechanical, electric, and instrumental failures [25, 26]. Alemzadeh and colleagues reported up to 2.7% of conversion rates due to instrumental and robotic malfunction [27].

In our experience, all instruments are tested on the surgical back table. The robotic instruments have the tips, and the protective sheets checked before being inserted into the patient. Especial attention must be taken with the vascular bulldog clamps because the pressure applied by each clamp differs among the brands, sizes, and the number of times used [28]. Before using in the patient, the clamps and appliers must be checked by the surgeon and tableside assistant. Having a bulldog clamp with inappropriate pressure leads to two different types of complications. Clamps with a loose grip and decreased pressure lead to a hemorrhagic state during the tumor enucleation, while clamps with a strong grip or opening issues lead to a more extended ischemic state, which impacts the renal function (Fig. 6).

2.7 Considerations for Vena Cava Thrombus Surgery

Renal surgery in patients with vena cava thrombus is one of the most challenging procedures in urology due to the increased intra- and postoperative complication rates compared to the standard partial nephrectomy [1]. Despite the potential blood loss during the surgery, these cases, depending on the thrombus level, must be faced by a high-volume

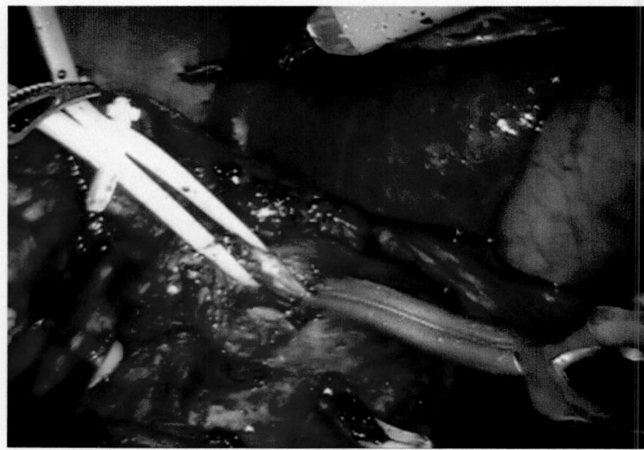

Fig. 6 Laparoscopic bulldog with opening issues during renal artery clamping

center with a multidisciplinary surgical team including vascular and cardiac surgery.

Our consideration for this type of surgery regard the IVC thrombectomy. Before opening the vena cava, the thrombus must have its limits identified with intraoperative ultrasound, and an appropriate IVC clamping with vessel loops must be performed to avoid embolism of any fragment. After the thrombus removal, the IVC interior walls are checked for tumoral infiltration. In these cases, the infiltration is removed, and a bovine patch is placed to repair the IVC wall. Finally, before releasing the tourniquet, the IVC is filled with saline solution to avoid gas embolism.

3 Postoperative Complications Related with the Robotic Approach

Some of the complications related with robotic approach may be experienced during the postoperative period, and they should be properly identified in order to optimize their management.

3.1 Acute Kidney Injury

Acute Kidney Injury (AKI) is a common occurrence after partial nephrectomy and is a significant risk factor for chronic kidney disease. RAPN have been demonstrated to reduce the risk of AKI [29], but this finding may be related to the shorter ischemia time of robotic surgery or to the selective clamping of only arteries in RAPN [30]. Therefore, prospective evidence is needed to confirm these findings from retrospective analyses. Within the context of patients treated with robot-assisted approach, age, gender, BMI, diabetes, nephrometric scores, and baseline estimated glomerular filtration have been demonstrated to be strongly associated with the risk of experiencing AKI in the postoperative time [31]. The data corroborate the importance of patient selection to reduce the risk of AKI. Moreover, when considering ischemia time, this preoperative information can aid in the early identification of patients who would potentially benefit from an early multidisciplinary consultation.

3.2 Venous Thromboembolism (VTE) Complications

Deep venous thrombosis (DVT) and pulmonary embolism are postoperative complications strongly related to oncological surgeries. Although there are many risk factors inherent to the patients, positioning and prolonged operative time can remarkably influence thromboembolic events [32, 33]. Surgical features, such as lymph node dissection, can increase the incidence of DVT/pulmonary embolism up to sevenfold, while minimally invasive surgery seems to have lower risk of thromboembolism than open approaches [34].

While comorbidities and most of the surgical features related to VTE are not modifiable, VTE prophylaxis management is of utmost relevance. Early ambulation, sequential compression devices, and chemoprophylaxis are helpful measures in patients at risk of VTE without contraindications [32]. A randomized study showed that 4-week anticoagulation prophylaxis has advantages in relation to 1-week administration after major abdominal surgeries [35]. Single preoperative chemoprophylaxis has also shown benefits without increasing the risk of bleeding in patients [36].

3.3 Rhabdomyolysis

Clinically relevant rhabdomyolysis can occur in patients exposed to prolonged robotic procedures, particularly at the beginning of the procedure learning curve. Serum creatine kinase (CK) increases after surgery peak at 18 h after the procedure, but CK elevation in isolation should not be used to predict positioning injury [37]. Prolonged Trendelenburg position, high body mass index, peripheral vascular disease, and comorbidities increase the risk of muscle injuries [38, 39]. Serum CK dosage is indicated for these patients and for those with pain in the back, thigh, or gluteals after surgery. Serum CK levels of >1000 IU/L or myoglobinuria confirms a rhabdomyolysis diagnosis, which increases the postoperative renal failure risk. Hypervolemic diuretic therapy and management of metabolic acidosis are required in such situations [37].

3.4 Ocular Complications

A steep Trendelenburg position combined with pneumoperitoneum can cause increased intraocular pressure, reduced ocular perfusion, and possibly visual impairment caused by ischemic optic neuropathy. Permanent vision loss is a rare but important complication [40, 41]. In the context of renal surgery, the risk of ocular complications is reduced due to the limited use of steep Trendelenburg, while pneumoperitoneum still remains a notable risk factor. Therefore, limiting operative time, adequate intraoperative blood pressure monitoring, and transparent occlusive dressing as opposed to standard eye tape may play a role in minimizing the risk of postoperative ocular complications [40].

3.5 Port-Site Hernias

Port-site hernias are a late access-related complication, which occur in <1% of robot-assisted procedures. There is a higher incidence with >10 mm port sites, although 8 mm robotic and even 5 mm port-site hernias have been described. Cutting trocars have been associated with larger fascial defects; thus, blunt-tipped obturators have been preferred. Port-site with >10 mm closure is the best way to avoid hernias, although some studies have shown low incidence of hernia in non-midline port-sites of <12 mm [42].

3.6 Skin Lesions

Most skin lesions are positioning related. The combination of general anesthesia and prolonged immobilization is a combination of known risk factors which increase the risk of decubitus pressure lesions. Moreover, inadequate fixation and patient slippage might potentiate it and lead to severe decubitus and trocar-site lesions. Therefore, fixation of the patient on the table with a gel mattress, restraints, and body and shoulder straps may prevent such complications [43].

3.7 Postoperative Complication Assessment: Is there a Quality Control?

During the past decade, it has been proposed to introduce standardized systems for reporting complications [44–47]. Although these recommendations, few studies demonstrated a weakness in the literature for grading and reporting of complications following partial nephrectomy [48]. For instance, it was found that only six studies (2.9%) fulfilled all the criteria proposed by the European Association of Urology (EAU) for reporting complications. Therefore, the EAU recommended to use a 14-criteria template to collect and report complications after urological surgery [49]. A recent systematic review described that, after publication of the EAU guideline recommendations on outcome reporting, there was mainly better adherence to all the criteria [50]. Overall, there was underreporting (<50%) for 6 of the 14 criteria after publication of the EAU guidelines. Moreover, they found statistically significant improvements in the inclusion of mortality rates and causes of death, definitions of complications, severity grade, postoperative complications tabulated either by grade or complication type, and inclusion of risk factors in analyses. As previously reported, the vast majority of studies did not investigate who collected the data and the percentage of patients lost to follow-up. Despite a causal link between the introduction of EAU guidelines for reporting complications and the improvement of quality assessment after renal surgery cannot be proven (particularly in non-European center), the introduction of standardized guideless may have influenced the methodology of researchers for collecting and reporting complications after robotic renal surgery.

Of note, most complications may happen at the beginning of a surgeon learning curve; therefore, console and team training outside the OR represent a crucial step to reduce the risk of experiencing complications related to robotic approach. Indeed, it has been agreed during international multi-specialty consensus meeting that basic device training and basic skills training are fundaments steps to be achieved when starting with a robotic surgery program [51].

4 Conclusion

Patients' selection, adequate positioning, mentorship training during the learning curve, and avoiding last-longing procedures are key steps to prevent robot-assisted-related complications.

Considering the importance of team training and communication, the assistant has a fundamental role and should undergo a similar pattern of basic training. This said, we believe that team training and standardization of the surgical technique is crucial to minimize the risk of complications. From a clinical point of view, complex renal surgery should be always performed in a high-volume center where urological department is supported by other highly experienced specialties, such as vascular and general surgery, which can help in managing intra- and postoperative complications.

References

1. Seetharam Bhat KR, Moschovas MC, Onol FF, et al. Robotic renal and adrenal oncologic surgery: a contemporary review. Asian J Urol. 2021;8(1):89–99. https://doi.org/10.1016/j.ajur.2020.05.010.
2. Van Poppel H, Da Pozzo L, Albrecht W, Matveev V, Bono A, Borkowski A. A prospective, randomised EORTC intergroup phase 3 study comparing the oncologic outcome of elective nephron-sparing surgery and radical nephrectomy for low-stage renal cell carcinoma. Eur Urol. 2011;59:543–52.
3. Scosyrev E, Messing EM, Sylvester R, Campbell S, Van Poppel H. Renal function after nephron-sparing surgery versus radical nephrectomy: results from EORTC randomized trial 30904. Eur Urol. 2014;65:372–7.
4. Sampat A, Parakati I, Kunnavakkam R, Glick DB, Lee NK, Tenney M, et al. Corneal abrasion in hysterectomy and prostatectomy: role of laparoscopic and robotic assistance. Anesthesiology. 2015;122:994–1001.
5. Sundi D, Reese AC, Mettee LZ, Trock BJ, Pavlovich CP. Laparoscopic and robotic radical prostatectomy outcomes in obese and extremely obese men. Urology. 2013;82(3):600–5. https://doi.org/10.1016/j.urology.2013.05.013.
6. Potretzke AM, Kim EH, Knight BA, Anderson BG, Park AM, Sherburne Figenshau R, Bhayani SB. Patient comorbidity predicts hospital length of stay after robot-assisted prostatectomy.

J Robot Surg. 2016;10(2):151–6. https://doi.org/10.1007/s11701-016-0588-6.
7. Chitlik A. Safe positioning for robotic-assisted laparoscopic prostatectomy. AORN J. 2011 Jul;94(1):37–45. https://doi.org/10.1016/j.aorn.2011.02.012.
8. Barnett JC, Hurd WW, Rogers RM Jr, Williams NL, Shapiro SA. Laparoscopic positioning and nerve injuries. J Minim Invasive Gynecol. 2007 Sep–Oct;14(5):664–72. https://doi.org/10.1016/j.jmig.2007.04.008.
9. Shveiky D, Aseff JN, Iglesia CB. Brachial plexus injury after laparoscopic and robotic surgery. J Minim Invasive Gynecol. 2010;17(4):414–20. https://doi.org/10.1016/j.jmig.2010.02.010.
10. Sotelo RJ, Haese A, Machuca V, Medina L, Nunez L, Santinelli F, et al. Safer surgery by learning from complications: a focus on robotic prostate surgery. Eur Urol. 2016;69:334–44.
11. Ahmad G, Gent D, Henderson D, O'Flynn H, Phillips K, Watson A. Laparoscopic entry techniques. Cochrane Database Syst Rev. 2015;2:CD006583. https://doi.org/10.1002/14651858.CD006583.
12. Horovitz D, Feng C, Messing EM, Joseph JV. Extraperitoneal vs transperitoneal robot-assisted radical prostatectomy in the setting of prior abdominal or pelvic surgery. J Endourol. 2017;31:366–73.
13. Tourinho-Barbosa RR, Tobias-Machado M, Castro-Alfaro A, Ogaya-Pinies G, Cathelineau X, Sanchez-Salas R. Complications in robotic urological surgeries and how to avoid them: a systematic review. Arab J Urol. 2018;16(3):285–92. https://doi.org/10.1016/j.aju.2017.11.005.
14. Sutton PA, Awad S, Perkins AC, Lobo DN. Comparison of lateral thermal spread using monopolar and bipolar diathermy, the harmonic scalpel and the Ligasure. Br J Surg. 2010 Mar;97(3):428–33. https://doi.org/10.1002/bjs.6901.
15. Canes D, Aron M, Nguyen MM, Winans C, Chand B, Gill IS. Common bile duct injury during urologic laparoscopy. J Endourol. 2008;22(7):1483–4. https://doi.org/10.1089/end.2007.0351.
16. Dal Moro F, Crestani A, Valotto C, Guttilla A, Soncin R, Mangano A, Zattoni F. Anesthesiologic effects of transperitoneal versus extraperitoneal approach during robot-assisted radical prostatectomy: results of a prospective randomized study. Int Braz J Urol. 2015;41(3):466–72. https://doi.org/10.1590/S1677-5538.IBJU.2014.0199.
17. Hong JY, Kim JY, Choi YD, Rha KH, Yoon SJ, Kil HK. Incidence of venous gas embolism during robotic-assisted laparoscopic radical prostatectomy is lower than that during radical retropubic prostatectomy. Br J Anaesth. 2010;105(6):777–81. https://doi.org/10.1093/bja/aeq247.
18. Lebowitz P, Yedlin A, Hakimi AA, Bryan-Brown C, Richards M, Ghavamian R. Respiratory gas exchange during robotic-assisted laparoscopic radical prostatectomy. J Clin Anesth. 2015;27(6):470–5. https://doi.org/10.1016/j.jclinane.2015.06.001.
19. Putman SS, Bishoff JT. Visceral and gastrointestinal complications of laparoscopic and robotic urologic surgery. In: Ghavamian R, editor. Complications of laparoscopic and robotic urologic surgery. New York: Springer; 2010. p. 73–90.
20. Bertolo R, Autorino R, Fiori C, Amparore D, Checcucci E, Mottrie A, Porter J, Haber GP, Derweesh I, Porpiglia F. Expanding the indications of robotic partial nephrectomy for highly complex renal tumors: urologists' perception of the impact of hyperaccuracy three-dimensional reconstruction. J Laparoendosc Adv Surg Tech A. 2019;29(2):233–9. https://doi.org/10.1089/lap.2018.0486.
21. Dionigi G, Boni L, Rovera F, Dionigi R. Dissection and hemostasis with hydroxylated polyvinyl acetal tampons in open thyroid surgery. Ann Surg Innov Res. 2007;1(3):2007. https://doi.org/10.1186/1750-1164-1-3.
22. Richter F, Schnorr D, Deger S, Trk I, Roigas J, Wille A, Loening SA. Improvement of hemostasis in open and laparoscopically performed partial nephrectomy using a gelatin matrix-thrombin tissue sealant (FloSeal). Urology. 2003;61(1):73–7.
23. Rouach Y, Delongchamps NB, Patey N, Fontaine E, Timsit MO, Thiounn N, Mejean A. Suture or hemostatic agent during laparoscopic partial nephrectomy? A randomized study using a hypertensive porcine model. Urology. 2009;73(1):172–7. https://doi.org/10.1016/j.urology.2008.08.477.
24. Gill IS, Ramani AP, Spaliviero M, Xu M, Finelli A, Kaouk JH, Desai MM. Improved hemostasis during laparoscopic partial nephrectomy using gelatin matrix thrombin sealant. Urology. 2005;65(3):463–6. https://doi.org/10.1016/j.urology.2004.10.030.
25. Lavery HJ, Thaly R, Albala D, Ahlering T, Shalhav A, Lee D, Fagin R, Wiklund P, Dasgupta P, Costello AJ, Tewari A, Coughlin G, Patel VR. Robotic equipment malfunction during robotic prostatectomy: a multi-institutional study. J Endourol. 2008;22(9):2165–8. https://doi.org/10.1089/end.2007.0407.
26. Borden LS Jr, Kozlowski PM, Porter CR, Corman JM. Mechanical failure rate of da Vinci robotic system. Can J Urol. 2007;14(2):3499–501.
27. Alemzadeh H, Raman J, Leveson N, Kalbarczyk Z, Iyer RK. Adverse events in robotic surgery: a retrospective study of 14 years of FDA data. PLoS One. 2016;11(4):e0151470. https://doi.org/10.1371/journal.pone.0151470.
28. Lee HJ, Box GN, Abraham JB, Elchico ER, Panah RA, Taylor MB, Moskowitz R, Deane LA, McDougall EM, Clayman RV. Laboratory evaluation of laparoscopic vascular clamps using a load-cell device: are all clamps the same? J Urol. 2008;180(4):1267–72. https://doi.org/10.1016/j.juro.2008.06.018.
29. Tachibana H, Kondo T, Yoshida K, Takagi T, Tanabe K. Lower incidence of postoperative acute kidney injury in robot-assisted partial nephrectomy than in open partial nephrectomy: a propensity score-matched study. J Endourol. 2020;34(7):754–62. https://doi.org/10.1089/end.2019.0622.
30. Schuler TD, Perks AE, Fazio LM, et al. Impact of arterial and arteriovenous renal clamping with and without intrarenal cooling on renal oxygenation and temperature in a porcine model. J Endourol. 2008;22:2367–72.
31. Martini A, Sfakianos JP, Paulucci DJ, et al. Predicting acute kidney injury after robot- assisted partial nephrectomy: implications for patient selection and postoperative management. Urol Oncol. 2019;37:445–51.
32. Jordan BJ, Matulewicz RS, Trihn B, Kundu S. Venous thromboembolism after nephrectomy: incidence, timing and associated risk factors from a national multi-institutional database. World J Urol. 2017;35:1713–9.
33. Abel EJ, Wong K, Sado M, Leverson GE, Patel SR, Downs TM, et al. Surgical operative time increases the risk of deep venous thrombosis and pulmonary embolism in robotic prostatectomy. JSLS. 2014;18:282–7.
34. Tyritzis SI, Wallerstedt A, Steineck G, Nyberg T, Hugosson J, Bjartell A, et al. Thromboembolic complications in 3,544 patients undergoing radical prostatectomy with or without lymph node dissection. J Urol. 2015;193:117–25.
35. Rasmussen MS, Jorgensen LN, Wille-Jorgensen P, Nielsen JD, Horn A, Mohn AC, et al. Prolonged prophylaxis with dalteparin to prevent late thromboembolic complications in patients under-going major abdominal surgery: a multicenter randomized open- label study. J Thromb Haemost. 2006;4:2384–90.
36. Selby LV, Sovel M, Sjoberg DD, McSweeney M, Douglas D, Jones DR, et al. Preoperative chemoprophylaxis is safe in major oncology operations and effective at preventing venous thromboembolism. J Am Coll Surg. 2016;222:129–37.
37. Mattei A, Di Pierro GB, Rafeld V, Konrad C, Beutler J, Danuser H. Positioning injury, rhabdomyolysis, and serum creatine kinase-concentration course in patients undergoing robot-assisted radical

prostatectomy and extended pelvic lymph node dissection. J Endourol. 2013;27:45–51.
38. Karaoren G, Bakan N, Kucuk EV, Gumus E. Is rhabdomyolysis an anaesthetic complication in patients undergoing robot-assisted radical prostatectomy? J Minim Access Surg. 2017;13:29–36.
39. Gezginci E, Ozkaptan O, Yalcin S, Akin Y, Rassweiler J, Gozen AS. Postoperative pain and neuromuscular complications associated with patient positioning after robotic assisted laparoscopic radical prostatectomy: a retrospective non-placebo and non-randomized study. Int Urol Nephrol. 2015;47:1635–41.
40. Gkegkes ID, Karydis A, Tyritzis SI, Iavazzo C. Ocular complications in robotic surgery. Int J Med Robot Comput. 2015;11:269–74.
41. Kan KM, Brown SE, Gainsburg DM. Ocular complications in robotic-assisted prostatectomy: a review of pathophysiology and prevention. Minerva Anestesiol. 2015;81:557–66.
42. Il KD, Woo SH, Lee DH, Kim IY. Incidence of port-site hernias after robot-assisted radical prostatectomy with the fascial closure of only the midline 12-mm port site. J Endourol. 2012;26:848–51.
43. Chitlik A. Safe positioning for robotic-assisted laparoscopic prostatectomy. AORN J. 2011;94:37–48.
44. Dindo D, Clavien PA. Quality assessment of partial nephrectomy complications reporting: time to get the head out of the sand. Eur Urol. 2014;66:527–8.
45. Martin RC 2nd, Brennan MF, Jaques DP. Quality of complication reporting in the surgical literature. Ann Surg. 2002;235:803–13.
46. Dindo D, Demartines N, Clavien PA. Classification of surgical complications: a new proposal with evaluation in a cohort of 6336 patients and results of a survey. Ann Surg. 2004;240:205–13.
47. Tobias-Machado M, Moschovas MC. Inguinal lymphadenectomy. In: Sotelo R, Arriaga J, Aron M, editors. Complications in robotic urologic surgery. Cham: Springer; 2018. https://doi.org/10.1007/978-3-319-62277-4_32.
48. Mitropoulos D, Artibani W, Biyani CS, et al. Quality assessment of partial nephrectomy complications reporting using EAU standardised quality criteria. Eur Urol. 2014;66:522–6.
49. Mitropoulos D, Artibani W, Graefen M, et al. Reporting and grading of complications after urologic surgical procedures: an ad hoc EAU guidelines panel assessment and recommendations. Eur Urol. 2012;61:341–9.
50. Cacciamani GE, Medina LG, Tafuri A, Gill T, Baccaglini W, Blasic V, Glina FPA, De Castro Abreu AL, Sotelo R, Gill IS, Artibani W. Impact of implementation of standardized criteria in the assessment of complication reporting after robotic partial nephrectomy: a systematic review. Eur Urol Focus. 2020;6(3):513–7. https://doi.org/10.1016/j.euf.2018.12.004.
51. Vanlander AE, Mazzone E, Collins JW, Mottrie AM, Rogiers XM, van der Poel HG, Van Herzeele I, Satava RM, Gallagher AG. Orsi consensus meeting on European robotic training (OCERT): results from the first multispecialty consensus meeting on training in robot-assisted surgery. Eur Urol. 2020;78(5):713–6. https://doi.org/10.1016/j.eururo.2020.02.003.

Intraoperative Complications in Urologic Robotic Surgeries

Marcio Covas Moschovas, Marta Anton-Juanilla, and David Bouchier-Hayes

1 Introduction

Since the Food and Drug Administration (FDA) cleared the first robotic surgery in the USA in 2000, several authors have described the outcomes and benefits of this technology in urologic procedures [1–5]. Despite some advantages over laparoscopy and open surgery, robotic technology is not devoid of complications. In this scenario, Alemzadeh et al. reported a retrospective study accessing the nationwide complication rates of robotic surgery in the MAUDE (Manufacture and User Facility Device Experience) database, collected by the FDA. In this study, the author identified 10.624 (0.6%) complication events among 1,745,000 robotic surgeries performed by several specialties from 2000 to 2013 [6]. Urology represented 15% of all complications reported in this period.

Recently, despite the increasing number of robotic procedures performed annually, other authors have reported similar rates of outcomes and complications associated with this type of surgery [7]. In this scenario, this chapter aims to describe different types of intraoperative complications of the robotic approach to urologic surgeries.

2 Robotic Platform and Instrument Malfunction

According to some reports in the literature, the robotic malfunction rates range from 0.4% to 4.6% and include software-related, mechanical, electric, and instrumental failures [8, 9]. Borden et al. reported 2.6% (9 surgeries) of robotic technology failure in a series of 350 radical prostatectomies [9]. Among these cases, six malfunction episodes happened before surgery and three during the procedure. The most common issues reported were setup and arm malfunction. Kozlowski et al. also described issues related to robotic technology in 4.6% of the cases. Overall, the robotic malfunction rates reported by current studies range from 0.4% to 8%, with an average of 3%, while the conversion rates related to these issues can reach up to 2.7%. The most common problems reported by these studies were fallen pieces, broken instruments, arcing tip covers, system errors, and imaging issues [6].

3 Patient Positioning and Cutaneous Lesion Considerations

In our concept, laparoscopic and robotic surgery begins on the correct patient positioning with appropriate mattress and pad protection in all articulations and body contacts with the table. In addition, special attention must be taken to protect the patient's face and eyes.

Several authors have reported in the literature complications related to inappropriate positioning, especially in cases of prolonged operative times and obese patients [10, 11]. In these cases, skin lesion is the most common issue, which is prevented by the initial process of patient positioning and by a final checking before the sterile draping procedure [12]. The operative time length has been described as a risk factor for nerve injury caused by the positioning. According to these studies, for each additional hour of surgery, the nerve injury increases up to 100-fold [13, 14]. Common nerve injuries include the brachial nerve plexus due to hyperabduction in kidney surgery, ulnar nerve injury due to elbow compression against the table corner, radial nerve injury due to hand and wrist compression, and femoral nerve injury due to the lithotomy position in radical prostatectomies and cystectomies.

The robotic arm movement outside of the body is another source of skin lesions. In cases that the trocars are not placed correctly, the working angle is only achieved with an extra angulation of the arms outside of the body. In these situations, the tableside assistant must monitor these movements during the whole procedure to prevent these collisions [15].

M. C. Moschovas (✉)
AdventHealth Global Robotics Institute, Celebration, FL, USA

University of Central Florida, UCF, Orlando, USA

M. Anton-Juanilla · D. Bouchier-Hayes
Galway Clinic, Galway, Ireland

P. Wiklund et al. (eds.), *Robotic Urologic Surgery*, https://doi.org/10.1007/978-3-031-00363-9_51

The CO_2 insufflation is also a potential factor for skin lesions, especially in the scrotum. The gas distention can dissect the scrotal tissues during the surgery leading to an intraoperative scrotal swelling, which causes cutaneous itching and sometimes painful sensations in the postoperative period [16].

All patients undergoing robotic surgery with prolonged operative times have higher risks of rhabdomyolysis, especially during the surgeon's learning period. Some risk factors for this type of complication include the steep Trendelenburg position, obesity, previous peripheral vascular disease, and comorbidities such as cardiac insufficiency [17]. Patients with these clinical characteristics and postoperative muscular pain should have serum CK levels checked in the postoperative period.

Finally, ocular injury is another type of complication related to inappropriate positioning. Some authors described that the chances of corneal abrasion in robotic surgery reach up to 6.5-fold compared to open surgery [18]. In addition, the association between Trendelenburg and pneumoperitoneum increases the intraocular pressure, which could lead, in the worst scenarios, to ischemic neuropathy and vision loss [19, 20].

4 Port Placement Considerations

4.1 Assessment of Surgical Field

Initially, the abdominal wall status and body habitus should be assessed, and special attention should be paid to scars from previous surgeries, extensive midline incisions, or umbilical hernia repairs, which may have had the placement of surgical mesh. In addition, a note should be taken of any umbilical or paraumbilical hernias, as the bowel may be very close to the skin incision and initial entry into the abdomen.

In obese patients, the use of extra-long bariatric trocars may need to be contemplated. It should be noted that any abdominal cavity may have bowel and (or) omentum adherent to the abdominal wall, often secondary to an unrecognized intra-abdominal inflammatory process, even if there is no history of previous surgery.

4.2 Abdominal Access Techniques

There are two commonly used methods for obtaining initial entry into the abdominal cavity to establish an initial pneumoperitoneum: the Veress needle technique and Hasson's technique. Both are routinely employed, and each one has its proponents. This initial point of entry is probably the most dangerous moment of trocar insertion, as it is not done under direct view.

4.2.1 Veress Needle Technique

This technique relies on using a specialized insertion needle with a unique valve system on it, which is passed in a blind puncture method, allowing for initial CO_2 insufflation of the abdominal cavity. The Veress needle has a two-cylinder design consisting of an outer short and a long inner component. The inner cylinder has a retractable blunt tip, which retracts, deploying the outer sharp edge when contacting resilient structures, allowing passage through the abdominal wall. A "click" may be audible when the blunt tip has re-engaged after passage through the abdominal fascia. This, in conjunction with tactile feedback, allows the surgeon to determine when to stop needle advancement [21].

Once the Veress needle is in place, before starting insufflation, several maneuvers can be used to confirm proper positioning (e.g., needle aspiration, injection and recovery, "drop test," and the initial intraperitoneal pressure test). It is usually advised to place the Veress needle far from previous surgical scars. For Bianchi et al., the bowel perforation rate with the blind access technique was 0.33% [22].

When the Veress needle perforates an intra-abdominal organ and no enteric content or a hollow viscus is observed, conservative treatment may be an option [23]. Usually, when the Veress needle is in the bowel, asymmetrical abdominal distension will appear, and the insufflation must be stopped immediately. The management will depend on the severity of the injury. Laparoscopic intracorporeal suturing techniques or open surgery based on the experience of the operating surgeon are valid approaches.

Once the pneumoperitoneum is established, the primary trocar must be inserted. As there is no direct visual guidance, it is responsible for most trocar-induced bowel injuries [24]. Thus, the first step with the camera is the abdominal cavity inspection for detecting potential injuries.

Trocar insertion in upper abdominal accesses may also result in gastric perforation. Therefore, fasting for 8 h before surgery and inserting an oro- or nasogastric tube can minimize this risk. The needle should never be moved or "waggled" around, as that can convert a minor vascular or visceral injury into a larger one, which can become a significant life-threatening emergency.

4.2.2 Hasson Open Technique

This is an open cutdown technique, which decreases (but does negate) the risk of blind entry into an abdominal viscera [25]. The initial incision should be planned above the umbilicus, approximately 20 cm from the root of the penis. The skin is incised, and the dissection is performed by planes until reaching the peritoneum layer below the rectus abdominis muscle. The peritoneum is then opened, and the surgeon's finger is passed into the opening to check for visceral adhesions. In sequence, the trocar is placed without the obturator, and the CO_2 insufflation is commenced.

Initially, a low flow of 5 L/min is recommended, while an assessment of intra-abdominal pressure is made. Care should be taken with a rapid increase in pressure due to cardiorespiratory issues or evidence of a pulmonary gas embolus. Upon full insufflation, the robotic camera is inserted carefully in a freehand manner, and a full laparoscopy is performed. Then, all trocars are placed under visualization.

It is important to note that this technique usually provides an incision bigger than the trocar caliber. Thus, especially in the Xi robot, which has 8 mm trocars, CO_2 leakage can happen around the trocar. In these cases, performing an aponeurotic suture (U shape) provides an appropriate CO_2 sealing.

4.2.3 Insertion of Additional Trocars

After placing the first trocar and inserting the camera, the remaining ports are placed using similar principles under direct vision. The 8 mm robotic ports should be positioned between 7 and 10 cm from each other to minimize clashing of robotic arms. These arms should also be 10–20 cm from the target organ. The ruler and marking pen are used here to measure the appropriate distances and mark potential insertion sites [26].

Finally, trocar placement is one part of the procedure that has to be done in part without the benefit of direct vision, and injuries to large vessels, bowel, and other abdominal contents can have catastrophic consequences and turn a routine procedure into potentially disastrous outcomes. Thus, it is worthwhile to have a standardized trocar insertion technique associated with the ability to respond to the variabilities that each step may pose.

5 Pneumoperitoneum Considerations

Pneumoperitoneum insufflation (PI) is crucial in laparoscopic and robotic surgeries to provide the appropriate space for performing the procedure. However, this process is not devoid of complications. The initial access to the abdominal cavity with Veress needle puncture must be performed cautiously due to potential bowel or vascular injury, especially in patients with previous abdominal surgeries (higher chances of adhesions) and low BMI (shorter space between the skin and aortocaval space).

Another consideration regards the prolonged operative time with intra-abdominal CO_2 insufflation due to increased hypercapnia and metabolic acidosis ricks, especially in smokers and patients with chronic obstructive pulmonary disease (COPD). In such cases, some authors have described pneumoperitoneum insufflation with helium gas as an alternative to CO_2 [27–29].

Finally, the rate of CO_2 insufflation is also important due to the increased risk of embolic events, hypotension, and vagal response. Monitoring the rapid increase of intra-abdominal pressure is crucial, mainly when operating patients with cardiovascular diseases and morbid obesity due to the asystole and ventilation issues during the surgery [11].

6 Thermal Injury

The robotic platform usually provides two sources of intraoperative energy: monopolar and bipolar. Stray energy can be transferred from the instruments to the camera, other instruments, and trocar by different mechanisms. For this reason, all instruments must have the insulation sleeve as a security measure for minimizing stray energy [16].

Surgical technique refinement is also another way of minimizing thermal injuries. Before activating the pedal energy (monopolar or bipolar), the surgeon needs to certify that the instruments are not in contact with each other and that the arm is not touching the bowel, vessels, or adjacent structures; only the tip of the instrument must be in contact with the bleeding tissue to be cauterized. Having a thermal injury outside of the operative view is challenging because it usually has a clinical impact a couple of days after surgery (5–10 days); patients typically complain of abdominal pain and ileus symptoms (constipation and vomits).

7 Visceral and Vascular Injury Considerations

Visceral and vascular injuries are rare events in laparoscopic and robotic surgeries. Some authors described that the likelihood of these complications could reach up to 0.1%, with vascular injury more common. Some risk factors include prior abdominal surgery, which increases the rates of adhesions and changes the intra-abdominal anatomy. In these cases, it is advised to perform the trocar placement with Hasson's technique or Palmer's point access [30, 31]. In addition, patients with low BMI have a smaller distance between the skin and aortocaval space, which is easier for vascular lesions while placing the Veress needle or trocar.

In both situations (visceral or vascular injuries), the management and repair must be performed immediately, even if that requires converting to open surgery or even canceling the main procedure. Depending on the type of injury or severity, it is advised to have a specialist reviewing the lesion (vascular or general surgeon) before the procedure is finished.

Some considerations during the vascular injury regard the assistant role in these episodes. Due to extensive bleeding, the assistant must associate the blood suction with the vessel compression. The most important initial step is the compression to minimize blood loss; then performing suction will clear the field for surgical repair. Performing suction without local compression increases blood loss and aggravates the patient clinical scenario. Special attention must be taken while increasing the pneumoperitoneum pressure in bleeding episodes to avoid gas embolization. Consider using laparoscopic bulldog clamps and vessel loops in big vessels, such as aorta and vena cava injuries, to minimize the blood loss and optimize the lesion visualization during the repairing process.

7.1 Bowel Injury Caused by Electrocautery and Mechanical Effects

Thermal damage can get unrecognized during the surgery and cause serious complications. Frequently, it results from monopolar electrosurgical current activated unintentionally outside the operational field or unwanted energy transfer during tissue dissection. Monopolar energy causes more lateral thermal spread and produces the highest temperatures than bipolar electrocautery, the harmonic scalpel, and LigaSure [22]. Thermal injury is usually more extensive than expected, and conservative management can result in acute perforation during the postoperative period. Intraoperative repair is usually significantly safer. If an enterotomy is required, all bowel edges must be refreshed, and all affected tissue removed before the primary repair [22]. The injured site should be drained, and the patient must be prescribed antibiotic treatment [24].

Furthermore, robotic arms with no tactile feedback can cause mechanical bowel injuries. These lesions can be sharp or blunt and mainly occur outside the operative field. Therefore, all tissue handling and instrument insertion must be performed under direct view.

Mechanical bowel injuries are managed with intracorporeal suturing. Bowel resection and a diverting colostomy are rarely required, and if there is an extensive injury or a bowel resection is necessary, a general surgeon must be consulted. Unrecognized bowel injuries usually present as sepsis and acute abdominal pain in the postoperative period. Other signs and symptoms are leukopenia or leukocytosis, fever, orifice pain trocar, ileus, nausea, or vomiting. In these scenarios, a CT scan usually supports the diagnosis. In cases with high suspicion, a diagnostic laparoscopy should be performed.

7.2 Spleen and Liver Injuries

Most splenic lesions (0.3%) happen during left upper urinary tract surgeries when the retroperitoneum is exposed to mobilize the spleen [21]. On the other hand, liver injury is uncommon, although the true incidence is difficult to estimate because minor injuries are not usually reported.

Compression and cautery are usually enough to manage minor injuries to both organs [23]. Splenectomy due to a severe injury with massive bleeding is rare. Open surgical repair of the liver can be necessary in cases of uncontrolled bleeding [21]. Bile duct injuries appear in the right adrenalectomy and partial nephrectomy. Prompt recognition and cholangiography to stage the damage direct the appropriate treatment, whether endoscopic or surgical.

7.3 Pancreatic Injury

Pancreatic injury is also a rare complication (incidence 0.2%) but can have substantial morbidity. The organ is damaged typically during left adrenalectomy or left renal surgery. The best advice to prevent this complication is a careful dissection of the upper renal pole, between the tail of the pancreas and Gerota's fascia [22].

Although most superficial lesions are managed conservatively with parenteral nutrition, somatostatin administration, and drainage, a major pancreatic duct injury may require distal pancreatectomy. In this scenario, a general surgeon consultation is always advised [24].

7.4 Rectal Injury

Rectal injury is the most common intestinal complication during radical prostatectomy, but it can also occur during radical cystectomy. The incidence rate is 0.17% for robot-assisted radical prostatectomy and 1% for robot-assisted radical cystectomy [32, 33]. These lesions convert the surgery from clean to contaminated, increasing the risk of wound infection, pelvic abscess, recto-urinary fistula, sepsis, or even death [26].

Some factors, such as previous prostate or rectal surgery, radiotherapy, pelvic fracture, or hormonal therapy, might distort surgical planes leading to challenging dissections and increasing the risk of rectal injury [34]. Other factors include a locally advanced disease, non-nerve-sparing extrafascial-wide excision, and blunt dissection.

Surgeon expertise is an essential factor in avoiding complications. According to the learning curve of a single-center analysis, 150 to 200 cases were needed to decrease complications as bowel injury [35]. For Guiote et al., hospitals with more than 100 robot-assisted radical cystectomies per year also have lower complication rates [33].

Management of rectal injury depends on its presentation. Once the rectal wall and muscular layers are identified, a continuous absorbable suture is performed. Several ways of rectal repair have been described. Some surgeons close the defect in two planes, while others use only one layer of barbed suture. Longitudinal closure may be preferred over a transverse or Heineke-Mikulicz technique to minimize anastomotic tension since the rectal luminal diameter is usually sufficient to obviate significant narrowing [22].

The rectal repair can be further reinforced by overlaying an omental flap from the transverse colon. Obtaining an omental flap might sometimes be challenging in patients undergoing transperitoneal RARP because of the steep Trendelenburg position. Therefore, a full-layer peritoneal graft obtained from the pelvic sidewall can alternatively be used as a third layer to cover the area of RI repair [36].

The repair integrity is checked by filling the pelvic cavity with sterile saline and the rectum with air. In addition, methylene blue can be injected into the rectum, while the surgeon observes the anastomosis. At the end of the procedure, the abdomen is drained, and the patient is prescribed broad-spectrum antibiotics [23].

Although a routine diverting colostomy has been recommended in the past, nowadays, it is only reserved for cases of massive fecal spillage, previous radiotherapy, extensive rectal injury (>2 cm) with cautery application, or a tense suture line [26]. Recent literature continues to advocate primary closure for rectal injury. Kheterpal et al. described a single-surgeon series of 4400 RARP, including 10 intraoperative rectal injuries [37]. All lesions were closed with a two-layer suture and only in one case required diverting ileostomy.

If the diagnosis of the rectal injury is delayed, the early postoperative symptoms manifest as lower abdominal pain, fever, abnormal white blood cell count, and sepsis [23]. In such cases, investigation with a Gastrografin enema, retrograde urethrography, or CT scan might confirm the diagnosis.

8 Compartment Syndrome (CS)

Compartment syndrome (CS) is an uncommon but possibly underappreciated potential complication of RARP, especially in complex cases or initial learning curve, where operative time is extensive. The underlying cause of CS is the increasing pressure in the muscle compartments surrounded by inelastic fascia due to swelling or edema. This condition leads to an eventual increase in pressure in the compartment above perfusion pressure, which potentially disrupts the oxygenated blood flow and, in the worst scenarios, causes tissue necrosis [38]. The CS pathophysiology describes a rise of the internal compartment pressure to above 30 mmHg, although it can occur at lower pressures.

Lower limb compartment syndrome (LLCS) following RARP can be devastating, including loss of motor function, foot drop, permanent disability and mobility restriction, lower limb amputation, renal failure from rhabdomyolysis, and death.

Some authors described the CS incidence as reaching up to 0.29% [38]. This rate equates to three cases per thousand, so it is possible that most moderate to high volume surgeons may come across it once in their career. LLCS is often related to lithotomy position due to excessive pressure on the calf muscles by the weight of the leg. Trendelenburg positioning can also contribute to LLCS in the setting of RARP [38]. Predisposing factors include the following:

1. Extended time in lithotomy over 4 h increases the risk of LLCS, but it can occur in cases that last less than an hour.
2. Blood loss/hypovolemia
3. Hypotension
4. Obesity
5. Muscular, tight calves
6. Smoking
7. Peripheral vascular disease
8. Compression of iliac vessels such as during lymphadenectomy.

8.1 CS Clinical Presentation

LLCS usually manifests in the first few hours after surgery, but the symptoms may present later in some cases. Pain is usually the first major complaint, which is out of proportion to the injury and usually increases on passive stretching. The tissue may also feel tense and "woody." The traditional conglomeration of symptoms is described by the "the Five P's," including pain, pulselessness, paresthesia, pallor, and paralysis [39]. However, these may be late signs, and pain should be considered a cardinal sign, although this may be confused with the pain from deep vein thrombosis and may be masked by epidural analgesia use. Paresthesia or loss of sensation in the first interdigital web space of the foot is also related to the CS. The diagnosis is clinical, but measuring intracompartmental pressures using either a transducer-tipped catheter or a conventional fluid-filled system is also helpful.

8.2 CS Surgical Intervention

There is no universal agreement on the precise intracompartmental pressure at which intervention should be considered. The decision to operate should be made in conjunction with clinical findings, although a value of >30 mm Hg usually shows that surgical decompression is needed. Alternatively, the perfusion pressure of the compartment is used, or compartment delta pressure, which is the diastolic pressure minus the intracompartmental pressure. If this value is less than 30 mmHg, there is an imminent risk of anoxia and ischemia, which requires intervention [40]. Serial creatine kinase levels sequentially elevated occur with increasing muscle damage [41]. In such cases, renal function should be serially assessed as renal impairment may occur secondary to rhabdomyolysis [42].

The procedure of choice for LLCS is urgent fasciotomy of the compartments of the below-knee compartments to allow the release of pressure. This should be done as soon as possible and usually requires the intervention of orthopedic, trauma, plastic, or general surgery depending on what expertise is available. It is vital to open the anterior compartment as this is the one most commonly affected, but more extensive fasciotomy with the opening of other compartments is often needed. Repeat inspections of the muscle bellies under anesthesia are usually required, and skin grafts are often employed to close the resultant defect [43].

The risk of CS is lowered by reduced operative time and keeping the legs in a flat position instead of using stirrups and the lithotomy position. There is no significant association of the use of mechanical thromboprophylaxis and compartment syndrome [44, 45].

9 Conclusion

Robotic surgery has evolved in the past 20 years. However, like any other type of surgical procedure, this approach is not devoid of complications. In this chapter, we have described the most common types of complications reported in the current literature. The main concept, common to all episodes of complications, is the immediate identification and repair of accidental lesions. In our experience, appropriate team training, surgical technique standardization, and high volume are crucial factors for increasing expertise and proficiency while minimizing surgical complications in robotic surgery.

References

1. Covas Moschovas M, Helman T, Reddy S, Bhat S, Rogers TP, Sandri M, Noel J, Patel V. Minimally invasive lymphocele drainage using the da Vinci® single port platform: step-by-step technique of a prostate cancer referral center. J Endourol. 2021;35(9):1357–64. https://doi.org/10.1089/end.2020.1175.
2. Noël J, Moschovas MC, Sandri M, Bhat S, Rogers T, Reddy S, Corder C, Patel V. Patient surgical satisfaction after da Vinci® single-port and multi-port robotic-assisted radical prostatectomy: propensity score-matched analysis. J Robot Surg. 2021;18:1–9. https://doi.org/10.1007/s11701-021-01269-6.
3. Moschovas MC, Timóteo F, Lins L, de Castro NO, Seetharam Bhat KR, Patel VR. Robotic surgery techniques to approach benign prostatic hyperplasia disease: a comprehensive literature review and the state of art. Asian J Urol. 2021 Jan;8(1):81–8. https://doi.org/10.1016/j.ajur.2020.10.002.
4. Covas Moschovas M, Bhat S, Rogers T, Thiel D, Onol F, Roof S, Sighinolfi MC, Rocco B, Patel V. Applications of the da Vinci single port (SP) robotic platform in urology: a systematic literature review. Minerva Urol Nephrol. 2021;73(1):6–16. https://doi.org/10.23736/S0393-2249.20.03899-0.
5. Giedelman C, Covas Moschovas M, Bhat S, Brunelle L, Ogaya-Pinies G, Roof S, Corder C, Patel V, Palmer KJ. Establishing a successful robotic surgery program and improving operating room efficiency: literature review and our experience report. J Robot Surg. 2021;15(3):435–42. https://doi.org/10.1007/s11701-020-01121-3.
6. Alemzadeh H, Raman J, Leveson N, Kalbarczyk Z, Iyer RK. Adverse events in robotic surgery: a retrospective study of 14 years of FDA data. PLoS One. 2016;11(4):e0151470. https://doi.org/10.1371/journal.pone.0151470.
7. Muaddi H, Hafid ME, Choi WJ, Lillie E, de Mestral C, Nathens A, Stukel TA, Karanicolas PJ. Clinical outcomes of robotic surgery compared to conventional surgical approaches (laparoscopic or open): a systematic overview of reviews. Ann Surg. 2021;273(3):467–73. https://doi.org/10.1097/SLA.0000000000003915.
8. Lavery HJ, Thaly R, Albala D, Ahlering T, Shalhav A, Lee D, Fagin R, Wiklund P, Dasgupta P, Costello AJ, Tewari A, Coughlin G, Patel VR. Robotic equipment malfunction during robotic prostatectomy: a multi-institutional study. J Endourol. 2008;22(9):2165–8. https://doi.org/10.1089/end.2007.0407. PMID: 18811574
9. Borden LS Jr, Kozlowski PM, Porter CR, Corman JM. Mechanical failure rate of da Vinci robotic system. Can J Urol. 2007;14(2):3499–501.
10. Sundi D, Reese AC, Mettee LZ, Trock BJ, Pavlovich CP. Laparoscopic and robotic radical prostatectomy outcomes in obese and extremely obese men. Urology. 2013;82(3):600–5. https://doi.org/10.1016/j.urology.2013.05.013.
11. Potretzke AM, Kim EH, Knight BA, Anderson BG, Park AM, Sherburne Figenshau R, Bhayani SB. Patient comorbidity predicts hospital length of stay after robot-assisted prostatectomy. J Robot Surg. 2016;10(2):151–6. https://doi.org/10.1007/s11701-016-0588-6.
12. Chitlik A. Safe positioning for robotic-assisted laparoscopic prostatectomy. AORN J. 2011 Jul;94(1):37–45. https://doi.org/10.1016/j.aorn.2011.02.012.
13. Barnett JC, Hurd WW, Rogers RM Jr, Williams NL, Shapiro SA. Laparoscopic positioning and nerve injuries. J Minim Invasive Gynecol. 2007 Sep–Oct;14(5):664–72. https://doi.org/10.1016/j.jmig.2007.04.008.
14. Shveiky D, Aseff JN, Iglesia CB. Brachial plexus injury after laparoscopic and robotic surgery. J Minim Invasive Gynecol. 2010;17(4):414–20. https://doi.org/10.1016/j.jmig.2010.02.010.
15. Sotelo RJ, Haese A, Machuca V, Medina L, Nunez L, Santinelli F, et al. Safer surgery by learning from complications: a focus on robotic prostate surgery. Eur Urol. 2016;69:334–44.
16. Tourinho-Barbosa RR, Tobias-Machado M, Castro-Alfaro A, Ogaya-Pinies G, Cathelineau X, Sanchez-Salas R. Complications in robotic urological surgeries and how to avoid them: a systematic review. Arab J Urol. 2018;16(3):285–92. https://doi.org/10.1016/j.aju.2017.11.005.
17. Karaoren G, Bakan N, Kucuk EV, Gumus E. Is rhabdomyolysis an anaesthetic complication in patients undergoing robot-assisted radical prostatectomy? J Minim Access Surg. 2017;13:29–36.
18. Sampat A, Parakati I, Kunnavakkam R, Glick DB, Lee NK, Tenney M, et al. Corneal abrasion in hysterectomy and prostatectomy: role of laparoscopic and robotic assistance. Anesthesiology. 2015;122:994–1001.
19. Gkegkes ID, Karydis A, Tyritzis SI, Iavazzo C. Ocular complications in robotic surgery. Int J Med Robot Comput. 2015;11:269–74.
20. Kan KM, Brown SE, Gainsburg DM. Ocular complications in robotic-assisted prostatectomy: a review of pathophysiology and prevention. Minerva Anestesiol. 2015;81:557–66.

21. Putman SS, Bishoff JT. Visceral and gastrointestinal complications of laparoscopic and robotic urologic surgery. In: Ghavamian R, editor. Complications of laparoscopic and robotic urologic surgery. New York: Springer; 2010. p. 73–90.
22. Sutton PA, Awad S, Perkins AC, Lobo DN. Comparison of lateral thermal spread using monopolar and bipolar diathermy, the harmonic scalpel and the Ligasure. Br J Surg. 2010;97(3):428–33. https://doi.org/10.1002/bjs.6901.
23. Velilla G, Redondo C, Sánchez-Salas R, Rozet F, Cathelineau X. Visceral and gastrointestinal complications in robotic urologic surgery. Actas Urol Esp (Engl Ed). 2018;42(2):77–85. https://doi.org/10.1016/j.acuro.2016.12.010.
24. Canes D, Aron M, Nguyen MM, Winans C, Chand B, Gill IS. Common bile duct injury during urologic laparoscopy. J Endourol. 2008;22(7):1483–4. https://doi.org/10.1089/end.2007.0351.
25. Hasson HM. A modified instrument and method for laparoscopy. Am J Obstet Gynecol. 1971;110(6):886–7. https://doi.org/10.1016/0002-9378(71)90593-x.
26. Yee DS, Ornstein DK. Repair of rectal injury during robotic-assisted laparoscopic prostatectomy. Urology. 2008;72(2):428–31. https://doi.org/10.1016/j.urology.2007.12.022.
27. Dal Moro F, Crestani A, Valotto C, Guttilla A, Soncin R, Mangano A, Zattoni F. Anesthesiologic effects of transperitoneal versus extraperitoneal approach during robot-assisted radical prostatectomy: results of a prospective randomized study. Int Braz J Urol. 2015;41(3):466–72. https://doi.org/10.1590/S1677-5538.IBJU.2014.0199.
28. Hong JY, Kim JY, Choi YD, Rha KH, Yoon SJ, Kil HK. Incidence of venous gas embolism during robotic-assisted laparoscopic radical prostatectomy is lower than that during radical retropubic prostatectomy. Br J Anaesth. 2010;105(6):777–81. https://doi.org/10.1093/bja/aeq247.
29. Lebowitz P, Yedlin A, Hakimi AA, Bryan-Brown C, Richards M, Ghavamian R. Respiratory gas exchange during robotic-assisted laparoscopic radical prostatectomy. J Clin Anesth. 2015;27(6):470–5. https://doi.org/10.1016/j.jclinane.2015.06.001.
30. Ahmad G, Gent D, Henderson D, O'Flynn H, Phillips K, Watson A. Laparoscopic entry techniques. Cochrane Database Syst Rev. 2015;2:CD006583. https://doi.org/10.1002/14651858.CD006583.
31. Horovitz D, Feng C, Messing EM, Joseph JV. Extraperitoneal vs transperitoneal robot-assisted radical prostatectomy in the setting of prior abdominal or pelvic surgery. J Endourol. 2017;31:366–73.
32. Wedmid A, Mendoza P, Sharma S, Hastings RL, Monahan KP, Walicki M, Ahlering TE, Porter J, Castle EP, Ahmed F, Engel JD, Frazier HA 2nd, Eun D, Lee DI. Rectal injury during robot-assisted radical prostatectomy: incidence and management. J Urol. 2011;186(5):1928–33. https://doi.org/10.1016/j.juro.2011.07.004.
33. Guiote I, Gaya JM, Gausa L, Rodríguez O, Palou J. Complications from robot-assisted radical cystectomy: where do we stand? Actas Urol Esp. 2016;40(2):108–14. https://doi.org/10.1016/j.acuro.2015.03.002.
34. Mandel P, Linnemannstöns A, Chun F, Schlomm T, Pompe R, Budäus L, Rosenbaum C, Ludwig T, Dahlem R, Fisch M, Graefen M, Huland H, Tilki D, Steuber T. Incidence, risk factors, management, and complications of rectal injuries during radical prostatectomy. Eur Urol Focus. 2018;4(4):554–7. https://doi.org/10.1016/j.euf.2017.01.008.
35. Ou YC, Yang CR, Wang J, Yang CK, Cheng CL, Patel VR, Tewari AK. The learning curve for reducing complications of robotic-assisted laparoscopic radical prostatectomy by a single surgeon. BJU Int. 2011;108(3):420–5. https://doi.org/10.1111/j.1464-410X.2010.09847.x.
36. Canda AE, Tilki D, Mottrie A. Rectal injury during radical prostatectomy: focus on robotic surgery. Eur Urol Oncol. 2018;1(6):507–9. https://doi.org/10.1016/j.euo.2018.07.007.
37. Kheterpal E, Bhandari A, Siddiqui S, Pokala N, Peabody J, Menon M. Management of rectal injury during robotic radical prostatectomy. Urology. 2011;77(4):976–9. https://doi.org/10.1016/j.urology.2010.11.045.
38. Simms MS, Terry TR. Well leg compartment syndrome after pelvic and perineal surgery in the lithotomy position. Postgrad Med J. 2005;81(958):534–6. https://doi.org/10.1136/pgmj.2004.030965.
39. Andrews LW. Neurovascular assessment. Adv Clin Care. 1990;5(6):5–7.
40. Frink M, Hildebrand F, Krettek C, Brand J, Hankemeier S. Compartment syndrome of the lower leg and foot. Clin Orthop Relat Res. 2010;468(4):940–50. https://doi.org/10.1007/s11999-009-0891-x.
41. Nilsson A, Alkner B, Wetterlöv P, Wetterstad S, Palm L, Schilcher J. Low compartment pressure and myoglobin levels in tibial fractures with suspected acute compartment syndrome. BMC Musculoskelet Disord. 2019;20(1):15. https://doi.org/10.1186/s12891-018-2394-y.
42. Zutt R, van der Kooi AJ, Linthorst GE, Wanders RJ, de Visser M. Rhabdomyolysis: review of the literature. Neuromuscul Disord. 2014;24(8):651–9. https://doi.org/10.1016/j.nmd.2014.05.005.
43. Tillinghast CM, Gary JL. Compartment syndrome of the lower extremity. In: Mauffrey C, Hak DJ, Martin III MP, editors. Compartment syndrome: a guide to diagnosis and management [internet]. Cham: Springer; 2019.
44. Gelder C, McCallum AL, Macfarlane AJR, Anderson JH. A systematic review of mechanical thromboprophylaxis in the lithotomy position. Surgeon. 2018;16(6):365–71. https://doi.org/10.1016/j.surge.2018.03.005.
45. Tobias-Machado M, Moschovas MC. Inguinal lymphadenectomy. In: Sotelo R, Arriaga J, Aron M, editors. Complications in robotic urologic surgery. Cham: Springer; 2018. https://doi.org/10.1007/978-3-319-62277-4_32.

Technical Advances in Robotic Renal Surgery

Stefano Puliatti, Carlo Andrea Bravi, Pieter De Backer, and Erdem Canda

1 Introduction

The surgical discipline revolves around the use of medical technologies and where the initial medical devices were just scalpels; today's armamentarium consists of complex technologies. Laparoscopy is one of the areas where technical breakthroughs have impacted the way patients are treated. In nearly 30 years, it has become the standard of care in many indications [1, 2]. Despite this success, laparoscopic surgery is limited by the prolonged learning curve, the 2D vision, the limited range of motion of the laparoscopic instruments, and the unsatisfactory movement ergonomics [3]. In 1999, a new surgical system (da Vinci Surgical System, InSite Vision Systems, Intuitive Surgical Inc., Mountain View, CA, USA) was developed and initially used by cardiac surgeons at the University Hospital of Frankfurt, Germany. However, this system is not an autonomous robot, but a robotic assistance system for laparoscopic surgery that addressed the limits of laparoscopy. This system was then used for the first time in the urological field, in the same center, for a series of ten radical prostatectomies [4]. Since then, the robotic approach changed the landscape of urological surgery, ultimately crowning itself as the gold standard over other alternatives (open and laparoscopic surgery) in different procedures, including renal surgery [2, 5]. Several innovations facilitated the acceptance and diffusion of this technology, allowing for the implementation of both pre- and intraoperative performance.

S. Puliatti (✉)
Department of Urology, Onze Lieve Vrouw Hospital, Aalst, Belgium

ORSI Academy, Melle, Belgium

Department of Urology, University of Modena & Reggio Emilia, Modena, Italy

C. A. Bravi
Department of Urology, Onze Lieve Vrouw Hospital, Aalst, Belgium

ORSI Academy, Melle, Belgium

Unit of Urology, Division of Experimental Oncology, Urological Research Institute (URI), IRCCS San Raffaele Scientific Institute, Vita-Salute San Raffaele University, Milan, Italy

P. De Backer
Department of Urology, Onze Lieve Vrouw Hospital, Aalst, Belgium

ORSI Academy, Melle, Belgium

Department of Urology, Ghent University Hospital, Ghent, Belgium

E. Canda
Department of Urology, School of Medicine, Koç University, Istanbul, Turkey

2 Preoperative Planning

2.1 Three-Dimensional (3D) Models

In the era of precision surgery, a comprehensive and patient-specific understanding of surgical anatomy is the cornerstone of procedural planning, especially in oncologic surgery [6]. Conventionally, surgical roadmaps are created based on cross-sectional imaging studies, mainly computed tomography (CT), magnetic resonance imaging (MRI), positron emission tomography/CT (PET), and/or single photon emission CT [7]. However, this may render a suboptimal evaluation of the patient's anatomy as it is based on bidimensional images; thus, it requires sophisticated cognitive processing to conceptualize a 3D reconstruction from the 2D images, and subsequently relate such information to the repositioned patient [8]. Hence, it comes as no surprise that nowadays technological advances such as 3D printing and/or 3D virtual models of target organs have been applied with increasing interest in surgical planning [6–11].

Porpiglia et al. [6] used the Polyjet® technology to produce a 3D printed model of the prostate or kidney of 18 patients undergoing live surgery (robot-assisted laparoscopic prostatectomy [RALP] or minimally invasive partial nephrectomy) in a urology meeting. These models were used by surgeons to discuss the case with the patient and to eluci-

P. Wiklund et al. (eds.), *Robotic Urologic Surgery*, https://doi.org/10.1007/978-3-031-00363-9_52

date the optimal surgical plan with the attendees. Following the surgery, 144 attendees were asked to fill in a questionnaire, which showed that this tool is convenient for surgical planning and patient education [6]. Similarly, von Rundstedt et al. expanded the use of renal models beyond surgical decision-making into preoperative rehearsal and training. Interestingly, the authors reported no significant difference between resection times and tumor volumes of the models and the actual tumors, demonstrating the usefulness of this as a training tool [9].

Three-dimensional visualization techniques have been particularly applied for the surgical planning of robot-assisted partial nephrectomy (RAPN) (Fig. 1) [7–12]. Different nephrometry scores (based on bidimensional CT scans) are commonly used to predict perioperative outcomes of patients receiving RAPN. Thus, 3D virtual models were proposed to improve the prediction of surgical complexity in patients with renal masses [11]. In fact, such models reduced the predicted anatomical complexity of renal masses using different nephrometry scores compared to the 2D images [8, 12]. Interestingly, when the CT scans of 20 complex renal masses were showed to 108 attendees of the sixth Techno-urology Meeting (overall, 542 views), RAPN was selected in only 47.2% of the views. Subsequently, the attendees viewed the 3D virtual models of the same patients, and the indication for RAPN increased to 74.5% [7]. Furthermore, the use of these models allowed for an increased rate of selective arterial clamping, resulting in significantly fewer patients with complex renal masses receiving total ischemia during RAPN (80.6% versus 23.8%; $p < 0.001$) [10]. Very recently, new predictive 3D models are finding their way into clinical trials, in which the surgeon gets a suggestion on the clamping strategy, allowing him to upfront estimate the ischemic and perfused zones of the tumor bed [13]. This way, the surgeon should be able to make a better estimation on the benefit of a clamped, an unclamped, or a selective clamped approach.

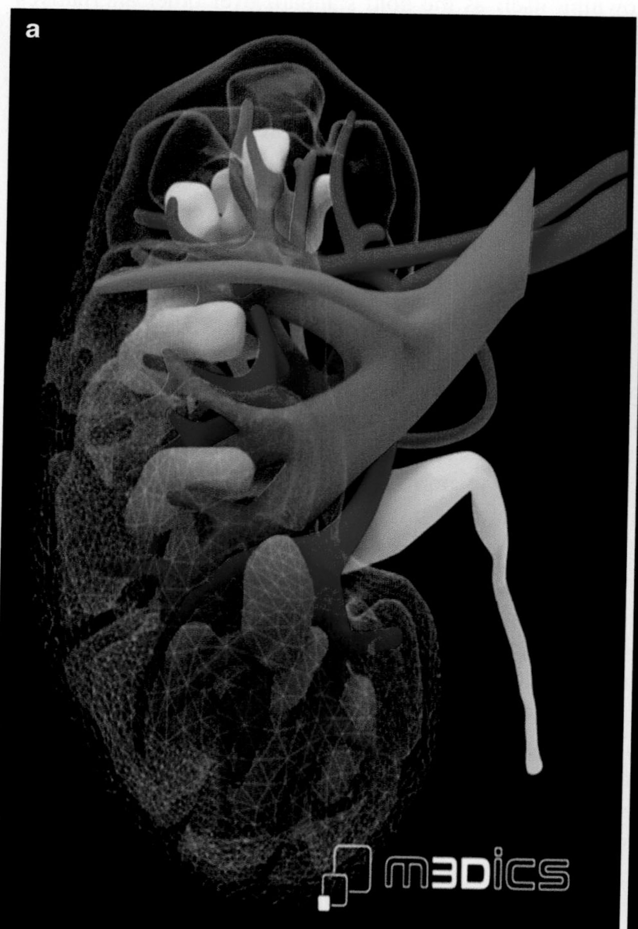

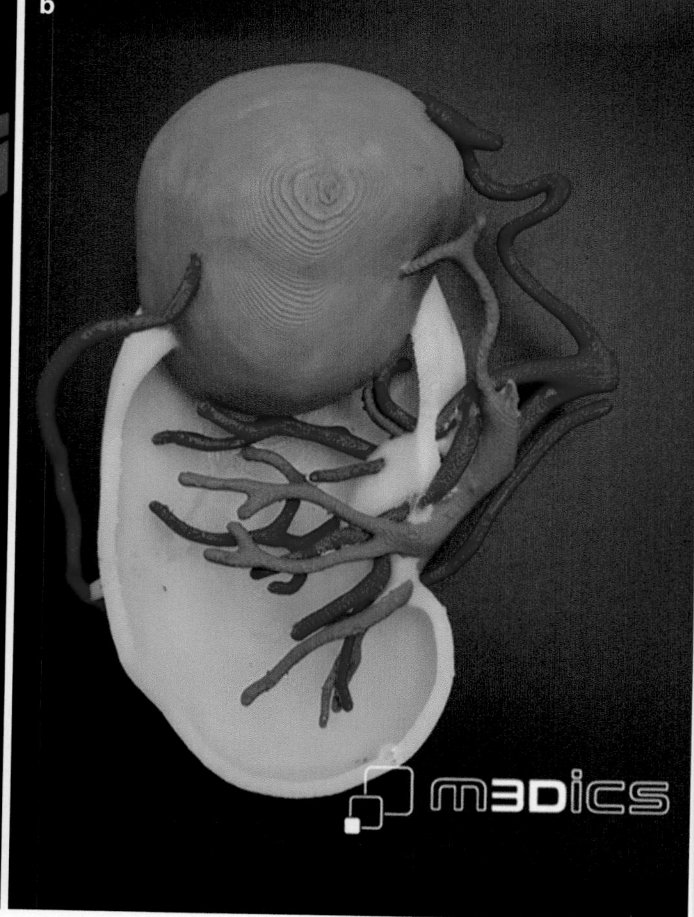

Fig. 1 (**a**) Virtual 3D reconstruction of the kidney showing a small tumor in the middle zone and kidney vasculature (arteries in red and veins in blue). (**b**) Printed 3D model showing upper pole tumor and the renal vasculature. These pictures are provided by and published with permission from MEDICS®

2.2 Hologram

Holographic reconstruction is the use of light waves to reconstruct a 3D floating projection of a specific object. Generally, it integrates the advantages of 3D reconstruction with the immersive experience, interactivity, and flexibility of digitalization. There is only one report in the literature comparing the holographic reconstruction of renal tumors to conventional CT scans demonstrating a higher level of interobserver agreement and shorter time of evaluation for the holographic images [14]. Generally, further investigations are needed to draw definitive conclusions on the value of the 3D visualization technology in urological practice.

3 Intraoperative Guidance

3.1 Three-Dimensional Augmented Reality (AR)

The ability to use the 3D virtual models as surgical roadmaps in surgical planning has led to increased interest in using these advanced techniques for intraoperative navigation. Three-dimensional representations of anatomical structures reconstructed from the preoperative CT or MRI were superimposed over the anatomy in vivo to allow intraoperative guidance by creating an augmented reality view that depicts both the surgical anatomy and scan data [15–17]. Initially employed in robotic radical prostatectomy, Hyperaccuracy 3D™ model AR-models can be applied during RAPN of complex renal masses in order to identify intraparenchymal structures and guide the surgical resection (Fig. 2). Canda et al. similarly published their initial experience on the use of 3D virtual reality (VR) tumor navigation during robotic prostate cancer surgery incorporating both multiparametric prostate MR and Ga68 PSMA PET images and suggested that this approach was particularly useful in high-risk prostate cancer cases [18]. Porpiglia et al. [15] demonstrated that this technology was associated with lower rates of global ischemia and higher tumor enucleation than intraoperative ultrasound (US) guidance. Moreover, the AR technology was associated with less violation of the collecting system and lower drop of the estimated renal plasma flow at 3 months [15].

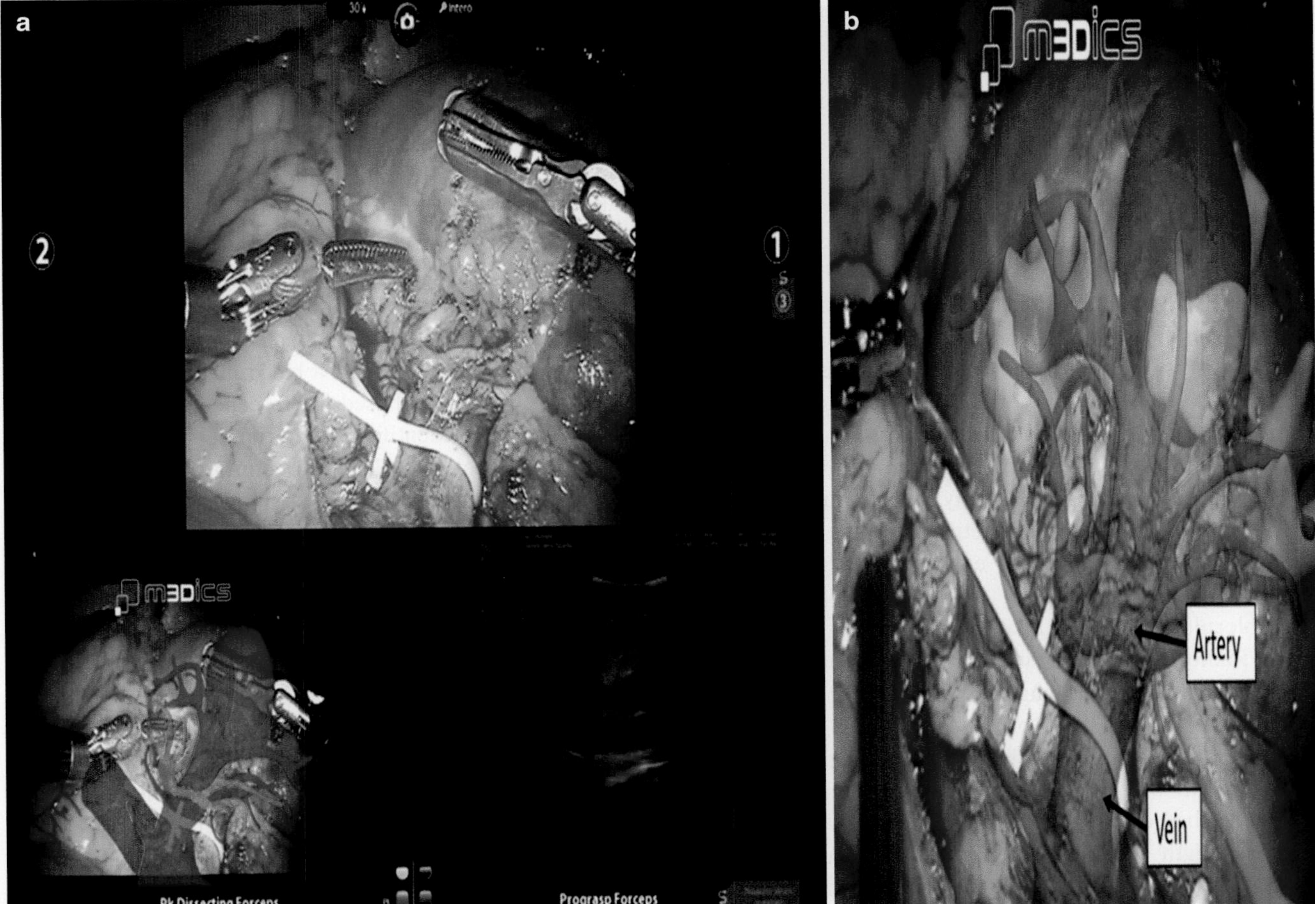

Fig. 2 (**a**) Augmented reality superimposition during RAPN. (**b**) Zoomed image of augmented reality superimposition during RAPN, showing the precise location of the tumor and the vasculature of the kidney. These pictures are provided by and published with permission from MEDICS®

3.2 Virtual Reality (VR) Surgical Navigation

These surgical navigation systems are based on the 3D reconstruction derived from preoperative imaging and use the anatomical landmarks to align the endoscopic view to the VR one [19]. The main difference between these systems and AR models is that the images are not superimposed over the real anatomical endoscopic view in the da Vinci console [19, 20]. On the contrary, in a feasibility study, the endoscopic view from recorded short videos was superimposed over the VR view to give a more realistic view and ensure a better alignment [20]. Among possible applications, it can be used for intraoperative real-time orientation and guidance of the procedure like, for instance, it may support the surgeon in the identification of the renal artery during RAPN [19, 20]. In general, the VR navigation systems may improve the surgeon's skills [19].

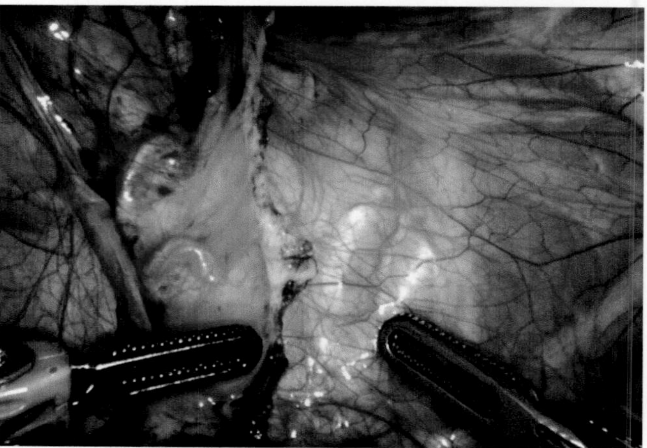

Fig. 3 Firefly® mode in the da Vinci robotic platform. This picture is provided by and published with permission from Intuitive®

3.3 Image-Guided Surgery

The concept of image-guided surgery is not new to urologists. It represents the base for different endoscopic surgeries such as percutaneous nephrolithotomy. Still, innovation within imaging modalities has allowed their integration in laparoscopic and robotic surgeries.

There are two main types of image-guided surgery that are listed below:

1. Morphological Imaging Guidance

   Ultrasound represents a key surgical modality for this technology. The introduction of robotic drop-in US probes and the ProGrasp forceps allows direct control of the probe by the surgeon at the console and facilitated the intraoperative use of US imaging during RAPN [21, 22]. This probe may be used to guide the enucleation of small renal masses (including totally endophytic tumors) and decrease warm ischemia times [21]. Furthermore, Alenezi et al. described an innovative technique of "sequential selective occlusion angiography," which utilizes contrast-enhanced US for intraoperative mapping of renal and tumor vasculature, thus enabling efficient selective clamping [22].
2. Molecular Imaging Guidance

   Radio-guided surgery allows the integration and translation of molecular imaging in surgery. The introduction of laparoscopic gamma probes has enabled the adaptation of this technology in minimally invasive surgery [23, 24].

   Visualizing fluorescent dyes using fluorescence imaging are based on the concept that the emission of higher wavelength light energy can be detected using high-resolution cameras (such as the Firefly® mode in the da Vinci robotic platform) and coded into a pseudocolored image as an output (Fig. 3) [25]. Indocyanine green (ICG) is one of the most commonly used fluorescent dyes in urological practice, as it can be detected using the near-infrared light spectrum (NIRF) [26]. This technology has gained great interest in the urological field for different indications such as angiographic agent during RAPN [25–28], or as a flushing agent during robot-assisted ureteral reconstruction [29, 30]. As regards partial nephrectomy, it is well known that the off-clamp approach can improve renal function. However, it may also increase the operative blood loss and disturb the view during resection that can potentially result in positive surgical margins. On the contrary, the on-clamp approach may prolong the ischemia time and potentially increase the perfusion/reperfusion injury. These factors combined have driven an increasing interest in selective arterial clamping to limit the ischemia to the involved renal tissues as much as possible [27]. ICG-based fluorescence imaging was proposed to help identify the arterial supply to the tumor, which may allow selective clamping and improve the functional outcomes [25]. Diana et al. [26] presented the largest series available to date which included 318 patients undergoing ICG-guided RAPN, showing that ICG-guided surgery is a promising tool in deciding the type of clamping (selective or global clamping). Several other authors supported this finding [25, 27]. Moreover, Mattevi et al. [27] compared 42 patients undergoing non-selective clamping with 20 patients undergoing NIRF-ICG-guided selective arterial clamping during RAPN, demonstrating a greater glomerular filtration rate loss in patients undergoing nonselective clamping RAPN (21.5% versus 5.5%, $p = 0.046$). Likewise, Simone et al. [28] proposed the use of the ICG guidance as an alternative to US in totally endophytic tumors. In this regard, a mixture of ICG-lipidol (to delay the ICG washout from the kidney) can be delivered in the arterial branches supplying the tumor to facilitate its identification and subsequent enucleation.

Another interesting application of ICG is to evaluate the blood flow to the remaining parenchymal tissue after renorrhaphy, particularly in patients with chronic kidney disease [26]. Furthermore, the ICG-guided approach to RAPN can potentially be used for reducing positive surgical margins as ICG tends to accumulate in normal parenchymal tissues (hyperfluorescent), while malignant tissues do not store ICG (hypofluorescent) [25, 26, 28].

During robot-assisted ureteral reconstruction, retrograde or antegrade ICG injection through a ureteral catheter or nephrostomy tube may help to overcome two main challenges, that is, the identification of the ureter (especially in the case of fibrosis or inflammation) and the identification of ureteral stricture margins that have notably lower vascularity. This would, in turn, facilitate a complete excision of required ureteral segment, reducing the risk of recurrence while preserving as much of the healthy ureter as possible [29, 30]. Furthermore, it can guide the identification and dissection of the ureter during robotic reimplantation of ureteroileal anastomotic stricture [29].

3.4 Intraoperative Pathology

The main aim of oncological surgery is the complete resection of tumors without compromising postoperative oncological and functional outcomes. For this reason, there is increased interest among urologists in new technologies that can provide a real-time pathological examination of surgical margins such as confocal laser endomicroscopy (CLE) [31], ex-vivo fluorescence confocal microscopy (FCM) [32, 33], and Raman spectroscopy [34].

Ex vivo fluorescence confocal microscopy VivaScope® 2500M-G4 (MAVIG GmbH, Munich, Germany; Caliber I.D.; Rochester, NY, USA) is a new technology that utilizes two lasers to allow digital pathological examination of the freshly excised tissues in the reflectance (785 nm) and fluorescence (488 nm) modalities, revealing images that resemble hematoxylin and eosin (H&E) staining in just a few minutes [35, 36].

Similarly, CLE Cellvizio (Mauna Kea Technologies, Paris, France) is capable of providing an in vivo high-resolution histopathological imaging by employing a 488 nm laser with fluorescein. This technology can be potentially used in vivo for the identification of identify vessels, nerves, and connective tissues [31]. Likewise, Pinto et al. [34] presented a preliminary study integrating an in vivo dual excitation Raman spectroscopy (680 and 785 nm) during RALP. Raman spectroscopy is an emerging technology that can be used in molecular tissue characterization, allowing the ex vivo differentiation between prostatic and extraprostatic tissues. Although the first applications of all these technologies were performed in prostate surgery, they are compatible with the robotic system, and as such, their application to renal surgery is similarly feasible.

Canda et al. recently published their technique on RAPN that enables cold ischemia with application of ice pieces and intraoperative frozen section evaluation [37].

3.5 Artificial Intelligence

This technology is based on computational analysis of the endoscopic views to provide additional information that might be camouflaged to the naked eye and assess surgical performance [38–41]. Amir-Khalili et al. [38] proposed the use of machine learning algorithms to guide the vascular dissection during RAPN as it is capable of detecting the faint motion of connective tissue surfaces resulting from the pulsation of blood vessels hidden below them. However, this was an experimental study, and it was applied only on recorded RAPN cases. Yet, this technique may be affected by the image's "noise" and cannot identify deeply hidden vasculature [39]. Thus Nosrati et al. [39] combined the advantages of visual cues and machine learning to improve the accuracy of this technology, where they used the preoperative imaging studies to identify the patient-specific 3D position and deformations of different structures in combination with the visual cues.

First feasibility studies also show promising results of the use of machine learning/AI models in predicting intraoperative and 30-day postoperative events in RAPN, although more validation is required [35].

3.6 Instruments

One of the main limitations of robotic surgery (particularly during pelvic or multiquadrant surgery) is the inability to change the patient's position without undocking the robot, which may prolong the operative time. The TruSystem 7000dV Operating Table (TS7000dV, TRUMPF Medizin Systeme GmbH & Co. KG, Saalfeld, Germany) overcame this limitation by adding coordinated motion of both the table and the robotic instruments, thus allowing a change in the patient's position mid-procedure without undocking [42].

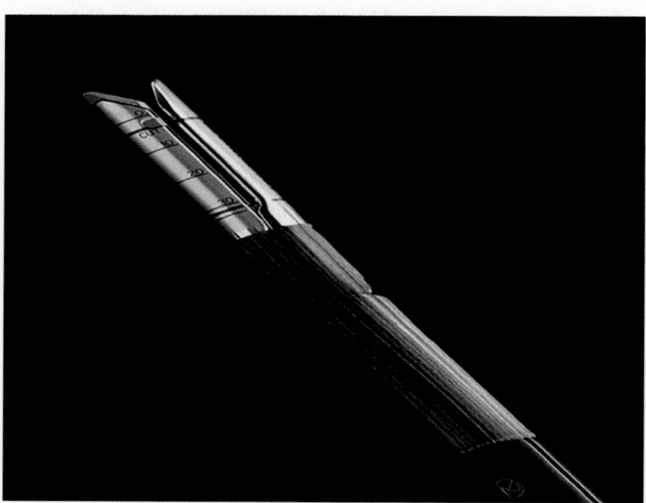

Fig. 4 Figure of the EndoWrist® Stapler, Intuitive Surgical Inc., Sunnyvale, California, USA. This picture is provided by and published with permission from Intuitive®

The robotic stapler (EndoWrist® Stapler, Intuitive Surgical Inc., Sunnyvale, California, USA) is another instrument that might facilitate robotic surgeries because it offers several advantages compared to the traditionally used laparoscopic staplers (Endo GIA™ Stapler, Medtronic, Dublin, Ireland and Ethicon Stapler, © Johnson & Johnson Medical) such as tremor reduction and a higher degree of freedom of movement (Fig. 4). This robotic stapler has been used safely in ten patients undergoing robotic living-donor nephrectomies without any related complications [36].

One of the interesting innovations in the last few years is the magnetic retraction system Levita™ Magnetic Surgical System (LMSS) (Levita Magnetics, San Mateo, CA), which may ease some of the concerns related to reduced working space in laparoscopic or robotic surgery. The LMSS works by attaching a spring-loaded grasper, characterized by a small magnetic end, to the targeted tissue, subsequently controlling it using an external stronger magnet [43]. Steinberg et al. [38] assessed the feasibility of this technology in 15 patients undergoing single-port RALP showing that it was able to improve tissue exposure during the different surgical steps. Similarly, Fulla et al. [43] reported the safety and feasibility of the magnetic retraction technology during minimally invasive renal surgeries.

4 Robotic Platforms

da Vinci Single-Port (SP) Robotic System

More than a decade ago, laparoendoscopic single-site surgery (LESS) was proposed as a promising alternative to conventional minimally invasive surgery. Later on, this technology was adopted by robotic surgeons to perform robotic LESS (R-LESS); however, it did not gain wide acceptance due to the associated technical limitations, including external collisions between robotic arms and difficult assistant access [39, 40]. Recently, the da Vinci SP device (Intuitive Surgical, Sunnyvale, CA, USA) has revived interest in single-site surgery with a system that has been specifically designed to overcome the limitation of R-LESS through its articulating camera and wristed surgical instruments (Fig. 5) [39–41]. Several studies evaluated the new SP robotic system in urological procedures including partial nephrectomy [39, 40, 44, 45], radical nephrectomy [39], and pyeloplasty [45]. While da Vinci SP system initially has been trialed with robotic radical prostatectomy, there is increasing evidence on SP-RAPN. The mean size of the renal tumors treated with this robotic system ranged from 2.6 cm [44] to 3.4 cm [39], and the operative time ranged from 153 to 244 min [45]. The reported warm ischemia time ranged from 25 min [40] to 27.5 min [44]. Only one patient throughout the included studies required conversion to open surgery because of significant abdominal adhesions [39]. The hospitalization period ranged from 1 to 5 days [45]. Interestingly, Na et al. [44] made a comparison between the da Vinci Xi single-site partial nephrectomy and the da Vinci SP-RAPN, reporting that the SP surgical system was able to overcome the technical limitations of R-LESS.

New Robotic Platforms

Over the last two decades, Intuitive Surgical has dominated the global surgical robotics' market with different generations of the da Vinci surgical system, while competitors were struggling due to patenting issues. However, the landscape of robotic surgery started to change over the last few years with the introduction of several new surgical robotic systems in clinical practice [46–50]. The REVO-I robot (Meere Company Inc., Yongin, Republic of Korea) design is similar to the da Vinci robots. It consists of an open console, four robotic arms attached to an operation cart, high-definition vision cart, and reusable robotic instruments [47]. Similarly, the Micro Hand S, Chinese robotic system, was developed in 2013, and it is similar to the da Vinci robotic system. It has not been used in urological practice yet [50].

Another new robotic system is the Versius Surgical System (CMR surgical, Cambridge, UK), consisting of separate wheeled carts for each instrument, all of which are controlled by a game-controller handgrip and visual feedback on the surgeon's open console (Fig. 6). This system has been used in a preclinical urological trial in human cadavers to perform renal and prostate surgeries [46]. Similarly, the Senhance® robotic system (TransEnterix Surgical Inc., Morrisville, NC, USA) (previously known as Telelap ALF-X) consists of four independent robotic arms that can be

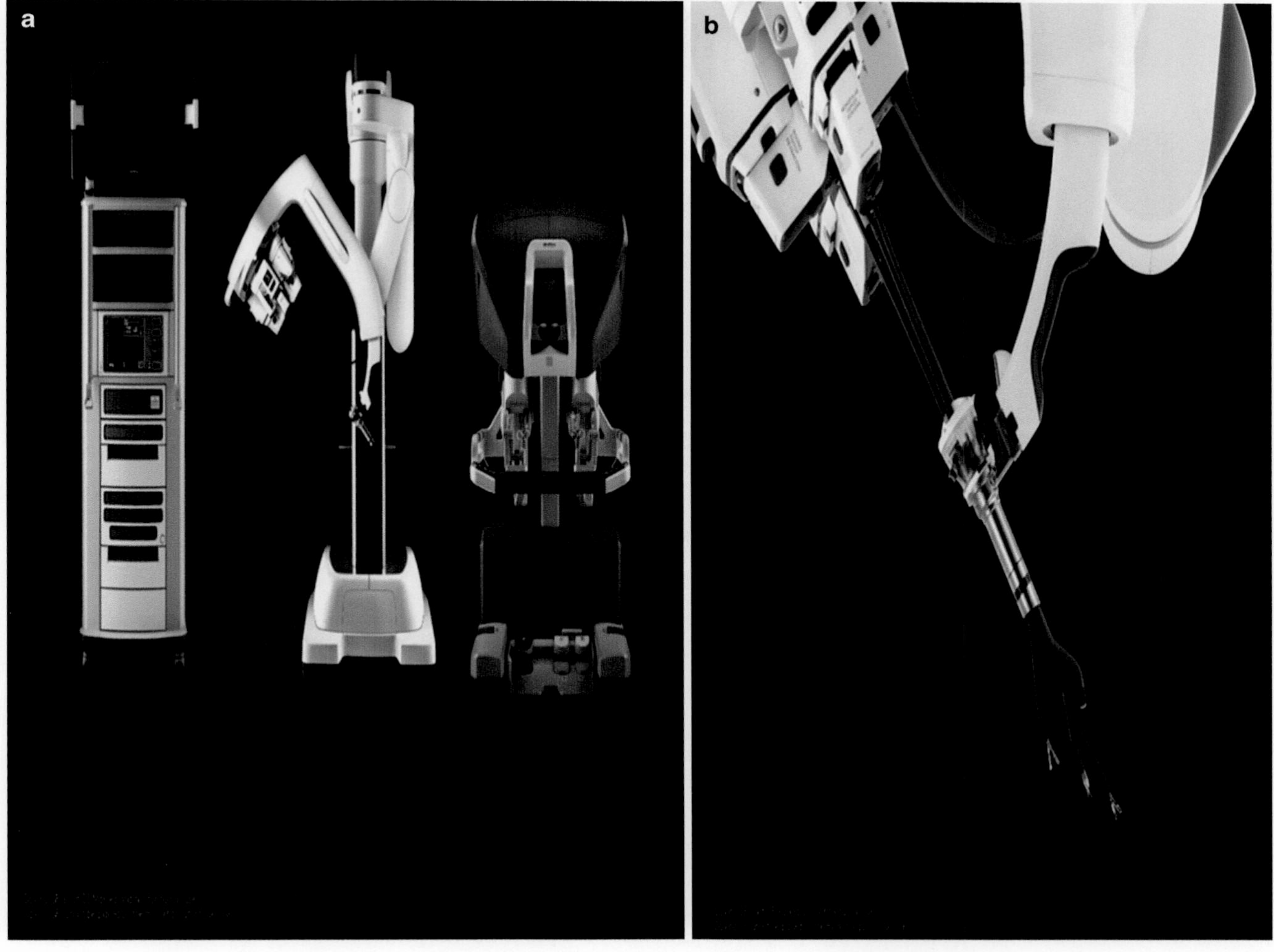

Fig. 5 (**a**) Image of the different components of da Vinci SP device (Intuitive Surgical, Sunnyvale, CA, USA). (**b**) A close-up image of the da Vinci SP arms. This picture is provided by and published with permission from Intuitive®

manipulated by laparoscopic handles at the surgeon's console (Fig. 7). Notably, this system offers the advantage of haptic feedback, and as such, surgeons do not have to rely solely on visual feedback [48]. Samalavicius et al. [48] reported the safety and efficacy of this robotic system in the largest series of patients undergoing different surgeries (31 urological, 39 abdominal, and 30 gynecological procedures) with only three patients requiring conversion to either laparoscopic or open approaches due to technical difficulties.

Although clinical studies are not yet available, several other surgical robots are at an advanced stage of development including the Hugo robot (Medtronic-Covidien, Dublin, Ireland), Medicaroid (Kobe, Japan), Avatera (Avateramedical, Jena, Germany), Verb Surgical (Johnson & Johnson, Inc., New Jersey, USA), and Virtuoso Surgical system (Nashville, TN, USA) [51]. In the near future, it will be possible to evaluate the applicability and results of using these platforms in renal surgery.

5 Training and New Technologies

A significant driver of the development of new technologies is the simple fact that less invasive procedures (i.e., minimally invasive surgery (MIS), surgical robotics, endovascular interventions, etc.) are better tolerated by patients who may not be suitable candidates for open surgical procedures (e.g., transcatheter aortic valve implantation procedures). The introduction of these technologies has however been accompanied by an increased frequency of complications, many life-threatening, particularly during the early experiences. In the 1990s, a series of high-profile adverse medical events [52, 53] as well class actions [54, 55] against one of the leading manufacturers of surgical robots drew the attention of the general public and authorities (e.g., Food and Drug Administration) to issues of clinical training. Urologists have been enthusiastic and early adopters of new, innovative, and less invasive technologies. However, in the last three

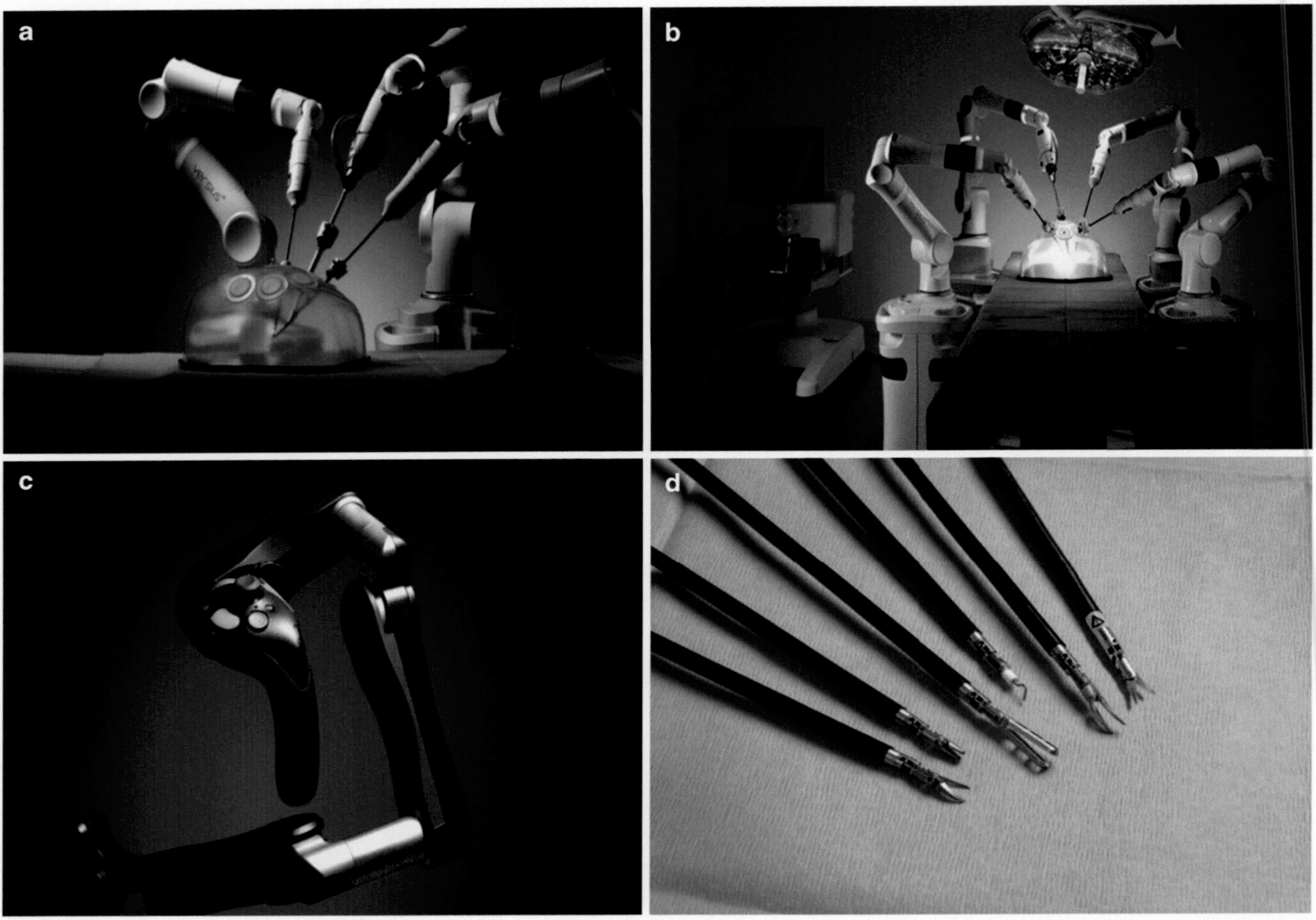

Fig. 6 Versius Surgical System (CMR surgical, Cambridge, UK). (**a**) Image of the entire robot. (**b**) Simulation of the robot in action. (**c**) Control joystick. (**d**) Different instruments of the robot. These pictures are provided by and published with permission from CMR surgical, Cambridge, UK

decades, they have underscored the imperative of quality-assured training as part of the successful rollout and adoption of these technologies. Mindful of these adverse events, corporate medicine (e.g., institute of medicine) has championed an outcome-based approach to skills training. The trainee (no matter how senior) must demonstrate a quantitatively defined performance benchmark before training progression and before using the device clinically. In this sense, proficiency-based progression training produces trainees that perform significantly (i.e., 60%) better in the operating room in comparison to trainees graduating from conventional training programs [56]. This approach to training derives the performance metrics from experienced and proficient practitioners, and after satisfactory validation, the metrics are used to set performance benchmarks which trainees must demonstrate before training progression [57]. Users and manufacturers of new and potentially high-risk devices/procedures (e.g., carotid artery stenting with embolic protection [58], mechanical thrombectomy for ischemic stroke [59], surgical robotics [60], etc.) find this training approach appealing because it quality assures the skill level of the trainee at the completion of training. Furthermore, it has the potential to produce more homogeneous performance levels to use new devices [61]. No matter how innovative or revolutionary a robotic technology is, it is merely a tool to augment the efforts of the clinician themselves. Tools will not perform optimally when users do not really know how to use them due to lack of training of interest. Like all tools, their impact is in the hands of the user.

6 Conclusions

Technological innovation and urology have a historically privileged relationship. The innovations introduced in the field of robotic renal surgery have shown to deliver substantial improvements, both in preoperative planning and intraoperative guidance. Moreover, new surgical platforms have recently appeared on the market showing encouraging results, opening a new chapter of competition, and pushing further advancements in the field of robotic surgery in urology.

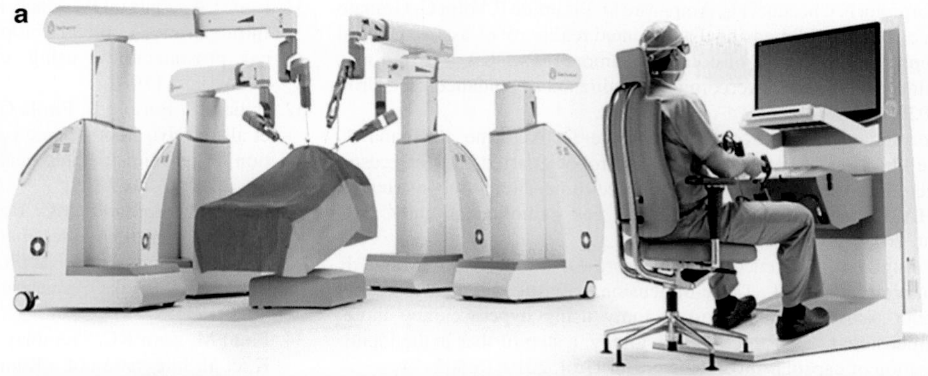

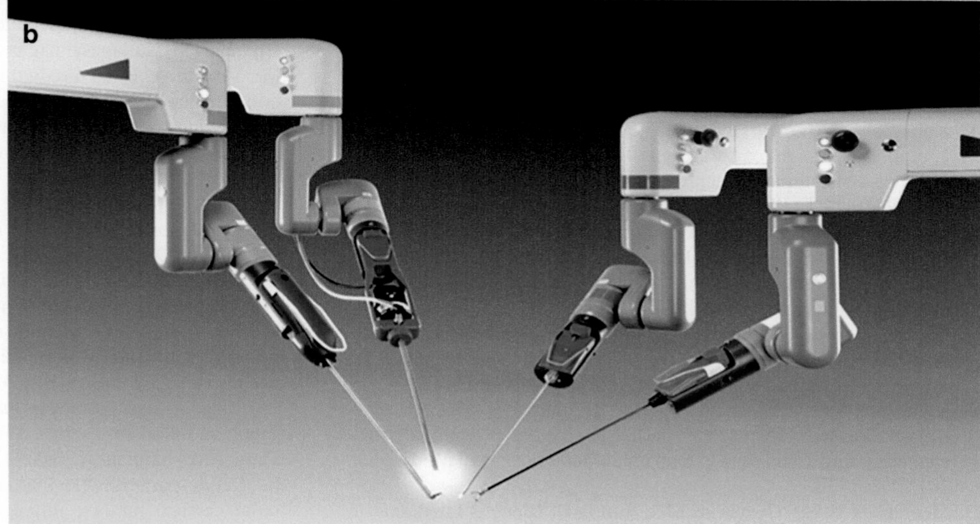

Fig. 7 Senhance® Robotic System (TransEnterix Surgical Inc., Morrisville, NC, USA). (**a**) Different components of the robot. (**b**) Zoom up on the robotic arms. These pictures are provided by and published with permission from TransEnterix Surgical Inc.

References

1. Ozkara H, Watson LR. Laparoscopic surgery in urology. Int Urol Nephrol. 1992;24:461–4.
2. El Sherbiny A, Eissa A, Ghaith A, Morini E, Marzotta L, Sighinolfi MC, et al. Training in urological robotic surgery. Future perspectives. Arch Esp Urol. 2018;71:97–107.
3. Kockerling F. Robotic vs. standard laparoscopic technique - what is better? Front Surg. 2014;1:15.
4. Binder J, Kramer W. Robotically-assisted laparoscopic radical prostatectomy. BJU Int. 2001;87:408–10.
5. Gettman M, Rivera M. Innovations in robotic surgery. Curr Opin Urol. 2016;26:271–6.
6. Porpiglia F, Bertolo R, Checcucci E, Amparore D, Autorino R, Dasgupta P, et al. Development and validation of 3D printed virtual models for robot-assisted radical prostatectomy and partial nephrectomy: urologists' and patients' perception. World J Urol. 2018;36:201–7.
7. Bertolo R, Autorino R, Fiori C, Amparore D, Checcucci E, Mottrie A, et al. Expanding the indications of robotic partial nephrectomy for highly complex renal tumors: Urologists' perception of the impact of hyperaccuracy three-dimensional reconstruction. J Laparoendosc Adv Surg Tech A. 2019;29:233–9.
8. Porpiglia F, Amparore D, Checcucci E, Manfredi M, Stura I, Migliaretti G, et al. Three-dimensional virtual imaging of renal tumours: a new tool to improve the accuracy of nephrometry scores. BJU Int. 2019;124:945–54.
9. von Rundstedt FC, Scovell JM, Agrawal S, Zaneveld J, Link RE. Utility of patient-specific silicone renal models for planning and rehearsal of complex tumour resections prior to robot-assisted laparoscopic partial nephrectomy. BJU Int. 2017;119:598–604.
10. Porpiglia F, Fiori C, Checcucci E, Amparore D, Bertolo R. Hyperaccuracy three-dimensional reconstruction is able to maximize the efficacy of selective clamping during robot-assisted partial nephrectomy for complex renal masses. Eur Urol. 2018;74:651–60.
11. Huang Q, Gu L, Zhu J, Peng C, Du S, Liu Q, et al. A three-dimensional, anatomy-based nephrometry score to guide nephron-sparing surgery for renal sinus tumors. Cancer. 2020;126(Suppl 9):2062–72.
12. Rocco B, Sighinolfi MC, Menezes AD, Eissa A, Inzillo R, Sandri M, et al. Three-dimensional virtual reconstruction with DocDo, a novel interactive tool to score renal mass complexity. BJU Int. 2020;125:761–2.
13. De Backer SV, C. Van Praet, S. Vandenbulcke, M. Lejoly, S Vanderschelden, C. Debbaut, A Mottrie, K. Decaestecker Selective arterial clamping in robot assisted partial nephrectomy using 3D nearest distance perfusion zones. J Endourol 2021. 35(9):1357-1364
14. Antonelli A, Veccia A, Palumbo C, Peroni A, Mirabella G, Cozzoli A, et al. Holographic reconstructions for preoperative planning before partial nephrectomy: a head-to-head comparison with standard CT scan. Urol Int. 2019;102:212–7.

15. Porpiglia F, Checcucci E, Amparore D, Piramide F, Volpi G, Granato S, et al. Three-dimensional augmented reality robot-assisted partial nephrectomy in case of complex Tumours (PADUA ≥ 10): a new intraoperative tool overcoming the ultrasound guidance. Eur Urol. 2020;78:229–38.
16. Porpiglia F, Checcucci E, Amparore D, Autorino R, Piana A, Bellin A, et al. Augmented-reality robot-assisted radical prostatectomy using hyper-accuracy three-dimensional reconstruction (HA3D) technology: a radiological and pathological study. BJU Int. 2019;123:834–45.
17. Porpiglia F, Checcucci E, Amparore D, Manfredi M, Massa F, Piazzolla P, et al. Three-dimensional elastic augmented-reality robot-assisted radical prostatectomy using hyperaccuracy three-dimensional reconstruction technology: a step further in the identification of capsular involvement. Eur Urol. 2019;76:505–14.
18. Canda AE, Aksoy SF, Altinmakas E, Koseoglu E, Falay O, Kordan Y, et al. Virtual reality tumor navigated robotic radical prostatectomy by using three-dimensional reconstructed multiparametric prostate MRI and 68Ga-PSMA PET/CT images: a useful tool to guide the robotic surgery? BJUI Compass. 2020;1:108–15.
19. Kobayashi S, Cho B, Huaulme A, Tatsugami K, Honda H, Jannin P, et al. Assessment of surgical skills by using surgical navigation in robot-assisted partial nephrectomy. Int J Comput Assist Radiol Surg. 2019;14:1449–59.
20. Mehralivand S, Kolagunda A, Hammerich K, Sabarwal V, Harmon S, Sanford T, et al. A multiparametric magnetic resonance imaging-based virtual reality surgical navigation tool for robotic-assisted radical prostatectomy. Turk J Urol. 2019;45:357–65.
21. Gunelli R, Fiori M, Salaris C, Salomone U, Urbinati M, Vici A, et al. The role of intraoperative ultrasound in small renal mass robotic enucleation. Arch Ital Urol Androl. 2016;88:311–3.
22. Alenezi A, Motiwala A, Eves S, Gray R, Thomas A, Meiers I, et al. Robotic assisted laparoscopic partial nephrectomy using contrast-enhanced ultrasound scan to map renal blood flow. Int J Med Robot. 2017;13:e1738.
23. Meershoek P, van Oosterom MN, Simon H, Mengus L, Maurer T, van Leeuwen PJ, et al. Robot-assisted laparoscopic surgery using DROP-IN radioguidance: first-in-human translation. Eur J Nucl Med Mol Imaging. 2019;46:49–53.
24. Maurer T, Robu S, Schottelius M, Schwamborn K, Rauscher I, van den Berg NS, et al. (99m)Technetium-based prostate-specific membrane antigen-radioguided surgery in recurrent prostate cancer. Eur Urol. 2019;75:659–66.
25. Gadus L, Kocarek J, Chmelik F, Matejkova M, Heracek J. Robotic partial nephrectomy with indocyanine green fluorescence navigation. Contrast Media Mol Imaging. 2020;2020:1287530.
26. Diana P, Buffi NM, Lughezzani G, Dell'Oglio P, Mazzone E, Porter J, et al. The role of intraoperative indocyanine green in robot-assisted partial nephrectomy: results from a large, multi-institutional series. Eur Urol. 2020;78:743–9.
27. Mattevi D, Luciani LG, Mantovani W, Cai T, Chiodini S, Vattovani V, et al. Fluorescence-guided selective arterial clamping during RAPN provides better early functional outcomes based on renal scan compared to standard clamping. J Robot Surg. 2019;13:391–6.
28. Simone G, Tuderti G, Anceschi U, Ferriero M, Costantini M, Minisola F, et al. "Ride the green light": indocyanine green-marked off-clamp robotic partial nephrectomy for totally endophytic renal masses. Eur Urol. 2019;75:1008–14.
29. Tuderti G, Brassetti A, Minisola F, Anceschi U, Ferriero M, Leonardo C, et al. Transnephrostomic Indocyanine green-guided robotic ureteral reimplantation for benign ureteroileal strictures after robotic cystectomy and intracorporeal neobladder: step-by-step surgical technique, perioperative and functional outcomes. J Endourol. 2019;33:823–8.
30. Lee Z, Moore B, Giusto L, Eun DD. Use of indocyanine green during robot-assisted ureteral reconstructions. Eur Urol. 2015;67:291–8.
31. Lopez A, Zlatev DV, Mach KE, Bui D, Liu JJ, Rouse RV, et al. Intraoperative optical biopsy during robotic assisted radical prostatectomy using confocal endomicroscopy. J Urol. 2016;195:1110–7.
32. Puliatti S, Bertoni L, Pirola GM, Azzoni P, Bevilacqua L, Eissa A, et al. Ex vivo fluorescence confocal microscopy: the first application for real-time pathological examination of prostatic tissue. BJU Int. 2019;124:469–76.
33. Rocco B, Sighinolfi MC, Bertoni L, Spandri V, Puliatti S, Eissa A, et al. Real-time assessment of surgical margins during radical prostatectomy: a novel approach that uses fluorescence confocal microscopy for the evaluation of peri-prostatic soft tissue. BJU Int. 2020;125:487–9.
34. Pinto M, Zorn KC, Tremblay JP, Desroches J, Dallaire F, Aubertin K, et al. Integration of a Raman spectroscopy system to a robotic-assisted surgical system for real-time tissue characterization during radical prostatectomy procedures. J Biomed Opt. 2019;24:1–10.
35. Bhandari M, Nallabasannagari AR, Reddiboina M, Porter JR, Jeong W, Mottrie A, et al. Predicting intra-operative and postoperative consequential events using machine-learning techniques in patients undergoing robot-assisted partial nephrectomy: a Vattikuti collective quality initiative database study. BJU Int. 2020;126:350–8.
36. Perkins SQ, Giffen ZC, Buck BJ, Ortiz J, Sindhwani P, Ekwenna O. Initial experience with the use of a robotic stapler for robot-assisted donor nephrectomy. J Endourol. 2018;32:1054–7.
37. Canda AE, Ozkan A, Arpali E, Koseoglu E, Kiremit MC, Kordan Y, et al. Robotic assisted partial nephrectomy with cold ischemia applying ice pieces and intraoperative frozen section evaluation of the mass: complete replication of open approach with advantages of minimally invasive surgery. Cent Eur J Urol. 2020;73:234–5.
38. Steinberg RL, Johnson BA, Meskawi M, Gettman MT, Cadeddu JA. Magnet-assisted robotic prostatectomy using the da Vinci SP robot: an initial case series. J Endourol. 2019;33:829–34.
39. Fang AM, Saidian A, Magi-Galluzzi C, Nix JW, Rais-Bahrami S. Single-port robotic partial and radical nephrectomies for renal cortical tumors: initial clinical experience. J Robot Surg. 2020;14:773–80.
40. Shukla D, Small A, Mehrazin R, Palese M. Single-port robotic-assisted partial nephrectomy: initial clinical experience and lessons learned for successful outcomes. J Robot Surg. 2021;15:293–8.
41. Dobbs RW, Halgrimson WR, Madueke I, Vigneswaran HT, Wilson JO, Crivellaro S. Single-port robot-assisted laparoscopic radical prostatectomy: initial experience and technique with the da Vinci((R)) SP platform. BJU Int. 2019;124:1022–7.
42. Morelli L, Palmeri M, Simoncini T, Cela V, Perutelli A, Selli C, et al. A prospective, single-arm study on the use of the da Vinci(R) table motion with the Trumpf TS7000dV operating table. Surg Endosc. 2018;32:4165–72.
43. Fulla J, Small A, Kaplan-Marans E, Palese M. Magnetic-assisted robotic and laparoscopic renal surgery: initial clinical experience with the Levita magnetic surgical system. J Endourol. 2020;34:1242–6.
44. Na JC, Lee HH, Yoon YE, Jang WS, Choi YD, Rha KH, et al. True single-site partial nephrectomy using the SP surgical system: feasibility, comparison with the Xi single-site platform, and step-by-step procedure guide. J Endourol. 2020;34:169–74.
45. Kaouk J, Aminsharifi A, Sawczyn G, Kim S, Wilson CA, Garisto J, et al. Single-port robotic urological surgery using purpose-built single-port surgical system: single-institutional experience with the first 100 cases. Urology. 2020;140:77–84.
46. Thomas BC, Slack M, Hussain M, Barber N, Pradhan A, Dinneen E, et al. Preclinical evaluation of the versius surgical system, a new robot-assisted surgical device for use in minimal access renal and prostate surgery. Eur Urol Focus. 2021;7:444–52.
47. Chang KD, Abdel Raheem A, Choi YD, Chung BH, Rha KH. Retzius-sparing robot-assisted radical prostatectomy using the

Revo-i robotic surgical system: surgical technique and results of the first human trial. BJU Int. 2018;122:441–8.
48. Samalavicius NE, Janusonis V, Siaulys R, Jasenas M, Deduchovas O, Venckus R, et al. Robotic surgery using Senhance((R)) robotic platform: single center experience with first 100 cases. J Robot Surg. 2020;14:371–6.
49. Chaddha U, Kovacs SP, Manley C, Hogarth DK, Cumbo-Nacheli G, Bhavani SV, et al. Robot-assisted bronchoscopy for pulmonary lesion diagnosis: results from the initial multicenter experience. BMC Pulm Med. 2019;19:243.
50. Yi B, Wang G, Li J, Jiang J, Son Z, Su H, et al. The first clinical use of domestically produced Chinese minimally invasive surgical robot system "Micro Hand S". Surg Endosc. 2016;30:2649–55.
51. Rassweiler JJ, Autorino R, Klein J, Mottrie A, Goezen AS, Stolzenburg JU, et al. Future of robotic surgery in urology. BJU Int. 2017;120:822–41.
52. Walshe K, Offen N. A very public failure: lessons for quality improvement in healthcare organisations from the Bristol Royal Infirmary. Qual Health Care. 2001;10:250–6.
53. Van Der Weyden MB. The Bundaberg hospital scandal: the need for reform in Queensland and beyond. Med J Aust. 2005;183:284–5.
54. Pradarelli JC, Thornton JP, Dimick JB. Who is responsible for the safe introduction of new surgical technology?: an important legal precedent from the da Vinci surgical system trials. JAMA Surg. 2017;152:717–8.
55. Nik-Ahd F, Souders CP, Zhao H, Houman J, McClelland L, Chughtai B, et al. Robotic urologic surgery: trends in litigation over the last decade. J Robot Surg. 2019;13:729–34.
56. Mazzone E, Puliatti S, Amato M, Bunting B, Rocco B, Montorsi F, et al. A systematic review and meta-analysis on the impact of proficiency-based progression simulation training on performance outcomes. Ann Surg. 2020;274(2):281–9.
57. Gallagher AG, Ritter EM, Champion H, Higgins G, Fried MP, Moses G, et al. Virtual reality simulation for the operating room: proficiency-based training as a paradigm shift in surgical skills training. Ann Surg. 2005;241:364–72.
58. Gallagher AG, Cates CU. Approval of virtual reality training for carotid stenting: what this means for procedural-based medicine. JAMA. 2004;292:3024–6.
59. Liebig T, Holtmannspotter M, Crossley R, Lindkvist J, Henn P, Lonn L, et al. Metric-based virtual reality simulation: a paradigm shift in training for mechanical thrombectomy in acute stroke. Stroke. 2018;49:e239–e42.
60. Satava RM, Stefanidis D, Levy JS, Smith R, Martin JR, Monfared S, et al. Proving the effectiveness of the fundamentals of robotic surgery (FRS) skills curriculum: a single-blinded, multispecialty, multi-institutional randomized control trial. Ann Surg. 2020;272:384–92.
61. Vanlander AE, Mazzone E, Collins JW, Mottrie AM, Rogiers XM, van der Poel HG, et al. Orsi consensus meeting on European robotic training (OCERT): results from the first multispecialty consensus meeting on training in robot-assisted surgery. Eur Urol. 2020;78:713–6.

Outcomes of Robotic Radical and Partial Nephrectomy

Shirin Razdan and Ketan K. Badani

1 Overview

Since the advent of the first laparoscopic nephrectomy in 1990 by Clayman et al., the use of the robotic platform has revolutionized the performance of minimally invasive renal surgery. Robotic surgery allows for a magnified, three-dimensional (3D) view with reduced tremor and articulating robotic instruments that offer a greater range of motion compared to traditional laparoscopic instruments. The greatest improvement arguably is seen in the ease by which intracorporeal suturing can be performed. Over the last decade, the robotic platform as allowed partial nephrectomy to become more feasible due to improved visualization and hilar dissection, as well as expedient tumor excision and renorrhaphy. More recently the retroperitoneal approach has also become a popular option, with surgeons relying on the retroperitoneal approach for posterior and lateral tumors as well as in those patients with hostile abdomens. In this chapter we review the literature on outcomes and complications after robotic radical, partial, and retroperitoneal partial nephrectomy.

2 Robotic Radical Nephrectomy

The first transabdominal laparoscopic nephrectomy was performed by Clayman et al. for a renal tumor. The authors utilized a morcellator to deliver a 190 gram kidney through a 1 cm incision [1]. The first retroperitoneal laparoscopic nephrectomy was performed in 1993 by Gaur et al., utilizing the assistance of a dissecting balloon [2]. The first experience with robotic assisted radical nephrectomy was done experimentally in pigs in 2000 [3]. Bilateral nephrectomy was performed in five pigs, with one side being performed robotically and the other laparoscopically. The robotic approach required significantly longer total operative and actual surgical times, but blood loss, complication rates, and adequacy of surgical resection were comparable between the two groups. The first robotic nephrectomy in a human was described in 2001 and was performed in a 77-year-old female with a nonfunctioning, hydronephrotic right kidney secondary to a chronic ureteropelvic junction obstruction [4]. The surgery was performed with the assistance of the Zeus robotic surgical system with an operative time of 200 min and estimated blood loss (EBL) of less than 100 mL.

The first reported series of robotic radical nephrectomy was performed in 2005 and established the safety and feasibility of the procedure. Of five patients, only one patient was converted to hand-assist laparoscopy due to bleeding from the renal vein. Median operative time was 321 min, EBL 150 mL, hospital stay 3 days, and tumor size 66 cm^3 [5]. Since then, numerous retrospective studies have been performed to compare outcomes of the robotic approach with both open and laparoscopic. In 2006, Nazemi et al. compared robotic, open, laparoscopic with and without hand-assist radical nephrectomy [6]. There was no significant difference in patient or tumor characteristics. The robotic approach resulted in significantly longer surgical times than open approach, whereas robotic and laparoscopic approaches had comparable total operative time given longer setup times. EBL, requirement for patient-controlled analgesia (PCA), and hospital length of stay were longer in the open group. Rogers et al. performed another retrospective study examining their outcomes for 42 consecutive patients who underwent robotic radical or simple nephrectomy [7]. Mean operative console time was 158 min, mean EBL was 223 mL, mean tumor size was 5.1 cm, and mean hospital stay was 2.4 days. There was a 2.6% complication rate due to one morbidly obese patient having a wound dehiscence. In those patients who underwent radical nephrectomy, there were no positive margins. There was no evidence of tumor recurrence at a mean (range) follow-up of 15.7 (1–51) months.

More recently, an expansive multi-institution retrospective study was performed to compare outcomes of robotic

S. Razdan (✉) · K. K. Badani
Department of Urology, Icahn School of Medicine at Mount Sinai Hospital, New York, NY, USA

P. Wiklund et al. (eds.), *Robotic Urologic Surgery*, https://doi.org/10.1007/978-3-031-00363-9_53

and laparoscopic radical nephrectomy for large (≥ cT2) renal masses [8]. From 2004 to 2017, a total of 941 patients underwent surgery. Patients undergoing robotic radical nephrectomy RRN had higher median BMI (27.6 vs. 26.5, $p < 0.01$) as well as longer operative times (185.0 vs. 126 min, $p < 0.001$). However, length of stay was shorter for the robotic approach (3.0 vs. 5.0 days, $p < 0.001$), although robotic cases were more likely to present with more advanced disease—higher pathologic staging (pT3–4 52.5 vs. 24.2%, $p < 0.001$) and rate of nodal disease (pN1 5.4 vs. 1.9%, $p < 0.01$). The authors also examined the trend in robotic usage, finding that in the study period, robotic radical nephrectomy had annual increase of 11.75%, whereas laparoscopic radical nephrectomy had an annual decline of 5.39%. The increased use of the robotic platform for numerous urologic procedures not limited to renal surgery has allowed surgeons to become very comfortable with its usage, most likely accounting for the preference seen in this modality for patients with more advanced disease.

Helmers et al. queried their institution's renal mass registry to compare outcomes between robotic and laparoscopic radical nephrectomy, as well as hospital costs [9]. They found total operative time, intraoperative complications, and length of stay equivalent between both approaches. The robotic approach was associated with significantly higher EBL (50 mL vs. 100 mL, $p = 0.041$) as well as conversion to alternate surgical approach (0% vs. 11.1%, $p < 0.001$). Along the same lines as the aforementioned study by Anele et al., these authors found robotic cases were more likely to include a lymph node dissection (12.6% vs. 24.2%, $p = 0.031$), again a tribute to the comfort many surgeons feel with the robotic platform, allowing for more complex dissection and surgery on more advanced disease. Although robotic radical nephrectomy incurred higher costs than laparoscopic surgery, the difference was not significant ($14,913 vs. $16,265, $p = 0.171$).

A population-based analysis comparing robotic and laparoscopic radical nephrectomy using the SEER database was performed in 2017 [10]. Between the years 2008 and 2012, 241 patients over the age of 65 underwent a robotic radical nephrectomy for localized renal cell carcinoma, while 574 patients underwent the standard laparoscopic approach. Using a propensity score matched analysis, the researchers found no significant difference in adverse event rate, length of stay, overall survival, and cancer-specific survival at 3 years. The robotic cohort did incur higher hospitalization costs compared to the laparoscopic group ($53,681 vs. $44,161, $p < 0.01$).

In the prospective setting, Hemal et al. compared robotic and laparoscopic radical nephrectomy for patients with T1–T2 renal tumors [11]. In their cohort of 30 patients, 15 underwent either procedure. Patients who underwent a robotic procedure had significantly longer operative times (221 vs.175 min); otherwise, there was no difference between the two approaches when comparing EBL, complication rate, blood transfusion rate, hospitalization, and analgesic requirement. There was no recurrence in either group at a mean follow-up time of 8.3 months in the robotic group and 9.1 months in the laparoscopic group.

A systematic review was recently published in 2020 comparing robotic radical nephrectomy with laparoscopic and open nephrectomy [12]. A total of 12 studies were included in the meta-analysis, incorporating 64,221 patients. Weighted mean differences (WMD) were calculated. When comparing robotic to open surgery, the robotic platform allowed for shorter length of stay (WMD -3.06 days; $p = 0.002$), fewer overall complications (OR 0.56; $p < 0.001$), lower EBL (WMD −702 ml; $p = 0.01$), and higher total hospital costs (WMD US$4520; $p = 0.004$). When compared to the laparoscopic approach, robotic radical nephrectomy resulted in statistically significant longer operative time (WMD 37.44 min; $p = 0.03$), shorter length of stay (WMD −0.84 days; $p = 0.02$), and higher total costs (WMD US$4700; $p < 0.001$). There were no significant differences in terms of transfusion rate, complication rate, conversion to open, or perioperative mortality rate.

The above studies, particularly the systematic review and meta-analysis, suggest that robotic radical nephrectomy is a safe and efficacious modality of treatment compared to laparoscopic and open radical nephrectomy, although associated with longer operative times and cost.

3 Robotic Partial Nephrectomy

Nephron sparing surgery is the accepted surgical standard for management of small renal masses [13, 14]. It has been shown to have equivalent oncologic outcomes to radical nephrectomy, and the minimally invasive approach has proven to result in improved patient convalescence and decreased morbidity when compared to the open approach [15–17].

The first study describing robotic partial nephrectomy was published in 2004 by Gettman et al. [18] In their series of 13 patients with mean tumor size of 3.5 cm, 11 patients underwent a transperitoneal robotic partial, while the remaining two underwent a retroperitoneal partial. Eight of the partial nephrectomies were performed after placement of an intraarterial cooling balloon catheter that fully occluded the renal artery. In these patients, the mean cold ischemia time (CIT) was 33 min, while in the remaining five patients who underwent more traditional renal artery and vein clamping, warm ischemia time (WIT) was 22 min. Mean operative time was 215 min and EBL 170 mL. There was no conversion to alternate surgical approach, and the only complication was one patient with ileus. Mean length of stay was 4.3 days. There was no recurrence observed at 2–11 months of follow-up.

Subsequent studies describing the robotic partial experience found decreasing rates of WIT and total operative time [19–22]. Most common complications included need for blood transfusion and conversion to open or laparoscopic approach. This early experience with robotic partial nephrectomy found that the robotic platform allowed for shorter WIT and decreased blood loss when compared to the laparoscopic approach, likely due to improved hilar visualization and wrist articulation allowing for precise clamping and unclamping of the renal vessels, with quick and efficacious resection of the target tumor and subsequent renorrhaphy [23].

Similar to the trend seen with robotic radical nephrectomy, robotic partial nephrectomy has been increasingly utilized for more complex renal tumors. Khalifeh et al. retrospectively reviewed the charts of 500 patients who underwent robotic or laparoscopic partial nephrectomy at their institution [24]. While patient demographics were similar, the robotic group had a significantly higher Charlson Comorbidity Index (3.75 vs. 1.26) and more complex tumors (RENAL score 7.2 vs. 5.98). The authors found that robotic partial nephrectomy engendered shorter operative and WIT, fewer intraoperative and postoperative complications, and lower positive margin rate when compared to laparoscopic partial nephrectomy. Thus, they argued that robotic partial nephrectomy allows for a "higher overall trifecta rate" (WIT less than 25 min, negative surgical margins, and no perioperative complications), thereby placing it as the standard approach for minimally invasive partial nephrectomy.

Wu et al. performed a propensity-matched analysis of 237 patients who underwent robotic or laparoscopic partial nephrectomy [25]. In their cohort, patients who underwent a robotic procedure had lower EBL (156 vs. 198 mL, $p = 0.025$), a shorter WIT (22.8 vs. 31 min, $p < 0.001$), higher proportion of malignant lesions (88.4 vs. 67.5%; odds ratio [OR]: 2.6; 95% confidence interval [CI]: 1.2–5.67; $p = 0.023$), and lower intraoperative complication rate (1.3 vs. 11.7%; OR 0.1, 95% CI 0.01–0.81; $p = 0.018$). They also found that early functional outcomes were greater in the robotic group, with smaller decline in estimated glomerular filtration rate (eGFR) (-4.8 ± 17.9 and -12.2 ± 16.6; $p = 0.018$).

A prolific group out of France published prospective studies comparing robotic partial nephrectomy with both open and laparoscopic nephrectomy [26, 27]. When compared to the laparoscopic approach, robotic partial nephrectomy resulted in lower WIT, EBL, total operative time, use of hemostatic agents, and length of stay. When compared to the open approach, robotic surgery was also associated with lower EBL and length of stay, albeit equivalent WIT, operative time, complication rate, and effect on renal function. The researchers also concluded that robotic partial nephrectomy, particularly in T1b or higher tumors, provided acceptable short-term cancer-specific survival rates (2 year progression free survival 90.5%) with acceptable morbidity [28].

Given the recent explosion in the literature on the subject of robotic partial nephrectomy outcomes, numerous systematic reviews have been performed to better synthesize the available data [29, 30]. Xu et al. queried 19 studies that compared robotic partial nephrectomy to open partial nephrectomy [31]. On meta-analysis they found that robotic partial resulted in significantly improved postoperative complication rates (risk ratio [RR] = 0.60, 95% confidence interval [CI] = 0.46, 0.78, $p = 0.0002$), lower need for transfusion (RR = 0.64, 95% CI = 0.41, 0.98, $p = 0.04$), less EBL (weighted mean difference [WMD] = −98.82, 95% CI = −125.64, −72.01, $p < 0.00001$), and shorter length of stay (WMD = −2.64, 95% CI = −3.27, −2.00, $p < 0.00001$). On the contrary, open partial nephrectomy had improved operative time (WMD = 18.56, 95% CI = 2.13, 35.00, $p = 0.03$) and WIT (WMD = 3.65, 95% CI = 0.75, 6.56, $p = 0.01$). Positive surgical margin rate (RR = 0.87, 95% CI = 0.56, 1.34, $p = 0.52$) and short-term eGFR change (WMD = −1.56, 95% CI = −3.41, 0.28, $p = 0.10$) were equivalent between the two approaches.

A more recent systematic review by Tsai et al. examined 34 studies comparing outcomes of robotic and open partial nephrectomy encompassing 60,808 patients [32]. Similar to Xu et al., they found improved EBL and transfusion rates as well as lower complication rates. Open partial still held the advantage in terms of total operative time. Aboumarzouk et al. performed a systematic review of robotic versus laparoscopic partial nephrectomy [33]. On meta-analysis of 717 patients, the authors found no significant difference in total operative time, EBL, or conversion to open. However, the patients undergoing robotic partial nephrectomy had significantly shorter WIT. There was no difference in length of stay, complication rate, or rate of positive surgical margins. Choi et al. also performed a systematic review of 23 studies comparing robotic with laparoscopic partial nephrectomy. There were no significant differences in complication rates, operative time, EBL, or positive surgical margin rate. Robotic partial nephrectomy resulted in lower rate of conversion to open, shorter WIT, smaller decrease in eGFR, and shorter length of stay.

The above data shows a definite trend toward increased usage of the robotic platform for partial nephrectomy. Robotic technology allows for improved WIT, allowing for preservation of renal function postoperatively, with equivalent complication rates to open and laparoscopic approaches. When comparing robotic to open approach, the increased operative time of the robotic approach and possible increased WIT have to be balanced against the increased length of stay of patients who undergo open surgery. When compared to laparoscopic approach, robotic partial is clearly preferred in terms of WIT, conversion to open, and maintenance of eGFR postoperatively.

4 Robotic Retroperitoneal Partial Nephrectomy

The retroperitoneal approach to the kidney has emerged as a viable option for those patients with posterior and laterally located tumors. It has the benefit of avoiding the peritoneal cavity and has a role in those patients with multiple prior abdominal surgeries who may have hostile anatomy precluding transperitoneal approach. The first minimally invasive retroperitoneal approach was described by McDougall et al. in 1996, when they described their series of 33 patients who underwent laparoscopic nephrectomy for benign disease, 23 via transperitoneal approach, and 10 via retroperitoneal approach. They found faster resumption of regular diet and decreased need for analgesia for tumors smaller than 100 grams in patients who underwent retroperitoneal approach [34]. The 2000s brought the advent of robotic technology, and its attendant improved wrist articulation and 3D visualization. Subsequent studies on robotic retroperitoneal partial nephrectomy found decreased hospital length of stay, EBL, and shorter operative time [35–38].

Abaza et al. in their initial series showed that there is negligible learning curve when making the transition from transperitoneal to retroperitoneal approach, with patients undergoing robotic retroperitoneal partial nephrectomy having equivalent tumor characteristics, operative time, WIT, and positive margin rates [39]. The retroperitoneal group had statistically lower EBL and shorter length of stay. There were only two attempts at retroperitoneal approach that had to be converted to transperitoneal due to morbid obesity affecting access.

Stroup et al. performed a retrospective review of 404 patients who underwent transperitoneal and retroperitoneal robotic partial nephrectomy with the aim of determining how many achieved the "pentafecta"—a composite of negative margin, no 30-day complications, ischemia time $\leq$ 25 min, return of eGFR to >90% from baseline at last follow-up, and no chronic kidney disease upstaging. They found that pentafecta rates were not significantly different between the transperitoneal and retroperitoneal approaches (33.9% vs. 43.3%, $p = 0.526$). The retroperitoneal approach afforded a shorter operative time [40]. The pentafecta was again examined by Choi et al. in their cohort of 523 patients who underwent transperitoneal or retroperitoneal robotic partial nephrectomy [41]. They also found no significant difference in attainment of the pentafecta between the two approaches. However, retroperitoneal approach had shorter operative time, WIT, and EBL, albeit at the expense of greater eGFR decline postoperatively.

There have been three systematic reviews performed to integrate the available literature on robotic retroperitoneal partial nephrectomy compared to the transperitoneal approach. Xia et al. performed a systematic review of four studies totaling 449 patients [42]. They found no differences between retroperitoneal or transperitoneal approach in terms of tumor size, tumor laterality, RENAL nephrometry score, and tumor pathology. The retroperitoneal approach trended toward shorter operative time. Pavan et al. performed a systematic review of seven case-control studies totaling 1379 patients [43]. On their meta-analysis, they found that the retroperitoneal group was more likely to have posteriorly/laterally located tumors and be larger. Additionally, operating time (WMD 20.17 min; 95% CI 6.46–33.88; $p = 0.004$) and EBL (WMD 54.57 mL; 95% CI 6.73–102.4; $p = 0.03$) were significantly lower in the retroperitoneal group. Length of stay was significantly shorter in the retroperitoneal group as well (WMD 0.46 days; CI 95% 0.15–0.76; $p = 0.003$). There was no difference between the retroperitoneal and transperitoneal group in complication rate, WIT, or positive surgical margin rate. Most recently, McLean et al. performed a systematic review of three publications comparing transperitoneal and retroperitoneal partial nephrectomy for posterior tumors, finding the only significant difference was a shorter length of stay for the retroperitoneal group, with otherwise equivalent complication rate, WIT, EBL, and positive surgical margin rate [44].

All in all, the retroperitoneal approach appears to be a technically feasible procedure for surgeons who are already familiar with the robotic transperitoneal approach. It may result in faster operative times with shorter length of stay compared to transperitoneal partial nephrectomy, the latter outcome likely secondary to avoidance of peritoneal irritation.

5 Conclusion

In the preceding chapter we presented a broad recap of the available literature on outcomes of robotic radical, partial, and retroperitoneal partial nephrectomy. The current national trend is toward increased utilization of robotic technology, with more recent systematic reviews available that allow us to understand comparative efficacy with the laparoscopic and open approaches. There does not appear to be a drawback in functional or oncologic outcomes or complication rate with the robotic approach, with comparably acceptable outcomes of intraoperative parameters such as operative time, WIT, and EBL. The available literature overwhelmingly supports the adoption of robotics for the surgical treatment of renal masses.

References

1. Clayman RV, Kavoussi LR, Soper NJ, et al. Laparoscopic nephrectomy: initial case report. J Urol. 1991;146:278.
2. Gaur DD, Agarwal DK, Purohit KC. Retroperitoneal laparoscopic nephrectomy: initial case report. J Urol. 1993;149:103.
3. Gill IS, Sung GT, Hsu TH, et al. Robotic remote laparoscopic nephrectomy and adrenalectomy: the initial experience. J Urol. 2000;164:2082.
4. Guillonneau B, Jayet C, Tewari A, et al. Robot assisted laparoscopic nephrectomy. J Urol. 2001;166:200.
5. Klingler DW, Hemstreet GP, Balaji KC. Feasibility of robotic radical nephrectomy: initial results of single-institution pilot study. Urology. 2005;65:1086.
6. Nazemi T, Galich A, Sterrett S, et al. Radical nephrectomy performed by open, laparoscopy with or without hand-assistance or robotic methods by the same surgeon produces comparable perioperative results. Int Braz J Urol. 2006;32:15.
7. Rogers C, Laungani R, Krane LS, et al. Robotic nephrectomy for the treatment of benign and malignant disease. BJU Int. 2008;102:1660.
8. Anele UA, Marchioni M, Yang B, et al. Robotic versus laparoscopic radical nephrectomy: a large multi-institutional analysis (ROSULA Collaborative Group). World J Urol. 2019;37:2439.
9. Helmers MR, Ball MW, Gorin MA, et al. Robotic versus laparoscopic radical nephrectomy: comparative analysis and cost considerations. Can J Urol. 2016;23:8435.
10. Golombos DM, Chughtai B, Trinh QD, et al. Adoption of technology and its impact on nephrectomy outcomes, a U.S. population-based analysis (2008–2012). J Endourol. 2017;31:91.
11. Hemal AK, Kumar A. A prospective comparison of laparoscopic and robotic radical nephrectomy for T1-2N0M0 renal cell carcinoma. World J Urol. 2009;27:89.
12. Crocerossa F, Carbonara U, Cantiello F, et al. Robot-assisted radical nephrectomy: a systematic review and meta-analysis of comparative studies. Eur Urol. 2020;80(4):428–39.
13. Fergany AF, Hafez KS, Novick AC. Long-term results of nephron sparing surgery for localized renal cell carcinoma: 10-year followup. J Urol. 2000;163:442.
14. Becker F, Siemer S, Humke U, et al. Elective nephron sparing surgery should become standard treatment for small unilateral renal cell carcinoma: long-term survival data of 216 patients. Eur Urol. 2006;49:308.
15. Dash A, Vickers AJ, Schachter LR, et al. Comparison of outcomes in elective partial vs radical nephrectomy for clear cell renal cell carcinoma of 4-7 cm. BJU Int. 2006;97:939.
16. Margulis V, Tamboli P, Jacobsohn KM, et al. Oncological efficacy and safety of nephron-sparing surgery for selected patients with locally advanced renal cell carcinoma. BJU Int. 2007;100:1235.
17. Gill IS, Kavoussi LR, Lane BR, et al. Comparison of 1,800 laparoscopic and open partial nephrectomies for single renal tumors. J Urol. 2007;178:41.
18. Gettman MT, Blute ML, Chow GK, et al. Robotic-assisted laparoscopic partial nephrectomy: technique and initial clinical experience with DaVinci robotic system. Urology. 2004;64:914.
19. Michli EE, Parra RO. Robotic-assisted laparoscopic partial nephrectomy: initial clinical experience. Urology. 2009;73:302.
20. Benway BM, Bhayani SB, Rogers CG, et al. Robot assisted partial nephrectomy versus laparoscopic partial nephrectomy for renal tumors: a multi-institutional analysis of perioperative outcomes. J Urol. 2009;182:866.
21. DeLong JM, Shapiro O, Moinzadeh A. Comparison of laparoscopic versus robotic assisted partial nephrectomy: one surgeon's initial experience. Can J Urol. 2010;17:5207.
22. Ellison JS, Montgomery JS, Wolf JS Jr, et al. A matched comparison of perioperative outcomes of a single laparoscopic surgeon versus a multisurgeon robot-assisted cohort for partial nephrectomy. J Urol. 2012;188:45.
23. Zhang X, Shen Z, Zhong S, et al. Comparison of peri-operative outcomes of robot-assisted vs laparoscopic partial nephrectomy: a meta-analysis. BJU Int. 2013;112:1133.
24. Khalifeh A, Autorino R, Hillyer SP, et al. Comparative outcomes and assessment of trifecta in 500 robotic and laparoscopic partial nephrectomy cases: a single surgeon experience. J Urol. 2013;189:1236.
25. Wu Z, Li M, Song S, et al. Propensity-score matched analysis comparing robot-assisted with laparoscopic partial nephrectomy. BJU Int. 2015;115:437.
26. Masson-Lecomte A, Bensalah K, Seringe E, et al. A prospective comparison of surgical and pathological outcomes obtained after robot-assisted or pure laparoscopic partial nephrectomy in moderate to complex renal tumours: results from a French Multicentre Collaborative Study. BJU Int. 2013;111:256.
27. Masson-Lecomte A, Yates DR, Hupertan V, et al. A prospective comparison of the pathologic and surgical outcomes obtained after elective treatment of renal cell carcinoma by open or robot-assisted partial nephrectomy. Urol Oncol. 2013;31:924.
28. Masson-Lecomte A, Yates DR, Bensalah K, et al. Robot-assisted laparoscopic nephron sparing surgery for tumors over 4 cm: operative results and preliminary oncologic outcomes from a Multicentre French Study. Eur J Surg Oncol. 2013;39:799.
29. Shen Z, Xie L, Xie W, et al. The comparison of perioperative outcomes of robot-assisted and open partial nephrectomy: a systematic review and meta-analysis. World J Surg Oncol. 2016;14:220.
30. Grivas N, Kalampokis N, Larcher A, et al. Robot-assisted versus open partial nephrectomy: comparison of outcomes. A systematic review. Minerva Urol Nefrol. 2019;71:113.
31. Xia L, Wang X, Xu T, et al. Systematic review and meta-analysis of comparative studies reporting perioperative outcomes of robot-assisted partial nephrectomy versus open partial nephrectomy. J Endourol. 2017;31:893.
32. Tsai SH, Tseng PT, Sherer BA, et al. Open versus robotic partial nephrectomy: systematic review and meta-analysis of contemporary studies. Int J Med Robot. 2019;15:e1963.
33. Aboumarzouk OM, Stein RJ, Eyraud R, et al. Robotic versus laparoscopic partial nephrectomy: a systematic review and meta-analysis. Eur Urol. 2012;62:1023.
34. McDougall EM, Clayman RV. Laparoscopic nephrectomy for benign disease: comparison of the transperitoneal and retroperitoneal approaches. J Endourol. 1996;10:45.
35. Choo SH, Lee SY, Sung HH, et al. Transperitoneal versus retroperitoneal robotic partial nephrectomy: matched-pair comparisons by nephrometry scores. World J Urol. 2014;32:1523.
36. Hughes-Hallett A, Patki P, Patel N, et al. Robot-assisted partial nephrectomy: a comparison of the transperitoneal and retroperitoneal approaches. J Endourol. 2013;27:869.
37. Maurice MJ, Kaouk JH, Ramirez D, et al. Robotic partial nephrectomy for posterior tumors through a retroperitoneal approach offers decreased length of stay compared with the transperitoneal approach: a propensity-matched analysis. J Endourol. 2017;31:158.
38. Arora S, Heulitt G, Menon M, et al. Retroperitoneal vs transperitoneal robot-assisted partial nephrectomy: comparison in a multi-institutional setting. Urology. 2018;120:131.
39. Abaza R, Gerhard RS, Martinez O. Feasibility of adopting retroperitoneal robotic partial nephrectomy after extensive transperitoneal experience. World J Urol. 2020;38:1087.
40. Stroup SP, Hamilton ZA, Marshall MT, et al. Comparison of retroperitoneal and transperitoneal robotic partial nephrectomy for Pentafecta perioperative and renal functional outcomes. World J Urol. 2017;35:1721.

41. Choi CI, Kang M, Sung HH, et al. Comparison by Pentafecta criteria of transperitoneal and retroperitoneal robotic partial nephrectomy for large renal tumors. J Endourol. 2020; 34:175.
42. Xia L, Zhang X, Wang X, et al. Transperitoneal versus retroperitoneal robot-assisted partial nephrectomy: a systematic review and meta-analysis. Int J Surg. 2016;30:109.
43. Pavan N, Derweesh I, Hampton LJ, et al. Retroperitoneal robotic partial nephrectomy: systematic review and cumulative analysis of comparative outcomes. J Endourol. 2018;32:591.
44. McLean A, Mukherjee A, Phukan C, et al. Trans-peritoneal vs. retroperitoneal robotic assisted partial nephrectomy in posterior renal tumours: need for a risk-stratified patient individualised approach. A systematic review and meta-analysis. J Robot Surg. 2020;14:1.

Part IV

Bladder

Surgical Anatomy and Clinical Relevance to Robot-Assisted Cystectomy and Urinary Diversion

Bastian Amend, Panagiotis Mourmouris, Peter Wiklund, Arnulf Stenzl, and Stavros I. Tyritzis

1 Introduction

Proceeding from open to endoscopic surgery and continuing to robot-assisted surgery does not change the anatomical facts, but visual perspective on anatomical structures and landmarks changes literally. The technical evolution has enhanced and modified the angle of view of topographic relations between anatomical structures and the attention to details. Variable magnification and full high-definition stereoscopic view along with the possibility of tremor reduction feature and precise preparation facilitated these real-time insights into human pelvic anatomy. The following chapter addresses the macroscopic and microscopic anatomy of the lower urinary tract, ureters, and bowel with regard to special needs of a surgeon performing robot-assisted radical cystectomy with urinary diversion. In addition to basic anatomical knowledge, this chapter highlights the topographic anatomy of the female and male pelvis, the urethral sphincter mechanisms, visceral vascularization, and genitourinary tract innervation. Whereas macroscopic anatomy is extensively investigated and knowledge is established, microscopic anatomy, especially the complex pelvic neural network and the structure and topography of the rhabdosphincter, is still in the spotlight of scientific investigations. The prostate and the periprostatic nerve courses are excluded and focused on in another chapter, but regarding nerve-sparing radical cystectomy in male patients' understanding of the well-described periprostatic, autonomous nerve course is also essential. The incorporation of novel insights into urological practice, along with traditional anatomical knowledge, will improve our patients' treatment outcomes following robotic pelvic surgery.

B. Amend · A. Stenzl (✉)
Department of Urology, Eberhard Karls University, Tuebingen, Germany

P. Mourmouris
2nd University Urological Department, Athens University Medical School, SISMANOGLIO Hospital, Athens, Greece

P. Wiklund
Section of Urology, Department of Molecular Medicine and Surgery, Karolinska Institute, Stockholm, Sweden

Department of Urology, Icahn School of Medicine, Mount Sinai Health System, New York, NY, USA

S. I. Tyritzis
Department of Molecular Medicine and Surgery, Karolinska Institutet, Stockholm, Sweden

4th Urological Department-HYGEIA Hospital, Athens, Greece

2 The Anterior Abdominal Wall: Anatomical Landmarks

For laparoscopic and robot-assisted surgery, identifying the distinct anatomical structures of the anterior abdominal wall is essential. Trocar insertion and the early steps of intrapelvic preparation necessitate anatomical landmark orientation. Figure 1 shows a projection of the principal structures onto the skin of the anterior abdominal wall, whereas Fig. 2 shows a realistic and outlined laparoscopic view of the male pelvis

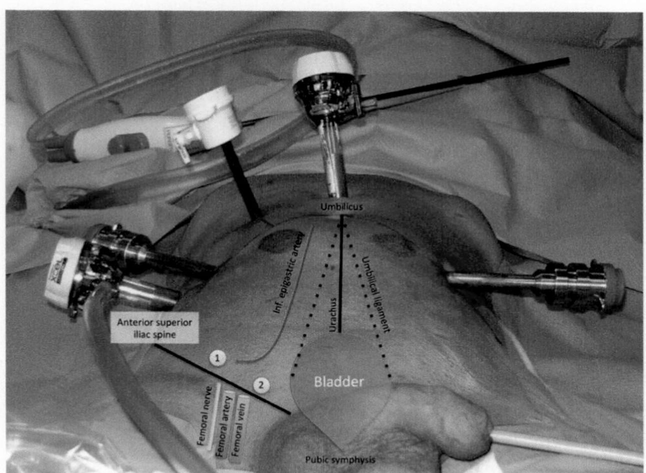

Fig. 1 Anatomical landmarks projected on the external abdominal wall (internal inguinal ring (*1*), external inguinal ring (*2*), trocar positioning for robot-assisted radical cystectomy)

P. Wiklund et al. (eds.), *Robotic Urologic Surgery*, https://doi.org/10.1007/978-3-031-00363-9_54

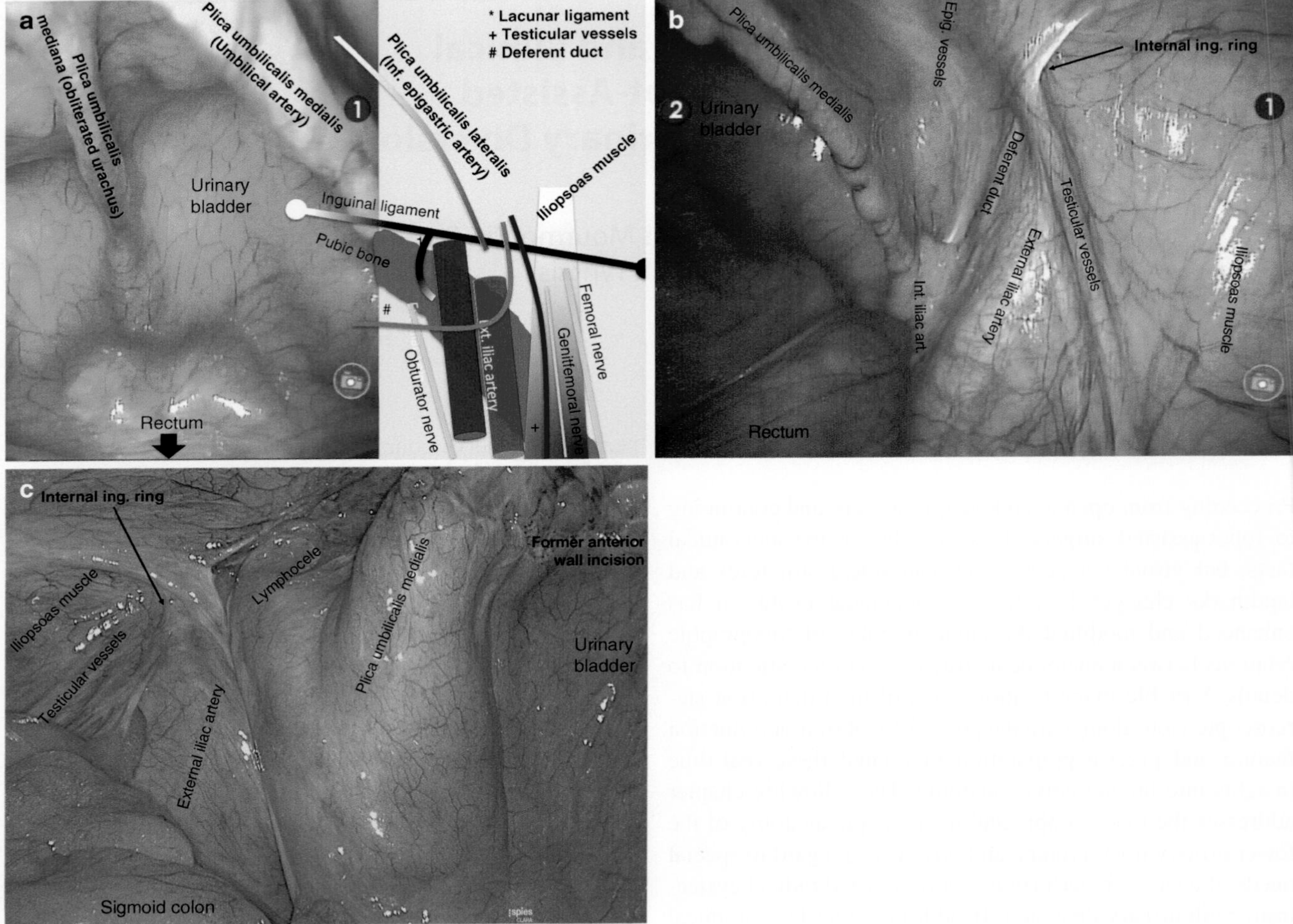

Fig. 2 (**a**) Intrapelvic anatomical landmarks. *Left*: laparoscopic view into the male pelvis (camera trocar insertion below the umbilicus). *Right*: anatomical structures of the inguinal region and the internal abdominal wall [additional annotation: deferent duct (#, *orange*), testicular vessels (+, *violet*), lacunar ligament (*)]; (**b**) Anatomical landmarks in the pelvis; (**c**) "Regeneration/Refixation" of the anterior abdominal wall after complete detachment during robot-assisted radical prostatectomy (laparoscopic view during laparoscopic lymphocele fenestration)

at the start of robot-assisted pelvic surgery. The anterior abdominal wall is divided into five tissue folds. The median umbilical ligament, which raises the median umbilical fold between the apex of the urinary bladder and the umbilicus, is derived from the former embryonic urachus (which connects the urinary bladder to the embryonic allantois) and is situated between the transversalis fascia and the peritoneum. The remnants of the fetal umbilical arteries are accommodated by the medial umbilical folds on both sides of the median umbilical fold. The excavation in the middle is known as the supravesical fossa. During cystectomy, the medial umbilical ligaments serve as guiding structures to identify the upper vesical pedicle, which includes the superior vesical artery. The lateral umbilical folds are formed by both inferior epigastric arteries. The location of the hernia passage to the lateral umbilical fold is used to classify hernias. The medial inguinal fossa, located medial to the lateral umbilical fold, is where direct inguinal hernias pass. The lateral inguinal fossa is related to the deep inguinal ring, which serves as the entrance to the inguinal canal. An indirect inguinal hernia could accompany spermatic cord components through the inguinal canal. The inguinal ligament is formed by the aponeurosis of the oblique external abdominal muscle and connects the pubic tubercle to the anterior superior iliac spine. Furthermore, the iliopectineal arch subdivides the space below the inguinal ligament. The iliopsoas muscle and the femoral nerve are found laterally in the muscular lacuna, while the external iliac vessels are found medially in the vascular lacuna. The lacunar ligament, which connects the inguinal ligament to the superior pubic ramus and is directly medial to the external iliac vein, represents the caudal extent after lymphadenectomy for prostate or bladder

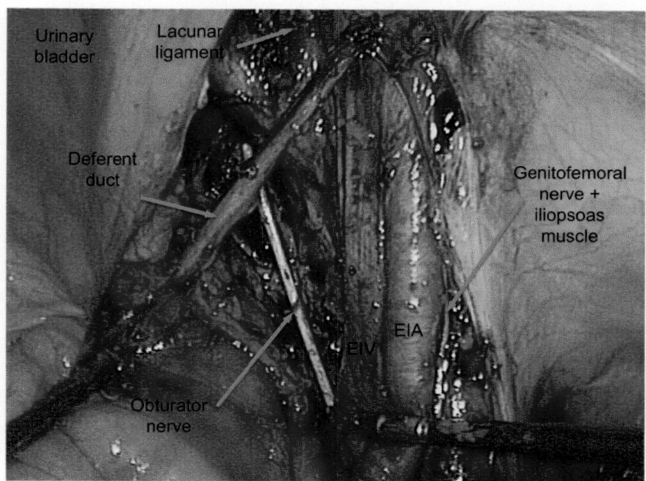

Fig. 3 Intrapelvic view after laparoscopic lymphadenectomy for prostate cancer; *EIV* external iliac vein, *EIA* external iliac artery. The lacunar ligament represents the distal extent of pelvic lymphadenectomy

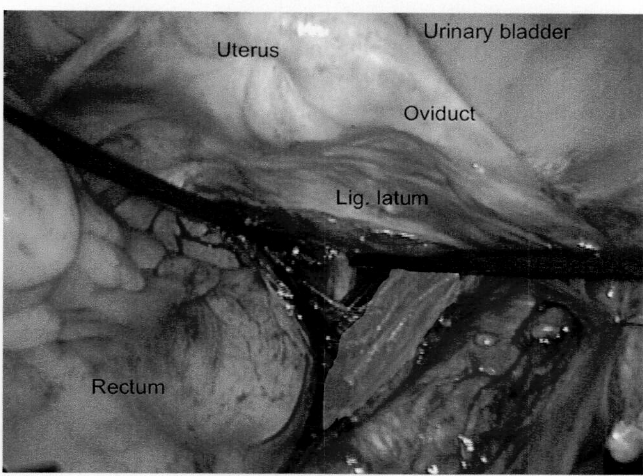

Fig. 4 Laparoscopic insight into the female pelvis during sacrocolpopexy. The rectovaginal fold, which includes the inferior hypogastric plexus (right side), is highlighted in lucent blue

cancer (Fig. 3). Interestingly, the anatomy has been restored with distinct anatomic features even after total detachment of the anterior abdominal wall after pelvic surgery. Figure 2c shows a lymphocele on the left pelvic axis after a robot-assisted radical prostatectomy [1–3].

3 Anatomical Topography of the Female Pelvis

The female pelvic bone has a flat sacral promontory and wide-open iliac wings. The urinary bladder, ureters, uterus, vagina, ovaries, oviducts, and rectum are the main organs of the peritoneal and subperitoneal pelvic cavity. The upper half of the urinary bladder, the uterus, the adnexa, and the anterior wall of the rectum are all covered by the parietal peritoneum, resulting in a variety of peritoneal conditions. The rectouterine excavation (Douglas' fold) and the vesicouterine excavation are caused by the uterus location between the urinary bladder and the rectum. The uterus is held in place by several ligaments: the cardinal ligaments (transverse cervical ligaments) include the uterine arteries, the uterine venous plexus, and portions of the distal third of the ureters and link the cervix to the lateral pelvic wall. Although it is not a ligament in the physical sense, the bilateral peritoneal duplication between the uterus and the pelvic wall in cranial continuation to the cardinal ligaments is known as ligamentum latum (broad ligament). The ovarian vessels are contained by the suspensory ligaments, which attach the ovaries to the lateral wall of the pelvis. The ovarian ligaments align the ovaries to the uterus in the opposite direction; supplementary vessels coming from the uterine arteries are included in these structures (ovarian branches of the uterine artery). The round ligaments connect the deep inguinal rings to the uterine horns. The rectouterine folds define the boundaries of the rectouterine excavation; they are made up of fibrous tissue and smooth muscle fibers, as well as they include the route of the inferior hypogastric plexus (Fig. 4). The pelvic fascia (endopelvic fascia), which is split into the parietal and visceral layers, comprises the superior layer of the fascia of the pelvic diaphragm and covers the boundaries of the subperitoneal space (also known as cavum retzii). The pubovesical ligaments (condensation of fibrous tissue and no ligaments in the anatomical sense) connect the urinary bladder to the symphysis pubis, with lateral connections to the superior layer of the fascia of the pelvic diaphragm [1–4].

4 Anatomical Topography of the Male Pelvis

In male humans, the pelvic bone is thinner and characterized by a larger protrusion of the sacral promontory, resulting in a heart-shaped pelvic entrance. The urinary bladder, ureters, prostate, seminal vesicles, deferent ducts, and rectum are all part of the pelvis. The rectovesical excavation is the lowest part of the abdominal cavity between the urinary bladder and the rectum (Fig. 5). The inferior hypogastric plexus is included in the rectovesical fold, which borders the excavation laterally (Fig. 6a). By elevating a peritoneal fold, the deferent ducts form the paravesical fossa. The current literature contains inconsistencies in the description and nomenclature of the subperitoneal fascias, particularly when examining the periprostatic fascia and the rectoprostatic septum, which separates the urinary bladder and the rectum beginning at the rectovesical excavation ("cul-de-sac"). Like female anatomy, the pelvic fascia is made up of two layers: a parietal layer that covers the lateral wall of the pelvis and a visceral layer (clinically known as "endopelvic fascia") that covers the pelvic organs. The tendinous arch of pelvic fascia is the intersection of two layers. It is still unknown if the prostate's own fascia divides the gland. The absence of a fascia in the apical area of the prostate, as well as the creation of the so-called puboprostatic ligaments by an aggregation of the endopelvic fascia, indicates that the visceral layer of the pelvic fascia and the fascia of the prostate correlate. Muscle fibers (smooth or striated) may also have a role in the architecture of the puboprostatic ligaments. Similarly, the configuration of the Denonvilliers fascia remains unknown in the literature. The rectoprostatic septum is defined in anatomical nomenclature as a membranous separation between the rectum and the ventral urinary bladder with the prostate. From the lowest point of the rectovesical excavation to the pelvic floor, the fascia arose from two layers of a peritoneal cul-de-sac. Currently, it is considered that the rectoprostatic septum is composed of two former peritoneal layers that cannot be separated bluntly in the majority of individuals. It is thought that writers illustrating fascia separation procedures are referring to the gap between Denonvilliers fascia and the rectal fascia propria (a part of the visceral layer of the pelvic fascia) [1–3, 5–10].

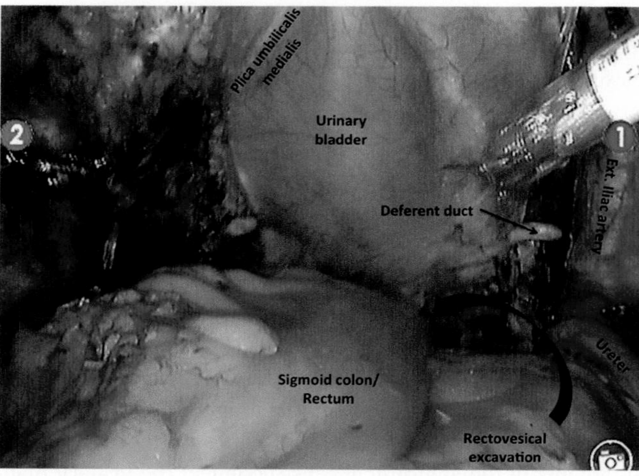

Fig. 5 Anatomical landmarks during robot-assisted laparoscopic cystectomy after the first step of lymphadenectomy

5 Ureter and Periureteral Space

The ureter can be identified after incising the posterior peritoneal layer just over the iliac vessel (landmark: bifurcation of the common iliac artery) crossing with the uterine artery in the female and medially to the junction of the medial umbilical ligament and the internal iliac artery in males. The ureter is then running down to its final third crossing posteriorly to the superior vesical pedicle. The ureter is supplied by branches of renal, gonadal, common iliac, internal iliac, vesical, and uterine arteries and also directly from branches of the abdominal aorta. It is important for the surgeon to remember that the vascularization of the ureter is commonly medially for its abdominal part whereas for the pelvic ureter is situated laterally. Also, there is a good longitudinal anastomosis between all the above mentioned branches that facilitates the transection and anastomosis in any level. The distal ureter is situated in females inside the transverse cervical ligament (which also contains the uterine arteries and

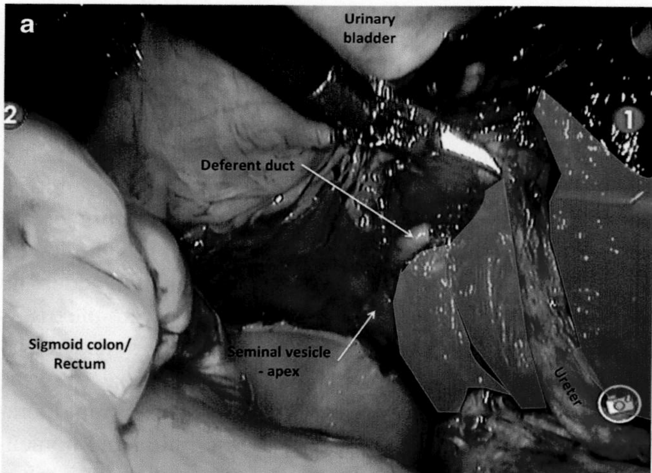

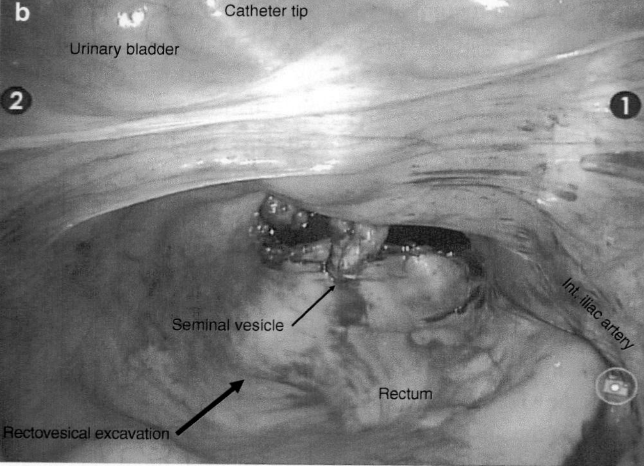

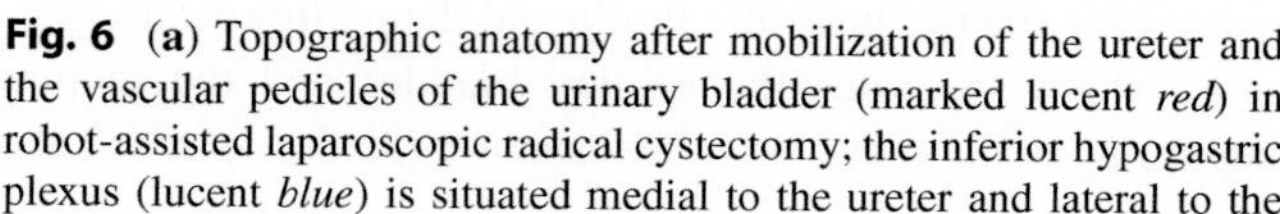

Fig. 6 (**a**) Topographic anatomy after mobilization of the ureter and the vascular pedicles of the urinary bladder (marked lucent *red*) in robot-assisted laparoscopic radical cystectomy; the inferior hypogastric plexus (lucent *blue*) is situated medial to the ureter and lateral to the apex of the seminal vesicle; (**b**) Rectovesical excavation with crosswise peritoneal incision for retroprostatic preparation; the inferior hypogastric plexus is located lateral to the seminal vesicles (small arrow) and the internal iliac artery

veins), whereas in the males medial to the ureter and lateral to the apex of the seminal vesicle lies the inferior hypogastric plexus. The anatomy of the ureter and periureteral space is of great importance for various reasons. The length of the ureter as a factor influencing functional outcomes of robot-assisted radical cystectomy via anastomotic stricture occurrence is still debatable [11, 12], but surgeons must preserve as much ureteral length as possible. However, the most important factor seems to be the preservation of adequate periureteral fatty tissue. Excision of a possible compromised section of the ureter can effectively prevent stricture formation [13]. In addition, preoperative imaging helps to identify regularly occurring ureteral abnormalities: ectopic ureter, ureter duplication (fissus/duplex), retrocaval ureter, or crossed renal dystopia. In case of ureteral stenting, the surrounding tissue is often characterized by periureteral fibrotic reaction.

6 Macroscopic and Microscopic Anatomy of the Urinary Bladder

The urinary bladder is a distensible, muscular organ that collects urine and allows for regulated micturition. The apex, corpus, fundus, and collum (with the trigone) are the macroscopic divisions of the urinary bladder (Fig. 7). Between 300 and 500 cm³ is the typical filling volume. The trigone is distinguished by an interureteric crest raised between the obliquely descending ureters. The mucosa (transitional cells), the submucosa, the detrusor muscle (three layers), and the surrounding adipose and connective tissue constitute the urinary bladder wall (Fig. 7). In the trigone region, the mucosa adheres directly to the submucosa; however, the other sections of the urinary bladder show a loose relationship between these two layers. There are three layers to the detrusor muscle: an exterior and internal longitudinal muscle

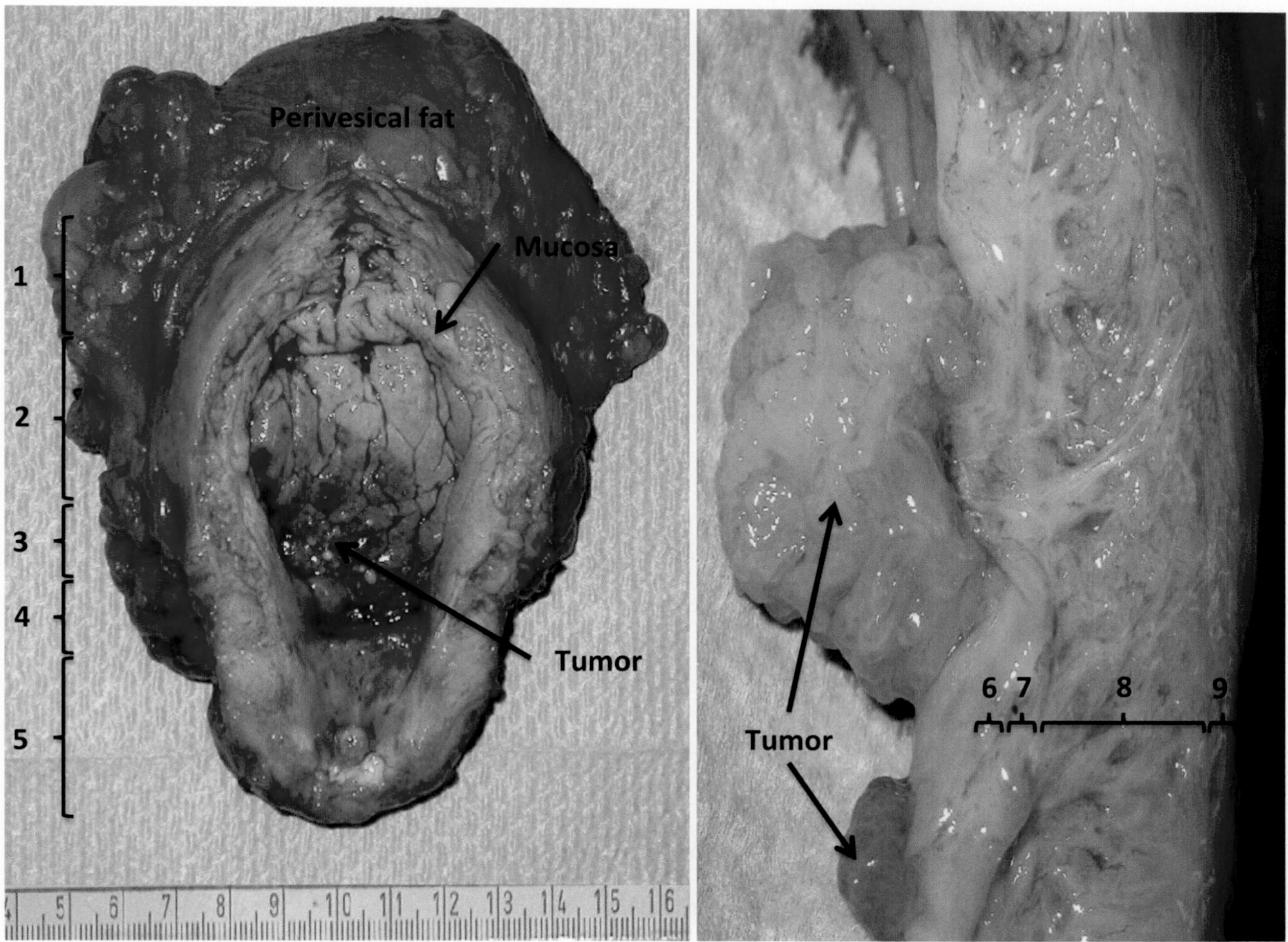

Fig. 7 Macroscopic anatomy of the urinary bladder. *Left*: male cystectomy specimen ventrally incised; *1* apex, *2* corpus, *3* fundus, *4* collum/trigone, *5* Prostate with verumontanum. *Right*: Cross section of cystectomy specimen with muscle bladder cancer; *6* mucosa, *7* submucosa, *8* detrusor muscle (three layers), *9* adventitia with perivesical fat tissue or serosa (peritoneum)

layer, as well as an interjacent circular layer. The circular layer does not reach the trigone or the bladder neck. The longitudinal muscle fibers of both ureters, in combination with the expanding longitudinal fibers of both ureters, extend below the bladder neck and reach the muscular layers of the urethra, creating the Waldeyer's sheath of the ureterovesical junction. These structures reach the seminal colliculus point in male humans.

Table 1 summarizes the arterial blood supply to the pelvis and, in particular, the genitourinary tract. The superior vesical artery and the inferior vesical artery are the two major branches of each of the internal iliac arteries that supply the urinary bladder (clinically the superior and inferior vesical pedicle). The superior vesical artery arises from a shared branch with the previous umbilical artery and passes through the medial umbilical ligament. The inferior vesical artery develops from a branch of the middle rectal artery. The inferior vesical artery is the most common source of prostatic branches. The urinary bladder's venous drainage is controlled by a series of distinct venous plexuses on both sides

Table 1 Pelvic vascularization: main arteries with origin, branches, and supplied organs [1]

Artery	Origin	Main branches	Blood supply to (lead structure)
Testicular/ovarian	Abdominal aorta	–	Testes (spermatic cord)/ovaries (suspensory ligament)
Inferior mesenteric	Abdominal aorta	Left colic art.	Descending colon
		Sigmoid branches	Sigmoid colon
		Superior rectal art.	Rectum
Middle sacral	Abdominal aorta	–	Sacral nerves, coccygeal glomus
Common iliac	Abdominal aorta	External iliac art.	(Ureter crosses iliac bifurcation)
		Internal iliac art.	
External iliac	Common iliac art.	Inferior epigastric art.	Rectus abdominis muscle (lateral umbilical fold)
		Deep circumflex iliac art.	Surrounding muscles/structures
		Femoral art.	Leg (vascular lacuna)
Internal iliac	Common iliac art.	See below	See below
Iliolumbar	Internal iliac art. (parietal branch)	…	Iliopsoas and quadratus lumborum muscle, spinal cord
Lateral sacral	Internal iliac art. (parietal branch)	…	Erector spinae muscles
Obturator	Internal iliac art. (parietal branch)	Pubic branch	Surrounding tissue (anastomosis to inferior epigastric art.—corona mortis)
		Anterior branch	Anterior adductor muscles
		Posterior branch	Posterior adductor muscles
		Acetabular branch	Femur head
Superior gluteal	Internal iliac art. (parietal branch)	–	Gluteal muscles (suprapiriform foramen)
Inferior gluteal	Internal iliac art. (parietal branch)	–	Gluteal muscles (infrapiriform foramen), hip external rotators, ischial nerve
Umbilical	Internal iliac art. (visceral branch)	Obliterated distal part	(Medial umbilical fold)
		Superior vesical art.	Urinary bladder, prostate, ureter
		Art. of the vas deferens	Vas deferens
Inferior vesical	Internal iliac art. (visceral branch)	–	Urinary bladder, prostate, seminal vesicles/vagina
Uterine	Internal iliac art. (visceral branch)	Vaginal branch	Vagina
		Arcuate vessels	Uterus (broad ligament)
		Ovarian branch	Ovary (ovarian ligament)
		Tubal branch	Uterine tube
Middle rectal	Internal iliac art. (visceral branch)	–	Rectum and surrounding organs
Internal pudendal	Internal iliac art. (visceral branch)	Inferior rectal art.	Rectum
		Perineal art.	Perineum
		Posterior labial/scrotal branch	Labia/scrotum
		Art. of the bulb of vestibule/penis	Urethra, bulb of vestibule/corpus spongiosum
		Dorsal art. of clitoris/penis	Corpus cavernosum clitoridis/glans penis
		Deep art. of clitoris/penis	Corpus cavernosum clitoridis/penis

… indicates different small branches, *art.* artery

of the vesical base. These venous vessels have significant communication with the prostatic venous plexus in male humans and the vaginal venous plexus in females.

The proper functioning of the urinary bladder to manage urine storage, continence, and micturition is facilitated by a sophisticated neurological system. For a precise procedure, interactions between separate reflex circuits and arbitrary actions are required. Lower urinary tract innervations are enhanced by both the autonomous and somatic neural systems, making bladder filling and emptying possible. Table 2 shows the nerves and plexus of the pelvis in detail, as well as their neurological functions.

Through the inferior hypogastric plexus, parasympathetic and sympathetic nerve fibers reach the urinary bladder and surrounding organs (pelvic plexus). The inferior hypogastric plexus is derived from the superior hypogastric plexus, which crosses the distal ureter and the common iliac artery on both sides and enters the pelvis proximally and medially (Fig. 8). As previously stated, the inferior hypogastric plexus is a component of the rectouterine or rectovesical fold (Figs. 4 and 6b). In a sagittal orientation, the plexus extends laterally to the rectum, the vagina (in females, Fig. 9), the bladder neck, and the seminal vesicles (in men) (Fig. 10). It appears that nerve fibers inside the plexus can be assigned to innervated destinations. The front section is responsible of urogenital innervations, whereas the posterior part directs to the rectum. The perivesical extent and trajectory of autonomous nerve fibers are less understood. According to detailed descriptions of periprostatic nerve characteristics, a significant number of nerves congregate lateral and anterior to the seminal vesicles at the level of the urine bladder neck (Fig. 11). To define nerve courses proximal to the bladder neck in terms of nerve-sparing methods, more research is needed.

The inferior hypogastric plexus sympathetic fibers are derived from two superior retroperitoneal sympathetic chains known as sacral splanchnic nerves, which travel topographically through the superior hypogastric plexus. Sympathetic excitations cause the detrusor muscle to be inhibited and the smooth muscle sphincter cells at the bladder neck and urethra to be stimulated, resulting in urinary bladder filling. Parasympathetic fibers from the sacral spinal cord (S2–S5)

Table 2 Main nerve pathways of the pelvis [1]

Nerve	Spinal origin	Intermediary trunk	Innervation
Iliohypogastric	L1	Lumbar plexus	M: transversus abdominis and internal oblique muscle S: hip and lower abdominal wall
Ilioinguinal	L1	Lumbar plexus	M: abdominal muscles S: inguinal region, penile root, proximal medial femoral skin, scrotum/labia majora
Genitofemoral	L1/2	Lumbar plexus	M: cremaster muscle S: tunica vaginalis, tunica dartos, hiatus saphenus
Lateral femoral cutaneous nerve	L2/3	Lumbar plexus	M: – S: anterolateral femoral skin
Femoral nerve	L2/3/4	Lumbar plexus	M: iliopsoas/pectineus/sartorius/quadriceps femoris muscle S: anteromedial femoral skin, anteromedial crural skin, medial forefoot skin
Obturator	L2/3/4	Lumbar plexus	M: external obturator/pectineus/adductor brevis/adductor longus et magnus et minimus/gracilis muscle S: distal medial femoral skin
Inferior gluteal	L4/L5/S1	Lumbosacral plexus	M: gluteus maximus muscle S: –
Posterior femoral cutaneous	S1/2/3	Sacral plexus	M: – S: gluteal skin, posterior scrotal/labial skin
Ischial	L4/S1/S2/S3	Lumbosacral plexus	M: ischiocrural and forefoot muscles S: crural and forefoot skin (except medial)
Pudendal	(S2)/S3/S4	Sacral plexus	M: levator ani muscle, external urethral sphincter and urogenital diaphragm S: skin above the ischial tuberosity, labia (majora and) minora and clitoris, penile skin with glans and prepuce
Coccygeal	S5/Co1	Coccygeal plexus	M: – S: anococcygeal skin
Sacral splanchnic	Sympathetic trunk	Superior hypogastric plexus	Sympathetic: urinary bladder, internal sphincter complex, ejaculation reflex
Pelvic splanchnic	S2/S3/S4	Inferior hypogastric plexus—prostatic plexus—cavernous nerve	Parasympathetic: erectile function

M motoric, *S* sensory

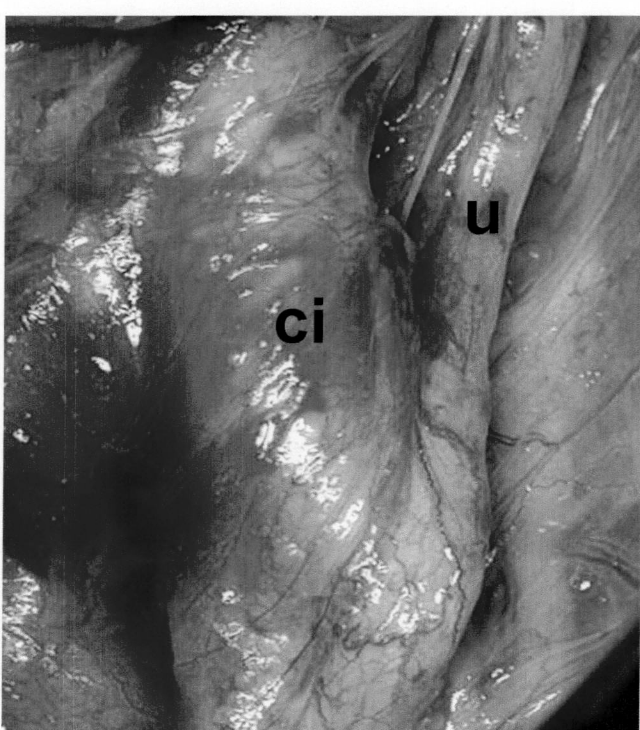

Fig. 8 Nerve course of the sympathetic fibers deriving from the superior hypogastric plexus (*ci* common iliac artery, *u* ureter) (Schilling et al. [14])

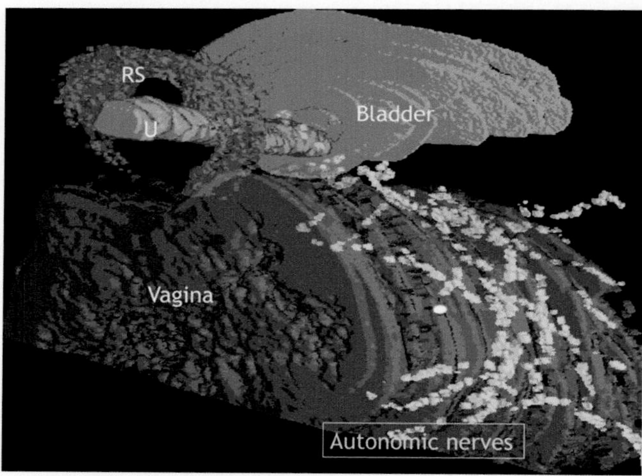

Fig. 9 Fetal female pelvic study illustrates 3D distribution pattern of autonomic nerves between the rhabdosphincter, the urethra, the urinary bladder, and the vagina (Colleselli et al. [15])

emerge via the foramina of the sacral bone and go to the bladder through the inferior hypogastric plexus. The parasympathetic neural system controls both urinary bladder sensibility (and, presumably, proximal urethral sensation) and detrusor muscle contraction. A new article uses three-

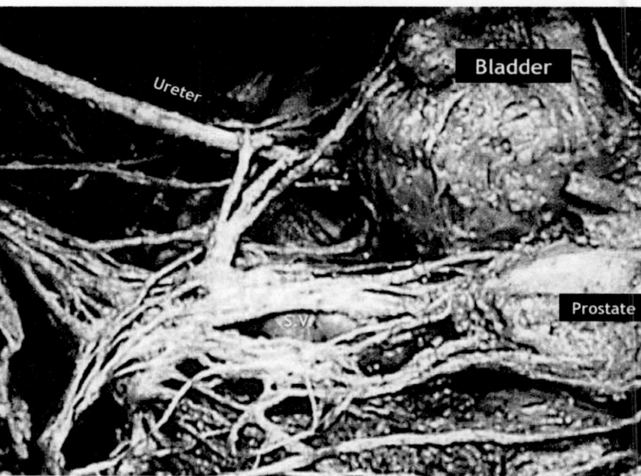

Fig. 10 Human male cadaver study to illustrate topographical relation of the complex intrapelvic nerve plexus to the urinary bladder, the ureter, the male adnexa, and the prostate. The superior vesical artery crosses the ureter almost orthogonally (Colleselli et al. [15])

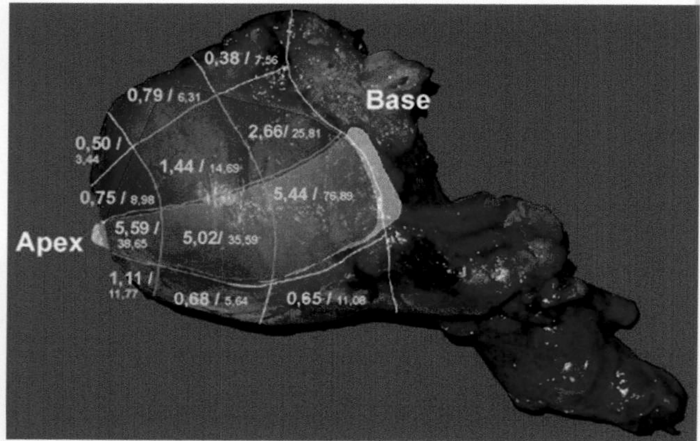

Fig. 11 Prostate specimen after non-nerve-sparing radical prostatectomy indicating mean nerve counts of extraprostatetic nerve fibers (>200 μm/<200 μm). Orange field marks the accumulation of periprostatic nerves/bundle (Sievert et al. [16])

dimensional nerve mapping to show the nerve entry into the urinary bladder wall at the level of the bladder neck and the trigone. The pudendal nerve is a somatic nerve that innervates the striated portions of the external urethral sphincter, among other muscles as well as sensibility of the skin of the perineum and partly the external genitals. The pudendal nerve exits the pelvis by encircling the ischial spine and passing via the pudendal canal (Alcock's canal) at the bottom of the inferior pubic bone after distributing the lumbosacral plexus. Stimulation causes the external urethral sphincter and neighboring segments of the levator muscle to contract more intensely. The process of filling and emptying involves complex linkages on many areas of the central nervous system, including the Onuf's nucleus (found in the sacral region of the spinal cord), the periaqueductal gray, the pontine micturition center, and the frontal lobe of the cerebrum [1–3, 14, 16–19].

7 Anatomic Abnormalities of the Urinary Bladder

Depending on the treated condition and the guideline-based extent of preoperative staging diagnostics, unexpected intrapelvic anatomic abnormalities or changes have not been disclosed in all situations. The following changes in human pelvic anatomy should be anticipated on a more or less regular basis. There are two types of urinary bladder diverticula: congenital and acquired. The most common bilateral para-ureteral diverticulum (Hutch diverticulum) is congenital and causes vesicoureteral reflux in the majority of cases (Fig. 12). Acquired diverticula arise because of infravesical occlusion and can grow to be very large. Only a few occurrences of urachal obliterations were determined to be abnormal. There are four types of malformations: (1) persistent urachus with continuous urine leakage, (2) urachal cyst located along the medial umbilical ligament, (3) umbilical-urachus sinus with obliteration toward the urinary bladder, and (4) vesicourachal diverticulum with obliteration toward the umbilicus. Ureteroceles, ectopic placements, and refluxive diseases are further examples of ureteric orifices (Fig. 12) [1, 2, 20].

8 Pelvic Floor

The pelvic diaphragm and the urogenital diaphragm are two separate fibromuscular layers that form the inferior pelvic aperture. The coccygeal muscle and the levator ani muscle constitute the pelvic diaphragm, which is formed up of the following components, which are called according to their origins and insertions: the pubococcygeal muscle, the iliococcygeal muscle, and the puborectalis muscle. The superior layer of the levator ani fascia is formed by the endopelvic fascia, while a distinct layer covers the caudal section; the levator ani muscle's pelvic insertion is known as the tendinous arch of levator ani. In men, the levator ani muscle creates an archway-shaped entry for the anus and urethra and, in females, the anus, vagina, and urethra. The sacral plexus (S3 and S4) provides the majority of the innervation, with some nerve fibers reaching the puborectalis muscle through the pudendal nerve. Although the contributions of shape topography and pelvic diaphragm contraction to anal continence appear to be demonstrated, it is still unknown to what degree these anatomical structures also impact urine continence. The pelvic diaphragm and the striated external urethral sphincter are muscularly independent, according to recent publications, but a connective tissue link creating a tendinous connection originating from the inferior portion of the external urethral sphincter in females has been shown. These interactions lead the authors to believe that urinary continence requires a healthy pelvic diaphragm.

The urogenital diaphragm is not recognized by anatomical nomenclature, and its precise anatomical and histomorphological structure is unknown. According to anatomical atlases, the urogenital diaphragm is made up of the deep transverse perineal muscle (which is less developed in females) and a superior and inferior urogenital fascia. The conventional image of the urogenital diaphragm is completed by the superficial transverse perineal muscle entering at the perineal body (central tendon of the perineum), the striated external urethral sphincter, and the surrounding connective tissue. Although some publications claim to have discovered a deep transverse perineal muscle, most subsequent investigations have been unable to confirm this claim. The

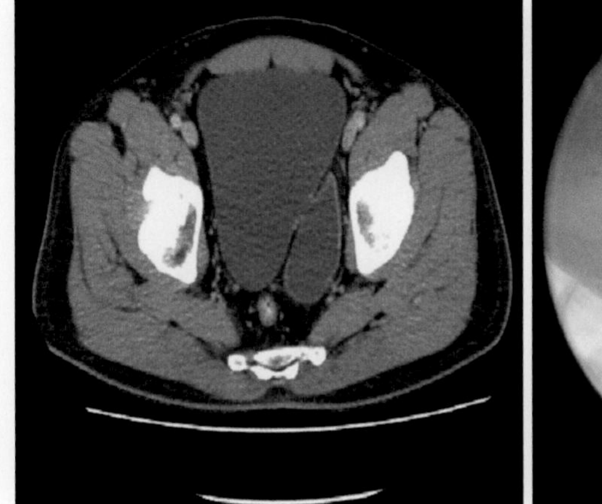
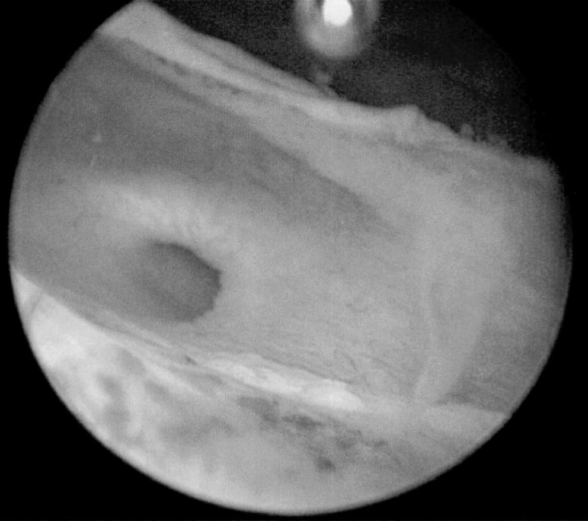
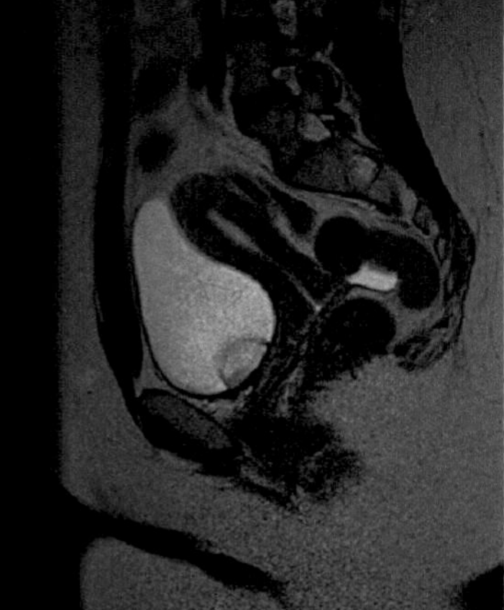

Fig. 12 *Left:* male patient CT-scan with a para-ureteral diverticulum; *middle and right:* left ureteric orifice after transurethral resection of an obstructive ureterocele with an ectopic orifice at the bladder neck in a female patient (endoscopic view after resection and sagittal CT-scan)

external urethral sphincter, the perineal body, the inferior pubic bone, and the superficial transverse perineal muscle are all embedded in the urogenital diaphragm, which is made up of layers of connective tissue. Directly under the urogenital diaphragm are the internal pudendal artery and the pudendal nerve. The bulbourethral glands (Cowper's glands) are located in the urogenital diaphragm, laterally to the membranous urethra [1, 2, 21–27].

9 Male Urethra

The intramural periprostatic urethra at the bladder neck, the prostatic urethra, the membranous urethra, and the spongy urethra compose up the male urethra. Transitional cells form the mucosa of the proximal sections, while a gradual shift from stratified columnar to stratified squamous cells characterizes the distal region near the navicular fossa. The muscle layer is split into three sections: an inner longitudinal, a middle circular, and an outer longitudinal stratum that is poorly defined. The bulbourethral artery enters the spongy urethra at the level of the penile bulb and receives blood from the internal pudendal artery [1–3].

10 Female Urethra

From the urinary bladder neck to the vaginal vestibule, the female urethra measures around 4 cm. An inner longitudinal and a surrounding circularly orientated stratum compose up the muscle layer. Figure 13 depicts the female urethra's innervations and blood supply, which are provided by the internal pudendal artery and the pudendal nerve. Females have a smooth transition from the bladder neck to the proximal urethra, unlike males who have a clear boundary between the bladder neck and the prostatic urethra. A transurethral catheter balloon is used intraoperatively to aid in the optimal identification of the anatomical resection line in order to maintain continence (short proximal urethra) and minimize urine retention (long proximal urethra) [1–3].

11 Sphincter Mechanisms

In the past, urinary continence was attributed to the voluntary, striated external urethral sphincter (rhabdosphincter) in the urogenital diaphragm and the autonomous, smooth internal sphincter (lissosphincter) in the bladder neck. The anatomical and functional knowledge of the sphincter complex has changed dramatically as a result of extensive research (Fig. 14). Although the precise anatomical formation and interaction are debated, three components of the sphincter complex are widely accepted: the smooth detrusor muscle fibers of the bladder neck, including the trigone, the intrinsic smooth muscle fibers of the urethral wall, and the external urethral sphincter.

11.1 The Bladder Neck Component

Various authors have disputed the presence of an isolated, circularly orientated smooth muscle sphincter at the internal urethral orifice during the previous two centuries, even though numerous anatomical atlases still depict a typical inner urinary bladder sphincter. In fact, at the bladder outlet, a complex network of smooth muscle strands forms, with detrusor muscle fibers condensing toward the trigone, longitudinal fibers originating from the ureteral orifices, and

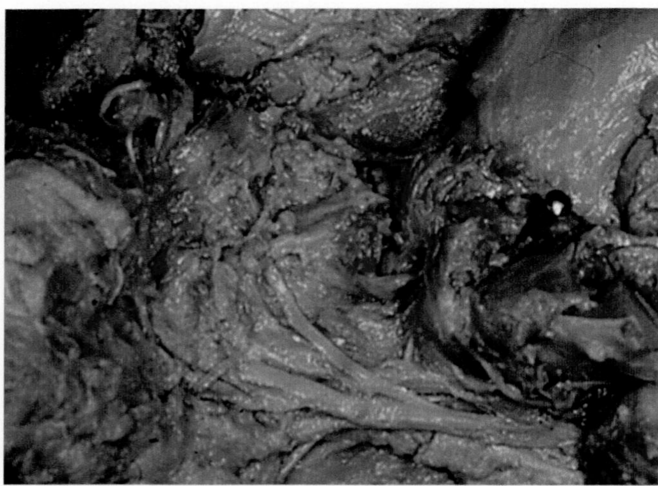

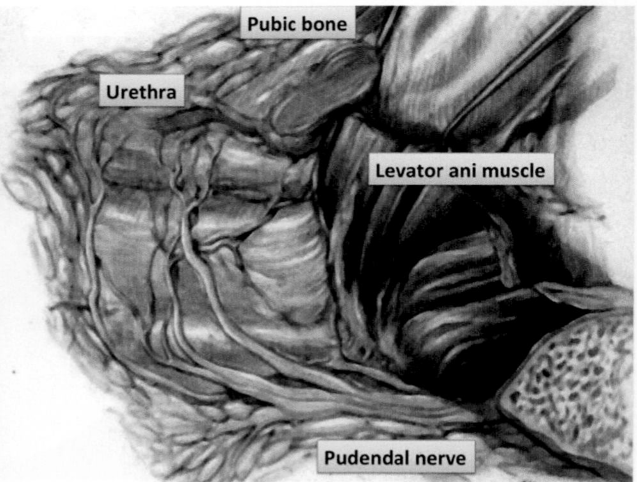

Fig. 13 Human female cadaver study illustrating the pudendal nerve arising from the Alcock's canal to innervate the distal third of the urethra including branches to the rhabdosphincter (Colleselli et al. [15]; additional annotations have been made for clarification)

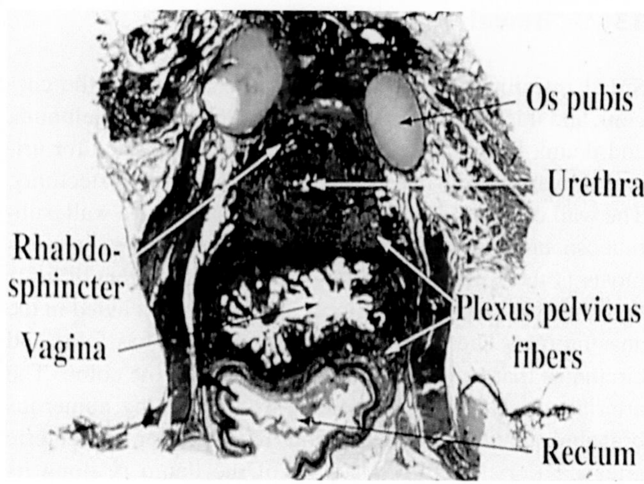

Fig. 14 Fetal female pelvis illustrating the omega-shaped rhabdosphincter surrounding the urethra and the topographical location of pelvic plexus (Colleselli et al. [15])

smooth intrinsic fibers of the urethral wall forming a muscular compartment innervated by the autonomic nervous system. Muscle fibers arising from the ureteral orifices distend downward into the verumontanum in male individuals.

11.2 The Urethral Wall Component

The smooth muscle fibers of the urethral wall are integrated continuously from the bladder neck component into the urethral closure mechanism. The urethral muscular element consists of inner longitudinal and surrounding circular oriented muscle fibers. Inconsistently, an outer longitudinal muscular layer has been described. Also, these smooth muscle fibers receive autonomic innervations (Fig. 14).

11.3 The External Urethral Sphincter

To present, there is no widely recognized anatomical and functional understanding of the external urethral sphincter complex. There is agreement on the three-dimensional profile of the external urethral sphincter, which is characterized as omega or horseshoe shaped in both male and female individuals (Fig. 14). As a result, muscle fibers are seen in the anterior and lateral parts of the urethra. By connecting the posterior muscular ends of the external urethral sphincter, fibrous tissue completes the horseshoe form dorsally. The external urethral sphincter is debated as to whether it is a component of the urogenital diaphragm and hence buried in the doubtfully existent deep transverse perineal muscle. The external urethral sphincter is increasingly being recognized as a separate entity maintained by a fibrous link to the surrounding tissue, particularly the pelvic diaphragm and puborectalis muscle. Similarly, the vertical extent and histological composition of the external urethral sphincter are being studied in depth. The striated muscle fibers of the pronounced anterior portion of the sphincter are thought to disseminate under the puboprostatic ligaments over the anterior face of the prostate in male humans. The striated muscle fibers' communication with components of the urine bladder neck is yet unknown. Parts of the striated external sphincter were only discovered in the two distal thirds of the urethra in females. For a long time, it has been well recognized that striated muscle fibers play a major role in the formation of the external sphincter. In terms of function, the external sphincter must always maintain continence by maintaining a static closure pressure, as well as during stress episodes when the need for urethral constriction increases fast. Two possible explanations for achieving continence are the existence of two specialized striated muscle fibers, "slow twitch fibers" for basal pressure and "fast twitch fibers" for rapid pressure increases, as well as the existence of a smooth muscle component ("lissosphincter") located within the main part of striated fibers (named the internal urethral sphincter). The axons for somatic innervation of the voluntary striated external sphincter are found in the pudendal nerve (Fig. 14). It is currently unknown if autonomous fibers derived from the inferior hypogastric plexus, which may have an influence following nerve sparing ablative pelvic surgery, are involved in sphincter innervation [1–3, 7, 15, 21, 23, 24, 26–29].

12 Lymph Node Dissection

The extended lymph node dissection is a surgical step of paramount importance to the oncological outcome of the procedure. The template of the lymph node dissection has to be precise, and there are anatomical landmarks that define it. The upper border of an extended template is defined by the crossing of the common iliac artery. The medial border is defined by the umbilical ligament, the lateral border by the genitofemoral nerve, and the distal end by the lacunar ligament (Fig. 15).

Relevant to the lymph nodes in patients with bladder cancer are the juxtavisceral nodes (anterior, lateral, posterior, subvesical) which are located on the corresponding site of the urinary bladder, the external iliac, the internal iliac, and the common iliac nodes. The juxtavisceral nodes collect lymph fluid from the bladder and transport it to the external, internal iliac, and the presacral lymph nodes.

The external iliac nodes are subdivided into three distinctive chains:

- Lateral external iliac chain which is situated between psoas muscle and lateral side of the external iliac artery.

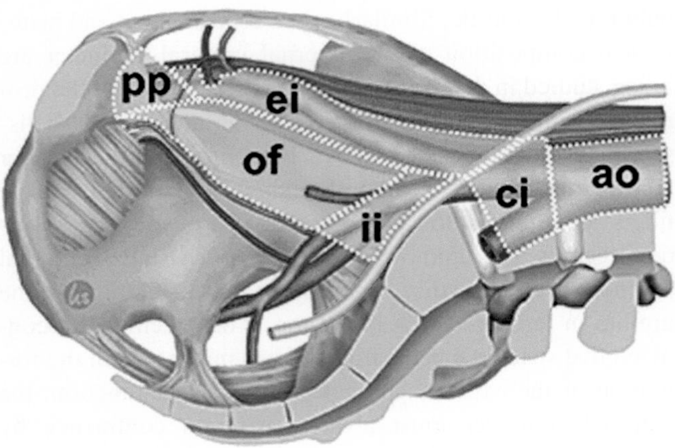

Fig. 15 Definition of anatomic region for pelvic lymphadenectomy (Schiling et al. [14]) [preaortic (ao), common iliac (ci), internal iliac (ii), external iliac (ei), obturator foramen (of) and preperitoneal (pp)]

- Middle external iliac chain which is situated in the medial side of the external iliac artery.
- Medial external iliac chain which is situated against the lateral pelvic wall above the obturator nerve. This chain is well known in most of surgeons as obturator nodes even though anatomically the true obturator nodes are significantly lower in the obturator fossa.

The internal iliac nodes are surrounding the internal iliac vessels. These nodes receive lymph fluid from all afferent vessels of major pelvic organs, and their chain follows cranially hypogastric lamina and passes underneath the common iliac vein and drain in the intermediate group of common iliac nodes.

The common iliac nodes are situated around the common iliac vessels, which are divided topographically in three smaller groups:

- The lateral situated between common iliac artery and psoas muscle
- The middle situated on the posterior side of the common iliac artery
- The medial situated just below the aortic bifurcation

These nodes are of great importance in controlling bladder cancer, and their excision is mandatory during radical cystectomy. There are studies reporting common iliac node involvement in nearly 20% of cancer patients [30]. The extend of the lymph node dissection has been extensively studied and found to be much greater than originally thought and must include lymph nodes up to aortic bifurcation [31]. Surgical anatomy of lymph nodes is clinically important especially for identification of the correct ones along with the appropriate numbers since ten lymph nodes are being proposed as the minimum number of lymph nodes required for optimal cancer control [32].

13 Bowel

Small intestine extends between the pylorus and the caecum, and it is 3–5 m long. It consists of duodenum, jejunum, and ileum. From these parts, only the ileum is used for urinary diversion during robot-assisted radical cystectomy. The wall of the intestine divides in serosa, muscle wall, submucosa, and mucosa. The important layer for bowel anastomosis is the submucosa since it is the basic strength layer that can hold staples and sutures and must be included in the anastomosis. The wall of the small intestine has folds and circulates that can aid in distinguish it from the colon. The arterial supply of small intestine is achieved by numerous branches that are derived from the superior mesenteric artery. The richest blood supply of the ileum is along its mesenteric border, whereas the poorer is in its antimesenteric border. This has a significant impact on every ileal anastomosis (ileo-ileal, ureteroileal, urethroileal), which needs to be done in the antimesenteric border in order to maintain arterial integrity.

The required length of the ileum depends on the type of urinary diversion. If an ileal conduit is decided, then 12–15 cm of terminal ileum must be prepared, whereas for neobladder the required length is 40–60 cm, depending of the type of orthotopic neobladder. The ileum is harvested at least 20 cm from the ileocecal valve. The length should not only be too short in order to prevent tension of the stoma but also not too long in order to avoid residual urine volume and urinary infections [33] in the ileal conduit. Especially in obese patient a wide incision of the aboral mesentery is necessary. In fact, the depth of mesenterial incision of the aboral end defines the possible length of abdominal wall transition. For neobladder diversion, the ileal length does not seem to influence the final outcome of the procedure [34]. Furthermore, the length of the mesentery can greatly impact the tension-free anastomosis between the urethra and the neobladder; thus surgeons should choose the segment of ileum with the longest mesentery in order to ensure that it reaches effortlessly the urethral stump [35].

14 Summary

Robot-assisted pelvic surgery allows for a stereoscopic and more comprehensive view of anatomical features that would be impossible to see with the naked eye during open surgery. As a result, surgeons who use robots benefit from submacroscopic and microscopic anatomical expertise to achieve the best oncological and functional outcomes for their patients. The unique vascular and neurological structures having the most pronounced influence on urine continence and erectile function must be given special attention.

References

1. Benninghoff D. Anatomy. 16th ed. München: Urban & Fischer Verlag; 2003.
2. Campbell MF, Wein AJ, Kavoussi LR. In: Wein AJ, Kavoussi LR, et al., editors. Campbell-Walsh urology. 9th ed. Philadelphia: W.B. Saunders; 2007.
3. Netter FH. Atlas of human anatomy. 1st ed. Stuttgart: Thieme; 1997.
4. Otcenasek M, Baca V, Krofta L, Feyereisl J. Endopelvic fascia in women: shape and relation to parietal pelvic structures. Obstet Gynecol. 2008;111(3):622–30.
5. Shapiro E, Hartanto V, Perlman EJ, Tang R, Wang B, Lepor H. Morphometric analysis of pediatric and nonhyperplastic prostate glands: evidence that BPH is not a unique stromal process. Prostate. 1997;33(3):177–82.
6. Stolzenburg JU, Rabenalt R, Do M, Schwalenberg T, Winkler M, Dietel A, et al. Intrafascial nerve-sparing endoscopic extraperitoneal radical prostatectomy. Eur Urol. 2008;53(5):931–40.
7. Stolzenburg JU, Schwalenberg T, Horn LC, Neuhaus J, Constantinides C, Liatsikos EN. Anatomical landmarks of radical prostatecomy. Eur Urol. 2007;51(3):629–39.
8. van Ophoven A, Roth S. The anatomy and embryological origins of the fascia of Denonvilliers: a medico-historical debate. J Urol. 1997;157(1):3–9.
9. Wimpissinger TF, Tschabitscher M, Feichtinger H, Stackl W. Surgical anatomy of the puboprostatic complex with special reference to radical perineal prostatectomy. BJU Int. 2003;92(7):681–4.
10. Young HH. The radical cure of cancer of the prostate. Surg Gynecol Obstet. 1937;64:472–84.
11. Richards KA, Cohn JA, Large MC, Bales GT, Smith ND, Steinberg GD. The effect of length of ureteral resection on benign uretero-intestinal stricture rate in ileal conduit or ileal neobladder urinary diversion following radical cystectomy. Urol Oncol. 2015;33(2):65.e1–8.
12. Ahmed YE, Hussein AA, May PR, Ahmad B, Ali T, Durrani A, et al. Natural history, predictors and management of ureteroenteric strictures after robot assisted radical cystectomy. J Urol. 2017;198(3):567–74.
13. Richards KA, Steinberg GD. Perioperative outcomes in radical cystectomy: how to reduce morbidity? Curr Opin Urol. 2013;23(5):456–65.
14. Schilling D, Horstmann M, Nagele U, Sievert KD, Stenzl A. Cystectomy in women. BJU Int. 2008;102(9 Pt B):1289–95.
15. Colleselli K, Stenzl A, Eder R, Strasser H, Poisel S, Bartsch G. The female urethral sphincter: a morphological and topographical study. J Urol. 1998;160(1):49–54.
16. Sievert KD, Hennenlotter J, Laible I, Amend B, Schilling D, Anastasiadis A, et al. The periprostatic autonomic nerves–bundle or layer? Eur Urol. 2008;54(5):1109–16.
17. Baader B, Baader SL, Herrmann M, Stenzl A. Autonomic innervation of the female pelvis. Anatomic basis. Urologe A. 2004;43(2):133–40.
18. Baader B, Herrmann M. Topography of the pelvic autonomic nervous system and its potential impact on surgical intervention in the pelvis. Clin Anat. 2003;16(2):119–30.
19. Purves JT, Spruill L, Rovner E, Borisko E, McCants A, Mugo E, et al. A three dimensional nerve map of human bladder trigone. Neurourol Urodyn. 2017;36(4):1015–9.
20. Hutch JA. Saccule formation at the ureterovesical junction in smooth walled bladders. J Urol. 1961;86:390–9.
21. Fritsch H, Lienemann A, Brenner E, Ludwikowski B. Clinical anatomy of the pelvic floor. Adv Anat Embryol Cell Biol. 2004;175:III–IX, 1–64.
22. Nakajima F, Takenaka A, Uchiyama E, Hata F, Suzuki D, Murakami G. Macroscopic and histotopographic study of the deep transverse perineal muscle (musculus transversus perinei profundus) in elderly Japanese. Ann Anat. 2007;189(1):65–74.
23. Oelrich TM. The urethral sphincter muscle in the male. Am J Anat. 1980;158(2):229–46.
24. Oelrich TM. The striated urogenital sphincter muscle in the female. Anat Rec. 1983;205(2):223–32.
25. Shafik A, Sibai OE, Shafik AA, Shafik IA. A novel concept for the surgical anatomy of the perineal body. Dis Colon Rectum. 2007;50(12):2120–5.
26. Stein TA, DeLancey JO. Structure of the perineal membrane in females: gross and microscopic anatomy. Obstet Gynecol. 2008;111(3):686–93.
27. Wallner C, Dabhoiwala NF, Deruiter MC, Lamers WH. The anatomical components of urinary continence. Eur Urol. 2008;
28. Koraitim MM. The male urethral sphincter complex revisited: an anatomical concept and its physiological correlate. J Urol. 2008;179(5):1683–9.
29. Strasser H, Ninkovic M, Hess M, Bartsch G, Stenzl A. Anatomic and functional studies of the male and female urethral sphincter. World J Urol. 2000;18(5):324–9.
30. Smith JA Jr, Whitmore WF Jr. Regional lymph node metastasis from bladder cancer. J Urol. 1981;126(5):591–3.
31. Roth B, Wissmeyer MP, Zehnder P, Birkhäuser FD, Thalmann GN, Krause TM, et al. A new multimodality technique accurately maps the primary lymphatic landing sites of the bladder. Eur Urol. 2010;57(2):205–11.
32. Wright JL, Lin DW, Porter MP. The association between extent of lymphadenectomy and survival among patients with lymph node metastases undergoing radical cystectomy. Cancer. 2008;112(11):2401–8.
33. Colombo R, Naspro R. Ileal conduit as the standard for urinary diversion after radical cystectomy for bladder cancer. Eur Urol Suppl. 2010;9(10):736–44.
34. Mischinger J, Abdelhafez MF, Rausch S, Todenhöfer T, Neumann E, Aufderklamm S, et al. Perioperative morbidity, bowel function and oncologic outcome after radical cystectomy and ileal orthotopic neobladder reconstruction: Studer-pouch versus I-pouch. Eur J Surg Oncol. 2018;44(1):178–84.
35. Almassi N, Zargar H, Ganesan V, Fergany A, Haber G-P. Management of challenging urethro-ileal anastomosis during robotic assisted radical cystectomy with intracorporeal neobladder formation. Eur Urol. 2016;69(4):704–9.

Imaging in Bladder Cancer Surgery

Valeria Panebianco, Emanuele Messina,
Hebert Alberto Vargas, and James Catto

1 Introduction

1.1 Bladder Anatomy

The urinary bladder is a muscular hollow organ, part of the urinary system, representing the reservoir of the urine received from the ureters. It acts also as an active organ because it expels urine into the urethra, through contraction of the detrusor muscle. Because of its structure, when it is completely distended, the bladder can accept up to 400–600 mL of urine [1, 2].

Its shape and location differ depending on the amount of the urine stored: When the bladder is empty, it has a pyramid shape, and it is located in the lower pelvis; when it is full, it presents a round or oval shape, and it extends into the abdomen. Anatomically, the bladder can be divided into four parts: a base (also known as fundus) located posteriorly and inferiorly, an anterior-superior apex (also known as dome), a body (the main part of the bladder located between the apex and the fundus), and a neck, which gives origin to the urethra [2]. A specific area of the bladder is called the trigone, and it is a triangular area of smooth mucosa; the superolateral angles are formed by the ureteral orifices, and the inferior angle is formed by the internal urethral orifice. This area is important because urine enters the bladder through the left and right ureters and exits via the urethra [3].

The bladder mucosa is represented by urothelium, a pseudostratified columnar epithelium formed by three different kinds of cells: apical umbrella, medial, and basal cells (with multiple possible shapes). The lamina propria is constituted from a highly vascularized connective tissue, and it lies underneath the mucosa. The muscularis propria, also indicated as detrusor muscle, surrounds the former layer and is formed by three layers of smooth muscle tissue: The middle one is circular, while the inner and the outer are longitudinal. The adventitia is the outermost layer and is made up of mesenchymal tissue that envelops the bladder and establishes contact with the surrounding tissues [4].

V. Panebianco (✉) · E. Messina
Department of Radiological Sciences, Oncology and Pathology, Sapienza University of Rome, Rome, Italy

H. A. Vargas
Department of Radiology, Memorial Sloan-Kettering Cancer Center, New York, NY, USA

J. Catto
Academic Urology Unit, University of Sheffield, Sheffield, UK

1.2 Bladder Cancer

Bladder cancer (BCa) is the seventh most frequent cancer diagnosed in men globally, while it is the tenth when both genders are taken into account [5]. Every year around 550,000 new BCa diagnoses are made [1].

Urothelial cell carcinoma is the most common histologic variety of BCa, representing more than 90% of all cases; other less common types include squamous cell carcinoma, adenocarcinomas, and lymphomas [1]. BCa can show different morphologies, which could also succeed one another during the tumor progression and growth. These tumors can be represented by exophytic polypoid masses or sessile infiltrative lesions, whereas carcinoma in situ (CIS) grows horizontally and is extremely invasive.

A crucial predictive and prognostic factor is represented by the invasion of the muscularis propria (pT2). In fact, muscle-invasive BCa (MIBC) presents an extremely poorer prognosis, compared to non-muscle-invasive BCa (NMIBC) [6]. This point assigns a key role to pathologic and radiologic assessment of muscle invasion, with a significant impact on treatment strategies [1].

2 Bladder Cancer Diagnosis

2.1 From Symptom to Imaging

The most frequent presenting symptom of BCa is macrohematuria. CIS can cause lower urinary tract symptoms, par-

P. Wiklund et al. (eds.), *Robotic Urologic Surgery*, https://doi.org/10.1007/978-3-031-00363-9_55

ticularly irritative voiding. Microhematuria, dysuria, increased urinary frequency, pelvic discomfort, and signs related to urinary tract blockage are other possible manifestations of MIBC, even if they rarely appear at the onset [5].

All the international guidelines agree that the first step in case of macrohematurai should be physical examination, which can be supported by the use of ultrasound (US). Imaging techniques will help on the detection of bladder abnormalities, even if the final diagnosis always implicates cystoscopy.

Imaging presents especially a supportive role, even if it is essential in the staging phase in case of muscle-invasive and metastatic BCa. In fact, computed tomography (CT) and magnetic resonance imaging (MRI) are essential to investigate the eventual presence of metastasis and lymph nodes involvement. In this scenario, a recent new score has been published, Node Reporting and Data System (Node-RADS), which tackles the lack of consensus in the radiologic evaluation of cancer-related lymph node involvement and fulfills the growing request for standardized reporting. This scoring can be deduced both from CT and MRI images [7].

Moreover, the exclusive use of imaging techniques (i.e., CT urography, US, or MRI) does not permit the diagnose of carcinoma in situ (CIS) [5].

2.2 Ultrasound

US shows intermediate sensitivity in the identification of a wide variety of anomalies of upper and lower urinary tract. In fact, it can be used as a supplement tool to physical examination. It can aid to characterize intraluminal bladder masses and renal masses and to detect hydronephrosis, but it cannot exclude every possible cause of hematuria [5, 8, 9]. Furthermore, US cannot confidently rule out the presence of upper tract urothelial carcinoma and take the place of a CT urography. Consequently it cannot represent the only imaging tool to investigate the possible cause of hematuria [5].

2.3 CT Urography

In case of suspected BCa, CT with and without contrast media intravenous injection should always include the study of the excretory phase, obtaining CT urography (CTU). This technique has the aim to investigate the urinary tract, searching the presence of papillary tumors, which usually appears as filling defects and/or hydronephrosis [5].

Before the CTU acquisition, the patient should undergo oral hydration, with up to 1 L of water, during the previous 20–60 min. This precaution will permit a better definition of the ureters and of the bladder. When this preparation is not possible, because of patients' intolerance or impossibility, diuresis can be stimulated with a slow intravenous drip infusion of 0.9% saline (maximum 500 mL) before and during the CTU [10].

The injection of furosemide before contrast media infusion does not present wide consensus, even if it is proved that it could improve CTU quality and performance. Within minutes after the administration, furosemide causes hyperdiuresis, which speeds up the opacification of the urinary system and amplifies the distension and consequently the visualization of the ureters and of the bladder. It also causes a dilution of the excreted contrast media, diminishing streaking artifacts and ameliorating ureteral and bladder wall visualization and filling defect identification. A consensus conference from the French Society of Genitourinary Imaging suggests the intravenous administration of 20 mL of furosemide before contrast media injection [11].

Concerning contrast media injection, two possible approaches are possible: the single bolus technique and the split bolus technique. The first one requests a classic single bolus injection of contrast media, followed by different scans, decided by the radiologist. In particular, it will be necessary to acquire the renal parenchymal phase and then the excretory one. Each phase is scanned separately, increasing radiation dose while improving images quality thanks to the greater volume of contrast media. Conversely, with the split bolus technique, a first lower dose of contrast will be injected, and after a specific delay, the remaining volume will be administrated. Consequently, with a single scan, both the renal parenchyma phase and the excretory one will be obtained in the same image. The advantage will be to reduce the radiation dose; however this could lead to a lower urinary tract distension and a weaker renal parenchyma enhancement [12].

2.4 Multi-parametric Magnetic Resonance Imaging (mpMRI)

Multi-parametric magnetic resonance imaging (mpMRI) shows an extremely powerful potential in the detection, description, and classification of BCa, even if it is not yet widely introduced in the international guidelines ruling BCa diagnostic workup. Its application led to the introduction of VI-RADS, a useful tool which permitted to standardize mpMRI of the bladder technique and reporting [5, 13].

2.5 International Guidelines

2.5.1 European Association of Urology (EAU)

When any diagnostic imaging approach detects a bladder mass, cystoscopy, biopsy, and/or resection should be performed, to achieve histological diagnosis and staging.

Imaging techniques (such as US, CT, MRI) show high sensitivity for the identification of bladder tumors; in fact, when they are indisputably positive for bladder masses, diagnostic flexible cystoscopy could be skipped, proceeding straight to rigid cystoscopy and transurethral resection of bladder tumor (TURBT) [5, 14].

Imaging plays a key role in the staging process for muscle-invasive bladder cancer (MIBC), furnishing prognosis information and helping in the decision of the most proper treatment [5].

In case of diagnosed MIBC, CT of the chest, abdomen, and pelvis should always be performed for a correct staging. CT is necessary for a correct pulmonary evaluation, in case of lung metastases, while CT and MRI present comparable performances for the research of abdominal and pelvic metastasis. CT urography technique should also be executed for an appropriate urothelial assessment. When CT urography cannot be performed because of contraindications, for example, related to contrast administration or radiation exposure, MRI urography should replace it. CT and MRI should always be requested to stage locally advanced or metastatic disease, when radical treatment is necessary [5].

Unless the patient presents symptoms or signs implying possible bone or brain metastases, a bone scan and further brain imaging are not typically recommended. Furthermore, MRI shows higher sensitivity and specificity than bone scintigraphy in the detection of bone metastases [5].

2.5.2 American Urological Association/Society of Urodynamics, Female Pelvic Medicine and Urogenital Reconstruction (AUA/SUFU)

According to the 2012 AUA guidelines, CT urography and cystoscopy are always suggested when microscopic hematuria occurs in patients over 35 years of age. The 2020 update of these guidelines highlights the necessity of risk-based stratification of patients with microhematuria. Low-risk patients should follow shared decision-making with the physician, considering the possibility of repeating urinalysis within 6 months or directly perform cystoscopy and renal US; intermediate risk patients should undergo cystoscopy and renal US; high-risk patients should be investigated with cystoscopy and CT urography. The risk-based stratification is founded on several major risk factors, such as the patient's age, previous episodes of microhematuria, and smoke history [15].

When CT urography is contraindicated, MRI urography should replace it [15].

2.5.3 National Comprehensive Cancer Network (NCCN)

Patients with micro- or macrohematuria should always undergo cystoscopy, to investigate the possible presence of a bladder mass. In case of cystoscopy confirmation, a TURBT should be executed, to obtain the final diagnosis and to establish the extent of the tumor.

Before TURBT, CT or MRI (with and without contrast media injection) of the abdomen and pelvis is suggested to better define the anatomy of the lesion and to demarcate the depth of invasion. In particular CT or MRI urography should also be performed in case of hematuria to investigate the upper urinary tract: without specific contraindications, CT should be preferred [16].

2.5.4 National Institute for Health and Care Excellence (NICE)

CT or MRI should be performed before TURBT, in patients with suspicion of MIBC at cystoscopy. When MIBC or high-risk NMIBC is diagnosed and a radical treatment is indicated, CT or MRI staging is necessary, also with the acquisition of the excretory phase for a detailed study of a possible upper urinary tract involvement. In these cases, CT of the thorax should also be executed to investigate eventual pulmonary metastasis. In this kind of patients, or when there is a high risk of metastatic disease (i.e., T3b tumor), fluorodeoxyglucose positron emission tomography (FDG PET) CT should be utilized.

CT of the abdomen, pelvis, and chest should be used for the follow-up, in particular 6, 12, and 24 months both after radical cystectomy and radical radiotherapy, to investigate possible local and distant recurrence [17].

3 MRI of the Bladder

The principal role of MRI is the local tumor staging [18]. Clinical staging of BCa is paramount to plan the most suitable treatment for every patient. Moreover, the differentiation between NMIBC and MIBC is mandatory, because it changes the treatment planning: NMIBC (stage T1) are treated with TURBT, whereas MIBC (stage T2 or higher) are treated with radical cystectomy or with radiotherapy and palliative chemotherapy [19].

At the moment, MRI represents the best imaging technique for BCa regional staging, and the main advantages are its superior contrast resolution of soft tissues, the absence of ionizing radiation, and its ability to evaluate tumor infiltration grade in the bladder wall and the perivesical extension.

The use of mpMRI of the bladder is crucial: it combines anatomical and functional sequences that improve the accuracy of tumor detection and local tumor staging compared to conventional imaging alone. Moreover it also helps to monitor post-therapy response, and it identifies potential local disease recurrence [20]. We can thus obtain multiplanar images with high spatial and contrast resolution, with morphological

T2-weighted imaging (T2WI) and additional information with functional sequences such as diffusion-weighted imaging (DWI) and dynamic contrast-enhanced (DCE) MRI [21].

3.1 Bladder MRI Anatomy and MRI Semeiotics

MRI does not permit to visualize every histological layer of bladder wall. On T2WI, urine can be distinguished from the bladder wall because of the high signal intensity (SI) of urine and the low intensity of the bladder wall. The inner layer (mucosa), composed of urothelium and lamina propria, cannot be visualized, while the muscularis propria (detrusor muscle) appears as a low signal intensity line on T2WI. Also, on DWI, the inner layer is not seen, while muscularis propria appears as an intermediate SI line, and on apparent diffusion coefficient (ADC) maps, urine appears hyperintense, and bladder wall is of intermediate SI. With DCE, the inner layer presents early enhancement, and it appears as a high SI line, while muscularis propria is seen as a low SI line that enhances slowly and progressively [22].

Intravesical lesions can be endophytic with intramural growth, exophytic with endoluminal growth, flat (non-mass effect), and mixed forms. The exophytic lesions can be papillary or sessile; the papillary lesions can be pedunculated (with a stalk) or not-pedunculated: papillary tumors with a stalk generally have a better prognosis than papillary tumors without a stalk or broad sessile cancers [23]. The tumor size is generally related to the grade of the tumor: high grade BCa are generally the largest tumors. Concerning tumor location, many studies have shown that most new tumors arise from the lateral walls of the bladder, while the others take origin from the trigone, neck, and ureteral orifices. In particular, bladder neck cancers show a significantly higher frequency of muscle invasion.

Using DCE and DWI imaging, we can improve the accuracy of diagnosis. Intravesical lesions with a T2 SI intermediate to urine and muscle, with high DWI signal and low signal at ADC map, and post-contrast early enhancement at DCE MRI, should be reported as a lesion suspected for BCa [24].

The first thing to describe in morphological sequences is the muscularis propria, to discern MIBC from NMIBC: The muscularis propria is a continuous hypointense line in T2WI in NMIBC, while in MIBC there is an interruption of this low SI muscular line, suggesting muscle invasion. This means that when the radiologist acknowledges the preservation of the low SI of the muscle, a stage T1 can be assessed. On the other hand, when there is an interruption of muscular line, indicating muscle-invasive cancer, a stage T2 would be indicated. In stage T3 lesions there is not only interruption of detrusor line but also extension to perivesical fat, while stage T4 implicates extension of the tumor to adjacent organs.

In DWI the tumor presents an hyperintense signal at high *b*-value (and an hypointense signal at ADC map). In particular, in stage T1 the hyperintense signal is seen only within lumen of bladder, in stage T2 it is seen within the bladder wall, in stage T3 it disrupts the bladder wall, and in T4 it extends to adjacent organs.

In DCE imaging, BCa presents an early enhancement. When the tumor enhancement does not disrupt the low SI of detrusor, it indicates a stage T1, while stage T2 shows muscle invasion with an interrupted hypointense muscle line. In stage T3 there is an early enhancement extended to perivesical fat, and in stage T4 the lesion enhancement is seen also into adjacent organs [25] (Table 1).

Table 1 TNM classification of bladder cancer, 2017

T-Primary tumour	Description	N-Lymph Nodes	Description
Tx	The tumour cannot be evaluated	Nx	Lymph nodes cannot be evaluated
T0	The tumour is not evident	N0	No evidence of regional lymphadenopathies
Ta	Non invasive papillary carcinoma	N1	Metastasis in a single lymph node (hypogastric, obturator, external iliac, presacral)
Tis	Flat tumour: carcinoma in situ	N2	Metastasis in a multiple lymph nodes (hypogastric, obturator, external iliac, presacral)
T1	Tumour invades mucosa and submucosa	N3	Metastasis in common iliac lymph nodes
T2	Tumour invades muscolaris propria T2 a: Superficial muscle T2 b: Deep muscle	**M-Distant metastasis**	**Description**
		M0	No evidence of distant metastasis
T3	Tumour invades perivesical tissue T3 a: Microscopically T3 b: Macroscopically	M1	Metastasis M1 a: Metastasis in non regional lymph nodes M1 b: Other distant metastasis
T4	Tumour invades adjacent organs T4 a: Prostate, seminal vesicles, uterus or vagina T4 b: Pelvic and abdominal wall		

3.2 MRI Acquisition Protocol

Before MRI examination, appropriate bladder distention is required to avoid a misdiagnosis of BCa or an overstaging in case of insufficient bladder filling; moreover, an overdistension of the bladder may cause a motion artifact and complicate the diagnosis.

The patient must empty the bladder 1–2 h before imaging and then drink 500–1000 mL of water half an hour before the examination. Real-time MRI images can be used to determine adequate bladder filling. In addition, an antispasmodic agent can be administered to reduce bowel movement artifacts, if there are no contraindications.

MRI (1.5 or 3.0T) is recommended to achieve high spatial resolution and signal-to-noise ratio with a multichannel phased array external surface coil. The protocol image acquisition consists of T2WI fast-spin-echo (FSE) or turbo-spin-echo sequences (TSE) with at least two planes of multiplanar (axial, coronal, and sagittal) and with a slice thickness of 3–4 mm, DWI with high *b* value (800–1000 s/mm^2) and with an ADC map, and DCE-MRI, administering a gadolinium-based contrast agent and preferring a 3D acquisition to obtain higher spatial resolution. Pre-contrast image (T1-weighted) should also be acquired [13] (Table 2).

3.3 VI-RADS

The promising performance of mpMRI of the bladder and its spread led to the conception and designing of the VI-RADS score [13]. This new scoring system has the aim to standardize the approach to imaging and reporting of mpMRI for bladder cancer and to define the risk of BCa muscle invasion. The score is based on *T*2WI (weighted images), DCE-MRI, and DWI findings. In particular, for each sequence, five categories can be identified: structural categories (SC) for T2WI, contrast-enhanced (CE) categories for DCE sequences, diffusion-weighted (DW) categories for DWI, and ADC map.

3.3.1 T2WI Categories

1. *SC 1*: Continuous low SI line (muscularis propria is intact), the lesion should be <1 cm, exophytic with or without stalk and/or thickened inner layer.
2. *SC 2*: continuous low SI line (muscularis propria is intact), the lesion should be >1 cm, exophytic with stalk and/or high SI inner layer, when present, or sessile/broad-based with high SI thickened inner layer, when present.
3. *SC 3*: No evidence of category 2 characteristics, exophytic tumor without stalk, or sessile/broad-based tumor without high SI thickened inner layer; no clear interruption of low SI muscularis propria.
4. *SC 4*: Clear interruption of low SI line (infiltration to muscularis propria).
5. *SC 5*: Extension of tumor to extravesical fat and extravesical tissues.

3.3.2 DCE-MRI Categories

1. *CE 1*: The muscularis propria does not show early enhancement (with lesions corresponding to SC 1).
2. *CE 2*: The muscularis propria does not show early enhancement, but there is evidence of early enhancement of inner layer (with lesions corresponding to SC 2).
3. *CE 3*: No evidence of category 2 findings (with lesions corresponding to SC category 3) and no evident interruption of low SI muscularis propria.
4. *CE 4*: Tumor early enhancement involving focally the muscularis propria.
5. *CE 5*: Tumor early enhancement involving the entire bladder wall and exceeding to the extravesical fat.

3.3.3 DWI/ADC Categories

1. *DW 1*: Continuous and intermediate SI of the muscularis propria on DWI with lesion <1 cm, hyperintense on DWI and hypointense on ADC, with or without stalk and/or low SI thickened inner layer on DWI.

Table 2 MRI parameters setting

	3T			1.5T		
Parameters	T2	DWI	DCE	T2	DWI	DCE
TR (ms)	4690	2500–5300	3.8	5000	4500	3.3
TE (ms)	119	61	1.2	80	88	1.2
FA (fleep angle)	90	90	15	90	90	13
FOV (cm)	23	32	27	23	27	35
Matrix	400 × 256/320	128 × 128	192 × 192	256 × 189/256	128 × 109	256 × 214
Slice thickness (mm)	3–4	3–4	1	4	4	2
Slice gap (mm)	0–0.4	0.3–0.4	0	0–0.4	0–0.4	0
Number of excitations	2–3	4–10	1	1–2	10–15	1
B values	–	0–800–1000–2000	–	–	0–800–1000	–

2. *DW 2*: Continuous and intermediate SI of the muscularis propria on DWI with lesion >1 cm, hyperintense on DWI and hypointense on ADC, with low SI stalk and/or low SI thickened inner layer on DWI, or broad-based/sessile tumor with low/intermediate SI thickened inner layer on DWI.
3. *DW 3*: No evidence of category 2 findings (with lesions corresponding to SC category 3) and no clear interruption of low SI muscularis propria.
4. *DW 4*: High SI on DWI and low SI on ADC map involving focally the muscularis propria.
5. *DW 5*: High SI on DWI and low SI on ADC map involving the entire bladder wall and exceeding to the extravesical fat.

3.3.4 Definitive VI-RADS Score

The final score is based on these categories, on T2WI for the morphology and on DWI/DCE for the definitive decision about muscular invasion. The dominant sequence is DWI; if the DWI is not optimal, the DCE will aid to obtain the final decision. In conclusion, there are five final VI-RADS scoring categories, and each one corresponds to a different probability of muscle invasion.

- *VI-RADS 1*: SC, CE, and DW category 1 suggest that muscle invasion is highly unlikely.
- *VI-RADS 2*: SC, CE, and DW category 2 or CE and DW category 2 and SC category 3 suggest that muscle invasion is unlikely (Fig. 1).
- *VI-RADS 3*: SC, CE, and DW category 3 and SC category 3 or CE category or DW category 3 and the other sequence belong to category 2; VI-RADS 3 suggest that the muscle invasion is equivocal.
- *VI-RADS 4*: at least SC and/or DW and CE category 4, the remaining category 3 or 4, SC category 3 plus DW and/or CE category 4, and SC category 5 plus DW and/or CE category 4. It indicates that muscle invasion is likely (Fig. 2).
- *VI-RADS 5*: At least SC plus DW and/or CE category 5; the remaining category 4 or 5. It suggests that muscle invasion and the extension to adjacent organs are very likely (Fig. 3).

4 MRI Future Perspectives for Bladder Cancer

VI-RADS and mpMRI of the bladder might be exploited for different further applications.

The use of VI-RADS is now especially dedicated to the pre-TURBT workup and before intravesical BCG (Bacillus Calmette-Guerin) injection. Preoperative MRI and VI-RADS score give interesting and useful information in the evaluation of treatment response, indicating when BCa requires a more aggressive approach. Furthermore, in cases of high-risk NMIBC, VI-RADS score may play a useful role also for disease risk stratification and as an indicator of whether a secondary excision of the tumor is necessary. The high risk of tumor recurrence and the frequent necessity for a secondary tumor resection stimulate its application as a follow-up diagnostic tool [1].

4.1 Surveillance in Non-muscle-Invasive Bladder Cancer

MRI may constitute a solid noninvasive substitute to cystoscopy for follow-up, resulting in lower disease-related expenditures, particularly representing a promising and powerful tool in NMIBC surveillance [1].

The bladder wall structural alterations must be considered in this context. Wall thickening can be induced by fibrosis and inflammation as result of the treatment and might be misinterpreted as BCa recurrence/residue on T2-weighted imaging (T2WI). To solve these problems, functional sequences, particularly DCE-MRI and DWI, have proven to be accurate in distinguishing BCa from these findings [1]. To minimize overstaging caused by posttreatment structural modifications, MRI should be performed at least 2 weeks after TURBT and BCG administration and at least 2 days after cystoscopy or withdrawal of a Foley catheter [13].

4.2 MRI Before and After Bladder Cancer Treatment

MRI and VI-RADS scoring may be extremely helpful in case of MIBC, to stage tumors that will benefit from neoadjuvant chemotherapy, to detect lesions that will take advantage from bladder-sparing surgery and chemoradiation, and schedule therapeutic TURBT [1].

The VI-RADS score could be effective to predict BCa aggressiveness and its response to therapy, and it could represent a clinical predictor of posttreatment outcomes. On this scenario, MRI functional sequences have been shown to be accurate in assessing and predicting tumor aggressiveness [1]. For example, ADC value has been appointed as a potential biomarker, indicating a potential cutoff value of $0.86 \cdot 10^{-3}$ mm^2/s, to distinguish clinically aggressive from less aggressive phenotypes [26].

BCa response to therapy may be assessed by MRI in a variety of clinical scenarios, including before, during, and after treatment. More specifically, DWI-MRI has been indicated as a biomarker to predict MIBC chemoradiation sensitivity [27]. Furthermore, it has been demonstrated that resistant BCas show more diversified spatial representation

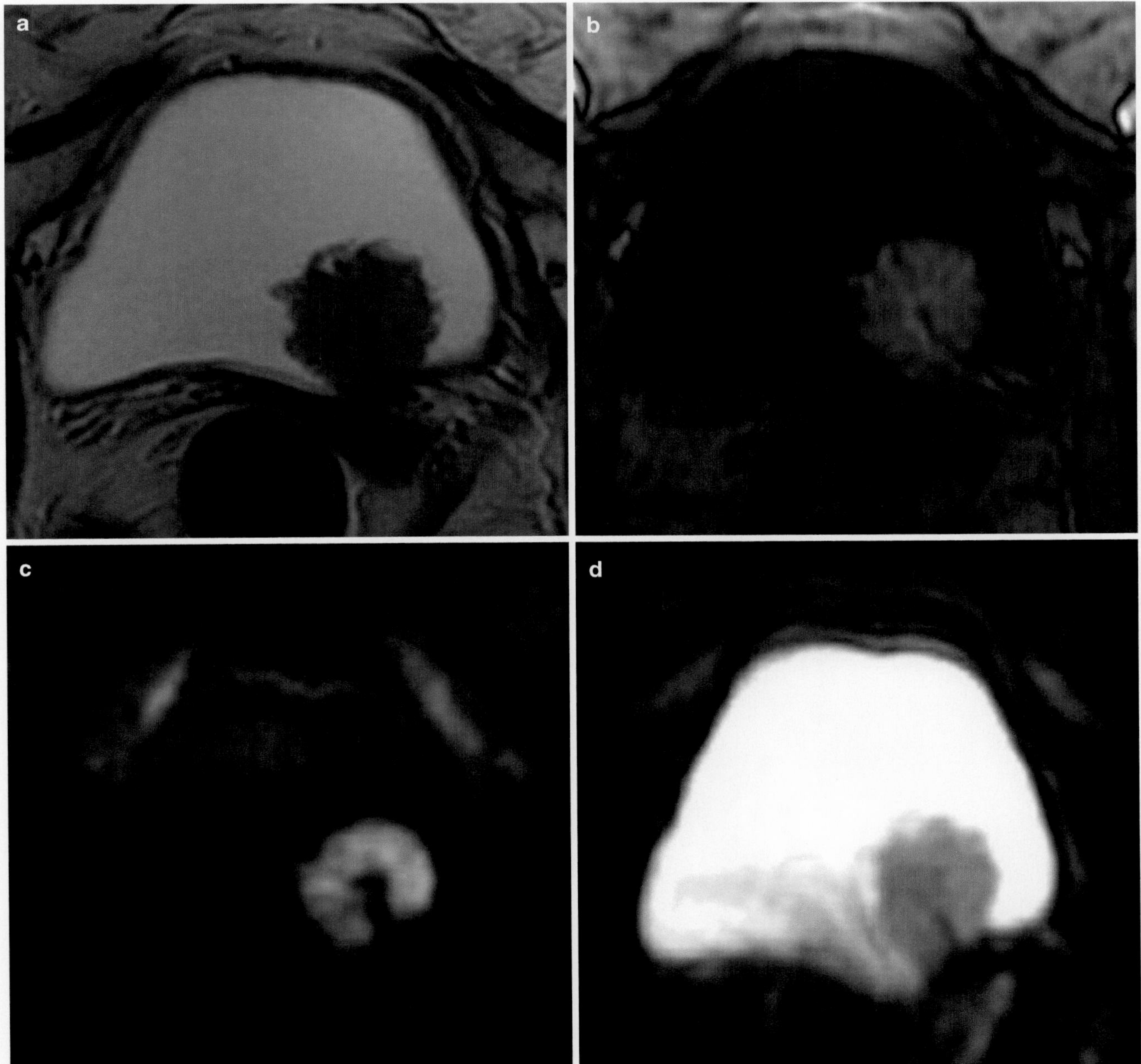

Fig. 1 A 62-year-old female patient with positive US. (**a**) T2WI (axial plane) shows an exophytic and pedunculated mass, >1 cm in size, at the level of the posterior bladder wall, near the left ureteral orifice, with intermediate SI not extending through the muscularis propria. T2WI assigned as VIRADS category 2. (**b**) DCE imaging shows early and heterogeneous enhancement of the lesions, not extending through the muscularis propria. DCE assigned as VI-RADS category 2. (**c, d**) DWI (b = 2000) and ADC map show significant restricted diffusion, not extending through the muscularis propria. DWI assigned as VIRADS category 2. Definitive VI-RADS score was 2

of ADC values, furnishing useful information in the pre-neoadjuvant chemotherapy (NACT) [28]. MRI has been proved to produce extremely useful results also in the study of BCa before and after immunotherapy [29].

MRI has been proved to be a powerful tool in the stratification of patients affected by BCa, especially during chemotherapy. In fact it can predict treatment failure, with the consequent reduction of morbidity and costs, already with the only use of T2WI [30]. With the addition of DCE sequences, MRI performance becomes extremely strong, assigning to DCE a key role in the detection of chemotherapy responders [1]. MRI is definitively a promising tool in the evaluation of patients affected by MBIC treated with NACT, indicated their response to therapy [31].

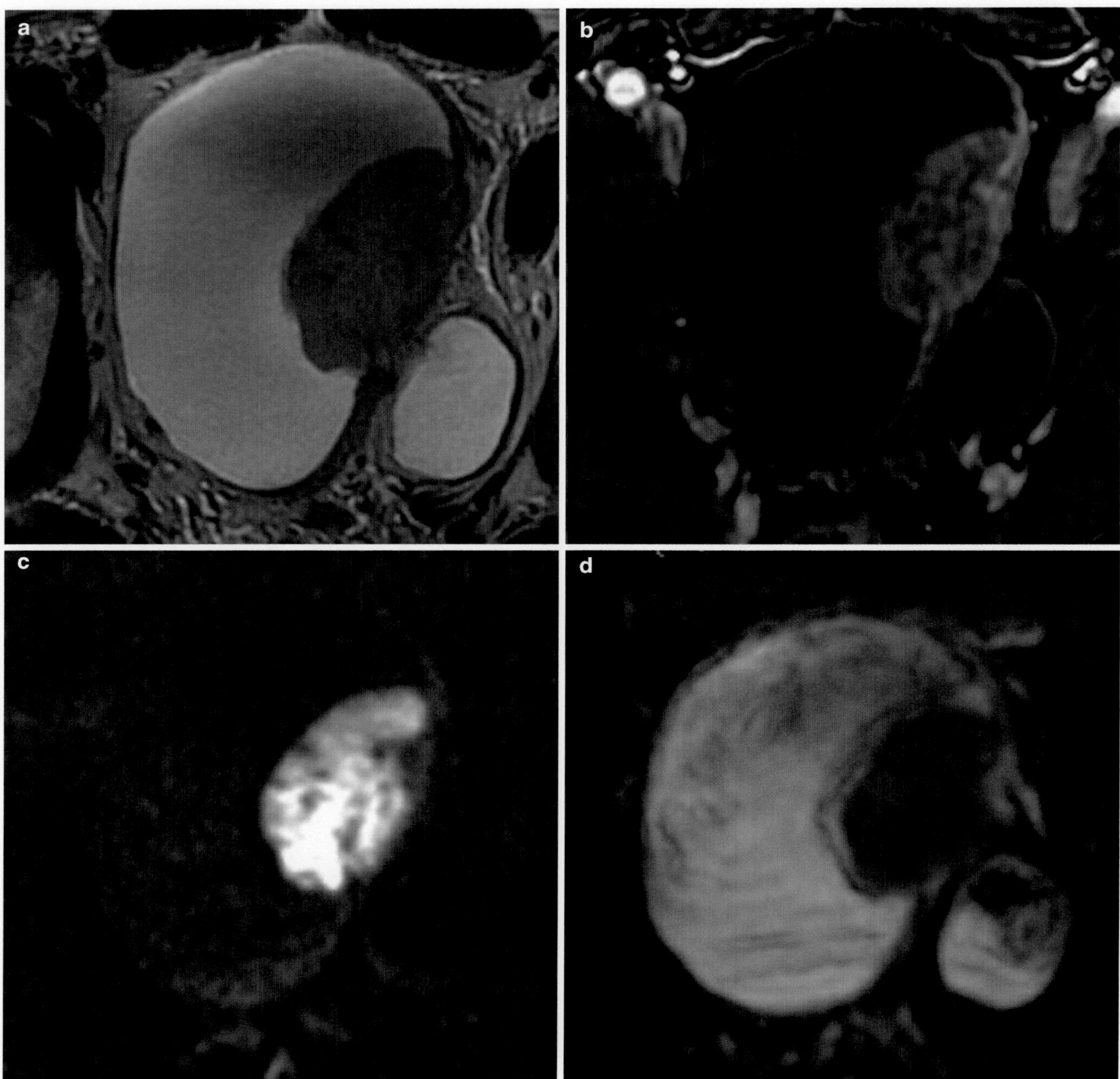

Fig. 2 A 68-year-old male patient presenting with macroscopic hematuria, with further positive cystoscopy. (**a**) T2WI (axial plane) shows an exophytic and sessile mass >1 cm in size at the level of the posterolateral left bladder wall, with an adjacent diverticulum, with intermediate SI extending through the muscularis propria and invading the perivesical fat tissue. T2WI assigned as VIRADS category 5. (**b**) DCE imaging shows early and heterogeneous enhancement of the lesion, extending through the muscularis propria. DCE assigned as VI-RADS category 4. (**c**, **d**) DWI (b = 2000) and ADC map show a lesion with significant restricted diffusion, extending through the muscularis propria. DWI assigned as VIRADS category 4. Definitive VI-RADS score was 4

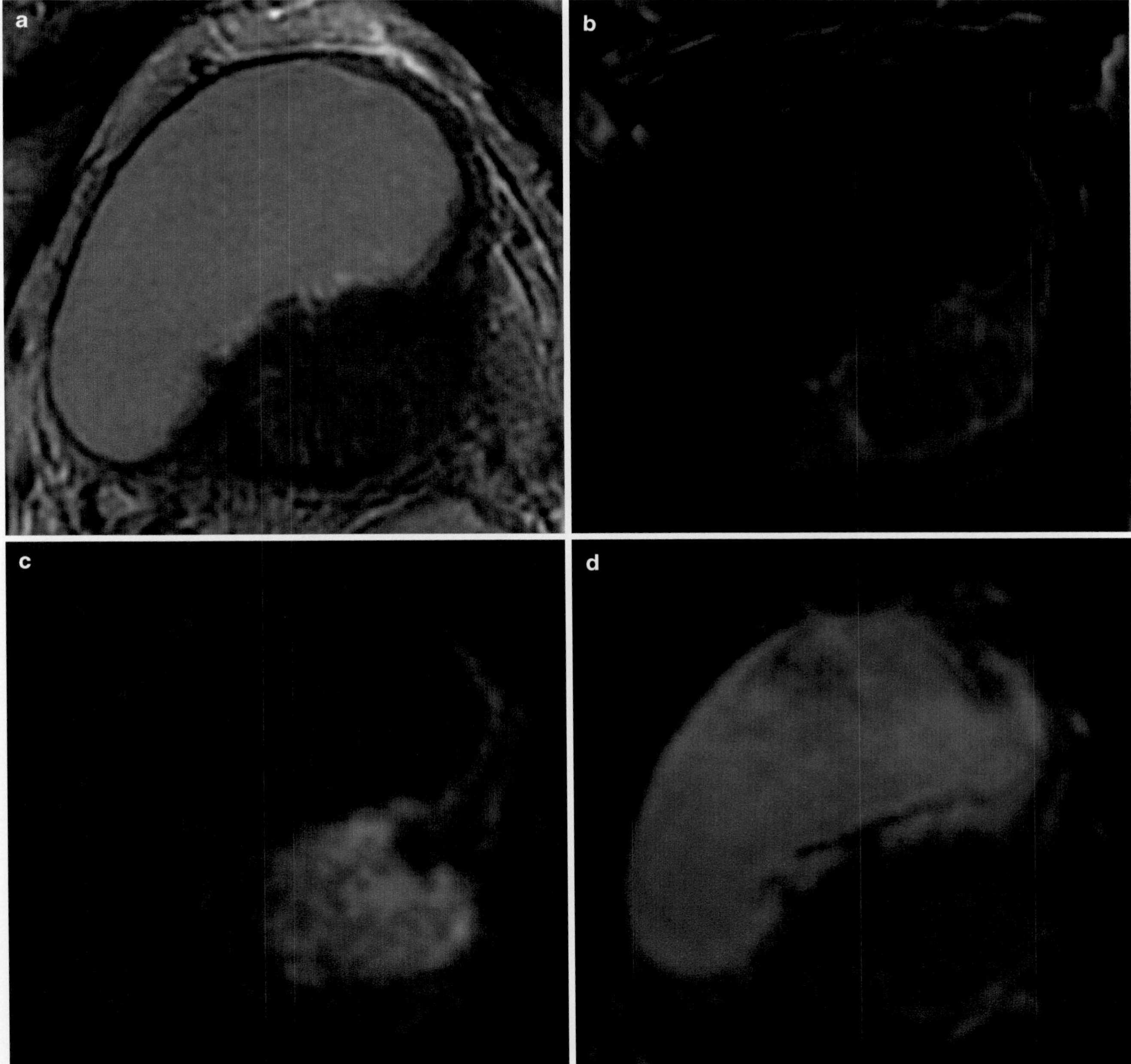

Fig. 3 A 71-year-old male patient presenting with macroscopic hematuria, with further positive cystoscopy. (**a**) T2WI (axial plane) shows a sessile mass >1 cm in size at the level of the posterolateral left bladder wall, with intermediate SI extending through the muscularis propria, invading the perivesical fat tissue. T2WI assigned as VIRADS category 5. (**b**) DCE imaging shows early and heterogeneous enhancement of the lesion, extending through the muscularis propria, invading the perivesical fat tissue. DCE assigned as VI-RADS category 5. (**c**, **d**) DWI ($b = 2000$) and ADC map show a lesion with significant restricted diffusion, extending through the muscularis propria, invading the perivesical fat tissue. DWI assigned as VIRADS category 5. Definitive VI-RADS score was 5

The use of DCE-MRI has been indicated also as an important biomarker during post-radical cystectomy follow-up [32].

Additionally, the VI-RADS score proved to be a reliable tool to stratify patients according to risk with a personalized management. Indeed, VI-RADS 5 score proved to be an independent factor for significant delay to the execution of radical cystectomy, in particular to a time to cystectomy >3 months from the diagnosis of MIBC obtained with TURBT, time which is correlated to reduced survivals. VI-RADS might be used to reduce the reliance and morbidity of TURBT for MIBC detection and also to assist urologists in the identification of patients that may need immediate radical surgery [1, 33].

References

1. Panebianco V, Pecoraro M, Del Giudice F, et al. VI-RADS for bladder cancer: current applications and future developments. J Magn Reson Imaging JMRI. 2020; https://doi.org/10.1002/jmri.27361.
2. Sam P, Nassereddin A, LaGrange CA. Anatomy, abdomen and pelvis, bladder detrusor muscle. Treasure Island, FL: StatPearls; 2021.
3. Shermadou ES, Rahman S, Leslie SW. Anatomy, abdomen and pelvis, bladder. Treasure Island, FL: StatPearls; 2021.
4. Bolla SR, Jetti R. Histology bladder. Treasure Island, FL: StatPearls; 2020. http://www.ncbi.nlm.nih.gov/books/NBK540963/
5. EAU Guidelines. Edn. presented at the EAU Annual Congress Milan 2021. ISBN 978-94-92671-13-4.
6. Herr H. Preventable cancer deaths associated with bladder preservation for muscle invasive bladder cancer. Urology. 2019;130:20–1. https://doi.org/10.1016/j.urology.2019.04.032.
7. Elsholtz FHJ, Asbach P, Haas M, et al. Introducing the Node Reporting and Data System 1.0 (Node-RADS): a concept for standardized assessment of lymph nodes in cancer. Eur Radiol. 2021; https://doi.org/10.1007/s00330-020-07572-4.
8. Choyke PL. Radiologic evaluation of hematuria: guidelines from the American College of Radiology's appropriateness criteria. Am Fam Physician. 2008;78:347–52.
9. Hilton S, Jones LP. Recent advances in imaging cancer of the kidney and urinary tract. Surg Oncol Clin N Am. 2014;23:863–910. https://doi.org/10.1016/j.soc.2014.06.001.
10. CT Urography Working Group of the European Society of Urogenital Radiology (ESUR), Van Der Molen AJ, Cowan NC, et al. CT urography: definition, indications and techniques. A guideline for clinical practice. Eur Radiol. 2008;18:4–17. https://doi.org/10.1007/s00330-007-0792-x.
11. On behalf of the "French Society of Genitourinary Imaging Consensus group," Renard-Penna R, Rocher L, et al. Imaging protocols for CT urography: results of a consensus conference from the French Society of Genitourinary Imaging. Eur Radiol. 2020;30:1387–1396. https://doi.org/10.1007/s00330-019-06529-6
12. Wong VK, Ganeshan D, Jensen CT, Devine CE. Imaging and management of bladder cancer. Cancers. 2021;13:1396. https://doi.org/10.3390/cancers13061396.
13. Panebianco V, Narumi Y, Altun E, et al. Multiparametric magnetic resonance imaging for bladder cancer: development of VI-RADS (Vesical Imaging-Reporting And Data System). Eur Urol. 2018;74:294–306. https://doi.org/10.1016/j.eururo.2018.04.029.
14. Blick CGT, Nazir SA, Mallett S, et al. Evaluation of diagnostic strategies for bladder cancer using computed tomography (CT) urography, flexible cystoscopy and voided urine cytology: results for 778 patients from a hospital haematuria clinic. BJU Int. 2012;110:84–94. https://doi.org/10.1111/j.1464-410X.2011.10664.x.
15. Barocas DA, Boorjian SA, Alvarez RD, et al. Microhematuria: AUA/SUFU Guideline. J Urol. 2020;204:778–86. https://doi.org/10.1097/JU.0000000000001297.
16. Flaig TW, Spiess PE, Agarwal N, et al. Bladder cancer, version 3.2020, NCCN Clinical Practice Guidelines in Oncology. J Natl Compr Canc Netw. 2020;18:329–54. https://doi.org/10.6004/jnccn.2020.0011.
17. NICE (National Institute for Health and Care Excellence) Guideline. Bladder cancer: diagnosis and management. 2015.
18. Juri H, Narumi Y, Valeria P, Osuga K. Staging of bladder cancer with multiparametric MRI. Br J Radiol. 2020;93:20200116. https://doi.org/10.1259/bjr.20200116.
19. Verma S, Rajesh A, Prasad SR, et al. Urinary bladder cancer: role of MR imaging. RadioGraphics. 2012;32:371–87. https://doi.org/10.1148/rg.322115125.
20. de Haas RJ, Steyvers MJ, Fütterer JJ. Multiparametric MRI of the bladder: ready for clinical routine? Am J Roentgenol. 2014;202:1187–95. https://doi.org/10.2214/AJR.13.12294.
21. Panebianco V, Barchetti F, de Haas RJ, et al. Improving staging in bladder cancer: the increasing role of multiparametric magnetic resonance imaging. Eur Urol Focus. 2016;2:113–21. https://doi.org/10.1016/j.euf.2016.04.010.
22. Narumi Y, Kadota T, Inoue E, et al. Bladder wall morphology: in vitro MR imaging-histopathologic correlation. Radiology. 1993;187:151–5. https://doi.org/10.1148/radiology.187.1.8451403.
23. Panebianco V, De Berardinis E, Barchetti G, et al. An evaluation of morphological and functional multi-parametric MRI sequences in classifying non-muscle and muscle invasive bladder cancer. Eur Radiol. 2017;27:3759–66. https://doi.org/10.1007/s00330-017-4758-3.
24. Zhou G, Chen X, Zhang J, et al. Contrast-enhanced dynamic and diffusion-weighted MR imaging at 3.0T to assess aggressiveness of bladder cancer. Eur J Radiol. 2014;83:2013–8. https://doi.org/10.1016/j.ejrad.2014.08.012.
25. Makboul M, Farghaly S, Abdelkawi IF. Multiparametric MRI in differentiation between muscle invasive and non-muscle invasive urinary bladder cancer with vesical imaging reporting and data system (VI-RADS) application. Br J Radiol. 2019;92:20190401. https://doi.org/10.1259/bjr.20190401.
26. Kobayashi S, Koga F, Yoshida S, et al. Diagnostic performance of diffusion-weighted magnetic resonance imaging in bladder cancer: potential utility of apparent diffusion coefficient values as a biomarker to predict clinical aggressiveness. Eur Radiol. 2011;21:2178–86. https://doi.org/10.1007/s00330-011-2174-7.
27. Yoshida S, Koga F, Kawakami S, et al. Initial experience of diffusion-weighted magnetic resonance imaging to assess therapeutic response to induction chemoradiotherapy against muscle-invasive bladder cancer. Urology. 2010;75:387–91. https://doi.org/10.1016/j.urology.2009.06.111.
28. Nguyen HT, Mortazavi A, Pohar KS, et al. Quantitative assessment of heterogeneity in bladder tumor MRI diffusivity: can response be predicted prior to neoadjuvant chemotherapy? Bladder Cancer Amst Neth. 2017;3:237–44. https://doi.org/10.3233/BLC-170110.
29. Necchi A, Bandini M, Calareso G, et al. Multiparametric magnetic resonance imaging as a noninvasive assessment of tumor response to neoadjuvant pembrolizumab in muscle-invasive bladder cancer: preliminary findings from the PURE-01 study. Eur Urol. 2020;77:636–43. https://doi.org/10.1016/j.eururo.2019.12.016.
30. Barentsz JO, Berger-Hartog O, Witjes JA, et al. Evaluation of chemotherapy in advanced urinary bladder cancer with fast dynamic contrast-enhanced MR imaging. Radiology. 1998;207:791–7. https://doi.org/10.1148/radiology.207.3.9609906.

31. Choueiri TK, Jacobus S, Bellmunt J, et al. Neoadjuvant dose-dense methotrexate, vinblastine, doxorubicin, and cisplatin with pegfilgrastim support in muscle-invasive urothelial cancer: pathologic, radiologic, and biomarker correlates. J Clin Oncol Off J Am Soc Clin Oncol. 2014;32:1889–94. https://doi.org/10.1200/JCO.2013.52.4785.
32. Donaldson SB, Bonington SC, Kershaw LE, et al. Dynamic contrast-enhanced MRI in patients with muscle-invasive transitional cell carcinoma of the bladder can distinguish between residual tumour and post-chemotherapy effect. Eur J Radiol. 2013;82:2161–8. https://doi.org/10.1016/j.ejrad.2013.08.008.
33. Del Giudice F, Leonardo C, Simone G, et al. Preoperative detection of Vesical Imaging-Reporting and Data System (VI-RADS) score 5 reliably identifies extravesical extension of urothelial carcinoma of the urinary bladder and predicts significant delayed time to cystectomy: time to reconsider the need for primary deep transurethral resection of bladder tumour in cases of locally advanced disease? BJU Int. 2020;126:610–9. https://doi.org/10.1111/bju.15188.

Step-by-Step Approach to Robot-Assisted Male Cystectomy

J. Palou, F. D'Hont, M. Annerstedt, and A. Piana

1 Introduction

Open radical cystectomy (ORC) with pelvic lymph node dissection and urinary diversion is considered the gold standard treatment for nonmetastatic muscle invasive bladder cancer and for recurrent noninvasive disease [1]. However, due to its high complexity and rate of complications, the robot-assisted radical cystectomy (RARC) has gained popularity as a minimally invasive alternative to the standard approach, bringing to potential advantages in terms of lower intraoperative blood loss, postoperative blood transfusions, and morbidity, leading to a shorter hospital stay [2, 3]. Despite a definitive high-level evidence supporting RARC is still lacking, as reported from the main randomized control trials (RCTs) comparing OKT with RARC [4–7], this approach has the potential to achieve excellent postoperative results in terms of early recovery of sexual function. In fact, due to the enhanced three-dimensional (3D) visualization and high precision movements, the robotic approach seems to give significant advantages when performing a nerve-sparing surgery [8, 9].

1.1 Robotic Instruments Used

- Large needle driver
- Monopolar curved scissor
- Vessel Sealer®/SynchroSeal®
- Fenestrated bipolar forceps (or Cadiere forceps)
- 0° 3D laparoscope

1.2 Patient Positioning and Trocar Placement

Patient positioning changes according to the robotic system employed. If Da Vinci X® is used, the patient is placed in the dorsal lithotomy position, with arms tucked to the side and legs opened. Leg attachment is then lowered, and the patient is placed in 30-degree Trendelenburg position. A Foley catheter is placed on a sterile operative field.

The first incision is made 2 cm above the umbilicus according to Hasson's technique, in order to place the optic trocar. The pneumoperitoneum is created insufflating CO_2 continuously. The AirSeal system may be used to provide a stable pressure with constant smoke evacuation. All remaining trocars are placed under direct vision along a horizontal line which pass 1 cm under the umbilicus considering possible slight differences in trocar placement among different authors; two robotic trocars are placed on the left side, with a distance of at least 8 cm and not less than 2 cm from the iliac crest; another robotic trocar is placed on the right side. A 15 mm assistant trocar is placed 8 cm away from the right robotic trocar; an ulterior 5 mm assistant trocar is placed between the optical and the robotic trocar on the right side (Fig. 1). Surgery is performed under low insufflation pressure (8 mmHg).

The da Vinci X® system is docked between the patients' legs with the robotic arms oriented in a cephalad direction. The primary assistant operates from the patient's right.

da Vinci Xi® system is docked on the patient's right. The primary assistant operates from the patient's left.

Supplementary Information The online version contains supplementary material available at [https://doi.org/10.1007/978-3-031-00363-9_56].

J. Palou · A. Piana (✉)
Urology Department, Fundació Puigvert, Autonomous University of Barcelona, Barcelona, Spain

F. D'Hont
Department of Urology, Onze-Lieve-Vrouwziekenhuis, Aalst, Belgium

M. Annerstedt
Department of Urology, Stockholm Urology Clinic, Stockholm, Sweden

P. Wiklund et al. (eds.), *Robotic Urologic Surgery*, https://doi.org/10.1007/978-3-031-00363-9_56

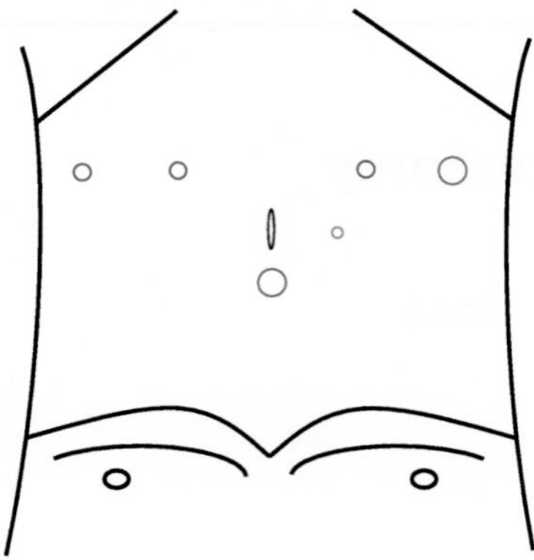

○ 12 mm camera port ○ 8 mm robotic trocar ○ 12 mm assistant trocar
○ 5 mm assistant trocar

Fig. 1 Trocar placement (daVinci® X, Si, Xi)

1.3 Pelvic Lymph Node Dissection

Pelvic lymph node dissection could be performed before or after the cystectomy according to the surgeon's preference. The procedure is described in Chap. 65.

2 Non-nerve-Sparing RARC in Male: Surgical Technique

- **Dissection of the Ureters**

The procedure is begun by incising the peritoneum over the right ureter as the sigmoid colon is often attached to the left side wall. A longitudinal incision is made just medial to the ureter, which is mobilized from just above the crossing of the iliac vessels down to the ureterovesical junction, where the umbilical ligament can be seen just lateral of the ureter. Once the right ureter is completely mobilized, the sigmoid colon is released to allow access to the left iliac vessels and left ureter. The left ureter is dissected free of its attachments up to the level of the psoas muscle. This should be done before dividing the ureter as proximal dissection can be difficult once the ureter is divided.

During the complete dissection, special attention is needed to maintain adequate periureteral tissue. Note that too much or too aggressive dissection proximal on the ureter can result in devitalization of the ureter and may contribute to anastomotic stricture. Sometimes, individual vessels from the common iliac or distal aorta can be seen and preserved (Fig. 2, Video 1).

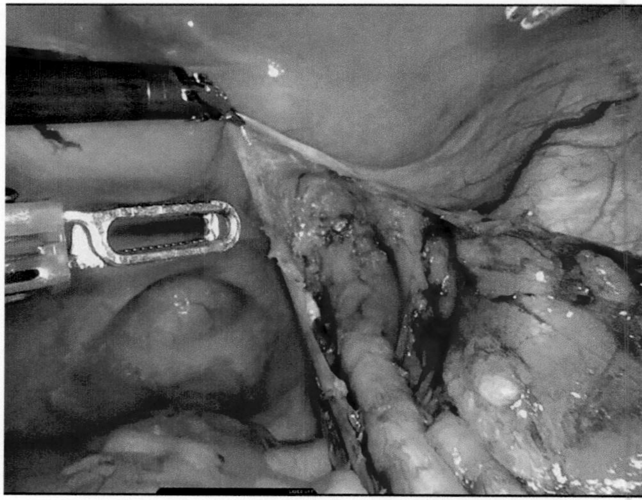

Fig. 2 Dissection of the right ureter. The ureter is mobilised from just above the crossing of the iliac vessels down to the ureterovesical junction, where the umbilical ligament can be seen just lateral of the ureter

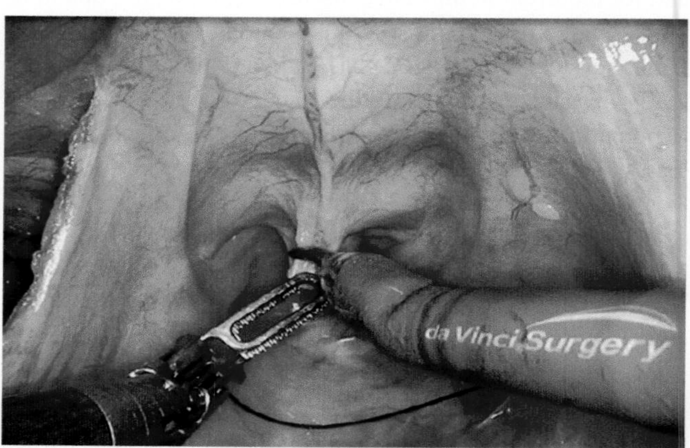

Fig. 3 Incision of the peritoneum just above its reflection over the rectum

- **Posterior Dissection**

The aim of this step is to mobilize the posterior bladder and prostate from the rectum. The posterior dissection starts with the incision of the peritoneum just above its reflection over the rectum, connecting the incision with previously incisions for both ureters (Fig. 3). The seminal vesicles are freed, which can be done mainly bluntly. Further dissection to the base of the seminal vesicles exposes Denonvilliers fascia. This multilayered fascia is opened, and a plane is developed between the fascia (still attached to the prostate) and the rectum until the rectourethralis muscle is seen. Proceeding anteriorly, the yellow pre-rectal fat is followed to avoid rectal

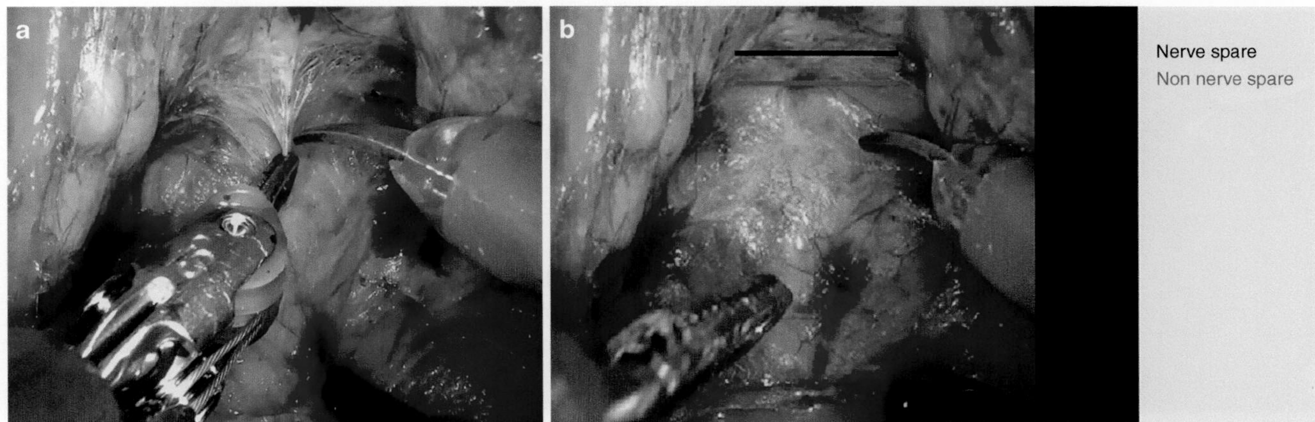

Fig. 4 (**a**) Denonvillers fascia exposure. (**b**) Dissection layers of Denonvillers fascia: above (black line) during a nerve sparing procedure; below (red line) during a non nerve sparing procedure

injury. Once the rectum is freed on the midline, extend the dissection further laterally to the neurovascular pedicle of the prostate. In this way, the rectum becomes completely exposed (Fig. 4, Video 2).

- **Lateral Dissection**

The goal of this step is to develop the space between bladder/prostate and sidewall. This will also facilitate the exposure of the bladder pedicle. The peritoneum, which was already incised for the dissection of the ureters, is progressively incised following the genitofemoral nerve and continued laterally from the medial umbilical ligaments. The vas deferens is divided, which allows the bladder to be retracted medially and facilitates further exposure. It is important not to drop the bladder at this point. With mainly blunt dissection, an avascular plane between bladder (medially) and lymph nodes (laterally) can be identified. Care must be taken not to injure the obturator nerve. The peri-vesical space is developed distally, up to the level of the endopelvic fascia and proximally to the origin of the umbilical ligament, which is clipped with a Hem-o-lok® at the base. This clip can also be used later on as a repair during later lymphadenectomy (Fig. 5). The endopelvic fascia, which forms the superior layer of the levator ani fascia, is incised, and the lateral surface of the prostate can be identified until the apex of the prostate (Fig. 6, Video 3).

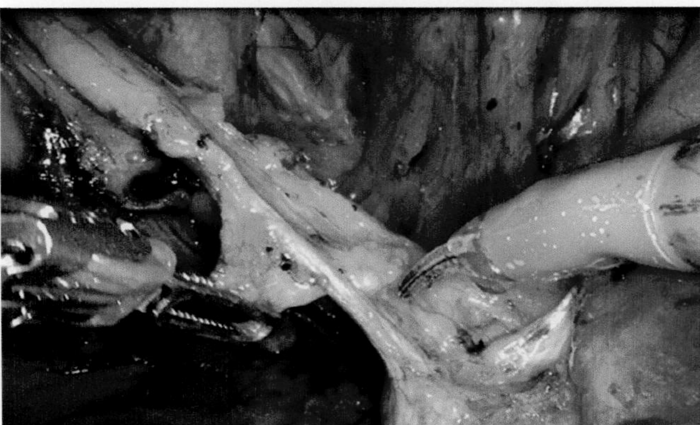

Fig. 5 Identification of the origin of the umbilical ligament, which is clipped at the base

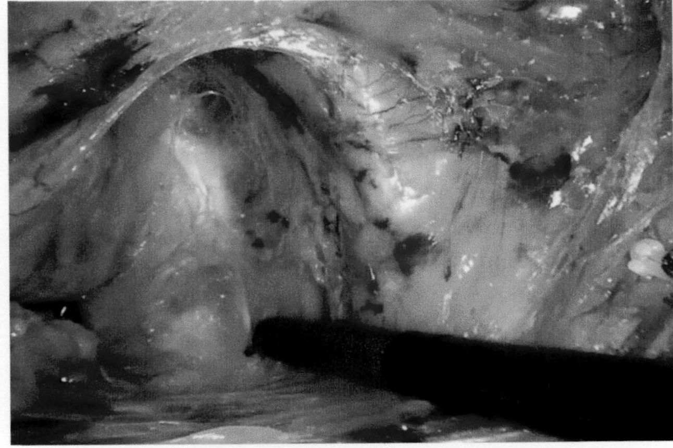

Fig. 6 Incision of the endopelvic fascia to expose the lateral surface of the prostate

- **Securing the Bladder Pedicles**

Once the bladder pedicles are completely dissected, the ureters are divided between clips (Fig. 7). A stay suture (4 cm) is placed on the proximal clip for an easier identification and manipulation. The distal margins are sent for frozen sections, if indicated. The transection of the pedicle is performed with the Vessel Sealer® or SynchroSeal™ system.

To have a good exposure, the fourth arm retracts the umbilical ligament toward the umbilicus. As the superior vesical artery descends in most of the cases from a common branch

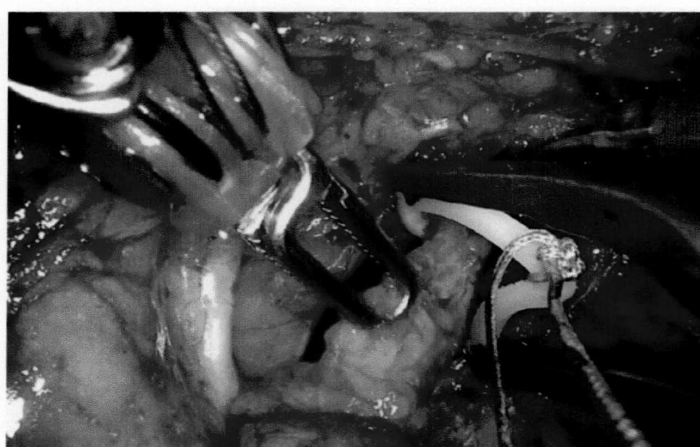

Fig. 7 The left ureter is divided using clips

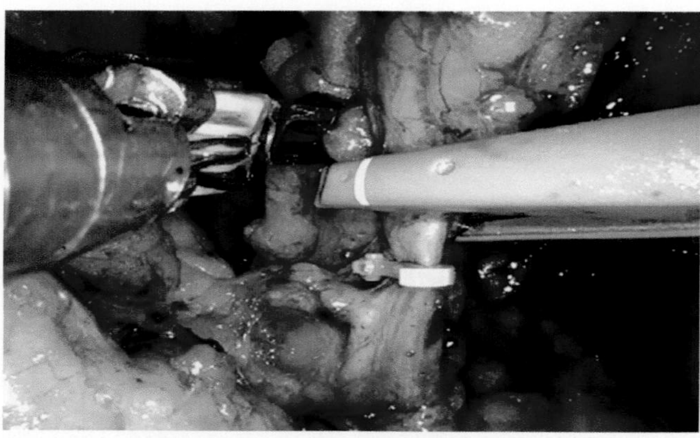

Fig. 8 Dissection of the right umbilical ligament at its origin. A clip is placed at the base and the ligament is sealed and cut

with the former umbilical artery proceeding in the medial umbilical ligament, sealing and cutting above the previously placed clip is the first step (Fig. 8).

The internal iliac arteries are followed downward, and the inferior vesical artery is sealed and cut. To facilitate the dissection, especially in obese patients with wide pedicels, a space can be created just under the clipped ureter. The pedicle can then be divided in a lateral vascular segment and a more medial neurovascular segment (Fig. 9). In a non-nerve spare procedure, use the seminal vesicle as a guide to progress dissection. The neurovascular bundle on the posterolateral side of the prostate is easily dissected with the vessel sealer down to the prostatic apex. Make sure that the previously done posterior dissection extends laterally enough to prevent any rectal injury. Furthermore, the already incised endopelvic fascia helps to expose the pedicle at the prostatic base. At the level of the prostatic base, dissection is done posterior to the prostate. Closer to the apex, the bundle is dissected more lateral to the prostate, again to prevent any rectal injury (Fig. 10).

- **Section of Urachus and Anterior Plane**

The urachus, just below the umbilicus, and the median umbilical ligaments are coagulated and cut. The bladder is dropped down to gain access to the space of Retzius. Staying in the correct plane, the pubic bone is followed until the dorsal vein complex (DVC) and puboprostatic ligaments are identified.

- **Prostate Apex**

The DVC is divided with cold scissors. Arterial bleedings can be secured with monopolar coagulation. If extensive blood loss occurs, the intra-abdominal pressure can be increased to 15 mmHg. The anterior contour of the prostate is followed until the apex is reached and the urethra is identified. The DVC is secured with a continuous hemostatic V-Loc™ suture. The most important concept is to proceed with the urethral dissection, once there is a good visualization of the apex and the bleeding is under control (Video 4).

- **Dissection of Urethra**

At this point, the membranous urethra is completely isolated. Depending on underlying disease and type of diversion, the urethra can be dissected at different levels.

- Maximum sparing of the urethra is performed when a neobladder is planned. Frozen section of the urethra may be taken, if indicated. The catheter is withdrawn, and a large clip is placed at the level of the apex, as high as possible into the prostatic urethra in order to prevent tumor spillage and to preserve as much as possible the sphincteric area of the urethra.
- If a simultaneous urethrectomy is planned, the urethra can be dissected further trough the pelvic floor to create a maximal urethral length. This will facilitate the urethrectomy.
- When an ileal conduit is planned, the membranous urethra is isolated for 2–3 cm. The catheter is withdrawn, and a large clip is placed at the level of the apex. A second clip is placed on the urethra at the level of the pelvic floor. The urethra is cut between the clips, and the specimen is immediately placed in an Endobag® (Fig. 11).

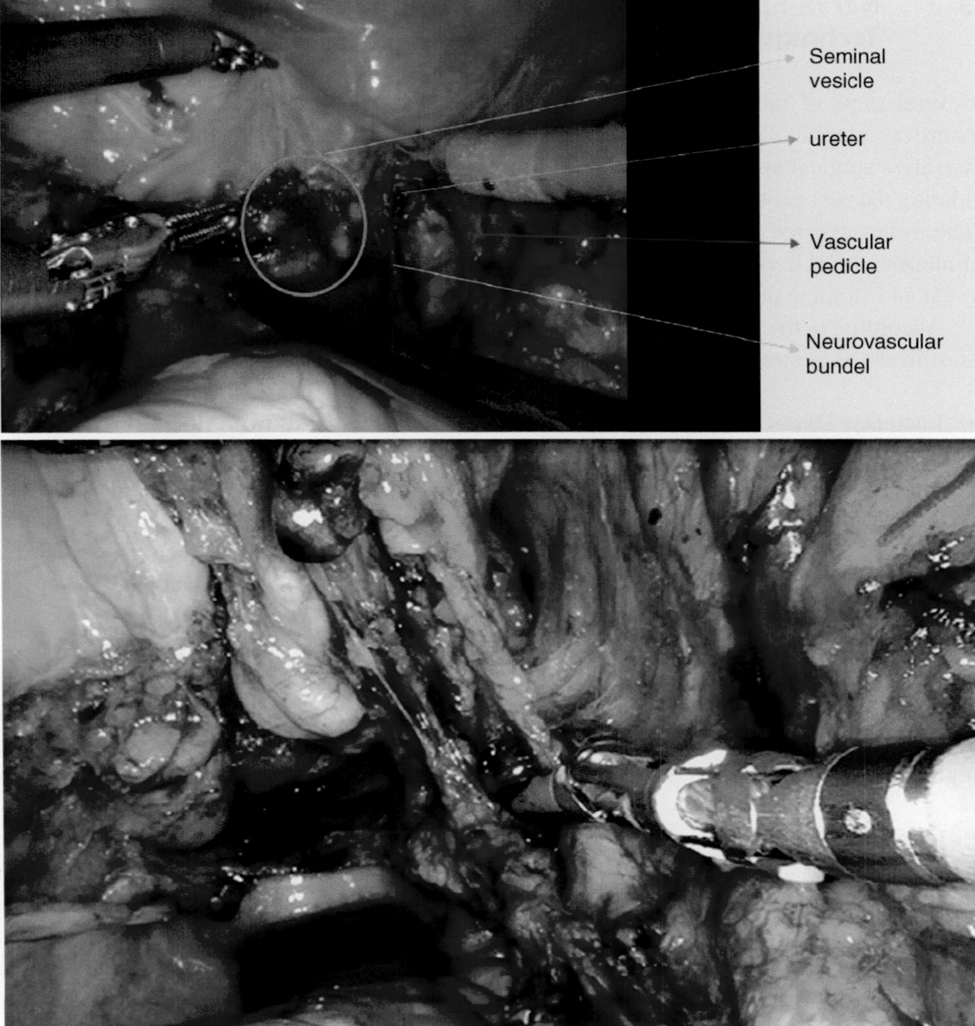

Fig. 9 To facilitate the dissection (especially in obese patients with wide pedicels), a space can be created just under the clipped ureter. The pedicle can then be divided in a lateral vascular segment and a more medial neurovascular segment

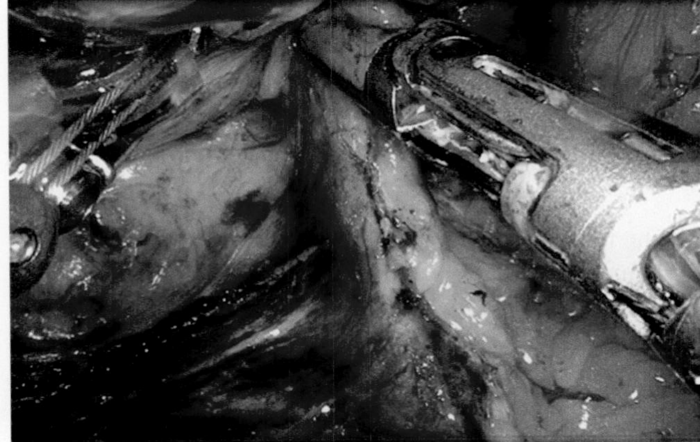

Fig. 10 Dissection of the right neurovascular bundle of the prostate. Important that the rectum is dissected completely free to prevent any injury

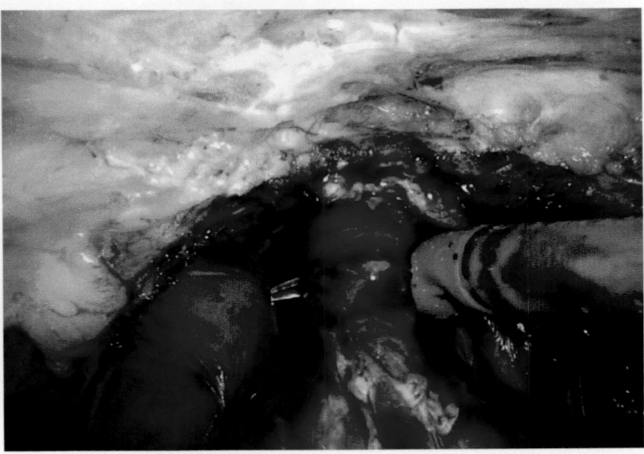

Fig. 11 Dissection of the urethra

3 Nerve-Sparing RARC in Male: Surgical Technique

Several steps of radical cysto-prostatectomy are at risk of neurovascular bundle (NVB) damage. For this reason, a conservative surgical approach is carried out by identifying and sparing the peri-prostatic neurovascular structures (Video 5). The robot-assisted approach allows an enhanced three-dimensional (3D) visualization, with dramatically improvement and surgical precision.

According to the surgeon's preference, the dissection may start from the posterior plane or from the iliac ureters.

- **Posterior Dissection**

The posterior peritoneum is opened at the level of pre-rectal space, and by a carefully dissection of the posterior wall of the bladder, the seminal vesicles are identified. At this point, it is possible to keep dissecting posteriorly until the prostate. If the posterior dissection is carried out, vas deferens can be tied up and cut. Then it is important to perform a dissection of the seminal vesicles separating them internally, from the external and lateral pedicle of the bladder. This maneuver allows the section of the lateral pedicles at higher level and thus preserves the bundles (Fig. 12).

- **Identification of the Ureters and Lateral Dissection**

Once the robot is docked, the camera is oriented toward the pelvis. The posterior peritoneum on the right side is opened at the level of iliac vessels, and the right ureter is identified. The right iliac vessels and ureter are easier to locate and dissect, due to less intrusion of the colon. A vase-loop is passed around the ureter and closed with a Hem-o-lok®. At this level, extreme attention has to be paid in order to preserve as much peri-ureteral tissue as possible, with the aim of preserving ureter's vascularization, avoiding subsequent stenosis. During the dissection of the pre-vesical ureter, the umbilical artery, the superior vesical artery, and the lateral umbilicus-vesical ligament are identified and dissected. Later on, the inferior vesical artery and vein are identified and cut. At the end of this procedure, two Hem-o-lok® are placed on the terminal tract, and the ureter is cut just before the intravesical segment. A distal ureteral margin should be sent for a frozen section, if indicated. Subsequently, sigmoid mobilization is performed to create the left space, allowing the left ureter dissection, that will be carried out with the same modality. The left ureter is transposed to the right retrosigmoid space besides the right ureter after this dissection or later on. It is better to do it after the bilateral lymphadenectomy, which facilitates this maneuver because of the clear anatomical space developed.

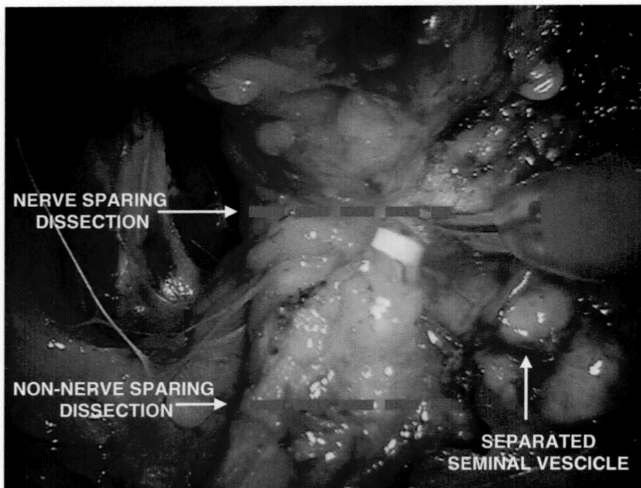

Fig. 12 Seminal vescicles are separated internally, from the external and lateral pedicle of the bladder. This manoeuver allows the section of the lateral pedicles at higher level, and thus preserving the bundles

- **Lateral Dissection**

Once the posterior plan has been developed, the dissection continues laterally until the endopelvic fascia, which has to be separated from levator ani muscles. The procedure continues distally to the apex and laterally, maintaining a plane of incision immediately alongside the prostatic fascia, to expose the neurovascular triangle between Denonvilliers fascia, lateral pelvic fascia, and the prostate. At this point, prostatic pedicles can be identified. Due to the absence of prostate cancer, an intra-fascial nerve-sparing approach can be performed, leaving no fascial layer overlying the prostatic tissue but keeping a layer of Denonvilliers fascia on the surface of the rectal wall (Fig. 13). In order to avoid thermal injuries, a sharp dissection at this level and the use of clips are recommended. Moreover, as it happens for radical prostatectomy, care must be taken to avoid excessive traction to the bundle, because of the fragility of the nerves.

- **Bladder Pedicles**

The lateral pedicles can be taken down using a 5–10 mm LigaSure™ device (Tyco Healthcare) at high level of the dissection, but when getting closer to space of the bundles created after the dissection of the seminal vesicles, it is better to use Hem-o-lok clips taking every vessel separately.

- **Section of Urachus and Anterior Plane**

At this point, the anterior peritoneum is incised. The urachus and the median umbilical ligaments are cut with monopolar scissors. The bladder is dropped down to gain access to the space of Retzius. At the level of Santorini plexus, a suture

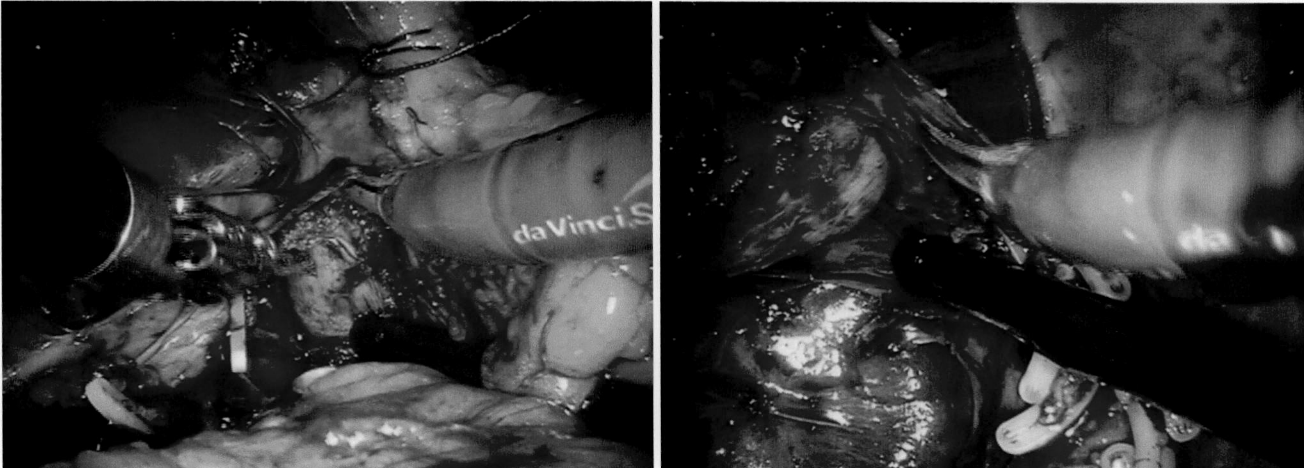

Fig. 13 Lateral detachment of the periprostatic fascia and isolation of NVB

is performed to limit bleeding from venous sinus. An anatomic dissection of the apex as we do in radical prostatectomy is important. Different techniques can be considered, but the surgical field has to be bloodless when performing the final dissection of the apex of the prostate. Considering that accessory pathways of neural net may run close to the anterior urethra, a deep placement of the dorsal venous (DVP) stitch may increase the risk of neural damage. This can be avoided by placing the stitch prior to disconnection of the apex, when the venous complex can be better visualized. At this point, it is possible to dissect the anterior space until the urethra, where a Hem-o-lok® is placed, as high as possible, internally in the prostatic urethra, before its section to avoid tumor seeding. A frozen section can be taken from the proximal portion of the divided urethra if indicated.

- **End of the Demolitive Phase**

At this point, the demolitive phase is completed, and the hemostasis is carefully performed. The specimen can be extracted in a retrieval bag through a 5–6 cm infraumbilical or periumbilical incision.

4 Conclusions

Robot-assisted radical cystectomy may offer several advantages compared to the standard open technique, due to its mini-invasiveness. Moreover, in case of young men who desire to preserve their sexual function, some of the critical surgical steps seem to significantly beneficiate from a minimally invasive approach. It is known that a nerve-sparing technique improves continence in radical prostatectomy; thus it is better to use this technique, if oncologically feasible, in patients undergoing radical cystectomy and a neobladder. The oncological and functional results of the nerve-sparing robot-assisted radical cystectomy corroborate the role of this approach.

References

1. Professionals S-O. EAU Guidelines: muscle-invasive and metastatic bladder cancer. Uroweb. https://uroweb.org/guideline/bladder-cancer-muscle-invasive-and-metastatic/. Accessed 25 May 2021.
2. Novara G, Catto JWF, Wilson T, et al. Systematic review and cumulative analysis of perioperative outcomes and complications after robot-assisted radical cystectomy. Eur Urol. 2015;67(3):376–401. https://doi.org/10.1016/j.eururo.2014.12.007.
3. Musch M, Janowski M, Steves A, et al. Comparison of early postoperative morbidity after robot-assisted and open radical cystectomy: results of a prospective observational study. BJU Int. 2014;113(3):458–67. https://doi.org/10.1111/bju.12374.
4. Prospective randomized controlled trial of robotic versus open radical cystectomy for bladder cancer: perioperative and pathologic results – ClinicalKey. https://www.clinicalkey.com/#!/content/playContent/1-s2.0-S0302283809010288?returnurl=https:%2F%2Flinkinghub.elsevier.com%2Fretrieve%2Fpii%2FS0302283809010288%3Fshowall%3Dtrue&referrer=https:%2F%2Fpubmed.ncbi.nlm.nih.gov%2F. Accessed 25 May 2021.
5. Desai MM, Gill IS. "The devil is in the details": randomized trial of robotic versus open radical cystectomy. Eur Urol. 2015;67(6):1053–5. https://doi.org/10.1016/j.eururo.2015.01.017.
6. Parekh DJ, Reis IM, Castle EP, et al. Robot-assisted radical cystectomy versus open radical cystectomy in patients with bladder cancer (RAZOR): an open-label, randomised, phase 3, non-inferiority trial. Lancet. 2018;391(10139):2525–36. https://doi.org/10.1016/S0140-6736(18)30996-6.
7. Khan MS, Gan C, Ahmed K, et al. A single-centre early phase randomised controlled three-arm trial of open, robotic, and laparoscopic radical cystectomy (CORAL). Eur Urol. 2016;69(4):613–21. https://doi.org/10.1016/j.eururo.2015.07.038.
8. Collins JW, Tyritzis S, Nyberg T, et al. Robot-assisted radical cystectomy: description of an evolved approach to radical cystectomy. Eur Urol. 2013;64(4):654–63. https://doi.org/10.1016/j.eururo.2013.05.020.
9. Nyame YA, Zargar H, Ramirez D, et al. Robotic-assisted laparoscopic bilateral nerve sparing and apex preserving cystoprostatectomy in young men with bladder cancer. Urology. 2016;94:259–64. https://doi.org/10.1016/j.urology.2016.04.026.

Step-by-Step Approach to Robot-Assisted Female Cystectomy, Anterior Exenteration, and Pelvic Organ Preserving Approaches

Zachary Dovey and Peter Wiklund

1 Background

In their lifetime, women will have a 0.27% or 1 in 400 risk of being diagnosed with bladder cancer, approximately four times less than men, with the highest incidences in Europe, Syria, Egypt, Israel, and the United States [1, 2]. The standard treatment for localized muscle invasive bladder cancer (MIBC), as well as carefully selected higher-risk non-muscle invasive bladder cancer (NMIBC), is radical cystectomy [3], which includes removal of the bladder and urethra, bilateral extended pelvic lymphadenectomy (EPLND), and urinary diversion. This procedure has significant morbidity (up to a 60% complication rate) and a recognized mortality (1–4%) [4, 5]. Robotic approaches to radical cystectomy evolved from "minimally invasive" and laparoscopic surgery, with the Intuitive Da Vinci gaining FDA approval in 2000. Menon et al. [6] published the first description of robot-assisted radical cystectomy (RARC), and since then the technique has evolved significantly, with a wealth of studies comparing its outcomes to those of open radical cystectomy (ORC). The randomized controlled RAZOR trial is the largest of these to date, demonstrating non-inferiority of RARC. When comparing ORC to RARC at 3 years follow-up, disease-free survival (DFS) (65.4% vs. 68.4%), overall survival (OS) (68.5% vs. 73.9%), complication rates (69% vs. 67%), and outcomes related to quality of life (QOL) were not significantly different [7]. Moreover, a recent Cochrane systematic review of five other relevant RCTs found no difference between oncological outcomes, complication rates, and quality of life results for RARC and ORC, other than possibly lower transfusion rates and shorter hospital stay (LOS) for RARC [8].

Z. Dovey
Department of Urology, Icahn School of Medicine at Mount Sinai, New York, NY, USA

P. Wiklund (✉)
Department of Urology, Icahn School of Medicine at Mount Sinai, New York, NY, USA

Department of Urology, Karolinska University Hospital Solna, Solna, Sweden

Whichever approach is used, standard radical cystectomy in females requires removal of the bladder and urethra, an EPLND as well as removal of the gynecological organs (ovaries, fallopian tubes, uterus, and anterior vaginal wall) in what is termed anterior pelvic exenteration. With a view to improving postoperative sexual function, pelvic organ prolapse (POP) RARC can be undertaken in carefully selected patients, allowing preservation of the ovaries, fallopian tubes, uterus, anterior vaginal wall, and urethra [9]. The rationale for this is reinforced by evidence that these organs are involved histologically in up to only 7.5% of patients, and the procedure may be done in conjunction with robotic intracorporeal neobladder (RIN) to further improve postoperative functional outcomes and body image. This chapter will discuss in detail patient selection, patient preparation, and the step-by-step technique for RARC with anterior pelvic exenteration as well as with POP. Following this, outcomes of each will be presented, where possible comparing female RARC directly with female ORC, as well as outlining the importance of enhanced recovery after surgery (ERAS) protocols, the influence of experience, and surgical learning curves, as well as novel approaches to RARC, wherever possible with specific reference to female patients.

2 Patient Selection

Patient selection is crucial when considering patients for RARC, and surgeon and operating team experience are an important part of the decision-making process. An ideal robotic case has an ECOG score of 0, no extravesical disease with T2 clinical staging, a BMI of less than 30, no history of abdominal pelvic irradiation or surgery, and no significant past medical history of note. Surgeon experience with the potential for prolonged operative times and Trendelenburg influences how stringently these factors are applied, and as the console surgeon and operative team gain experience, more complex cases may be chosen. Factors considered as relative contraindications, regardless of surgeon experience,

P. Wiklund et al. (eds.), *Robotic Urologic Surgery*, https://doi.org/10.1007/978-3-031-00363-9_57

may be significant past cardiac or pulmonary disease compromising the safety of anesthesia, morbid obesity, and prior abdomino-pelvic surgery, trauma, or irradiation [10].

When planning POP RARC with or without RIN, the surgeon will have to consider additional factors. The main risk is inadequate excision of tumor with a concomitant increase in the local recurrent rate, which may primarily arise from inaccuracies in staging prior to surgery. Preoperatively patients under consideration of POP RARC should have full gynecological and sexual histories, with a detailed discussion of goals for sexual function and fertility longer term once recovered from surgery. Specific contraindications include any evidence of more extensive local disease, such as radiological evidence of T3 disease on clinical staging including hydronephrosis or nodal involvement, palpable tumor and tumors at the bladder base, trigone or neck at the time of primary trans urethral resection of bladder tumor (TURBT), or CIS on TURBT histology [9]. Similarly, patients who carry BRCA1/2 mutations or have Lynch syndrome have an increased future risk of gynecological malignancies and so would be relatively contraindicated for POP RARC [11]. When planning RIN with POP RARC, additional considerations are liver and renal failure which may result in longer-term metabolic problems, tumor involving the urethral margin (which may be excluded with an intraoperative negative frozen section of urethral margin tissue), cognitive impairment causing compliance issues with postoperative training protocols, physical disability preventing the ability to intermittently self-catheter and urethral sphincter injuries that would cause incontinence [12]. Once a decision about the robotic approach has been made, patients should undergo their surgery as soon as possible and definitely within 3 months. Both US SEER database analysis as well as a more recent meta-analysis have confirmed delays in surgery for bladder cancer beyond 3 months result in inferior longer-term survival outcomes [13, 14].

In order to facilitate the selection process, all patients should have a full medical and surgical history, physical examination, and diagnostic workup including hematology, biochemistry, urine microbiology, and cytology as well as CT or MRI of the chest, abdomen, and pelvis. Informed decision-making is important, and patients should be counseled regarding the pros and cons of the different technical approaches for bladder removal and urinary diversion, before the final procedure is chosen. The use of enhanced recovery after surgery (ERAS) protocols for patient preparation pre surgery and recovery afterward is now an accepted part of robotic cystectomy programs for women and men, and this is discussed in a separate section below.

3 Patient Positioning and Port Placement

Accurate positioning of the patient and port placement will facilitate smooth step by step progress through the procedure and limit the technical problems for each step. After induction of general anesthesia, a nasogastric tube is inserted for the period of the operation to remove any gastric contents that may accumulate. Patients are placed in 30 degrees of Trendelenburg to bring the bowel out of the pelvis, with a foam cushion under them and if necessary padded shoulders at the head of the operating table to prevent sliding. The legs are fixed up in stirrups and lifted apart with hips and knees flexed to allow the robot to come forward between them. To further keep the patient stable on the table, a soft chest strap may be applied, and the arms may be strapped to the side of the body or held on arm boards. Once positioning is complete, it is crucial to check all pressure points to prevent subsequent pressure necrosis injuries and compartment syndrome. For port placement, the Karolinska method will be described [15]. Prepping and draping is done from the lower sternum to superior thigh, including the perineum and vagina, and a urethral catheter is inserted and left on free drainage. A midline 12 mm camera port is inserted 5 cm above the umbilicus using the open Hasson technique to prevent bowel injury, and all subsequent ports are inserted under direct vision, with the camera placed intra-abdominally. Pressure is set slightly higher at 18 mmHg while the ports are being placed and then reduced to 12 mmHg when the surgery starts. Two 8 mm robotic instrument ports are placed 8–10 cm away from and on each side of the umbilicus, at the lateral edge of the rectus sheath. A 12 mm assistant aspiration post triangulates between the right instrument and camera port high enough up toward the inferior edge of the rib cage to prevent clashing during the operation. A second 12 mm assistant port is placed on the right side, level with the anterior axillary line, 2–3 cm above the anterior superior iliac spine. The final 15 mm robotic instrument port mirrors the right lateral assistant port over the left anterior axillary line, again 2–3 cm above the anterior superior iliac spine. With a lumen of 15 mm, an 8 mm robotic instrument port can telescope through it, and during the bowel division and re-anastomosis, this can be replaced by a handheld GI stapler. The proximal positioning of the ports for RARC when compared to robotic prostatectomy allows for easier presacral dissection during the EPLND and easier suturing technique for the afferent limb of the uretero-ileal anastomosis.

4 RARC with Anterior Exenteration

There are some fundamental modules or steps for RARC which have been widely accepted and are beneficial for many reasons. They allow the operating surgeon to benchmark his or her progress through the procedure and facilitate a focus on each task and the instrument movements that are necessary for each module. This not only limits technical difficulties and thus potential complications but also provides a structure for learning and progress on the learning curve, inevitably helping to reduce operating time. By contributing to the educational process, modules also help with mentoring, and as new methods and techniques emerge, having a clear procedural structure already in place helps with their introduction [15]. For standard RARC, these may be common to men and women, but the nuances specific to women and anterior exenteration are described in detail below.

Dissection of the Ureters (Fig. 1) In female RARC it is valuable to orientate oneself with the position of the gynecological organs at the beginning of the operation. The ureters enter the pelvis over the bifurcation of the common iliac arteries and can generally be found once the peritoneum is incised overlying this point. This may be obscured on the left by the sigmoid colon, potentially with the addition of adhesions, necessitating adhesiolysis and sigmoid instrument retraction with the fourth arm. Once the peritoneum is incised, dissecting just medial to pelvic wall may help to find the ureters, which are followed and dissected distally toward the uretero-vesical junction (UVJ). During this process it's important not to overmanipulate the ureters and prevent any injury to their blood supply that may increase the risk of subsequent ischemic stricture. With the distal dissection, the infundibulo-pelvic (IP) suspensory ligament and adnexa may be lifted superiorly, and the uterine artery may be seen crossing over the ureter from lateral to medial. Once the UVJ is identified, the ureter is doubly clipped with two hem-o-loks with a stay suture on the distal clip, just proximal to the junction itself, and then the ureter is divided between the clips.

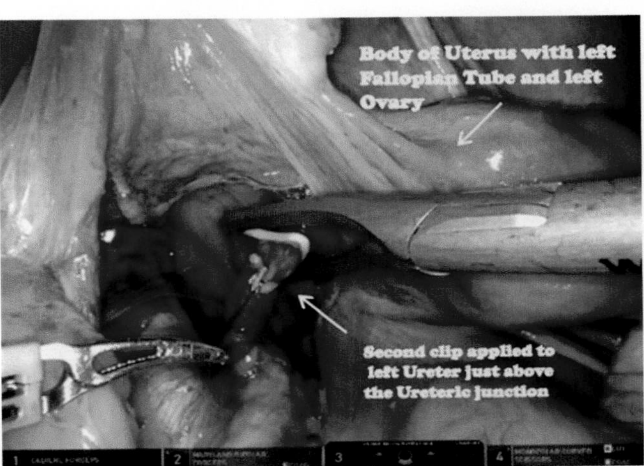

Fig. 1 Second Clip applied to distal left ureter, just above the left vesico-ureteric junction

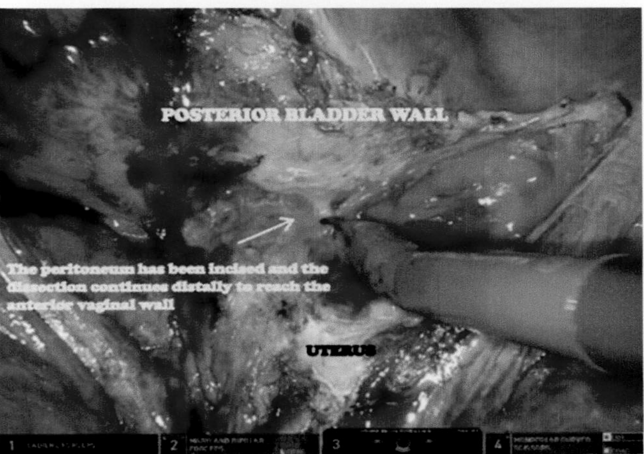

Fig. 2 Incision of peritoneum and dissection into plane between posterior bladder wall and body of the uterus and cervix

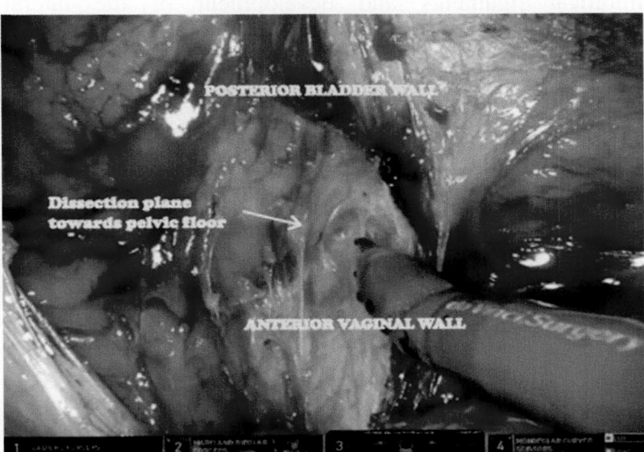

Fig. 3 Distal dissection into plane between posterior bladder wall and anterior vaginal wall, towards the pelvic floor, during a POP RARC approach

Posterior Dissection (Figs. 2 and 3) If the approach is non-organ preserving, this part of the operation starts with an inverted U-shaped incision in the midline of the posterior peritoneum below the bladder, with the limbs of the inverted U extending proximally on each side toward the bifurcation of the common iliac vessels. The uterus is placed under traction by the fourth robotic arm, and the dissection continues distally opening the plane between the body of uterus and cervix and posterior bladder wall toward the fornix of the vagina. If it has not already been done, the IP ligament is ligated and divided using a LigaSure, as are the ovarian and uterine pedicles. To identify the junction of the cervix with the vagina, a sponge on a stick may be placed and manipulated within the vagina by the bedside assistant. Positioning of the fourth robotic arm and uterus is an important aspect of removal of the gynecological organs, also helped by the bedside assistant moving the sponge within the vagina. This clearly identifies the position of the vaginal posterior fornix, which can then be incised through the overlying peritoneum. This incision passes caudally down the anterolateral aspect of the vagina, so the anterior vaginal wall, uterus, and ovaries are removed with the specimen.

Lateral Dissection (Figs. 4 and 5) The lateral dissection begins with incision of the peritoneum lateral to the medial umbilical ligaments and development of the lateral paravesical space, which can be opened up down to the pelvic floor and endopelvic fascia. The space medial and lateral to the medial umbilical ligament can be connected, and the round ligament divided. The bladder can then be lifted under traction with the fourth robotic arm, pulling the superior bladder pedicle away from the external iliac vessels and rectum. The superior bladder pedicle is then divided by LigaSure, and as the dissection continues down to the pelvic floor, the inferior pedicle and any small perforating arteries are dealt with in the same way.

Bladder Drop and Dissection of the Urethra (Figs. 6, 7, 8, 9, 10 and 11) The median umbilical ligaments and urachus are divided proximally, and the bladder is then dissected off the under surface of the anterior abdominal wall. The dissection continues in the midline down to the pubis, with most of the lateral dissection having already been completed as

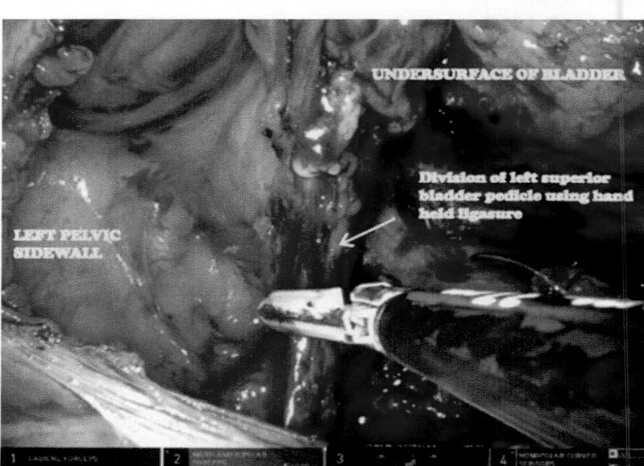

Fig. 5 Division of the right superior bladder pedicle, using a ligasure which is hand held by the surgical bedside assistant

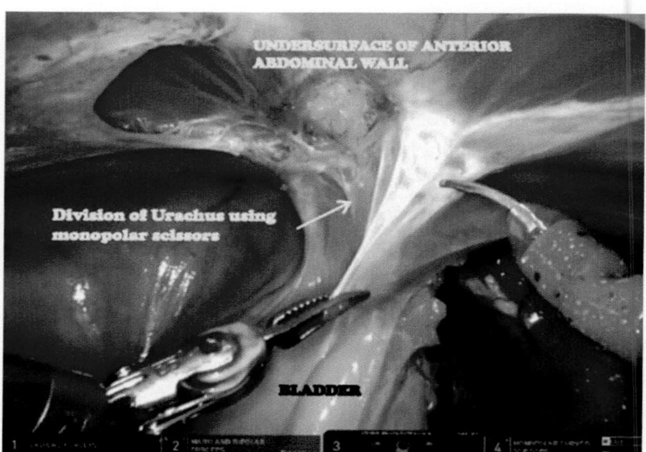

Fig. 6 Urachal division

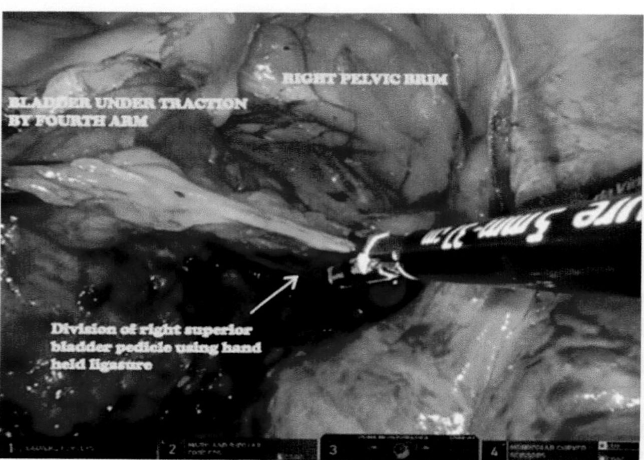

Fig. 4 Division of the left superior bladder pedicle, using a ligasure which is hand held by the surgical bedside assistant

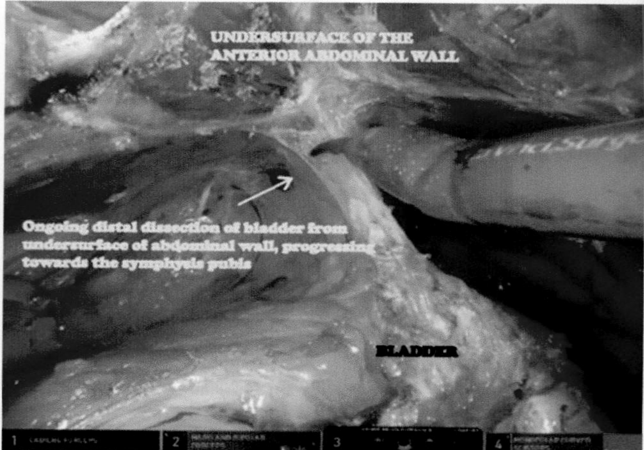

Fig. 7 Dissection of bladder from abdominal wall continuing distally towards the pelvis

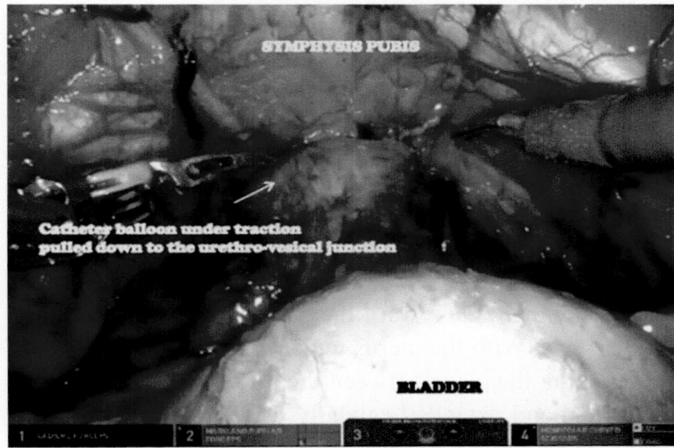

Fig. 8 Demonstration of the vesico-urethral junction by pulling down the catheter balloon down during a POP RARC approach

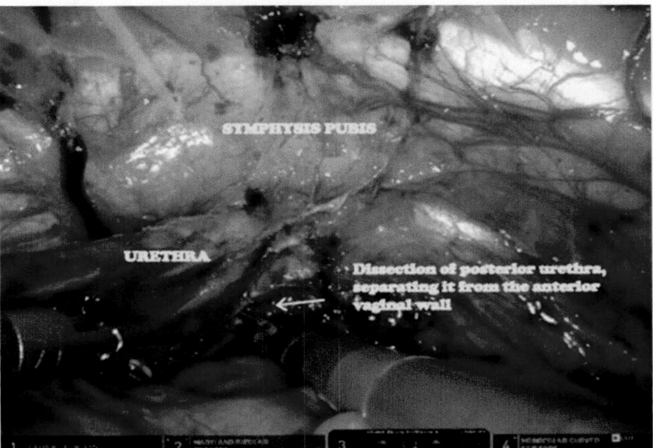

Fig. 9 Dissection of the urethra, including dissection posteriorly between the wall of the posterior urethra and anterior wall of the vagina for the POP RARC approach

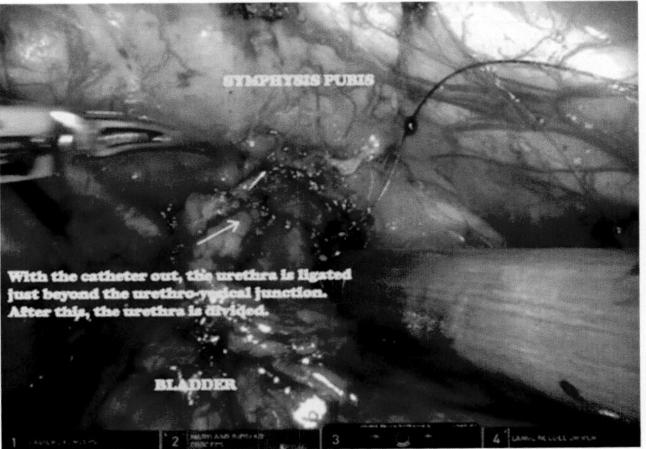

Fig. 10 Urethral ligation just beyond the junction between the bladder and urethra, aiming to maximise distal urethral stump length during POP RARC

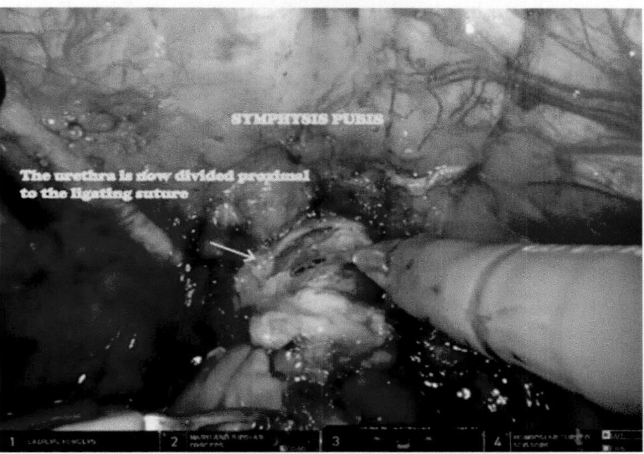

Fig. 11 Urethral transection, aiming to maximise distal urethral stump length during POP RARC

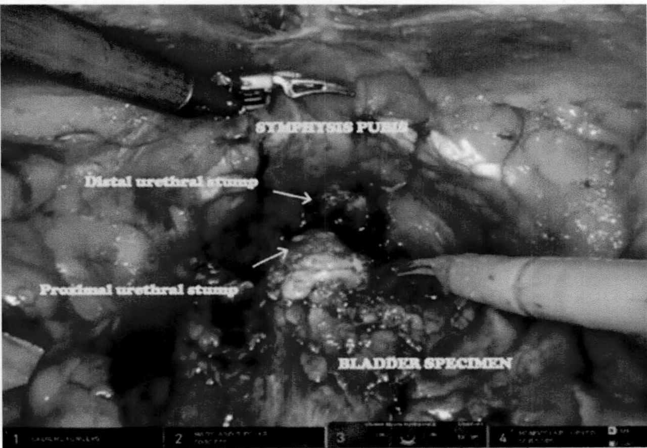

Fig. 12 Bladder specimen with proximal and distal urethral stumps, following POP RARC. In cases where Orthotopic Neobladder is being considered, a tissue sample is taken form the urethral margin for frozen section. A positive margin would be a contraindication for Neobladder

above. At this point it is helpful if the bedside assistant places the urinary catheter under traction, which pulls the catheter balloon down, and helps to identify the bladder neck and vesicourethral junction. The dorsal vein complex (DVC) over the female urethra can be divided and hemostasis achieved with cautery alone for most patients, although sometimes a hemostatic suture is required. The urethra is then dissected and excised with the anterior vaginal wall ensuring the urethrectomy is complete.

EPLND, Specimen Removal and Urinary Diversion (UD) (Fig. 12) A detailed discussion of EPLND and UD is beyond the scope of this chapter, suffice to say most surgeons would perform the EPLND prior to the UD. The anatomical borders for the EPLND dissection template are well described and include removing all lymph node tissue within the area bounded by the genitofemoral nerve laterally, the pelvic floor and internal iliac vessels inferiorly, the circumflex iliac vessels distally, and proximally up to the aortic bifurcation over the presacral area. Any venous injuries may be better dealt with by applied pressure using an intra-abdominal swab and surgical rather than any attempts at suturing, which may be more technically challenging and has potential to make the vessel injury worse. The cystectomy specimen and lymph node packets are placed into large and individual small bags, respectively, and may be removed through vaginotomy, or through the camera port incision. If removed through the camera port incision at the end of the procedure, this should be done carefully to prevent any injury to the mesentery of the conduit.

Regardless of the modality of UD, the left ureter is carefully brought across to the right side of the abdomen beneath the sigmoid mesentery, and a handheld GI stapler is brought into the abdomen through the 15 mm left lateral trocar. At the same time, a robotic bowel grasper and robotic cadiere instrument are exchanged with the robotic instruments on the second and third arms, allowing the bowel work to begin. If a RIN is planned, a tissue sample is taken from the distal urethral stump for frozen section to ensure no cancerous urethral involvement, which would be a contraindication to proceeding.

Other technical variations that may be considered if RIN is planned after standard RARC include avoiding overlapping suture lines between the vaginal remnant and neobladder-urethral anastomosis and placing an omental flap between the vagina and anastomosis, both of which may reduce the risk of neobladder-vaginal fistula [11]. Finally, a modified sacrocolpopexy may also be done not only to prevent prolapse of the vaginal remnant through the weakened pelvic floor but also to reduce the risk of urinary retention caused by loss of mechanical support from the gynecological organs and angulation at the neobladder-urethral anastomosis. This requires suturing a mesh to the vaginal remnant, which is then fixed proximally to the sacral promontory [11].

5 RARC with POP

The ureteric dissection does not differ for POP RARC, but there are technical differences relating to preservation of the gynecological organs as well as in the posterior and urethral dissection, notwithstanding that POP RACR is commonly performed with RIN as the modality of UD. For RIN, preservation of the gynecological organs will provide mechanical support to the overlying neobladder, and by reducing the angle at the urethral anastomosis potentially lowers the risk of urinary retention. Maximizing urethral stump length is also important for RIN, and analogous to nerve sparing during a robotic prostatectomy, preservation of the autonomic nerves that run lateral to the vagina may contribute to recovery of sexual and urinary function [11].

Posterior Dissection in POP RARC (Figs. 2 and 3) The dissection begins in the same way with an inverted U-shaped incision in the posterior peritoneum below the bladder across the midline, with the limbs of the U extending proximally on either side toward the bifurcation of the common iliac vessels. With the uterus under traction from the fourth robotic arm, the plane between the posterior bladder wall is developed and extended caudally down toward the cervix. Once the vagina is reached, care is taken to ensure the anterior vaginal wall is kept intact. The paravaginal tissues are notably vascular, and it is important to prevent any nervous or vaginal injury when using cautery, the latter of which would require a repair, resulting in unwanted suture lines in the vagina. As the dissection continues distally toward the pelvic floor, the posterior bladder and anterior vaginal wall are separated completely down to the bladder neck and urethra.

Preservation of the Gynecological Organs During dissection of the posterior plane, the uterine and ovarian ligaments are left intact. This includes the IP suspensory ligament, the round ligament and pedicle of the ovaries, and the cardinal ligaments containing the uterine arteries, all of which would otherwise have been ligated and divided with a LigaSure. Further manipulation of the uterus to help open up the plane between posterior bladder and anterior vaginal walls is done with the fourth robotic arm, but dissection around the posterior and lateral aspects of the uterus is minimized, as is dissection of the lateral vaginal walls and endopelvic fascia.

6 Evidence Acquisition

Evidence was derived from searches of Web of Science, Scopus, and PubMed databases using three separate search terms "robot assisted" AND "cystectomy," "da Vinci radical cystectomy" and "robot*" AND "cystectomy." A total of 2354 references were retrieved and categorized under the broad headings of comparative and case series, as well as those focused on learning curves, ERAS, and nerve sparing or pelvic organ preservation. Studies with an emphasis on laparoscopic surgery and duplicates were excluded, and those reporting on functional and oncological outcomes were included. The remaining 71 references were then reviewed to extract information focused specifically on female RARC.

7 RARC with Anterior Exenteration Outcomes

In general, oncological and functional outcomes for patients following RARC are not stratified by gender. However, some studies were found where outcomes were reported by gender (or were simply case studies and series and the results reported on an individual basis), or where gender was used as a predictor variable in the analysis of perioperative surgical, functional, and oncological outcomes.

7.1 RARC with Anterior Exenteration: Perioperative Outcomes and Complications (See Table 1)

Pruthi et al. [16] first presented on a case series of 12 women (mean age 67.9 years), undergoing RARC with pelvic exenteration [nine with ileal conduit (ECUD) and three with robotic intracorporeal neobladder (RIN)]. Mean estimated blood loss (EBL) and operating time (OT) were 221 ml and 4.6 h, respectively. There were no positive surgical margins, and the mean number of lymph nodes was 19 (range 12–34). Two postoperative complications were encountered in two patients, though the Clavien-Dindo classification or severity of these complications was not disclosed. The mean LOS was 4.8 days. A follow-up study compared outcomes for females ($n = 10$) to men operated upon during the same time period ($n = 20$) [17]. There was no significant difference in blood loss, OT, or mean time to flatus, bowel movement, or discharge. However, when compared to a second group of men ($n = 20$) who were operated on during the previous year, female patients were found to have significantly shorter OTs (4.6 h vs. 5.9 h; $p < .001$) and less blood loss (215 ml vs. 330 ml; $p = .012$) as well as a shorter time to bowel movement (2.4 days vs. 2.8 days; $p = .057$). These improvements likely reflected improvements in the learning curve for the operating surgeons.

Table 1 Perioperative and pathological outcomes comparing men and women from studies where sufficient information is provided to permit informed comparisons with minimal confounding factors

Reference	Cohort	Diversion	Mean operating time	Blood loss (ml)	Lymph nodes removed (range)	Length of stay	Positive surgical margins
Pruthi [16]	12 women; mean age = 67.9 years	Ileal conduit = 9 (75%) Neobladder = 3 (25%)	4.6 h	221	19 (12–34)	4.8 days	0
Pruthi [17]	10 female; mean age = 68.4 years 40 male; mean age = 62.8 years (cysto-prostatectomy)	Females: Ileal conduit = 7 (70%) Neobladder = 3 (30%) Males: Ileal conduit = 23 (57.5%) Neobladder = 17 (42.5%)	Female = 4.6 h Male[a] = 4.4 h	Female = 215 Male[a] = 233	Female = 19 (12–34) Male = 18 (8–37)	Female = 4.9 days Male[a] = 4.4 days	Female = 0 Male = 0
Kwon [18]	5 female 12 male	Ileal conduit = 14 Neobladder = 4 – No information on gender distribution	Female = 6.0 h Male = 6.45 h	Female = 210 Male = 211	n/a	Female = 20.1 days Male = 22.2 days	Female = 0 Male = 0
Kang [19]	22 female 82 male	Female Ileal conduit = 13 (59.1%) Neobladder = 9 (40.9%) Total cohort Ileal conduit = 60 (57.7%) Neobladder = 44 (42.3%) Female cohort similar to total cohort, so it follows distribution of diversion types are similar between male and female	Female = 8.3 h Male = 7.9 h	Female = 591 Male = 515	Female = 16.0 Male = 19.1	Female = 20.0 days Male = 17.7 days	Female = 0 Male = 0
Yuh [20]	32 female 164 male	Females: Ileal conduit = 15 (46.9%) Neobladder = 0 (0%) Continent cutaneous = 17 (53.1%) Males: Ileal conduit = 47 (28.7%) Neobladder = 86 (52.4%) Continent cutaneous = 31 (18.9%)				Females 1–7 days = 5 (15.6%) 8–14 days = 22 (68.8%) >14 days = 5 (15.6%) Males 1–7 days = 50 (30.5%) 8–14 days = 82 (50.0%) >14 days = 32 (19.5%)	

[a] Data from male cohort of 20 from same time as females. Other 20 males were done earlier and make up learning curve

One of the first studies to report actual differences in procedural and postoperative outcomes between males ($n = 12$) and females ($n = 5$) was that by Kwon et al. [18]. Ileal conduits were performed in 13 cases, while the other four patients obtained neobladders, though how these were distributed across gender was not disclosed. They examined the differences in mean OT, EBL, time to oral intake and ambulation, and LOS. They found no significant differences in any of these categories between men and women (p-values between 0.241 and 0.552).

A multicenter Korean study summarized by Kang et al. [19] also compared results between males ($n = 82$) and females ($n = 22$). Of the 22 women, 13 had ECUD, while 9 had RIN (a similar distribution of UD was noted in the male group). The mean age of the women was 66.1 years, and median OT and EBL was 567 min and 591 ml, respectively. The median number of lymph nodes was 16, and all surgical margins were negative. The authors statistically analyzed differences between the men and women for age, BMI, OT, pelvic lymph node dissection time, urinary diversion time, EBL, LOS, time to flatus, number of lymph nodes, and the mean follow-up time. They found no difference between the male and female patients, with p-values for all these factors ranging between 0.186 (LOS) and 0.644 (OT).

Yuh et al. [20] studied a cohort of 32 females and 164 males. Of the females, 47% received an ileal conduit, but none received neobladders. The remaining were cutaneous continent UDs. Fifty-two percent of the males underwent RIN and a further 19% ileal conduits. The remaining 19% were cutaneous continent diversions. For LOS, 15.6% of females were discharged within 1–7 days, compared to 30.5% for males. Approximately 69% of females were discharged between 8 and 14 days, compared to 50% for the men. LOS greater than 14 days were similar at 15.6% for females and 19.5% for men.

The data presented in Table 1 provides no strong evidence to suggest that there is a difference between perioperative outcomes between males and females when diversion types are accounted for to the greatest extent possible. Some study differences are observed in operating times and length of stays, but these may be due to learning curve issues and local hospital discharge guidelines, respectively. Also, when reporting operating times, it is not always clear whether the reported value includes the time required for lymph node dissection. No positive surgical margins were reported in any of the studies.

With regard complications (see Table 2), there appears to be no significant evidence that females are more prone to

Table 2 Summary of available oncological and functional outcomes following RARC with anterior exenteration in females as compared to males

Reference	Cohort	Diversion	Complications	Survival	Continence outcomes	Sexual outcomes
Pruthi [16]	12 women; mean age = 67.9 years	Ileal conduit = 9 (75%) Neobladder = 3 (25%)	2/12 (17%) Grade unidentified			
Pruthi [17]	10 female; mean age = 68.4 years 40 male; mean age = 62.8 years (Cysto-prostatectomy)	Females: Ileal conduit = 7 (70%) Neobladder = 3 (30%) Males: Ileal conduit = 23 (57.5%) Neobladder = 17 (42.5%)	Females = 20% Males = 30% – Not found to be statistically significantly different			
Yuh [20]	32 female 164 male	Females: Ileal conduit = 15 (46.9%) Neobladder = 0 (0%) Continent cutaneous = 17 (53.1%) Males: Ileal conduit = 47 (28.7%) Neobladder = 86 (52.4%) Continent cutaneous = 31 (18.9%)	Gender not found to be a predictor of all complications or only major complications in univariate or multivariate analysis Incidence of transfusion: Women = 21/32 (66%) Men = 65/164 (40%)	90 day survival rate: Women = 30/32 (94%) Men = 158/164 (96%)		

Table 2 (continued)

Reference	Cohort	Diversion	Complications	Survival	Continence outcomes	Sexual outcomes
Johar [21]	189 female 750 male	Ileal conduit = 613 (68%) Continent = 294 (32%)	Predictors of any complication—multivariate analysis, pre-operative variables only: Gender *p*-value = .605 (gender not significant predictor) Predictors of Clavien III–V complication—multivariate analysis, pre-operative variables only: Gender *p*-value = .097 (gender a weak predictor) Odds ratio (female/male) = 0.67 (0.42–1.07)	Predictors of 90-day mortality—multivariate analysis, pre-operative variables only: Gender *p*-value = .766 (gender not significant predictor)		
Nazmy [22]	33 female 176 male	Female: Ileal conduit = 15 (45%) Indiana pouch = 18 (55%) Male: Ileal conduit = 52 (30%) Indiana pouch = 33 (19%) Orthotopic bladder substitute = 91 (51%)	Predictors of urinary tract infection—multivariate analysis: Gender *p*-value = 0.09 (gender a weak predictor) Odds ratio (Female/Male) = 2.48 (0.87–7.06) Predictors of any complication—multivariate analysis, pre-operative variables only: Gender *p*-value = 0.6 (gender not significant predictor) Predictors of Clavien III–V complication—multivariate analysis, pre-operative variables only: Gender *p*-value = .7 (gender not significant predictor) Predictors of anemia—multivariate analysis, pre-operative variables only: Gender *p*-value = .1 (gender a weak predictor) Odds ratio (female/male) = 2.32 (0.80–6.74)			
Sung [23]	RARC 4 female 31 male ORC 19 female 85 male	RARC Ileal conduits = 13 (37%) Neobladder = 22 (63%) ORC Ileal conduits = 81 (78%) Neobladder = 19 (18%) Other = 4 (4%)	Predictors for Grade II or greater complications—multivariate: Gender *p*-value = .028 Odds ratio (female/male) = 4.06			
Tyritzis [24]	8 female; mean age = 55.6 2 with organ sparing 62 male; mean age = 60.3 41 with nerve sparing	All neobladders			12 month day: Women 2/3 (66%) Men 16/18 (89%) Men (nerve-spared) 30/34 (88%) 12 month night: Women 2/3 (66%) Men 13/16 (81%) Men (nerve-spared) 25/34 (73%)	Sexually active: Women 4/8 (50%) Men (nerve-spared) 27/32 (84%)

(continued)

Table 2 (continued)

Reference	Cohort	Diversion	Complications	Survival	Continence outcomes	Sexual outcomes
Canda [25]	2 female 25 male	Female Neobladder = 2 (100%) Male Neobladder = 21 (84%) Ileal conduit = 4 (16%)			Minimum 5 month follow-up— Daytime: Women 0/2 (0%) Men 8/12 (66.6%)	
Smith [26]	49 female 178 male	168 Ileal conduit (74%) 58 Neobladder (26%)	None: Female = 37 (60%) Male = 122 (69%) Clavien I–II: Female = 11 (22%) Male = 42 (24%) Clavien III–V Female = 1 (2%) Male = 14 (8%) Logistic regression analysis: Gender not a predictor of complications ($p = .2148$)			

complications following RARC than males. Only in the study by Sung et al. [23] was gender found to be a significant predictor of complications (in this case Clavien II or greater). Their cohort was 139 patients (35 RARC, 104 ORC, with 4 females in the RARC group and 19 in the ORC group). The odds ratios (OR) for grade II or greater complications were 2.44 (1.02–5.84) for ORC versus RARC ($p = .045$) and 4.06 (1.12–14.11) for females over males ($p = .028$). By contrast, Johar et al. [21] found a weak gender-specific difference in complications in a large cohort of 189 females and 750 males but actually in favor of females (OR female/male = 0.67 [0.42–1.07]). Nazmy et al. [22] in their study of 33 females [45% ECUD, 55% Continent Cutaneous Diversion (Indiana Pouch)] and 176 males (30% ECUD, 19% Continent Cutaneous Diversion (Indiana Pouch), 51% RIN) found a weak increase in risk for females for urinary tract infection and anemia requiring transfusion following RARC (OR = 2.48 and 2.32, respectively).

7.2 RARC with Anterior Exenteration: Oncological and Survival Outcomes (See Tables 1 and 2)

There is a paucity of data on pathological outcomes between men and women, where available lymph node yield and margin status are presented in Table 1. In their follow-up study comparing men and women, Pruthi et al. [17] did note that 50% of females had a pathological outcome of less than or equal T2N0 (compared to 70% for men); 30% had T3N0 (15% for men) and 20% TxN+ (15% for men). Their male data included a cohort of 20 men that had been operated upon prior to any of the women, and thus outcomes may have been comprised the operating surgeon's inexperience and learning curve.

Attempts to compare complication and survival outcomes between women and men are summarized in Table 2. Again, there are some confounding factors that must be considered, and as in the previous section, in some cases it was impossible to stratify the type of UD by gender. However, many of these studies employ multivariate logistic regression analyses that include UD as one of the variables, and so UD would be accounted for.

In the few studies with comparable survival data, there is no evidence that gender is significant. Yuh et al. [20] noted similar 90-day survival rates between men and women, even though a much higher fraction of men underwent the more complex neobladder procedure. In their multivariate logistic regression analysis of 90-day mortality, Johar et al. [21] did not find that gender was a significant factor ($p = .766$).

7.3 RARC with Anterior Exenteration Outcomes: Functional Outcomes (See Table 2)

Although formal statistical analyses were not provided, it does appear continence rates are higher for males. In their study, Tyritzis et al. [24] focused only on patients that underwent RIN (patients assessed were 3 women, 18 men, and 34 men who underwent nerve sparing RARC). They found 12 months day continence rate for women was 66%, compared to 89% for men and 88% for nerve-spared men. With regard to nighttime continence, 66% of women compared to 81% of men and 73% of nerve-spared men were dry at night. The study by Canda et al. [25] also showed similar results in 2 women and 12 men undergoing RARC with RIN. At minimum 5 months follow-up, neither of the women achieved daytime continence, while 66% of the men reported continence during the day. The study by Tyritzis et al. [24] was also the only one where data reporting on sexual activity allowed any comparison between men and women, finding men were more sexually active following RARC (84% compared to 50%).

8 Female POP RARC Outcomes

As has been discussed, the potential criticism of female POP RARC is underestimating disease stage prior to the procedure, resulting in inadequate excision with a negative influence of longer-term oncological outcomes. Nevertheless, a recent systematic review examining 197 female POP open cystectomy (ORC) patients with follow-up between 1 and nearly 13 years showed disease-free survival (DFS) of 87–100% and cancer-specific survival (CSS) of 70–100% [9]. This compares favorably to a larger multicenter series of standard ORC without preservation of the gynecological organs in 888 patients (167 of whom were female), which demonstrated DFS and CSS at 5 years follow-up of 58% and 66% [27]. Similarly, with neobladder as the modality of UD, local urethral recurrence rates for the standard ORC and POP ORC also compare favorably at 0.6–4.3% and 0–13% [9, 28–30]. However, transferring these outcomes from open to POP RARC as a technique has been less well studied with a paucity of series in the literature examining functional and oncological outcomes.

The first report of organ preservation during RARC in women was provided by Menon et al. in 2004 [31]. This was a case series study of three female patients, aged 59–66 all with preoperative tumor stage T3b. The chosen UD was different for each (W and T-pouch neobladder and Ileal conduit). Final histopathology ranged from PT1 to PT3a with all surgical margins negative. There were no in-hospital complications reported, no open conversions and LOS ranged from 5 to 8 days. These findings supported the view the technique was safe and technically feasible, although it clearly required more study before widespread use.

More recently, Tuderti et al. [32] reported a retrospective case series of 11 female patients undergoing organ sparing RARC with RIN (Padua type). Their mean age and BMI were 47.1 years and 23.1, respectively. Ten of the patients had ASA scores of 2 or less prior to surgery. The median OT and LOS was 255 min and 7 days, respectively. No major complications (Clavien-Dindo grade III or higher) were reported. Four patients suffered from lower grade, Clavien-Dindo grade I-II, complications. The mean lymph node count was 26.2, and no positive surgical margins were reported. At median follow-up of 28 months, 1-year recurrence-free, cancer-specific, and overall survival were all 100%. The probability of daytime and nighttime continence recovery was determined as 90.9% and 86.4%, respectively. Results from the EORTC-QLQ-C30 survey indicated that the global health status/quality of life and physical and emotional functioning items improved significantly over time (all $p \leq 0.04$). Of the 11 patients, 8 (72.7%) remained sexually active at the 12-month evaluation.

In a video publication demonstrating their technique, Goh et al. [33] also summarized their method and results in a case series of four females of median age and BMI of 67 years and 27, respectively, so older and potentially at higher risk when compared to the previous study of Tuderti et al. [32] Median OT was 396 min, and media lymph node yield was 63. All surgical margins were negative, and the median LOS was 12 days. One patient required a blood transfusion, but no long-term outcomes or functional outcomes were described.

Apart from the better functional outcomes and if combined with RIN, improved body image and ovarian sparing will preserve estrogen levels, lowering the risk of long-term osteoporosis as well as the potential cognitive and cardiovascular issues related to chronic estrogen depletion. If RIN is the chosen modality of UD, the gynecological organs will also provide mechanical support to the neobladder, reducing the angle of the neobladder-urethral anastomosis and reducing the risk of postoperative neobladder retention [34]. Although a small number of series, the findings suggest that female POP RARC and RIN is not only safe and technically feasible but also may improve sexual activity and continence outcomes at rates similar to organ sparing ORC. A recent systematic review sanctioned by the EAU and incorporated into the European Association of Urology (EAU) guidelines for muscle invasive bladder cancer (MIBC) suggested female POP ORC and neobladder offered the potential for improve potency and continence [34], and from a technical viewpoint, these findings would also support use of the robotic approach.

9 ERAS

The concept of "Enhanced Recovery after Surgery" (ERAS) was developed in colorectal surgery in the late 1990s. It actually refers to detailed activities relevant to patient's preparation before surgery outlining pre-, peri-, and post-surgery protocols all aimed at speeding up and improving recovery [35]. Investigating the physiology of surgical recovery and the stress response to surgical trauma, it became clear that catabolic processes induced by the hormonal response to surgical stress, mediated by inflammatory and metabolic pathways, may have a negative impact on surgical recovery [35]. To prevent the negative effects of this catabolic stress response, a number of pre- and postoperative protocols were devised. Robotic surgery, as a minimally invasive approach, contributes to ERAS programs by limiting surgical trauma. According to the Karolinska ERAS pathway, patient education regarding in-hospital care pathways, complications, and surgical recovery are an important part of the preoperative process, as is medical optimization, including cessation of smoking and dietary advice to optimize preoperative nutritional status. At the authors center, patients are recommended for clear fluids and loading with carbohydrates the day before surgery, with no specific additional bowel prep. In the OR, epidural analgesia is avoided, antibiotics are administered at induction according to AUA guidelines, and pneumatic calf compression with heparin at induction is used for thromboprophylaxis. Postoperatively patients are managed initially on the intensive care unit, but the emphasis is on early feeding and mobilization, with multimodal analgesia with a view to minimizing the use of opioids. On discharge, thromboprophylaxis is prescribed for another 3 weeks. To date there is little information regarding effectiveness of ERAS protocols specific to female RARC, and further study is required in this area.

10 Learning Curves

All modalities of RARC, especially if RIN is the planned modality of UD, require great technical expertise. As a result, surgical mentoring and trainee learning curves for RARC are an important part of the procedure's introduction into robotic programs, notwithstanding the potential negative influence of less experienced robotic cystectomy on functional and oncological outcomes.

There are a few studies that have examined learning curves using sequential case numbers and surgical experience by volume as variables, with an additional analysis of patient gender (Porreca et al; Calderon et al.; Hellenthal et al.) [36–39]. In the study by Porreca et al. [36], they used a sequential case number model assessing 90-day postoperative complication rates but found gender not to be significant on univariate analysis ($p = 0.7$). Similarly, Calderon et al. [37] examined any complications and major complications using surgical experience as one of the predictor variables with gender once again not showing significance. Although there is a paucity of data, the published evidence suggests that female RARC may be learnt without any negative influence on perioperative outcomes, but further study is required. Overall, those groups who studied learning curve analysis, not only for female RARC but for RARC as a whole, emphasized learning should be modular and take place within an experienced mentor and team in an established robotic program. Moreover, the educational approach should be multimodal combining experience gained in the OR with theoretical lectures and a detailed modular examination of technical videos where the procedure is performed by experts [36].

11 Novel Approaches to RARC

As female RARC becomes more widespread in established programs with more technical advances in robotic surgery, new indications and approaches are emerging. These include single port RARC, palliative RARC, salvage RARC, and RARC in the elderly. Once again there are limited studies on these approaches that have specific reference to gender, but there is some emerging data.

Female Elderly RARC. Mortezavi et al. [40] examined the postoperative complications in octogenarians following RARC with ICUD. There cohort consisted of 1726 patients <80 years of age and 164 >80 years of age. By analyzing predictors of any complication and specifically major complications with Clavien-Dindo classification greater than III, they found that gender was a nonsignificant predictor in either. By further examining cancer-specific, other cause, and all-cause mortality, once again gender was not found to be a significant factor. In another study of RARC in octogenarians, Elsayed et al. [41] found that females were more prone to readmissions following RARC with an odds ratio of 2.10 (1.30–3.50; $p < .01$), but gender was not a significant factor for recurrence-free survival, disease-specific survival, or overall survival.

Single port RARC. In the evolution of minimally invasive approaches, single port robotic systems are now being used in a number of high volume robotic programs. In one of the earliest reports of single port RARC, Kaouk et al. [42] presented a case series of four patients, two of whom were females. One was a 70-year-old female who presented with a pT2 tumor and underwent single port RARC with extracorporeal urinary diversion. The OT was 496 min with an EBL of 100 ml. A total of nine lymph nodes were retrieved (all negative), and the final pathology was pT4aN0. LOS that was 5 days with only one Clavien-Dindo grade I 30-day complication was reported (nausea and vomiting). The second was a 71-year-old female with a pT1 tumor. OT was 420 min, EBL was 100 ml, 18 lymph nodes were retrieved (all negative), and the final pathology was pTisN0. She was discharge 5 days post procedure and did not report any 30 day complications.

These favorable reports of female RARC in novel settings require further study.

12 Conclusion

Female RARC with standard anterior exenteration and pelvic organ preservation, as well as both ileal conduit and intracorporeal neobladder as modalities of urinary diversion, is increasingly widespread. The techniques for each of these approaches in females are now well established, and applying a step-by-step modular approach as described facilitates smooth progress through the operation as well as facilitating learning. Reviewing the literature reveals, apart from some evidence of an increase risk in urinary tract infection and perioperative anemia requiring transfusion, there is no gender-specific increase risk of adverse perioperative outcomes. Similarly, for either standard or POP female RARC, if neobladder is the modality of urinary diversion, females may have an increased risk of long-term incontinence, but otherwise there are no gender-specific differences in functional or oncological outcomes reported. With regard to female POP RARC, the published evidence suggests it is feasible and, when patients are carefully selected, has the potential to improve functional outcomes without compromising oncological outcomes. Although there is a paucity of learning curve analyses specific to female RARC, the data available shows female RARC can be taught in high volume robotic programs without adversely influencing outcomes. Moreover, as high volume robotic programs gain experience, single port RARC and RARC in elderly patients over 80 is becoming more widespread, with early reports of favorable results.

References

1. Bray F, Ferlay J, Soerjomataram I, Siegel RL, Torre LA, Jemal A. Global cancer statistics 2018: GLOBOCAN estimates of incidence and mortality worldwide for 36 cancers in 185 countries. CA Cancer J Clin. 2018;68:394–424.
2. Richters A, Aben KKH, Kiemeney LALM. The global burden of urinary bladder cancer: an update. World J Urol. 2020;38:1895–904.
3. Liss MA, Kader AK. Robotic-assisted laparoscopic radical cystectomy: history, techniques and outcomes. World J Urol. 2013;31:489–97.
4. Shabsigh A, Korets R, Vora KC, et al. Defining early morbidity of radical cystectomy for patients with bladder cancer using a standardized reporting methodology. Eur Urol. 2009;55:164–76.
5. Morgan TM, Barocas DA, Chang SS, Phillips SE, Salem S, Clark PE, Penson DF, Smith JA, Cookson MS. The relationship between perioperative blood transfusion and overall mortality in patients undergoing radical cystectomy for bladder cancer. Urol Oncol Semin Orig Investig. 2013;31:871–7.
6. Menon M, Hemal AK, Tewari A, Shrivastava A, Shoma AM, El-Tabey NA, Shaaban A, Abol-Enein H, Ghoneim MA. Nerve-sparing robot-assisted radical cystoprostatectomy and urinary diversion. BJU Int. 2003;92:232–6.
7. Parekh DJ, Reis IM, Castle EP, et al. Robot-assisted radical cystectomy versus open radical cystectomy in patients with bladder cancer (RAZOR): an open-label, randomised, phase 3, non-inferiority trial. Lancet. 2018;391:2525–36.
8. Rai BP, Bondad J, Vasdev N, et al. Robotic versus open radical cystectomy for bladder cancer in adults. Cochrane Database Syst Rev. 2019; https://doi.org/10.1002/14651858.CD011903.pub2.
9. Veskimäe E, Neuzillet Y, Rouanne M, et al. Systematic review of the oncological and functional outcomes of pelvic organ-preserving radical cystectomy (RC) compared with standard RC in women who undergo curative surgery and orthotopic neobladder substitution for bladder cancer. BJU Int. 2017;120:12–24.
10. Chan KG, Guru K, Wiklund P, et al. Robot-assisted radical cystectomy and urinary diversion: technical recommendations from the Pasadena Consensus Panel. Eur Urol. 2015;67:423–31.
11. Truong H, Maxon V, Goh AC. Robotic female radical cystectomy. J Endourol. 2021;35:S-106–15.
12. Maqboul F, Thinagaran JKR, Dovey Z, Wiklund P. The contemporary status of robotic intracorporeal neobladder. Mini-Invasive Surg. 2021; https://doi.org/10.20517/2574-1225.2021.54.
13. Gore JL, Lai J, Setodji CM, Litwin MS, Saigal CS. Mortality increases when radical cystectomy is delayed more than 12 weeks. Cancer. 2009;115:988–96.
14. Russell B, Liedberg F, Khan MS, Nair R, Thurairaja R, Malde S, Kumar P, Bryan RT, Van Hemelrijck M. A systematic review and meta-analysis of delay in radical cystectomy and the effect on survival in bladder cancer patients. Eur Urol Oncol. 2020;3:239–49.
15. Collins JW, Tyritzis S, Nyberg T, Schumacher M, Laurin O, Khazaeli D, Adding C, Jonsson MN, Hosseini A, Wiklund NP. Robot-assisted radical cystectomy: description of an evolved approach to radical cystectomy. Eur Urol. 2013;64:654–63.
16. Pruthi RS, Stefaniak H, Hubbard JS, Wallen EM. Robot-assisted laparoscopic anterior pelvic exenteration for bladder cancer in the female patient. J Endourol. 2008;22:2397–402.
17. Pruthi RS, Stefaniak H, Hubbard JS, Wallen EM. Robotic anterior pelvic exenteration for bladder cancer in the female: outcomes and comparisons to their male counterparts. J Laparoendosc Adv Surg Tech. 2009;19:23–7.
18. Kwon S-Y, Kim BS, Kim T-H, Yoo ES, Kwon TG. Initial experiences with robot-assisted laparoscopic radical cystectomy. Korean J Urol. 2010;51:178.
19. Kang SG, Kang SH, Lee YG, et al. Robot-assisted radical cystectomy and pelvic lymph node dissection: a multi-institutional study from Korea. J Endourol. 2010;24:1435–40.
20. Yuh BE, Nazmy M, Ruel NH, Jankowski JT, Menchaca AR, Torrey RR, Linehan JA, Lau CS, Chan KG, Wilson TG. Standardized analysis of frequency and severity of complications after robot-assisted radical cystectomy. Eur Urol. 2012;62:806–13.
21. Johar RS, Hayn MH, Stegemann AP, et al. Complications after robot-assisted radical cystectomy: results from the International Robotic Cystectomy Consortium. Eur Urol. 2013;64:52–7.
22. Nazmy M, Yuh B, Kawachi M, Lau CS, Linehan J, Ruel NH, Torrey RR, Yamzon J, Wilson TG, Chan KG. Early and late complications of robot-assisted radical cystectomy: a standardized analysis by urinary diversion type. J Urol. 2014;191:681–7.
23. Sung HH, Ahn J-S, Il SS, Jeon SS, Choi HY, Lee HM, Jeong BC. A comparison of early complications between open and robot-assisted radical cystectomy. J Endourol. 2012;26:670–5.
24. Tyritzis SI, Hosseini A, Collins J, Nyberg T, Jonsson MN, Laurin O, Khazaeli D, Adding C, Schumacher M, Wiklund NP. Oncologic, functional, and complications outcomes of robot-assisted radical cystectomy with totally intracorporeal neobladder diversion. Eur Urol. 2013;64:734–41.
25. Canda AE, Atmaca AF, Altinova S, Akbulut Z, Balbay MD. Robot-assisted nerve-sparing radical cystectomy with bilateral extended pelvic lymph node dissection (PLND) and intracorporeal urinary diversion for bladder cancer: initial experience in 27 cases. BJU Int. 2012;110:434–44.
26. Smith AB, Raynor M, Amling CL, et al. Multi-institutional analysis of robotic radical cystectomy for bladder cancer: perioperative out-

comes and complications in 227 patients. J Laparoendosc Adv Surg Tech. 2012;22:17–21.
27. Shariat SF, Karakiewicz PI, Palapattu GS, et al. Outcomes of radical cystectomy for transitional cell carcinoma of the bladder: a contemporary series from the Bladder Cancer Research Consortium. J Urol. 2006;176:2414–22.
28. Ali-El-Dein B, Mosbah A, Osman Y, El-Tabey N, Abdel-latif M, Eraky I, Shaaban AA. Preservation of the internal genital organs during radical cystectomy in selected women with bladder cancer: a report on 15 cases with long term follow-up. Eur J Surg Oncol. 2013;39:358–64.
29. Akkad T, Gozzi C, Deibl M, Müller T, Pelzer AE, Pinggera GM, Bartsch G, Steiner H. Tumor recurrence in the remnant urothelium of females undergoing radical cystectomy for transitional cell carcinoma of the bladder: long-term results from a single center. J Urol. 2006;175:1268–71.
30. Gakis G, Ali-El-Dein B, Babjuk M, Hrbacek J, Macek P, Burkhard FC, Thalmann GN, Shaaban A-A, Stenzl A. Urethral recurrence in women with orthotopic bladder substitutes: a multi-institutional study. Urol Oncol Semin Orig Investig. 2015;33:204.e17–23.
31. Menon M, Hemal AK, Tewari A, Shrivastava A, Shoma AM, Abol-Ein H, Ghoneim MA. Robot-assisted radical cystectomy and urinary diversion in female patients: technique with preservation of the uterus and vagina. J Am Coll Surg. 2004;198:386–93.
32. Tuderti G, Mastroianni R, Flammia S, Ferriero M, Leonardo C, Anceschi U, Brassetti A, Guaglianone S, Gallucci M, Simone G. Sex-sparing robot-assisted radical cystectomy with intracorporeal padua ileal neobladder in female: surgical technique, perioperative, oncologic and functional outcomes. J Clin Med. 2020;9:577.
33. Goh AC, Abreu A, Mercado M, Sotelo R, Fernandez G, Aron M, Gill IS, Desai M. Female organ-sparing robotic cystectomy: a step-by-step anatomic approach. Videourology. 2014;28:vid.2013.0099.
34. Abdul-Muhsin HM, Woods ME, Castle EP. Robot assisted anterior pelvic exenteration for bladder cancer in female. Cham: Springer International; 2018. p. 733–42.
35. Kehlet H. Multimodal approach to control postoperative pathophysiology and rehabilitation. Br J Anaesth. 1997;78:606–17.
36. Porreca A, Mineo Bianchi F, Romagnoli D, et al. Robot-assisted radical cystectomy with totally intracorporeal urinary diversion: surgical and early functional outcomes through the learning curve in a single high-volume center. J Robot Surg. 2020;14:261–9.
37. Posada Calderon L, Al Hussein Al Awamlh B, Shoag J, Patel N, Nicolas JD, Scherr DS. The role of surgical experience in patient selection, surgical quality, and outcomes in robot-assisted radical cystectomy. Urol Oncol Semin Orig Investig. 2021;39:6–12.
38. Hellenthal NJ, Hussain A, Andrews PE, et al. Surgical margin status after robot assisted radical cystectomy: results from the International Robotic Cystectomy Consortium. J Urol. 2010;184:87–91.
39. Hellenthal NJ, Hussain A, Andrews PE, et al. Lymphadenectomy at the time of robot-assisted radical cystectomy: results from the International Robotic Cystectomy Consortium. BJU Int. 2011;107:642–6.
40. Mortezavi A, Crippa A, Edeling S, et al. Morbidity and mortality after robot-assisted radical cystectomy with intracorporeal urinary diversion in octogenarians: results from the European Association of Urology Robotic Urology Section Scientific Working Group. BJU Int. 2020; https://doi.org/10.1111/bju.15274.
41. Elsayed AS, Aldhaam NA, Brownell J, et al. Perioperative and oncological outcomes of robot-assisted radical cystectomy in octogenarians. J Geriatr Oncol. 2020;11:727–30.
42. Kaouk J, Garisto J, Eltemamy M, Bertolo R. Step-by-step technique for single-port robot-assisted radical cystectomy and pelvic lymph nodes dissection using the da Vinci ® SP™ surgical system. BJU Int. 2019;124:707–12.

Robot-Assisted Intracorporeal Ileal Conduit

Carl J. Wijburg, Stephan Buse, and Erdem Canda

1 Introduction

The use of intracorporeal urinary diversion has increased from 9% in 2005 to 95% in 2018. Although the technique may seem to be more complicated because of the intracorporeal robot-assisted laparoscopic bowel handling, high volume centers show shorter operative times and no difference in high-grade complications as compared to the extracorporeal technique [1]. *High-grade complications decreased with time and can be as low as 10%* [2]. *A transition from extracorporeal to intracorporeal urinary diversion is safe and reduces operative time, blood loss, and uretero-enteric stricture rates* [3].

A recent meta-analysis also showed lower blood loss and less need for blood transfusion, shorter operative times, and comparable complications rates for the intracorporeal technique [4]. *We provide here a step-by-step description of intracorporeal robot-assisted ileal conduit.*

2 Patient Positioning

Patient positioning is depending on the robotic system and the sex of the patient.

Details are described in Chap. 20 (RARC). In short, male patients are positioned in 25–30 degrees Trendelenburg. da Vinci Si or X-system can be located between the legs in lithotomy position. Alternatively, side docking with legs straight is also possible. For da Vinci Xi-system, the male patients can be positioned with straight legs and 25–30 degrees Trendelenburg.

In female patients, lithotomy positioning and 25–30 degrees Trendelenburg are always the preferred approach. The choice between side docking or robot position between the legs will depend on the robotic system. Side docking is advisable in the case of a simultaneous urethrectomy.

During the bowel-handling part of iRARC, Trendelenburg tilt can be reduced to 15–25 degrees. If table motion is available, undocking the robot is not needed, and the Trendelenburg can be adjusted to an optimal minimum number of degrees.

3 Instruments

For the bowel handling part in particular, it is crucial to be aware of the force of the instruments and how traumatic they can be for vulnerable organs like the ileum. Therefore, we advise *not* to use needle drivers, ProGrasp, and Maryland bipolar forceps for the bowel handling. Special bowel instruments like *Small Graptors* are preferable for bowel handling. For bowel and tissue handling, the Cadiere forceps is a safe and useful instrument. Not only the type of instrument but also the atraumatic surgical technique plays an important role. To prevent iatrogenic trauma to the bowel, care should be taken to grab as much as possible the fatty tissue close to the bowel, instead of the bowel itself.

4 Trocar Placement

For trocar placement during cystectomy, please refer to Chap. 20 (RARC). For intracorporeal conduit, based on our experience, guiding the stapler from the left side will ensure better maneuverability inside the abdomen. Depending on surgical preferences the additional robotic arm will be either on the right-hand side or on the left-hand side.

4.1 Two Robotic Arms on the Left

If two robotic arms on the *left* side were used during the cystectomy, the most lateral of these two arms should be used for the robotic stapler (SureForm). This also applies if

C. J. Wijburg (✉)
Rijnstate Hospital, Arnhem, The Netherlands

S. Buse
Alfried Krupp Krankenhaus, Essen, Germany

E. Canda
Koç University Hospital, Istanbul, Turkey

P. Wiklund et al. (eds.), *Robotic Urologic Surgery*, https://doi.org/10.1007/978-3-031-00363-9_58

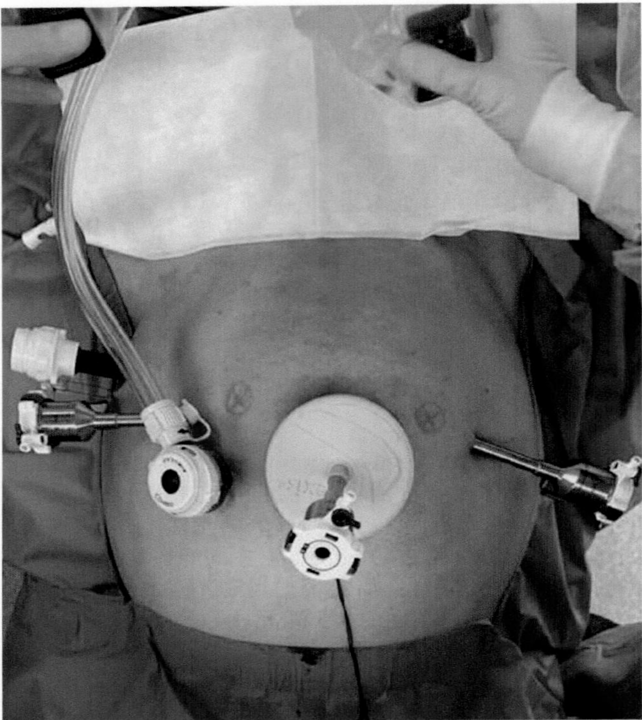
Fig. 1 Trocar placement two robotic arms on the left side of the patient, port-through-port

another stapling device is used. The stapler should then be inserted from the most lateral (15 mm) trocar (2 cm medial and 2–4 cm superior to the left anterior superior iliac spine). An 8 mm-sized robotic trocar for the first arm goes through the 15 mm-sized port (port through port), and at the time of ileal stapling, first arm is undocked with the 8-mm port, and ileal staplers go through the 15 mm-sized port. In addition, an Alexis port (C8501, S 2.5–6 cm) can be inserted above the umbilicus, and the 8-mm-sized camera robotic port for the third arm goes through the Alexis port (Fig. 1). The Alexis port might be used in order to extract the cystoprostatectomy specimen in male patients.

4.2 Two Robotic Arms on the Right

The use of two robotic arms on the *right* side during the cystectomy (see Fig. 2) will require redocking of arm number 1 to reach the most lateral left position for the stapling device.

To use the robotic stapler, arm number 1 is undocked with the 8 mm trocar left in place. The 12 mm robotic trocar is then docked on arm number 1 and inserted through the 15 mm port. The camera is now inserted in arm number 3 and the left-hand instrument in arm number 2. Now the surgeon has a robotic stapler most lateral to the left and bowel handling instruments in arm number 2 and 4.

In case of the use of laparoscopic bowel staplers, the robotic arms can stay in place, and the bowel stapler is inserted through the 15 mm port.

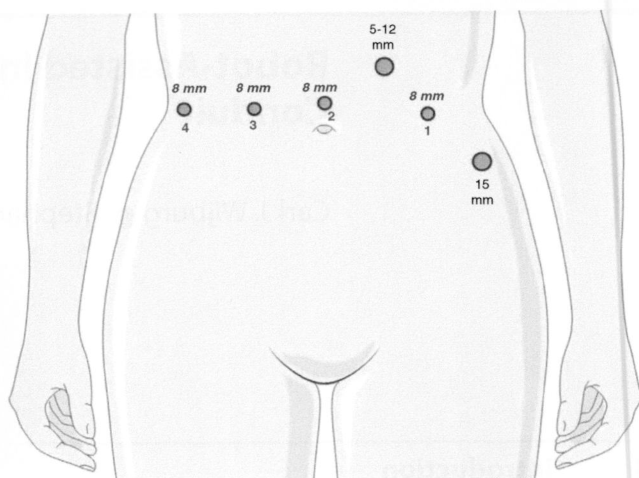

Fig. 2 Trocar placement two robotic arms on the right side of the patient

5 Staplers

Different laparoscopic stapling devices are available on the market with continuously improving techniques. In addition, the length of the staplers can differ. It is advisable to have knowledge of the technique, the length, and the depth of the staplers that will be used. For example, both bowel staplers and vascular staplers should be available.

The robotic stapling device is available in 45 mm or 60 mm. The 60 mm is preferred, because the ileal-ileal anastomosis needs to be closed, for which at least one filling with the length of 60 mm is necessary. An advantage of the robotic stapler is that the surgeon has full control of the angle and positioning of the stapler and the firing process.

6 Step by Step: Bowel Handling and FireFly

First, the ileocecal junction is identified. About 20 cm proximal of this junction, the bowel is stapled with a 60 mm firing, perpendicular to the bowel (Fig. 3). In obese patients, a longer section of meso is necessary to extract the ileal conduit at the end of the operation. One extra firing of 45 mm or 60 mm with a vascular stapler may then be used. To preserve the good vascularity of the ileum, it is of utmost importance to place the stapler perpendicular to the bowel. To ensure that vascularity is maintained, we suggest the following approach: close the stapler without firing it. Now (if available) use the FireFly technique. Inject 2–4 ml Verdye solution (indocyanine green, ICG) and check the perfusion of bowel and ureters. If there is good perfusion of the bowel, one can fire the stapler. Should the perfusion not appear optimal (Fig. 4), then open again and reposition the stapler and check perfusion again. This not only can prevents serious bowel-related

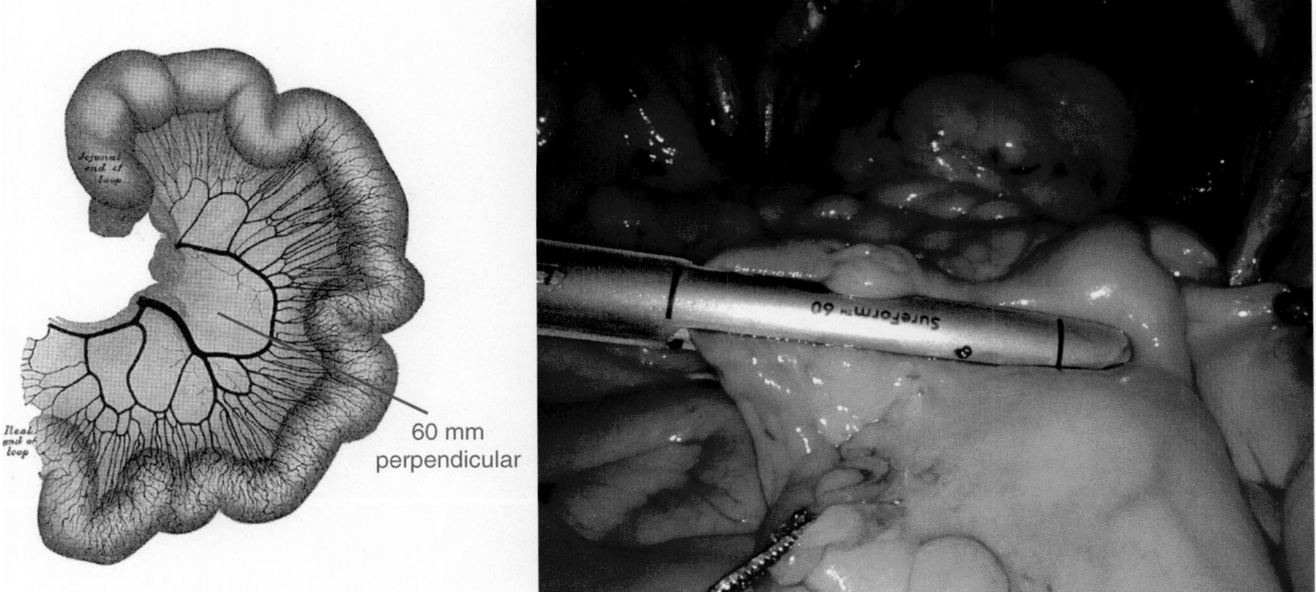

Fig. 3 Bowel stapling

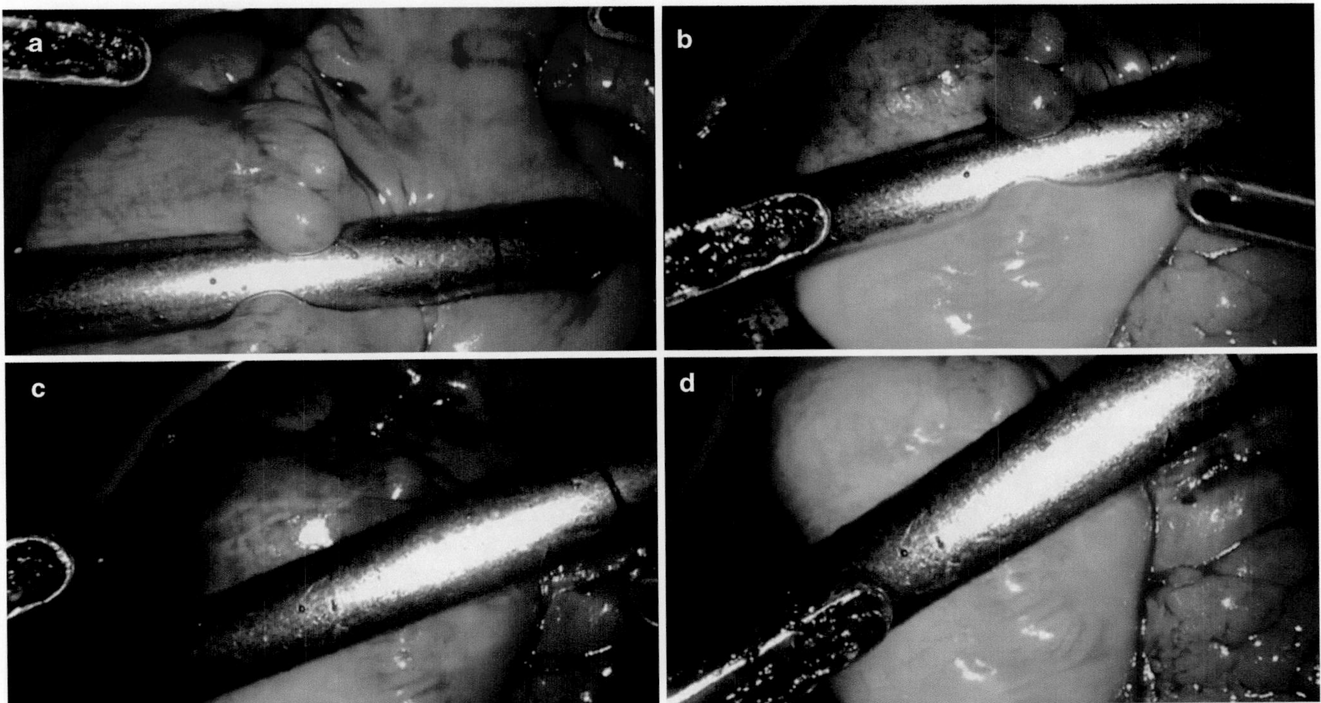

Fig. 4 Check bowel perfusion with FireFly technique (**a**) stapler is placed and closed, perpendicular to the bowel (**b**) Verdye is injected intraveneously. With the FireFly technique, good perfusion (green) is shown only in the lower part (**c** and **d**) stapler is opened, perfusion of the bowel is restored and stapler is replaced and closed

complications but also prevents uretero-enteric strictures. As shown in Fig. 5, the perfusion of the ureters can be checked easily, and the place of the uretero-enteric anastomosis can be adjusted as needed.

The length of bowel needed for the formation of an ileal conduit depends on the adiposity of the patient. In most patients about 15 cm should be enough. Again, we suggest stapling the oral side of the ileal conduit (perpendicular) with 60 mm. Before the start of the ileal-ileal anastomosis, the distal part of the ileum (proximal from the last staples) can be excised with another 60 mm bowel or vascular stapler, Fig. 6.

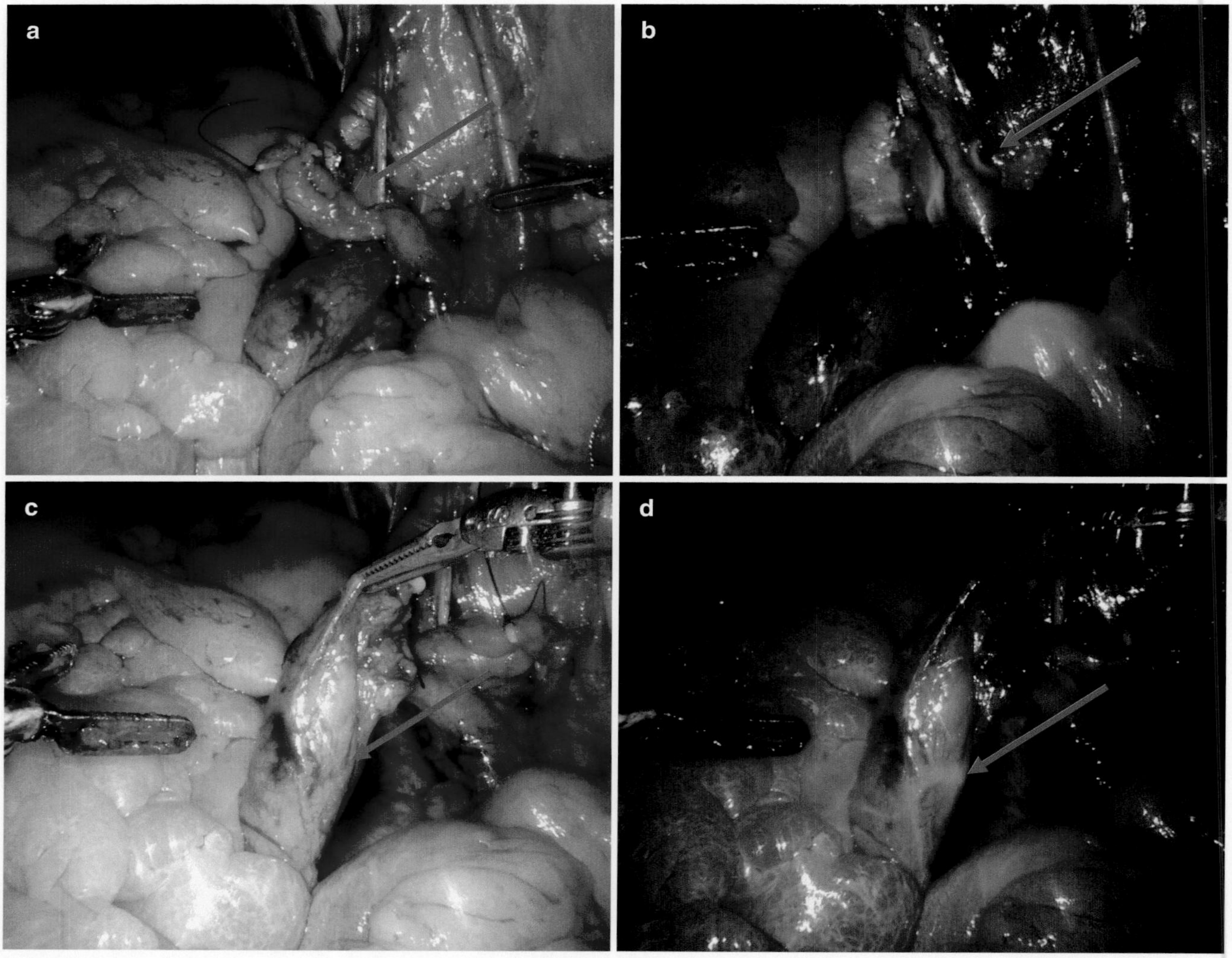

Fig. 5 Check ureter perfusion with FireFly technique (**a**) normal view of right ureter (**b**) perfusion of right ureter is checked with FireFly (**c**) normal view of left ureter (**d**) perfusion of left ureter is checked with FireFly

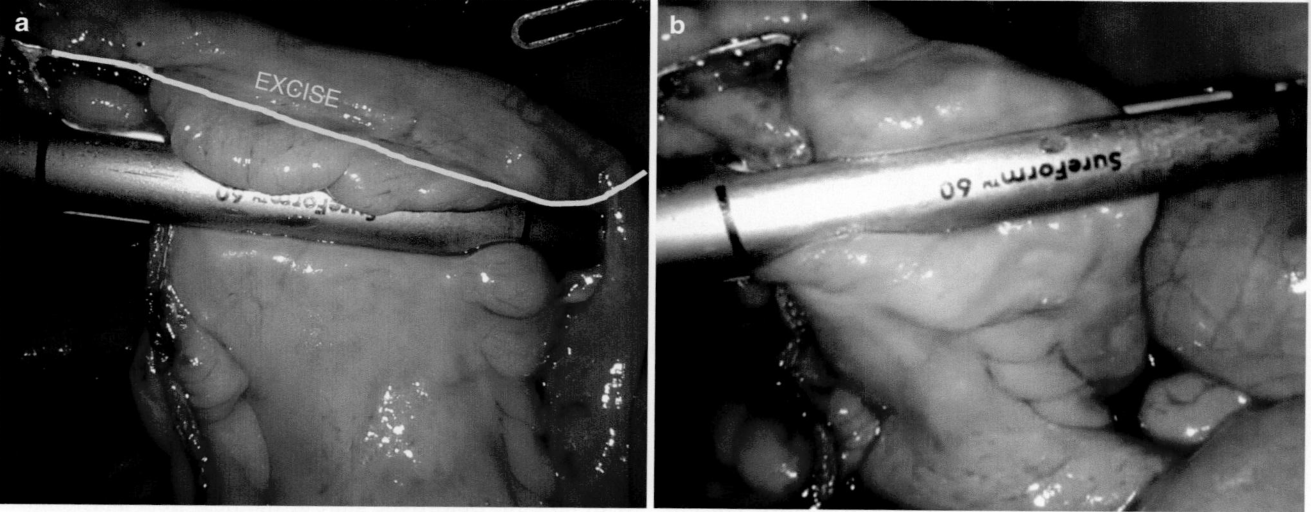

Fig. 6 Excise proximal part of the bowel (**a**) staple close and parallel to the bowel (**b**) excise proximal part of the bowel with stapler

6.1 Side-to-Side Anastomosis Ileum

The last step is the formation of a side-to-side ileal-ileal anastomosis. First a small hole in the bowel is made, close to the staples, on the antimesenteric side. The next step consists of the insertion of one limb of a 60 mm bowel stapler in the lumen of each ileum (Fig. 7a, b). Make sure that only the antimesenteric ileum border is included between the limbs of the stapler. Each limb must be inserted completely, to ensure that a wide ileal-ileal anastomosis is created (Fig. 7c, d). A second 60 mm stapler can be used, if the opening appears to be too small (Fig. 7e). The last step is to transversely close the opening of the two ileal parts with a 60 mm bowel stapler (Fig. 7f). The complete side-to-side ileal-ileal anastomosis is checked for its width and integrity. With a 3/0 absorbable suture, the top and the corner of the anastomosis can be reinforced. The mesentery gap between the anastomosis needs no reconstruction.

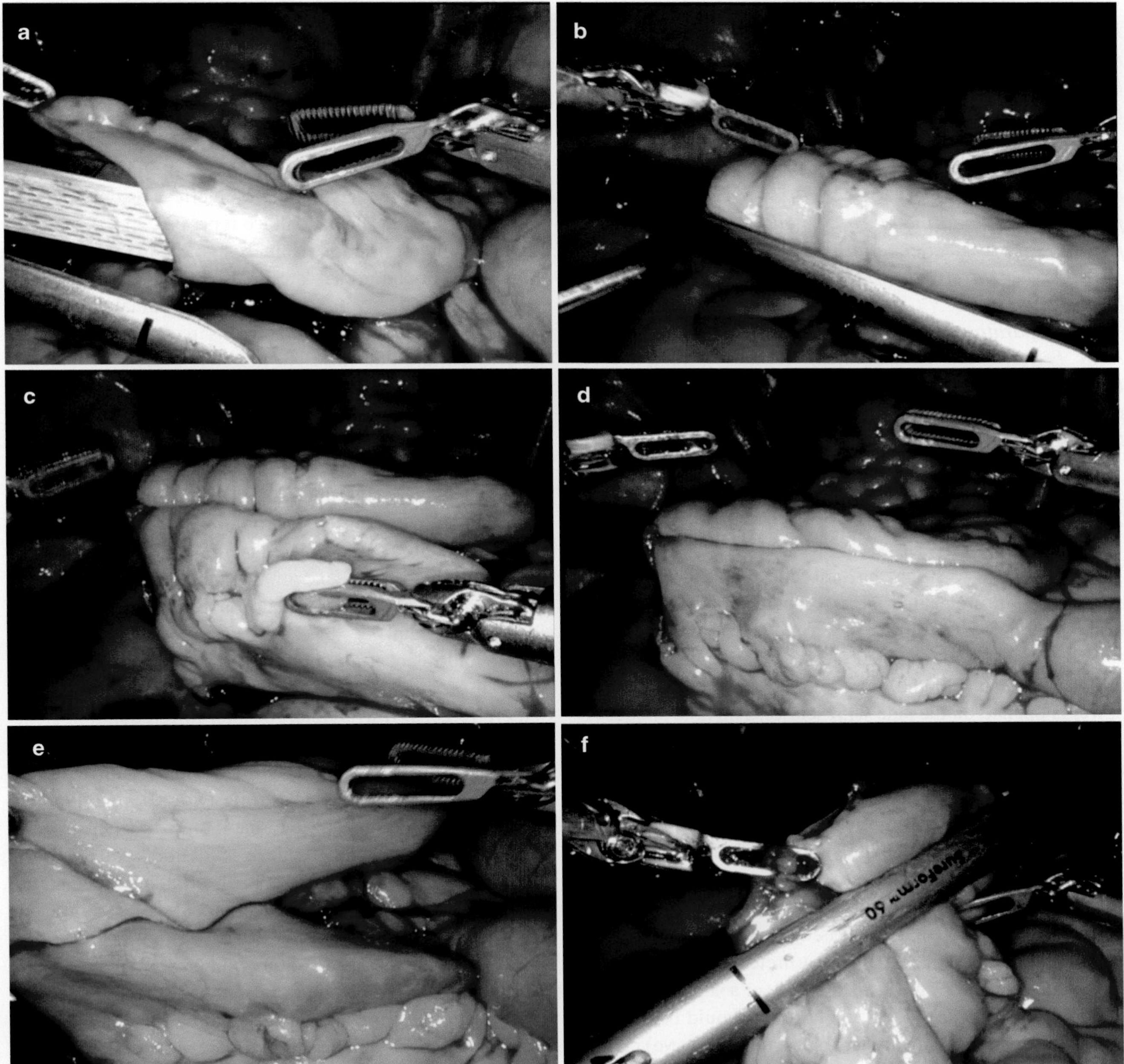

Fig. 7 Step-by-step and side-to-side stapled ileal anastomosis. (**a, b**) insertion first limb of 60 mm stapler in distal ileal loop. (**c, d**) insertion second limb of 60 mm staler in proximal ileal loop. (**e**) extend side-side anastomosis with 45 or 60 mm stapler. (**f**) close the opening of the two ileal parts with a 60 mm bowel stapler

7 Step-by-Step: Uretero-enteric Anastomosis Techniques

The most commonly used techniques for uretero-enteric anastomosis are Bricker (side-to-side, separate) and Wallace (conjoined, side-to-side end). Care should be taken to prevent uretero-enteric strictures, which occur in 3–15% of the patients. One population-based retrospective study compared stricture rates after open radical cystectomy (ORC) with RARC, performed between 2009 and 2014 [5]. *The stricture incidence after 1-year follow-up was higher for RARC (15%) vs. ORC (9.5%). A stricture was defined as the need for an intervention. The study could not differentiate between intra- and extracorporeal reconstruction technique.*

A single center observational study of a large intracorporeal cohort showed a stricture rate of 6.5% at a median time of 165 days after surgery [6]. *Strictures occurred in 8.3% of patients with an orthotopic neobladder and in 5.4% of patients with an ileal conduit urinary diversion. There was no difference in stricture rates between monofilament or barbed suture.*

A comparative study showed no difference in stricture rates between the Bricker and Wallace technique [7]. *Indocyanine green (ICG) fluorescence to assess distal ureter perfusion during intracorporeal reconstruction may reduce the risk of ischemic uretero-enteric stricture* [8].

7.1 Bricker Technique

The first step is to bring the oral side of the ileal conduit toward the left ureter that is passed under the mesosigmoid from the left to the right (Fig. 8a). With a V-Lock barbed absorbable suture, the stapled meso of the ileum is attached to the peritoneum of the mesosigmoid (Fig. 8b). Then the bowel is opened on the side with scissor. The hole should be as large as 2–3 cm in length (Fig. 8c). Thereafter, the ureter is opened on the avascular side and spatulated for 2–3 cm (Fig. 8d). With a double-armed absorbable barbed suture (like FillBlock), a circular ureter-bowel anastomosis is made. The suture is started on the left side, outside-in of the bowel and then to the corner of the spatulated ureter, inside-out of the ureter (Fig. 8e, f). It is continued with the dorsal caudal side taking care that the suture is tight enough but without excessive traction (Fig. 9a). Now a ureter stent is inserted, either a double J or single J stent Ch7-8, or a straight Ch8-10 silicon drain (Fig. 9b). The straight drain should be fixed to the bowel with a rapid absorbable suture (Fig. 9c). After closing the cranial side of the anastomosis, the ureter is transected, and its distal part is sent to the pathologist (Fig. 9d). Finally, the anastomosis of the left ureter is closed and completed.

To start the anastomosis of the right ureter, the ileal conduit is flipped cranially, and a hole is opened in the bowel on the caudal/right side (Fig. 9e, f). The right ureter is straightened, incised transversely, and spatulated for 2–3 cm. The same technique described for the left ureter is then used. When both ureters are implanted in the ileal conduit, the conduit is covered with the peritoneum of the mesosigmoid, to prevent traction on the conduit and ureters. This may also prevent herniation of small bowel underneath the left ureter (Fig. 10).

7.2 Wallace Technique

An alternative approach to uretero-enteric anastomosis is the creation of a ureter plate (Wallace type, Fig. 11). After passing the left ureter through the mesosigmoid to the right, both previously clipped ureters are hold using the fourth robotic arm in front of the orifice of the inner inguinal ring on the patient's right side. It is crucial to ensure that the ureters are not crossed and that the right ureter is placed on the right side. Using the fourth arm, both ureters are then incised over a length of 2–3 cm. To create the posterior plate, both dorsal sections of the ureters are sutured using a running 4-0 or 5-0 monofilament absorbable suture. Care should be taken to put the suture knot *outside* the plate. Both stapled ends of the bowel are cut with scissors. Through the ileum conduit part, mono- or double J catheters are inserted into the ureters from the aboral to the oral end of the ileum (the anastomosis between Wallace plate and ileum is conducted on the oral side of the conduit).

To avoid dislocation during removal of the guidewire, it proved useful to hold the stent in place by grasping it using a Cadière forceps. If available, for later differentiation, stents of different color may be used.

To perform the anastomosis of the plate with the ileum conduit, suture is prepared by tying two 4-0 monofilament absorbable sutures, 18 cm long back to back using a round half-circle needle as to achieve a double-armed suture. Alternatively with a double-armed absorbable barbed suture (like FillBlock). The first running suture is started immediately left of the mesentery (7 o'clock position) from the outside and is led to the inside of the right ureter at the proximal end of spatulation. The suture is continued in counterclockwise direction keeping an outside-in direction on the enteric tissue and an inside-out direction for the ureteral plate. Every three bites the suture is carefully tightened to bring the edges

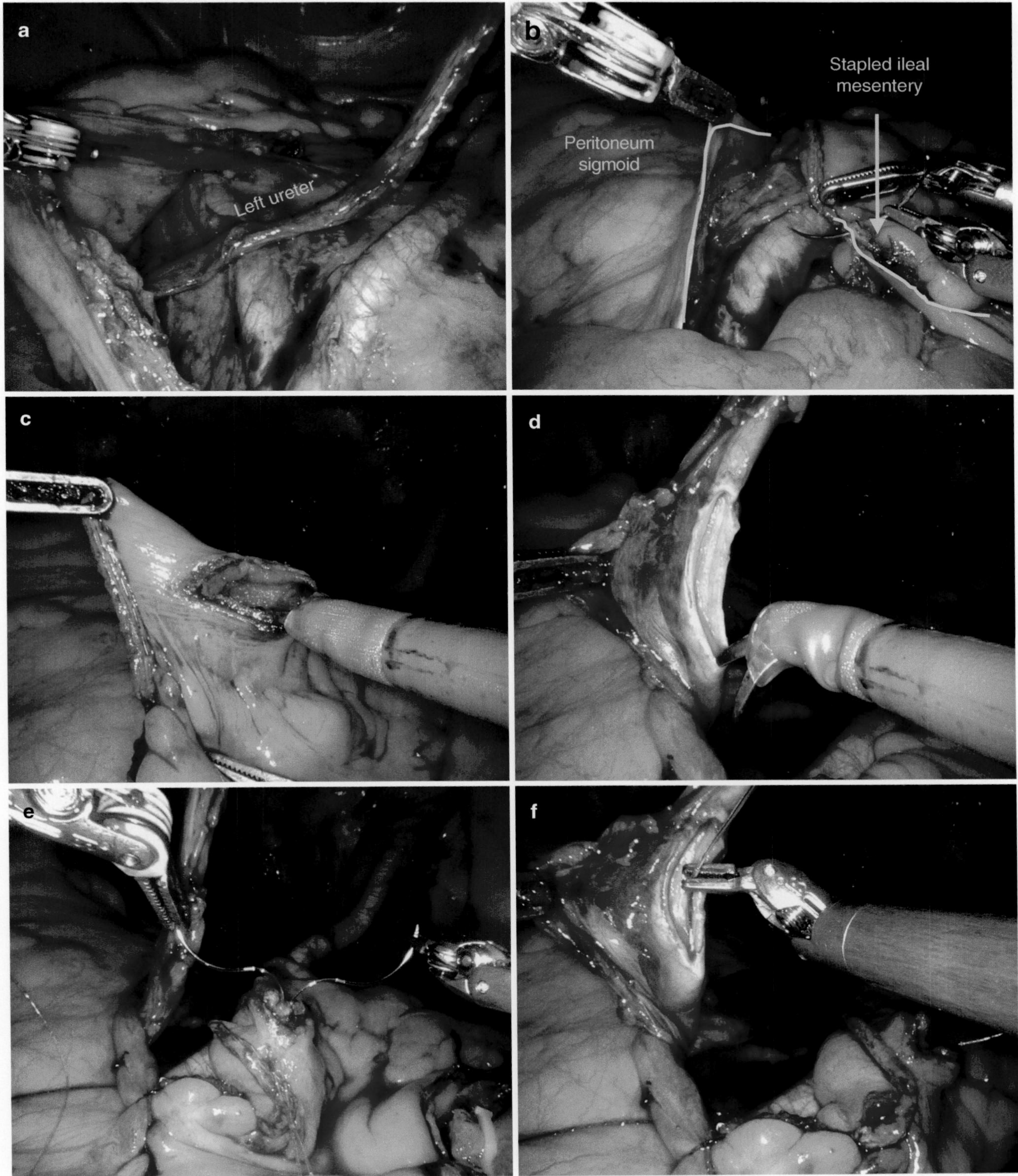

Fig. 8 Step-by-step uretero-enteric anastomosis left ureter. (**a**) Transpose left ureter under the mesosigmoid from the left to the right. (**b**) stapled meso of the ileum is attached to the peritoneum of the mesosigmoid. (**c**) bowel is opened 2–3 cm. (**d**) left ureter is opened on the avascular side and spatulated for 2–3 cm. (**e**, **f**) circular ureter-bowel anastomosis is made

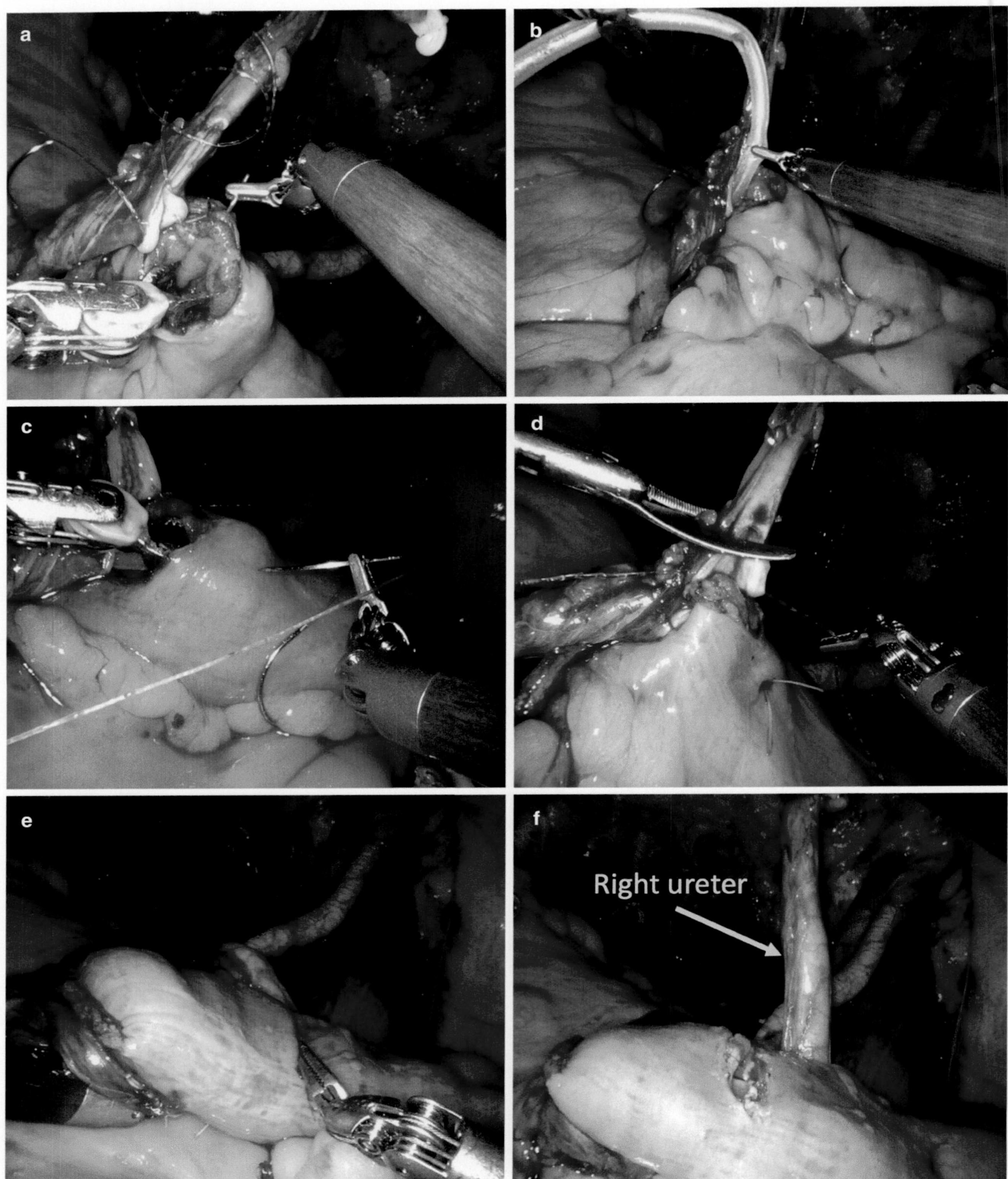

Fig. 9 Step-by-step ureteroenteric anastomosis right ureter and stent placement . (**a**) ureter-bowel anastomosis, dorsal caudal side. (**b**) insertion of ureter stent, either a double J or single J stent Ch7-8, or a straight Ch8-10 silicon drain. (**c**) straight drain fixed to the bowel with a rapid absorbable suture. (**d**) After closing the cranial side of the anastomosis, the ureter is transected, and its distal part is sent to the pathologist. (**e**, **f**) To start the anastomosis of the right ureter, the ileal conduit is flipped cranially, and a hole is made in the bowel on the caudal/right side

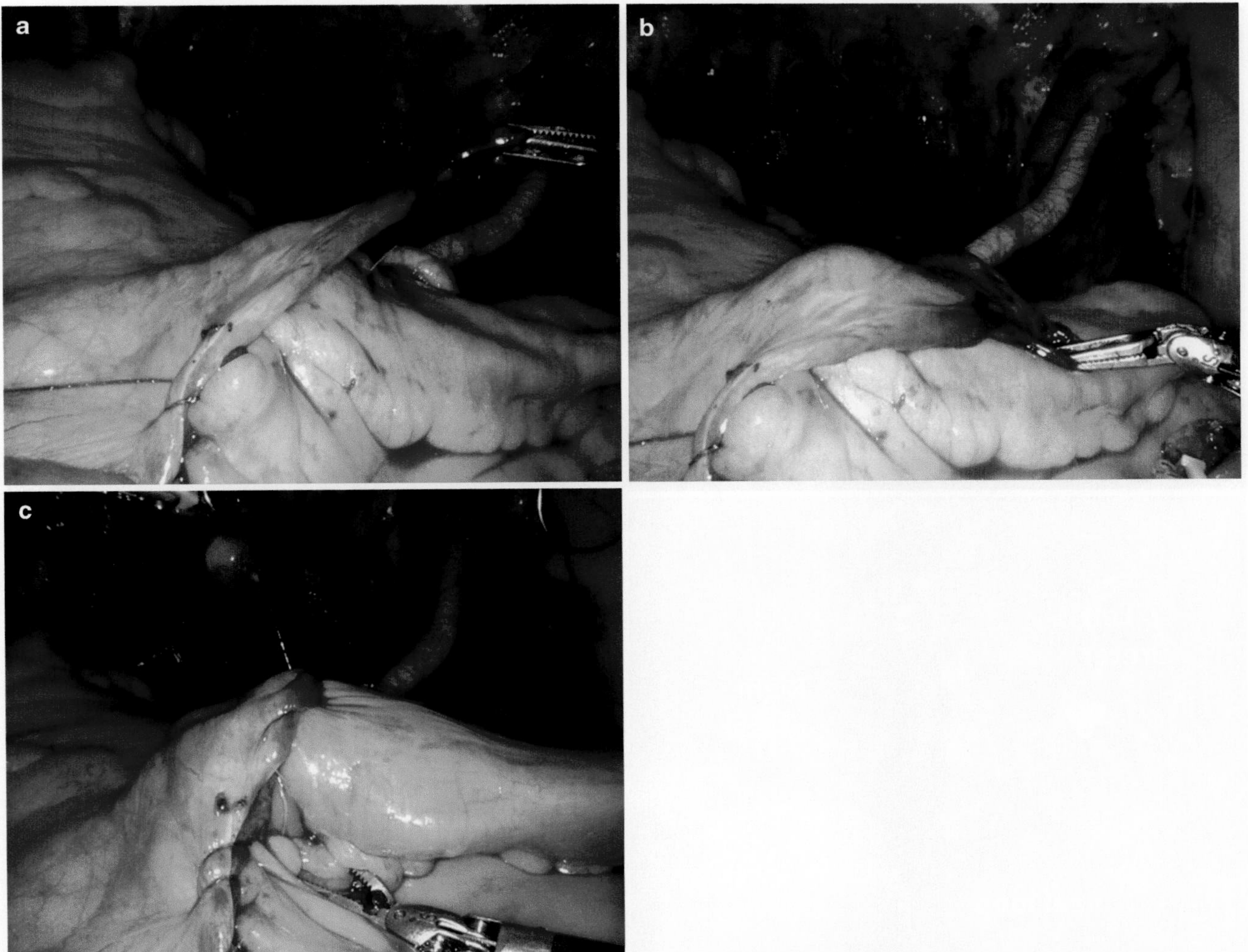

Fig. 10 Retroperitonialisation of oral side of ileal conduit. (**a–c**) the conduit is covered with the peritoneum of the mesosigmoid

to each other. This first running suture is continued until a 12 o'clock position is reached. The second suture is now started clockwise from 7 to 12 o'clock using the same technique of outside-in on the enteric and inside-out of the ureteral part of the anastomosis. Care should be applied to avoid suturing the ureteral stents. Once both sutures are at the 12 o'clock position, they are tied to each other to complete the uretero-enteric anastomosis.

8 Step by Step: Extraction Ileal Conduit and Stoma Formation

Skin is excised at the preoperatively marked preferred stoma site, the fascia of the abdominal wall is incised for each 4–5 cm in the length and transversely, the fibers of the musculus abdominis is spread, and the peritoneum entered. Care should be taken that the opening is as wide as two fingers, and then a bowel clamp is placed on the distal side of the ileal conduit to extract it.

All instruments are extracted, the abdomen is deflated, the robot is undocked, and the trocars are removed. To extract the cystectomy specimen, the incision of the 15 mm trocar on the left side is enlarged. Alternatively, the specimen can be extracted using a Pfannenstiel incision. In women, transvaginal extraction is also a possibility. The incision is then closed stratum by stratum as usual. Alternatively, as described above, a supra-umbilical Alexis port might be used in order to extract the cystoprostatectomy specimen in male patients.

Work is then resumed on the ileal conduit: The ileum is fixed to the fascia and/or to the skin, opened by excising the staples line, and the lumen is everted. The straight splints (single J or silicon drains) are led out of the conduit. If double J stents are used, or if the splints cannot be reached with

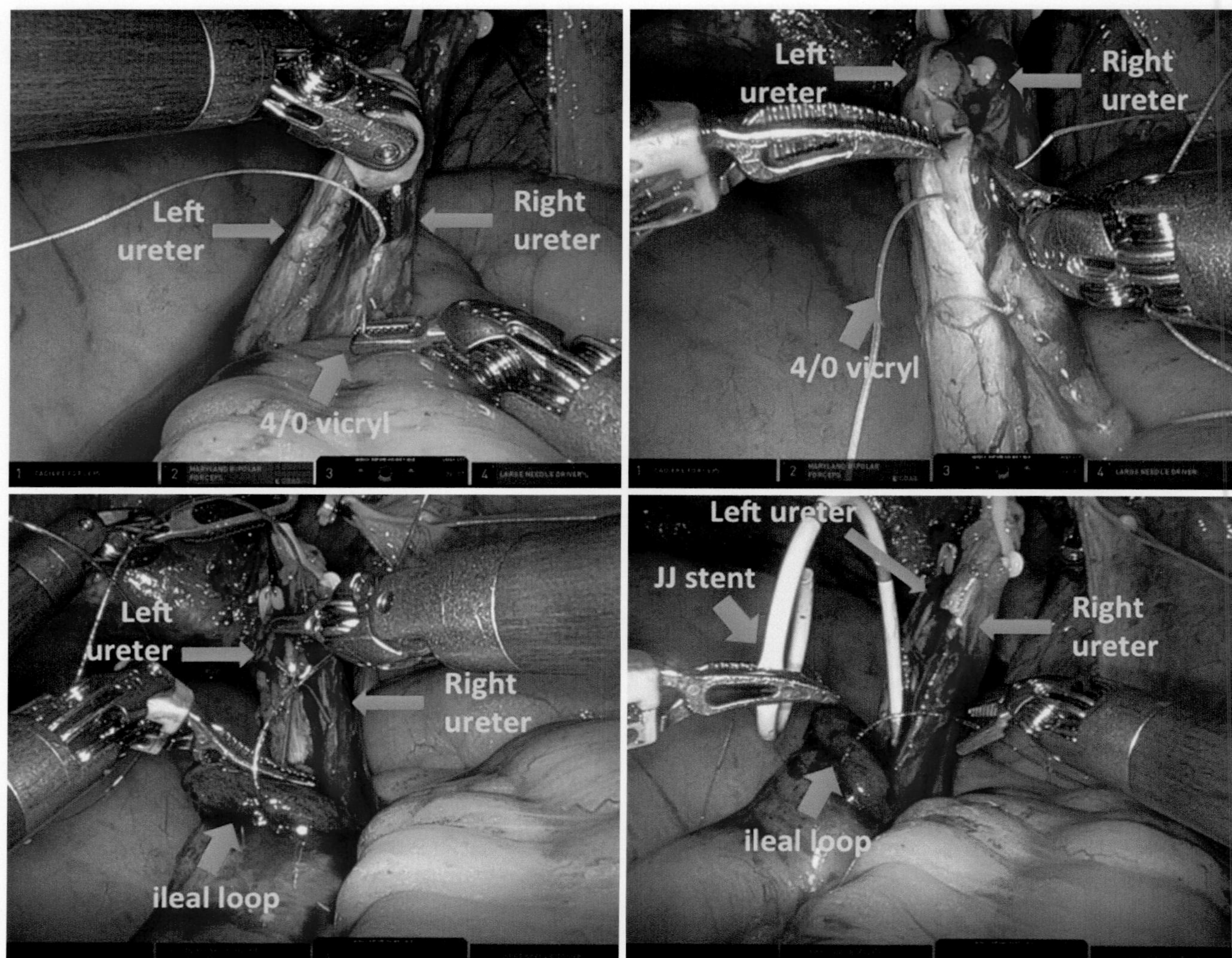

Fig. 11 Construction of Wallace type side-to-side uretero-uretero anastomosis

a finger, a catheter can be placed in the stoma with 3–5 cc in the balloon, for about 3 days.

Although often double J stent can be removed with a finger in the conduit, single J or straight drains used as ureter stent are preferred over double J stents, because they do not require flexible cystoscopy in the conduit for extraction.

9 Tips and Tricks

The uretero-enteric anastomosis can be checked for possible leakage at the end of the procedure. Instead of removing trocars as described above, all ports are left in place. After completion of the conduit, the abdomen is insufflated with CO_2, and sterile serum is given through the stoma opening while the anastomosis is visualized. Should leakage be detected, additional sutures are applied?

References

1. Hussein AA, Elsayed AS, Aldhaam NA, Jing Z, Peabody JO, Wijburg CJ, et al. A comparative propensity-score matched analysis of perioperative outcomes of intracorporeal versus extracorporeal urinary diversion after robot-assisted radical cystectomy: results from the International Robotic Cystectomy Consortium. BJU Int. 2020; https://doi.org/10.1111/bju.15083.
2. Hussein AA, May PR, Jing Z, Ahmed YE, Wijburg CJ, Canda AE, et al. Outcomes of intracorporeal urinary diversion after robot-assisted radical cystectomy: results from the International Robotic Cystectomy Consortium. J Urol. 2017; https://doi.org/10.1016/j.juro.2017.12.045.

3. Tan TW, Nair R, Saad S, Thurairaja R, Khan MS. Safe transition from extracorporeal to intracorporeal urinary diversion following robot-assisted cystectomy: a recipe for reducing operative time, blood loss and complication rates. World J Urol. 2019;37:367–72. https://doi.org/10.1007/s00345-018-2386-4.
4. Tanneru K, Jazayeri SB, Kumar J, Alam MU, Norez D, Nguyen S, et al. Intracorporeal versus extracorporeal urinary diversion following robot-assisted radical cystectomy: a meta-analysis, cumulative analysis, and systematic review. J Robot Surg. 2020:1–13. https://doi.org/10.1007/s11701-020-01174-4.
5. Goh AC, Belarmino A, Patel NA, Sun T, Sedrakyan A, Bochner BH, et al. A population-based study of ureteroenteric strictures after open and robot-assisted radical cystectomy. Urology. 2020;135:57–65. https://doi.org/10.1016/j.urology.2019.07.054.
6. Hosseini A, Dey L, Laurin O, Adding C, Hoijer J, Ebbing J, et al. Ureteric stricture rates and management after robot-assisted radical cystectomy: a single-centre observational study. Scand J Urol. 2018:1–5. https://doi.org/10.1080/21681805.2018.1465462.
7. Liu L, Chen M, Li Y, Wang L, Qi F, Dun J, et al. Technique selection of bricker or wallace ureteroileal anastomosis in ileal conduit urinary diversion: a strategy based on patient characteristics. Ann Surg Oncol. 2014;21:2808–12. https://doi.org/10.1245/s10434-014-3591-z.
8. Ahmadi N, Ashrafi AN, Hartman N, Shakir A, Cacciamani GE, Freitas D, et al. Use of indocyanine green to minimise uretero-enteric strictures after robotic radical cystectomy. BJU Int. 2019;124:302–7. https://doi.org/10.1111/bju.14733.

Robot-Assisted Intracorporeal Neobladder: The Karolinska Standardized Technique

Justin W. Collins, Abolfazl Hosseini, and Peter Wiklund

Abbreviation

e-PLND	Extended pelvic lymph node dissection
ERP	Enhanced recovery protocol
ICUD	Intra-corporeal urinary diversion
RARC	Robot-assisted radical cystectomy

1 Introduction

Radical cystectomy with extended pelvic lymphadenectomy (ePLND) and urinary diversion still represents the gold standard treatment for muscle invasive bladder cancer and high-risk bladder cancer unresponsive to intravesical treatments. Irrespective of surgical approach RC remains a complex multistep surgery, being associated with a high rate of complications [1, 2]. With the purpose of further reducing morbidity, minimally invasive approaches have been described, and the 2020 EAU guidelines [3] consider robot-assisted radical cystectomy (RARC) as a viable alternative to open radical cystectomy (ORC). Concluding current evidence indicates RARC has longer operative time (1–1.5 h) and major costs but shorter length of hospital stay (1–1.5 days) and less blood loss compared to ORC [4]. Surgeons' experience and institutional volume are considered the key factor for outcome of both RARC and ORC [5]. Laparoscopic radical cystectomy never gained wide acceptance in the urological community due to long operative time and the technical difficulties related to both ePLND and urinary diversion reconfiguration. With the introduction of robot-assisted laparoscopic surgery, RARC has emerged as a more viable alternative to both open and laparoscopic approaches to radical cystectomy [6, 7].

To date, the RARC experience is increasing worldwide, minimizing surgical insult, and aiming to result in reductions in postoperative morbidity while offering improved ergonomics for the surgeon [8]. Several meta-analyses have demonstrated that RARC decreases blood loss and reduces overall complication rates, resulting in reduced transfusion rates, shorter time to normal diet, and length of stay [4, 9], without compromising oncologic safety as compared to open surgery [10]. Several urinary diversions have been described, but only limited randomized clinical trials performed by few super-specialized tertiary referral centers have demonstrated the advantages offered by intracorporeal urinary diversion (ICUD). The potential advantages of a complete intracorporeal procedure are less intraoperative blood loss, decreased bowel manipulation and exposure, reduced insensible losses, decreased morbidity from smaller incisions, reduced postoperative analgesic requirements, shorter hospital stay, and earlier return to normal activities [7].

In this paper we describe our standardized approach with modifications to technique for intracorporeal neobladder formation performed since December 2003 [6].

2 Materials and Methods

In this chapter, we describe our standardized approach to modified Studer intracorporeal neobladder formation performed from 2003 identifying potential hazard steps and identifying strategies to help avoid complications [6]. Particularly attention has been placed in patient selection, preoperative preparation, enhanced recovery protocol (ERP), operative setup including patient positioning, and the equipment required.

J. W. Collins (✉) · A. Hosseini · P. Wiklund
Departments of Molecular Medicine and Surgery, Section of Urology, Karolinska Institute, Stockholm, Sweden

P. Wiklund et al. (eds.), *Robotic Urologic Surgery*, https://doi.org/10.1007/978-3-031-00363-9_59

2.1 Patient Selection, Inclusion, and Exclusion Criteria

The selection process includes preoperative investigation to ensure fitness for surgery as well as specific counseling about robotic technology. The exclusion criteria for RARC include the following: (a) bulky tumors with persisting signs of locally advanced/frozen pelvis cancer, cT4 disease after neo-adjuvant chemotherapy; (b) history of extensive abdominal surgery; (c) the presence of contraindications to laparoscopy and steep Trendelenburg position (30°): ASA score >3, severe cardiac and/or lung insufficiency; and (d) relative contraindications that include avoiding bulky tumors (cT3-4) early in the learning curve, extensive lymph node involvement, age >75 years, and body mass index (BMI) >30.

In the absence of contraindications and following appropriate discussion, patients chose between an open procedure and RARC with totally intracorporeal orthotopic ileal neobladder or ileal conduit.

2.2 Preoperative Preparation and Enhanced Recovery Protocol

In order to reduce perioperative stress response and to aid faster patient recovery, we routinely apply an enhanced recovery protocol (ERP) [2, 11]. There is also evidence for decreased financial costs associated with ERAS for radical cystectomy [12]. Our multidisciplinary team routinely suggests the patient preoperative regarding smoking cessation, appropriate weight loss, and physical activity. Medical comorbidities are addressed, and cardiopulmonary testing is completed where indicated. Social issues are identified, and discharge planning is agreed before admission. The ERP protocol advises no preoperative mechanical bowel preparation, and premedication includes omeprazole and metoclopramide with the avoidance of anxiolytics preoperatively. Postoperatively avoidance of the use of opiate-based analgesia, early postoperative nasogastric and drainage tubes removal as well as early feeding and patient mobilization aid early bowel recovery. All patients have a stoma site marked the day before surgery. One dose of broad-spectrum intravenous antibiotics is administered at the start of the procedure [11].

2.3 Operative Setup

After induction of general anesthesia and nasogastric tube and sterile urinary catheter insertion, patient is placed in lithotomy position with arms adducted and padded. The lower limb calves are wrapped with Flowtron pneumatic compression stockings and then placed and secured within stirrups where they can be abducted and slightly lowered on spreader bars. The table is placed in the 25–30° Trendelenburg position. Standard, Si, and Xi da Vinci robotic systems (Intuitive Surgical, Sunnyvale, CA, USA) have been used, respectively. The technique has evolved with experience from 2003, and the technique described in this chapter has been used since 2008. A 0° lens is used for the majority of cases. Standard robotic instruments are: Maryland Bipolar Forceps, Large Needle Driver, Monopolar Curved Scissors, Cadiere forceps, and bowel graspers. Among other standard laparoscopic surgical equipment, essential additional instruments are required: LigaSure ® (Covidien plc, Dublin, Ireland), surgical endoscopic clip applicators, laparoscopic Endo-Catch bags, and laparoscopic stapler with 60 and 45 mm cartridges for intestinal stapling.

2.4 Surgical Technique

2.4.1 Trocar Configuration

RARC is commonly performed via a six-port laparoscopic approach. A 5-cm supraumbilical optical port position is placed with Hasson technique; the other ports are placed in view of the camera. A pneumoperitoneum pressure of 18 mmHg during the port placement can be helpful in creating additional tension on the abdominal wall. Two robotic ports are placed symmetrically and level with the umbilicus on the left and right side, lateral to the rectus sheath. A third robotic instrument port is placed just above and medial to the left anterior superior iliac spine through a 15-mm port thereby enabling laparoscopic stapling by the assistant when the third robotic port is temporarily disconnected. Two assistant 12-mm ports are placed on either side of the right robotic instrument port (Fig. 1). The pneumopertioneum can then be reduced to 10–12 mmHg.

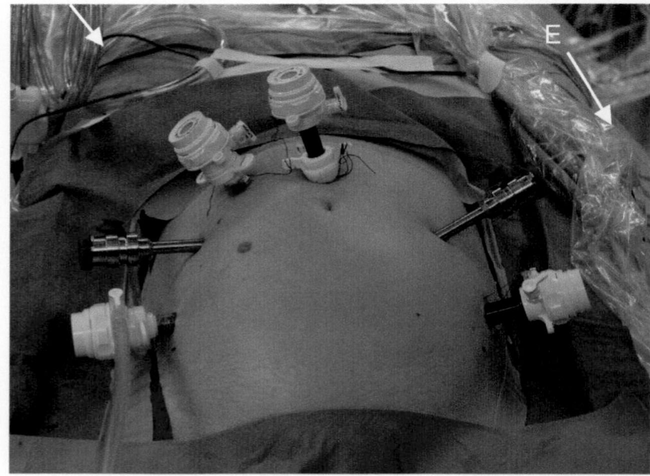

Fig. 1 Port configuration. Karolinska six-port approach

2.4.2 Orthotopic Neobladder, Intracorporeal Technique

Step 1: Development of periureteral space, clipping, and division of ureters

The ureters are identified, and the peritoneum covering them is carefully opened. The ureters are dissected out toward the bladder, holding them by the peri-ureteric tissue and maintaining adequate peri-ureteral tissue. Avoid excessive dissection of the peri-ureters, as this causes increased risk of strictures. Close to the ureterovesical junction, they are divided between two Hem-o-lok clips. The Hem-o-lok clips on the ureter end are knotted at their corner with a suture to facilitate the handling of the ureter: a direct manipulation of the ureter with the robotic instruments during construction of the urinary diversion should be avoided in order to prevent ureteric trauma and later strictures. The distal ureteric margin will be sent for frozen section in case of CIS in the bladder.

Step 2: Passing the left ureter to the right side under the mesosigmoid

After completion of RARC and ePLND, the presacral area under the mesosigmoid is already prepared, as the lymph nodes below the aortic bifurcation are removed at both sides [6]. The robotic Cadiere forceps are passed under the sigmoid from the right to the left side. The left ureter is grasped by the stay suture and brought to the right side. In this step careful attention should be paid to move the instrument in a horizontal direction in order to avoid damage to the vessels or nerves that lie posteriorly.

Step 3: Identifying and selection of terminal ileum

An ileal loop of 50–55 cm is required to form the ileal neobladder, and this harvested loop should be at least 20–25 cm from the ileo-caecal junction. A section of ileum is identified 35–40 cm from the ileo-caecal junction and brought down to the urethra. The ileum is sufficiently mobilized to reach down to the urethra without tension. A 20F opening is made on the antimesenteric side of ileum, using cold robotic scissors (Fig. 2a).

In case of a short mesentry or fatty mesentry, the ileum can be difficult to mobilize sufficiently to come down into the pelvis, therefore undermining the ability to complete a neobladder. To obtain precious millimeters to get the ileum down to the urethra, different solutions can be attempted:

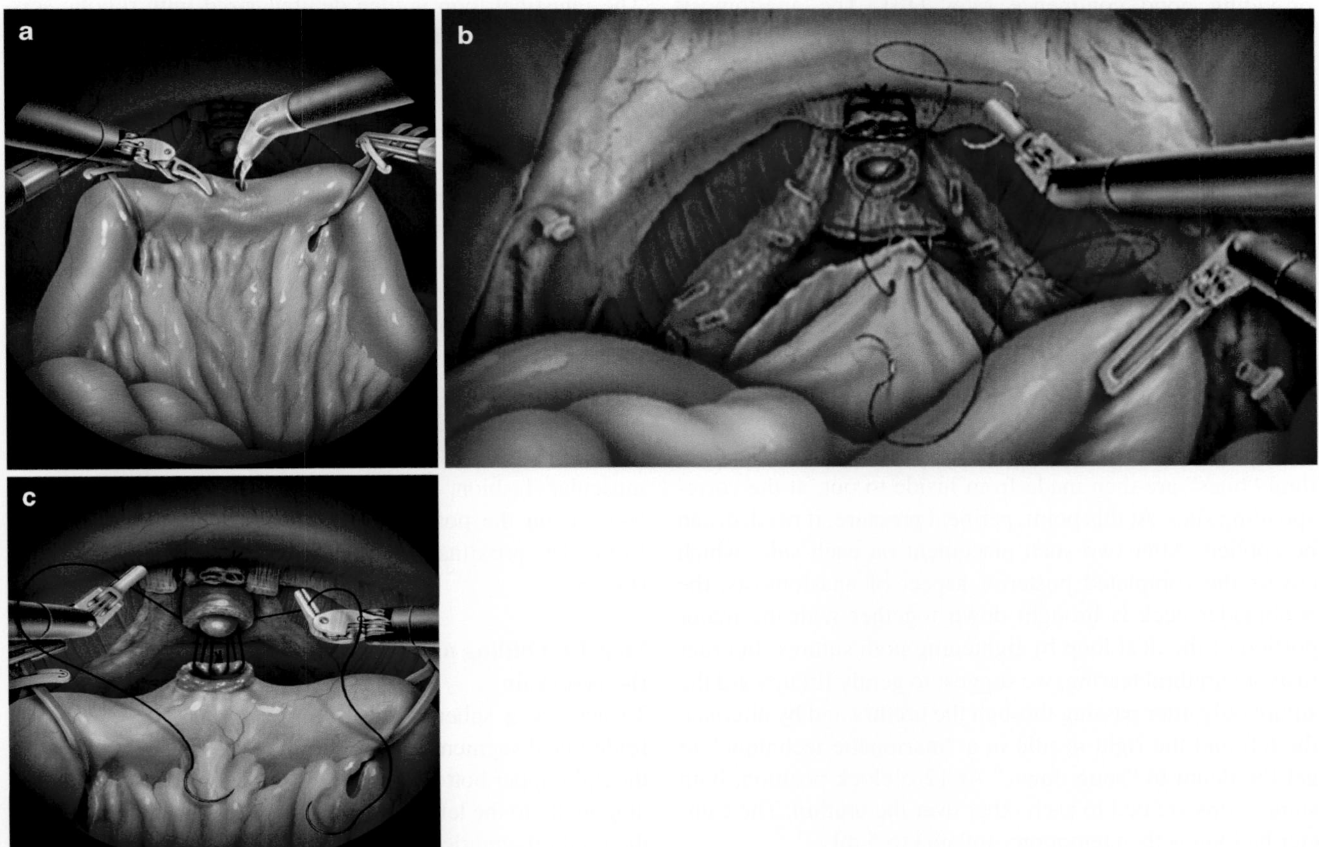

Fig. 2 Urethro-neovesical anastomosis. (**a**) Neo urethra opening: A 20F opening is made on the antimesenteric side of ileum, using cold robotic scissors. (**b**) Modified posterior Rocco's repair: The posterior reconstruction begins by suturing the rhabdosphincter to the remaining Denonvilliers' fascia in a running fashion. (**c**) Urethro-neovesical anastomosis

- Complete dissection of all adhesions.
- Detachment of the cecum and the first part of the ascending colon.
- Superficial incision of the peritoneal layer on the mesentry in a line parallel with the ileum, making sure that the incision is not damaging the mesenteric vessels below.
- Reducing Trendelenburg.
- To assist the manipulation and positioning of the ileum, two vessel loops are passed around the intestine through the mesentery either side of the section of ileum loop to be anastomosed to the urethra.

Step 4: Posterior reconstruction
Our evolved technique now includes a modified posterior Rocco's repair [13] with a barbed suture with two needles (2.0 Quill SRS; Angiotech, Reading, PA) suturing the rhabdosphincter and the median fibrous raphe to the remaining Denonvilliers' fascia in a running fashion. The resulting reconstructed plane is then fixed to the posterior aspect of the ileum at the level of opening for the ileal-urethral anastomosis (neobladder neck) approximately 8 mm dorsocephalad. Putting traction on this suture, the opening for the neobladder neck descends toward the urethral stump (Fig. 2b). The posterior reconstruction during RARC is safe and feasible, providing good continence rates [13]. The anastomosis between the neobladder and urethra can then be made without tension, and this maneuver also ensures an uncomplicated catheter placement, and the neobladder will be placed correctly in the small pelvis during the whole procedure.

Step 5: Urethro-neovesical anastomosis
The anastomosis between ileum and urethra is then performed according to the van Velthoven technique, with two 16 cm 2-0 Quill® suture, allowing for 10-12 suture passes (Fig. 2c) [14]. The running suture is commenced by placing both needles from outside to in through the new "bladder neck," one needle at the 5:30 o'clock and the other at the 6:30 o'clock position, so that the "middle" sits at the 6 o'clock position on the posterior neobladder neck. The urethral "bites" are then made from inside to out, at the corresponding sites. At this point, perineal pressure, if needed, can be applied. After two such placement on each side, which covers the completed posterior aspect of anastomosis, the neobladder neck is brought down together with the major portion of the ileal loop by tightening both sutures. In order to avoid urethral tearing, we suggest to gently lift upward the suture only after passing through the urethra and by alternate the left and the right needle in a "marionette technique" to get the ileum to "snug down." At 12 o'clock position, both suture arms are tied to each other over the urethra. The catheter balloon is then temporary inflated to 5 mL.

Step 6: Section of ileum segment and commencing the orthotopic reservoir
The orthotopic neobladder is fashioned from a 50–55 cm segment of terminal ileum (Fig. 3a). After the urethral–ileum anastomosis, an ileal inverse U-shaped loop is obtained (Fig. 3b). The Endo-GIA stapler is inserted by the bedside assistant through the left hybrid 15 mm trocar and a charge of 60 mm fired twice over the ileum (Fig. 3c), to select an ileal segment going from 35 to 40 cm from the ileo-caecal valve and 15 cm from the urethral–enteric anastomosis and 40 cm from the urethral–enteric anastomosis, to obtain the afferent reservoir loop. The selected point included not more than 3–4 cm of the ileal mesentery.

Step 7: Restoring continuity of the ileum (side-to-side entero-enteric anastomosis)
A side-to-side ileum anastomosis is performed by opening a 1-cm hole at the antimesenteric bowel border just next to the staple line. The continuity of the bowel is restored by inserting through these holes, the jaws of the stapler, and fired twice with 60 mm firing (Fig. 3d–f). The transverse opening is then closed by an additional 60 mm firing of the stapler.

Step 8: Detubularization of ileum
The intestinal loop is then detubularized with robotic scissors along the anti-mesenteric border apart from the last 12–14 cm of the distal 40 cm of the isolated ileal segment (Fig. 4).

Careful attention has to be paid at level of the anastomosis, where the incision can be performed closer to the mesenteric border, by keeping a safe distance from the anastomosis. The left ileum loop will be preserved, as the proximal isoperistaltic afferent limb for the ureteral anastomosis.

Step 9: Construction of the posterior wall of the reservoir
The posterior part of the reservoir is closed using a multiple running self-anchoring suture (V-Loc® closure device, Covidien V-Loc 180 3-0®, Mansfield, MA, US) in a seromuscular fashion. After applying traction sutures every 5–7 cm on the posterior aspect the running suturing start from the proximal aspect of the detubularized bowel (Fig. 3a).

Step 10: Folding and constructing the anterior wall of the reservoir
To achieve a spherical reservoir consisting of four cross-folded ileal segments, similar to the Studer neobladder [15], the right upper bottom of the U is folded over approximating diagonally to the left limb of reservoir loop, at 7–10 cm from the urethral–enteric anastomosis (Fig. 3a). The distal half of

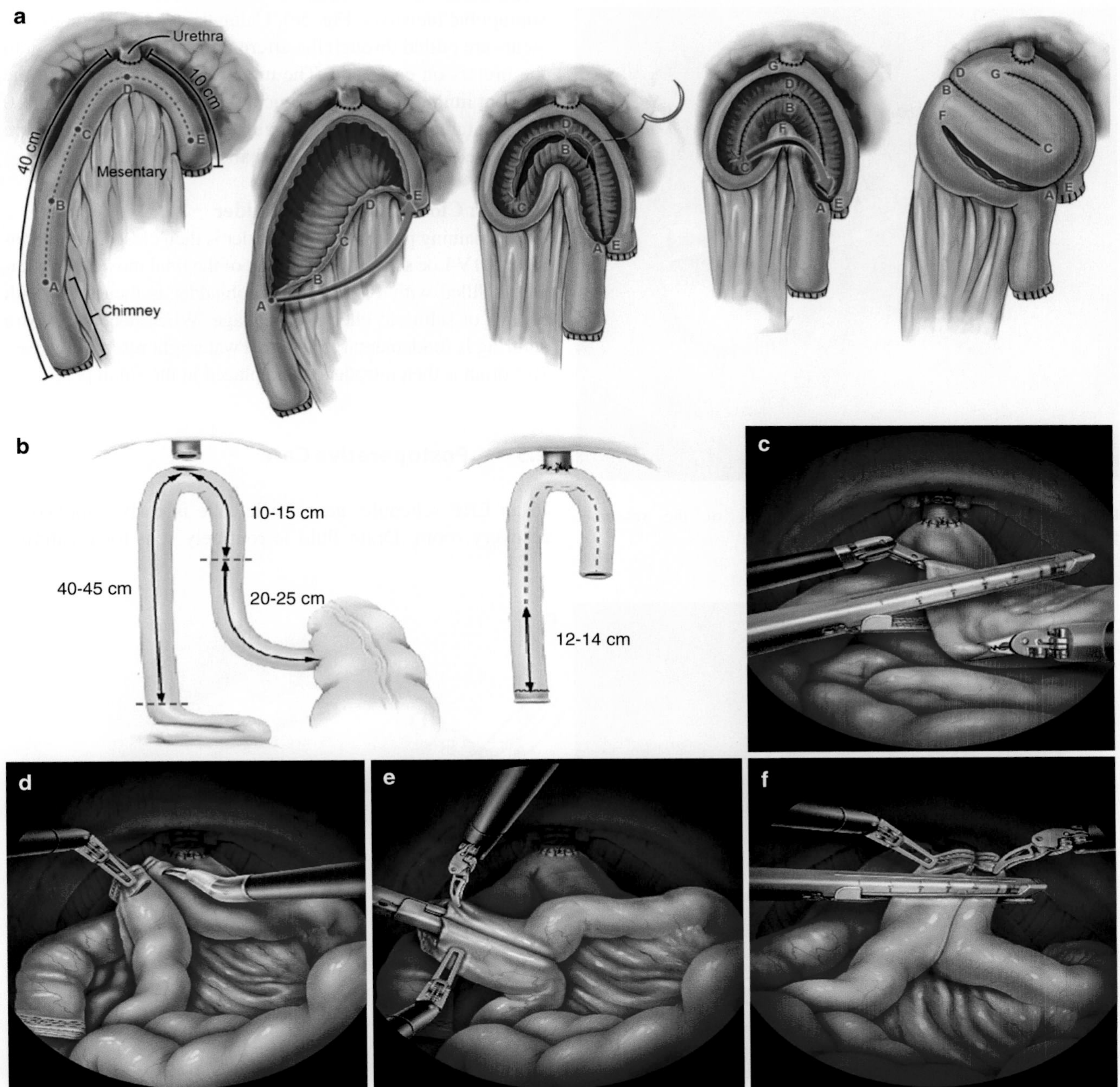

Fig. 3 Forming the modified Studer neobladder. (**a**) The orthotopic neobladder is fashioned from a 50–55 cm segment of terminal ileum. (**b**) The ileal inverse U-shaped loop is obtained after urethro-enteric anastomosis and intestinal stapling. (**c**) Endoscopic view of Endo GIA stapler and ileum. (**d**) The selected point incised for insertion of the stapler to avoid the stapling the mesentery. (**e**) Restoring continuity of the ileum (side-to-side entero-enteric anastomosis). (**f**) Ileum is closed with further stapling

the anterior part of the reservoir is then sutured, while the proximal half is temporary left open, to let ureteric stents passing through the abdominal wall.

Step 11: The uretero-enteric anastomosis

At this point, the staple line of the afferent reservoir loop is excised, and a Wallace technique is adopted for the uretero-enteric anastomosis: while the fourth arm holding still the ties attached to Hem-o-lok clips, the ureters are aligned. Following ureter incision and spatulation for 2 cm (Fig. 5a), the posterior walls of ureters are sutured side to side with a 15-cm running 5-0 PDS suture (Synature, Covidien) (Fig. 5b). Bilateral single-J, 70-cm 7.2 Fr ureteric stents are introduced with the Seldinger technique through two separate 4-mm

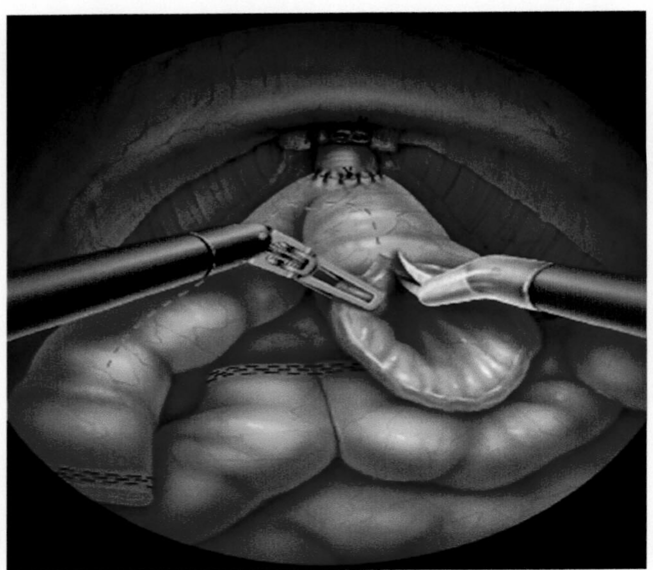

Fig. 4 Construction of the posterior wall of the reservoir. Detubularization of ileum

suprapubic incisions (Fig. 5c). Using the Cadiere forceps, the stents are pulled through the afferent limb and pushed up into the ureters on each side. The ureters are then sutured to the afferent limb of the Studer pouch, using two-times 16 cm 3-0 Quill suture [16]. After the entero-ureteric anastomoses are completed, the stents are sutured and fixed to the skin.

Step 12: Closure of the neobladder

The remaining part of the neobladder is then closed with a running 3-0 V-Loc suture. The balloon of the final indwelling catheter is filled with 10 mL. The neobladder is then filled with 50 mL of saline to check for leakage. When necessary extra suturing is fundamental to secure a watertight reservoir. A passive drain is then introduced and placed in the small pelvis.

2.5 Postoperative Care

In an ERP schedule, nasogastric tube is early removed in recovery room. Drain fluid is routinely sent for creatinine

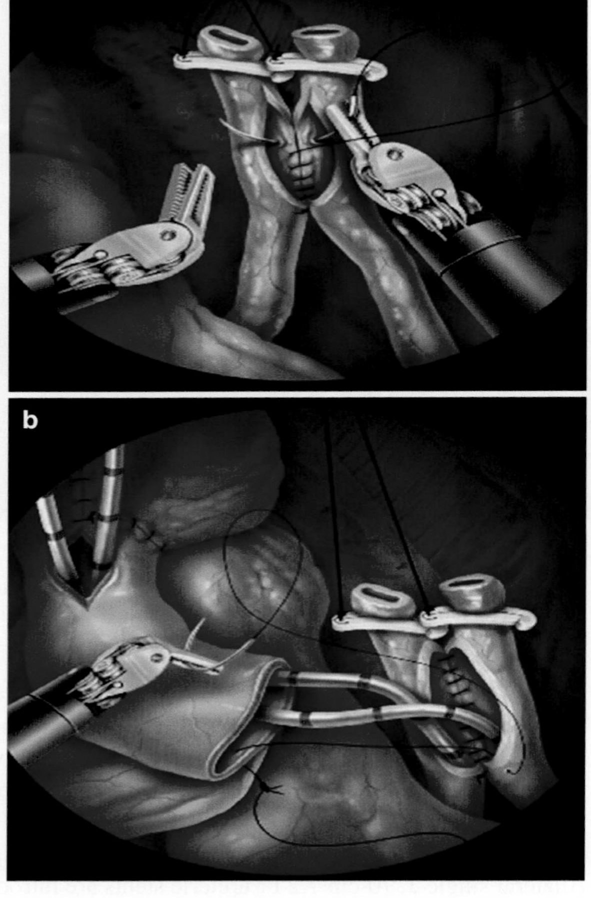

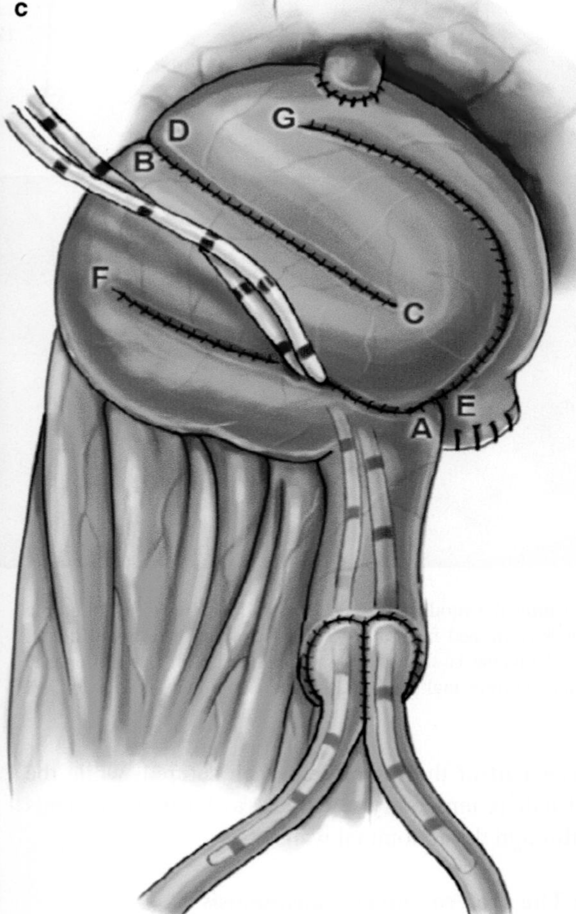

Fig. 5 The uretero-enteric anastomosis (Wallace I). (**a**) Ureter incision and spatulation for 2 cm. Posterior walls of ureters are sutured side-to-side with a 15-cm running 5-0. (**b**) Bilateral single-J, 40-cm ureteric stents inserted into each ureter. (**c**) The ureters are then sutured to the afferent limb of the Studer pouch, using two-times 16 cm 3-0 Quill suture

analysis on postoperative day (POD) 1, and the drain can be removed from POD 1 if fluid indicates serum creatinine levels. Both compression stockings and low molecular weight heparin are routinely administered for 3–4 weeks postoperatively. Single J's will be removed POD 14. Indwelling catheter will be removed 3 weeks postoperatively.

3 Conclusions

A totally intracorporeal RARC with urinary diversion is gaining popularity as a realistic alternative to open surgery. RARC with intracorporeal neobladder performed in experienced robotic centers have reported functional and complication rates comparable to open series with the potential advantages over open approach, which include reduced blood loss and length of stay [17].

However, totally intracorporeal RARC represents a complex multistep procedure, and we highlight the importance of adequate planning and proper mentoring while commencing this procedure, initiation of an ERP, and establishment of a dedicated RARC team with continual auditing of results [6].

References

1. Stenzl A, Cowan NC, De Santis M, et al. Treatment of muscle-invasive and metastatic bladder cancer: update of the EAU Guidelines. Eur Urol. 2011;59:1009–1. https://doi.org/10.1016/j.eururo.2011.03.023.
2. Collins JW, Adding C, Hosseini A, Nyberg T, Pini G, Dey L, Wiklund PN. Introducing an enhanced recovery programme to an established totally intracorporeal robot-assisted radical cystectomy service. Scand J Urol. 2016;50(1):39–46. https://doi.org/10.3109/21681805.2015.1076514. Epub 2015 Aug 25.
3. Witjes JA, Bruins HM, Cathomas R, Compérat E, Cowan NC, Efstathiou JA, Fietkau R, Gakis G, Hernández V, Lorch A, Milowsky MI, Ribal MJ, Thalmann GN, van der Heijden AG, Veskimäe E. European Association of Urology Guidelines on muscle-invasive and metastatic bladder cancer: summary of the 2020 Guidelines. Eur Urol. 2021;79:82. https://uroweb.org/guideline/bladder-cancer-muscle-invasive-and-metastatic
4. Tang K, Xia D, Li H, Guan W, Guo X, Hu Z, Ma X, Zhang X, Xu H, Ye Z. Robotic vs. open radical cystectomy in bladder cancer: a systematic review and meta-analysis. Eur J Surg Oncol. 2014;
5. Dell'Oglio P, Mazzone E, Lambert E, Vollemaere J, Goossens M, Larcher A, Van Der Jeugt J, Devos G, Poelaert F, Uvin P, Collins J, De Naeyer G, Schatteman P, D'Hondt F, Mottrie A. The effect of surgical experience on perioperative and oncological outcomes after robot-assisted radical cystectomy with intracorporeal urinary diversion: evidence from a referral centre with extensive experience in robotic surgery. Eur Urol Focus. 2021;7(2):352–8. https://doi.org/10.1016/j.euf.2020.01.016.
6. Collins JW, Tyritzis S, Nyberg T, Schumacher M, Laurin O, Khazaeli D, et al. Robot-assisted radical cystectomy: description of an evolved approach to radical cystectomy. Eur Urol. 2013;64:654–63.
7. Hosseini A, Mortezavi A, Sjöberg S, Laurin O, Adding C, Collins J, Wiklund PN. Robot-assisted intracorporeal orthotopic bladder substitution after radical cystectomy: perioperative morbidity and oncological outcomes – a single-institution experience. BJU Int. 2020;126(4):464–71. https://doi.org/10.1111/bju.15112. Epub 2020 Jun 5.
8. Yu D, Dural C, Morrow MM, et al. Intraoperative workload in robotic surgery assessed by wearable motion tracking sensors and questionnaires. Surg Endosc. 2017;31(2):877–86.
9. Li K, Lin T, Fan X, Xu K, Bi L, Duan Y, Zhou Y, Yu M, Li J, Huang J. Systematic review and meta-analysis of comparative studies reporting early outcomes after robot-assisted radical cystectomy versus open radical cystectomy. Cancer Treat Rev. 2013;39(6):551–60.
10. Snow-Lisy DC, Campbell SC, Gill IS, Hernandez AV, Fergany A, Kaouk J, Georges-Pascal Haberw-Lisy DC, Campbell SC, Gill IS, Hernandez AV, Fergany A, Kaouk J, Haber. Robotic and laparoscopic radical cystectomy for bladder cancer: long-term oncologic outcomes. Eur Urol. 2014;65(1):193–200. https://doi.org/10.1016/j.eururo.2013.08.021.
11. Collins JW, Patel H, Adding C, et al. Enhanced recovery after robot-assisted radical cystectomy: EAU Robotic Urology Section Scientific Working Group Consensus View. Eur Urol. 2016;70(4):649–60.
12. Brooks NA, Kokorovic A, McGrath JS, Kassouf W, Collins JW, Black PC, Douglas J, Djaladat H, Daneshmand S, Catto JWF, Kamat AM, Williams SB. Critical analysis of quality of life and cost-effectiveness of enhanced recovery after surgery (ERAS) for patient's undergoing urologic oncology surgery: a systematic review. World J Urol. 2020. https://doi.org/10.1007/s00345-020-03341-6.
13. Rocco B, Luciani LG, Collins J, Sanchez-Salas R, Adding C, Mattevi D, Hosseini A, Wiklund P. Posterior reconstruction during robotic-assisted radical cystectomy with intracorporeal orthotopic ileal neobladder: description and outcomes of a simple step. J Robotic Surg. 2021;15:355–61. https://doi.org/10.1007/s11701-020-01108-0.
14. Van Velthoven RF, Ahlering TE, Peltier A, Skarecky DW, Clayman RV. Technique for laparoscopic running urethrovesical anastomosis:the single knot method. Urology. 2003;61(4):699–702.
15. Wiklund NP, Poulakis V. Robotic neobladder. BJU Int. 2011;107(9):1514–37.
16. Hosseini A, Dey L, Laurin O, Adding C, Hoijer J, Ebbing J, Collins JW. Ureteric stricture rates and management after robot-assisted radical cystectomy: a single-centre observational study. Scand J Urol. 2018;52(4):244–8.
17. Hosseini A, Ebbing J, Collins J. Clinical outcomes of robot-assisted radical cystectomy and continent urinary diversion. Scand J Urol. 2019;53(2–3):81–8. https://doi.org/10.1080/21681805.2019.1598486.

Robotic Intracorporeal Neobladder: UCLH Experience

Emmanuel Weyne, Wei Shen Tan, John Kelly, and Ashwin Sridhar

1 Introduction

Radical cystectomy remains the golden standard for the treatment of muscle-invasive bladder cancer and selected high risk non-muscle-invasive bladder cancer [1]. Over the last decade, robot-assisted radical cystectomy (RARC) is increasingly being utilized. The intended benefits for the patient include lower wound-related complications, decreased intraoperative blood loss, lower blood transfusion rates, shorter hospital stay, and faster recovery after surgery [2].

To date, randomized trials between open and RARC have showed equivocal perioperative outcomes with the exception of blood loss and blood transfusion rates, and this has been reaffirmed in meta-analysis [3–6]. These trials were limited by extracorporeal construction urinary diversions and surgeons early in their learning curve. It is postulated that intracorporeal constructed diversion is deemed to have an even higher benefit for the patient in terms of recovery and hospital length of stay. The iROC trial, randomizing patients to open radical cystectomy versus robotic cystectomy with intracorporeal urinary diversion, intends to address this hypothesis and has completed patient accrual [7].

Following radical cystectomy, two types of urinary diversion can be constructed: a non-continent ileal conduit or a continent urine reservoir either in a form of orthotopic (neobladder) or heterotopic (Mitrofanoff or Monti). The choice of urinary diversion depends on bladder cancer disease characteristics, patient characteristics, patient choice, and patient motivation.

2 Patient Selection

In our institution, all patients are seen in a multidisciplinary bladder clinic before surgery consisting of an evaluation with the surgeon, anesthetist, urinary diversion nurse, and oncology specialist nurse. Anesthetic review includes cardiopulmonary exercise tolerance (CPET) testing to assess preoperative risk.

All patients opting for neobladder as a urinary diversion are taught and must be able to successfully perform intermittent self-catherization before surgery. Patients undergo a clinical exam under anesthesia and rigid cystoscopy with biopsy to exclude disease involvement of the prostatic urethra. Relative contraindications to neobladder diversion are impaired renal function, bladder neck or prostatic urethra involvement, salvage surgery and extensive anterior bladder disease in women. In our center, a preoperative MRI of the bladder is routinely performed which aids with visualizing and planning the cystectomy. The MRI helps to exclude occult prostate malignancy which can interfere with extensive erectile nerve sparing. Furthermore, it assesses potential involvement of the distal ureter and relationship of the tumor to the anterior vaginal wall in women.

Our preoperative protocol before cystectomy has been previously described in detail and follows enhanced recovery after surgery (ERAS) principles [8].

3 Operative Setup

In our institution, we use a da Vinci X (Intuitive Surgical) robotic platform. The patient is installed on an anti-slip surface (Xodus Medical, Pittsburgh, PA, USA) mat to prevent sliding down in Trendelenburg positioning, with the arms tucked to the sides. The level of Trendelenburg is modified based on patient tolerance. Our standard is to aim for 26° head down. If the patient cannot tolerate the Trendelenburg

E. Weyne
Department of Uro-Oncology and Robotic Urology, University College London Hospitals, London, UK

Department of Urology, AZ St Blasius Hospital, Dendermonde, Belgium

W. S. Tan · J. Kelly · A. Sridhar (✉)
Department of Uro-Oncology and Robotic Urology, University College London Hospitals, London, UK

P. Wiklund et al. (eds.), *Robotic Urologic Surgery*, https://doi.org/10.1007/978-3-031-00363-9_60

position, we will perform a side dock procedure with a break at the level of the hips to keep the legs flat but the upper body down. A nasogastric tube is inserted and will be removed at the end of the surgery. Flowtron© intermittent pneumatic compression stockings are applied around the lower limbs to prevent lower limb compartment syndrome and minimize risk of lower limb deep venous thrombosis. A Bair Hugger (3M, St Paul, MN, USA) is used to prevent hypothermia.

A six-port configuration is used for transperitoneal robotic surgery (Fig. 1). A Hassan technique is used to insert a camera port about one hand width cranial to the umbilicus and to create a pneumoperitoneum. The position of the camera port is typically more cranial compared to a radical prostatectomy configuration. This allows for better manipulation of the bowel during the creation of the urinary diversion and allows for a more extensive lymphadenectomy template. Subsequently, two 8 mm robotic ports are inserted at the level of the umbilicus just lateral to the rectus abdominis muscle. A 15 mm AirSeal port (ConMed, New York, USA) is placed in the right iliac fossa, about two fingers above the bony projection of the anterior superior iliac spine. The use of the AirSeal port prevents changes in pneumoperitoneum during the procedure. A 15 mm robotic port is placed in the left iliac fossa to allow for the use of a robotic bowel stapler. Special care is taken to position this port caudal and lateral enough. This will facilitate faster introduction of the robotic stapler by the bedside assistant and allows to staple the bowel without the need for extreme angulation with the stapling device. A 5 mm suction port is placed cranially and triangulated between the camera port and right lateral port.

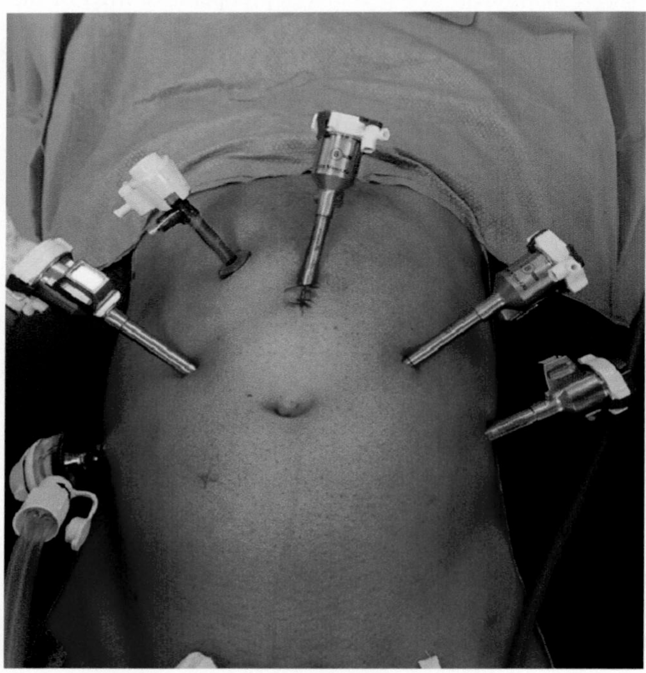

Fig. 1 Trocar positioning

4 Special Attention Points During Cystectomy to Facilitate Neobladder Creation

The detailed technique of the exenterative part of a robotic radical cystectomy is extensively discussed in other chapters. In this chapter, we will focus on the technique of constructing an orthotopic neobladder. We do like to stress some important points during the cystectomy that will facilitate the subsequent steps during the reconstructive phase of the surgery.

In female patients, a female organ-sparing cystectomy is performed sparing ovaries and uterus. This allows for better support of the native tissues and reduces the risk of vaginal prolapse which is frequently seen after en-bloc anterior pelvic exenteration. Furthermore, this technique limits the risk of fistula formation between the vagina and neobladder, as the vagina is conserved. For the same reason, the specimen is delivered through a Pfannenstiel incision in women undergoing a neobladder urinary diversion. This is in contrast to the transvaginal delivery of the specimen in women undergoing cystourethrectomy and ileal conduit. Typically, the Pfannenstiel incision is slightly more cranial to avoid injury to the neobladder when delivering the specimen. An oncological contraindication for female organ sparing cystectomy is anterior or extensive trigonal bladder cancer disease. Full urethral sparing is essential for early urinary continence recovery in women, and this means not opening the endopelvic fascia during the exenterative bit of the surgery. The distal bladder limit is at the vesicourethral junction.

In male patients, special attention is paid to preserve maximal urethral length during the apical dissection of the prostate and urethra. If needed, part of the apical prostate is preserved to maintain a lengthy urethral stump and to stabilize the apical sphincter mechanism. In men with good preoperative erectile function and non-extensive bladder cancer disease who are keen on preserving their erectile function after surgery, a prostatic capsule sparing cystectomy is an option. Preoperative MRI is used to exclude the presence of prostate cancer. In a prostate capsule-sparing cystectomy, the posterior dissection is continued in the plane above the seminal vesicles and vas deferens. The prostatic tissue is enucleated within the prostatic capsule (Millin's plane). This will allow maximal sparing of the cavernous nerves on the dorsolateral side of the prostate (Fig. 2). Nerve-sparing radical cystectomy has a proven beneficial impact on urinary continence after orthotopic neobladder construction [9].

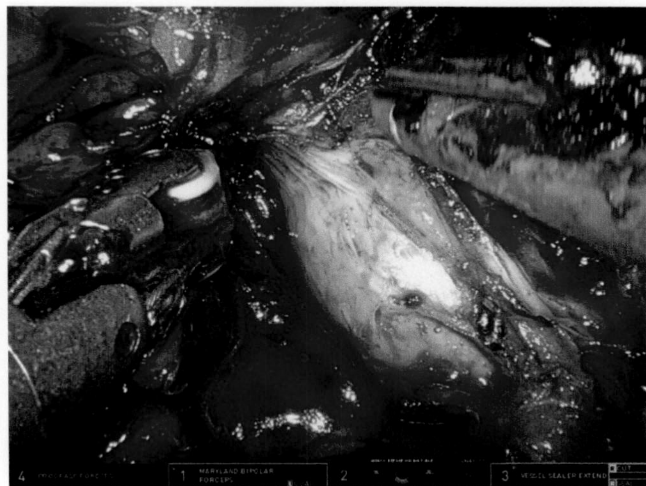

Fig. 2 Prostate capsule-sparing cystectomy: the prostatic adenoma is enucleated within the prostatic capsule (Millin's plane)

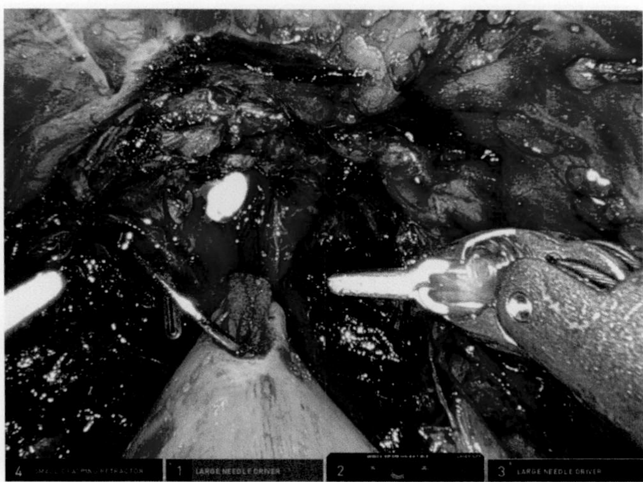

Fig. 3 Posterior wall of urethral-intestinal anastomosis

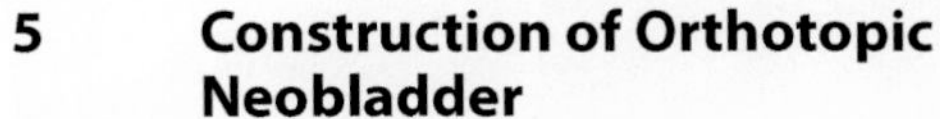

5 Construction of Orthotopic Neobladder

After completion of the radical cystectomy and bilateral pelvic lymph node dissection, the specimens are placed in the left upper quadrant above the spleen to free up space within the pelvis before constructing the neobladder. The cords of the endobags are hitched with a clip to the left lateral peritoneum. The left and right ureters would have already been clipped to the right lateral peritoneum.

5.1 Rocco Stitch and Urethral-Intestinal Anastomosis

The most dependent part of the ileum is brought down to the pelvis toward the urethra. If required, Trendelenburg positioning can be reduced to avoid too much tension on the small bowel's mesentery. The further steps of the neobladder have been modified over the years. These changes aim to obtain a neobladder shape closest to a spherical configuration on leak test and long-term follow-up. On the right side of the urethral-ileal anastomosis, 10 cm of ileum will be isolated to be incorporated into the neobladder, whereas on the left side 35–40 cm of the ileum is incorporated to construct the neobladder. One should pay attention that there is enough length left on the terminal ileum for the bowel anastomosis. A robotic small bowel grasper is used to minimize trauma to the small bowel during manipulation.

Using a 9 in. 3.0 Filbloc® (Assut Europe) with 5/8 neeldle, a Rocco suspension stitch is placed between the periurethral Denonvilliers fascia 1 cm proximal of the urethra and the small bowel near the posterior mesenteric limit. A longer suture will have enough length to allow parachuting down of the small bowel. After three consecutive sutures, a hole is made in the small bowel to create the bowel anastomosis with the urethra cranial to the Rocco. While making the neobladder opening, care should be taken to allow enough small bowel width to allow for detubularizing. The detubularizing incision is made on the mesenteric edge opposite to the Rocco edge. The first suture line is tightened to complete the Rocco anastomosis. The same suture is used to continue the urethral-ileal anastomosis (Fig. 3). After completion of the posterior wall of the anastomosis, the bowel is opened on the mesenteric side to pass through the urinary catheter. After completing one-halve of the anastomosis, a second Filbloc suture is used. Starting at the 6 o'clock position, the other halve of the anastomosis is completed.

5.2 Isolation of Small Bowel for Neobladder

On the right side, 10 cm of ileum will be isolated to be incorporated into the neobladder, whereas on the left side 35–40 cm of the ileum is incorporated to construct the neobladder. The jaws of the small bowel grasper can be used as a measuring tool. This measures 5 cm in length. The small bowel is divided at the appropriate length. Attention is paid to leave sufficient length to the terminal ileum to avoid disturbances in vitamin B12 uptake and allow for a tension-free small bowel anastomosis.

A robotic vessel sealer is used to divide the bowel (Fig. 4). Cutting mode is used on the bowel for transection and sealing mode to divide the subsequent mesentery. A wedge of small bowel and mesentery is discarded distal to the neobladder to create space between the neobladder and the small bowel anastomosis, as well as to ensure adequate vascular supply to the segment of bowel re-anastomosed. By the use

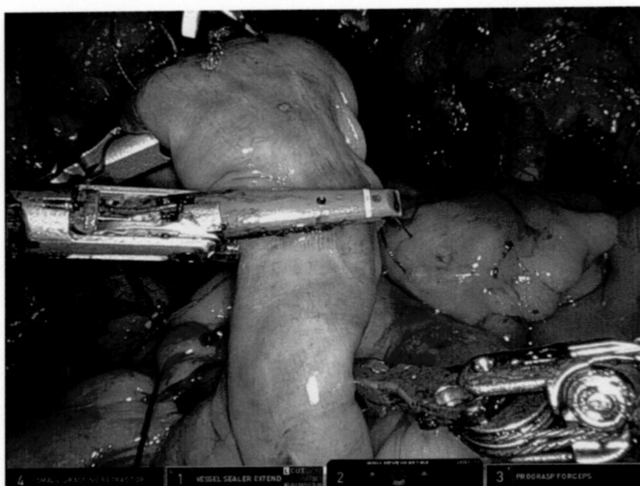

Fig. 4 Isolation of bowel loop with vessel sealer

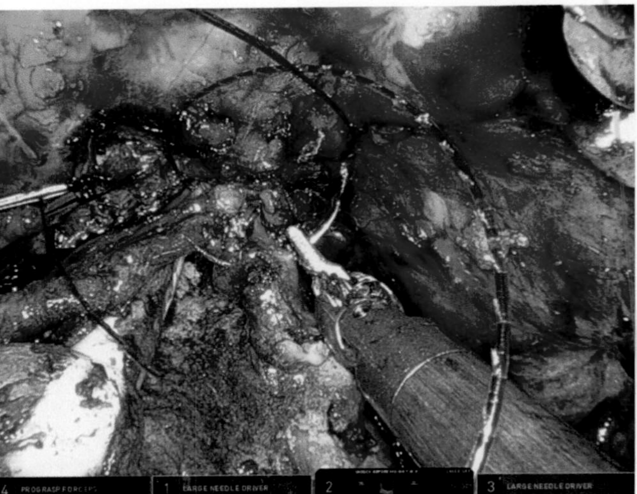

Fig. 5 Closure anterior apex neobladder

of a robotic stapler, the bowel continuity is re-established with a side-to-side anastomosis. Two consecutive 60 mm staplers are used on the antimesenteric wall of the bowel. This is followed by another 60 mm stapler transversally.

5.3 Construction of the Neobladder

The UCLH neobladder consists of a pyramid shape which is obtained by hitching the anterior side of the neobladder to the anterior abdominal wall [10].

To start off, the antimesenteric side of the isolated bowel is opened on each side at the proximal site and continued distally to the previous incision above the urethra in order to detubularize the bowel. On the left side, the proximal 5–10 cm is spared to create the chute. The fourth arm is used to hold the chute. The assistant grabs the opposite side of the bowel and pushes down the posterior bowel wall with the tip of the suction during the incision of the bowel loop.

The posterior closure of the neobladder is made by using multiple 6 in. 2.0 Filbloc sutures with a half curved needle. The closure is started 10 cm to the left of the urethral-ileal anastomosis such that the posterior closure is performed horizontally between to equal limbs (20 cm each). Attention is paid to take equal steps on each limb to avoid asymmetry.

The closure of the anterior wall starts at the apex just proximal to the urethral-ileal anastomosis (Fig. 5). This reduces the stretch of the mesentery, chute, and the ureteroileal anastomosis. After this is closed to the level of the pubis, the remaining anterior wall is closed along the horizontal axis (like the posterior wall). Before preparing to fold the neobladder by hitching it to the anterior abdominal wall, a suture can be placed to stabilize the apex of the neobladder. This is done by placing a Vicryl 3.0 suture on each side between the apex of the neobladder and the endopelvic fascia. The anterior wall of the neobladder is hitched to the anterior abdominal wall and secured by additional anterior holding sutures (Fig. 6).

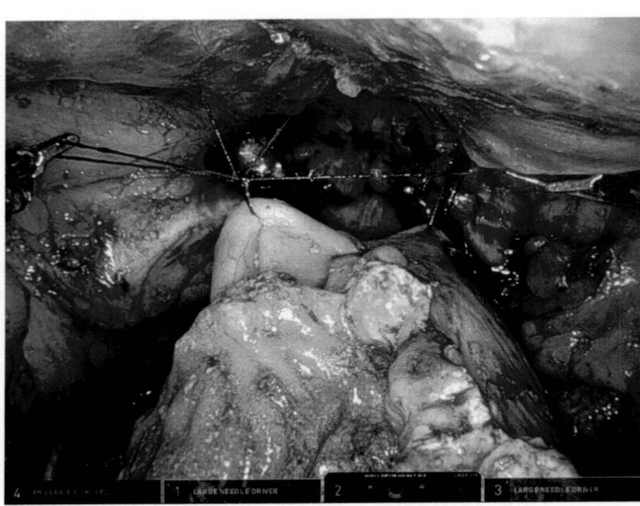

Fig. 6 Hitching of the anterior wall of the neobladder to obtain a pyramidic shape

5.4 Ureteroileal Anastomosis

Two separate incisions are made on the top of the afferent limb of the neobladder to implant the ureters individually. The left ureter is tunneled under the sigmoid mesentery, and the right ureter is brought under the neobladder mesentery. The ureter is spatulated and then anastomosed in a continuous fashion with two separate sutures PDS 4.0. After completing the posterior half of the anastomosis, a single J stent on a guidewire is inserted in the ureter. After

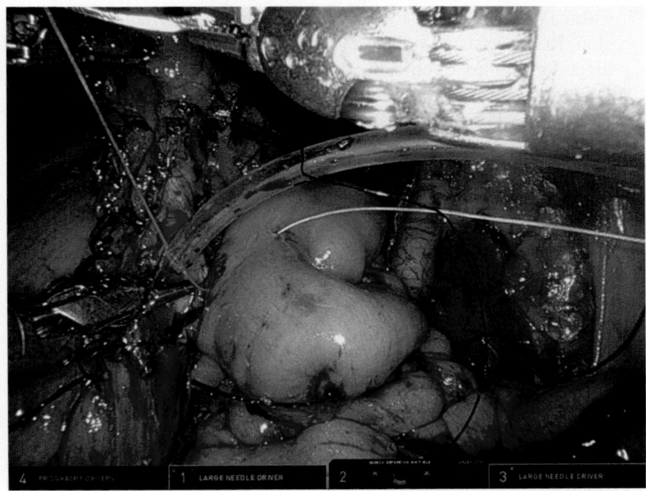

Fig. 7 Ureteric stent in ureteroileal anastomosis being fixed with Vicryl Rapide 3.0 to prevent accidental pulling during procedure

positioning the tip of the ureteric stent in the kidney, the stent is fixed to the bowel with a suture point of Vicryl Rapide 3.0 (Fig. 7). After this, the end of the ureteric stent will be passed through from the ureterointestinal anastomosis and then through an opening made on either side of the chute near the mesentery (left on the left side and right on the right). The anastomosis is then finished off, and the peritoneum of the ureter is placed over the anastomosis as a second layer to limit chances of leakage and to improve vascularization.

The neobladder is closed, paying special attention to tightly close the area around the exit point of the ureteric stents in order to avoid urinary leakage. The stents are picked up with an artery clip through the abdominal wall. This is at the site where a precautionary stoma site has been marked on the abdominal wall that should an ileal conduit be necessary (Fig. 1 "cross mark").

5.5 Finishing Off the Procedure

A leak test is performed by filling the neobladder with saline. The neobladder is partly retroperitonialized, by placing sutures between the medial side of the neobladder and lateral edge of incised peritoneum using Vicryl 3.0. Another suture is used to bury the transverse staple line of the transverse side-to-side bowel anastomosis. This is to minimize the risk of fistulation of the bowel anastomosis to the neobladder due to the presence of the stapler line. Where omentum is available, it should be used to drape around the neobladder. A 20 Fr passive drains are placed inside the pelvis, around the neobladder. The specimens are delivered through a Pfannenstiel incision which is typically placed slightly more cranial to avoid injury to the neobladder.

5.6 Postoperative Care

Patients routinely will be monitored for in an intensive care unit for the first 24 h post-surgery. An early recovery after surgery (ERAS) protocol is initiated [8]. The nasogastric tube is removed at the end of the surgery. Antibiotics are continued for 24 h. In cases with high intraperitoneal fecal spillage, antibiotics are administered for 5 days. For the first 3 days postoperatively, patients are prescribed intravenous metoclopramide three times daily, and chewing gum is used as a gastroprokinetic to minimize the risks of postoperative ileus. Patients can commence free fluids a few hours following surgery, and oral feeding is started the day after surgery if tolerated and in the absence of signs of nausea. Low molecular weight heparin is administered 6 h postoperatively and is continued daily for 4 weeks postoperatively. The urethral catheter is flushed daily to ensure good drainage of the neobladder and avoid blockage due to mucous built up. Patients are admitted to hospital for 1 day for a cystogram to confirm no evidence of leakage prior to the removal of ureteric and urethral catheter 3 weeks postoperatively.

5.7 Postoperative Outcomes

Between 2011 and 2016, a total of 60 intracorporeal neobladder cases were performed at UCLH. Median patient age was 55.6 years (IQR: 48.7–61.9). Fifty-four (90%) patients were male, and 12 patients (20.0%) had an American Society of Anesthesiologists (ASA) ≥III. Median hospital length of stay was 10 days (IQR: 7–13) with a 30- and 90-day readmission rate of 13.3% (n = 8) and 28.3% (n = 17), respectively.

Median operating time was 398.0 min (IQR: 328.5–473.8) 30-day, and 90-day major complication rate was 13.3% (n = 8) and 16.7% (n = 10), respectively. Postoperative ileus was reported in 14 patients (23.3%). At 90-day follow-up, infection and gastrointestinal-related complications were most common and were reported by 46.7% (n = 28) and 36.7% (n = 22) of patients, respectively. Perioperative blood transfusion rate was 6.7% (n = 4).

References

1. Witjes JA, Bruins HM, Cathomas R, Compérat EM, Cowan NC, Gakis G, et al. European Association of Urology Guidelines on Muscle-invasive and metastatic bladder cancer: summary of the 2020 guidelines. Eur Urol. 2021;79(1):82–104.
2. Wijburg CJ, Michels CTJ, Hannink G, Grutters JPC, Rovers MM, Alfred Witjes J, et al. Robot-assisted radical cystectomy versus open radical cystectomy in bladder cancer patients: a multicentre comparative effectiveness study. Eur Urol. 2021;79(5):609–18.
3. Khan MS, Omar K, Ahmed K, Gan C, Van Hemelrijck M, Nair R, et al. Long-term oncological outcomes from an early

phase randomised controlled three-arm trial of open, robotic, and laparoscopic radical cystectomy (CORAL). Eur Urol. 2020;77(1):110–8.

4. Bochner BH, Dalbagni G, Marzouk KH, Sjoberg DD, Lee J, Donat SM, et al. Randomized trial comparing open radical cystectomy and robot-assisted laparoscopic radical cystectomy: oncologic outcomes. Eur Urol. 2018;74(4):465–71.
5. Parekh DJ, Reis IM, Castle EP, Gonzalgo ML, Woods ME, Svatek RS, et al. Robot-assisted radical cystectomy versus open radical cystectomy in patients with bladder cancer (RAZOR): an open-label, randomised, phase 3, non-inferiority trial. Lancet. 2018;391(10139):2525–36.
6. Tan WS, Khetrapal P, Tan WP, Rodney S, Chau M, Kelly JD. Robotic assisted radical cystectomy with extracorporeal urinary diversion does not show a benefit over open radical cystectomy: a systematic review and meta-analysis of randomised controlled trials. PLoS ONE. 2016;11(11):e0166221.
7. Catto JWF, Khetrapal P, Ambler G, Sarpong R, Khan MS, Tan M, et al. Robot-assisted radical cystectomy with intracorporeal urinary diversion versus open radical cystectomy (iROC): protocol for a randomised controlled trial with internal feasibility study. BMJ Open. 2018;8(8):e020500.
8. Tan WS, Lamb BW, Sridhar A, Briggs TP, Kelly JD. A comprehensive guide to perioperative management and operative technique for robotic cystectomy with intracorporeal urinary diversion. Urologia. 2017;84(2):71–8.
9. Furrer MA, Studer UE, Gross T, Burkhard FC, Thalmann GN, Nguyen DP. Nerve-sparing radical cystectomy has a beneficial impact on urinary continence after orthotopic bladder substitution, which becomes even more apparent over time. BJU Int. 2018;121(6):935–44.
10. Tan WS, Sridhar A, Goldstraw M, Zacharakis E, Nathan S, Hines J, et al. Robot-assisted intracorporeal pyramid neobladder. BJU Int. 2015;116(5):771–9.

Step-by-Step Approach to Intracorporeal Urinary Diversion, Ileal Conduit, and W-Neobladder: The Roswell Park Technique

Umar Iqbal, Ahmed Aly Hussein, and Khurshid A. Guru

1 Introduction

In the initial era of robot-assisted radical cystectomy (RARC), urologic surgeons mainly focused on developing surgical techniques that optimize oncological outcomes. There is growing body of evidence supporting the non-inferiority of oncologic and perioperative outcomes of robot-assisted radical cystectomy (RARC) compared to open cystectomy [1–3]. RARC has been shown to provide some perioperative benefits such as reduced blood loss, transfusion need, pain, faster bowel recovery, and shorter hospital stay [4]. The attention shifted to more focus on the potential additional benefits of intracorporeal urinary diversion (ICUD). Several advantages of ICUD have been proposed, including reduced third space fluid loss, blood loss, perioperative transfusions, faster bowel function recovery, shorter hospital stay, and earlier convalescence [5] .

In centers of excellence, up to 97% of diversions are now performed intracorporeally [6]. The Pasadena Consensus Panel recommends building experience in a graduated manner, starting first with ileal conduits and shifting gradually to the more complex neobladders [7]. Several techniques have been proposed for intracorporeal neobladder after RARC. Herein, we describe the construction of ICUD (ileal conduit and neobladder) with step-by-step instructions and illustrations.

1.1 Choice of Urinary Diversion

ICUD is appropriate for most patients except those with decreased cardiac and pulmonary compliance. These patients may not be able to tolerate the steep Trendelenburg position for a prolonged time that is needed for ICUD. However, the newer Xi model of da Vinci® Surgical System and AirSeal® has mitigated this by decreasing the need for steep Trendelenburg angle to more manageable levels. For the neobladder construction, the absolute and relative contraindications are summarized in Table 1. Additionally, patient preference and surgeon comfort with the procedure are important driving factors for the selection of diversion type and approach for each patient [8].

Table 1 Absolute and relative contraindications for neobladder construction [8]

Absolute contraindication	Relative contraindication
Tumor involvement of distal urethral margin in men	Advanced age
Tumor infiltration of bladder neck in women	Inflammatory bowel disease
Damaged rhabdosphincter	Locally advanced disease
Poor renal function with creatinine >2 mg/dL	Prior pelvic irradiation
Impaired hepatic function	Multiple prior abdominal surgeries
Severe intestinal disease, for example, Crohn's	Adjuvant chemotherapy planned/anticipated
Intellectual disability, noncompliant patient	
Unwillingness or inability to perform intermittent self-catheterization	

1.2 Preoperative Preparation

Enhanced recovery after surgery (ERAS) pathway has previously been shown to achieve quicker recovery and enhance patient satisfaction. The ERAS pathway includes components like skipping mechanical or chemical bowel preparation, early ambulation and oral feeding, appropriate fluid management, drugs like Alvimopan, and avoidance of epidurals. It has been shown to decrease complications, shorten length of stay, and reduce readmissions [9]. The "NEEW" (Nutrition, Exercise, patient Education and Wellness) pathway, which in addition incorporates physical prehabilitation, nutrition, and social work, has been suggested as a further improvement to ERAS and was shown to improve short-term

U. Iqbal · A. A. Hussein · K. A. Guru (✉)
Department of Urology, Roswell Park Comprehensive Cancer Center, Buffalo, NY, USA

P. Wiklund et al. (eds.), *Robotic Urologic Surgery*, https://doi.org/10.1007/978-3-031-00363-9_61

perioperative outcomes [10]. Additionally, mechanical bowel preparation and oral antibiotics should be avoided. Anticoagulant therapy should be used before and up to 4 weeks after surgery [11].

2 Surgical Technique

Instruments used are summarized in Table 2.

2.1 Positioning and Port Placement

Patient is placed in dorsal lithotomy position with adequate padding of all pressure points. The patient's arms are adducted and padded, and the table is placed in Trendelenburg position at 30 degrees. A 22 Fr Foley catheter and a rectal tube are placed. A Veress needle is used to achieve pneumoperitoneum. The standard insufflation or the AirSeal® may be used (the latter can be useful especially in female patients) [12]. A standard six-port transperitoneal approach is used. The 8 mm camera port is first placed an inch above and to the left of the umbilicus. The abdominal cavity is then inspected. All other ports are introduced under vision. Three 8 mm robotic trocars are introduced in addition to 15 mm assistant port and a 5 mm suction port. An additional 15 mm short suprapubic port is placed to facilitate bowel anastomosis toward the end of the procedure. Placing the ports an inch higher may facilitate bowel manipulation during intracorporeal urinary diversion (Fig. 1).

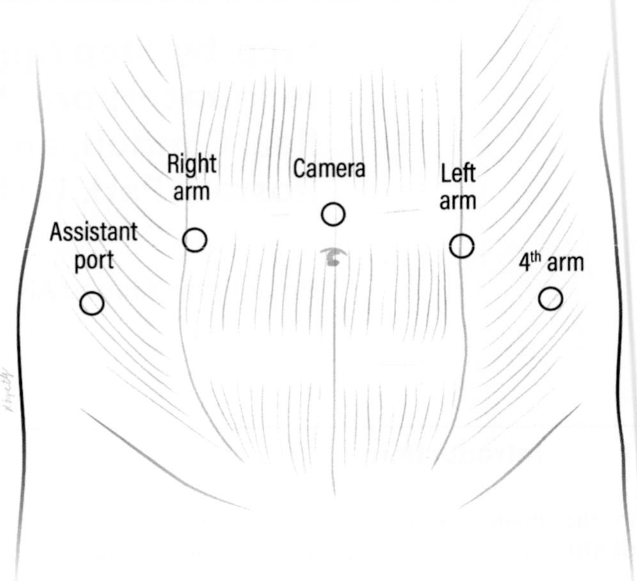

Fig. 1 Port configuration (Credit for Surgical Complications after Robot-Assisted Radical Cystectomy chapter, Techniques of Robotic Urinary Tract Reconstruction: A Complete Approach, 2021. Publisher: Springer. Editors: Michael Stifelman, Lee Zhao, Daniel Eun and Chester Koh)

2.2 Technique of Intracorporeal Ileal Conduit: The "Marionette" Technique [13]

- **Isolation of the Bowel Segment**

A 12–15 cm bowel segment is identified approximately 15–20 cm proximal to the ileocecal valve. A silk suture on a straight Keith needle is introduced through the abdominal wall and passed through the small bowel (at the distal end of the conduit) and back through the abdominal wall as a "marionette stitch." The marionette stitch is not tied and is used for dynamic retraction by the bedside assistant (Fig. 2).

Table 2 Instruments and sutures used

Robotic instruments • Fenestrated bipolar (or Maryland) forceps. • Monopolar scissors (or hook). • Cobra forceps. • Large needle drivers x 2.
Sutures Marionette stitch: 1-0 Silk suture on Keith needle; Uretero-ileal anastomosis: 4/0 Vicryl® Neobladder Sutures: 3/0 V-Loc®; Ureterovesical anastomosis: 3/0 V-loc®; Mesenteric defect: 3–0 Silk; Stoma: 3/0 Vicryl®; Stent fixation: 2-0 chromic sutures.
Endo GIA® stapler, Hem-o-lok® clip, AirSeal insufflator
Laparoscopic scissors, suction device, graspers, Hem-o-lok® clip appliers

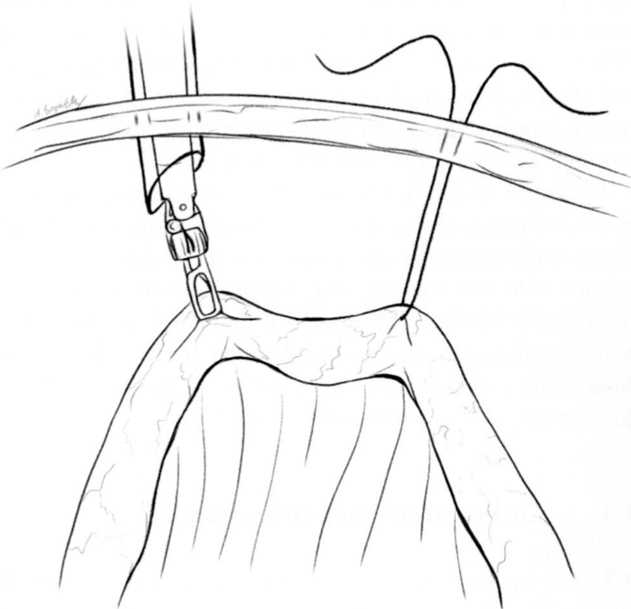

Fig. 2 Marionette stitch (Credit for Surgical Complications after Robot-Assisted Radical Cystectomy chapter, Techniques of Robotic Urinary Tract Reconstruction: A Complete Approach, 2021. Publisher: Springer. Editors: Michael Stifelman, Lee Zhao, Daniel Eun and Chester Koh)

Indocyanine green (ICG) can be injected, and the FireFly® technology may be used to ensure adequate blood supply of the bowel segment used for the conduit, as well as for the distal ureters. The bowel can be manipulated utilizing the fourth arm and the marionette stitch. The hook cautery (or the hot scissors) is used to develop two mesenteric windows in the mesentery while ensuring a wide base to maintain adequate blood flow to the conduit. An Endo GIA® stapler is used to divide the conduit from the rest of the ileum (Fig. 3).

- **Preparation of the Conduit and the Ureter**

A buttonhole enterotomy is made using scissors at the proximal end of the conduit (one or two enterotomies based on the ureteral reimplantation technique). Then, using the fourth arm to hold the Hem-o-lok® clip on the distal end of the clipped ureter, the ureter is spatulated generously (Fig. 4).

- **Uretero-Ileal Anastomosis**

The left ureter is crossed toward the right side through the sigmoid mesentery. Caution should be used to avoid twisting of the ureter. The direction of the Hem-o-lok clip on the distal end of the ureter can help maintain orientation. Excessive ureteral dissection should be avoided, and care should be taken to ensure enough periureteral tissue to maintain vascularity.

(a) Wallace Technique

Both ureters are aligned together using the fourth arm. The adjacent edges of the ureters are sutured together in a running side-to-side fashion to form the Wallace plate. This is followed by uretero-ileal anastomosis to a single enterotomy using 4/0 Vicryl® suture in a continuous (or interrupted) end-to-side fashion (Fig. 5).

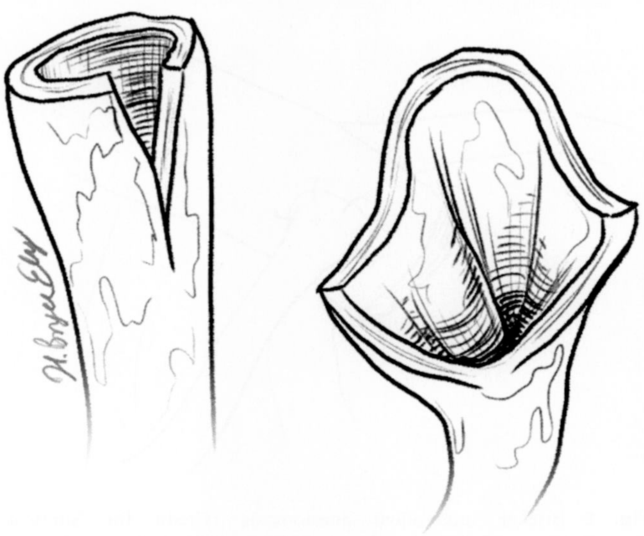

Fig. 4 Ureteral spatulation

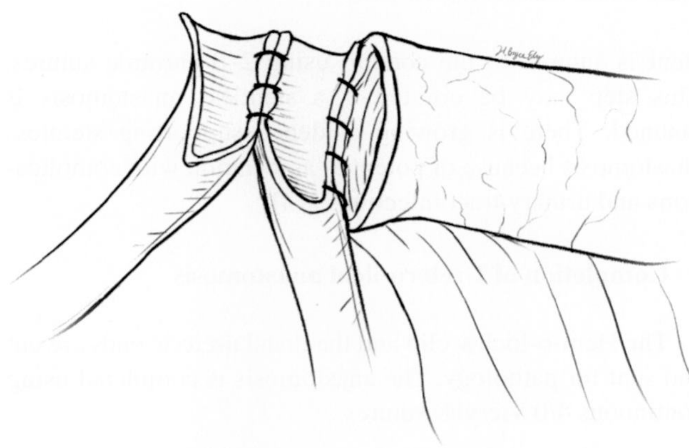

Fig. 5 Wallace ureteroileal anastomosis (Credit for Surgical Complications after Robot-Assisted Radical Cystectomy chapter, Techniques of Robotic Urinary Tract Reconstruction: A Complete Approach, 2021. Publisher: Springer. Editors: Michael Stifelman, Lee Zhao, Daniel Eun and Chester Koh)

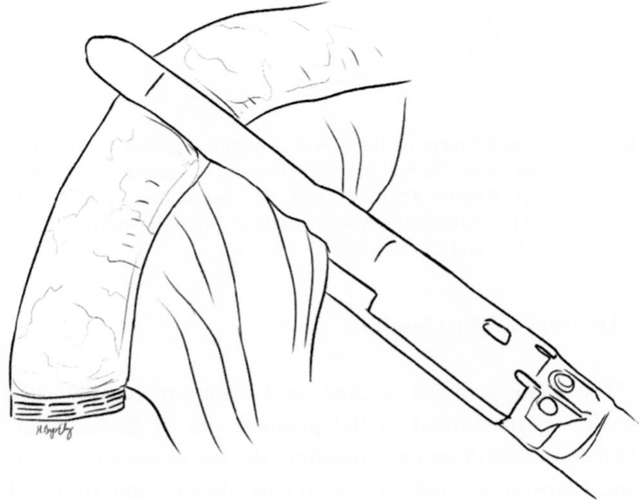

Fig. 3 Isolation of the conduit (Credit for Surgical Complications after Robot-Assisted Radical Cystectomy chapter, Techniques of Robotic Urinary Tract Reconstruction: A Complete Approach, 2021. Publisher: Springer. Editors: Michael Stifelman, Lee Zhao, Daniel Eun and Chester Koh)

(b) Bricker

Each ureter is sutured on its corresponding enterotomy on the conduit in an end-to-side fashion (Fig. 6).

Before completion of the uretero-ileal anastomosis, an 8.5 Fr single J stent or a feeding tube is passed. A metal laparoscopic suction tube is gently advanced through the distal enterotomy up to the anastomosis, guided by the robotic needle driver, to allow passage of stent into the ureter. The

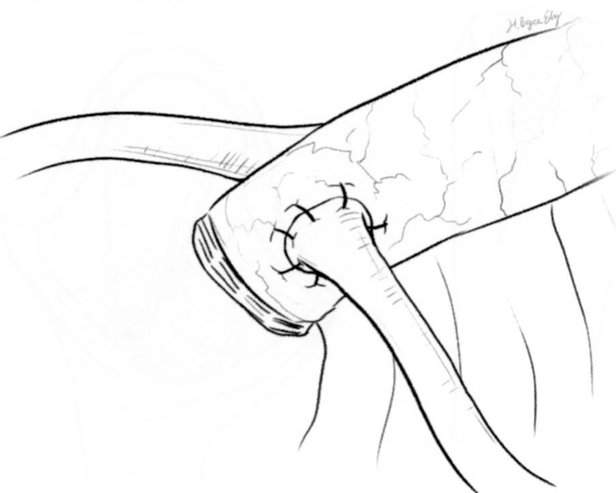

Fig. 6 Bricker ureteroileal anastomosis (Credit for Surgical Complications after Robot-Assisted Radical Cystectomy chapter, Techniques of Robotic Urinary Tract Reconstruction: A Complete Approach, 2021. Publisher: Springer. Editors: Michael Stifelman, Lee Zhao, Daniel Eun and Chester Koh)

stent is sutured to the conduit using 2–0 chromic sutures. This step may be omitted if a stentless anastomosis is planned. There is growing evidence supporting stentless anastomosis because of potential association with complications and urinary tract infections [14].

- **Completion of Uretero-ileal anastomosis**

The Hem-o-lock® clip and the distal ureteric ends are cut and sent for pathology. The anastomosis is completed using continuous 4/0 Vicryl® sutures.

- **Retroperitonealization of the Conduit**

The peritoneal fold adjacent to the conduit is used to cover the proximal end of the conduit and the uretero-ileal anastomosis (Fig. 7). We found this helpful to support the anastomosis, contain potential leakage, and prevent strictures.

- **Re-establishment of the Bowel Continuity**

An extra 15 mm short suprapubic port is placed. The fourth arm is used to approximate the two sides of the divided ileum together in a side-to-side fashion. Using the monopolar hook, two enterotomies are made on the proximal and distal ileal limbs. Ensuring that the anti-mesenteric sides of the bowel are properly aligned, two sequential side-to-side bowel re-anastomosis are performed using a 60 mm Endo GIA® stapler. This is followed by closure of the intestinal stump using another load applied transversely (Fig. 8). This is followed by closure of the mesenteric defect using silk sutures to avoid internal hernia.

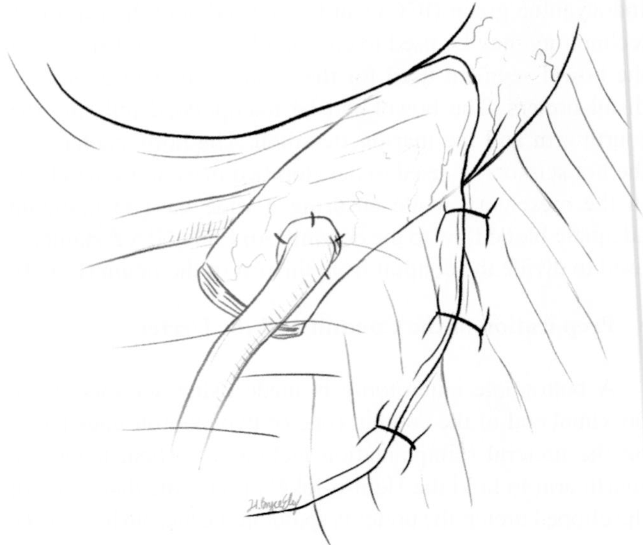

Fig. 7 Reperitonealization of the conduit (Credit for Surgical Complications after Robot-Assisted Radical Cystectomy chapter, Techniques of Robotic Urinary Tract Reconstruction: A Complete Approach, 2021. Publisher: Springer. Editors: Michael Stifelman, Lee Zhao, Daniel Eun and Chester Koh)

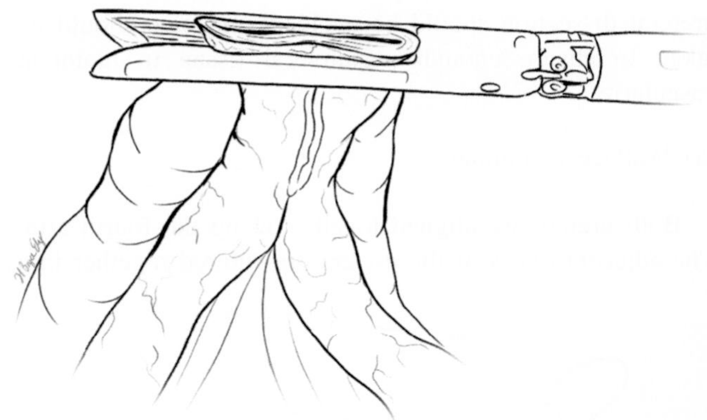

Fig. 8 Re-establishment of the bowel continuity (Credit for Surgical Complications after Robot-Assisted Radical Cystectomy chapter, Techniques of Robotic Urinary Tract Reconstruction: A Complete Approach, 2021. Publisher: Springer. Editors: Michael Stifelman, Lee Zhao, Daniel Eun and Chester Koh)

- **Delivery of the Conduit**

The robot remains docked, and a circumferential skin incision is performed in the planned site of the conduit. Dissection continues until reaching the rectus sheath. A cruciate incision is made in the rectus sheath, and four 3/0 Vicryl® anchoring sutures are placed at the corners of the cruciate incision. A clamp is introduced through the cruciate incision to grasp the marionette stitch and deliver the conduit through the rectus muscle to the skin surface. About five centimeters of the conduit are delivered above the skin surface. The conduit is anchored to the fascia using the stay suture. The conduit is everted and sutured to the skin by a series of four interrupted 3/0 Vicryl sutures, starting from the edge of the conduit, to the body of the conduit at the junction between the distal 2/3 and proximal 1/3, then finally to the skin. Simultaneous tightening of all the sutures everts the conduit. Lastly, the conduit edge is sutured to the skin surface. Drain is placed through one of the port sites, and a large hematuria catheter is left as a pelvic drain.

2.3 Technique of Intracorporeal W Neobladder

We have previously described our W neobladder technique [15]. In the current discussion, we will focus and highlight the modifications that we have adopted since then.

- **Stay Sutures and the W Configuration**

A 45 cm bowel segment is identified approximately 15–20 cm proximal to the ileocecal valve, and a W configuration is set up and maintained in place by stay sutures. There are four "limbs" of the W configuration, each two adjacent limbs make a "trough" for each side of the W. The most dependent parts of the right and left troughs are maintained in place with sutures to the Foley's catheter using 2/0 silk sutures. The catheter will act as a dynamic retractor until the neobladder-urethral anastomosis is performed (Fig. 9). The sutures maintain the W orientation and facilitate manipulation of the bowel and construction of the neobladder. They mark the end of the pouch and the beginning of the chimney on each side.

- **Detubularization of the Bowel**

The right trough is detubularized using hot scissors along the anti-mesenteric border. Detubularization can be done while providing traction using the assistant's laparoscopic suction device. One trough is opened at a time to avoid spillage of the intestinal contents and maintain orientation. Traction by the bedside assistant using the Foley catheter and by the fourth arm on the proximal trough sutures helps to stretch the bowel segment. The adjacent bowel edges of the detubularized right trough are sutured together in a running fashion using 3/0 V-Loc® sutures. Suturing is done in a continuous fashion with tightening every three throws. The same steps are repeated for the left trough (Fig. 10).

- **Construction of the Posterior Plate**

The right and left trough are sutured together in the midline to form the posterior plate of the neobladder (Fig. 11).

- **Neobladder-Urethral Anastomosis**

At this time, biopsy from the urethral end should be taken if not previously performed. The traction sutures are released

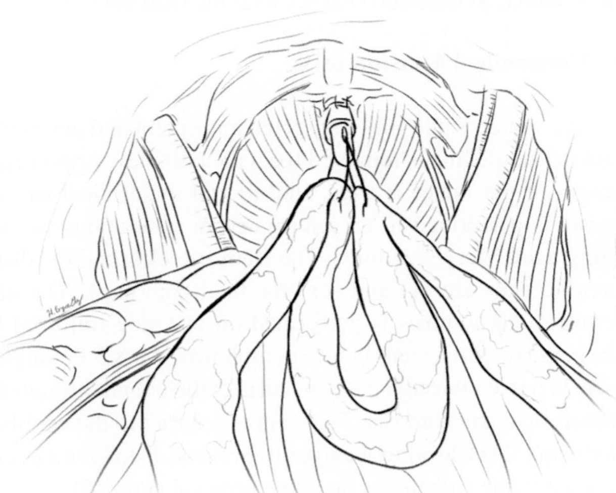

Fig. 9 Formation of W configuration (Credit for Surgical Complications after Robot-Assisted Radical Cystectomy chapter, Techniques of Robotic Urinary Tract Reconstruction: A Complete Approach, 2021. Publisher: Springer. Editors: Michael Stifelman, Lee Zhao, Daniel Eun and Chester Koh)

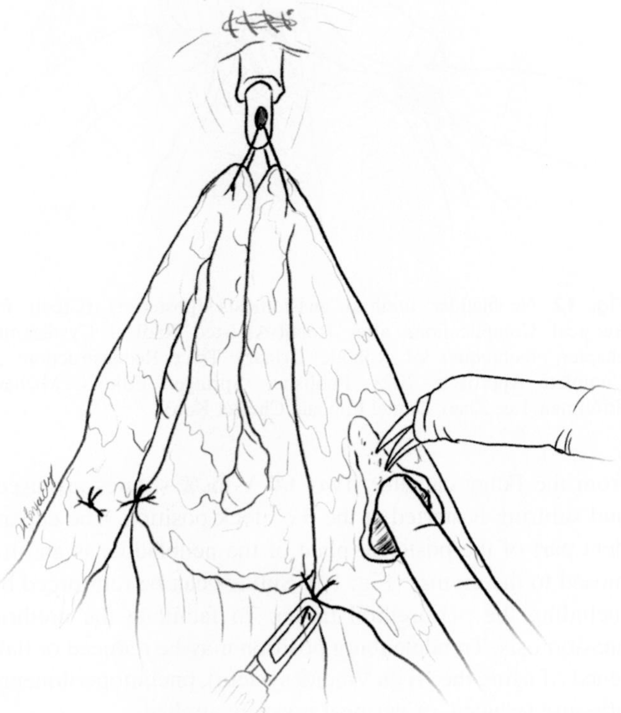

Fig. 10 Detubularization of the bowel

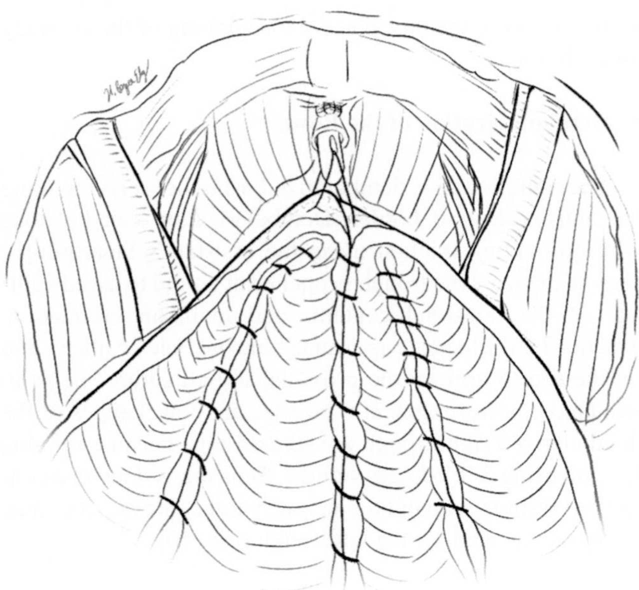

Fig. 11 Posterior plate of W neobladder (Credit for Surgical Complications after Robot-Assisted Radical Cystectomy chapter, Techniques of Robotic Urinary Tract Reconstruction: A Complete Approach, 2021. Publisher: Springer. Editors: Michael Stifelman, Lee Zhao, Daniel Eun and Chester Koh)

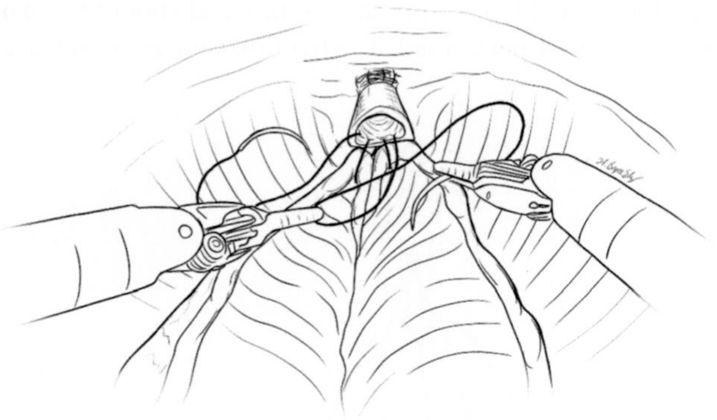

Fig. 12 Neobladder urethral anastomosis (posterior) (Credit for Surgical Complications after Robot-Assisted Radical Cystectomy chapter, Techniques of Robotic Urinary Tract Reconstruction: A Complete Approach, 2021. Publisher: Springer. Editors: Michael Stifelman, Lee Zhao, Daniel Eun and Chester Koh)

from the Foley catheter. Two 3/0 V-loc® sutures are used, and suturing is started at the 6 o'clock position. The dependent part of the posterior plate of the neobladder is anastomosed to the urethra (Fig. 12). Sutures can be reinforced by including the periurethral tissue. To facilitate the urethral anastomosis, Trendelenburg position may be reduced or flattened (if using the Xi da Vinci® system), pneumoperitoneum pressure reduced, or perineal pressure applied.

The urethral-neobladder sutures are continued anteriorly over a 22 Fr hematuria catheter until the 12 o'clock position, folding the right and left edges around the urethra. Suturing

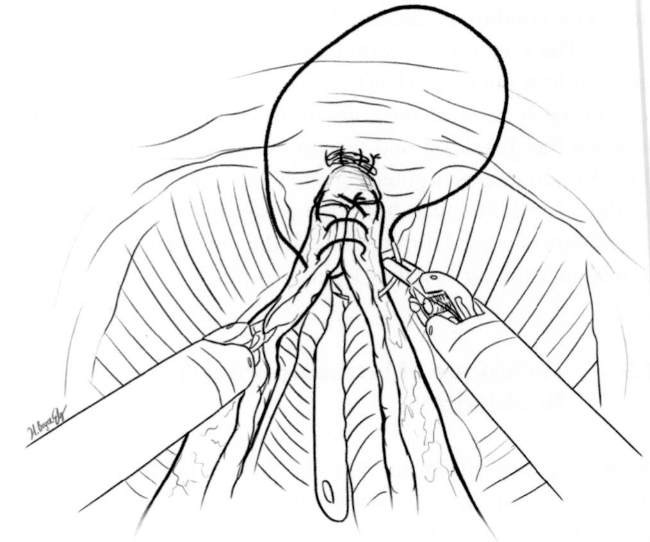

Fig. 13 Neobladder urethral anastomosis (anterior) (Credit for Surgical Complications after Robot-Assisted Radical Cystectomy chapter, Techniques of Robotic Urinary Tract Reconstruction: A Complete Approach, 2021. Publisher: Springer. Editors: Michael Stifelman, Lee Zhao, Daniel Eun and Chester Koh)

is completed, closing the caudal 2/3 of the anterior surface of the neobladder (Fig. 13).

- **Bowel Division**

Ten centimeters are left for each chimney proximal to the stay sutures. An Endo GIA® vascular stapler is used to divide the neobladder from the bowel on each side (Fig. 14). Bowel continuity can be restored now or after construction of the neobladder, as described earlier with the ileal conduit.

- **Ureteroileal Anastomosis**

The ureter is partially transected and spatulated anteriorly, and the staple line is removed from the chimney. Appropriate length of the ureter is used. End-to-end ureteroileal anastomosis is performed in an interrupted or continuous fashion using a 4/0 Vicryl® sutures. The Hem-o-lock® and the distal ureteric ends are cut and sent for final pathology. The ureteroileal anastomosis is performed on one side followed by the passage of the stent before completion. An 8.5 Fr single J stent is passed through the hematuria catheter and through the ureteroileal anastomosis. The stent is secured to the neobladder using 2/0 Chromic® catgut to prevent dislodgement and sutured to the catheter to facilitate removal (Fig. 15).

- **Closure of the Anterior Plate of the Neobladder**

The remaining suture from the anterior wall is lifted by the fourth arm. The rest of the anterior wall is closed like a "cigarette box," giving the neobladder a globular configuration (Fig. 16).

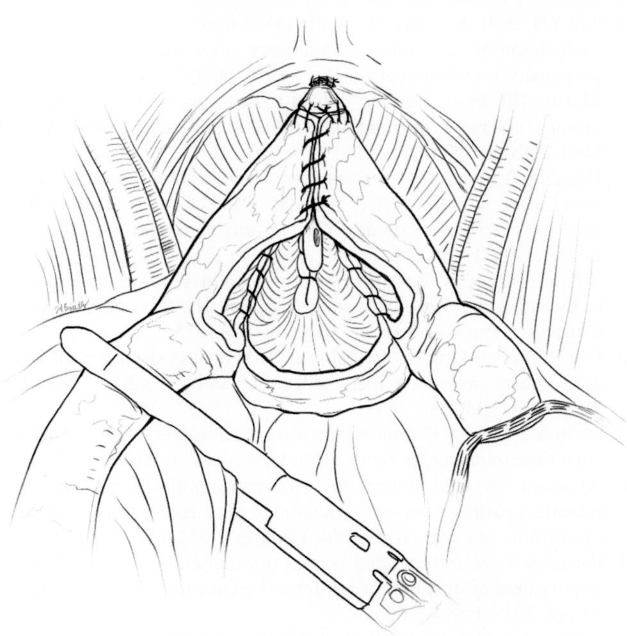

Fig. 14 Bowel division (Credit for Surgical Complications after Robot-Assisted Radical Cystectomy chapter, Techniques of Robotic Urinary Tract Reconstruction: A Complete Approach, 2021. Publisher: Springer. Editors: Michael Stifelman, Lee Zhao, Daniel Eun and Chester Koh)

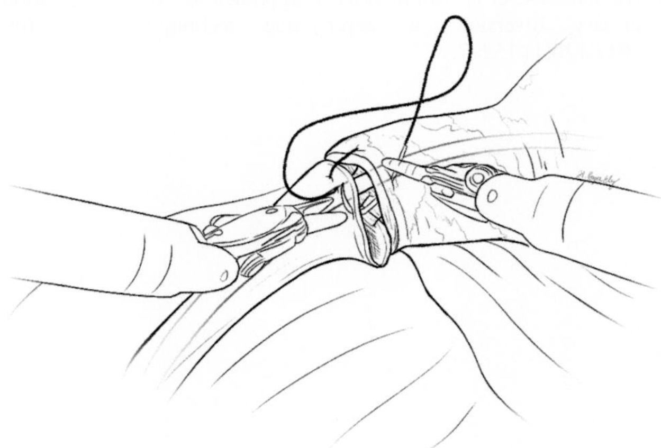

Fig. 15 Ureteroileal anastomosis (Credit for Surgical Complications after Robot-Assisted Radical Cystectomy chapter, Techniques of Robotic Urinary Tract Reconstruction: A Complete Approach, 2021. Publisher: Springer. Editors: Michael Stifelman, Lee Zhao, Daniel Eun and Chester Koh)

- **Omental Coverage**

The omentum is pulled and anchored to cover the anterior aspect of the neobladder without tension (Fig. 17). Drain is left to drain the pelvis.

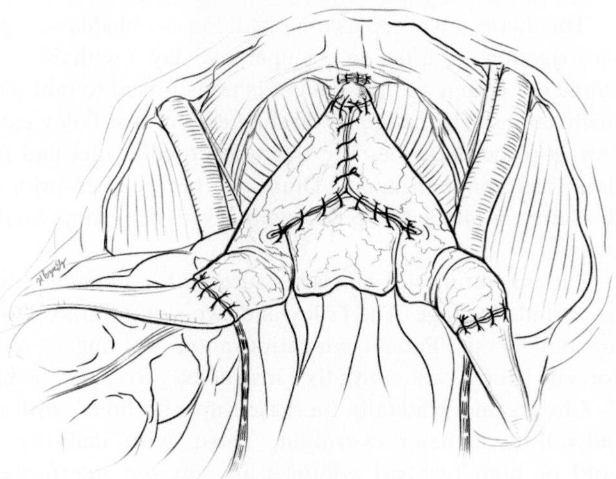

Fig. 16 Anterior plate of the neobladder (Credit for Surgical Complications after Robot-Assisted Radical Cystectomy chapter, Techniques of Robotic Urinary Tract Reconstruction: A Complete Approach, 2021. Publisher: Springer. Editors: Michael Stifelman, Lee Zhao, Daniel Eun and Chester Koh)

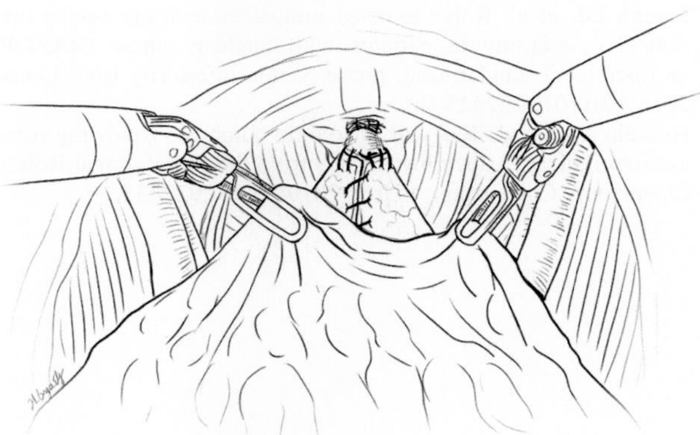

Fig. 17 Omental coverage (Credit for Surgical Complications after Robot-Assisted Radical Cystectomy chapter, Techniques of Robotic Urinary Tract Reconstruction: A Complete Approach, 2021. Publisher: Springer. Editors: Michael Stifelman, Lee Zhao, Daniel Eun and Chester Koh)

2.4 Postoperative Management

The patient is encouraged to ambulate on postoperative day 1 provided there are no contraindications. A clear liquid diet and prophylactic anticoagulation are started. For ileal conduits, Foley catheter is removed. For female patients, any vaginal packing is also removed. Daily complete blood count (CBC) and comprehensive metabolic panel (CMP) are drawn, and all lab values are trended and replaced as needed.

The diet is advanced as tolerated. For neobladders, regular irrigation is started on postoperative day 3 with 50 cc of saline q 8 hours, and the patient is transitioned to oral pain medications. The patient is discharged with the Foley catheter in place once they are tolerating regular diet and the drain has minimal output. Drain can be removed prior to discharge or on the first postoperative visit depending on the output.

Patients return 4 weeks after surgery for a pouchogram to exclude leakage. The Foley and two stents sutured to it are pulled out. Patient education about voiding is reinforced. They are initially instructed to void every 2–3 hours and gradually increased up to 5 hours with an indwelling catheter overnight. Those with inability to void or high residual volumes are advised intermittent self-catheterization.

References

1. Bochner BH, et al. Randomized trial comparing open radical cystectomy and robot-assisted laparoscopic radical cystectomy: oncologic outcomes. Eur Urol. 2018;74(4):465–71.
2. Parekh DJ, et al. Robot-assisted radical cystectomy versus open radical cystectomy in patients with bladder cancer (RAZOR): an open-label, randomised, phase 3, non-inferiority trial. Lancet. 2018;391(10139):2525–36.
3. Hussein AA, et al. Ten-year oncologic outcomes following robot-assisted radical cystectomy: results from the International Robotic Cystectomy Consortium. J Urol. 2019;202(5):927–35.
4. Tan YG, et al. Benefits of robotic cystectomy compared with open cystectomy in an enhanced recovery after surgery program: a propensity-matched analysis. Int J Urol. 2020;27(9):783–8.
5. Murthy PB, et al. Robotic radical cystectomy with intracorporeal urinary diversion: beyond the initial experience. Transl Androl Urol. 2020;9(2):942.
6. Hussein AA, et al. Outcomes of intracorporeal urinary diversion after robot-assisted radical cystectomy: results from the International Robotic Cystectomy Consortium. J Urol. 2018;199(5):1302–11.
7. Wilson TG, et al. Best practices in robot-assisted radical cystectomy and urinary reconstruction: recommendations of the Pasadena Consensus Panel. Eur Urol. 2015;67(3):363–75.
8. Lee RK, et al. Urinary diversion after radical cystectomy for bladder cancer: options, patient selection, and outcomes. BJU Int. 2014;113(1):11–23.
9. Melnyk M, et al. Enhanced recovery after surgery (ERAS) protocols: time to change practice? Can Urol Assoc J. 2011;5(5):342.
10. Aldhaam NA, et al. Impact of perioperative multidisciplinary rehabilitation pathway on early outcomes after robot-assisted radical cystectomy: a matched analysis. Urology. 2021;147:155–61.
11. Klaassen Z, et al. Extended venous thromboembolism prophylaxis after radical cystectomy: a call for adherence to current guidelines. J Urol. 2018;199(4):906–14.
12. Sroussi J, et al. Low pressure gynecological laparoscopy (7 mmHg) with AirSeal® System versus a standard insufflation (15 mmHg): a pilot study in 60 patients. J Gynecol Obstet Hum Reprod. 2017;46(2):155–8.
13. Ahmed YE, et al. Robot-assisted radical cystectomy in men: technique of spaces. J Endourol. 2018;32(S1):S-44–8.
14. Aldhaam NA, et al. Detailed analysis of urinary tract infections after robot-assisted radical cystectomy. J Endourol. 2021;35(1):62–70.
15. Hussein AA, et al. Robot-assisted approach to 'W'-configuration urinary diversion: a step-by-step technique. BJU Int. 2017;120(1):152–7.

Step-by-Step Approach to Extracorporeal Urinary Diversion in Robot-Assisted Cystectomy

Yasmeen Jaber, Timothy G. Wilson, and Kevin Chan

1 Introduction

Robot-assisted radical cystectomy (RARC) has established itself as a standard treatment for muscle invasive bladder cancer which to date has shown comparable perioperative and oncologic outcomes to the gold standard of open radical cystectomy [1–6]. The primary morbidity associated with radical cystectomy remains the urinary diversion [7]. Significant achievements in perioperative morbidity have been achieved in the recent past with the implementation of extended recovery after surgery protocols, cessation of mechanical bowel preparation, integration of Alvimopan, and restrictive deferred hydration [8–16].

However, future improvements in perioperative and functional outcomes with RARC will ultimately rest on our ability to refine and optimize urinary diversion [17–19]. Forward progress in urinary diversion requires techniques that are reproducible and achieve consistent evidence-based results. Extracorporeal urinary diversion (ECUD) in the setting of RARC was first described by Menon et al. and since inception has consistently demonstrated non-inferiority compared to the gold standard in prospective randomized controlled trials [1, 2, 20].

As it stands today, intracorporeal urinary diversion (ICUD) adds complexity to an already complex surgery [21]. Although some retrospective data suggest equivalence in skilled hands, with the potential for faster convalescence and decreased evaporative fluid losses, level one evidence has yet to be elucidated [21, 22]. It is also worth noting the importance of proficiency in multiple forms of urinary diversions. Proficiency in one, but not all forms, may lead to implicit bias during diversion counseling and determination, thus limiting patient options. This highlights the need for ECUD training for trainees. It is our belief that it is incumbent upon all practicing reconstructive urologists to be well versed and comfortable with ECUD.

Herein we will discuss important patient factors for diversion selection, provide a step-by-step approach to the different extracorporeal urinary diversions that may be performed in the setting of robot-assisted laparoscopic radical cystectomy (RARC), and report on specific risks, complication rates, and long-term data associated with each reconstruction technique. Specifically, we will discuss in detail the extracorporeal techniques of a Studer orthotopic neobladder, Indiana pouch continent cutaneous urinary diversion, and ileal conduit urinary diversion.

2 Perioperative Considerations

Oncologic indications for radical cystectomy include urothelial and non-urothelial carcinoma of the bladder with invasion into the muscularis propria, as well as high-risk, non-muscle invasive disease refractory to prior therapy. All patients should undergo appropriate cardiac and medical clearance. Patients must be physiologically able to tolerate pneumoperitoneum and prolonged Trendelenburg for the RARC.

The type of urinary tract reconstruction is determined after meticulous preoperative evaluation of the patient with particular interest in the patient's comorbidities, support system, dexterity, and neurologic status. An important component of the preoperative evaluation is a discussion regarding the patient's priorities and tolerance, both psychologically and physically, for potential complications. It is important that patients are counseled and demonstrate understanding of all potential risks and complications prior to surgery. Patients must also be informed that intraoperative findings may dictate a change in the planned form of urinary diversion. No randomized data exist regarding the superiority of one type of diversion over another, so oftentimes, in the absence of

Y. Jaber · K. Chan
City of Hope National Cancer Center Duarte, Duarte, CA, USA

T. G. Wilson (✉)
The St. John's Cancer Institute, Santa Monica, CA, USA

P. Wiklund et al. (eds.), *Robotic Urologic Surgery*, https://doi.org/10.1007/978-3-031-00363-9_62

absolute and relative contraindications, the diversion decision comes down to patient preferences and surgeon biases and experience.

Broadly, urinary diversions can be classified into incontinent, ileal or colonic conduits and continent, orthotopic, and cutaneous. Diversions using the anal sphincter as the continence mechanism are best served as historic reference and will not be discussed in this chapter. It is important to note that regardless of diversion selected lifelong follow-up is necessary for all patients [23, 24].

In this chapter, we describe the extracorporeal technique of the ileal conduit, the Studer orthotopic neobladder, and the Indiana pouch continent cutaneous urinary diversions. However, there are various other types of orthotopic and continent cutaneous urinary diversions that can easily be applied and translated to the extracorporeal techniques we describe. RARC is detailed in another chapter; however briefly we will touch on positioning, port placement, and broad robotic preparation.

3 Patient Positioning, Port Placement, and Robotic Preparation

The patient should be placed in the dorsal lithotomy or split-leg position when the da Vinci® standard, S, or Si robotic platform is employed. Male patients can remain in the supine position when the da Vinci® XI robotic platform is employed. An exaggerated Trendelenburg position is utilized to allow for adequate exposure of the pelvis and lower retroperitoneum. Care should be taken to adequately pad all pressure points, especially the posterior lower extremity, to avoid a peroneal nerve palsy.

Port placement is similar to that for robot-assisted laparoscopic radical prostatectomy, with the ports placed further cephalad to allow for a more extended lymph node dissection. Port placement can be varied according to surgeon preference.

Extracorporeal urinary diversion mirrors open surgical technique regardless of the type of urinary diversion being performed. However, in the setting of robotic cystectomy, there are maneuvers that can aid in allowing the incision to remain the size of the extraction site and optimize surgical efficiency by utilizing the advantages of robotics and laparoscopy for key portions of the operation.

During the RARC, the ureters are divided between two extra-large Weck Hem-o-lok® clips. The clips have a pre-tied 8-cm, dyed, or undyed suture to denote left and right. The clips are placed on the ureter through the right iliac 12-mm bedside assistant's port in a right to left orientation. This allows us to identify any twists in the ureter at the time of the ureteroileal anastomosis. The ureteral suture tags are placed aside, out of the operative field, during the completion of the cystectomy.

Once the cystectomy and lymph node dissection are complete, there are a number of final steps performed prior to undocking the robot. The left ureter is brought under the sigmoid mesentery by guiding the attached suture with a laparoscopic needle driver. At this time one may choose to use the Carter-Thomason® Suture Passer to pass a suture through the 12 mm assistant port in preparation for closure. The remaining diversion-specific preparatory steps will be discussed further in the respective sections later within the chapter.

4 Ileal Conduit Extracorporeal Urinary Diversion

The primary goal in selecting a urinary diversion is to minimize the potential for, perioperative and oncologic, complications while maximizing quality of life. The decision process warrants careful consideration of issues related to cancer stage, comorbidities, age, and patient desires. The ileal conduit is the least complicated diversion. The relative simplicity enables less time under anesthesia and decreased postoperative complications. As a result, the ileal conduit has largely become the default diversion and primary choice for patients with contraindications to continent diversion.

5 Robotic Preparation

As discussed previously, the left ureter is transposed to the right abdomen through the sigmoid mesenteric window. Both ureters remain clipped and tagged as described above. An additional identification tag, using 2–0 silk, is placed through the terminal ileum. We then use a laparoscopic needle driver, through the assistant port, to take hold of the three tags. The needle driver remains intracorporeal and is secured to the drape with a peon. This allows for all three components to be readily available for the urinary diversion. The robotic instruments are then removed, and the robot is undocked.

6 Ileal Harvest

Several sites can be used for the specimen extraction and subsequent extracorporeal urinary tract reconstruction including periumbilical midline (incorporating the camera port), infraumbilical midline, Pfannestiel, and McBurney (incorporating right-sided port site for ileal conduits) [25]. We routinely use a 6-cm midline incision just below the umbilicus (Fig. 1). With the abdomen still insufflated, we open the rectus fascia and peritoneum. The insufflation is turned off, and the specimen is extracted using an Endo Catch™ II 15-mm specimen pouch (Covidien, Mansfield, MA). A wound retractor is then placed to aid in exposure. One may opt to use an Alexis wound retractor (Applied Medical, Rancho Santa Margarita, CA) or a CleanCision™ (Prescient Surgical, San Carlos, CA) (Fig. 2). The sutures for the right ureter, left ureter, and terminal ileum are delivered through the incision with the aid of the laparoscopic needle driver. The ureters are then placed in their correct anatomic orientation, using both visual and manual evaluation to check for twisting or crossing of the ureters.

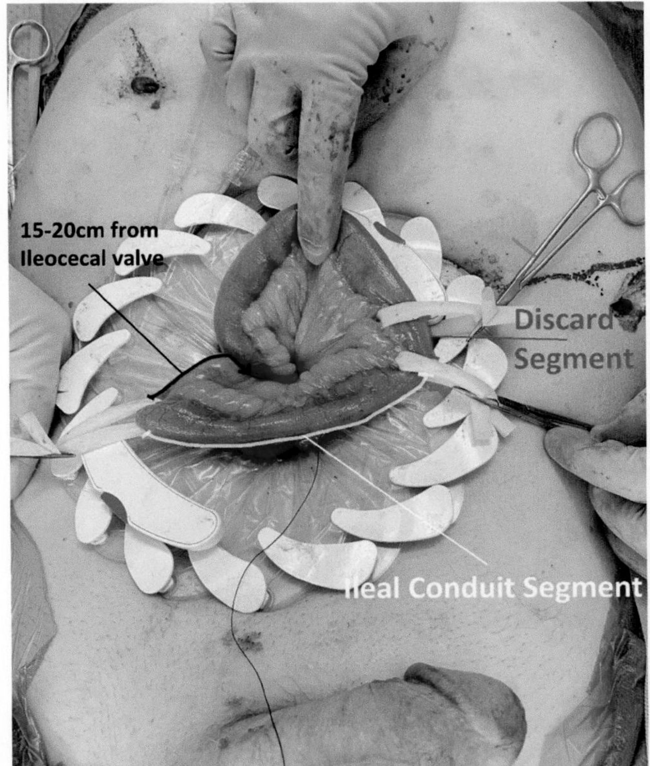

Fig. 1 This picture shows the midline incision just below the umbilicus with a CleanCision™ wound retractor. The ileal segment is brought through the incision, and the ileal harvest measurements are completed. The Penrose drains demarcate the ileal segment to be used as well as the discard segment

At this point it is our practice to complete real-time indocyanine green angiography using the PINPOINT fluorescence imaging platform (Stryker Corp., Kalamazoo, MI, USA, previously Novadaq, Mississauga, ON, Canada) to assess ureteral perfusion. With the assistance of our anesthesia colleagues, 3 ml of ICG, followed by 10 ml of saline, is administered intravenously. After approximately 30–45 seconds, a perfusion assessment is performed using the PINPOINT® Fluorescence Imaging System. The imaging displays ICG photon emission detected in the tissue. Dark images result from low photon emission indicating poor perfusion, while bright imaging results from abundant photon emission indicating good perfusion. A suture is then used to mark the distal-most extent of ureteral perfusion for each ureter (Fig. 3). Eventually, the ureter will be divided proximal to this suture to ensure adequate blood supply to the anastomosis. It is important to note that ICG perfusion assessment is best done prior to dividing the bowel for the urinary diversion. This allows for tailoring of the bowel segment length in situations where a large portion of ureter needs to be excised due to poor perfusion [26].

After the ureteral perfusion assessment, the ileum is identified with the assistance of the 2–0 silk tag and brought through the incision. The terminal ileum is then stapled and divided using a GIA stapler approximately 15 cm proximal to the ileocecal valve (Fig. 1). The mesentery at this location is divided for approximately 8–10 cm at the plane of Treves. This can be performed with the LigaSure device or suture ligations of crossing mesenteric vessels, using 3–0 silk sutures. A segment of ileum is then measured to create the

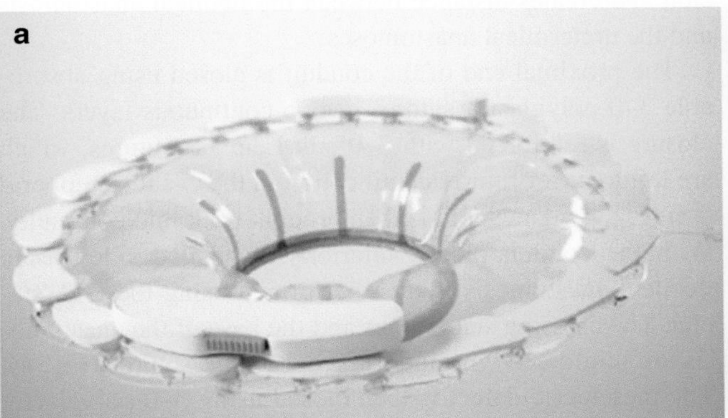

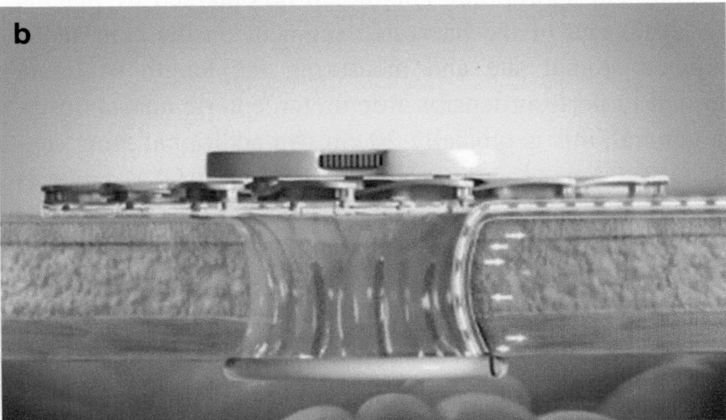

Fig. 2 (**a**) Image of antibiotic wound protector. (**b**) Cross-sectional image of antibiotic wound protector inside wound. Antibiotic flows from superficial to deep portions of the wound (dotted white line)

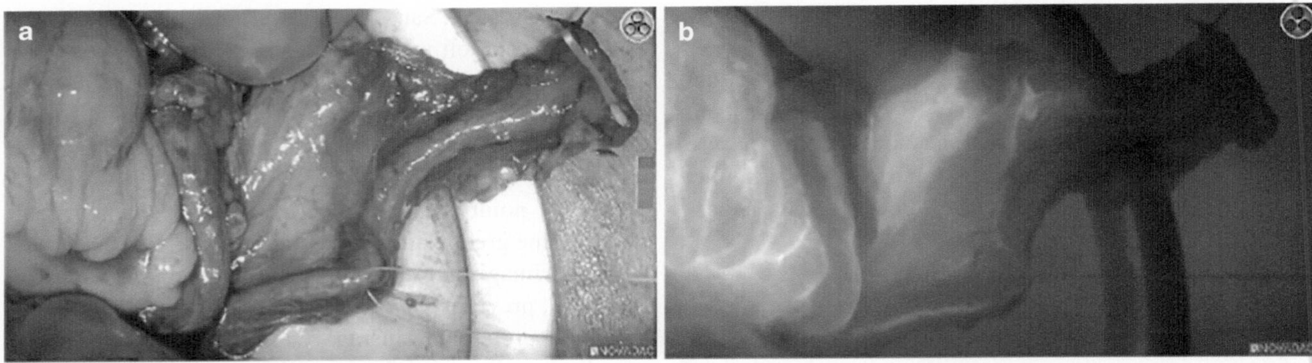

Fig. 3 Evaluation of ureteral perfusion using ICG and Novadaq platform. A suture is placed to mark the ureter where we identified the margin of good perfusion. (**a**) White luminescence demonstrates flow. (**b**) Blue coloration indicates good perfusion

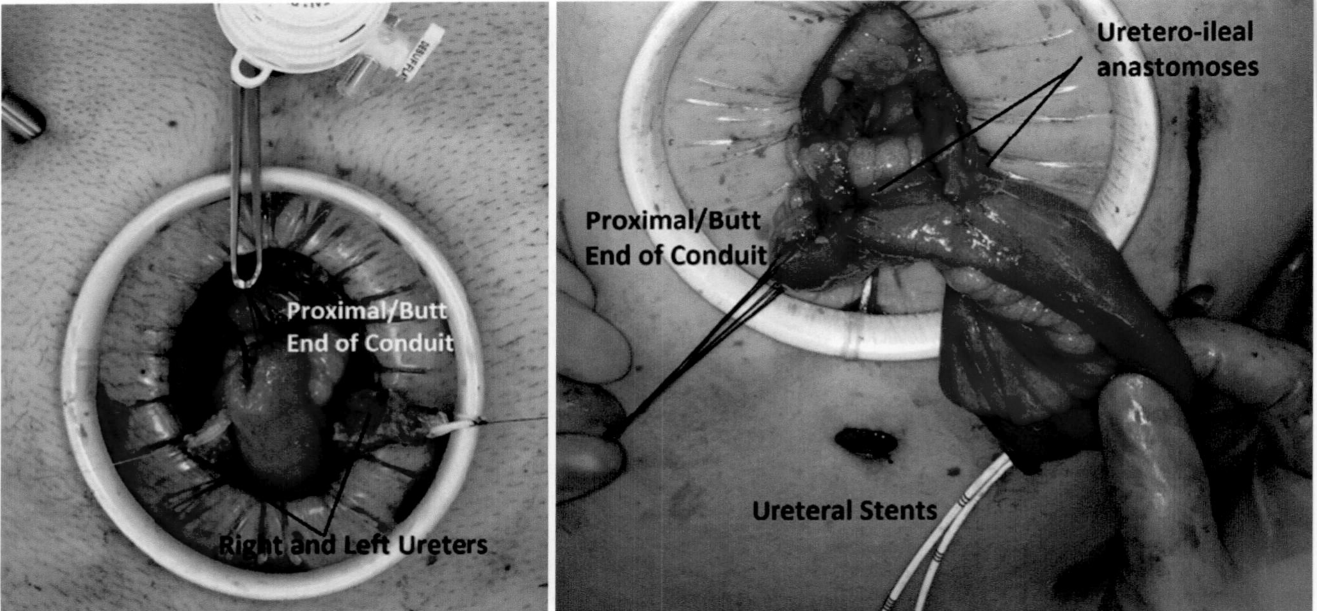

Fig. 4 The proximal conduit can be seen with the silk Lembert sutures. The ureters can be seen with Weck clips prior to anastomoses on the left and just after anastomoses on the right. Ureteral stents are seen exiting the stomal end of conduit

conduit. An appropriate length can be obtained by placing the distal end of the harvested segment on the skin at the planned stomal site and measuring the length of ileum needed to perform tension-free ureteroenteric anastomoses. In general, this is typically 20 cm. An additional 5-cm segment of ileum is then marked for excision. A GIA stapler is used to staple and divide the ileal segment at the determined distal and proximal ends. The stapled proximal and distal ileal segments are tagged with a 3–0 silk. These silk tags assist in alignment during the side-to-side ileoileal anastomosis. Using Bovie electrocautery, the proximal 5-cm discard segment is then excised and discarded (Fig. 1). This 5-cm discard serves two purposes. It reduces mesenteric tension and creates distance between the ileoileal anastomosis and the ureteroileal anastomoses.

The proximal end of the conduit is closed using absorbable 3–0 polyglactin sutures in two continuous layers. The closure is reinforced with 3–0 silk Lembert sutures, which are left long for future identification in the event of reoperation (Fig. 4). The ileum is then brought back into continuity. With the conduit placed inferiorly, a stapled side-to-side ileoileal anastomosis is then performed using the GIA stapler. The crossing staple lines and the base of the anastomosis are reinforced with interrupted 3–0 silk sutures (Fig. 4). The mesenteric defect is then closed using 3–0 polyglactin suture in continuous fashion.

7 Ureteroileal Anastomoses

For the left ureter, a small enterotomy is made sharply adjacent to the proximal end of the conduit using Metzenbaum scissors. The mucosal edges are then everted using 4–0 chromic sutures in the four quadrants of the enterotomy. The left ureter is then brought adjacent to the planned anastomosis site. The excess ureter is excised proximal to the tag placed during ICG and sent as a final specimen. The ureteroileal anastomosis is then performed in end-to-side, spatulated fashion using interrupted or continuous 4–0 polyglactin or monofilament absorbable suture (Fig. 4). Halfway through a single-J urinary diversion stent is placed across the ureteroileal anastomosis and brought out the distal end of the conduit. The remaining anastomotic stitches are subsequently completed. Care should be taken to create a watertight anastomosis with a no touch technique. The procedure is then replicated for the right ureteroenteric anastomosis.

8 Ileal Conduit Stoma Creation

A circle of skin approximately 2.5 cm in diameter is excised at the previously marked planned stoma site. The subcutaneous tissue is divided using cautery, and a cruciate incision is made in the anterior rectus fascia. The peritoneum is then incised. To avoid strangulation of the conduit, the fascial incision should be wide enough to accommodate two fingerbreadths. If the small bowel mesentery is compliant, a rosebud stoma can be created, but if the small bowel mesentery is shortened and noncompliant, a modified Turnbull stoma should be created.

For a rosebud stoma, the distal end of the conduit is brought through the incision with the mesentery along the superior aspect. The conduit is secured to the fascia at four locations using a 0 polyglactin suture through a seromuscular layer of the conduit. The distal staple line is then excised. The stoma is then matured using 2–0 polyglactin sutures through the distal edge of the stoma, then through the seromuscular layer of the conduit at the level of the skin, and then lastly through the dermis. The stomal mucosa is everted as these sutures are tightened. The intervening gaps can then be filled in with additional 2–0 polyglactin sutures (Fig. 5). For a modified Turnbull stoma, a segment of conduit several centimeters proximal to the distal end is brought through the incision. The conduit is secured to the fascia at four locations using 0 polyglactin suture through a seromuscular layer. A semilunar incision is then created through the conduit, and the stoma is then matured at the functional limb using 2–0 polyglactin sutures as described above.

A red Robinson catheter is placed into the conduit and secured at the stomal level, along with the two ureteral stents.

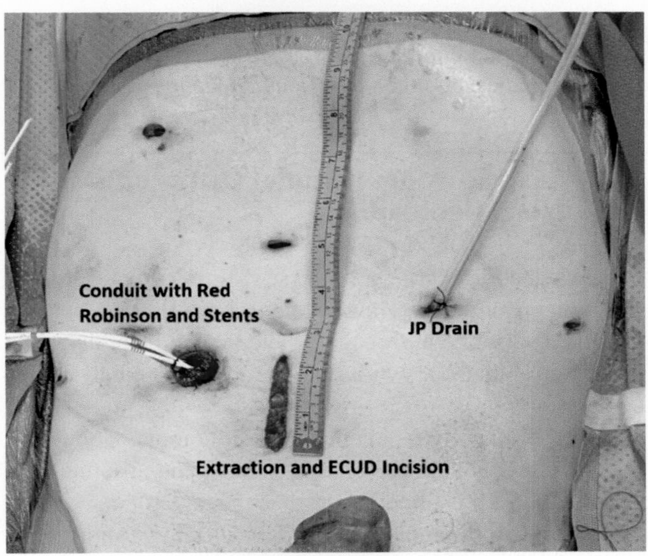

Fig. 5 The 6-cm extraction and ECUD incision are shown here. The stoma can be seen with the Robinson catheter secured at the stomal level, along with the two ureteral stents. A 19-Fr round Blake drain is then placed through the left pararectus port site

A 19-Fr round Blake drain is then placed through the left pararectus port site, traversing the pelvis and ending adjacent to the ureteroileal anastomoses at the proximal end of the conduit (Fig. 5). The incisions are irrigated thoroughly. The fascia and skin are then closed at the midline incision, and all port sites are closed. A urostomy appliance is placed over the stoma and placed to gravity drainage.

9 Postoperative Care

The hospital stay typically ranges from 5 to 7 days. An ERAS protocol is followed with early oral feeding and minimal narcotic administration. Prior to stent removal a JP creatinine is obtained. In the absence of concern for urinary leak, the stents and red Robinson catheter are removed once the patient is unequivocally tolerating a diet and experiencing return of bowel function. Typically, this occurs between postoperative days 4–6. The drain is removed when the output is less than 600 mL/24 h.

10 Ileal Conduit-Specific Complications

The ileal conduit is the default diversion for patients with significant medical comorbidities. The greater prevalence of morbidity in these patients leads to a rate of surgical complications that approaches that of the continent diversions performed in healthier patients. The most common complications reported are pyelonephritis, ureteric obstruction, urinary calculi, and stomal complications [27]. Metabolic and absorptive aberrancies are much less frequent [23].

11 Extracorporeal Studer Orthotopic Ileal Neobladder

Patient selection is critical to the success of orthotopic, continent diversions. The primary goal is always cancer control, and the decision to pursue an orthotopic continent diversion should not interfere with the curative potential of the surgery.

When evaluating a patient for an orthotopic neobladder, one must take into consideration relative and absolute contraindications. It is important to note that age is not a contraindication to orthotopic neobladder diversion. Appropriate physical and cognitive capacity is imperative. This is true not only for orthotopic neobladders but also for all continent diversions. Unlike conduit diversions, all continent diversions require active patient participation and understanding to ensure proper maintenance and use. If hindrances to participation exist, such as limited dexterity and understanding, a continent diversion should not be undertaken.

In conjunction with physical and mental impairment, absolute contraindications for continent diversions include impaired renal and hepatic function. Patients with impairment in renal and hepatic function are at risk for reabsorption of urinary waste products including creatinine, urea, and ammonia. These waste products are subsequently absorbed by the intestinal segment and enter systemic circulation, increasing the burden on renal and hepatic clearance. This increased metabolic burden can potentiate the preexisting impairment.

The final absolute contraindication to an orthotopic neobladder is urethral disease. This includes urethral dysfunction as well as malignant involvement [23, 28].

12 Robotic Preparation

Several key steps performed with the robot still docked facilitate an expeditious creation of the orthotopic urinary diversion. As discussed previously, the left ureter is transposed to the right abdomen through the sigmoid mesenteric window. Both ureters remain clipped and tagged as described above. An additional identification tag, using 2–0 silk, is placed on the terminal ileum.

During the RARC as the urethra is divided, we place a 9-in. 2–0 Vicryl™ (Ethicon, New Brunswick, NJ) suture at the 6 o'clock position of the urethra. This suture serves as the initial ureteral stitch in the urethral anastomosis. The needle remains intracorporeally, in the periosteum of the pubic bone, so that it can be easily found when the robot is redocked for the anastomosis.

Once the cystectomy and lymph node dissection are complete, a 16-Fr red Robinson catheter, with an 8-cm 0 silk suture pre-tied to the end, is placed in the urethra. The red Robinson catheter will assist in bringing the assembled neobladder down into the pelvis later in the case. The two ureteral sutures, the ileal suture, and the red Robinson suture are then placed into the assistant's laparoscopic needle driver by the console surgeon. The needle driver remains intracorporeal and is secured to the drape with a peon. This allows all four components to be readily available and identifiable for the urinary diversion when the robot is undocked, and the infraumbilical midline incision is opened. The robotic instruments are removed, the ports are kept in place, and the robot is undocked. The ports will be utilized later when the robot is re-docked for the urethral anastomosis.

13 Ileal Harvest and Neobladder Formation

The robot is undocked but kept sterile to be used later for the urethral anastomosis. The insufflation is turned off, and all port sites are kept in place. The patient remains in Trendelenburg position to keep the small bowel out of the way during the neobladder construction.

As discussed above, one may choose from a variety of incision types. We prefer to use a 7-cm midline infraumbilical incision for extracorporeal Studer neobladders, as this is the shortest length that accommodates a constructed neobladder. After the rectus fascia and peritoneum are opened, the specimen is extracted using an Endo Catch™ II 15-mm specimen pouch (Covidien, Mansfield, MA). A wound retractor is then placed to aid in exposure. The sutures for the right ureter, left ureter, terminal ileum, and red Robinson are delivered through the incision with the aid of the laparoscopic needle driver. The ureters are then placed in their correct anatomic orientation, using both visual and manual evaluation to check for twisting or crossing of the ureters. At this point it is our practice to complete real-time indocyanine green angiography using the PINPOINT fluorescence imaging platform (Stryker Corp., Kalamazoo, MI, USA, previously Novadaq, Mississauga, ON, Canada) to assess ureteral perfusion as discussed above (Fig. 3).

After the ureteral perfusion assessment, the ileum is identified with the assistance of the 2–0 silk tag and brought through the incision. The terminal ileum is then stapled and divided using a GIA stapler approximately 15 cm proximal to the ileocecal valve. The mesentery at this location is divided for approximately 8–10 cm at the plane of Treves.

A 60-cm segment of ileum is then measured to create the neobladder (Fig. 6).

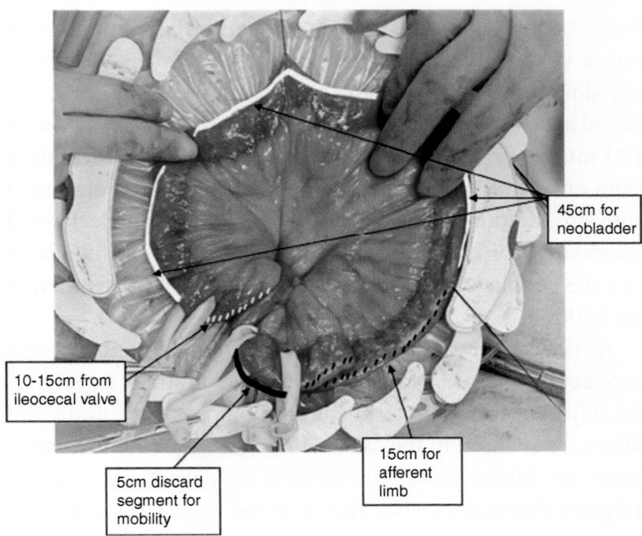

Fig. 6 Ileal segment for Studer Pouch neobladder

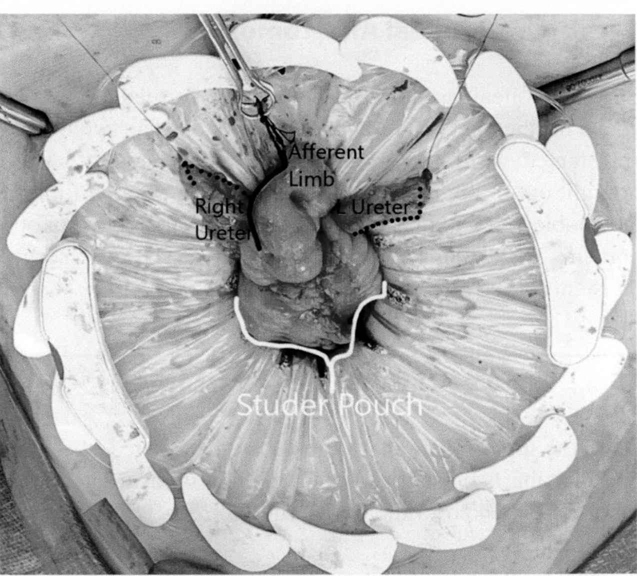

Fig. 7 Neobladder constructed with bilateral ureters adjacent to afferent limb where they will be anastomosed

An additional 5-cm segment of ileum is then marked for later excision. A GIA stapler is then used to staple and divide the ileal segment at the determined distal and proximal ends. The stapled proximal and distal ileal segments that are to be anastomosed are tagged with a 3–0 silk. These silk tags assist in alignment during the side-to-side ileoileal anastomosis. Using Bovie electrocautery, the proximal 5-cm discard segment is then excised from the diversion segment of ileum. As with the ileal conduit, this 5-cm discard serves to reduce mesenteric tension and create distance between the end of the afferent limb of the neobladder and the ileoileal anastomosis.

The proximal end of the neobladder is closed in two running layers using absorbable 3–0 polyglactin suture. The closure is reinforced with 3–0 silk Lembert sutures, which are left long for future identification in the event of reoperation. The ileum is then brought back into continuity. With the ileal segment to be used for the neobladder placed inferiorly, a stapled side-to-side bowel anastomosis is then performed using the GIA stapler. The crossing staple lines and the base of the anastomosis are reinforced with interrupted 3–0 silk sutures. The mesenteric defect is then closed using 3–0 polyglactin suture in continuous fashion.

The most proximal 15-cm of ileum from the neobladder segment is marked and delineated as the afferent limb. The remaining 45 cm of ileum from the neobladder segment is then detubularized using cautery along the antimesenteric edge. The detubularized segment is then placed in a U-shaped configuration, and the medial edges are sewn together using continuous 3–0 polyglactin sutures.

These sutures should be placed in close enough proximity to ensure a watertight closure, incorporating a larger seromuscular bite and a smaller mucosal bite to allow for adequate inversion of the mucosa. The pouch is then folded on itself in Heineke-Mikulicz fashion, and the remaining edges are sewn to close the pouch using 3–0 polyglactin suture, with the same technique as described above (Fig. 7).

Once the pouch is completed, two 0 polyglactin sutures, one dyed and one undyed, are used to mark the 6 o'clock and 12o'clock positions, relative to the anticipated anastomotic location on the neobladder. A figure of eight suture is utilized at the 6 o'clock to allow for traction to be placed on this suture to aid in the urethral anastomosis. These stitches will be used to orient the console surgeon robotically and will also serve as handles for the console surgeon's fourth arm. An additional polyglactin suture is used to secure the neobladder and the tip of the urethral red Robinson catheter. This stitch will act as a handle for the bedside assistant later in the case. It is important to note that the neovesical-urethral anastomotic location is not committed to until the robot is re-docked and the neobladder has been brought down to the pelvis. Once the neobladder has been brought into the pelvis, one should evaluate lie, exposure, and point of minimal tension. All three factors should be considered when determining the location on the pouch for the urethral anastomosis.

The neobladder is then placed into the pelvis with only the afferent limb and bilateral ureters exposed at the infraumbilical midline incision (Fig. 7) in preparation for the ureteroileal anastomoses.

14 Ureteroileal Anastomoses

The ureteroileal anastomoses are then performed as detailed above for the ileal conduit urinary diversion. The two ureters are stented with single-J urinary diversion stents that are brought out through a 1-mm incision in the afferent limb of the neobladder and placed beside the right pararectus robotic port site. A 3–0 plain gut purse-string suture is used to secure the stents at the afferent limb.

15 Neovesical-Urethral Anastomosis

Once the ureteroileal anastomoses are completed, the midline incision is closed, and the abdomen is insufflated. The robot is re-docked to the ports, and the robotic instruments are replaced.

The redundant sigmoid colon is moved out of the pelvis, and the neobladder is then brought down toward the pelvis by the console surgeon using the pre-placed suture handles and the fourth arm. The assistant can aid in the maneuver by placing gentle traction on the red Robinson catheter attached to the 6 o'clock position of the neobladder.

The posterior urethral plate reconstruction is then performed in similar fashion to a Rocco reconstruction [29]. First, the musculofascial plate of the rectourethralis is approximated to the cut edge of Denonvilliers' fascia in figure-of-eight fashion using 9 inch 3–0 V-Loc absorbable suture. The needle is kept on the suture for the second part of the Rocco reconstruction. The neobladder is then brought down to the pelvis by applying gentle traction on the red Robinson catheter and the 6 o'clock suture of the neobladder. Once in the pelvis, the neobladder is held in place using the robotic fourth arm and the 6 o'clock suture. Care should be taken to ensure that the fourth arm is not resting in such a way that it compresses the external iliac vessels.

Next, the musculofascial plate of the rectourethralis is approximated to the posterior neobladder, approximately 2 cm posterior to the planned urethral aperture, using 3–0 V-Loc suture still attached to the first part of the Rocco reconstruction.

The suture on the red Robinson catheter is cut, and this catheter is removed. The urethral aperture is then created sharply or with cautery using the cutting current.

The previously placed 3–0 polyglactin 6 o'clock posterior urethral stitch is then utilized to reapproximate the posterior urethral plate to the neobladder aperture. If tension is appreciated when tying this stich down, additional interrupted sutures can be used to reapproximate the posterior urethral plate. Two 3–0 absorbable barbed sutures that are looped together are then brought in and are placed in the neobladder neck on each side of the 3–0 polyglactin suture and then in their corresponding location in the posterior urethra. Each suture is used to complete the urethra-neovesical anastomosis, along each side up to the 12 o'clock position. The completed anastomosis is tested by irrigating the neobladder with 120 ml of normal saline. Any visible area of extravasation from either the neobladder or the anastomosis is reinforced with an additional 3–0 Vicryl™ or 3–0 absorbable barbed sutures. A new two-way 18-Fr hematuria catheter is placed into the neobladder, and 15 mL of sterile water is instilled in the balloon.

A 19-Fr round Blake drain is brought through the left pararectus port site and placed along the urethral anastomosis, adjacent to the ureteroileal anastomoses. The drain and stents are secured to the skin. The remaining robotic instruments are removed, and the robot is undocked. All ports are irrigated thoroughly. The fascia at the 12-mm robotic port site is closed. All remaining skin incisions are closed. The stents are cut approximately 5 cm, and an ostomy appliance is placed over them.

16 Postoperative Care

The hospital stay typically ranges from 5 to 7 days. An ERAS protocol is followed with early oral feeding and minimal narcotic administration. Prior to stent removal a JP creatinine is obtained. In the absence of concern for urinary leak, the stents and red Robinson catheter are removed once the patient is unequivocally tolerating a diet and experiencing return of bowel function. Typically this occurs between postoperative days 4–6. The drain is removed when the output is less than 600 mL/24 h. The neobladder Foley catheter is hand-irrigated every 4 h and kept in place for 3 weeks. A cystogram is performed to ensure no leakage before catheter removal. Patients are taught clean intermittent catheterization at their catheter removal visit and instructed to perform timed catheterizations if retention is suspected until residuals are consistently minimal.

17 Orthotopic Neobladder-Specific Complications

Continent orthotopic urinary diversions involve multiple suture lines and longer operative times than ileal conduits. As such, they are subject to a higher incidence of urinary leaks, fecal leak, prolonged ileus, and wound infection in the early postoperative period. Similarly, any continent reservoir is at greater risk of rupture than an incontinent diversion [23]. Other orthotopic neobladder-specific complications include hypercontinence, incontinence, and ureteral anastomotic stricture. Generally, continence rates in the literature vary but with a general trend toward higher continence rates in experienced hands. In fact, some institutions have reported daytime continence rates greater than 90% and nocturnal continence rates greater than 80% [30].

The corollary complication is hypercontinence after orthotopic neobladder. Urinary retention, and the need for intermittent catheterization, is more frequently seen in females with orthotopic neobladders. It is believed that this hypercontinence is due in part to posterior prolapse of the neobladder [31].

Lastly, specific to all continent diversions is the increased risk of resorptive metabolic derangements due to prolonged urinary dwell times.

18 Extracorporeal Indiana Pouch Urinary Diversion

Continent cutaneous urinary diversion remains an important option for those patients who are not candidates for orthotopic urinary diversion due to urethral disease. Aside from the urethral contraindications, the requirements and contraindications for cutaneous continent diversions are much the same as that discussed for orthotopic neobladders.

Appropriate physical and cognitive capacity is imperative as continent cutaneous diversions require active patient participation and understanding to ensure proper maintenance and use. Specifically, the ability and willingness to perform regimented timed intermittent catheterization is mandatory. If hindrances to participation exist, such as limited dexterity and understanding, a continent diversion should not be undertaken.

19 Robotic and Laparoscopic Preparation

As discussed previously the left ureter is transposed to the right abdomen through the sigmoid mesenteric window. Both ureters remain clipped and tagged as described above. The sutures on the two ureters are secured with a laparoscopic needle driver that is in the right iliac port. At this point, the robot is undocked, and the patient is positioned flat, with the right side up. An 8 cm incision is made for specimen extraction, and the specimen is extracted as detailed above. Using the existing port configuration, a hand-assist gel port and Alexis wound retractor (Applied Medical, Rancho Santa Margarita, CA) are placed in the extraction incision. The abdomen is re-insufflated and hand-assisted, and laparoscopic mobilization of the right colon is then performed. Using monopolar shears, the ascending colon is then mobilized by continuing the peritoneal incision lateral to the colon along the white line of Toldt. The colon and colonic mesentery are then dissected medially. The hepatic flexure is taken down using cautery. This mobilization is continued to the mid transverse colon.

20 Ileocolonic Harvest

After the right colon mobilization, the abdomen is desufflated, and the gel port is removed. The Alexis wound retractor is kept in place for exposure. The sutures for the left ureter and right ureter are delivered through the incision. At this point it is our practice to complete real-time indocyanine green angiography using the PINPOINT fluorescence imaging platform to assess ureteral perfusion as discussed above (Fig. 3).

After the ureteral perfusion assessment, the ileum is identified and then stapled and divided using a GIA stapler, approximately 15 cm proximal to the ileocecal valve. The mesentery at this location is divided for approximately 8–10 cm at the plane of Treves.

A 31-cm segment of ascending colon is then measured starting at the appendix; this segment will be used to create the colonic reservoir. The colon is then stapled and divided at this location using a GIA stapler (Fig. 8). The ileocolonic anastomosis is then performed with the future Indiana pouch segment inferior to the bowel anastomosis. A stapled side-to-side bowel anastomosis is then performed. The crossing staple lines and the base of the anastomosis are reinforced with interrupted 3–0 silk sutures. The mesenteric trap is then closed using a 3–0 polyglactin suture in continuous fashion.

The colonic portion of the Indiana pouch is then detubularized using cautery along its antimesenteric surface. This incision is continued around the appendix.

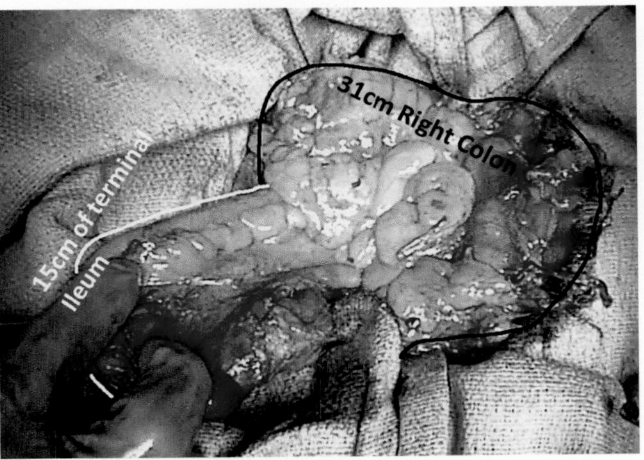

Fig. 8 Ileocolonic harvest for Indiana Pouch

21 Catheterizable Limb Formation

The creation of the catheterizable limb is performed with colon segment completely opened. The staple line on the ileal segment of the Indiana pouch is excised. A 14-Fr red Robinson catheter is then advanced through the ileal segment and into the pouch itself, serving as a tapering guide. Allis clamps are used to tension the ileal segment against the red Robinson catheter along its antimesenteric edge. A GIA stapler is then used to excise this excess ileum along the catheter. The staple line should continue up to approximately 1–2 cm from the ileocecal valve; multiple staple loads may be required (Fig. 9). The base of the ileocecal valve is imbricated over the catheter, using three Lembert style 3–0 silk sutures. These imbricating stiches are placed in a seromuscular layer equally spaced around the ileocecal valve, superiorly, anteriorly, and inferiorly. The catheter is then removed and replaced, ensuring ease of catheterization.

22 Pouch Formation

As described in the ileocolonic harvest section, the colonic portion of the Indiana pouch has been detubularized using cautery along its antimesenteric edge. The mesoappendix and the appendix have been removed. The detubularized colonic segment is then folded on itself in Heineke-Mikulicz fashion, and the edges are sewn together using 3–0 polyglactin suture. These sutures should be placed in close enough proximity to ensure a watertight closure, incorporating a larger seromuscular bite and a smaller mucosal bite to allow for adequate inversion of the mucosa.

Once completed, the pouch is then filled with 300 mL of normal saline to confirm the presence of a watertight pouch and continence at the ileal segment. The pouch is then emptied.

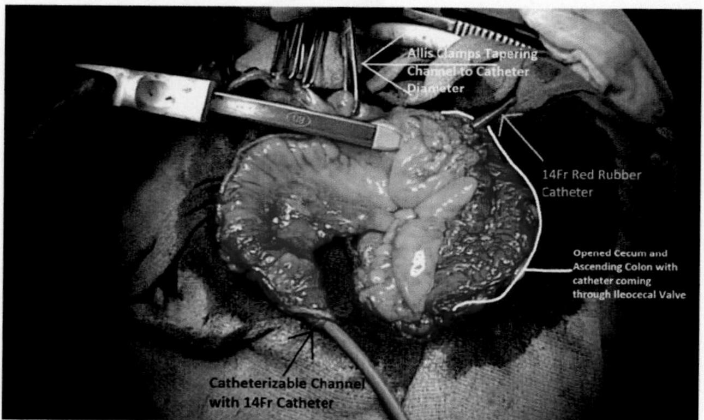

Fig. 9 Indiana pouch and catheterizable limb formation

23 Ureteroenteric Anastomoses

Once the pouch is created and the continence mechanism is completed, we proceed with the ureteral anastomoses. The right side of the Indiana pouch is then rotated counterclockwise 90°. A small enterotomy is made sharply along the left aspect of the Indiana pouch, at least 1 cm away from any suture line. The mucosal edges of the enterotomy are then everted using 4–0 chromic sutures in four quadrants. The left ureter is then brought adjacent to the planned anastomosis site. The excess ureter is excised and sent as a specimen. The uretero-colonic anastomosis is then performed as detailed earlier. Either interrupted or continuous fashion using 4–0 polyglactin or monofilament absorbable suture may be used. Halfway through the anastomosis, a single-J urinary diversion stent is placed across the anastomosis and brought out through a stab incision in the right anterior aspect of the pouch. After which, the remainder of the anastomosis is then completed. Care should be taken to create a watertight anastomosis, using a "no touch" technique on the ureteral mucosa. The procedure is then repeated with the right ureter. The stents are then secured to the pouch using a 4–0 plain gut purse-string suture. Stents are then externalized at the right iliac port site.

24 Suprapubic Catheter Placement

A 24-Fr Foley catheter is brought into the abdomen through the right upper quadrant port site. A separate 1-cm incision may be used if the port site is too cranial. It should be noted that the term suprapubic is used as a historical term for this catheter, as the location is not at within the suprapubic region. When determining the suprapubic site on the skin, it should be determined in relation to location of the catheterizable channel. The distance and orientation between two sites on the pouch should match the corresponding sites on the skin. Once the sites have been determined, the catheter is placed into the Indiana pouch in Stamm fashion using 3–0 polyglactin sutures. The suprapubic catheter balloon is then filled with 10 ml of sterile water. The suprapubic catheter is then pulled taut. The pouch is then anchored to the anterior abdominal wall in Stamm fashion using 2–0 polyglactin sutures. The catheter is secured at the skin using a 0 silk suture.

25 Creation of Catheterizable Channel

A small disk of skin is then excised at the right pararectus port site. The fascia at this location is bluntly dilated to one fingerbreadth. The stoma location can also be at the umbilicus depending on patient preference. The limb is then

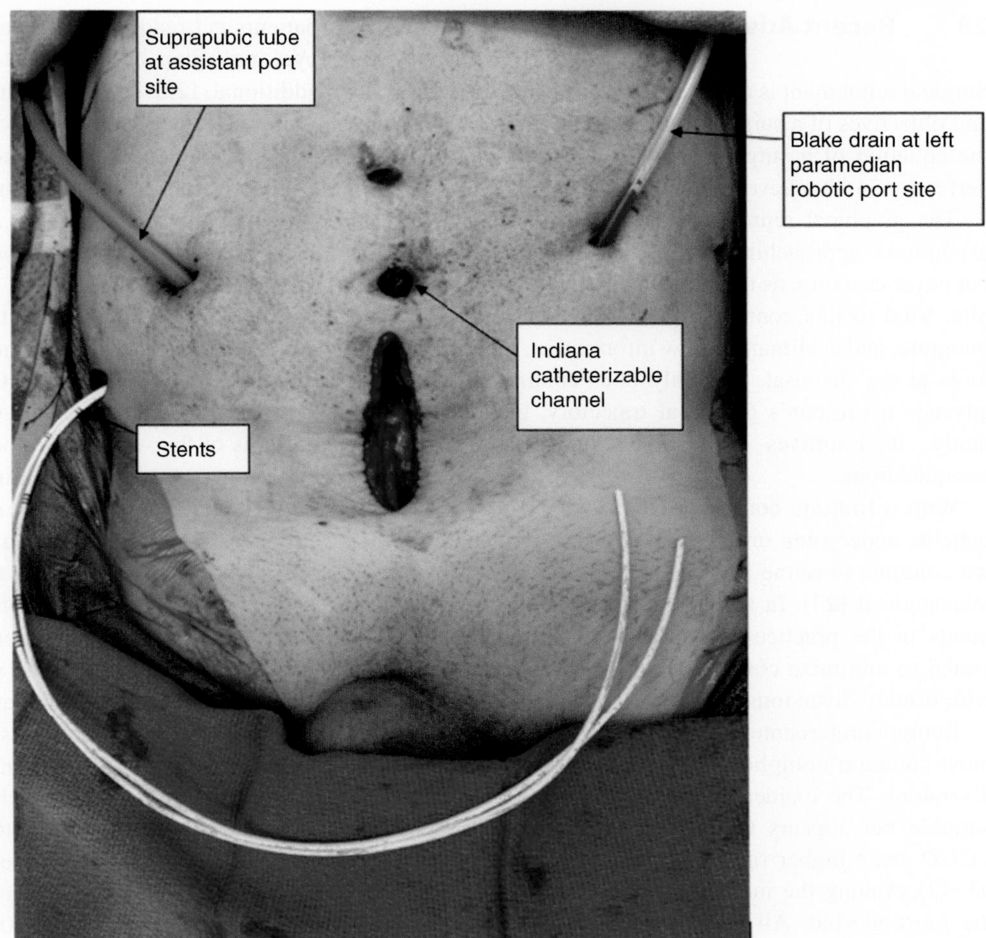

Fig. 10 Completed umbilical Indiana stoma with port sites and drain sites

brought through this incision until the excess limb is outside the skin. The excess is then excised 1 cm above the level of the skin and discarded using cautery. Our goal is to excise as much redundant ileal segment as possible to create an easily catheterizable channel. Catheterization is then performed again to ensure ease. The stoma is secured to the skin using interrupted 3–0 polyglactin sutures, full thickness through the stoma, and subcuticular at the skin. A 19-Fr Blake drain is placed in the pelvis and adjacent to the uretero-colonic anastomoses. The drain is externalized at the left pararectus port site. The fascia and skin are then closed at the midline incision. All remaining port sites are irrigated and then closed (Fig. 10). The suprapubic tube and stents are placed to gravity drainage. A Vaseline gauze is used to cover the stoma which is left uncatheterized.

26 Postoperative Care

Similar to the neobladder, the hospital stay typically ranges from 5 to 7 days. As with the neobladder, regular pouch irrigations, every 4 hours, are required until the suprapubic catheter is removed. An ERAS protocol is followed with early oral feeding and minimal narcotic administration. Prior to stent removal a JP creatinine is obtained. In the absence of concern for urinary leak, the stents are removed once the patient is unequivocally tolerating a diet and experiencing return of bowel function. Typically this occurs between postoperative days 4–6. The drain is removed when the output is less than 600 mL/24 h. The suprapubic Foley catheter is hand-irrigated every 4 h and kept in place for 3 weeks. A cystogram is performed to ensure no extravasation before catheter removal. The stomal dressing is changed daily.

27 Indiana Pouch-Specific Complications

Complications include many of those discussed for the orthotopic neobladder. However, additional complications seen in continent cutaneous diversions, which are not seen in orthotopic diversions, relate to the efferent limb. The most prevalent of these complications reported in recent studies is stomal stenosis, the second of which is difficulty with catheterization [32].

28 Recent Advancements in ECUD

Surgical refinement is a continuous variable among the goals and objectives of a surgeon. This continuous variable moves the equation of a surgeon incrementally closer to surgical perfection, without ever achieving it.

The graphical representations of the best surgeons are asymptotic, approaching ever nearer to the line of perfection but never crossing, as the potential for growth is always infinite. Vital to this continued growth is the ability to adapt, integrate, and acclimate to new information, technology, and tools at our disposal. Not only does continued refinement advance a surgeon's graphical trajectory, but most importantly it improves patient outcomes and decreases complications.

With a lifetime complication risk of up to 36% for all patients undergoing urinary diversions, it is mandatory that we continue to refine surgical techniques and perioperative management [23]. In this section we will discuss advancements in the practices and techniques of ECUD that are aimed to minimize common complications seen in patients with urinary diversions.

Benign ureteroenteric strictures (UES) are among the most common complications seen in patients with urinary diversions. The incidence reported in the literature is quite variable but appears to be between 1.3% and 16.8% for ECUD, even higher rates can be seen for ICUD [2, 7, 27, 33–43]. Among the most common complications, UES are the most morbid. All UES require at least one operative intervention. However, it is not infrequent that multiple interventions are required. UES are also the leading cause of renal dysfunction after urinary diversion [36, 44]. Although the pathophysiology has yet to be definitively elucidated, it is largely believed that UES development is a consequence of ureteral devascularization and ischemia, leading to scar formation [38, 39]. The associated morbidity of UES has led to many observational investigations on causality and mitigating factors including extracorporeal versus intracorporeal, running versus interrupted anastomosis, and touch versus no-touch technique. The results within the literature are varied regarding those factors; however the use of a promising new technology, indocyanine green (ICG) with near-infrared fluorescence for intraoperative vascular evaluation, appears to have a consistent and significant UES reduction benefit. The technique has been used for at our institution for over five years with a clinically evident decrease in UES. In fact, we found that our UES went from 7.5% in the non-SPY group ($p = 0.01$) to 0% in the SPY group [26, 45].

Another common complication seen in RARC patients is infection. Approximately 31.9% of radical cystectomy patients get readmitted for early infection including sepsis, pyelonephritis, abscess, UTI, bacteremia, and C.Diff. An additional 12.2% get readmitted for surgical site infection [46]. The effect of this high complication rate in this population cannot be understated as hospital readmission, additional procedures, and economic burden all negatively impact patient quality of life [47]. As a result we have adopted a new ECUD retractor, CleanCision™ (Prescient Surgical, San Carlos, CA). CleanCision™ is a wound retraction device that combines barrier protection and continuous antibiotic irrigation to the surgical wound (Fig. 7). We utilize a solution of 2 gm of cefazolin and 240 mg of gentamicin in 1 L of normal saline that flows to gravity into the superficial to deep portions of the wound into the dispersive sponge system of the retractor, providing continuous and consistent delivery throughout the duration of the surgery. A retrospective review at our institution has shown a decrease in 30-day infectious complication rate from 30.4 to 6.5% ($p = 0.003$) since we started utilizing CleanCision. This pattern persisted on 90-day infectious complication rates as well.

The last complications we would like to discuss is diminished renal function. This patient population is at risk for increased renal function loss, with continuous decline of 1.0 mL/min/1.73 m2 per year. There are multiple contributing factors to this decline including the site of anastomosis, reservoir/conduit outflow, stones, and chronic infection. Makino et al. identified ureteroenteric stricture as the sole risk factor associated with early renal function deterioration [odds ratio (OR) 4.22, $p = 0.037$]. Diabetes mellitus (OR 8.24, $p = 0.015$) and episodes of pyelonephritis (OR 4.89, $p = 0.038$) were also independently associated with the gradual decline in the late postoperative period [48]. Many of these contributing factors are reversible, or can have a minimized impact, if identified early with frequent and careful surveillance. It is our practice to follow our patients lifelong. The first week after discharge patients are sent home with intravenous hydration of 1 L per day and home health nursing checks for a minimum of one week. Their first visit is at the end of the first week at home, and their second visit is one week thereafter. Prior to each visit the patient obtains labs, which allow continued metabolic, hemodynamic, and renal monitoring. At six week postoperative visit, the patient receives labs and a renal ultrasound for upper tract evaluation. The patient continues to follow every six months with CT and labs for two years, after which the patient is seen every 6 months with alternating imaging, CT and renal US with CXR, and labs. At any point upper tract dilation is identified, and we order a nuclear medicine MAG3 and a loopogram. We maintain a low threshold for intervention if obstruction is suspected.

29 Conclusion

In conclusion, it is prudent upon urologists to continue to adapt and improve technique to further better patient outcomes. Ultimately, future improvements in operative and functional outcomes with RARC will ultimately rest on our ability to refine and optimize the urinary diversion. Forward progress will require techniques that are reproducible and achieve consistent evidence-based results. We should strive to continue to integrate technology and push the forefront, safely, building upon the original core principles and operative steps first described for urinary diversions.

References

1. Parekh DJ, Reis IM, Castle EP, Gonzalgo ML, Woods ME, Svatek RS, Weizer AZ, Konety BR, Tollefson M, Krupski TL, Smith ND, Shabsigh A, Barocas DA, Quek ML, Dash A, Kibel AS, Shemanski L, Pruthi RS, Montgomery JS, Weight CJ, Sharp DS, Chang SS, Cookson MS, Gupta GN, Gorbonos A, Uchio EM, Skinner E, Venkatramani V, Soodana-Prakash N, Kendrick K, Smith JA Jr, Thompson IM. Robot-assisted radical cystectomy versus open radical cystectomy in patients with bladder cancer (RAZOR): an open-label, randomised, phase 3, non-inferiority trial. Lancet. 2018;391(10139):2525–36. https://doi.org/10.1016/S0140-6736(18)30996-6.
2. Bochner BH, Dalbagni G, Sjoberg DD, Silberstein J, Keren Paz GE, Donat SM, Coleman JA, Mathew S, Vickers A, Schnorr GC, Feuerstein MA, Rapkin B, Parra RO, Herr HW, Laudone VP. Comparing open radical cystectomy and robot-assisted laparoscopic radical cystectomy: a randomized clinical trial. Eur Urol. 2015;67(6):1042–50. https://doi.org/10.1016/j.eururo.2014.11.043.
3. Bochner BH, Dalbagni G, Marzouk KH, Sjoberg DD, Lee J, Donat SM, Coleman JA, Vickers A, Herr HW, Laudone VP. Randomized trial comparing open radical cystectomy and robot-assisted laparoscopic radical cystectomy: oncologic outcomes. Eur Urol. 2018;74(4):465–71. https://doi.org/10.1016/j.eururo.2018.04.030.
4. Nix J, Smith A, Kurpad R, Nielsen ME, Wallen EM, Pruthi RS. Prospective randomized controlled trial of robotic versus open radical cystectomy for bladder cancer: perioperative and pathologic results. Eur Urol. 2010;57(2):196–201. https://doi.org/10.1016/j.eururo.2009.10.024.
5. Khan MS, Omar K, Ahmed K, Gan C, Van Hemelrijck M, Nair R, Thurairaja R, Rimington P, Dasgupta P. Long-term oncological outcomes from an early phase randomised controlled three-arm trial of open, robotic, and laparoscopic radical cystectomy (CORAL). Eur Urol. 2020;77(1):110–8. https://doi.org/10.1016/j.eururo.2019.10.027.
6. Yuh B, Wilson T, Bochner B, Chan K, Palou J, Stenzl A, Montorsi F, Thalmann G, Guru K, Catto JW, Wiklund PN, Novara G. Systematic review and cumulative analysis of oncologic and functional outcomes after robot-assisted radical cystectomy. Eur Urol. 2015;67(3):402–22. https://doi.org/10.1016/j.eururo.2014.12.008.
7. Nazmy M, Yuh B, Kawachi M, Lau CS, Linehan J, Ruel NH, Torrey RR, Yamzon J, Wilson TG, Chan KG. Early and late complications of robot-assisted radical cystectomy: a standardized analysis by urinary diversion type. J Urol. 2014;191(3):681–7. https://doi.org/10.1016/j.juro.2013.10.022.
8. Frees SK, Aning J, Black P, Struss W, Bell R, Chavez-Munoz C, Gleave M, So AI. A prospective randomized pilot study evaluating an ERAS protocol versus a standard protocol for patients treated with radical cystectomy and urinary diversion for bladder cancer. World J Urol. 2018;36(2):215–20. https://doi.org/10.1007/s00345-017-2109-2.
9. Ziegelmueller BK, Jokisch JF, Buchner A, Grimm T, Kretschmer A, Schulz GB, Stief C, Karl A. Long-term follow-up and oncological outcome of patients undergoing radical cystectomy for bladder cancer following an enhanced recovery after surgery (ERAS) protocol: results of a large randomized, prospective, single-center study. Urol Int. 2020;104(1–2):55–61. https://doi.org/10.1159/000504236.
10. Vlad O, Catalin B, Mihai H, Adrian P, Manuela O, Gener I, Ioanel S. Enhanced recovery after surgery (ERAS) protocols in patients undergoing radical cystectomy with ileal urinary diversions: a randomized controlled trial. Medicine (Baltimore). 2020;99(27):e20902. https://doi.org/10.1097/MD.0000000000020902.
11. Lin T, Li K, Liu H, Xue X, Xu N, Wei Y, Chen Z, Zhou X, Qi L, He W, Tong S, Jin F, Liu X, Wei Q, Han P, Gou X, He W, Zhang X, Yang G, Shen Z, Xu T, Xie X, Xue W, Cao M, Yang J, Hu J, Chen F, Li P, Li G, Xu T, Tian Y, Wang W, Song D, Shi L, Yang X, Yang Y, Shi B, Zhu Y, Liu X, Xing J, Wu Z, Zhang K, Li W, Liang C, Yang C, Li W, Qi J, Xu C, Xu W, Zhou L, Cai L, Xu E, Cai W, Weng M, Su Y, Zhou F, Jiang L, Liu Z, Chen Q, Pan T, Liu B, Zhou Y, Gao X, Qiu J, Situ J, Hu C, Chen S, Zheng Y, Huang J. Enhanced recovery after surgery for radical cystectomy with ileal urinary diversion: a multi-institutional, randomized, controlled trial from the Chinese bladder cancer consortium. World J Urol. 2018;36(1):41–50. https://doi.org/10.1007/s00345-017-2108-3.
12. Karl A, Buchner A, Becker A, Staehler M, Seitz M, Khoder W, Schneevoigt B, Weninger E, Rittler P, Grimm T, Gratzke C, Stief C. A new concept for early recovery after surgery for patients undergoing radical cystectomy for bladder cancer: results of a prospective randomized study. J Urol. 2014;191(2):335–40. https://doi.org/10.1016/j.juro.2013.08.019.
13. Wuethrich PY, Burkhard FC, Thalmann GN, Stueber F, Studer UE. Restrictive deferred hdration combined with preemptive norepinephrine infusion during radical cystectomy reduces postoperative complications and hospitalization time: a randomized clinical trial. Anesthesiology. 2014;120(2):365–77. https://doi.org/10.1097/ALN.0b013e3182a44440.
14. Lee CT, Chang SS, Kamat AM, Amiel G, Beard TL, Fergany A, Karnes RJ, Kurz A, Menon V, Sexton WJ, Slaton JW, Svatek RS, Wilson SS, Techner L, Bihrle R, Steinberg GD, Koch M. Alvimopan accelerates gastrointestinal recovery after radical cystectomy: a multicenter randomized placebo-controlled trial. Eur Urol. 2014;66(2):265–72. https://doi.org/10.1016/j.eururo.2014.02.036.
15. Large MC, Kiriluk KJ, DeCastro GJ, Patel AR, Prasad S, Jayram G, Weber SG, Steinberg GD. The impact of mechanical bowel preparation on postoperative complications for patients undergoing cystectomy and urinary diversion. J Urol. 2012;188(5):1801–5. https://doi.org/10.1016/j.juro.2012.07.039.
16. Aslan G, Baltaci S, Akdogan B, Kuyumcuoğlu U, Kaplan M, Cal C, Adsan O, Turkolmez K, Ugurlu O, Ekici S, Faydaci G, Mammadov E, Turkeri L, Ozen H, Beduk Y. A prospective randomized multicenter study of Turkish Society of Urooncology comparing two different mechanical bowel preparation methods for radical cystectomy. Urol Oncol. 2013;31(5):664–70. https://doi.org/10.1016/j.urolonc.2011.03.009.
17. Xu R, Zhao X, Zhong Z, Zhang L. No advantage is gained by preoperative bowel preparation in radical cystectomy and ileal conduit: a randomized controlled trial of 86 patients. Int Urol Nephrol. 2010;42(4):947–50. https://doi.org/10.1007/s11255-010-9732-9.
18. Hashad MM, Atta M, Elabbady A, Elfiky S, Khattab A, Kotb A. Safety of no bowel preparation before ileal urinary diversion. BJU Int. 2012;110(11 Pt C):E1109–13. https://doi.org/10.1111/j.1464-410X.2012.11415.x.

19. Menon M, Hemal AK, Tewari A, et al. Nerve-sparing robot-assisted radical cystoprostatectomy and urinary diversion. BJU Int. 2003;92:232.
20. Nix J, Smith A, Kurpad R, et al. Prospective randomized controlled trial of robotic versus open radical cystectomy for bladder cancer: perioperative and pathologic results. Eur Urol. 2010;57:196.
21. Koie T, Ohyama C, Makiyama K, Shimazui T, Miyagawa T, Mizutani K, Tsuchiya T, Kato T, Nakane K. Utility of robot-assisted radical cystectomy with intracorporeal urinary diversion for muscle-invasive bladder cancer. Int J Urol. 2019;26(3):334–40. https://doi.org/10.1111/iju.13900.
22. Murthy PB, Campbell RA, Lee BH. Intracorporeal urinary diversion in robotic radical cystectomy. Urol Clin North Am. 2021;48(1):51–70. https://doi.org/10.1016/j.ucl.2020.09.005.
23. Lee RK, Abol-Enein H, Artibani W, Bochner B, Dalbagni G, Daneshmand S, Fradet Y, Hautmann RE, Lee CT, Lerner SP, Pycha A, Sievert KD, Stenzl A, Thalmann G, Shariat SF. Urinary diversion after radical cystectomy for bladder cancer: options, patient selection, and outcomes. BJU Int. 2014;113(1):11–23. https://doi.org/10.1111/bju.12121.
24. Daneshmand S, Svatek RS, Singh P, Woldu S. American Urological Association. 2021, March 1. https://university.auanet.org/core/oncology-adult/bladder-neoplasms-muscle-invasive-bladder-cancer/index.cfm
25. Chan KG, Guru K, Wiklund P, et al. Robot-assisted radical cystectomy and urinary diversion: technical recommendations from the Pasadena consensus panel. Eur Urol. 2015;67:423–31.
26. Shen JK, Jamnagerwalla J, Yuh BE, Bassett MR, Chenam A, Warner JN, Zhumkhawala A, Yamzon JL, Whelan C, Ruel NH, Lau CS, Chan KG. Real-time indocyanine green angiography with the SPY fluorescence imaging platform decreases benign ureteroenteric strictures in urinary diversions performed during radical cystectomy. Ther Adv Urol. 2019;11:1756287219839631. https://doi.org/10.1177/1756287219839631.
27. Madersbacher S, Schmidt J, Eberle JM, et al. Long-term outcome of ileal conduit diversion. J Urol. 2003;169:985–90.
28. Qu LG, Lawrentschuk N. Orthotopic neobladder reconstruction: patient selection and perspectives. Res Rep Urol. 2019;11:333–41. https://doi.org/10.2147/RRU.S181473.
29. Rocco F, Gadda F, Acquati P, et al. Personal research: reconstruction of the urethral striated sphincter. Arch Ital Urol Androl. 2001;73(3):127–37.
30. Kessler TM, Burkhard FC, Perimenis P, et al. Attempted nerve sparing surgery and age have a significant effect on urinary continence and erectile function after radical cystoprostatectomy and ileal orthotopic bladder substitution. J Urol. 2004;172:1323–7.
31. Ali-El-Dein B, Gomha M, Ghoneim MA. Critical evaluation of the problem of chronic urinary retention after orthotopic bladder substitution in women. J Urol. 2002;168:587–92.
32. Holmes DG, Thrasher JB, Park GY, Kueker DC, Weigel JW. Long-term complications related to the modified Indiana pouch. Urology. 2002;60(4):603–6. https://doi.org/10.1016/s0090-4295(02)01945-3.
33. Anderson CB, Morgan TM, Kappa S, et al. Ureteroenteric anastomotic strictures after radical cystectomy does operative approach matter? J Urol. 2013;189:541.
34. Richards KA, Cohn JA, Large MC, et al. The effect of length of ureteral resection on benign ureterointestinal stricture rate in ileal conduit or ileal neobladder urinary diversion following radical cystectomy. Urol Oncol Semin Orig Investig. 2015;33:65.e1.
35. Studer UE, Burkhard FC, Schumacher M, et al. Twenty years experience with an ileal orthotopic low pressure bladder substituted lessons to be learned. J Urol. 2006;176:161.
36. Hautmann RE, de Petriconi RC, Volkmer BG. 25 years of experience with 1,000 neobladders: long-term complications. J Urol. 2011;185:2207.
37. Hollowell CMP, Christiano AP, Steinberg GD. Technique of Hautmann ileal neobladder with chimney modification: interim results in 50 patients. J Urol. 2000;163:47–51.
38. Katkoori D, Samavedi S, Adiyat KT, et al. Is the incidence of uretero-intestinal anastomotic stricture increased in patients undergoing radical cystectomy with previous pelvic radiation? BJU Int. 2009;105:795.
39. Large MC, Cohn JA, Kiriluk KJ, et al. The impact of running versus interrupted anastomosis on ureterointestinal stricture rate after radical cystectomy. J Urol. 2013;190:923.
40. Lawrentschuk N, Colombo R, Hakenberg OW, et al. Prevention and management of complications following radical cystectomy for bladder cancer. Eur Urol. 2010;57:983.
41. Shimko MS, Tollefson MK, Umbreit EC, et al. Long-term complications of conduit urinary diversion. J Urol. 2011;185:562.
42. Reesink DJ, Gerritsen SL, Kelder H, van Melick HHE, Stijns PEF. Evaluation of Ureteroenteric anastomotic strictures after the introduction of robot-assisted radical cystectomy with Intracorporeal urinary diversion: results from a Large tertiary referral center. J Urol. 2021;205(4):1119–25. https://doi.org/10.1097/JU.0000000000001518.
43. Ahmed YE, Hussein AA, May PR, Ahmad B, Ali T, Durrani A, Khan S, Kumar P, Guru KA. Natural history, predictors and Management of Ureteroenteric Strictures after robot assisted radical cystectomy. J Urol. 2017;198(3):567–74. https://doi.org/10.1016/j.juro.2017.02.3339.
44. Hautmann RE, de Petriconi R, Kahlmeyer A, et al. Preoperatively dilated ureters are a specific risk factor for the development of ureteroenteric strictures after open radical cystectomy and ileal neobladder. J Urol. 2017;198:1098.
45. Doshi CP, Wozniak A, Quek ML. Near-infrared fluorescence imaging of ureters with intravenous Indocyanine green during radical cystectomy to prevent Ureteroenteric anastomotic strictures. Urology. 2020;144:220–4. https://doi.org/10.1016/j.urology.2020.06.026.
46. Chappidi MR, Kates M, Stimson CJ, Johnson MH, Pierorazio PM, Bivalacqua TJ. Causes, timing, hospital costs and perioperative outcomes of index vs nonindex hospital readmissions after radical cystectomy: implications for regionalization of care. J Urol. 2017;197(2):296–301. https://doi.org/10.1016/j.juro.2016.08.082.
47. Badia JM, Casey AL, Petrosillo N, Hudson PM, Mitchell SA, Crosby C. Impact of surgical site infection on healthcare costs and patient outcomes: a systematic review in six European countries. J Hosp Infect. 2017;96(1):1–15.
48. Makino K, Nakagawa T, Kanatani A, Kawai T, Taguchi S, Otsuka M, Matsumoto A, Miyazaki H, Fujimura T, Fukuhara H, Kume H, Homma Y. Biphasic decline in renal function after radical cystectomy with urinary diversion. Int J Clin Oncol. 2017;22(2):359–65. https://doi.org/10.1007/s10147-016-1053-2.

Single-Port Robot-Assisted Radical Cystectomy

Reza Mehrazin, Eric H. Kim, Etienne Lavallee, and Mutahar Ahmad

1 Introduction

Robot-assisted radical cystectomy (RARC) has been demonstrated to have non-inferior oncologic outcomes when compared to open radical cystectomy in several studies, with RARC providing a reduction in rates of perioperative blood transfusion and reducing hospital stay [1–3]. With the development of the da Vinci® Single-Port (SP) platform (Intuitive Surgical, Sunnyvale, CA), SP RARC has been increasingly performed. The safety and feasibility of SP RARC with intracorporeal ileal conduit was first demonstrated by Kaouk et al. and Zhang et al. [4–6]. In initial series including patients with intracorporeal urinary diversion, SP RARC was non-inferior to conventional multiport (MP) RARC [7, 8].

The SP platform has distinct advantages over MP for RARC, including less incisions, camera flexibility, and robot patient-cart maneuverability for multi-quadrant surgery (e.g., pelvic for the cystectomy and right lower quadrant for the bowel harvest). However, the design differences in the SP instruments that allow for single point of entry, including the more proximal location of the instrument joint, require specific considerations when performing SP RARC. In this chapter, we describe the surgical steps and specific considerations of SP RARC and intracorporeal urinary diversion.

R. Mehrazin (✉)
Icahn School of Medicine at Mount Sinai, New York, NY, USA

E. H. Kim
Washington University School of Medicine, St. Louis, MO, USA

E. Lavallee
Department of Urology, Laval University, Quebec, Canada

M. Ahmad
Hackensack Meridian School of Medicine, New Jersey, NJ, USA

2 Single-Port Robotic Radical Cystecomy and Extended Pelvic Lymph Node Dissection

2.1 Patient Positioning, Port Placement, and Robot Docking

Patients are placed in either supine or dorsal lithotomy position with arms tucked and all pressure points padded. The Pink Pad® (Xodus Medical, New Kensington, PA) is used to secure patients to the table, and the table is placed in 20–25 degrees Trendelenburg during the cystectomy and lymph node dissection. Trendelenburg can be reduced to 15–20 degrees during the urinary diversion if necessary. For SP RARC, adequate working space (10–25 cm from target anatomy) can be obtained with the SP robotic trocar placed either 1.) directly into the abdomen through a 2.7 cm incision or 2.) through a GelPOINT access platform (Applied Medical, Rancho Santa Margarita, CA) using an open Hasson technique [9]. Patient body habitus and prior surgical history should be considered when deciding between these approaches for SP robotic trocar placement. For intracorporeal urinary diversions, a dedicated 12–15 mm assistant port is added for the Endo GIA™ stapler (Medtronic, Minneapolis, MN) [10, 11]. As such, we use of the 12 mm AirSeal® access port and system (CONMED, Largo, FL) through an additional incision (e.g., SP "plus 1"). Typically, the SP robotic trocar is placed 3–4 cm above the umbilicus, and the assistant port is placed in the left lower quadrant or the right mid-abdominal ostomy site. Alternatively, the SP trocar can be placed through the ostomy site, and the assistant port can be placed through the left lower quadrant. In female patients, the vaginal cuff can also be used as an entry point for instruments and staplers. This technique can enable single-incision surgery for radical cystectomy in females. Once the patient has been placed into Trendelenburg position, the robot is docked from either the patient's right or left side. The pitch limit is then set to avoid inadvertent pressure against the patient's upper body.

P. Wiklund et al. (eds.), *Robotic Urologic Surgery*, https://doi.org/10.1007/978-3-031-00363-9_63

2.2 Ureteral Dissection

Beginning with the camera up (12 o'clock), we adjust the camera to recreate a 30 degree down view. The fenestrated bipolar is placed in the 9 o'clock position (e.g., left hand), and the monopolar scissors and Cadiere forceps are placed in either the 3 o'clock or 6 o'clock position. The ureter is identified where it crosses the iliac artery. The overlying peritoneum is grasped and incised lateral to the expected trajectory of the ureter. Using the Cadiere forceps, the cut edge of the peritoneum is grasped and brought medially, and the ureter is dissected meticulously using mostly blunt dissection and occasional electrocautery when perforating vessels from the internal iliac artery are seen. The periureteral tissues are preserved, and direct manipulation of the ureter is minimized to avoid inadvertent injury. The ureter is traced down to the bladder, beyond the level of the medial umbilical ligaments. Once the intramural tunnel of the ureter is visualized, the distal ureter can be grasped to provide counter traction for Weck® Hem-o-lok® clip (Teleflex, Morrisville, NC) placement near the ureterovesical junction. The ureter is then sharply divided proximal to the clip, and a distal segment of the ureter is removed and sent for frozen section. The dissection is then repeated for the contralateral ureter.

2.3 Posterior Bladder and Pedicle Dissection

On occasion, we have noted that visualization of the posterior bladder and the pedicles can be achieved with the camera up (12 o'clock) and the angle adjusted to recreate a 0 degree or 15 degree up view. In other cases, supplemental anterior retraction of the posterior bladder is required, and leaving the camera up causes internal instrument collisions. If this is the case, we have adjusted the camera down (6 o'clock) with the Cadiere forceps up (12 o'clock). Once adequate visualization is achieved and retraction can be performed while minimizing internal collisions, attention is turned to the posterior peritoneum. In the male patient, the seminal vesicles and vas deferens are exposed in a similar fashion to the posterior approach to a radical prostatectomy; however, these structures are not dissected. With retraction of these structures cranially and anteriorly, Denonvilliers' fascia is opened sharply, and the posterior prostate is dissected bluntly in a similar fashion as a radical prostatectomy. In the female patient, the cervix or vaginal cuff (if status-post hysterectomy) is identified by using a sponge stick in the vagina. The peritoneum is opened at this level and the vaginal canal is intentionally entered with electrocautery. Either the anterior vaginal wall is retracted anteriorly with the specimen (non-vaginal sparing), or the anterior vaginal wall is dissected away from the posterior bladder (vaginal sparing).

The posterior plane of dissection described above is extended by working medial to lateral using mostly blunt dissection. To define the bladder pedicle, the medial umbilical ligament is once again identified, and the space lateral to the medial umbilical ligament is bluntly dissected to the level of the endopelvic or endocervical fascia. In the male patient, the vas deferens is divided lateral to the medial umbilical ligament. In the female patient, if concurrent hysterectomy, oophorectomy, and salpingectomy are being performed, the gonadal vessels are identified and clipped; the infundibulopelvic, round, and broad ligaments are divided with bipolar electrocautery. The medial umbilical ligament is clipped and divided. The bladder pedicle is now exposed both medially and laterally. With the bladder retracted cranially, anteriorly, and away from the pedicle to be divided, the pedicle can be controlled with either 1.) a carefully placed load of the Endo GIA stapler, 2.) sequential clips, or 3.) bipolar electrocautery. Once the dissection has been carried distally, the endopelvic or endocervical fascia can be opened sharply, and nerve-sparing can be performed using clips or bipolar electrocautery to control the prostatic pedicles. For males, careful apical dissection is important so as not to disturb the striated muscle. Careful dissection and preservation of the tissue near the apex of the prostate helps to promote postoperative continence. Similarly, the bladder neck can be dissected from the distal vaginal canal in female patients with bipolar electrocautery (vaginal sparing). In females undergoing neobladder reconstruction, preservation of the anterior vagina below the urethra and trigone is important to help with postoperative continence. Uterine sparing can also be performed as necessary or when desired.

2.4 Anterior Dissection

If the camera was moved to the down (6 o'clock) position, continue with this instrument arrangement until the median and proximal medial umbilical ligaments are divided from the anterior abdominal wall and the pubic bone can be visualized. For the anterior bladder and apical dissection, we have found that the camera up (12 o'clock) position with variable camera adjustments between 0 degrees and 30 degree down view is optimal. The space of Retzius is developed in similar fashion as in MP cystectomy. The endopelvic and endocervical fascia can be opened sharply at this point if they were not opened previously and the puboprostatic or pubovesical ligaments can be divided. The dorsal venous complex (DVC) can be divided with either 1.) bipolar electrocautery, 2.) monopolar electrocautery, 3.) a carefully placed load of the Endo GIA stapler, or 4.) using a suture to ligate the DVC. The pelvic floor is swept away laterally from the prostate (or bladder neck) with blunt dissection. Once the rectourethralis muscle (in males) or the distal anterior vagina (in females) is dissected away from the posterior urethra, the Cadiere forceps are used to retract the specimen cranially, and the anterior urethra can be opened. If a neobladder is planned, a generous urethral stump should be saved, and a frozen section should be performed to ensure a negative urethral margin. The Foley catheter should now be visualized and a clip can be applied to the exposed catheter to ensure the balloon does not deflate once the catheter is cut. We recommend having the assistant divide the Foley catheter intraabdominally, distal to the clip, using the laparoscopic scissors to avoid dulling the robotic scissors, which will be important during the ureteral reconstructions during urinary diversion.

2.5 Specimen Extraction

We have noted that the Inzii® 12/15 mm specimen retrieval bag (Applied Medical) is particularly useful as it fits through the 12 mm AirSeal® access port without encumbering the insufflation pressure and providing 1600 mL capacity. Additionally, once deployed, the specimen retrieval bag can be carefully manipulated open to deposit lymph node specimens and re-closed. The specimen retrieval bag is set aside in a male patient for later extraction through the SP robotic trocar site after undocking or through a separate midline incision. In female patients, specimen extraction is performed through the vaginal cuff with an empty ring forceps. The vaginal cuff is then closed in either a "clam-shell" configuration for non-vaginal sparing cases or horizontally for vaginal sparing cases, using a 2-0 V-Loc™ suture (Medtronic) in running fashion.

2.6 Lymph Node Dissection

We recommend switching to or continuing in the camera up (12 o'clock) position with a 15 to 30 degree down view. The same lymph node dissection templates as discussed in previous chapters by XX for MP RARC can be achieved during SP RARC. The standard template is bounded by the genitofemoral nerve laterally, Cooper's ligament distally, the obturator nerve posterior-medially, and the common iliac artery at or near its bifurcation proximally. The extended template includes the common iliac lymph node packets taken to the bifurcation of the aorta or the inferior mesenteric artery proximally as well as presacral packets posterior to the rectosigmoid mesentery [12]. In the case of extended template dissection, use of a GelPOINT access platform for the SP robotic trocar will be necessary to provide the minimum 10 cm working distance to the target anatomy. The use of judicious monopolar electrocautery, rather than continuous application of electrocautery while the instrument is in motion, is strongly recommended during the lymph node dissection. Specifically, an internal collision of the active arm, such as the monopolar scissors against the camera, with continued motion will cause the monopolar scissors to "roll" over the camera with a sudden movement of the active arm. This risk of SP instrument arm "roll" over an adjacent instrument arm can risk inadvertent vascular injury, particularly if the monopolar electrocautery is active. Thus, we recommend when at all possible judicious "point" monopolar or the use of bipolar electrocautery.

After completing the lymphadenectomy and before moving on to the reconstructive part of the surgery, the left ureter is passed behind the sigmoid mesentery and brought to the right side of the abdomen in preparation for the ureterointestinal anastomosis.

3 Intracorporeal Urinary Diversion

3.1 Neobladder

The ileum is identified, with a 45–50 cm segment needed for the creation of a neobladder. A coarse measurement is performed using the length of the robotic instruments. The ileum is harvested about 15–20 cm proximal to the ileocecal junction. 3-0 silk stitches are placed at the distal and proximal ends of the intended ileal segment to be used. These stay sutures are established to serve as markers and to be used as handles for bowel manipulation. The stapler is introduced through the 12 mm trocar. Alternatively, in women, it can be introduced through the vagina.

After the ileal segment is transected on either side, a side-to-side bowel anastomosis is performed to reestablish bowel continuity. Small openings in both ends of the free bowel are made to accommodate the stapler. 3-0 silk stay sutures are left in place near the openings to aid with bowel grasping. About 6 cm from the bowel's free ends, another 3-0 silk stitch is placed to bring the two bowel segments together and to be used as a handle. Each jaw of the stapler is passed through an open end of the bowel to create the anastomosis. The free bowel's distal end is stapled close and buttressed with 3-0 silk stitches. In females, the vaginal orifice is closed with a 3-0 barbed suture after completing the stapling.

We create an off-center U pouch with a chimney as initially described and illustrated by Studer [13] and more recently adapted for intracorporeal reconstruction [14, 15]. We begin with the posterior urethral anastomosis at the apex of the bowel segment. After the posterior urethral anastomosis is complete, we detubularize the ileum while preserving a 10 cm segment proximally to serve as the chimney. The posterior aspect of the detubularized ileum is sutured with a 30 barbed suture and then folded to create a spherical pouch. A 22 Fr silicone catheter is placed before the anterior bladder wall closure is completed in order to ensure its good positioning. Once the pouch is made, we complete the anterior urethral anastomosis. The ureteroileal anastomosis is then performed at the chimney of the U pouch using the Wallace technique. The distal ends of the ureters are spatulated and sutured together with 4-0 Monocryl in a running fashion. The end of the ileum is cut and the combined ureters are sutured to the ileum on either side with 4-0 Monocryl. Prior to closure of the final backwall of the ureter, a wire with double JJ stent is advanced through the assistant port and placed in each ureter. The curl is left in the neobladder. Finally, we irrigate the neobladder with 120–180 cc of normal saline to check for any leaks.

3.2 Ileal Conduit

For ileal conduit, we use many of the same techniques with a few key differences to accommodate the differences in urinary diversion. We identify 15 cm of ileum for use in the ileal conduit. We use the same techniques with silk stitches to mark the segments intended for the urinary diversion. Once the ileum is resected, the bowel anastomosis matches the technique used in neobladder. The ureterointestinal anastomosis and stent placement are performed as described for neobladders. The stents will be pulled at bedside at 4 weeks, or if not visible or through the conduit, cystoscope can be used to find the stent for removal in the office.

The other end of the ileum is suture with a long 3-0 silk which serves as a tag. For male patients, the 12 mm robotic assistant trocar is placed at the site of the intended ostomy at the beginning of the case. For female patients, a 12 mm assistant trocar is optional as the vaginal cuff opening can be used for bowel stapling. If using an assistant in females, a grasper is placed through the trocar situated at the ostomy site and the tag is grasped tightly. The robot is undocked, and the ileal conduit is pulled through the ostomy site via the trocar. Alternatively, if the robotic port was placed at the ostomy site, the conduit can be grasped directly with the robotic instruments and extracted en bloc. The ileal conduit is then matured in a standard fashion using 3-0 Vicryl sutures. We place 3 Vicryl sutures along the anti-mesenteric border through the fascia and deep tissue of the stoma. We then place sutures circumferentially at the skin and edge of ileum to complete the stoma.

3.3 Indiana Pouch

The creation of the Indiana pouch has a few differences and key benefits when utilizing the single-port robotic system. The Indiana pouch is created using the ileocecal valve as the continence mechanism. In total, this requires about 60 cm of ascending colon and transverse colon which is utilized for the pouch and about 12 cm of terminal ileum which is used for the stoma. We have performed robotic Indiana pouches in association with radical cystectomy. In multiport cases, the robot is docked near the umbilicus and pointed in the direction of the pelvis. After completion of the radical cystectomy, the cecum and initial portion of the ascending colon are mobilized along the line of Toldt. This process is mimicked with the single-port robot.

In multiport robots, the next step involves undocking the robot, flipping the robot toward the head, placing the patient in reverse Trendelenburg, and then redocking the robot. With the single-port robot, none of these steps are required given the ability of the robot to reposition on its own. With the single-port robot, the proximal ascending colon is mobilized, and the single-port robot can be repositioned intracorporeally to march up the colon to continue the dissection. The mobilization of the ascending colon continues 60 cm from the cecum. This process requires dissection of the hepatocolic ligament and progression beyond the hepatic flexure to the initial portion of the transverse colon. The transverse colon is typically very mobile and does not require extensive dissection.

Once the colon is fully mobilized, creation of the Indiana pouch begins. The next steps can be done intracorporeally or extracorporeally. For urologists transitioning to the single-port robot, we advocate starting with extracorporeal approach as this allows for a smoother transition to the new system. With proper experience and support, the entire process can be performed intracorporeally.

The bowel anastomosis is performed similarly to the neobladder anastomosis as described above. We make one adjustment when making the bowel anastomosis between the large bowel and small bowel. For a small bowel anastomosis, we fire one 60 cm load to create the connection between the two free ends. With the large to small bowel anastomosis, we fire two loads to create a larger anastomosis. With removal of the ileocecal valve, there is concern for abdominal symptoms including diarrhea, but in our experience and reported literature, there are no significant differences in long term quality of life [16].

To create the pouch, the colon is divided along its antimesenteric border and then folded over to detubularize it. The ends of the pouch are then sutured together with running 3-0 barbed suture. Attention is then turned to the small bowel and ileocecal valve to create a continent catheterizable stoma. The small bowel lumen is too large for a catheterizable channel and requires imbrication to get it to the appropriate size. A Foley is placed within the small bowel lumen and a stapler is then placed along the antimesenteric border to imbricate the small bowel. This requires multiple loads to complete the imbrication across the segment of small bowel. We continue the imbrication until the final load reaches and includes the cecum. We further imbricate and tighten the tissue near the valve with a simple 3-0 Vicryl suture to help maintain the long-term continence of the pouch.

Finally, we turn our attention to the ureteral anastomosis. We perform a Bricker anastomosis of the ureter to the end of the cecum. The anastomosis can be tunneled if a nonrefluxing anastomosis is required. We use 4-0 Monocryl to complete each individual ureteral anastomosis. Prior to completion of the anastomosis, a double JJ stent is placed in the ureter and pouch. Once the ureteral anastomosis is complete, we place a 20 Fr Malecot catheter directly through the pouch and then through the skin. This is used as the main catheter for daily irrigation.

Once the intracorporeal work is complete, we mature the stoma at the umbilicus. We use the single-port incision to guide the stoma to the umbilicus and make a small incision at the umbilicus to accommodate the stoma. When placing the initial incision for the single-port robot, we make sure to be at least 2 cm from the umbilicus to provide room for the stoma site. The stoma is matured similar to the stoma for the ileal conduit as noted above. The Malecot catheter is passed through the skin at a separate location from the single-port incision and stoma site. A 14 Fr catheter is placed through the stoma and capped. Finally, the single-port incision site is closed.

We found this combination of drainage catheters and stoma catheters provides optimal function and comfort for the patient. We use double JJ stents which eliminates the need for stents to come out of the body and be placed to a urostomy appliance. We use a large caliber Malecot catheter which is utilized for daily irrigation to minimize mucus buildup. We finally utilize a small lumen catheter in the stoma which can help the stoma heal and be used as a backup catheter for drainage if there are any issues with the Malecot catheter. We remove the Malecot catheter after 4 weeks and 24 hours later remove the stoma catheter. We find that leaving the stoma catheter for an additional 24 hours helps to close the opening in the pouch that was utilized for the Malecot catheter. The stents are also removed at 4 weeks via cystoscopy.

3.4 Postoperative Outcome

In another submitted publication, we discuss many of the benefits and drawbacks of the single-port system for urinary diversion. In our early experience, we have noted no major differences in complication rates between multiport urinary diversion and single-port urinary diversion. When looking specifically at PO and IV narcotic use, SP cystectomy patients required fewer narcotics than their MP counterparts which was statistically significant. A review of the colorectal literature demonstrates that the return of bowel function strongly correlates with the amount of morphine used. The transition from ORC to MP has already demonstrated benefits to the return of bowel function. Lower opioid usage after SP cystectomy might contribute toward further improving the return of bowel function.

3.5 Other Considerations

There remain significant challenges when using SP modality. Due to its recent implementation, there still exists a learning curve when using the SP. Previous studies have commented on the ergonomic challenges arising from using an SP modality while occupying a large extraperitoneal space. Anecdotally, we have noted similar challenges when first utilizing the SP robotic system. We posit that a surrogate measure for technical difficulty during surgery is operative time, and while we found no difference in our operative time between SP versus MP, more data is needed.

Technical challenges exist when utilizing the SP surgical system. These challenges are related to the limited workspace when using the robotic arms, as large movements across the field are grossly limited. This limitation reduces the traction the fourth arm can provide as it needs to remain within the confines of the working space. Additionally, all four arms need to be moved in tandem, which contrasts with the MP system, where the fourth arm can be left behind to retract while the surgeon operates outside of the visual workspace. Thus, the surgeon must pay greater attention to robotic arm positioning in situ while using the SP system for radical cystectomy. In our early experience with the SP robotic system, we often utilize an additional port for suction and traction to mitigate this added cognitive load.

Another difficulty associated with the SP robot is the clashing of the instruments, which we believe is amplified in the SP system compared to the MP system due to the introduction of the proximal elbow and the small working field. Our observation is that the instruments often clash at the proximal elbow which is commonly outside the surgeon's view. We predict this to be possibly hazardous during surgery as clashing may cause rapid and potentially dangerous movements of the arms; however, further studies are needed. The surgeon must pay attention to the on-screen navigator, which shows where the instruments are within the working field.

While we hypothesized that there would be a learning curve with the SP system, our early data shows that we could maintain our operative times. Our data could not measure cognitive load, and we have not found an adequate surrogate endpoint to measure this challenge. Further evaluation is warranted.

3.6 Conclusion

The single-port robotic system can be utilized when performing urinary diversion. While some considerations are specific to the SP platform, the surgical steps mimic the multiport approach. The single-port system has many technical differences, but none are uniquely applicable to urinary diversion. In our experience, we find the single-port robotic system to be an effective tool for urinary diversion.

References

1. Bochner BH, et al. Randomized trial comparing open radical cystectomy and robot-assisted laparoscopic radical cystectomy: oncologic outcomes. Eur Urol. 2018;74(4):465–71.
2. Parekh DJ, et al. Robot-assisted radical cystectomy versus open radical cystectomy in patients with bladder cancer (RAZOR): an open-label, randomised, phase 3, non-inferiority trial. Lancet. 2018;391(10139):2525–36.
3. Sathianathen NJ, et al. Robotic assisted radical cystectomy vs open radical cystectomy: systematic review and meta-analysis. J Urol. 2019;201(4):715–20.
4. Kaouk J, et al. Step-by-step technique for single-port robot-assisted radical cystectomy and pelvic lymph nodes dissection using the da Vinci((R)) SP surgical system. BJU Int. 2019;124(4):707–12. https://doi.org/10.1111/bju.14744.
5. Kaouk J, et al. Single-port robotic intracorporeal ileal conduit urinary diversion during radical cystectomy using the SP surgical system: step-by-step technique. Urology. 2019;130:196–200.
6. Zhang M, et al. Single port robotic radical cystectomy with intracorporeal urinary diversion: a case series and review. Transl Androl Urol. 2020;9(2):925–30.
7. Gross JT, et al. Initial experience with single-port robot-assisted radical cystectomy: comparison of perioperative outcomes between single-port and conventional multiport approaches. J Endourol. 2021;35(8):1177–83.
8. Palka JK, Henning GM, Gross JT, Kim EH. Single-port robot-assisted laparoscopic radical cystectomy with intracorporeal ileal conduit. Videourology. 2021;35(4) https://doi.org/10.1089/vid.2020.0133.
9. Hasson HM. A modified instrument and method for laparoscopy. Am J Obstet Gynecol. 1971;110(6):886–7.
10. Ahmed K, et al. Analysis of intracorporeal compared with extracorporeal urinary diversion after robot-assisted radical cystectomy: results from the International Robotic Cystectomy Consortium. Eur Urol. 2014;65(2):340–7.
11. Hussein AA, et al. Outcomes of intracorporeal urinary diversion after robot-assisted radical cystectomy: results from the International Robotic Cystectomy Consortium. J Urol. 2018;199(5):1302–11.
12. Hwang EC, et al. Extended versus standard lymph node dissection for urothelial carcinoma of the bladder in patients undergoing radical cystectomy. Cochrane Database Syst Rev. 2019;5:CD013336.
13. Studer UE, et al. Three years' experience with an ileal low pressure bladder substitute. Br J Urol. 1989;63(1):43–52.
14. Jonsson MN, et al. Robot-assisted radical cystectomy with intracorporeal urinary diversion in patients with transitional cell carcinoma of the bladder. Eur Urol. 2011;60(5):1066–73.
15. Abreu AL, et al. Robotic radical cystectomy and intracorporeal urinary diversion: the USC technique. Indian J Urol. 2014;30(3):300–6.
16. Germani P, et al. Ileocecal valve syndrome and vitamin b12 deficiency after surgery: a multicentric prospective study. Updat Surg. 2021;73(2):569–80.

Complications of Robot-Assisted Radical Cystectomy

Ralph Grauer, John P. Sfakianos, Reza Mehrazin, and Peter Wiklund

1 Overall Complication Rates of Robot-Assisted Radical Cystectomy

RARC has a morbidity rate reported to range from 30% to 70%, even at high-volume, tertiary referral centers; RARC also carries a 15–25% rate of high-grade complications, defined as Clavien-Dindo (CD) III–V [1–4]. The breadth of complications associated with RARC is very similar to that of its open counterpart, yet there are reported differences in the rates of these complications. We report complication frequency by etiology from large, retrospective multi-institutional studies (Table 1). These complications data come from studies that contain RARC with both extracorporeal and intracorporeal urinary diversions. Direct comparisons of complication rates in extracorporeal versus intracorporeal approaches are discussed below.

Table 1 Types and frequencies of complications associated with robot-assisted radical cystectomy

Etiology[a]	Frequency	References
Infectious	23%–60%	[3–7]
Gastrointestinal	22%–31%	[3–7]
Genitourinary	8%–22%	[3, 4, 6, 7]
Cardiac	4%–10%	[3–6]
Vascular	6%–11%	[3, 4, 6]
Wound	2%–13%	[3, 4]
Pulmonary	3%–13%	[3, 4, 6]
Neurological	2%–7%	[3, 4, 7]

[a] Infectious includes urinary tract infection, sepsis, intrabdominal infection, wound infection, and pneumonia; gastrointestinal includes anastomotic bowel leak, colitis, intestinal perforation, ileus, small bowel obstruction, bowel ischemia, ulcer, and diarrhea; genitourinary includes acute kidney injury, urinary fistula, and ureteral stricture; cardiac includes arrythmia and acute coronary syndrome; vascular includes pulmonary embolism, thromboembolic event, deep vein thrombosis, bleeding, anemia, and lymphocele; wound includes wound dehiscence and disruption; pulmonary includes aspiration, pulmonary edema, pleural effusion, and respiratory failure; neurological includes delirium, stroke, seizure, and transient ischemic attack.

2 Predictors of Complications

Preoperative predictors for complications are important if they reveal modifiable risk factors. We must function to optimize preoperative condition ahead of surgery to mitigate the likelihood of complications. Several studies incorporate a multivariable analysis predicting the occurrence of postoperative complications following RARC [1, 3–5, 8, 9]. Zhang et al. found predictors of increased 90-day major complications were age, the Charlson Comorbidity Index (CCI) and operative time. Johar et al. also found age, BMI, current smoking status, and the receipt of neoadjuvant therapy to be associated with any complication as well as major complications [4]. Kauffman et al. found preoperative renal insufficiency and intraoperative intravenous (IV) fluids of >5000 mL were significantly associated with postoperative complications of any grade, with respective odds ratios of 4.2 and 4.1; age of ≥65 years, operative blood loss of ≥500 mL, and intraoperative IV fluids of >5000 mL predicted CD grade III-V complications, with respective ORs of 12.7, 9.7, and 42.1 [5]. Smith et al. similarly found increased age to be predictive of CD complication grades. Naturally, these factors tended to correlate to poor preoperative health reserve—the preoperative predictors of major complications are displayed in Table 2. We see three of the five most common variables are possibly modifiable: BMI, smoking status, and CCI. Thus, the commonsense notion that preoperative patients should stop smoking, lose weight, and optimize medical conditions to avoid complications is supported by data. Unfortunately, the time to surgery following diagnosis in bladder cancer is short—the patient does not have time to adopt such modifications to a measurable effect, besides smoking cessation.

R. Grauer (✉) · J. P. Sfakianos · R. Mehrazin · P. Wiklund
Department of Urology, Icahn School of Medicine at Mount Sinai, New York, NY, USA

P. Wiklund et al. (eds.), *Robotic Urologic Surgery*, https://doi.org/10.1007/978-3-031-00363-9_64

Table 2 Preoperative predictors on multivariable analysis of major (Clavien-Dindo III-V) robotic-assisted radical cystectomy postoperative complications

Variable	Odds ratio (95% CI)	p-value	Reference[a]
Age (10-yr intervals)	1.47 (1.15–1.88)	0.002	[1, 4, 5, 8, 9]
CCI	1.13 (1.03–1.23)	0.007	[1]
BMI (kg/m^2)	1.04 (1.01–1.08)	0.014	[4, 9]
Current smoker	1.63 (1.02–2.60)	0.042	[4, 9]
Neoadjuvant chemotherapy	1.87 (1.12–3.10)	0.016	[4, 9]

[a] Multiple references listed indicates variable was found to be statistically significant within each study

3 Bias in Comparing Complication Rates Using Multi-Institutional and Non-prospective Data

Pooled studies and meta-analyses that integrate multi-institutional data form the strongest level of evidence. The premise that the component studies are consistent in measuring relevant criteria allows the drawing of robust conclusions. In 2012, to bolster consistency, the European Association of Urology (EAU) Ad Hoc Panel proposed a 14-item standardized tool for reporting and grading complications after urological surgical procedures [10]. However, a 2021 systematic review that examined the impact of this reporting tool found low adherence and heterogeneity in adverse event assessment and reporting; this inconsistency could lead to an underestimation of perioperative complications, precluding sound comparison of complication rates between studies [11]. Thus, the strongest level of evidence will come from studies that directly compare complication rates within a study as opposed to across studies, preserving validity. Bias also exists in non-prospectively collected data and single instructional data. Due to the lack of standardization in non-prospective studies, internal reliability is affected—it becomes more difficult to ascribe cause and effect to interventions and outcomes. Single intuitional/regional practices affect the external validity of studies. Institutional inertia and established postoperative pathways confound certain outcomes such hospital length of stay and return of bowel function. With this intellectual skepticism in mind, we present the various complication rates as well as selected perioperative outcomes reported in the literature for open radical cystectomy (ORC) versus RARC with intracorporeal urinary diversion (ICUD) or extracorporeal approach to urinary diversion (ECUD).

4 Complication Rates: Open Versus Robot-Assisted Radical Cystectomy

Seven prospective randomized controlled trials (RCTs) within six articles have compared ORC and RARC [6, 12–16]. The largest (n = 302) was the RAZOR study, a non-inferiority trial with the primary endpoint of 2-year progression-free survival that also analyzed secondary endpoints that included proportion of patients requiring intraoperative blood transfusions and surgical complications at 90 days. The proportion of patients who required postoperative blood transfusions was significantly lower in the RARC group, though there was no difference in major or minor CD complications between groups at 90 days [6]. In the second largest study (n = 118), Bochner et al. examined complications between ORC and RARC in the setting of an RCT and found lower intraoperative blood loss for RARC but no advantage for 90-day major (CD III–V) or minor complication rates [12]. These two RCTs, as well as the remaining five, are included in a recent meta-analysis that evaluates the efficacy and safety of ORC versus minimally invasive radical cystectomy (both RARC and laparoscopic cystectomy) [17]. Shi et al. found that RARC showed longer operating time, less estimated blood loss, lower blood transfusion rate, shorter time to regular diet, and shortened length of hospital stay compared to ORC; there was no significant difference in the complication rates between both groups, pooled OR 0.75 (95% CI, 0.54–1.03; p = 0.07) [17]. Though a benefit in morbidity rates was not shown in these RCTs, exclusive extracorporeal reconstruction was performed in all RARC groups—leaving the possibility of a difference between totally intracorporeal approaches and ORC, as the reconstructive phase of radical cystectomy is the primary driver of perioperative morbidity [18].

5 Complication Rate: Extracorporeal Versus Intracorporeal Urinary Diversions

The reconstructive phase, whereby a urinary diversion is created, of the RARC is the primary factor in perioperative morbidity. It is postulated the ICUD may be more beneficial in terms of perioperative complications, especially gastrointestinal (GI) ones, as the bowel experiences less exposure to ambient air and remains at body temperature throughout the procedure [18]. There exists no RCT comparing ECUD to ICUD, and there is only one prospective study explicitly comparing the two robotic approaches in terms of perioperative complications [19]. Bertolo et al. compared perioperative and oncological outcomes in these two approaches with ileal conduit ($n = 126$). They found no differences in overall or major (CD III–V) postoperative complications during admission or at 30- and 90-days postoperatively [19]. However, several retrospective studies of prospectively maintained databases compare ICUD to ECUD, though are subject to the aforementioned bias [1, 3, 7, 9, 20–26]. One of the largest of these studies, and the only to provide direct evidence for evaluating the relative perioperative complications rates of open radical cystectomy, intracorporeal RARC, and extracorporeal RARC, comes from a large, single-institution three-way comparison trial [1]. Though retrospective, the study's sample size was 948, including 272, 301, and 375 patients treated with ORC, ICUD, and ECUD, respectively. They found 30-day and 90-day overall and major (CD III–V) complication rates of ICUD (30-day major, 10.0%; 90-day major, 16.9%) were lower than those of ECUD (17.9%, 24.8%) and ORC (21.0%, 26.1%), $p = 0.002, 0.015$; there were no significant differences in readmission rates or oncologic outcomes [1].

The International Robotic Cystectomy Consortium (IRCC) has published multiple papers assessing the differences in perioperative outcomes between ICUD and ECUD via their multi-institutional, prospectively maintained database [3, 9, 25]. These studies aggregate multi-institutional data in a productive way, but there is high variability in reported complications between centers—perhaps biasing the interpretation of these data [11]. The study with the largest sample size ($n = 2125$) found that ICUD resulted in a higher overall complication rate at month one after RARC as compared to ECUD (31% vs 19%, $p < 0.001$); this difference became insignificant at 90 days [25]. The ICUD group also had higher rate of CD III-V complication (13% vs 10%, $p = 0.02$), though incidence of high-grade complications after ICUD decreased from 25% in 2005 to 6% in 2015 ($p < 0.001$), while it remained stable for ECUD at 13–14% [25]. This effect is thought to be due to the protracted learning curve of the ICUD approach as well as increased technique standardization. Thus, at the most recent time point, ICUD may offer an advantage in terms of major complication rate, though this statistical analysis was not performed. Data comparing each approach including ORC is provided in Table 3.

Few studies report the rates of re-operation, and they are unilaterally retrospective in nature. Johar et al. reported a reoperation rate of 5.6% ($n = 53$) within 30 days of RARC, agnostic to diversion approach; they identify fascial dehiscence ($n = 12$), small bowel obstruction ($n = 8$), and urine leak ($n = 7$) as the top three causes [4]. Ahmed et al. examined this same endpoint at 30 days and compared the rates between ECUD and ICUD. They reported 32 (6%) and 12 (8%) reoperations in the groups, respectively ($p = 0.42$). It appears both procedures carry similar reoperation risk, though more data on this subject is required.

Two recent meta-analyses integrated the above data to explore differences in perioperative complications for ICUD versus ECUD [27, 28]. Katayama et al. combined 12 studies to form a sample size of 3067 patients that met inclusion criteria; they found no significant difference between ICUD and ECUD in overall and major complications, regardless of the period (short-term [≤30 days] or midterm [>30 days]).

Table 3 Rates of patients experiencing major (CD III-V) postoperative complications and readmission for any reason in selected studies that include a comparison between ICUD, ECUD, and open technique for radical cystectomy. The table is split by the studies that report 30–90-day complications and those that report total < 90-day complications

	Major complication rates, n (%)								
	< 30 days			30–90 days			Readmission (<90 days)		
Study	Open	ECUD	ICUD	Open	ECUD	ICUD	Open	ECUD	ICUD
Bertolo (2018)[b]	–	1 (1)	1(2)	–	0 (0)	1 (2)	–	11 (17)	9 (15)
Lenfant (2018)	–	2 (6)	7 (10)	–	6 (18)	9 (12)	–	–	–
Carrion (2019)	–	4 (21)	6 (37)	–	–	–	–	6 (27)	4 (21)
Zhang (2020)[a]	57 (21)	67 (18)	31 (10)	71 (26)	93 (25)	51 (17)	92 (34)	108 (29)	85 (28)
Mistretta (2021)	–	9 (21)	11 (19)	–	11 (25)	16 (28)	–	–	–

	Major complication rates, n (%)					
	< 90 days			Readmission (<90 days)		
Study	Open	ECUD	ICUD	Open	ECUD	ICUD
Bochner (2015)[b]	12 (21)	13 (22)	–	–	–	–
Khan (2016)[b]	4 (20)	7 (35)	–	–	–	–
Parekh (2018)[b]	34 (22)	33 (22)	–	–	–	–
Ahmed (2014)[a]	–	115 (18)	34 (18)	–	121 (19)	22 (12)
Hussein (2018)[a]	–	99 (10)	141 (13)	–	90 (8)	103 (9)
Shim (2020)	–	57 (21)	11 (13)	–	–	–
Hussein (2020)[a]	–	39 (12)	66 (14)	–	11 (6)	49 (19)

[a] Statistically significant difference detected
[b] Prospective study

However, subgroup analysis revealed that ICUD performed by high-volume center had a significantly lower risk of major complications at both short- and midterm time points (OR 0.57, 0.66; $p = 0.008$, 0.02, respectively) [27]. Patients who underwent ICUD were found to have lower blood loss and were less likely to receive to receive blood transfusions, even at low-volume centers. Tanneru et al. performed a meta-analysis on six studies to examine the complications in ECUD versus ICUD as well as a cumulative analysis on 83 studies that reported perioperative outcomes in either approach. Within the meta-analysis, ICUD and ECUD had comparable complication rates at <30 days (RR 1.19, 95% CI 0.71–2.0; $p = 0.5$); similar rates were also reported in the cumulative analysis, 59% (range: 31%–86%) and 44% (range: 29%–78%), in the ICUD and ECUD groups, respectively. Similarly, there was no difference in complication rates at 30 and 90 days between ICUD and ECUD, (RR 0.91; 95% CI 0.71–1.15, $p = 0.4$). However, in the cumulative analysis, the rate of GI complications was lower in ICUD (9.3%) group versus ECUD (13.4%)—an important consideration in hospital stay prolongation. Additionally, they report that most ICUD used ileal conduit (78%) versus neobladder (22%), though robust data are lacking for complication comparison. Overall, these meta-analyses suggest there is value in the centralization/specialization of urological surgery, as it will make the postoperative morbidity advantages of ICUD more pronounced in expert care—a fact acknowledged by the EAU guidelines [29].

Nevertheless, there still exists a need for a randomized controlled trial comparing these three approaches to radical cystectomy to draw the most robust conclusions about perioperative outcomes. A trial in the United Kingdom comparing RARC with ICUD and ORC (iROC; clinicaltrials.gov: NCT03049410) is pending. In addition, specific types of urinary diversion (neobladder versus ileal conduit) via intracorporeal and extracorporeal approaches still require comparison in the setting of a RCT.

6 Perioperative Outcomes

Historically, robotic-assisted surgery has tended to outperform its open counterpart in perioperative outcomes. We examine operative time, the use of pain medication, the time to return of bowel function, hospital length of stay (LOS), and quality of life (QOL) outcomes as important drivers of cost and patient satisfaction.

6.1 Operative Time

Operative time is an important perioperative outcome as it relates to patient and payer surgical cost—which directly informs the adoptability and long-term viability of procedures. In a cost analysis comparing RARC and ORC, Martin et al. found the direct procedure cost was most sensitive to operative time—however, this model was agnostic to differences in complication rates. Thus, an effective surgery is synergized by also being efficient. ORC has been shown to be quicker operation than RARC by either approach. The RAZOR study found ORC ($n = 152$) to have a median operative time of 361 minutes and RARC ($n = 150$) to last a median of 428 minutes, $p = 0.0005$ [6]. Similar statistical differences between ORC and RARC have been reported in other smaller, prospective studies, retrospective studies, and a recent metanalysis by Shi et al. [1, 13, 14, 17, 30]. Despite the longer operative time in RARC, it is important not to draw conclusion about total cost, as other perioperative outcomes such as hospital LOS and complication rate are important factors. Within RARC, there is conflicting evidence regarding the relative operative duration of ICUD versus ECUD approaches. Though some studies have noted a statistically significant advantage in ECUD by <30 minutes, two recent meta-analyses suggest equivalent operative duration between approaches [27, 28]. The meta-analysis by Tanneru et al. posited no difference between ICUD and ECUD, but their cumulative analysis supported a difference within the ICUD approach based on the type of urinary diversion used. From the 83 studies included, the mean ICUD operative times for neobladder and ileal conduit were 428 ± 42 min and 313 ± 54 min, respectively; this compared to ECUD's 426 ± 72 min and 428 ± 181 min, respectively [28]. Hussein et al. leveraged the prospectively maintained IRCC database ($n = 972$) for a comparative propensity score-matched analysis of perioperative outcome between ICUD and ECUD approaches. Interestingly, they reported that ICUD operative times were shorter than ECUD (355 vs 401, $p < 0.01$) [3]. These results suggest that higher-volume institutions with experienced surgeons can shorten the time for ICUD, making it the preferred approach with respect to operative time. Despite these data, it is important to remember institutional variation in the amount of trainee teaching, in the operating room setup, and in the accuracy of recording procedure time can bias results.

6.2 Analgesia and Bowel Function Return

The usage of pain medication, specifically narcotics, in the postoperative setting directly impacts the return of normal bowel function. In turn, this can lead to sooner discharges and cost savings. Therefore, reducing postoperative pain via minimally invasive techniques can have a multiplicative effect on procedure expenditure. Nix et al. prospectively compared postoperative analgesia in a RCT between ORC and RARC in 41 patients. They reported significantly less morphine equivalent units in the robotic group versus the open group (89.0 mg, 147.4, $p = 0.004$) [13]. Similarly, another prospective study ($n = 40$) explicitly comparing postoperative pain in ORC versus RARC found that morphine sulfate equivalents differed significantly between both groups, despite having similar average pain scores [31]. Nix et al. also found statistically significantly sooner flatus and bowel movement in the robotic group by one day; this could be driven by narcotic use. This finding has been corroborated by a meta-analysis by Shi et al., reporting a mean difference of 1 day, in favor of robotic surgery. Data is lacking comparing pain and analgesia use between ICUD and ECUD approaches. In comparing both robotic approaches with respect to return of normal bowel function, it is hypothesized that ICUD results in the fastest return of function due to less bowel manipulation and less exposure to ambient temperature and air—an effect that has been documented in non-urological, laparoscopic literature [32]. In the most recent meta-analysis comparing ECUD and ICUD, Katayama et al. find ICUD to have benefit in the occurrence of ileus (OR = 0.72, 95% CI 0.5—1.03, $p = 0.07$), significant at $\alpha = 0.10$ but not at $\alpha = 0.05$.

6.3 Hospital Length of Stay

Hospital LOS in the postoperative setting is directly correlated to narcotic use and hence also time to return of bowel function. Thus, given the advantage RARC holds over ORC in these metrics, it stands to reason that patients that underwent robotic surgery would have shorter LOS. In the setting of a meta-analysis, Shi et al. show that minimally invasive radical cystectomy has shorter LOS than open surgery (mean difference = −0.93, 95% CI -1.32 to −0.54). Both approaches of robotic surgery, ICUD and ECUD, have not been shown to be significantly difference with respect to LOS, in a recent meta-analysis [27].

6.4 Quality of Life Scores

Patient QOL scores highlight tradeoffs involved in treatment. They inform the importance of understanding the impact of interventions on patients' life activities. Three RCTs study the health-related QOL scores between ORC and RARC, two of which use FACT-VCI questionnaire and one used the EORTC QLQ-C30 [6, 12, 33]. These questionnaires inquired on the dimensions of urinary, bowel, and sexual function, as well as body image, physical, social, emotional, and functional well-being. There were no differences between groups in each of these studies at baseline, 3 months, 6 months, 9 months, and at 1 year—except for the RAZOR trial, which picked up a 2.5 points lower score in the ORC arm for physical well-being at 6 months. A recent meta-analysis that combines these 3 RCTs and examines 31 nonrandomized studies also found no differences in QOL measures [33]. Though these data show no difference, QOL benefit in robotic surgery occurs in the short-term (<3 months), a measure not yet investigated. The pending iROC study will produce data investigating short-term and 12-month QOL outcomes. Data is lacking comparing QOL outcomes in ICUD and ECUD approaches.

7 Conclusions

Radical cystectomy is a morbid procedure, regardless of whether it is performed robotically or open, with complication rates ranging between 30 and 70%. Several RCTs have demonstrated equivalence in perioperative complications between open technique and robot-assisted procedure with extracorporeal urinary diversion. There is reason to believe that robotic approach with intracorporeal urinary diversion provides a benefit in perioperative morbidity, as there are less intestinal manipulation and exposure to ambient air and temperature—though this claim is unsubstantiated by randomized clinical trials. Several multi-institutional studies have credited ICUD with an advantage in complication rate, after a protracted learning curve—though these results carry bias as there still exists space for improved standardization of reporting outcomes. We anticipate the iROC trial to mature soon comparing ICUD to ORC, yet there is still a need for a three-armed RCT comparing ORC, ECUD, and ICUD. Moreover, there still is ongoing research regarding the optimal type of urinary diversion in this setting. A desire for better quality of life, enhanced recovery, and minimized cost will drive physicians and payers to research the best surgical approach to radical cystectomy. We eagerly await the results of these future studies.

References

1. Zhang JH, Ericson KJ, Thomas LJ, Knorr J, Khanna A, Crane A, et al. Large single institution comparison of perioperative outcomes and complications of open radical cystectomy, intracorporeal robot-assisted radical cystectomy and robotic extracorporeal approach. J Urol. 2020;203(3):512–21. https://doi.org/10.1097/JU.0000000000000570.
2. Novara G, Catto JW, Wilson T, Annerstedt M, Chan K, Murphy DG, et al. Systematic review and cumulative analysis of perioperative outcomes and complications after robot-assisted radical cystectomy. Eur Urol. 2015;67(3):376–401. https://doi.org/10.1016/j.eururo.2014.12.007.
3. Hussein AA, Elsayed AS, Aldhaam NA, Jing Z, Peabody JO, Wijburg CJ, et al. A comparative propensity score-matched analysis of perioperative outcomes of intracorporeal vs extracorporeal urinary diversion after robot-assisted radical cystectomy: results from the International Robotic Cystectomy Consortium. BJU Int. 2020;126(2):265–72. https://doi.org/10.1111/bju.15083.

4. Johar RS, Hayn MH, Stegemann AP, Ahmed K, Agarwal P, Balbay MD, et al. Complications after robot-assisted radical cystectomy: results from the International Robotic Cystectomy Consortium. Eur Urol. 2013;64(1):52–7. https://doi.org/10.1016/j.eururo.2013.01.010.
5. Kauffman EC, Ng CK, Lee MM, Otto BJ, Portnoff A, Wang GJ, et al. Critical analysis of complications after robotic-assisted radical cystectomy with identification of preoperative and operative risk factors. BJU Int. 2010;105(4):520–7. https://doi.org/10.1111/j.1464-410X.2009.08843.x.
6. Parekh DJ, Reis IM, Castle EP, Gonzalgo ML, Woods ME, Svatek RS, et al. Robot-assisted radical cystectomy versus open radical cystectomy in patients with bladder cancer (RAZOR): an open-label, randomised, phase 3, non-inferiority trial. Lancet. 2018;391(10139):2525–36. https://doi.org/10.1016/S0140-6736(18)30996-6.
7. Mazzone E, D'Hondt F, Beato S, Andras I, Lambert E, Vollemaere J, et al. Robot-assisted radical cystectomy with intracorporeal urinary diversion decreases postoperative complications only in highly comorbid patients: findings that rely on a standardized methodology recommended by the European Association of Urology Guidelines. World J Urol. 2021;39(3):803–12. https://doi.org/10.1007/s00345-020-03237-5.
8. Smith AB, Raynor M, Amling CL, Busby JE, Castle E, Davis R, et al. Multi-institutional analysis of robotic radical cystectomy for bladder cancer: perioperative outcomes and complications in 227 patients. J Laparoendosc Adv Surg Tech A. 2012;22(1):17–21. https://doi.org/10.1089/lap.2011.0326.
9. Ahmed K, Khan SA, Hayn MH, Agarwal PK, Badani KK, Balbay MD, et al. Analysis of intracorporeal compared with extracorporeal urinary diversion after robot-assisted radical cystectomy: results from the International Robotic Cystectomy Consortium. Eur Urol. 2014;65(2):340–7. https://doi.org/10.1016/j.eururo.2013.09.042.
10. Mitropoulos D, Artibani W, Graefen M, Remzi M, Rouprêt M, Truss M, et al. Reporting and grading of complications after urologic surgical procedures: an ad hoc EAU guidelines panel assessment and recommendations. Eur Urol. 2012;61(2):341–9. https://doi.org/10.1016/j.eururo.2011.10.033.
11. Dell'Oglio P, Andras I, Ortega D, Galfano A, Artibani W, Autorino R, et al. Impact of the implementation of the EAU guidelines recommendation on reporting and grading of complications in patients undergoing robot-assisted radical cystectomy: a systematic review. Eur Urol. 2021; https://doi.org/10.1016/j.eururo.2021.04.030.
12. Bochner BH, Dalbagni G, Sjoberg DD, Silberstein J, Keren Paz GE, Donat SM, et al. Comparing open radical cystectomy and robot-assisted laparoscopic radical cystectomy: a randomized clinical trial. Eur Urol. 2015;67(6):1042–50. https://doi.org/10.1016/j.eururo.2014.11.043.
13. Nix J, Smith A, Kurpad R, Nielsen ME, Wallen EM, Pruthi RS. Prospective randomized controlled trial of robotic versus open radical cystectomy for bladder cancer: perioperative and pathologic results. Eur Urol. 2010;57(2):196–201. https://doi.org/10.1016/j.eururo.2009.10.024.
14. Khan MS, Gan C, Ahmed K, Ismail AF, Watkins J, Summers JA, et al. A single-centre early phase randomised controlled three-arm trial of open, robotic, and laparoscopic radical cystectomy (CORAL). Eur Urol. 2016;69(4):613–21. https://doi.org/10.1016/j.eururo.2015.07.038.
15. Bochner BH, Dalbagni G, Marzouk KH, Sjoberg DD, Lee J, Donat SM, et al. Randomized trial comparing open radical cystectomy and robot-assisted laparoscopic radical cystectomy: oncologic outcomes. Eur Urol. 2018;74(4):465–71. https://doi.org/10.1016/j.eururo.2018.04.030.
16. Parekh DJ, Messer J, Fitzgerald J, Ercole B, Svatek R. Perioperative outcomes and oncologic efficacy from a pilot prospective randomized clinical trial of open versus robotic assisted radical cystectomy. J Urol. 2013;189(2):474–9. https://doi.org/10.1016/j.juro.2012.09.077.
17. Shi H, Li J, Li K, Yang X, Zhu Z, Tian D. Minimally invasive versus open radical cystectomy for bladder cancer: a systematic review and meta-analysis. J Int Med Res. 2019;47(10):4604–18. https://doi.org/10.1177/0300060519864806.
18. Satkunasivam R, Wallis CJ, Nam RK, Desai M, Gill IS. Contemporary evidence for robot-assisted radical cystectomy for treating bladder cancer. Nat Rev Urol. 2016;13(9):533–9. https://doi.org/10.1038/nrurol.2016.139.
19. Bertolo R, Agudelo J, Garisto J, Armanyous S, Fergany A, Kaouk J. Perioperative outcomes and complications after robotic radical cystectomy with intracorporeal or extracorporeal ileal conduit urinary diversion: head-to-head comparison from a single-institutional prospective study. Urology. 2019;129:98–105. https://doi.org/10.1016/j.urology.2018.11.059.
20. Lenfant L, Verhoest G, Campi R, Parra J, Graffeille V, Masson-Lecomte A, et al. Perioperative outcomes and complications of intracorporeal vs extracorporeal urinary diversion after robot-assisted radical cystectomy for bladder cancer: a real-life, multi-institutional french study. World J Urol. 2018;36(11):1711–8. https://doi.org/10.1007/s00345-018-2313-8.
21. Carrion A, Piñero A, Raventós C, Lozano F, Díaz F, Morote J. Comparison of perioperative outcomes and complications of robot assisted radical cystectomy with extracorporeal vs intracorporeal urinary diversion. Actas Urol Esp (Engl Ed). 2019;43(6):277–83. https://doi.org/10.1016/j.acuro.2019.01.006.
22. Pyun JH, Kim HK, Cho S, Kang SG, Cheon J, Lee JG, et al. Robot-assisted radical cystectomy with total intracorporeal urinary diversion: comparative analysis with extracorporeal urinary diversion. J Laparoendosc Adv Surg Tech A. 2016;26(5):349–55. https://doi.org/10.1089/lap.2015.0543.
23. Shim JS, Kwon TG, Rha KH, Lee YG, Lee JY, Jeong BC, et al. Do patients benefit from total intracorporeal robotic radical cystectomy?: a comparative analysis with extracorporeal robotic radical cystectomy from a Korean multicenter study. Investig Clin Urol. 2020;61(1):11–8. https://doi.org/10.4111/icu.2020.61.1.11.
24. Tan TW, Nair R, Saad S, Thurairaja R, Khan MS. Safe transition from extracorporeal to intracorporeal urinary diversion following robot-assisted cystectomy: a recipe for reducing operative time, blood loss and complication rates. World J Urol. 2019;37(2):367–72. https://doi.org/10.1007/s00345-018-2386-4.
25. Hussein AA, May PR, Jing Z, Ahmed YE, Wijburg CJ, Canda AE, et al. Outcomes of intracorporeal urinary diversion after robot-assisted radical cystectomy: results from the International Robotic Cystectomy Consortium. J Urol. 2018;199(5):1302–11. https://doi.org/10.1016/j.juro.2017.12.045.
26. Mistretta FA, Musi G, Collà Ruvolo C, Conti A, Luzzago S, Catellani M, et al. Robot-assisted radical cystectomy for non-metastatic urothelial carcinoma of urinary bladder: a comparison between intracorporeal versus extracorporeal orthotopic ileal neobladder. J Endourol. 2021;35(2):151–8. https://doi.org/10.1089/end.2020.0622.
27. Katayama S, Mori K, Pradere B, Mostafaei H, Schuettfort VM, Quhal F, et al. Intracorporeal versus extracorporeal urinary diversion in robot-assisted radical cystectomy: a systematic review and meta-analysis. Int J Clin Oncol. 2021;26(9):1587–99. https://doi.org/10.1007/s10147-021-01972-2.
28. Tanneru K, Jazayeri SB, Kumar J, Alam MU, Norez D, Nguyen S, et al. Intracorporeal versus extracorporeal urinary diversion following robot-assisted radical cystectomy: a meta-analysis, cumulative analysis, and systematic review. J Robot Surg. 2021;15(3):321–33. https://doi.org/10.1007/s11701-020-01174-4.
29. Bruins HM, Veskimäe E, Hernández V, Neuzillet Y, Cathomas R, Compérat EM, et al. The importance of hospital and surgeon volume as major determinants of morbidity and mortality after radical

cystectomy for bladder cancer: a systematic review and recommendations by the European Association of Urology Muscle-invasive and Metastatic Bladder Cancer Guideline Panel. Eur Urol Oncol. 2020;3(2):131–44. https://doi.org/10.1016/j.euo.2019.11.005.

30. Soria F, Moschini M, D'andrea D, Abufaraj M, Foerster B, Mathiéu R, et al. Comparative effectiveness in perioperative outcomes of robotic versus open radical cystectomy: results from a multicenter contemporary retrospective cohort study. Eur Urol Focus. 2020;6(6):1233–9. https://doi.org/10.1016/j.euf.2018.11.002.
31. Guru KA, Wilding GE, Piacente P, Thompson J, Deng W, Kim HL, et al. Robot-assisted radical cystectomy versus open radical cystectomy: assessment of postoperative pain. Can J Urol. 2007;14(6):3753–6.
32. Salimath J, Jones MW, Hunt DL, Lane MK. Comparison of return of bowel function and length of stay in patients undergoing laparoscopic versus open colectomy. JSLS. 2007;11(1):72–5.
33. Messer JC, Punnen S, Fitzgerald J, Svatek R, Parekh DJ. Health-related quality of life from a prospective randomised clinical trial of robot-assisted laparoscopic vs open radical cystectomy. BJU Int. 2014;114(6):896–902. https://doi.org/10.1111/bju.12818.

Robotic-Assisted Radical Cystectomy Outcomes

Abolfazl Hosseini and Ashkan Mortezavi

1 Introduction

Outcome assessment of radical cystectomy with pelvic lymph node dissection and subsequent urinary diversion can be subdivided into three categories: 1. perioperative outcome including complications and early postoperative mortality, 2. quality of life and functional outcome in case of continent bladder substitution, and 3. oncological outcome. Significant efforts have been made in the last decades to achieve improvements across all of these areas. These measures included centralization of bladder cancer treatment to high-volume centers [1], introduction of enhanced recovery after surgery protocols [2], and standardization of surgical technique [3], together with the implementation of robot-assisted laparoscopic radical cystectomy (RARC) with or without intracorporeal urinary diversion (ICUD). While the oncological outcome is largely influenced by the ablative surgery, the perioperative and functional outcome are generally affected by the reconstructive part. Therefore, a differentiation between the hybrid approach of RARC followed by extracorporeal urinary diversion (ECUD) and a fully minimal invasive technique of RARC with ICUD for outcome assessment is fundamental.

2 Perioperative Outcome

Relevant perioperative and short-term postoperative parameters for evaluation of a surgical technique are estimated blood loss, transfusion rates, operation time, intra- and postoperative complications, and hospital length of stay. Five randomized clinical trials with a total of 541 patients have assessed some of these parameters prospectively, although all patients in these studies received an ECUD. The first report was by Nix et al. from the United States (University of North Carolina) who randomized 41 patients [4]. Although the primary endpoint was lymph node yield in a noninferiority setting, secondary endpoints also included perioperative parameters. In 2013, Parekh et al. followed with results on perioperative and oncological outcome from their pilot RCT including 40 patients in the United States; purpose of the study was to establish the feasibility of a RCT for RARC vs. ORC [5]. The same author reported 5 years later results of the randomized open versus robotic cystectomy (RAZOR) trial [6] from 15 US centers with 302 patients compromising more than half of the total population included in the available five RCTs. This was the first trial not only reporting perioperative outcome but also oncological follow-up data. Bochner et al. had already presented their perioperative outcome data of the MSKCC RCT three years earlier in 2015 including 118 patients [7] when they gave an update also on oncological outcome in the same year (2018) [8]. The only study from outside the USA was the Cystectomy Open Robotic and Laparoscopic (CORAL) single center trial from the UK [9]. After a first report on perioperative outcome, a follow-up report on long-term oncological outcome followed in 2019 [10]. This was also the only trial performing a three-way comparison of ORC, RARC, and a laparoscopic approach. Results of all the abovementioned RCTs on perioperative outcome are presented in Table 1. All five RCTs reported a significantly longer operation time and a lower estimated blood loss for RARC (all $p < 0.05$), although there was a large variability [4–6, 8, 10]. Only two studies provided transfusion rates, with both showing an advantage (less transfusions) in the RARC cohort [5, 6]. Three studies did not find a significant difference in length of stay [4, 5, 8]. Two trials, including the largest RCT (RAZOR), reported a shorter hospitalization time for RARC patients [6, 10]. A meta-analysis including data from all the abovementioned trials concluded that the mean estimated blood loss favored RARC (difference − 281 ml, 95% CI -435 to −125) and

A. Hosseini (✉)
Department of Molecular Medicine and Surgery, Karolinska Institute and Department of Pelvic Surgery, Karolinska University Hospital, Stockholm, Sweden

A. Mortezavi
Department of Urology, University Hospital Basel, Basel, Switzerland

P. Wiklund et al. (eds.), *Robotic Urologic Surgery*, https://doi.org/10.1007/978-3-031-00363-9_65

Table 1 Prospective randomized controlled trials comparing robot-assisted radical cystectomy (RARC) with extracorporeal urinary diversion (ECUD) with open radical cystectomy (ORC). *OP* operation, *estim.* Estimated. N represents the number of analyzed cases. [1]intraoperative, [2]perioperative

Study	Modality	N		OP time (min)	Estim. blood loss (ml)	Transfusion rate (%)	Length of stay (days)
Nix 2009 [4]	RARC	21	Median	252	258	–	5
	ORC	20		210	575	–	6
Parekh 2013 [5]	RARC	20	Median	300	400	40%	6
	ORC	20		286	800	50%	6
Bochner 2015 [7] (MSKCC)	RARC	60	Mean	464	500	–	8
	ORC	58		330	681	–	8
Khan 2015 [9] (CORAL)	RARC	20	Mean	389	585	–	12
	ORC	20		293	808	–	14
Parekh 2018 [6] (RAZOR)	RARC	150	Median	428	300	13%[1] / 24%[2]	6
	ORC	152		361	700	34%[1] / 45%[2]	7

Table 2 Perioperative outcome parameters of large retrospective and prospective not randomized cohort/comparative effectiveness studies. Results presented as median. *OP* operation, *Estim.* estimated, *ICUD* intracorporeal urinary diversion, *ECUD* extracorporeal urinary diversion. 1: 94% ICUD. 2: 88% ICUD. N represents the number of analyzed cases. *All results from the inverse probability weighted population

Study	Modality	N	OP time (min)	Estim. blood loss (ml)	Transfusion rate (%)	Length of stay (days)
Hussein (IRCC), 2018 [15]	ICUD	1031	357	300	5	9
	ECUD	1094	400	350	13	8
Zhang (Cleveland), 2020 [16]	ICUD	301	396	300	16.9	6
	ECUD	375	421	400	24.3	7
	ORC	272	332	700	38.6	8
Mortezavi (Sweden), 2021	ICUD[1]	874	320	150	7.7	9
	ORC	1554	323	700	38.7	13
Wijburg (Netherlands)*, 2021 [17]	ICUD[2]	180	330	300	9.2	8
	ORC	168	229	600	14	11

mean operation time was shorter for ORC (difference 75 min, 95% CI 26–123). Hospital length of stay favored RARC but did not reach statistical significance (0.5 d, 95% CI -1.15 to 0.14) [11]. Multiple retrospective reports comparing RARC with ECUD and with ORC have reproduced these findings from the prospective RCTs [12].

No prospective RCT has been performed so far to compare a completely intracorporeal approach to an open approach. It has been proposed that ICUD might have potential benefits compared to ECUD; the obvious advantages of the totally intracorporeal technique are the protection of bowel inside the abdomen (faster return of function), reducing hypothermia and loss of fluids through dehydration, less bleeding, no need for extensive ureteral dissection, which may cause ureteral strictures, and further reduction of the surgical trauma. However, evidence exists almost exclusively from small retrospective single center trials [12–14]. Recently, four groups reported results including large and multicenter populations undergoing RARC with ICUD, although only one was prospective (Table 2).

One of the largest sources of retrospective outcome data on RARC with ICUD and ECUD has been the International Robotic Cystectomy Consortium (IRCC) [15]. The IRCC database was established in 2006, initially with four participating institutions. In an analysis in 2018, Hussein et al. retrospectively reviewed the records of 2432 patients from a total of 29 institutions who were included in the IRCC database. ICUD was performed in 51% of the cases. The rate increased from 9% of all urinary diversions in 2005 to 97% in 2015. On multivariable analysis, higher annual cystectomy volume (OR 1.02, 95% CI 1.01–1.03, $p < 0.002$), the year of RARC (2013–2016 OR 68, 95% CI 44–105, $p < 0.001$), and American Society of Anesthesiologists score less than 3 (OR 1.75, 95% CI 1.38–2.22, $p < 0.001$) were associated with undergoing ICUD. These patients demonstrated shorter operative time (357 vs. 400 min), less blood loss (300 vs. 350 ml), fewer blood transfusions (5% vs. 13%, all $p < 0.001$), but longer lengths of stay (9 vs. 8 days, $p < 0.001$) compared with ECUD.

Zhang et al. performed a three-way comparison of ORC, ECUD, and ICUD, all performed at their institution between 2011 and 2018 [16]. A total of 948 patients were analyzed, well balanced between the three groups. Operative time was lower for ICUD (396 min) compared to ECUD (421 min). However, it was lowest for ORC (332 min). Estimated blood loss was lower for ICUD than for ECUD and ORC (300 vs. 400 and 700 ml, respectively). All pairwise comparisons between surgical approaches for operative time and estimated blood loss were statistically significant. Intraoperative transfusion rates were lowest for ICUD compared to ECUD and ORC (16.9% vs. 24.3% and 38.6%, respectively, $p < 0.001$). Pairwise comparisons of transfusion requirements between ICUD and ORC and between ECUD and

ORC were statistically significant ($p < 0.001$). However, this difference did not reach statistical significance for ICUD vs. ECUD. Contrary to the IRCC report, length of stay was shortest for ICUD compared to ECUD and ORC (6 vs. 7 and 8 days, respectively, $p < 0.001$).

In our own analysis (Mortezavi et al., unpublished data), we used nationwide population-based data to compare outcomes after RARC vs. ORC in a cohort comprising >97% of the national bladder cancer cases in Sweden over a time period of eight years (2011–2018). To account for possible selection bias, observed differences in baseline characteristics between patients who received ORC vs. RARC were addressed using propensity score matching. The matched cohort consisted of 2428 patients (1554 [64%] ORC and 874 [36%] RARC) from 24 different hospitals in Sweden with balanced preoperative parameters. The vast majority of the procedures were classified as ICUD (94%). Notably, operation time was comparable between the groups (320 min vs. 323 min, $p = 0.5$, Table 2). RARC was associated with lower estimated blood loss (150 ml vs. 700 ml, $p < 0.001$) and intraoperative transfusion rate (7.7% vs. 38.7%, OR = 0.13, $p < 0.001$). Patients undergoing RARC had a shorter length of stay (9d vs. 13d, $p < 0.001$).

Just recently, one-year results of the RACE (Radical Cystectomy Evaluation) study from the Netherlands were reported [17]. This is an ongoing prospective comparative effectiveness study at 19 Dutch centers recruiting a total of 348 participants. Patients entered the nearest hospital, and surgeons did not select a technique based on patient or tumor characteristics. Ten centers performed RARC, nine performed ORC, and two of the participating centers performed both techniques. All but one RARC center performed ICUD leading to a fully minimal invasive approach rate of 88%. To address potential systematic differences between two groups, inverse probability of treatment weighting (IPW) with the pretreatment variables was used. In comparison with RARC, the ORC group showed higher median estimated blood loss (600 vs. 300 ml, $p < 0.01$), shorter median skin-to-skin operating time (229 vs. 330 min, $p < 0.01$), and longer median length of stay (11 vs. 8 d, $p < 0.01$). No statistically significant differences were found regarding transfusion rates (14% vs. 9.2%, $p = 0.17$).

3 Complications

Complications are a critical issue for complex procedures such as radical cystectomy. Rates have been reported extensively for ORC showing a high risk for complications (>60%), including a substantial risk for high-grade (Clavien-Dindo III-V) complications (13–40%) and 30–/90-day mortality (up to 7%) [18, 19]. These rates are dependent on the treated patient population, on peri- and postoperative protocols, and specially on hospital and surgeon experience and volumes. Several studies have demonstrated improved performance in high-volume centers by high-volume surgeons. For a newly introduced technique such as RARC, this has to be taken into consideration. This is particularly the case for the available RCTs, since in contrast to RARP, these trials were conducted at the very beginning of this technical development. Therefore, it is remarkable that in none of these studies, a higher rate of complications was observed for RARC compared to the prior routinely performed technique of ORC. Nix et al. did not observe a significant difference in the total number of complications ($p = 0.3$) and also when comparing the groups using the Clavien-Dindo system ($p = 0.3$) [4]. Ileus was the most observed complication in both groups. However, the RARC cohort demonstrated a more rapid return of bowel function as evidenced by time to flatus ($p = 0.001$) and bowel movement ($p = 0.001$). Patients in the RARC arm also required less in-house analgesia (milligrams of morphine equivalents) compared with their open counterparts (89 vs. 147 mg; $p = 0.019$). Notably, only a limited number of orthotopic bladder substitutions were performed in this RCT (Table 3). In their first RCT, Parekh

Table 3 Prospective randomized controlled trials comparing complication rates between robot-assisted radical cystectomy (RARC) with extracorporeal urinary diversion (ECUD) and with open radical cystectomy (ORC). *OBS* orthotopic bladder substitution, *CC* continent cutaneous reservoir, *FU* follow-up time (for complications), *d* days, *BM* bowel movement. 1, Only complications graded as grade II or higher (Clavien-Dindo); 2, Clavien-Dindo grade III-V; 3, Time to oral solids. N represents the number of analyzed cases

Study	Modality	N	OBS/CC	FU	Any complication	High-grade complication[2]	Mortality	Time to BM
Nix 2009 [4]	RARC	21	7%	NA	33%	NA	0%	3.2
	ORC	20	6%		50%	NA	5%	4.3
Parekh 2013 [5]	RARC	20	NA	NA	25%[1]	NA	NA	4[3]
	ORC	20	NA		25%[1]	NA	NA	5.5[3]
Bochner 2015 [7] (MSKCC)	RARC	60	55%	90d	63%[1]	21%	0%	NA
	ORC	58	60%		65%[1]	21%	1.7%	NA
Khan 2015 [9] (CORAL)	RARC	20	10%	90d	55%	35%	NA	4[3]
	ORC	20	15%		70%	20%	NA	7.5[3]
Parekh 2018 [6] (RAZOR)	RARC	150	25%	90d	67%	22%	NA	NA
	ORC	152	20%		69%	22%	NA	NA

et al. only reported complications graded as Clavien II or higher, and no data on diversion type was available [5]. No difference in the complication rate was detected ($p = 0.5$). Both studies did not provide the follow-up time for complications, which is an important to enable comparability between studies. Bochner et al. reported all Clavien-Dindo grade II-V complications observed in the first 90 postoperative days without finding a difference between the groups (intention to treat (ITT) analysis, 62% and 66% of RARC and ORC patients, difference: −4%; 95% CI, −21 to 13%; $p = 0.7$) [7]. Overall, 21% of patients experienced high-grade complications (grade III-V), with no differences observed between treatment groups (difference: 1.0%; 95% CI, −14 to 16%; $p = 0.9$). When patients were analyzed based on actual surgical procedure received rather than ITT, similar results were observed (Table 3). The types of complications observed were similar in the two groups, with infectious complications the most commonly classified. The only statistically significant difference identified was a higher rate of wound complications in the ORC arm. Khan et al. (CORAL) reported almost identical 30- and 90-day complication rates, although the classification by system showed that multiple complications occurred between day 30 and 90. This observation suggests that patients with a late complication usually also experience complications in the early postoperative stage (30 days), and these events do not have an impact on the overall per patient complication rate. This is in line with the clinical experience that cystectomy patients regularly experience infectious complications or ureteric strictures late in the postoperative course. There were no statistically significant differences between the RARC and ORC arm for all grades and for high-grade complications. Lastly, in the large RAZOR trial, no significant differences in overall (grades I–V) and major (grades III–IV) were identified between the treatment groups. The most common adverse events were urinary tract infection (35% in the RARC group vs. 26% in the ORC group) and postoperative ileus (22% in the RARC group vs. 20% in the ORC).

Radical cystectomy is a two-step procedure, namely, the removal of the bladder/lymph nodes and subsequently the reconstruction and urinary diversion. The majority of the postoperative complications are associated with the reconstructive part, challenging any potential difference in complications between ORC and RARC with ECUD since the technical approach for diversion is identical. The question arises whether the fully minimal invasive approach of ICUD can lead to a lower rate of adverse events, such as ileus, leakages (bowel and urine), hernia, and cardiovascular events, or if we are making an already challenging procedure more complex prolonging the operation time and potentially the complication rate. So far, no level 1 evidence exists for this comparison, although the rate for ICUD has significantly increased from 2% in 2005 to 81% in 2016 and to a lesser extent for intracorporeal orthotopic bladder substitutions (iOBS) with a rate increase from 7% in 2005 to 17% in 2016 (IRCC) [15]. While reporting this significant increase in utilization of ICUD after RARC, Hossein et al. observed that patients treated with ICUD experienced complications more often (57% vs. 43%, $p < 0.001$), especially in the first 30 days after RARC (31% vs. 19%, $p < 0.001$). However, the incidence of high-grade complications after ICUD decreased significantly with time from 25% in 2005 to 6% in 2015 ($p < 0.001$) while it remained stable for ECUD at 13% in 2005 and 14% in 2015 ($p = 0.76$). ECUD was associated with more overall readmissions (34% vs. 26%, $p = 0.003$, Table 4). A history of abdominal surgery was the only significant factor associated with high-grade complications (OR 1.52, 95% CI 1.06–2.15, $p = 0.02$).

Zhang et al. found in their retrospective large single-center three-way comparison that 30-day overall and high-grade complication rates of ICUD were lower than those of ECUD and ORC (Table 3) [16]. This pattern persisted on subsequent 90-day analysis with ICUD demonstrating an advantage of high-grade complications compared to ECUD and ORC ($p = 0.015$). Pairwise comparisons between the robotic approaches (ICUD vs. ECUD) differed in high-grade but not overall complications at 30 and 90 days. All compari-

Table 4 Large retrospective and prospective not randomized cohort/comparative effectiveness studies comparing complication rates of robot-assisted radical cystectomy with extracorporeal urinary diversion (ECUD), intracorporeal urinary diversion (ECUD), and open radical cystectomy (ORC). Results presented as median. *OP* operation, *Estim.* estimated. 1: 94% ICUD. 2: 88% ICUD. N represents the number of analyzed cases. *All results from the inverse probability weighted population

Study	Modality	N	OBS/CC	FU	Any complication	High-grade complication[2]	Mortality	Readmission
Hussein (IRCC), 2018 [15]	ICUD	1031	21%	NA	57%	13%	3%	26%
	ECUD	1094	23%		43%	10%	3%	34%
Zhang (Cleveland), 2020 [16]	ICUD	301	15%	90d	44.2%	16.9%	NA	28.2%
	ECUD	375	29%		48.3%	24.8%	NA	28.8%
	ORC	272	25%		54.8%	26.1%	NA	33.8%
Mortezavi (Sweden), 2021	ICUD[1]	874	20%	90d	50.9%	17.2%	2.7%	34.3%
	ORC	1554	9%		50.5%	23.9%	4.2%	26.1%
Wijburg* (Netherlands) 2021 [17]	ICUD[2]	180	16%	90d	56%	16%	3.4%	24%
	ORC	168	17%		63%	15%	2.4%	21%

sons between ICUD and ORC remained statistically significant. ICUD was associated with lower rate of ileus than ECUD and ORC (21.3% vs. 27.5% and 31.3%, respectively, $p = 0.023$). The total parenteral nutrition requirement was 5.6% of ICUD, 11.7% of ECUD and 18.0% of ORC cases ($p < 0.001$) supporting the findings for ileus. The most frequent complications observed were gastrointestinal, infectious, acute kidney injury, and acute blood loss anemia regardless of the surgical approach. Notably, the ICUD group had the lowest rate for OBS, potentially influencing the complication rates. However, a subgroup analysis for only ileal conduit diversions demonstrated a lower complication rate for ICUD than for ECUD and ORC for the 30 and 90-day time points. On univariable analysis patient age, Charlson Comorbidity Index and operative time were positive predictors of a higher 90-day major complication rate, while the ICUD approach was a negative predictor. These four factors remained significant on multivariable analysis.

In the Swedish population-based cohort study, the overall 90-day complication rate was comparable in both groups. However, ICUD was associated with a significantly lower high-grade complication rate compared with ORC (17.2% vs. 23.9%, OR = 0.66, 95%CI: 0.54–0.82; $p < 0.001$). Notably, the groups were well balanced regarding the preoperative parameters (including ASA score), while the rate for OBS was more than twice as high in the ICUD group than in the ORC cohort. However, we observed a higher 90-day rehospitalization rate in the robotic group (34.3% vs. 26.1%, OR = 1.48, 95%CI: 1.23–1.77; $p < 0.001$). Regarding classification of adverse events, infectious complications were more common in the RARC group, while lymphoceles and events concerning the cardiovascular/respiratory system or the abdominal wall/stoma occurred more frequently in the ORC group.

The only available prospective trial comparing complication rates between RARC with ICUD and ORC is the Dutch comparative effectiveness study using inversed probability of treatment weighting by Wijburg et al. (RACE) [17]. Within 90 days, 63% of ORC and 56% of ICUD patients experienced at least one complication (any grade), resulting in a risk difference of—6.4% (95% CI −17 to 4.5). Regarding major complications, the rates were 15% for ORC and 16% for RARC (risk difference 0.9%, 95% CI −7.0 to 8.8). However, the ORC group had a higher rate of ICU admissions (48% vs. 25%, risk difference 24%, 95% CI 13–34%) and higher use of total parenteral nutrition (33% vs. 16%, risk difference 17%, 95% CI 7.5–27%). No differences were found regarding median time to defecation and unplanned readmissions.

While there are increasing numbers of series reporting data on complications after RARC with intra- and extracorporeal ileal conduit, limited data is available on complications in the subgroup of patients with iOBS. The largest iOBS series included 158 patients from Sweden reporting a 90-day high-grade complication rate of 23% [20]. The lowest rates for high-grade complications were reported from Japan [21] and France [22] with 4.5% and 7.5%, respectively. However, these patients were highly selected in terms of age and other baseline parameters. Therefore, these results were in contrast to rates reported by other groups ranging between 25.0% and 27.5% [23–26]. Simone et al. could show a trend toward a decrease in the overall complication rate (first 15 cases: 66.6%, last 15 cases: 26.7%, $p = 0.07$) and in the high-grade complication rate (first 15 cases: 26.7%, last 15 cases: 6.6%, $p = 0.07$) in the chronology of a learning curve [24]. Simultaneously, he performed a propensity score matched comparison of perioperative complications (30-day) between 64 iOBS and 46 open OBS cases. The open cases experienced a higher incidence of perioperative complications (91.3% vs. 42.2%, $p = 0.001$), most of which represented by the need for blood transfusions [27]. High-grade complications were observed in both groups with a comparable frequency (RARC 6.3% vs. ORC 2.2%, $p = 0.31$), although significantly lower than rates reported by other groups. Overall, the comparability of iOBS with intracorporeal ileal conduits in terms of complication rates remains challenging; most iOBS series report a per patient rate for 0–30 days and 30–90 days without providing a 90-day overall per patient rate, as done by the majority of the abovementioned trials (Table 5).

4 Functional Outcomes

The assessment of the functional outcome after RARC is in most studies limited to urinary continence after orthotopic bladder substitution (OBS). A fully intracorporeal reconstruction of an OBS (iOBS), with detubularization of the isolated bowel segment and subsequent reconfiguration of the reservoir, is challenging and time-consuming. Consequently, the ileal conduit has been the most common intracorporeal urinary diversion after RARC. The number of studies reporting on functional outcome after iOBS is therefore limited.

Irrespective of how an orthotopic neobladder is reconstructed after RARC, it should have a good capacity with low pressure, enable spontaneous micturition, preserve kidney function in the long term, and most important of all it should be continent. In a systematic review of reported functional outcomes by the Pasadena Consensus Panel in 2015, the number of patients evaluated for continence after RARC with iOBS was <200. This number increased in the last five years to a total of 647, brought together in a recent systematic review performed by Daza et al. [29] (Table 6). However, the cases are reported from 12 different cites with the largest series reporting less than 100 cases. Additionally, the authors identified widespread differences in patient selection, methods of data collection, and outcome assessments.

Table 5 Characteristics and complication rates of selected large intracorporal neobladder series

Publication	Desai et al. [23]	Schwentner et al. [26]	Simone et al. [24]	Gok [28]	Hosseini et al. [20]
	Multicenter	Multicenter	Single center	Multicenter	Single center
Year of publication	2014	2015	2016	2019	2020
No. of patients	132	62	45	98	158
Male/female	114 (86.4%)/ 18 (13.6%)	50 (80.6%)/ 12 (19.4%)	32 (71.1%)/ 13 (28.9%)	92 (93.9%)/ 6 (6.1%)	134 (85%)/ 24 (15%)
Shape of neobladder	Globular/ amorphous	Amorphous	Triangular + neobladder neck	Amorphous	Amorphous
Afferent limb	Yes	Yes	None	Yes	Yes
Method of ileal detubularization	Scissors	Scissors	Stapler	Scissors	Scissors
Neobladder construction	Sewn	Sewn	Stapler	Sewn	Sewn
Ureteroileal anastomosis	Bricker/Wallace	Wallace	Modified split-nipple	Wallace	Wallace
Conversion to ECUD	2.9%	0%	0%	–	3%
Short-term complication rate (30d)					
Overall	47%	50%[a]	N = 14[b]	51.0%	63%
High-grade (III-V)	15%	25.8%[a]	N = 0[b]	20.4%	18%
Long-term complication rate (30–90d)					
Overall	27%	–	N = 19[b]	13.3%	24%
High-grade (III-V)	13%	–	N = 5[b]	7.1%	5%
FU time for specific complications	0–90d	ØFU 37.3 mo	0–90d	0–90d	0–90d
Bowel complications	3.8%[1] 1.5%[2] 1.5%[3]	–	20%[1] 5%[3]	6.0%[1]	1%[1] 0.6%[2]
Neobladder leak	4.5%	–	10%	7.1%	9.4%
Ureterointestinal anastomosis stricture	3.8%	8.3%	5%	5.0%	2.5%
Stone formation in the neobladder	2.3%	–	10%	–	1.8%

[1] Bowel obstruction/ileus, [2]Bowel anastomotic leak, [3]Neobladder-bowel fistula
[a] Unknown follow-up time
[b]Authors describe numbers of complications not the complication rate assigned to each case based on the highest grade recorded for the period. High-grade complications: Clavien-Dindo grade III-IV. *FU* follow-up

Table 6 Urinary continence rate in RARC with totally intracorporeal orthotopic bladder substitution

Study	N	Daytime continence	Nighttime continence	Nerve- sparing*	Sexual function
Atmaca 2015 [34]	32 (13***)	84.6%	46.1%	93.7%	IIEF 13.6
Gok 2019 [28]	98 (61**)	60.6%	40.9%	95.7%	IIEF 20.6
Porreca 2019 [32]	51	90.2%	70.6%	50%	31%**
Jonsson 2011 [36]	36	83%	66%	NA	NA
Goh 2012 [37]	15	75%	NA	NA	NA
Tyritzis 2013 [30]	70	89% (m), 67% (f)	73% (m) 67% (f)	64.2%	81%**
Tan 2015 [38]	20	95%	65%	NA	NA
Asimakopoulos 2016 [22]	40	100%	72.5%	100%	21.9
Satkunasivam 2016 [35]	28	16.7% pad free 84% <2 pads	NA	NA	NA
Simone 2018 [24]	45	73.2% (m: 84%, f: 46%)	55.5% (m: 62%, f: 38%)	NA	NA
Sim 2015 [31]	73	89.2%	67.6%	m: 63.4% f: 78.9%	NA
Schwentener 2015 [26]	62	88%	55.1%	93.5%	NA

NA Not available, *Uni- or bilateral, ** Erection sufficient for penetration, *** no of patients available for functional assessment. m, male; f, female

4.1 Continence

Several factors have been identified to have an impact on continence after RARC with iOBS such as age, baseline urinary function, level of motivation, intact innervation to urethral sphincter, and urethral length analogue to open OBS [27]. Additionally, there are technical aspects known from former historic series including internal pressure and capacity of the urinary reservoir, and also time since surgery.

Only a few series have reported on patient cohorts adequately sized for review and statistical analysis. One of the first series of RARC with iOBS was from Tyritzis et al. in 2013 with 70 patients who observed 12-mo daytime continence rates of 89% in men and 67% in women and 12-month night-time continence rates of 73% in men and 67% in female patients [30]. Definition for continence was generally no pad or using one safety pad per day. Following this, four other reports have been available with more than 50 patients in their cohort; a study by Gok et al. included 98 patients undergoing iOBS (Studer pouch) with a follow-up of 24 months. With functional outcome being available for 61 patients, full continence was achieved in 60.6% (0–1 pad), 22.9% had a mild incontinence (1–2 pads), 9.8% moderate (3 pads), and 6.5% severe daytime incontinence (>3 pads) [28]. Nighttime continence was good in 40.9% (dry), fair (dry+1 awakening) in 42.6%, and poor (wet, leakage, urge incontinence) in 16.3% of the cohort. Schwentener et al. included 62 patients in their retrospective study and observed day and nighttime continence (up to 1 pad) of 88% and 55.1% after 12 months, respectively [26]. Similarly, Sim et al. reported a daytime continence rate (no pads) of 89.2% and nighttime of 67.6% in 73 patients receiving an iOBS [31]. In the most recent study by Porreca et al., 51 of the 100 patients included received an iOBS [32]. The overall day and nighttime continence were 90.2% and 70.6%, respectively.

Although the results across the studies reported by high-volume centers seem to be consistent and reproducible, evidence is poor when comparing results to the open technique. In larger contemporary series of open OBS daytime, continence rates range between 87 and 98% and nighttime continence rates between 70 and 95% (iOBS: 61–100% and 41–72.5%) [33]. Atmaca et al. reported a comparable daytime continence with no pad use (75% and 84.6%, $p = 0.6$) after 42 open OBS and 32 iOBS cases [34]. Satkunasivam et al. performed an in-depth analysis of the functional outcome, although the included number of patients was low. They compared 28 patients with iOBS with 79 open OBS cases and demonstrated no difference in the number of pads used, rate of pad-free continence, frequency of mucus leakage, and Bladder Cancer Index questionnaire score [35]. Rates of intermittent self-catheterization were 10.7% in patients receiving robotic surgery and 6.3% in those whose surgeries were open. Urodynamic data from 12 male patients with iOBS showed no detrusor overactivity, normal compliance, and a mean capacity of 514 mL. However, some of the parameters showed an inferior outcome in the iOBS group; for example, timing of pad use (day or night) tended toward both day and night use for the robotic iOBS (78%) compared to the open OBS group (50%; $p = 0.005$). The robotic iOBS group reported the use of larger pads during daytime ($p < 0.001$) and nighttime ($p = 0.007$) compared to the open OBS group. The degree of daytime pad wetness was worse in the robotic iOBS group than in the open OBS group ($p = 0.002$), but wetness was comparable at night ($p = 0.1$). Major limitation is the dissimilar follow-up time of 9.4 moths for the robotic cohort and 62.1 months for the open cohort.

4.2 Sexual Function

Data over sexual function after RARC and iOBS is also limited, and evaluation methods are not clearly defined in the published cohorts. Some series of RARC with iOBS have evaluated erectile function postoperatively with varying results.

In a series of 40 patients that underwent RARC with seminal vesicle sparing approach and iOBS, the authors reported that erectile function returned to normal, defined as an IIEF score greater than 17, in 31 of 40 patients (77.5%) within 3 months while 29 of 40 patients (72.5%) returned to the preoperative IIEF score within 12 months [35]. Gok et al. reported for men with mild dysfunction prior to surgery ($n = 8$) a mean a postoperative IIEF score of 11.1 +/−4.6 and for patients without preoperative sexual dysfunction ($n = 23$), mean score of 20.6 +/−7.4 [28]. Atmaca et al. reported that those with no erectile dysfunction prior to the surgery had better erectile function or higher IIEF scores postoperatively than those with mild dysfunction [34]. These patients also were dependent on PDE5 inhibitors. Although the rate of nerve sparing was higher in the RARC group compared to the open surgery group, the latter one reported better IIEF scores postoperatively (22 vs. 13.6, $n = 13$, $p > 0.05$). In one of the earlier reports by Tyritzis et al., 41 of 62 men (66%) underwent unilateral or bilateral nerve sparing RARC and 81% of patients were potent with or without using PDE5-I at 12 months follow-up [30]. All women in this cohort underwent nerve-sparing surgery, which involves preservation of the autonomic nerves at the anterior vaginal wall at the 10 and 2 o'clock position. Four out of six women remained sexually active postoperatively. Until now, no data on the impact of RARC on female sexual function has been available.

4.3 Quality of Life

Most reported studies have focused on perioperative and oncological outcomes, which are the primary goals of any oncological surgery. Although there is a consensus that quality of life may be as important as survival duration, this domain remains significantly unexplored [39]. And again, the majority of available evidence is for RARC with ECUD leaving the potential benefits of a fully minimal invasive approach on quality of life unanswered. However, all available RCTs reporting HRQoL comparison between RARC with ECUD and ORC have shown no significant differences.

Messer et al. reported on health-related quality-of-life (HRQoL) results of the abovementioned RCT by Parekh et al. in 2013 [5, 40]. Patients completed the Functional Assessment of Cancer Therapy–Vanderbilt Cystectomy Index (FACT–VCI) questionnaire preoperatively and then at 3, 6, 9, and 12 months postoperatively. The FACT–VCI consists of 45 items scored from 0 to 4 with higher scores indicating a better HRQoL. Univariate analysis showed a return to baseline scores at 3 months postoperatively in all measured domains with no statistically significant difference among the various domains between the RARC and the ORC cohorts. Multivariate analysis showed no difference in HRQoL between the two approaches in any of the various domains with the exception of a slightly higher physical well-being score in the RARC group at 6 months.

Bochner et al. used a different questionnaire for assessment of HRQoL [7]. Patients completed the validated European Organisation for Research and Treatment of Cancer (EORTC) Quality of Life Questionnaire Core 30 (QLQ-C30) survey. Similarly, they did not observe any difference between RARC and ORC arms in the HRQoL change from baseline to 3 and 6 mo for any EORTC QLQ-C30 item analyzed.

In the CORAL trial, HRQoL was assessed by the Functional Assessment of Cancer Therapy- Bladder (FACT-Bl) scale v.4, covering physical well-being, functional well-being, emotional well-being, social/family well-being, and additional questions specific to bladder cancer [9]. One questionnaire was analyzed per patient (average 8 mo postoperatively). There were no statistically significant relationships in HRQoL according to surgical arm.

In the large RAZOR trial, outcomes were assessed at baseline, 3 and 6 months after surgery using FACT-VCI [6]. No significant differences were identified between the treatment groups at any timepoint for all FACT-VCI endpoints. In the RARC and ORC group, the mean estimated score for emotional wellbeing was significantly higher at 3 months and 6 months than at baseline ($p < 0.05$). Both groups had significant improvement in mean total FACT-VCI score 6 months after surgery compared with baseline.

Very limited HRQoL data for RARC with ICUD has been reported so far. Wijburg et al. measured HRQoL in their prospective trial at baseline and after cystectomy at 30, 90, 180, and 365 days using FACT-Bl-Cys (formerly FACT-VCI) and Bladder Cancer Index (BCI). Regarding HRQoL, both the BCI and the FACT-Bl-Cys did not show statistically significant differences between RARC (88% ICUD) and ORC at any time point. The mean scores were lowest at 30 days, but at 90 days, both measures returned to the mean baseline score.

Just recently, an interim analysis of 1-year HRQoL data from an ongoing RCT conducted in Italy was reported [39]. Results from patient-reported questionnaire EORTC generic QLQ-C30 and bladder cancer-specific instruments (QLQ-BLM30) were collected at baseline and 1 year after surgery. A total of 51 patients (24 RARC, 27 ORC) were assessed. In the RARC group, all diversions were performed intracorporeal. The most commonly used urinary diversion was the orthotopic Padua ileal bladder for both approaches (RARC 77% vs. ORC 71%; $p = 0.438$). Overall, both groups reported significant worsening of body image and physical and sexual functions (all $p \leq 0.012$). Patients receiving ORC were more likely to report significant 1-year impairment of role functioning, fatigue, dyspnea, constipation, diarrhea, financial difficulties, and abdominal bloating and flatulence (all $p \leq 0.048$). By contrast, no other statistically significant difference except for impairment of urinary symptoms and problems ($p = 0.018$) was observed for the RARC group, suggesting a faster return to normal activities of daily living. This difference may be explained by the lower compliance of a robotic OBS.

5 Oncological Outcomes

Despite the apparent advantages of RARC, debate remains as to whether minimally invasive surgery negatively impacts survival outcomes, potentially due to inadequate resection, suboptimal lymph node dissection, or alteration of recurrence patterns due to "tumor seeding" related to the pneumoperitoneum or insufflation [41–43]. However, growing evidence supports the non-inferiority of RARC in terms of oncological outcome (Table 7) [44]. Individual and pooled results from three prospective randomized clinical trials (RCT) involving 460 patients have confirmed that RARC and ORC are comparable in terms of the positive surgical margin rate, number of removed lymph nodes, progression-free survival (PFS), cancer-specific (CSS) and overall survival (OS) [6, 8, 10, 45]. Two RCTs did not report survival outcome but positive surgical margin (PSM) rates and lymph node (LN) yield; both did not observe a statistically significant difference for these early indicators of oncological outcome ($p > 0.05$ for PSM and LN yield) [4, 5].

The RAZOR trial [6], which is the largest single RCT, compared the two-year PFS between RARC and ORC. Recruiting 302 patients in a 1:1 randomization between RARC and ORC, a non-inferiority of RARC compared to ORC in terms of 2y PFS was observed (72.3% vs. 71.6%, *p*

Table 7 Progression-free survival rates from prospective randomized controlled trials comparing RARC and ORC. 1: mean, 2: median. *RARC* robot-assisted radical cystectomy, *y* year, *ORC* open radical cystectomy, *PFS* progression-free survival, *PSM* positive surgical margin, *LNY* lymph node yield, *Ext* extended, *Stan.* standard

Study	Modality	N	PFS		PSM	LNY
Nix 2009 [17]	RARC	21	–	–	0%	19^1
	ORC	20		–	0%	18^1
Parekh 2013 [5]	RARC	20	–	–	5%	11^2
	ORC	20		–	5%	23^2
Bochner 2018 [8] (MSKCC)	RARC	60	5y	64%	3.3%	Ext: 31.9^1 Stan: 19.5^1
	ORC	58		59%	5.2%	Ext: 30.0^1 Stan: 18.9^1
Khan 2019 [10] (CORAL)	RARC	20	5y	58%	15%	16.3^1
	ORC	20		60%	10%	18.8^1
Parekh 2018 [6] (RAZOR)	RARC	150	2y	72.3%	6%	23.3^1
	ORC	152		71.6%	5%	25.7^1

non-inferiority = 0.001). Bochner et al. [8] compared oncological outcome of RARC and ORC after 5 years in their RCT including 118 patients. Lymph node yield and positive surgical margin rate demonstrated no significant differences based on technique (p = 0.5 and p = 0.6). No differences were observed in PFS (64% RARC, 59% ORC; p = 0.4), cancer-specific survival (CSS, p = 0.4), and overall survival (p = 0.8). In the CORAL trial, a total of 60 patients were randomized 1:1:1 to ORC, RARC, and laparoscopic radical cystectomy [10]. Lymph node yield and positive surgical margin rates were comparable. The 5-yr PFS was 60%, 58%, and 71%; 5-yr CSS was 64%, 68%, and 69%; and 5-yr OS was 55%, 65%, and 61% for ORC, RARC, and LRC, respectively. There was no significant difference in PFS, CSS, and OS between the three surgical arms. Finally, Satkunasivam et al. performed recently a meta-analysis based on data from these RCTs. They found no difference between RARC and ORC in oncologic outcome, including PFS (HR 0.89, 95% CI 0.64–1.24), surgical margin rates (OR 1.00, 95% CI 0.48–2.11), or lymph node dissection yield (mean difference 1.98, 95% CI 5.2 to 1.25) [11].

Besides RCTs of RARC with ECUD, a limited number of large single and multicenter studies assessing the oncological outcome of RARC with ICUD have been reported (Table 8). In contrast to the prior reports, the prospective comparative effectiveness study from 19 Dutch centers reported a significantly higher PSM rate of 18% for ORC compared to only 5.6% for RARC (difference − 12, 95% CI -20 to 5.2), $p < 0.01$) after adjusting for potential baseline differences by means of propensity score-based inverse probability of treatment weighting [17]. The authors did not have an explanation for this not only in comparison but also

Table 8 Oncological outcome parameters of large retrospective and prospective not randomized cohort/comparative effectiveness studies. *PSM* positive surgical margin, *LNY* lymph node yield. N represents the number of analyzed cases. 1, 88% ICUD; 2, 60% ICUD; 3, 94% ICUD; 4, 100% ICUD

Study	Modality	N	Oncological outcome		PSM	LNY (median)
Wijburg (Netherlands), 2021 [17]	RARC[1]	180	1y (PFS)	76%	5.6%	15
	ORC	168		75%	18%	13
Elsayed (IRCC), 2020 [46]	RARC[2]	2107	5y (PFS)	66%	6%	17 (mean)
			5y (OS)	60%		
Mortezavi (Sweden), 2021	RARC[3]	874	5y (OS)	61%	NA	20
	ORC	1554		58%	NA	14
Collins (ERUS), 2017 [47]	RARC[4]	717	2y	75%	4.8%	18

in absolute terms high PSM rate in the ORC group. Furthermore, the median number of removed lymph nodes was significantly higher in the RARC group compared to ORC (15 vs. 13, difference 2.3, 95% CI 0.5–4.2, p = 0.001). Although these early indicators of oncological safety were in favor of RARC, no impact on the short-term oncological outcome could be observed so far. After a follow-up of 12 months, the PFS rates of 75% for ORC and 76% for RARC were comparable (p = 0.8).

One of the largest sources of oncological outcome data on RARC is the IRCC registry. An updated analysis in 2020 with focus on oncological outcome included 2107 patients (60% ICUD) and revealed a 1y and 5y PFS rate of 82% and 66% after a median follow-up time 26 months, respectively. The 1y and 5y OS rate was 88% and 60%, respectively [46]. The PSM rate and mean LN yield were comparable to large open series (Table 8).

In our own large population-based cohort study of bladder cancer in Sweden we observed after propensity score matching for baseline parameters a higher overall mortality after ORC than after RARC with ICUD. The overall-survival benefit was 2% in the first year and increased to around 7% after seven years (hazard ratio 0.83, 95% CI: 0.72–0.96; p = 0.01). We assume that a combination of multiple effects of the minimal invasive approach may have enabled the overall-survival benefit. Besides the observed lower Clavien-Dindo grade V complication rate for RARC (0.8% vs. 1.8%, p = 0.06), estimated blood loss, blood transfusions, higher lymph node yield, and CD III/IV complications were strong predictors of all-cause mortality in the cox analysis; RARC with ICUD had a beneficial effect on all of them.

The EAU Robotic Urology Section (ERUS) Scientific Working Group performed a similar analysis on recurrence rates of 717 patients at 9 institutions who all underwent RARC with ICUD. They observed a PSM rate of 4.8%. PFS rates at 1y and 2y are 80.2% and 74.6%, respectively [47].

These rates are similar compared to the previously discussed RCTs and prior large ORC series [48].

Analogue to functional outcome, oncological outcome for RARC with iOBS is scarce. Recently, follow-up data on the largest iOBS cohort from Sweden was reported [20]. After following 158 patients for a median of 34 months, the 5y PFS, CSS, and OS rates were 70%, 72%, and 71%, respectively.

Although prospective and retrospective trials have reported favorable and comparable recurrence rates after RARC, conflicting evidence exists regarding the recurrence patterns. It has been hypothesized that the lack of tactile feedback, the pneumoperitoneum pressure, and port placement may lead to an inadequate intra-abdominal cancer control. In particular, a retrospective review of 383 consecutive patients who underwent ORC ($n = 120$) or RARC ($n = 263$) observed within 2 years of surgery has a higher incidence of peritoneal carcinomatosis and extraperitoneal lymph node recurrences in patients undergoing RARC, although there was no difference in the total number of local recurrences (ORC 15/65 [23%] vs. RARC 24/136 [18%]). Similarly, the number of distant recurrences did not differ between the groups (26/73 [36%] vs. 43/147 [29%]) [43]. The potential for differences in recurrence patterns was also observed by Bochner et al. [8]. The pattern of first recurrence demonstrated a non-statistically significant increase in metastatic sites for those undergoing ORC (sub-HR [sHR]: 2.21; 95% CI: 0.95–5.11; $p = 0.064$) and a greater number of local/abdominal sites in the RARC-treated patients (sHR: 0.34; 95% CI: 0.12–0.93; $p = 0.035$). However, these observations could not be confirmed in other reported cohorts and studies, and the assessment of different recurrence patterns after cystectomy remains methodologically difficult. The ERUS scientific working group series identified in their RARC cohort of 717 patients bone, lung, and liver as the most frequent location for distant and pelvic lymph nodes for local recurrence [49]. This is consistent with the pattern of recurrences seen in previous studies of ORC and in autopsy series [50]. They did not observe "unusual recurrence patterns"; five patients (0.7%) were diagnosed with peritoneal carcinomatosis and two patients (0.3%) with port site (abdominal wall) metastasis, which are both of low incidence and consistent with published open series. Slightly higher but comparable rates have been reported by the IRCC [46]; in their recent update, port site metastases and peritoneal carcinomatosis were both observed in 1.2% of the patients. An overall local recurrence rate of 11%, despite a significant number of patients with extravesical disease and variant histology, was lower than prior reports. Finally, a systematic literature review in 2016 could only identify four cases of port site metastasis after RARC [51].

Although retrospective in these large cohorts, no evidence of an unusual recurrence pattern after RARC was observed. The RCT iROC will most likely be sufficiently powered to shed more light on this issue.

References

1. Bagi P, Nordsten CB, Kehlet H. Cystectomy for bladder cancer in Denmark during the 2006–2013 period. Dan Med J. 2016;63(4):748.
2. Collins JW, Patel H, Adding C, Annerstedt M, Dasgupta P, Khan SM, et al. Enhanced recovery after robot-assisted radical cystectomy: EAU robotic urology section scientific working group consensus view. Eur Urol. 2016;70(4):649–60.
3. Collins JW, Tyritzis S, Nyberg T, Schumacher M, Laurin O, Khazaeli D, et al. Robot-assisted radical cystectomy: description of an evolved approach to radical cystectomy. Eur Urol. 2013;64(4):654–63.
4. Nix J, Smith A, Kurpad R, Nielsen ME, Wallen EM, Pruthi RS. Prospective randomized controlled trial of robotic versus open radical cystectomy for bladder cancer: perioperative and pathologic results. Eur Urol. 2010;57(2):196–201.
5. Parekh DJ, Messer J, Fitzgerald J, Ercole B, Svatek R. Perioperative outcomes and oncologic efficacy from a pilot prospective randomized clinical trial of open versus robotic assisted radical cystectomy. J Urol. 2013;189(2):474–9.
6. Parekh DJ, Reis IM, Castle EP, Gonzalgo ML, Woods ME, Svatek RS, et al. Robot-assisted radical cystectomy versus open radical cystectomy in patients with bladder cancer (RAZOR): an open-label, randomised, phase 3, non-inferiority trial. Lancet. 2018;391(10139):2525–36.
7. Bochner BH, Dalbagni G, Sjoberg DD, Silberstein J, Keren Paz GE, Donat SM, et al. Comparing open radical cystectomy and robot-assisted laparoscopic radical cystectomy: a randomized clinical trial. Eur Urol. 2015;67(6):1042–50.
8. Bochner BH, Dalbagni G, Marzouk KH, Sjoberg DD, Lee J, Donat SM, et al. Randomized trial comparing open radical cystectomy and robot-assisted laparoscopic radical cystectomy: oncologic outcomes. Eur Urol. 2018;74(4):465–71.
9. Khan MS, Gan C, Ahmed K, Ismail AF, Watkins J, Summers JA, et al. A single-Centre early phase randomised controlled three-arm trial of open, robotic, and laparoscopic radical cystectomy (CORAL). Eur Urol. 2016;69(4):613–21.
10. Khan MS, Omar K, Ahmed K, Gan C, Van Hemelrijck M, Nair R, et al. Long-term oncological outcomes from an early phase randomised controlled three-arm trial of open, robotic, and laparoscopic radical cystectomy (CORAL). Eur Urol. 2020;77(1):110–8.
11. Satkunasivam R, Tallman CT, Taylor JM, Miles BJ, Klaassen Z, Wallis CJD. Robot-assisted radical cystectomy versus open radical cystectomy: a meta-analysis of oncologic, perioperative, and complication-related outcomes. Eur Urol Oncol. 2019;2(4):443–7.
12. Kimura S, Iwata T, Foerster B, Fossati N, Briganti A, Nasu Y, et al. Comparison of perioperative complications and health-related quality of life between robot-assisted and open radical cystectomy: a systematic review and meta-analysis. Int J Urol. 2019;26(8):760–74.
13. Bertolo R, Agudelo J, Garisto J, Armanyous S, Fergany A, Kaouk J. Perioperative outcomes and complications after robotic radical cystectomy with intracorporeal or extracorporeal ileal conduit urinary diversion: head-to-head comparison from a single-institutional prospective study. Urology. 2019;129:98–105.
14. Lenfant L, Verhoest G, Campi R, Parra J, Graffeille V, Masson-Lecomte A, et al. Perioperative outcomes and complications of intracorporeal vs extracorporeal urinary diversion after robot-assisted radical cystectomy for bladder cancer: a real-life, multi-institutional French study. World J Urol. 2018;36(11):1711–8.

15. Hussein AA, May PR, Jing Z, Ahmed YE, Wijburg CJ, Canda AE, et al. Outcomes of intracorporeal urinary diversion after robot-assisted radical cystectomy: results from the International Robotic Cystectomy Consortium. J Urol. 2018;199(5):1302–11.
16. Zhang JH, Ericson KJ, Thomas LJ, Knorr J, Khanna A, Crane A, et al. Large single institution comparison of perioperative outcomes and complications of open radical cystectomy, intracorporeal robot-assisted radical cystectomy and robotic extracorporeal approach. J Urol. 2020;203(3):512–21.
17. Wijburg CJ, Michels CTJ, Hannink G, Grutters JPC, Rovers MM, Alfred Witjes J, et al. Robot-assisted radical cystectomy versus open radical cystectomy in bladder cancer patients: a multicentre comparative effectiveness study. Eur Urol. 2021;79(5):609–18.
18. Novara G, De Marco V, Aragona M, Boscolo-Berto R, Cavalleri S, Artibani W, et al. Complications and mortality after radical cystectomy for bladder transitional cell cancer. J Urol. 2009;182(3):914–21.
19. Novara G, Catto JW, Wilson T, Annerstedt M, Chan K, Murphy DG, et al. Systematic review and cumulative analysis of perioperative outcomes and complications after robot-assisted radical cystectomy. Eur Urol. 2015;67(3):376–401.
20. Hosseini A, Mortezavi A, Sjoberg S, Laurin O, Adding C, Collins J, et al. Robot-assisted intracorporeal orthotopic bladder substitution after radical cystectomy: perioperative morbidity and oncological outcomes – a single-institution experience. BJU Int. 2020;126(4):464–71.
21. Koie T, Ohyama C, Yoneyama T, Nagasaka H, Yamamoto H, Imai A, et al. Robotic cross-folded U-configuration intracorporeal ileal neobladder for muscle-invasive bladder cancer: initial experience and functional outcomes. Int J Med Robot. 2018;14(6):e1955.
22. Asimakopoulos AD, Campagna A, Gakis G, Corona Montes VE, Piechaud T, Hoepffner JL, et al. Nerve sparing, robot-assisted radical cystectomy with intracorporeal bladder substitution in the male. J Urol. 2016;196(5):1549–57.
23. Desai MM, Gill IS, de Castro Abreu AL, Hosseini A, Nyberg T, Adding C, et al. Robotic intracorporeal orthotopic neobladder during radical cystectomy in 132 patients. J Urol. 2014;192(6):1734–40.
24. Simone G, Papalia R, Misuraca L, Tuderti G, Minisola F, Ferriero M, et al. Robotic intracorporeal Padua ileal bladder: surgical technique, perioperative, oncologic and functional outcomes. Eur Urol. 2018;73(6):934–40.
25. Tan WS, Lamb BW, Tan MY, Ahmad I, Sridhar A, Nathan S, et al. In-depth critical analysis of complications following robot-assisted radical cystectomy with intracorporeal urinary diversion. Eur Urol Focus. 2017;3(2–3):273–9.
26. Schwentner C, Sim A, Balbay MD, Todenhofer T, Aufderklamm S, Halalsheh O, et al. Robot-assisted radical cystectomy and intracorporeal neobladder formation: on the way to a standardized procedure. World J Surg Oncol. 2015;13(3):1–6.
27. Simone G, Tuderti G, Misuraca L, Anceschi U, Ferriero M, Minisola F, et al. Perioperative and mid-term oncologic outcomes of robotic assisted radical cystectomy with totally intracorporeal neobladder: results of a propensity score matched comparison with open cohort from a single-centre series. Eur J Surg Oncol. 2018;44(9):1432–8.
28. Gok B, Atmaca AF, Canda AE, Asil E, Koc E, Ardicoglu A, et al. Robotic radical cystectomy with intracorporeal Studer pouch formation for bladder cancer: experience in ninety-eight cases. J Endourol. 2019;33(5):375–82.
29. Daza J, Jones T, Raven M, Charap A, Sfakianos JP, Mehrazin R, et al. Functional outcomes after robotic radical cystectomy with intracorporeal diversion: a systematic review. Bladder Cancer. 2020;6:329–42.
30. Tyritzis SI, Hosseini A, Collins J, Nyberg T, Jonsson MN, Laurin O, et al. Oncologic, functional, and complications outcomes of robot-assisted radical cystectomy with totally intracorporeal neobladder diversion. Eur Urol. 2013;64(5):734–41.
31. Sim A, Balbay MD, Todenhofer T, Aufderklamm S, Halalsheh O, Mischinger J, et al. Robot-assisted radical cystectomy and intracorporeal urinary diversion – safe and reproducible? Cent European J Urol. 2015;68(1):18–23.
32. Porreca A, Mineo Bianchi F, Romagnoli D, D'Agostino D, Corsi P, Giampaoli M, et al. Robot-assisted radical cystectomy with totally intracorporeal urinary diversion: surgical and early functional outcomes through the learning curve in a single high-volume center. J Robot Surg. 2020;14(2):261–9.
33. Lee RK, Abol-Enein H, Artibani W, Bochner B, Dalbagni G, Daneshmand S, et al. Urinary diversion after radical cystectomy for bladder cancer: options, patient selection, and outcomes. BJU Int. 2014;113(1):11–23.
34. Atmaca AF, Canda AE, Gok B, Akbulut Z, Altinova S, Balbay MD. Open versus robotic radical cystectomy with intracorporeal Studer diversion. JSLS. 2015;19(1):e201400193.
35. Satkunasivam R, Santomauro M, Chopra S, Plotner E, Cai J, Miranda G, et al. Robotic intracorporeal orthotopic neobladder: urodynamic outcomes, urinary function, and health-related quality of life. Eur Urol. 2016;69(2):247–53.
36. Jonsson MN, Adding LC, Hosseini A, Schumacher MC, Volz D, Nilsson A, et al. Robot-assisted radical cystectomy with intracorporeal urinary diversion in patients with transitional cell carcinoma of the bladder. Eur Urol. 2011;60(5):1066–73.
37. Goh AC, Gill IS, Lee DJ, de Castro Abreu AL, Fairey AS, Leslie S, et al. Robotic intracorporeal orthotopic ileal neobladder: replicating open surgical principles. Eur Urol. 2012;62(5):891–901.
38. Tan WS, Sridhar A, Goldstraw M, Zacharakis E, Nathan S, Hines J, et al. Robot-assisted intracorporeal pyramid neobladder. BJU Int. 2015;116(5):771–9.
39. Mastroianni R, Tuderti G, Anceschi U, Bove AM, Brassetti A, Ferriero M, et al. Comparison of patient-reported health-related quality of life between open radical cystectomy and robot-assisted radical cystectomy with intracorporeal urinary diversion: interim analysis of a randomised controlled trial. Eur Urol Focus. 2021; https://doi.org/10.1016/j.euf.2021.03.002.
40. Messer JC, Punnen S, Fitzgerald J, Svatek R, Parekh DJ. Health-related quality of life from a prospective randomised clinical trial of robot-assisted laparoscopic vs open radical cystectomy. BJU Int. 2014;114(6):896–902.
41. Ost MC, Patel KP, Rastinehad AR, Chu PY, Anderson AE, Smith AD, et al. Pneumoperitoneum with carbon dioxide inhibits macrophage tumor necrosis factor-alpha secretion: source of transitional-cell carcinoma port-site metastasis, with prophylactic irrigation strategies to decrease laparoscopic oncologic risks. J Endourol. 2008;22(1):105–12.
42. Albisinni S, Fossion L, Oderda M, Aboumarzouk OM, Aoun F, Tokas T, et al. Critical analysis of early recurrence after laparoscopic radical cystectomy in a large cohort by the ESUT. J Urol. 2016;195(6):1710–7.
43. Nguyen DP, Al Hussein Al Awamlh B, Wu X, O'Malley P, Inoyatov IM, Ayangbesan A, et al. Recurrence patterns after open and robot-assisted radical cystectomy for bladder cancer. Eur Urol. 2015;68(3):399–405.
44. Yuh B, Wilson T, Bochner B, Chan K, Palou J, Stenzl A, et al. Systematic review and cumulative analysis of oncologic and functional outcomes after robot-assisted radical cystectomy. Eur Urol. 2015;67(3):402–22.
45. Rai BP, Bondad J, Vasdev N, Adshead J, Lane T, Ahmed K, et al. Robotic versus open radical cystectomy for bladder cancer in adults. Cochrane Database Syst Rev. 2019;4:CD011903.
46. Elsayed AS, Gibson S, Jing Z, Wijburg C, Wagner AA, Mottrie A, et al. Rates and patterns of recurrences and survival outcomes after robot-assisted radical cystectomy: results from the International Robotic Cystectomy Consortium. J Urol. 2021;205(2):407–13.

47. Collins JW, Hosseini A, Adding C, Nyberg T, Koupparis A, Rowe E, et al. Corrigendum re: "Early recurrence patterns following totally intracorporeal robot-assisted radical cystectomy: results from the EAU robotic urology section (ERUS) scientific working group" [Eur Urol 2017;71:723-6]. Eur Urol. 2017;72(3):e80.
48. Hautmann RE, de Petriconi RC, Pfeiffer C, Volkmer BG. Radical cystectomy for urothelial carcinoma of the bladder without neoadjuvant or adjuvant therapy: long-term results in 1100 patients. Eur Urol. 2012;61(5):1039–47.
49. Collins JW, Hosseini A, Adding C, Nyberg T, Koupparis A, Rowe E, et al. Early recurrence patterns following totally intracorporeal robot-assisted radical cystectomy: results from the EAU robotic urology section (ERUS) scientific working group. Eur Urol. 2017;71(5):723–6.
50. Wallmeroth A, Wagner U, Moch H, Gasser TC, Sauter G, Mihatsch MJ. Patterns of metastasis in muscle-invasive bladder cancer (pT2-4): an autopsy study on 367 patients. Urol Int. 1999;62(2):69–75.
51. Khetrapal P, Tan WS, Lamb B, Nathan S, Briggs T, Shankar A, et al. Port-site metastases after robotic radical cystectomy: a systematic review and management options. Clin Genitourin Cancer. 2017;15(4):440–4.

Robotic Surgery Applications for Benign Bladder Diseases

H. John, N. Abo Youssef, and A. Ploumidis

1 Robot-Assisted YV Plasty (RAYV) for Recurrent Bladder Neck Stenosis

N. Abo Youssef and H. John

1.1 Introduction

The transurethral surgery of the prostate due to benign prostatic hyperplasia (BPH) is the gold standard after failed or refused medical therapy [1]. The well-known complication of a bladder neck stenosis (BNS) occurs rarely but most frequently described after transurethral resection of the prostate. According to the International Consultation on Urological Diseases (ICUD), the term “bladder neck stenosis (BNS)” is recommended to use when the prostate is still in situ [2]. In cases where BNS occurs after radical/total prostatectomy, the condition should be described as “vesicourethral anastomotic stenosis (VUAS).” In the present chapter, we focus on the technique of the robot-assisted YV plasty for recurrent BNS as an individualized treatment option.

1.2 Etiology

The fully pathophysiological mechanisms of bladder neck stenosis remain unknown. As showed by Barboglu et al., smoking, coronary artery disease, hypertension, and diabetes contribute to VUAS; it appears obvious to transfer these unfavorable predictors in the same way to BNS [3]. The altered microvascular blood supply in the bladder neck in combination with the local iatrogenic ischemia/wounds could favor the scar formation [4]. Several risk factors are described to be associated with BNS: small prostate volume, higher International Prostate Symptom Score storage scores (IPSS), preoperative uncontrolled infection, unsuitable resectoscope, large resection loop, extensive resection of the bladder neck, long surgical time, and recatherization after surgery. The incidence of BNS after transurethral resection of the prostate (TUR-P) is described between 0.3 and 9.2% [5–7]. It occurs typically early within the first 2 years post-operation after transurethral therapy [4]; thereby, no significant difference between monopolar and bipolar resection technique has been shown [8]. Other techniques such as photo vaporization of the prostate reported similar rates of BNS [9].

1.3 Treatment Options

An initial treatment step for the primary BNS is the widely accepted endoscopic procedure. It ranges from a simple dilatation, bladder neck resection (TUR-BN), bladder neck incision (TUI-BN), stent placement, bipolar plasma vaporization, injection of mitomycin C to various kinds of laser-type incision. The success rates of the most common option of the TUR-BN and TUI-BN are reported approximately 90% [10]. C. M. Rosenbaum et al. and other studies showed a declined success rate [11]. However, highly repeated BNS are rare and complex. Reconstructive surgery as a further treatment option should be discussed with the patient. First described by Young in 1953 [12], the latest YV plasty with the transposition of a well-vascularized bladder wall flap into the completely transected anterior area of the bladder neck is gaining more popularity—especially in the area of robotic urology.

Supplementary Information The online version contains supplementary material available at [https://doi.org/10.1007/978-3-031-00363-9_66].

H. John (✉)
Klinik für Urologie, EBU Certified Training Centre, Urologisches Tumorzentrum, Kantonsspital Winterthur, Winterthur, Switzerland

N. Abo Youssef
Klinik für Urologie, EBU Certified Training Centre, Kantonsspital Winterthur, Winterthur, Switzerland

A. Ploumidis
Department of Urology, Athens Medical Center, Athens, Greece

P. Wiklund et al. (eds.), *Robotic Urologic Surgery*, https://doi.org/10.1007/978-3-031-00363-9_66

1.4 Patient Selection and Preoperative Preparation

A diagnostic cystoscopy has to be performed prior to surgery to confirm and assess the bladder neck stenosis. At least two unsuccessful endoscopic treatments should be performed before confirming the indication of a YV pasty. Patients are given a single broad-spectrum antibiotic within 60 minutes of skin incision. An indwelling bladder catheter is placed if possible, alternatively a single-use catheter.

1.5 Surgical Technique

Patients are placed in a supine 15° Trendelenburg position with abducted legs. All pressure points should be padded. After setting a pneumoperitoneum with 12 mmHg over the 8 mm paraumbilical camera port, a total of four ports are inserted according to the scheme of the radical prostatectomy (da Vinci Xi® system): two left lateral 8 mm worksite ports and one 8 mm working port on the right side. The port distance should range between 6 and 10 cm along a line perpendicular to the target anatomy. Furthermore, a 5 mm assistant port and a 12 mm VersaPort™ is inserted in the right lower quadrant (not between da Vinci ports) (Fig. 1).

According to the radical prostatectomy [13], the extraperitoneal approach offers some advantages (e.g., better pulmonal ventilation due to reduced Trendelenburg position, open dissection planes after previous intraperitoneal surgery [14]). However, the standard transperitoneal approach should be chosen if there are some contraindication for the extraperitoneal approach such as hernia mesh implants or pelvic kidney. In the following section, the technique refers to the extraperitoneal approach.

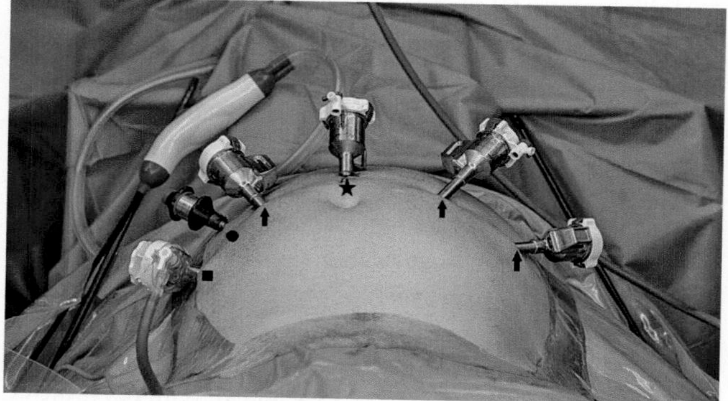

Fig. 1 ★ camera port, ↑ 8 mm worksite port, ■ 12 mm VersaPort™, • 5 mm trocar

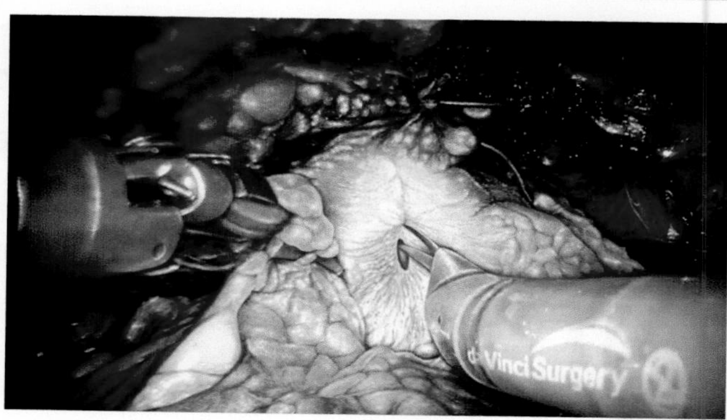

Fig. 2 Incision of the vesicoprostatic stenosis

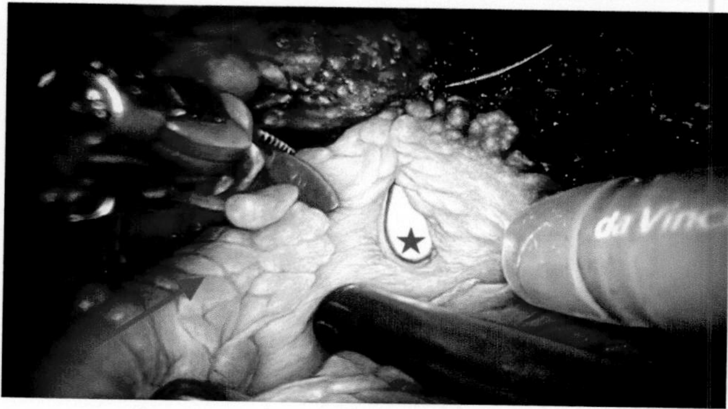

Fig. 3 The stenotic area of the bladder neck and intraprostatic urethra is widely open. ↗ bladder wall, ★ tip of indwelling catheter

1.6 Operative Technique

As a first step, the prevesical fat is removed and the perivesical space cleaned. The bladder neck is located, and the ventral part of the prostate is exposed. Carefully the pelvic floor around the prostate is exposed. The anterior prostatic venous plexus can be ligated to avoid bleeding. An anterior longitudinal incision in hot and cold scissor-incision technique is performed starting from the bladder neck and ventral vesico-prostatic junction down through the stenotic area (Figs. 2 and 3). The caudal extension of the incision is performed at the height of the seminal colliculus. As the dorsal bladder base and ureteral ridges are not touched, ureteral stents are not routinely necessary. The cut is enlarged to an inverted Y-shaped manner (Fig. 4). As a result, a well-vascularized and tension-free flap is created, which offers the possibility of reconstructing a wide bladder neck and an anterior prostatic urethra with vital tissue. Therefore, the tip of the inverted V-flap is brought and fixed to the base point of the inverted Y-incision distal of the stricture (Fig. 5). This is an essential step to keep the reconstruction

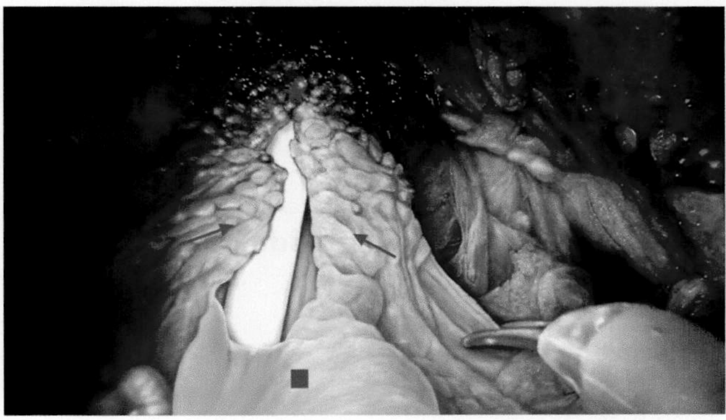

Fig. 4 The incision is prolonged into the bladder as an inverted Y in order to create a flap. ★ prostatic capsule, → bladder wall, ■ flap

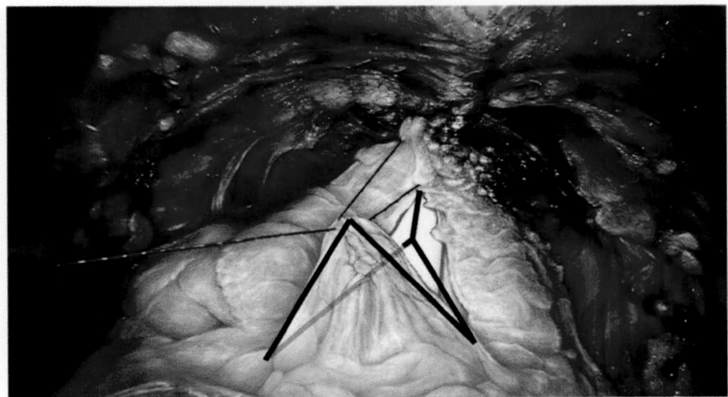

Fig. 5 The tip of the flap is fixed at the base point of the inverted Y incision with a 3–0 barbed suture

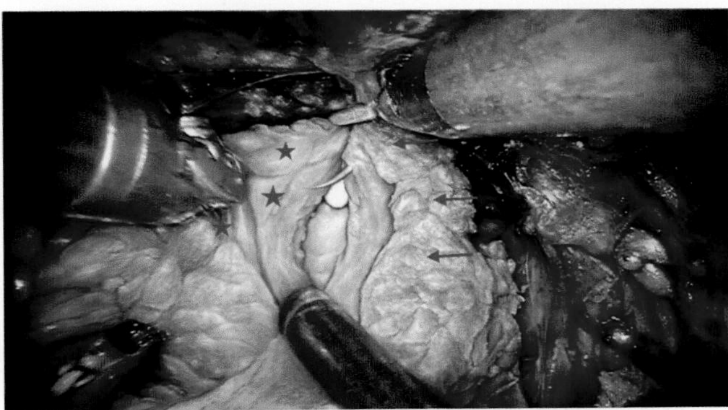

Fig. 6 Closure of the right inverted Y side of the bladder flap. ★ right side of the bladder flap, ← prostatic capsule

symmetric. Both sides of the inverted V shape are then closed with running sutures using a V-Loc™ 3–0 (Figs. 6 and 7). Thereafter, a new indwelling catheter 20 Fr foley is placed. To test the leak tightness, the bladder should be filled with 200 ml of sterile normal saline. There is no necessity of a pelvic drain.

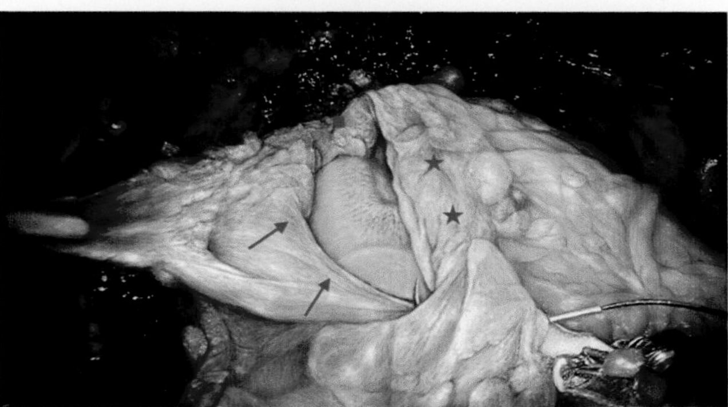

Fig. 7 Closure of the left side of the bladder flap by an ascending continuous suture. ★ left side of the bladder flap, → bladderwall, ■ prostatic capsule

1.7 Postoperative Management

Patients suffer from full diet and mobilization on day 1 postoperatively. The transurethral catheter can be removed on the fifth postoperative day after exclusion of a urinary extravasation in the cystourethrogram. Spontaneous micturition is observed with urinary diary and the residual volume controlled by ultrasound.

1.8 Discussion

Bladder neck stenosis (BNS) ranges from a simple contracture to recurrent stenoses, which are refractory to repeated surgical treatments. The primary surgical technique, including the necessity of the application of thermal, cryo, or radiation energy, the occurrence of urinary infections, or the delayed wound healing – all may play an important role in the development of BNS. Today, there exists a variety of surgical possibilities to treat BNS such as dilatation, transurethral resection, cold knife incision, diversion, open reconstruction, adjuvant agents during transurethral surgery, and more. The treatment of choice remains unclear and provides the opportunity of discussion based on the complex underlying disease. Cindolo et al. argue that the lack of well-designed studies makes it reasonable to leave the choice of BNS treatment technique to the surgeon's own judgement [15]. J. Kranz et al. reported that most patients who have undergone an endoscopic therapy are treated successfully in up to 65% after the first TUR. However, there was a success rate of only 25% after more than three transurethral procedures [16]. To higher the chances of success in complex bladder neck stenosis, the reconstruction of the bladder neck should be discussed into account of the patient age and comorbidities. The open surgical approach is weakly recommended due to the necessity of a relatively large and morbid median laparotomy, which is needed to gain an acceptable exposure of the surgical field [17]. A robot-assisted minimally invasive surgical procedure provides once again several advantages: wider range of motion near the bladder neck, enhanced visualization especially to define the anatomical borders of the external sphincter, less blood loss, etc.

Reiss et al. propose for patients with BNS the so-called T plasty, which is basically a modified YV plasty for recurrent BNS, with a reported high success rate in all ten patients (defined as no need for further instrumentation); thereby, two vascularized flaps are used to reconstruct the bladder neck in comparison to one flap with the YV technique. The argument creating a wider bladder neck with less tension and thus theoretically to reduce the risk of recurrence remains doubtful. A group from Kliniken Essen-Mitte, around M. Musch et al. in Germany showed in a case series including 12 patients treated with RAYV a treatment success of more than 80% during a median follow-up of 23.2 months. No intraoperative or major postoperative complications were observed [17]. Another case series with a retrospective evaluation of 24 patients who underwent an open YV plasty showed a significant improvement of postoperative Qmax, post-void urine residual, and IPSS score [18].

We are currently in our institution in process conducting a case series with at least 30 patients who received RAVY due to BNS. In general, we prefer an extraperitoneal access as there is no need for a large dissection area in the intraperitoneal cavity, preventing any intraperitoneal complications and drawbacks. While an extraperitoneal approach in BNS procedure is very suitable, we recommend a transperitoneal access in patients with vesicourethral anastomotic stenosis. We always incise the prostatic capsule and full-thickness bladder wall with hot and cold scissors, which is at least as efficient as a blade fixed in a needle holder. Finally, we suture the inverted V flap in continuous suture technique with a barbed suture, which allows a stable flap position. The use of indocyanine green in the da Vinci fluorescence imaging mode helps us to confirm blood flow in the tip of the inverted V bladder flap. In patients with long stricture zones, including the external sphincter and consecutive possible stress urinary incontinence, an artificial sphincter system can be placed in the future if necessary.

1.9 Conclusion

After repetitive endourological attempts to cure BNS, a new reconstructive procedure must be offered to the patient as a definitive solution. The robot-assisted inverted YV plasty of the bladder neck with interposition of a well-vascularized bladder flap into the edges of the opened bladder neck and prostatic stricture seems to be a promising concept with good early postoperative results.

2 Robotic-Assisted Bladder Diverticulectomy

A. Ploumidis

2.1 Introduction

Bladder diverticula (BD) are herniations of the bladder urothelium and lamina propria through a defect of the bladder wall. Because they lack muscularis propria lining and contain only a few scattered muscle fibers, they are unable to contract efficiently during voiding. Subsequently failing to empty their content causes urinary stasis and high residual volume in the bladder [19].

Although BD are usually asymptomatic, they may cause LUTS, urinary tract infections, formation of bladder calculi within the BD, and sensation of incomplete bladder emptying, all of which are associated with the urinary stasis [20, 21]. In rare cases, they may compress the ureter causing ureteral obstruction and hydronephrosis [22]. Furthermore, an increased risk of bladder cancer due to chronic inflammation within the BD has been noticed [23].

BD are classified as congenital and acquired. The former is commonly seen in the pediatric population, while the latter is usually secondary to obstruction and high voiding pressure and is typically encountered in older adults. In this chapter, we are mainly going to address BD in adults secondary to bladder outlet obstruction such as urethral stricture, bladder neck contracture, benign prostatic enlargement, etc. [24–26].

Bladder diverticulectomy is indicated in large symptomatic cases and was first described in 1987 by Czerny et al. [27]. In 1992, Parra et al. reported the first laparoscopic bladder diverticulectomy (LBD), while the first robotic bladder diverticulectomy (RBD) followed in Berger et al. in 2006 [28, 29]. Since then, many RBD case series have been described with good functional results, and RBD can be offered sequentially after other procedures that address the underlying bladder outlet obstruction (BOO), such as robotic simple prostatectomy (RSP), TURP, PVP, HOLEP, robotic radical prostatectomy, etc. [30–35] or alone as part of a second staged procedure where the obstruction has already been managed on the first stage.

2.2 Preoperative Evaluation and Preparation

Cystoscopy is the mainstay of the preoperative evaluation especially when surgery is considered. It can give information about the number, size, location of the BD relative to the ureteral orifices, concomitant stones, or transitional cell carcinoma (TCC).

Other imaging studies such as ultrasonography, computed tomography, voiding cystourethrogram (VCUG) can give further details for the upper and lower urinary tracts as far as reflux, hydronephrosis, and underlying LUTS is concerned.

Urine cytology should be offered to all patients given the higher probability of TCC in the BD. Urinalysis, negative urine culture, and informed consent preoperatively are mandatory.

2.3 Operating Room Configuration and Patient Positioning

Under general anesthesia, the patient is placed in a dorsal lithotomy position with the legs supported on Allen stirrups and the hands tucked to the sides. All pressure points are well padded. The perineum and abdomen are prepared and draped for cystoscopic evaluation and for trocar placement. A single perioperative dose of broad-spectrum antibiotic prophylaxis is administered.

2.4 Endoscopic Preparation

We suggest a cystoscopic evaluation before the robotic operation especially in the beginning of the learning curve. Apart from visualizing the BD, a Councill-tip catheter can be placed over a wire inside the diverticulum. Selective distention of the diverticulum by installation of fluid through the catheter can aid the identification and dissection of the diverticulum during surgery [36–38]. Others have suggested intraoperative transillumination of the BD with the flexible cystoscope placed inside the BD [39, 40].

Furthermore, most of the times the BD is located anterolateral to the ipsilateral ureteral orifice and in close proximity. Placement of a ureteral catheter or a stiff hydrophilic wire that can be manipulated by the assistant could aid in the identification of the ureter and avoid subsequent injury. After cystoscopy, a bladder catheter is placed.

If the cystoscopy has already been done in the office setting and the surgeon feels adequate confident of identifying both BD and ipsilateral ureter, this part of the procedure can be omitted [30].

It is important to emphasize that if an endoscopic procedure for BOO (such as TURP, HOLEP, or GreenLight laser) is performed sequentially to RBD, it should be performed before RBD to avoid the potential risk of bladder perforation on the suture line due to the irrigation fluid. For the same reason, the bladder and prostatic bed should be thoroughly checked at the end of the endoscopic procedure for blood clots and for free prostatic tissue to avoid potential blockage of the output of the catheter during continuous irrigation postoperatively.

2.5 Trocar Placement and Instrumentation

Our technique uses a four-arm robotic configuration with an addition of one or two laparoscopic ports for the bedside assistant. A 12 mm or 8 mm robotic camera trocar (depending if the da Vinci Si or Xi system [Intuitive Surgical] is being used) is placed supraumbilical. Two 8 mm robotic trocars are placed 8 cm lateral to the camera trocar on each side of the rectus abdominis muscle. The fourth robotic trocar is placed 8 cm to the right of the right lateral robotic port and at least two fingerbreadths above the anterior superior iliac spine (ASIS). When the da Vinci Si is used, the trocars are placed more in an arc configuration where with the da Vinci Xi, they are placed more in a straight line. A 12 mm assisting trocar is placed between and slightly higher the camera port and the left lateral robotic trocar. If needed, an additional 5 mm trocar can be placed lateral to the left robotic trocar and at least two fingerbreadths higher than the ASIS.

This trocar configuration is similar to that of robotic simple prostatectomy (RSP) (and radical prostatectomy); since in our experience, most of the times RBD is offered sequentially to this operation. On the contrary to what was mentioned above for sequential endoscopic procedures for BOO, in the case of a combined pure robotic procedure, we believe that it is preferable to start with the RBD followed by the RSP. The reason for this is that in some cases RSP could be accompanied by slight hemorrhage, which will hinder the good visibility needed for the dissection of the BD if an intravesical approach is decided.

Our preference is to place the fourth robotic arm on the side of the dominant hand of the surgeon (right iliac fossa for a right-handed surgeon). The reason for this is that especially during RBD the surgeon will need to continuously change between two grasping tools (left robotic arm and fourth arm) in order to lift a large diverticulum and one grasping tool and the scissors (left and right robotic arm) in order to perform blunt and sharp dissection (Fig. 8).

Finally, the patient is placed in a steep Trendelenburg position (25–30%), and side docking of the robot will facilitate intraoperative cystoscopy if needed.

We usually use three robotic instruments: Hot Shears monopolar [Intuitive Surgical] curved scissors, Fenestrated Bipolar [Intuitive Surgical] forceps, and a large needle driver

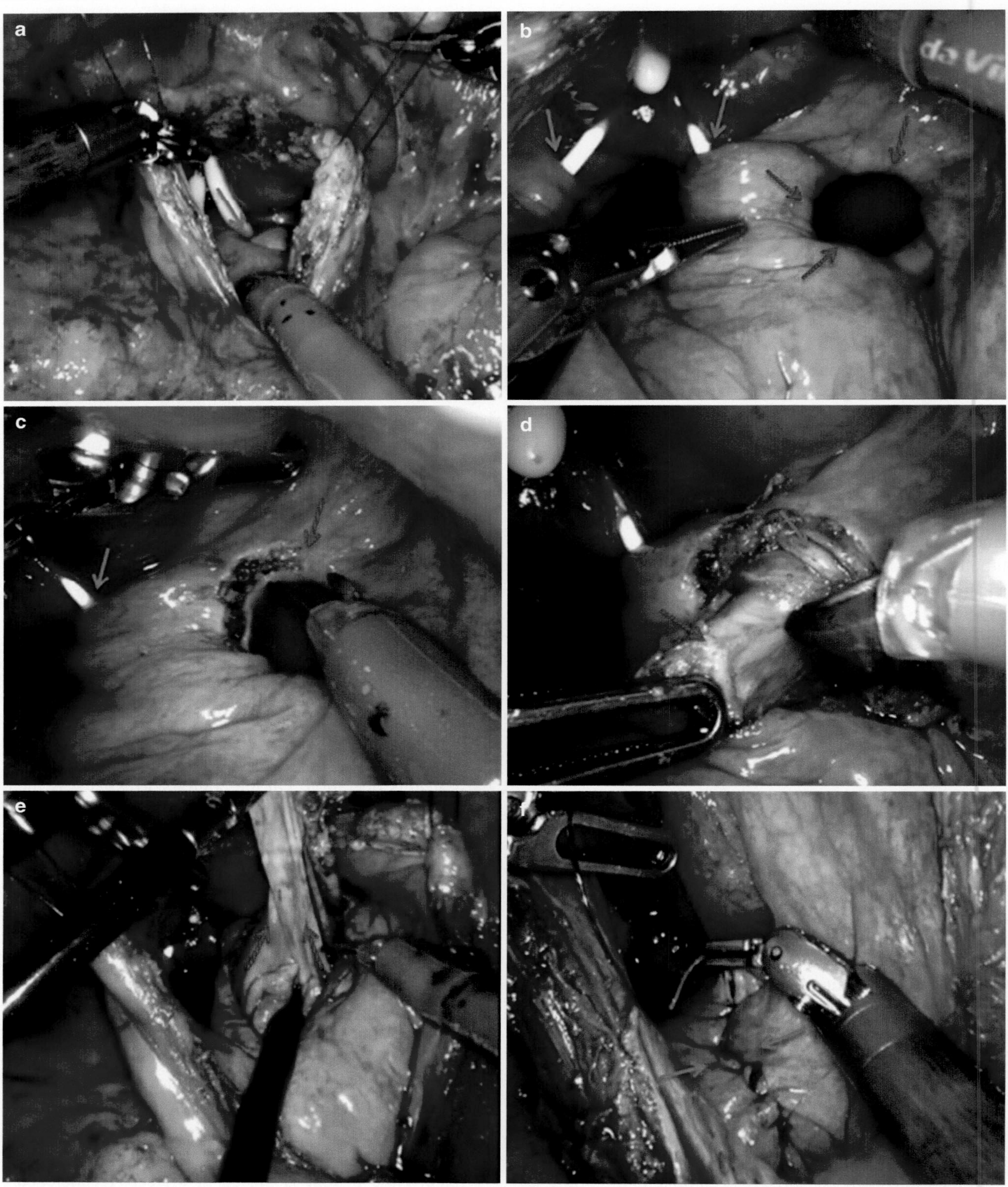

Fig. 8 (**a**) Longitudinal cystotomy on the anterior wall of the bladder with two stay sutures for exposure. The Councill-tip catheter is seen (blue arrow) leading to the BD. (**b**) The two ureteral catheters are seen (blue arrows) with the BD (green arrows) close to the right ureteral orifice. (**c**) The edges of the opening of the BD (green arrows) are scored with monopolar cautery so that the mucosa of the BD is incised from the mucosa of the rest of the bladder. (**d**) Dissection into the avascular plane between the diverticulum (green arrow) and the fibrous capsule formed around it. (**e**) The assistant (or the fourth arm) is lifting the BD to aid in the dissection. (**f**) Suturing the bladder opening in two layers

[Intuitive Surgical]. A ProGrasp forceps [Intuitive Surgical] can be used in the fourth arm instead for the large needle holder if robotic instrument consumption is not an issue. A 30-degree lens is used although the operation can be done with a zero degree lens.

2.6 Procedure

During RBD, essentially the surgeon is mimicking the open technique; thus, mainly two approaches can be performed: the intravesical where the bladder is opened and the BD is dissected and inverted within the bladder and the extravesical where the BD is dissected from outside the bladder and only when the BD neck is identified it is incised. If RBD is combined with RSP, an intravesical approach is preferred since with the same bladder incision both operations can be performed. Some authors suggest a purely extravesical approach when the BD is not in proximity to the ureter [40].

2.6.1 Intravesical Approach

The bladder is released from the anterior abdominal wall and the space of Retzius is exposed in similar manner as in radical prostatectomy. After filling the bladder with 120 cc normal saline through the indwelling catheter, a longitudinal cystotomy is done close to the prostate-vesical junction. Two extracorporeal stay sutures are placed on either side of the bladder incision with the aim to keep the bladder open and ensure adequate exposure. The two ureteral orifices are identified in case ureteral catheters are not placed and the BD is visualized with the Councill-tip catheter inside. Subsequently the edge of the opening of the BD is scored with monopolar cautery so that the mucosa of the BD is incised from the mucosa of the rest of the bladder. The surgeon lifts the urothelium of the BD on one side and with pinpoint coagulation and blunt dissection searches for the avascular plane between the diverticulum and the fibrous capsule formed around it. This plane of dissection once found is continued around the edges of the ostium of the BD before proceeding to further deeper dissection. Once the BD is adequately dissected, the fourth arm (or the bedside assistant) can lift it so it is constantly under tension. With blunt and sharp dissection, the plane can be easily advanced while further pealing of the BD can be done with the scissors slightly open. Once the BD is completely removed, the opening of the bladder is sutured with 3.0 V-Loc suture in two layers in a continuous fashion (Fig. 8) (Video 1).

Subsequently, the surgeon can proceed with the RSP as previously described if a combined operation for BOO is planned [41]. Finally, the initial opening of the bladder is closed in one or two layers with 3.0 V-Loc (Covidien) suture in a continuous fashion.

Alternatively, instead of dropping down the bladder from the abdominal wall, some authors suggest a cystotomy at the fundus of the bladder and extending this incision into the neck of the BD [42]. Further dissection can be done as described.

2.6.2 Extravesical Approach

The bladder is filled through the indwelling catheter. Since the BD is expected to be posteriorly or posterolaterally to the bladder, it can be recognized as a bulge over the peritoneum. At this site, monopolar scissors is used to incise the peritoneum and expose the fundus of the BD. Once identified, the diverticulum is grasped by the bedside assistant or the fourth arm and firm tension is used. At this point, identification of the ureter could be a safe option especially in cases when large a BD is close to the ureter. Furthermore, a combination of sharp and blunt dissection circumferentially and in close proximity to the BD with pinpoint coagulation when needed is applied. Progressively, the dissection of the BD from its surrounding fibrotic tissue is advanced till the BD neck is identified. Once identified, the BD neck is incised anteriorly with electrocautery, and the bladder is inspected from the inside to identify potential proximity to the ureteral orifice. The incision of the BD neck is not fully carried out, and before complete removal of the BD, suturing of the edges of the bladder is initiated with a 3.0 V-Loc (Covidien) suture. The reason for this is to take advantage of the tension applied on the BD to fully expose the opening of the bladder and ensure a better approximation. Finally, the BD is fully removed and the opening of the bladder sutured in a running fashion (Fig. 9) (Video 2).

2.7 Postoperative Management

In case RBD is combined with RSP, continuous irrigation through the catheter can be used preferably with a low flow rate. On the first postoperative day, the patient can ambulate and start a regular diet. At the same time, the drain can be removed if there is no fluid collection coming out. In case of noticeable output from the drain, continuous irrigation if used must be stopped and the subsequent fluid collection must be checked for creatinine. If the creatinine level is higher than serum creatinine, then urine leakage should be suspected and the patient should undergo imaging studies to rule out bladder perforation or even ureteral injury. Parenteral analgesics can be changed to oral ones as soon as possible, and subcutaneous heparin and compression stocking are used during the hospitalization period and till the patient is fully ambulatory. If the postoperative period is uneventful, the patient can be discharged the second postoperative day with the catheter connected to a leg bag. The catheter can be

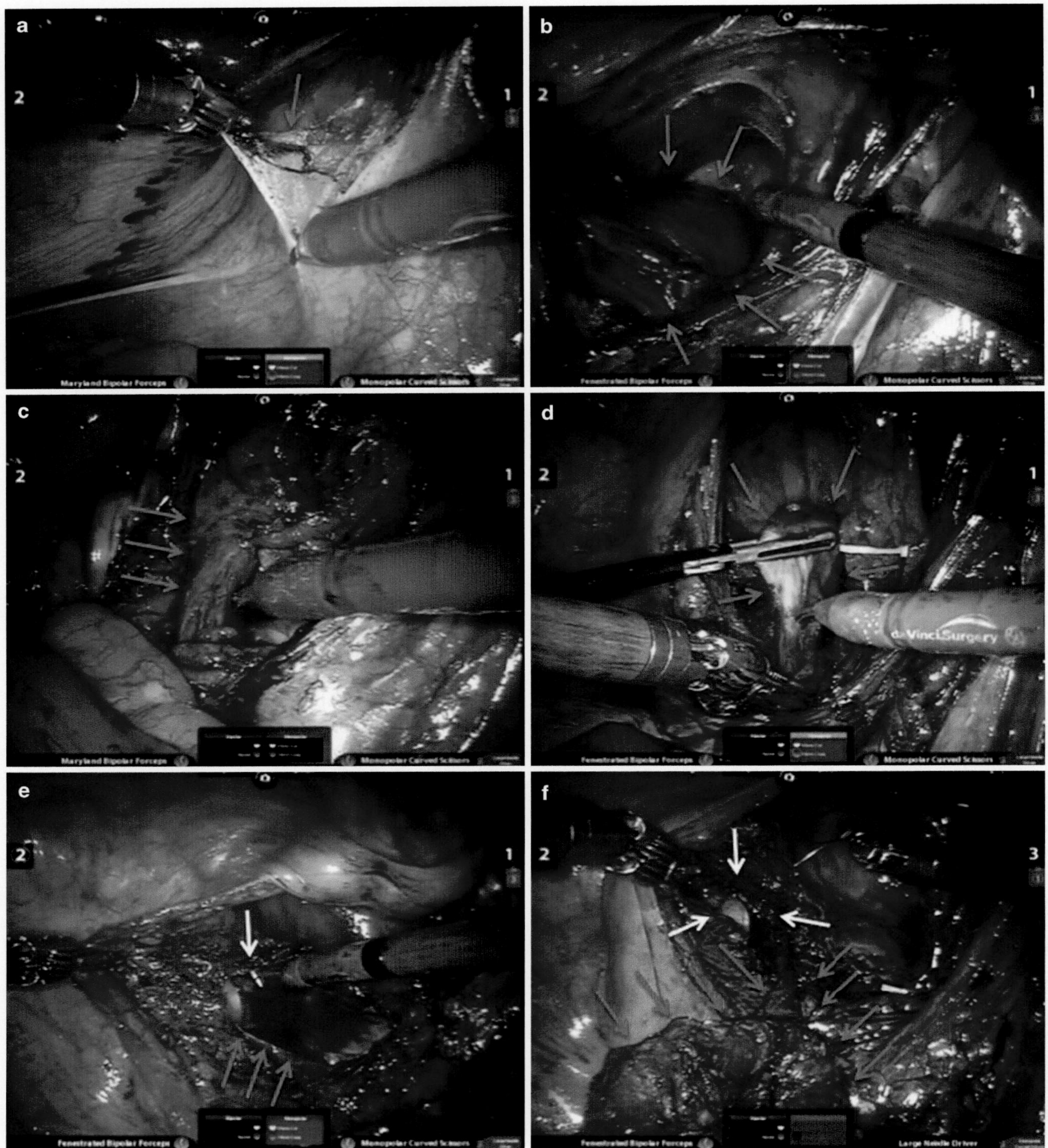

Fig. 9 (**a**) Vertical incision lateral to the medial umbilical ligament (blue arrow). (**b**) Identification of the BD (blue arrow) after filling the bladder with normal saline. (**c**) Dissection of the ipsilateral ureter in case of large BD in close approximation. (**d**) The assistant (or the fourth arm) is lifting the BD exerting steady traction to aid dissection. (**e**) Opening of the BD neck and identification of the ureteric catheter (white arrow) close to the BD as well as the bladder catheter (green arrow). (**f**) Suturing the opening of the bladder (white arrow) before fully incising the BD (blue arrow) for better exposure of the bladder opening

removed after 7 days, while a cystogram can be suggested but is not routinely required. Follow-up will include abdominal ultrasound and/or cystogram to evaluate post is post void residual.

Tips and Tricks

- Place a ureteral catheter on the ipsilateral ureteral orifice if the BD is close to it in order to avoid inadvertent injury of the ureter.
- Place a Councill-tip catheter over a wire inside the BD. Selective distention with saline of the BD will aid its identification and dissection.
- Place the fourth robotic arm on the side of the dominant hand of the surgeon (right iliac fossa for a right-handed surgeon) in order to interchange between two grasping tools and one grasping tool and the scissors.
- Side docking of the robot in case of intraoperative cystoscopy.
- Endoscopic procedures for BOO when performed sequentially to RBD should be performed before RBD to avoid the potential risk of bladder perforation on the suture line due to the irrigation fluid. On the contrary, if RBD is combined with RSP, the former should be done first to avoid a hemorrhagic surgical field.
- In case of urine collection in the drain, ureteral injury should be excluded.

References

1. Gravas S, Cornu JN, Gacci M, Gratzke C, Herrmann TRW, Mamoulakis C, Rieken M, Speakman MJ, Tikkinen KAO. Management of non-neurogenic male lower urinary tract symptoms (LUTS), incl. Benign prostatic obstruction (BPO). European Association of Urology, (European Association of Urology Guidelines); 2019.
2. Latini JM, McAninch JW, Brandes SB, Chung JY, Rosenstein D. SIU/ICUD consultation on urethral strictures: epidemiology, etiology, anatomy, and nomenclature of urethral stenoses, strictures, and pelvic fracture urethral disruption injuries. Urology. 2014;83(3, Supplement):S1–7.
3. Borboroglu PG, Sands JP, Roberts JL, Amling CL. Risk factors for vesicourethral anastomotic stricture after radical prostatectomy. Urology. 2000;56(1):96–100.
4. Chen YZ, Lin WR, Chow YC, Tsai WK, Chen M, Chiu AW. Analysis of risk factors of bladder neck contracture following transurethral surgery of prostate. BMC Urol. 2021;21(1):59.
5. Lee YH, Chiu AW, Huang JK. Comprehensive study of bladder neck contracture after transurethral resection of prostate. Urology. 2005;65(3):498–503. discussion
6. Michielsen DP, Coomans D. Urethral strictures and bipolar transurethral resection in saline of the prostate: fact or fiction? J Endourol. 2010;24(8):1333–7.
7. Rassweiler J, Teber D, Kuntz R, Hofmann R. Complications of transurethral resection of the prostate (TURP)--incidence, management, and prevention. Eur Urol. 2006;50(5):969–79. discussion 80
8. Tang Y, Li J, Pu C, Bai Y, Yuan H, Wei Q, et al. Bipolar transurethral resection versus monopolar transurethral resection for benign prostatic hypertrophy: a systematic review and meta-analysis. J Endourol. 2014;28(9):1107–14.
9. Cornu JN, Ahyai S, Bachmann A, de la Rosette J, Gilling P, Gratzke C, et al. A systematic review and meta-analysis of functional outcomes and complications following transurethral procedures for lower urinary tract symptoms resulting from benign prostatic obstruction: an update. Eur Urol. 2015;67(6):1066–96.
10. Pansadoro V, Emiliozzi P. Iatrogenic prostatic urethral strictures: classification and endoscopic treatment. Urology. 1999;53(4):784–9.
11. Rosenbaum CM, Vetterlein MW, Fisch M, Reiss P, Worst TS, Kranz J, et al. Contemporary outcomes after transurethral procedures for bladder neck contracture following endoscopic treatment of benign prostatic hyperplasia. J Clin Med. 2021;10(13):2884.
12. Young BW. The retropubic approach to vesical neck obstruction in children. Surg Gynecol Obstet. 1953;96(2):150–4.
13. John H, Schmid DM, Fehr JL. Extraperitoneal radical prostatectomy Da Vinci. Actas Urologicas Espanolas. 2007;31(6):580–6.
14. Erdogru T, Teber D, Frede T, Marrero R, Hammady A, Seemann O, et al. Comparison of transperitoneal and extraperitoneal laparoscopic radical prostatectomy using match-pair analysis. Eur Urol. 2004;46(3):312–9. discussion 20
15. Cindolo L, Marchioni M, Emiliani E, DEF P, Primiceri G, Castellan P, et al. Bladder neck contracture after surgery for benign prostatic obstruction. Minerva urologica e nefrologica/Ital J Urol Nephrol. 2017;69(2):133–43.
16. Kranz J, Reiss PC, Salomon G, Steffens J, Fisch M, Rosenbaum CM. Differences in recurrence rate and de novo incontinence after endoscopic treatment of vesicourethral stenosis and bladder neck stenosis. Front Surg. 2017;4:44.
17. Musch M, Hohenhorst JL, Vogel A, Loewen H, Krege S, Kroepfl D. Robot-assisted laparoscopic Y-V plasty in 12 patients with refractory bladder neck contracture. J Robot Surg. 2018;12(1):139–45.
18. Sayedahmed K, El Shazly M, Olianas R, Kaftan B, Omar M. The outcome of Y-V plasty as a final option in patients with recurrent bladder neck sclerosis following failed endoscopic treatment. Cent Eur J Urol. 2019;72(4):408–12.
19. Rao R, Nayyar R, Panda S, et al. Surgical techniques: robotic bladder diverticulectomy with the da Vinci-S surgical system. J Robot Surg. 2007;1(3):217–20.
20. Melekos MD, Asbach HW, Barbalias GA. Vesical diverticula: etiology, diagnosis, tumorigenesis, and treatment. Analysis of 74 cases. Urology. 1987;30(5):453–7.
21. Cacciamani G, De Luyk N, De Marco V, Sebben M, Bizzotto L, De Marchi D. Maria Angela Cerruto, Salvatore Siracusano, Antonio Benito Porcaro & Walter Artibani: robotic bladder diverticulectomy: step-by-step extravesical posterior approach – technique and outcomes. Scand J Urol. 2018;52(4):285–90.
22. Livne PM, Gonzales ET Jr. Congenital bladder diverticula causing ureteral obstruction. Urology. 1985;25(3):273–6.
23. Idrees MT, Alexander RE, Kum JB, et al. The spectrum of histopathologic findings in vesical diverticulum: implications for pathogenesis and staging. Human Pathol. 2013;44(7):1223–32.
24. Kelalis PP, McLean P. The treatment of diverticulum of the bladder. J Urol. 1967;98(3):349–52.
25. Blane CE, Zerin JM, Bloom DA. Bladder diverticula in children. Radiology. 1994;90(3):695–7.
26. Preciado-Estrella DA, Cortés-Raygoza P, Morales-Montor JG, Pacheco-Gahbler C. Multiple bladder diverticula treated with robotic approach-assisted with cystoscopy. Urol Ann. 2018;10(1):114–7.

27. Flasko T, Toth G, Benyo M, Farkas A, Berrczi C. A new technical approach for extraperitoneal laparoscopic bladder diverticulectomy. J Laparoendosc Adv Surg Tech A. 2007;17(5):659–61.
28. Fox M, Power RF, Bruce AW. Diverticulum of the bladder – presentation and evaluation of treatment of 115 cases. Br J Urol. 1962;34(September):286–98.
29. Parra RO, Boullier JA. Endocavitary (laparoscopic) bladder surgery. Semin Urol. 1992;10(November (4)):213–21.
30. Ploumidis A, Skolarikos A, Sopilidis O, et al. Sequential robotic-assisted bladder diverticulectomy and radical prostatectomy. Technique and review of the literature. Int J Surg Case Rep. 2013;4(1):81–4.
31. Porpiglia F, Tarabuzzi R, Cossu M, et al. Sequential transurethral resection of the prostate and laparoscopic bladder diverticulectomy: comparison with open surgery. Urology. 2002;60(6):1045–9.
32. Kural AR, Atug F, Akpinar H, et al. Robot-assisted laparoscopic bladder diverticulectomy combined with photoselective vaporization of prostate: a case report and review of literature. J Endourol. 2009;23(8):1281–5.
33. Shah HN, Shah RH, Hegde SS, Shah JN, Bansal MB. Sequential holmium laser enucleation of the prostate and laparoscopic extraperitoneal bladder diverticulectomy: initial experience and review of literature. J Endourol. 2006;20(May (5)):346–50.
34. Skolarikos A, Alivizatos VI, Chalikopoulos G, Papachristou D, Deliveliotis CC. Con- comitant radical prostatectomy and bladder diverticulectomy: functional and oncological outcome. Eur Urol Suppl. 2007;6(2):152.
35. Magera JS Jr, Childs MA, Frank I. Robot-assisted laparoscopic transvesical diverticulectomy and simple prostatectomy. J Robot Surg. 2008;2(3):205–8.
36. Myer EG, Wagner JR. Robotic assisted laparoscopic bladder diverticulectomy. J Urol. 2007;178(6):2406–10.
37. Khonsari S, Lee DI, Basillote JB, et al. Intraoperative catheter management during laparoscopic excision of a giant bladder diverticulum. J Laparoendosc Adv Surg Tech A. 2004;14(1):47–50.
38. Ashton A, Soares R, Kusuma VRM, Moschonas D, Perry M, Patil K. Robotic assisted bladder diverticulectomy: point of technique to identify the diverticulum. Robot Surg. 2019;13(1):163–6.
39. Macejko AM, Viprakasit DP, Nadler RB. Cystoscope- and robot- assisted bladder diverticulectomy. J Endourol. 2008;22(10):2389–92.
40. Altunrende F, Autorino R, Patel NS, White MA, Khanna R, Laydner H, Yang B, Haber G-P, Kaouk JH, Stein RJ. Robotic bladder diverticulectomy: technique and surgical outcomes. Int J Urol. 2011;18:265–71.
41. Pokorny M, Novara G, Geurts N, Dovey Z, De Groote R, Ploumidis A, Schatteman P, de Naeyer G, Mottrie A. Robot-assisted simple prostatectomy for treatment of lower urinary tract symptoms secondary to benign prostatic enlargement: surgical technique and outcomes in a high-volume robotic centre. Eur Urol. 2015;68(3):451–7.
42. Thüroff JW, Roos FC, Thomas C, Kamal MM, Hampel C. Surgery illustrated–surgical atlas robot-assisted laparoscopic bladder diverticulectomy. JU Int. 2012;110(11):1820–36.

Robotic-Assisted Surgery in Urinary Fistulas

H. John, D. Pushkar, M. Randazzo, and J. Rassweiler

1 Vesicovaginal Fistulas

M. Randazzo and H. John

1.1 Definition and Types of VVF

The English translation of the Latin word "fistula" means pipe, duct, or tube, and it stands for an abnormal anatomical junction between two hollow organs. Thus, the vesicovaginal fistula (VVF) is defined as the anatomical connection of the dorsal bladder wall with the anterior vaginal wall. The fistula is usually permanent as a result of a necrosis of both organ walls due to an ischemic condition or direct injury during surgery.

There are two different types of VVF: 1) VVF after surgery and 2) VVF due to prolonged child birth. The first one usually occurs in resourced countries by an iatrogenic unperceived injury of the dorsal bladder wall during hysterectomy or sometimes sling placement for incontinence with an estimated incidence of 0.3–2% [1]. Other more rare causes include pelvic irradiation or malignant disease [2]. The second form of VVF is more likely to occur in less-resourced countries: The most frequent condition is a cephalopelvic disproportion during child birth with prolonged labor. This disproportion then causes a prolonged pressure with consecutive ischemia of the vaginal wall. Some authors call the first type of VVF "iatrogenic" and the second one "ischemic" [3], although an unperceived injury by electrocautery during surgery might also lead to an ischemic vaginal wall in the first type.

Generally, type 2 VVF (prolonged labor) has a broad ischemic area from the cephalopelvic disproportion, which usually leads to the formation of a larger fistula. These VVF may also be located deeper in the pelvis and sometimes include a urethral loss, rectovaginal fistula formation, as well as an anal sphincter incompetence or even osteitis pubis [4].

1.2 Prevalence of VVF

The overall prevalence of VVF in lower-resourced countries is higher than in higher-resourced countries. In African countries, such as Ethiopia, the prevalence is estimated to 1.5 per 1000 women [5] indicating the limited access to obstetric intervention [6]. In some other countries, such as Pakistan, there is a switch with a rising trend for type 1 (iatrogenic) and a decreasing one for type 2 VVF (prolonged labor) [3].

The urinary leakage through the vagina is the typical manifestation of a VVF with the degree of incontinence being proportional to the size of the fistula [7]. The vagina may become inflammated and ulcerated [8], which is why VVF should always be treated—although there might be a continent urinary situation in extremely rare situations [9].

Taken together, VVF usually create hygienic, social, infectious, psychological, and sexual problems.

1.3 Etiology of VVF

The etiology of VVF has impact on the surgical approach. Whenever urinary discharge through the vagina after hysterectomy or obstetric surgery is appearing, a VVF should be

Supplementary Information The online version contains supplementary material available at [https://doi.org/10.1007/978-3-031-00363-9_67].

H. John (✉)
Klinik für Urologie, EBU Certified Training Centre, Urologisches Tumorzentrum, Kantonsspital Winterthur, Winterthur, Switzerland

D. Pushkar
Department of Urology MSMSU, Urologist General of Russia, Moscow, Russia

M. Randazzo
Urologie Zentrum, Klinik Hirslanden Aarau, Schänisweg, Aarau, Switzerland

J. Rassweiler
Department of Urology, SLK Klinken Heilbronn, Heilbronn, Germany

P. Wiklund et al. (eds.), *Robotic Urologic Surgery*, https://doi.org/10.1007/978-3-031-00363-9_67

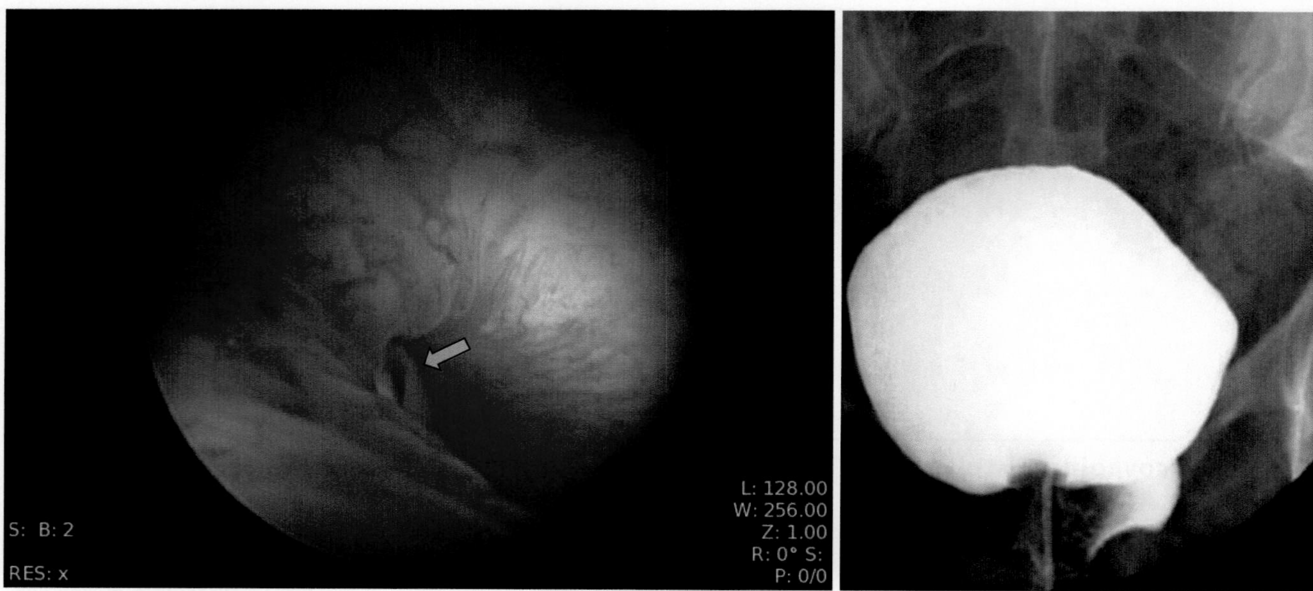

Fig. 1 Simple vesicovaginal fistula with single fistula tract (left figure, arrow) and corresponding cystogram (right)

suspected [10, 11]. Compared to VVF provoked by prolonged labor, iatrogenic fistulas are located higher in the pelvis and are therefore supratrigonal. The mechanism for a VVF consists of a thermal injury leading to a necrosis of the posterior bladder wall. Once the process of necrosis has started, an inflammatory process leads to production of collagen and perifistula fibrosis. This damage might occur during mobilization of the vagina, e.g., during hysterectomy. The reported incidence varies from 0.02 to 1.2% depending on the approach to hysterectomy [12, 13]. Thus, surgery is the most important risk factor for VVF in well-resourced countries [14]. In a recent review, 62.7% of postoperative VVF were due to hysterectomy performed by any route, 12.7% were associated by other types of pelvic surgery such as colorectal, urological, or gynecological procedures, whereas 13% were developed after radiotherapy [14]. Other reasons include infection, foreign bodies, or pelvic malignancy [15].

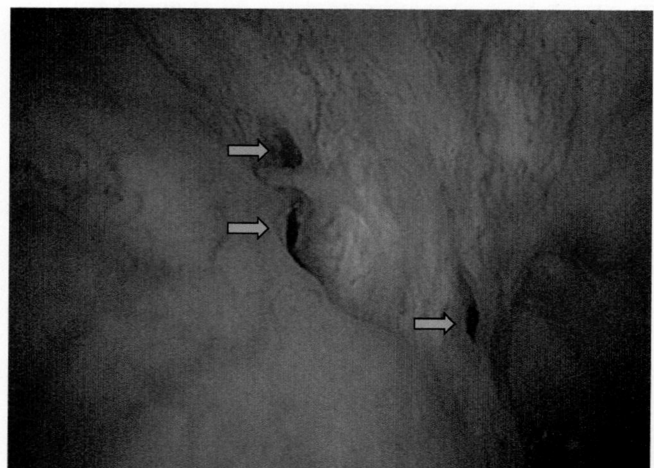

Fig. 2 Complex vesicovaginal fistula with multiple fistula tracts on the left bladder wall (arrows)

1.4 Preoperative Imaging

The correct fistula identification is the most crucial step in their management. The workup includes the pelvic examination with speculum and cystoscopy (Fig. 1). In some cases, a fistula tract might be seen during clinical examination or by cystoscopy, although VVF can be very difficult to diagnose. When imaging modalities are not available, a "double-dye test" might be helpful to better understand the fistula location [16]. The preoperative understanding is of paramount importance in order to understand the number of fistula ("hidden fistula"), their size, location, their distance to the ureteral orifices, as well as possible fistula branching. Although the majority of VVF are caused by iatrogenic injury, prolonged labor, or radiation, VVF caused by malignancy should be ruled out by tissue biopsy. In addition, a CT scan with cystogram is helpful in exactly locating the fistula. On MRI images, VVF usually shows a wall enhancement if the tissue is active or in a healing process [17], and sometimes, a healing VVF has a central granulation tissue [18].

Patients with multiple fistulas (Fig. 2) should always prompt the suspicion of hidden fistula. Whether MRI is helpful in detecting these hidden fistulas remains unclear so far.

VVF should be graded according to their location ("supratrigonal" or "trigonal"), size, and etiology. However, the most challenging step often remains the location of the fistula during surgery. Often, the fistula is located at the trigone close to the ureteral orifice [19].

1.5 Classification of VVF

Table 1 summarizes current VVF classification systems. Several attempts have been made for a risk stratification according to their risk to relapse—recurrent VVF is the most common complication after fistula repair. There are currently a couple of risk scores or classifying systems, but the clinical usefulness remains to be discussed. Older systems like the one by Lawson [20] simply include the rough location of the fistula (such as "juxtaurethral" or "juxtavaginal"). More recent classification systems such as Goh [21] include the distance from the external urinary meatus to the distal edge of the fistula (from >3.5 cm to <1.5 cm), the diameter, as well as the degree of fibrosis. Waaldijk includes the size, involving of the urethra, and the closing mechanism (type I not involving closing mechanism versus type II involving closing mechanism, [22]). It is reasonable that a more extended VVF with an increased perifocal fibrosis, the involvement of other anatomical structures (such as the urethra), or VVF after irradiation has a greater risk of recurrence than those without "risk factors." Notably, most of the current classification systems have a poor to fair performance with an area under the curve of 0.60 to 0.63 [23]. In addition, there are other important clinical, metabolic, technical, and anatomical variables that might need to be involved in a classification system. There is also evidence that moderate to severe perifistula fibrosis as well as the presence of multiple fistula have been reported to negatively affect the recurrence rate of VVF [24]. The size of the fistula seems to be another risk factor: Some studies have reported lower success rates for fistula >1 cm [25] or > 3 cm [26], while other authors found no difference for fistula size but for bladder capacity, urethra involvement, fibrosis, and prior surgery [27]. From a practical point of view, the ability to mobilize local tissue for a tension-free cover of the lesion is probably one of the most important factors influencing the success rate. Commonly reported recurrence rates vary between 0 and 30%.

Factors influencing the success rate of VVF repair include size, location, prior fistula repair, clinical experience, and skills of the surgeon, perifistula fibrosis which depends on the etiology and clinical course of VVF, and the quality of the surrounding tissue, such as the peritoneum or sigmoidal epiploic appendices.

VVF due to irradiation and malignant condition is usually more difficult to treat. One of the most frequent malignant conditions is cervical cancer. The incidence depends on the tumor stage and the involvement of the bladder and varies between 3 and 48% 3 to 25 months after irradiation [28–30].

Complex VVF are characterized by either multiple previous surgeries, a large size or in case of multiple fistulas, or a demanding underlying disease (Fig. 2). Some of complex VVF have a high degree of perifistula inflammation and fibrosis, whereas others lack of interposition tissue. Some complex VVF are located low in the pelvis and might involve the urethra. Other complex VVF include those after malignancy such cervical cancer with an altered pelvic anatomy after previous surgery. Pelvic irradiation or endometriosis can complicate treatment and needs to be considered for the surgical approach. MRI might be a useful diagnostic tool for complex fistula. These VVF often show a wall enhancement or sometimes central granulation tissue on MRI [17, 18].

Table 1 Current VVF classification systems

Author
Lawson
Goh
Waaldijk
Panzi
Sims
Mahfouz
Moir
Mc Connachie
Bird
Gray
Hamlin and Nicholson
Arrowsmith
Tafesse
WHO

1.6 Surgical and Robotic Approach to VVF (Video 1)

The transabdominal approach was first described by von Dittel in 1893 [31]. In 1980, O'Conor once described the transabdominal, suprapubic, extraperitoneal access with a cystostomy [32]. This approach allowed a good mobilization of the bladder and exposition of the Retzius space. The first published laparoscopic repair of VVF was in 1994 by Nezhat [33]. The first robotic repair was published in 2005 [34]. Meanwhile, there is a variety of studies on robotic VVF repair with different techniques. There is a standardized algorithm for the robotic management since 2020 [35, 36]. JJ placement should always be performed in order to protect the ureters during surgery [37–39]. Some are convinced of putting a flap onto the excised fistula [40], while others are not [41]. Even the repair with fibrin sealant has been described [42]. Finally, the surgical approach (e.g., vaginal or abdominal, laparoscopic, or with robotic assistance) is often chosen according to location, complexity, and surgeon's preference [43]. Thus, there is a variety in techniques for the management of VVF.

1.7 Step-by-Step Procedure for Robotic VVF Repair

The first robotic-assisted repair was published in 2005 [34]. During the last couple of years, several reports for robotic VVF repair have been published [34, 37–39, 42, 44–48]. Since then, several case series have been published with a reported success rate of 100% in most series [38–40, 45, 49, 50].

The quality of dissection on the one side and the correct suture on the other side are crucial steps along with a urine drainage after surgery. Table 2 depicts the principle steps of robotic VVF repair.

1.8 Step-by-Step Procedure

The patient is placed in a low lithotomy position. Most surgeons agree to administer a single-shot antibiotic prophylaxis (e.g., 2 g cefazolin intravenously at the start of anesthesia). Cystoscopy is firstly performed to identify the fistula. During cystoscopy, a Fogarty catheter or a guidewire can be placed in the fistula. Ureteral stents should be placed in order to protect the ureteric orifices. The operation might also be started with the colposcopy in lithotomy position and the insertion of a 5-F Fogarty catheter through the fistula into the bladder using a vaginal speculum. For easier identification of the vagina and dissection of the vesicovaginal space, a gauze sponge stick might be inserted into the vagina. The operation is then continued in a low lithotomy position with a 25° Trendelenburg tilt. For a standardized patient positioning, a goniometer can be used. The abdomen and the vagina are disinfected using povidone-iodine. After establishing the pneumoperitoneum via the 12-mm camera port, all ports are installed according to the scheme of radical prostatectomy: One 8-mm da Vinci port left and right to the umbilicus, one 12-mm Versaport™ in the right lower quadrant (3-cm craniomedial of the anterior iliac spine), and one 5-mm port is installed right of the camera port 3 cm proximally (Fig. 3). The fourth arm might be useful for holding the bladder upward during dissection of the vesicovaginal space.

Table 2 Principle steps of VVF repair

Perform cystoscopy; consider JJ placement if required
Mark VVF by placing a guidewire or 5 Fr catheter into the VVF. If possible, extract guidewire/catheter through the vagina
Separate the bladder and vagina. Expose the fistula track by exposing the guidewire
Excise the fibrotic tissue to obtain histological specimen
Suture healthy tissue in a tension-free manner, multiple layers close the vagina and bladder
Test water tightness of the bladder
Tissue interposition such as the peritoneal flap, omentum, or appendix epiploica
Insert bladder catheter

Sharp and blunt dissection is then performed in order to expose the vesicovaginal space or the vaginal stump in case of post hysterectomy. A good exposition of the vesicovaginal space is crucial in order to visualize the fistula marked with a guidewire. The bladder might subsequently be opened for preparation toward the fistula in order to finally resect the fistula completely including perifistula scar and inflammation tissue (Fig. 4). The next and most important step is the

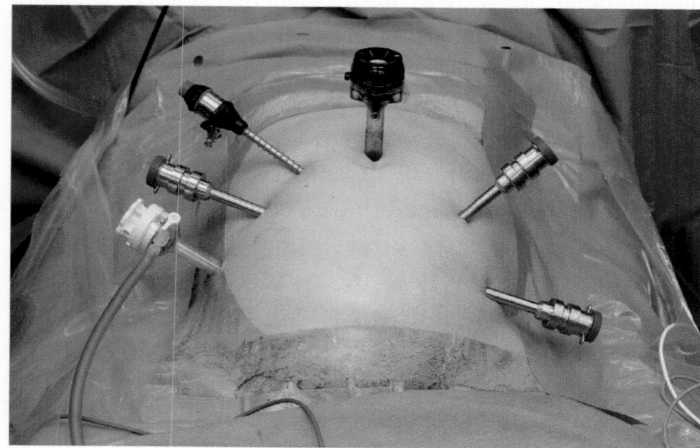

Fig. 3 Port placment for robotic fistula repair

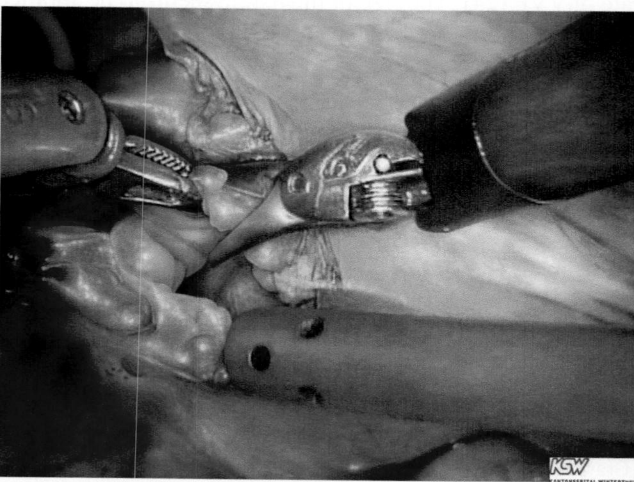

Fig. 4 Complete resection of the fibrotic scar tissue around the fistula tract

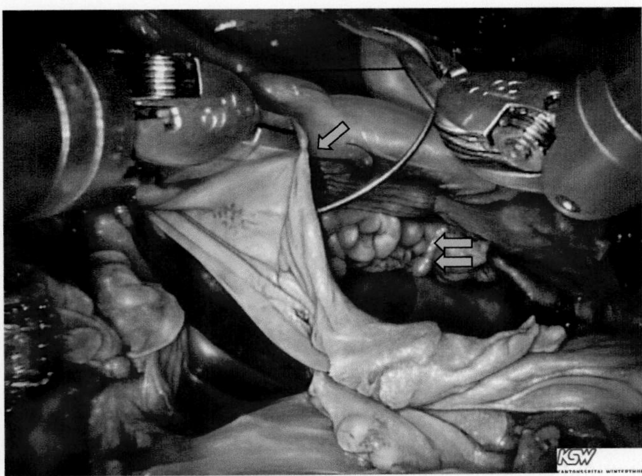

Fig. 5 The peritoneal flap (arrow) is used to cover the space between the bladder and the vagina (colporrhaphy, double arrows)

mobilization of the bladder wall circumferentially to provide a tension-free closure. This is of utmost importance in order to prevent fistula recurrence. Before closure of the bladder, a flap is mobilized such as the adjacent peritoneum to use it as a vital layer between the vaginal and bladder sutures (Fig. 5). The suture of the vagina is performed using 2–0 Vicryl®. The bladder is finally closed using 4–0 Biosyn® in two layers. After performing a final leakage test of the bladder, all the ports are removed.

1.9 Interposition Tissue

There is no randomized study comparing VVF repair with and without interposition tissue. Some few authors report no flap interposition [19, 41, 51]. A variety of intraabdominal interposition tissues can be used in order to cover the fistula area. These include peritoneal, omental, pedicled rectus myofascial flaps, buccal flaps [52], or perisigmoid epiploic tissue [40]. Even a buccal mucosal graft has been described [53]. In addition, robotic repair offers additional reconstructive procedures such as bladder augmentation or ureteral reconstruction if needed. The robotic approach often includes VVF repair with a peritoneal flap inlay [54–56]. With the aggressive surgical approach for pelvic malignancies such as ovarian cancer, omentum might be missing in these patients. Tumor debulking often includes wide excision of the peritoneum with dissection of the bladder and ureters. Thus, in some patients, pedicled rectus myofascial flaps or perisigmoid epiploic tissue or even no flap might be used as interposition tissue [57].

1.10 Leakage of Pneumoperitoneum

One of the problems encountered in robotic VVF repair is the leak of pneumoperitoneum after opening of the bladder and vagina. To reduce air leakage, a sponge stick or a wet swab gauze might be inserted into the vagina. Other methods include the AirSeal® valve-less trocar system which in general offers a more stable pneumoperitoneum [58].

1.11 Timing of Fistula Repair

There is no consensus on the optimal timing for surgery of VVF. In addition, the type, etiology, and duration of the fistula as well as the metabolic situation of the patient need to be considered. Most fistula won't close spontaneously and require operative closure. Nevertheless, spontaneous fistula closure has been reported in patients with "small" fistula after prolonged labor [59]. The EAU Guidelines on Urinary Incontinence suggest catheterization [60]. Historical data suggest a spontaneous fistula closure of up to 20% [61]. The ERUS Reconstructive Panel recommends a trial with catheter for attempting a conservative management of up to 12 weeks. There is no minimum timing for surgical treatment (robotic VVF repair) from initial diagnosis in order for the edema to resolve.

1.12 Intraoperative Diagnosis of the VVF and Protective JJ Placement

Cystoscopy is the standard to visualize the VVF. A 5-F catheter or a guidewire can be placed through the VVF in order to mark the fistula channel and the inflammatory tissue to be excised. The panel recommends placements of ureteral stents preoperatively, especially in fistulas close to the ureteral orifices.

Some authors reported for fistula identification the use of intraoperative combined cystoscopy with the cystoscope focusing on the fistula while the robotic camera light is switched off [62].

1.13 Postoperative Management

The wound drain, if even placed, should be removed after 24 h if there is no evidence of bleeding or urinary leakage. The indwelling Foley catheter is left in the bladder for 10 to 14 days with open drainage; cystography is then performed prior to the catheter removal. However, there is evidence that 7-day bladder catheterization is non-inferior to 14 day catheterization [63]. Sexual intercourse is prohibited for 4 weeks, and the ureteral catheters are cystoscopically removed after 4 weeks.

1.14 Robotic Repair of VVF: Special Comments

Basically, there are two techniques in addressing the repair robotically. One is going directly in between the bladder and the vagina and finding directly the VVF. The other technique opens the bladder in a higher point (away from the fistula) with or without continuing this opening up until the fistula tract (O'Conor technique) thus giving a wider exposure, and the dissection starts from normal tissue and advancing to scared tissue. Both techniques have their advantages and disadvantages. But the most important factor is the surgeon's experience.

The transvaginal approach has the advantage of a low patient morbidity, low blood loss, minimal postoperative pain, and low postoperative bladder irritability [64–66].

For VVF situated low in the pelvis, such as deep obstetric fistula, the vaginal approach might be feasible. Some authors report similar success rates by vaginal techniques compared to abdominal approaches using a peritoneal flap, with or without a labial Martius flap [65, 67]. The main exclusion criteria for the transvaginal approach are 1) major circumferential induration of the fistula, 2) a high fistula location where the transvaginal approach gives too little exposure, 3) fistula involving ureters, or 3) the patient's wish for the transabdominal approach [64, 68]. Combined transabdominal and transvaginal procedures have also been reported [69].

However, when a safe transvaginal fistula repair cannot be granted, the transabdominal approach is always an option. This technique provides most space for exact and wide preparation of the bladder and vaginal wall and easier identification of the scar and fistula tissue. Therefore, an abdominal approach provides a safe basis for complete excision of the inflamed fistula tissue, wide bladder wall mobilization, and tension-free bladder closure. More recent techniques have become less morbid than the historical transvesical O'Conor procedure even though there are "mini" variations [70, 71].

The technical advantages of the robotic approach are furthermore underlined by its low morbidity; we observe that patients after robotic VVF repair recover immediately after surgery as compared to the open operation. The most difficult steps during the procedures are likely the ones that keep urologic surgeons away from the laparoscopic approach. It is the tricky preparation of previously damaged tissue and the suturing. This is where the robotic surgery gives the utmost assistance as it provides an optimal exposure to the fistula area and in particular the possibility for a wide excision of the fistula tissue.

The perifistula anatomy can exactly be exposed and therefore the access to interpolate the tissue is easy to achieve. In contrast, access through the vagina as a natural orifice gives less working space to prepare precisely, not to mention that many high fistulas are difficult to reach.

In a few cases, ureters can be affected by the fistula or have to be partially resected. In these cases, the operation can also be performed by the robotic approach, while a transvaginal access is futile. Moreover, the robotic system offers a precise and easy suturing of the interposition tissue.

Some authors used flaps such as epiploic appendix of the sigmoid colon [39], epiploic appendix of the sigmoid colon or a peritoneal flap [45], omentum [38], or fibrin glue [34]. A similar functional result in all these different ways might be assumed, but randomized controlled trials are lacking. Major importance remains the separation of the suture lines of the bladder and vagina and tension-free water-tight bladder closure.

2 Rectovesical Fistulas

J. Rassweiler

2.1 Frequency Origin and Early Management of Rectovesical Fistula

Rectal injury with subsequently developing rectovesical fistula may occur in 0.4–4.9% following retropubic, laparoscopic, or robotic-assisted radical prostatectomy. Previous transurethral resection of the prostate represents a risk factor [72–78].

Other reasons include previous irradiation, brachytherapy, the application of high-intensity focused ultrasound, and rectal surgery, respectively [79–82]. Prostatic abscess perforated spontaneously into the rectum is an uncommon reason for urorectal fistula [83–86]. However, under these circumstances especially, a prostate-rectal fistula occurs. This requires different treatment modalities, such as (robot-assisted) laparoscopic radical prostatectomy [78, 86, 87].

Early management should focus on colostomy, even if there have been reports on conservative management using IV nutrition and placement of single J stent [77, 78, 88]. Such results have been achieved with specially designed nutrition solutions. Following complete healing of the vesicourethral anastomosis plus a period of 90–100 days, surgical repair can be planned. In case of associated complications like sepsis or pelvic abscess formation, this interval might be prolonged.

2.2 Surgical Management of Rectovesical Fistula

Transanal closure of the fistula using an endoscopic single-port technique [89–91] has been reported; however, our own experience was not satisfactory. Open surgical repair usually involves major surgical procedures using different approaches (transabdominal, perineal, posterior sagittal). Most of them are associated with major risk of impotence or fecal and urinary incontinence [92–100] (Table 3).

Since the beginning of this century, different laparoscopic and robotic-assisted techniques for repair of such fistula have been published [78, 101–104]. This included transperitoneal, transvesical approaches, as well as a combination of both techniques [101]. The approach depends on the extent and localization of the fistula. Evidently, the situation is different if the fistula occurs after a transurethral resection.

Table 3 Surgical approaches for recto-vesical fistula (modified from Dal Moro 2006)

Approach	Comment
Open surgery	
Transabdominal	Poor exposure
	Availability of tissue to interpose
	Familiar approach to surgeons
Perineal	Good exposure
	Risk of impotence
	Interposition of connective tissue
	Familiar approach to urologists
Anterior transanorectal	Minimal blood loss
	Risk of impotence
Perianal	Poor exposure
	Difficult maneuverability of instruments
	Low risk of wound infection
Laterosacral	Excellent exposure
	Risk of incontinence and impotence
Posterior sagittal transrectal	Excellent exposure
(York-Mason)	Unfamiliar approach to urologist
Minimally invasive surgery	
Transanal microsurgery	Technique requires special instruments
	No tissue to interpose
	No risk of impotence or incontinence
	Minimal morbidity
Transvesical mini-laparocopy	Difficult technique
	No tissue to interpose
	Risk of bowel injury by port placement
	No risk of impotence or incontinence
Transperitoneal robotic assisted	Optimal exposure
Laparoscopy	All kinds of tissue to interpose
	Low risk of impotence and incontinence
	Reduced morbidity

2.3 Patient Preparation

Preoperative diagnosis should include rectoscopy and cystoscopy to clarify the actual anatomy and to exclude associated findings (i.e., urinary stones, tumors). During cystoscopy, the ureter close to the fistula should be stented to prevent any injury during the repair and prevent obstruction due to postoperative edema (Fig. 6). The fistula can be catheterized with a 4 F ureteral catheter if it is difficult to identify endoscopically. The patient should be pre-treated with antibiotics (i.e., cephalosporine) and urine culture should be negative.

For a better identification of the rectum, a rectal balloon catheter can be inserted (Fig. 7) once the patient is in the lithotomy position. Alternatively, the assistant should be prepared to insert the finger into the rectum. For this purpose, a rectal shield like in the TURP set is helpful to maintain sterility without changing gloves. We use a transperitoneal approach with trocar arrangement similar to robotic-assisted radical prostatectomy (RALP). This can be accomplished with a 3 or 4 arm setting with the da Vinci Xi system (earlier versions) (Fig. 8).

2.4 Operative Technique (Video 2)

The first step is the opening of the previously dissected Retzius space to take the bladder down until the pubic bone (Fig. 9a). Thereafter, we dissect the bladder neck from both sides to identify the rectum (Fig. 9b). Then the bladder is opened and the fistula is recognized (Fig. 10a). This allows better isolation of the lateral bladder wall from the rectum. Then, we incise the fistula canal and open the rectum (Fig. 10b) and complete the isolation of the rectal wall from the bladder.

Once the rectum is sufficiently dissected, we start with the closure of the rectum using a continuous double-layer suture (PDS, RB-1 needle, 15 cm) (Fig. 11). There are two options to cover the anastomosis: If the Omentum majus is long enough to create an omental flap. Here, the da Vinci Xi system is very helpful, because the camera can be changed to all ports. However, another alternative represents the use of a free peritoneal graft from the bladder peritoneum, which is sutured to the rectum (Fig. 12). Both techniques act as a tissue layer to minimize the risk of recurrence of the fistula.

The final step is the closure of the bladder wall using a continuous V-Loc suture (3–0, SH needle, 15 cm) (Fig. 13a). Finally, the partially incised urethro-vesical anastomosis is closed by interrupted sutures (4–0 Vicryl, RB1 needle, 10 cm) (Fig. 13b). It is important to place a well-draining catheter (20 F silicone) to avoid any tension on these sutures.

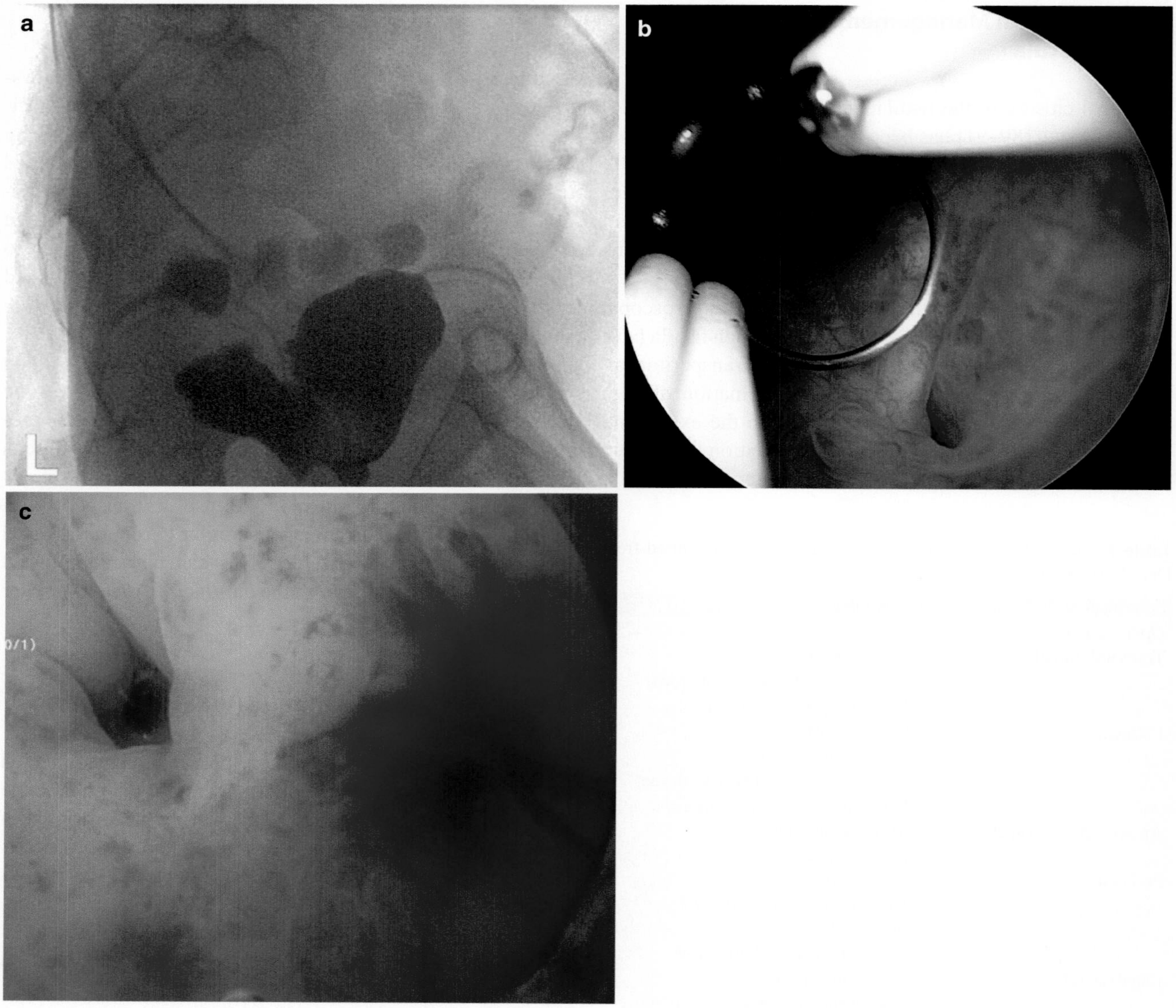

Fig. 6 Diagnostic work-up for vesico-rectal fistula. (**a**) Cystography prior to the surgery with contrast-filled bladder and rectum. (**b**) Cystoscopy showing the entrance of the fistula lateral to the left orifice. (**c**) Colonoscopy showing the exit of the fistula in the rectum

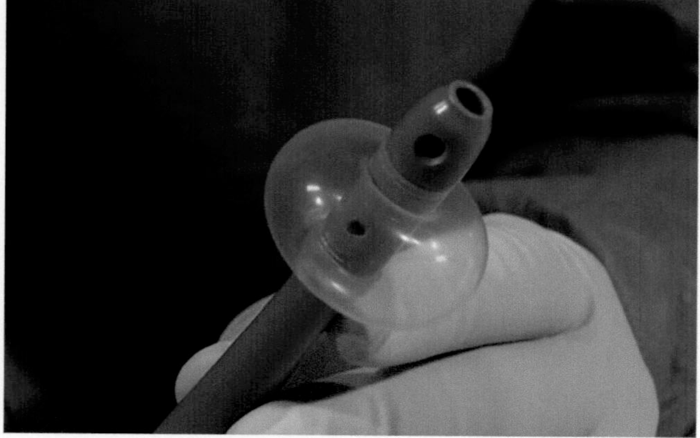

Fig. 7 Rectal-balloon catheter for better identification of the rectal wall

Then we readapt the bladder peritoneum to the pubic bone to cover the anastomosis. Finally, a drain is placed lateral to the bladder neck following checking the tightness of the bladder and anastomosis (Fig. 13c).

2.5 Follow-Up

We remove the drain when the secretion is below 100 cc usually on the third day. In case of urine extravasation, which might occur, the drain is kept longer. A cystography to demonstrate complete healing of the bladder neck and the absence of the fistula is mandatory before the removal of the catheter (Fig. 14). After 4–6 weeks, we remove the DJ stent. Closure of the colostomy can be accomplished 8–12 weeks later.

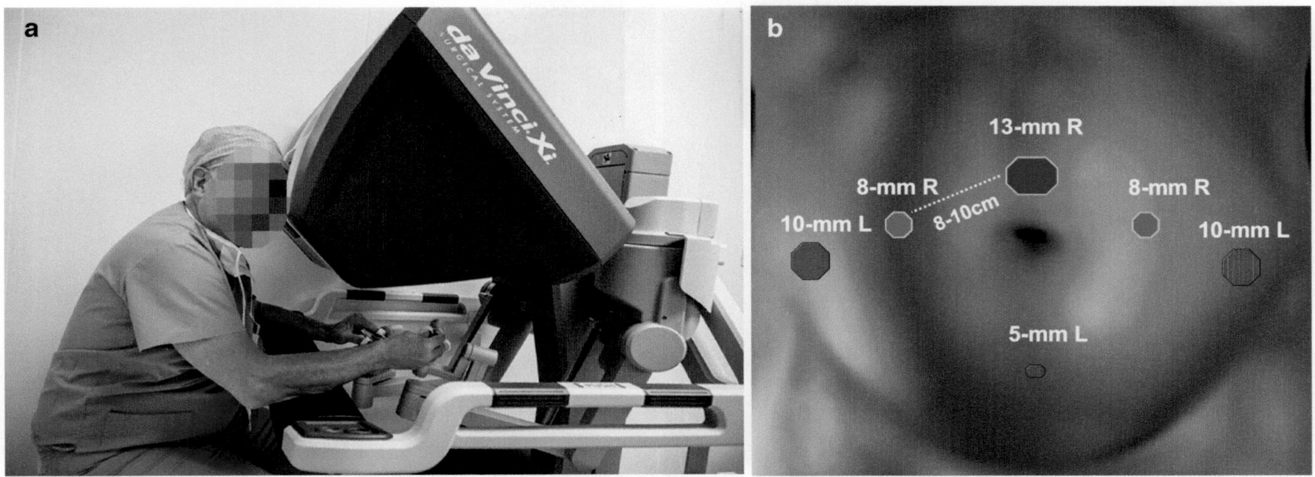

Fig. 8 Da Vinci XI-System as preferred device (**a**) Console with the possibility to turn the 30°-optic. (**b**) Position of trocars. Left 10 mm trocar can be changed to an 8 mm-port for the 4th arm

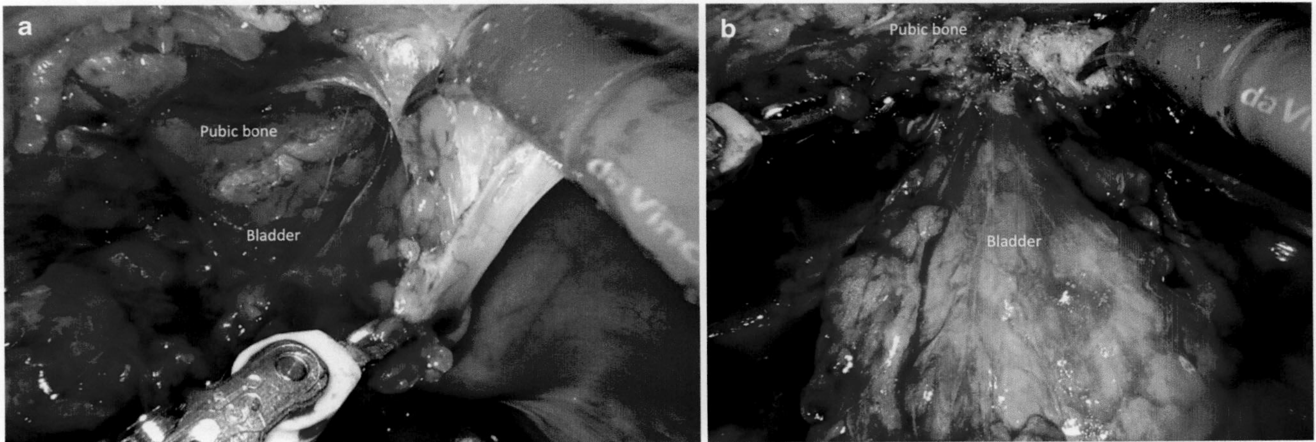

Fig. 9 Exposure of the bladder neck. (**a**) Opening of Retzius' space. (**b**) Dissection of the bladder neck

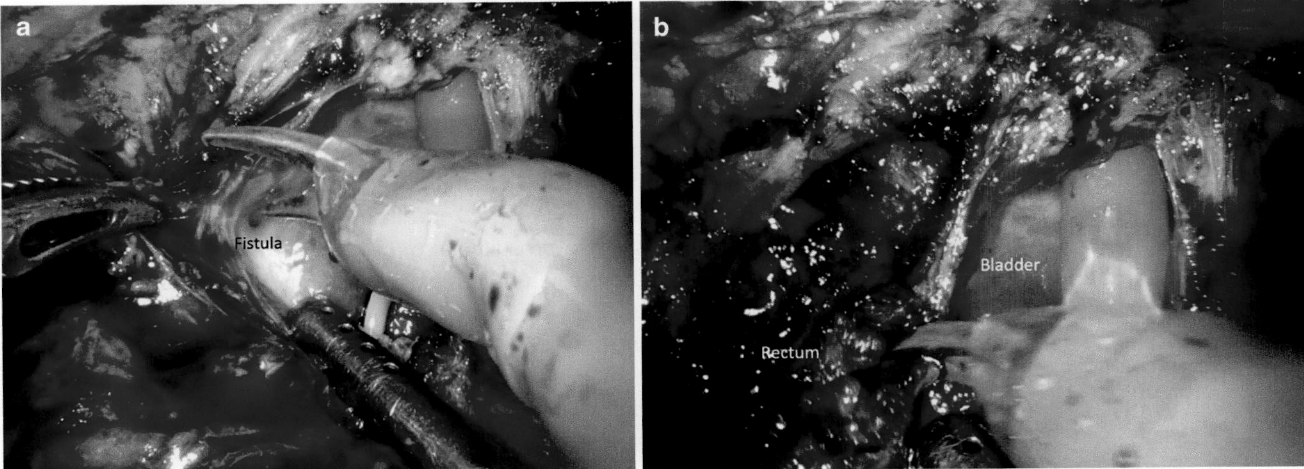

Fig. 10 Identification of the fistula (**a**) Opening of the bladder with indwelling DJ-stent. (**b**) Incision of the fistula until the rectum

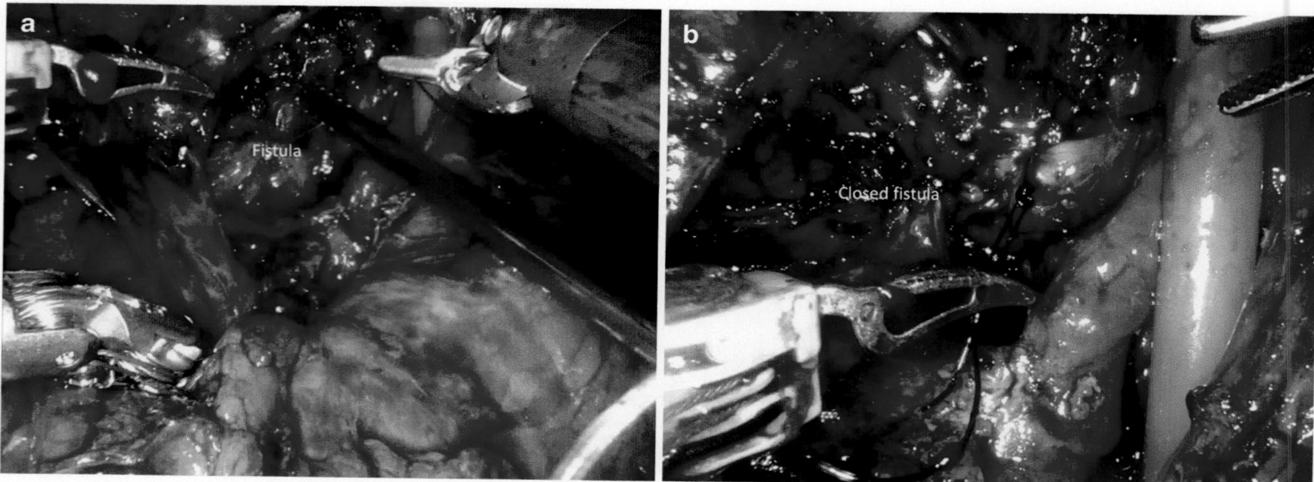

Fig. 11 Dissection and closure of rectum. (**a**) Dissection of the rectum from the bladder with identified rectal fistula. (**b**) Closure of the fistula with a double-layer continuous PDS-suture

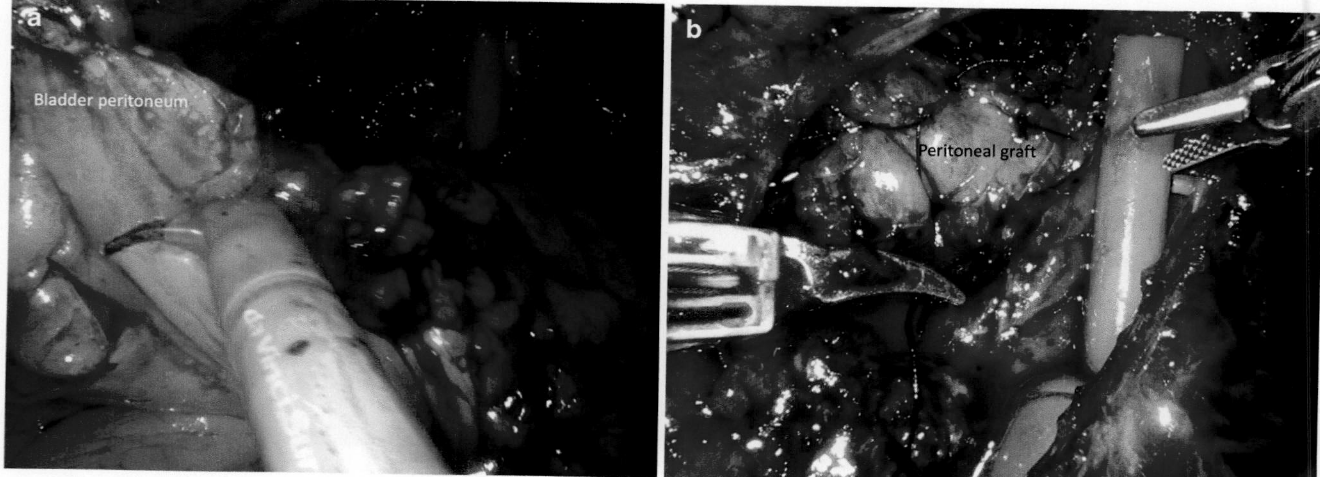

Fig. 12 Free-peritoneal graft (**a**) Harvesting the graft from the bladder peritoneum. (**b**) Fixation of the graft over the sutured rectum using interrupted Vicryl-sutures

2.6 Alternative Robotic-Assisted Techniques for Vesicorectal Fistula

Following radical prostatectomy, usually the fistula is located close to the bladder neck lateral to the respective orifice (Fig. 5a). However, following rectal surgery or treatment of a local recurrence by high-intensity focused ultrasound, this might differ. In such situation, bivalving of the bladder similar to the technique used for the management of vesicovaginal fistula might be appropriate [36, 78]. Another alternative represents the combined lateral and transvesical approach [104].

2.7 Management of Rectoprostatic Fistula

In case of a fistula between the prostate and the rectum, mainly occurring after extended TURP, brachytherapy combined with percutaneous irradiation, and the use of high-intensity focused ultrasound, we prefer a robotic-assisted salvage prostatectomy [78, 87]. After complete removal of the prostate, the rectal fistula can be optimal identified and closed with interposition of an omental flap, free peritoneal graft, or even a tunica vaginalis graft (Fig. 15).

The advantage of this approach is also to guarantee optimal healing of the urethro-vesical anastomosis.

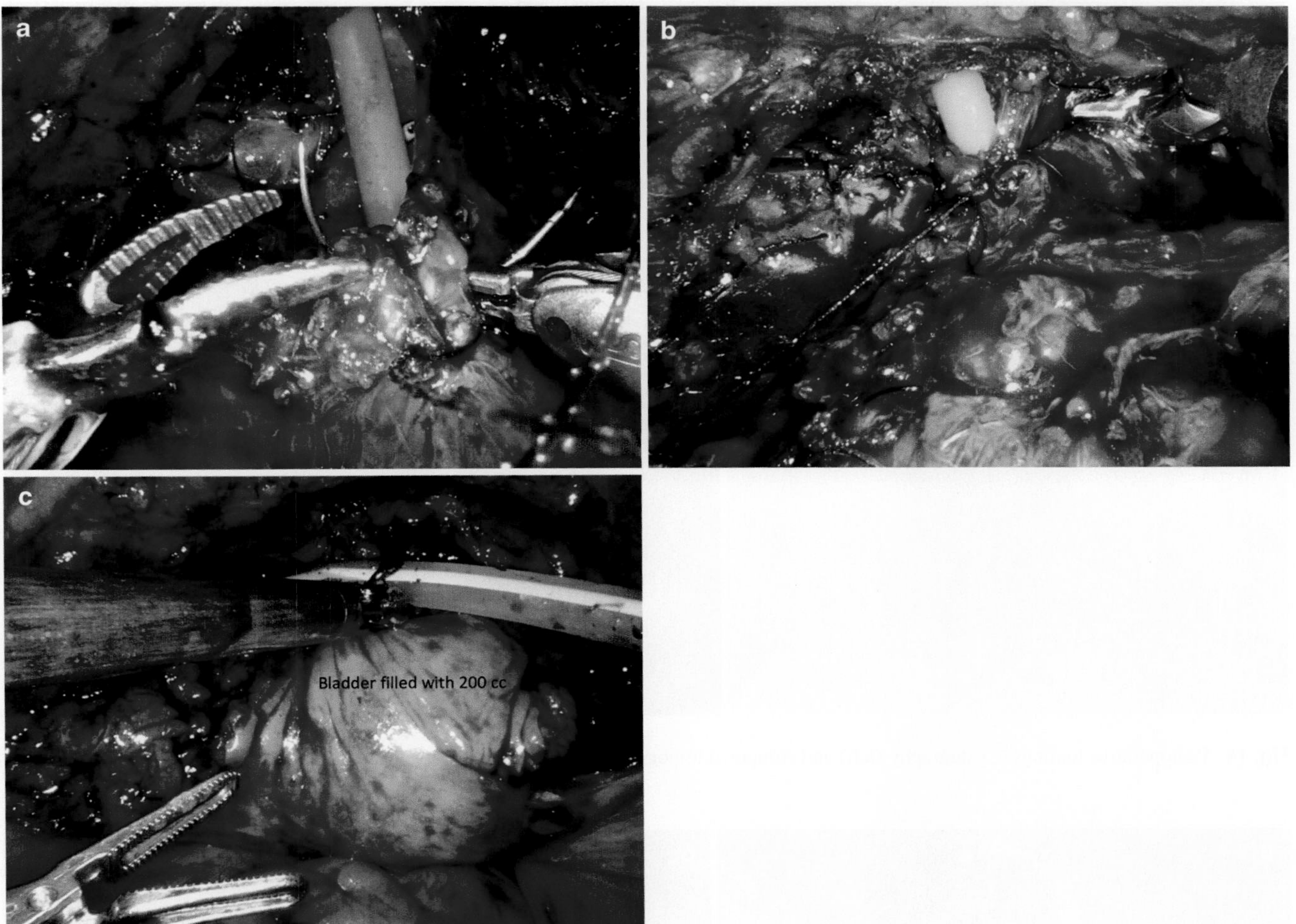

Fig. 13 Closure of the bladder and bladder neck. (**a**) Closure of the bladder using a continuous V-lock-suture. (**b**) Closure of the urethra-vesical anastomosis by interrupted Vicryl-sutures. (**c**) Re-adaptation of the bladder peritoneum and placement of drain

2.8 Discussion

Iatrogenic urorectal fistulas are rare but devastating complication that mostly develop after transurethral resection of the prostate or radical prostatectomy [72–77]. Based on the underlying anatomy, urorectal fistula can be classified distinguishing between rectovesical and recto-prostatic fistula. Moreover, urorectal fistulas can be differentiated between benign, infectious or traumatic, and malignancy-related complex fistulas such as neoplastic, surgical, and radiogenic (Table 4). For the latter, the situation even more complicated and accordingly is the success rate slow.

Conservative approaches, consisting of urinary diversion, wide spectrum antibiotics, and parenteral nutrition, may allow cure in certain iatrogenic fistulas. Success rates as high as 25–53% have been reported in the literature [86, 87] and were based on specific nutrition solutions [77, 88]. It has to be emphasized that they have to include all essential vitamins (i.e., B12, C). However, most of them required finally surgical interventions especially if the fistula remained in 3–6 months [77, 78].

Another "conservative approach" option is fecal diversion via a colostomy or ileostomy plus urinary diversion via a bladder catheter. Indeed, we feel that this should be the first approach not only when there have been previous failed repairs, complex fistulae, a history of radiotherapy or pelvic sepsis, or in the absence of bowel preparation [74, 78]. The combination of fecal diversion and urinary diversion minimizes the risk of further complications, such as septicemia. Additionally, it allows healing of the developed fistula or associated structures like the vesicourethral anastomosis after radical prostatectomy (Fig. 16). Ideally, the fistula may heal completely [69]. Nevertheless, this approach guarantees optimal wound healing even if the fistula persists.

Successful operative treatment of an urorectal fistula is often challenging [76]. Several procedures have been described, which include different approaches and different flap types and techniques. However, there has been no con-

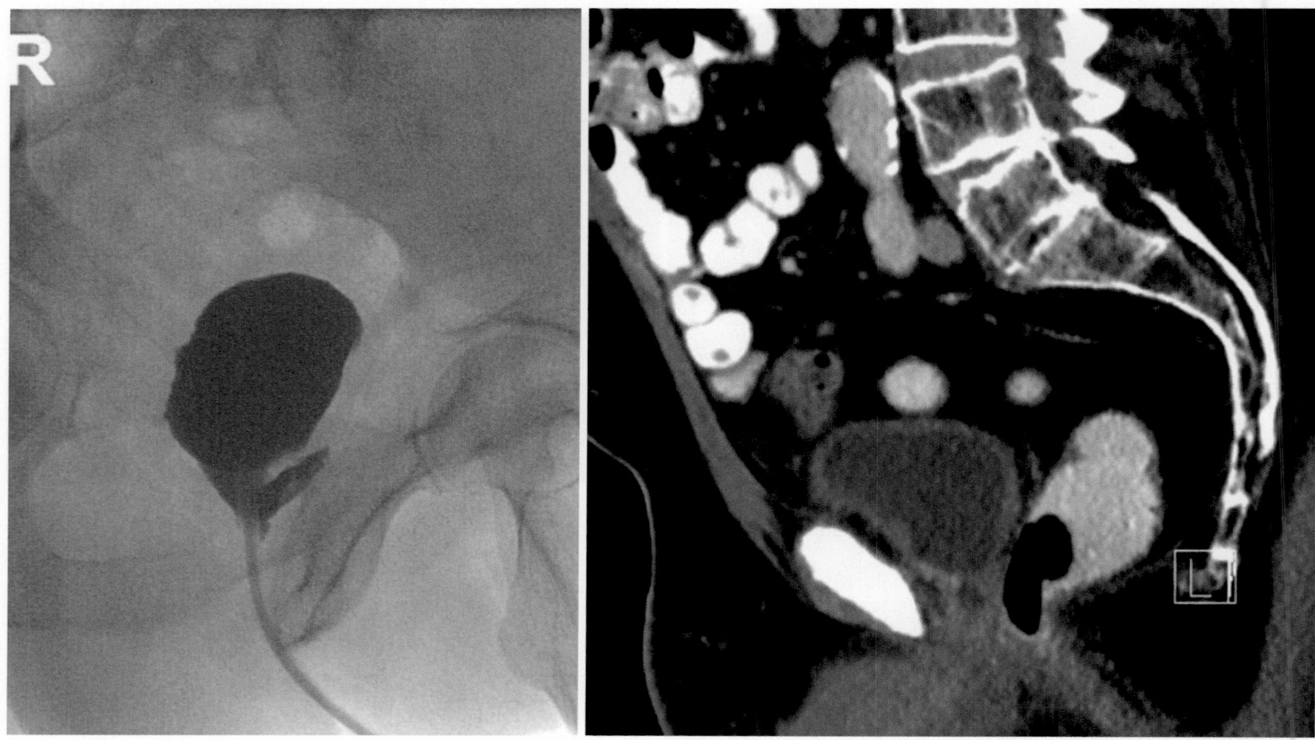

Fig. 14 Postoperative findings. Cystography (left) and computed tomography (right) demonstrate closure of the fistula

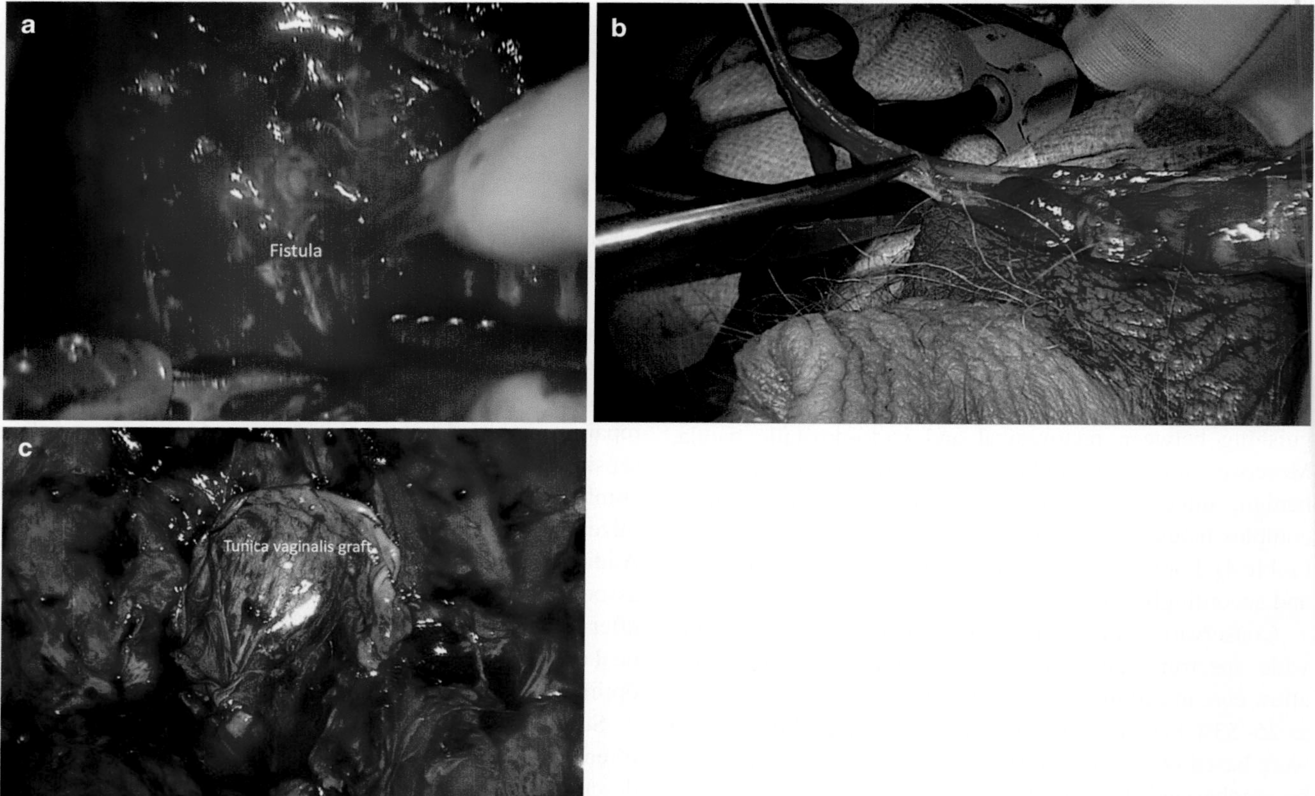

Fig. 15 Use of tunica vaginalis to cover the suture of the rectum following robot-assisted salvage prostatectomy. (**a**) Demonstration of fistula. (**b**) Harvesting of tunica vaginalis. (**c**) Covered suture of the rectum with a free-graft of tunica vaginalis

Table 4 Classification of uro-rectal fistula

Criteria	Cause	Comment
Anatomy		
Recto-vesical fistula	Radical prostatectomy	TURP is risk factor
	Rectal surgery	Transabdominal
		Robot-assisted approach
Recto-prostatic fistula	TUR P	Robot-assisted salvage prostatectomy
	Brachytherapy	
	(plus radiotherapy)	
	High intensity focal	
	Ultrasound (HIFU)	
	Radiotherapy	
	Rectal surgery	
	Prostatic abscess	
Cause of fistula		
Benign	TUR P	Robot-assisted salvage prostatectomy
	Trauma	
	Infectious	
Malignancy-related	Radical prostatectomy	Transabdominal robot-assisted approach
	Brachytherapy	
	HIFU	
	Radiotherapy	
	Rectal surgery	

sensus on the best method of repair. Even if we were able to successfully apply the transvesical approach [101], we have completely switched to the robot-assisted surgical fistula repair, since it offers optimal exposure of the fistula and allows to apply all basic surgical principles including excision and debridement of the fistula tract to healthy vascular tissue and separation of the rectal and bladder suture lines with tissue interposition [36]. The six degrees of freedom and the optimal 3D vision with the ability to turn the 30° lens upside down (using the da Vinci Xi system) offer additional advantages over the previously used laparoscopic approach [36].

Especially for fistulas in irradiated fields with ischemic fibrosis and radiation changes around the fistula, the procedure is technically difficult and the probability of successful closure is low [77–82]. Munoz et al. reported on 23 patients with complex fistulas, using different surgical approaches, and their success rate was only 25% (six patients) by the first operation [74].

Open salvage prostatectomy was reported before in the literature specially the postirradiation urorectal fistulas. Mundy and Andrich have advocated that a good exposure following a salvage radical prostatectomy for closure of the rectal defect and interposition of an omental flap before the vesicourethral anastomosis was advantageous. However, they found the salvage radical prostatectomy not easy to perform in this group of patients with complex fistulas associated with a high rate of postoperative incontinence [76]. Thus, the role and value of salvage prostatectomy in these difficult and complex cases is still to be determined.

We have promising experiences with robotic-assisted laparoscopic salvage prostatectomy for urethrorectal fistula. Based on more than 5000 cases, we are able to transfer the basic principles of preservation of continence, such as the preservation of the puboprostatic collar, dissection of a long urethral stump, and a vesicourethral anastomosis with posterior and anterior reconstruction to minimize the side effects of the salvage prostatectomy. Herein, the advantage of the Heilbronn technique includes that the posterior dissection is performed on the rectum at an early step of the operation which has allowed us a good exposure of the rectum and better dissection of the anterior rectal wall and the fistula tract [87].

A very important step is the interposition of tissue between the suture lines, basically to cover the suture of the rectum. Best choice is an omental flap, in contrast to vesicovaginal fistula, a peritoneal flap can hardly be created [36]. However, a free peritoneal graft from the bladder peritoneum is easy to harvest. If this is not possible, a tunica vaginalis graft might be unseful. In very complicated cases, muscular flaps (i.e., gracilis or rectus) can be applied but require an open surgical approach [98, 99].

2.9 Conclusions

Robot-assisted laparoscopic urorectal fistula repair seems to be safe, feasible, and efficacious alternative to the open abdominal approach with the advantages of magnification, homeostasis, decreased postoperative pain, shorter hospital stay, and fast recovery. Although it is not possible to draw a strict conclusion with the limited number of patients reported in the literature, we recommend this minimally invasive surgery in the management of urorectal fistulas, particularly in centers with experience. Further randomized studies are warranted to compare the outcomes of laparoscopy versus open urorectal fistula repair.

3 Ureterovaginal Fistulas

D. Pushkar

3.1 Introduction

Descriptions of urinary fistulas may be found in the ancient writings of Hippocrates. Nowadays, specialists all over the world encounter fistulas as a result of surgery, radiation, or

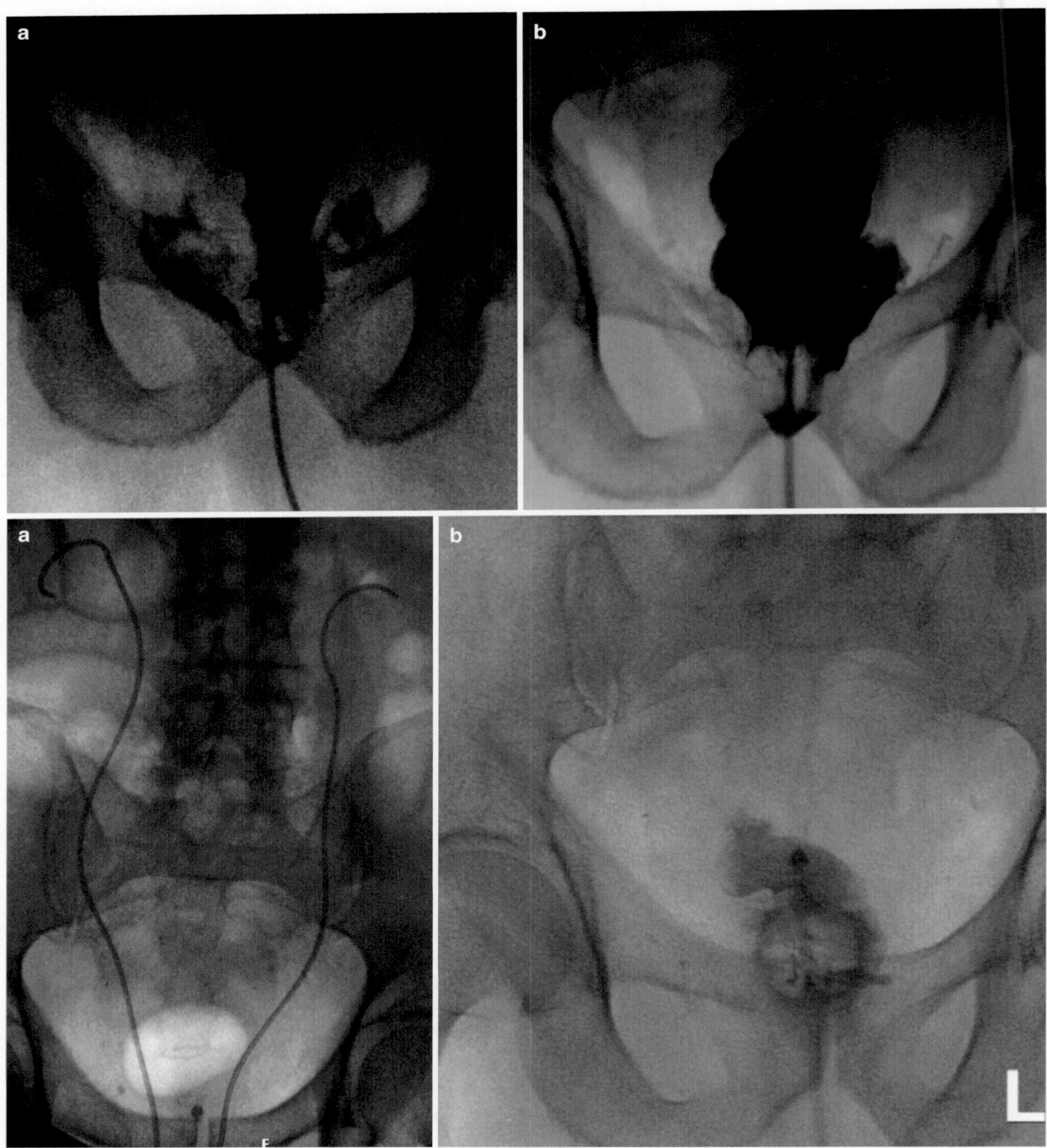

Fig. 16 Early "conservative" management of vesico-rectal fistula with insufficiency of the urethra-vesical anastomosis. (**a**) Cystography on 6th postoperative day shows massive extravastion, but no vesico-rectal fistula. (**b**) Cystography on 12th postoperative day demonstrates vesico-rectal fistula. (**c**) Placement of two Single-J-stents followed by colostomy. (**d**) Cystography after 6 weeks: Complete healing of the urethra-vesical anastomosis, but persistence of the vesico-rectal fistula

any other intervention to the human organism for varying medical conditions. Fistula repair may be really challenging, and success is common only in experienced hands. According to the WHO (World Health Organization) data, approximately two million women suffer from obstetric fistula in developing regions (especially Africa) and up to 100,000 cases occur annually worldwide.

The ureterovaginal fistula (UVF), the most common ureteral fistula, is a rare occurrence with a 5% incidence in the developed countries. Despite this, UVF has become more common with the development of advanced options for pelvic disease. Genitourinary fistulas rank among the most serious complications in gynecology. They are debilitating for the patient and challenging for the surgeon to correct.

This section reviews the etiology, symptoms, diagnosis, prevention, and the management of ureterovaginal fistulas.

3.2 Etiology

The ureter is vulnerable to injury during pelvic surgery as it courses through the retroperitoneum. The formation of UVF depends on injury to the ureter that can destroy its wall or result in delayed necrosis leading to urine extravasation [105]. Injury may be acute or delayed in onset. Acute ureteral injury is immediately apparent (iatrogenic trauma—suture ligation, ureter incision or transection, crushing). A delayed change is seen mostly in heat therapy, cryoablation therapy, or radiation [106].

The anatomical course of the ureter is the cornerstone to understanding the sites of injury. The ureter travels caudally through the retroperitoneum, along the anterior psoas muscle, posterior to the colonic mesentery, and lateral to the gonadal vein [107]. Approximately 80 to 90% of injuries occur in the distal portion where it passes beneath the uterine vessels [108].

UVF may occur as a complication of colorectal surgery, vascular surgery, other urologic procedures, and obstetric care, but most arise following gynecologic surgery. The incidence of iatrogenic ureteral injuries during gynecologic surgery is 0.04–4.3%, and these numbers probably underestimate the true incidence [109, 110]. Most UVF are caused by one procedure—hysterectomy. The incidence is estimated to be 0.04% for abdominal hysterectomy, 0.02% for vaginal hysterectomy [12], and 0.8–4.3% for laparoscopic hysterectomy [12, 111–113]. With the introduction of laparoscopy and minimally invasive techniques, the incidence of iatrogenic gynecologic ureteral injuries is increasing [12, 114]. Rates are slightly higher following pelvic reconstructive surgery, ranging between 2% and 11% [115]. Most ureteric injuries resulting from gynecological surgery occur during procedures that surgeons describe as uncomplicated and routine and where the pelvic anatomy is normal [116]. Many injuries are missed at the time of operation and discovered only when they become symptomatic [117].

Risk factors for the development of UVF include endometriosis, obesity, pelvic inflammatory disease, radiation therapy, and pelvic malignant disease [117]. Most ureterovaginal fistulas occur during procedures for benign indications [118], usually hysterectomy, but also cesarean section, pelvic organ prolapse repair, and other pelvic operations during which surgical injury of the distal third or pelvic portion of the ureter occurs.

3.3 Symptoms

Ureterovaginal fistulas most commonly manifest with a sudden onset of persistent urinary incontinence 1 to 4 weeks after surgery [118]. This complication may be associated with or preceded by flank pain, nausea, prolonged ileus, or fever related to a urinoma or renal obstruction [69]. Flank pain is usually limited by postoperative analgesic. These patients maintain normal voiding patterns as the bladder continues to be filled by the contralateral kidney.

The type of ureteral injury does often determine the timing of manifestation. Partial excisions of the ureter usually lead to urinary extravasation and related symptoms δ 48 h postoperatively. Ischemic injuries (ligation, clamping, partial ligation) may initially be associated with obstruction, followed by stricture formation, necrosis, and fistula formation. Therefore, presentation may not occur for 1 to 3 weeks. In radiated patients, ureterovaginal fistulas appear late, approximately 5 weeks postoperatively [107].

3.4 Diagnosis

A complete history and physical examination are necessary in evaluating for UVF. These actions are not so important as in patients with vesicovaginal fistulas (VVF). A tampon test using a combination of phenazopyridine and diluted methylene blue provides preliminary evidence of a VVF or a ureterovaginal fistula. Patients are given phenazopyridine, which colors the urine orange. A tampon inserted into the vagina before the phenazopyridine is administered. The bladder is also filled with diluted methylene blue before placement of the tampon. The patient then ambulates for 15–30 min. If the tampon is orange, a ureterovaginal fistula and VVF are likely. If the tampon turns blue, this finding supports a VVF. Certainly, this classic and old-fashioned test is imprecise. A ureterovaginal fistula cannot be confirmed without imaging.

Radiologic examination should include a CT urogram and a cystoscopy with retrograde pyelogram. Ureterovaginal fistulas are unique in their association with urinoma or ureteral obstruction, and therefore upper tract imaging with CT is valuable in patients who present with flank pain, fever, nausea, or prolonged ileus. These patients may need percutaneous drainage of a urinoma or abscess.

3.5 Prevention

Many ureteral iatrogenic injuries occur during blind cauterization or clipping to rich hemostasis or dissection without considering the location and direction of the ureteral blood supply. A good understanding of the anatomy and careful dissection without blind attempts at control during times of significant bleeding is essential for preventing ureterovaginal fistula formation. The use of the intraoperative stents to determine the course of the ureter for dissecting large tumors has been controversial over the years. Stenting definitely adds time and cost to the procedure. In spite of the fact that no objective evidence indicates that ureteral stenting decreases ureteral complication rates, [107] sometimes it may be very useful in preventing trauma and fistula formation.

3.6 Management

Management of a ureterovaginal fistula depends on time of diagnosis, location, nature, and extent of injury. Intraoperative detection and repair are ideal, with excellent results and fewer complications. At that time, the tissues are typically in their best condition. In general, minimally invasive techniques for repair are favored over open repair except in cases of extensive ureteric damage, complete transection, or significant delay in recognition of injury. Ligation of the ureter is usually managed with immediate intraoperative removal of the ligature or surgical clip and observation because damage is usually minimal as a result of the inclusion of other tissue. If there is a doubt about ureteral integrity, a stent should be placed. If recognition of the condition is delayed, retrograde pyelogram and an attempt at stent should be performed. A successfully placed stent is maintained for up to 6 weeks [119, 120].

There have been divergent opinions regarding the initial conservative management of ureterovaginal fistula, since prolonged delay can lead to ureteral stricture, infection, and potentially irreversibly compromised renal function [121, 122]. Patients eligible for nonsurgical management include those with unilateral injury, absence of upper tract infection of the involved kidney, presence of ureteral continuity, normality of the infralesional ureter, and reliability to follow-up [123, 124]. Recent success rates of ureteral stent insertion in the setting of complex injuries or fistula have been reported to be as high as 55–76% [125, 126]. However, in the largest case series, consisting of 84 patients, a ureteric catheter could be passed in just 9% of cases [127]. When stenting is possible, fistula resolution rates are >63%, and the risk of subsequent ureteral stricture is between 6% and 38% [125–129].

When retrograde stenting fails, antegrade stenting through a percutaneous nephrostomy tract is often successful. Schmeller et al. reported 11 patients with UVFs treated only by percutaneous nephrostomy, of which 6 (55%) had persistent fistula while another 2 (18%) had stricture [130]. Al-Otaibi treated 3 patients, initially by percutaneous nephrostomy alone, and all had persistent fistulas [130]. Patients who present with sepsis are better managed with nephrostomy tube placement and simultaneous drainage of present urinoma [107]. Most ureteric injuries during vaginal surgery are ligation injuries that result from attempts to achieve hemostasis and are detected after the operation. In all these cases, ureteric patency should be assessed with intravenous indigo carmine before completion of the procedure. If an afflux of indigo carmine is not noted, the ureter may be kinked or ligated [131, 132]. Complete ureteric obstruction during cystocele, enterocele, or bladder neck suspension surgery is managed with the removal of offending sutures and confirmation of efflux. If any doubt exists about the integrity of the ureter, a retrograde pyelogram may be done and a stent placed. Following vaginal hysterectomy or vaginal vault reconstruction, obstructing ureteral sutures are typically not removed and the ureter is reimplanted [119].

When the conservative approach fails, surgical intervention becomes necessary. General principles of ureteric reconstruction include ureteral mobilization preserving adventitia, debridement of devitalized tissue, mucosa-to-mucosa spatulation (tension free, watertight), ureteric drainage, and isolation of anastomosis (omental or peritoneal coverage) [119, 133, 134]. Historically, nephrectomy was the treatment of choice during ureteral injury. Surgical techniques for ureterovaginal fistula repair, including the Boari–Ockerblad bladder flap and psoas hitch for ureteroneocystostomy, permit renal preservation. In 2005, the first laparoscopic technique was performed [135], and recently, robotic-assisted repair has been described as a feasible and safe procedure. Traditional recommendation was that repair of fistulas with delayed presentation should not be attempted for 3–6 months. However, fistulas diagnosed less than 2 weeks postoperatively can be immediately repaired because inflammation is minimal in the range of 2 to 6 weeks. Some controversy exists, but most surgeons proceed with operative repair at 6 weeks.

3.7 Robotic Repair of Ureterovaginal Fistula

3.7.1 Preoperative Preparation

All patients planned for ureteral reconstruction undergo a 2-day bowel prep, with clear liquid diet starting 48 h prior to surgery and whole bowel irrigation via osmotically balanced solutions.

Patients receive an extensive informed consent regarding all possible options of ureteral reconstruction: ileal ureter, Boari flap, psoas hitch, transureteroureterostomy, uretero-calicostomy, ureteral reimplantation, nephrectomy, and auto-transplant. All possible operative interventions, including open, endoscopic, laparoscopic, and robotic, are thoroughly discussed with and fully understood by the patient during the informed consent. In addition to bleeding, transfusion, and infection, patients undergoing robotic ureteral reconstruction must be aware of the potential for conversion to open surgery.

3.7.2 Surgical Room Setup

The anesthesiologic team is located at the head of the patient. The da Vinci Si robot is docked between the legs of the patient. The da Vinci Xi system is located in a side docking position. The bedside assistant is to the right of the patient, and the same localization is used for the scrub nurse.

3.7.3 Patient Positioning

The target is situated in the deep pelvis; thus, the patient should be placed in the same position as for the radical prostatectomy – supine with legs in low dorsal lithotomy with arms placed alongside the body. Trendelenburg table pads are used to prevent the patient from moving in steep Trendelenburg position. It is better to avoid strapping the patient's chest in order to facilitate its adequate ventilation. Special accuracy should be applied to the patient positioning for minimization of brachial plexus injuries.

3.7.4 Trocar Configuration

Trocar configuration is similar to that of radical prostatectomy with minimal modification depending on the trauma side. It is the standard five-port transperitoneal approach.

For the da Vinci Si system, five trocars are used as follows. A 12-mm camera port placed in the midline 3–4 cm above the umbilicus (1–2 cm higher than for radical prostatectomy). The two 8-mm robotic working trocars are placed 10 cm lateral to the camera port on a line between the first trocar and the iliac spine on each side. The fourth port is placed 7 cm lateral to the robotic working trocar on the straight line on the contralateral to the injured ureter side. A 12-mm assistant port is placed between two working robotic trocars on the contralateral to the injured ureter side.

For the da Vinci Xi system, five trocars are used as follows. Camera port is placed in the midline 3–4 cm above the umbilicus (1–2 cm higher than for radical prostatectomy). The two robotic working trocars are placed laterally to the camera along the pararectus line, at the level of the first port. The fourth port is placed 7 cm lateral to the robotic working trocar on the straight line on the contralateral to the injured ureter side. A 12-mm assistant port is placed between two working robotic trocars on the contralateral to the injured ureter side.

3.7.5 Instrumentation and Equipment List

Equipment
- Da Vinci Si or Xi system
- EndoWrist curved monopolar scissors
- EndoWrist bipolar Maryland grasper
- EndoWrist ProGrasp forceps
- EndoWrist needle drivers (2)
- 0^0 and 30^0 robotic lens

Trocars (da Vinci Si)
- 12-mm trocars (2)
- 8-mm robotic trocars (3)

Trocars (da Vinci Xi)
- 12-mm trocar (1)
- Robotic trocars (3).

Recommended sutures
- 3–0 barbed suture on SH needles
- 2–0 barbed suture on SH needle
- 3–0 Monocryl suture on SH needle

Instruments used by the assistant
- Laparoscopic needle driver
- Laparoscopic scissors
- Suction irrigator device
- Hem-o-lok clip applier

3.7.6 Step-by-step Technique

Step 1: Adhesiolysis

In some cases, UVF may appear as a result of injury during abdominal surgery. In such patients, the presence of colostomy is not a rare situation and is not a contraindication for robotic procedure. Adhesiolysis, either laparoscopic or robotic, with gentle and sharp dissection should be performed to facilitate safe trocar placement. Then, the colon must be reflected cranially in order to facilitate the approach to the deep pelvis. The steep Trendelenburg position also helps with it. Release of bowel adhesions also avoids inadvertent bowel injury during the procedure and reduces tension on the bladder or vagina, promoting a tension-free anastomosis.

Step 2: Exposure of the ureter

Surgeon instrumentation (for right-handed surgeon)

Right arm: curved monopolar scissors
Left arm: Maryland bipolar grasper
Fourth arm: ProGrasp

Endoscope lens: 30⁰ down

The posterior peritoneum is incised longitudinally at the level of the iliac vessels and the ureter is identified and isolated. The peritoneum is then incised over the ureter until the damaged segment is identified. In all cases of reimplantation, the ureter must be dissected all the way to the bladder wall. Care must be taken during dissection in close proximity to vagina.

Step 3: Division of the ureter and dissection of damaged part

Surgeon instrumentation (for right-handed surgeon)

Right arm: curved monopolar scissors
Left arm: Maryland bipolar grasper
Fourth arm: ProGrasp

Endoscope lens: 30⁰ down

The ureter is then transected just proximal to the damaged part and spatulated. Sometimes it is necessary to put a Hem-o-lok clip on the bladder cuff. It is also possible to put a 3–0 Monocryl suture on it.

Step 4: Bladder mobilization

Surgeon instrumentation (for right-handed surgeon)

Right arm: curved monopolar scissors
Left arm: Maryland bipolar grasper
Fourth arm: ProGrasp

Endoscope lens: 30⁰ down

Next, the bladder is mobilized from the anterior abdominal wall, using the same technique as is used for radical prostatectomy. The peritoneum is incised lateral to the medial umbilical ligament and the Retzius space is entered and dissected to the pubic bone if necessary. Some surgeons perform a psoas hitch during this step. The reason for that is an opinion that this maneuver minimizes tension at the anastomosis and keeps the path of the ureter lateral and away from the bowel. While fixing the posterior bladder wall to the psoas muscle, it is necessary to remember and avoid genitofemoral nerve.

Step 5: Ureteroneostomy and Boari Flap techniques and ureteral stent placement

Surgeon instrumentation (for right-handed surgeon)

Right arm: curved monopolar scissors, needle driver
Left arm: Maryland bipolar grasper, needle driver
Fourth arm: ProGrasp

Endoscope lens: 30⁰ down

Next, a small area of the bladder is isolated at the lateral dome, and 1–1.5 cm incision is made into the bladder wall and mucosa (metal bougie inside the bladder may help a lot to identify the right spot). With the opened bladder and spatulated ureter, it is possible to start anastomosis using 3–0 barbed suture on double needles. After the first stitch on the posterior part of the anastomosis ureteral, JJ stent is placed and interrupted sutures completed the mucosal anastomosis. The bladder is then filled with 300 mL of normal saline, and the ureteral reimplantation site is assessed to verify that there is no leakage or tension. Additional sutures may be placed if necessary. A second anastomotic layer is performed using sutures between the serosa of the bladder and the adventitia of the ureter. The peritonization is then performed using 3–0 barbed suture. Drainage tube is placed.

For Boari flap technique, the bladder is mobilized as distal as possible ipsilaterally to the structured ureter. It is very important not to transect the vascular supply of the bladder. The Boari flap is formed by an incision with a 2:1 proportion in length and width. The ureter is spatulated and implanted through a submucosal tunnel in the apex of the Boari flap. Then the ureter is retracted through the submucosal tunnel and the ureteral adventitia is sutured to the mucosa of the flap. At this point, a JJ stent is inserted in the ureter over a guidewire. The flap is then tabularized in two layers. The bladder opening is then closed in two layers. The bladder is then filled with 150–200 mL saline to exclude any extravasation. A drainage tube is inserted.

Step 6: Exiting the abdomen

The operative field is examined under low pressure and hemostasias is achieved. All trocars are removed under a direct laparoscopic view. A Bersi needle is used in all cases for closing the port's incision.

3.7.7 Postoperative Management

Patients typically remain in the hospital for 2–3 days. On the first day, a clear diet begins. Drain is removed on the first post-op day after the US investigation and once its output is less than 50 ml. The urethral catheter remains indwelling for 10–14 days and is removed in the office. The stent is removed with the local office cystoscopy in 4–6 weeks. Appropriate imaging studies are obtained in 3–6 months postoperatively (Figs. 17, 18, 19, 20, 21, and 22).

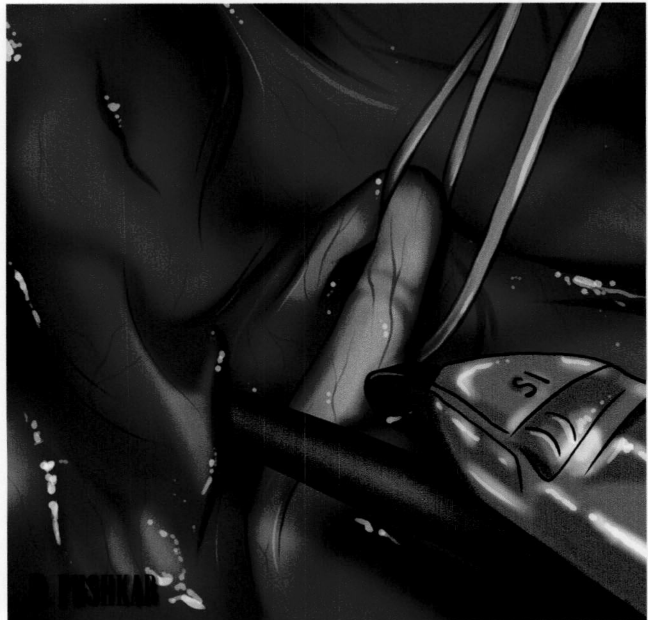

Fig. 17 Dissection of the ureter

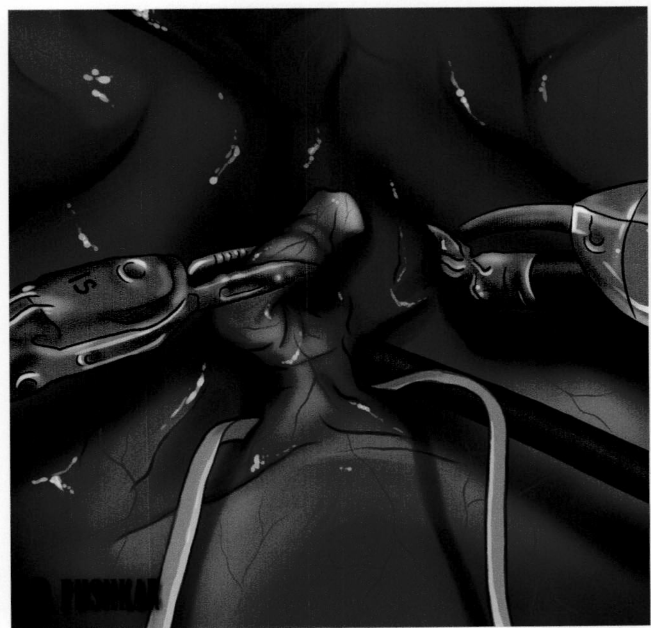

Fig. 18 Excision of the ureter

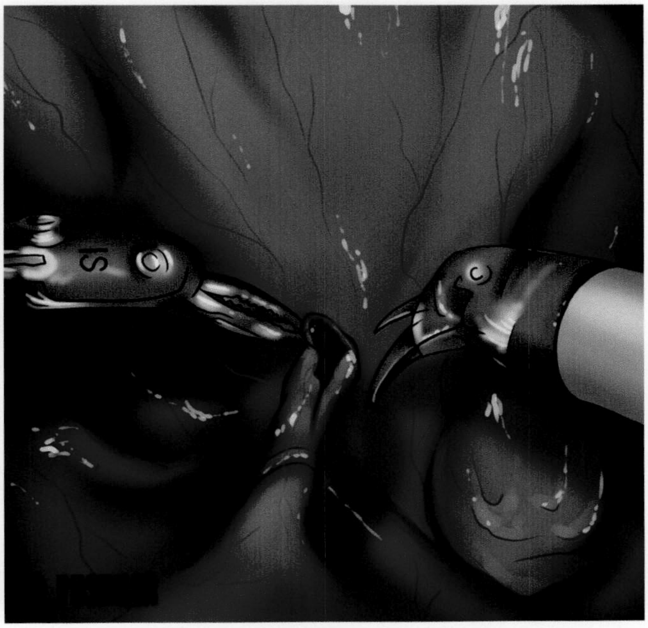

Fig. 19 Spatulation of the ureter

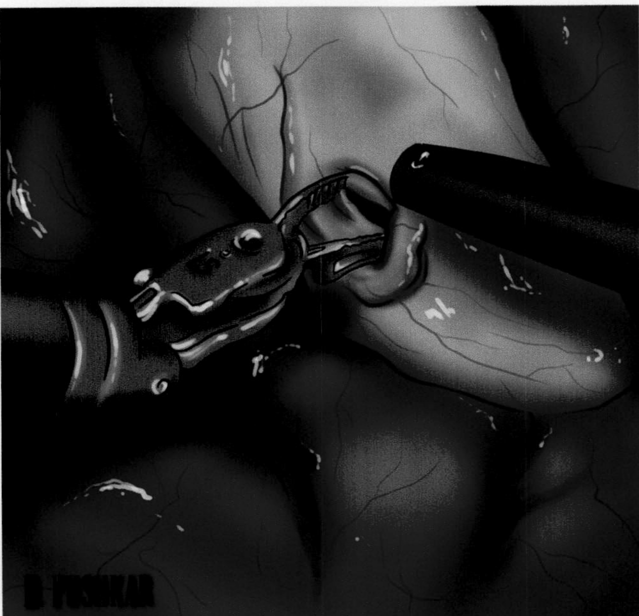

Fig. 20 Excision of the bladder

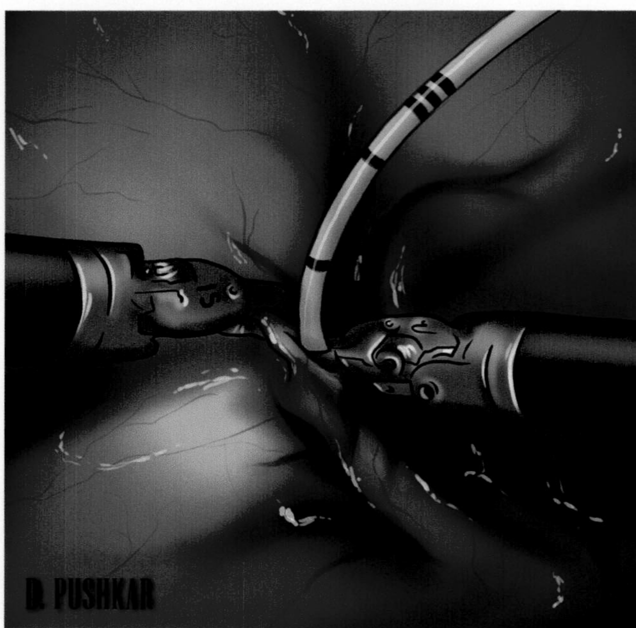

Fig. 21 Double J stenting

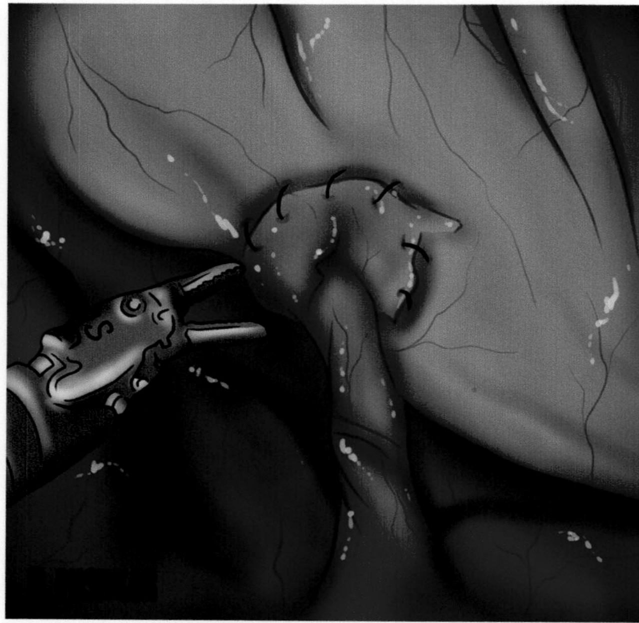

Fig. 22 Ureterocystoanastomosis

References

1. Hilton P. Vesico-vaginal fistula: new perspectives. Curr Opin Obstet Gynecol. 2001;13(5):513–20.
2. Bodner-Adler B, et al. Management of vesicovaginal fistulas (VVFs) in women following benign gynaecologic surgery: a systematic review and meta-analysis. PLoS One. 2017;12(2):e0171554.
3. Tasnim N, et al. Rising trends in iatrogenic urogenital fistula: a new challenge. Int J Gynaecol Obstet. 2020;148(Suppl 1):33–6.
4. Arrowsmith S, Hamlin EC, Wall LL. Obstructed labor injury complex: obstetric fistula formation and the multifaceted morbidity of maternal birth trauma in the developing world. Obstet Gynecol Surv. 1996;51(9):568–74.
5. Muleta M, et al. Obstetric fistula in rural Ethiopia. East Afr Med J. 2007;84(11):525–33.
6. Hilton P. Trends in the aetiology of urogenital fistula: a case of 'retrogressive evolution'? Int Urogynecol J. 2016;27(6):831–7.
7. Angioli R, et al. Guidelines of how to manage vesicovaginal fistula. Crit Rev Oncol Hematol. 2003;48(3):295–304.
8. Sims JM. On the treatment of vesico-vaginal fistula. 1852. Int Urogynecol J Pelvic Floor Dysfunct. 1998;9(4):236–48.
9. Toledo LG, et al. Continent vesicovaginal fistula. Einstein (Sao Paulo). 2013;11(1):119–21.
10. Hilton P, Ward A. Epidemiological and surgical aspects of urogenital fistulae: a review of 25 years' experience in Southeast Nigeria. Int Urogynecol J Pelvic Floor Dysfunct. 1998;9(4):189–94.
11. Forsgren C, et al. Hysterectomy for benign indications and risk of pelvic organ fistula disease. Obstet Gynecol. 2009;114(3):594–9.
12. Harkki-Siren P, Sjoberg J, Tiitinen A. Urinary tract injuries after hysterectomy. Obstet Gynecol. 1998;92(1):113–8.
13. Hilton P, Cromwell DA. The risk of vesicovaginal and urethrovaginal fistula after hysterectomy performed in the English National Health Service--a retrospective cohort study examining patterns of care between 2000 and 2008. BJOG. 2012;119(12):1447–54.
14. Hillary CJ, et al. The Aetiology, treatment, and outcome of urogenital fistulae managed in well- and low-resourced countries: a systematic review. Eur Urol. 2016;70(3):478–92.
15. Redman JF. Female urologic diagnostic techniques. Urol Clin North Am. 1990;17(1):5–8.
16. Raghavaiah NV. Double-dye test to diagnose various types of vaginal fistulas. J Urol. 1974;112(6):811–2.
17. Hyde BJ, et al. MRI review of female pelvic fistulizing disease. J Magn Reson Imaging. 2018;48(5):1172–84.
18. Hosseinzadeh K, Heller MT, Houshmand G. Imaging of the female perineum in adults. Radiographics. 2012;32(4):E129–68.
19. Matei DV, et al. Robot-assisted Vesico-vaginal fistula repair: our technique and review of the literature. Urol Int. 2017;99(2):137–42.
20. Lawson JB. Tropical gynaecology birth-canal injuries. Proc R Soc Med. 1968;61(4):368–70.
21. Goh JT. A new classification for female genital tract fistula. Aust N Z J Obstet Gynaecol. 2004;44(6):502–4.
22. Waaldijk K. Surgical classification of obstetric fistulas. Int J Gynaecol Obstet. 1995;49(2):161–3.
23. Frajzyngier V, Ruminjo J, Barone MA. Factors influencing urinary fistula repair outcomes in developing countries: a systematic review. Am J Obstet Gynecol. 2012;207(4):248–58.
24. Zhou L, et al. Factors influencing repair outcomes of vesicovaginal fistula: a retrospective review of 139 procedures. Urol Int. 2016;99(1):22–8.
25. Ayed M, et al. Prognostic factors of recurrence after vesicovaginal fistula repair. Int J Urol. 2006;13(4):345–9.
26. Ockrim JL, et al. A tertiary experience of vesico-vaginal and urethro-vaginal fistula repair: factors predicting success. BJU Int. 2009;103(8):1122–6.
27. Barone MA, et al. Determinants of postoperative outcomes of female genital fistula repair surgery. Obstet Gynecol. 2012;120(3):524–31.
28. Hata M, et al. Radiation therapy for stage IVA uterine cervical cancer: treatment outcomes including prognostic factors and risk of vesicovaginal and rectovaginal fistulas. Oncotarget. 2017;8(68):112855–66.

29. Mabuchi S, et al. Chemoradiotherapy followed by consolidation chemotherapy involving paclitaxel and carboplatin and in FIGO stage IIIB/IVA cervical cancer patients. J Gynecol Oncol. 2017;28(1):e15.
30. Moore KN, et al. Vesicovaginal fistula formation in patients with stage IVA cervical carcinoma. Gynecol Oncol. 2007;106(3):498–501.
31. Von Dittel L. Abdominale Blasenscheidenfistel-Operation. Wien. Klin. Wochenschr. 1893;6:449–452.
32. O'Conor VJ Jr. Review of experience with vesicovaginal fistula repair. J Urol. 1980;123(3):367–9.
33. Nezhat CH, et al. Laparoscopic repair of a vesicovaginal fistula: a case report. Obstet Gynecol. 1994;83(5 Pt 2):899–901.
34. Melamud O, et al. Laparoscopic vesicovaginal fistula repair with robotic reconstruction. Urology. 2005;65(1):163–6.
35. Randazzo M, et al. Best practices in robotic-assisted repair of Vesicovaginal fistula: a consensus report from the European Association of Urology Robotic Urology Section Scientific Working Group for Reconstructive Urology. Eur Urol. 2020;78(3):432–42.
36. Randazzo M, Lengauer L, Rochat CH, Ploumidis A, Kröpfl D, Rassweiler J, Buffi NM, Wiklund P, Mottrie A, John H. Corrigendum re "best practices in robotic-assisted repair of Vesicovaginal fistula: a consensus report from the European Association of Urology Robotic Urology Section Scientific Working Group for Reconstructive Urology" [Eur Urol 2020; 78: 432-42]. Eur Urol. 2021;79(2):e63.
37. Jairath A, et al. Robotic repair of vesicovaginal fistula - initial experience. Int Braz J Urol. 2016;42(1):168–9.
38. Sundaram BM, Kalidasan G, Hemal AK. Robotic repair of vesicovaginal fistula: case series of five patients. Urology. 2006;67(5):970–3.
39. Schimpf MO, et al. Vesicovaginal fistula repair without intentional cystotomy using the laparoscopic robotic approach: a case report. JSLS. 2007;11(3):378–80.
40. Dutto L, O'Reilly B. Robotic repair of vesico-vaginal fistula with perisigmoid fat flap interposition: state of the art for a challenging case? Int Urogynecol J. 2013;24(12):2029–30.
41. Martini A, et al. Robotic vesico-vaginal fistula repair with no omental flap interposition. Int Urogynecol J. 2016;27(8): 1277–8.
42. Machen GL, et al. Robotic repair of vesicovaginal fistulas using fibrin sealant. Can J Urol. 2017;24(2):8740–3.
43. Miklos JR, Moore RD, Chinthakanan O. Laparoscopic and robotic-assisted vesicovaginal fistula repair: a systematic review of the literature. J Minim Invasive Gynecol. 2015;22(5): 727–36.
44. Engel N and John H. Laparoscopic robot assisted vesico-vaginal fistula repair with peritoneal flap inlay. Eur Urol Suppl. 2008;179(4):666.
45. Hemal AK, Kolla SB, Wadhwa P. Robotic reconstruction for recurrent supratrigonal vesicovaginal fistulas. J Urol. 2008;180(3):981–5.
46. Kelly E, Wu MY, MacMillan JB. Robotic-assisted vesicovaginal fistula repair using an extravesical approach without interposition grafting. J Robot Surg. 2017;12(1):173–6.
47. Bora GS, et al. Robot-assisted vesicovaginal fistula repair: a safe and feasible technique. Int Urogynecol J. 2017;28(6):957–62.
48. Agrawal V, et al. Robot-assisted laparoscopic repair of vesicovaginal fistula: a single-center experience. Urology. 2015;86(2):276–81.
49. Sears CL, Schenkman N, Lockrow EG. Use of end-to-end anastomotic sizer with occlusion balloon to prevent loss of pneumoperitoneum in robotic vesicovaginal fistula repair. Urology. 2007;70(3):581–2.
50. Pietersma CS, et al. Robotic-assisted laparoscopic repair of a vesicovaginal fistula: a time-consuming novelty or an effective tool? BMJ Case Rep. 2014;2014:610.
51. Miklos JR, Moore RD. Laparoscopic extravesical vesicovaginal fistula repair: our technique and 15-year experience. Int Urogynecol J. 2015;26(3):441–6.
52. Salup RR, et al. Closure of large postradiation vesicovaginal fistula with rectus abdominis myofascial flap. Urology. 1994;44(1):130–1.
53. Hadzi-Djokic J, et al. Buccal mucosal graft interposition in the treatment of recurrent vesicovaginal fistula: a report on two cases. Taiwan J Obstet Gynecol. 2015;54(6):773–5.
54. Kurz M, Horstmann M, John H. Robot-assisted laparoscopic repair of high vesicovaginal fistulae with peritoneal flap inlay. Eur Urol. 2012;61(1):229–30.
55. John H. Vesikovaginale Fistel: Rekonstruktive Techniken. Urol Urogynäkol. 2005;12:35–6.
56. John H. Therapie der vesikovaginalen Fistel in Westafrika und Europa. Urol Urogynäkol. 2016;18:16–8.
57. Zhou L, et al. Factors influencing repair outcomes of vesicovaginal fistula: a retrospective review of 139 procedures. Urol Int. 2017;99(1):22–8.
58. Horstmann M, et al. Prospective comparison between the AirSeal(R) system valve-less trocar and a standard versaport plus V2 trocar in robotic-assisted radical prostatectomy. J Endourol. 2013;27(5):579–82.
59. Waaldijk K. The immediate management of fresh obstetric fistulas. Am J Obstet Gynecol. 2004;191(3):795–9.
60. Nambiar AK, et al. EAU guidelines on assessment and nonsurgical management of urinary incontinence. Eur Urol. 2018;73(4):596–609.
61. Latzko W. Postoperative vesicovaginal fistulas. Am J Surg. 1942;58:211.
62. Sotelo R, et al. Laparoscopic repair of vesicovaginal fistula. J Urol. 2005;173(5):1615–8.
63. Barone MA, et al. Breakdown of simple female genital fistula repair after 7 day versus 14 day postoperative bladder catheterisation: a randomised, controlled, open-label, non-inferiority trial. Lancet. 2015;386(9988):56–62.
64. Blaivas JG, Heritz DM, Romanzi LJ. Early versus late repair of vesicovaginal fistulas: vaginal and abdominal approaches. J Urol. 1995;153(4):1110–2. discussion 1112-3
65. Eilber KS, et al. Ten-year experience with transvaginal vesicovaginal fistula repair using tissue interposition. J Urol. 2003;169(3):1033–6.
66. Nagraj HK, Kishore TA, Nagalaksmi S. Early laparoscopic repair for supratrigonal vesicovaginal fistula. Int Urogynecol J Pelvic Floor Dysfunct. 2007;18(7):759–62.
67. Raz S, et al. Transvaginal repair of vesicovaginal fistula using a peritoneal flap. J Urol. 1993;150(1):56–9.
68. Kumar S, Kekre NS, Gopalakrishnan G. Vesicovaginal fistula: an update. Indian J Urol. 2007;23(2):187–91.
69. Lee RA, Symmonds RE, Williams TJ. Current status of genitourinary fistula. Obstet Gynecol. 1988;72(3 Pt 1):313–9.
70. Chibber PJ, Shah HN, Jain P. Laparoscopic O'Conor's repair for vesico-vaginal and vesico-uterine fistulae. BJU Int. 2005;96(1):183–6.
71. Rizvi SJ, et al. Modified laparoscopic abdominal vesico-vaginal fistula repair—"Mini-O'Conor" vesicotomy. J Laparoendosc Adv Surg Tech A. 2010;20(1):13–5.
72. Prasad ML, Nelson R, Hambrick E. York Mason procedure for repair of postoperative rectoprostatic urethral fistula. Dis Colon Rectum. 1983;26(11):716–20.
73. Harpster LE, Rommel FM, Sieber PR. The incidence and management of rectal injury associated with radical pros-

tatectomy in a community-based urology practice. J Urol. 1995;154(4):1435–8.
74. Munoz M, Nelson H, Harrington J. Management of acquired rectourinary fistulas: outcome according to cause. Dis Colon Rectum. 1998;41:1230–8.
75. Quazza JE, Firmin F, Cossa JP. Recto-urethral fistula following prostatectomy: surgical repair using a combined perineal and laparoscopic approach. Procedure and results of two cases. Prog Urol. 2009;19(6):434–7.
76. Mundy AR, Andrich DE. Urorectal fistulae following the treatment of prostate cancer. BJU Int. 2010;107:1298–3.
77. Hruza M, Weiß HO, Pini G, Gözen AS, Schulze M, Teber D, Rassweiler JJ. Complications in 2200 consecutive laparoscopic radical prostatectomies: standardised evaluation and analysis of learning curves. Eur Urol. 2010;58:733–41.
78. Goezen AS, Malkoc E, Yousef I, Rassweiler J. Laparoscopic urorectal fistula repair: value of the salvage prostatectomy and review of current approaches. J Endourol. 2012;26:1171–6.
79. Jordan GH, Lynch DF, Warden SS. Major rectal complications following interstitial implantation of 125iodine for carcinoma of the prostate. J Urol. 1985 Dec;134(6):1212–4.
80. Davis JW, Schellhammer PF. Prostatorectal fistula 14 years following brachytherapy for prostate cancer. J Urol. 2001;165(1):189.
81. Shah SA, Cima RR, Benoit E. Rectal complications after prostate brachytherapy. Dis Colon Rectum. 2004;47(9):1487–92.
82. Mao Q, Luo J, Fang J, Jang H. Management of radiation-induced rectovesical fistula in a woman using ileum – case report and review of the literature. Medicine. 2017;96:46. e8553
83. Sadamoto Y, Araki Y, Harada N. A case of rectoprostatic fistula due to prostatic abscess visualized by barium enema. Br J Radiol. 1999 Oct;72(862):1016–7.
84. Mitchell RJ, Blake JR. Spontaneous perforation of prostatic abscess with peritonitis. J Urol. 1972;107(4):622–3.
85. Singh I, Mittal G, Kumar P. Delayed post–traumatic prostate-urethro rectal fistula: Transperineal rectal sparing repair-point of technique. Int J Urol. 2006;13(1):92–4.
86. Bauer HW, Sturm W, Schmiedt E. Surgical correction of recto-prostatic fistula. Urology. 1984;24(5):452–5.
87. Rassweiler JJ, Weiss H, Heinze A, Elmussareh M, Fiedler M, Goezen AS. Bladder neck sclerosis following prostatic surgery – which therapy when? Urologe A. 2017;56:1129–38.
88. Yan S, Sun H, LiZ LS, Han B. Conservative treatment of rectovesical fistula after leakage following laparoscopic radical resection of rectal cancer. J Int Med Res. 2020;48:1–5.
89. Parks AG, Motson RW. Peranal repair of rectoprostatic fistula. Br J Surg. 1983;70:725–6.
90. Kanehira E, Tanida T, Kamel A, Nakagi M, Iwasaki M, Shimizu H. Transanal endoscopic microsurgery for surgical repair of rectal fistula following radical prostatectomy. Surg Endosc. 2015;29:851–5.
91. Kanehira E, Tanida T, Kamel Kanehira A, Kodai T, Obana Y, Iwasaki M, Sagawa K. A new technique to repair vesicorectal fistula: overlapping rectal muscle plasty by transanal endoscopic surgery. Urol Int. 2021;105:309–15.
92. Elmajian DA. Surgical approaches to repair of rectourinary fistulas. AUA Update Series. 2000;19:42.
93. Visser BC, Mc Aninch JW, Welton ML. Rectourethral fistulae: the perineal approach. J Am Coll Surg. 2002 Jul;195(1):138–43.
94. Garofalo TE, Delaney CP, Jones SM. Rectal advancement flap repair of rectourethral fistula: a 20-year experience. Dis Colon Rectum. 2003 Jun;46(6):762–9.
95. Noldus J, Fernandez S, Huland H. Rectourinary fistula repair using the Latzko technique. J Urol. 1999;161(5):1518–20.
96. Venable DD. Modification of the anterior perineal transanorectal approach for complicated prostatic urethrorectal fistula repair. J Urol. 1989;142(2 Pt 1):381–4.
97. Dafnis G, Wang YH, Borck L. Transsphincteric repair of rectourethral fistulae following laparoscopic radical prostatectomy. Int J Urol. 2004;11(11):1047–9.
98. Zmora O, Potenti FM, Wexner SD. Gracilis muscle transposition for iatrogenic rectourethral fistula. Ann Surg. 2003;237(4): 483–7.
99. Zinman L. Managing complex rectourethral fistulas. Contemp Urol. 2005;17:30–8.
100. Dal Moro F, Mancini M, Pinto F, Zanovello N, Bassi PF, Pagano F. Successful repair of iatrogenic rectourinary fistulas using the posterior sagittal transrectal approach (York-Mason): 15-year experience. World J Surg. 2006;30:107–13.
101. Gozen AS, Teber D, Moazin M. Laparoscopic transvesical urethrorectal fistula repair: a new technique. Urology. 2006;67(4):833–6.
102. Sotelo R, Garcia A, Yaime H. Laparoscopic rectovesical fistula repair. J Endourol. 2005;19(6):603–7.
103. Sotelo R, de Andrade R, Carmona O. Robotic repair of rectovesical fistula resulting from open radical prostatectomy. Urology. 2008;72(6):1344–6.
104. Yeung LL, Mason J, Dersch J. Robotic Rectovesical Fistula Repair. In: Su LM, editor. Atlas of robotic urologic surgery. Cham: Springer; 2017. https://doi.org/10.1007/978-3-319-45060-5_24.
105. Rovner ES. Urinary tract fistula. In: Wein AJ, Kavoussi LR, Novick AC, Partin AW, Peters CA, editors. Campbell-Walsh urology. 9th ed. Philadelphia: Saunders; 2007. p. 2322.
106. Elliott SP, McAninch JW. Ureteral injuries: external and iatrogenic. Urol Clin North Am. 2006;33:55–66.
107. Rodriguez L, Payne CK. Management of urinary fistulas. In: Taneja SS, Smith RB, Ehrlich RM, editors. Complications of urologic surgery: prevention and management. 3rd ed. Philadelphia: WB Saunders; 2001. p. 186.
108. Mattingly RF, Borkowf HI. Acute operative injury to the lower urinary tract. Clin Obstet Gynaecol. 1978;5:123–49.
109. Gilberti C, Germinale F, Lillo M, et al. Obstetrics and gynaecological ureteric injuries: treatment and results. Br J Urol. 1996;77:21–6.
110. Drake MJ, Noble JG. Ureteric trauma in gynecologic surgery. Int Urogynecol J. 1998;9:108–17.
111. Jelovsek JE, Chiung C, Chen G, Roberts SL, Paraiso MF, Falcone T. Incidence of lower urinary tract injury at the time of total laparoscopic hysterectomy. JSLS. 2007;11:422–7.
112. Tamussino KF, Lang PF, Breinl E. Ureteral complications with operative gynecologic laparoscopy. Am J Obstet Gynecol. 1998;178:967–70.
113. Harmanli OH, Tunitsky E, Esin S, Citil A, Knee A. A com- parison of short-term outcomes between laparoscopic supracervical and total hysterectomy. Am J Obstet Gynecol. 2009;201:536. e1–7.
114. Assimos DG, Patterson LC, Taylor CL. Changing incidence and etiology of iatrogenic ureteral injuries. J Urol. 1994;152:2240–6.
115. Kim JH, Moore C, Jones JS, Rackley R, Daneshgari F, Goldman H, et al. Management of ureteral injuries associated with vaginal surgery for pelvic organ prolapse. Int Urogynecol J Pelvic Floor Dysfunct. 2006;17:531–5.
116. Brandes S, Coburn M, Armenakas N, McAninch J. Diagnosis and management of ureteric injury: an evidence-based analysis. BJU Int. 2004;94:277–89.
117. Symmonds RE. Ureteral injury associated with gynecologic surgery: prevention and management. Clin Obstet Gynecol. 1976;19:623–44.
118. Mandal AK, Sharma SK, Vaidyanathan S, et al. Ureterovaginal fistula: summary of 18 years of experience. Br J Urol. 1990;65:453–6.
119. Brandes S, Coburn M, Armenakas N, et al. Diagnosis and management of ureteric injury: an evidence-based analysis. BJU Int. 2004;94:277–89.

120. Kim J-H, Moore C, Jones JS, et al. Management of ureteral injuries associated with vaginal surgery for pelvic organ prolapse. Int Urogynecol J. 2006;17:531–5.
121. Peterson DD, Lucey DT, Fried FA. Nonsurgical management of ureterovaginal fistula. Urology. 1974;4:677–80.
122. Goodwin WE, Scardino PT. Vesicovaginal and ureterovaginal fistulas: a summary of 25 years of experience. J Urol. 1980;123:370–4.
123. Hulse CA, Sawtelle WW, Nadig PW, Wolff HL. Conservative management of ureterovaginal fistula. J Urol. 1968;99:42–9.
124. Alonso Gorrea M, Fernandez Zuazu J, Mompo Sanchis JA, Jimenez-Cruz JF. Spontaneous healing of ureterogenital fistulas: selection criteria. Eur Urol. 1986;12:322–6.
125. Al-Otaibi KM. Ureterovaginal fistulas: the role of endoscopy and a percutaneous approach. Urol Ann. 2012;4:102–5.
126. Rajamaheswari N, Chhikara AB, Seethalakshmi K. Management of ureterovaginal fistulae: an audit. Int Urogynecol J. 2013;24:959–62.
127. Kumar A, Goyal NK, Das SK, Trivedi S, Dwivedi US, Singh PB. Our experience with genitourinary fistulae. Urol Int. 2009;82:404–10.
128. Elabd S, Ghoniem G, Elsharaby M, Emran M, Elgamasy A, Felfela T, et al. Use of endoscopy in the management of postoperative ureterovaginal fistula. Int Urogynecol J Pelvic Floor Dysfunct. 1997;8:185–90.
129. Selzman AA, Spirnak JP, Kursh ED. The changing management of ureterovaginal fistulas. J Urol. 1995;153:626–8.
130. Schmeller NT, Gottinger H, Schuller J, Marx FJ. Percutaneous nephrostomy as primary therapy of ureterovaginal fistula. Urologe A. 1983;22:108–12.
131. Selzman AA, Spirnak JP. Iatrogenic ureteral injuries: a 20 year experience in treating 165 injuries. J Urol. 1996;155:878–81.
132. Blandy JP, Badenoch DF, Fowler CG, et al. Early repair of iatrogenic injury to the ureter or bladder after gynecological surgery. J Urol. 1991;146:761–5.
133. Presti JC, Carroll PR, McAninch JW. Ureteral and renal pelvic injuries from external trauma: diagnosis and management. J Trauma. 1989;29:370–4.
134. Velhamos GC, Dergiannis E, Wells M, et al. Penetrating ureteral injuries: the impact of associated injuries on management. Am Surg. 1996;62:461–7.
135. Ramalingam M, Senthil K, Venkatesh V. Laparoscopic repair of ureterovaginal fistula: successful outcome by laparoscopic ureteral reimplantation. J Endourol. 2005;10:1174–6.

Part V

Pediatric Surgery

Robotic Surgery Applications in Pediatric Urologic Patients: Physiology and Special Considerations

Christina Kim and Chester J. Koh

1 Physiology of Minimally Invasive Surgery

Minimally invasive surgery (MIS) has become a common approach for many urologic surgeries. Initially this was applied to adults but has expanded into the pediatric population for many years.

We will highlight the physiologic effects of pneumoperitoneum and positioning used in MIS. We will also review special considerations when performing MIS in children.

Most of the physiologic changes with laparoscopy and robotic surgery are due to the increased intra-abdominal pressure (IAP) when carbon dioxide (CO2) insufflates the abdominal cavity. Higher IAP directly and indirectly influences the respiratory, cardiac, cerebral, and renal systems.

1.1 Cardiovascular Changes

A rise in IAP affects both arterial and venous blood flow. Cardiac output (CO) and respiratory regulation are altered as well. Most of these changes appear similar in children compared to adults.

Specifically, as IAP rises, there is an increase in mean arterial pressure (MAP), systemic vascular resistance (SVR), and central venous pressure (CVP). At higher IAP pressures, there is a decrease in cardiac output (CO) and stroke volume (SV).

The increased MAP and SVR is multifactorial. As IAP rises, there is a catecholamine release and activation of the renin-angiotensin system. This can increase mean arterial pressure and systemic vascular resistance seen with higher IAP [1]. Additionally, there is compression of both the arterial and venous vessels.

Changes in cardiac output appear variable at different pressures. When IAP is less than 5 mmHg, there is compression of the splanchnic vasculature. This leads to a greater venous return to the right atrium and an increase in cardiac output. But at higher IAP (15 mmHg), there can be lower cardiac output due to inferior venal cava (IVC) and aortic compression, pooling of blood in the lower extremities, and a subsequent rise in arterial resistance.

There are limited studies in the physiologic changes in children undergoing MIS. One study of 13 children (6–36 months old) looked at hemodynamic changes associated with laparoscopic fundoplication. Patients were positioned with head elevated 10 degrees and insufflation pressure of 5 mmHg. Multiple parameters were measured: cardiac index (CI), stroke volume index (SVI), heart rate (HR), and mean arterial pressure (MAP). During insufflation, end-tidal CO2 tension (PetCO2), cardiac index (CI), heart rate (HR), and MAP all increased. But there were no changes in SVI or arterial oxygen saturation. The authors concluded that low insufflation pressure (5 mmHg) did not decrease CI in young patients [2].

Another study looked at 33 pediatric patients undergoing laparoscopic fundoplication. They did not see significant cardiovascular changes if IAP was <10 mmHg [3].

If CO2 insufflation causes hypercarbia, acidosis can occur. With acidosis, there can be lower cardiac contractility, systemic vasodilation, and a greater chance of arrhythmias. Also, pneumoperitoneum can lead to a robust vagal reflex. A vagal reflex can cause bradycardia. If this occurs during initial insufflation, the team needs to be ready for emergent desufflation [4, 5].

Overall, the use of MIS in pediatric patients has shown favorable results, even if there is a history of congenital heart disease (CHD). A meta-analysis looking at patients with CHD who underwent laparoscopic surgery included a total of 2502 patients who underwent open surgery (OS) and 1182 with laparoscopic surgery (LS). Cardiac risk was similar in

C. Kim
Shriners Children's New England, Springfield, MA, USA

C. J. Koh (✉)
Division of Pediatric Urology, Department of Surgery, Texas Children's Hospital, Houston, TX, USA

Scott Department of Urology, Baylor College of Medicine, Houston, TX, USA

P. Wiklund et al. (eds.), *Robotic Urologic Surgery*, https://doi.org/10.1007/978-3-031-00363-9_68

both populations. Patients who had LS were more likely to have undergone prior cardiac surgery. The LS group had shorter hospitalizations and lower overall complication rates (specifically lower pulmonary, bleeding, and wound complications). The two groups had similar rates of postoperative cardiac arrest [6].

1.2 Respiratory Effect

Higher IAP can displace the diaphragm leading to lower total lung capacity and increased peak inspiratory pressures. This can result in atelectasis, higher airway pressures, and reduced lymphatic drainage. A lower functional residual capacity and atelectasis may cause a mismatch of ventilation and perfusion. These respiratory changes can lead to collapse of the alveoli with subsequent hypoxemia.

A study in 1995 looked at 126 children (11 months-13 years old) undergoing laparoscopic inguinal hernia explorations. These patients were categorized in three groups based on age (Group 1, ages 11 months-2 years; Group 2, ages 2–5 years; and Group 3: ages 5–13 years). All patients showed an increase in airway pressure and PetCO2 during laparoscopy with little difference between the groups. But the time lag from CO2 insufflation to PetCO2 change was fastest in youngest patients and slowest in oldest patients. However, body temperature and hemodynamics were not significantly altered in any of the groups [7].

A study in 2003 looked at effects of carbon dioxide (CO2) insufflation in both extraperitoneal and intraperitoneal laparoscopic cases. 29 children had retroperitoneal surgery and 33 patients had intraperitoneal surgery with a mean age of 7.2 years and 3.8 years, respectively. In these cases, mean retroperitoneal insufflation of 12 mmHg lead to significant increases in end-tidal CO2 (ETCO2), respiratory rate (RR), and peak airway pressure (PAP). The rise in ETCO2 was notably higher when patients were in a left lateral decubitus position. Mean intra-abdominal insufflation of 11 mmHg led to a rise in ETCO2, RR, and PAP. It also led to a lower O2 saturation level. Although there were no intraoperative complications seen with these hemodynamic changes, it is important to recognize these effects [8].

This same group did a prospective study of retroperitoneal surgery between 2003 and 2004. 18 consecutive patients followed the same anesthetic protocol. Mean age was 79.4 months and mean insufflation pressure was 12 mmHg. ETCO2, RR, PAP, mean arterial pressure (MAP), and heart rate (HR) were recorded before, during, and after CO2 insufflation. Data was collected at 1–2 minute intervals. There were significant changes in ETCO2, PAP, and MAP after CO2 insufflation. But these variables trended back to baseline after the laparoscopic procedure was done [9].

CO2 is rapidly absorbed and highly soluble s o insufflation can lead raise CO2 levels due to direct absorption. Some studies have shown an inverse correlation between age and the higher CO2 levels. Infants continue to have a rise in CO2 levels, whereas adults hit a plateau [10]. This may be due to infant peritoneal cavities being proportionally larger and better perfused. Also, the peritoneum in children can absorb more gases relative to adults due to a shorter distance between the capillaries and the peritoneum. Lastly, children typically have a higher absorptive area relative to body weight. Some of these respiratory changes can be offset by increasing minute ventilation or increasing positive end expiratory pressure (PEEP). The ventilatory rate may need to be increased by over 60% to balance end-tidal CO2 levels [11].

1.3 Renal Effects

The effects of IAP on renal function have been attributed to multiple factors. This includes increased compression of the renal vein and renal parenchyma, increased renal vascular resistance, increased antidiuretic hormone production, and secondary effects of decreased cardiac output [12]. The renal effects appear to be most notable when IAP is >15 mmHg. Since most pediatric MIS cases are done with IAP <12 mmHg, these renal changes are not as likely to manifest. But there are many notable renal changes linked to MIS.

Pneumoperitoneum appears to stimulate the renin-angiotensin-aldosterone system. This increases renin, aldosterone, and anti-diuretic hormone levels. These hormonal changes can cause salt retention, water retention, and oliguria [13]. Higher IAP can cause a pressure dependent decrease in renal blood flow, glomerular filtration, and urinary output. Studies have shown these changes are all reversible.

The impact of the renin-angiotensin-aldosterone system was challenged in a 2002 study comparing open and laparoscopic gastric bypass surgery. They found similar levels of ADH, aldosterone, and renin in both groups [14].

When patients have normal renal function, the renal effects seen with MIS are typically transient. Oliguria is likely related to compression of both the renal parenchyma and the renal vein [12, 15].

A study of 8 pediatric patients (0–12 months old) looked at renal function when laparoscopic IAP was 8 mmHg. In this study, 88% developed anuria during the operative case. All patients had resumption of urinary production postoperatively. This production reached its maximum 5 hours after desufflation [16].

Gomez et al. looked at 30 children with normal renal function undergoing laparoscopic surgery. They measured renal blood flow by Doppler ultrasound before surgery, every 15 minutes during surgery, and 24 hours after surgery. Blood and urine samples were collected before surgery and 24 hours after surgery. Although urine output decreased within 45 minutes of pneumoperitoneum in all patients, there was significant recovery of urine production 5–6 hours later (in both infants and older children). There was temporary anuria in most of the infants and oliguria in one third of the older children. However, there was no significant change in renal blood flow, levels of cystatin C, creatinine, or urea nitrogen. In this study, the volume of intraoperative intravenous fluids did not correlate with urine production. The authors concluded that urine output changes seen during MIS are reversible and intravenous fluid management should not be dictated by the urine production [16].

Another study looked at 29 patients having laparoscopic surgery. Information was recorded 15 minutes before, during, and 15 minutes after pneumoperitoneum insufflation and deflation. Pneumoperitoneum levels varied based on age: 0–1 month had <6 mmHg; 2–12 months had <8 mmHg; 1–2 years old had <10 mmHg, and 2–8 years old had <12 mmHg. Surgeons used the lowest pressure to allow adequate visualization. All patients had normal renal function and near-infrared spectroscopy (NIRS) probes were used to measure renal regional oxygen saturation (rSO2). There were no significant drops in rSO2 between preinsufflation, insufflation, and desufflation. Also, there was no significant association between urine output and fluid input. The authors concluded that renal hypoxia did not occur during laparoscopy when age-appropriate IAP was used [17].

Most pediatric studies looked at patients with normal renal function. If patients have preoperative renal dysfunction, deterioration of renal function after MIS is always possible.

1.4 Cerebral Effect

Cerebral hemodynamics are affected by the cardiovascular system, abdominal pressure, and the position of the patient. The relationship is likely due to compression of the lumbar venous plexus with impaired venous drainage. Also, higher IAP can impair reabsorption of cerebrospinal fluid. CO2 insufflation also appears to directly affect cerebral blood flow [18].

In 2011, Karsli et al. evaluated 18 retroperitoneal and 18 transperitoneal laparoscopic surgeries in children. Their team measured ETCO2, middle cerebral arterial blood flow velocity, heart rate, and mean arterial blood pressure. The middle cerebral blood flow was measured with transcranial Doppler ultrasound. Data was collected before, during, and after CO2 insufflation (mean 12 mmHg). In the transperitoneal group, there was a rapid increase in middle cerebral arterial blood flow velocity, mean arterial pressure, and ETCO2 during the first 8 minutes of pneumoperitoneum. ETCO2 continued to increase after 8 minutes, but the MAP and middle cerebral arterial blood flow velocity hit a plateau after 8 minutes. However, in the retroperitoneal group, the middle cerebral flow velocity and ETCO2 progressively increased throughout intraabdominal insufflation. The authors believe the smaller absorptive surface in retroperitoneal surgery explained these hemodynamic differences [19].

A study in 2020 looked at cerebral and renal oxygenation during laparoscopic procedures. This study evaluated 25 infants (mean age 40 days and weight 4.0 kg). The regional oxygen saturation (rSO2) was measured during laparoscopic pyloromyotomy. Parameters were compared at the time of incision and the end of pneumoperitoneum. Both cerebral and renal rSO2 decreased at the end of laparoscopy, but there was only a statistically significant change in cerebral rSO2. There was an increase in cerebral tissue oxygen extraction. However, the values did not decrease below those seen before induction of anesthesia [20].

Cerebral blood flow and intracranial pressure may be increased with higher IAP. So, if a patient has reduced intracranial compliance, a laparoscopic approach should be avoided. Patients with head injuries have a higher risk since they may have compromised regulation of intracranial pressures [21].

1.5 Insufflation Gas

When choosing the gas used for insufflation, CO2 is the primary gas used for MIS. It is noncombustible, relatively inexpensive, and highly soluble in blood. Its solubility minimizes the risk of embolism. Other gas agents (e.g., room air, nitrogen, helium, and oxygen) have been associated with significant problems [22].

A study in 2003 looked at the pattern of CO2 elimination during laparoscopic surgery in infants and children. In this study, 20 children underwent laparoscopic surgery and 19 children underwent laparotomy for elective intra-abdominal surgery. Indirect calorimetry was used to measure CO2 elimination as well as PeCO2. These variables were measured before CO2 insufflation, during pneumoperitoneum, and after desufflation. After desufflation, CO2 elimination decreased toward the preinsufflation values, but did not return to those baseline levels. PeCO2 peaked at 1 hour and then decreased in response to ventilatory adjustments. The total CO2 insufflated had a positive correlation with patient age. CO2 elimination was age related and had negative correlation to weight. These results suggested CO2 elimination was higher in the younger and smaller patients. Also, younger patients absorbed proportionally more CO2 than older patients during pneumoperitoneum. The increase in CO2 elimination after desufflation may be related to a higher venous return from the lower extremities after releasing the intra-abdominal pressure during desufflation. The authors concluded that it is important to use close monitoring during laparoscopy and the immediate postoperative period [23].

In 1994, an adult study compared hemodynamic effects of CO_2 and nitrous oxide (N_2O). Insufflation went up to 20 mmHg. CO_2 insufflation led to increase in MAP, systemic vascular resistance index, and CVP. There was not a change in HR with insufflation. This differed from N_2O insufflation which correlated with decreased MAP and no change in vascular resistance. Overall, both gases were associated with cardiovascular depression. But mean arterial pressure was better preserved with CO_2 [24].

Studies on adults have looked at the use of heated and humidified CO_2 for pneumoperitoneum. This has been associated with lower postoperative pain, lower analgesic dosage, and lower risk of postoperative hypothermia. Therefore, its use should be strongly considered when performing robotic and laparoscopic procedures [25].

1.6 Trendelenburg Position

Trendelenburg position can lead to lower lung capacity and increased peak inspiratory pressures. Although the Trendelenburg position increases SVR and heart rate, it can increase venous return to the heart, leading to an increase in cardiac output. Reverse Trendelenburg can have the reverse effects due to reduced venous return to the heart and lower cardiac filling pressure.

Oztan et al. looked at 44 children who had appendectomy (22 laparoscopic and 22 open). They measured cerebral oxygenation, heart rate, mean arterial pressure, end-tidal CO_2 pressure, and peripheral oxygen saturations. Measurements were taken at multiple times during induction, after open incisions were made, and after positional changes. There were no significant changes in cerebral oxygenation, MAP, $ETCO_2$, $PETCO_2$, and pneumoperitoneum. Therefore, Trendelenburg position did not appear to alter hemodynamic values. The authors felt laparoscopic surgery in Trendelenburg can be safely done without altering regional brain oxygenation levels [26].

1.7 Abdominal Wall Elasticity

A child's abdomen stretches up to 17% after induction of pneumoperitoneum. The degree of stretch tapers as the intra-abdominal pressure approaches peak pressure. Older children have a lower longitudinal abdominal elasticity but have higher transverse abdominal elasticity.

In 2020, Zhou et al. looked at 163 children undergoing laparoscopic surgery. These patients had pre-stretching of their abdomen using IAP of 0, 4, 6, 8, 10, and 12 mmHg. Regardless of age, pre-stretching led to increased elasticity over the transverse and lower sagittal abdominal wall. This can lead to a larger working space. Given the space limitations in pediatric robotic surgery, this can be extremely helpful [27].

Vlot et al. performed abdominal stretching in a porcine model. They stretched the abdominal cavities between 5 and 15 mmHg and used computed tomography (CT) to measure volumes and linear dimensions. By pre-stretching the abdominal wall, they achieved similar surgical field exposure at lower IAPs. The concept of pre-stretching may have potential benefit in human subjects [28].

1.8 Inflammation

A study in 2019 looked at the inflammatory stress response between laparoscopic and open inguinal hernia repairs in children. A total of 32 patients were randomly divided into one of the two surgical approaches. Mean age was 4.5 years. Blood samples were obtained in three different time frames. Specific lab values of white blood cell count (WBC), C-reactive protein (CRP), and tumor necrosis factor alpha (TNF-alpha) were measured. There were significant increases in all levels with surgery, but a significantly higher level was seen with the open approach. This may be attributed to a variety of factors. The operative time was significantly shorter with the laparoscopic approach. Regardless, the laparoscopic technique showed a lower stress response when compared to an open hernia approach [29].

Oxidative stress can be induced by reactive oxygen species (ROS). Since the pneumoperitoneum can temporarily compromise splanchnic blood flow, there is reperfusion after deflation. Baysal et al. looked at the oxidative-antioxidative status in pediatric patients undergoing laparoscopic surgery. Blood samples were collected and centrifuged to separate the plasma. Then plasma total antioxidative status (TAS), total oxidant status (TOS), and oxidative stress index (OSI) were all measured. When compared to levels at induction, the levels of TOS and OSI were higher at the end of surgery. But TAS was lower. The authors concluded that the ROS generated during laparoscopic surgery may cause oxidative stress and consume plasma antioxidants. This may be a result of ischemia-reperfusion secondary to insufflation-deflation associated with pneumoperitoneum [30].

1.9 Metabolic Response

Neonates differ from adults in their metabolic response to laparoscopic surgery. Immediately after surgery, neonates have a small increase in oxygen consumption and resting energy expenditure. However, this returns to normal levels within 24 hours. The conservative rise in energy expenditure may be secondary to energy diverted from growth and into tissue repair.

Older children appear similar to adults with a drop in resting energy expenditure immediately after surgery but with no late hypermetabolism.

Postoperative changes are likely influenced by intraoperative thermoregulation and metabolism. Minimally invasive surgery (MIS) may keep postoperative metabolic processes at a physiologic level or simply maintain thermoregulation. If so, this can help maintain preoperative metabolic processes [23].

1.10 Conclusions: Physiology Associated with Robotic Surgery Applications in Pediatric Urologic Patients

Most pediatric MIS cases are done at lower IAP (<12 mmHg). Regardless of the pressure used, MIS causes a variety of physiologic changes in the cardiac, respiratory, renal, and cerebral systems. However, these physiologic changes appear reversible.

Many studies of MIS in children have shown favorable outcomes. Despite excellent outcomes, it is important for the surgeon and anesthesia team to be aware of these physiologic changes so they can provide the safest environment for the patient.

2 Special Considerations

Special considerations exist with the use of robot-assisted laparoscopic surgery in children due to their smaller anatomy when compared to the adult population as well as the different types of urologic conditions that are surgically addressed in children.

2.1 Small Working Spaces

One special consideration in small children and especially in infants is the smaller working space in these patients that leads to a perception of increased difficulty and associated reluctance to perform robotic surgery in infants and small children. Robot-assisted laparoscopic pyeloplasty (RALP) is the most common robotic surgical procedure in the field of pediatric urology for the treatment of ureteropelvic junction obstruction (UPJO). The treatment goals are to prevent deterioration of the affected kidney's renal function from the effects of urinary tract obstruction, and minimally invasive surgery offers numerous potential benefits over conventional open surgery that includes reduced blood loss, pain medication usage, infection risk, and shorter recovery times [31–36]. However, in a nationwide inpatient sample data of US children's hospitals between 2005 and 2010, the percentage of RALP in infants was only 2.9% of the total number of pediatric RALP cases, while infants comprised 39.9% of the pediatric patients undergoing open pyeloplasties [32]. As a result, there are limited reports of infant RALP since many consider it to be a challenging procedure [37–40].

The limited adoption of RALP in infants may stem from the perception that there is increased operative difficulty than with RAL pyeloplasty in older children, since a typical infant's small size usually correlates with a smaller operative working space. This may lead to difficulties with port placement and can dissuade robotic surgeons from performing RALP in infants. Furthermore, minimally invasive surgery (robotic and conventional laparoscopic surgery) has been performed with caution in infants because of the perceived risks to hemodynamic and respiratory functions in small infants as well as the established long experience and high success rates associated with open surgery in this age group [41, 42].

However, we previously reported that infant RALP with 5 mm instruments is feasible, safe, and effective, with similar outcomes when compared to RALP in older children with larger working spaces [43]. In this study, the total operative times as well as console times were similar between the infant and older children groups, which suggests similar levels of operative difficulty in these groups. One of the most important steps of infant RALP is appropriate robotic port placement, since infants have a relatively shorter and wider abdominal wall surface area as well as relatively distended bowel when compared to older children. While the recommended distances between the camera port and each instrument port is usually at least 4 cm, this can be difficult to apply in infants due to their small body habitus. To overcome this difficulty, the inferior instrument port is often placed in the inferior midline region. In addition, with the smaller working space in infants, wide side-to-side movements can be difficult in infants and should be avoided. RALP usually requires only a single area of anatomic access (the ureteropelvic junction and proximal ureter). Of note, we found that the operative time for dissection to UPJO as well as anastomosis time were longer in the older pediatric age group (>10 years old) in comparison to the other age groups. We hypothesized that the larger anatomy of the older patients required more dissection than in infants and may have led to the longer operative times for these portions of the procedure. In addition, since the indication for operation in the older pediatric age groups was mostly related to the presence of UPJO-related symptoms (flank pain/abdominal pain – 11 of 15 pyeloplasties, 73.3%) rather than worsening hydronephrosis, there may have been less dilation of the renal pelvis than in the infant group, which may have increased the level of difficulty of the dissection around the UPJO in the older pediatric age group.

Additional operative recommendations may help to overcome the complexities of infant RALP. Clashing of the robotic arms and the robotic instruments within the smaller working space can be reduced by limiting the depth of port insertion inside the peritoneal cavity. However, this may increase the risk of port dislodgement as well as lead to increased camera lens fogging since a larger amount of the camera scope is exposed to the external environment. Increasing the gas insufflation flow rates up to 2–3 L/min or higher to expand the abdominal cavity has previously been recommended, [40] but this should be used with caution to avoid potential respiratory difficulties that may occur if the intra-abdominal pressures are increased.

2.2 Lack of Small Pediatric-Sized Instruments

A limited selection of instruments was available in the 5 mm size as compared to the instruments in the 8 mm size that included the lack of a bipolar energy source with the 5 mm dissectors, where the primary cautery instrument was the hook cautery. However, the monopolar hook cautery was often beneficial for pediatric procedures, since it allowed for atraumatic handling of the delicate tissues in pediatric patients with the use of the blunt tip of the hook. Curved scissors with cautery also were not available in the 5 mm size, where only "cold" scissors were available. However, this again was sufficient for pediatric procedures such as RALP since minimal blood loss was routinely encountered. In addition, the 5 mm instruments have a longer articulated wrist distance where some surgeons believed that a slightly longer working distance was necessary, which may not be available in infant cases. However, this did not materialize as a challenge in the infant cases in our experience, since we did not see longer operative times with these cases when compared to previously reported cases of infant RALP using 8 mm robotic instruments [38–40].

Unfortunately, there has been decreasing availability of small pediatric-sized robotic instruments with the discontinuation of the 5 mm instrument product line for the da Vinci Si system (Intuitive Surgical, Sunnyvale, California) in late 2020 as well as the planned discontinuation of maintenance services for the da Vinci Si system in early 2024. In addition, since only 8 mm instruments are available with the da Vinci Xi system, pediatric-sized robotic instruments (5 mm) are now limited to institutions and their current inventory which cannot be restocked.

The benefit of the smaller pediatric-sized (5 mm) instruments and especially in the infant population was the avoidance of larger scars that were associated with the 8 mm instruments, especially when these procedures were performed safely and effectively with the limited selection of 5 mm instruments without the need for conversion to an open procedure or conversion to the 8 mm instruments.

Despite benefits seen in the pediatric population with pediatric devices, pediatric patients and their device needs continue to be underserved with the discontinuation of pediatric-sized robotic instruments as an example. While it is well known that "children are not small adults," a persistent shortage of pediatric medical devices that can accommodate the unique anatomy and physiology of pediatric patients continues to exist. As a result, pediatric clinicians and surgeons are often using adult devices in an off-label manner [44]. There are multiple factors that contribute to this public health problem, including the smaller pediatric population when compared to the adult population, less attractive financial projections with pediatric device development, the relatively high cost and low enrollment numbers with pediatric clinical studies relative to the market size as well as the perceived increased risk with pediatric device development and the limited funding sources that are available to pediatric device innovators [45]. With advocacy by key stakeholders including the American Academy of Pediatrics to address this shortage, Congress passed the Pediatric Medical Device Safety and Improvement Act in 2007, which included the creation of the US Food and Drug Administration (FDA) Pediatric Device Consortia (PDC) Grant program. The PDC program allows consortia at tertiary care children's hospitals and academic institutions to support pediatric device innovators in the development of novel pediatric medical devices throughout the pediatric device life cycle with local, regional, and national institutional and innovation partners [46, 47]. Figure 1 lists the five current FDA P50 grant-supported pediatric device consortia.

To increase the pipeline of pediatric clinicians and surgeons with pediatric device development experience, the collaboration of biomedical engineers with pediatric clinicians and surgeons has been encouraged by the consortia via capstone engineering design programs and medical product development-focused Master's programs that are available at all accredited engineering schools in the USA [48]. Capstone engineering design programs that are partnered with tertiary care children's hospitals and the regional engineering universities allow for prototype development during an academic year (September to April) and enable pediatric clinicians and surgeons with busy clinical schedules to create novel pediatric device prototypes with their engineering team partners to address unmet pediatric device needs.

Once a prototype is created, the later stages of device development and especially the preclinical, clinical, and commercialization steps can be supported by federal grant funding such as the Small Business Innovation Research

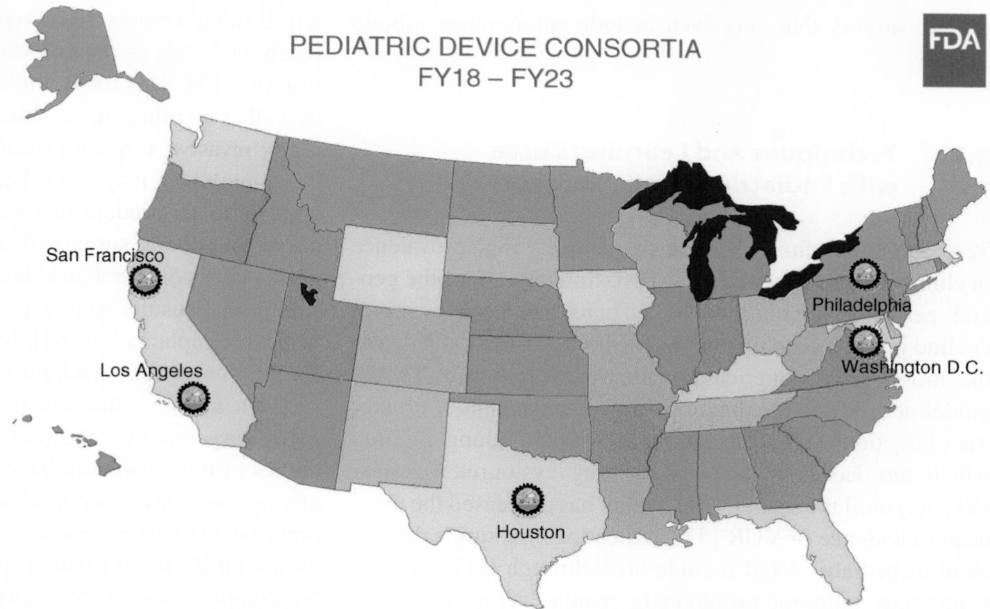

Fig. 1 The five current FDA P50 grant-supported pediatric device consortia that support pediatric device innovators

(SBIR) (R43/R44) and Small Business Technology Transfer (STTR) (R41/42) programs that are available through the National Institutes of Health (NIH) and the National Science Foundation (NSF) [44]. While engineering faculty are often aware of the NSF SBIR and STTR funding opportunities, clinical faculty may not be aware of these federal grant programs in the NIH due to the traditional emphasis on R01 basic science funding. While federal grant funding is difficult to obtain, pediatric faculty have been awarded NIH SBIR or STTR funding for various pediatric/fetal devices, including several at our institutions: 1) ureteral stent electromagnetic removal device for pediatric patients, 2) uterine wall membrane anchor device for the prevention of preterm premature rupture of the membranes in fetoscopic surgery, 3) pediatric urinary sphincter device for neurogenic bladder, 4) pediatric polymeric heart valves, and 5) vaginal stent for neo-vagina creation in female pediatric patients [44]. In comparison to NIH basic science research funding, the SBIR/STTR grants are often more reachable for pediatric clinicians and surgeons with partnership with qualified small business concerns than with NIH R01 funding, since the Impact Score paylines of SBIR/STTR grants at many NIH Institutes are often above 25. While also improving the academic record of faculty member toward promotion with this type of federal grant funding, this non-dilutive funding source for pediatric device development provides needed funding to pediatric device innovators during the early stages of development when funding is often in short supply.

In addition, new device innovation including new robotic systems also may help to address the pediatric device shortage in minimally invasive surgery. With a long history of minimally invasive/laparoscopy surgery in children since its first use for non-palpable testicles in the 1960s, widespread adoption of minimally invasive surgery has occurred within the field of pediatric urology and has even replaced open surgery in some situations as the gold standard [49]. With the benefits of smaller surgical scars and decreased hospital lengths of stay, robotic surgery has expanded minimally invasive surgery to complex reconstructive cases due to the improved surgeon dexterity with the robotic instruments, visualization, and sensory feedback (visual). The introduction of the da Vinci Surgical System (Intuitive Surgical, Inc., Sunnyvale, CA) in 1999 [50] led to key improvements for surgeons such as 3D visualization, 7-degree range of motion, tremor elimination, a fourth arm for retraction in limited cases, as well as teaching capabilities with dual-console systems and skill simulators. Emerging robotic platforms may provide new capabilities for robotic surgeons with continued reduction in the number of incisions to a single port platform and possibly even no incisions in the future. In addition, the combination of virtual reality technology and robotic surgery may lead to a completely new future for robotic surgery that may even include autonomous robotic surgery.

2.3 Techniques and Learning Curve with Pediatric Robotic Surgery

Vesicoureteral reflux (VUR) has a relatively high prevalence in children, where it occurs in approximately 1% of the general pediatric population [51]. There has been a recent decline in the screening and diagnostic tests for VUR due to the most recent American Academy of Pediatrics (AAP) guidelines [52] on the diagnosis and management of urinary tract infections (UTIs) in febrile infants and young children which has led to a delay of voiding cystourethrography (VCUG) until the second UTI, which has decreased the diagnostic incidence of VUR [53]. Indications for surgical treatment of pediatric VUR include breakthrough UTI while on continuous antibiotic prophylaxis, renal scarring, and worsening or unresolving VUR. Despite the reduction in VCUG studies, the historically high utilization of surgical intervention for VUR has led to the introduction of minimally invasive surgical options including robot-assisted laparoscopic ureteral reimplantation (RALUR) which has become more prevalent over the past decade but still remains relatively uncommon in many pediatric centers. Bowen et al. previously analyzed the use of pediatric open, laparoscopic, and robot-assisted laparoscopic ureteral reimplantation in the USA from 2002 to 2012 [54]. The number of ureteral reimplantations annually decreased by 14.3% during this time period, but the minimally invasive ureteral reimplantations increased from 0.3% in 2000 to 6.3% in 2012. Of the minimally invasive ureteral reimplantations, 81.2% were robot-assisted laparoscopic.

Traditionally, open ureteral reimplantation has been considered the gold standard surgical intervention for VUR [55] in addition to the endoscopic option for subureteric injections. However, over the past 2 decades, minimally invasive techniques such as robotic surgery has increasingly been utilized for the treatment of pediatric surgical conditions [56, 57] as robotic surgical systems have provided surgeons with three-dimensional vision, 10x magnification, and fully articulating endo-wrists suitable for dissection and suturing. As a result, minimally invasive surgery options have become increasingly available for many complex reconstructive procedures in pediatric urology such as RALUR which can be a relatively high-volume procedure for a pediatric robotic surgery program due to the high incidence of VUR in the pediatric population.

However, differences in outcomes and especially in the rate of perioperative complications have been noted among pediatric centers where many centers have reported favorable outcomes and safety profiles for RALUR) [58–61], while other centers have reported outcomes that did not reach the levels associated with traditional open reimplantation [62, 63]. This likely indicates differences in techniques as well as learning curve issues with this relatively new minimally invasive surgical procedure. While RALUR's technical complexity may have been underestimated initially, it appears to be prudent that surgeons early in their learning curve for robotic surgery should defer RALUR procedures until a later point in their robotic experience. It is of note that suboptimal results were reported initially with open extravesical reimplantation [64], but since then, has been associated with widespread adoption worldwide.

Even though extravesical RALUR has been utilized by many surgeons over the past 1.5 decades, the surgical outcomes of this procedure have been reported with variability among previously reported series. In 2008, Casale et al. reported their extravesical RALUR experience of 41 children with VUR [58] with a reflux resolution rate of 97.6%. No complications were reported except for one febrile UTI episode which occurred in the patient with persistent VUR postoperatively. In 2012, a subsequent RALUR case series by this group with an increased number of 150 children with bilateral VUR and at least 2 years of postoperative follow-up [60] was associated with a 99.3% reflux resolution rate based on postoperative VCUG and no patients with novo voiding dysfunction or urinary retention. Other subsequent series also reported similar favorable outcomes of RALUR. In 2011, Smith et al. compared surgical outcomes of 25 extravesical RALUR patients with those of 25 open cross-trigonal ureteral reimplantation patients [59] with an overall success rate was 97% for RALUR compared to 100% for open reimplantation but with a reduced mean length of stay (33 vs 53 hours) and reduced pain medication usage in the RALUR group. In 2015, Silay et al. reported the outcomes of 72 children (91 ureters) who underwent extravesical RALUR [61] with complete resolution of VUR in 97.9% with only two patients (2.7%) developing temporary postoperative urinary retention that self-resolved within 2 weeks.

Other series have reported favorable reflux resolution rates with RALUR but with uncommon but significant complications. In 2011, Marchini et al. reported 20 cases of extravesical RALUR with a reflux resolution rate of 100% but with 2 cases (10%) of ureteral injury [65]. In 2014, Akhavan et al. reported the outcomes of 78 extravesical RALUR in 50 patients [66]. The reflux resolution rate was 92.3% based on postoperative VCUG, but the overall complication rate was 10% that included ureteral obstruction in 2 patients and ureteral injury in 1 patient, with ureteral stent placement required in these three patients.

Two other series have reported suboptimal success rates with relatively high complication rates. In 2015, Grimsby et al. reported on the experience at two institutions with extravesical RALUR [62]. Of the 61 patients (93 ureters) who underwent RALUR, VUR resolution was noted in only 44 of 61 patients (72%), while 6 major complications (10%) were also noted including ureteral obstruction or ureteral leak. In 2016, Herz et al. reported the outcomes of extravesical RALUR in 54 children with a total of 72 ureters [63]. Overall surgical success was 85.2% of ureters and overall complication was 11% including ureteral obstruction (7.4%) or ureteral injury (3.7%).

As with any new surgical treatment, variability in the reported surgical outcomes can occur at different institutions and this includes extravesical RALUR. Variabilities in the patient populations and in surgeon experience are likely, where the reported success rates after RALUR at different institutions may have been affected by case selection as well as by a surgeon's learning curve. Similar to the adoption of robot-assisted laparoscopic pyeloplasty (RALP), the operative time of RALP significantly decreased as surgeons progressed through their learning curve with reductions in operative time and the potential for major complications, and this is expected for RALUR as well [67].

Another consideration is the underestimated complexity of the extravesical RALUR procedure. Some of the most important principles for operative success with RALUR are based on principles commonly taught for all open reimplantation surgery such as a no-touch rule for handling the ureter, low cautery settings, and careful use of the robotic instruments that do not lead to inadvertent injury to the ureter and bladder. These may not be fully appreciated by a surgeon early in their robotic experience when there is a minimally invasive approach with no haptic (sensory) feedback. Similar to open reimplantation, essential surgical steps for RALUR include the mobilization of the ureter proximally for approximately 4 to 5 cm to achieve a sufficient length for reimplantation as well as minimal usage of cautery and ureteral handling during distal ureteral dissection to preserve the delicate periureteral tissues and blood supply to the ureter.

Similar to the trifecta of outcomes for prostate cancer surgery (cancer control, urinary continence, and preservation of erectile function), a similar trifecta for VUR surgery can be equivalent success rates, equivalent hospital charges, and low complication rates similar to those of the gold standard, open ureteral reimplantation. RALUR has been established as a viable option for the surgical management of VUR, but it is well understood that the favorable outcomes and low complication rates for RALUR need to be comparable to open ureteral reimplantation for all surgeons and centers. Educational opportunities such as robotic hands-on course and expanded training during residency/fellowship training should help to standardize RALUR techniques to those that are associated with comparable outcomes to open reimplantation. Furthermore, multi-institutional collaborations are in progress that are identifying technical factors that hopefully will lead to widespread best practices for RALUR. In addition, we expect that the further advances in robotic technology will benefit the pediatric field and especially for complex procedures such as RALUR. However, the impetus to improve pediatric medical devices is difficult because of the smaller pediatric population and therefore smaller number of pediatric procedures when compared to the adult population [47].

References

1. Rostrup MBT, Stokland O. Plasma catecholamines and haemodynamic changes during pneumoperitoneum. Acta Anaesthesiol Scand. 1998;42:343–7.
2. De Waal EE, Kalkman CJ. Haemodynamic changes during low-pressure carbon dioxide pneumoperitoneum in young children. Paediatr Anaesth. 2003;13(1):18–25.
3. Mattioli G, Montobbio G, Pini Prato A, Repetto P, Carlini C, Gentilino V, et al. Anesthesiologic aspects of laparoscopic fundoplication for gastroesophageal reflux in children with chronic respiratory and gastroenterological symptoms. Surg Endosc. 2003;17(4):559–66.
4. Terrier G. Anaesthesia for laparoscopic procedures in infants and children: indications, intra- and post-operative management, prevention and treatment of complications. Curr Opin Anaesthesiol. 1999;12(3):311–4.
5. Brady M, Kinn S, O'Rourke K, Randhawa N, Stuart P. Preoperative fasting for preventing perioperative complications in children. Cochrane Database Syst Rev. 2005;2:CD005285.
6. Kim JSZ, Englum BR, Allori AC, Adibe OO, Rice HE, Tracy ET. Laparoscopy is safe in infants and neonates with congenital heart disease: a national study of 3684 patients. J Laparoendosc Adv Surg Tech A. 2016;26(10):836–9.
7. Hsing CH, Hseu SS, Tsai SK, Chu CC, Chen TW, Wei CF, et al. The physiological effect of CO2 pneumoperitoneum in pediatric laparoscopy. Acta Anaesthesiol Sin. 1995;33(1):1–6.
8. Halachmi S, El-Ghoneimi A, Bissonnette B, Zaarour C, Bagli DJ, McLorie GA, et al. Hemodynamic and respiratory effect of pediatric urological laparoscopic surgery: a retrospective study. J Urol. 2003;170(4 Pt 2):1651–4. discussion 4
9. Lorenzo AJ, Karsli C, Halachmi S, Dolci M, Luginbuehl I, Bissonnette B, et al. Hemodynamic and respiratory effects of pediatric urological retroperitoneal laparoscopic surgery: a prospective study. J Urol. 2006;175(4):1461–5.
10. McHoney M, Corizia L, Eaton S, Kiely EM, Drake DP, Tan HL, et al. Carbon dioxide elimination during laparoscopy in children is age dependent. J Pediatr Surg. 2003;38(1):105–10. discussion-10
11. Pennant JH. Anesthesia for laparoscopy in the pediatric patient. Anesthesiol Clin North Am. 2001;19(1):69–88.
12. McDougall EM, Monk TG, Wolf JS Jr, Hicks M, Clayman RV, Gardner S, et al. The effect of prolonged pneumoperitoneum on renal function in an animal model. J Am Coll Surg. 1996;182(4):317–28.
13. Sodha S, Nazarian S, Adshead JM, Vasdev N, Mohan SG. Effect of pneumoperitoneum on renal function and physiology in patients undergoing robotic renal surgery. Curr Urol. 2016;9(1):1–4.
14. Nguyen NT, Perez RV, Fleming N, Rivers R, Wolfe BM. Effect of prolonged pneumoperitoneum on intraoperative urine output during laparoscopic gastric bypass. J Am Coll Surg. 2002;195(4):476–83.
15. Razvi HA, Fields D, Vargas JC, Vaughan ED Jr, Vukasin A, Sosa RE. Oliguria during laparoscopic surgery: evidence for direct renal parenchymal compression as an etiologic factor. J Endourol. 1996;10(1):1–4.

16. Gomez Dammeier BH, Karanik E, Gluer S, Jesch NK, Kubler J, Latta K, et al. Anuria during pneumoperitoneum in infants and children: a prospective study. J Pediatr Surg. 2005;40(9):1454–8.
17. Westgarth-Taylor C, de Lijster L, van Bogerijen G, Millar AJ, Karpelowsky J. A prospective assessment of renal oxygenation in children undergoing laparoscopy using near-infrared spectroscopy. Surg Endosc. 2013;27(10):3696–704.
18. Halverson AL, Barrett WL, Iglesias AR, Lee WT, Garber SM, Sackier JM. Decreased cerebrospinal fluid absorption during abdominal insufflation. Surg Endosc. 1999;13(8):797–800.
19. Karsli C, El-Hout Y, Lorenzo AJ, Langer JC, Bagli DJ, Pippi Salle JL, et al. Physiological changes in transperitoneal versus retroperitoneal laparoscopy in children: a prospective analysis. J Urol. 2011;186(4 Suppl):1649–52.
20. Kamata M, Hakim M, Walia H, Tumin D, Tobias JD. Changes in cerebral and renal oxygenation during laparoscopic pyloromyotomy. J Clin Monit Comput. 2020;34(4):699–703.
21. Spinelli G, Vargas M, Aprea G, Cortese G, Servillo G. Pediatric anesthesia for minimally invasive surgery in pediatric urology. Transl Pediatr. 2016;5(4):214–21.
22. Cheng YLJ, Xiong X, Wu S, Lin Y, Wu T. Gases for establishing pneumoperitoneum during laparoscopic abdominal surgery. Cochrane Database Syst Rev. 2013;1:CD009569.
23. McHoney M, Eaton S, Pierro A. Metabolic response to surgery in infants and children. Eur J Pediatr Surg. 2009;19(5):275–85.
24. Rademaker BM, Odoom JA, de Wit LT, Kalkman CJ, ten Brink SA, Ringers J. Haemodynamic effects of pneumoperitoneum for laparoscopic surgery: a comparison of CO2 with N2O insufflation. Eur J Anaesthesiol. 1994;11(4):301–6.
25. Sajid MS, Mallick AS, Rimpel J, Bokari SA, Cheek E, Baig MK. Effect of heated and humidified carbon dioxide on patients after laparoscopic procedures: a meta-analysis. Surg Laparosc Endosc Percutan Tech. 2008;18(6):539–46.
26. Oztan MO, Aydin G, Cigsar EB, Sutas Bozkurt P, Koyluoglu G. Effects of carbon dioxide insufflation and Trendelenburg position on brain oxygenation during laparoscopy in children. Surg Laparosc Endosc Percutan Tech. 2019;29(2):90–4.
27. Zhou R, Cao H, Gao Q, Guo Y, Zhang Q, Wang Z, et al. Abdominal wall elasticity of children during pneumoperitoneum. J Pediatr Surg. 2020;55(4):742–6.
28. Vlot J, Slieker JC, Wijnen R, Lange JF, Bax KN. Optimizing working-space in laparoscopy: measuring the effect of mechanical bowel preparation in a porcine model. Surg Endosc. 2013;27(6):1980–5.
29. Jukic M, Pogorelic Z, Supe-Domic D, Jeroncic A. Comparison of inflammatory stress response between laparoscopic and open approach for pediatric inguinal hernia repair in children. Surg Endosc. 2019;33(10):3243–50.
30. Baysal Z, Togrul T, Aksoy N, Cengiz M, Celik H, Boleken ME, et al. Evaluation of total oxidative and antioxidative status in pediatric patients undergoing laparoscopic surgery. J Pediatr Surg. 2009;44(7):1367–70.
31. Sutherland RW, Chung SK, Roth DR, Gonzales ET. Pediatric pyeloplasty: outcome analysis based on patient age and surgical technique. Urology. 1997;50:963–6.
32. Monn MF, Bahler CD, Schneider EB, Whittam BM, Misseri R, Rink RC, et al. Trends in robot-assisted laparoscopic pyeloplasty in pediatric patients. Urology. 2013;81:1336–41.
33. Akhavan A, Merguerian PA, Larison C, Goldin AB, Shnorhavorian M. Trends in the rates of pediatric pyeloplasty for ureteropelvic junction obstruction over 19 years: a PHIS database study. Adv Urol. 2014;2014:142625.
34. Barbosa JA, Kowal A, Onal B, Gouveia E, Walters M, Newcomer J, et al. Comparative evaluation of the resolution of hydronephrosis in children who underwent open and robotic-assisted laparoscopic pyeloplasty. J Pediatr Urol. 2013;9:199–205.
35. Sukumar S, Roghmann F, Sood A, Abdo A, Menon M, Sammon JD, et al. Correction of ureteropelvic junction obstruction in children: national trends and comparative effectiveness in operative outcomes. J Endourol. 2014;28:592–8.
36. Cundy TP, Harling L, Hughes-Hallett A, Mayer EK, Najmaldin AS, Athanasiou T, et al. Meta-analysis of robot-assisted vs conventional laparoscopic and open pyeloplasty in children. BJU Int. 2014;114:582–94.
37. Kutikov A, Nguyen M, Guzzo T, Canter D, Casale P. Robot assisted pyeloplasty in the infant-lessons learned. J Urol. 2006;176:2237–9. discussion 2239-40
38. Dangle PP, Kearns J, Anderson B, Gundeti MS. Outcomes of infants undergoing robot-assisted laparoscopic pyeloplasty compared to open repair. J Urol. 2013;190:2221–6.
39. Bansal D, Cost NG, Bean CM, Vanderbrink BA, Schulte M, Noh PH. Infant robot-assisted laparoscopic upper urinary tract reconstructive surgery. J Pediatr Urol. 2014;10:869–74.
40. Avery DI, Herbst KW, Lendvay TS, Noh PH, Dangle P, Gundeti MS, et al. Robot-assisted laparoscopic pyeloplasty: multi-institutional experience in infants. J Pediatr Urol. 2015;11:139e1-5.
41. Pennant JH. Anesthesia for laparoscopy in the pediatric patient. Anesthesiol Clin North Am. 2001;19:69–88.
42. Kutikov A, Resnick M, Casale P. Laparoscopic pyeloplasty in the infant younger than 6 months--is it technically possible? J Urol. 2006;175:1477–9.
43. Baek M, Silay MS, Au J, Huang GO, Elizondo RA, Janzen N, Seth A, Roth DR, Koh CJ. Does the use of 5 mm instruments affect the outcomes of robot-assisted laparoscopic pyeloplasty in smaller working spaces? A comparative analysis of infants and children. J Pediatr Urol. 2018;14(6):537.e1–6.
44. Sun RC, Kamat I, Byju AG, Wettergreen M, Heffernan MJ, Willson R, Haridas B, Koh CJ. Advancing Pediatric medical device development via non-dilutive NIH SBIR/STTR grant funding. J Pediatr Surg. 2021;56(11):2118–23.
45. Joseph PD, Craig JC, Caldwell PH. Clinical trials in children. Br J Clin Pharmacol. 2015;79(3):357–69.
46. Ulrich LC, Joseph FD, Lewis DY, et al. FDA's pediatric device consortia: national program fosters pediatric medical device development. Pediatrics. 2013;131(5):981–5.
47. Grant M, Stanasel I, Koh CJ. Pediatric medical device consortia: a novel pathway for pediatric device development for pediatric urologists and other pediatric specialists. Urol Pract. 2015;2(4):206–10.
48. Sack BS, Elizondo RA, Huang GO, et al. Pediatric medical device development by surgeons via capstone engineering design programs. J Pediatr Surg. 2018;53(3):493–8.
49. Gobbi D, Midrio P, Gamba P. Instrumentation for minimally invasive surgery in pediatric urology. Transl Pediatr. 2016;5(4):186–204.
50. Rassweiler JJ, Teber D. Advances in laparoscopic surgery in urology. Nat Rev Urol. 2016;13(7):387–99.
51. Arant BS Jr. Vesicoureteric reflux and renal injury. Am J Kidney Dis. 1991;17:491–511.
52. Roberts KB, Subcommittee on Urinary Tract Infection, Steering Committee on Quality Improvement and Management. Urinary tract infection: clinical practice guideline for the diagnosis and management of the initial UTI in febrile infants and children 2 to 24 months. Pediatrics. 2011;128:595–610.
53. Capone MA, Balestracci A, Toledo I, Martin SM. Diagnosis of vesicoureteral reflux according to the 1999 and 2011 guidelines of the Subcommittee on Urinary Tract Infection of the American Academy of Pediatrics. Arch Argent Pediatr. 2016;114:129–34.
54. Bowen DK, Faasse MA, Liu DB, Gong EM, Lindgren BW, Johnson EK. Use of pediatric open, laparoscopic and robot-assisted laparoscopic ureteral reimplantation in the United States: 2000 to 2012. J Urol. 2016;196:207–12.

55. Elder JS, Peters CA, Arant BS Jr, Ewalt DH, Hawtrey CE, Hurwitz RS, et al. Pediatric vesicoureteral reflux guidelines panel summary report on the management of primary vesicoureteral reflux in children. J Urol. 1997;157:1846–51.
56. Song SH, Kim KS. Current status of robot-assisted laparoscopic surgery in pediatric urology. Korean J Urol. 2014;55:499–504.
57. Cundy TP, Shetty K, Clark J, Chang TP, Sriskandarajah K, Gattas NE, et al. The first decade of robotic surgery in children. J Pediatr Surg. 2013;48:858–65.
58. Casale P, Patel RP, Kolon TF. Nerve sparing robotic extravesical ureteral reimplantation. J Urol. 2008;179:1987–9.
59. Smith RP, Oliver JL, Peters CA. Pediatric robotic extravesical ureteral reimplantation: comparison with open surgery. J Urol. 2011;185:1876–81.
60. Kasturi S, Sehgal SS, Christman MS, Lambert SM, Casale P. Prospective long-term analysis of nerve-sparing extravesical robotic-assisted laparoscopic ureteral reimplantation. Urology. 2012;79:680–3.
61. Silay MS, Baek M, Koh CJ. Robot-assisted laparoscopic extravesical ureteral reimplantation in children: top-down suturing technique without stent placement. J Endourol. 2015;29:864–6.
62. Grimsby GM, Dwyer ME, Jacobs MA, Ost MC, Schneck FX, Cannon GM, et al. Multi-institutional review of outcomes of robot-assisted laparoscopic extravesical ureteral reimplantation. J Urol. 2015;193:1791–5.
63. Herz D, Fuchs M, Todd A, McLeod D, Smith J. Robot-assisted laparoscopic extravesical ureteral reimplant: a critical look at surgical outcomes. J Pediatr Urol. 2016;12:402.e1–9.
64. Hendren WH. Ureteral reimplantation in children. J Ped Surg. 1968;3:649–64.
65. Marchini GS, Hong YK, Minnillo BJ, Diamond DA, Houck CS, Meier PM, et al. Robotic assisted laparoscopic ureteral reimplantation in children: case matched comparative study with open surgical approach. J Urol. 2011;185:1870–5.
66. Akhavan A, Avery D, Lendvay TS. Robot-assisted extravesical ureteral reimplantation: outcomes and conclusions from 78 ureters. J Pediatr Urol. 2014;10:864–8.
67. Lee RS, Retik AB, Borer JG, Peters CA. Pediatric robot assisted laparoscopic dismembered pyeloplasty: comparison with a cohort of open surgery. J Urol. 2006;175:683–7.

Robotic Pediatric Renal Surgery

Daniel E. Nassau, Miguel Castellan, Pasquale Casale, and Pablo Gomez III

1 General Principles of Robotic Renal Surgery

By now, this book has comprehensively highlighted the numerous applications and advantages that have come to light after more than 20 years since the inception of the first robotic surgical system. As the field has matured, it has become increasingly apparent that the advantages offered by the robotic surgical system are further enhanced when it is utilized in confined, difficult to access spaces, particularly if detailed, meticulous surgical technique is warranted, such as the one required during reconstructive surgery in the pediatric population. In this chapter, we will review the general principles, patient selection, positioning, trocar sites, and preferred robotic instruments as they apply to its use on renal reconstructive and extirpative surgery. Given the author's background, specific emphasis will be placed in reviewing the applications as they pertain to the field of pediatric urology, although these techniques certainly translate to the adult patient population. We will tackle a variety of techniques and review data associated with robotic pyeloplasty, revision robotic pyeloplasty, and the synchronous treatment of nephrolithiasis while undergoing robotic renal surgery; we will touch upon the "bail-out" procedures such as ureterocalicostomy; and we will finish by reviewing robotic heminephrectomy in the pediatric population.

Supplementary Information The online version contains supplementary material available at [https://doi.org/10.1007/978-3-031-00363-9_69].

D. E. Nassau · M. Castellan
Nicklaus Children's Hospital, University of Miami, Miami, FL, USA

P. Casale · P. Gomez III (✉)
AdventHealth for Children, Walt Disney Pavilion, Orlando, FL, USA

2 Patient Selection for Robotic Renal Surgery

One of the most important aspects and predictors of success for robotic surgical procedures is one that it is often ignored or undervalued. Patient selection is critical, particularly in the pediatric population. It sounds obvious, but the first step prior to offering patient robotic surgery as a surgical treatment alternative, the surgeon must recognize his/her own limitations and should disclose his/her experience and results as well as complications to the patient. The basis of a healthy patient-surgeon relationship has its base in the absolute trust and transparency of both involved parties. Often, complications arise when one embarks on surgical endeavors that exceed our comfort zone. Complications are inherent to any surgical approach, but it is our belief that surgical introspection minimizes those risks. The disclosure of potential complications to the patient and patient's family is fundamental, and if those complications arise, early recognition and the ability to address and repair these complications truly cement the surgeon's mastery of such surgical intervention. The role of correct patient selection cannot be overstated, as one cannot embark in the wrong path without ever starting such path.

Comorbidities: Recognizing significant comorbidities in anticipation of potential robotic-assisted laparoscopic surgery is a determining factor. Significant cardiac and pulmonary pathology may preclude the patient's ability to tolerate pneumoperitoneum. A "hostile" abdomen following previous, often multiple, intra-abdominal surgeries may significantly impact the ability to place the trocars and gain access into the abdomen. Furthermore, intestinal adhesions and synechiae increase the likelihood of inadvertent bowel injury. Hematologic conditions and blood dyscrasia may preclude patients from undergoing such procedures. Active sepsis is also viewed as a contraindication to robotic, minimally invasive surgery.

Age: Age is a relative contraindication for robotic surgical procedures. In the pediatric population, robotic surgery in

P. Wiklund et al. (eds.), *Robotic Urologic Surgery*, https://doi.org/10.1007/978-3-031-00363-9_69

healthy children is frequently performed in children over 12 months old. Experienced surgeons lower age limits and are not infrequent to offer robotic surgery for children at 6 months of age. The authors of this chapter have performed robotic surgery in children as young as 4 months of age but warn colleagues that these age group pose significant challenges, both physiological and anatomical, and do not advise the routine performance of robotic surgery and children less than 6 months of age. Age may not be the only factor; body habitus is fundamental as well. In a study by Finkelstein et al., a pubo-xyphoid distance of at least 15 cm and a distance of 13 cm between the two anterior-superior iliac spines were found to be suitable for selecting infants undergoing robotic procedures [1].

3 Patient Positioning and Preoperative Steps Prior to Robotic Renal Surgery

Optimal patient positioning is of paramount importance when performing any surgical intervention, but it is particularly important when performing minimally invasive surgery. When positioning a patient, important variables to be considered should include body habitus, laterality, operating table capabilities (i.e., kidney rest) robotic system being used, room setup, the need for gastric and bladder emptying during the procedure, pressure point padding, prevention of position-associated nerve injury, and the potential intraoperative need for position modification such as Trendelenburg, reverse Trendelenburg, and "airplane."

Prior to incision, insertion of an orogastric/nasogastric tube for gastric emptying as well as a Foley catheter for bladder emptying minimize the risk of stomach and bladder perforation during access. The size of the Foley catheter varies according to the age of the patient, with the infant typically using an 8 French catheter, whereas in older prepubertal, a 10 French is most commonly used. In the adolescent population, a 12–14 French is preferred. If the renal surgery is uneventful, the orogastric or nasogastric tube can be discontinued at the end the procedure, while the Foley catheter typically is kept overnight for accurate fluid management and to allow for overnight bedrest. Prophylactic antibiotics is typically preferred for upper urinary tract surgery, and currently other's preference is a first-generation cephalosporin such as intravenous cefazolin at 25 milligrams/kilogram prior to incision.

Specific to renal robotic surgery, we position the patient in modified lateral decubitus, 30–45°, with the affected side facing upward. Some surgeons utilize the kidney rest and flex the table similarly to the position utilized for an open surgical repair approach for renal surgery; however, for laparoscopic transabdominal surgery, these may not be necessary. The patient should be at the edge of the bed so that the abdomen protrudes, thereby facilitating mobility of the robotic instruments. An axillary roll is placed in its size varies according to age. The lower leg nearest to the operating table is flexed at the level of the knee in 90 degrees while the other leg is straight, both separated by adequate padding using a pillow or foam depending on the age. The arm nearest to the operating table is placed in an armrest; axillary roll is placed. The contralateral upper limb can either rest in the patient's flank with attention for it not to impinge in the surgical field, or alternatively he can be secured in a "hugging position" with the use of an elevated arm rest. All pressure points are carefully padded, and the patient is secured to the operating table in multiple points (lower extremities, pelvis, thorax, and head) utilizing 3-inch heavy tape (i.e., silk tape) over surgical towels to avoid direct adhesion to the skin or by Velcro straps. The bed is "test tilted" replicating the expected intraoperative maneuvers (Trendelenburg, "airplane") to assure the patient is secure.

4 Trocar Site for Robotic Renal Surgery

Historically, in the first three generations of the da Vinci robotic surgical system, the da Vinci, da Vinci S and in da Vinci Si, trocar triangulation and distance played important roles. Those systems offered 5 mm and 8 mm trocars, with the 5 mm trocars having a very limited arsenal of surgical instruments. Furthermore, although the 5 mm instruments were narrower, they required significantly more intra-abdominal space to maneuver given their intrinsic articulation and lack of endo-wrist action. In the latest model, the Da Vinci Xi system, the 5 mm trocars have disappeared and only 8 mm trocars/instruments exist, and trocar triangulation is no longer required as it has been replaced by a linear trocar configuration. This linear configuration has enabled multi-quadrant surgical procedures be performed without the need for undocking. Also, the Xi's patient side-cart's capabilities have dramatically improved, now allowing for easier docking, extended instrument reach, and guided targeting. Although the manufacture's recommended minimal distance between trocars is 8 cm, a distance that is often not available for those of us performing pediatric surgery, especially in infants. Distances of 4.5 cm above are often sufficient.

It is also worth mentioning alternate trocar placement sites. In an attempt to maximally conceal the trocar incisions, Gargollo et al. elegantly described the hidden incision endoscopic surgery (HIdES) technique where all trocars are located at the level of the Pfannenstiel incision without a visible abdominal scar [2]. This technique has occasionally been used by then authors successfully for upper urinary tract surgery.

5 Robotic Instruments Helpful in Robotic Renal Surgery

There is a constellation of available surgical instruments and ultimately its selection boils down to surgeon preference. We won't expand into all available instruments but would like to mention a few of our preferred instruments for pediatric robotic renal surgery. The Debakey forceps offer excellent grasping force for the initial dissection. If thermal energy is required, the Maryland bipolar forceps are an excellent alternative. We often use the curved monopolar scissors as part of the arsenal. For fine dissection, the bipolar fine tissue graspers offer and excellent alternative while minimizing tissue damage. The black diamond forceps are another alternative but have higher crushing pressure and lack thermal energy. For suturing, the large suture-cut needle driver is an excellent option and reduces the surgical time as the surgeon can cut its own sutures without the need of instrument exchange. For vascular control, the "vessel sealer" offers excellent hemostasis and so does the harmonic scalpel. The clip appliers in different sizes can be useful particularly for small- to medium-sized vessels.

6 Robotic Pyeloplasty

Ureteropelvic junction obstruction (UPJO) is one of the most common forms of hydronephrosis in pediatric patients. UPJO can present at any age depending on the underlying etiology, whether due to an intrinsic malformation (typically presenting perinatally) or an extrinsic compression on the UPJ (typically symptomatic older patients) or a combination thereof [3]. In the Unites States, owing to the widespread use of screening fetal ultrasonography (US), congenital hydronephrosis is estimated to occur in 1–5% of pregnancies, of which UPJO accounts for 10–30% [4, 5]. UPJO is slightly more common on boys than girls and occurs on the left side 67% of the time and may be bilateral in up to 10% of cases [6].

A significant decrease in flow of urine from the renal pelvis into the proximal ureter due to a UPJO will cause hydronephrosis which can lead to pain and/or kidney damage. Diagnosis is often made using a combination of US and, given the increased radiation, less preferred computed tomography (CT) and, confirmed with diuretic renography, most commonly in the form of a nuclear medicine technetium-99 m mercaptoacetyltriglycerine (^{99m}Tc-MAG3) renal scan [7]. In recent years, the use of magnetic resonance urography (MRU) has largely replaced the use of MAG3 renal scans in our practice. Using the free software developed by the Children's Hospital of Philadelphia [8], MRU achieves excellent diagnostic accuracy by providing differential renal function and drainage time while also providing far superior images than the MAG3 scan. Surgical intervention is recommended if there is a significant difference in renal function (<40% of the affected side), bilateral severe or solitary kidney UPJO, cyclic pain with or without vomiting, worsening obstruction, presence of concomitant nephrolithiasis, or recurrent urinary tract infections despite antibiotic prophylaxis [9].

Historically, UPJO was surgically corrected by an open dismembered pyeloplasty which remains the gold standard. However, as the benefits of minimally invasive surgery in the pediatric population have become apparent, there has been a shift toward a laparoscopic approach since the first laparoscopic pyeloplasty (LPP) was performed in 1995 [9]. Unfortunately, owing to the delicate suturing required in a relatively confined space for pediatric pyeloplasty, LP had a steep learning curve. Robotic assistance during laparoscopic surgery overcomes some of these challenges because of the robotic system's features which include three-dimensional vision, tremor cancellation, and seven degrees of instrument movement which mimics surgeon hand movements during open surgery [10]. The combination of these features makes robotic-assisted laparoscopic surgery ideal for pediatric patients given the limited working space. In fact, given the familiarity of the LPP to pediatric urologists, the first pediatric robotic surgery was indeed a robotic pyeloplasty (RPP) in 2002, and it is currently the most commonly performed robotic procedure in the pediatric population [9].

6.1 Procedure

After the induction of general endotracheal anesthesia, the procedure typically begins with the patient in the modified lateral decubitus position. Two authors (PG and PC) rarely perform cystoscopy and retrograde pyelogram since it rarely changes the surgical plan when well-performed preoperative radiological studies are available. If cystoscopy is to be performed, the patient will start in a dorsal lithotomy position in order to perform a retrograde pyelogram (RGP) of the affected side to delineate the anatomy. Performing a RGP prior to RPP may help identify a complicating factor such as a ureteral polyp, nephrolithiasis, or a long stenosed ureteral segment that can help with operative planning during the procedure. In some practices (MC and DN), a retrograde ureteral stent (with or without a string) is placed after the RGP. Alternatively, a double J ureteral stent can be placed in an antegrade fashion during the reconstruction of the UPJ or a nephrostomy/nephroureteral tube can be placed as well either prior to the procedure or concurrently. There have also been recent reports of a "drainless" RPP, in which a ureteral stent is omitted from the procedure without any significant short-term complications [11]. Both PC and PG do not routinely place stents if the RPP is uneventful. If a stent is to be placed, we prefer the antegrade approach where the JJ stent is placed through a small 14G Angiocath inserted transabdominally by the bedside assistant. Our current indications for JJ stent placement include children under 6 months of age; massive reduction of the renal pelvis; abnormal anatomy such as malrotated kidney with a posteriorly deviated UPJO; tension of the anastomosis, typically secondary to significant loss of ureteral length secondary to fibroepithelial polyps; and solitary kidney.

A Foley catheter is typically left in place during the procedure and overnight. If a retrograde stent has been placed intraoperatively, some authors (MC) prefer to occlude the urethral catheter during the procedure as bladder distention helps to maintain renal pelvis distention. The catheter is open to drainage once the anatomy has been adequately identified.

In transperitoneal RPP (our preference), robotic ports are placed as described above. A retroperitoneoscopic technique has also been described in the pediatric population with comparable outcomes [12]. Unfortunately, although the UPJ can be rapidly identified using a retroperitoneal approach, decreased space of the operative field has limited its uptake, and as such, a transperitoneal approach is performed most commonly. Prior to docking the robotic patient cart, the operating table rotated toward the contralateral side to aide in order to displace the peritoneal contents away from the UPJ.

Robotic dissection begins by accessing the retroperitoneum. The white line of Toldt is incised in order to reflect the colon medially, and the proximal ureter or renal pelvis is identified. Alternatively, a trans-mesenteric incision can be made when the renal pelvis is easily identified through the mesentery (Fig. 1). After identifying the ureter, UPJ, and renal pelvis in the retroperitoneum, the proximal ureter is mobilized toward the UPJ with judicious use of electrocautery. Often, the gonadal vessels are identified overlying the ureter and may require medial reflection after a window is created between the vessels and the ureter, in order to avoid injury. As the UPJ is approached, a lower pole crossing renal vessel may be identified as a cause an extrinsic compression UPJO. If a crossing vessel is identified, we begin dissection and mobilization of the renal pelvis before addressing the ureter and UPJ underneath the artery.

Once adequate dissection of the ureter and renal pelvis is achieved, a transabdominal traction stitch through the renal pelvis is often utilized to aide in the UPJ reconstruction. In our practice MC), a 4–0 polypropylene (Prolene) suture on a straight Keith needle is passed through the skin percutaneously into the abdomen just superior to the renal pelvis by the bedside assistant. The stitch is then placed in the renal pelvis and passed back out through the abdominal wall and clamped at the skin level at the desired level of traction (Fig. 2). Alternatively, using a manually straightened SH needle has been described [13].

The Anderson-Hynes dismembered pyeloplasty is the most used reconstructive robotic technique due to its versatility and ability to be utilized for many different UPJ configurations [14]. The UPJ is transected, followed by wide spatulation of the renal pelvis and proximal ureter in order to

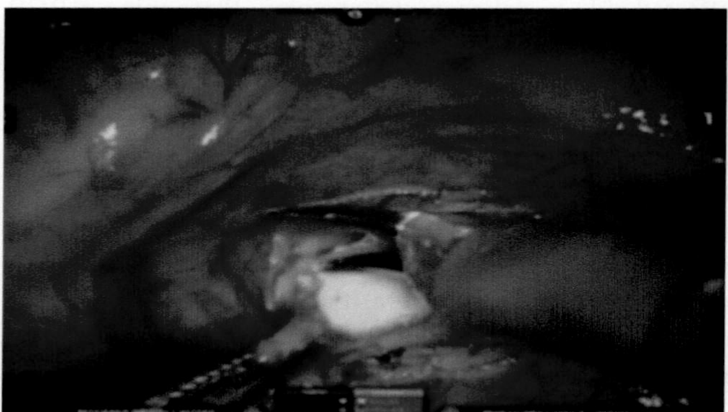

Fig. 1 Transmesenteric approach for a left robotic pyeloplasty. The mesentery is incised revealing the renal pelvis underneath

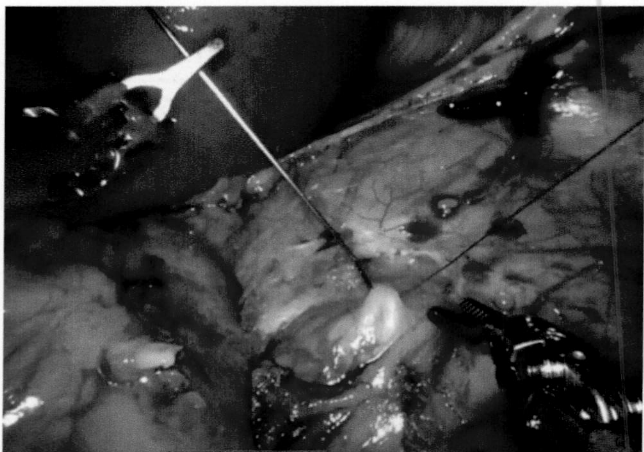

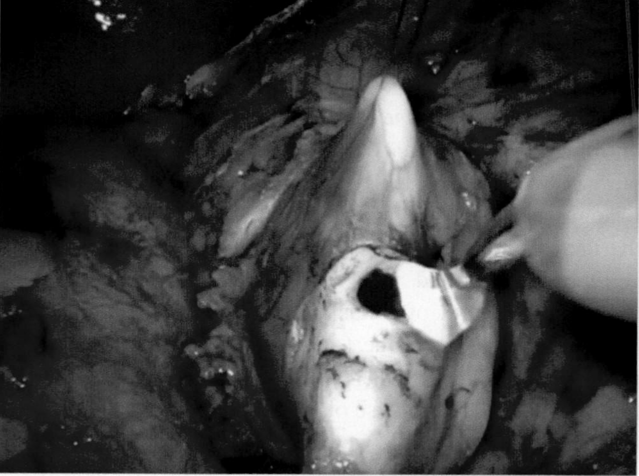

Fig. 2 Placement of a percutaneous stitch to be used for traction on the renal pelvis

facilitate a wide anastomosis of healthy ureter. After transection, if a stenotic UPJ segment is identified, this can be removed; however, this can preferentially be done after the anastomosis is completed as it can be used as a handle to aide with suturing. When a crossing vessel is present, the renal pelvis and proximal ureter should be brought anterior to the vessels. The proximal ureter is typically spatulated laterally to maintain the medial blood supply. A running or interrupted fine absorbable suture on a tapered needle is used for the anastomosis, beginning at the most dependent portion of the renal pelvis to the spatulated ureter. We use two 5–0 or 6–0, depending on patient size, poliglecaprone (Monocryl) (MC) suture on an RB1 needle 12-14 cm in length. PG prefers to use 5–0 PDS in an RB1 needle. We begin by placing and tying both sutures at 6 o'clock in the most dependent portion of the anastomosis and then run each individually, typically beginning with the lateral edge, followed by the medial edge (Fig. 3). Any stenotic or poorly vascularized proximal ureter is removed, and any remaining renal pelvis defects are closed primarily. Additionally, renal pelvis reduction can also be performed. At the conclusion of the procedure, a surgical drain is typically not necessary; however, if desired, a perirenal Penrose drain can be used, sutured to the skin at one of the dependent port sites or through the lateral abdominal wall near the repair. Suction drains (Jackson-Pratt) around the anastomosis are discouraged.

If a ureteral stent is desired and not already in place, an antegrade ureteral stent can be placed after one of the edges has been closed, usually passed in over a wire through the superior abdominal port or through the previously described 14 gauge angiocath. After the wire is removed, similarly to an already indwelling ureteral stent, the proximal curl can be placed with the robotic arm into the renal pelvis before completing the anastomosis. Another technique is passing the ureteral stent through a large angiocatheter placed percutaneously through the abdominal wall in the direction of the ureter [13] (Fig. 4). Visualizing urine reflux through the ureteral stent confirms the distal end of the stent is in the proper

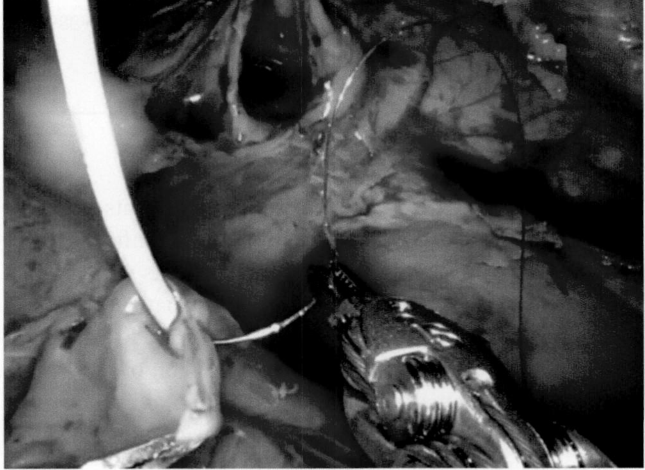

Fig. 3 Anastomosis for dismembered robotic Anderson-Hynes robotic pyeloplasty, a second stitch is placed next to this stitch for the other edge

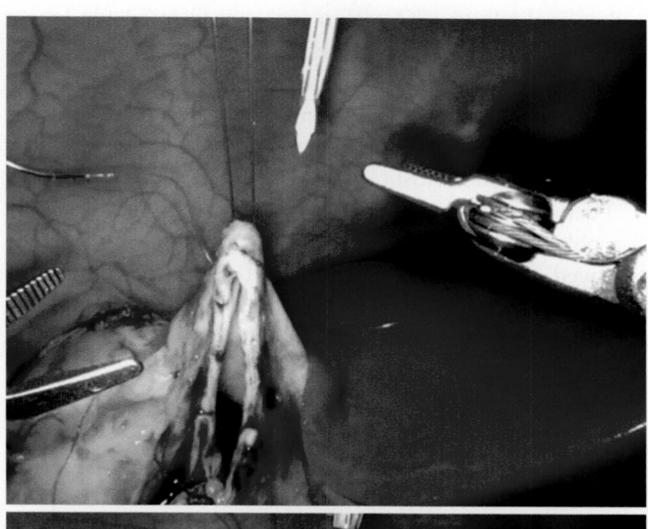

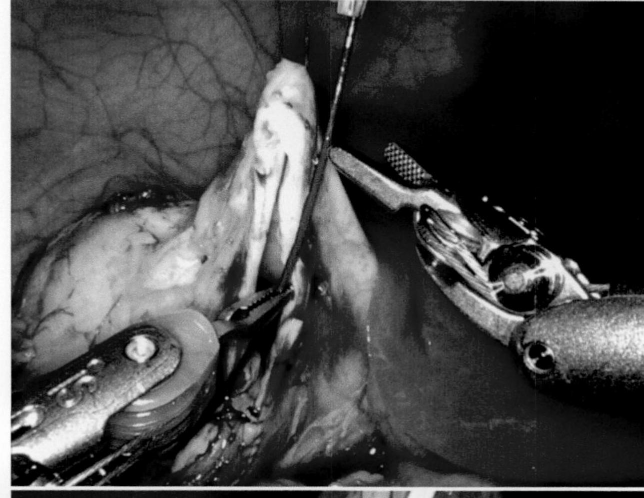

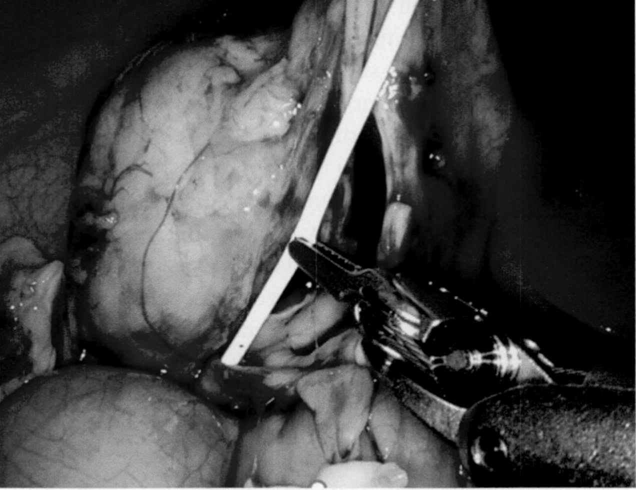

Fig. 4 Percutaneous placement of ureteral stent through large-bore angiocatheter

position, but if the bladder is empty from foley catheter drainage, this may not occur.

Although used less commonly, non-dismembered pyeloplasty techniques have also been described using on a laparoscopic platform. For intrinsic UPJ deficits, a Foley YV for a flap pyeloplasty (PC preference) can be used for longer segments or even in the presence of a crossing vessel if a modified Hellstrom technique is also used [13, 15]. Laparoscopic Fenger plasty has also been described for short stenotic segments, in which a pelviotomy is created and a Heineke-Mikulicz closure is performed [16].

Postoperatively patients typically are admitted overnight for observation with a Foley catheter in place which is removed on postoperative day one. If renal function allows, the patients are managed on the floor with standing intravenous acetaminophen and Toradol without the use of narcotics. If the child is able to ambulate, tolerate diet, and void without difficulty, they are discharged on postoperative day one, with plans for follow-up and stent removal in 4–8 weeks. Typically, a baseline renal ultrasound is obtained 4–6 weeks after stent removal and repeated at 6 months and a year postoperatively. Success rates range between 94 and 100% with a recent long-term follow-up reporting an 8-year failure-free rate of 91.5% [9, 13, 17].

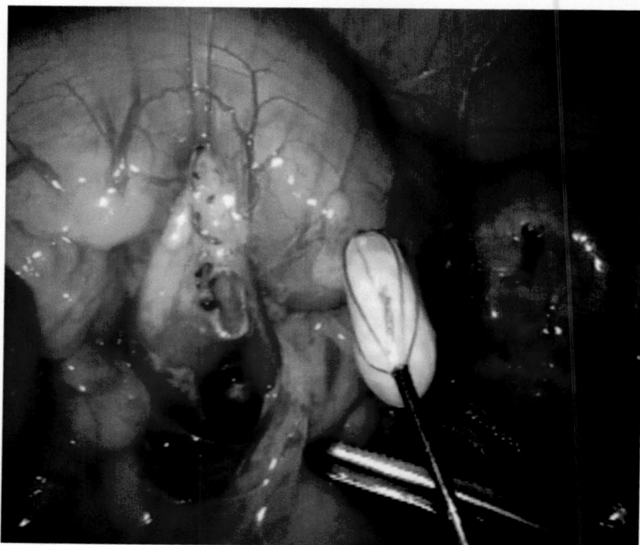

Fig. 5 Pyelolithotomy with stone basket extraction

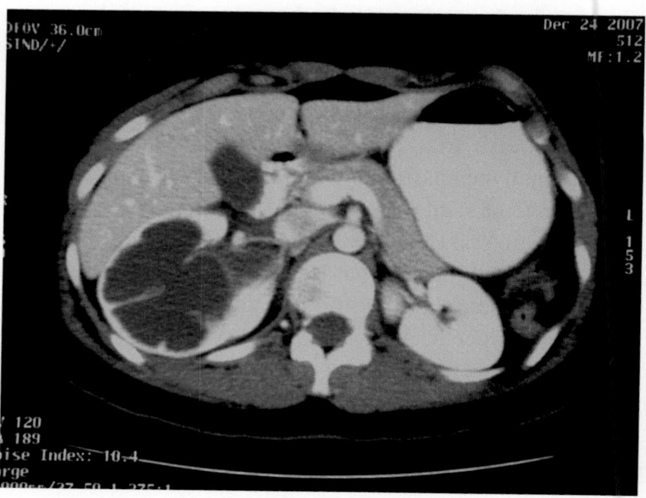

Fig. 6 Representative CT scan showing a completely exaggerated intrarenal collecting system

6.2 Complex RPP

Enhanced three-dimensional visualization and instruments able to make fine wrist movements makes the robotic platform ideal for treating complex UPJO, such as concurrent renal stones, ureteral polyps, or revision pyeloplasty. If pyelolithotomy is required, the renal pelvis should be opened in order to accommodate the robotic instruments, and the stones can be gently manipulated out renal pelvis and placed in a specimen bag. Alternatively, a flexible ureteroscope can be introduced through a trocar and placed into the renal pelvis with the robotic arm, and a basket can be used to remove any visualized ureteral stones (Fig. 5). Ureteral polyps can be removed in a similar fashion. If a ureteral polyp is observed after transection of the UPJ, the segment of the ureter containing the polyp can be removed or the polyp can be removed from its stalk and sent for histological analysis.

Revision or redo pyeloplasty can be especially challenging due to fibrosis around the UPJ and/or long stenotic ureteral segments that require repair. For long ureteral segments, wide spatulation with renal pelvis and ureteral mobilization with or without concomitant nephropexy may be required. For segments that are not amenable to dismembered or non-dismembered approaches, buccal mucosal onlay grafting or appendiceal substitution (on the right side) may be required [18, 19]. Ureterocalicostomy, especially with a concurrent lower pole caliectasis, is another option after failed pyeloplasty.

7 Robotic Ureterocalicostomy

Ureterocalicostomy is a potential option in patients with ureteropelvic junction (UPJ) obstruction and significant lower pole caliectasis. It is often reserved for patients with a failed pyeloplasty with a minimal pelvis or for patients with an exaggerated intrarenal pelvis. Initially described by Neuwrit in 1932, ureterocalicostomy involves excision of the hydronephrotic lower renal pole parenchyma and anastomosis of the dismembered ureter directly to the lower pole calyx providing urinary drainage [20] (Fig. 6).

Robotic surgery has become mainstream for various ablative and reconstructive renal applications in the pediatric population. Various purely laparoscopic and robotic pyeloplasty techniques have been described, including non-dismembered Fenger plasty, dismembered Anderson-Hynes plasty, and flap pyeloplasty [14, 21–23]. The robotic and laparoscopic ureterocalicostomy techniques have been described in the adult population [24, 25]. Robotic ureterocalicostomy was first described in children with 9 patients between the ages of 3 to 15 years (mean age 6.5 years) who underwent transperitoneal robotic ureterocalicostomies for an ureteropelvic junction obstruction [26]. Of the nine, six had recurrent UPJO after a primary pyeloplasty. The remaining 3 had an exaggerated intrarenal collecting system with minimal or no appreciable renal pelvis for reconstruction.

A transperitoneal approach is implemented as previously described in the literature [27, 28]. The colon is reflected in all cases exposing the massively dilated kidney (Fig. 7). The ureter is transected and ligated with absorbable sutures at the level of the renal pelvis or crossing vessels if the pelvis was not readily accessible. The ureter is spatulated prior to trans-section (Fig. 8). The most dependent lower pole calyx is amputated with a hot shears (Fig. 9). The posterior anastomosis can be performed with absorbable (5–0 polyglycolic acid) sutures in running fashion (Fig. 10). A 4.8 French double-pigtail ureteral stent is placed in an antegrade fashion via a 14 gauge angiocath over a guidewire (Fig. 11). The anterior anastomosis is performed in an interrupted manner allowing visualization and approximation of the renal collecting system to the ureteral mucosa without placing tension on the renal parenchyma (Fig. 12).

Pediatric robotic urology continues to evolve. Patients in need of extirpative or reconstructive urological procedures can benefit from the advantages of minimally invasive tech-

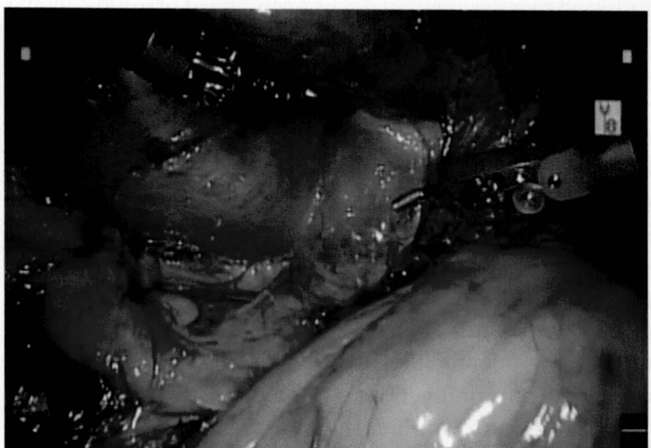

Fig. 7 Colonic mobilization was utilized to allow complete exposure of the kidney and access to the hilum

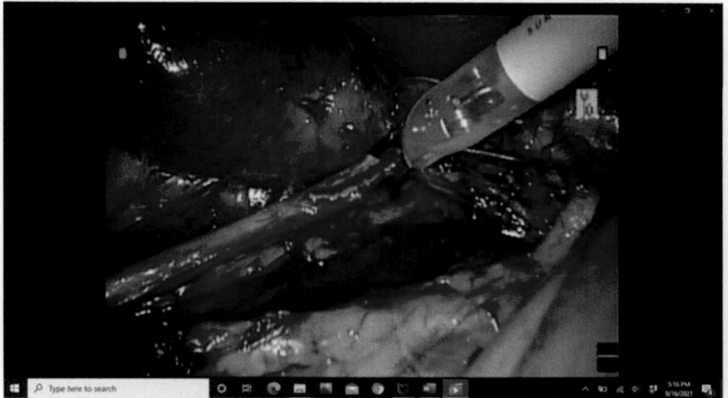

Fig. 8 Ureteral spatulation prior to full transaction helps prevent disorientation and spiraling of the ureter

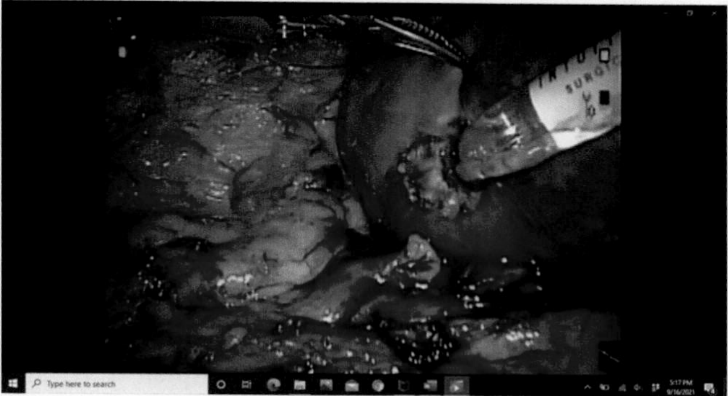

Fig. 9 Lower pole inferior calyx amputation

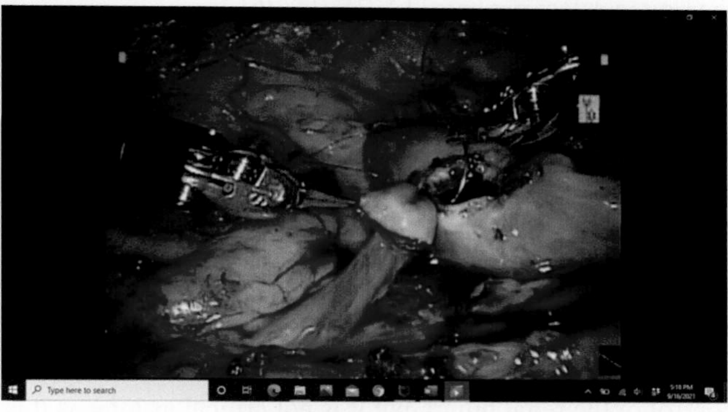

Fig. 10 The posterior anastomosis

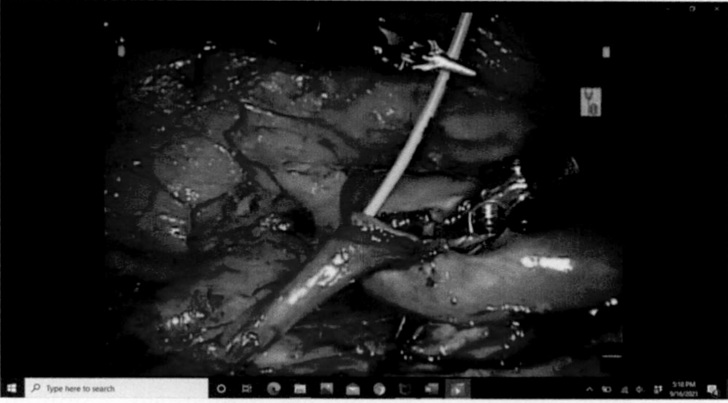

Fig. 11 Stent placement

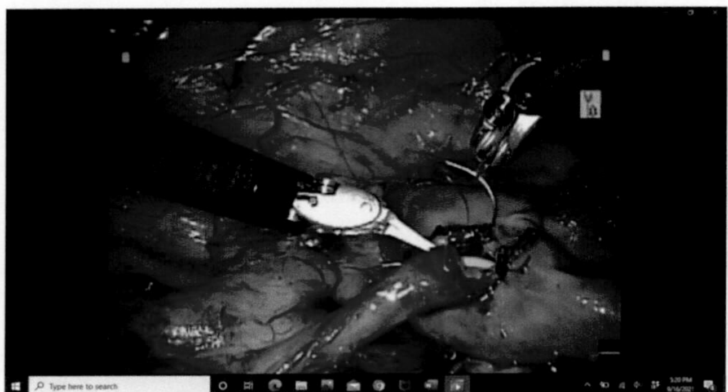

Fig. 12 The anterior anastomosis

niques. In addition to adrenalectomy and simple or radical nephrectomy, dismembered and flap pyeloplasty, ureteroneocystostomy, nephroureterectomy, partial nephrectomy, and ureteroureterostomy, bladder augmentation and catheterizable channels are being performed robotically in children [23]. Treatment of symptomatic intrarenal or recurrent ureteropelvic junction obstruction has been traditionally performed via open surgery through a flank incision or transabdominally, necessitating an extended hospital stay and convalescence. Today minimally invasive laparoscopic and robotic treatments have emerged at the forefront with some centers offering these approaches preferentially as first line therapy in select patients [14, 21–23, 26].

Persistent symptomatic, significant ureteropelvic junction obstruction in which surgical repair has failed represents a unique and difficult clinical situation. Excellent results have been reported for laparoscopic dismembered pyeloplasty after failed endopyelotomy in adults, but this data is lacking in children [29]. The essential steps of robotic ureterocalicostomy technique are based on the open procedure and do not differ from that practice. Therefore, a generous amount of lower pole renal parenchyma overlying the most inferior, dependent dilated calix is routinely excised. One can gain control of the renal hilum, but it is not critical as long as it is circumferentially mobilized and visualized. A tension-free ureterocaliceal anastomosis is formed by ureteral mobilization and spatulation. Recurrent obstruction is the most commonly reported complications of ureterocalicostomy [30]. Recurrent obstruction might occur secondary to scarring at the ureterocalicostomy site due to a segment of ischemic renal parenchyma or ureter. This complication can be minimized by generous excision of the renal parenchyma at the anastomotic site and a tension-free anastomosis [20].

8 Heminephroureterectomy

Duplex renal collecting systems are a relatively common congenital anomaly. The superior renal moiety is most frequently associated with obstruction, usually from an ectopic ureter or ureterocele, and the inferior renal moiety with vesicoureteral reflux. Both renal units can be affected with resultant loss of function. Nonfunctioning moieties of a duplicated system can be treated by superior or inferior moiety partial nephrectomy [31]. This procedure was first described laparoscopically in 1993 by Jordan and Winslow [32] and has been reported with increasing frequency since then [33–40]. Laparoscopically heminephroureterectomy was described to be performed transperitoneally or retroperitoneally in a similar manner to nephrectomy. Later, robotic-assisted laparoscopic (RAL) approaches have been described, most commonly using the transperitoneal approach [41–44].

9 Transperitoneal Approach: Surgical Technique

Surgical positioning and technique can be performed in a manner similar to the nephrectomy. If both ureters are similar in caliber, patients underwent cystoscopy with retrograde ureteropyelography of the duplex system and, in some cases, followed by placement of a 4 Fr open-ended ureteral catheter into the functioning moiety (for intraoperative identification of the normal ureter), secured to a Foley catheter. Patients were then repositioned in the 45 degrees modified flank position. Three 8 mm robotic trocars are placed, most of the times in the midline, and an additional 5 mm laparoscopic trocar can be used for assistance if necessary, with peritoneal insufflation to 10–12 mmHg. After docking the robot, the ipsilateral colon was reflected medially, and both ureters of the duplicated system were identified medial to the lower pole of the kidney (Fig. 13). The ureter of the functioning moiety was identifiable by the previously placed ureteral catheter. The nonfunctioning moiety ureter was dissected cephalad toward its hilum (Fig. 14). In cases of a nonfunctioning superior moiety, care was taken not to injure the inferior moiety vasculature as it crossed anterior to the supe-

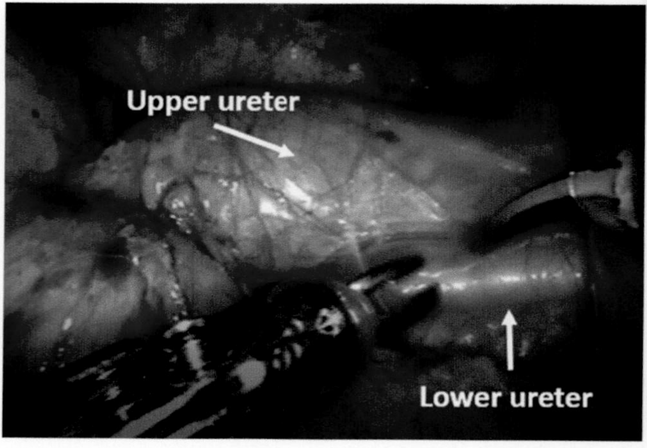

Fig. 13 Identification of both ureters

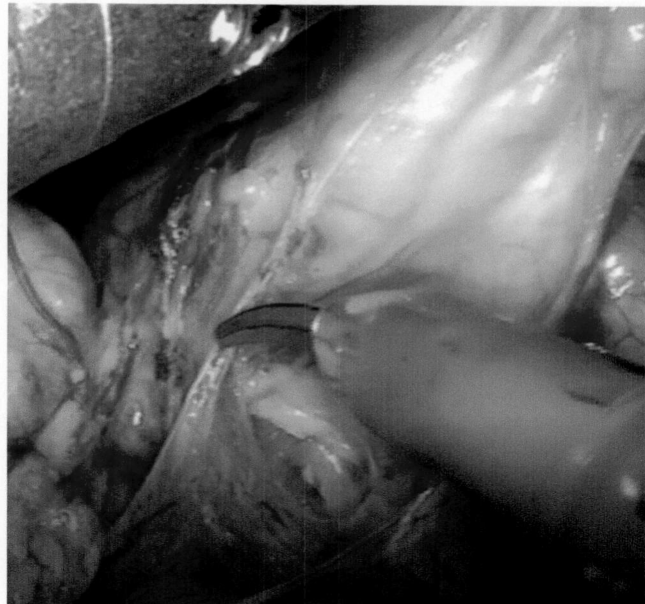

Fig. 14 Dissection continue below the obstructed upper pole ureter

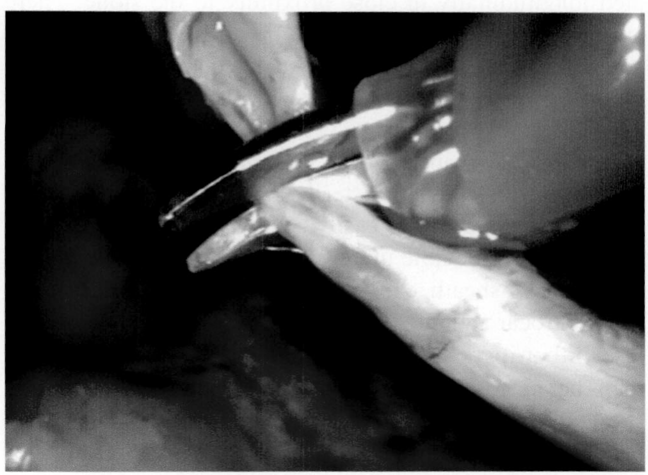

Fig. 15 Transection of upper pole ureter

rior moiety ureter. The dilated nonfunctioning ureter is then divided proximally (Fig. 15), allowing decompression of the dilated nonfunctioning renal moiety. In cases of a nonfunctioning superior moiety, the divided proximal superior moiety ureter is passed beneath the inferior moiety vasculature (Fig. 16). The hilum of the affected renal pole is dissected, only with selective vascular dissection of the nonfunctional moiety. The vasculature of the nonfunctioning moiety is ligated (Fig. 17) using either clips or silk ligature. In cases of severely atrophic vasculature, vessels can be simply divided by monopolar or harmonic dissector (Ethicon, Somerville, NJ, US). During lower pole HN, the lower pole ureter was identified and dissected free from the upper pole ureter and investing Gerota's fascia. We identified the blood vessels to both moieties before ligation and separation of the lower pole. In either the case of a nonfunctioning superior or inferior moiety, the proximal ureter is used for retraction and mobilization of the affected moiety. The demarcation between the functioning and nonfunctioning moieties is then visualized (Fig. 18) and divided using the robotic vessel sealer or the laparoscopic harmonic electrocautery device (Fig. 19). The distal ureteric stump is traced down as far as is necessary in the pelvis, taking great care to isolate and preserve the normal ureter. The ureter is ligated prior to transection when there is associated VUR. Specimens were brought out through the umbilical port.

Robot-assisted laparoscopic heminephrectomy with ureterectomy is a proven treatment of nonfunctioning duplex kidney units in children and infants. The versatility of the articulating instrument and tridimensional vision of the robotic system help in the dissection of the affected moiety hilum and parenchyma.

10 Robotic Platform for Nephrolithiasis

Over the last several decades, minimally invasive techniques for the treatment of nephrolithiasis has widely replaced open stone surgery [45]. In children, most kidney and ureteral stones are treated similarly to adults, making use of extracorporeal shockwave lithotripsy (ESWL) or endoscopic management either by ureteroscopy (URS) or percutaneous Nephrolithotomy (PCNL). For this reason, nephrolithiasis is an uncommon indication for robotic surgery; however, in the pediatric population, endoscopic stone management can be challenging due to anatomic size limitations, making laparoscopic or robotic-assisted approaches suitable alternatives in certain patients. Given the decreased morbidity compared to open stone surgery, laparoscopic surgery in stone disease has increased over the last few decades [46]. The achievable learning curve to become proficient in robotic surgery as well as the advantages previously discussed make it a desirable option for challenging stone management, especially when stone disease coincides with a congenital condition that requires reconstruction, such as a UPJO or a calyceal diverticulum [47].

Prior to robotic surgery for nephro- or ureterolithiasis a sterile urine culture is imperative. Broad-spectrum antibiotics should be administered preoperatively given the potential for urine spillage during the procedure. For obstructive stones, a ureteral stent may have been placed prior to the procedure, and if not, depending on surgeon preference, a retrograde or antegrade stent can be placed at the time of surgery. The patient should be positioned in a modified flank position with the ports placed to triangulate the stone's location within the upper urinary tract. For renal

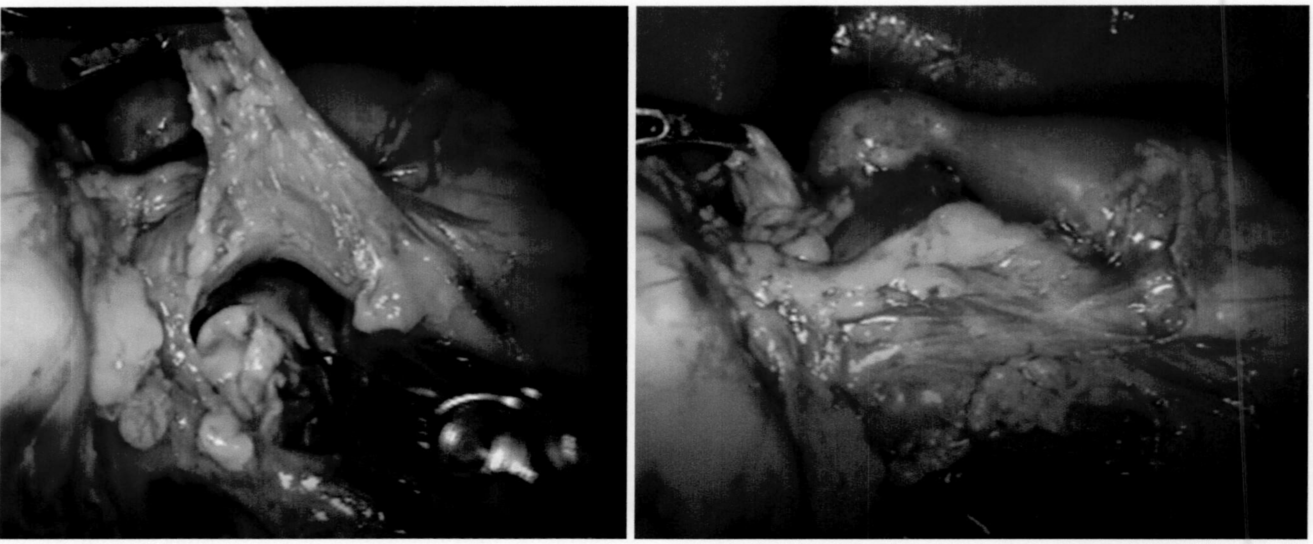

Fig. 16 The divided proximal superior moiety ureter is passed beneath the inferior moiety vasculature

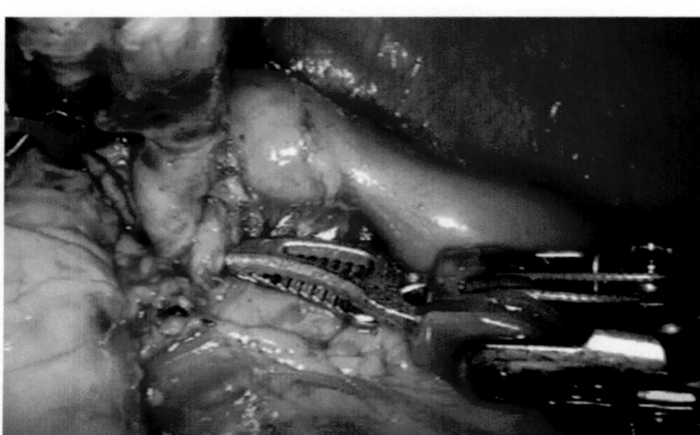

Fig. 17 The vasculature of the nonfunctioning moiety is identified and ligated

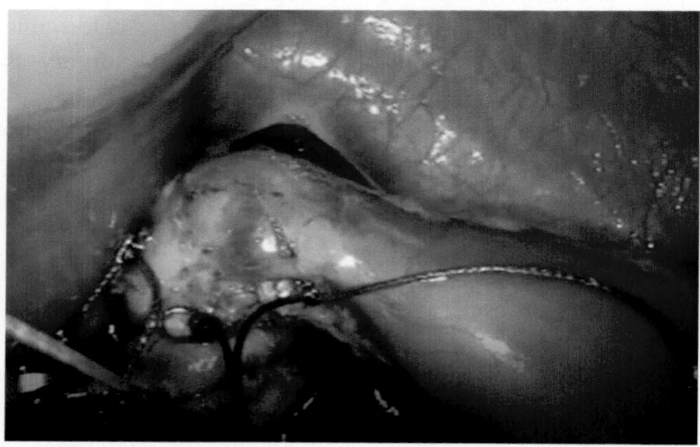

Fig. 18 Identification and demarcation between the functioning and nonfunctioning moieties

pelvis stones, a pelviotomy should be made away from the UPJ, and for ureteral stones, a ureterotomy should be created longitudinally in close proximity to the stone. There are different techniques that can be utilized to remove the stone. If the stone(s) is easily visualized and can be manipulated by the robotic instruments, a grasping forceps can be used to remove the stone(s). The retrieved stones can be placed within a laparoscopic specimen or homemade bag even a cut finger from a sterile glove has been described [48]. If the stone cannot easily be removed with the robotic instruments, a flexible ureteroscope with or without a ureteral access sheath can be inserted through an existing robotic trocar and directed into the renal pelvis or ureter. A laser lithotripsy or a basket stone extraction (Fig. 5) can then be performed through the ureteroscope. After the stone(s) have been removed, the ureter or renal pelvis can be closed with a fine absorbable suture in a running or interrupted fashion, similarly to as described earlier in the chapter. A suction or passive drain is not typically left in place unless there is concern for contaminated urine intraabdominal spillage [47].

Large renal stones >2 cm as well as partial or complete staghorn calculi can present a particular challenge in the pediatric population, usually requiring a PCNL. For stones not amenable or have failed PCNL/ESWL, robotic surgery may be a viable option, especially since it has been associated with less blood loss and postop analgesia requirements compared to PCNL in adults [49, 50]. For large stones, patient selection is crucial, as complete staghorn calculi will be more challenging with the robotic platform compared with partial staghorn stones [51]. For complete staghorn

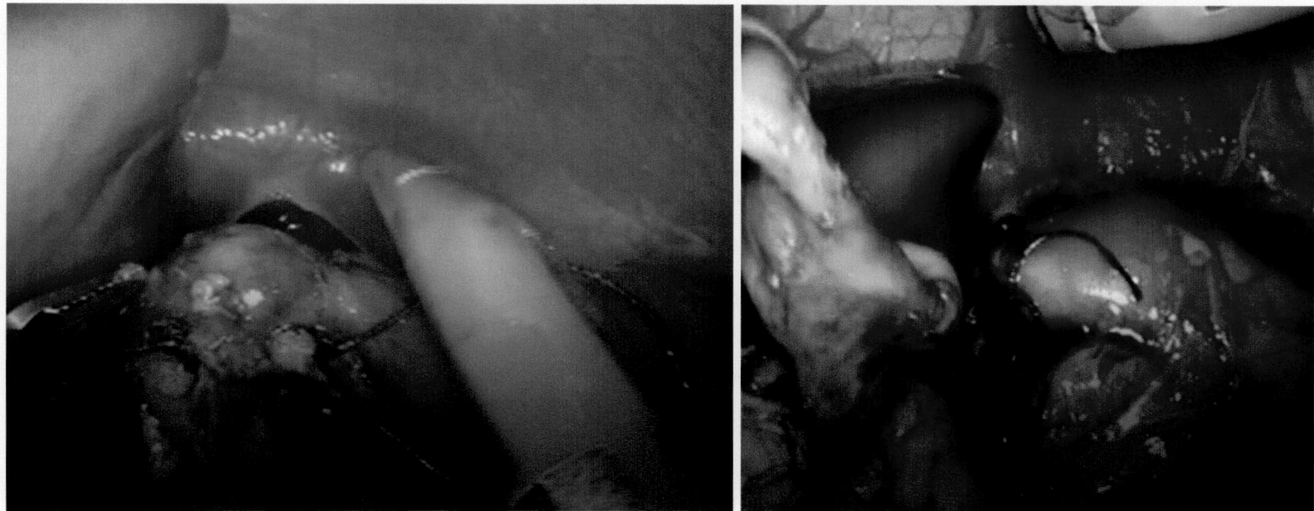

Fig. 19 Resection of affected moiety with adequate vascularization of the normal renal unit

stones, an robotic anatrophic nephrolithotomy has been described and could be considered as a last resort given its morbidity; however, this should be reserved for the most experienced robotic surgeons [52].

Robotic surgery for stone disease is most applicable when there is a concomitant condition that is amenable to reconstruction such as a UPJO or calyceal diverticulum. As described earlier, renal pelvic stones secondary to a UPJO can be removed robotically after dividing the UPJ and before the ureteropelvic reconstruction. Calculi within a calyceal diverticulum, laparoscopic, or robotic approach is considered first-line treatment for stones >3 cm within an anterior diverticulum by some authors [53]. Prior to robotic calyceal diverticulectomy, cystoscopic insertion of an open-ended ureteral (Pollack) catheter may be placed in order to instill retrograde dye for infundibular identification. The patient is then positioned in the modified flank position and the retroperitoneum is accessed as previously described. Gerota's fascia is incised and the diverticulum located. The nonfunctional renal parenchyma overlying the diverticulum is incised and resected and the stone is removed. Any functional parenchyma is fulgurated and the infundibulum is sewn closed with a water-tight absorbable suture. For large cavities, an omental patch can be placed within the cavity.

Although there is a paucity of data about robotic surgery for nephrolithiasis in the pediatric population, the versatility of the robotic platform and ease of accessing and reconstructing the upper urinary tract, with an attainable learning curve, makes it an exciting technology for challenging stone management in children.

References

1. Finkelstein JB, Levy AC, Silva MV, Murray L, Delaney C, Casale P. How to decide which infant can have robotic surgery? Just do the math. J Pediatr Urol. 2015;11(4):170.e1–4.
2. Gargollo PC. Hidden incision endoscopic surgery: description of technique, parental satisfaction and applications. J Urol. 2011;185(4):1425–31.
3. Kohno M, Ogawa T, Kojima Y, Sakoda A, Johnin K, Sugita Y, et al. Pediatric congenital hydronephrosis (ureteropelvic junction obstruction): medical management guide. Int J Urol. 2020;27(5):369–76.
4. Nguyen HT, Herndon CDA, Cooper C, Gatti J, Kirsch A, Kokorowski P, et al. The Society for Fetal Urology consensus statement on the evaluation and management of antenatal hydronephrosis. J Pediatr Urol. 2010;6(3):212–31.
5. Mallik M, Watson AR. Antenatally detected urinary tract abnormalities: more detection but less action. Pediatr Nephrol Berl Ger. 2008;23(6):897–904.
6. Park JM, Bloom DA. The pathophysiology of UPJ obstruction: current concepts. Urol Clin North Am. 1998;25(2):161–9.
7. Gopal M, Peycelon M, Caldamone A, Chrzan R, El-Ghoneimi A, Olsen H, et al. Management of ureteropelvic junction obstruction in children—a roundtable discussion. J Pediatr Urol. 2019;15(4):322–9.
8. Khrichenko D, Darge K. Functional analysis in MR urography - made simple. Pediatr Radiol. 2010;40(2):182–99.
9. Morales-López RA, Pérez-Marchán M, Pérez Brayfield M. Current concepts in pediatric robotic assisted pyeloplasty. Front Pediatr. 2019;7:4.
10. Orvieto MA, Large M, Gundeti MS. Robotic paediatric urology. BJU Int. 2012;110(1):2–13.
11. Fichtenbaum EJ, Strine AC, Concodora CW, Schulte M, Noh PH. Tubeless outpatient robotic upper urinary tract reconstruction in the pediatric population: short-term assessment of safety. J Robot Surg. 2018;12(2):257–60.
12. Olsen LH, Rawashdeh YF, Jorgensen TM. Pediatric robot assisted retroperitoneoscopic pyeloplasty: a 5-year experience. J Urol. 2007;178(5):2137–41.

13. Bilgutay AN, Kirsch AJ. Robotic ureteral reconstruction in the pediatric population. Front Pediatr. 2019;7:85.
14. Lee RS, Retik AB, Borer JG, Peters CA. Pediatric robot assisted laparoscopic dismembered pyeloplasty: comparison with a cohort of open surgery. J Urol. 2006;175(2):683–7.
15. Laparoscopic pyeloplasty with cephalad translocation of the crossing vessel – a new approach to the Hellström technique [Internet]. [cited 2021 Sep 23]. Available from https://www.ncbi.nlm.nih.gov/pmc/articles/PMC4414101/
16. Janetschek G, Peschel R, Bartsch G. Laparoscopic Fenger Plasty. J Endourol. 2000;14(10):889–93.
17. Hopf HL, Bahler CD, Sundaram CP. Long-term outcomes of robot-assisted laparoscopic pyeloplasty for ureteropelvic junction obstruction. Urology. 2016;1(90):106–11.
18. Zampini AM, Nelson R, Zhang JJH, Reese J, Angermeier KW, Haber G-P. Robotic salvage pyeloplasty with buccal mucosal Onlay graft: video demonstration of technique and outcomes. Urology. 2017;1(110):253–6.
19. Ahn JJ, Shapiro ME, Ellison JS, Lendvay TS. Pediatric robot-assisted redo pyeloplasty with buccal mucosa graft: a novel technique. Urology. 2017;1(101):56–9.
20. Ross JH, Streem SB, Novick AC, Kay R, Montie J. Ureterocalicostomy for reconstruction of complicated Pelviureteric junction obstruction. Br J Urol. 1990;65(4):322–5.
21. Peters CA. Laparoscopic and robotic approach to genitourinary anomalies in children. Urol Clin North Am. 2004;31(3):595–605, xi.
22. Gutt CN, Oniu T, Mehrabi A, Kashfi A, Schemmer P, Büchler MW. Robot-assisted abdominal surgery. Br J Surg. 2004;91(11):1390–7.
23. Casale P. Robotic pediatric urology. Expert Rev Med Devices. 2008;5(1):59–64.
24. Gill IS, Cherullo EE, Steinberg AP, Desai MM, Abreu SC, Ng C, et al. Laparoscopic ureterocalicostomy: initial experience. J Urol. 2004;171(3):1227–30.
25. Korets R, Hyams ES, Shah OD, Stifelman MD. Robotic-assisted laparoscopic ureterocalicostomy. Urology. 2007;70(2):366–9.
26. Casale P, Mucksavage P, Resnick M, Kim SS. Robotic ureterocalicostomy in the pediatric population. J Urol. 2008;180(6):2643–8.
27. Passerotti CC, Nguyen HT, Eisner BH, Lee RS, Peters CA. Laparoscopic reoperative pediatric pyeloplasty with robotic assistance. J Endourol. 2007;21(10):1137–40.
28. Lee RS, Passerotti CC, Cendron M, Estrada CR, Borer JG, Peters CA. Early results of robot assisted laparoscopic lithotomy in adolescents. J Urol. 2007;177(6):2306–9. discussion 2309-2310
29. Jarrett TW, Chan DY, Charambura TC, Fugita O, Kavoussi LR. Laparoscopic pyeloplasty: the first 100 cases. J Urol. 2002;167(3):1253–6.
30. Selli C, Carini M, Turini D, Masini G, Costantini A. Experience with ureterocalyceal anastomosis. Urology. 1982;20(1):7–12.
31. Peters CA, Schlussel R, Mendelsohn C. Ectopic ureter, ureterocele, and ureteral anomalies. In: Wein AJ, Kavoussi LR, Novick AC, Partin AW, Peters CA, editors. Campbell-Walsh urology. 10th ed. Philadelphia: Saunders Elsevier; 2011. p. 3236–66.
32. Jordan GH, Winslow BH. Laparoendoscopic upper pole partial nephrectomy with ureterectomy. J Urol. 1993;150(3):940–3.
33. Horowitz M, Shah SM, Ferzli G, Syad PI, Glassberg KI. Laparoscopic partial upper pole nephrectomy in infants and children. BJU Int. 2001;87(6):514–6.
34. Janetschek G, Seibold J, Radmayr C, Bartsch G. Laparoscopic heminephroureterectomy in pediatric patients. J Urol. 1997;158(5):1928–30.
35. Valla J-S, Breaud J, Carfagna L, Tursini S, Steyaert H. Treatment of ureterocele on duplex ureter: upper pole nephrectomy by retroperitoneoscopy in children based on a series of 24 cases. Eur Urol. 2003;43(4):426–9.
36. Robinson BC, Snow BW, Cartwright PC, De Vries CR, Hamilton BD, Anderson JB. Comparison of laparoscopic versus open partial nephrectomy in a pediatric series. J Urol. 2003;169(2):638–40.
37. El-Ghoneimi A, Farhat W, Bolduc S, Bagli D, McLorie G, Khoury A. Retroperitoneal laparoscopic vs open partial nephroureterectomy in children. BJU Int. 2003;91(6):532–5.
38. Lee RS, Retik AB, Borer JG, Diamond DA, Peters CA. Pediatric retroperitoneal laparoscopic partial nephrectomy: comparison with an age matched cohort of open surgery. J Urol. 2005;174(2):708–11. discussion 712
39. Piaggio L, Franc-Guimond J, Figueroa TE, Barthold JS, González R. Comparison of laparoscopic and open partial nephrectomy for duplication anomalies in children. J Urol. 2006;175(6):2269–73.
40. Wang DS, Bird VG, Cooper CS, Austin JC, Winfield HN. Laparoscopic upper-pole heminephrectomy for ectopic ureter: surgical technique. J Endourol. 2003;17(7):469–73.
41. Pedraza R, Palmer L, Moss V, Franco I. Bilateral robotic assisted laparoscopic heminephroureterectomy. J Urol. 2004;171(6 Pt 1):2394–5.
42. Olsen LH, Jørgensen TM. Robotically assisted retroperitoneoscopic heminephrectomy in children: initial clinical results. J Pediatr Urol. 2005;1(2):101–4.
43. Lee RS, Sethi AS, Passerotti CC, Retik AB, Borer JG, Nguyen HT, et al. Robot assisted laparoscopic partial nephrectomy: a viable and safe option in children. J Urol. 2009;181(2):823–8. discussion 828-829
44. Mason MD, Anthony Herndon CD, Smith-Harrison LI, Peters CA, Corbett ST. Robotic-assisted partial nephrectomy in duplicated collecting systems in the pediatric population: techniques and outcomes. J Pediatr Urol. 2014;10(2):374–9.
45. Müller PF, Schlager D, Hein S, Bach C, Miernik A, Schoeb DS. Robotic stone surgery – current state and future prospects: a systematic review. Arab J Urol. 2018;16(3):357–64.
46. Humphreys MR. The emerging role of robotics and laparoscopy in stone disease. Urol Clin North Am. 2013;40(1):115–28.
47. Ballesteros N, Snow ZA, Moscardi PRM, Ransford GA, Gomez P, Castellan M. Robotic Management of Urolithiasis in the pediatric population. Front Pediatr. 2019;7:351.
48. Meggiato L, Cattaneo F, Zattoni F, Dal Moro F, Beltrami P, Zattoni F. Complex cystine kidney stones treated with combined robot-assisted laparoscopic pyelolithotomy and intraoperative renoscopy. Urologia. 2018;85(2):76–8.
49. Singh V, Sinha RJ, Gupta DK, Pandey M. Prospective randomized comparison of retroperitoneoscopic pyelolithotomy versus percutaneous nephrolithotomy for solitary large pelvic kidney stones. Urol Int. 2014;92(4):392–5.
50. Pedro RN, Buchholz N. Laparoscopic and robotic surgery for stone disease. Urolithiasis. 2018;46(1):125–7.
51. Badani KK, Hemal AK, Fumo M, Kaul S, Shrivastava A, Rajendram AK, et al. Robotic extended pyelolithotomy for treatment of renal calculi: a feasibility study. World J Urol. 2006;24(2):198–201.
52. Ghani KR, Rogers CG, Sood A, Kumar R, Ehlert M, Jeong W, et al. Robot-assisted anatrophic nephrolithotomy with renal hypothermia for managing staghorn calculi. J Endourol. 2013;27(11):1393–8.
53. Koopman SG, Fuchs G. Management of stones associated with intrarenal stenosis: infundibular stenosis and caliceal diverticulum. J Endourol. 2013;27(12):1546–50.

Robotic Reconstructive Surgery of Ureter in the Pediatric Population

Alaa El-Ghoneimi, Ana Bujons, Amrita Mohanty, and Mohan S Gundeti

1 Part I: Robot-Assisted Laparoscopic Ureteral Reimplantation: "LUAA" Gundeti Technique, Description, and Outcomes

Within pediatric urology, utilization of the minimally invasive robotic-assisted laparoscopic (RAL) approach has increased over time due to its many technical and clinical benefits and is now regularly performed at centers across the world. Despite the rise in popularity of RAL, there is little standardization of its technique in ensuring best outcomes for patients. Gundeti et al. described the LUAA technique in an effort to optimize results for robot-assisted laparoscopic extravesical ureteral reimplantation (RALUR-EV). In this chapter, we aim to share technical details of the "LUAA" technique, which emphasizes the length of detrusor tunnel (L), utilization of U stitch at the UVJ (ureterovesical junction) (U) for advancement, placement of the ureteral apical stay stitch (A) at the summit of the tunnel, and inclusion of ureteral adventitia in detrusorrhaphy (A). A full video describing the LUAA Gundeti technique can be found in the electronic supplementary material of the text (Video 1).

Supplementary Information The online version contains supplementary material available at [https://doi.org/10.1007/978-3-031-00363-9_70].

A. El-Ghoneimi
University of Paris, Paris, France

Department of Pediatric Urology, University Hospital Robert Debré, APHP, Paris, France

National Reference Center for Rare Urinary Tract Malformations (MARVU), Paris, France

A. Bujons
Department of Pediatric Urology, Fundació Puigvert, Barcelona, Spain

A. Mohanty (✉) · M. S Gundeti
The University of Chicago Pritzker School of Medicine, Chicago, IL, USA

Pediatric Urology, Section of Urology Department of Surgery, Comer Children's Hospital, The University of Chicago Medical Center, Chicago, IL, USA

1.1 Indications

Indications for surgery include VUR (vesicoureteral reflux) grades 3–5 with breakthrough urinary tract infections, non-resolution beyond age five, increasing severity of reflux, and deteriorating renal function. Surgery is performed after the toilet training period, preferably after two years.

1.2 Preoperative Preparation

Preoperative assessment involved obtaining a complete medical and surgical history and identifying any comorbidities. Emphasis should be placed on investigating patient's previous abdominal or pelvic surgical history, underlying disease processes, additional ureteral pathologies, and bladder bowel dysfunction (BBD), which may further complicate surgery.

In preparation for surgery, preoperative imaging should be obtained to evaluate the current renal status of the patient and factors that may impede the operation. Preoperative evaluation of VUR includes VCUG (voiding cystourethrogram), ultrasound scan (USS), and dimercaptosuccinic acid (DMSA) scan to detect any evidence of renal scaring. Optimization of BBD should be obtained prior to surgery. Any indicated cystoscopy should be performed before the docking of the robot though it is not routinely performed or required.

1.3 Technical Description

1. Following written informed consent and administration of general anesthesia, patient is placed in semi-lithotomy position with legs separated and arms tucked to the sides.
2. A urethral catheter is placed in the sterile field and the patient is painted and draped.

P. Wiklund et al. (eds.), *Robotic Urologic Surgery*, https://doi.org/10.1007/978-3-031-00363-9_70

3. An open Hassan technique is used for transperitoneal placement of an 8/12-mm umbilical port for the camera, along with two 5/8-mm robotic trocars placed on the midclavicular line supraumbilically and a 5-mm assistant port on the left side placed equally between the umbilicus and midclavicular ports (Fig. 1).

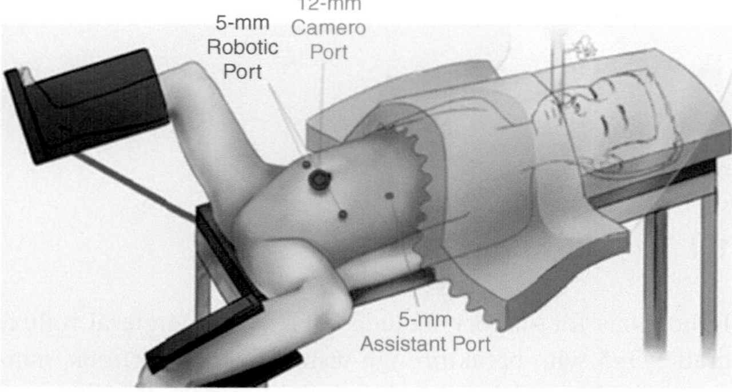

Fig. 1 Positioning and placement of ports for patient (adapted from Gundeti et al., *European Urology* [1])

4. The robot is docked between the legs while the patient's head is lowered to about 5 degrees (Trendelenburg). Often, this can be performed with XI side dock.
5. An 8-mm precise bipolar is used in the left hand along with a monopolar scissor in the right hand for dissection. Additional needle drivers are used for suturing. We prefer not to use 5-mm pediatric instruments in a narrow space like the pelvis, as these instruments lack articulation.
6. Upon entering the pelvis, the urinary bladder must be localized and the ureter identified as it transverses over the iliac vessels at the pelvic brim. Peritoneum covering the ureter is incised. The ureter is then mobilized to the vas deferens or uterine artery, maintaining an adequate layer of its adventitia in an effort to preserve its vascularity. Umbilical tape is brought around the ureter to loop it, ensuring atraumatic handling of the ureter (Fig. 2a, b).
7. A peritoneal window is created distal to the vas deferens or uterine artery, advancing the ureter below. Dissection near the ureterovesical junction (UVJ) continues close to

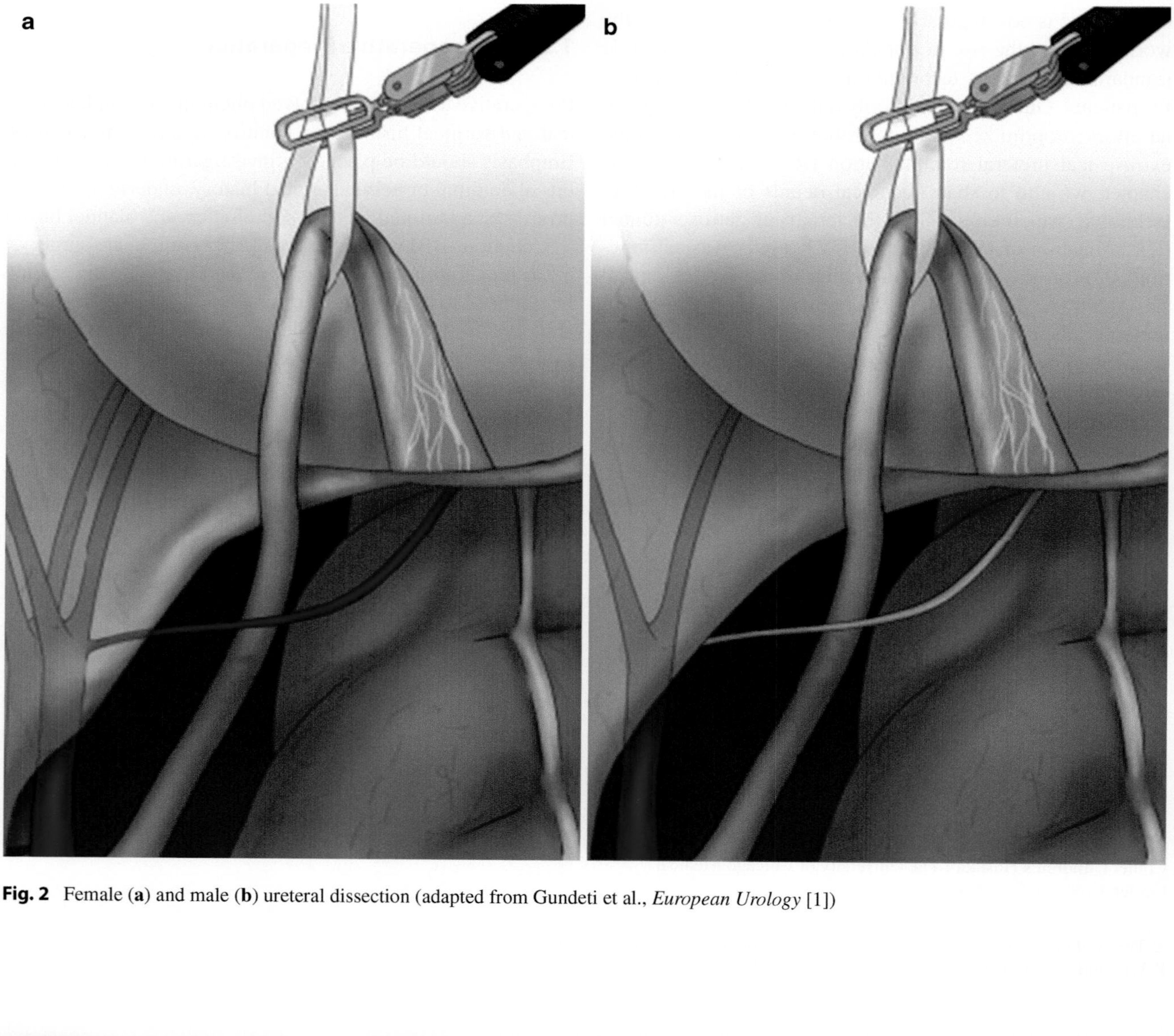

Fig. 2 Female (**a**) and male (**b**) ureteral dissection (adapted from Gundeti et al., *European Urology* [1])

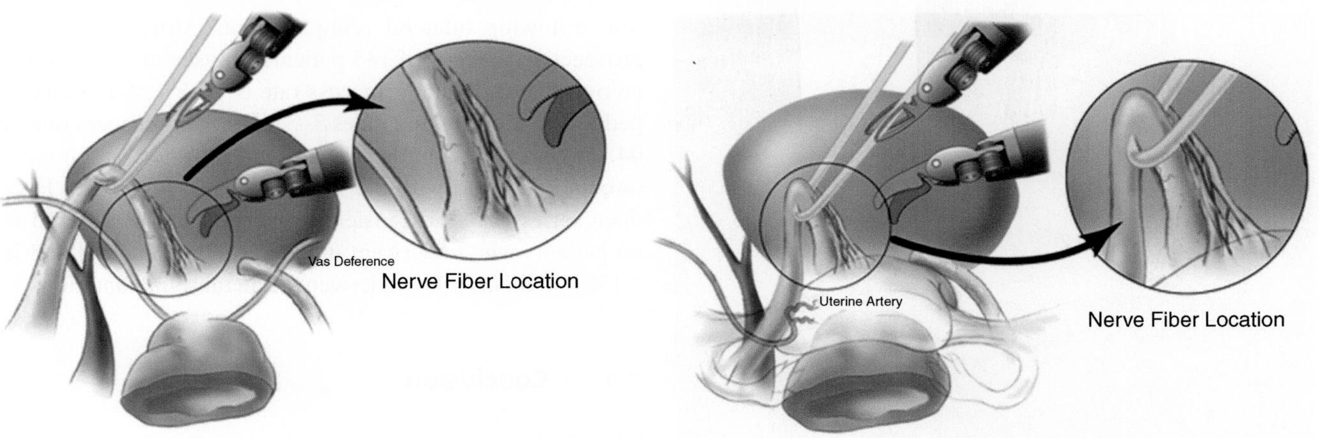

Fig. 3 Nerve localization dorsomedially of the distal ureter (adapted from Dangle et al., *Journal of Pediatric Urology* [2])

the ureter, with careful attention to preserving the neurovascular bundle situated dorsomedially (Fig. 3). Often, there is a need to take the uterine artery for proper mobilization, and diligent care should be demonstrated for this.

8. A 60 ml of sterile saline is introduced into the bladder to facilitate the detrusorotomy while a transabdominal stay stitch with 2′0 Vicryl is used to hitch the bladder.
9. A detrusorotomy of 4–5 cm <u>L</u>ength is recommended, regardless of preoperative VUR grade or age of patient. It is of utmost importance to perform a detrusorotomy that aligns with the UVJ to prevent angulation.
10. Carefully ensuring that the UVJ and detrusorotomy are in a straight line, a Y dissection is completed at the UVJ in an effort to preserve the vascularity and neurovascular bundle. Careful effort should be taken to minimize the use of diathermy in this area.
11. Detrusoraphy starts firstly with the <u>*U*</u> stitch (advancement stitch), which is placed at the distal end of the detrusorotomy, advancing the ureter by taking the detrusor at the 5 o'clock position and subsequently adding ureteral adventitia at the 6 o'clock position and detrusor at the 7 o'clock position (Fig. 4). This is executed using the 4′0 PDS and tied carefully.
12. The further detrusorraphy is performed with a running stitch of 4′0 PDS that incorporates the <u>A</u>dventitia of the ureter in every alternate stitch (Fig. 5).
13. <u>A</u>pical stay stitch (5–0 PDS) is placed at the apex of the detrusor tunnel through the ureteral adventitia and detrusor following completion of the detrusorraphy to both keep the alignment of the ureter inside the tunnel and prevent slippage.
14. Careful attention should be provided to ensure that the neotunnel is not too tight. To confirm it is not too tight, one prong of the needle holder can be placed in the tunnel apex at the completion of the detrusorraphy. Completion is shown in Fig. 6.

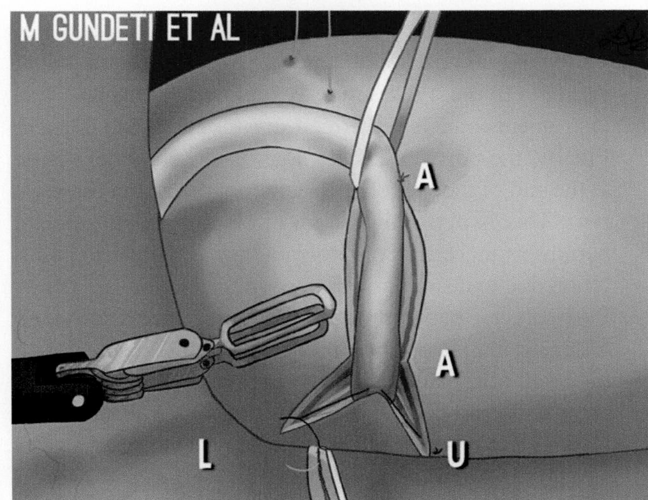

Fig. 4 (L)ength of detrusor tunnel, (U) stitch, and (A)pical alignment (adapted from Gundeti et al., *European Urology* [1])

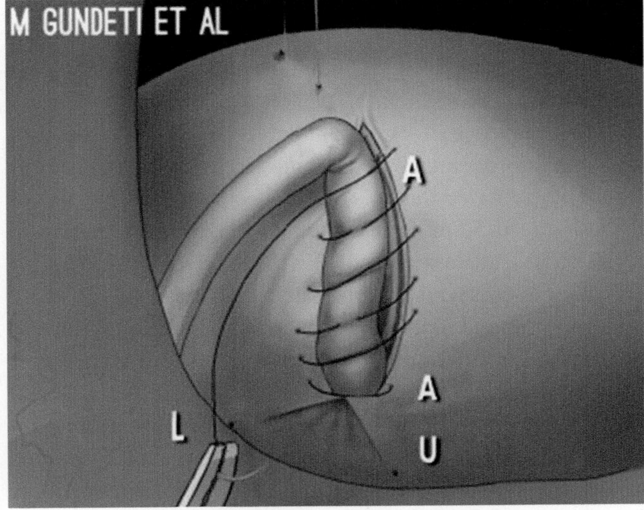

Fig. 5 Suturing of detrusor tunnel with adventitial incorporation of the ureter (A) (adapted from Gundeti et al., *European Urology* [1])

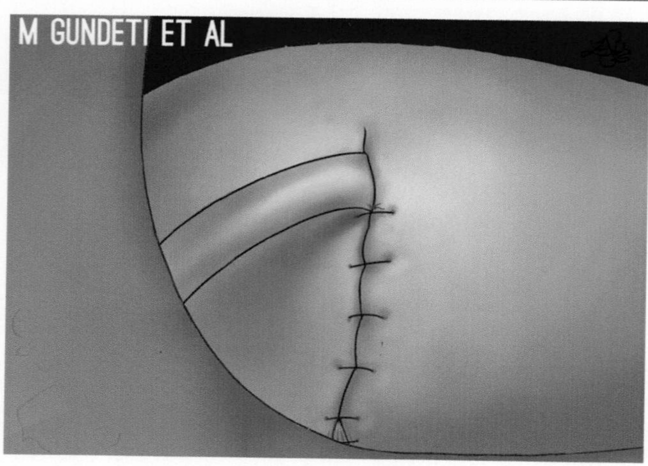

Fig. 6 Completed detrusorraphy (adapted from Gundeti et al., *European Urology* [1])

15. Following completion of the detrusorraphy, the bladder is emptied, the hitch suture is removed, the needle and instrument count is performed, and the robot is undocked.
16. Finally, the port site fascial layer is closed under vision at the end of the procedure, including the 5-mm assistant port. This is performed in an effort to prevent omental hernias as these are common among our pediatric population due to a smaller diameter of the bowel.
17. Post-surgery, patients with unilateral reimplantation are observed in the hospital for one night while patients with bilateral reimplantation are observed for two nights. Prior to formal discharge, the catheter is removed, and a bladder scan is performed to ensure adequate bladder emptying. Appropriate instructions are given for timed voiding and bowel function. Prophylaxis is continued until VCUG is performed.

1.4 Outcomes

The first follow-up is at one month with USS, and VCUG is completed at four months postoperatively, with success defined as absence of VUR. Gundeti et al. [1] observed considerable improvements in outcomes from RALUR-EV over time. They reported that this current technique, with usage of a standardized 5-cm detrusor tunnel length, demonstrates a RALUR-EV success rate of 87% (range of 72–97%) for pediatric patients with predominately high-grade VUR. There were no ureteral complications at median follow-up of 30 months. Furthermore, Boysen et al. [3] in their multicenter study found that with usage of this technique, among 260 patients undergoing RALUR-EV, radiographic resolution was seen in 87.9% of patients. There was an overall complication rate of 9.6% with no grade 4 or 5 complications. Around 3.9% of patients studied had transient urinary retention following bilateral reimplantation. More recently, in prospective analysis of 143 patients, Boysen et al. [4] found an overall radiographic success rate of 93.8%. Additionally, pediatric patients with grades 3–5 VUR had a success rate of 94.1%. Ureteral complications requiring intervention were rare and occurred with the same incidence found in a large open series (2.5%). Transient urinary retention occurred in no patients who underwent unilateral reimplantation and in 7.1% of patients who underwent bilateral reimplantation.

1.5 Conclusion

With the increasing popularity of robotic technology within the field of pediatric urology, it is critical that there is standardization of techniques to ensure the best possible outcomes for patients. Research indicates considerable improvements in outcomes from usage of the LUAA technique. The outlined technique and its studied outcomes provided in this chapter will hopefully assist surgeons in performing the RALUR-EV procedure. Definitive conclusions cannot be made surrounding the success rate of this technique because of its variance with surgeon experience and complexity of patient anatomy and disease processes. Regardless, we hope to facilitate an overall improvement in success rates by sharing a standard technique to serve as a guide in improving outcomes.

2 Part II: Robot-Assisted Ureteroureterostomy in Pediatric Patients

Ureteral duplication anomalies have been widely reported in the pediatric literature. The ureter of the upper moiety is frequently associated with ectopic insertion, which can result in incontinence, obstruction, or vesicoureteral reflux (VUR). Various methods for the management of ureteral duplication anomalies have been proposed. In cases with adequate upper pole function, preservation of this moiety is preferred. Ureteral reimplantation, ureteropyelostomy, and ureteroureterostomy have all been described as reconstructive alternatives [5–8].

Ureteroureterostomy is a commonly employed strategy for the management of a duplicated ureteral system, and this approach minimizes the risk to a healthy ureter as might be seen in a common sheath ureteral reimplantation. End-to-side ureteroureterostomy can be performed proximally or distally depending on surgeon preference [9]. We use a distal approach, eliminating the risk of hilar vessel injury [10].

Ureteroureterostomy was first described by Foley in 1928 [11]. In 1952, Kuss performed this operation on an ectopic ureter, and it became a widely used procedure for the treatment of these congenital malformations [12].

In the last ten years, expert laparoscopists have shown that performance of this complex reconstruction in a minimally invasive fashion is feasible and offers certain advantages. Moreover, it has been reported that suturing and tissue handling in a limited space can be performed more easily with a robot compared with conventional laparoscopy.

2.1 Preoperative Assessment

Children must have a negative culture before surgery, and we usually administer a dose of cefazolin chemoprophylaxis before the intervention.

2.2 Patient Positioning

The patient is first placed in a lithotomy position to perform a cystoscopy for the placement of a double J catheter in the ureter of the ipsilateral lower pole. This allows intraoperative identification of the lower hemisystem ureter. Only if ureteroureterostomy is performed for VUR will the double J catheter be placed in the upper pole. After the cystoscopy has been performed, a Foley catheter is placed, and the patient is placed in a modified flank position with the side of surgical interest facing upward. It is very important that all pressure points are carefully padded. The ipsilateral arm is secured at the patient's side, which helps prevent robotic arm injuries to the child.

2.3 Port Placement

For the Xi, the camera and working ports are identical, allowing placement of the camera through any port. Robotic working ports are then placed under direct vision. For the Si, 8- and 5-mm robotic ports and instruments are available. However, limitations of the 5-mm instrumentation include lack of bipolar electrocautery and restriction of monopolar cautery to the hook instrument. Furthermore, the wristed motion of the 5-mm instruments is more proximal than that of the 8-mm instruments, which may limit surgeon motion in situations where intracorporeal space is limited. For these reasons, the use of the 8-mm instruments is to be preferred: this allows for a greater selection of instrumentation, including monopolar and bipolar cautery for a variety of instruments and fine needle drivers.

In children, we prefer to perform intraperitoneal access using the Hasson technique. We place the trocars as follows: Port placement begins with an umbilical incision and placement of an 8-mm robotic camera trocar. Then, two 8-mm robotic ports and a 5-mm laparoscopic assistant port are placed below the line of a Pfannenstiel incision (Fig. 7).

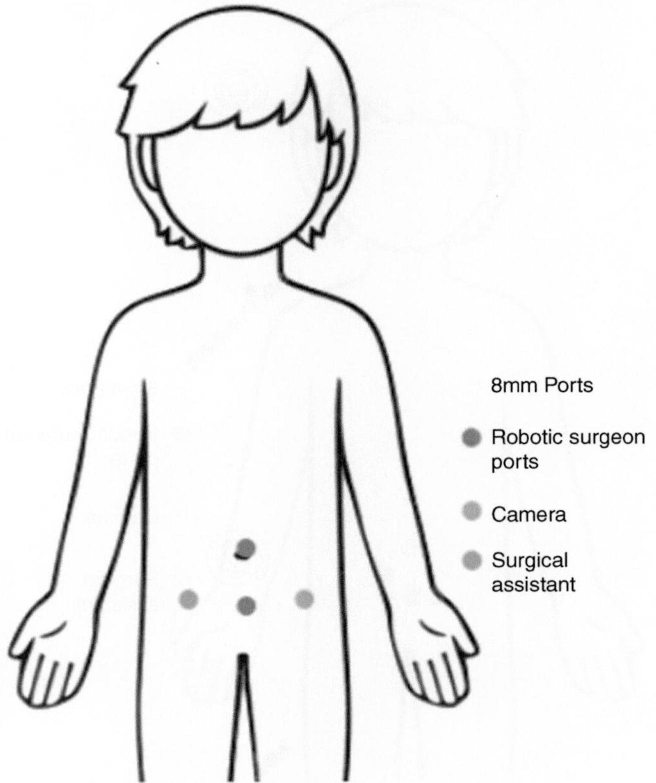

Fig. 7 Preferred option for trocar placement: An 8-mm robotic camera trocar is placed in the umbilicus. Two 8-mm working ports and a 5-mm assistant port are placed below the Pfannenstiel incision

Another possible option for trocar placement is as follows: Port placement begins with an umbilical incision and placement of an 8-mm robotic camera trocar. Then, two 8-mm working ports are placed under direct vision above and below the midline, lateral to the ipsilateral rectus muscle at the level of the anterior superior iliac spine and subcostal margin. Following placement of the three robotic ports, a laparoscopic 5-mm trocar can be placed for the assistant (Fig. 8).

We usually place the assistant port to help with suctioning, passing sutures, or holding tissues. Sometimes, in children, it is not possible to separate the trocars by 7–8 cm, and they have to be much closer.

2.4 Approach

The ureter of the upper pole is mobilized; it is usually much more dilated than that of the lower pole and can be easily identified in most cases. In addition, the lower pole has a double J catheter (Fig. 9). Once the ureters have been identified at the pelvic edge, they are approached below the pelvic brim, and the trocar positions are shifted. The ureter is then dissected from the lower hemisystem (Fig. 10), in the area

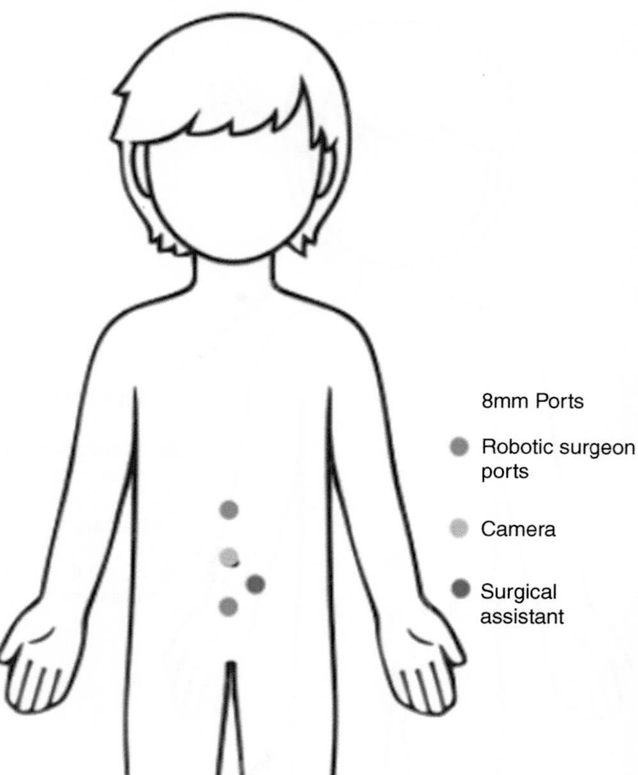

Fig. 8 Alternative option for trocar placement: An 8-mm robotic camera trocar is placed in the umbilicus. Two 8-mm working ports are placed under direct vision above and below the midline. An assistant port can be placed

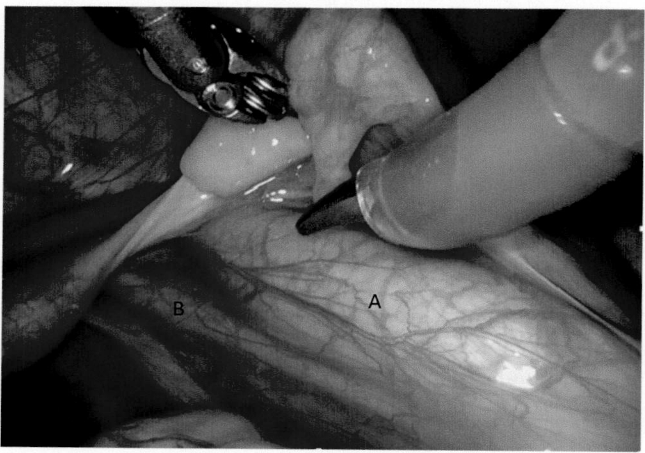

Fig. 9 The dilated upper ureter (A) and the lower ureter (B) are identified

where the anastomosis will be performed, to minimize any damage to the ureter (Fig. 11). The anastomosis is done at the level of the distal ureter, where it crosses the iliac vessels.

This is followed by a cross section of the ureter of the upper pole (in cases of ectopic ureteral insertion or uretero-

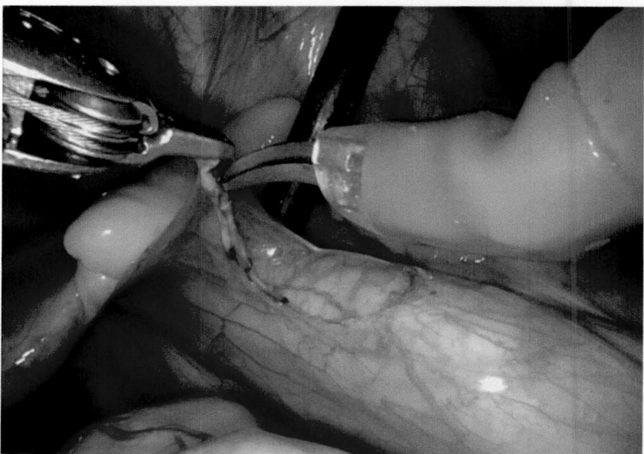

Fig. 10 The upper ureter is dissected and transected

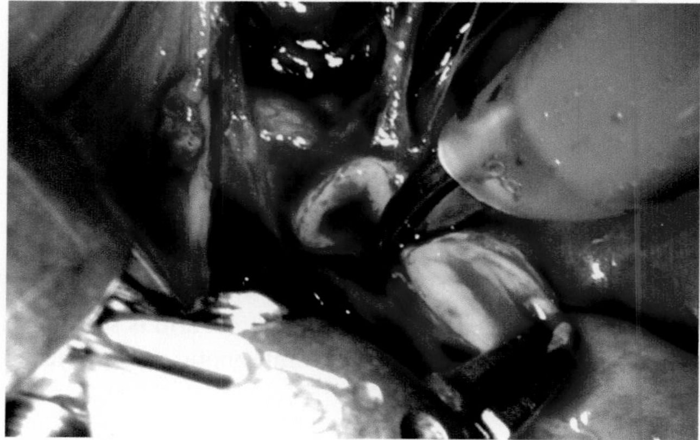

Fig. 11 The upper ureter is dissected and transected

cele) or of the ureter of the lower pole if the operation is performed for VUR. The ureterotomy is made as long as the width of the donor ureter using Potts scissors. Although there may be disparity in size between the two ureters, we have found that this does not influence our results.

An end-to-side anastomosis is then performed. In our center, we prefer to perform a running suture with 6–0 polyglactin, completing first the posterior edge and then the anterior edge of the anastomosis (Figs. 12 and 13).

After the anastomosis has been completed, the distal ureteral stump is resected, taking care to avoid injury to the normal ureter as well as to the Müllerian and Wolffian structures. Removal of the distal ectopic ureteral stump is important because this may be a reservoir for infection even if it does not reflux (Fig. 14).

The robot is undocked and the ports are removed under vision. The fascia of all ports is closed to prevent herniation. We do not routinely place a drain. The skin can be closed with a 5/0 monofilar absorbable synthetic subcuticular stitch. The Foley catheter is removed the day after the surgery, and the ureteral catheter is removed four weeks later.

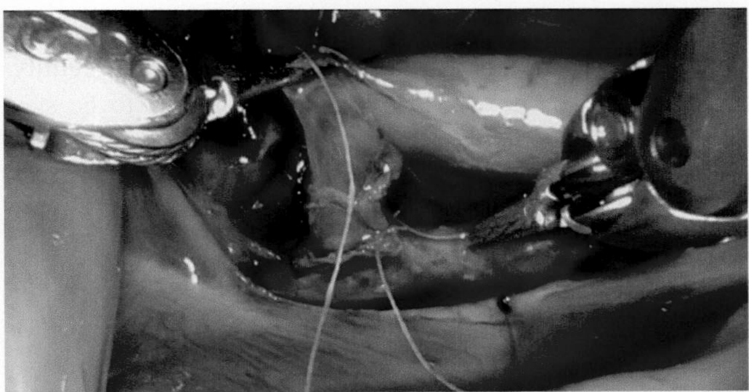

Fig. 12 End-to-side anastomosis with a running 6–0 polyglactin suture

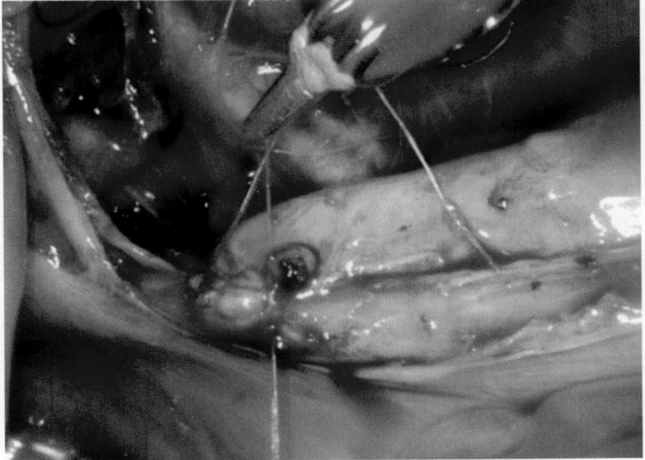

Fig. 13 End-to-side anastomosis with a running 6–0 polyglactin suture

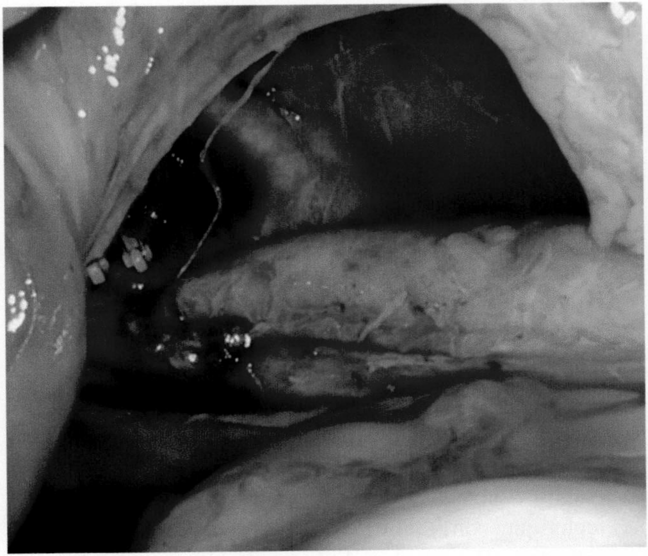

Fig. 14 Removal of the distal ureter stump

2.5 Follow-Up

We usually perform renovesical ultrasound one month after removal of the double J catheter and again three months later if there have been any changes. Later, we do an annual control with ultrasound.

2.6 Postoperative Complications and Outcomes

Intraoperative complications are those that can occur in robotic or laparoscopic intraperitoneal surgery. The postoperative complications due to ureteroureterostomy include urinary leakage from the anastomosis, which has been observed in up to 14% of open surgery cases [13], urinary tract infections, paralytic ileus, stenosis, persistence of hydronephrosis, and stump VUR [14]. The possible complication of "yo-yo" reflux R has not been observed in the cases published in the literature. There are no large series of complications in the literature on robotic ureteroureterostomy.

Passerotti et al. published the first series of three robotic cases with proximal ureteral strictures in nonduplicated systems in 2008 [15]. Leavitt et al. published the first five cases of children undergoing ipsilateral robotic ureteroureterostomy for ureteral duplication with a distal approach and with UTI (urinary tract infection) as a complication [16]. Lee et al. [17] reported the advantages of a robotic platform in 25 pediatric patients compared with 19 patients who underwent open surgery. They showed comparable operative time, estimated blood loss, and complication rate, but the robotic group had slightly shorter hospitalization and higher rates of improved hydronephrosis or drainage in initial follow-up imaging. In a series of 24 patients, Ellison and Lendvay observed similar results to the aforementioned authors, including comparable operative times and length of stay. Median follow-up was 16 months. Two patients had postoperative UTI, and one patient required a revision open ureteroureterostomy due to a recurrent stricture ~1 year following the initial procedure.

2.7 Conclusion

Robotic ureteroureterostomy is a safe and effective procedure with outcomes comparable to the traditional open approach. Several reports have demonstrated positive short-term results. However, follow-up times are limited. More prospective studies are required to establish the long-term efficacy of this procedure.

3 Part III: Robot-Assisted Ureteral Mitrofanoff Procedure, Description, and Outcomes

3.1 Introduction

The continent cystostomy technique was first described by Mitrofanoff in 1980 [18]. It consists of fashioning a catheterizable channel with a flap-valve continence mechanism,

in order to be both continent to promote storage and accessible to allow low-pressure emptying. The conduit for catheterization is the appendix in the majority of cases. The use of ureter as an alternative to appendix was published since 1984 by Monfort et al. [19], and its efficiency has been demonstrated by many publications with long-standing comparable results to the appendix [20–25].

Minimal invasive approach is commonly used for Mitrofanoff procedure either by standard laparoscopic or robotic assisted [1, 26]. The robotic-assisted approach for extravesical reimplantation has been proven and its efficiency and is written in details in this chapter. If the ipsilateral nonfunctioning kidney has a high-grade reflux, an efficient reimplantation procedure must be proceeded to avoid the major complication of incontinent channel. The robotic approach for such challenging cases, combining nephrectomy and reimplantation of the ureter to be used as CIC (clean intermittent catheterization) channel, seems to us as an efficient and alternative to open surgery.

3.2 Indications

Indications for Mitrofanoff procedures are in patients who have significant bladder dysfunction associated with an intact urethral sensation or having already had bladder neck or urethral surgery.

The specific indication for using the ureter as continent catheterization channel is the case of nonfunctioning kidney without the need for bladder augmentation.

3.3 Preoperative Preparation

Preoperative assessment involved obtaining a complete medical and surgical history and identifying any comorbidities.

Before the Mitrofanoff procedure is considered, urodynamic evaluation is done for each patient to study bladder compliance, detrusor activity, and bladder capacity.

This evaluation is mandatory to confirm the indication of isolated Mitrofanoff procedure without bladder augmentation.

The child and his family are seen by the pediatric urology nurse and psychologist. Determining the placement of the skin stoma (iliac or umbilical) is an important step and should be understood by the child and his/her family. Training with models is of extreme importance to be sure that the child and his family are capable of doing CIC; this preoperative information and training are mandatory to avoid postoperative difficulties to catheterize.

No preoperative intestinal preparation is needed.

Any indicated cystoscopy should be performed before the docking of the robot though it is not routinely performed or required.

3.4 Technical Description

18. Following written informed consent and administration of general anesthesia, patient is placed in dorsal position and arms tucked to the sides.
19. A urethral catheter is placed in the sterile field and the patient is painted and draped.
20. Skin stoma flap is designed.
21. An open technique is used for transperitoneal placement of an 8-mm port for the camera (30°), midway between the umbilicus and xiphoid processes on the midline if the umbilicus is chosen for stoma site; otherwise, the first access incision is done through the umbilicus for the camera. Our preference is not to use the stoma site for any trocar insertion to reduce an excessive trauma to the skin.
22. Three 8-mm robotic trocars are placed on an oblique line opposite to the nephrectomy site; this configuration is designed to be able to do the nephrectomy and the reimplantation of the ureter without re-docking the robot (Da Vinci Xi). An extra laparoscopic 5-mm trocar is inserted for assistant 5-mm instruments and connected to AirSeal°. All trocars are inserted under laparoscopic control (Fig. 15).
23. The robot is docked on the left side of the table (the side of the nephrectomy).
24. An 8-mm precise bipolar is used in the left hand along with a monopolar scissor in the right hand for dissection. Additional needle drivers are used for suturing. A holding forceps is used on the fourth arm for exposure.
25. The first step is abdominal exploration to identify the bladder, the appendix for eventual future use, and any intra-abdominal adhesions are freed (in multi-operated children).
26. Nephrectomy is done according to standard robotic technique; on the described case, the left colon is reflected. The renal pedicle is identified and fully dissected. The ureter is transected just below the UPJ (uteropelvic junction), and care is taken not to devascularize the ureter. The renal vessels are ligated and sec-

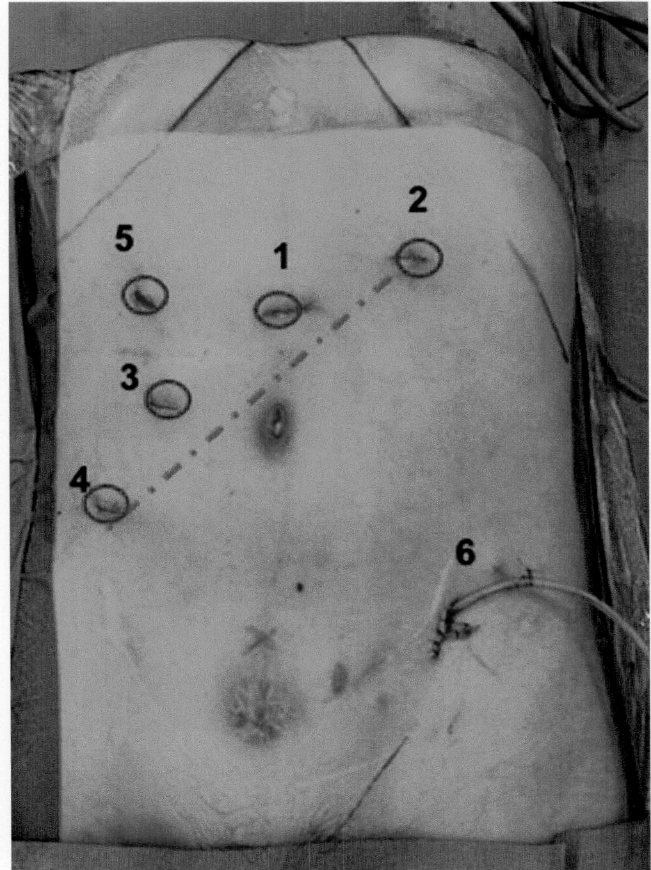

Fig. 15 Trocars position for both nephrectomy and extravesical ureteral reimplantation and creation of skin stoma for CIC. A 14- year-old boy, multi-operated of ureters and bladder. 1) Camera robotic port, 30°, 8 mm. 2) 2,3,4: robotic 8-mm trocars. 3) 5, accessory 5-mm AirSeal trocar. 4) 6, Y skin flap incision to anastomose with spatulated reimplanted ureter

tioned, using either robotic vessel seal or endocorporeal ligature or clips according to the surgeon's preference and the size of the vessels.

27. Reimplantation: The table is tilted in Trendelenburg, 18°, and rotated for 5°. Filling of the bladder will help in identifying it.
28. Steps for an extravesical reimplantation are the same as the technique described in the chapter of extravesical reimplantation with the following specific points related to the use of the ureter as CIC channel:
    (a) Most of these children are already operated on their bladders and had failed ureterovesical reimplantation with dilated ureters. Care must be taken in limiting the dissection to the detrusotomy especially at the area of the terminal ureter (Fig. 16).
    (b) There is no need to put any loop as the ureter is totally free and its upper end is handled directly by a traction suture (Fig. 17).

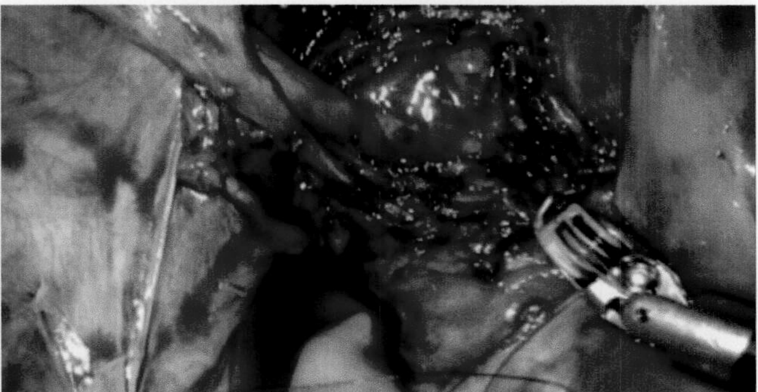

Fig. 16 Detrusotomy, with careful dissection of the terminal ureter, especially in redo cases to keep the ureter viable with its adventitia

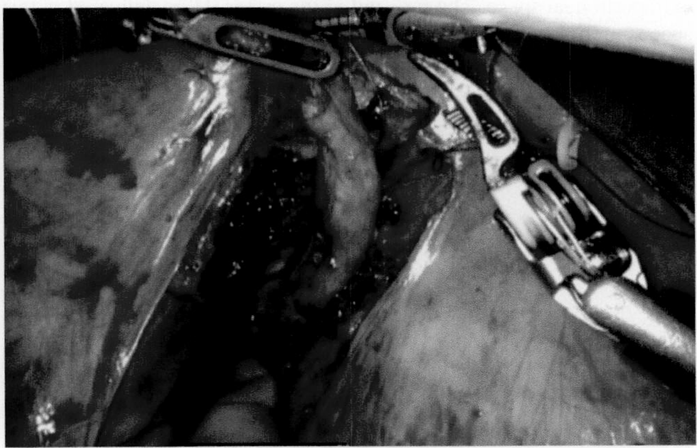

Fig. 17 The distal ureter is positioned in the detrusotomy extramucosal tunnel before starting the detrusorraphy

    (c) The bladder is hanged by sutures to the abdominal wall for exposure.
    (d) The detrusorraphy over the ureter can be as tight as possible to avoid any stoma incontinence secondary to residual reflux, ureteral tapering to be avoided. Detrusorraphy is done by interrupted Vicryl 4–0 sutures, to be able to replace any suture if there is difficulty during the catheterization at the end of procedure.
    (e) The free end of the ureter is brought through the inguinal incision by an extraperitoneal pathway to keep the bladder and the ureter in extraperitoneal space (Fig. 18).
    (f) At the end of detrusorraphy and the exteriorization of the ureter, it is crucial to full the bladder and to try the same catheter as that will be used for CIC. The ureter must be as short as possible to avoid any kinking. If any difficulty is encountered, the detrusorraphy or the length of the ureter must be revisited. Care was taken to ensure absence of twisting.
    (g) Following completion of the detrusorraphy, the bladder is emptied, the hitch suture is removed, and

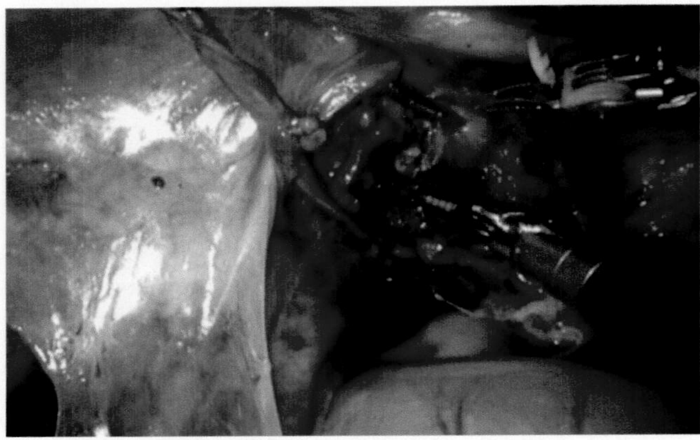

Fig. 18 A forceps is introduced by the skin stoma and remains in the extraperitoneal space. The free end of the ureter (U) is delivered in this space anterior to the vas (V)

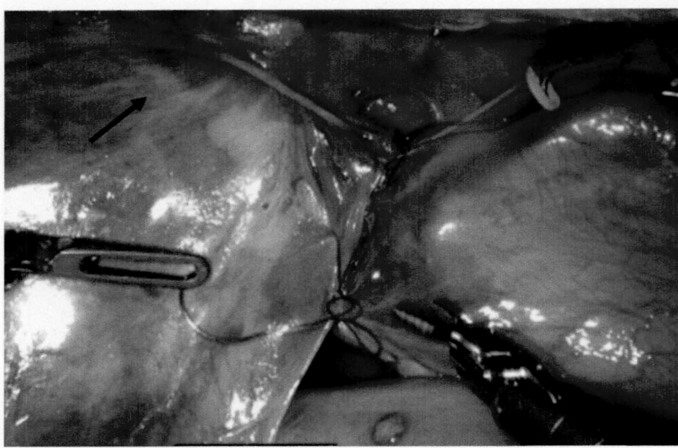

Fig. 19 The pelvic peritoneum is sutured to keep the ureter (arrow) in the extraperitoneal space

the peritoneum is closed to keep the bladder and the ureter in extravesical space (Fig. 19). Needle and instrument count is performed, and the robot is undocked.

(h) The ureter is sutured to the skin flap (Fig. 20), and an indwelling catheter is left in the ureteral stoma, without a balloon.
(i) Finally, the port site fascial layer is closed under vision at the end of the procedure, including the 5-mm assistant port. A local anesthesia is injected in each trocar incision.
(j) Post-surgery, patients are allowed for free diet and mobilized as soon as possible. They are discharged according to their medical underlying status and their pain management.
(k) The patient will be back on the outpatient clinic for catheter removal at day 10, and the first CIC will be done at the outpatient clinic.

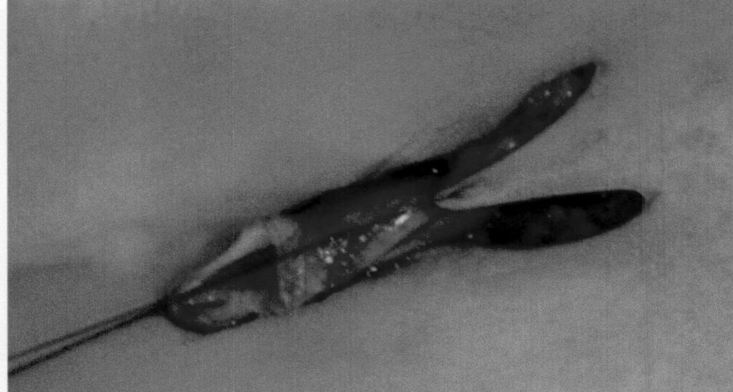

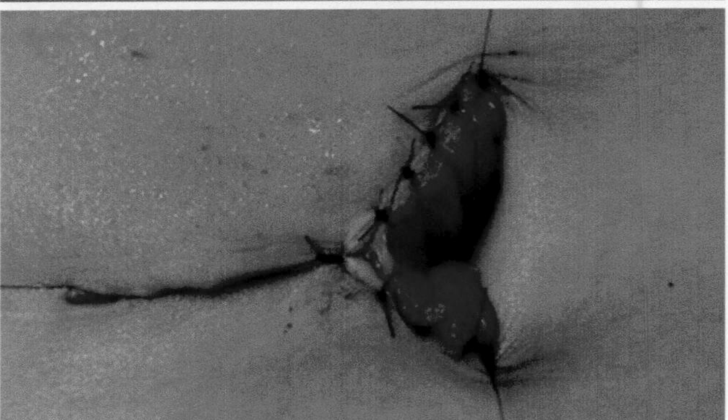

Fig. 20 The ureter is delivered through an inguinal incision, extraperitoneal approach. The "V" skin flap is sutured to the spatulated ureter

3.5 Outcomes

There are many publications describing the ureteral Mitrofanoff, all of them were done by open surgery. Van Savage et al. [21] have reported 12 cases; the ureteral conduit was catheterizable in 84% of patients compared to 94% for the appendix, and continence was achieved in 97%. Mor et al. [22] have reported a large series of 22 cases, 3 had stenosis and 5 had incontinent stoma, and only 1 needed replacement by the appendix. Pain at the bladder neck was reported in one patient. The largest series was reported by Radojicic et al. [23], 35 children had catheterizable reimplanted ureters, 3 needed stoma revision for stenosis, and 3 had incontinent stoma. Landa Juárez et al. [25] had reported laparoscopic ureteral Mitrofanoff associated with ureterocystoplasty in four children with excellent results for all of them.

Our experience with standard minimal invasive isolated ureteral Mitrofanoff is limited to eight cases. Six of them had retroperitoneoscopic nephrectomy associated with open extravesical and ureteral Mitrofanoff. The last two cases were done entirely by minimal invasive for high-grade refluxing ureter, one umbilical and the other one iliac (robotic). Our preliminary results, even limited to a few number of cases, are encouraging as none of our patients needed revision for stenosis or leak from the ureteral stoma after a mean follow-up of 23 months.

3.6 Conclusion

Robotic-assisted ureteral Mitrofanoff, in our limited experience, allowed us to combine nephrectomy and extravesical reimplantation in a single setting without the need of re-docking the robot in a multi-operated 14-year-old child. This minimal invasive procedure was efficient and can be applied in complex case with high-grade reflux. It is of specific interest in patients who are waiting for renal transplantation, and minimal invasive surgery would allow reduction of abdominal wall scaring.

The outlined simple technique and its favorable outcome provided in this chapter will hopefully assist surgeons in performing the robotic-assisted ureteral Mitrofanoff in very selected indications.

References

1. Gundeti MS, Boysen WR, Shah A. Robot-assisted laparoscopic extravesical ureteral reimplantation: technique modifications contribute to optimized outcomes. Eur Urol. 2016;70(5):818–23. https://doi.org/10.1016/j.eururo.2016.02.065.
2. Dangle PP, Razmaria AA, Towle VL, Frim DM, Gundeti MS. Is pelvic plexus nerve documentation feasible during robotic assisted laparoscopic ureteral reimplantation with extravesical approach? J Pediatr Urol. 2013;9(4):442–7. https://doi.org/10.1016/j.jpurol.2012.10.018.
3. Boysen WR, Ellison JS, Kim C, et al. Multi-institutional review of outcomes and complications of robot-assisted laparoscopic extravesical ureteral reimplantation for treatment of primary vesicoureteral reflux in children. J Urol. 2017;197(6):1555–61. https://doi.org/10.1016/j.juro.2017.01.062.
4. Boysen WR, Akhavan A, Ko J, et al. Prospective multicenter study on robot-assisted laparoscopic extravesical ureteral reimplantation (RALUR-EV): outcomes and complications. J Pediatr Urol. 2018;14(3):262.e1–6. https://doi.org/10.1016/j.jpurol.2018.01.020.
5. Casale P, Kojima Y. Robotic-assisted laparoscopic surgery in pediatric urology: an update. Scand J Surg. 2009;98(2):110–9.
6. Chacko JK, Koyle MA, Mingin GC, Furness PD. Ipsilateral ureteroureterostomy in the surgical management of the severely dilated ureter in ureteral duplication. J Urol. 2007;178(4):1689–1692.7.
7. Ewalt D, Glenski W, Bernier P. Ureterocele associated with ureteral duplication and a nonfunctioning upper pole segment: management by partial nephroureterectomy alone. J Urol. 1995;154(2):723–6.
8. Jelloul L, Valayer J. Ureteroureteral anastomosis in the treatment of reflux associated with ureteral duplication. J Urol. 1997;157(5):1863–5.
9. Merguerian PA, Taenzer A, Knoerlein K, McQuiston L, Herz D. Variation in management of duplex system intravesical ureteroceles: a survey of pediatric urologists. J Urol. 2010;184(4):1625–30.
10. Prieto J, Ziada A, Baker L, Snodgrass W. Ureteroureterostomy via inguinal incision for ectopic ureters and ureteroceles without ipsilateral lower pole reflux. J Urol. 2009;181(4):1844–50.
11. Foley F, Uretero-ureterostomy. As applied to the obstructions of the duplicated upper urinary tract. J Urol. 1928;20(1):109–20.
12. Kuss R. Chirurgie plastique et reparatrice de la vie excretice du rein. Indications et techniques operatoires. Masson et Ce Editeurs. 1954;1:98–103.
13. Lashley DB, McAleer IM, Kaplan GW. Ipsilateral ureteroureterostomy for the treatment of vesicoureteral reflux or obstruction associated with complete ureteral duplication. J Urol. 2001;165(2):552–4. https://doi.org/10.1097/00005392-200102000-00067.
14. Pantuck A, Barone J, Rosenfeld D, Fleisher M. Occult bilateral ectopicvaginal ureters causing urinary incontinence: diagnosis by computed tomography. Abdom Imaging. 1996;21(1):78–80.
15. Passerotti CC, Diamond DA, Borer JG, Eisner BH, Barrisford G, Nguyen HT. Robot-assisted laparoscopic ureteroureterostomy: description of technique. J Endourol. 2008;22(4):581–6.
16. Leavitt DA, Rambachan A, Haberman K, DeMarco R, Shukla AR. Robot-assisted laparoscopic ipsilateral ureteroureterostomy for ectopic ureters in children: description of technique. J Endourol. 2012;26(10):1279–83.
17. Lee NG, Corbett ST, Cobb K, Bailey GC, Burns AS, Peters CA. Bi-institutional comparison of robot-assisted laparoscopic versus open ureteroureterostomy in the pediatric population. J Endourol. 2015;29:1237–41. https://doi.org/10.1089/end.2015.0223.
18. Mitrofanoff P. Trans-appendicular continent cystostomy in the management of the neurogenic bladder. Chir Pediatr. 1980;21:297–305.
19. Monfort G, Guys JM, Morisson LG. Appendicovesicostomy: an alternative urinary diversion in the child. Eur Urol. 1984;10(6):361–3. https://doi.org/10.1159/000463833.
20. Ashcraft KW, Dennis PA. The reimplanted ureter as a catheterizing stoma. J Pediatr Surg. 1986;21(12):1042–5. https://doi.org/10.1016/0022-3468(86)90004-7.
21. Van Savage JG, Khoury AE, McLorie GA, Churchill BM. Outcome analysis of Mitrofanoff principle applications using appendix and ureter to umbilical and lower quadrant stomal sites. J Urol. 1996;156(5):1794–7. https://doi.org/10.1097/00005392-199611000-00094.
22. Mor Y, Kajbafzadeh AM, German K, Mouriquand PD, Duffy PG, Ransley PG. The role of ureter in the creation of Mitrofanoff channels in children. J Urol. 1997;157(2):635–7.
23. Radojicic ZI, Perovic SV, Vukadinovic VM, Bumbasirevic MZ. Refluxing megaureter for the Mitrofanoff channel using continent extravesical detrusor tunneling procedure. J Urol. 2005;174(2):693–5. https://doi.org/10.1097/01.ju.0000164747.90562.59.
24. Liard A, Séguier-Lipszyc E, Mathiot A, Mitrofanoff P. The Mitrofanoff procedure: 20 years later. J Urol. 2001;165(6 Pt 2):2394–8. https://doi.org/10.1097/00005392-200106001-00045.
25. Landa Juárez S, Fernández AM, Castro NR, De La Cruz YH, Hernández CG. Laparoscopic ureterocystoplasty with Mitrofanoff system. J Laparoendosc Adv Surg Tech A. 2014;24(6):422–7. https://doi.org/10.1089/lap.2013.0290. Epub 2014 Jan 29
26. Blanc T, Muller C, Pons M, Pashootan P, Paye-Jaouen A, El Ghoneimi A. Laparoscopic Mitrofanoff procedure in children: critical analysis of difficulties and benefits. J Pediatr Urol. 2015;11(1):28.e1–8.

Robotic Vaginoplasty, Urinary, and Bowel Continent Procedures (Bladder Neck Reconstruction and Continent Catheterizable Channels)

Tanya W. Kristof, Clark E. Judge, Tony Da Lomba, and Mohan S Gundeti

Abbreviations

APV	appendicovesicostomy
AUS	artificial urinary sphincter
BMG	Buccal mucosal grafts
CAID	complete androgen insensitivity syndrome
CCC	continent catheterizable channel
CIC	clean intermittent catheterization
DVT	deep vein thrombosis
MACE	Malone antegrade colonic enema
MRKH	Mayer-Rokitansky-Küster-Hauser
OT	operative time
PDS	polydioxanone
TAP	transverse abdominis plane
UO	ureteral orifice
VP	ventriculoperitoneal
YDL	Young-Dees-Leadbetter

1 Vaginoplasty

1.1 Patient Selection

Possible candidates for vaginoplasty include children born with Mayer-Rokitansky-Küster-Hauser syndrome (also known as congenital vaginal agenesis or Mullerian aplasia), complete androgen insensitivity syndrome (CAIS), and cloacal exstrophy or who are trans-female. These patients typically present in adolescence. For patients with MRKH syndrome, first-line treatment has historically been vaginal dilation, although in some European countries, the first-line treatment is surgery with graft or local flaps, followed by vaginal dilation [1]. Buccal mucosal grafts (BMG) are a viable option as well and are preferred by some surgeons [2]. In either case, vaginoplasty using a segment of bowel is historically only offered after a patient has failed first-line options. While vaginal reconstruction utilizing bowel has historically been performed open, a few case reports have described the robotic approach using sigmoid [3, 4] and ileum [5]. The robotic approach appears to be safe and effective for surgeons comfortable with robotics and bowel surgery.

Typically, the use of the sigmoid colon versus ileum for the neovagina is determined by which segment of bowel will reach into the pelvis while minimizing tension, although surgeon preference and comfort play a large factor as well. Using the sigmoid colon has the benefit of less mucus production (although it can still be bothersome), a more caudal location, and a more durable mucosa. Ileum has the advantage of a lower risk of diversion colitis [1]. Here, we describe our technique for robotic vaginoplasty with ileum in a patient with MRKH syndrome after previous failed dilatation and BMG vaginoplasty.

1.2 Preoperative Preparation

A complete history and physical should be done for every patient, noting especially prior abdominal and perineal surgery, as well as previous bowel surgery and overall body habitus. If a patient is undergoing the procedure as part of gender-affirming surgery, then the surgeon should be communicating with the patient's multidisciplinary team of physicians to ensure everyone is on the same page. Patients are not typically given a mechanical or oral antibiotic bowel preparation.

1.3 Positioning and Port Placement

The patient is positioned in the low lithotomy position with a Trendelenburg of 10–15 degrees and arms tucked at the side

Supplementary Information The online version contains supplementary material available at [https://doi.org/10.1007/978-3-031-00363-9_71].

T. W. Kristof · C. E. Judge (✉) · T. Da Lomba · M. S Gundeti
University of Chicago, Chicago, IL, USA

P. Wiklund et al. (eds.), *Robotic Urologic Surgery*, https://doi.org/10.1007/978-3-031-00363-9_71

with palms up to prevent ulnar nerve injury. Foam padding should be used on all pressure areas and on the face to prevent injury. A 12 mm blunt tip balloon trocar is used for the camera port. We use the Hassan technique for this initial port, placed just superior to the umbilicus to ensure a minimum 10–12 cm pubo-umbilical distance is maintained. If the distance is adequate, then umbilicus itself can be used for primary port. The left port is placed 4–8 cm lateral to the umbilicus, and the right arm is placed 5–10 cm lateral to the umbilicus, depending on the size of the patient and working space available. If there is enough working space, an additional third arm lateral to the right arm is beneficial for traction and countertraction. A 5 mm assistant port is placed in the left upper quadrant, which is equidistant from the camera and left working port (Fig. 1).

1.4 Surgical Steps

Perioperative antibiotics are administered within 1 h of incision to all patients. The patient is draped and a Foley catheter is placed in the sterile field. Local anesthetic injection into the port sites or a transverse abdominis plane (TAP) block should be used prior to incision of port sites. The camera port is then placed via the open Hassan technique. Pneumoperitoneum is established to 12 mmHg with a low flow rate (~2 L/min). A diagnostic peritoneoscopy is performed to assess for scar tissue and any other abnormalities. The remaining robotic arm ports and assistant ports are then placed under direct visualization. Initially, a fenestrated bipolar arm is used in the left arm and robotic scissors in the right arm.

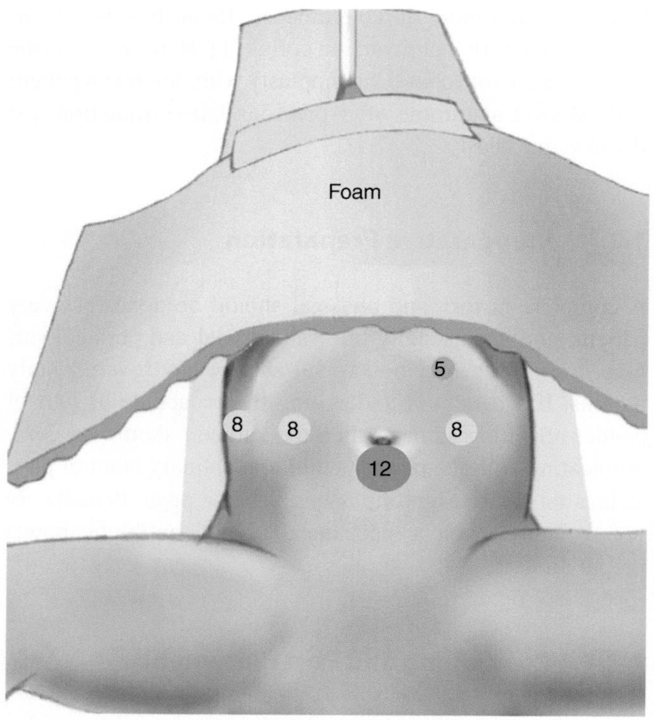

Fig. 1 Port placement for robotic vaginoplasty [5]

Attention is then turned to identification of the bowel segment that will become the neovagina. Using a marked piece of umbilical tape, a 10–15 cm segment of the terminal ileum is isolated. It is important that this is at least 15–20 cm proximal to the ileocecal valve and has good vascular pedicles. The ileal segment, however, also be able to reach down to the pelvis without too much tension. Once identified, a percutaneous stay suture is used to tack up the ileal segment on either end of the segment to be divided. Using the coagulation feature on the scissors, the ileum is divided at the proximal and distal ends. The corresponding mesentery is also divided. At this point, the robotic arms are replaced with needle driving robotic arms. Then, using a 4–0 PDS suture, the ileum is re-anastomosed in a single running layer, in an end-to-end fashion. The mesentery defect is also closed in a single running 4–0 PDS suture, making sure the future ileal neovagina is inferior to the re-anastomosed ileum. The ileal neovagina can also be harvested using an endo-GIA stapler if the surgeon is more comfortable with this modality.

Next, the abdominal end of the ileal neovagina is closed in a single running layer using 4–0 PDS suture. This step is not necessary if harvesting with the GIA stapler. The abdominal end of the ileal neovagina is then tacked to the posterior peritoneum to prevent prolapse. The neovagina should be temporarily brought down to its final pelvic location to ensure there is no mesenteric twisting. The fenestrated bipolar and robotic scissors are reinserted as the left and right arms, respectively. Attention is then turned to the peritoneum. A horizontal incision is created just posterior to the bladder using coagulation on the robotic scissors. Carefully paying attention to the rectum to prevent injury, the space between the rectum and bladder is then dissected. We retract the bladder anteriorly with a percutaneous stay suture. If there is significant scaring in this area due to a previous procedure, it can also be accessed with a Pfannenstiel incision and dissected in an open fashion.

Then the anastomosis is completed by dissecting from the vagina up to the robotic dissection area. The vaginal end of the ileal neovagina is elongated down to the posterior bladder dissection site (Fig. 2) and sutured to the labia minora by the hand from below to create the introital opening. We prefer 4–0 PDS suture for this step. In patients with previous graft or flaps, the vaginal end of the ileal neovagina is sutured to the previous graft from below (in our case, the existing BMG).

One of the robotic arm port sites can be used as a drain site. We place a 15fr Blake drain in the left arm port. The ports are all removed under direct visualization, and the fascia is closed using a 2–0 Vicryl stitch. The camera port is the last to be closed. The skin is then closed with subcutaneous and subcuticular suture and surgical glue. We do not leave a

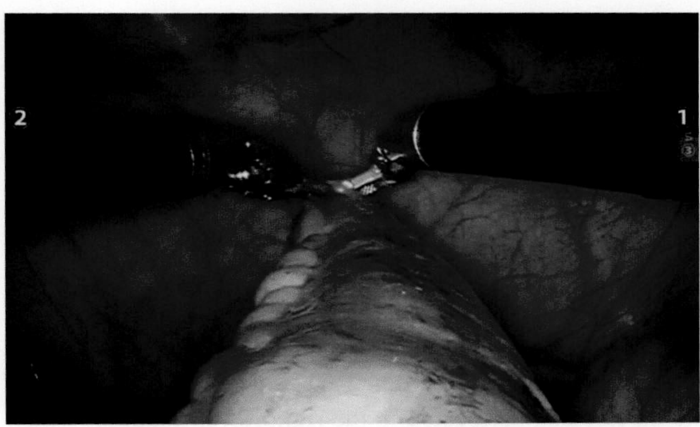

Fig. 2 Robotic view of assessing length of the ileal neovagina to ensure it reaches pelvic floor without mesenteric kinking or excess tension [5]

Table 1 Vaginoplasty brief surgical steps

• Low lithotomy with 10–15° Trendelenburg, arms tucked palms up
• Foley placed in sterile field
• Camera port supraumbilical, working aims 4–8 cm lateral, 5 mm assistant port in LUQ
• Fenestrated bipolar left arm, robotic scissors right arm
• Identify 10–15 cm segment of terminal ileum for neovagina—15 cm from ileocecal valve
• Divide ileum us well us corresponding mesentery
• Replace both arms with needle drivers
• Re-anastomose ileum
• Close abdominal end of ileal neovagina as well us mesenteric defect
• Replace fenestrated bipolar and robotic scissors
• Horizontal incision posterior to bladder and dissect down to vaginal opening
• Pull ileal neovagina down to vaginal opening and suture from below
• Remove ports under direct visualization, close fascia, leave a blake drain
• Pack neovagina with burrier ointment coated gauze

mold in the neovagina but do pack the area lightly with barrier ointment-coated gauze. A summary of the surgical steps is available in the following table (Table 1).

1.5 Postoperative Care

The Foley is maintained for 3–5 days postoperatively. The drain is removed prior to discharge so long as the output is less than 100 cc per day. Triple antibiotics are given for 24–48 h post-op. The vaginal pack is removed after 48–72 h. Routine postoperative care after robotic surgery applies to this pediatric population, including early diet advancement, limiting of narcotics, and early ambulation. After 4–6 weeks, an exam under anesthesia is performed to ensure proper healing and to assess appropriate graduated dilator size. Then graduated dilators are used to maintain introital opening patency for those not sexually active. Postoperative care should consist of occupational therapists, social workers, and a care coordinator to support the patient and caregivers.

1.6 Outcomes and Complications

Literature regarding the outcomes of vaginoplasty is heterogeneous, with many studies describing the procedure in the transgender and cloaca patient populations, in addition to those with MKRH syndrome and CAIS. For patients with MKRH syndrome or CAIS, open intestinal vaginoplasty has historically had good results with modest complication rates.

Lima et al. reported a series of 47 patients with mixed MKRH syndrome, CAIS, adrenogenital syndrome, and penile agenesis. Forty-six of the patients had vaginoplasty with sigmoid colon and one with ileum. All patients reported satisfactory aesthetics, but there was a significant complication profile. One patient had sigmoid flap necrosis, 8 (17%) patients had introital stenosis, 4 (8%) patients had neovagina prolapse, and 2 (4%) patients developed bowel obstructions. In total, 30% of patients required reoperation. Duration of follow-up was for a mean of 34 months (4–72 months) [6]. Karateke et al. published a series of 29 patients (27 sigmoid, 2 ileum) with MKRH syndrome with similarly high satisfaction rates, but a lower complication rate. One patient had a rectal injury intraoperatively, one patient with an ileal neovagina had bowel necrosis requiring an ileostomy, and two patients had wound infections. Notably, 52% (15/29) of patients had introital stenosis, but all of them resolved with finger dilation and none required reoperation [7]. For comparison, in the transgender population, the incidence of rectal injury ranges from 0.4 to 4.5% and introital stenosis from 2 to 12%, although this is thought to be directly correlated to cessation of manual dilation [8]. There are no comparable outcomes from robotic-assisted vaginoplasty to compare these to as there are only single case reports.

2 Continent Catheterizable Channels

Robotic-assisted laparoscopic approach for complex pediatric urologic cases such as continent catheterizable channels (CCCs) is increasingly being studied and improved. CCCs are utilized for the treatment of bladder and bowel dysfunction. Bladder dysfunction is most commonly secondary to neuropathic bladder from etiologies such as myelodysplasias, sacral agenesis, tethered cord, bladder exstrophy, prune belly syndrome, and trauma. Patients with a neuropathic bladder can have an array of medical consequences such as renal function deterioration and social consequences such as urinary incontinence. Additionally, if patients or their caregiver are not able to easily and adequately empty the bladder, the patients are at risk of urinary tract infections and bladder stones. Patients often utilize medical management first with or without clean intermittent catheterization (CIC). While CIC is an option for social continence in patients with incomplete emptying with or without an augmented bladder, using a CCC can be more comfortable for the patients than urethral catheterization and can decrease the rate of false passages and urethral strictures.

One type of CCC is the appendicovesicostomy (APV), first described by Mitrofanoff in 1980, which utilizes the appendix through a detrusor tunnel for a non-refluxing and convenient way to empty the bladder [9]. The model CCC is short and straight with a good blood supply, and the appendix is an ideal length and width for catheterization. The appendix has minimal function in digestion and elimination, making bowel recovery easy with a low risk of metabolic side effects. The first laparoscopic APV was described in 1993 and involved laparoscopic mobilization of the colon to reach the appendix followed by open anastomosis of the appendix to the bladder via a lower abdomen incision [10]. Hsu and Pedraza were among the first to complete the APV with a robotic-assisted laparoscopic procedure in 2004 [11, 12].

When no appendix is available or suitable for an APV, a tubularized 2 cm segment of ileum can be reconfigured into a Yang-Monti channel. This channel is a smaller caliber, longer intestinal tube adequate for catheterization. First described by Yang in 1993 and Monti in 1997, the Yang-Monti CCC is more technically challenging than APV but can provide additional length compared to the appendix [13, 14]. This was later modified by Casale et al. to create even more length, where a 3.5 cm segment of the ileum is partially transected to form a Z-shaped plate that is then re-tubularized to create a "spiral Monti" [15]. Two side-by-side Yang-Monti channels anastomosed together are called a "double Monti."

Similar to bladder incontinence, fecal incontinence negatively impacts pediatric quality of life. Underlying diseases that may cause negative fecal effects include anorectal malformations, Hirschsprung's disease, spina bifida, spinal injuries, cerebral palsy, and neuropathic disorders that are similar to those that cause neurogenic bladder. While initial dietary management and timed evacuation with a mix of stool softeners, laxatives, and/or bulking agents are used, many patients will require enemas for adequate colonic evacuation. Rectal administration of laxatives and enemas can be uncomfortable for the patients, requires increased caregiver demand, and can affect patient's independence long term. The Malone antegrade colonic enema (MACE) is a catheterizable channel that gives an alternative way to administer enemas to patients with neurogenic bowel. First introduced in 1990, a MACE provides a non-refluxing intestinal conduit for antegrade enema administration through the cecum [16, 17]. Although originally described by Malone to transect and reverse the appendix, most perform an orthotopic appendicovesicostomy, taking care to preserve the native appendiceal blood supply. Some of the first robotic MACE surgeries were reported by Lendvay et al. [18] and Thakre et al. [19].

Stoma site selection for any CCC depends on patient characteristics such as length of channel created, body habitus, and patient preference, as well as surgeon preference and experience. The stoma can be hidden in the umbilicus, which has the advantage of easy accessibility above the pant line as well as the minimal adipose tissue. However, there may be a longer intra-abdominal course with umbilical stomas. The stoma can also be located in the right lower quadrant which may have a shorter intraperitoneal course but is less hidden.

Additional CCCs have been described, including the use of ureter and bladder. However, these channels have a high rate of complication such as stricture or stenosis and a high rate of reoperation. These procedures are less common and will not be described in this chapter.

Goals of catheterizable channels for bladder management include urine drainage, renal protection, continence, and cosmesis. These channels are more convenient and socially acceptable for many patients, and it has been shown to increase patient compliance with a CIC regimen. A channel that can easily accommodate a 12–14F catheter is ideal. Goals of CCC for bowel management include predictability in timing of passing bowels, reducing constipation, independence with bowel regiments, and/or reducing fecal incontinent episodes. The use of robotic surgery for the creation of CCC prioritizes patient outcomes such as length of stay and faster bowel recovery. However, the use of robotics in the pediatric population must accommodate smaller working spaces and a high learning curve. Here, we describe our techniques for common robotic-assisted laparoscopic continent catheterizable channels in the pediatric population.

3 Anatomy of the Ileocecal and Appendiceal Region

The ileocecal valve lies at the junction of the ileum and the cecum, where insertion of the ileum forms a right angle to the cecum approximately 2 cm above the insertion of the appendix and just medial to the mesocolic tenia (Fig. 3). The terminal ileum intussuscepts 2–3 cm into the cecal lumen as a papilla, pushing the apex of the valve and the appendix to the left. The valve itself is two-layered, formed by continuation of the circular and longitudinal muscle of the cecal wall. This forms a papilla that is supplemented by complex veins and serves as a pressure equalizing valve to prevent reflux of cecal contents back into the ileum.

The vermiform appendix varies in length but is approximately 9 cm and is attached to the cecum 2 cm below the ileocecal junction. It is held by a triangular mesoappendix to

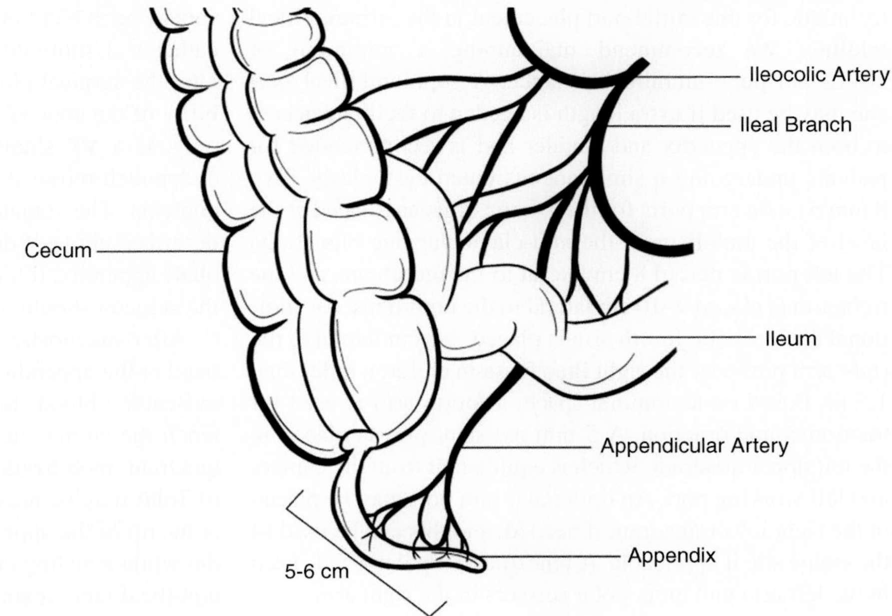

Fig. 3 Anatomy of the appendix and surrounding structure

the terminal part of the ileal mesentery. The appendix has four layers—mucous, submucous, muscular, and serous.

The ileocolic artery, a branch off the superior mesenteric artery, gives rise to the ascending colic artery, ileal artery, appendicular artery, and anterior and posterior cecal arteries and provides the bloody supply to the ileocecal and appendiceal regions. The appendicular artery may alternatively come from the cecal artery. The base of the appendix may be supplied by the anterior or cecal arteries as well. The ascending colic artery supplies the first part of the ascending colon.

4 Appendicovesicostomy

4.1 Patient Selection

Patient selection is critical for any CCC. An APV is used for bladder emptying when this cannot consistently be done via the native urethra. Patients must have a healthy appendix of reasonable length. The patient or a reliable caregiver must be able to perform catheterizations with adequate dexterity and consistency. Patients with a progressive neurologic condition should be counseled that long-term catheterization strategies may be adjusted pending their clinical course and upper motor dexterity. Specific to the robotic approach, multiple abdominal surgeries, ventriculoperitoneal (VP) shunt, and severe kyphoscoliosis may increase the likelihood of conversion to an open procedure due to extensive adhesions and difficulty achieving adequate pneumoperitoneum. Patients and their caregivers should be extensively counseled on the indications, operative expectations, and postoperative course prior to embarking on this procedure. Depending on the patient's bladder urodynamic findings, this procedure may be done in conjunction with an enterocystoplasty and/or bladder neck reconstruction for those with diminished bladder capacity and poor bladder compliance and/or bothersome urinary leakage.

4.2 Preoperative Preparation

A complete history and physical should be done for every patient, noting especially prior bowel surgery, prior abdominal surgery, and body habitus. A stoma site should be premarked accounting for patient's dexterity, body habitus, and abdominal folds. The umbilicus is often chosen due to relative absence of the adipose tissue and for overall aesthetic appearance. Patients are not typically given a mechanical or oral antibiotic bowel preparation. A preoperative urine culture is obtained, as it is important to treat any concomitant urinary tract infection prior to surgery. There is no role for radiologic studies for identification of the appendix.

4.3 Positioning and Port Placement

The patient is placed in low dorsal lithotomy position with a Trendelenburg of 10–15 degrees and arms tucked at the side. Foam padding should be used on all pressure areas and on the face to prevent injury. The patient is draped and a Foley catheter should be placed in the sterile field. Local anesthetic into the port sites or a TAP block should be used prior to incision of port sites. Ports include a 12 mm blunt tip balloon trocar for the camera port. We prefer utilization of the Hassan technique for this initial port placement in the infraumbilical midline. We recommend maintaining a minimum of 10–12 cm pubo-umbilical distance. A supraumbilical port site may be used if extra length is needed to facilitate access to both the appendix and bladder and is recommended for patients undergoing a simultaneous enterocystoplasty. Two 8 mm robotic arm ports for the robotic arms are placed at the level of the umbilicus in the mid-clavicular line bilaterally. The left port is placed 8 cm lateral to the umbilicus, and the right arm is placed 9–10 cm lateral to the umbilicus. An additional 8 cm robotic fourth arm is placed 7–8 cm lateral to the right arm port near the right iliac fossa in children taller than 1.5 m. Based on abdominal space, a fourth arm is used for traction/countertraction. A 5 mm assistant port is placed in the left upper quadrant, which is equidistant from the camera and left working port. An optional 5 mm port may be placed in the right lower quadrant if needed, and this can be used as the stoma site if applicable. A fenestrated bipolar arm is used in the left arm and monopolar scissors in the right arm.

4.4 Surgical Steps

Perioperative antibiotics are administered within 1 h of incision to all patients, generally cefazolin, gentamicin, and metronidazole. Vancomycin is used instead of cefazolin if a VP shunt is present. The Foley is placed. The 12 mm trocar is placed with an open Hassan technique. Pneumoperitoneum is established to 12 mmHg. A diagnostic peritoneoscopy is performed to identify the location and length of the appendix and its associated mesentery. In patients with a history of previous abdominal surgery or with a history of a VP shunt, pure laparoscopy may be useful for adequate adhesiolysis and peritoneoscopy prior to robot docking. The appendix should be 5–6 cm in length and able to accommodate a 10F catheter at minimum. The surgeon should be prepared to alter the surgical plan based on the appearance and accessibility of the appendix in accordance with the patient's anatomy. If a VP shunt is present, this can be placed in an endopouch retrieval bag to avoid contamination with bowel contents. The remaining robotic arms should be placed as described above if diagnostic peritoneoscopy shows an adequate appendix. If a Yang-Monti channel is indicated instead, the surgeon should alter the surgical approach as needed.

After diagnostic peritoneoscopy, the appendix is mobilized at the appendicular/cecal junction, keeping in mind its mesenteric blood supply. If the mesentery is too superior to reach the stoma site either at the umbilicus or right lower quadrant, mobilization of the ascending colon along the line of Toldt may be necessary (Fig. 4a). A stay suture is placed at the tip of the appendix to facilitate handling of the appendix while avoiding crush injury to the tissue. A premeasured umbilical tape or suture is used to intracorporeally measure the appendix. The appendix is then transected sharply using endoscissors (Fig. 4b). It can be helpful to make a window between the mesentery and cecum to preserve adequate mesenteric blood supply to the appendix. The addition of a cecal flap may reduce the risk of stomal stenosis and provide additional channel length. A cecal flap should be utilized for an appendix <4 cm to lengthen the appendix. The colonic defect is closed in one seromuscular layer using 4–0 or 5–0 PDS. Of note, if a concurrent MACE (described below) is indicated and the appendix is sufficiently long (10–12 cm), use the proximal 2–4 cm of the appendix for the ACE channel and the remaining distal appendix and its mesentery for the APV. If the appendix is short and a concurrent MACE is indicated, it is appropriate to use the appendix for the APV, and to perform a cecal flap tubularization for the MACE. If

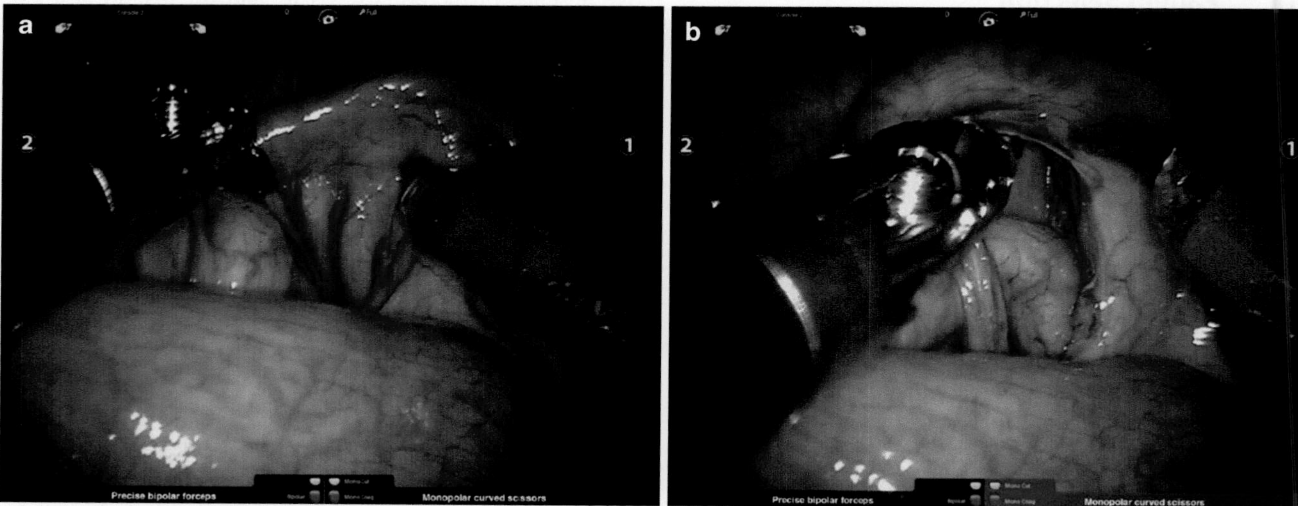

Fig. 4 (**a**) Mobilization of the appendix [20]. (**b**). Isolation of the appendix [20]

splitting the appendix between a MACE and APV, maintain vasculature for the APV as the proximal appendiceal stump can often be sustained via the colonic blood supply.

If no additional procedures are to be performed, the anterior aspect of the bladder is chosen for the anastomotic site with an extravesical approach (Fig. 4). This is technically easier than the posterior wall of the bladder and shortens the required length of the appendix. Utilization of a Keith needle to retract and the bladder dome can be helpful for visualization. The bladder is distended with 60–200 mL of sterile saline via the Foley catheter, with volumes depending on the patient's bladder capacity. A detrusorotomy is performed with electrocautery, taking care not to violate the bladder mucosa (Fig. 5). A 4 cm detrusorotomy is recommended for adequate anti-refluxing continence outcomes [17, 21, 22]. As the bladder physiologically fills, the intraluminal pressure in the channel along the 4 cm tunneling increases and compresses the channel, resulting in a lack of flow and a continence mechanism. The detrusorotomy is done in the midline bladder wall in a craniocaudal orientation if an umbilical stoma is to be performed. If a right lower quadrant stoma is desired, this may be carried out on the right posterolateral wall of the bladder in an oblique orientation.

The distal 1 cm tip of the appendix should be transected and spatulated using Potts scissors to produce an adequate lumen in preparation for the anastomosis to the bladder (Fig. 6). The first anastomotic suture is placed at the caudal apex of the detrusorotomy and then through the spatulated apical end of the distal tip of the appendix with 5–0 PDS (polydioxanone) suture. We recommend the use of black diamond robotic needle drivers as these allow facile manipulation of small needles and suture material. The bladder mucosa can then be incised 1 cm in length. The crotch of the spatulation is then anchored to the cranial end of the 1 cm defect in the bladder mucosa, opposite the apical stitch. An 8F feeding tube is placed through the appendix and into the bladder, and the appendicovesical anastomosis is completed

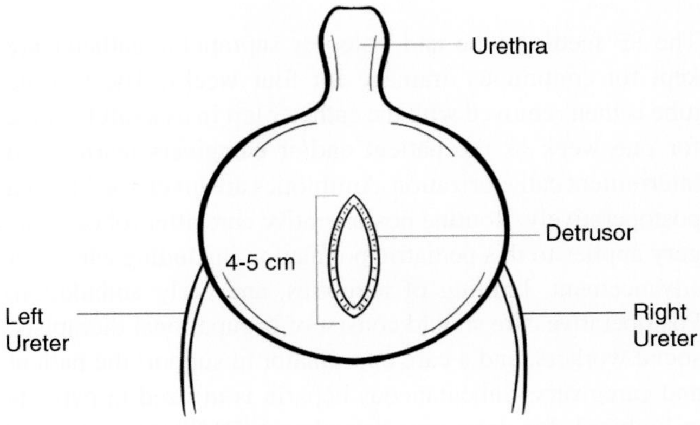

Fig. 5 Transection and spatulation of the appendix

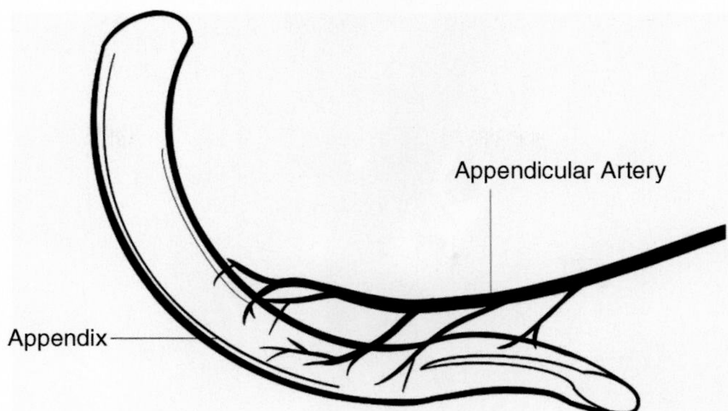

Fig. 6 Detrusor tunnel creation for the appendicovesicostomy anterior approach

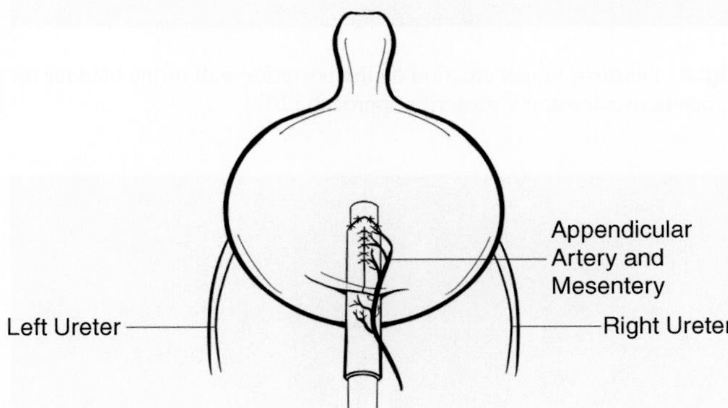

Fig. 7 Appendiceal anastomosis and detrusor imbrication for appendicovesicostomy anterior approach

with 4–0 PDS suture using an interrupted suture technique. The feeding tube can be sutured in place with absorbable suture to prevent migration. The appendix is then placed in the previously incised 4 cm trough, and the detrusor is imbricated over it with running 4–0 PDS suture. The APV is now ready to be brought to the skin surface for maturation (Fig. 7).

If performing a simultaneous bladder augmentation enterocystoplasty, a posterior wall with intravesical approach may be used. A cystotomy is performed on the posterior aspect of the bladder wall using electrocautery. The ureteral orifices are noted to avoid injury during tunneling. A stay stitch is then placed on the posterior wall of the bladder to ease manipulation. Electrocautery is used to make a small hiatus in the posterior bladder wall where the appendix will penetrate the bladder wall. A 4 cm submucosal tunnel is then made through which the appendix will be placed (Fig. 8). This may be especially difficult in a thick-walled bladder seen in many neurogenic bladder patients. A larger mucosal opening may be made to ease the dissection, which is later closed after the appendix is placed in the tunnel. Once tunneling is complete, the appendix is brought through the bladder wall and into the submucosal tunnel (Fig. 9). A 5–0 PDS suture is used to anchor the distal appendix and close the

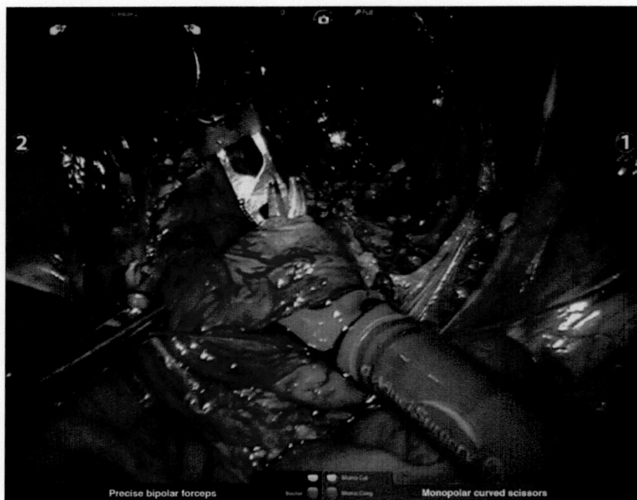

Fig. 8 Detrusor tunnel creation on the posterior wall of the bladder for appendicovesicostomy posterior approach [20]

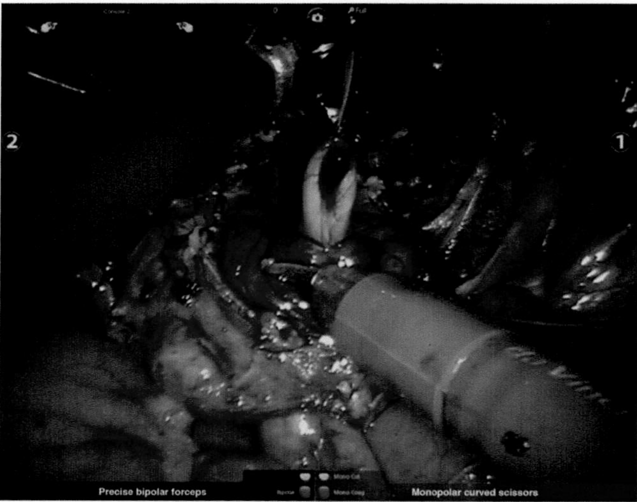

Fig. 9 Tunneling of the appendix through the detrusor muscle for implantation [20]

bladder mucosa. The distal appendix is then spatulated to open the lumen, and the crotch of the spatulation is anchored to the opposite end. An 8F feeding tube is then placed through the appendix and into the bladder, and the appendicovesical anastomosis is completed with 4–0 PDS suture using an interrupted suture technique (Fig. 10). The feeding tube can be sutured in place with absorbable suture to ensure it stays in place. Once the anastomosis is complete, the defect in the bladder mucosa should be closed. The serosa of the appendix can be incorporated in this closure to prevent migration of the channel. The completed tunnel is again measured using the pre-marked umbilical tape. Once the augmentation enterocystoplasty is performed, the APV is ready to be brought to the skin surface.

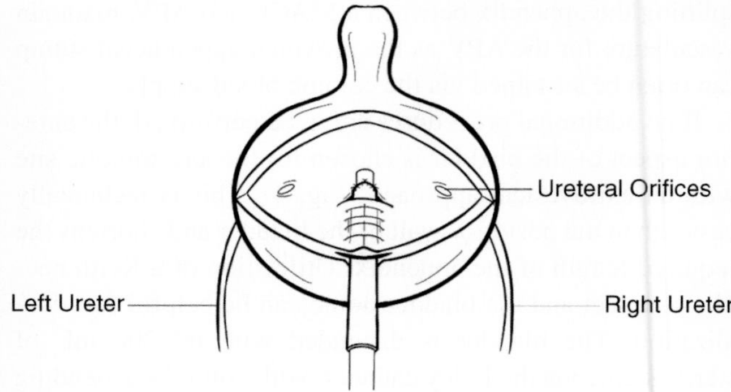

Fig. 10 Appendiceal intravesical anastomosis and detrusor imbrication for appendicovesicostomy posterior approach

If a Foley catheter is not used, a suprapubic catheter should be placed using Seldinger technique. If a concomitant augmentation is performed, dual catheter use is recommended. The proximal end of the appendix, with or without a cecal cuff, is brought through the umbilical port site or the right lower quadrant site using the respective port sites, taking care to ensure a straight trajectory from the bladder to skin. Appendix fixation to the abdominal wall is not necessary as no posterior support to the channel is needed. Stoma creation is done by spatulating the appendix and performing a cutaneous anastomosis via a V-, VQ-, or VQZ-flap. The remaining skin is approximated with interrupted 5–0 PDS sutures, and an 8F feeding tube is placed and secured to the stitch with the previous suture.

If an endopouch was used to hold the VP shunt, this should be removed. The ports are all removed and the fascia closed using a 2–0 Vicryl stitch under direct vision. The camera port is the last to be closed. The skin is then closed with subcutaneous and subcuticular suture and surgical glue. A summary of the surgical steps is available in the following table (Table 2).

4.5 Postoperative Care

The 8F feeding tube and Foley or suprapubic catheter are kept for continuous drainage for four weeks. The feeding tube is then removed with the catheter left in as a safety valve for one week as the patient and/or caregivers learn clean intermittent catheterization. Antibiotics are given for 24–48 h postoperatively. Routine postoperative care after robotic surgery applies to this pediatric population, including early diet advancement, limiting of narcotics, and early ambulation. Postoperative care should consist of occupational therapists, social workers, and a care coordinator to support the patient and caregivers. Subcutaneous heparin is utilized in patients at high risk for deep vein thrombosis (DVT), such as high BMI or immobility.

Table 2 Appendicovesicostomy (APV) brief surgical steps

• Low lithotomy with 10–15° Trendelenburg, arms tucked palms up
• Camera port supraumbilical, working arms 8 cm lateral, 4th arm 7–8 cm lateral to right arm near iliac fossa, 5 mm assistant port in RUQ
• Appendicular identification and mobilization. Taken with a cecal cuff if needed. Length should be 5–6 cm
• Cecal defect closure with 4- or 5–0 PDS suture
• Bladder detrusor anterior tunnel creation (if no augmentation enterocystoplasty) • Fill bladder with 60–200 cc saline depending on bladder capacity • Using electrocautery, incise detrusor to expose bladder mucosa, at least 4 cm (for continence) • Spatulate the distal appendix and incise the bladder mucosa 1 cm • Complete appendicovesical anastomosis with 4–0 PDS interrupted sutures over an 8F feeding tube • Place appendix in previously incised 4 cm trough and imbricate detrusor muscle over it with 4–0 PDS suture
• Bladder detrusor posterior tunnel creation (if concurrent augmentation entcrocystoplasty) • Using electrocautery, a cystotomy is performed on posterior wall of the bladder • Identify bilateral ureteral orifices • Using electrocautery, make a small hiatus for the appendicovesical anastomosis • Create a 4 cm submucosal tunnel and place appendix in the tunnel • Spatulate and suture distal appendix to bladder mucosa with 4–0 PDS interrupted sutures over an 8F feeding tube • Close the bladder mucosal defect
• Bring proximal appendix to umbilical or RLQ port sites
• Stoma maturation: create stoma by spatulating appendix and perform cutaneous flap anastomosis
• Secure 8F feeding tube with a stitch
• Remove ports, close fascia with 2–0 vicryl under direct vision and perform skin closure.

4.6 Outcomes and Complications

Data and outcomes of robotic-assisted laparoscopic APV are limited to retrospective series and single-center studies without case-controlled or randomized trials. Early outcomes support the safety and efficacy of this procedure with results comparable to the open approach. The robotic approach results in decreased days to return to diet compared to the open approach (4 vs 6 days) and a 50% reduction in the length of hospital stay (6.8 vs 13 days). While there is a longer operative time (OT) for the robotic approach overall, if no bladder augment is necessary and an extravesical anastomosis may be performed, the OT is similar [20].

Continence rates are comparable to the open approach, ranging from 91 to 95% continence compared to the quoted 91–98% continence with the open approach [20, 23–27]. Patients with postoperative urinary incontinence may have had a shorter tunneling length or have elevated bladder pressures. If a patient has elevated bladder pressures, management with anticholinergic medications, intravesical Botox therapy, or consideration of an augmented enteroplasty is warranted. For those with a short tunnel length, injection with dextranomer/hyaluronic acid (Deflux) often successfully achieves social continence for these patients.

Other important functional outcomes and complications for Mitrofanoff appendicovesicostomy include stomal stenosis, stomal prolapse, channel stricture, and false passage formation. Difficulty with catheterization can be due to stomal stenosis, channel redundancy, or awkward angulation of the channel. If stomal stenosis begins to occur and the patient or caregiver stops catheterizing, there is a risk of complete obliteration of the channel. Maintaining an open bladder neck allows for a safety valve in case of high bladder pressures or inability to catheterize. There is a 17–40% overall complication rate with a 5–28% surgical revision rate for Mitrofanoff appendicovesicostomy [28–30]. Stomal stenosis occurs in 5–10% of patients utilizing the robotic approach, which includes suprafascial and subfascial stenosis. Retrospective data indicates that there is no difference in complication rates between the open and robotic approaches [31].

5 Yang-Monti

5.1 Patient Selection

A Yang-Monti ileovesicostomy is used for the same indications as an APV but for patients who lack an appendix or the appendix cannot be used. For example, if the appendix length is too short even with a cecal flap or if the patient's body habitus is quite large, a Yang-Monti can provide the necessary additional length. The ileum is a preferred channel material due to its redundant physiologic nature and low complication rates. Like any CCC, a candidate for the Yang-Monti must have adequate dexterity for self-catheterization or have a reliable caregiver to do so. Patients and their caregivers should be extensively counseled on the indications, operative expectations, and postoperative course prior to embarking on this procedure. If a simultaneous bladder augmentation enterocystoplasty is performed, the Yang-Monti can be constructed from adjacent bowel for a single bowel anastomosis.

5.2 Preoperative Preparation

A complete history and physical should be done for every patient, noting prior bowel surgery, prior abdominal surgery, history of abdominal radiation, history of inflammatory bowel disease, and body habitus. A stoma site should be premarked accounting for patient's dexterity, body habitus, and abdominal folds. The umbilicus is often chosen due to relative absence of the adipose tissue and for cosmesis. Patients are not typically given a mechanical or oral antibiotic bowel preparation. A preoperative urine culture is obtained, as it is important to treat any concomitant urinary tract infection prior to surgery.

5.3 Positioning and Port Placement

The patient is placed in low dorsal lithotomy position with a Trendelenburg of 10–15 degrees and arms tucked at the side. Foam padding should be used on all pressure areas and on the face to prevent injury. The patient is draped and a Foley catheter should be placed in the sterile field. Local anesthetic into the port sites or a transverse abdominis plane (TAP) block should be used prior to incision of port sites. Ports include a 12 mm blunt tip balloon trocar for the camera port in the supraumbilical position. Two 8 mm robotic arm ports for the robotic arms are placed at the level of the umbilicus in the mid-clavicular line bilaterally. The left port is placed 8 cm lateral to the umbilicus, and the right arm is placed 9–10 cm lateral to the umbilicus. A 5 mm assistant port is placed in the left upper quadrant, which is equidistant from the camera and left working port. An additional 8 cm robotic fourth arm is placed 7–8 cm lateral to the right arm port in children taller than 1.5 m. Alternatively, an optional 5 mm working port may be placed in the right lower quadrant, and this can be used as the stoma site if applicable. A fenestrated bipolar arm is used in the left arm and monopolar scissors in the right arm.

5.4 Surgical Steps

Perioperative antibiotics are administered within 1 h of incision to all patients, generally cefazolin, gentamicin, and metronidazole. Vancomycin may be used instead of cefazolin if a VP shunt is present. Of note, if a VP shunt is present, this can be placed in an endopouch retrieval bag to avoid contamination with bowel contents. The Foley is placed. The 12 mm trocar is placed with an open Hassan technique. Pneumoperitoneum is established to 12 mmHg. The remaining robotic arms should be placed as described above.

A 2–3 cm segment of bowel, usually the ileum, is isolated on its mesentery. This segment should be at minimum 15–20 cm proximal to the ileocecal junction. A 2.0–2.5 cm segment of bowel will usually result in a tube of 6–7 cm in length when tubularized transversely (Fig. 11a). Using electrocautery, transect the segment of the ileum. Maintain adequate enteric blood supply by identifying and preserving the vascular arcades supplying the bowel segment. If a simultaneous augmentation enterocystoplasty or neobladder creation is to be performed, the Yang-Monti segment should be harvested from an adjacent section of the bowel in order to eliminate the need for an additional bowel anastomosis (Fig. 11).

The bowel is then opened longitudinally along its antimesenteric border with electrocautery scissors (Fig. 11b). Stay sutures may be placed on either end to facilitate easier handling and suturing. It is then re-tubularized transversely in two layers with absorbable suture (Fig. 11c). We recommend using running suture technique for the center of the channel and interrupted sutures on each end so that adjustments to channel length can be made without compromising the integrity of the closure.

The ileovesical anastomosis, stoma location and maturation, and skin closure are the same as the robotic APV procedure described earlier in this chapter (Fig. 11d). The use of a 14F Foley catheter in the new channel and either a urethral Foley or a suprapubic catheter is used. If an endopouch was used to hold the VP shunt, this should be removed. The ports are all removed and the fascia closed using a 2–0 Vicryl stitch under direct vision. The camera port is the last to be closed. The skin is then closed with subcutaneous and subcuticular suture and surgical glue.

5.5 Double Monti

If a longer channel than 6–7 cm is required, a double Monti may be performed. This involves two consecutive Monti segments as described above sutured together to form a 10–12 cm channel. The bowel segments should be incised near the mesentery to create a short side and a long side relative to the mesentery. The short sides can then be sutured together so that the mesenteric blood supply to the channel is in the middle of the channel, providing adequate length and maneuverability for the bladder and skin anastomoses.

5.6 Spiral Monti

An alternative to the double Monti is the spiral Monti. This uses a 3.5–4 cm segment of bowel isolated on its mesentery in the customary fashion (Fig. 12a). The segment is transversely divided in half for 80% of its circumference generally in the middle of the bowel segment, preserving the strip of bowel over the mesentery (Fig. 12b–c). There are then two "halves" of the bowel segment. The first segment is incised longitudinally near the mesentery on one side. The second segment is incised longitudinally near the mesentery on the opposite side (Fig. 12d–e). After unfolding the bowel, the middle corners along the mesentery are sutured together in the middle of the new spiral Monti tube (Fig. 12f–g). The resulting strips of bowel are sutured as previously described (Fig. 12h). A summary of the surgical steps is available in the following table (Table 3).

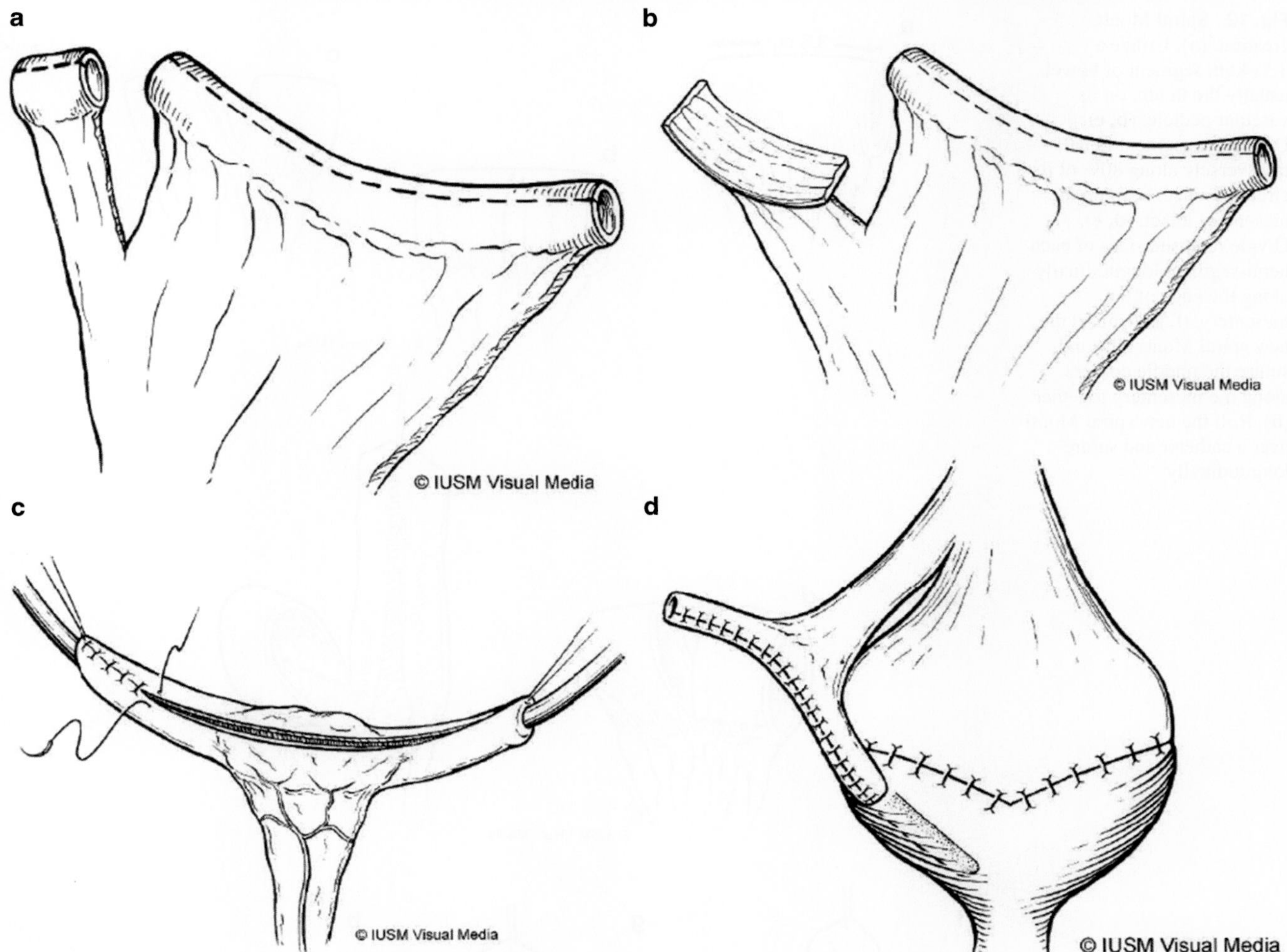

Fig. 11 Isolation and retubularization of a segment of the ileum. Shown with concomitant ileocystoplasty. (**a**). A 2.5–3 cm segment of bowel is isolated on a vascular pedicle adjacent to the segment of bowel being utilized for ileocystoplasty. (**b**). The Monti tube is opened longitudinally on the anti-mesenteric border. (**c**). The distal ends of the tube are sutured to create a longer channel with the mesentery in the middle. Complete this over a catheter. (**d**). Anastomose the Monti channel to the bladder with a minimum of 4 cm of the detrusor muscle imbricated over as an antirefluxing mechanism

5.7 Postoperative Care

The 14F catheter in the ileovesicostomy channel and the urethral Foley or suprapubic catheter are kept for continuous drainage for four weeks. The 14F catheter is then removed from the ileovesicostomy with the urethral Foley or suprapubic catheter left in as a safety valve for one week as the patient and/or caregivers learn clean intermittent catheterization. Antibiotics are given for 24–48 h postoperatively. Routine postoperative care after robotic surgery applies to this pediatric population, including early diet advancement, limiting of narcotics, and early ambulation. Postoperative care should consist of occupational therapists, social workers, and a care coordinator to support the patient and caregivers. Subcutaneous heparin is utilized in patients at high risk for DVT, such as high BMI or immobility.

5.8 Outcomes and Complications

Similar to APV, the Yang-Monti ileovesicostomy is safe and effective in both the open and robotic approaches [20]. Continence rates are similar to APV at around 95%. The advantages of robotic surgery of faster return to diet and decreased hospital length of stay are applicable to the Monti procedure as well. Unlike the APV, there is a bowel anastomosis, typically in the ileum, which has an increased risk of bowel leak and complication rates compared to the use of the appendix [32].

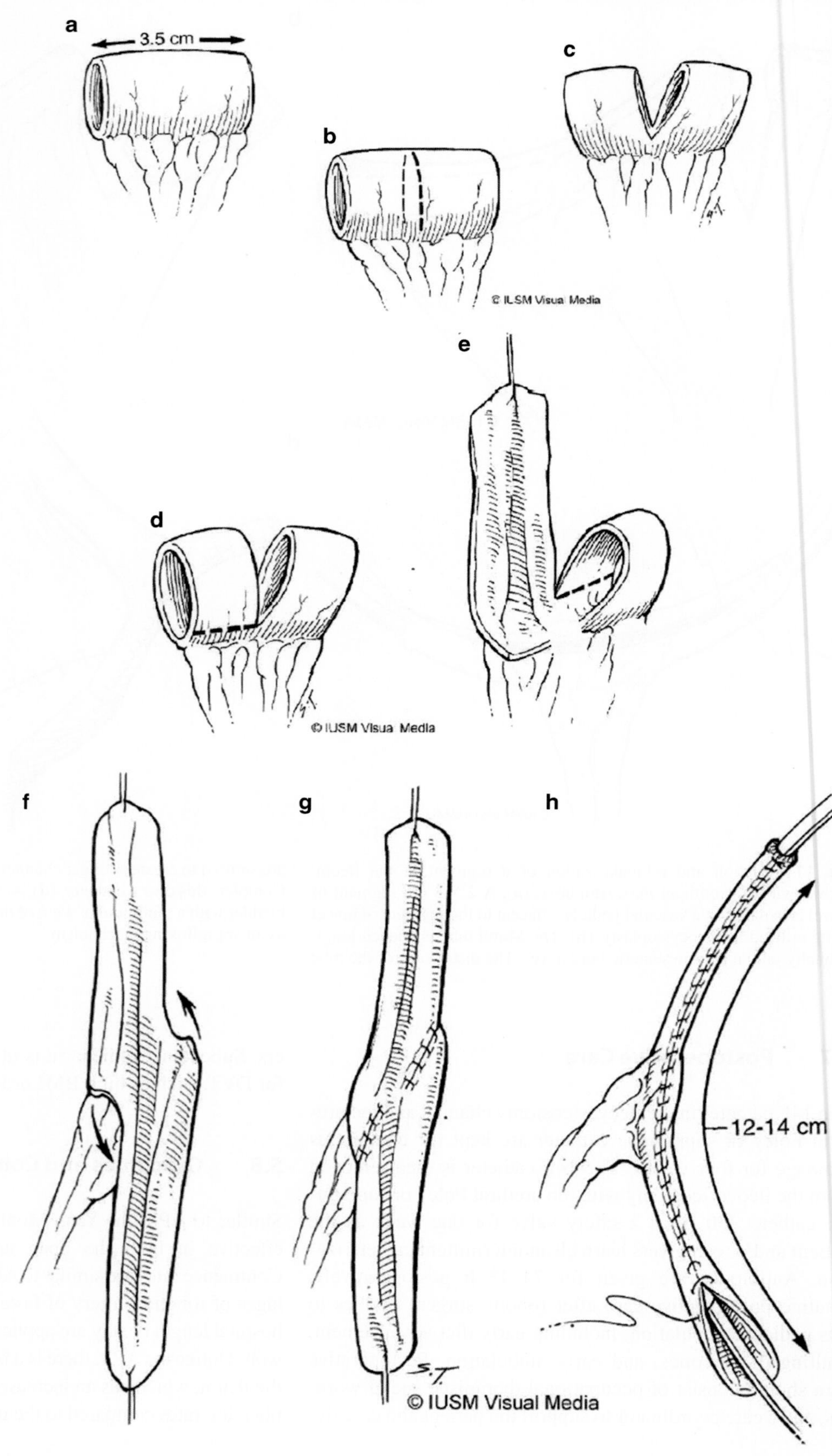

Fig. 12 Spiral Monti creation. (**a**). Utilize a 3.5–4 cm segment of bowel, usually the ileum, on its vascular pedicle. (**b, c**). Divide the segment in half transversely along 80% of its circumference, keeping the mesentery intact. (**d, e**). Divide opposite sides of each hemi-segment longitudinally along the edge of the mesentery. (**f, g**). Unfold the new spiral Monti tube and suture the middle corners along the mesentery together. (**h**). Roll the new spiral Monti over a catheter and suture longitudinally

Table 3 Yang-Monti brief surgical steps

• Low lithotomy with 10–15° Trendelenburg, arms tucked palms up
• Camera port supraumbilical, working arms 8 cm lateral, 4th arm 7–8 cm lateral to right arm near iliac fossa, 5 mm assistant port in RUQ
• 2–3 cm segment of ileum 15–20 cm proximal from ileocecal valve is isolated on its mesentery
• Use electrocautery' to open the bowel longitudinally along its anti-mesenteric border
• Retubularize transversely in two layers to create a 6–7 cm tube
• Bladder detrusor anterior tunnel creation (if no augmentation enterocystoplasty) • Fill bladder with 60–200 cc saline depending on bladder capacity' • Using electrocautery, incise detrusor to expose bladder mucosa at least 4 cm (for continence) • Spatulate the distal Monti and incise the bladder mucosa 1 cm • Complete anastomosis with 4–0 PDS interrupted sutures over an 8F feeding tube • Place Monti channel in previously incised 4 cm trough and imbricate detrusor muscle over it with 4–0 PDS suture
• Bladder detrusor posterior tunnel creation (if concurrent augmentation enterocystoplasty) • Using electrocautery, a cystotomy is performed on posterior wall of the bladder • Identify bilateral ureteral orifices • Using electrocautery, make a small hiatus for the anastomosis • Create a 4 cm submucosal tunnel and place Monti channel in the tunnel • Spatulate and suture distal Monti channel to bladder mucosa with 4–0 PDS interrupted sutures over an 8F feeding tube • Close the bladder mucosal defect
• Bring proximal Monti channel to umbilical or RLQ port sites
• Stoma maturation. Create stoma by spatulating the distal Monti channel and perform cutaneous flap anastomosis
• Secure 8F feeding tube with a stitch
• Remove ports, close fascia with 2–0 vicryl under direct vision and perform skin closure

Stomal stenosis rates are approximately 5–10%, which is similar to the APV [30, 33]. Diverticular pouch formation is more common in a Monti channel due to the generally increased length of the channel resulting in channel redundancy. There is a higher rate of diverticular pouch formation in the double Monti, resulting in difficulty with catheterization [34]. Overall revision rates are two times higher for a Monti than APV and four times higher for a spiral Monti, although Szymanski et al. reported similar revision rates. This discrepancy may be attributable to the higher subfascial revisions with Monti channels compared to APV but not in suprafascial revision. Subfascial complication rates, specifically, are highest for spiral Monti with an umbilical stoma at 32%, compared to 15% for conventional Monti channels [35]. Thus, when feasible, a single Yang-Monti configuration is preferred. Risk factors for complications requiring revision include age, weight, type of channel, and stoma location.

6 Malone Antegrade Colonic Enema

6.1 Patient Selection

Patients considered for a MACE should have intractable constipation who have failed multiple bowel evacuation regimens. The patient or a reliable caregiver must be able to perform catheterizations and antegrade enema delivery with adequate dexterity and consistency. Patients and their caregivers should be extensively counseled on the indications, operative expectations, and postoperative course prior to embarking on this procedure. Multiple abdominal surgeries resulting in intra-abdominal adhesions and severe kyphoscoliosis may increase the likelihood of conversion to an open procedure.

6.2 Preoperative Preparation

A complete history and physical should be done for every patient, noting especially prior bowel surgery, prior abdominal surgery, and body habitus. Patients are not typically given a mechanical or oral antibiotic bowel preparation as this does not improve outcomes.

6.3 Positioning and Port Placement

The patient is placed in the supine position with arms tucked at the sides. Foam padding should be used on all pressure areas and on the face to prevent injury. The patient is draped in sterile fashion. Local anesthetic into the port sites or a TAP block should be used prior to incision of port sites. Ports include a 12 mm blunt tip balloon trocar for the camera port in the infraumbilical midline. Two 8 mm robotic arm ports are placed in the midline in the sub-xyphoid and suprapubic positions. A fourth arm is placed in the right lower quadrant, which will be the site of the stoma. A fenestrated bipolar arm is used in the left arm and monopolar scissors in the right arm.

6.4 Surgical Steps

Perioperative antibiotics are administered within 1 h of incision to all patients, generally cefazolin, gentamicin, and metronidazole. Vancomycin may be used instead of cefazolin if a VP shunt is present. A Foley is placed. The 12 mm trocar is placed with an open Hassan technique. Pneumoperitoneum is established to 12 mmHg. If a VP shunt is present, it can be placed in an endopouch retrieval bag to avoid contamination with bowel contents. The remaining robotic arms should be placed as described above.

If utilizing an appendix for the MACE, the appendix is mobilized at the appendicular/cecal junction, keeping in mind that mobilization of the ascending colon along the line of Toldt may be necessary in order for the distal appendix to reach the skin. A stay suture may be placed at the tip of the appendix to facilitate handling of the appendix while avoiding crush injury to the tissue. A mesenteric window is made at the proximal end of the appendix, taking care not to compromise the blood flow to the appendix. While imbrication of the appendix is debated, we do not perform this, and our experience and data indicate that this step is not essential to prevent leak [36]. The appendix is then grasped using the stay suture and delivered through the laparoscopic port in the right lower quadrant or umbilicus for stoma maturation. For patients with a simultaneous APV or Yang-Monti, the right lower quadrant is the preferred location. The cecum is secured to the abdominal wall with absorbable monofilament suture. The stoma is matured via spatulation on the anti-mesenteric border and is sewn with 5–0 PDS monofilament absorbable suture. A 10F catheter is secured to stoma to be left in place for three weeks.

6.5 Split APV and ACE

For patients undergoing a simultaneous APV and ACE creation, the appendix may be used and split between the two procedures in those who have an appendix long enough. This is generally at 10–12 cm appendix. A minimum of 4 cm is necessary for the APV, with preference for 5–6 cm. The proximal 2–4 cm is then utilized for the ACE channel. The appendiceal artery and its arcades are prioritized for the distal appendix used for the APV as the proximal appendiceal stump can be sustained via collateral blood flow from the cecal blood supply. Once each appendiceal segment is isolated, each procedure proceeds as previously described.

6.6 Cecal Flap ACE

If no appendix is available due to history of appendectomy or concomitant APV with a short appendix, a cecal tube can be made for the ACE channel [37]. Incise the proximal cecum in a U-shape to form a cecal flap. The cecal flap should be 4 cm in length and 3 cm in width. Reapproximate the proximal cecum until a 10–12F hole remains adjacent to the cecal flap. Tubularize the flap around a 10F feeding tube. A 4–0 or 5–0 monofilament absorbable suture can be used. A stay suture can be used on the cecum in order to decrease manipulation of the cecal flap with robotic instruments. Once the tubularized cecal flap is formed, deliver the distal end through the laparoscopic port in the right lower quadrant or umbilicus for stoma maturation. The cecum is secured to the abdominal wall. The stoma is matured with 5–0 PDS monofilament absorbable suture. A 10F catheter is secured to stoma to be left in place for three weeks.

Stoma maturation and skin closure are the same as the robotic APV procedure described earlier in this chapter. If an endopouch was used to hold the VP shunt, this should be removed. The ports are all removed and the fascia closed using a 2–0 Vicryl stitch under direct vision. The camera port is the last to be closed. The skin is then closed with subcutaneous and subcuticular suture and surgical glue. A summary of the surgical steps is available in the following table (Table 4).

6.7 Postoperative Care

The 10F catheter is kept for three weeks. After removal, catheterization is taught to the patient and/or caregiver. Antegrade enemas are started once daily and increased thereafter as needed. Antibiotics are given for 24–48 h postoperatively. Routine postoperative care after robotic surgery applies to this pediatric population, including early diet advancement, limiting of narcotics, and early ambulation. Postoperative care should consist of occupational therapists, social workers, and a care coordinator to support the patient and caregivers. Subcutaneous heparin is utilized in patients at high risk for DVT, such as high BMI or immobility.

6.8 Outcomes and Complications

MACEs are commonly used to help achieve fecal continence. They are used in over 27% of adolescents with spina bifida and have success ranges ranging from 59 to 97% [38]. There is an approximately 81–91% continence rate with

Table 4 Malone antegrade colonic enema (MACE) brief surgical steps

• Low lithotomy with 10–15° Trendelenburg, arms tucked palms up
• Camera port supraumbilical, working arms in the midline in the sub-xyphoid and suprapubic positions, 4th arm in RLQ
• If utilizing the appendix, mobilize the appendix until it can reach the previously marked stoma site. Imbrication of the appendix is optional
• If no appendix is available, create a cecal flap by incising a 4 × 3 cm U-chape in the proximal cecum and tubularizing this around a 10F feeding tube with 4- or 5–0 PDS
• Secure the cecum to the abdominal wall
• Bring appendix or cecum to desired stoma location
• Stoma maturation via spatulation on the antimesentenc border and perform cutaneous flap anastomosis
• A 10F catheter is secured to the stoma for 3 weeks
• Remove ports, close fascia with 2–0 vicryl under direct vision and perform skin closure

MACE and a 90% improvement in patient-reported quality of life [20, 39, 40]. Complications include stomal stenosis (16–30%), continued fecal incontinence or fecal leaking (6–11%), difficult catheterization (4%), wound infection (3%), pain with enema administration (3%), and granulation tissue formation (<1%). MACE stomal stenosis tends to occur earlier than in other CCCs [26]. About 40% of patients with complications will require surgical revision. Decisional regret has been investigated, and 53% of patients and/or their parents have some form of regret, most of which was mild and owing to persistent fecal incontinence. Robotic and pure laparoscopic MACE surgeries are reported with excellent outcomes [20, 41–43].

7 Bladder Neck Reconstruction

7.1 Patient Selection

Possible candidates for bladder neck reconstruction are children with incompetent urethral sphincters and bothersome urinary leakage despite exhaustion of conservative measures. Whether or not a patient has adequate bladder capacity and compliance to maintain normal pressures determines whether or not they need a concomitant bladder augmentation. Etiologies include exstrophy, cloacal abnormalities, and neurogenic bladder secondary to spinal cord injury/neural tube defects. Patients typically undergo urodynamic study while on anticholinergic medication prior to surgery to determine if augmentation is necessary.

Other options to a bladder neck reconstruction include bulking agents injected at the bladder neck, artificial urinary sphincters (AUS), a bladder neck sling, bladder neck flap procedures, and closure of the bladder neck. Here, we describe our robotic bladder neck reconstruction technique, which is a modification of the Young-Dees-Leadbetter (YDL) technique.

7.2 Preoperative Preparation

A complete history, physical, and video urodynamic study should be done for every patient, especially noting prior surgery to the bladder or previous continence procedures. Patients are not typically given a mechanical or oral antibiotic bowel preparation. A preoperative urine culture is obtained, as it is important to treat any concomitant urinary tract infection prior to surgery.

7.3 Positioning and Port Placement

The patient is positioned in the low lithotomy position with a Trendelenburg of 10–15 degrees and arms tucked at the side with palms up to prevent ulnar nerve injury. Foam padding should be used on all pressure areas and on the face to prevent injury. An 8 mm (12 mm for Si robots) blunt tip balloon trocar is used for the camera port. We prefer the Hassan technique for this initial port, placed just superior to the umbilicus to ensure a minimum 10–12 cm pubo-umbilical distance is maintained. The left port is placed 8 cm lateral to the umbilicus, and the right arm is placed 9 cm lateral to the umbilicus. If the patient's size will not permit this, a distance of 4–5 cm between the camera and robotic arm ports is acceptable. An additional 8 cm robotic fourth arm is placed 7–8 cm lateral to the right arm port near the right iliac fossa in children taller than 1.5 m undergoing a concomitant CCC. A 5 mm assistant port (12 mm for cases with augmentation cystoplasty) is placed in the left upper quadrant, which is equidistant from the camera and left working port. An optional 5 mm port, or a third working arm, may be placed in the right lower quadrant if needed, and this can be used as the stoma site if applicable.

7.4 Surgical Steps

Perioperative antibiotics are administered within 1 h of incision to all patients, generally cefazolin. More broad antibiotics may be used if a VP shunt is present. Of note, if a VP shunt is present, this can be placed in an endopouch retrieval bag to avoid contamination with bowel contents (if undertaking simultaneous bowel surgery). First, the patient is draped and cystoscopy is performed. Using a pediatric cystoscope (size based on patient's age), bilateral ureteral stents are placed to later identify the ureteral orifices (UOs) during the procedure. Afterward, the patient is re-draped, and a 6fr Foley catheter is placed in the sterile field (larger Foleys are acceptable for bigger children). Local anesthetic into the port sites or a TAP block should be used prior to incision of port sites. The camera port is then placed via the open Hassan technique. Pneumoperitoneum is established to 12 mmHg. A diagnostic peritoneoscopy is performed to assess for scar tissue and any other abnormalities. The remaining robotic arm and assistant ports are then placed under direct visualization. Initially, a fenestrated bipolar arm is used in the left arm and robotic scissors in the right arm.

The bladder is then filled with 80 cc of saline. A vertical cystotomy is performed along the anterior portion of the bladder using the robotic scissors. A percutaneous stay suture is then placed on each lateral aspect of the cystotomy. Next, a "V"-shaped segment of the bladder mucosa is resected just below each ureteral orifice to create a long strip that will become the newly tubularized urethra. The mucosa excision is extended anteriorly to the level of the verumontanum, roughly 3 cm from the ureteral orifices (Figs. 13 and 14). Then, the arms are switched out for needle drivers. The mucosal layer of the newly tabularized urethra is sutured

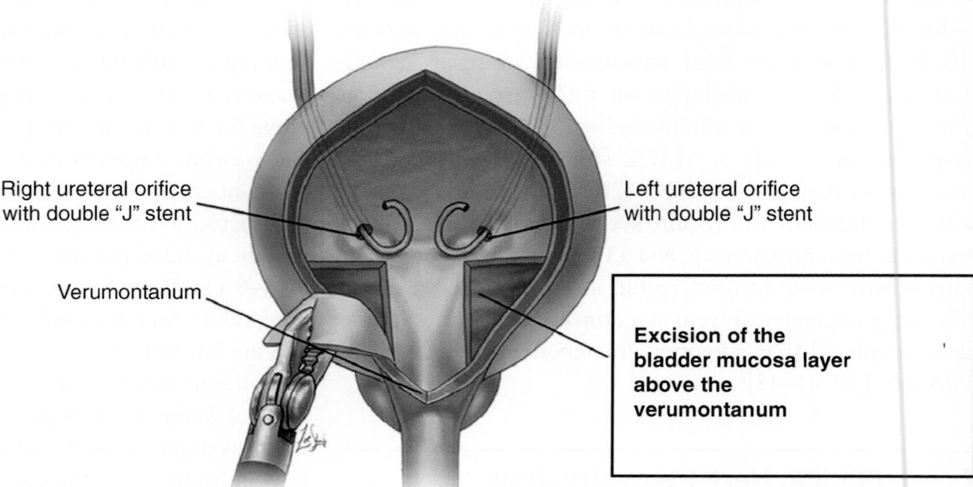

Fig. 13 Excision of the bladder neck mucosa [44]

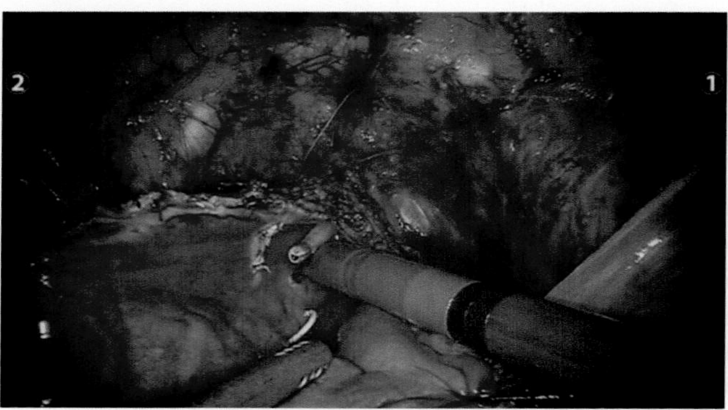

Fig. 14 Robotic view of bladder neck mucosa excision [44]

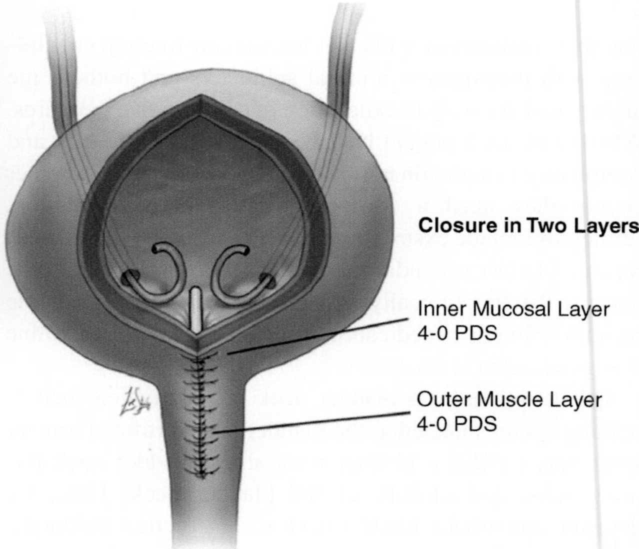

Fig. 15 Bladder neck closure over catheter [44]

with 4–0 PDS sutures in a running fashion from the verumontanum back toward the newly created bladder neck over the 6-French Foley catheter. The outer muscular layer is also closed with a 4–0 PDS suture in a continuous fashion, also starting from the verumontanum. The newly reconstructed bladder neck should be 3 cm in length (Figs. 15 and 16).

This procedure is nearly always accompanied by a urinary catheterizable channel (+/− bladder augmentation), often using the appendix. Once all other portions of the procedure are completed, the cystotomy (if it remains) is closed in a single layer using 3–0 Vicryl. A summary of the surgical steps is available in the following table (Table 5).

7.5 Postoperative Care

Duration of the Foley catheter is largely dependent on whether or not a concomitant catheterizable channel and SPT were placed. Often the Foley can be removed on POD1, and bladder drainage is maintained via the SPT or channel for at least four weeks (at which point CIC via a catheterizable channel can be initiated). The drain is removed prior to discharge so long as the output is less than 100 cc per day. Triple antibiotics are given for 24–48 h post-op. Routine postoperative care after robotic surgery applies to this pediatric population, including early diet advancement, limiting of narcotics, and early ambulation. Postoperative care should consist of occupational therapists, social workers, and a care coordinator to support the patient and caregivers.

7.6 Outcomes and Complications

True success rates of bladder neck repair operations are hard to find given that most studies are case series or retrospective

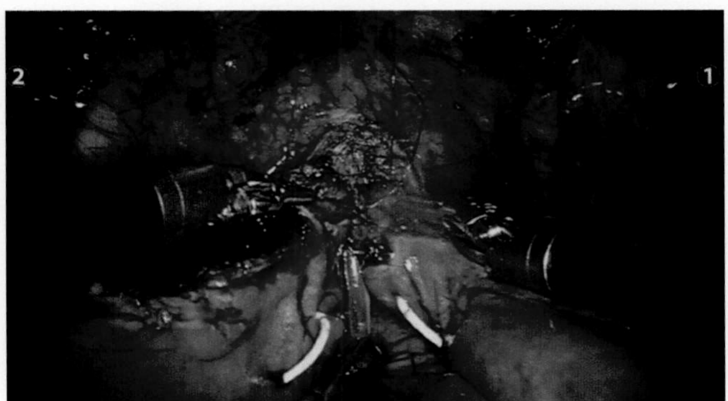

Fig. 16 Robotic view of bladder neck closure over catheter [44]

Table 5 Bladder neck reconstruction brief surgical steps

• Low lithotomy with 10–15° Trendelenburg, arms tucked palms up
• Cystoscopy to place bilateral ureteral stents for UO identification, foley then placed in sterile field
• Camera port supraumhilical, working arms 4–8 cm lateral, 5 mm assistant port in RUQ
• Additional robotic 4th arm 7–8 cm lateral to right arm if undergoing CCC
• Optional assistant port in in LUQ for augmentation cystoplasty
• Fenestrated bipolar right arm, robotic scissors left arm
• Fill bladder with 80 cc saline → vertical cystotomy along anterior aspect
• Percutaneous stay sutures on each lateral aspect of the cystotomy
• "V" shaped segment of bladder mucosa resected below each UO
• Extend excision anteriorly to level of verumontanum (3 cm from UOs)
• Needle drivers in fur each arm
• Mucosal closure of newly tubularized urethra with 4–0 PDS over foley, running from verumontanum back to bladder neck
• Muscle layer closure of urethra with 4–0 PDS. New length should be 3 cm in length
• Bladder augment/Catheterizable channel portion of the case
• Cystotomy closure in single layer using 3–0 vicryl
• Remote ports under direct visualization, close fascia, leave a blake drain

reviews and that there are various confounders, including differing primary diagnoses and concurrent procedures such as fascial slings, augmentation cystoplasty, and/or APV/Monti. Given those caveats, in the larger series, open bladder neck repair continence rates have historically been reported as 44–79% [45]. In the larger series, robotic repair continence rates range from 58 to 85% after the initial procedure [45]. Continence rates are even higher if a secondary or reoperation is included in the analysis.

Operative time tends to be longer for robotic bladder neck procedures, although again this is confounded by concurrent procedures. Robotic procedure time has been shown to decrease as the surgeon climbs the initial learning curve. Grimsby et al. retrospectively reported a mean OR time of 4.6 h for open bladder neck reconstruction versus 8.1 h for robotic reconstruction, although, again, OR times decreased with more experience in the robotic cohort [46]. None of those patients underwent augmentation cystoplasty. The literature for robotic bladder neck reconstruction shows OR times varying from 5.8 to 8.2 h [45].

Decreased blood loss, length of stay, improved cosmesis, and decreased postoperative bowel adhesions are thought to be reasons the robotic approach could be superior, although robust data on this is currently lacking. Gundeti et al. did report on 88 patients who underwent robotic APV (with bladder neck reconstruction in 39% and augmentation cystoplasty in 17%). They showed a 90-day complication rate of 30% with a mean estimated blood loss of 54 mL and a mean length of stay of 5.2 days [28]. The four patient case series by Bagrodia et al. had a mean estimated blood loss of 117.8 mL and mean length of stay of 3.6 days for patients undergoing robotic APV, LM BNR with BNS [47]. These numbers are in line with the open approach with a lower estimated blood loss. Full continence rates, complication profiles, and OR times are shown in the table (Tables 6 and 7).

Table 6 Outcomes and complications of robotic bladder neck reconstruction

Citation	Surgical approach	Continence rate	Complications	OR time
Gargollo [48]	RAL APV, LM (Leadbetter/Mitchell) BNR, BNS ($n = 38$)	82%	11% conversion to open 11% new VUR 5% bladder stones 21-month follow-up	5.8 h
Gargollo et al. [49]	RAL LM BNR w CCC, BNS ($n = 25$)	NR	16% conversion to open 4% ileus	9 h
Bagrodia and Gargollo [47]	RAL APV, LM BRN, BNS ($n = 4$)	100%	25% conversion to open 50% de novo VUR	7.75 h
Grimsby et al. [31]	RAL APV, some with concurrent BNR ($n = 39$)	NR	10% conversion to open 26% acute complications	NR
Grimsby et al. [46]	RAL BNR, BNS w CCC ($n = 19$)	58%	16% acute complications	8.1 h
Gundeti et al. [28]	RAL APV, 24% with concurrent BNR ($n = 88$)	85%	11% ileus	7.1 h

Table 7 Outcomes and complications of open bladder neck reconstruction

Article	Surgical approach	Continence rate	Complications	OR time
Cole [50]	Open YDL BNR ($n = 14$)	79%	NR	NR
Grimsby et al. [31]	Open APV, some with concurrent BNR ($n = 28$)	NR	29% acute complications	NR
Grimsby et al. [46]	Open BNR, BNS w CCC ($n = 26$)	44%	12% acute complications	4.6 h
Jawaheer and Rangecroft [51]	Open Pippi Salle, some with cystoplasty and APV ($n = 18$)	61%	39% required reoperation	NR

References

1. Nakhal RS, Creighton SM. Management of vaginal agenesis. J Pediatr Adolesc Gynecol. 2012;25(6):352–7.
2. Grimsby GM, Baker LA. The use of autologous buccal mucosa grafts in vaginal reconstruction. Curr Urol Rep. 2014;15(8):428.
3. Boztosun A, Olgan S. Robotic sigmoid vaginoplasty in an adolescent girl with Mayer-Rokitansky-Kuster-Hauser syndrome. Female Pelvic Med Reconstr Surg. 2016;22(5):e32–5.
4. Kim C, Campbell B, Ferrer F. Robotic sigmoid vaginoplasty: a novel technique. Urology. 2008;72(4):847–9.
5. Gundeti MS, Kumar R, Mohammad M. Robotic assisted ileo-vaginoplasty for vaginal atresia. J Pediatr Urol. 2021;S1477–5131(21):00024–3.
6. Lima M, Ruggeri G, Randi B, Dòmini M, Gargano T, La Pergola E, Gregori G. Vaginal replacement in the pediatric age group: a 34-year experience of intestinal vaginoplasty in children and young girls. J Pediatr Surg. 2010;45(10):2087–91.
7. Karateke A, Haliloglu B, Parlak O, Cam C, Coksuer H. Intestinal vaginoplasty: seven years' experience of a tertiary center. Fertil Steril. 2010;94(6):2312–5.
8. Pariser JJ, Kim N. Transgender vaginoplasty: techniques and outcomes. Transl Androl Urol. 2019;8(3):241–7.
9. Mitrofanoff P. Trans-appendicular continent cystostomy in the management of the neurogenic bladder. Chir Pediatr. 1980;21:297–305.
10. Jordan GH, Winslow GH. Laparoscopically assisted continent catheterizable cutaneous appendicovesicostomy. J Endorurol. 1993;7:517–20.
11. Hsu TH, Shortliffe LD. Laparoscopic Mitrofanoff appendicovesicostomy. Urology. 2004;64:802–4.
12. Pedraza R, Weiser A, Franco I. Laparoscopic appendicovesicostomy (Mitrofanoff procedure) in a child using the da Vinci robotic system. J Urol. 2004;171:1652–3.
13. Monti PR, Lara RC, Dutra MA, et al. New techniques for construction of efferent conduits based on the Mitrofanoff principle. Urology. 1997;49:112–5.
14. Yang WH. Yang needle tunneling technique in creating antireflux and continent mechanisms. J Urol. 1993;150:830–4.
15. Casale AJ. A long continent ileovesicostomy using a single piece of bowel. J Urol. 1999;162:1743–5.
16. Duckett JW, Snyder HM 3rd. Use of the Mitrofanoff principle in urinary reconstruction. Urol Clin North Am. 1986;13:271–4.
17. Malone P, Ransley P, Kiely E. Preliminary report: the antegrade continence enema. Lancet. 1990;336:1217–8.
18. Lendvay TS, Shnorhavorian M, Grady RW. Robotic-assisted laparoscopic Mitrofanoff appendicovesicostomy and antegrade continent enema colon tube creation in a pediatric spina bifida patient. J Laparoendosc Adv Surg Tech A. 2008;18:310–2.
19. Thakre AA, Yeung CK, Peters C. Robot-assisted Mitrofanoff and Malone antegrade continence enema reconstruction using divided appendix. J Endourol. 2008;22:2393–6. discussion 6
20. Galansky L, Andolfi C, Adamic B, Gundeti MS. Continent cutaneous Catheterizable channels in Pediatric patients: a decade of experience with open and robotic approaches in a single Center. Eur Urol. 2020;S0302–2838(20):30630–8.
21. Kaefer M, Retik AB. The Mitrofanoff principle incontinent urinary reconstruction. Urol Clin North Am. 1997;24:795–811.
22. Wille MA, Zagaja GP, Shalhav AL, Gundeti AS. Continence outcomes in patients undergoing robotic assisted laparoscopic Mitrofanoff appendicovesicostomy. J Urol. 2011;185:1438–43.
23. Cain MP, Casale AJ, King SJ, et al. Appendicovesicostomy and newer alternatives for the Mitrofanoff procedure: results in the last 100 patients at Riley Children's Hospital. J Urol. 1999;162:1749–52.
24. Creatsas G, Deligeoroglou E. Vaginal aplasia and reconstruction. Best Pract Res Clin Obstet Gynaecol. 2010;24(2):185–91.
25. Famakinwa JF, Rosen AM, Gundeti MS. Robot-assisted laparoscopic Mitrofanoff appendicovesicostomy technique and outcomes of extravesical and intravesical approaches. Eur Urol. 2013;64:831–6.
26. Thomas JC, Dietrich MS, Trusler L, et al. Continent catheterizable channels and the timing of their complications. J Urol. 2006;176:1816–20. discussion 1820
27. Welk BK, Afshar K, Rapoport D, et al. Complications of the catheterizable channel following continent urinary diversion: their nature and timing. J Urol. 2008;180:1856–60.
28. Gundeti MS, Petravick ME, Pariser JJ, Pearce SM, Anderson BB, Grimsby GM, Akhavan A, Dangle PP, Shukla AR, Lendvay TS, Cannon GM Jr, Gargollo PC. A multi-institutional study of perioperative and functional outcomes for pediatric robotic-assisted laparoscopic Mitrofanoff appendicovesicostomy. J Pediatr Urol. 2016;12(6):386.e1–5.
29. Harris CF, Cooper CS, Hutcheson JC, et al. Appendicovesicostomy: the Mitrofanoff procedure-a 15-year perspective. J Urol. 2000;163:1922–6.
30. Szymanski KM, Whittam B, Misseri R, et al. Long-term outcomes of catheterizable continent urinary channels: what do you use, where you put it, and does it matter? J Pediatr Urol. 2015;11(210):e1–7.
31. Grimsby GM, Jacobs MA, Gargollo PC. Comparison of complications of robot-assisted laparoscopic and open Appendicovesicostomy in children. J Urol. 2015;194(3):772–6.
32. Piagglio L, Myers S, Figueroa TE, et al. Influence of type of conduit and site of implantation on the outcome of continence catheterizable channels. J Pediatr Urol. 2007;3:230–4.
33. Whittam BM, Szymanski KM, Flack C, et al. A comparison of the Monti and spiral Monti procedures: a long-term analysis. J Pediatr Urol. 2015;11(134):e1–6.
34. Narayanaswamy B, Wilcox DT, Cuckow PM, et al. The Yang-Monti ileovesicostomy: a problematic channel? BJU Int. 2001;87:861–5.
35. Leslie JA, Cain MP, Kaefer M, et al. A comparison of the Monti and Casale (spiral Monti) procedures. J Urol. 2007;178:1623–7. discussion 1627
36. Chan YY, Gonzalez R, Kurzrock EA. Malone antegrade continence enema: Is cecal imbrication essential? J Pediatr Urol. 2018;14(6):546.e1–5.
37. Kudela G, Smyczek D, Springer A, Korecka K, Koszutski T. No appendix is too short-simultaneous Mitrofanoff Catheterizable vesicostomy and Malone antegrade continence enema (MACE) for children with spina bifida. Urology. 2018;116:205–7.

38. Kelly MS. Maole antegrade continence enemas vs. cecostomy vs. Transanal irrigation–what is new and how do we counsel our patients? Curr Urol Rep. 2019;20:41.
39. Graf JL, Strear C, Bratton B, Housley HT, Jennings RW. The antegrade continence enema procedure: a review of the literature. J Pediatr Surg. 1998;33:1294–6.
40. Mohamed H, Wayne C, Weir A, Partridge EA, Langer JC, Nasr A. Tube cecostomy versus appendicostomy for antegrade enemas in the management of fecal incontinence in children: a systematic review. J Ped Surg. 2020;55:1196–200.
41. Karpman E, Das S, Kurzrock EA. Laparoscopic antegrade continence enema (Malone) procedure: description and illustration of technique. J Endourol. 2002;16(6):325–8.
42. Webb HW, Barraza MA, Crump JM. Laparoscopic appendicostomy for management of fecal incontinence. J Pediatr Surg. 1997;32:457–8.
43. Zee RS, Kern NG, Herndon CDA. Robotic-assisted laparoscopic MACE. J Pediatr Urol. 2017;13:525–6.
44. Rodriguez MV, Wallace A, Gundeti MS. Robotic bladder neck reconstruction with Mitrofanoff Appendicovesicostomy in a neurogenic bladder patient. Urology. 2020;137:206–7. https://doi.org/10.1016/j.urology.2019.11.023. Epub 2019 Nov 30
45. Gargollo PC, White LA. Robotic-assisted bladder neck procedures in children with neurogenic bladder. World J Urol. 2020;38(8):1855–64.
46. Grimsby GM, Menon V, Schlomer BJ, Baker LA, Adams R, Gargollo PC, Jacobs MA. Long-term outcomes of bladder neck reconstruction without augmentation cystoplasty in children. J Urol. 2016;195(1):155–61.
47. Bagrodia A, Gargollo P. Robot-assisted bladder neck reconstruction, bladder neck sling, and appendicovesicostomy in children: description of technique and initial results. J Endourol. 2011;25(8):1299–305.
48. Gargollo PC. Robotic-assisted bladder neck repair: feasibility and outcomes. Urol Clin North Am. 2015;42(1):111–20.
49. Gargollo PC, Granberg C, Gong E, Tu D, Whittam B, Dajusta D. Complex robotic lower urinary tract surgery in patients with history of open surgery. J Urol. 2019;201(1):162–8.
50. Cole EE, Adams MC, Brock JW 3rd, Pope JC 4th. Outcome of continence procedures in the pediatric patient: a single institutional experience. J Urol. 2003;170(2 Pt 1):560–3. discussion 563
51. Jawaheer G, Rangecroft L. The Pippi Salle procedure for neurogenic urinary incontinence in childhood: a three-year experience. Eur J Pediatr Surg. 1999;9(Suppl 1):9–11.

Robotic Surgery to Approach Bladder Disorders in Pediatric Patients

Dana A. Weiss, Arun K. Srinivasan, and Aseem R. Shukla

1 Introduction

Following a long tradition of urology being an early adaptor of minimally invasive surgery (MIS), pediatric urologists also have been widely accepting new techniques to provide minimally invasive surgical options for children. As such, the robotic platform has been used in pediatric urology for well over a decade and has become nearly standard of care for some procedures, such as pyeloplasty. It also is widely used in ureteral reimplantation, although there remains some controversy for that procedure. Due to its more widespread usage, overall experience has increased, and experienced robotic surgeons are now performing more complex procedures on the bladder, including creating catheterizable channels, providing minimally invasive options for ileocystoplasty, and offering options for bladder neck reconstruction.

In general, the benefits of MIS include decreased pain, decreased length of stay in the hospital, and improved cosmesis, trading a single long incision for several smaller incisions. However, the benefits have had to be balanced with the drawbacks of long learning curves, higher cost, and increased operative times. These factors are often only temporary. All surgical intervention has a learning curve—it just depends on when that learning curve happens (in training or in practice). Long operative times have been listed as critiques for robotic reconstructive surgeries; however, like all things, experience improves time. The first laparoscopic nephrectomies took a long time. The first robotic prostatectomies took a long time. Similarly, the first robotic augmentations took a long time, but with perseverance and gaining expertise, all of these times decrease and the end result is a comparable if not optimal approach. The first open augmentations that a surgeon does in his/her practice also take longer than his/her mentors, but time is not the goal.

Another potential benefit of robotic surgery as compared to the traditional open approach is that there may be a decreased risk of adhesions. This was demonstrated in a porcine model, showing both decreased number of adhesions and increased density and complexity of the adhesions in the open augmentation group [1].

2 Bladder Diverticula

The first report of robot-assisted laparoscopic bladder diverticula excision was in 2009 [2]. The robotic platform offered the ease of intracorporal suturing over the previously described laparoscopic approach and thus combined the benefits of MIS with a focally directed excision of a bladder diverticula. We have found that robot-assisted laparoscopic approach allows excellent repair both as a stand-alone procedure and repair of paraureteric/periureteral diverticulum as part of anti-reflux procedure. We start the procedure with a cystoscopy to determine the relationship of the diverticulum to the ureteral orifices and, if close, place a stent in that ureter. Then, we proceed to surgically dissect the diverticulum with robot assistance. Filling the bladder intermittently helps identify the diverticulum (Fig. 1). One has to be careful to protect the ureters and the vas during the dissection. Once the stand-alone diverticulum is identified, it is dissected free from surrounding structures down to its neck. The diverticulum is then incised open and divided at the level of the neck. At the level of the neck, the bladder is then closed in two layers.

In the setting of the paraureteral or periureteral diverticulum, one can repair the diverticulum as part of ureteral reimplantation surgery. Once the ureter and diverticulum are dissected free as one entity, the detrussor tunnels are made as is normal for an extravesical ureteral reimplantation approach. Then, the diverticulum along with the ureter is reduced inside the bladder and anchored in place with an anchoring suture at the 12'o clock position. The rest of the detrusorraphy is completed in a routine fashion tunneling the ureter inside the detrusor tunnel. An alternative approach

D. A. Weiss (✉) · A. K. Srinivasan · A. R. Shukla
Division of Urology, Children's Hospital of Philadelphia, Philadelphia, PA, USA

P. Wiklund et al. (eds.), *Robotic Urologic Surgery*, https://doi.org/10.1007/978-3-031-00363-9_72

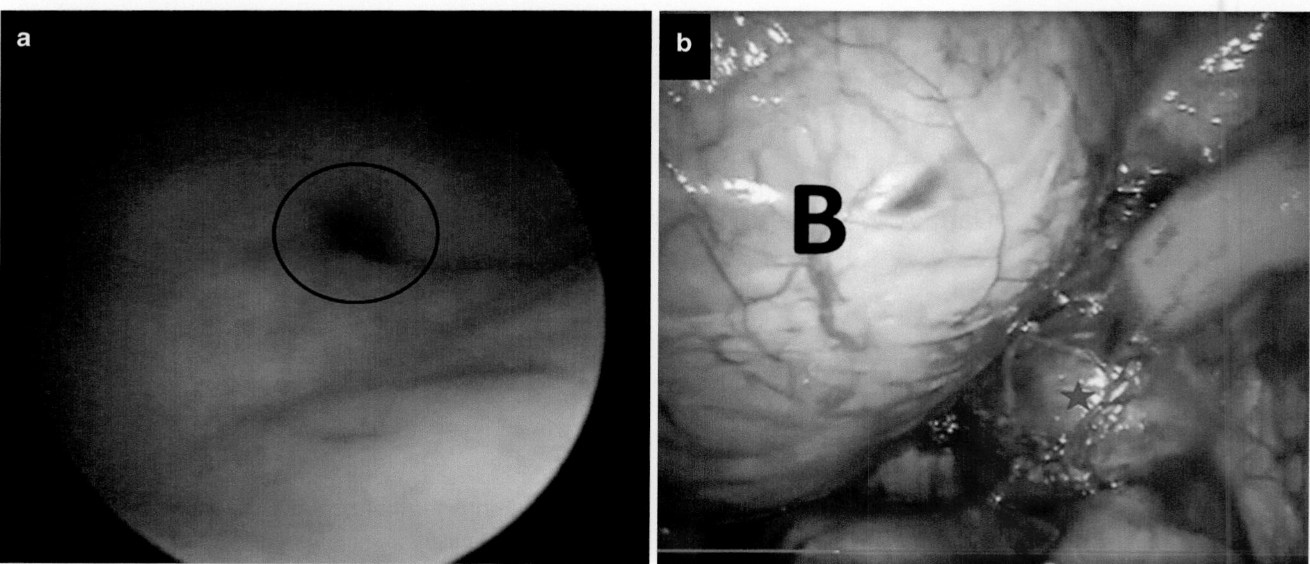

Fig. 1 (**a**) Bladder diverticulum from the inside bladder. (**b**) Diverticulum (blue star) filled and easily seen outside the bladder (B)

would be to perform a dismembered ureteral reimplant after excision of the diverticulum.

A series of 14 patients was presented in 2012, demonstrating an average hospital length of stay of 24.4 hours with the Foley catheter being removed the following day, and there were no short- or long-term complications [3]. Postoperative VCUGs (voiding cystourethrograms) demonstrated no evidence of the persistent diverticula. In this series, the ureters were protected with temporary indwelling ureteral catheters. This series was followed a year later by a case report of a diverticulectomy along with ureteral reimplantation for a paraureteral diverticulum [4]. In this case, the shared common wall of the inside of the diverticulum and the anterior ureter was left intact, and once the diverticulum was excised, the ureter was placed into a detrusor tunnel much like a standard extravesical reimplantation. This procedure has also been demonstrated in a recent video that is available [5].

3 Appendicovesicostomy/Continent Catheterizable Channels

Following on the heels of experience with robot-assisted laparoscopic ureteral reimplantation, as well as the longtime experience with laparoscopic appendectomies, a logical progression was the creation of appendicovesicostomy (APV) catheterizable channels via a robot-assisted approach. The completely laparoscopic appendicovesicostomy was first reported in 2004 [6].

Some concerns about the robotic approach to the APV is the risk of leakage from the stoma. In addition, the location of insertion of the channel into the bladder is controversial. Historically, a posterior insertion was thought to be better for clearance of the mucous and to prevent stones. However, technically, implantation anteriorly is easier, and it decreases the length of the appendix needed to reach the abdominal wall, thus enabling a longer tunnel which aids in the continence mechanism of the channel. There are no data to definitively advocate for one approach or the other. In a series of open channels in patients with bladder exstrophy, anterior channels had increased risk of infections and an increase, but not significantly, in stone formation [7]. This series however excluded patients with spina bifida due to decreased mobility and overall increase in risk of stone formation. In three robotic series, one in which both anterior and posterior implantations were constructed [8] and two in which only anterior implantation of the appendix was used, bladder stones were not reported in any children, so the comparison could not be made [9, 10].

The technique for RALM (robot-assisted laparoscopic Mitrofanoff) has been previously well described [11]. In summary, the appendix is first mobilized (Fig. 2). This is often easier done with a straight laparoscopic technique in order to enable a high dissection of the cecum if needed in order to gain length or to access a retrocecal appendix. The goal is to mobilize the cecum and right colon, if needed, in order that the appendix can easily reach from the bladder to the abdominal wall. After mobilizing the appendix, a cecal flap can be used as well in order to elongate the channel. Ideally, the appendix will be 5–6 cm in length at least and accommodate a 10–12F catheter. Once the appendix is mobilized and the appendiceal mesentery mobilized partly, a purse string suture is placed at the base of the appendix, and

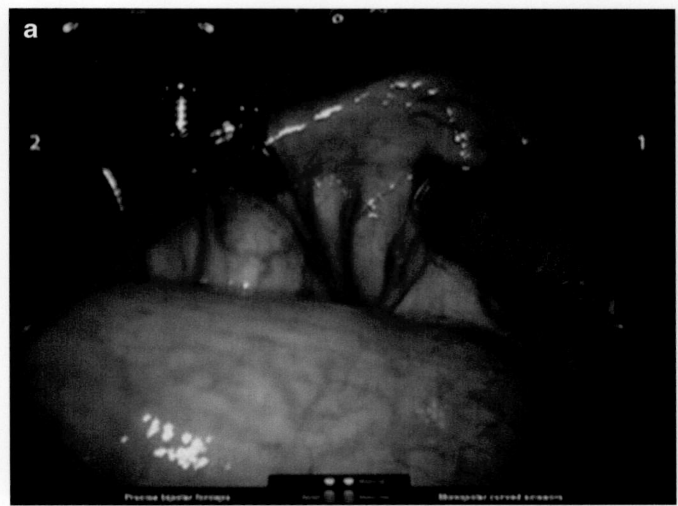

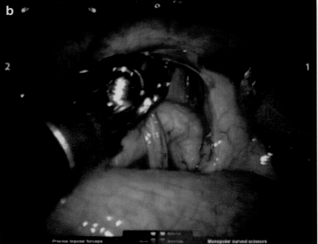

Fig. 2 (**a**) Appendix mobilization. (**b**) Split of the appendix. With permission, from Galansky L, Andolfi C, Adamic B, and Gundeti MS. Continent Cutaneous Catheterizable Channels in Pediatric Patients: A Decade of Experience with Open and Robotic Approaches in a Single Center. European Urology 2021; 79: 866–78. https://doi.org/10.1016/j.eururo.2020.08.013

it is separated from the cecum. The cecal opening is then oversewn. Alternatively, a laparoscopic stapler device can be utilized to divide the appendix. The appendiceal mesentery is further mobilized to gain length on the channel, and then the distal 1 cm is excised to open the lumen. In settings where the appendix is unavailable or inadequate, a Monti can be created (Fig. 3).

If an isolated APV is being created, the appendix is most often inserted into the anterior bladder wall, as this is an easier procedure than the posterior wall and has shorter distance to the abdominal wall for a short appendix. However, as mentioned above, this point is controversial.

Next, the bladder is distended, and a detrusorotomy is performed akin to that made during an extravesical reimplantation, with the goal of an approximately 4 cm tunnel. The tunnel can be created in the midline if going to the umbilicus or toward the right lateral posterior wall if the stoma will be in the right lower quadrant (RLQ). The appendix is spatulated, and a stitch (Fig. 4) is placed into the caudal most end of detrusorotomy and then through the distal apex of the spatulated appendix. The bladder mucosa is opened about 1 cm, and an 8F feeding tube is inserted through the appendix and into the bladder, to better delineate the bladder and appendix mucosa for the anastomosis. The anastomosis is then completed circumferentially, and the appendix is placed in the detrusor trough, which is closed over the top of it. At the proximal/cranial end, a stay suture is placed into the appendix and into tunnel to prevent slippage. Once this is completed, then the proximal, cecal end is brought through the umbilical port side or RLQ site, and the stoma is created (Fig. 5). Often a suprapubic tube will be placed as a safety drainage in case the tube does not drain well. Postoperatively, usually the catheter is kept in place for four weeks, and then it is removed and CIC (clean intermittent catheterization) is initiated.

The main criteria of comparison to the open approach have been incontinence, stomal stenosis, stomal prolapse, stricture of the channel, and creation of false passages. In a report of 18 patients with mean follow-up of 24.2 months after RALMA (robotic-assisted Mitrofanoff appendicovesicostomy), the overall stomal continence was 94.4%, and the patient with incontinence for a year was then treated with Deflux [9]. In this series, there were three stoma complications (two in stenosis, one in parastomal hernia). An updated report of the experience with open and robotic catheterizable channels, bladder neck surgery, and augmentations was presented recently. Fifty-one APVs were made (19 open, 32 robotic), 34 augmentations (16 open, 18 robotic), and 18 bladder necks (12 open, 6 robotic). The robotic approach had a quicker return to regular diet (4 vs. 6 days, $p = 0.0092$) and a nearly 50% reduction in LOS (length of stay) (6.8 vs. 13 d, $p = 0.0081$). No difference in rate of complications was found between open and robotic approaches (42.9 vs. 38.2%). Moreover, stomal continence rates were equal in both the open and robotic approaches, 91.4 vs. 91.2%, respectively [12].

4 Bladder Augmentation

Bladder augmentation has a long history for use in patients with high pressure and small capacity bladder storage, in order to increase capacity, improve compliance, and ultimately protect against renal deterioration. As with any major reconstruction like this, patient selection is the most important part of the surgical planning, because especially in chil-

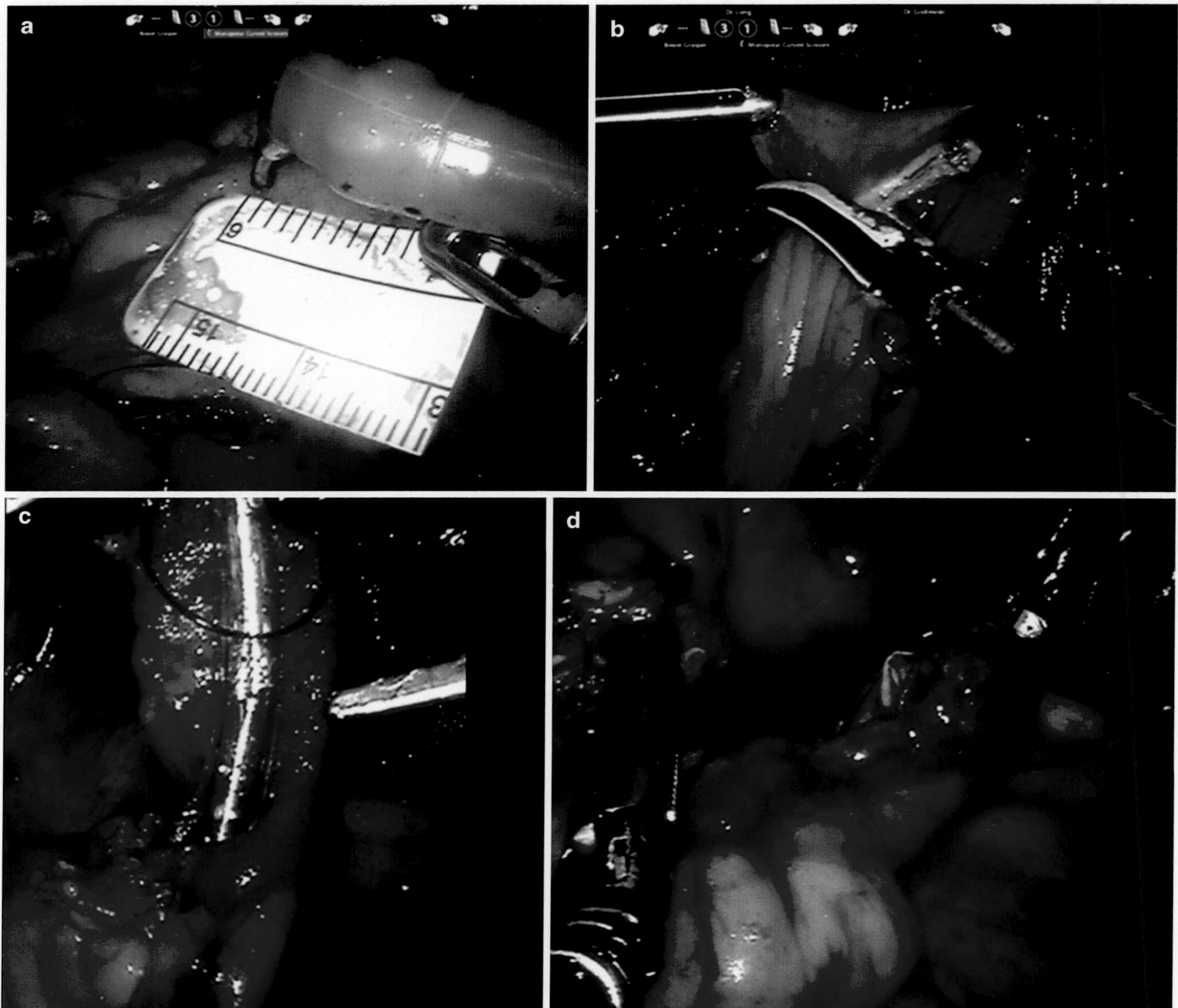

Fig. 3 (**a**) Creation of Monti starts with isolation of a 2 cm section of bowel. (**b**) Isolated bowel segment opened close to the mesenteric insertion on one side—not at the antimesenteric border. (**c**) With the fourth arm holding the feeding tube in place, the detubularized bowel segment is rolled to a tube. (**d**) The finished Monti channel

dren, the decision must be made with a child and family willing and able to perform the update that is required to prevent serious complications.

The advancement of robot-assisted reconstructive surgery in adults has naturally translated to the pediatric population. The first completely intracorporeal robotic-assisted laparoscopic augmentation ileocystoplasty and Mitrofanoff appendicovesicostomy (RALIMA) was reported in 2008 [13].

The largest series to date has come from Gundeti et al. in Chicago. The surgical technique has been described by the Chicago group and is described briefly below.

Perioperative preparation includes antibiotics (cefazolin, gentamicin, and metronidazole, with the addition of vancomycin if VP shunt is present). At the time, no mechanical or oral bowel prep is utilized other than the patient's routine bowel prep in the setting of the neurogenic bowel and bladder; however, the use of bowel preparations has gone through many iterations and continues to be reassessed.

The patient is positioned in low lithotomy, with the arms tucked. Cystoscopy is performed and bilateral double J stents are placed for ureteric identification. We do consider preemptive bladder Botox injection particularly in children with poor bladder compliance. A Foley catheter is placed on the

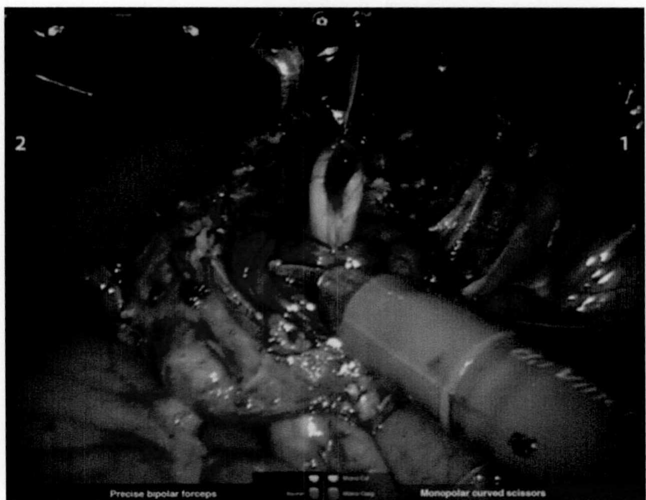

Fig. 4 Appendix spatulation. With permission, from Galansky L, Andolfi C, Adamic B, and Gundeti MS. Continent Cutaneous Catheterizable Channels in Pediatric Patients: A Decade of Experience with Open and Robotic Approaches in a Single Center. European Urology 2021; 79: 866–78. https://doi.org/10.1016/j.eururo.2020.08.013

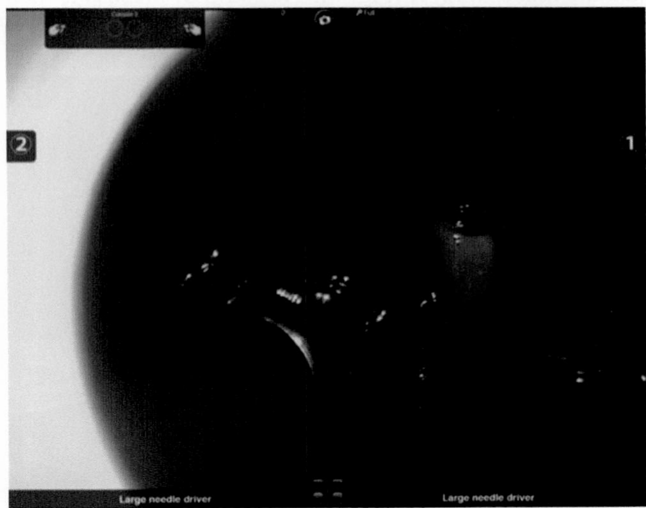

Fig. 5 Stoma maturation. With permission, from Galansky L, Andolfi C, Adamic B, and Gundeti MS. Continent Cutaneous Catheterizable Channels in Pediatric Patients: A Decade of Experience with Open and Robotic Approaches in a Single Center. European Urology 2021; 79: 866–78. https://doi.org/10.1016/j.eururo.2020.08.013

field. Next, ports are placed, including a 12 mm camera port, two 8 mm robotic ports, 10 mm assistant port in LUQ, and + − 5 mm port in RLQ to aid, and then can be a site of stoma if needed. The end of the ventriculoperitoneal shunt tubing can be placed in an Endopouch retrieval bag to prevent contamination.

The surgery is very similar to the open approach. A 20 cm segment of the ileum identified 15–20 cm away from the ileocecal junction is identified. A premeasured silk suture can be used to do this, and then stay sutures are placed on the two ends of the segment. The mesentery is then pulled down to the pelvis to make sure it reaches, and then windows are created and the mesentery and bowel are divided. In their report, the bowel-to-bowel anastomosis is performed in an end-to-end manner, but this can also be done with a stapler introduced through the assistant port.

If a catheterizable channel with appendix is planned, the appendix with a cecal cuff is then taken, as described previously. The appendix is then implanted into the posterior bladder wall before laying on the ileal patch.

The bladder is opened coronally from side to side, bivalving the bladder with an additional incision of the posterior plate in the midline ensuring safety of the vas deferens. The ileal segment is then incised on the antimesenteric border. The posterior ends of the segment are anastomosed to each edge of the cystotomy, and then the posterior edge is attached to the bladder with a running suture. The same is done on the anterior side.

When a catheterizable channel is performed along with bladder augmentation, it is better done in our opinion before the augment is done on the open bladder plate. We typically choose the right lateral half of the posterior bladder plate to perform an intravesical approach to create a submucosal tunnel for the appendix and perform the anastomosis.

An update of outcomes was presented in 2015, of 15 patients who underwent successful robotic-assisted laparoscopic ileocystoplasty (RALI), in comparison to 13 who underwent open procedure. Median operative time was definitely longer in RALI (623 vs. 287 min), but median length of stay was shorter (6 vs. 8 days), but there was no difference in narcotic use. Overall, there was no difference in surgical outcomes such as bladder capacity and complication rates [14].

5 Bladder Neck Surgery

5.1 AUS (Artificial Urinary Sphincter)

AUS has gone through an evolution, with an early interest in the surgery that could still allow for bladder emptying without catheterization, to a period of explantations for erosion and malfunctioning devices. While the overall success rates have been in the 70% range, beginning with an early report of 107 children with an overall success of 77%, the complications are steep. In this same series, the mean life of the sphincter was only 56 months, 19% were explanted, and at least one revision was required in 59% [15]. More recent success rates remained the same, approximately 70% success, with over 50% complication rate [16]. The first reported robotic insertion was by Moscardi et al. in 2017 in a six-year-old girl, but this report only had a three-month follow-up [17]. The robotic approach to placement is unlikely to change the overall efficacy and durability of the device and procedure, but further data will be needed to fully assess that. While not for every patient, for the properly selected patient, some families and some physicians find the product favorable.

5.2 Bladder Neck Sling

Similar to the AUS, the use of bladder neck slings in the neurogenic bladder population has showed only modest success and has the ability to lead to detrusor and subsequently renal deterioration. In a long-term follow-up of bladder neck procedures, only 15/43 (35%) were dry within one year [18]. As in all situations, the robotic platform is a tool to achieve the same surgical procedure, so the robotic approach to bladder neck slings is not expected to yield different results; however, it may make the placement easier and more approachable. Moreover, when a sling is done in conjunction with other procedures such as a BNR (bladder neck reconstruction) and APV, then the results will never truly be known.

5.3 Bladder Neck Reconstruction

The challenge with bladder neck reconstruction is that there is no one perfect technique. This then translates to the robotic approach, which attempts to recapitulate the open approach—and so the technique varies based on surgeon experience. Open BNR series have a range of continence from 50 to 79% in a single series of various approaches (Young-Dees-Leadbetter with or without sling, Pippi Salle, or Kropp's procedures) [19], so this has to be taken into account when assessing the robotic approach. The way we approach bladder neck repairs robotically is a variation of Pippi Salle's anterior bladder tube [20]. Ureteral stents are placed cystoscopically prior to starting. Dissection is done in the anterior aspect of the bladder down to the puboprostatic ligaments in the male and endopelvic fascia in females. A 2 cm wide 4 cm long anterior bladder wall section is demuscularized leaving just the mucosal layer (Fig. 6). This strip of mucosa is then

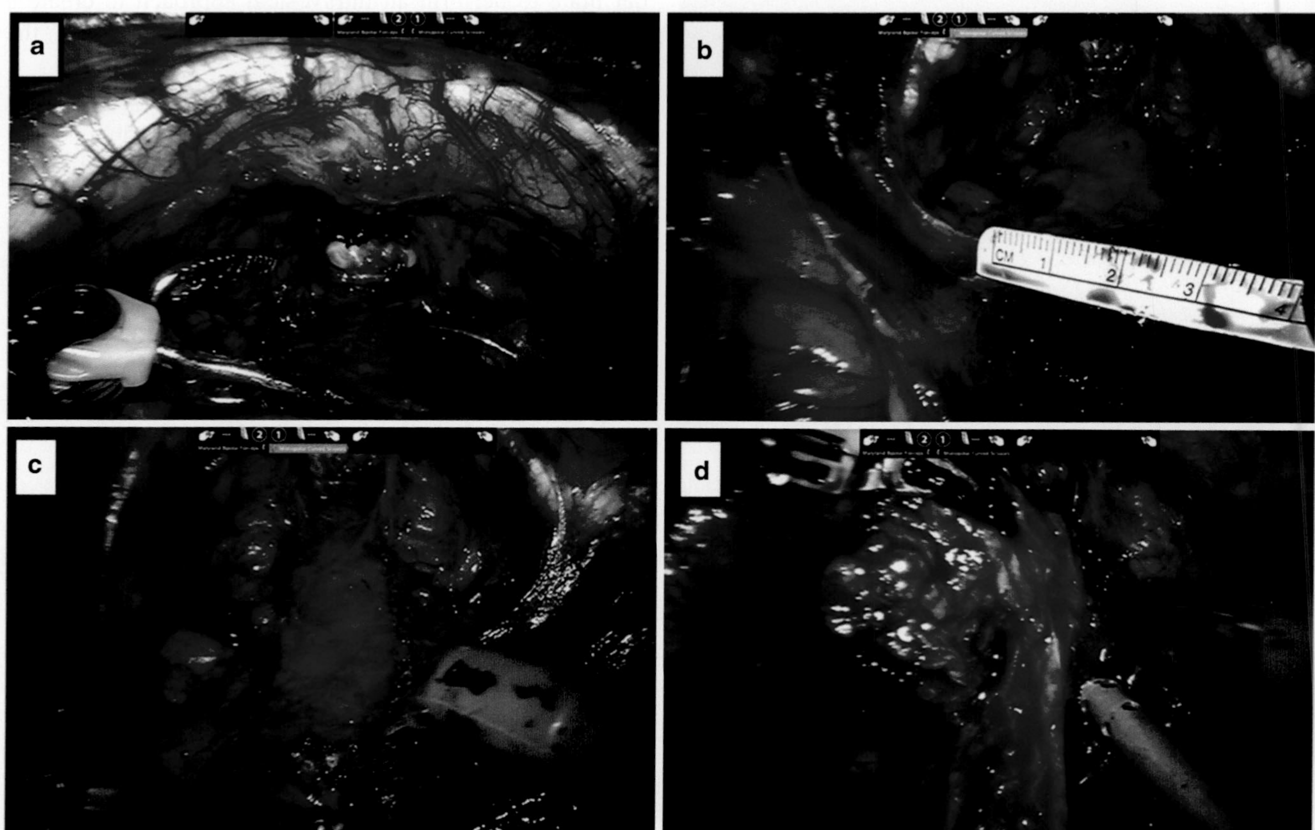

Fig. 6 (**a**) The bladder is taken down below the pubic symphysis to expose the bladder neck. (**b**) A ruler is introduced in order to measure the length of segment that will be rolled into a tube. (**c**) The anterior bladder wall is marked with cautery to delineate section of the bladder that will be opened for tubularization (**d**) Flap of the anterior bladder wall is a raised BNR with external dissection

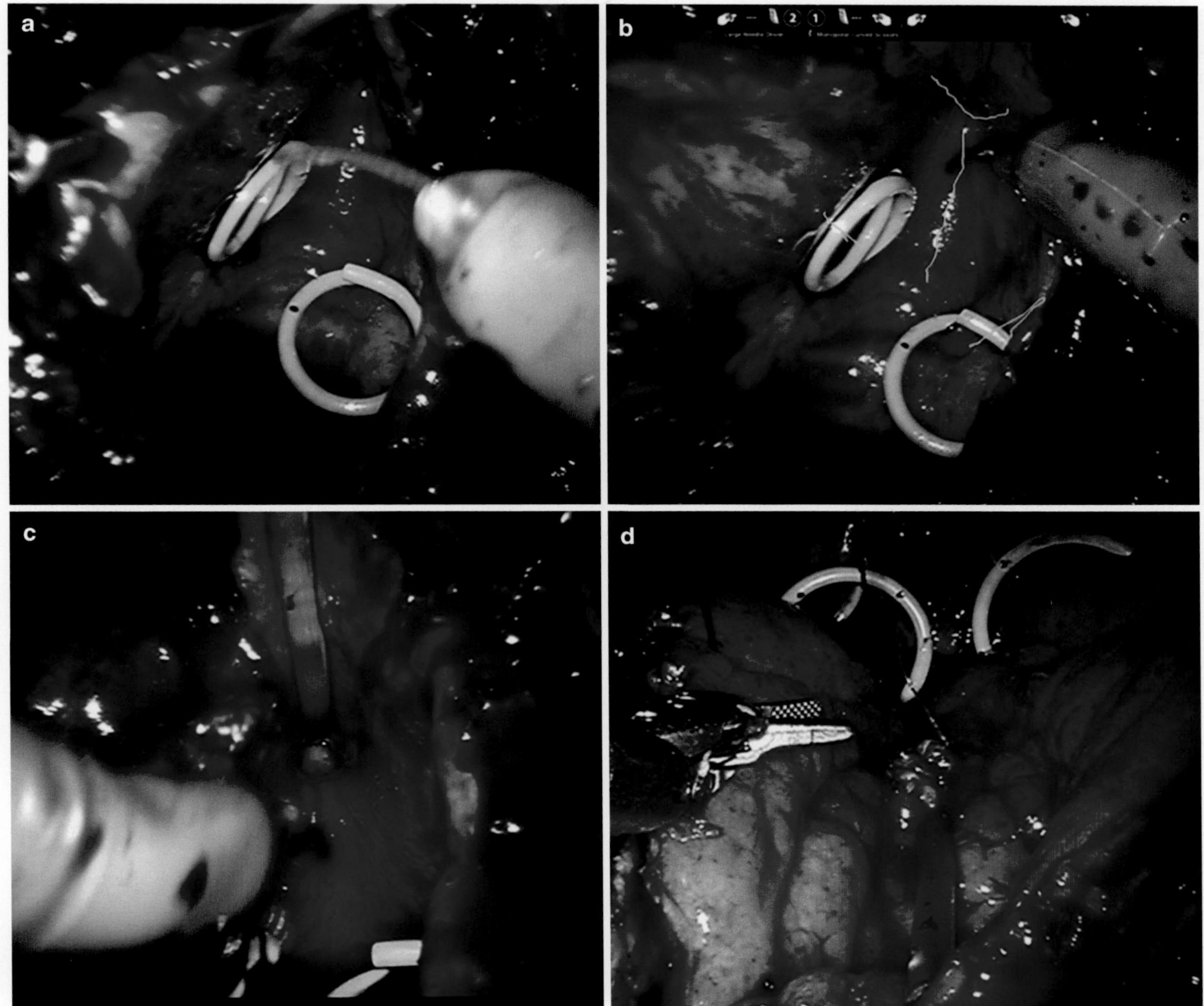

Fig. 7 (**a**) Bladder flap is opened and double J ureteral stents are visualized inside (**b**) Posterior bladder wall mucosal incision marked on monitor—this will be made in the midline between the ureteral orifices and half way around the bladder neck. (**c**) Bladder flap raised with the mucosa ready to be tubularized over 8F feeding tube. (**d**) Appearance of anterior bladder tube once buried into the posterior bladder wall mucosa

divided from the bladder in an inverted U shape and rolled into a tube over a feeding tube. This tube is then placed in a submucosal tunnel in the posterior wall of the bladder in between the ureteral orifices (Fig. 7).

A series comparing open and robotic BNR demonstrated longer operative time but no difference in length of stay, complications, or continence outcomes between approaches [21]. Some groups have combined a bladder sling with a BNR procedure; however, the utility of this is not known as the reported success of 82% in this cohort of 38 patients [22, 23] is consistent with an 85.2% continence in a cohort of 55 patients who underwent robotic APV, with 21 of them undergoing concomitant BNR, 17 urethral sling, and 15 augmentation [24].

5.4 Bladder Neck Closure

Bladder neck closure is the most aggressive of bladder outlet surgeries, yet it is the most successful and can be used as a secondary option after other options have failed. We do this with robot assistance using an anterior bladder approach and dividing the urethra from the bladder at the level of the bladder neck. At this level, the dorsal venous complex can be frequently spared. Key concepts of this procedure are to mobilize the bladder well away from the urethra, to perform a multilayered closure of both the urethra and bladder with inversion of the edges of the closure, and to place a barrier layer between the closed edges, like the rectal muscle flap based on the inferior epigastric artery or Alloderm. All these maneuvers are to prevent fistula formation that would lead to recurrent incontinence.

6 Summary

The robot-assisted laparoscopic approach is an excellent tool to perform complex bladder reconstruction. We truly believe that with continued evolution of instrumentation and technique, this will be a predominant way to perform complex bladder reconstruction in children.

References

1. Razmaria AA, Marchetti PE, Prasad SM, Shalhav AL, Gundeti MS. Does robot-assisted laparoscopic ileocystoplasty (RALI) reduce peritoneal adhesions compared with open surgery? BJU Int. 2014;113:468–75. https://doi.org/10.1111/bju.12284.
2. Meeks JJ, Hagerty JA, Lindgren BW. Pediatric robotic-assisted laparoscopic diverticulectomy. Urology. 2009;73:299–301. https://doi.org/10.1016/j.urology.2008.06.068.
3. Christman MS, Casale P. Robot-assisted bladder diverticulectomy in the Pediatric population. J Endourol. 2012;26:1296–300. https://doi.org/10.1089/end.2012.0051.
4. Noh PH, Bansal D. Pediatric robotic assisted laparoscopy for paraureteral bladder diverticulum excision with ureteral reimplantation. J Pediatr Urol. 2013;9:e28–30. https://doi.org/10.1016/j.jpurol.2012.06.011.
5. Koehne E, Desai S, Lindgren B. Robot-assisted laparoscopic diverticulectomy with ureteral reimplantation. J Pediatr Urol. 2020;16:508–9. https://doi.org/10.1016/j.jpurol.2020.06.009.
6. Hsu THS, Shortliffe LD. Laparoscopic Mitrofanoff appendicovesicostomy. Urology. 2004;64:802–4. https://doi.org/10.1016/j.urology.2004.04.059.
7. Berkowitz J, North AC, Tripp R, Gearhart JP, Lakshmanan Y. Mitrofanoff continent catheterizable conduits: top down or bottom up? J Pediatr Urol. 2009;5:122–5. https://doi.org/10.1016/j.jpurol.2008.11.003.
8. Nguyen HT, Passerotti CC, Penna FJ, Retik AB, Peters CA. Robotic assisted laparoscopic Mitrofanoff appendicovesicostomy: preliminary experience in a pediatric population. J Urol. 2009;182:1528–34. https://doi.org/10.1016/j.juro.2009.06.055.
9. Famakinwa O, Rosen A, Gundeti M. Robot-assisted laparoscopic Mitrofanoff Appendicovesicostomy technique and outcomes of extravesical and intravesical approaches. Eur Urol. 2013;64:831–6.
10. Wille MA, Zagaja GP, Shalhav AL, Gundeti MS. Continence outcomes in patients undergoing robotic assisted laparoscopic Mitrofanoff appendicovesicostomy. J Urol. 2011;185:1438–43. https://doi.org/10.1016/j.juro.2010.11.050.
11. Cohen AJ, Pariser JJ, Anderson BB, Pearce SM, Gundeti MS. The robotic appendicovesicostomy and bladder augmentation. Urol Clin N Am. 2015;42:121–30. https://doi.org/10.1016/j.ucl.2014.09.009.
12. Galansky L, Andolfi C, Adamic B, Gundeti MS. Continent cutaneous Catheterizable channels in pediatric patients: a decade of experience with open and robotic approaches in a single center. Eur Urol. 2021;79:866–78. https://doi.org/10.1016/j.eururo.2020.08.013.
13. Gundeti MS, Eng MK, Reynolds WS, Zagaja GP. Pediatric robotic-assisted laparoscopic augmentation Ileocystoplasty and Mitrofanoff appendicovesicostomy: complete intracorporeal—initial case report. Urology. 2008;72:1144–7. https://doi.org/10.1016/j.urology.2008.06.070.
14. Murthy P, Cohn JA, Selig RB, Gundeti MS. Robot-assisted laparoscopic augmentation Ileocystoplasty and Mitrofanoff Appendicovesicostomy in children: updated interim results. Eur Urol. 2015;68:1069–75. https://doi.org/10.1016/j.eururo.2015.05.047.
15. Simeoni J, Guys JM, Mollard P, Buzelin JM, Moscovici J, Bondonny JM, et al. Artificial urinary sphincter implantation for neurogenic bladder: a multi-institutional study in 107 children. Br J Urol. 1996;78:287–93. https://doi.org/10.1046/j.1464-410X.1996.06126.x.
16. Catti M, Lortat-Jacob S, Morineau M, Lottmann H. Artificial urinary sphincter in children—voiding or emptying? An evaluation of functional results in 44 patients. J Urol. 2008;180:690–3. https://doi.org/10.1016/j.juro.2008.04.039.
17. Moscardi PRM, Ballesteros N, Abd-El-Barr A-E-R, Salvitti M, Castellan M. Robotic-assisted laparoscopic artificial urinary sphincter and MACE procedure on a pediatric patient. J Pediatr Urol. 2017;13:527–8. https://doi.org/10.1016/j.jpurol.2017.06.011.
18. Noordhoff TC, van den Hoek J, Yska MJ, Wolffenbuttel KP, Blok BFM, Scheepe JR. Long-term follow-up of bladder outlet procedures in children with neurogenic urinary incontinence. J Pediatr Urol. 2019;15(35):e1–35.e8. https://doi.org/10.1016/j.jpurol.2018.08.018.
19. Cole EE, Adams MC, Brock JW, Pope JC. Outcome of continence procedures in the pediatric patient: a single institutional experience. J Urol. 2003;170:560–3. https://doi.org/10.1097/01.ju.0000078015.55801.52.
20. Bagli DJ, Khoury AE. Urethral lengthening with anterior Bladder Wall flap (Pippi salle procedure): modifications and extended indications of the technique. J Urol. 1997;158(2):585–90.
21. Grimsby GM, Jacobs MA, Menon V, Schlomer BJ, Gargollo PC. Perioperative and short-term outcomes of robotic vs open bladder neck procedures for neurogenic incontinence. J Urol. 2016;195:1088–92. https://doi.org/10.1016/j.juro.2015.11.043.
22. Gargollo PC. Robotic-assisted bladder neck repair. Urol Clin N Am. 2015;42:111–20. https://doi.org/10.1016/j.ucl.2014.09.013.
23. Gargollo PC, White LA. Robotic-assisted bladder neck procedures for incontinence in pediatric patients. Front Pediatr. 2019;7:172. https://doi.org/10.3389/fped.2019.00172.
24. Gundeti MS, Petravick ME, Pariser JJ, Pearce SM, Anderson BB, Grimsby GM, et al. A multi-institutional study of perioperative and functional outcomes for pediatric robotic-assisted laparoscopic Mitrofanoff appendicovesicostomy. J Pediatr Urol. 2016;12(386):e1–386.e5. https://doi.org/10.1016/j.jpurol.2016.05.031.

Miscellaneous Procedures (Prostatic Utricle/UG Sinus/Oncological/Renal Transplantation Applications)

Rohan Batra, Arvind Ganpule, Sheila Mallenahalli, and Pankaj P. Dangle

1 Background

Pelvic surgeries have evolved considerably in recent years—not only in technique but in outcomes as well. The traditional open procedures have since started to be replaced by robotic or laparoscopic approaches due to their considerable benefits. Open techniques are invasive and technically challenging due to the complex anatomy of the pelvic area. The potential risk involves damage to the pelvic plexus nerves, urethra, and external sphincter due to the close proximity of these structures [1]. This in turn could lead to complications with fertility and poor bladder control [2]. Open techniques do allow for greater visualization of the area but can be associated with greater complications due to the necessity of separating the bladder walls [3].

The robotic approach allows for three-dimensional magnification which provides a greater field of vision and more accurate visualization of the operative cavity [4, 5]. Its minimally invasive techniques, access to more complex anatomy, ability for great precision, and faster healing times have brought it to the forefront [6]. Robotic approaches were also shown to have lower rates of acute kidney injury (AKI) as compared to open procedures [7]. Furthermore, robotic techniques also provide the ability to eliminate user's tremors, allowing for more precise instrument handling [8]. Laparoscopic procedures have also been shown to not only reduce hospital stay but also to provide greater cosmetic satisfaction to patients and their families [3]. Furthermore, this technique allowed for a lower blood loss than other methods [9].

R. Batra
Muljibhai Patel Urological Hospital, Nadiad, India

A. Ganpule (✉)
Department of Urology, Division of Robotic and Laparoscopic Surgery, Muljibhai Patel Urological Hospital, Nadiad, India

S. Mallenahalli
School of Medicine, University of Alabama at Birmingham, Birmingham, AL, USA

P. P. Dangle
Department of Urology, School of Medicine, Indiana University, Indianapolis, IN, USA

Riley Children's Hospital, Indianapolis, IN, USA

2 Prostatic Utricle

One use of robotic pelvic surgery includes prostatic utricle (PU) cyst excisions. PUs are lesions that appear as midline diverticula between the bladder and the rectum, usually connecting to the prostatic urethra [2]. PUs also often characteristically have a tubular shape [9]. They are quite uncommon, presenting in up to 4% of newborns and 5% of urologic patients [2, 10]. Around 11–14% of PUs are associated with hypospadias, with a larger frequency in perineal hypospadias specifically [2]. They are thought to primarily arise from the failed regression of the Mullerian ducts in male prostatic urethra [11]. Their cranial section is derived from the Mullerian ducts while their caudal sections are derived from the urogenital sinus (UGS) and Wolffian ducts [1]. Due to their complex embryological origins, PUs often present in association with proximal hypospadias, cryptorchidism, renal agenesis, and disorders of sexual development [12, 13].

Due to the mixed urogenital sinus origin of the PU cyst, it can be lined with many different cell types such as transitional, cuboid, and squamous epithelium arising from the urogenital sinus, Wolffian ducts, and Mullerian ducts, respectively [10]. This lends this area to a predilection of metaplasia and thus dysplasia. Therefore, an oncologic risk exists for PUs and must be considered when managing surgically.

Although most PU cases present silently, upward of 29% can become symptomatic secondary to urine retention within the cyst [3]. This can cause recurrent urinary tract infections (UTI), pseudo-incontinence, and dysuria among other symptoms caused by mass effect on surrounding organs [1, 14]. A significant amount of large PUs, up to 12%, can be associated with decreased fertility rates. Once symptomatic, the next step in care is obtaining radiologic imaging studies to confirm the presences of the PU cyst. This can be done via

P. Wiklund et al. (eds.), *Robotic Urologic Surgery*, https://doi.org/10.1007/978-3-031-00363-9_73

ultrasound for an initial assessment or a T2 MRI (magnetic resonance imaging) for a more detailed view [2]. Once visualized by a voiding cystourethrogram, PUs can then be graded into different categories. Grade 0 is present only in the verumontanum, Grade 1 is below the bladder neck, Grade 2 is over the bladder neck, and Grade 3 is distal to the external sphincter [1, 10]. Higher PU grades are almost exclusively seen in the setting of severe hypospadias [1]. If the cyst is not fully filled at time of imaging, however, it can be missed and remain undetected. Following confirmation of the anatomic anomaly, surgical options can then be considered.

2.1 Surgical Approach

Due to the complex anatomy that a PU presents, it remains precedent for symptomatic PUs only to undergo surgical management [2]. Conservative symptomatic management is also available, such as transrectal ultrasound-guided aspiration or antimicrobial treatment; however, these may fail to resolve the underlying pathology [10]. Many surgical approaches have been attempted such as transperitoneal, sagittal, rectum retraction and perineal techniques [12]. However, the two primary surgical corrections for PUs are open transvesical excisions (OTE) and laparoscopic excisions. The OTE procedure begins with a ureteroscope being placed into the prostatic utricle, after which the ureters are dissected and the bladder is incised through the trigone. This allows for the utricle to be secured and trace its connection to the urethra. The utricle is then excised. A urethral stent tube is placed to create and close the stump [3]. This procedure has much more morbidity due to the nature of dissection involved.

For robot-assisted laparoscopic techniques, the patient is first placed into lithotomy position. Cystoscopy is then done using a guide wire to catheterize the prostatic utricle itself, traditionally using a Foley catheter with 1.5 mL balloon. An umbilical camera port is placed using the open Hassan technique, after which two more ports are placed on either side of the midclavicular line. Another assistant port just under the costal margin is placed on the left side. The robot is then docked after which a 30^0 down lens is inserted. The peritoneum is then incised and dissected behind the bladder into the Denonvilliers fascia between the anterior bladder and posterior rectum. In order to retract the bladder, a holding stitch is placed percutaneously through the bladder. The vas deferens, the prostatic utricle, and the seminal vesicles are then identified with continued dissection via the previously inserted Foley catheter. The cyst is incised anteriorly with a 30^0 up lens, opening the cyst cavity. The anterior wall is excised while the posterior wall was kept intact and approximated with 5–0 PDS suture. The posterior wall is kept intact when the anatomy does not preclude the complete excision due to the vas deferens or seminal vesicles being closely associated. If this is not the case, then the excision can be performed. Utmost precaution must be taken as the excision is performed close to the urethra to prevent the urethral stricture. A cystoscopy is then performed again to place another Foley catheter over a guide wire into the bladder. The ports were then closed to complete the procedure [15].

3 Oncology

In addition to surgical approaches for prostatic utricle repair, robotic surgery approaches can be used to excise malignant growths. The Society of Paediatric Oncology (SIOP) published a list of indications for laparoscopic nephrectomies including unilateral lesions, lesions that are small and central with clear negative margins, and the ability to sample lymph nodes [8]. For example, Wilms' tumor is the most common pediatric renal cancer, and unilateral lesions can be resected via laparoscopic methods. The precision and technical skill that accompany robotic techniques are especially imperative for Wilms' tumors because of the risk of intraoperatively seeding the other kidney [16]. Nephron-sparing surgeries (NSS) are preferred due to the ability of patients to retain some kidney function postoperatively rather than a full nephrectomy. Partial nephrectomies have also long been performed in the setting of pediatric renal cell carcinomas (RCC). This procedure is done due to the lack of medical therapies available to treat RCC [17]. For many pediatric RCC cases, surrounding lymph nodes are also removed to appropriately stage the disease.

Retroperitoneal lymph node dissection (RPLND) is a procedure that can also be used as a treatment for certain types of non-seminomatous germ cell tumors (NSGCT). Robotic techniques are ideal for this operation because they can be performed with a single dock. A supine position and transperitoneal approach are traditionally used to create a flap from the posterior peritoneum of the cecum and ligament of Treitz [18]. The robotic laparoscopic approach again provides greater dexterity of instruments in such a sensitive space as well as more satisfactory cosmetic outcomes [19]. However, these procedures are better done in collaboration with an adult urologist and are described further in later chapters.

It is also imperative that negative margins are obtained to ensure all of the tumors have been resected. Laparoscopic cases showed no difference in the ability to obtain negative margins versus open cases, and this is often done with the help of intraoperative ultrasound [7]. One other consideration for robotic partial nephrectomies is the decision of which vessels to clamp during surgery. Open techniques do indeed have better rates of clampless procedures as compared to robotic cases [7].

The same principles apply to cystic nephromas, a type of benign renal cysts. As it is a benign lesion, a more conservative approach is traditionally taken to treatment—hence the preference for laparoscopic techniques versus open techniques. The details are not discussed here as they are described in the adult section of this book. We suggest that as these procedures are uncommon, it may be beneficial to work with an adult urologist who is familiar with such cases on routine basis.

4 Urogenital Sinus

Urogenital sinuses (UGS) occur when the urethra and vagina fail to separate during development [20]. Surgical correction of UGS usually involves a clitoroplasy, labiaplasty, and vaginoplasty [21]. These procedures are very technically involved and complex due to the many anatomic structures needing to be manipulated. Robotic instruments are particularly useful when retracting the vagina and visualizing the fistula connection [22]. Vaginoplasty with bowel segments can be performed easily using the robotic approach [23]. The details have been described in this chapter.

5 Pediatric Renal Transplant

Robotic platform in the pediatric urology population was first described in 2002 for a pyeloplasty for an ureteropelvic junction obstruction. Renal transplantation is a standard of care in the adult as well as the pediatric populations in patients with end-stage renal disease (ESRD) [24]. In the last few years, outcomes of pediatric transplantation have improved due to improved immunosuppressive therapy, expanded living kidney donor transplantation programs and better pretransplant preparation of the recipient, and improved surgical techniques in kidney retrieval. Currently, the survival rates at one, five, and ten years posttransplant are 98, 95, and 91%, respectively [25]. Robot-assisted laparoscopic surgery has changed the scope of minimally invasive surgery. But the adaptation of robotic platform in children has been challenging [26]. This is due to the need for additional skill sets and specialized instrumentation required for the procedure.

The first adult robot-assisted kidney transplantation (RAKT) was performed by Giulianotti et al. [27] in 2010. In 2014, Menon et al. [28] standardized the transperitoneal approach with regional hypothermia maintenance during the rewarming time, albeit this was described in adults. In the following years, RAKT has become an increasingly common procedure in select high-volume centers. This can be attributed to promising results which have indicated RAKT to be a safe, feasible, and reproducible procedure [29, 30].

However, children are not "small adults" and results of adults cannot be plainly extrapolated to the pediatric population. Till date, RAKT experience remains limited in the pediatric population. The first full case report on pediatric (eight-year-old child) RAKT was published in 2019 by Decaestecker and team at the Ghent University Hospital, Belgium. It demonstrated that RAKT in children is technically feasible and safe and resulted in excellent graft function.

Bansal et al. released a comparative analysis of outcomes and long-term follow-up of pediatric RAKT with an open kidney transplantation counterpart [31]. Twenty-five patients were included in the study, 21 of whom underwent open renal transplantation and 4 underwent RAKT. A significantly higher rewarming ischemia time was noted in the RAKT group [31] but that may be attributable to the initial phase of the learning curve for the procedure, a phenomenon which was similarly observed in the initial phases of adult RAKT [29]. Perioperative analgesic requirements were significantly higher among the open renal transplantation groups as compared to the RAKT group. RAKT complications included transplant renal artery stenosis and subcapsular hematoma, but it was not exclusive to RAKT. Despite the limitations of this study, it demonstrated that pediatric RAKT is a feasible and safe procedure that results in excellent graft function [31].

In addition, Modi et al. [32] described a group of five children undergoing RAKT in 2013. All except one kidney were harvested from living donors. In two children, concomitant seminal vesicle cyst excision and nephrectomy were carried out. One child experienced spontaneous graft rupture on the third postoperative day requiring emergency exploration. Patel et al. [33] have compared outcomes of open versus robot-assisted pediatric renal transplant at a single center, involving 60 and 22 patients undergoing RAKT and OKT, respectively. Endpoints of their trial were feasibility of RAKT and creatinine value at 30 days posttransplantation. Both ureteric reimplantation time and intraoperative blood loss were significantly decreased in the RAKT group. In the RAKT group ($n = 60$), five patients had slow graft function, and seven patients lost graft during follow-up. Two patients had acute antibody-mediated rejection, four had chronic rejection, and one had de novo collapsing glomerulopathy with BKV nephropathy. Five patients from the RAKT group deceased during follow-up. In the OKT group ($n = 20$), two patients had slow graft function, two lost graft, and two deceased during follow-up. There was no significant observed difference in graft survival or overall survival [33].

Both Modi et al. and Patel et al. [32, 33] concluded that RAKT is feasible and safe.A pediatric robot-assisted kidney transplantation program is ongoing at Ghent, Belgium. Since the first pediatric RAKT case in 2018 [34], they have operated on an additional two children with good results. A pediatric robot-assisted kidney transplantation program is also ongoing at the Muljibhai Patel Urological Hospital, India, since 2014. Two children, one with 16 years and one with 18 years of age, have been operated with good results [35].

6 Challenges in Pediatric Transplant

There are a number of challenges in pediatric patients including increased abdominal pressure, hypothermia, increased carbon dioxide absorption, and the physiologic effects of Trendelenburg position. These may impair cardiovascular function and ventilation, induce cerebral vasodilatation, and negatively affect urine output [36]. Intra-abdominal pressures lower than 10 mmHg do not appear to induce any significant clinical hemodynamic effects, and pressures up to 12 mmHg seem to be well tolerated [37].

The decreased workspace in pediatric abdominal surgeries makes trocar placement a critical procedural component as it can lead to desufflation, bleeding risk, and organ damage. Poorly positioned trocars may generate a gas leak, provoking rapid desufflation and further decreasing the small workspace [38]. Pediatric abdominal cavities typically contain adjacent organs in proximity to each other, increasing the risk for damage to surrounding organs during surgical procedures. Trocar positioning is also important for maximization of robot dexterity within the already restricted pediatric abdominal cavity. The recommended 8 cm gap for collision avoidance between the robot arms in adult cases is often difficult in children due to workspace limitations. Also, there is no standardized trocar placement in robotic pediatric procedures due to variations in weight and height. Da Vinci Xi and X facilitate the docking procedure with easy connection of instruments and the increased movement ability of the patient cart. Additionally, while most robotic adult procedures involve four robot arms, the limited workspace in pediatric patients commonly only allows usage of three out of four robot arms (camera port and two robotic ports) [39, 40].

There are differences in both the aesthetic and functional outcomes of RAKT as compared to open renal transplant [31, 41, 42]. RAKT can give superior aesthetic outcomes, which are especially desired for young children [31]. Surgeons should discuss differences in clinical outcomes with the patient's parents, in addition to the resultant scarring of different approach modalities.

To date, an 8 kg cutoff value is the lowest weight allowed for consideration of robot-assisted minimally invasive surgery in children. For RAKT specifically, eight years of age is considered to be the minimum threshold, as most transplanted kidneys are adult-sized kidneys which are then transplanted into a smaller child [43].

In order to start a pediatric RAKT program, a team of surgeons experienced both in robotic-assisted surgery and kidney transplantation surgery, along with the full support of a pediatric nephrology and anesthesiology team, is recommended. A high level of robotic experience is recommended before initiating a RAKT program [44].

7 Specific Considerations

Contrary to the adult RAKT procedure, in pediatric RAKT, the graft renal vessels are anastomosed to the common iliac vessels instead of the external iliac vessels, in order to match the vessel size of the donor (adult-sized renal vessels) and recipient (pediatric-sized iliac vessels). We use a modified hypothermia jacket to keep the graft cool during the anastomosis (Figs. 1 and 2) [31]. It should be noted that according to the literature, renal blood flow and function are reduced in the presence of pneumoperitoneum, potentially leading to graft impairment [45]. But the potential damage to the graft as a result of pneumoperitoneum is not yet fully known, and a correlation between operative time (and thus exposure to

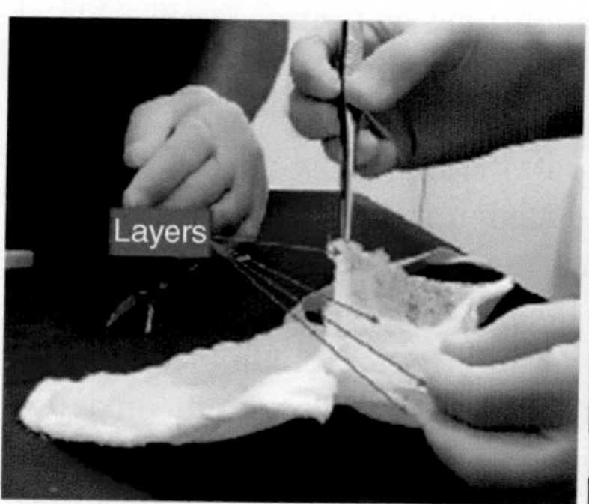

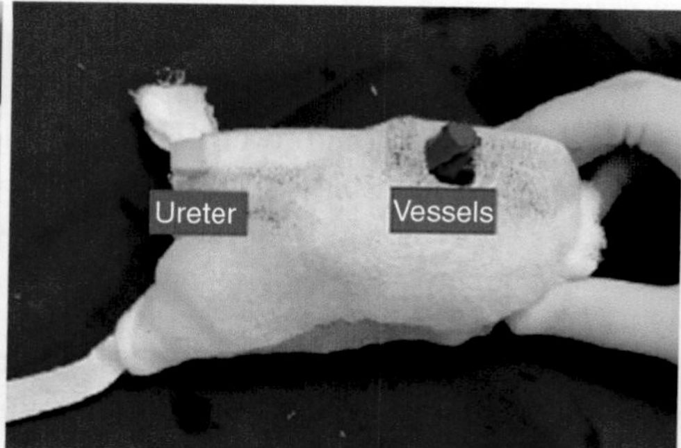

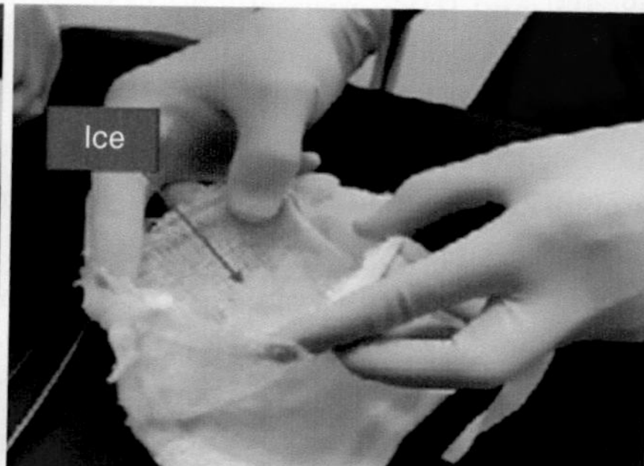

Fig. 1 Modified Hypothermia graft jacket

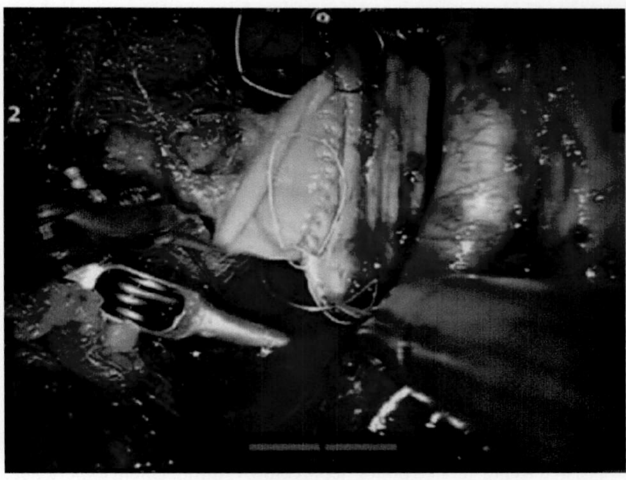

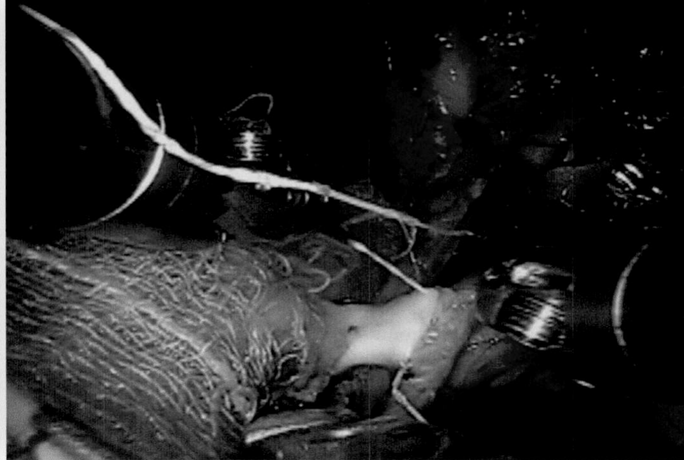

Fig. 2 Venous and arterial anastomosis (end to side)

pneumoperitoneum) and graft function in adult RAKT has not yet been identified [29]. We prefer a stable low pneumoperitoneum pressure of 8 mmHg for RAKT as of the moment of reperfusion to mitigate any potential adverse influence of higher pneumoperitoneum pressures [46, 47].

8 Conclusion

It is technically feasible to perform robotic or laparoscopic operations in the pediatric population for a variety of urologic pathologies including pediatric utricle, urogenital sinus, and malignancy resection. These minimally invasive procedures allow for greater precision of operating instruments, shorter hospital stays, shorter healing times, and greater cosmetic satisfaction. Thus, robotic techniques are often preferred over open techniques when performing pelvic surgery in children.

Although data on RAKT in children is less, it is a safe and feasible procedure and results in excellent graft function. It should only be performed by a RAKT team experienced in both robot-assisted laparoscopic surgery and transplantation surgery, fully supported by a team of pediatric nephrologists and anesthesiologists.

References

1. Meisheri IV, Motiwale SS, Sawant VV. Surgical management of enlarged prostatic utricle. Pediatr Surg Int. 2000;16(3):199–203. https://doi.org/10.1007/s003830050722.
2. Priyadarshi V, Singh JP, Mishra S, Vijay MK, Pal DK, Kundu AK. Prostatic utricle cyst: a clinical dilemma. APSP J Case Rep. 2013;4(2):16.
3. Jia W, Liu GC, Zhang LY, Wen YQ, Fu W, Hu JH, Xia HM. Comparison of laparoscopic excision versus open transvesical excision for symptomatic prostatic utricle in children. J Pediatr Surg. 2016;51(10):1597–601. https://doi.org/10.1016/j.jpedsurg.2016.06.004. Epub 2016 Jun 13
4. Goruppi I, Avolio L, Romano P, Raffaele A, Pelizzo G. Robotic-assisted surgery for excision of an enlarged prostatic utricle. Int J Surg Case Rep. 2015;10:94–6. https://doi.org/10.1016/j.ijscr.2015.03.024. Epub 2015 Mar 13
5. Masieri L, Sessa F, Cini C, Sessa M, Vanacore D, Tasso G, Pili A, Sforza S, Greco I, Campi R, Minervini A, Carini M. Robot-assisted nephron-sparing surgery for cystic nephroma in a pediatric patient: a case report. J Endourol Case Rep. 2019;5(1):7–9. https://doi.org/10.1089/cren.2018.0084.
6. Hong YK, Onal B, et al. Robot-assisted laparoscopic excision of symptomatic retrovesical cysts in boys and young adults. J Urol. 2011;186:2372–8.
7. Bravi CA, Larcher A, Capitanio U, Mari A, Antonelli A, Artibani W, Barale M, Bertini R, Bove P, Brunocilla E, Da Pozzo L, Di Maida F, Fiori C, Gontero P, Li Marzi V, Longo N, Mirone V, Montanari E, Porpiglia F, Schiavina R, Schips L, Simeone C, Siracusano S, Terrone C, Trombetta C, Volpe A, Montorsi F, Ficarra V, Carini M, Minervini A. Perioperative outcomes of open, laparoscopic, and robotic partial nephrectomy: a prospective multicenter observational study (The RECORd 2 Project). Eur Urol Focus. 2021;7(2):390–6. https://doi.org/10.1016/j.euf.2019.10.013. Epub 2019 Nov 12
8. Blanc T, Pio L, Clermidi P, Muller C, Orbach D, Minard-Colin V, Harte C, Meignan P, Kohaut J, Heloury Y, Sarnacki S. Robotic-assisted laparoscopic management of renal tumors in children: preliminary results. Pediatr Blood Cancer. 2019;66(Suppl 3):e27867. https://doi.org/10.1002/pbc.27867. Epub 2019 May 28
9. Chang C, Steinberg Z, Shah A, Gundeti MS. Patient positioning and port placement for robotic surgery. J Endourol. 2014;28:631–8.
10. Liu B, He D, Zhang D, Liu X, Lin T, Wei G. Prostatic utricles without external genital anomalies in children: our experience, literature review, and pooling analysis. BMC Urol. 2019;19(1):21. https://doi.org/10.1186/s12894-019-0450-z.
11. Bayne AP, Austin JC, Seideman CA. Robotic assisted retrovesical approach to prostatic utricle excision and other complex pelvic pathology in children is safe and feasible. J Pediatr Urol. 2021;S1477-5131(21):00376–4. https://doi.org/10.1016/j.jpurol.2021.08.004. Epub ahead of print
12. Mostafa IA, Woodward MN, Shalaby MS. Cystoscopic-assisted laparoscopic excision of prostatic utricle. J Pediatr Urol. 2018;14(1):77–8. https://doi.org/10.1016/j.jpurol.2017.09.024. Epub 2017 Oct 27

13. Dai LN, He R, Wu SF, Zhao HT, Sun J. Surgical treatment for prostatic utricle cyst in children: a single-center report of 15 patients. Int J Urol. 2021;28(6):689–94. https://doi.org/10.1111/iju.14543. Epub 2021 Mar 29
14. Hester AG, Kogan SJ. The prostatic utricle: an under-recognized condition resulting in significant morbidity in boys with both hypospadias and normal external genitalia. J Pediatr Urol. 2017;13(5):492.e1–5. https://doi.org/10.1016/j.jpurol.2017.01.019. Epub 2017 Mar 1
15. Nigam M, Dangle PP, Cohen AJ, Gundeti MS. Robot-assisted laparoscopic excision of prostatic utricle cyst. J Endourol Part B Videourol. 2014;28(5):10. https://doi.org/10.1089/vid.2014.0025.
16. Yadav P, Mahajan A, Kandpal DK, Chowdhary SK. Nephron-sparing surgery for syndromic Wilms' tumor: robotic approach. Urology. 2018;116:172–5. https://doi.org/10.1016/j.urology.2018.03.003. Epub 2018 Mar 20
17. Cost NG, Geller JI, DeFoor WR Jr, Wagner LM, Noh PH. A robotic-assisted laparoscopic approach for pediatric renal cell carcinoma allows for both nephron-sparing surgery and extended lymph node dissection. J Pediatr Surg. 2012;47(10):1946–50. https://doi.org/10.1016/j.jpedsurg.2012.08.017.
18. Mittakanti HR, Porter JR. Robotic retroperitoneal lymph node dissection for testicular cancer: feasibility and latest outcomes. Curr Opin Urol. 2019;29(2):173–9. https://doi.org/10.1097/MOU.0000000000000582.
19. Klaassen Z, Hamilton RJ. The role of robotic retroperitoneal lymph node dissection for testis cancer. Urol Clin North Am. 2019;46(3):409–17. https://doi.org/10.1016/j.ucl.2019.04.009. Epub 2019 May 21
20. Acién P, Acién M. The presentation and management of complex female genital malformations. Hum Reprod Update. 2016;22(1):48–69. https://doi.org/10.1093/humupd/dmv048. Epub 2015 Nov 3
21. Rink RC, Cain MP. Urogenital mobilization for urogenital sinus repair. BJU Int. 2008;102(9):1182–97. https://doi.org/10.1111/j.1464-410X.2008.08091.x.
22. Phillips MR, Linden AF, Vinocur CD, Hagerty JA. Robot-assisted repair of a urogenital sinus with an anorectal malformation in a patient with McKusick-Kaufman syndrome. J Pediatr Urol. 2019;15(5):481–3. https://doi.org/10.1016/j.jpurol.2019.08.001. Epub 2019 Aug 13
23. Gundeti MS, Kumar R, Mohammad M. Robotic assisted ileo-vaginoplasty for vaginal atresia. J Pediatr Urol. 2021;17(2):273–4. https://doi.org/10.1016/j.jpurol.2021.01.023. Epub 2021 Jan 26
24. Dharnidharka VR, Fiorina P, Harmon WE. Kidney transplantation in children. N Engl J Med. 2014;371(6):549–58.
25. Talley L, Stablein DM. North American pediatric renal trials and collaborative studies: NAPRTCS 2006 Annual Report.
26. Spinoit AF, Subramaniam R. Update on the minimally invasive approach in paediatric urology: remote help for human hands? Eur Urol Suppl. 2015;14(1):20–4.
27. Giulianotti P, Gorodner V, Sbrana F, Tzvetanov I, Jeon H, Bianco F, Kinzer K, Oberholzer J, Benedetti E. Robotic transabdominal kidney transplantation in a morbidly obese patient. Am J Transplant. 2010;10(6):1478–82.
28. Menon M, Sood A, Bhandari M, Kher V, Ghosh P, Abaza R, Jeong W, Ghani KR, Kumar RK, Modi P, Ahlawat R. Robotic kidney transplantation with regional hypothermia: a step-by-step description of the Vattikuti Urology Institute–Medanta Technique (IDEAL Phase 2a). Eur Urol. 2014;65(5):991–1000.
29. Breda A, Territo A, Gausa L, Tuğcu V, Alcaraz A, Musquera M, Decaestecker K, Desender L, Stockle M, Janssen M, Fornara P. Robot-assisted kidney transplantation: the European experience. Eur Urol. 2018;73(2):273–81.
30. Musquera M, Peri L, Ajami T, Campi R, Tugcu V, Decaestecker K, Stockle M, Fornara P, Doumerc N, Vigues F, Barod R. Robot-assisted kidney transplantation: update from the European Robotic Urology Section (ERUS) series. BJU Int. 2021;127(2):222–8.
31. Bansal A, Maheshwari R, Chaturvedi S, Bansal D, Kumar A. Comparative analysis of outcomes and long-term follow-up of robot-assisted pediatric kidney transplantation, with open counterpart. Pediatr Transplant. 2021;25(3):e13917.
32. Modi P, Pal B, Modi J, Sarmah A, Kumar S, Kute V, Modi M, Shah V, Trivedi H. Robotic assisted laparoscopic kidney transplantation in children-an initial experience: abstract# A356. Transplantation. 2014;15(98):501.
33. Patel D, Singla SK, Mishra A, Chauhan R, Patel H, Kute V, Saha A, Vala K, Modi P. Prospective non-randomized open label trial comparing outcome of open versus robotic pediatric kidney transplant at single Centre. Transplantation. 2020;104(S3):S23.
34. Spinoit AF, Moreels N, Raes A, Prytula A, De Groote R, Ploumidis A, De Bleser E, Randon C, Vanpeteghem C, Walle JV, Van Laecke E. Single-setting robot-assisted kidney transplantation consecutive to single-port laparoscopic nephrectomy in a child and robot-assisted living-related donor nephrectomy: initial Ghent experience. J Pediatr Urol. 2019;15(5):578–9.
35. Ganpule A, Patil A, Singh A, Desai M, Gill I, Sabnis R, Desai M. Robotic-assisted kidney transplant: a single center experience with median follow-up of 2.8 years. World J Urol. 2020;38(10):2651–60.
36. Tobias JD. Anaesthesia for minimally invasive surgery in children. Best Pract Res Clin Anaesthesiol. 2002;16(1):115–30.
37. Baroncini S, Gentili A, Pigna A, Fae M, Tonini C, Tognù A. Anaesthesia for laparoscopic surgery in paediatrics. Minerva Anestesiol. 2002;68(5):406–13.
38. Peters CA. Robotically assisted surgery in pediatric urology. Urol Clin. 2004;31(4):743–52.
39. Spinoit AF, Nguyen H, Subramaniam R. Role of robotics in children: a brave new world! Eur Urol Focus. 2017;3(2–3):172–80.
40. Tennankore KK, Kim SJ, Alwayn IP, Kiberd BA. Prolonged warm ischemia time is associated with graft failure and mortality after kidney transplantation. Kidney Int. 2016;89(3):648–58.
41. Blinman T. Incisions do not simply sum. Surg Endosc. 2010;24(7):1746–51.
42. Barbosa JA, Barayan G, Gridley CM, Sanchez DC, Passerotti CC, Houck CS, Nguyen HT. Parent and patient perceptions of robotic vs open urological surgery scars in children. J Urol. 2013;190(1):244–50.
43. Grammens J, Schechter MY, Desender L, Claeys T, Sinatti C, Vande Walle J, Vermassen F, Raes A, Vanpeteghem C, Prytula A, Silay MS. Pediatric challenges in robot-assisted kidney transplantation. Front Surg. 2021;8:63.
44. Decaestecker K, Territo A, Campi R, Van Parys B, Bevilacqua G, Desender L, Breda A. Robot-assisted kidney transplantation. In: Küçük S, Canda AE, editors. Medical robotics-new achievements. London: IntechOpen; 2020.
45. Demyttenaere S, Feldman LS, Fried GM. Effect of pneumoperitoneum on renal perfusion and function: a systematic review. Surg Endosc. 2007;21(2):152–60.
46. Warle MC, Berkers AW, Langenhuijsen JF, Van der Jagt MF, Dooper PM, Kloke HJ, Pilzecker D, Renes SH, Wever KE, Hoitsma AJ, van der Vliet JA. Low-pressure pneumoperitoneum during laparoscopic donor nephrectomy to optimize live donors' comfort. Clin Transpl. 2013;27(4):E478–83.
47. Aditianingsih D, Mochtar CA, Lydia A, Siregar NC, Margyaningsih NI, Madjid AS, Suwarto S. Effects of low versus standard pressure pneumoperitoneum on renal syndecan-1 shedding and VEGF receptor-2 expression in living-donor nephrectomy: a randomized controlled study. BMC Anesthesiol. 2020;20(1):1–7.

Part VI

Penile

Robotic-Assisted Video Endoscopic Inguinal Lymphadenectomy (R-VEIL) Technique and Outcomes for Penile Cancer

Marcos Tobias-Machado, Victor Enrique Corona-Montes, Marcio Covas Moschovas, Rene Javier Sotelo, and On behalf of Penile Cancer Collaborative Coalition

Abbreviations

PeC	penile cancer
ESMIL	endoscopic subcutaneous modified inguinal lymphadenectomy
VEIL	video endoscopic inguinal lymphadenectomy
R-VEIL	robotic video endoscopic inguinal lymphadenectomy
RA-VEIL	robotic-assisted video endoscopic inguinal lymphadenectomy
RAIL	robotic-assisted inguinal lymphadenectomy
L-VEIL	lateral video endoscopic inguinal lymphadenectomy
H-VEIL	hypogastric video endoscopic inguinal lymphadenectomy
ILND	inguinal lymph node dissection

On behalf of Penile Cancer Collaborative Coalition

M. Tobias-Machado (✉)
Department of Urology, Instituto do Cancer Arnaldo Vieira de Carvalho, São Paulo, Brazil

Faculdade de Medicina do ABC, Rede D'or São Luis, São Paulo, Brazil

V. E. Corona-Montes
Department of Urology, General Hospital of México/American British Council Hospital (A.B.C), México City, México

M. C. Moschovas
Faculdade de Medicina do ABC, Rede D'or São Luis, São Paulo, Brazil

AdventHealth Global Robotics Institute, Celebration, FL, USA

R. J. Sotelo
Section of Urologic Oncology, University of South California, Los Angeles, CA, USA

P. Wiklund et al. (eds.), *Robotic Urologic Surgery*, https://doi.org/10.1007/978-3-031-00363-9_74

1 General Aspects of Penile Cancer (PeC)

Penile cancer is a rare neoplasm in developed countries, with an estimated of less than 1% of cancers in the United States, approximately 2,100 new cases, and 400 deaths annually [1, 2]. According to the Global Cancer Observatory, the estimated number of incident cases is 34,475, with mortality of 15,138 patients of all ages [1]. However, in less developed areas of the world, such as Africa, Asia, and South America, it accounts for up to 10–20% of all malignancies in men and is considered a disease of older men, with an abrupt increase in incidence in the sixth decade (mean ages between 55 and 58 years old). This tumor is unusual in younger patients (<40 years old), although cases have been reported [3].

Multiple factors are associated with a risk of developing PeC, including genital warts (OR 7.6), penile tears (OR 5.2), chronic penile rash (OR 3.2), penile injuries (OR 3.5), phimosis (seven times higher risk), human papillomavirus (DNA identified in 50%), human immunodeficiency virus (4–8 times higher risk), tobacco exposure (three times more likely), and lichen sclerosis (balanitis xerotica obliterans) [4].

Robotic-assisted video endoscopic inguinal lymphadenectomy (R-VEIL), aside from its high cost, is a feasible technique when carried out in specialized centers because it provides reduced morbidity, adequate oncological results, blood loss, and hospital stay [5]. This technique has been adapted to minimally invasive surgery and, in comparison to the open inguinal lymphadenectomy, is preferred because of the high incidence of morbidity that stands at 50–90% in the open approach [6].

2 Inguinal Dissemination of Penile Cancer

Penile cancer usually disseminates to the inguinal lymph nodes, but only 1–2% of the patients will present distant metastases. In addition, approximately 20% of patients with clinically non-palpable inguinal nodes harbor occult metastases. The first draining lymph node group is found in the superficial and deep inguinal region (superomedial zone); the second lymph node group spread is in the ipsilateral pelvic area and retroperitoneum (para-caval/para-aortic lymph nodes) [7].

Patients included in the low-risk penile cancer group (Tis, Ta, T1G1, No LVI) have less than 16% metastatic rate to the lymph nodes, intermediate risk (T1G2) 17–50%, and high risk (T1G3, >T2, LVI) 68–73% metastatic rate [8].

Radical resection of inguinal metastases of PeC is the standard of treatment, and the most significant single predictor of survival in penile squamous cell carcinoma is the incidence and extent of lymph node involvement [3, 8]. The objective of the lymph node resection is to provide accurate pathology staging. If PeC is detected in the nodes, the natural history and pattern of metastasis change. Men found to have a single node involved (N1) had a 100% three-year disease-specific survival. The presence between one and three involved nodes predicts a five-year overall survival (OS) of 75.6%. From four to five nodes, the OS decreases to 8.4%, and more than five positive nodes is associated with 0% of survival rates in five years [8].

There is no controversy regarding oncological results offered by conventional radical inguinal lymphadenectomy. The dilemma lies in the high morbidity rate of this procedure, which is usually between 50% and 90% of overall complications with 10% of severe complications.

3 Inguinal Lymphadenectomy Indications in Penile Cancer

The treatment of regional lymph nodes is crucial and prognostic of patient survival. In these cases, radical lymphadenectomy is the treatment of choice, and a cure in disease confined to regional nodes can be achieved with this procedure. Regarding surgical morbidity, IL has selective indications considering the different risk groups [9, 10].

3.1 Patients with Clinically Normal Inguinal Lymph Nodes (cN0)

The micrometastatic disease occurs in up to 25% of the patients, and invasive lymph node staging is necessary. The indication for inguinal lymphadenectomy is intermediate (T1b, Grade 1 or 2) and high-risk tumors (T1b, Grade 3 or 4; any T2 or greater), which are considered to have elevated risks for lymphatic spread. The superficial inguinal lymphadenectomy is an option and will be completed (radical) if one pathological lymph node is found without extranodal extension. If the extranodal extension is present in more than two lymph nodes, inguinal and pelvic lymphadenectomy should be considered.

3.2 Patients with Palpable Unilateral or Bilateral Inguinal Nodes (cN1/cN2)

Metastatic disease is highly likely, and lymph node surgery is necessary (radical inguinal lymphadenectomy). Treatment should not be delayed in these patients because metastatic spread continues. If a high-risk primary lesion was identified, a complete inguinal lymphadenectomy and contralateral superficial lymphadenectomy should be performed. If ≥ 2 cm inguinal nodes are positive or ≥ 1 cm inguinal node is positive with extra nodal extension, an ipsilateral pelvic lymph node dissection should be performed.

3.3 Patients with Bulky Inguinal Nodes

In this scenario, the patients require multimodal treatment with chemotherapy protocols associated with surgery. Radical inguinal lymphadenectomy will be indicated after having a positive metastatic (fine needle aspiration) disease in unilateral mobile ≥ 4 cm lymph node. If ≥ 2 cm nodes are positive or have an extranodal extension, a pelvic lymphadenectomy should be performed and adjuvant chemotherapy considered. In cases that the lymph node is ≥4 cm and fixed, or mobile bilateral, neoadjuvant chemotherapy should be administrated after the fine needle aspiration positive finding, followed by inguinal and pelvic lymphadenectomy if an adequate response to chemotherapy is documented. For patients with nodes smaller than 3 cm (not palpable or palpable), either VEIL or R-VEIL is a suitable indication. For patients with bulk inguinal disease, open surgery is the gold standard.

3.4 Other Indications Beyond Penile Cancer

Vulvar cancer, anal cancer, melanoma, and other skin neoplasms have also been described as an indication of IL. In these situations, R-VEIL was reported with safety and efficacy.

4 Development of Minimally Invasive Inguinal Lymph Node Dissection (ILND)

Inguinal lymphadenectomy has been adapted to minimally invasive surgery to reduce the traditional open surgery morbidity. In 2002, Ian M. Thompson and Jay T. Bishop conceived the idea of an endoscopic and subcutaneous approach for inguinal lymph node dissection applying laparoscopic techniques. The endoscopic subcutaneous modified inguinal lymphadenectomy (ESMIL) procedure was described in a cadaveric model, identifying anatomical structures and overall feasibility [11].

In 2006, Tobias-Machado et al. reported the first successful VEIL experience in humans. In 2007, the same group published the landmark study comparing VEIL x open (one side for each technique) in ten patients showing reduced complications (20% vs. 70%), shorter hospitalization times, favorable cosmesis, and adequate short-term oncological outcomes. In the same year, Sotelo and colleagues published their initial experience with the same results [6, 12, 13].

Currently, the best evidence is a meta-analysis of 10 comparative studies with 290 procedures showing clear benefits for VEIL, especially regarding skin events, lymphedema, and severe complications. The robotic surgery application is recent in the literature and will need continued prospective evaluation compared to the standard laparoscopic endoscopic procedures.

This chapter describes the surgical technique for robotic-assisted video endoscopic inguinal lymphadenectomy (R-VEIL) in penile cancer, which has been modified since the origin of "the robotic era."

5 Endoscopic Anatomy of Femoral Triangle Region

Video endoscopic inguinal surgery has been described as a viable option in patients with low-volume inguinal disease. The most routinely utilized technique is retrograde, initiating at the vertex of the femoral triangle distally and progressing toward the inguinal ligament proximally. To perform this surgery with good results, it is essential to know and understand all aspects of endoscopic anatomy [12, 13].

The first significant anatomical landmarks to identify include the skin limits, Camper's fascia, and Scarpa's fascia. After this identification, a small incision is performed, and digital maneuvers will create the space for the trocar placement. In sequence, CO_2 gas insufflation and blunt optic dissection allow proper skin separation from the lymphatic and vascular elements located beneath it. The lateral limit of the femoral triangle is the sartorius muscle, the medial limit is the adductor longus muscle, and the superior limit is the inguinal ligament (IL) (Fig. 1).

Both fascias are externally palpable and easily identified. Crossing the medial limit, the saphena magna and the great

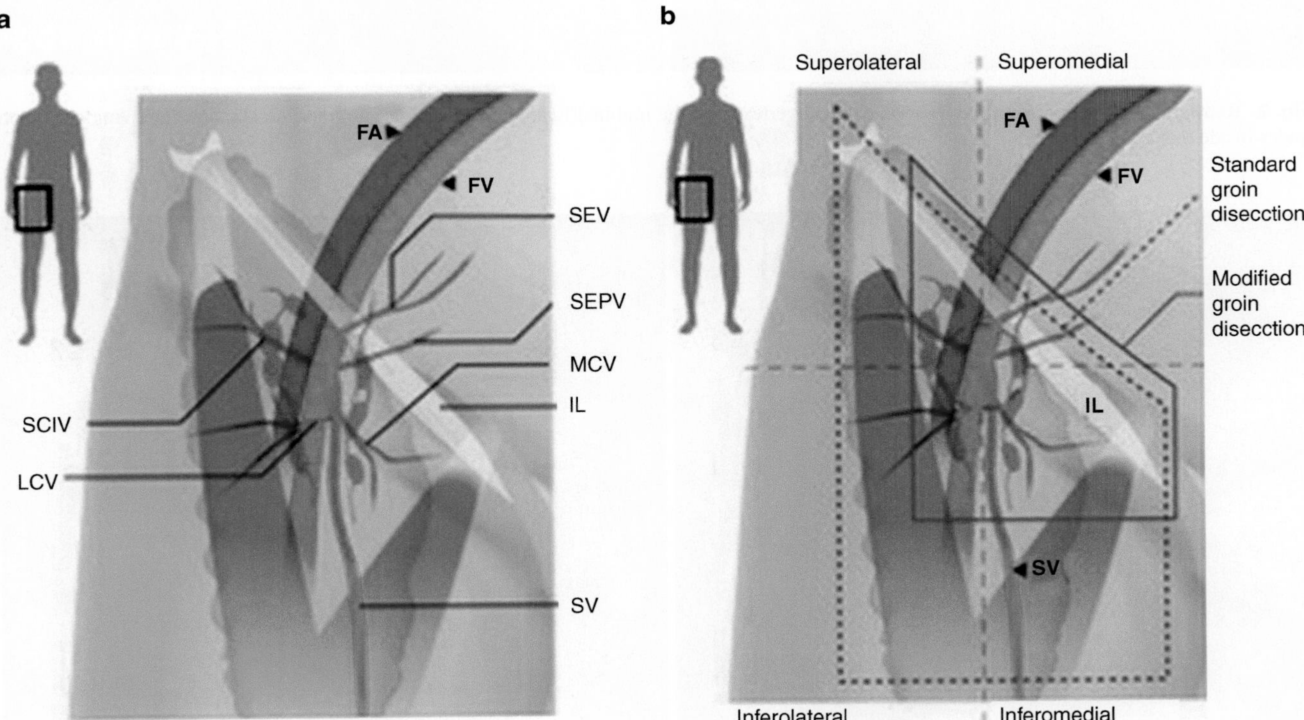

Fig. 1 FT, femoral triangle; IL, inguinal ligament; FA, femoral artery; SEV, superior epigastric vein; SEPV, superior epigastric posterior vein; SCIV, superior circumflex inferior vein; LCV, lateral cutaneous vein; SV, saphenous vein; MCV, medial cutaneous vein

saphenous vein are identified. In most patients with non-palpable lymph nodes, it is possible to spare the saphenous vein. Dissection under the Scarpa's fascia preserving subcutaneous adipose tissue, minimizing energy dissipation, is essential to prevent areas of skin devascularization. With progressive dissection, some lymph nodes are identified and separated from the skin to be included in the surgical specimen (Fig. 2).

Proximal dissection will lead to the fossa ovalis, also referred to as the saphenous hiatus, and identification of the accessory saphenous vein and other saphena tributaries. In normal conditions, seven tributaries drain to the femoral vein in the fossa oval (Fig. 1, schematic, and Fig. 3, endoscopic).

Externally, the junction between the saphenous and femoral is located approximately two fingerbreadths lateral and two fingerbreadths inferior to the pubic tubercle. The saphenous vein passes anteriorly through the fossa ovalis and elapses to the superficial inguinal region.

The fascia lata separates the inguinal lymph nodes into superficial and deep groups. The superficial inguinal lymph nodes are situated in the deep membranous layer of the superficial fascia of the thigh (Camper's fascia), approximately composed of 4 up to 25 nodes. The superficial inguinal nodes have been divided into the following five anatomical groups by Daseler [7, 14] (Fig. 3):

1. Superomedial nodes (I) around the superficial external pudendal and superficial epigastric veins
2. Superolateral nodes (II) around the superficial circumflex vein

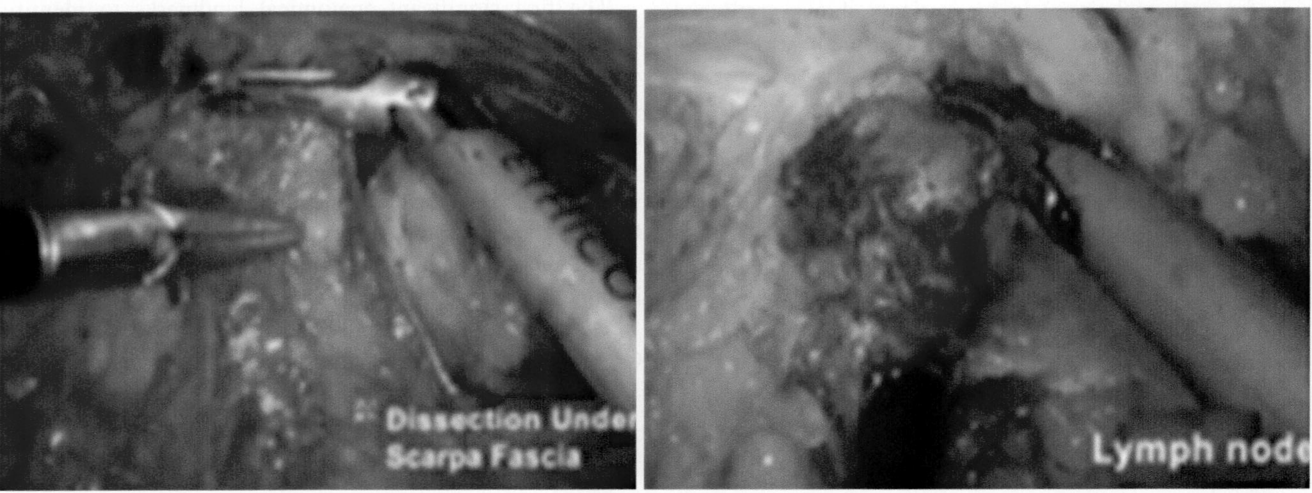

Fig. 2 Retrograde dissection from the femoral triangle vertex until the inguinal ligament preserving fat under the skin but removing all lymph nodes inside the template

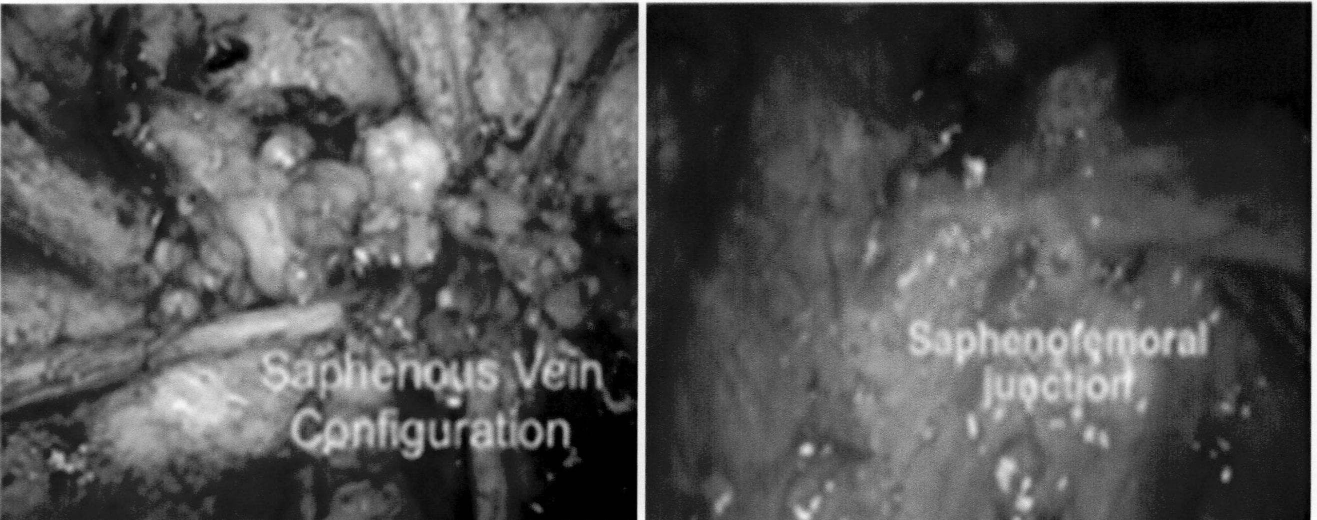

Fig. 3 Endoscopic view of tributaries of the saphena cross

3. Infero-lateral nodes (III) around the lateral femoral cutaneous and superficial circumflex veins
4. Inferomedial nodes (IV) around the greater saphenous vein
5. Central nodes (V) around the saphenofemoral junction

Most nodes are located above the fascia lata, specifically medial to the saphenous-femoral junction, and can be identified by their brown or green coloration. One must be careful to include all areolar tissues between the skin, inguinal cord, and saphenous vein. Preoperative ultrasound guidance and palpation may be helpful to mark the skin above the most prominent nodes.

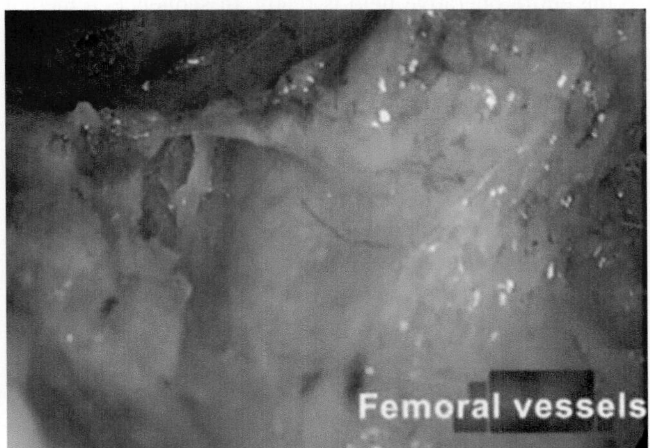

Fig. 4 The fascia lata is opened exactly in the area that covers the femoral artery to gain access to deep lymph nodes

Under the fascia lata, the structures that will be found in the femoral triangle are (from lateral to medial) the femoral nerve, femoral artery, femoral vein, and deep inguinal lymph nodes. The last three are inside the femoral sheath [7]. Sectioning the fascia lata over the pulse of the femoral artery is needed to access the deep node compartment where the deep inguinal nodes lie (Fig. 4). This includes all nodal and areolar tissues medial to the femoral vein and lateral to the adductor longus muscle. This resection is continued until Cloquet's node is identified (a more proximal node located inside the femoral channel). After this resection has been completed, the most critical structures of the femoral triangle have been identified.

The standard or full template of the inguinal lymph node dissection includes, according to Daseler, the superficial dissection and the deep inguinal nodes from the femoral triangle, limiting the dissection lateral to the femoral artery, which eliminates the risk of injury to the femoral nerve. This template incorporates the ligation of the saphenous vein as it emerges from the femoral vein [14].

In comparison, the modified template includes the superficial dissection of the 1, a portion of 2 and 5 lymph node groups. The inferior group nodes are not dissected; the deep dissection remains the same. The modified template was described to reduce the complication rate, which can also be accomplished by the minimally invasive approach. After total nodal resection, all anatomical landmarks can be identified (Fig. 5).

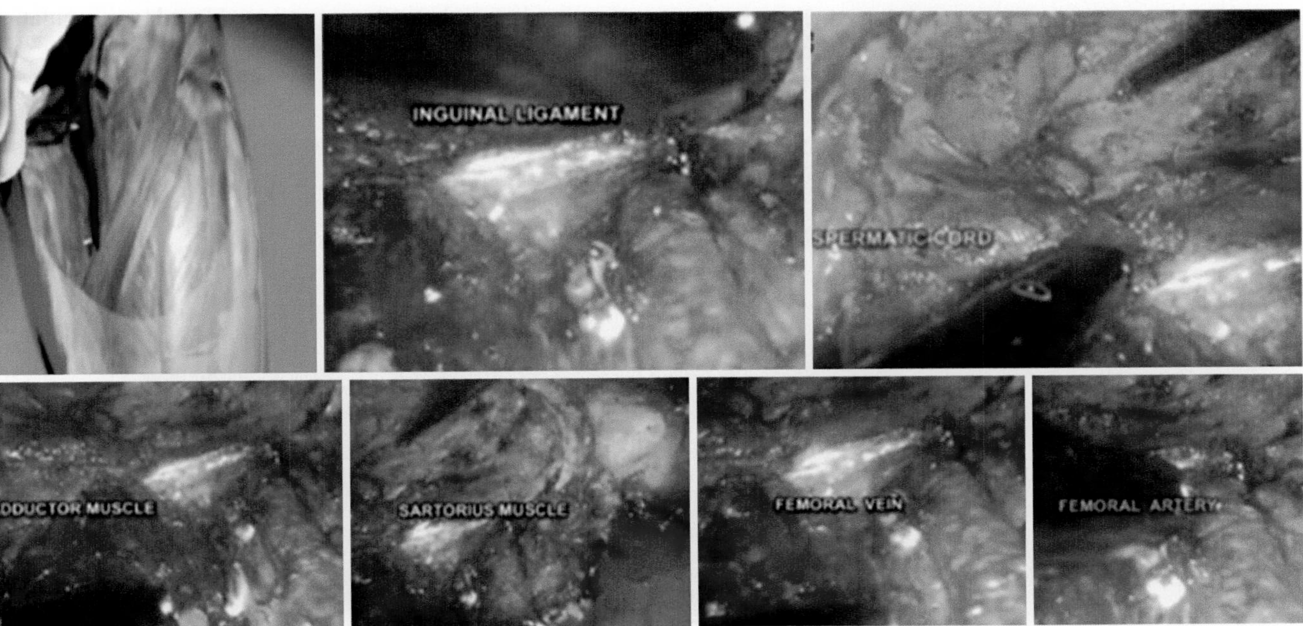

Fig. 5 Important structures preserved after resection of inguinal lymph nodes

6 Preoperative Patient Management

As previously described, for palpable disease, 30–50% of those nodes are secondary to associated inflammatory conditions. In general, we use four weeks of antibiotic therapy after penectomy and intraoperative prophylactic antibiotics to reduce postoperative inguinal infection. The most utilized broad-spectrum antibiotic is ampicillin with aminoglycoside or ciprofloxacin. The ideal time between penectomy and IL is six weeks.

As penile cancer patients generally have a high risk for thrombosis, we advocate routine low-molecular-weight heparin, starting the evening before surgery and continuing while the patient is in bed. Early ambulation is highly recommended as well. Heparin use may increase the risk of wound hematoma and serous wound drainage due to continued extravasation of the lymph.

In patients with a recent history of DVT (deep vein thrombosis) or pulmonary embolism (PE), a therapeutic dose of low-molecular-weight heparin followed by oral anticoagulants should be recommended.

7 R-VEIL Surgical Steps

7.1 Patient Positioning

The patient is placed on a low lithotomy position to allow bilateral groin dissection without repositioning the robot. The assistant stands lateral to the right leg for a right-sided dissection and between the legs for the left side. A Foley catheter is inserted in a sterile fashion after the inguinal and groin areas have been prepared and draped. Bony and soft tissue landmarks are marked on the skin surface, creating an inverted triangle in which the base is a line connecting the anterior superior iliac spine to the pubic tubercle along the course of the inguinal ligament. The lateral boundary is the sartorius muscle angling toward the apex. The medial limit is the adductor longus muscle, again extending toward the apex. These marks aid in correct trocar placement as well as in delineating the extent of dissection.

Positioning the robot is challenging during this surgery. At the beginning of our experience, we placed the robot on the right side of the table, considering it was an SI system, with not repositioning, just re-docking of the instruments. In the first step, we prepared the operating field, placing the patient in dorsal decubitus with the abduction of both legs, which are also dressed from the beginning to avoid time loss, so the entire operative field is ready. In sequence, a medial incision (3 cm) is performed in the femoral triangle, inside the sartorius muscle joint with the adductor longus.

A white subcutaneous layer is identified, which corresponds to the Scarpa's fascia. Sweeping finger dissection is used to dissect the potential space beneath the Scarpa's fascia to develop the skin flaps at the apex of the triangle in both directions and allow additional ports to be placed. We follow a digital dissection in the direction of the inguinal ligament. This blunt finger dissection is joined by movements to the left and right sides of the thigh and toward the upper limit as possible. The previous dissection is realized for the superficial plane of the lymphs (Fig. 6).

7.2 Trocar Placement and Docking

Once the space is created, we perform three additional incisions, and two robotic 8 mm ports are placed in triangulation with finger-guided techniques laterally and medially. One

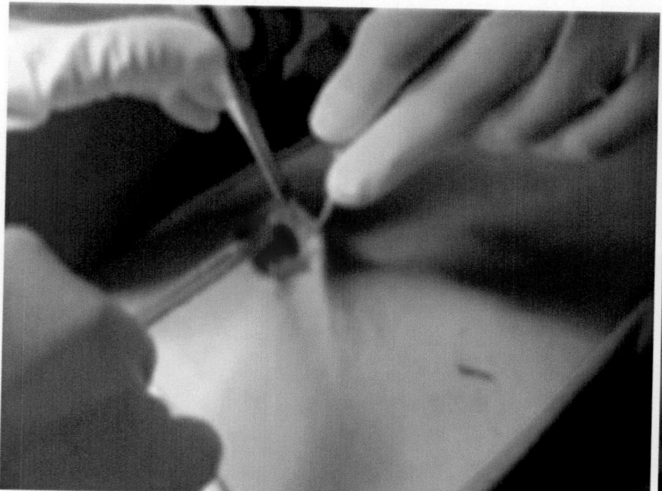

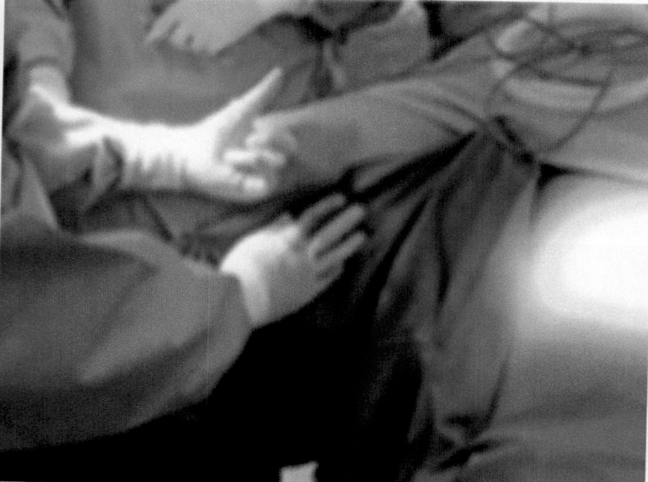

Fig. 6 Initial skin incision under the Scarpa's fascia distal for vertex of femoral triangle and finger dissection to create working space

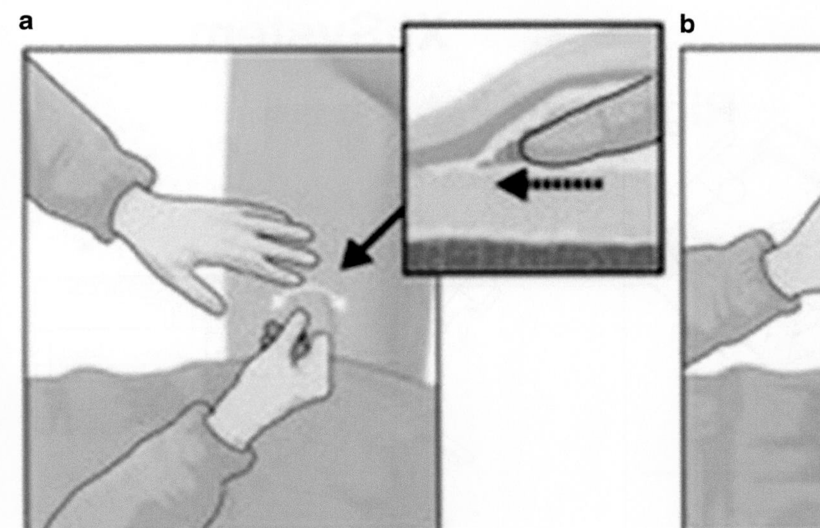

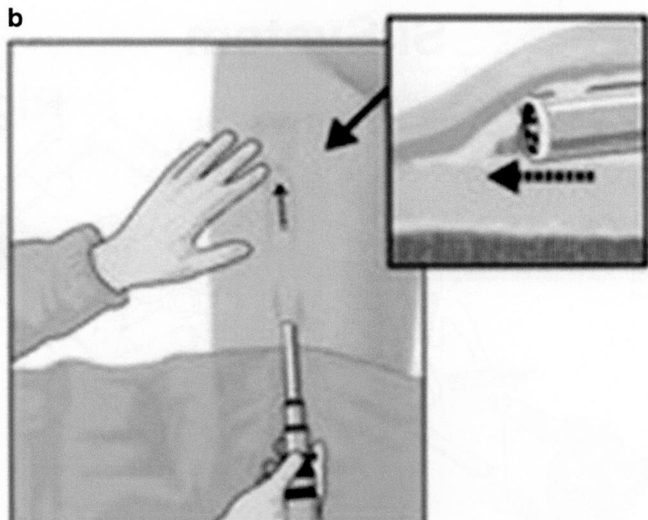

Fig. 7 Trocar placement and initial working space creation. Note that the skin is marked for femoral triangle limits and palpable or ultrasound located nodes to prevent that some node is not removed. Digital and optical dissections are done to create the space. Transillumination helps the surgeon to maintain dissection limits

additional 5–12 mm port between the scope and medial robotic port is an option for assistant aspiration, clipping, or stapling. A subcutaneous workspace is extended with the scope by sweeping the fat using the lens. This step aims to create a superficial subcutaneous flap under the Scarpa's fascia.

This description is done simultaneously, so both legs are ready for the robot docking. The da Vinci X or Xi provides smaller incisions and camera changing to another port, giving a faster and better position in the middle of the abducted legs of the patient. In all da Vinci systems, we use 0-degree lens, and once the ports are installed, the C02 insufflation is maintained at 10 mmHg (Fig. 7).

The robot is located at 45 degrees contralateral to the first procedure (right side) and ipsilateral to the patients in the second procedure (left side). The assistant is located lateral to the knees (Fig. 8).

7.3 Anterior, Posterior, and Lateral Dissection

Once the docking is completed, the 0-degree lens scope is placed, and all instruments are inserted under visualization. Several instruments can be used, including the bipolar Maryland, or forceps, in the left robotic arm and monopolar scissors in the right arm to dissect the membranous and lymphatic tissue deep to the Camper's fascia. Every effort is made to develop the anterior working space of the inguinal ligament, which is usually identified at the end of this dissection as a transverse structure with white fibers, marking the superior limit of the dissection.

A modern option is to utilize a robotic vessel sealer for dissecting and seal vessels up to 8 mm. Following the anatomical references of the femoral triangle, the packet of superficial nodes is located over the fascia lata (Fig. 9). Another suggestion for identifying and delineating the lymph nodes is fluorescence use. We usually inject 5–10 ml at the beginning of the procedure, at the peritumoral area, and minimally invasive resection can aid in removing suspicious nodes (Fig. 10).

With blunt dissection, the nodal tissue can be rolled inward on both sides. This maneuver is continued inferiorly and, on both sides, to define the inferior apex of the nodal packet. The saphenous vein is identified as it crosses the internal border of the dissection near the apex of the femoral triangle and, following the vein, leads the surgeon to the saphenous arch until its junction with the superficial femoral vein at the fossa ovalis. The dissection continues superiorly, where the packet is dissected away from the fascia lata with a combination of sharp and blunt dissection.

Typically, the nondominant hand lifts the packet, and the monopolar scissors in the dominant hand advance the dissection. After the fossa ovalis is encountered, the packet is dissected away at its superolateral and superomedial limits, narrowing it and pulling it away from the inguinal ligament. At this point, the superficial and deep plane of dissection joins and separates the package from the inguinal ligament. With the nodal packet circumferentially dissected except for its attachments to the saphenous arch, venous tributaries are clipped.

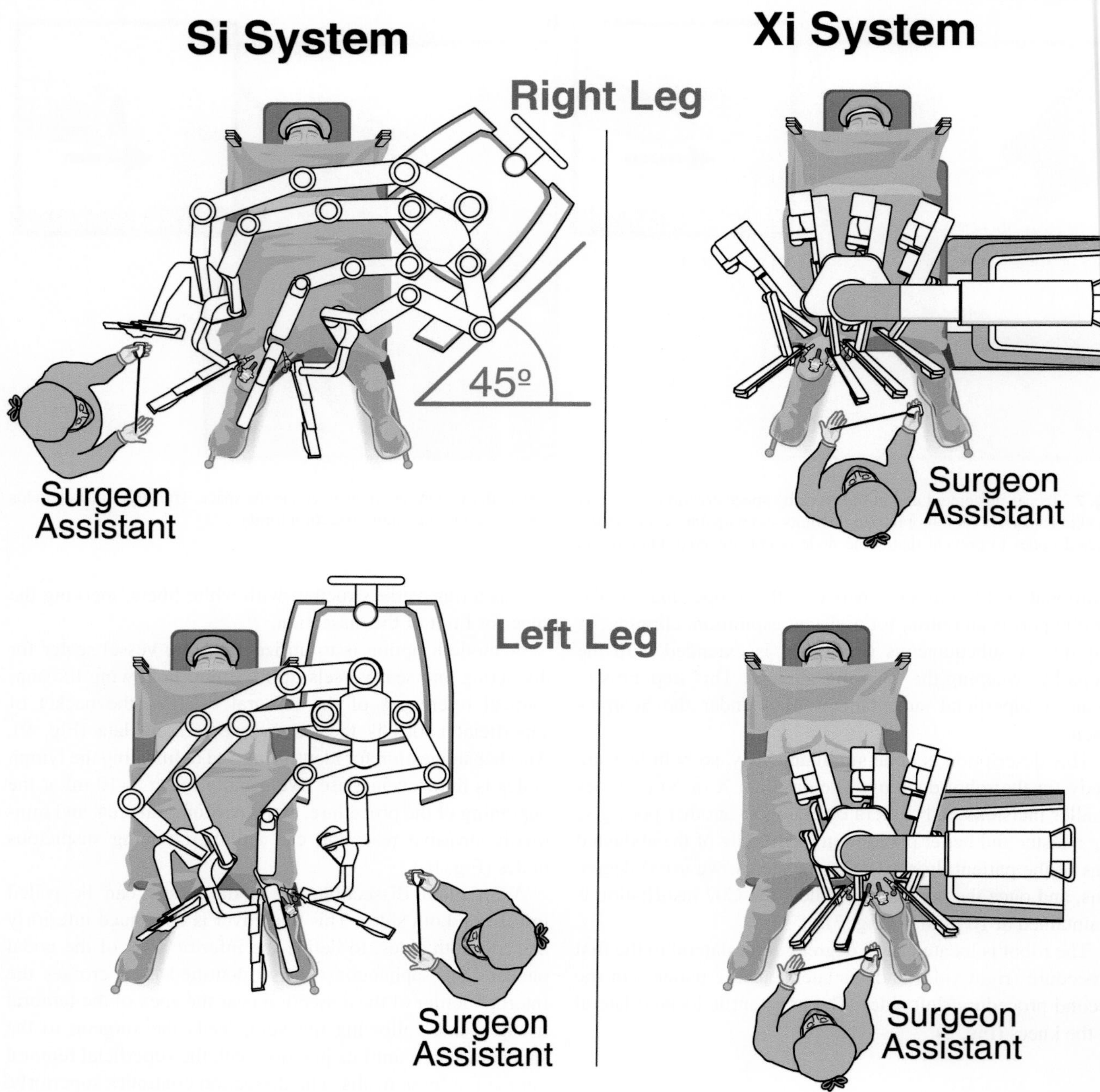

Fig. 8 Position of assistant and comparative docking for Si and Xi

Characteristic pulsations of the femoral artery serve as a nearby landmark. If possible, the packet will be released from the saphenous vein. If not, the vein can be ligated in the saphenous arch with Hem-o-lok clips. We must always attempt to preserve the saphenous vein whenever possible to reduce the risk of postoperative lymphedema.

When performing deep node dissection, we transected the fascia lata with each trocar staying laterally to the adductor longus and sartorius muscles to work below the fascia. The C02 insufflation creates a working space, so we follow the middle of the muscles to find the femoral nerve and vessels before removing the femoral nodes. Inferomedial dissection around the femoral vein enables resection of the deep inguinal nodes. This should be continued to the level of the femoral canal until the pectineus muscle is seen to ensure complete nodal retrieval. Afterward, we pull the trocars (without re-docking) to stay at the superficial space (Fig. 11).

In sequence, we lift and follow the superficial packet until the inguinal ligament, lateral to the saphenous vein, going higher to the saphenofemoral junction, accomplishing the superficial node's template. The saphenofemoral junction control can be performed by using metallic or 10 mm Hem-o-lok clips. The packet is placed in a bag and removed by the camera's initial incision or main port. In the end, a drain is placed in each leg through the 5 mm incision trocar.

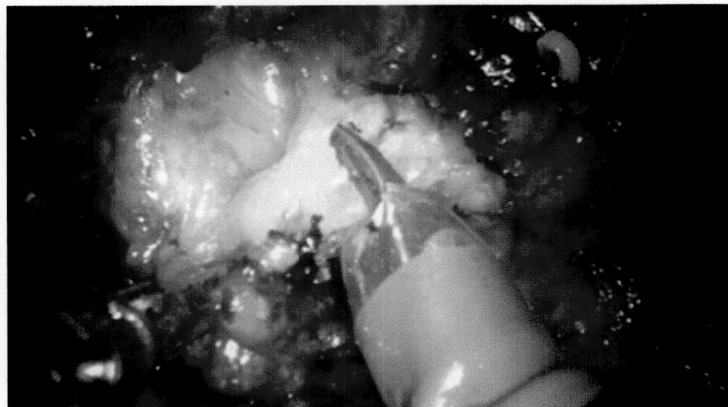

Fig. 9 Dissection of superficial package of nodes

8 Other Techniques

There are two technical variations described to perform VEIL. The first one is the lateral leg access (L-VEIL) described in only one comparative study that shows no clear advantages over the standard technique [15]. The other variation reported was the hypogastric subcutaneous approach (H-VEIL). In this technique, the advantages regard using fewer trocars to perform bilateral VEIL and the same trocars to operate pelvic nodes in the same procedure, if necessary. The disadvantage is that a simultaneous inguinal approach is not possible, and the area of skin dissection is more extended [16].

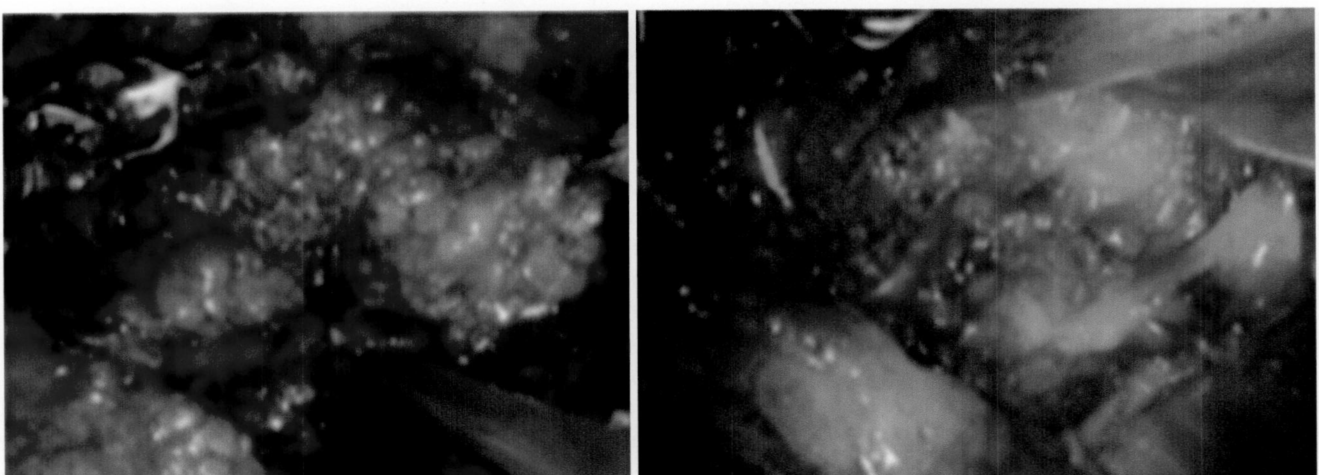

Fig. 10 Superficial nodal package observed with and without fluorescence. Note that nodes and lymphatic channels are more difficult to observe with normal vision

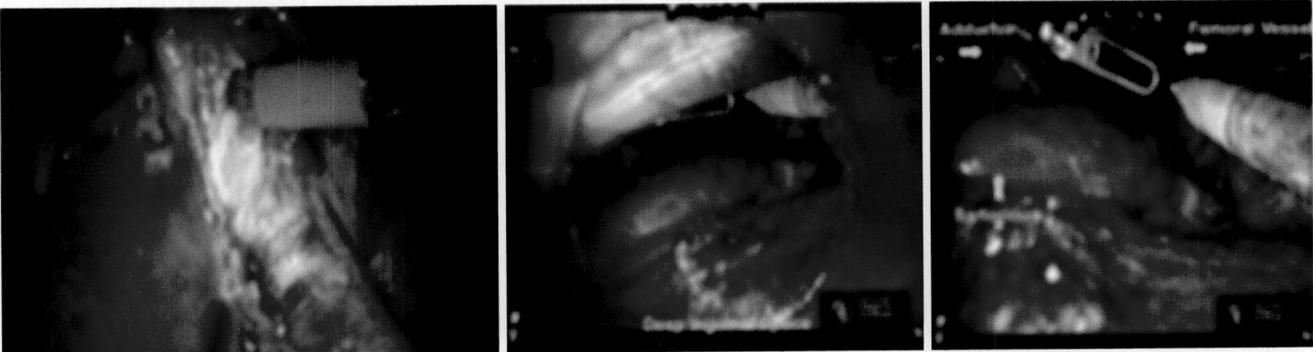

Fig. 11 Dissection of deep inguinal nodes. A: opening fascia lata over femoral artery pulsation. B: Dissection of deep inguinal space, femoral vessel, and deep nodes at femoral channel

9 Postoperative Care After Inguinal Lymphadenectomy

These patients present with high drainage of lymph fluid and should be recommended for hydration. Despite saturated fat restrictions, there are no other dietetic restrictions. We also recommend early or immediate ambulation after ILND.

The wound should be made as airtight as possible, suction drains can be used routinely, and applying pressure by heavy dressings on the thin flaps should be avoided due to higher chances of skin ischemia. Efforts to minimize lower extremity lymphedema include early ambulation and the use of elastic stockings and sequential compression devices. The patients are advised to wear individually fitted elastic socks for at least six months after surgery.

Lymphorrhea and seroma can be prevented by postoperative suction drainage and that the drains should be removed when the 24-hour output becomes less than 50 mL, usually between 3 and 15 days postoperatively. Prophylactic antibiotics should be continued for one week after surgery or until all drains have been removed. Colonization and spread of bacteria along these drains may increase the risk of infection if the drains stay in place for an extended period.

10 Our Data and Literature Analysis

Between 2015 and 2020, we performed 18 cases (36 limbs) of robotic inguinal lymph node dissection; the median age was 56 years old. All patients had a penile squamous cell carcinoma diagnosis confirmed by biopsy and partial or total penectomy. The TNM for the patients was T3N0M0G1-3. The mean operative time was 120 minutes. The mean blood loss was 40 ml. None of the patients were converted to an open approach.

The total mean number of dissected lymph nodes was nine for each limb. The presence of metastatic disease was 33%. Mean hospital stay was two days. The mean duration of the drainage was seven days, with rare cases prolonged to three weeks. The most frequent complication was lymphocele treated without hospitalization (Table 1). Finally, Fig. 12 illustrates some key points of a right-sided R-VEIL.

Table 1 Intra- and postoperative outcomes. *SCC* squamous cell carcinoma

No of Patients	18 (36 legs)
Age of patient (years)	(40–74) 56
Histological type	Penile SCC
Mean operative time (min)	(80–230) 120
Mean blood loss (ml)	(15–85) 40
Conversion to open	N (0)
Nr of dissected lymph nodes	6–15 (9)
Positive nodes	6/18 (33%)
Mean hospital stay (in days)	1–4 (2)
Main duration of drainage (in days)	3–21 (7)
Overall postoperative complications (%)	25%

11 Discussion

The robotic surgery approach to inguinal lymphadenectomy is recent in the literature. Compared to open procedures, minimally invasive surgery provides fewer complications, especially skin necrosis, without compromising oncologic control, which paves the way to utilize new technological advances as robotic-assisted video endoscopic inguinal lymphadenectomy (R-VEIL). The robotic technology allows for three-dimensional operative view, tremor filtering, and articulated instruments, improving visibility; identifying anatomical landmarks, dexterity, and ergonomics; and overcoming the VEIL limitations.

In this scenario, Josephson and associates were the first to describe the feasibility of a nonsimultaneous bilateral RAIL using the da Vinci S robotic system. In this case report, the authors presented a 37-year-old patient with penile squamous cell carcinoma, staged T3cN2. They removed ten lymph nodes in a full operative time of 120 minutes without complications [17].

In 2013, Matin et al. reported, in a prospective study, the oncologic efficacy of R-VEIL to stage the disease adequately, with an independent surgeon assessment by a direct visual evaluation of the dissection field through a small inguinal incision. They performed ten patients with penile squamous cell carcinoma. The median age was 62 years old, the stage was between T1 and T3, and a preclinical node stage was cN0–cN1. The author also reported a very similar level of node dissection with a mean of nine per limb, mean blood loss of 100 ml, and few complications [18]. Afterward, Sotelo's group performed the robotic-assisted VEIL in a 64-year-old patient with T3 stage and cN0. The author reported 33 nodes dissected in 360 minutes of operative time. This patient was described with postoperative lymphocele in the follow-up [19].

A few years later, Ahlawat et al. described different techniques of simultaneous bilateral RAIL without moving the robotic system across the operating room, with adequate reproducibility. The authors reported patients with a median age of 56 years old, T stage between T2 and T3 with nodes staging between clinical N0 and N2. Mean of 18 nodes were retrieved on the left and 14 on the right limbs. The operative time was 453 minutes with a blood loss of 147 ml, and one postoperative lymphocele was described. This technique allows bilateral staging in the same surgical time [20].

Russell and colleagues also described in 2017 the minimally invasive approach for robotic VEIL. The author compared the complications between R-VEIL and VEIL techniques (10% vs. 40%), although the group of VEIL patients was smaller. They performed 14 patients, mean age of 72 (62–76), clinical nodal stage from N0 to N2, and T1–T3. The mean number of dissected nodes was eight, and the operative time was 136.8 minutes. In this study, the most

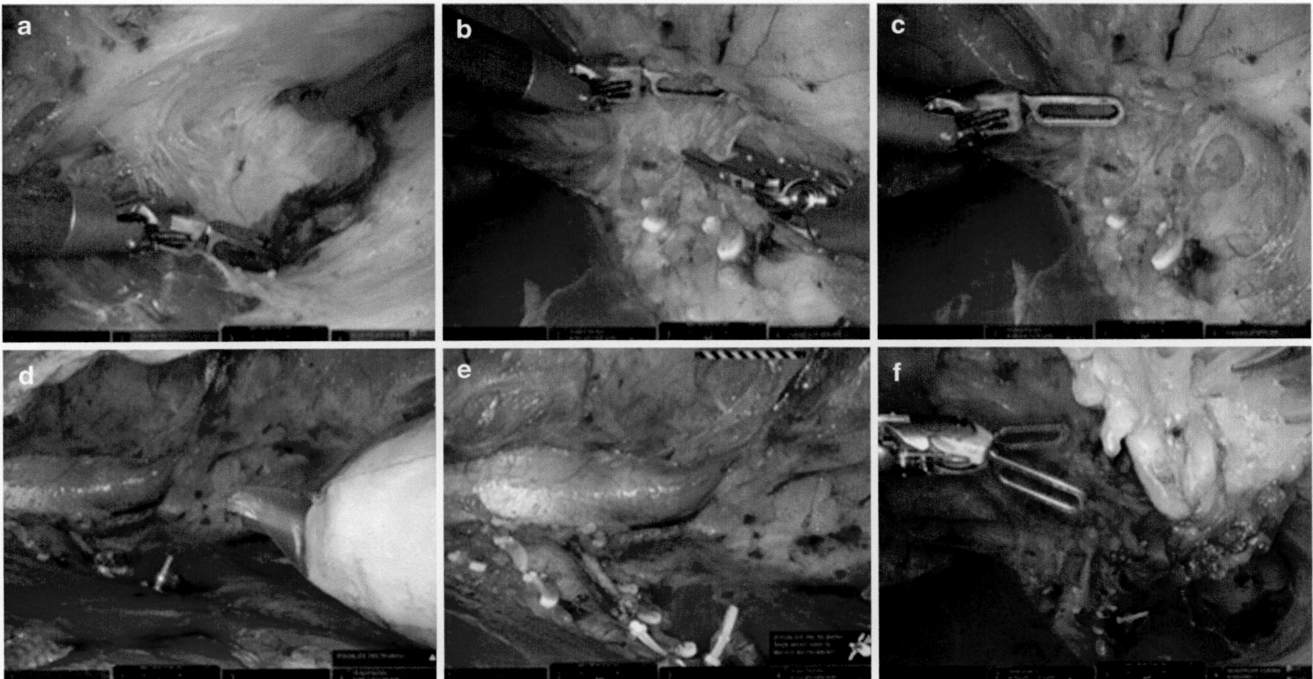

Fig. 12 (**a**) Dissection above the fascia lata searching for the inguinal ligament (the fascia above the sartorius muscle is opened). (**b**) Superficial lymphatics clipping at the fossa ovalis (clips applied over the femoral vessels). (**c**) Superficial lymph node dissection next to the sartorius limits after clipping the superficial lymphatics. (**d**) Exposure of the anatomical triangle floor with well-defined limits and lymph node template bagged. (**e**) External oblique muscle fascia and spermatic cord insertion. (**f**) Superficial lymph node dissection (medial to the saphena cross)

common complications were lymphocele, wound infection, and flap necrosis, similar to other authors [21].

Corona-Montes et al. described the first robotic-assisted inguinal lymph node dissection done in Mexico in 2015. The study reported a 73-year-old patient with penile squamous cell carcinoma (T3N0M0G1) and previous radical penectomy (four weeks) who underwent bilateral RAIL with the da Vinci Si preserving both saphenous veins. Afterward, this group published a series of 12 patients with penile squamous cell carcinoma. In addition, the same authors published a study with Machado et al. reporting 18 patients (36 limbs) who underwent REIL. The mean age was 56 years old, the operative time was 120 minutes (80–230), and the blood loss was 40 ml, with no conversions to open surgery. The node dissection resulted in 6/18 positive disease, and the mean hospitalization was two days (1–4). The time of drain placement was 7 days (ranging from 3 to 21). The most frequent complication was lymphocele [1, 5].

Sign et al. compared the outcomes of robotic and open inguinal approaches in one of the most recent series of R-VEIL in the literature. Fifty-one patients underwent R-VEIL, the median age was 58 years old, and 34 patients had clinical N0, 10 N1, and 7 N2. The pathological stage was pT2 in 51 % of the cases. Thirty-one patients had pathological pN0 31, 13 had pN1, 5 had pN2, and 2 had pN3 [22] (Table 2). The study reports a similar incidence of lymphocele, fewer lymphedemas, higher rates of skin preservation due to smaller incisions, and less traumatic tissue manipulation provided by the minimally invasive procedure. The three-dimensional view and the use of clips will theoretically be a reason to avoid lymphoceles and lymphedemas due to the proper closure of lymphatic vessels.

Most groups who have performed the robotic approach to inguinal lymph node dissection experienced a longer operative time, close to the times of VEIL, even with the faster installation of the endoscopic procedure. In addition, most publications were performed by groups with previous experience with VEIL. However, robotic experience allows efficiency by creating the space after robotic docking to avoid clashing and diminishing operating times.

Moreover, Hu et al. compared ten studies of VEIL technique, showing some advantages such as lower intraoperative blood loss, shorter hospital stay, a shorter period of drain use, and reduced percentage of wound infection, skin necrosis, and lymphedema [23].

Finally, despite the perioperative advantages of VEIL and R-VEIL over the open lymphadenectomy, the main discussion regards the oncological results compared with the open approach. In this scenario, better-designed studies with long-term follow-up are still awaited. The current data supports

Table 2 Literature reports of R-VEIL

Author	Year	Case report/ case series	Number of patients (no. of limbs)	Age (mean years)	Penile cancer (histologic)	T stage	Pre-LND cN stage	Lymph nodes dissected (n) – mean	Operative time (minutes)	Blood loss (mL)	Complications
Josephson et al.	2009	Case report	1 (2)	37	SCC◆	T3	cN2	10/9*	120/130*	100/50*	None
Matin et al.	2013	Case series	10 (20)	62 (58–69)	SCC◆	T1–T3	cN0–cN1	Left, 9; right, 9	180–240	100 (*mean*)	Cellulitis (1/10), wound breakdown (1/10), skin necrosis (1/10)
Sotelo et al.	2013	Case report	1 (2)	64	SCC◆	T3	cN0	33	360	100 (10–200)	Lymphocele
Ahlawat et al.	2016	Case series	3 (6)	56	SCC◆	T2–T3	cN1–cN2	Left, 18; right, 14	453	147 (*mean*)	Lymphocele (1/3)
Russel et al.	2017	Case series	14 (27)	72 (62–76)	SCC◆	T1–T3	cN0–cN2	8	136.8	50 (15–50)	(3/14) Lymphocele, wound infection, flap necrosis
Corona-Montes et al.	2018	Case series	12 (24)	58	SCC◆	T2–T3	cN1–cN2	12	110	59 (*mean*)	Lymphocele (2/12)
Singh et al.	2018	Case series	51 (102)	58 (50–68)	SCC◆	T1–T3	cN0–cN2	12	75/per limb	75 (*65–80*)	Edge necrosis, flap necrosis (2%), lymphocele (23%)

*R-VEIL performed in two separate procedures (*one OR time per limb*)
◆Squamous cell carcinoma of the penis

that robotic-assisted inguinal lymphadenectomy reduces morbidity with good oncological outcomes, less blood loss, and hospitalization time [24–27]. Aside from its high cost, it is a feasible technique when carried out in specialized centers.

12 Conclusions

Radical resection of penile cancer inguinal metastases is the standard treatment and the most significant single predictor of survival in penile squamous cell carcinoma. Open inguinal lymphadenectomy has shown increased morbidity and complication rates due to flap skin necrosis, more extended hospitalization, and infections. On the other hand, recent studies reported that patients who underwent robotic-assisted video endoscopic inguinal lymphadenectomy had fewer morbidity rates and debatable oncological outcomes. However, this technique is recent and needs better-designed studies to demonstrate its utility, even with the robotic surgery benefits described in the literature.

High costs, technology availability, and the learning curve to approach the femoral triangle and anatomical variations could be considered limitations of R-VEIL implementation. Further technological advances, refinements, and modifications in the minimally invasive lymph node dissection technique can reduce morbidity and complications while improving the quality of life of patients with penile cancer.

Conflict of Interest The authors declare no conflict of interest.

References

1. Global Cancer Observatory. Cancer Today [Internet]. 2018. Available from: https://gco.iarc.fr
2. Corona-Montes VE, Moyo-Martínez E, Almazán-Treviño L, Ríos-Dávila V, Santiago-Hernández Y, Mendoza-Rojas EE. Linfadenectomía inguinal robot asistida (LIRA) para cáncer de pene. Rev Mex Urol. 2015;75:292–6. https://doi.org/10.1016/j.uromx.2015.06.006.
3. Pettaway CA, Crook J, Pagliaro L. Tumor of the Penis. In: Wein A, Kavoussi L, Partin A, editors. Campbell-Walsh urology. 11th ed. Philadelphia: Elsevier; 2016. p. 846–78.
4. Daling JR, Madeleine MM, Johnson LG, Schwartz SM, Shera KA, Wurscher MA, et al. Penile cancer: importance of circumcision, human papillomavirus and smoking in in situ and invasive disease. Int J Cancer. 2005;116:606–16. https://doi.org/10.1002/ijc.21009.
5. Corona-Montes VE, Gonzalez-Cuenca E, Tobias-Machado M. Robotic-assisted inguinal lymphadenectomy (RAIL). In: Küçük S, Canda AE, editors. Medical robotics-new achievements. London: IntechOpen; 2019.
6. Tobias-Machado M, Tavares A, Ornellas AA, Molina WR, Juliano RV, Wroclawski ER. Video endoscopic inguinal lymphadenectomy: a new minimally invasive procedure for radical management of inguinal nodes in patients with penile squamous cell carcinoma. J Urol. 2007;177:953–7.; discussion 958. https://doi.org/10.1016/j.juro.2006.10.075.
7. Angermeier K, Sotelo R, Sharp D. Inguinal node dissection. In: Wein A, Kavoussi L, Partin A, editors. Campbell-Walsh urology. 11th ed. Philadelphia: Elsevier; 2016. p. 846–78.
8. Hegarty PK, Dinney CP, Pettaway CA. Controversies in ilioinguinal lymphadenectomy. Urol Clin North Am. 2010;37:421–34. https://doi.org/10.1016/j.ucl.2010.04.005.
9. Hakenberg OW. Penile cancer – European Association of Urology Guidelines [Internet]. 2018. https://uroweb.org/guideline/penile-cancer/. Accessed 08 Aug 2019.
10. Thomas A, Necchi A, Muneer A, Tobias-Machado M, Tran ATH, Van Rompuy AS, et al. Penile cancer. Nat Rev Dis Primers.

2021;7(1):11. https://doi.org/10.1038/s41572-021-00246-5. PMID: 33574340.

11. Bishoff JT, Lackland AFB, Basler JW, Teichman JM, Thompson IM. Endoscopic subcutaneous modified inguinal lymph node dissection (ESMIL) for squamous cell carcinoma of the penis. J Urol. 2003;169:78. abstract 301
12. Tobias-Machado M, Tavares A, Silva MNR, Molina WR, Forseto PH, Juliano RV, et al. Can video endoscopic inguinal lymphadenectomy achieve a lower morbidity than open lymph node dissection in penile cancer patients? J Endourol. 2008;22:1687–91. https://doi.org/10.1089/end.2007.0386.
13. Sotelo R, Sánchez-Salas R, Carmona O, Garcia A, Mariano M, Neiva G, et al. Endoscopic lymphadenectomy for penile carcinoma. J Endourol. 2007;21(4):364–7.
14. Daseler EH, Anson BJ, Reinmann AF. Radical excision of the inguinal and iliac lymph glands; a study based upon 450 anatomical dissections and upon supportive clinical observations. Surg Gynecol Obstet. 1948;87(6):679–94.
15. Nayak SP, Pokharkar H, Gurawalia J, Dev K, Chanduri S, Vijayakumar M. Efficacy and safety of lateral approach-video endoscopic inguinal lymphadenectomy (L-VEIL) over open inguinal block dissection: a retrospective study. Indian J Surg Oncol. 2019;10(3):555–62.
16. Wang H, Li L, Yao D, Li F, Zhang J, Yang Z. Preliminary experience of performing a video endoscopic inguinal lymphadenectomy using a hypogastric subcutaneous approach in patients with vulvar cancer. Oncol Lett. 2015;9(2):752–6.
17. Josephson DY, Jacobsohn KM, Link BA, Wilson TG. Robotic-assisted endoscopic inguinal lymphadenectomy. Urology. 2009;73:167–70. https://doi.org/10.1016/j.urology.2008.05.060.
18. Matin SF, Cormier JN, Ward JF, Pisters LL, Wood CG, Dinney CPN, et al. Phase 1 prospective evaluation of the oncological adequacy of robotic assisted video-endoscopic inguinal lymphadenectomy in patients with penile carcinoma. BJU Int. 2013;111:1068–74. https://doi.org/10.1111/j.1464-410X.2012.11729.x.
19. Sotelo R, Cabrera M, Carmona O, de Andrade R, Martin O, Fernandez G. Robotic bilateral inguinal lymphadenectomy in penile cancer, development of a technique without robot repositioning: a case report. Ecancermedicalscience. 2013;7:356. https://doi.org/10.3332/ecancer.2013.356.
20. Ahlawat R, Khera R, Gautam G, Kumar A. Robot-assisted simultaneous bilateral radical inguinal lymphadenectomy along with robotic bilateral pelvic lymphadenectomy: a feasibility study. J Laparoendosc Adv Surg Tech A. 2016;26:845–9. https://doi.org/10.1089/lap.2015.0611.
21. Russell CM, Salami SS, Niemann A, Weizer AZ, Tomlins SA, Morgan TM, Montgomery JS. Minimally invasive inguinal lymphadenectomy in the management of penile carcinoma. Urology. 2017;106:113–8.
22. Singh A, Jaipuria J, Goel A, Shah S, Bhardwaj R, Baidya S, et al. Comparing outcomes of robotic and open inguinal lymph node dissection in patients with carcinoma of the penis. J Urol. 2018;199(6):1518–25.
23. Hu J, Li H, Cui Y, Liu P, Zhou X, Liu L, et al. Comparison of clinical feasibility and oncological outcomes between video endoscopic and open inguinal lymphadenectomy for penile cancer: a systematic review and meta-analysis. Medicine. 2019;98(22):e15862.
24. Tobias-Machado M, Moschovas MC, Ornellas AA. History of minimally invasive inguinal lymphadenectomy. In: Delman K, Master V, editors. Malignancies of the groin. Cham: Springer; 2018. https://doi.org/10.1007/978-3-319-60858-7_1.
25. Tobias-Machado M, Almeida-Carrera RJ. Video endoscopic inguinal lymphadenectomy. In: Muneer A, Horenblas S, editors. Textbook of penile cancer. Cham: Springer; 2016. https://doi.org/10.1007/978-3-319-33220-8_15.
26. Tobias-Machado M, Moschovas MC. Inguinal lymphadenectomy. In: Sotelo R, Arriaga J, Aron M, editors. Complications in robotic urologic surgery. Cham: Springer; 2018. https://doi.org/10.1007/978-3-319-62277-4_32.
27. Correa WF, Tobias-Machado M, et al. Video-endoscopic inguinal lymphadenectomy. Eur Oncol. 2010;6(2):80–4. https://doi.org/10.17925/EOH.2010.06.02.80.

Robotic Surgery Applications in Female Pelvic Floor Reconstruction

Dmitry Y. Pushkar, Hugo H. Davila,
and Marcos A. Young Rodriguez

1 Introduction

Roughly 11% of females will have a surgical treatment for pelvic organ prolapse (POP) or urinary incontinence by the age of 80 [1]. Hysterectomy resulted in an 11.6% increase in the incidence of vaginal vault prolapse [2]. According to experts, one in nine women will undergo a hysterectomy. Hysterectomy leads to a median time to pelvic prolapse of 15.8 years (from 0.4 to 48.4 years) [3].

Although surgical repair of POP can be accomplished in a variety of ways, including transvaginal repair and placement of graft material via a vaginal approach, abdominal sacrocolpopexy has been considered the gold standard technique for repairing apical prolapse, with durable success rates ranging from 78 to 100% [4]. Suspension of the vaginal vault is an essential aspect of pelvic organ prolapse and surgical repair. Proper apical suspension protects the anterior and posterior vaginal walls from transabdominal forces that would otherwise push these tissues toward the introitus. Prolapse of the uterus or the vaginal vault occurs as a result of a weakened uterosacral-cardinal ligament that supports the vaginal apex. The traditional abdominal sacrocolpopexy includes a dissection of the vesicovaginal septum and the rectovaginal septum. The last may be carried to the levator muscle followed by securing the mesh at the anterior and posterior vaginal walls and the anterior longitudinal ligament of the sacrum.

After all, due to the invasiveness of the open approach, it has been replaced by laparoscopic sacrocolpopexy. The weaknesses of the laparoscopic approach are a longer operating time and the requirement for advanced laparoscopic skills. The da Vinci robotic system has enabled surgeons to overcome obstacles associated with laparoscopies, such as presacral and rectovaginal space dissection and a steep learning curve for laparoscopic suturing and knot-tying skills. Additionally, robotics has a three-dimensional vision system; wristed instrumentation, tremor filtering, and dexterity are all advantages of surgery. The first sacrocolpopexy performed with the assistance of a robot (RASC) was described by Di Marco in 2004 [5].

Robotic technology enables the pelvic surgeon to perform fine instrumentation for deep pelvic dissection while focusing on safety and efficiency. The advantage of wristed instrumentation is that it facilitates the transition from open to laparoscopic surgery by enhancing magnification, finer instrumentation, and facile suturing. The da Vinci camera's design, which enables three-dimensional visualization via two independent and parallel cameras, is a significant advantage over conventional two-dimensional laparoscopy. Additionally, the ergonomics of an adjustable seated console benefit the surgeon by reducing fatigue and enabling more precise maneuvers. Because the robotic technology mimics the surgeon's maneuvers in the console, it is more intuitive than standard laparoscopy. Knot tying is analogous to open surgery in that it enables the use of advanced reconstructive techniques. The addition of a fourth robotic arm enhances surgeon's efficiency even further, as it eliminates the need for the side surgeon to perform various steps during a typical POP repair.

The high cost of the robotic system and instruments and the associated maintenance are the main limitations of robotic procedures. It necessitates additional operating room time, which increases the cost of this surgical approach. Patient positioning requires collaboration with the anesthesiology team, which can add time to the setup process. Robotic-assisted POP surgery necessitates a steep Trendelenburg position, which may be detrimental in certain patients, including those with significant obesity, pulmonary disease, or gastroesophageal reflux, due to the increased risk of morbidity, increased airway pressures, and aspiration pneumonia. Standard laparoscopic sacrocolpopexy and open

D. Y. Pushkar (✉)
Urology Department, Moscow State University of Medicine and Dentistry, Moscow, Russia

H. H. Davila
Department of Surgery, Cleveland Clinic Indian River Hospital, Gifford, FL, USA

M. A. Young Rodriguez
Universidad de Panama, Panama City, Panama

P. Wiklund et al. (eds.), *Robotic Urologic Surgery*, https://doi.org/10.1007/978-3-031-00363-9_75

abdominal sacrocolpopexy do not require the same degree of Trendelenburg positioning and may be a better option for patients with the aforementioned comorbidities or significant retinal disease.

2 Etiology

The etiologies of the defects of the anatomic support of pelvic viscera include a combination of direct injury to the pelvic floor musculature, denervation of these muscles, and defects in the endopelvic fascia supportive ligaments. Childbirth and trauma could damage nerves, fascia, and pelvic floor musculature [6–8]. Some genetic disorders and variations of skeletal structure affect pelvic floor ligaments and muscles [9, 10]. Exacerbation of these defects can occur by menopausal estrogen deficiency, ageing, obesity, conditions increasing abdominal pressure (chronic cough, constipation), and heavy lifting. These risk factors may contribute to the deterioration of previously affected pelvic floor supporting mechanism. Together, the final result will be a pelvic floor dysfunction with distinct prolapse grades and variable symptoms and signs.

Most of the literature regarding risk factors for POP include age, parity and vaginal delivery, increased intrabdominal pressure (constipation, chronic pulmonary disease, obesity), occupational hazards, prior pelvic surgery, genetic syndromes, and variations in axial and pelvic skeletal structure [11]. Vaginal birth is the main etiological factor for POP [12–14]. There are data that link genetic syndromes of abnormalities of collagen to pelvic organ prolapse [15]. Variations in axial and pelvic skeletal structure can be associated with increased risks of POP. These include increasing degrees of thoracic kyphosis, a decrease in lumbar lordosis and in vertical orientation of the pelvic inlet, and an increase in the transverse diameter of the pelvic inlet [16, 17].

3 Epidemiology

POP prevalence in published studies usually underestimates the true prevalence of anatomic disease. Women typically do not seek medical care for prolapse until symptoms develop, and physicians generally do not offer surgical treatment until symptoms become bothersome; therefore, the number of women with POP who are managed without hospitalization and surgery and the number of women with POP who never seek medical care are unknown. Incidence and prevalence estimates based only on surgical procedure rates almost certainly underestimate the magnitude of POP [18]. Brubaker et al. report that the prevalence of prolapse to the level of the hymen varies from 2% to 48% [19]. Nygaard in 2008 describe 23.7% (95% CI, 21.2%–26.2%) of women had symptoms of at least one pelvic floor disorder. Of these, 15.7% (95% CI, 13.2%–18.2%) experienced urinary incontinence, 9.0% (95% CI, 7.3%–10.7%) experienced fecal incontinence, and 2.9% (95% CI, 2.1%–3.7%) experienced symptomatic pelvic organ prolapse [20]. Wu et al., in 2014, in a national survey, reported that 25.0% (95% CI 23.6, 26.3) of American women had one or more pelvic floor disorder. Urinary incontinence was the most common disorder reported, with a combined prevalence of 17.1% (95% CI 15.8, 18.4). The combined population-based prevalence was 9.4% (95% CI 8.6, 10.2) for fecal incontinence and 2.9% (95% CI 2.5, 3.4) for prolapse [21].

Virtually, all studies examining prolapse or surgery for prolapse show an increased prevalence with aging [22]. Diverse publications from all over the world recognize age as an important risk factor. In the United States, increased age by decade was associated with higher prevalence rates for all pelvic floor disorders. The proportion of women with one or more pelvic floor disorder dramatically increased from 6.3% (95% CI 5.0, 7.8) in women aged 20–29 to 31.6% (95% CI 28.3, 35.1) for women aged 50–59 years to 52.7% (95% CI 48.1, 57.2) for women 80 and older (+) [21, 22]. A population-based study from Jokhio et al. recognizes the relationship of POP with age and other risk factors in developing countries [23, 24]. This decrease in pelvic floor muscle strength was a significant independent determinant of the risk of POP, supporting an association between pelvic neuromuscular dysfunction, age, and prolapse [25].

Vaginal delivery is an important risk factor for POP [26]. In the prolapse epidemiology study, from Mant et al., parity was the strongest risk factor for the development of POP with an adjusted relative risk of 10.85 (4.65–33.81) [27]. In a Swedish study, Samuelson et al. found statistically significant associations of increasing parity and maximum birth weight with the development of POP [28].

Conditions increasing intrabdominal pressure, such as chronic pulmonary disease and constipation, are associated with POP. One case control study examined this and reported significantly more pulmonary diseases (such as asthma) in women < 45 years of age who developed prolapse (14%) compared to controls (2.4%) [29]. Evidence linking constipation to POP relates to data linking POP to pelvic floor denervation and neuropathy. While vaginal childbirth has been implicated as a major inciting event for pelvic neuropathy and prolapse, chronic constipation with repeated prolonged defecatory straining efforts has been shown to contribute to progressive neuropathy and dysfunction [30].

Obesity is another condition that is associated with chronically increased abdominal pressure [31]. Wu et al, adjusted for age in decades, race, education, poverty status, and other reproductive factors (parity, type of delivery), reported that the odds of having one or more pelvic floor disorder increased with being overweight (OR 1.3, 95% CI 1.1, 1.6) or obese (OR 1.6, 95% CI 1.3, 2.0) when compared to normal weight women in all models (+).

Occupational physical stress has been examined as a contributing factor for POP. A study using the Danish National Registry of Hospitalized Patients included over 28,000 assistant nurses (who are traditionally exposed to repetitive heavy lifting) aged 20–69, and they published that the odds ratio for the nurses compared to controls was 1.6 (1.3–1.9) for POP surgery and 1.6 (1.2–2.2) for disc surgery, suggesting that heavy lifting may contribute to POP [32].

Mant et al. reported that the POP surgical incidence rates were higher for women who had undergone a prior hysterectomy for reasons other than prolapse (29 per 10,000) and highest for women who had undergone hysterectomy for prolapse (158 per 10,000) [22]. Swift also demonstrated a significant association of POP with a prior history of hysterectomy or prolapse surgery [19].

4 Pelvic Organ Prolapse Classification

Pelvic organ prolapse has traditionally been classified by the degree of anatomical deformity, depending on the site of the defect and the presumed pelvic viscera that are involved. The large number of different grading systems that have been used is reflective of the difficulty in designing an objective, reproducible system of grading prolapses. Interobserver and intraobserver variability is often important and may lead to confusion.

We use the Pelvic Organ Prolapse Quantification (POP-Q) system. POP-Q system refers to an objective, site-specific system for describing, quantifying, and staging pelvic support in women [33]. The POP-Q system is approved by the International Continence Society (ICS), the American Urogynecologic Society (AUGS), and the Society of Gynecologic Surgeons for the description of female pelvic organ prolapse.

5 Pelvic Organ Prolapse Quantification (POP-Q)

1. Fixed point of reference. The hymen is the fixed point of reference used throughout the POP-Q system of quantitative prolapse description.
2. Defined points. The anatomic position of the six defined points (two on the anterior vaginal wall, two in the superior vagina, and two on the posterior vaginal wall) for measurement should be centimeters (cm) above or proximal to the hymen (negative number) or centimeters below or distal to the hymen (positive number) with the plane of the hymen being defined as zero (0). For example, a cervix that protruded 3 cm distal to the hymen would be + 3 cm. All points are measured on maximal straining (except total vaginal length).
3. Anterior vaginal wall:
   (a) Point Aa is a point located in the midline of the anterior vaginal wall three (3) cm proximal to the external urethral meatus. By definition, the range of position of Point Aa relative to the hymen is −3–+3 cm.
   (b) Point Ba is a point that represents the most distal (i.e., most dependent) position of any part of the upper anterior vaginal wall from the vaginal cuff or anterior vaginal fornix to Point Aa. By definition, Point Ba is at −3 cm in the absence of prolapse and would have a positive value equal to the position of the cuff (Point C) in women with total uterine prolapse or post-hysterectomy vaginal eversion (Fig. 1).
4. Superior vagina. These points represent the most proximal locations of the normally positioned lower reproductive tract. The two superior sites are as follows:
   (c) Point C is a point that represents either the most distal (i.e., most dependent) edge of the cervix or the leading edge of the vaginal cuff (hysterectomy scar) after total hysterectomy.
   (d) Point D is a point that represents the location of the posterior fornix in a woman who still has a cervix. It is included as a point of measurement to differentiate suspensory failure of the uterosacral-cardinal ligament “complex” from cervical elongation. When the location of Point C is significantly more positive than the location of Point D, this is indicative of cervical elongation which may be symmetrical or eccentric. Point D is omitted in the absence of the cervix.

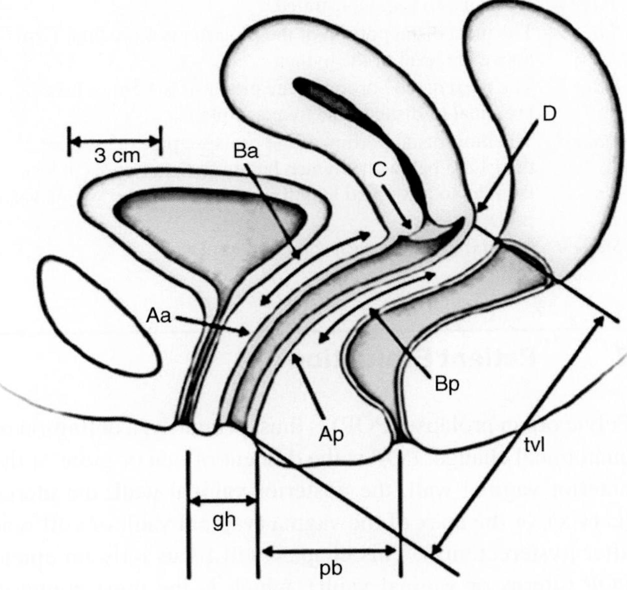

Fig. 1 Pelvic organ prolapse quantification points

5. Posterior vaginal wall:
   (e) Point Ap is a point located in the midline of the posterior vaginal wall three (3) cm proximal to the hymen. By definition, the range of position of Point Ap relative to the hymen is – 3–+3 cm.
   (f) Point Bp is a point that represents the most distal (i.e., most dependent) position of any part of the upper posterior vaginal wall from the vaginal cuff or posterior vaginal fornix to Point Ap. By definition, Point Bp is at −3 cm in the absence of prolapse and would have a positive value equal to the position of the cuff in a woman with total post-hysterectomy vaginal eversion.
6. Other landmarks and measurements:
   (g) The genital hiatus (GH) is measured from the middle of the external urethral meatus to the posterior margin of the hymen.
   (h) The total vaginal length (TVL) is the length of the vagina (cm) from the posterior fornix to the hymen when Point C or D is reduced to its full normal position.
   (i) The perineal body (PB) is measured from the posterior margin of the hymen to the mid-anal opening.

The position of Points Aa, Ba, Ap, Bp, C, and (if applicable) D with reference to the hymen should be measured (cm) and recorded. Once all the measurements are taken, the patients are assigned to the corresponding stage [34].

6 Stages of POP-Q System Measurement

Stage 0	No prolapse is demonstrated.
Stage 1	The most distal portion of the prolapse is more than 1 cm above the level of the hymen.
Stage 2	The most distal portion of the prolapse is 1 cm or less proximal or distal to the hymenal plane.
Stage 3	The most distal portion of the prolapse protrudes more than 1 cm below the hymen but no farther than 2 cm less than the total vaginal length (e.g., not all of the vagina has prolapsed).
Stage 4	Vaginal eversion is essentially complete.

7 Patient Evaluation

Pelvic organ prolapse (POP) is thus, primarily, a definition of anatomical change. POP is the descent of one or more of the anterior vaginal wall, the posterior vaginal wall, the uterus (cervix), or the apex of the vagina (vaginal vault or cuff scar after hysterectomy). This chapter will focus only on apical POP (uterus or vaginal vault), which is the most common prolapse.

8 Symptom Evaluation

POP symptoms are a departure from normal sensation, structure, or function, experienced by the woman in reference to the position of her pelvic organs. Symptoms are generally worse in situations when gravity might make the prolapse worse (e.g., after long periods of standing or exercise), and symptoms may be more noticeable at times of abdominal straining, for example, defecation. In our practice, the indication for robotic surgery is POP equal or greater than stage 2, life expectancy more than ten years, as well as associated symptoms based on the Pelvic Floor Distress Inventory-20 (PFDI-20). The PFDI-20 is comprised of three sections: (1) the Pelvic Organ Prolapse Distress Inventory-6 (POPDI-6) (range 0–300), (2) Urinary Distress Inventory-6 (UDI-6) (range 0–300), and (3) Colorectal-Anal Distress Inventory 8 (CRADI-8) (range 0–400). Subscales of the PFDI higher scores indicate worse symptoms (Table 1).

We use a frequency volume chart/bladder diary and number of pads in all patients before and after robotic surgery. The follow-up is at 2, 4, and 12 weeks, 6 and 12 months, and yearly after the first year. Our patients avoid any heavy lifting (> 4lbs), exercise (running, cycling, yoga, etc.), and intercourse for four weeks. All patient continues stool softer for six weeks.

8.1 Pelvic Exam and Signs of Pelvic Organ Prolapse

All examinations for POP should be performed with the woman's bladder empty (and if possible, an empty rectum). An increasing bladder volume has been shown to restrict the degree of descent of the prolapse [35]. The choice of the woman's position during examination, for example, left lateral, supine, and standing, or lithotomy is that which can best demonstrate POP in that patient and which the woman can confirm as the maximal extent she has perceived, for example, by the use of a mirror or digital palpation. The degree of prolapse may be worse after a lengthy time in the upright position.

During pelvic exam, the anterior vaginal wall (anterior compartment) prolapse, most commonly, might represent bladder prolapse. Higher-stage anterior vaginal wall prolapse will generally involve descent of the uterus or vaginal vault (apical compartment). The most common presentation of POP is apical and anterior compartment POP. Posterior vaginal wall (posterior compartment) prolapse, commonly, would represent rectal protrusion into the vagina (rectocele). Higher-stage posterior vaginal wall prolapse after prior hysterectomy will generally involve some vaginal vault (cuff scar) descent and possible enterocele formation. Enterocele formation can also occur in the presence of an intact uterus.

Table 1 Pelvic Floor Disability Index (PFDI-20)

Instructions: Please answer all of the questions in the following survey. These questions will ask you if you have certain bowel, bladder, or pelvic symptoms and, if you do, *how much they bother you*. Answer these by circling the appropriate number. While answering these questions, please consider your symptoms over the last 3 months. The PFDI-20 has 20 items and 3 scales of your symptoms. All items use the following format with a response scale from 0 to 4.		
Symptom scale: 0 = *not present* 1 = *not at all* 2 = *somewhat* 3 = *moderately* 4 = *quite a bit*		
Pelvic Organ Prolapse Distress Inventory 6 (POPDI-6)		
Do You...	No	Yes
1. Usually experience pressure in the lower abdomen?	0	1 2 3 4
2. Usually experience heaviness or dullness in the pelvic area?	0	1 2 3 4
3. Usually have a bulge or something falling out that you can see or feel in your vaginal area?	0	1 2 3 4
4. Ever have to push on the vagina or around the rectum to have or complete a bowel movement?	0	1 2 3 4
5. Usually experience a feeling of incomplete bladder emptying?	0	1 2 3 4
6. Ever have to push up on a bulge in the vaginal area with your fingers to start or complete urination?	0	1 2 3 4
Colorectal-Anal Distress Inventory 8 (CRAD-8) *Do You...*	No	Yes
7. Feel you need to strain too hard to have a bowel movement?	0	1 2 3 4
8. Feel you have not completely emptied your bowels at the end of a bowel movement?	0	1 2 3 4
9. Usually lose stool beyond your control if your stool is well formed?	0	1 2 3 4
10. Usually lose stool beyond your control if your stool is loose?	0	1 2 3 4
11. Usually lose gas from the rectum beyond your control?	0	1 2 3 4
12. Usually have pain when you pass your stool?	0	1 2 3 4
13. Experience a strong sense of urgency and have to rush to the bathroom to have a bowel movement?	0	1 2 3 4
14. Does part of your bowel ever pass through the rectum and bulge outside during or after a bowel movement?	0	1 2 3 4
Urinary Distress Inventory 6 (UDI-6) *Do You...*	No	Yes
15. Usually experience frequent urination?	0	1 2 3 4
16. Usually experience urine leakage associated with a feeling of urgency, that is, a strong sensation of needing to go to the bathroom?	0	1 2 3 4
17. Usually experience urine leakage related to coughing, sneezing or laughing?	0	1 2 3 4
18. Usually experience small amounts of urine leakage (that is, drops)?	0	1 2 3 4
19. Usually experience difficulty emptying your bladder?	0	1 2 3 4
20. Usually experience pain or discomfort in the lower abdomen or genital region?	0	1 2 3 4

Scoring the PFDI-20

Scale Scores: Obtain the mean value of all of the answered items within the corresponding scale (possible value 0 to 4) and then multiply by 25 to obtain the scale score (range 0 to 100). Missing items are dealt with by using the mean from answered items only

PFSI-20 Summary Score: Add the scores from the 3 scales together to obtain the summary score (range 0 to 300)

8.2 Supplementary Techniques During Pelvic Exam

The following are additional techniques during pelvic exam:

(a) Digital rectal-vaginal examination [36]: While the patient is straining and the prolapse is maximally developed. The aim is to try to differentiate between a high rectocele and an enterocele.
(b) Q-tip (urethral) testing [36]: Measurement of urethral axial mobility at rest and straining to assess degree of mobility.
(c) Evaluation of levator defects/trauma (3): Per-vaginal palpation for levator injury/defect/"avulsion" and evaluation of tenderness during palpation.
(d) Urinary incontinence signs (1 IUGA): urinary incontinence, stress (urinary) incontinence, and stress incontinence on prolapse reduction (occult stress incontinence).
(e) Vaginal/vulvar examination, vaginal atrophy, and urethral inspection/palpation (urethral mucosal prolapse, urethral caruncle, urethral diverticulum).
(f) Vaginal examination, bimanual pelvic examination, and perineal examination (perineal elevation, perineal descent).
(g) Rectal examination (anal sphincter tone and strength, anal sphincter tear, fecal impaction present/absent, other rectal lesions, anal lesions, other perianal lesions).

9 Additional Diagnostic Test

Urodynamics should be performed preoperatively, especially in case of overactive bladder symptoms, prior incontinence surgery, prior prolapse surgery, or disordered bladder emptying. The assessment of urethral function should be considered in the urodynamic investigation of stress urinary incontinence. In patients with pelvic prolapse, urodynamic investigations should be performed during prolapse reposition. We perform a pessary trial (two weeks) before robotic surgery to evaluate for occult stress incontinence. An alternative approach is to reduce the POP during urodynamic study to evaluate for stress urinary incontinence (SUI). We combined mid-urethral sling with robotic surgery when we documented SUI before surgery.

Anal manometry: The most common indications are fecal incontinence, distal constipation, and preoperative evaluation before sphincteroplasty or surgical rectocele repair. Patients complaining of fecal incontinence (FI) can be defined as the recurrent uncontrolled passage of fecal material for at least one-month duration in an individual with a developmental age of at least four years [37, 38]. Prevalence ranges from 7% to 15% in community-dwelling women and 18% to 33% in hospitals. Most patients are reluctant to mention this condition to a healthcare provider, so it should be actively questioned by the treating physician and is presumably significantly underestimated. We observed that a considerable percentage of patients with FI had clinical arguments for constipation, which could provoke incomplete rectal evacuation, fecal retention, and overflow incontinence. More than 80% of FI patients showed pelvic floor dyssynergia on anorectal manometry irrespective of the presence of constipation. The presence of a sphincter defect on anorectal ultrasound (US) (during pelvic floor ultrasound) was associated with more severe FI, manifesting as a higher Wexner score.

After open sacrocolpopexy, 13% women were classified as moderately severely FI. A self-reported obstetrical anal sphincter injury was associated with higher incontinence scores regardless of prolapse surgery. The Cleveland Clinic Incontinence Score was significantly higher in those women having had an obstetrical anal sphincter injury compared to those without. Therefore, obstetrical anal sphincter injury, and not sacrocolpopexy, is associated with fecal incontinence, and this needs to be documented before robotic surgery in patients with FI.

Cystoscopy is indicated in the evaluation of patients with voiding symptoms (storage or obstructive), gross or microscopic hematuria, evaluation of urologic fistulas, evaluation of urethral or bladder diverticula, and previous prolapses or anti-incontinence surgery.

10 Pelvic Floor Imaging

Pelvic floor ultrasound may assist the clinical assessment of POP or intercurrent pelvic floor diagnoses. The use of any of the different imaging modalities is, however, entirely optional such as ultrasound imaging two-dimensional or three-dimensional modalities: (a) transabdominal, (b) perineal, (c) transvaginal, and (d) transabdominal ultrasounds. Ultrasound evaluation may provide excellent information about bladder neck descent and mobility. The position of the bladder neck is at rest and on Valsalva. This is particularly important in patients with previous mid-urethral sling, periurethral bulking agents, and recurrent stress urinary incontinence and provides information about position of meshes, tapes, or implants. Other relevant indications for pelvic floor ultrasound are any suspicious of bladder abnormalities (tumor, foreign body) and urethral abnormality (diverticulum). Ultrasound measurement of bladder and detrusor wall thickness (DWT) is a potential noninvasive clinical tool for assessing the lower urinary tract. Post-void DWT is higher in women with overactive bladder and detrusor overactivity [39, 40].

Endovaginal or perineal three-dimensional ultrasound imaging: This allows to evaluate the levator ani muscles. The presence of levator ani trauma has been postulated to be associated with an increased risk of pelvic organ prolapse recurrence [41, 42]. This can be evaluated using a tomographic ultrasound imaging assessment of the levator ani muscles and three-dimensional ultrasound imaging of ballooning of the genital hiatus. The presence of ballooning of the genital hiatus (one-fourth excessive distensibility of the levator hiatus) on Valsalva maneuver has also been associated with the severity of urogenital prolapse. An area of more than 25 cm^2, 30 cm^2, 35 cm^2, and 40 cm^2 has been defined as mild, moderate, marked, and severe ballooning, respectively.

Magnetic resonance imaging (MRI) of the pelvic floor: MRI allows the detection of ligamentous and muscular pelvic floor structures in fine detail. Although it does not use ionizing radiation, it is a high-cost technique. Static MRI relies on static sequences and high spatial resolution images, to delineate the passive and active elements of the pelvic organ support system. Most commonly, images are acquired in axial, sagittal, and coronal planes. MRI has been proposed to be a useful method for diagnosing and staging POP. Several lines and levels of reference have been described in the literature. Other applications of MRI are the assessment of the levator ani muscles' morphology (size, thickness, volume) and detection of injuries/defects/"avulsion". We use imaging test either MRI or endovaginal US in selected patients, especially with history of previous pelvic floor surgery and recurrence POP.

Computed tomography (CT) of the pelvic floor is not routinely recommended for imaging the pelvic floor mainly due to irradiation and poor soft tissue contrast. However, multiplanar spiral CT may offer an accurate visualization of the pelvic floor soft and bony structures by reconstruction of axial images using 1-mm-thick slices without gaps, thus increasing the diagnostic accuracy of pelvic floor anatomical disorders (i.e., levator ani muscle trauma).

11 Robotic-Assisted Laparoscopic Surgeries for the Correction of Apical POP

In the Women's Health Initiative study, investigators found a 41% prevalence of pelvic organ prolapses (POP) during standard physical examination in postmenopausal women older than 60 years who had not had a hysterectomy [43]. Therefore, POP are common complains, and approximately 300,000 surgeries are performed annually to correct them in the United States, at a cost of more than $1 billion [44]. Sacrocolpopexy is considered the best approach, and robotic sacrocolpopexy (RS) has been adopted by many pelvic surgeons to minimize surgical morbidity and quicken patient recovery [45]. Sacrocolpopexy has been shown to have one of the highest long-term anatomic success rates (78–100%) among procedures for POP repair with minimal complications [46, 47]. However, after the FDA (Federal Drug Administration) prohibit the uses of vaginal mesh for the correction of POP, now many patients request "no-mesh surgery" even when long-term outcomes are better with mesh surgery.

12 Robotic-Assisted Single-Site Uterosacral Ligament Suspension

12.1 No-Mesh Technique

Since the initial report of single-port nephrectomy in 2007, urologists and gynecologists have successfully performed various procedures with laparoscopic single-site surgery (LESS) [48]. Further advancements in technology, such as new robotic single-site platforms and instrumentation, have broader application of this surgical technique. This approach enables surgeons to operate through a small incision in the patient's umbilicus, placing 3–4 instruments through this incision. This could be an alternative to mesh surgery, especially after the Federal Drug Administration (FDA) prohibit the uses of vaginal mesh in the repair of pelvic organ prolapses, and many patients present to our clinic with "mesh phobia" and demand a no-mesh surgical approach.

One of the most important publications evaluating no-mesh techniques was the Operations and Pelvic Muscle Training in the Management of Apical Support Loss (OPTIMAL) trial which was a 2 × 2 factorial trial comparing five-year outcomes in women undergoing vaginal apical prolapse repair without mesh [38]. This publication evaluated the two most common transvaginal procedures for apical POP, sacrospinous ligament fixation (SSLF) and uterosacral ligament vaginal vault suspension (ULS). By year five, the estimated surgical failure rate was 61% in the ULS group and 70% in the SSLF group. Compared with outcomes at two years, rates of surgical failure increased during the follow-up period, although prolapse symptom scores remained improved at five years. This data showed that no-mesh transvaginal approach may not be a good long-term surgical repair for POP.

Our group decided to merge the minimally invasive surgery advantages associated with robotic-assisted single-site (RASS) approach and the outcomes associated with ULS [49]. In this retrospective trial, RASS-ULS has similar operative times to laparo-endoscopic single-site (LESS) ULS and no differences in postoperative pain, at 6-month or at 12-month follow-up when compared with the LESS approach, although robotic surgical systems may accelerate the learning curve in single-site surgery. Anatomic support was 92% successful at 12 months in the LESS-ULS [49]. In a recent unpublished analysis of these patients at a two-year follow-up, we found a good anatomic support in 80% of the LESS-ULS vs. 95% RASS-ULS. We believe that this difference is related to the 5 ± 1 plications we did on the uterosacral ligaments, because RASS approach is easier to manipulate sutures in the tissue as compared to the LESS.

We demonstrated this finding in one of our previous publications; we evaluated the visibility and the extent of the cardinal/uterosacral ligaments during minimally invasive surgery (laparoscopic or robotic surgery) [50, 51]. Robotic technology has some advantages over vaginal and open abdominal surgery due to the high resolution of cameras, three-dimensional vision, and ten times magnification available during surgery and robotic instruments' dexterity. In this study, we measure the length of the uterosacral ligaments (UL) in their caudal-cranial extent which was 3.5 ± 0.5 cm (right side) and 2.58 ± 0.3 cm (left side). Measurements were performed on the same way for the cardinal ligaments, resulting in 5.1 ± 0.3 cm (both sides). The only significant difference was observed when comparing the right vs. left UL. This anatomic difference translates to 5 ± 1 plications on the right UL vs. 2 ± 1 on the left UL. In our anatomic evaluation, the right UL was significantly longer as compared to the left, and this allowed us to take three additional stitches on the right UTSL vs. left UTSL during robotic-assisted ULS. We believe that the main benefit of taking multiple plications on the UL during robotic surgery vs. vaginal approach may translate in better long-term support (95% good anatomic support at two years, unpublished data).

However, given the substantial added costs of robotic assistance, it is important for physicians, medical training programs, and health systems to consider the implications of widespread adoption of robotic technology and the relative use when compared with the conventional laparoscopy or vaginal surgery. With the new robotic single-site platforms, future investigations are warranted to discern the best applications for this technology in benign gynecologic and urologic surgeries.

13 Robotic-Assisted Laparoscopic Apical Suspension (RALAS-4) and RALAS Spiral

13.1 No-Mesh Technique

During sacrocolpopexy, identification of the presacral ligament can be difficult, particularly in obese patients. This area is surrounded by critical structures, such as the right ureter, where injuries happen in 1.0% of the procedures (0.8%–1.9%) [19]. The middle sacral vessels, the left iliac vein, and the caval bifurcation are also nearby the area where the mesh needs to be placed. Bleeding management can be particularly difficult in this area, and accidental lesions of these vessels can result in blood loss, which is described in 4.4% of the procedures (0.18%–16.9%) [51]. Awareness of these challenges may discourage the use of sacrocolpopexy, therefore, limiting the access of women with advanced apical prolapse to the most effective surgical strategy available. In addition, many patients demand no-mesh approach due to complications related to vaginal mesh. Our group continue exploring additional techniques without mesh and provide the best apical support; we described a surgical technique of robotic-assisted laparoscopic apical suspension (RALAS) using nonabsorbable sutures and described a new four-point technique (RALAS-4). In this technique, we used V-Loc 3-0, CV-23 (Covidien) sutures (absorbable) on the right and left UL, and these were reinforced with Gore-Tex 2-0, CV-2 (nonabsorbable, Gore Medical); these are the first two-point suspensions as we described previously. This was followed by the two-point anterior vaginal supports with Gore-Tex, Hem-o-lock (TeleFlex), and LAPRA-TY (Ethicon) for a total four-point apical support (Fig. 1). The two apical support sutures are taken from the vagina to the transversalis fascia and the level of the obliterated umbilical artery on the anterior abdominal wall (right/left) [53].

We believe this four-point support is more anatomical, due to the uterosacral ligaments and cardinal ligaments provided with four-point support at the apex. We incorporated an additional step (spiral technique) to our RALAS approach; we are exploring a supplementary anchoring point around the aponeurosis of the abdominal muscle, which may provide better long-term support [53]. These two sutures were taken from the vagina to the transversalis fascia (we changed the robotic camera for 30° up), 4 cm above the pubic bone and 4 cm lateral to the midline on the right and left. Now with the new spiral technique, we secured these sutures through the rectus abdominal muscle inside-outside-inside using a Carter-Thomason (cooper surgery) laparoscopic port closure system (Fig. 2). However, using these no-mesh approaches in our patients, we have seen an anatomic success of 88% at 12 months [44] and 80% at 24 months (unpublished data). It was due to these high recurrence rates that we decided to develop the spiral technique, to provide better long-term support. We found 95% good anatomic support at 12 months (unpublished data). During the initial three months, we have 30% of patients complaining urinary frequency and urgency, treated with medication and discontinued after three months. We believed this may be related to the anterior anchoring sutures and proximity with the bladder.

In our opinion, RALAS-4 spiral may represent an alternative to robotic or laparoscopic sacrocolpopexy. We are continuously collecting data for the evaluation of the long-term operative outcomes of this technique compared to our robotic sacrocolpopexy or sacrohysteropexy (Fig. 3).

14 New Technologies and Applications

Intraoperative ultrasound (IOUS) in pelvic and reconstructive surgery provides interactive and timely information during surgical procedures. Because the transducer is in direct contact with the organ being examined, high-resolution images can be obtained that are not degraded by air, bone, or overlying soft tissues. The role of intraoperative is in its infancy with anecdotal experience and literature involving predominantly case reports. Our group published a novel application of IOUS using three different probes, three-dimensional endovaginal US (EVUS), perineal pelvic floor US (pPFUS), and intra-abdominal laparoscopic US (ILUS), during robotic sacrocervicopexy [55]. IOUS imaging is particularly useful as this modality allows assessment of sacral promontory, right ureter, middle sacral artery/vein, pubocervical fascia (PF), rectovaginal septum (RVS), and tensioning of the mesh to the sacral promontory. Our technique of IOUS during robotic sacrocolpopexy appears to be feasible and safe. We found that the operative room time is longer with the IOUS approach but the sacral promontory was faster. When we did the pubocervical fascia plication, we accomplished better anterior compartment support at six months. We recently published our finding about IOUS and hypoechoic-hyperechoic defects (HHD) measuring a mean

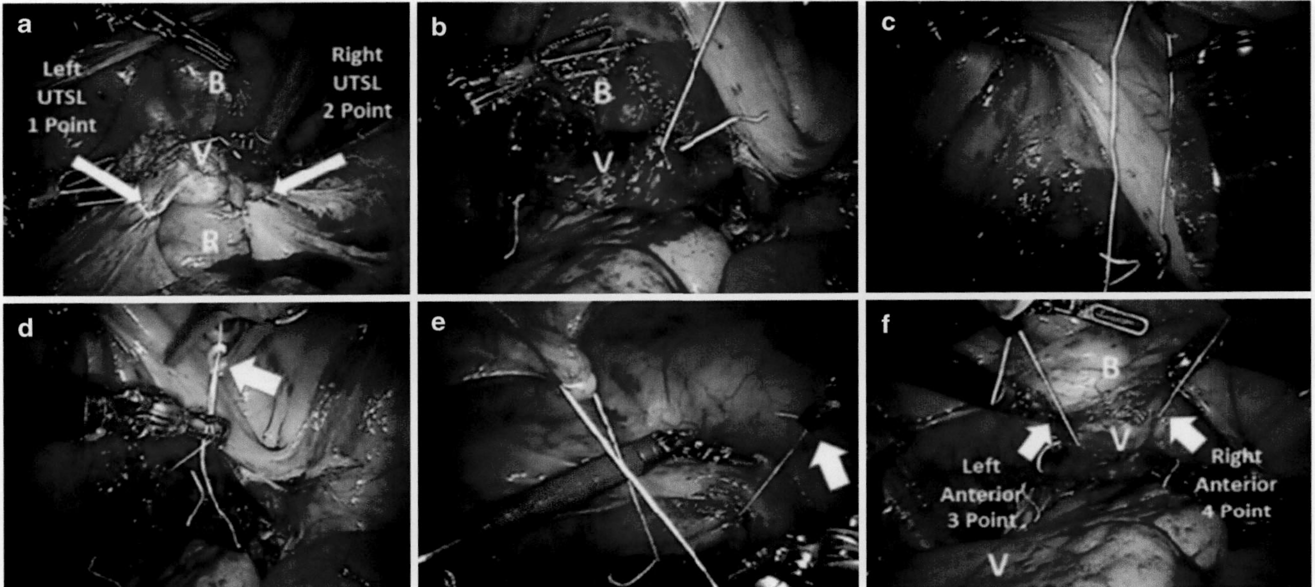

Fig. 2 Images during robotic-assisted laparoscopic apical suspension, four points (RALAS-4) after hysterectomy. (**a**) Right and left UTSL suspensions with V-loc and Gore-Tex (two-point suspension), white arrows; (**b**) demonstrates the right anterior vagina suture (Gore-Tex); (**c**) suture from the vagina to the anterior abdominal wall; (**d**) to keep the tension, we uses Hem-o-lock (TeleFlex), white arrow; (**e**) we used LAPRA-TY (Ethicon), white arrow, to hold the Hem-o-lock; (**f**) Right and left anterior vaginal suspensions (two-point suspension), white arrows; the locations of the bladder (B) and vagina (V) are shown

of 2.7 cm on three-dimensional EVUS evaluation of the anterior compartment which are associated with severe POP-Q of stage 3, supporting our theory that pubocervical fascia (PF) defects may present as HHD during EVUS. HHD seems to correlate with the number of PF plications during robotic surgery and a decreased length of the anterior vaginal mesh used during surgery. Therefore, EVUS may be an additional useful diagnostic test in the evaluation of patients with apical and anterior POP preoperatively and intraoperatively [56].

Augmented reality (AR) has been used for several years to train medical students on surgeries such as blood clot removal or penis implant surgery. However, moving from training to regular use in surgery is taking a bit longer to be adopted. AR is a novel technology used in partial nephrectomy that has the potential to increase the technical feasibility, accuracy, and safety of conventional intraoperative imaging. AR headset, visual data are directly projected to the operator's retina and overlaid onto the surgical field, thereby removing the requirement to shift attention to a remote display. Integrating CT scan or MRI information into the patient's surgical field, AR is being integrated to robotic surgery, and reconstructive pelvic surgery is an excellent indication.

Integration of three-dimensional printing and AR have been done with kidney models. A three-dimensional printed kidney model was created using multicolor, allowing a transparent kidney with coloring of the renal tumor, artery, vein, and ureter. The three-dimensional printed and AR models were used preoperatively and intraoperatively to assist in robotic partial nephrectomy. The application of three-dimensional printed and AR models is necessary in reconstructive pelvic surgery.

15 Step-by-Step Sacrocolpopexy

15.1 Patient's Positioning and Docking

Preoperative administration of antibiotics and sequential pneumatic devices is used to treat deep venous thrombosis. Following intubation, the patient is placed in the low lithotomy position, and straps are placed across the shoulders and chest in a crisscross pattern to secure the patient on the table. Arms are cushioned and tucked. A Foley catheter is placed after prepping and draping the abdomen, perineum, and vagina. Trocar placement is accomplished using a Veress needle or the Hassan technique, followed by insufflation to a 12–15 mmHg CO_2 pneumoperitoneum. The Da Vinci camera is introduced and the surgeon performs a general inspection. Depending on the surgeon's preference, a 0° or 30° down camera can be used. We prefer the 30° down scope because it allows for more detailed visualization of the sacral promontory in the presacral space.

The initial 12 mm camera port should be inserted no less than 15 cm and no more than 22 cm in the midline from the pubic symphysis. The patient is placed in a steep

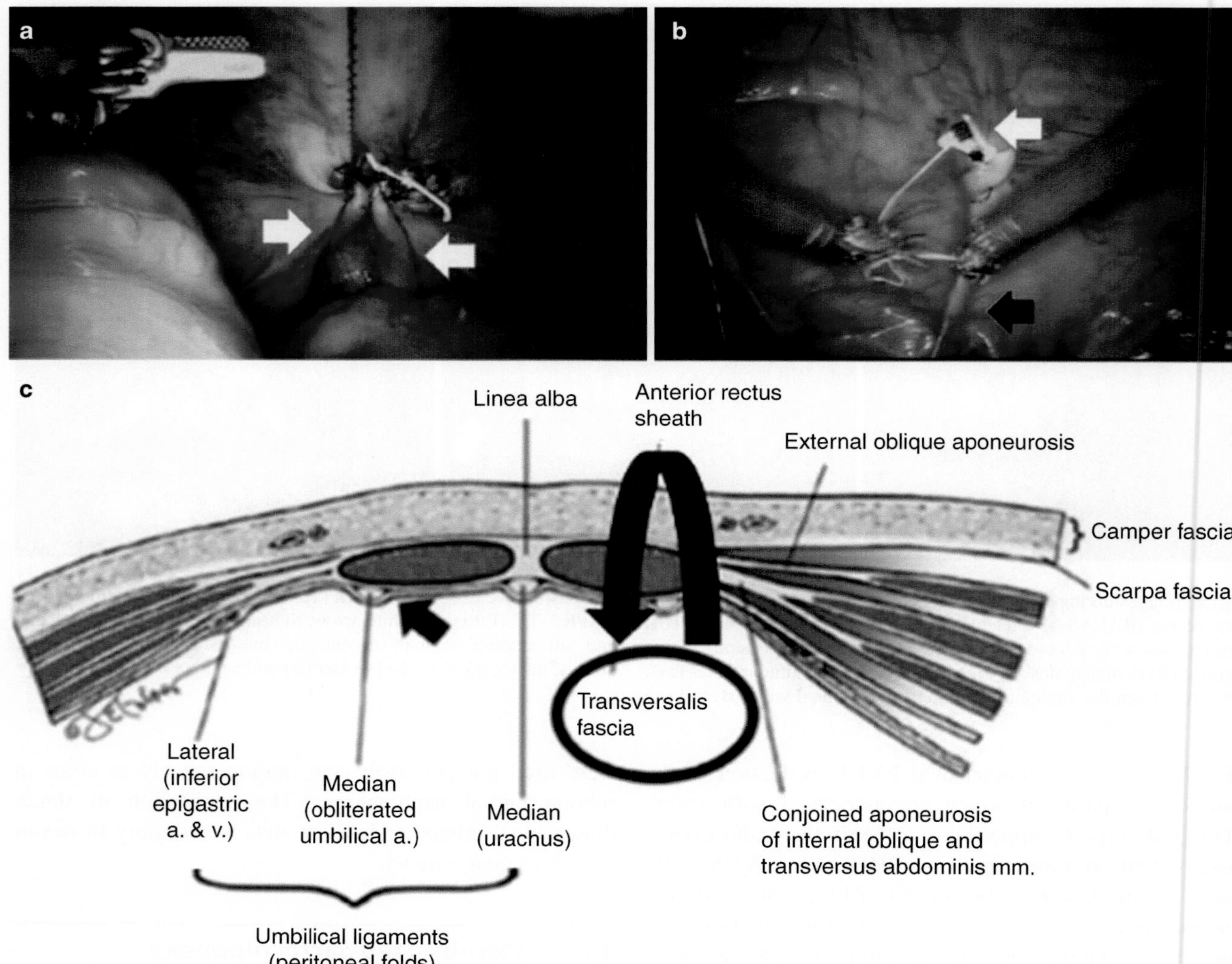

Fig. 3 Images during robotic-assisted laparoscopic apical suspension, four-point (RALAS-4) spiral technique. (**a**) Posterior view, after completing the right UTSL suspension, left UTSL is sutured to the right. White arrows: left/right UTSL. (**b**) Anterior view, apical suspension. Black arrow: suture behind the peritoneum. White arrow: Hem-o-lock (TeleFlex) and LAPRA-TY (Ethicon) to keep suture tension. (**c**) Diagram of the spiral technique. Black arrow: medial obliterated umbilical artery. Large black arrow: The direction of sutures through the rectus abdominal muscle inside-outside-inside using a Carter-Thomason (cooper surgery) laparoscopic port closure system

Trendelenburg tilt before the placement of lateral trocars. With complete insufflation (not to exceed 15 mm Hg), measurements are taken on the anterior abdomen to ensure proper placement of subsequent trocars and to avoid robotic arm collisions. Two lateral 8 mm ports are then positioned 10 cm inferolateral to the camera port, parallel to the ipsilateral anterior superior iliac spine (ports 1 and 2). A third 8 mm port is located 8–10 cm superolateral to port 2 (port 3), and a 12 mm assistant port is located 8 cm lateral to port 1 (port 1). The robot has been docked, and the ports have been secured.

After docking the robot, monopolar shears are inserted into port number 4 (right lower quadrant). A bipolar grasper is inserted into port number 3 (left mid-clavicular). A Prograsp or Cadiere forceps is inserted into port number 1 (left mid-clavicular), with the camera positioned in the supraumbilical port. The instruments in ports 1 and 3 are reversed for the left-handed surgeon. The Cadiere forceps are less traumatic when retracting the sigmoid mesentery, whereas the Prograsp forceps provide increased traction for manipulating the more robust pelvic structures. We recommend beginning with the Cadiere fenestrated forceps and switching to the Prograsp forceps only if the Cadiere is unable to retract tissues, such as the mesentery, adequately.

16 Exposure of Promontory

The procedure routinely starts by exposing the sacral promontory. If the surgeon cannot accomplish this step safely and promptly, a conversion to an open approach should be considered. The small bowel must be retracted cephalad, and the sigmoid colon is mobilized out of the pelvis and retracted laterally (to the patient's left) to visualize the sacral promontory. Both the small bowel and colon are typically easily retracted unless they are immobilized by adhesions. In this case, lysis of adhesions may be necessary until they are sufficiently retracted out of the operative field. Typically, the sacral promontory is visualized well after the sigmoid colon is moved laterally. The third robotic arm can be used to retract the colon and maintain the promontory's exposure. It should be kept out of the dissection field. After grasping the edge of the sigmoid, the third arm is moved to the left, parallel to the rectus muscle of the abdomen. The third arm should not obstruct the camera view in this position. The sacral promontory, aortic bifurcation, right and left common iliac vessels, and right ureter are the prominent anatomical landmarks for further dissection (Fig. 4). Alternatively, traction sutures (Vicryl, 2/0) can be placed through the sigmoid tenia in cases of a redundant sigmoid colon. Both ends of the strings are brought out of the abdominal cavity, through the skin from the left lower quadrant, where they are fixed with a small clamp. Adjusting the sigmoid colon's traction requires repositioning it to the left upper quadrant to maintain adequate exposure for the sacral dissection. The continuous suturing on the tenia can help gain sufficient traction and prevent tearing.

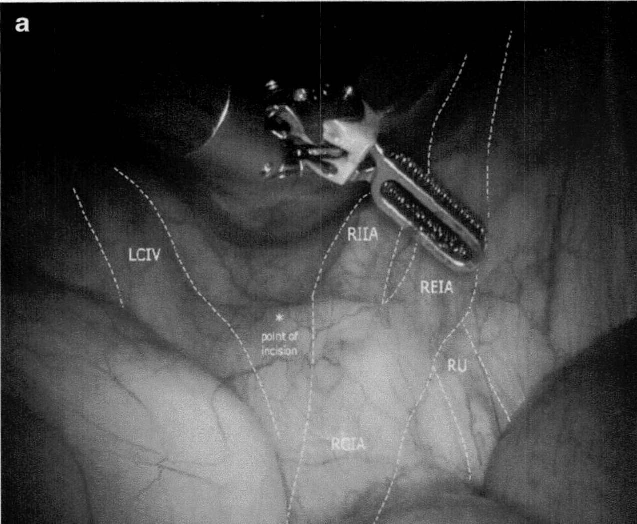

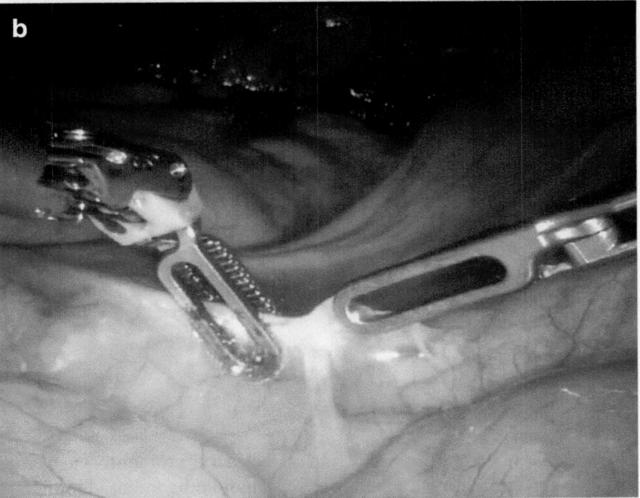

Fig. 4 (**a, b**) Identification of the promontory

16.1 Anatomical Landmarks

The sacral promontory is a protrusion of the S1 vertebra's upper anterior edge that serves as the pelvic cavity's border. Numerous anatomical landmarks are located on the same level in this area. The common iliac arteries divide into external and internal branches along with the promontory's projection; the ureters cross the left external iliac artery and the right common iliac artery. Just above this level, roughly in the projection of the L4 vertebra, is a bifurcation of the abdominal aorta and inferior vena cava, which lies behind and slightly to the right (Fig. 4).

In most cases, the sacral promontory is clearly prominent, and peritoneal dissection should begin here. In addition, the pulsating right common iliac artery is an important anatomical feature that aids in locating the promontory. However, if anatomic difficulties are encountered as a result of the fatty tissue or anything else obstructing visualization, the aortic bifurcation should be identified first.

Another valuable landmark for sacrocolpopexy is the right ureter. The sacral promontory is located about 3 cm medial to the right ureter at the level of the pelvic brim on average. Therefore, measuring 30 mm medial to the right ureter along the pelvic brim should allow the surgeon to identify the most likely location of the sacral promontory.

16.2 Nerve-Sparing Promontory Dissection

A fenestrated bipolar forceps on the left robotic arm and electrocautery scissors on the right robotic arm are usually used. The dissection begins with an incision in the lifted peritoneum and proceeds carefully caudally, away from the aortic bifurcation and right ureter. This protects the middle sacral vessels and, more importantly, the left common iliac

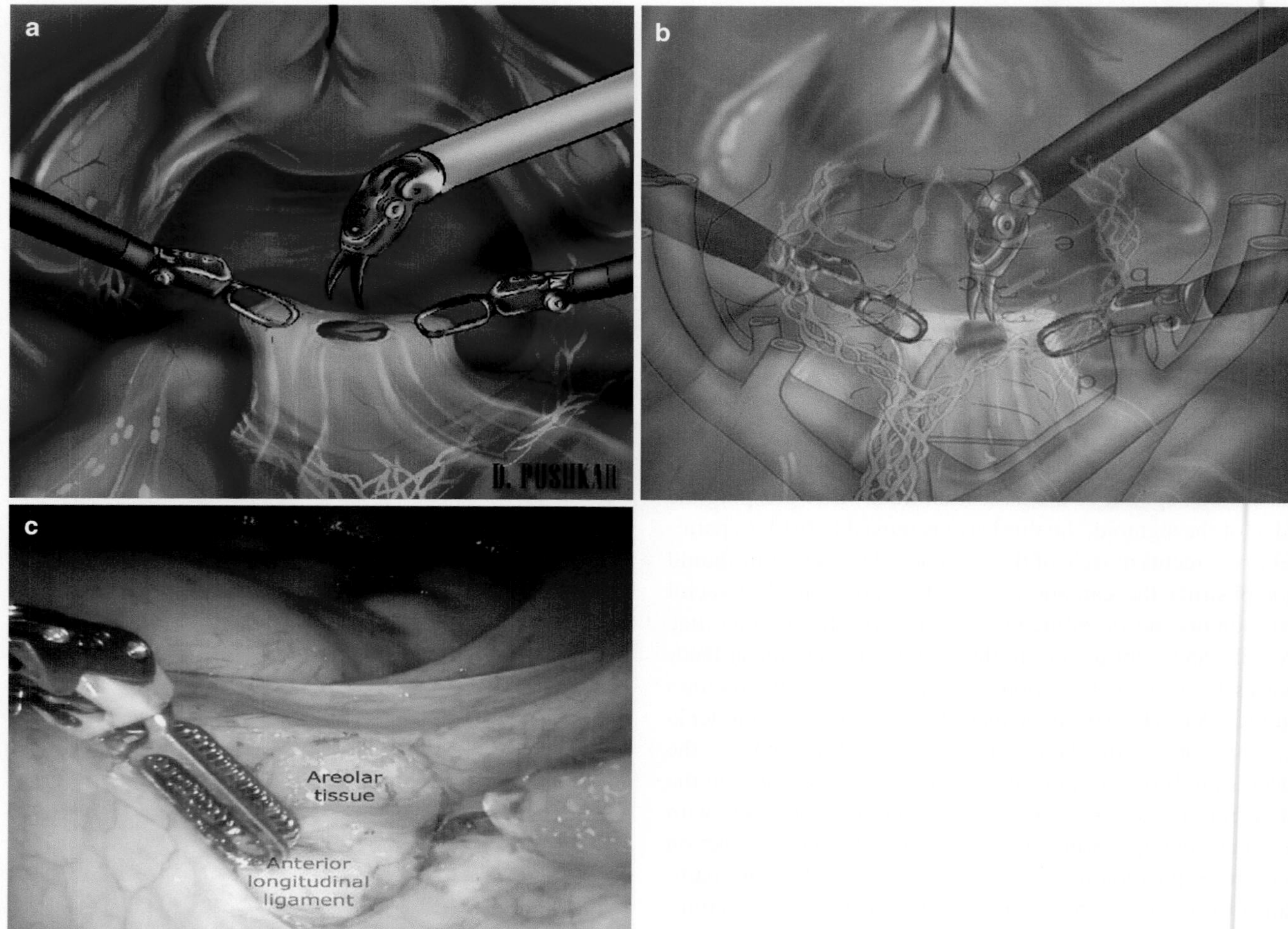

Fig. 5 (**a**) Nerve-sparing dissection of the sacral promontory; (**b**) right hypogastric plexus should be avoided. (**c**) Opening of the peritoneum on the level of promontory and anterior longitudinal ligament identification under the fatty areolar tissue

vein from injury. Next, dissection continues deeper until the longitudinal ligament is reached. At least two sutures should be placed in this dissection area. Along the way, if any apparent sacral vessels branch abnormally toward the patient's right side, they should be coagulated to avoid needle injuries later on. The most critical aspect of the dissection is determining the location of common iliac vein traces (Fig. 5).

The anterior longitudinal ligament is surrounded by the parietal peritoneum with loose areolar tissue and the presacral fascial layer. The hypogastric plexus and nerves pass through the presacral fascia. Therefore, it is critical to preserve nerve bundles during dissection of the promontory. According to anatomical studies, the hypogastric nerve plexus is typically located to the left of the median line (75% of cases), but it is also found in the middle in about a quarter of cases. Based on this feature, the incision should be made laterally to the middle line on the right, on the projection of the right common ileal artery. The underlying presacral fascia is separated from the hypogastric plexus, forming a 1.5–2 cm diameter opening. Then, the peritoneal incision is extended, creating a J-shaped incision to the level of the right uterosacral ligament while avoiding and leaving the right hypogastric nerve laterally. While the hypogastric plexus remains outside the dissection zone, one should remember that the plexus is divided into two sections at the level of the S1 vertebra, which means that the right hypogastric nerve can be damaged on its way from the promontory to the right uterosacral ligament. It usually runs parallel to the right uterosacral ligament and the right ureter. The plexus contains sympathetic innervation responsible for contracting the anal and urethral sphincters and proprioception nerves of the bladder, rectum, and uterus. As a result, the surgeon should avoid excessive coagulation during dissection of the peritoneum of the right side of the pelvis, opting instead for sharp and blunt separation.

16.3 Tips and Tricks

Almost always, the adipose tissue forms a protective layer over the ligament. Although, in obese patients, the significant adipose tissue covers the ligament. While the console surgeon becomes comfortable and familiar with the robotic approach, the side surgeon can assist by providing tactile feedback to ensure proper identification of the promontory. Hemostasis must be meticulously maintained throughout this dissection, as presacral vessels can cause significant bleeding. If bleeding occurs, the fenestrated bipolar forceps are ideal for squeezing the area while the assistant inserts a suction device. Dissection of the sacrum is continued until the periosteum is exposed. After completing the sacral dissection, peritoneal incision between the right ureter and the sigmoid colon angle should be made and extended caudally to the vaginal apex area. In some instances, this point is reached via a tunneling approach. Sometimes, a laparoscopic suction irrigator can be inserted into the space, followed by hydro dissection to create the tunnel.

17 Dissection of the Peritoneum

The peritoneal incision begins at the sacral promontory and expands in the J-shaped manner toward the pelvis, right to the sigmoid, and toward the vagina. To avoid damage to the ureter, care must be taken to visualize the right ureter during this dissection and to maintain a sufficient distance from it when coagulating.

To facilitate subsequent peritoneal closure over the mesh, the peritoneal edges should be separated as widely as possible. This is especially critical when dissecting distally in the pelvis. Bringing the left edge of the peritoneal opening over the mesh can be challenging if the peritoneum is not well mobilized in this area (Fig. 6).

18 Vesicovaginal Dissection

Vesicovaginal area dissection is a crucial part of sacrocolpopexy. The vesicovaginal space is exposed for dissection by superiorly retracting the bladder with the assistance of a robotic arm.

The use of a vaginal stenting device is essential to aiding dissection. A vaginal stent enables the assistant to manipulate the vagina for dissection and eventually aids in suture positioning. The vaginal probe is then advanced in a head-to-back direction. This identifies the approximate area of the tissue dissection plane (Fig. 7). Although an acute dissection in conjunction with electrocoagulation is typically required to initiate the dissection, once the tissue plane has been established, blunt dissection can be used.

When sacrocolpopexy is performed concurrently with hysterectomy, this tissue plane is already partially dissected. Moreover, when sacrocolpopexy is performed following prior hysterectomy, significant adhesions may exist, making detection of the tissue plane more problematic. The bladder frequently wholly covers the vaginal apex. When complex adhesions obscure the tissue plane, the bladder can be filled with fluid via a bladder catheter to identify the correct plane. Likewise, a cystoscope can be inserted into the bladder and the bladder outlined using transillumination. Any bladder damage that occurs during this dissection is easily repaired with absorbable sutures. In these cases, a bladder catheter should be retained postoperatively. The duration of catheter drainage and the need for a cystogram are determined by the surgeon and the repaired defect size.

18.1 Nerve-Sparing Anterior Dissection

When a significant cystocele is present, it is necessary to dissect the vesicovaginal space as far distally as possible to allow for distal mesh placement. When the mesh is posi-

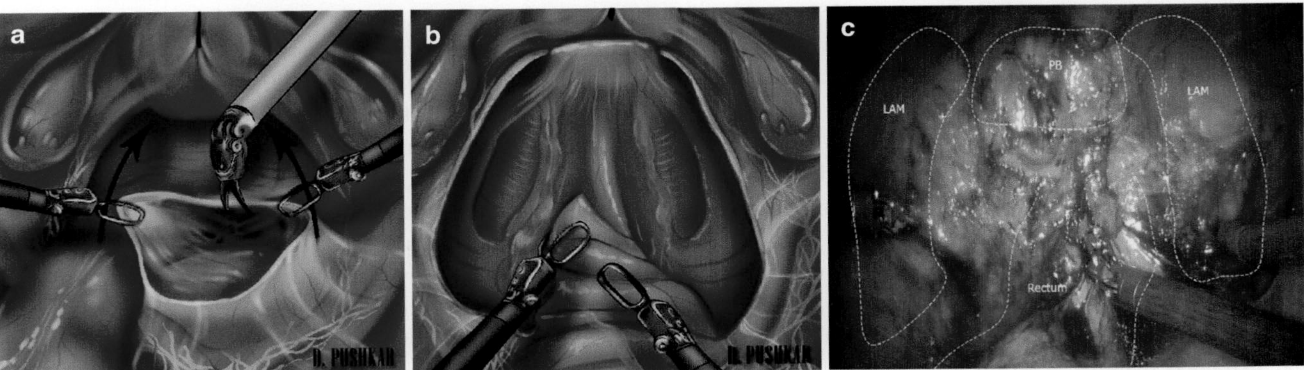

Fig. 6 (**a, b**) The opening of the peritoneum and posterior dissection; (**c**) – the levator ani muscle (LAM) and perineal body (PB) are identified

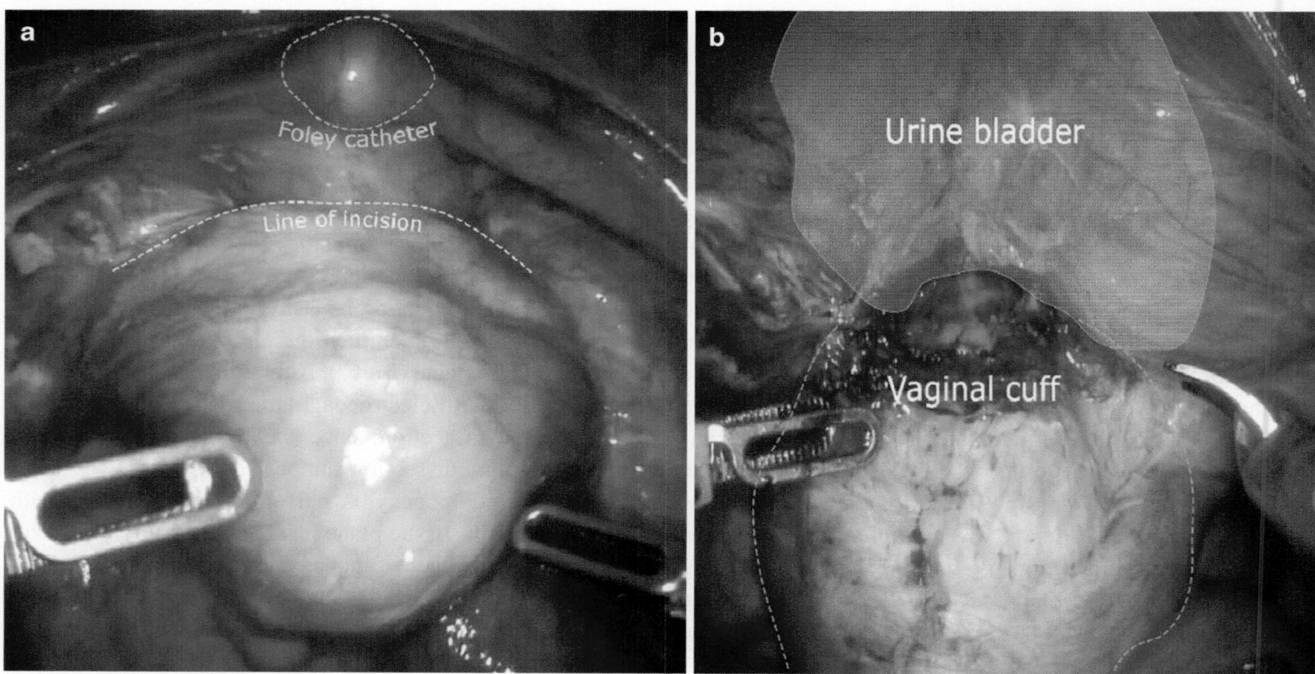

Fig. 7. (**a**) A line for the anterior dissection; (**b**) dissection between the bladder and the anterior vaginal wall started

tioned distally, even large cystoceles might be fixed without requiring additional transvaginal repair. The vesicovaginal space could be dissected entirely, resulting in a triangular-shaped area with an apex at the dorsal end of the bladder trigone and lateral limits defined by the superficial layer of vesicouterine ligaments. The descending branch of the uterine artery, the superficial vesical vein (an extension of the superficial uterine vein), and the cervicovesical vessels contribute to their formation. Significantly, an anatomical study showed that the avascular, easily cleavable vesicovaginal space accounted for one-half of the total vaginal length [54]. According to Shiozawa et al., during this dissection, no nerve structures were identified, though bladder nerve branches from the inferior hypogastric plexus were identified in the deep portion of the vesicouterine ligament [55].

19 Rectovaginal Dissection

Lastly, the rectovaginal incision is completed, allowing the posterior vaginal wall to be formed in coherence with the peritoneal opening. The rectovaginal space is opened to identify the puborectal/pubococcygeal levator ani muscles on both sides and the peritoneal body in the middle. Similar to the vesicovaginal area, the rectovaginal space is dissected and extended distally. A distal placement of the posterior vaginal mesh can address posterior compartment defects and prevent the need for concurrent posterior colporrhaphy. Additional caution is required during posterior vaginal wall detachment from the rectum to avoid any rectal injuries. As a result, the use of a vaginal probe can be helpful during this step.

Almost always, the cranial end of the perineal body can be reached by caudal blunt dissection without any significant vessels or tissue to be cut. The rectal fascia is easily separated from the pelvic parietal fascia that covers the puborectal and pubococcygeal parts of the levator ani muscle at this level, lateral to the posterior vaginal wall. During dissections, one could face the middle rectal vessels and the rectal nervous branch of the inferior hypogastric plexus that ran close to the puborectal/pubococcygeal levator ani muscle immediately beneath the rectal fascia [56]. When the rectovaginal space is wholly dissected, it results in an inverted V-shaped area. The lateral limits were defined by uterosacral and rectovaginal ligaments. The base is formed by the cranial end of the perineal body in the middle, left, and right puborectal/pubococcygeal portions of the levator ani muscle, which hugs both sides of the lateral vaginal walls. An apex is at the point of convergence of the left and right uterosacral ligaments. There is an avascular, easily cleavable rectovaginal area composing two-thirds of the total vaginal length in the craniocaudal direction [57].

20 Mesh Fixation

A permanent, synthetic mesh is used in the initial description of robotic sacrocolpopexy. Commercially available products from polypropylene are explicitly designed for POP repair. These products are available in a prefabricated "Y" shape or a soft polypropylene mesh sheet that can be cut to the desired size and configuration. We employ this type of mesh and cut it into two different strips to allow for differential tensioning of the anterior and posterior compartments. The first strip for the anterior vaginal wall is rectangular (7.5 × 5 cm) with a curved edge for the bladder neck. The posterior mesh should be cut in Y-manner from the soft mesh of 10 × 15 cm. The narrow end of the mesh is sutured at the promontory and the wide part is fixed to the levator ani; at the lowest position, there should be a cutout for the rectum. To fit the mesh properly, the surgeon constantly evaluates the total vaginal length preoperatively. Thus, the distance between the sacral promontory and the top point of adjusted prolapse will be the right length of the sacral part of the mesh. The width of the posterior mesh also should be anatomically based on the distance between levator ani muscles palpated vaginally, and its lower border should always be curved out to prevent any rectal compression by the mesh in the future.

Suturing both mesh strips to the anterior and posterior vaginal walls is followed by suturing them to the anterior longitudinal ligament overlying the sacral promontory. The assistant grasps both strips of mesh and adjusts each strip to the desired tension in collaboration with the surgeon. Because cell ingrowth into mesh occurs within 7–14 days, one could make a case for using absorbable sutures when placing mesh; however, there is a dearth of data on the use of absorbable sutures. In our practice, we prefer Ethibond® suture because its texture enables good knot tying.

One strip of polypropylene mesh is placed as far distally as possible on the anterior vaginal wall and secured in place with a suture. The vaginal probe is helpful in positioning the vaginal vault during suture placement. Five additional sutures are placed to form three rows of two sutures. Sutures should not be placed too deeply, as this may result in ligature or mesh exposure in the vagina. Although most reports indicate the use of six stitches, the actual number is likely to vary according to surgeon's preference. We usually fix the mesh to the cervix whenever it is present, as this provides the strong tissue to anchor.

The posterior strip of the mesh is then inserted in the peritoneal cavity and fixed upward. Firstly, it is sutured to the middle portion of puborectal muscles with a single nonabsorbable interrupted suture from both sides (Figs. 8 and 9). Then, it is set to the perineal body in the midline, to uterosacral ligaments laterally, and to the vaginal cuff/uterine cervix also using nonabsorbable sutures. A recent study of mesh deformation with the utilization of the finite element model of the female pelvic floor during abdominal sacrocolpopexy concluded that recommended distance between stitches of the posterior compartment should be about 3.5 cm and 2.5 cm for the anterior mesh [58]. The anterior mesh is fixed to the anterior vaginal wall upward from the bladder's trigone by nonabsorbable polyester interrupted sutures. Then, posterior and anterior strips are fixed together. The longer edge of the posterior mesh is used for the fixation to the sacral promontory.

If a "Y" mesh is used and the vaginal walls are subjected to asymmetric tension, the mesh can be plicated with a poly-

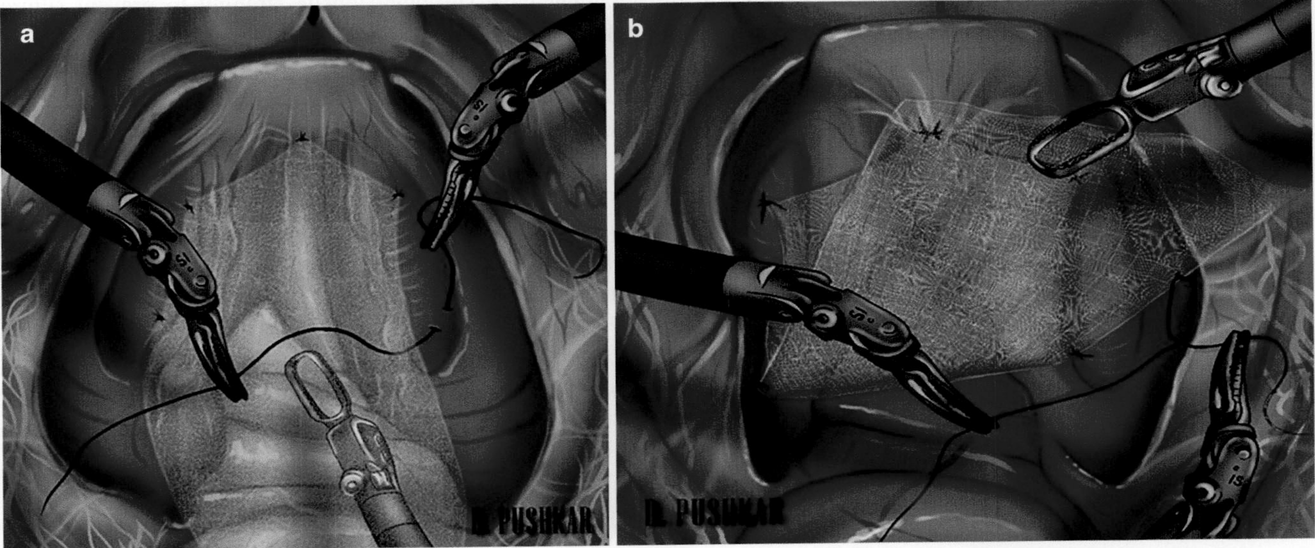

Fig. 8 (**a**) Mesh attachment to the perineal body and levator ani, (**b**) attachment to the perineal body and levator ani

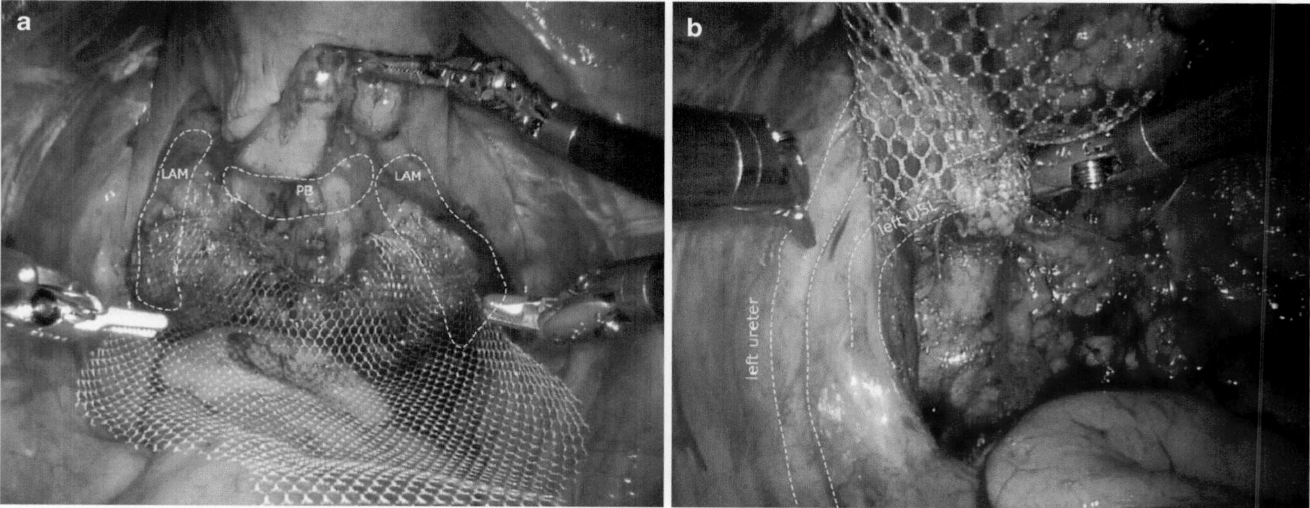

Fig. 9 (**a**) The posterior mesh is fixed to the levators and perineal body. (**b**) During fixation of the mesh to the uterosacral ligament, ureteral injuries should be avoided

propylene suture to correct the asymmetry. The vaginal probe should be removed or retracted to the mid-vagina while tensioning the mesh to prevent overcorrection of the prolapse. Unfortunately, there is no objective measure of mesh tension; however, the authors release tension if the mesh appears distorted following removal of the vaginal stent.

Once the desired tension is established, the assistant secures the mesh near the promontory and reintroduces the vaginal probe to relieve tension on the mesh during suturing. To secure the mesh in place, two sutures are typically inserted into the anterior longitudinal ligament.

The surgeon can secure the mesh strips to the ligament by threading both sutures through the mesh and ligament and then tying them down or by threading one suture through the mesh and ligament and immediately tying it down before threading the second suture. The latter has the advantage that once the first suture is secured, the assistant is no longer required to hold the mesh close to the promontory. The former has the advantage of exposing the ligament completely while placing both sutures without interference from the mesh. Regardless of technique, the suture should be threaded through the mesh before being inserted into the ligament. This allows the suture to be immediately tied down if any bleeding occurs. Ideally, any presacral vessels in the area of the dissection should have been cauterized previously to minimize bleeding during mesh suturing.

Some authors recommended that sutures be placed horizontally to maximize tensile strength and minimize the risk of suture pullout [58], but the authors do not hesitate to place sutures vertically when necessary to avoid vessel damage.

As we mentioned above, a surgeon should always keep in mind that the average thickness of the anterior longitudinal sacral ligament is no more than 2 mm. Sutures being placed too deep and entering the sacrum's periosteum is a common occurrence during suture placement. Deep fixation can cause a higher risk of pain, osteomyelitis, and spondylodiscitis formation during the postoperative period. That statement should also prevent using staples and tackers in that area because of deeper penetration of the ligament (5 mm) compared to 2–3 mm using nonabsorbable sutures. Also, according to some studies, tackers have lower biomechanical resistance than nonabsorbable sutures, and more than one staple is needed to avoid mesh snapping off [59].

Sutures adequately placed in the anterior longitudinal ligament have sufficient tensile strength to prevent suture pullout (Fig. 10).

21 Peritoneal Closure

Any excess mesh is excised after the mesh is secured to the anterior longitudinal ligament. Closure of the peritoneum prolongs the operation, but it may decrease the risk of bowel complications due to small bowel adhesion to the exposed mesh. It is accomplished with a running, locking Vicryl suture, beginning at the sacral promontory and progressing toward the vaginal cuff. The closure is tension-free as a result of the previous dissection. Additionally, any barbed suture can be used to close the peritoneum (Fig. 11).

Cystoscopy is required if there is any possibility of ureteral or bladder injury. To aid in the identification of ureteral efflux,

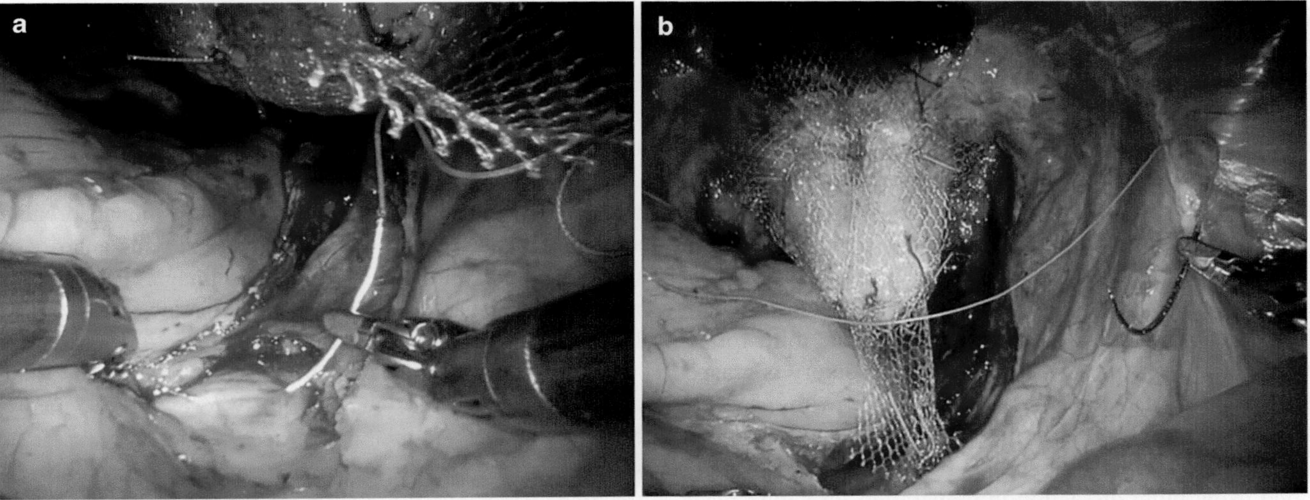

Fig. 10 (**a**) The mesh is fixed to the anterior longitudinal ligament of promontory; (**b**) the anterior mesh is fixed to the anterior longitudinal ligament of promontory

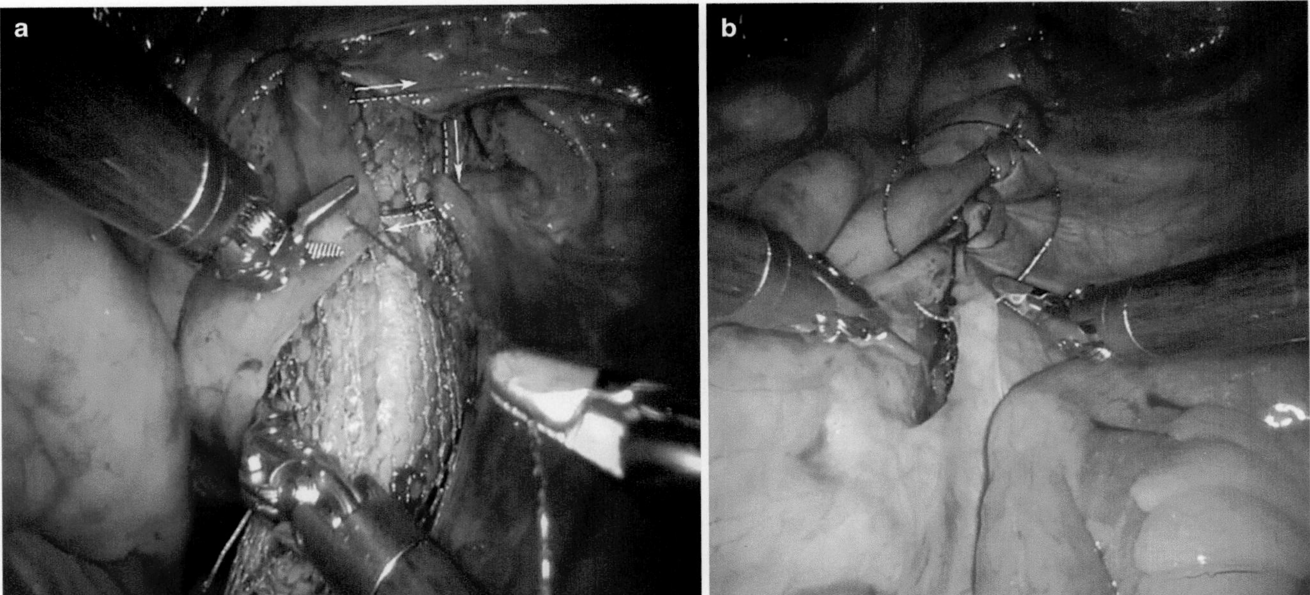

Fig. 11 (**a**, **b**) Mesh extraperitonization with absorbable barbed continuous suture

a preoperative oral dose of phenazopyridine or intraoperative intravenous administration, methylene blue, or sodium fluorescein can be used. Additionally, cystoscopy will confirm that no suture was accidentally placed in the bladder.

Postoperative vaginal examination is performed to ensure adequate apical support, to check for exposed mesh or sutures, and to determine if additional transvaginal anterior or posterior colporrhaphy is required. Apical support almost always improves the anatomic appearance of anterior prolapse, and concomitant anterior colporrhaphy is rarely needed. However, posterior defects frequently require concurrent repair, as sacrocolpopexy may not adequately address distal rectoceles. Therefore, on postoperative day one, the majority of patients are discharged home.

22 Robotic Sacrohysteropexy

Robotic sacrohysteropexy is an excellent minimally invasive option for women who desire uterine-sparing repair. The first robotic arm is equipped with monopolar endoshears, the second robotic arm is equipped with ProGrasp forceps or bipolar graspers, and the third robotic arm is equipped with a robotic tenaculum. The first step is to locate the sacral promontory. This requires sufficient retraction of the sigmoid colon toward the left pelvic sidewall, which can be accomplished using a bowel grasper forceps in the third robotic arm. The peritoneum that covers the promontory is grasped and incised with monopolar endoshears, with particular attention paid to the right ureter as it crosses the right iliac vessels. The anterior longitudinal ligament can then be identified using blunt dissection in preparation for suture placement. After fixation, the peritoneal incision can be extended caudally toward the posterior cervix and cul-de-sac to allow for extraperitonealization of the mesh. The side assistant is then asked to pass the mesh and sutures over the uterine side to begin mesh fixation. The polypropylene mesh is available in a Y-shape or as two longitudinal strips for anterior and posterior fixation.

Then, the robotic tenaculum is used to grasp the uterine fundus, and two openings in the broad ligament are prepared using monopolar or bipolar cautery. Each broad ligament is created with a 2–3 cm window to allow the mesh arms to pass anteriorly (Fig. 12).

The ventral deflection of the vaginal probe is used to demonstrate the anterior limit of the vaginal vault and guide the bladder's dissection from the vagina using a combination of monopolar and bipolar diathermy. The dissection is continued until the catheter balloon's outline is discernible. The anterior mesh is now sutured to the vaginal vault at the apex and along with the lateral aspects with nonabsorbable sutures. The mesh's two "tails" can be seen lying anterior to the uterus and fallopian tubes in this image. The anterior mesh's two tails are drawn through the windows in the broad ligaments and joined to the posterior mesh.

We prefer Ethibond sutures for mesh fixation because they are monofilament and thus less likely to extrude vaginally. Suturing the mesh to the posterior cervix with a total of four sutures is followed by anterior passage of the Y arms through the broad ligaments (Fig. 13). The mesh is then attached anteriorly to the cervix alone or the cervix and anterior vaginal wall, depending on the severity of the cystocele. Finally, the mesh is secured against the sacral promontory while the console or side surgeon inspects the vagina to determine the degree of prolapse reduction. Adjustments to the mesh tensioning can be made to eliminate prolapse. The mesh is then sutured sequentially to the sacral promontory using 3–4 sutures. To ensure proper mesh tensioning, it is beneficial to have the side surgeon assist with the knot tying of the first suture. After trimming the mesh, the peritoneum is closed by a continuous suture placed anteriorly in the peritoneum overlying the bladder and cervix to cover the mesh in that location.

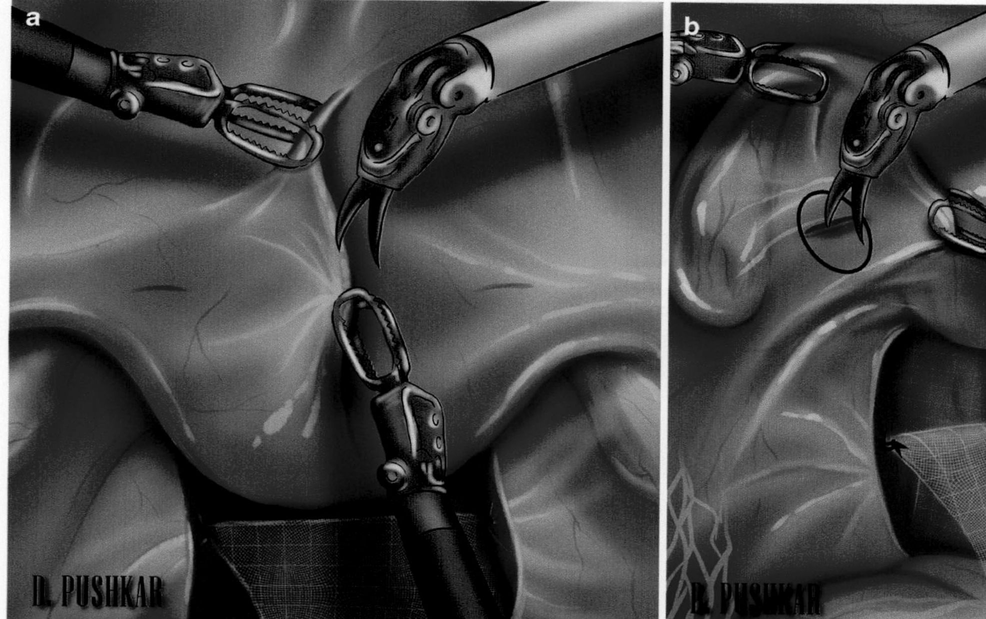

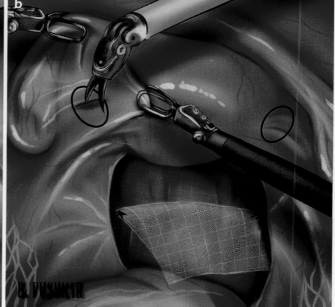

Fig. 12 (a) Anterior dissection during robotic hysterosacropexy is similar to sacrocolpopexy. (b) Openings in broad ligaments are cleated for the passage of the arms of anterior mesh

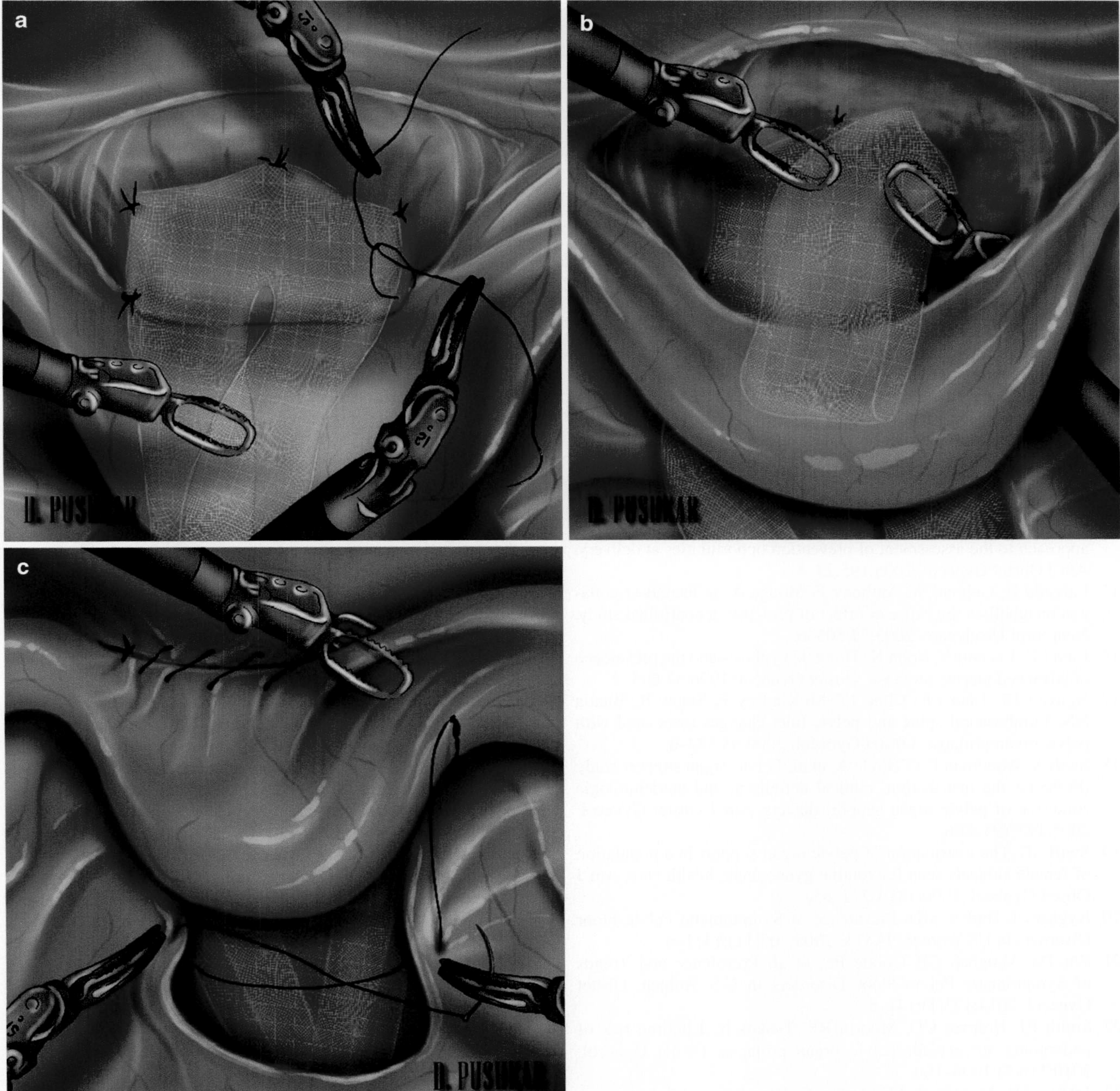

Fig. 13 (**a**) Anterior mesh is fixated to the vaginal wall; (**b**) arms of anterior mesh is passed through broad ligaments. (**c**) Peritoneal closure after sacrohysteropexy

Acknowledgments Thanks to Alexander Popov and George Kasyan for reviewing and preparing the chapter for publication. Thanks to Larisa Borchaninova for her comprehensive illustrations of surgical procedures.

References

1. Olsen AL, Smith VJ, Bergstrom JO, et al. Epidemiology of surgically managed pelvic organ prolapse and urinary incontinence. Obstet Gynecol. 1997;89:501.
2. Marchionni M, Bracco GL, Checcucci V, et al. True incidence of vaginal vault prolapse. Thirteen years of experience. J Reprod Med. 1999;44:679.
3. Elliott DS. Diagnosis and management of apical prolapse. In: Goldman HB, Vasavada SP, editors. Female urology: a practical clinical guide. Totowa, NJ: Humana Press Inc; 2007. p. 297–305. Chapter 21.
4. Gilleran JP, Johnson M, Hundley A. Robotic-assisted laparoscopic mesh sacrocolpopexy. Ther Adv Urol. 2010;2:195–208.
5. Di Marco DS, Chow GK, Gettman MT, et al. Robotic-assisted laparoscopic sacrocolpopexy for treatment of vaginal vault prolapse. Urology. 2004;63:373–6.

6. Akeel NY, Gurland B, Hull T. Pelvic floor disorders related to urology and gynecology. In: Beck DE, Steele SR, Wexner SD, editors. Fundamentals of anorectal surgery. Cham: Springer; 2019. p. 571–82.
7. Dietz HP. Pelvic organ prolapse: a review. AFP. 2015;44(7):446–52.
8. Dietz H. Pelvic floor trauma in childbirth. Aust NZ J Obstet Gynaecol. 2013;53:220–30.
9. McIntosh LJ, Mallett VT, Frahm JD, Richardson DA, Evans MI. Gynecologic disorders in women with Ehlers-Danlos syndrome. J Soc Gynecol Invest. 1995;2:559–64.
10. Jackson SR, Avery NC, Tarlton JF, Eckford SD, Abrams P, Bai- ley AJ. Changes in metabolism of collagen in genitourinary prolapse. Lancet. 1996;347:1658–61.
11. Dietz H. The aetiology of prolapse. Int Urogynecol J. 2008;19:1323–9.
12. Gyhagen M, Bullarbo M, Nielsen TF, Milsom I. Prevalence and risk factors for pelvic organ prolapse 20 years after childbirth: a national cohort study in singleton primiparae after vaginal or caesarean delivery. Br J Obstet Gynaecol. 2013;120:152–60.
13. Glazener C, Mac Arthur C, Bain C, et al. Epidemiology of pelvic organ prolapse in relation to delivery mode history at 12 years after childbirth: a longitudinal cohort study. Neurourol Urodyn. 2010;29:819–20.
14. Patel D, Xu X, Thomason AD, Ransom SB, Ivy JS, DeLancey JO. Childbirth and pelvic floor dysfunction: an epidemiologic approach to the assessment of prevention opportunities at delivery. Am J Obstet Gynecol. 2006;195:23–8.
15. Laborda E, Gelman W, Anthony F, Monga A. Is increased collagen metabolism the cause or effect of prolapse: a controlled study. Neurourol Urodynam. 2003;22:505–6.
16. Lind LR, Lucente V, Kohn N. Thoracic kyphosis and the prevalence of advanced uterine prolapse. Obstet Gynecol. 1996;87:605–9.
17. Nguyen JK, Lind LR, Choe JY, McKindsey F, Sinow R, Bhatia NN. Lumbosacral spine and pelvic inlet changes associated with pelvic organ prolapse. Obstet Gynecol. 2000;95:332–6.
18. Swift S, Woodman P, O'Boyle A, et al. Pelvic organ support study (POSST): the distribution, clinical definition, and epidemiologic condition of pelvic organ support defects. Am J Obstet Gynecol. 2005;192:795–806.
19. Swift SE. The distribution of pelvic organ support in a population of female subjects seen for routine gynecologic health care. Am J Obstet Gynecol. 2000;183:L277–85.
20. Nygaard I, Barber MD. Prevalence of Symptomatic Pelvic Floor Disorders in US Women. JAMA. 2008;300(11):1311–6.
21. Wu JM, Vaughan CP, Goode PS, et al. Prevalence and Trends of Symptomatic Pelvic Floor Disorders in U.S Women. Obstet Gynecol. 2014;123(1):141–8.
22. Smith FJ, Holman CD, Moorin RE, Tsokos N. Lifetime risk of undergoing surgery for pelvic organ prolapse. Obstet Gynecol. 2010;116(5):1096–100.
23. Jokhio AH, Mohsin R, MacArthur C. Prevalence of pelvic organ prolapse in women, associated factors and impact on quality of life in rural Pakistan: population- based study. BMC Women's Health. 2020;20:82.
24. Walker GJA, Gunasekera P. Pelvic organ prolapse and incontinence in developing countries: review of prevalence and risk factors. Int Urogynecol J. 2011;22:12.
25. Dietz H. Prolapse worsens with age, doesn't it? Aust N Z J Obstet Gynaecol. 2008;48:587–91.
26. Dixit P, Shek K, Dietz H. How common is pelvic floor muscle atrophy after vaginal childbirth? Ultrasound Obstet Gynecol. 2014;43:83–8.
27. Mant J, Painter R, Vessey M. Epidemiology of genital prolapse: observations from the Oxford Family Planning Association Study. Br J Obstet Gynaecol. 1997;104:579–85.
28. Samuelsson EC, Victor FTA, Tibblin G, Svärdsudd KF. Signs of genital prolapse in a Swedish population of women 20 to 59 years of age and possible related factors. Am J Obstet Gynecol. 1999;180:299–305.
29. Rinne KM, Kirkinen PP. What predisposes young women to genital prolapse? Eur J Obstet Gynecol Reprod Biol. 1999;84:23–5.
30. Lowenstein E, Ottesen B, Gimbel H. Incidence and lifetime risk of pelvic organ prolapse surgery in Denmark from 1977 to 2009. Int Urogynecol J. 2015;26:49–55.
31. Young N, Kamisan Atan I, Dietz H. Obesity: how much does it matter for female pelvic organ prolapse? In: RCOG World Congress. RCOG: Brisbane; 2015.
32. Jorgensen S, Hein HO, Gyntelberg F. Heavy lifting at work and risk of genital prolapse and herniated lumbar disc in assistant nurses. Occup Med. 1994;44:47–9.
33. Haylen BT, Maher CF, Barber MD, Camargo S, Dandolu V, Digesu A, Goldman HB, Huser M, Milani AL, Moran PA, Schaer GN, Withagen MI. An International Urogynecological Association (IUGA) /International Continence Society (ICS) joint report on the terminology for female pelvic organ prolapse (POP). Int Urogynecol J. 2016;27(2):165–94.
34. Persu C, Chapple CR, Gutue S, Geavlete P. Pelvic Organ Prolapse Quantification System (POP-Q) – a new era in pelvic prolapse staging. J Med Life. 2011;4(1):75–81.
35. Singh K, Jakab M, Reid WM, Berger LA, Hoyte L. Three-dimensional magnetic resonance imaging assessment of levator ani morphologic features in different grades of prolapse. Am J Obstet Gynecol. 2003;188(2, 2):910–915–915.
36. Nichols DH, Randall CL. Vaginal surgery. In: Types of prolapse. 4th ed. Baltimore: Williams & Wilkins; 1996. p. 101–18. Chapter 5.
37. Petros PE, Ulmsten UI. An integral theory of female urinary incontinence. Experimental and clinical considerations. Acta Obstet Gynecol Scand Suppl. 1990;153:7–31. (Review)
38. Davila HH, Gallo T, Bruce L, Landrey C. Robotic and laparoendoscopic single-site utero-sacral ligament suspension for apical vaginal prolapse: evaluation of our technique and perioperative outcomes. J Robot Surg. 2017;11(2):171–7.
39. Hendrix SL, Clark A, Nygaard I, Aragaki A, Barnabei V, McTiernan A. Pelvic organ prolapse in the women's health initiative: gravity and gravidity. Am J Obstet Gynecol. 2002;186(6):1160–6.
40. Olsen AL, Smith VJ, Bergstrom JO, Colling JC, Clark AL. Epidemiology of surgically managed pelvic organ prolapse and urinary incontinence. Obstet Gynecol. 1997;89:501–6.
41. Subak LL, Waetjen LE, van den Eeden S, Thom DH, Vittinghoff E, Brown JS. Cost of pelvic organ prolapse surgery in the United States. Obstet Gynecol. 2001;98:646–51.
42. Nygaard IE, McCreery R, Brubaker L, Connolly AM, Cundiff G, Weber AM, et al. Abdominal sacrocolpopexy: a comprehensive review. Obstet Gynecol. 2004;104:805–23.
43. Serati M, Bogani G, Sorice P, Braga A, Torella M, Salvatore S, Uccella S, Cromi A, Ghezzi F. Robot-assisted sacrocolpopexy for pelvic organ prolapse: a systematic review and meta-analysis of comparative studies. Eur Urol. 2014;66(2):303–18.
44. Culligan PJ, Lewis C, Priestley J, et al. Long-term outcomes of robotic assisted laparoscopic sacrocolpopexy using lightweight Y-mesh. Female Pelvic Med Reconstr Surg. 2020;26(3):202–6. https://doi.org/10.1097/SPV.0000000000000788.
45. Wu JM, Vaughan CP, Goode PS, et al. Prevalence and trends of symptomatic pelvic floor disorders in US women. Obstet Gynecol. 2014;123(1):141–8.
46. Nygaard I, Brubaker L, Zyczynski HM, et al. Long-term outcomes following abdominal sacrocolpopexy for pelvic organ prolapse. JAMA. 2013;309(19):2016–24.
47. Davila HH, Abdelhameed S, Malave-Huertas D, et al. Ultrasonography and robotic-assisted laparoscopic sacrocervico-

pexy with pubocervical fascia reconstruction: comparison with standard technique. J Robot Surg. 2020;14(5):759–66.

48. Jelovsek EJ, Barber MD, Brubaker L, Norton P, Gantz M, Richter HE, Weidner A, Menefee S, Schaffer J, Pugh N, Meikle S, NICHD Pelvic Floor Disorders Network. Effect of uterosacral ligament suspension vs sacrospinous ligament fixation with or without perioperative behavioral therapy for pelvic organ vaginal prolapse on surgical outcomes and prolapse symptoms at 5 years in the optimal randomized clinical trial. JAMA. 2018;319(15):1554–65.
49. Umek WH, Morgan DM, Ashton-Miller JA, DeLancey JO. Quantitative analysis of uterosacral ligament origin and insertion points by magnetic resonance imaging. Obstet Gynecol. 2004;103:447–51. https://doi.org/10.1097/01.AOG.0000113104.22887.cd.
50. Davila HH, Di Natale R, Bruce L, Goodman L, Gallo T. Anatomic evaluation of uterosacral and cardinal ligament during robotic and laparoscopic surgery for pelvic organ prolapse. Open J Obstet Gynecol. 2017;7:1216–27. https://doi.org/10.4236/ojog.2017.712124.
51. Nygaard IE, McCreery R, Brubaker L, et al. Pelvic Floor Disorders Network. Abdominal sacrocolpopexy: a comprehensive review. Obstet Gynecol. 2004;104:805–23. https://doi.org/10.1097/01.AOG.0000139514.90897.07.
52. Davila HH, Bruce L, Goodman L, Gallo T. Robotic assisted laparoscopic apical suspension. Description of a 4 points technique (RALAS-4): first case reported. Open J Obstet Gynecol. 2017;7:944–50. https://doi.org/10.4236/ojog.2017.79095.
53. Davila HH, Brown K, Dara P, Bruce L, Goodman L, Gallo T. Robotic-assisted laparoscopic apical suspension: description of the spiral technique. J Robot Surg. 2019;13(3):519–23. https://doi.org/10.1007/s11701-018-0879-1. Epub 2018 Oct 3
54. Ercoli A, Campagna G, Delmas V, Ferrari S, Morciano A, Scambia G, Cervigni M. Anatomical insights into sacrocolpopexy for multicompartment pelvic organ prolapse. Neurourol Urodyn. 2016;35(7):813–8. https://doi.org/10.1002/nau.22806. Epub 2015 Jul 5
55. Shiozawa T, Huebner M, Hirt B, Wallwiener D, Reisenauer C. Nerve-preserving sacrocolpopexy: anatomical study and surgical approach. Eur J Obstet Gynecol Reprod Biol. 2010;152(1):103–7. https://doi.org/10.1016/j.ejogrb.2010.05.009. Epub 2010 Jun 9
56. Kiyomatsu T, Ishihara S, Murono K, Otani K, Yasuda K, et al. Anatomy of the middle rectal artery: a review of the historical literature. Surg Today. 2017;47(1):14–9. https://doi.org/10.1007/s00595-016-1359-8. Epub 2016 Jun 3
57. Shiozawa T, Huebner M, Hirt B, et al. Nerve-preserving sacrocolpopexy: anatomical study and surgical approach. Eur J Obstet Gynecol Reprod Biol. 2010 Sep;152(1):103–7. https://doi.org/10.1016/j.ejogrb.2010.05.009.
58. Jeanditgautier E, Mayeur O, Brieu M, et al. Mobility and stress analysis of different surgical simulations during a sacrocolpopexy, using a finite element model of the pelvic system. Int Urogynecol J. 2016;27(6):951–7. https://doi.org/10.1007/s00192-015-2917-0. Epub 2016 Jan 11
59. White AB, Carrick KS, Corton MM, et al. Optimal location and orientation of suture placement in abdominal sacrocolpopexy. Obstet Gynecol. 2009;113(5):1098–103. https://doi.org/10.1097/AOG.0b013e31819ec4ee.
60. Boukerrou M, Orazi G, Nayama M, et al. Technique de la promontofixation: suspension au promontoire par fils ou Tackers? [Promontofixation procedure: use of non-absorbable sutures or Tackers?]. J Gynecol Obstet Biol Reprod (Paris). 2003;32(6):524–8. French

Robot-Assisted Retroperitoneal Lymph Node Dissection (RPLND)

Ralph Grauer, Scott Eggener, and John P. Sfakianos

1 Introduction

Testicular cancer is a relatively rare disease, projected to affect 6.0 men per 100,000 in 2021 in the United States, but its incidence has trended up over the last 30 years [1, 2]. In addition, it is the most common solid malignancy in men aged 20–34 and will be diagnosed in an estimated 9400 men in 2021 in the United States alone [2]. Testicular germ cell tumors (GCT) comprise 95% of all neoplastic testis tumors and are divided into two subtypes: seminoma and nonseminoma (NSGCT (nonseminomatous germ cell tumor)) [3]. Radical orchiectomy is the crux of diagnosis and therapy for any testicular mass suspected to be malignant. Both seminoma and nonseminoma subtypes have excellent oncological cure rates. Even NSGCT, the more aggressive subtype, has a five-year survival rate of over 80%–90% in the setting of advanced/metastatic disease [4].

For NSGCT, clinical staging is typically complete when pathologic information from the radical orchiectomy specimen is combined with radiologic and serologic studies, thus informing postoperative management. Following staging, high cure rates can be achieved with surveillance, platinum-based chemotherapy, retroperitoneal pelvic lymph node dissection (RPLND), and sometimes a combination of these therapies. RPLND is an important part of the post-radical orchiectomy clinical management in several settings.

2 Indications

In the United States, primary RPLND is most commonly performed in NSGCTs with normal serum tumor markers after orchiectomy for high-risk clinical stage (CS) I patients or in low-volume CS IIA/IIB patients [5]. In the former, RPLND serves to investigate occult metastases especially in the setting of lymphovascular invasion or > 50% embryonal carcinoma in the orchiectomy specimen. RPLND provides staging information and has therapeutic intent with high cure rates. Other clinical settings where RPLND is used include the presence of a > 1-cm retroperitoneal mass post-primary chemotherapy for NSGCT, salvage RPLND after induction and salvage chemotherapy, reoperative RPLND, and other less common clinical scenarios. There is emerging data that RPLND may have a role in the setting of low-volume metastatic seminoma as an alternative to radiation or chemotherapy, with 87% two-year recurrence-free survival, providing potential advantages compared to chemotherapy and radiation [6]. Another clinical trial, PRIMETEST, supports primary RPLND as an option in stage IIA/IIB seminoma to reduce long-term toxicity and secondary malignancy caused by radiation therapy. They report 77% two-year recurrence-free survival, with four of five recurrences occurring out of field [7].

While there are many potential clinical indications for RPLND, and it is important for clinicians to understand other options, the technical aspects of RPLND are common across settings. After initial radical orchiectomy, the goal of the RPLND is both prognostic and therapeutic as it cures many patients and can inform surveillance regimens or subsequent treatment recommendations. The efficacy and safety of open RPLND are well established [8]. However, there is morbidity associated with the open approach; most major complications relate to small bowel obstruction and atelectasis [9]. In an attempt to decrease the morbidity associated with the procedure, modified dissection templates and nerve-sparing techniques were developed to preserve antegrade ejaculation [10, 11]. Similarly, minimally invasive techniques such as laparoscopic (L-) and robot-assisted (RA-) RPLND have been increasingly performed over the past decade with the goal of minimizing morbidity while replicating the disease-free survival rates of open surgery.

R. Grauer · J. P. Sfakianos (✉)
Department of Urology, Icahn School of Medicine at Mount Sinai, New York, NY, USA

S. Eggener
Department of Urology, University of Chicago Medicine, Chicago, IL, USA

P. Wiklund et al. (eds.), *Robotic Urologic Surgery*, https://doi.org/10.1007/978-3-031-00363-9_76

3 Laparoscopic and Robot-Assisted RPLND

Traditionally, RPLND has been performed through a large open transabdominal incision. Advancements in minimally invasive approaches over the past 30 years have made laparoscopic and robot-assisted techniques a more attractive treatment option to patients and surgeons alike [12]. L-RPLND was introduced as a staging procedure in 1992 and more recently (and appropriately) has been utilized for curative purposes in both pre- and post- chemotherapy treatments. Compared to its open counterpart, L-RPLND has been suggested to be safe with decreased perioperative morbidity—including decreased postoperative pain, hastening convalescence and return to normal bowel function, assuaging incision cosmesis concerns, and improving postoperative quality of life scores [9, 10, 13–16]. However, concerns surrounding lower lymph node yield, protracted learning curve, indiscriminate use of adjuvant chemotherapy, and unknown long-term oncologic outcomes exist.

RA-RPLND emerged in 2006 as a potential alternative to the laparoscopic approach with the advantage of a shorter learning curve, improved dexterity, visualization, and ergonomics [11]. Ultimately, to prove true clinical equipoise to its open counterpart, RA-RPLND must reach benchmarked rates of infield and out-of-field recurrence as well as complication rates. Early studies on RA-RPLND have suggested equivalent surgical and oncologic effectiveness when compared to the open approach, but direct comparisons are limited by study size, variable patient cohorts, and different follow-up lengths. Overall, studies report median length of stay from 1.5 to 2 days, operative time of 200–300 minutes, EBL of 100 mL, lymph node yields >20, and negligible risk for blood transfusions (Table 1) [12–16]. For comparison, open RPLND series have reported median length of stays of 3–8 days, EBLs of 200 mL, and operative time of 150–200 minutes with lymph node yield of 25–30 [17–19]. Postoperative complication rates for RA-RPLND compare favorably to a large series of open RPLND—with Clavien-Dindo (CD) minor (I–III) and major (III–IV) complications ranging from 8%–30% to 2%–5%, respectively [15, 16, 20]. A 2018 systematic review of the RA-RPLND has corroborated these data and supports equivalent perioperative outcomes as compared to open surgery in addition to shorter hospital stays, lower EBL, and improved cosmesis [21].

Only three studies with over 40 patients have been published on primary RA-RPLND, which offer the strongest (but still suboptimal) data about recurrence rates (Table 2) [15, 16, 20]. Pearce et al. examined outcomes of RA-RPLND in 47 patients across 4 centers with CS I-IIA NSGCT [20]. Median follow-up was 16 months, and the 2-year recurrence-free survival rate was 97%—with the single recurrence arising out of field. Compared to historical open RPLND data, there was better cosmetic results, less postoperative morbidity and mortality, and fewer complications. Taylor et al.'s multi-institutional retrospective study included 47 patients with CS I-IIA NSGCT [15]. They reported infield recurrence rate of 2% and out-of-field recurrence rate of 6% at a median follow-up of 15 months. Rocco et al. reported a two-center retrospective analysis of 58 patients with CS I–IIA NSGCT that underwent RA-RPLND with a median follow-up of 47 months and a 2-year recurrence-free survival of 91%; all recurrences were out of field [16]. These reported rates of safety and oncologic compare favorably to open surgery, though no prospective randomized controlled trial or long-term data exists. In 2015, Harris et al. reported a comparative analysis of robotic and laparoscopic RPLND [22]. Both techniques had statistically similar operative times of

Table 1 Perioperative and morbidity outcomes of primary RA-RPLND in the three largest published studies

Study	No. patients	Median OR time (min)	Conversions to open *n*, (%)	Median EBL (mL)	Median length of stay (days)	Major complications (CD III–CD V) *n*, (%)	Antegrade ejaculation *n*, (%)
Pearce (2017)	47	235	1 (2)	50	1	2 (4)	47 (100)
Taylor (2020)	49	288	0 (0)	100	1	2 (4)	31 (74)
Rocco (2020)	58	319	1 (2)	100	2	1 (2)	44 (81)

Table 2 Oncologic outcomes of primary RA-RPLND in the three largest published studies

Study	No. patients	Median follow-up (months)	Median node yield	pN+ *n*, (%)	Adjuvant chemotherapy *n*, (%)	Recurrence-free survival
Pearce (2017)	47	16	26	8 (17)	5 (11)	97%
Taylor (2020)	49	15	32	21 (43)	9 (18)	92%
Rocco (2020)	58	47	26	17 (29)	5 (9)	91%

~4.5–5 hours, EBL of ~100 mL, median lymph node yield of 20–30, and similar rates of complications [22]. The authors concluded that R-RPLND is comparable to L-RPLND but it is unclear whether R-RPLND offers any measurable benefits over standard laparoscopy, perhaps besides an easier learning curve.

The application of RA-RPLND in the post-chemotherapy setting has also been studied and found in expert centers to be feasible and safe and have excellent recurrence-free survival rates [23–32]. Of the studies that included exclusively post-chemotherapy patients, few had accrual of more than 10 patients [23–25, 30, 32]; they included 11, 12, 13, 30, and 45 patients. A recent systematic analysis integrates data from these largest studies via a weighted mean approach [33]. Compared to the primary RPLND cohort, median EBL was greater, and hospital length of stay (LOS) was longer, reaching ~200 mL and 2–4 days. The rates of recurrence-free survival from these studies were 90% at median follow-up of 15 months, 100% in 23 months, 100% in 31 months, 100% in 4 months, and 98% at 2 years, respectively [30, 33]. The rates of antegrade ejaculation were 85%–90% [33]. Notably, the rate of major CD III–IV complications was 7% in this setting, similar to previously reported rates in laparoscopic (8%) and open (6%) surgery in the same clinical context [34]. Another review article that pooled many smaller studies reported a major complication rate of 14% [27].

In addition, RA-RPLND may represent a cost-equivalent option to open surgery with decreased hospital length of stay (LOS) [35]. Bhanvadia et al. compared perioperative outcomes and performed a cost analysis between the open and robot-assisted RPLND, pooling 319 and 44 cases, respectively, from a national all-payer inpatient care database—the US Nationwide Inpatient Sample (NIS). They found that patients who underwent open surgery had more than twice the LOS compared to RA-RPLND [median (IQR): 1.5 (1–3) days vs. 4 (3–6) days, $p < 0.01$]. Overall hospitalization costs were equivalent between R-RPLND and O-RPLND [median (IQR): R-RPLND vs. O-RPLND; $15,681 ($12,735–$21,596) vs. $16,718 ($11,799–$24,403), $p = 0.48$] [35]. They also performed a multivariable linear regression model to predict total hospitalization cost: robot-assisted surgery incrementally contributed $4457 ($p < 0.01$, 95% CI ($1134–$7779) and each day of hospitalization contributed $2431 ($p < 0.01$, 95% CI ($1960–$2903); the need for blood transfusion contributed $7721 ($p < 0.01$, 95% CI ($2673–$12,769) to overall cost; and other complications did not significantly affect cost [35]. Age, year, race, BMI, Charlson comorbidity index, median income, insurance status, hospital bed size, hospital teaching status, and discharge disposition did not affect total cost [35]. Their results suggest that the cost-equivalence/cost-saving is driven by the decreased LOS. For many patients undergoing RA-RPLND, discharge within 24 hours is safe. This suggests that RA-RPLND is a cost-saving procedure as compared to open, ceteris paribus—all other things being equal.

4 Robot-Assisted RPLND Surgical Technique

Mechanical bowel preparation the day prior to surgery to decompress the bowel is routine, but optional. Historically, some surgeons advocated for a low-fat diet up to two weeks prior to the surgery, to avoid chylous ascites, though conclusive data is not available. More contemporary approaches recommend a high-fat diet up to two weeks prior to surgery to allow for improved visualization of lymphatic channels, followed by a low-fat diet immediately postoperatively. Preoperative sperm banking should be encouraged if future fertility is desired.

Nerve-sparing techniques as well as unilateral modified templates for dissection exist for the preservation of antegrade ejaculation. Nerve sparing preserves the sympathetic fibers within a given template, whereas modified templates limit contralateral dissection in the region of nerves essential for ejaculatory function. Nerve sparing aims to preserve the sympathetic chain (autonomic preganglionic fibers that synapse with sympathetic ganglia adjacent to the great vessels) and the postganglionic fibers emanating from the sympathetic chain at each vertebral level (traveling anterior to the aorta and posterior to IVC) and coalescing to form the superior hypogastric plexus. A detailed understanding of the neuroanatomy is essential for any RPLND surgeon. Unilateral modified templates are an option for men with stage I NSGCT, without suspicious lymphadenopathy or suggestion of bilateral/widespread tumor dissemination. There are several versions of modified templates, but they share common regions. The 2019 AUA guidelines recommend that right-sided modified templates (Fig. 1) include, at a minimum, right common iliac, paracaval, precaval, retrocaval, interaortocaval, preaortic, and retro-aortic; the omission of para-aortic lymph nodes above the inferior mesenteric artery (IMA) is controversial [36]. The same guidelines suggest that left-sided modified templates (Fig. 2) include left common iliac, para-aortic, preaortic, and retro-aortic; the inclusion of interaortocaval nodes above the IMA is debated [36]. If metastatic disease is suspected in any nodes, then a full bilateral template (Fig. 3) is performed.

During surgery, patients are most commonly placed either in a modified flank position or supine in Trendelenburg, based on surgeon's preference. In the flank position, ports are placed in a similar fashion to robotic renal surgery, but often more medially and/or inferiorly; for unilateral modified templates, the camera port is placed superolateral to the umbilicus, and the two 8-mm robotic arm ports are placed

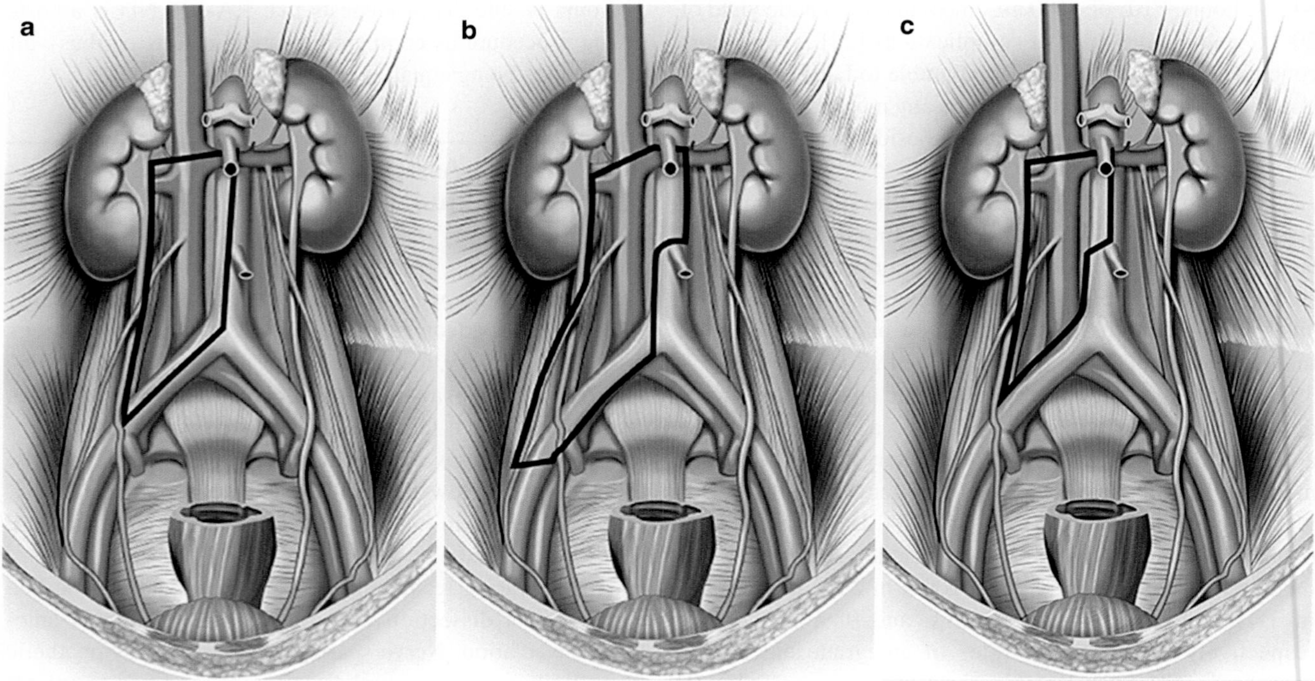

Fig. 1 (**a, b, c**) are representative variations of modified right template boundaries

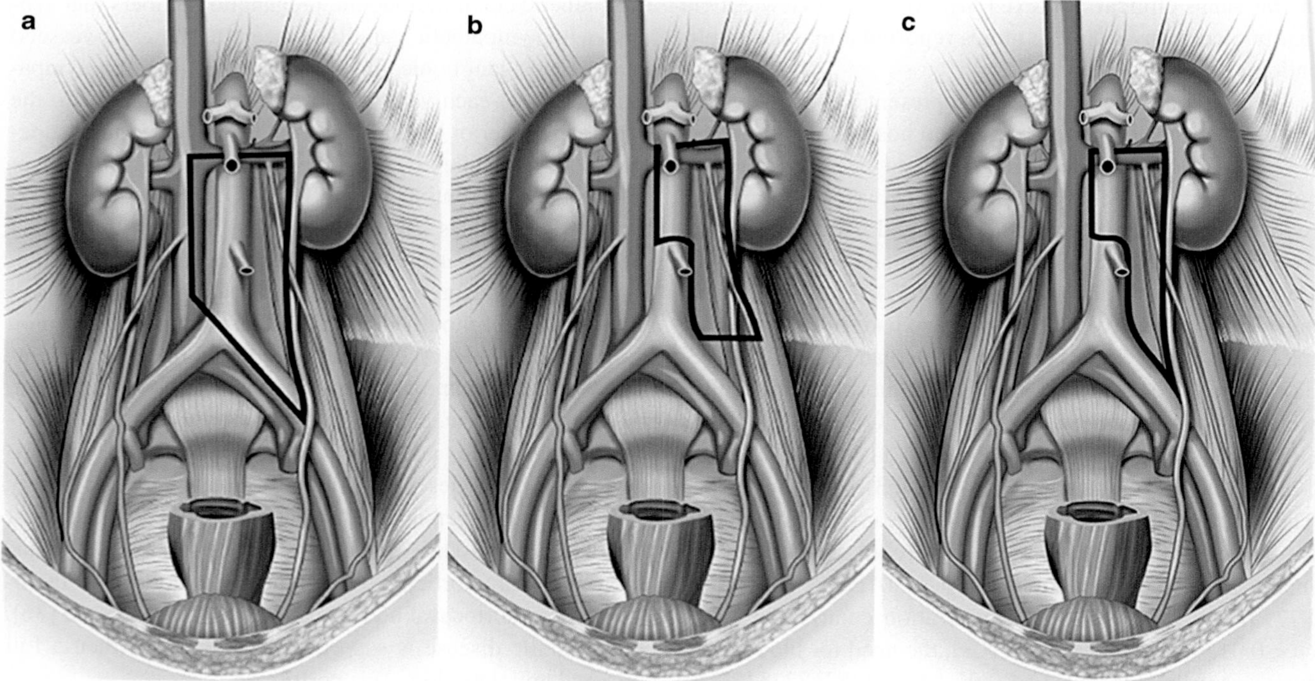

Fig. 2 (**a, b, c**) are representative variations of modified left template boundaries

inferior and superior lateral to the umbilicus. The fourth arm has many potential locations. A 12-mm assistant port is placed below the umbilicus. A 5-mm trocar port can be placed for liver retraction during right-sided procedures (Fig. 4). In supine positioning, the camera port is placed 3 cm inferolateral to the right of the umbilicus; the 8-mm robotic arm ports are placed bilaterally, near the level of the umbilicus; the fourth arm is placed outside of the robotic arm

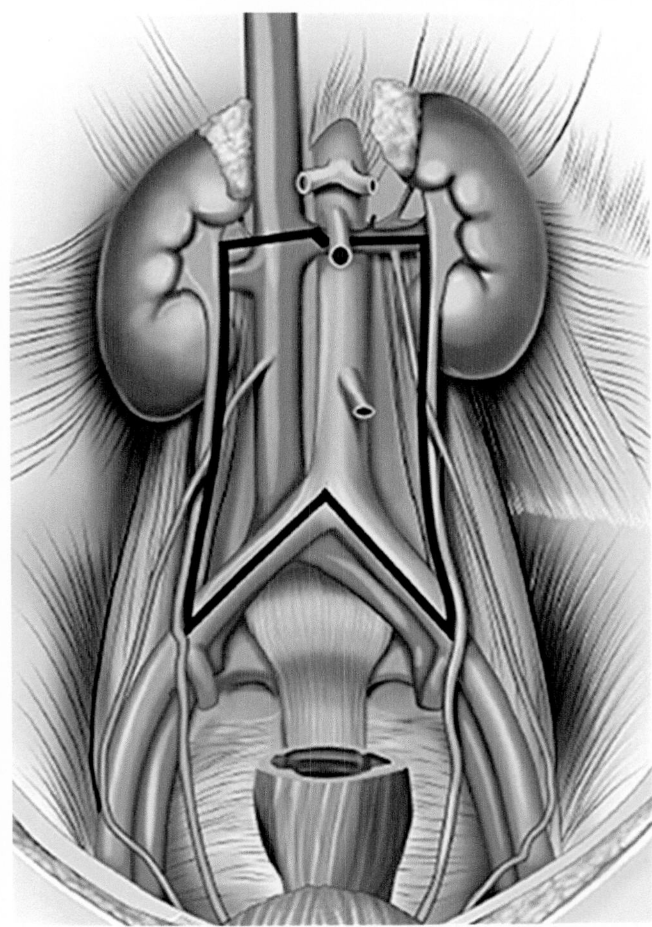

Fig. 3 Bilateral RPLND boundaries

that is contralateral to the operative side. A 12-mm assistant port can be placed contralateral to the fourth arm (Fig. 5). An additional supine technique has been described in which the trocars are placed similar to a robot-assisted prostatectomy but near the costal margin; the robot is docked cranially, and the dissection field is reversed [12]. In every technique, the use of a fourth arm is typical for improved retraction and visualization. However, to free up the use of the fourth arm, improved visualization can be achieved through the use of Keith needles to attach the cut edge of the posterior peritoneum onto the anterior abdominal wall. With the latest robotic technology, a full bilateral dissection can be performed without repositioning the patient or redocking the robot.

The surgical steps of the procedure are analogous to its open and laparoscopic counterparts. Briefly, a right-sided RA-RPLND begins with an incision along the white line of Toldt to medialize the colon, and then the second portion of the duodenum is kocherized and the IVC is identified. The gonadal vein and associated lymphatics are identified, mobilized, and appropriately ligated inferiorly to the ipsilateral inguinal ring and the spermatic cord stump; all structures are removed. The nodal tissue within the aforementioned template is completely excised. Careful attention to the sympathetic chain fibers that intertwine with the lymphatic tissue is warranted—the "split-and-roll" technique should be used in an athermal manner. It is important to identify and safely divide lumbar vessels to access and remove all lymphatic tissues lateral and posterior to the great vessels. A left-sided RA-RPLND is analogous to the right side, with the differ-

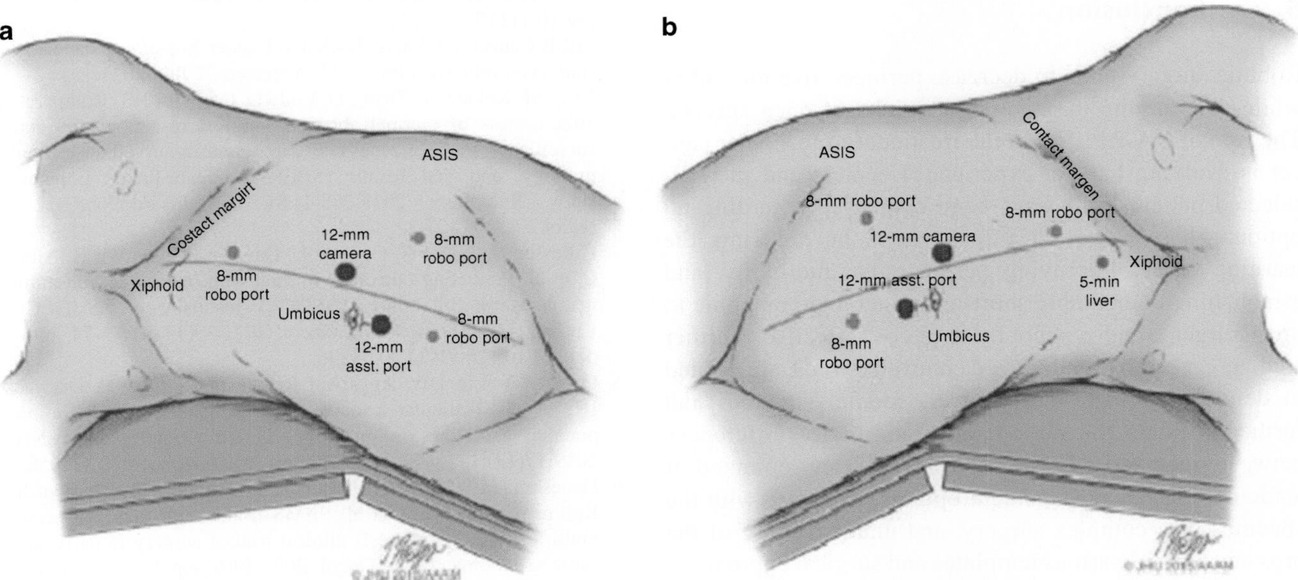

Fig. 4 The port placement locations for supine positioning are shown for both left and right RPLND

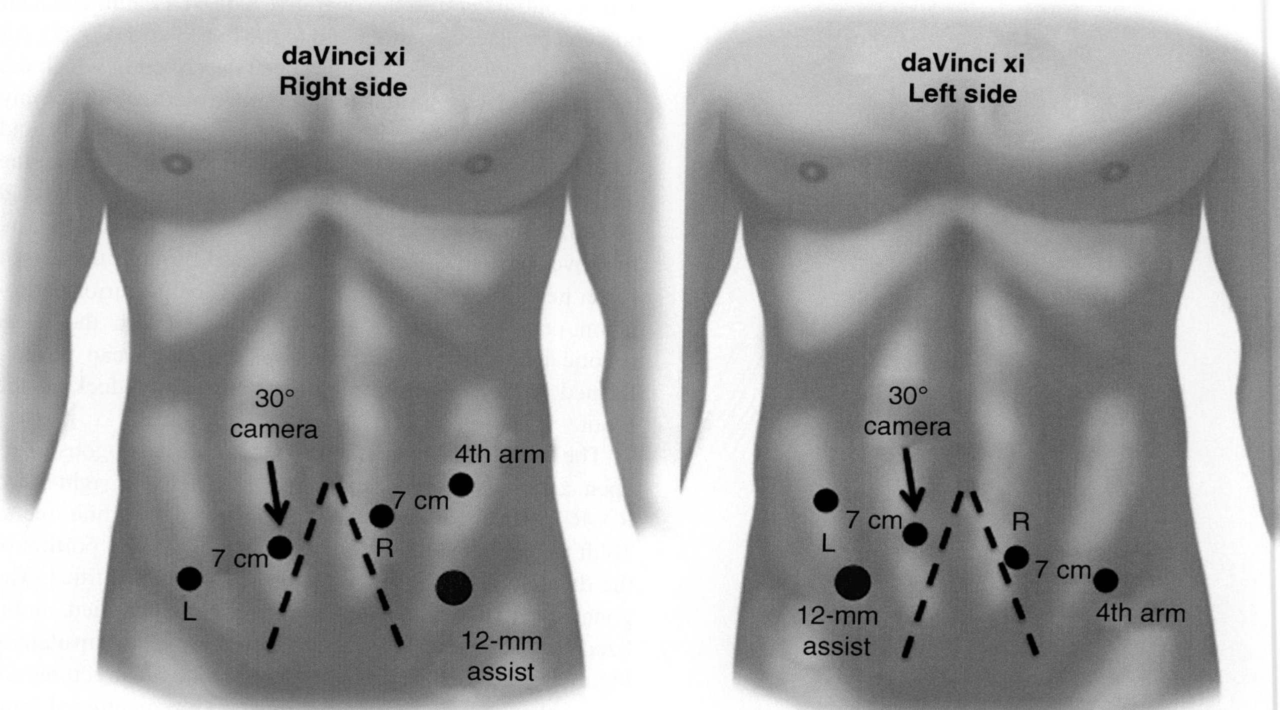

Fig. 5 The port placement locations of the camera, left and right robotic arm, the fourth arm, and the assistant port are showing for both left and right RPLND

ence being the dissection template. In cases of suspected nodal involvement or if a patient is CS II preoperatively, then a bilateral template is adopted.

5 Conclusion

Robotic surgery aims to decrease perioperative morbidity while maintaining the oncologic results of open surgery. The role of RA-RPLND in the treatment of testicular cancer is evolving but—at experienced centers and in well-selected patients who have been counseled regarding all options—has suggested effectiveness in reducing the learning curve, improving perioperative morbidity, and establishing comparable short-term oncologic outcome to open surgery, and potentially it is cost-effective. Further studies, especially randomized controlled trials, are needed to define the longer-term cancer-specific outcomes and further evaluate the perioperative morbidity differences between open and robot-assisted RPLND. A command of testicular cancer, management options, expertise with the specifics of a complex surgery, and understanding of the pros and cons of various templates and surgical approaches are essential to deliver high-quality care to these highly curable and typically young patients with testicular cancer.

References

1. Pishgar F, Haj-Mirzaian A, Ebrahimi H, Saeedi Moghaddam S, Mohajer B, Nowroozi MR, et al. Global, regional and national burden of testicular cancer, 1990-2016: results from the Global Burden of Disease Study 2016. BJU Int. 2019;124(3):386–94. https://doi.org/10.1111/bju.14771.
2. SEER Cancer Stat Facts: Testicular Cancer. https://seer.cancer.gov/statfacts/html/testis.html. 2021. Accessed 22 July 2021.
3. Xing M, Kokabi N, Zhang D, Ludwig JM, Kim HS. Comparative effectiveness of thermal ablation, surgical resection, and active surveillance for T1a renal cell carcinoma: a surveillance, epidemiology, and end results (SEER)-Medicare-linked population study. Radiology. 2018;288(1):81–90. https://doi.org/10.1148/radiol.2018171407.
4. Gillessen S, Sauvé N, Collette L, Daugaard G, de Wit R, Albany C, et al. Predicting outcomes in men with metastatic nonseminomatous germ cell tumors (NSGCT): results from the IGCCCG Update Consortium. J Clin Oncol. 2021;39(14):1563–74. https://doi.org/10.1200/JCO.20.03296.
5. Gilligan T, Lin DW, Aggarwal R, Chism D, Cost N, Derweesh IH, et al. Testicular cancer, version 2.2020, NCCN clinical practice guidelines in oncology. J Natl Compr Cancer Netw. 2019;17(12):1529–54. https://doi.org/10.6004/jnccn.2019.0058.
6. Daneshmand S, Cary C, Masterson TA, Einhorn L, Boorjian SA, Kollmannsberger CK, et al. SEMS trial: result of a prospective, multi-institutional phase II clinical trial of surgery in early metastatic seminoma. J Clin Oncol. 2021;39(6_suppl):375. https://doi.org/10.1200/JCO.2021.39.6_suppl.375.
7. Albers P, Hiester A, Siemer RG, Lusch A. The PRIMETEST trial: interim analysis of a phase II trial for primary retroperitoneal lymph node dissection (RPLND) in stage II A/B seminoma patients

without adjuvant treatment. J Clin Oncol. 2019;37(7_suppl):507. https://doi.org/10.1200/JCO.2019.37.7_suppl.507.

8. Donohue JP, Thornhill JA, Foster RS, Rowland RG, Bihrle R. Primary retroperitoneal lymph node dissection in clinical stage a non-seminomatous germ cell testis cancer. Review of the Indiana University experience 1965–1989. Br J Urol. 1993;71(3):326–35.
9. Poulakis V, Skriapas K, de Vries R, Dillenburg W, Ferakis N, Witzsch U, et al. Quality of life after laparoscopic and open retroperitoneal lymph node dissection in clinical Stage I nonseminomatous germ cell tumor: a comparison study. Urology. 2006;68(1):154–60.
10. Rassweiler JJ, Scheitlin W, Heidenreich A, Laguna MP, Janetschek G. Laparoscopic retroperitoneal lymph node dissection: does it still have a role in the management of clinical stage I nonseminomatous testis cancer? A European perspective. Eur Urol. 2008;54(5):1004–15. https://doi.org/10.1016/j.eururo.2008.08.022.
11. Davol P, Sumfest J, Rukstalis D. Robotic-assisted laparoscopic retroperitoneal lymph node dissection. Urology. 2006;67(1):199. https://doi.org/10.1016/j.urology.2005.07.022.
12. Stepanian S, Patel M, Porter J. Robot-assisted laparoscopic retroperitoneal lymph node dissection for testicular cancer: evolution of the technique. Eur Urol. 2016;70(4):661–7. https://doi.org/10.1016/j.eururo.2016.03.031.
13. Williams SB, Lau CS, Josephson DY. Initial series of robot-assisted laparoscopic retroperitoneal lymph node dissection for clinical stage I nonseminomatous germ cell testicular cancer. Eur Urol. 2011;60(6):1299–302. https://doi.org/10.1016/j.eururo.2011.03.009.
14. Cheney SM, Andrews PE, Leibovich BC, Castle EP. Robot-assisted retroperitoneal lymph node dissection: technique and initial case series of 18 patients. BJU Int. 2015;115(1):114–20. https://doi.org/10.1111/bju.12804.
15. Taylor J, Becher E, Wysock JS, Lenis AT, Litwin MS, Jipp J, et al. Primary robot-assisted retroperitoneal lymph node dissection for men with Nonseminomatous germ cell tumor: experience from a multi-institutional cohort. Eur Urol Focus. 2020;7(6):1403–8. https://doi.org/10.1016/j.euf.2020.06.014.
16. Rocco NR, Stroup SP, Abdul-Muhsin HM, Marshall MT, Santomauro MG, Christman MS, et al. Primary robotic RLPND for nonseminomatous germ cell testicular cancer: a two-center analysis of intermediate oncologic and safety outcomes. World J Urol. 2020;38(4):859–67. https://doi.org/10.1007/s00345-019-02900-w.
17. Heidenreich A, Albers P, Hartmann M, Kliesch S, Kohrmann KU, Krege S, et al. Complications of primary nerve sparing retroperitoneal lymph node dissection for clinical stage I nonseminomatous germ cell tumors of the testis: experience of the German Testicular Cancer Study Group. J Urol. 2003;169(5):1710–4. https://doi.org/10.1097/01.ju.0000060960.18092.54.
18. Masterson TA, Carver BS, Abel EJ, Pettus JA, Bosl GJ, Sheinfeld J. Impact of age on clinicopathological outcomes and recurrence-free survival after the surgical management of nonseminomatous germ cell tumour. BJU Int. 2012;110(7):950–5. https://doi.org/10.1111/j.1464-410X.2012.10947.x.
19. Beck SD, Peterson MD, Bihrle R, Donohue JP, Foster RS. Short-term morbidity of primary retroperitoneal lymph node dissection in a contemporary group of patients. J Urol. 2007;178(2):504–6.; discussion 6. https://doi.org/10.1016/j.juro.2007.03.123.
20. Pearce SM, Golan S, Gorin MA, Luckenbaugh AN, Williams SB, Ward JF, et al. Safety and early oncologic effectiveness of primary robotic retroperitoneal lymph node dissection for nonseminomatous germ cell testicular cancer. Eur Urol. 2017;71(3):476–82. https://doi.org/10.1016/j.eururo.2016.05.017.
21. Tselos A, Moris D, Tsilimigras DI, Fragkiadis E, Mpaili E, Sakarellos P, et al. Robot-assisted retroperitoneal lymphadenectomy in testicular cancer treatment: a systematic review. J Laparoendosc Adv Surg Tech A. 2018;28(6):682–9. https://doi.org/10.1089/lap.2017.0672.
22. Harris KT, Gorin MA, Ball MW, Pierorazio PM, Allaf ME. A comparative analysis of robotic vs laparoscopic retroperitoneal lymph node dissection for testicular cancer. BJU Int. 2015;116(6):920–3. https://doi.org/10.1111/bju.13121.
23. Kamel MH, Jackson CM, Moore JT, Heshmat SM, Bissada NK. Post-chemotherapy robotic retroperitoneal lymph node dissection (RRPLND) in testicular cancer. J Robot Surg. 2012;6(4):359–62. https://doi.org/10.1007/s11701-012-0345-4.
24. Singh A, Chatterjee S, Bansal P, Bansal A, Rawal S. Robot-assisted retroperitoneal lymph node dissection: feasibility and outcome in postchemotherapy residual mass in testicular cancer. Indian J Urol. 2017;33(4):304–9. https://doi.org/10.4103/iju.IJU_8_17.
25. Overs C, Beauval JB, Mourey L, Rischmann P, Soulié M, Roumiguié M, et al. Robot-assisted post-chemotherapy retroperitoneal lymph node dissection in germ cell tumor: is the single-docking with lateral approach relevant? World J Urol. 2018;36(4):655–61. https://doi.org/10.1007/s00345-018-2177-y.
26. Ray S, Pierorazio PM, Allaf ME. Primary and post-chemotherapy robotic retroperitoneal lymph node dissection for testicular cancer: a review. Transl Androl Urol. 2020;9(2):949–58. https://doi.org/10.21037/tau.2020.02.09.
27. Ruf CG, Krampe S, Matthies C, Anheuser P, Nestler T, Simon J, et al. Major complications of post-chemotherapy retroperitoneal lymph node dissection in a contemporary cohort of patients with testicular cancer and a review of the literature. World J Surg Oncol. 2020;18(1):253. https://doi.org/10.1186/s12957-020-02032-1.
28. Ohlmann CH, Saar M, Pierchalla LC, Zangana M, Bonaventura A, Stöckle M, et al. Indications, feasibility and outcome of robotic retroperitoneal lymph node dissection for metastatic testicular germ cell tumours. Sci Rep. 2021;11(1):10700. https://doi.org/10.1038/s41598-021-89823-y.
29. Annerstedt M, Gudjonsson S, Wullt B, Uvelius B. Robot-assisted laparoscopic retroperitoneal lymph node dissection in clinical stage II testicular cancer. J Robot Surg. 2008;2(3):189–91. https://doi.org/10.1007/s11701-008-0093-7.
30. Blok JM, van der Poel HG, Kerst JM, Bex A, Brouwer OR, Bosch JLHR, et al. Clinical outcome of robot-assisted residual mass resection in metastatic nonseminomatous germ cell tumor. World J Urol. 2021;39(6):1969–76. https://doi.org/10.1007/s00345-020-03437-z.
31. Hiester A, Nini A, Arsov C, Buddensieck C, Albers P. Robotic assisted retroperitoneal lymph node dissection for small volume metastatic testicular cancer. J Urol. 2020;204(6):1242–8. https://doi.org/10.1097/JU.0000000000001301.
32. Li R, Duplisea JJ, Petros FG, González GMN, Tu SM, Karam JA, et al. Robotic postchemotherapy retroperitoneal lymph node dissection for testicular cancer. Eur Urol Oncol. 2019;4(4):651–8. https://doi.org/10.1016/j.euo.2019.01.014.
33. Rodrigues GJ, Guglielmetti GB, Orvieto M, Seetharam Bhat KR, Patel VR, Coelho RF. Robot-assisted retroperitoneal lymphadenectomy: the state of art. Asian J Urol. 2021;8(1):27–37. https://doi.org/10.1016/j.ajur.2020.09.002.
34. Subramanian VS, Nguyen CT, Stephenson AJ, Klein EA. Complications of open primary and post-chemotherapy retroperitoneal lymph node dissection for testicular cancer. Urol Oncol. 2010;28(5):504–9. https://doi.org/10.1016/j.urolonc.2008.10.026.
35. Bhanvadia R, Ashbrook C, Bagrodia A, Lotan Y, Margulis V, Woldu S. Population-based analysis of cost and peri-operative outcomes between open and robotic primary retroperitoneal lymph node dissection for germ cell tumors. World J Urol. 2021;39(6):1977–84. https://doi.org/10.1007/s00345-020-03403-9.
36. Stephenson A, Eggener SE, Bass EB, Chelnick DM, Daneshmand S, Feldman D, et al. Diagnosis and treatment of early stage testicular cancer: AUA guideline. J Urol. 2019;202(2):272–81. https://doi.org/10.1097/JU.0000000000000318.

Index

P. Wiklund et al. (eds.), *Robotic Urologic Surgery*, https://doi.org/10.1007/978-3-031-00363-9

C

N

O

P

Q

R

V